MW01174598

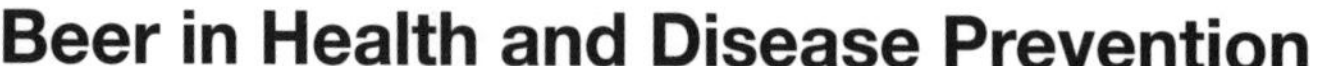

Beer in Health and Disease Prevention

Beer in Health and Disease Prevention

Edited by

Victor R. Preedy
Department of Nutrition and Dietetics
King's College London
London, UK

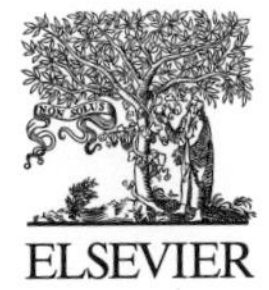

AMSTERDAM • BOSTON • HEIDELBERG • LONDON • OXFORD • NEW YORK
PARIS • SAN DIEGO • SAN FRANCISCO • SINGAPORE • SYDNEY • TOKYO

Academic Press is an imprint of Elsevier

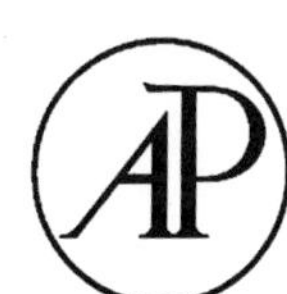

Academic Press is an imprint of Elsevier
30 Corporate Drive, Suite 400, Burlington, MA 01803, USA
525 B Street, Suite 1900, San Diego, California 92101-4495, USA
32 Jamestown Road, London NW1 7BY, UK

British Library Cataloguing in Publication Data
A catalogue record for this book is available from the British Library

Library of Congress Cataloguing in Publication Data
A catalogue record for this book is available from the Library of Congress

ISBN 978-0-12-373891-2

For information on all Academic Press publications
visit our website at www.elsevierdirect.com

Typeset by Charon Tec Ltd., A Macmillan Company. (www.macmillansolutions.com)

Printed and bound in the USA

09 10 11 10 9 8 7 6 5 4 3 2 1

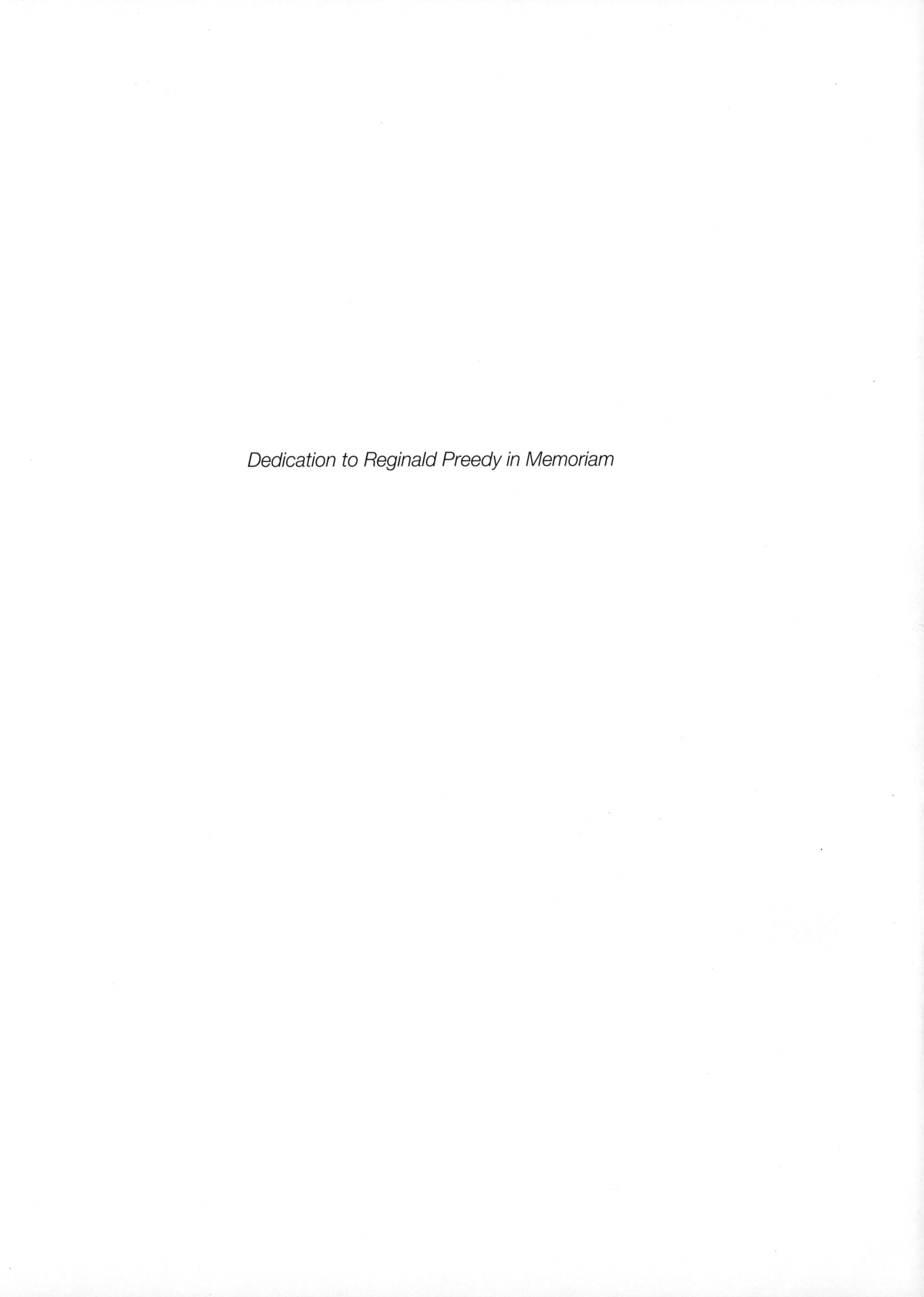

Dedication to Reginald Preedy in Memoriam

CONTENTS

†deceased

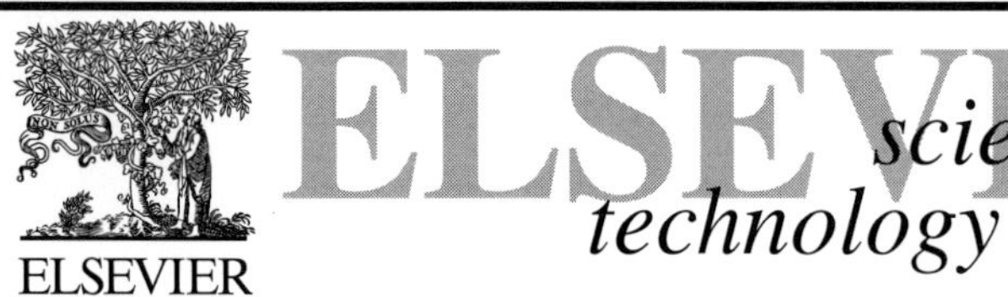

For additional, exclusive online chapters please go to the inside back cover of this book to reveal your own personal identification number to access these chapters, and then visit:
http://www.beerinhealthanddisease.com
Please note: When the personal identification number has been revealed, this book cannot be returned.

Technical support
Technical support for this product is available between 7.30am and 7.00pm CST, 1.30pm to 1.00am UK, Monday through Friday. Before calling be sure that your computer meets the minimum system requirements to run this software. Inside the US and Canada, please call 1-800-401-9962; Inside the UK, 0-0800-6929-0100;
Rest of the World call +1-314-872-8370. You may also fax your questions to +1-314-997-5080 or contact Technical support by email at online.help@elsevier.com

Beer in Health and Disease Prevention
Edited by Victor R. Preedy

List of Contributors

FUMIYOSHI ABE, Extremobiosphere Research Center, and Agency for Marine-Earth Science and Technology, 2-15 Natsushima-cho, Yokosuka 237-0061, Japan

GIOVANNI ADDOLORATO, Institute of Internal Medicine, Catholic University of Rome, L. go A. Gemelli 8, I-00168 Rome, Italy

PETER ALDRED, School of Science and Engineering, Institute of Food and Crop Science, Ballarat, Australia

R. ALLER, Institute of Endocrinology and Nutrition, Medicine School and Unit of Investigation, Hospital Rio Hortega, University of Valladolid, Valladolid, Spain

PAULO ALMEIDA, Department of Chemistry, Faculty of Science, University of Porto, Porto, Portugal

JESÚS-ROMÁN MARTÍNEZ ÁLVAREZ, Spanish Society of Dietetics and Food Science, Faculty of Medicine, Ciudad Universitaria 28040 Madrid, Spain

A.V. NIEUW AMERONGEN, Section of Oral Biochemistry, Department of Basic Dental Sciences, Academic Centre for Dentistry (ACTA), Amsterdam, The Netherlands

MOGENS L. ANDERSEN, Food Chemistry, Department of Food Science, University of Copenhagen, Rolighedsvej 30, Frederiksberg C DK-1958, Denmark

HITOSHI AOSHIMA, Applied Molecular Bioscience, Graduate School of Medicine, Yamaguchi University 1677-1 Yoshida, Yamaguchi 753-8512, Japan

SAKAE ARIMOTO-KOBAYASHI, Graduate School of Medicine, Dentistry and Pharmaceutical Sciences, Okayama University, 1-1-1 Tsushima, Okayama 700-8530, Japan

ALEMAYEHU ASFAW, Department of Chemistry, University of Oslo, Oslo, Norway

ERICA WEINTRAUB AUSTIN, Edward R. Murrow School of Communication, Washington State University, Pullman, WA, USA

WERNER BACK, Lehrstuhl für Technologie der Brauerei I, Weihenstephaner Steig 20, Freising-Weihenstephan D-85354, Germany

SEUNG JOON BAEK, Laboratory of Environmental Carcinogenesis, Department of Pathobiology, College of Veterinary Medicine, University of Tennessee, 2407 River Drive, Knoxville, TN 37996, USA

WANDA BAER-DUBOWSKA, Department of Pharmaceutical Biochemistry, Poznań University of Medical Sciences, Swieckiego 4, 60780 Poznań, Poland

AQUILES A. BARROS, Requimte/Departamento de Química, Faculdade de Ciências, da Universidade Do Porto, Rua do Campo Alegre 687, Porto 4169-007, Portugal

HANS BECKER, Pharmakognosie und Analytische Phytochemie, der Universitat des Saarlandes, Saarbrúcken D 66041, Germany

BAKAN BÉNÉDICTE, INRA Unité Biopolymères, Interactions, Assemblages, Nantes cedex, France

STEFANIE BERWANGER, Pharmakognosie und Analytische Phytochemie der Universität des Saarlandes, Saarbrücken, Germany

STEFAN BLEICH, Department of Psychiatry and Psychotherapy, University Hospital Erlangen, Germany

JEFFREY B. BLUMBERG, Antioxidants Research Laboratory, Jean Mayer USDA Human Nutrition Research Center on Aging, Tufts University, Boston, MA, USA

JERINA BOELENS, Department of Hematology, Ghent University Hospital, Ghent, Belgium

GREGOR BOHR, Pharmakognosie und Analytische Phytochemie, der Universität des Saarlandes, Saarbrücken, Germany

MARC BRACKE, Laboratory of Experimental Cancer Research, Department of Radiotherapy and Nuclear Medicine, Ghent University Hospital, De Pintelaan 185, Gent B-9000, Begium

H.S. BRAND, Department of Oral Biochemistry, Academic Centre for Dentistry Amsterdam (ACTA), Amsterdam, van der Boechorststraat 7, Amsterdam 1081 BT, The Netherlands

M.L. BRUINS, Section of Oral Biochemistry, Department of Basic Dental Sciences, Academic Centre for Dentistry (ACTA), Amsterdam, The Netherlands

STEFANO BUIATTI, Department of Food Science, University of Udine, Via Marangoni 97, 33100 Udine, Italy

RODRIGO R. CATHARINO, Thomson Mass Spectrometry Laboratory, Institute of Chemistry, State University of Campinas, Campinas, SP 13083-970, Brazil

M. LUISA CERVERA, Department of Analytical Chemistry, Edificio de Investigacion, University of Valencia, E-46100 Burjassot, Valencia, Spain

CHUNG-YEN CHEN, Antioxidants Research Laboratory, Jean Mayer USDA Human Nutrition Research Center on Aging, Tufts University, 711 Washington Street, Boston, MA 02111, USA

QIAO QIAO CHEN, Unidade de Nutrição e Metabolismo, Faculdade de Medicina da Universidade de Lisboa, Lisboa, Portugal

YUONNES CHEN, Edward R. Murrow School of Communication, Washington State University, Pullman, WA, USA

GIUSEPPE COMI, Department of Food Science, University of Udine, Via Marangoni 97, 33100 Udine, Italy

SONIA CORTACERO-RAMÍREZ, Department of Analytical Chemistry, Faculty of Sciences, University of Granada, Granada, Spain

L. DAENEN, Centre for Malting and Brewing Sciences, Catholic University of Leuven, Kasteelpark, Arenberg 22, PO Box 02463, Heverlee 3001, Belgium

L. De COOMAN, Laboratory of Enzyme and Brewing Technology, KaHo St-Lieven, Gent, Belgium

D.A. De LUIS, Institute of Endocrinology and Nutrition, University of Valladolid Medical School, c/Los perales 16 (URB Las Acenas), Simancas E-47130, Valladolid, Spain

D.P. De SCHUTTER, Department of Microbial and Molecular Systems, Centre for Malting and Brewing Science, Catholic University of Leuven, Kasteelpark, Arenberg 22, PO Box 02463, Heverlee 3001, Belgium

MAX L. DEINZER, Department of Chemistry, Oregon State University, Gilbert Hall 153, Corvallis, OR 97330, USA

F. DELVAUX, Department of Microbial and Molecular Systems, Centre for Malting and Brewing Science, Catholic University of Leuven, Kasteelpark, Arenberg 22, PO Box 02463, Heverlee 3001, Belgium

RALF DEMMEL, Department of Clinical Psychology, University of Muenster, Fliednerstr. 21, Muenster 48149, Germany

G. DERDELINCKX, Department of Microbial and Molecular Systems, Centre for Malting and Brewing Science, Catholic University of Leuven, Kasteelpark, Arenberg 22, PO Box 02463, Heverlee 3001, Belgium

ESTERA SZWAJCER DEY, Pure and Applied Biochemistry, Lund University, Lund, Sweden

M.E. DÍAZ-RUBIO, Department of Metabolism and Nutrition, CSIC, Ciudad Universitaria, C/Jose Antonio Novais 10, 28040 Madrid, Spain

J. RICHARD DICKINSON Cardiff School of Biosciences, Cardiff University, PO Box 915, Cardiff CF10 3TL, UK

MARION DIDIER, INRA, Unite Biopolymeres, Interactions, Assemblages, rue de la Geraudiere, Nantes BP71627 44316, Cedex 03, France

FRIEDHELM DIEL, IUG and University of Applied Sciencies, Hochschule Fulda, Fb:Oe, Marquardstrasse 35, Fulda D-36039, Germany

SUSANNE DIEL, Institut für Umwelt und Gesundheit (IUG) and University of Applied Sciences, FB:Oe, Biochemistry, Fulda, Germany

REINHARD A. DILLER, Institute of Technology of Biogenic Resources, Technical University of Munich, Straubing, Germany

ZODWA DLAMINI, Faculty of Health Sciences, School of Anatomical Sciences, University of the Witwatersrand, 7 York Road, Johannesburg 2193, South Africa

AGNIESZKA DOBROWOLSKA-ZACHWIEJA, Department of Gastroenterology and Human Nutrition, Poznań University of Medical Sciences, Poznań, Poland

JEAN-PIERRE DUFOUR, Department of Food Science, University of Otago, Dunedin, New Zealand

MARCOS N. EBERLIN, Thomson Mass Spectrometry Laboratory, Institute of Chemistry, State University of Campinas, UNICAMP, Campinas, SP, Brazil

KATHARINA E. EFFENBERGER, Department of Tumor Biology, Center of Experimental Medicine, University Medical Center Hamburg-Eppendorf, Martinistreet 52, Hamburg D-20246, Germany

GRAHAM EYRES, Department of Food Science, University of Otago, PO Box 56, Dunedin, New Zealand

PAOLO FANTOZZI, Italian Brewing Research Centre, CERB (Centro di Eccellenza per la Ricerca sulla Birra), University of Perugia, Via S. Costanzo, 06126 Perugia, Italy

JUSTIN A. FEGREDO, Department of Nutrition and Dietetics, King's College London, Franklin Wilkins Building, 150 Stamford Street, London SE1 9NH, UK

PETER FEICK, Department of Medicine II (Gastroenterology, Hepatology and Infectious Diseases), University Hospital of Heidelberg at Mannheim, Mannheim, Germany

ALBERTO FERNÁNDEZ-GUTIÉRREZ, Department of Analytical Chemistry, Faculty of Sciences, University of Granada, Granada, Spain

ISABEL M.P.L.V.O. FERREIRA, REQUIMTE, Servico de Bromatologia, Faculdade de Farmacia, Universidade do Porto, R. Anibal Cunha, Porto 4050-047, Portugal

ANNA FERRULLI, Institutes of Internal Medicine, Catholic University of Rome, Rome, Italy

MARTA FONTANA, Department of Agriculture and Environmental Sciences, University of Udine, Via delle Scienze 208, 33100 Udine, Italy

GLEN P. FOX, Plant Science-Wheat, Barley and Oats, PO Box 2282, Toowoomba Qld, 4350, Australia

JOSÉ Da CRUZ FRANCISCO, Pure and Applied Biochemistry, Lund University, Lund, Sweden

NORBERT FRANK, German Cancer Research Center (DKFZ) Chemoprevention, Im Neuenheimer Feld, Heidelberg, Germany

ANDREAS FRANKE, Department of Medicine II (Gastroenterology, Hepatology and Infectious Diseases), University Hospital of Heidelberg at Mannheim, Mannheim, Germany

GARY FREEMAN, BRI, Lyttel Hall, Nutfield, Surrey, UK

CORAZON FRIAS, Department of Pediatric Oncology/ Hematology, University Medical Center Charité, Campus Virchow, Berlin, Germany

SONJA FRÖLICH, Institut für Pharmazie (Pharmazeutische Biologie), Freie Universität Berlin, Berlin, Germany

DIETMAR FUCHS, Division of Biological Chemistry, Innsbruck Medical University, Ludwig Boltzmann Institute of AIDS-Research, Fritz Pregl Strasse 3, A-6020 Innsbruck, Austria

ANDRZEJ GAMIAN, Institute of Immunology and Experimental Therapy, Polish Academy of Sciences, Wrocław; Department of Medical Biochemistry, Wrocław Medical University, Wrocław, Poland

S. GARCÍA-FALCÓN, Nutrition and Bromatology Group, Department of Analytical and Food Chemistry, Food Science and Technology Faculty, University of Vigo, Ourense Campus, Ourense, Spain

SALVADOR GARRIGUES, Department of Analytical Chemistry, Edificio de Investigacion, University of Valencia, 50 Dr. Moliner Street, Burjassot E-46100, Valencia, Spain

ANTONIO GASBARRINI, Institutes of Pathology, Catholic University of Rome, Rome, Italy

GIOVANNI GASBARRINI, Institutes of Internal Medicine, Catholic University of Rome, Rome, Italy

CLARISSA GERHÄUSER, Deutsches Krebsforschungszentrum (DKFZ), Abteilung Toxikologie und Krebsrisikofaktoren, Workgroup Chemoprevention, Im Neuenheimer Feld 280, Heidelberg D-69120, Germany

ANDREAS GERLOFF, Department of Medicine II (Gastroenterology, Hepatology and Infectious Diseases), University Hospital of Heidelberg at Mannheim, Mannheim, Germany

ANDREA GHISELLI, National Research Institute for Food and Nutrition Research, Via Ardeatina, Rome, Italy

A.M. GIL, Department of Chemistry, University of Aveiro, Campus de Santiago, Aveiro 3810-193, Portugal

I. GOÑI, Unidad Asociada Nutrición y Salud Gastrointestinal (UCM-CSIC), Dpt. Nutrición I. Facultad de Farmacia, Ciudad Universitaria, Madrid, Spain

STANISLAVA GORJANOVIĆ, Institute of General and Physical Chemistry, Studentski trg 12-16/V, PO Box 551, 11001 Belgrade, Serbia

MIGUEL de la GUARDIA, Department of Analytical Chemistry, Edificio de Investigacion, University of Valencia, E-46100 Burjassot, Valencia, Spain

N.P. GUERRA, Nutrition and Bromatology Group, Department of Analytical and Food Chemistry, Food Science and Technology Faculty, University of Vigo, Ourense Campus, Ourense, Spain

LUIS F. GUIDO, Requimte/Departamento de Química, Faculdade de Ciências, da Universidade Do Porto, Rua do Campo Alegre 687, Porto 4169-007, Portugal

SANJAY GUPTA, Department of Urology, Case Western Reserve University, University Hospitals Case Medical Center and Case Comprehensive Cancer Center, Cleveland, OH, USA

LINDA HELLBORG, Department of Cell and Organism Biology, Lund University, Biologihuset Solvegatan 35, Lund S-223 62, Sweden

GÜNTER HENZE, Department of Pediatric Oncology/ Hematology, University Medical Center Charité, Campus Virchow, Berlin, Germany

MARÍA PURIFICACIÓN HERNÁNDEZ-ARTIGA, Department of Analytical Chemistry, Faculty of Sciences, University of Cadiz, Apdo. 40, Puerto Real 11510, Cadiz, Spain

JAVIER HERNÁNDEZ-BORGES, Department of Analytical Chemistry, Nutrition and Food Science, University of La Laguna, Avda, Astrofisico Fco. Sánchez s/n°, 38071 La Laguna, Tenerife, Canary Islands, Spain

MARIA HERWALD, Institut für Umwelt und Gesundheit (IUG) and University of Applied Sciences, FB:Oe, Biochemistry, Fulda, Germany

THOMAS HILLEMACHER, Department of Psychiatry and Psychotherapy, University of Erlangen-Nuremberg, Schwabachanlage 6, Erlangen D-91054, Germany

SHEIKH JULFIKAR HOSSAIN, Applied Molecular Bioscience, Graduate School of Medicine, Yamaguchi University 1677-1 Yoshida, Yamaguchi 753-8512, Japan

PAUL HUGHES, School of Life Sciences, International Centre for Brewing and Distilling, Heriot-Watt University, Riccarton, Edinburgh EH14 4AS, UK

STACEY J.T. HUST, Edward R. Murrow School of Communication, Communication Addition 101, PO Box 642520, Washington State University, Pullman, WA 99164-2520, USA.

KEVIN HUVAERE, Food Chemistry, Department of Food Science, University of Copenhagen, Frederiksberg C, Denmark

GIUSEPPE IACOMINO, Institute of Food Sciences, National Research Council, Avellino, Italy

EWA IGNATOWICZ, Department of Pharmaceutical Biochemistry, Poznań University of Medical Sciences, ul. Swiecickiego 4, 60780 Poznań, Poland

KATSUMI IKEDA, Department of Health and Bio-pharmaceutical Sciences, School of Pharmacy and Pharmaceutical Sciences, Mukogawa Women's University, Nishinomiya, Japan

PAVEL JANDERA, Department of Analytical Chemistry, Faculty of Chemical Technology, University of Pardubice, Nam. Cs. Legii 565, Pardubice CZ-532 10, Czech Republic

KRISTINA JENETT-SIEMS, Institut für Pharmazie, Freie Universitat Berlin, Konigin-Luise- Str. 2-4, D-14195 Berlin, Germany

RAVIN JUGDAOHSINGH, MRC Human Nutrition Research, Elsie Widdowson Laboratory, Fulbourn Road, Cambridge CB1 9NL, UK

MASATO KAWASAKI, Research Laboratories for Brewing, Technology Development Department, Production Division, Kirin Brewery Co., Limited, 1-17-1 Namamugi, Tsurumi-ku, Yokohama 230-8628, Japan

WILLIAM C. KERR, Alcohol Research Group, 6475 Christie Avenue, Suite 400, Emeryville, CA 94608, USA

IGOR KHMELINSKII, Universidade do Algarve, FCT, DQBF, Campus de Gambelas, Faro, Portugal

YOSHINOBU KISO, Institute for Health Care Science, Suntory Limited, Wakayamadai, Shimamoto-cho, Mishima-gun, Osaka, Japan

HIROFUMI KODA, Institute for Health Care Science, Suntory Limited, Wakayamadai, Shimamoto-cho, Mishima-gun, Osaka, Japan

M. KOMAITIS, Laboratory of Food Chemistry, Agricultural University of Athens, Iera Odo 75, Athens 118 55, Greece

KEIJI KONDO, Central Laboratories for Frontier Technology, Research Section for Applied Food Science, Kirin Brewery Co., Ltd.,Takasaki, Gunma, Japan

VIOLETTA KRAJKA-KUŹNIAK, Department of Pharmaceutical Biochemistry, Poznań University of Medical Sciences, Swieckiego 4, 60780 Poznań, Poland

ROBERTO KRATKY, Department of Food Science, University of Udine, Via Marangoni, 97, 33100 Udine, Italy

L. DARREN KRUISSELBRINK, School of Recreation Management and Kinesiology, Acadia University, 550 Main St., Wolfville, NS B4P 2R6, Canada

ALAN K.H. LAI, Department of Nutrition and Dietetics, King's College London, London, UK

M. LEDOCHOWSKI, Department of Internal Medicine, Innsbruck Medical University, Innsbruck, Austria

SEONG-HO LEE, Department of Pathobiology, College of Veterinary Medicine, University of Tennessee, Knoxville, TN, USA

LORENZO LEGGIO, Institutes of Internal Medicine, Catholic University of Rome, Rome, Italy

HUI-JING LI, Department of Chemistry, Oregon State University, Corvallis, OR, USA

KRIENGSAK LIRDPRAPAMONGKOL, Department of Biochemistry, Faculty of Science, Mahidol University and Laboratory of Biochemistry, Chulabhorn Research Institute, Bangkok, Thailand

ALEX G. LITTLE, Department of Surgery, Boonshoft School of Medicine, Wright State University, Dayton, OH, USA

C. LÓPEZ-MACÍAS, Nutrition and Bromatology Group, Department of Analytical and Food Chemistry, Food Science and Technology Faculty, University of Vigo, Ourense Campus, Ourense, Spain

SUZANNE LORET, Department of Biology, Faculty of Sciences, University of Namur (FUNDP), Rue de Bruxelles 61, B-5000 NAMUR, Belgium

ZACHARENIA LOUKOU, General Chemical States Laboratory, Kavala Division, Karaoli Square, Kavala, Greece

VALENTIN LOZANOV, Department of Chemistry and Biochemistry, Medical University of Sofia, Sofia 1431, Bulgaria

SOFIE LUST, Department of Hematology, Ghent University Hospital, Ghent, Belgium

JEAN ROBERT MABIALA-BABELA, Centre Hospitalier Universitaire,Service de Pediatrie Nourrissons, Brazzaville BP 32, Congo

MARISA MANZANO, Department of Food Science, University of Udine, Via Marangoni 97, 33100 UDINE, Italy

OMBRETTA MARCONI, Italian Brewing Research Centre, CERB (Centro di Eccellenza per la Ricerca sulla Birra), University of Perugia, Via S. Costanzo, 06126 Perugia, Italy

PEDRO MARQUES-VIDAL, Institut Universitaire de Medecine Sociale et Preventive, 17, rue du Bugnon, Lausanne CH-1005, Switzerland

PEDRO MARQUES-VIDAL, Unidade de Nutrição e Metabolismo, Instituto de Medicina Molecular, Faculdade de Medicina da Universidade de Lisboa, Av. Professor Egas Moniz, Lisboa 1649-028, Portugal

COLIN R. MARTIN, Psychology Group, School of Health and Human Services, Faculty of Health Leeds Metropolitan University, Civic Quarter, Leeds LS1 3HE, UK

E. MARTÍNEZ-CARBALLO, Nutrition and Bromatology Group, Department of Analytical and Food Chemistry, Food Science and Technology Faculty, University of Vigo, Ourense Campus, Ourense, Spain

ALPHONSE MASSAMBA, Centre Hospitalier et Universitaire, Service de Pediatrie Nourrissons, Brazzaville, Congo

HEIDI MAYER, Italian Brewing Research Centre, CERB (Centro di Eccellenza per la Ricerca sulla Birra), University of Perugia, Via S. Costanzo, 06126 Perugia, Italy

ZUKILE MBITA, University of the Witwatersrand, Wits Medical School, Johannesburg, South Africa

ADELE Mc KINNEY, School of Psychology, Life and Health Sciences, University of Ulster, Magee Camous, Derry BT48 7JL, Northern Ireland, UK

NIALL McCRAE, Health Services Research Department, Institute of Psychiatry, Denmark Hill, De Crespigny Park, PO Box 26, London SE5 8AF, UK

GARRY MENZ, School of Science and Engineering, Institute of Food and Crop Science, Ballarat, Australia

RACHEL MEYNELL, Department of Nutrition and Dietetics, King's College London, Franklin Wilkins Building, 150 Stamford Street, London SE1 9NH, UK

DOLORES BELLIDO MILLA, Department of Analytical Chemistry, Faculty of Sciences, University of Cádiz, Cádiz, Spain

STUART R. MILLIGAN, Division of Reproduction and Endocrinology, School of Biomedical Sciences, King's College London, Guy's Campus, Room 2.11N Hodgkin Building, London Bridge, London SE1 1UL, UK

LUIGI MONTANARI, Italian Brewing Research Centre, CERB (Centro di Eccellenza per la Ricerca sulla Birra), University of Perugia, Via S. Costanzo, 06126 Perugia, Italy

FRANCISCO J. MORALES, Consejo Sup. de Invest. Cie., Instituto del Frio (CSIC), Jose Antonio Novais 10, Madrid E-28040

YUJI MORIWAKI, Division of Endocrinology and Metabolism, Department of Internal Medicine, Hyogo College of Medicine, Mukogawa-cho 1-1, Nishinomiya Hyogo 663-8501, Japan

KENNETH J. MUKAMAL, Division of General Medicine and Primary Care, Beth Israel Deaconess Medical Center, 330 Brookline Avenue, Boston, MA 02215, USA

RENÉ J.L. MURPHY, School of Recreation Management and Kinesiology, Acadia University, Wolfville, NS, Canada

MAOURA NANADOUM, Laboratoire de Recherche sur les Substances Naturelles, Faculté des Sciences, Exactes et Appliquées BP, N'Djaména 1027, Tchad

MIRELLA NARDINI, Free Radical Research Group, National Institute for Food and Nutrition (INRAN), Via Ardeatina, 546, 00178 Rome, Italy

FAUSTA NATELLA, National Research Institute for Food and Nutrition Research, Via Ardeatina, Rome, Italy

SIMÓN NAVARRO, Department of Agricultural Chemistry, Geology and Pedology, School of Chemistry, University of Murcia, Campus Universitario de Espinardo, Murcia E-30100, Spain

JENNIFER NICOLAI, Department of Clinical Psychology, University of Münster, Münster, Germany

HAJIME NOZAWA, Central Laboratories for Frontier Technology, Kirin Brewery Co. Ltd., 3 Miyahara, Takasaki, Gunma 370-1295, Japan

FRITZ OFFNER, Department of Hematology, Ghent University Hospital, Ghent, Belgium

L.M. PASTRANA-CASTRO, Nutrition and Bromatology Group, Department of Analytical and Food Chemistry, Food Science and Technology Faculty, University of Vigo, Ourense Campus, Ourense, Spain

DOUGLAS E. PAULL, Department of Surgery, Wright State University School of Medicine, VA Medical Center, 4100 W. Third St. #112, Dayton, OH 45428, USA

ANDREA PAVSLER, Department of Food Science, University of Udine, Via Marangoni 97, 33100 Udine, Italy

C. PEHL, Department of Gastroenterology, Academic Teaching Hospital Bogenhausen, Englschalkinger Street 77, Munich 81935, Germany

JARA PÉREZ-JIMÉNEZ, Department of Metabolism and Nutrition, CSIC, Ciudad Universitaria, Madrid, Spain

BRUCE E. PINKLETON, Edward R. Murrow School of Communication, Washington State University, Pullman, WA, USA

JURE PISKUR, Department of Cell and Organism Biology, Lund University, Biologihuset Solvegatan 35, Lund S-223 62, Sweden

PAWEL POHL, Division of Analytical Chemistry, Faculty of Chemistry, Wroclaw University of Technology, Wybrzeze Stanislawa Wyspianskiego 27, 50-370 Wroclaw, Poland

SAM POSSEMIERS, Laboratory of Microbial Ecology and Technology (LabMET), Ghent University, Gent, Belgium

JACQUES POURQUIE, UMR Microbiologie et Genetique Moleculaire, CNRS/INA-PG/INRA, CBAI BP 01, 78 850, Thiverval Grignon, France

JONATHAN J. POWELL, MRC Human Nutrition Research, Elsie Widdowson Laboratory, Fulbourn Road, Cambridge CB1 9NL, UK

VICTOR R. PREEDY, Department of Nutrition and Dietetics, King's College London, Franklin-Wilkins Building, 150 Stamford Street, London SE1 9NH, UK

C. PROESTOS, Laboratory of Food Chemistry, Agricultural University of Athens, Iera Odos, Athens, Greece

ARAM PROKOP, Department of Pediatric Oncology/ Hematology, University Medical Center Charité, Campus Virchow, Berlin, Germany

SANDRA RAINIERI, Department of Agricultural Sciences, University of Modena and Reggio Emilia, Via J. F. Kennedy, 17, 42100 Reggio Emilia, Italy

RAJKUMAR RAJENDRAM, Nutritional Sciences Research Division, School of Life Sciences, King's College, and Departments of General Medicine and Intensive Care, John Radcliffe Hospital, Oxford OX3 0JH, UK

BRITTANY B. RAYBURN, Division of Maternal-Fetal Medicine, Department of Obstetrics and Gynecology, School of Medicine, University of New Mexico, Albuquerque, NM, USA

WILLIAM F. RAYBURN, Department of Obstetrics and Gynecology, University of New Mexico School of Medicine, MSC 10 5580, 1 University of New Mexico, Albuquerque, NM 87131, USA

HERBERT M. RIEPL, Institute of Technology for Biogenic Resources, Technical University of Munich, Petersgasse 18, Straubing D-94315, Germany

JOSÉ RODRIGUES, Departamento de Quimica, Faculdade de Ciencias, Universidade Do Porto, Rua do Campo Alegre, 687, Porto 4169-007, Portugal

MIGUEL ÁNGEL RODRIGUEZ-DELGADO, Department of Analytical Chemistry, Nutrition and Food Science, University of La Laguna, Avda, Astrofisico Fco. Sánchez s/n°, 38071 La Laguna, Tenerife, Canary Islands, Spain

OLIVER ROSE, Department of Pediatric Oncology/ Hematology, University Medical Center Charité, Campus Virchow, Berlin, Germany

NEIL E. ROWLAND, Department of Psychology, University of Florida, Center Drive, PO Box 112250, Gainesville, FL 32611-2250, USA

GIAN LUIGI RUSSO, Istituto di Scienze dell'Alimentazione, Consiglio Nazionale delle Ricerche, Via Roma 52 A/C, 83100 Avellino, Italy

IKUO SAIKI, Division of Pathogenic Biochemistry, Department of Bioscience, Institute of Natural Medicine and the 21st Century COE Program, University of Toyama, Toyama, Japan

D. SAISON, Department of Microbial and Molecular Systems, Centre for Malting and Brewing Science, Catholic University of Leuven, Kasteelpark, Arenberg 22, PO Box 02463, Heverlee 3001, Belgium

SHUSO SAKUMA, Production Division, Quality Assurance Department, Quality Assurance Center for Alcoholic Beverages, Kirin Brewery Co., Limited, 1-17-1 Namamugi, Tsurumi-ku, Yokohama 230-8628, Japan

HIROAKI SAKURAI, Division of Pathogenic Biochemistry, Department of Bioscience, Institute of Natural Medicine and the 21st Century COE Program, University of Toyama, Toyama, Japan

PAT SANDRA, Research Institute for Chromatography, Kennedypark 26, Kortrijk B-8500, Belgium

FULGENCIO SAURA-CALIXTO, Department of Metabolism and Nutrition, CSIC, Ciudad Universitaria, C/ Jose Antonio Novais 10, 28040 Madrid, Spain

ALEXANDRA C.H.F. SAWAYA, Program for Post-graduate Studies in Pharmacy, Bandeirante University of São Paulo, UNIBAN, São Paulo, SP, Brazil

CRISTINA SCACCINI, National Research Institute for Food and Nutrition Research, Via Ardeatina, Rome, Italy

H. SCHENNACH, Central Institute of Blood Transfusion and Immunology, University Hospital, Innsbruck, Austria

TANKRED SCHEWE, Institut fuer Biochemie und Molekularbiologie I, Universitaetsklinikum Duesseldorf, Postfach 101007, Duesseldorf D-40001, Germany

K. SCHROECKSNADEL, Division of Biological Chemistry, Biocentre, Innsbruck, Austria

CAROLA SCHUBERT, Institut für Pharmazie (Pharmazeutische Biologie), Freie Universität Berlin, Berlin, Germany

ANTONIO SEGURA-CARRETERO, Department of Analytical Chemistry, Faculty of Sciences, University of Granada, Granada E-18071, Spain

H. SEIDL, Department of Gastroenterology, Academic Teaching Hospital Bogenhausen, Englschalkinger Street 77, Munich 81935, Germany

JOSÉ SERRANO, Department of Metabolism and Nutrition, CSIC, Ciudad Universitaria, Madrid, Spain

TAKAYUKI SHIBAMOTO, Department of Environmental Toxicology, University of California, Davis, CA 95616, USA

SANJEEV SHUKLA, Department of Urology, Case Western Reserve University and University Hospitals Case Medical Center, Cleveland, OH, USA

HELMUT SIES, Institut fuer Biochemie und Molekularbiologie I, Duesseldorf, Germany

EWA SIKORSKA, Faculty of Commodity Science, Poznań University of Economics, al. Niepodleglosci 10, 60-967 Poznań, Poland

MAREK SIKORSKI, Faculty of Chemistry, A. Mickiewicz University, Poznań, Poland

J. SIMAL-GÁNDARA, Nutrition and Bromatology Group, Department of Analytical and Food Chemistry, Food Science and Technology Faculty, University of Vigo, Ourense Campus, Ourense, Spain

MANFRED V. SINGER, Department of Medicine II (Gastroenterology, Hepatology and Infectious Diseases), University Hospital of Mannheim, Theodor-Kutzer-Ufer 1–3, Mannheim D-68167, Germany

EDUARDO V. SOARES, Departamento de Engenharia Química, Instituto Superior de Engenharia do Instituto Politécnico do Porto, Rua Dr António Bernardino de Almeida, 431, Porto 4200-072, Portugal

RAJAVENTHAN SRIRAJASKANTHAN, Neuroendocrine Unit, Centre of Gastroenterology, Royal Free Hospital, Floor 10, Pond Street, London NW3 2QG, UK

KOJI SUZUKI, Analytical Technology Laboratory, Asahi Breweries Ltd., Midori 1-121 Moriya-shi Ibaraki-ken 302-0106, Japan

JISNUSON SVASTI, Department of Biochemistry, Faculty of Science, Mahidol University and Laboratory of Biochemistry, Chulabhorn Research Institute, Bangkok, Thailand

HANNA SZAEFER, Department of Pharmaceutical Biochemistry, Poznań University of Medical Sciences, Swieckiego 4, 60780 Poznań, Poland

IDOLO TEDESCO, Institute of Food Sciences, National Research Council, Avellino, Italy

HIROYASU TOBE, Department of Materials Science and Engineering, Kochi National College of Technology, Monobe B 200-1, Nankoku-city, Kochi 783-8508, Japan

DOMENICA TONELLI, Department of Physical and Inorganic Chemistry, Faculty of Industrial Chemistry, University of Bologna, Viale Risorgimento 4, 40136 Bologna, Italia

A.TORRADO-AGRASAR, Nutrition and Bromatology Group, Department of Analytical and Food Chemistry, Food Science and Technology Faculty, University of Vigo, Ourense Campus, Ourense, Spain

FRANCO TUBARO, Department of Chemical Sciences and Technology, University of Udine, Via Cotonificio 108, Udine 33100, Italy

VICTORIA VALLS-BELLÉS, Department of pediatrics, Faculty of Medicine, University of Valencia Victoria Valls Bellés, Avda. Blasco Ibañez, Valencia

BARBARA VANHOECKE, Laboratory of Experimental Cancer Research, Department of Radiotherapy and Nuclear Medicine, Ghent University Hospital, De Pintelaan 185, B-9000 Ghent, Belgium

GERD VANHOENACKER, Research Institute for Chromatography, Kennedypark, Kortrijk, Belgium

E.C.I. VEERMAN, Section of Oral Biochemistry, Department of Basic Dental Sciences, Academic Centre for Dentistry (ACTA), Amsterdam, The Netherlands

NURIA VELA, Department of Agricultural Chemistry, Geology and Pedology, School of Chemistry, University of Murcia, Campus Universitario de Espinardo, Murcia, Spain

H. VERACHTERT, Centre for Malting and Brewing Sciences, Catholic University of Leuven, Kasteelpark, Arenberg 22, PO Box 02463, Heverlee 3001, Belgium

WILLY VERSTRAETE, Laboratory of Microbial Ecology and Technology (LabMET), Ghent University, Gent, Belgium

K.J. VERSTREPEN, Centre for Malting and Brewing Sciences, Catholic University of Leuven, Kasteelpark, Arenberg 22, PO Box 02463, Heverlee 3001, Belgium

ANTONIO LUIS VILLARINO-MARÍN, Spanish Society of Dietetics and Food Science, Faculty of Medicine, Ciudad Universitaria 28040 Madrid, Spain

JOE A. VINSON, Department of Chemistry, Loyola Hall, University of Scranton, 800 Linden Street, Scranton, PA 18510, USA

GÜNTER VOLLMER, Institut für Zoologie, Molekulare Zellphysiologie und Endokrinologie, Zellescher Weg 20b, Room 253/254, 01217 Dresden, TU-Dresden, Dresden 01062, Germany

FRANK VRIESEKOOP, Microbiology and Fermentation Technology, School of Science and Engineering, University of Ballarat, PO Box 663, Ballarat, VIC 3353, Australia

CAROLINE WALKER, BRI, Lyttel Hall, Nutfield, Surrey, UK

S. GOYA WANNAMETHEE, Department of Primary Care and Population Sciences, Royal Free and University College Medical School, Rowland Hill St., London NW3 2PF, UK

JOHANNES WESTENDORF, Institute of Pharmacology and Toxicology, Center of Experimental Medicine, University Medical Center-Hamburg Eppendorf, Hamburg, Germany

GRETHE WIBETOE, Department of Chemistry, University of Oslo, PO Box 1033, Oslo, Norway

TOM Van De WIELE, Laboratory Microbial Ecology and Technology, Ghent University, Coupure Links 653, B-9000 Gent, Belgium

C. WINKLER, Division of Biological Chemistry, Biocentre, Innsbruck, Austria

HELEN WISEMAN, Department of Nutrition and Dietetics, King's College London, London, UK

MAX C.Y. WONG, Department of Nutrition and Dietetics, King's College London, London, UK

OWEN L. WOODMAN, Discipline of Cell Biology and anatomy, School of Medical Sciences, RMIT University, PO Box 71, Bundoora Vic 3083, Australia

SASCHA WUNDERLICH, Lehrstuhl für Technologie der Brauerei I, Weihenstephaner Steig 20, Freising-Weihenstephan D-85354, Germany

JIN-WEN XU, Division of Pathophysiology, Department of Pharmacy, School of Pharmacy and Pharmaceutical Sciences, Mukogawa Women's University, Nishinomiya 663-8179, Japan

HIROAKI YAJIMA, Central Laboratories for Frontier Technology, Kirin Brewery Co., Ltd., 1-13-5, Fukuura, Kanazawa-ku, Yokohama 236-0004, Japan

TETSUYA YAMAMOTO, Division of Endocrinology and Metabolism, Department of Internal Medicine, Hyogo College of Medicine, Mukogawa-cho 1-1, Nishinomiya, Hyogo 663-8501, Japan

ARUTO YOSHIDA, Central Laboratories for Key Technology, Kirin Brewery Co., Ltd., 1-13-5 Fukuura, Yokohama 236-0004, Japan

CHARLES Y.F. YOUNG, Department of Urology, Mayo Clinic/Foundation, Guggenheim Building 502, 200 First Street SW, Rochester, MN 55905, USA

PAOLA ZANOLI, Dipartimento di Scienze Biomediche, Sezione di Farmacologia, Via Campi 287, I-41100 Modena, Italy

MANUELA ZAVATTI, Department of Biomedical Sciences, Section of Pharmacology and National InterUniversity Consortium for the Study of Natural Active Principles (CINSPAN), University of Modena and Reggio Emilia, Modena, Italy

FENG ZHAO, Central Laboratories for Frontier Technology, Research Section for Applied Food Science, Kirin Brewery Co., Ltd., Takasaki, Gunma, Japan

MAŁGORZATA ZIELINSKA-PRZYJEMSKA, Department of Pharmaceutical Biochemistry, Poznań University of Medical Sciences, Swiecickiego 4, 60-780 Poznań, Poland

OLIVER ZIERAU, Molekulare Zellphysiologie und Endokrinologie, Institut für Zoologie, Technische Universität Dresden, Dresden, Germany

ANASTASIA ZOTOU, Laboratory of Analytical Chemistry, Department of Chemistry, Aristotle University of Thessaloniki, Thessaloniki 54124, Greece.

PREFACE

Evidence for the brewing of beer dates back to over 8,000 years and since then, its pattern and consumption has changed considerably: from a beverage of warriors to a cheap and affordable commodity. Like most alcoholic drinks, it has been prone to abuse and in some countries, the high per capita consumption of beer has led to considerable health risks. However, current science indicates that, in moderate or low amounts, the consumption of beer may be beneficial to good health.

Beer in Health and Disease Prevention addresses the need for a single, coherent volume presenting this spectrum of information. The book is composed of four main sections:

1. General aspects of beer and constituents
2. General effects on metabolism and body systems
3. Specific effects of selective beer-related components
4. Assay methods and techniques used for investigating beer and related compounds

Studying specific instances where beer consumption may have a positive impact on health, this book presents a comprehensive overview of both beer and its constituents, and their relationship to disease. For example, some cancers like bladder cancers and the incidence of cardiovascular disease are reported to be lower in moderate beer drinkers. These findings have led to the suggestion that beer contains substances that may be protective against disease. This has been shown to be true to the extent that compounds derived from beer and hops are protective against damaged cells. Xanthohumol and isoxanthohumol are just two examples of potential anticancer agents.

Furthermore, there is a considerable body of emerging evidence to show that the antioxidant capacity of beers is high. It has been argued by some that the total antioxidants ingested in some beer drinkers equates to that consumed by red wine drinkers. However, beer is a complex beverage with well over 1,000 identifiable compounds and there is a continual drive to identify and characterize new compounds that might also have potential pharmacological effects.

However, beer may also contain carcinogenic compounds, such as nitrosamines, even asbestos fibers from beer filters. All this requires a holistic understanding of beer and beer-related science from brewing to the isolation beer-related compounds.

This book is designed to provide insight into the possibilities of the role of beer in health maintenance as well as prevention of diseases. Contributors are authors of international and national standing, leaders in the field and trend-setters. Emerging fields of science and important discoveries relating to beer have been incorporated in *Beer in Health and Disease Prevention*, and this resource will be essential reading for nutritionists, pharmacologists, health care professionals, research scientists, cancer workers, cardiologists, pathologists, molecular or cellular biochemists, general practitioners as well as those interested in beer or alcohol studies in general.

Victor R. Preedy

FOREWORD

In recent years few issues have hit the public health agenda as hard as alcohol abuse. Excessive alcohol consumption carries an attributable risk to public disorder, violent crime, road traffic accidents, hospital admissions and social instability. The government purse, filled by every taxpayer, is increasingly called upon for alcohol-related health care and law enforcement. The public face of alcohol consumption comprises bars, clubs, pubs and various social and sporting events – and synonymous with these is beer. So from where does a sincere, scientific book arrive entitled *Beer in Health and Disease Prevention*? The answer, in large part, lies in the now famous J-shaped curve that links alcohol ingestion to risk for a number of diseases. In short, moderate alcohol consumers not only appear to have better long-term health outcomes than excessive alcohol consumers but they can also fare better than abstainers. In other words, for some diseases, the graph relating alcohol intake to morbidity has a J shape with the nadir corresponding to moderate alcohol consumption. Study after study has shown this; most famously for cardiovascular disease but additionally, for example, for bone disease, cognitive decline, Type II diabetes and even overall mortality. On balance, beer appears at least as effective as wine at protecting against disease, when either are enjoyed in moderation, and our research has suggested that this effect may not only be attributable to beer's ethanol content but also to cereal and hop-related components such as silicic acid (silicon) and certain phenolics. But there are two significant issues with the J-shaped curve: the first is one of scientific endeavor and the second of social implication.

The observation that moderate alcohol consumers enjoy better health than abstainers may be confounded by co-linear patterns of behavior, social class and education. Put simply, the argument is that moderate consumers are moderate individuals who enjoy moderate life styles (exercise, balanced diet, low prevalence of smoking, high education and general health awareness). In contrast, continues the argument, abstainers of alcohol also miss out elsewhere, including exercise, diet balance and health education. This debate is not easily resolved. In most areas of medical science an "intervention study" would allow consensus to be reached but ethically and practically it is all but impossible to supplement abstainers with alcohol in moderation to see if this leads to an improvement in long-term health. Thus, we must reply on population survey studies, with their inherent limitations noted above. A major step in addressing whether the "moderate alcohol-better health" picture is confounded or not is the identification of underlying mechanisms. If biological pathways exist that explain the observations, then greater confidence can be drawn from the survey data. *Beer in Health and Disease Prevention* provides extensive data on the underlying science that can link moderate ethanol consumption, or other components of beer, to biological responses thus explaining some of the epidemiological observations. It also provides a framework around which further scientific studies can be built and, therefore, paves the way in providing quantification or "attributable benefit" to the associations.

However, if the J-shaped curve is proven beyond reasonable doubt what then do governments and health organizations do with the data? Will this not simply fuel further excessive drinking? It, of course, depends on how the message is handled and the context in which it is delivered. The message of abstention (or less-is-better) is not working in certain quarters. The concept that responsible drinking could be well regarded in all circles of society while irresponsible drinking becomes socially unacceptable, again at all levels, has its merit. Industry, governments, health organizations, alcohol organizations and health care professionals will need to pull together with respect to taxation, acceptable beverage types and marketing strategies, serving sizes, alcohol content, sales policies, definition of moderation, and public dissemination of responsible drinking messages. As such the J-shaped curve may have a role to play in addressing one of the most pressing public health issues of our time. Beer has probably been around, in one form or another, since Neolithic times. It has, over millennia, provided clean, uninfected hydration and nutrition for many populations when water supplies and some foods have failed in this respect. It gently crosses geography, creed and culture and is enjoyed by hundreds of millions of people across the world. *Beer in Health and Disease Prevention* not only pushes our thinking on the breadth of the alcohol–health debate, but it is also a timely reminder to society of the more gentle face of Janus when it comes to the complex, ancient but humble pint.

Professor Jonathan J. Powell
Head of Section (Micronutrient Status Research) and
Visiting Chair of Medicine (KCL)
MRC Human Nutrition Research
Elsie Widdowson Laboratory
Cambridge, UK
Jonathan.powell@mrc-hnr.cam.ac.uk

Part I

General Aspects of Beer and Constituents

(i) Beer Making, Hops and Yeast

1

Overview of Manufacturing Beer: Ingredients, Processes, and Quality Criteria

Sascha Wunderlich and Werner Back Lehrstuhl für Technologie der Brauerei I, Freising-Weihenstephan, Germany

Abstract

Brewers worldwide produce beer at an advanced technological level while keeping in mind the importance of tradition. The basic ingredients are water, malted barley, hops, and yeast, as it is fixed in Germany by the legislation governing commercial brewing, the *Reinheitsgebot* (Purity Law) (BGB1, 1993). Brewing technologies worldwide are based on this recipe, although brewers in other countries have more flexibility, for example in selection of starch supply. Nevertheless, barley is commonly used as the source of starch but it has to be malted to dissolve starch in the grains prior to brewing. Malting steps are steeping, germination, and kilning. Enzymes digest grain contents during these processes and prepare starch for further processes. Heating during kilning produces coloring and flavoring substances. Further enzymes convert the starch of milled malt to fermentable sugars during mashing. This procedure results in wort that is boiled. Hops are added in this stage of boiling. Yeast converts sugars to alcohol during fermentation of cooled wort. After maturation and storage, beer is filtered and stabilized to inhibit quality deficiencies. These may be turbidity, decrease of flavor stability, or decrease of foam stability. Each production step influences decisively the resulting beer. So, an enormous variety of beers is possible that are all tasty, thirst-quenching and healthy.

List of Abbreviations

4-VG	Vinylguaiacol
°dH	Degree of hardness
DMS	Dimethyl sulfite
DMS-P	Dimethyl sulfite precursor
FAN	Free amino nitrogen
POC	Phenolic off-flavor
PVPP	Polyvinylpolypyrrolidon

Introduction

Beer is one of the oldest cultural achievements of mankind and one of the most popular beverages all over the world. From the technological point of view, beer has four main properties based on its contents and manufacturing processes. It is (i) pure, (ii) wholesome, (iii) valuable, and (iv) it displays a variety of styles and genres:

(a) The purity is guaranteed by the natural ingredients: hops, malt, yeast, and water. No pathogenic germs are found in beer because of the pH-value, presence of hop substances, the anaerobic environment, the alcohol content and also the fact that yeast metabolizes nearly all fermentable sugars. Therefore, other micro-organisms experience a food shortage. Additionally, the manufacturing process is a clarifying process. Mashing, lautering, boiling, fermentation, and filtration separate harmful or exogenous substances.

(b) Beer is wholesome because of the variability and the balance of its contents. For example, 1 l of beer has low carbohydrate contents and fewer calories than the equivalent amount of apple juice or milk. It contains no preserving agents but valuable amino acids at a moderate acidity. Generally, its alcohol content is in a physiologically advantageous relation to its water content.

(c) Beer is a valuable source of vitamins (especially in form of B-complexes), minerals and antioxidants. Beer is, *inter alia*, an excellent source of bio-available silicon. Further, gallic acid, quercetin, xanthohumol, and Maillard products like pronyl-lysine have been implicated in contributing to the wholesome nature of beer.

(d) All over the world more than 100 beer varieties are produced, from Pilsener to lager and wheat beer, as well as non-alcoholic varieties. Differences are based on the careful selection of raw materials and variations of the brewing process. Selected contents can be emphasized by special manufacturing methods (Back, 2005a; Bamforth, 2004).

Raw Materials

Water, malt, hops, and yeast are the four main ingredients for manufacturing beer. Quality and suitability of these ingredients is absolutely vital for a tasty and beneficial

Beer in Health and Disease Prevention
ISBN: 978-0-12-373891-2

product, as they are for cooking. Purchasing of raw materials for the brewery needs to strictly observe predefined quality criteria. These criteria are as variable as the different types of beer on the market (Kunze, 1999; Heyse, 2000; Bamforth, 2003; Briggs *et al.*, 2004).

Water

Water is the main component of beer and so breweries often stress the purity and originality of their brewing liquor. Water quality for brewing beer is often determined by legislation. It has to be potable, pure, and free of pathogens, as measured by chemical and microbial analyses. Additionally, there are ancillary quality requirements for water used for brewing. The pH-value is especially important because different production steps only take place optimally at defined pH-values. Substantial amounts of ions are released from malt during mashing. These ions react with water ions that cause changes in the pH-value. Alkaline earth metals (in first order Ca^{2+} and Mg^{2+}) are important for the aspect of hardness in brewing liquor. Others like K^+ often play a minor role. Generally, Ca^{2+} and Mg^{2+} are responsible for decreasing the pH-value. It is increased by hydrogen carbonate ions. Reactions with primary, secondary, and tertiary phosphates originating from malt inhibit this effect, but partly can also stimulate it. The relationship of pH-value increasing and decreasing ions finds its expression in the residual alkalinity of brewing water. It describes the effect that 3.5 mol Ca^{2+} or 7 mol Mg^{2+} can compensate the pH-value increasing effect of 1 mol hydrogen carbonate ions.

$$\text{Residual alkalinity} = \text{total alkalinity} - (\text{hardness of } Ca^{2+} + 0.5 \times \text{hardness of } Mg^{2+})/3.5$$

Total alkalinity represents hardness of carbonates, which is the content of carbonate and hydrogen carbonate ions. The contribution of carbonates to a conventional water pH-value below 8.2 is marginal and can be neglected. Traditionally, residual alkalinity is given in country-specific degrees of hardness. For example, in Germany 1 degree of hardness (°dH) is 10 CaO mg/l or 0.36 mmol/l. In mash, an increased pH-value can be expected with increasing residual alkalinity. An increase of the residual alkalinity of 10 °dH is accompanied by an increase of the pH-value of 0.3 as a guideline in Germany. Water with a residual alkalinity of 0 does not influence the pH-value in mash. It acts in a similar way to distilled water. A residual alkalinity $<$5 °dH (better below 2 °dH) is recommended for pale brews. Dark brews can take a residual alkalinity $<$10 °dH, which complements the more flavorsome character of dark beer. Most water has to be conditioned for brewing. This happens, for example by ion exchange using synthetic resins or by the addition of brewing gypsum ($CaSO_4$). In the latter case, the evolving K_2SO_4 is unfavorable from a sensory point of view. Amounts exceeding 30 mg $CaSO_4$/hl should be avoided. Other mineral ions also influence the brewing process or taste. Sulfate, for example, can cause a hard and dry taste but favors a hop bouquet. Iron and manganese contents of more than 0.2 mg/l result in an unfavorable color and taste. Calcium protects α-amylase from early inactivation during mashing. Zinc stimulates yeast growth and fermentation; these processes are inhibited by nitrates (Narziss, 1992; Heyse, 2000).

Barley and other cereals

Generally, barley (*Hordeum vulgare*) is – after water – quantitatively the second most important ingredient for beer. Brewers admire barley because it prospers even in adverse growing conditions. Germination may be easily adjusted during malting. Enzymes and other brewing technology-relevant substances that are produced are favorable from a process point of view. Two-row barley is preferred in Germany for its extract content. In general, barley with more rows has less developed grains but higher protein content and enzymatic strength. This is advantageous for adjunct brewing (brewing outside Germany).

Other crops like wheat, rye, triticale, spelt, and emmer are also suitable for brewing. Mostly they are added to barley malt. Bavarian wheat beer needs wheat as an adjunct in excess of 50%. Recently, first trials in assessing alternative cereals and pseudo-cereals like sorghum for their suitability in malting were conducted. They resulted in brews with novel sensory and health aspects (Back, 2005a). Alternative starch suppliers (malt substitutes) are interesting for their availability, profitability, and their special color and aroma contribution. Often raw materials, like unmalted barley, wheat, rice, or corn are used. Sometimes starch, saccharine, glucose, and corresponding syrups are also used (Bamforth, 2003; Briggs *et al.*, 2004). Their application is regulated in every country. In Germany, the use of malt substitutes is prohibited according to the *Reinheitsgebot* (the Purity Law governing commercial brewing). The United States allows an input of unmalted cereals of up to 34% and an input of sugars or syrups of up to 2.5% of the total grist (Back, 2005a).

Grain Contents *Starch* is the most important content in grain for brewers. It is produced during photosynthesis and is stored as starch granules in the endosperm (Figure 1.1). About 63% of the grain's dry weight is starch. It is a food source for the embryo until it is a self-sufficient producer of metabolites. Starch consists of amylose (20–25%) and amylopectin (75–80%) that are α-(1,4) glycosidic bonds of glucose molecules. Amylopectin is a more complex molecule than amylase and can absorb water into its macromolecular structure for easier enzymatic degradation. Amylose does not agglutinate. Thus, enzymatic degradation is therefore more difficult.

Cellulose is the crude fiber that represents about 6% of the grain's dry weight. It is mostly detected in the grain covering husks (Figure 1.1). Traces are also found in the embryo, pericarp, and testa. It consists of glucose molecules as β-(1,4) glycosidic bonds. Cellulose is flavor neutral. It does not dissolve

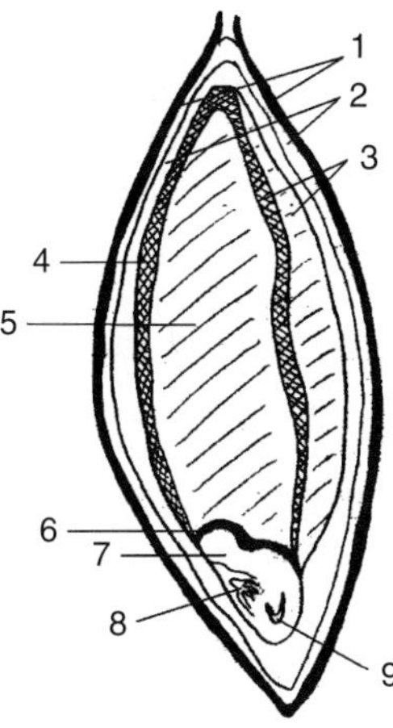

Figure 1.1 Grain morphology: 1–3 coating (1: husk, 2: pericarp and testa, 3: furrow); 4 and 5 endosperm (4: protein (gluten) layer, 5: starch granules); 6–9 embryo (6: epithelium, 7: shield, 8: acrospire, 9: root).

in water and survives the malting and brewing process intact. In husks cellulose is strengthened by lignin. It acts as a filter during lautering. *Hemicelluloses* mostly occur in membranes of starch granules in the endosperm, where they act as structural substances. They can also be found in husks to a lesser degree (Figure 1.1). Hemicelluloses are soluble in bases. The hot water soluble fractions are *gums*. Hemicelluloses and gums are polysaccharides and consist of glucose, hexurone acids and pentosans. β-Glucan is the most important factor in barley that influences the viscosity of wort and beer. *Protein* content in barley ranges between 8% and 13.5%. One-third may end up in the final beer. Protein is found in the embryo and mostly in the endosperm (Figure 1.1). It is divided into four fractions: albumins, soluble in distilled water; globulins, soluble in weak hydrochloric acid; prolamins, soluble in alcoholic solutions; and gutelins, soluble in weak bases. Prolamins and gutelins are storage proteins. Albumins and globulins are important for foam and colloidal characteristics of beer. *Minerals* originate in the embryo and the aleurone layer in the endosperm (Figure 1.1). They constitute 3% of the grain dry weight and are organically bound to about 80%. The most important minerals are silicon, potassium, and phosphorus as part of nucleic acids and phytin acid. Free phosphates influence the pH-value of the mash and downstream during fermentation. *Lipids* also occur in the embryo and the aleurone layer (about 3% grain dry weight). They may affect the taste and foam stability of beer. Especially, sterols may be regarded as pacemakers for starting fermentation. Barley and malt are rich in *vitamins*. These are mostly located in the embryo but also in the aleurone layer (Figure 1.1). Cereals also contain vitamin C, as do virtually all aerobically respiring forms of life. Most of the vitamins found belong to the B-complexes though. Vitamins can be nurtured and enhanced during malting. *Polyphenols* have numerous impacts on brewing. They influence color, foam, taste, and haze formation in beer. Husks, pericarp, and testa contain polyphenols in amounts between 0.1% and 0.3% grain dry weight (Figure 1.1). Some phenolic carbon acids act in larger amounts as inhibitors for germination (cumarin, vanillic acid, ferulic acid). In smaller amounts they can also stimulate it. Ferulic acid, additionally, is involved in the typical wheat beer aroma by its metabolite 4-vinylguaiacol. Monomer polyphenols originating from flavan, like delphinidin and catechin (anthocyanogens), are able to fix oxygen. They are transformed into protein precipitating, polymer condensation products that can cause haze problems (Briggs, 1998; Narziss, 1999; Heyse, 2000; Bamforth, 2003).

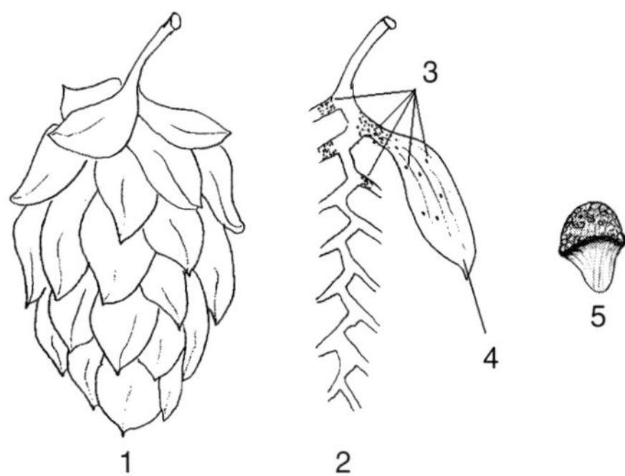

Figure 1.2 Hop morphology, 1: hop cone, 2: axis, 3: lupulin glands, 4: leaf, 5: lupulin gland.

Hop

Hop (*Humulus lupulus L.*) gives beer its typical bitterness and hop aroma. Traditionally, it is also added during brewing because of its preserving effects. Further, hop contains pharmacologically active substances, for example it is said to be soporific, or sleep inducing. All over the world hop is cultivated between the 35th and 55th parallels of latitude, north and south. The largest cultivation areas are in Germany (Hallertau, Elbe-Saale, Tettnang, Spalt) and the United States (Washington, Oregon, Idaho). In hop gardens, or hop fields, only unfertilized female plants are grown. They develop cones from their blossoms (Figure 1.2). Of interest to the brewer are lupulin glands, with the exception of the tannins. Lupulin glands are located between spindle and bracts (Figure 1.2).

Hop Contents Three groups of substances are especially interesting from the brewing technological point of view: hop resins, flavoring agents, and polyphenols. Hop resins constitute about 10–20% of the hop dry weight. They represent the sum of all bittering substances. Their important components are the α- and β-acids, whose bittering potential differs markedly. α-Acids are transformed into iso-α-acids during boiling. These iso-α-acids and their derivates have significant bittering potential. β-Acids have a low solubility in wort and beer. Thus, they contribute only a little to bitterness. Hop resins enhance physiological digestibility, foam stability, and bacteriostatic nature of wort and beer over and above the bittering potential.

Hop possesses approximately 0.4–2.0% flavoring agents per dry weight. These are essential oils that are responsible for the hop aroma and bouquet. More than 300 volatile substances have been identified up to now. Polyphenols (4–14% hop dry weight) also impact on beer quality. Additionally, low molecular polyphenols show antioxidative properties among their benefits. The hop polyphenol xanthohumol has been identified as a possible anticarcinogenic agent (Piendl, 2000; Back, 2005a). Amounts of polyphenols and composition depend on hop variety, cultivation area, and climatic conditions (Narziss, 1992).

Hop Products for the Brewery Brewers often stick to selected hop products because it gives their beer its special and predictable character. Generally, a differentiation is made between aroma hop and bitter hop. Flavor hops have lower α-acid contents but higher contents of essential oils. The flavor of each of these hop varieties has its own quality. Bitter hops have higher α-acid contents but lower contents of essential oils. Then there are different hop products. Breweries rarely use hop cones these days but pellets and hop extracts. Pellets are made from raw hops that are dried, ground, mixed, and pelletized. Hop extracts result from extraction with ethanol or carbon dioxide. After the extraction procedure, solvents are removed as far as possible. The resulting residue is a resin-like sticky substance. Extracted substances differ in their chemical make-up according to which solvent was used in extraction. In isomerized products α-acids are already transformed into iso-α-acids. These products can be added during wort boiling (kettle products) or before filtration (downstream products). It is possible to bitter a beer post-brewhouse or to give a hop aroma with special oils or emulsions. Special extracts can also be used for enrichment of hop substances, for example xanthohumol. Other products inhibit light-struck flavor or can be used to enhance foam. It should be noted that these special products have different sensory properties. An ancillary dosage regime is recommended (Narziss, 1992; Heyse, 2000).

Yeast

The following are the main criteria for a good brewing yeast: fermentation behavior (bottom or top fermentation), flocculation (powdery or flocculent yeast), fermentation performance (fermentation rate, degree of fermentation), production, and degradation of side products (aroma development, diacetyl removal), as well as intensity of propagation. Generally, yeasts are *Saccharomyces* yeasts and many breweries have their own yeast strains. In speciality beers different yeasts like *Brettanomyces* yeasts may also be used (Bamforth, 2003; Briggs *et al.*, 2004; Back, 2005b; Narziss, 2005). In the brewery, bottom fermenting yeast mostly is cultivated at 8–14°C. Pilsener or lager is general representatives of this genre. Top fermenting yeast mostly is cultivated at 15–26°C. Temperature increases during fermentation and creates a fruity, estery flavor (e.g. Bavarian wheat beer). Appropriate yeast propagation and fast fermentation are essential for good quality brewing. Yeast has to be at an optimal nutritional state and conditions for metabolism have to be optimized accordingly.

Yeast Nutrition All malt wort is the ideal nutrient solution for yeast. *Carbohydrates* occur as utilizable sugars (fructose, glucose, sucrose, maltose, maltotriose). *Nitrogen* is important for synthesis of proteins and therefore essential for yeast propagation and fermentation. In wort, nitrogen mostly occurs in amino acids, peptides, and proteins. Concentrations of 900–1,200 mg/l total soluble nitrogen are considered to be sufficient. A rate of 20–25% should occur as free amino nitrogen (FAN). Different amino acids are utilized at different rates. This is important when an amino acid (e.g. valine) is slowly taken up but is immediately needed for propagation. The amino acid has to be synthesized by the yeast itself. By-products like alpha-aceto-lactate (diacetyl precursor) are synthesized that may have an impact on beer quality. Yeasts need minerals for enzyme activation (mostly potassium for kinases and dehydrogenates) and propagation (magnesium > 40 mg/l). Magnesium acts as a link between phosphate structures and enzymes (phosphorylation) and is also needed for enzyme activation. Calcium helps propagation and slows down degeneration. Sodium is needed for potassium transport and enzyme synthesis. Trace elements like iron, zinc, manganese, and copper are also involved in cell construction and enzyme reactions. Propagation, fermentation activity, and flocculation decreases, if yeast is depleted in zinc levels. Yeast can be enriched by repeated generations in zinc rich wort because of accrual. Additionally, sufficient manganese content is positive for yeast metabolism. It is considered as a potentially substituting element for zinc. Oxygen is needed for synthesis of sterols (mostly ergosterol) and fatty acids (e.g. palmitic acid, oleic acid), although respiration is considered unimportant for yeast. Most of the oxygen is immediately esterified. So a sterol pool is built up for yeast propagation. Oxygen is also part of porphyrin synthesis, regulation of gene expression, and the development of mitochondria. Aeration with 8–12 mg O_2/l is considered as sufficient for standard gravity worts. Further nutrients that are needed in small amounts and are present in all malt wort are vitamins (mostly biotin, pantothenic acid, nicotinic acid, thiamine for synthesis of coenzymes), purines, pyrimidines, nucleosines, nucleotides (RNA and DNA synthesis), fatty acids (lipid synthesis), sulfur (for cysteine and methionine synthesis), and phosphorus (in phospholipids, for phosphorylation) (Heyse, 2000; Briggs *et al.*, 2004; Back, 2005a; Narziss, 2005).

Yeast Metabolism Alcoholic fermentation is the main metabolic pathway during brewing. Ethanol and CO_2 originate from glucose. The so named "Crabtree-effect" inhibits aerobic metabolism in the presence of oxygen due to glucose repression. Further quality-determining beer contents are produced during fermentation besides alcohol and CO_2, for example diacetyl, higher alcohols, esters, vinylguaiacol (4-VG), and SO_2. Higher alcohols like 2- or 3-methyl butanol and 2-phenyl ethanol may strongly influence the beer aroma. Mostly alcoholic, floral to solvent-like flavor notes are ascribed to higher alcohols. Esters are the most important aroma component in top fermented beers. They give fruity flavor notes and are divided into two groups: (i) acetate ester that result from acetyl-CoA and alcohol and (ii) fatty acid ester that result from fatty acids and ethanol. Important representatives are ethyl-acetate and isoamyl-acetate. 4-VG is a phenolic substance that mostly characterizes wheat beer. The origin of phenolic substances is regulated via POC (phenolic off-flavor) gene. It occurs in every yeast but is not expressed in bottom fermenting yeast. 4-VG results from ferulic acid. SO_2 is a natural antioxidant that is produced during fermentation. It contributes to flavor stability in beer. Sulfate originated from wort is enzymatically reduced to sulfite. This is used for amino acid synthesis or is released from cells. Reserve carbohydrates (glycogen, trehalose) are created at the beginning of nutrient shortage. They are said to be important for starting the fermentation, especially when repitching yeast (Heyse, 2000; Back, 2005a).

Demands on Yeast for Brewing Yeast for fermentation should be at peak condition. It has to have a high viability and vitality. Viability is the alive–dead rate of yeast cells. Vitality characterizes physiological condition of alive cells. In breweries different strategies are used to ensure optimal yeast condition. Brewers have to decide whether pure culture yeast or (also) repitched yeast is used. Repitched yeast characterizes yeast that has had prior exposure to fermenting wort (sometimes repeatedly). There are also different methods for yeast propagation before starting fermentation. The resulting yeast is always examined for viability and vitality (Heyse, 2000; Briggs *et al.*, 2004; Back, 2005a).

Making Beer

The production of beer includes malting and brewing. It is a value chain in which every step has an impact on the quality properties of the resulting beer.

Malting

Barley is a natural product. Its composition differs depending on variety, growing area, climate, harvesting conditions, preselection, and so on. Barley is rarely directly delivered from fields to maltings. Grain merchants normally act as go-betweens being responsible for pre-cleaning the crop and having samples analyzed in a laboratory.

Demands on Barley by the Maltster At first the maltster conducts a visual assessment of the crop at hand. This requires some experience, but often it is decisive in terms of the acceptance or rejection of a batch besides other analyses. Visual assessment values odor, color, homogeneity, brilliance, and husk quality. Additionally, it gives the counts of half grains, seeds of weeds, and alien elements that reduce the price. Crops with pest infestation, like grain weevil or grain moth, should definitely be rejected. Visual assessment may also discover grain defects that mostly result from adverse weather before cropping. Such a defect is, for example sprouting that occurs after seasons with hot weather during maturation. It accelerates the end of dormancy. Considerable precipitation causes germination of the grain just at the ear of the grain plant. Such grains are often dead and show an increased rate of microbial infection. There are percentage limits for grain defects that justify rejection. Other important criteria are germinative capacity, water content, and protein content. They are determined at delivery to the maltings by rapid tests. Germinative capacity is the percentage of alive to dead grains and should be $>95\%$ in rapid tests; $>96\%$ after cleaning and sorting in storage. Non-germinating grains retained as raw during malting may become infected by mildew and bacteria. Higher molecular β-glucan is dissolved from such grains during mashing. This can cause lautering and filtration problems downstream. Additionally, there may be a shortage of FAN. This may cause an insufficient fermentation and concomitant reduction in beer quality. Further non-germinating grains show a lower saccharification. So, only low final attenuations may be recorded. Water content should be no more than 13%. The higher the water content, the higher the respiration losses. Mildew infection may be the result. Grains with higher water content have to be dried. Protein content should be between 9.5% and 10% (water-free), so that beer can be brewed that shows resilience to long distance delivery or has better colloidal stability. Lower protein contents result in reduced foam stability, body, or flavor stability. Additionally, yeast nutrition may be reduced in assimilable nitrogen that may cause unfavorable fermentation by-products. Protein content varies between 10% and 11% (in the case of very bright beers of the Pilsener type). Protein contents between 11% and 11.5% are sufficient for conventional beers. Protein contents in the range of 11–12% are suitable for dark malt brews containing Münchner malt and darker due to its color and flavor. Barley that has a higher protein content may be the cause of colloidal instability in beer. These require an intensive, heavily malting with increased losses. Another criterion is the purity of the grade of barley. This is determined after cleaning and sorting. Grains should have diameters >2.2 mm, better >2.5 mm (full barley) at a rate of $>90\%$. Malting with grains of different sizes results in heterogeneous malt because small grains have increased protein contents and germinate faster compared to larger ones. In a brewery, heterogeneous malt causes problems during processing and reduces beer quality (Briggs, 1998; Narziss, 1999; Heyse, 2000; Back, 2005a).

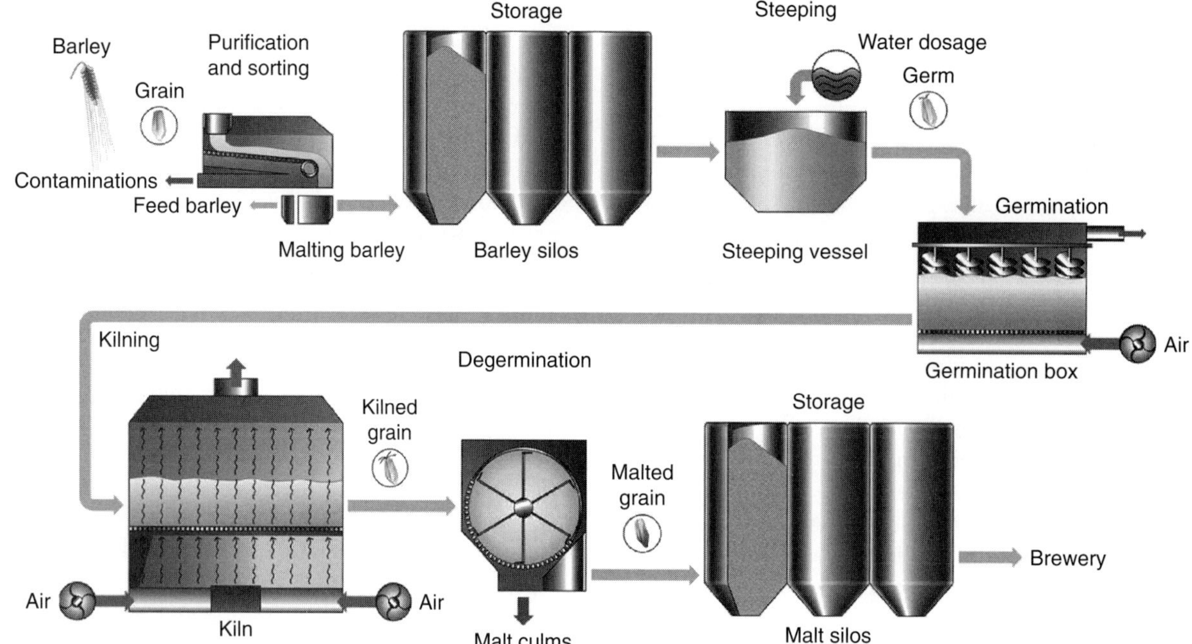

Figure 1.3 Malting process schematically. *Source*: Modified from Gesellschaft für Öffentlichkeitsarbeit, Deutscher Brauerbund.

Storage The crop is stored in aerated and cooled silos. Barley needs a time frame between 4 and 8 weeks after storage until it can be reprocessed. Grain is protected against early germination at the stem during this dormancy. Maturity of germination is determined via germinative energy prior to further processing. It is the percentage rate of grains that would germinate at the time of examination and should be >96% (Narziss, 1998; Heyse, 2000; Back, 2005a).

Malting Process Malting is the artificially induced germination of a crop. The maltster's aim is controlled dissolution of grain. Enough enzymes have to be activated and produced, so grain contents are homogeneously dissolved. Kilning follows steeping and germination to fix substantial translations and to create typical malt character (Figure 1.3).

Steeping and Germination Barley needs sufficient oxygen, heat, and humidity for germination. Water input induces changes in grain. Water content in grain of between 42% and 48% has to occur for the desired substantial translations within a defined time frame. Germination temperatures range between 14°C and 18°C. Oxygen is essential for respiration, otherwise the embryo dies. CO_2 has to be removed. At first, development of the embryo is visible at the root germ and acrospire (Figure 1.2). The main root breaks through the grain and emerges between husks (chit). Further side roots emerge (fork). Acrospire grows between pericarp, testa, and back husk. Reserving substances are degraded by enzymes and transferred into soluble forms in endosperm. Other substances are produced for energy supply and tissue. Solution processes increase, thus the grain becomes more and more brittle. Steeping and germination may differ depending on technical equipment, crop variety, and annual set. Six days are considered to be optimum for steeping and germination.

Biochemical Processes During Malting Following and regulating degradation of the three main groups of substances are the most important criteria during the malting and brewing process. These groups are starch (amylolysis), proteins (proteolysis), and structural substances (cytolysis). Further degradation processes are lipid and phosphate degradation.

Substances in starch granules coatings are degraded during *cytolysis*. This is the prerequisite for facilitating digestion of starch granules by enzymes during mashing. Insufficient cytolysis results in yield losses and release of higher molecular β-glucan. Proteins are transformed into soluble low, medium, and high molecular substances during *proteolysis*. Insufficient degradation results in shortage of assimilable nitrogen for yeast. Consequences may be problems during fermentation and maturation like production of unfavorable side products (mostly diacetyl). High molecular protein is missed at excessive proteolysis that reduces foam and flavor stability. Starch is digested by amylolytic enzymes during *amylolysis*. α- and β-Amylases are the most important representatives.

Enzymes that are important for malting and mashing are displayed in Table 1.1. Different enzymes are subdivided into endo- and exo-peptidases. Hydrolytic enzymes like α-amylase, limit dextrinase, and endo-peptidase are produced during germination (*de novo*). This enzyme induction is provided by gibberellins acid and gibberellins A1.

Table 1.1 Occurrence of important enzymes during malting and mashing

				Malting					Mashing	
	Enzyme	Substrate	Product	Barley	Green malt	Cured malt	Optimum temperature (°C)	Optimum pH	Optimum temperature (°C)	Optimum pH
Zytolysis	β-Glucan-solubilase	Matrix bound β-glucan	Soluble high molecular β-glucan	++	+++	++	62	4.6–7.0	62–65	6.8
	Endo-1,3-β-glucanase	Soluble high molecular β-glucan	Low molecular β-glucan, cellobiose, lamiaribiose	0	+++++	++++	60	4.6–5.5	<60	4.6
	Endo-1,4-β-glucanase	Soluble high molecular β-glucan	Low molecular β-glucan, cellobiose, lamiaribiose	+	++++	+++	40–45	4.5–4.8	40–45	4.5–4.8
	Exo-β-glucanase	Cellobiose, lamiaribiose	Glucose	+	++++	–	<40	4.5	<40	4.5
Proteolysis	Endo peptidase	Proteins	Peptides, free amino acids	+(+)	+++++	++++	40–55	5.0–5.2	45–50	3.9–5.5
	Carboxy peptidase	Proteins, peptides	Free amino acids	+	++++	+++	50–60	5.2	50	4.8–5.6
	Amino peptidase	Proteins, peptides	Free amino acids	++	+++	++	40–45	7.2	45	7.0–7.2
	Dipeptidase	Dipeptides	Free amino acids	+(+)	+++	+++	40–50	7.7–8.2	45	8.8
Amylolysis	α-Amylase	High and low molecular α-glucan	Melagosaccharids, oligosaccharids	0	++++	+++	70–75	5.6–5.8	65–75	5.6–5.8
	β-Amylase	α-Glucan	Maltose	+(+)	++++	++	60–65	5.4–5.6	60–65	5.4–5.6
	Maltase	Maltose	Glucose	+(+)	+++	++	34–40	6.0	35–40	6.0
	Limit dextrinase	Limit dextrine	Dextrine	(+)	+++	++	55–60	5.5	55–60	5.1
Further relevant enzymes	Lipase	Lipids, lipid hydro peroxides	Glycerine + free long chain fatty acids, fatty acid hydro peroxides	0	+++	+	15–18		55–60	6.8–7.0
	Lipoxygenase	Free long chain fatty acids	Fatty acid hydro peroxides	(+)	++++	–	12–15		45–55	6.5–7.0
	Polyphenoloxidase	Polyphenols	Oxidized polyphenols	++	+++	++	15		60–65	6.5–7.0
	Peroxidase	Organic + inorganic substrates	Free radicals	(+)	++	+	15		>60	6.2
	Phosphatase	Organically bound phosphate	Inorganic phosphate	+(+)	++++	++	15	5.6–6.1	50–53	5.0

Source: Back (2005a, b) and Narziss (1992, 1999).

These growth promoters (hormones) are led from embryo via shield to aleuronic epithelium. There and in shield enzymes are released. Endo-peptidase stimulates release of endo-β-glucanase and endo-xylanase. Other enzymes like acidic phosphatase are not released from aleurone but activated by water intake. Enzyme capacity and thus speed of dissolution processes is increased by addition of, for example, gibberellin acid, although this is not permitted in Germany under the *Reinheitsgebot*.

Kilning Malt Kilning removes water, fixes substantial translations, and creates typical malt colors and aromas. Green malt loses its raw grain character. Kilning is subdivided into withering and curing. Water content of from 45% to 10% is reduced at low temperatures during withering. Curing needs temperatures in a range between 80°C and 105°C. Duration and intensity of withering and curing depends on strived malt. Drying continues until water content reaches 3.5–4% in pale malts and 1.5–2% in dark malts. An amount of 100 kg barley results in about 160 kg green malt and about 80 kg cured malt after drying. The volume of green malt should be conserved. Essential chemical transformations take place during kilning. Growing is ongoing at temperatures below 40°C and water content above 20% (growing phase). Enzymes cause dissolution of the grain and the amount of degradation products increases. Further enzymatic degradation occurs at temperatures between 40°C and 70°C (enzymatic phase). Degradation processes stop with decreasing water content. The embryo's growth is discontinued and degradation products accumulate. Losses of enzymes increase with increasing humidity and temperature of malt. Coagulation and reduced dispersion of colloidal nitrogen substances occurs at temperatures >70°C (chemical phase). Properties of β-glucan change by production of low molecular substances at low viscosity. Intensive Maillard reaction takes place at temperatures >95°C. Color and aroma components arise from low molecular substances (sugars and amino acids). Dimethyl sulfite (DMS) is an important quality criterion in malt. It is a sulfur-containing, odor- and taste-intensive substance. The higher the curing temperature, the lower the contents of DMS precursors (DMS-P). Thus, dark malt has lower contents of DMS-P. Reduction of DMS-P in pale malts results from low temperatures for a longer time thus increased coloring is inhibited. Homogeneous inferior malt may be brewed to a pleasing beer by an adapted brewing process. In contrast, mixtures of high- and low-quality malt are insufficient. Radicles are removed after kilning because it rapidly adsorbs water again. Additionally, it causes bitter taste and increased coloring. Afterwards the malt is stored. Further physical and chemical changes during storage facilitate the reprocessing of malt (Briggs, 1998; Kunze, 1999; Narziss, 1999; Back, 2005a).

Different Malts Production of pale malt significantly differs from production of dark malt. Barley for dark malt needs higher protein content and more intensive handling (high degree of steeping, higher germination temperatures) for grain dissolution and enrichment of precursors for coloring and aroma. The moisture of green malt is slowly reduced during withering of dark malt. Thus, dissolution is ongoing and enough educts arise for Maillard reaction. High curing temperatures (>95°C) result in a typical dark malt aroma. Inverse processes are used for pale malt. Water in green malt is rapidly reduced by fresh air. Curing temperatures range between 76°C and 80°C for pale color and conserving enzymes.

There are many special malts and kilned raw grain that are similarly produced. All of them have a special impact on beer character:

- Pale or dark wheat malt is used for wheat beer at grist ratios >50%. Flavor precursors get into wort and result in typical wheat beer aroma by top fermentation.
- Caramel malt awards beer a mouthfilling, malty character, and dark color. They are used in grist ratios between 2% and 10%.
- Roasted malt is added in grist ratios between 0.5% and 5%. It gives dark color and roasting flavor.
- Roasted barley, roasted rye, and others originate from unmalted, but roasted crops. Resulting beers have a roasting, raw grain-like character. They are mostly used for stout and ale (Briggs, 1998; Narziss, 1999; Heyse, 2000).

Brewing process

There are four main steps during the brewing process: (i) wort preparation that includes mashing and boiling, (ii) fermentation, (iii) maturation, and (iv) filtration and/or stabilization (Figure 1.4).

Milling Prior to mashing malt has to be milled. Therefore, dust, stones, and metals are removed from malt to avoid damage at the milling cylinder or dust explosion. Generally malt mixtures are used for one brew. Milling increases reactive surfaces for enzymes, thus malt ingredients are easier to dissolve. Husk should be saved because it serves as filtration layer during lautering. In some breweries, mash filter is used as an alternative to the lauter tun in which no husk or coarse pieces are necessary. Malt can be fine milled in a hammer mill. The quality of milling has an impact on mashing and lautering and thus on quality of the resulting beer. For example, undissolved malt should be milled finer than well-dissolved malt because physical and enzymatic degradation processes are eased then (Narziss, 1992; Kunze, 1999; Briggs *et al.*, 2004).

Mashing Grist is mixed with water during mashing. Enzymes dissolute malt substances. Processes are regulated by temperature and its residence time (rest), pH-value, and water grist ratio (affusion). Generally, the same enzymatic processes take place as during malting; amylolysis, proteolysis, and cytolysis (section "Biochemical processes during malting" in Chapter 3).

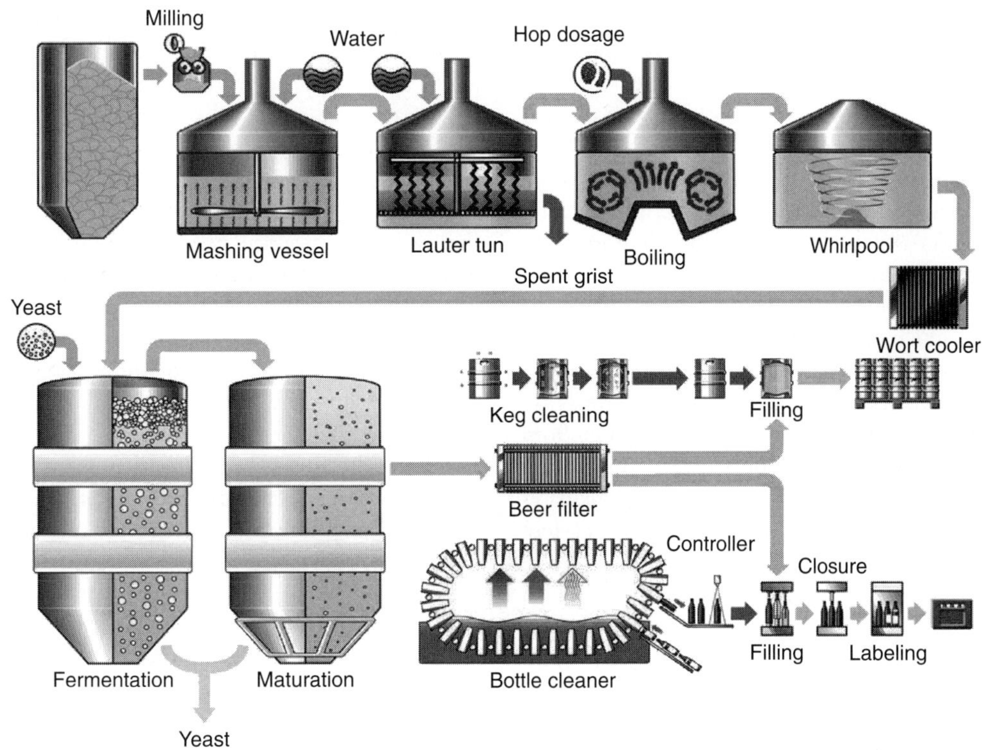

Figure 1.4 Brewing process schematically. *Source*: Modified from Gesellschaft für Öffentlichkeitsarbeit, Deutscher Brauerbund.

Amylolysis Starch occurs as amylose and amylopectin. Their dissolution proceeds in three steps: (1) gelatinizing starch, (2) liquefaction, and (3) saccharification. Starch molecules adsorb water during gelatinizing. They first swell and later explode. Gelatinizing temperature depends on the type of corn and occurrence of amylases. Starch originated from malt gelatinizes at 60°C with the presence of amylases. Other starch suppliers like rice, corn, rye, sorghum, etc., have different optimum temperatures for gelatinization. Availability, economy, and special color or flavor contribution increase interest in so-called adjuncts. Often they are used in raw, unmalted form. Special technologies like cereal cookers or addition of enzymes may be necessary for conversion to sugar. Pre-gelatinized products are used, too. Countries have fixed different maximum amounts of adjuncts for beer production. In United States, for example 34% of grist load may be unmalted cereals. In Germany use of adjuncts is prohibited. Gelatinized starch is mostly digested by amylases during liquefaction. α-Amylase splits α-1,4 bonds of amylose and amylopectin. Starch cracks from the inside and larger fragments result. Viscosity decreases at the same time and new reactive surfaces are created for β-amylase. Dextrins are broken down to maltose during saccharification.

Brewers control starch breakdown by 0.2 N iodine tincture. This iodine test is based on the coloring effect of iodine solution. Starch and larger dextrins result in blue to red color. Sugar and small dextrins show no color. In this case, mash is "iodine normal."

Proteolysis In contrast to low-ordered starch molecules, proteins occur in mash as a mix of different sized molecular groups. There are high molecular substances as well as amino acids. Enzymes for proteolysis are divided in endo- and exo-peptidases and are characterized by different effective optima. Endo-peptidases break down proteins from the inner and increase soluble nitrogen content. Exo-enzymes attack ends of protein chains and set free amino acids. Some proteins precipitate already during mashing as a result of temperature and pH-value. Dissolution processes of proteins are accelerated during mashing compared to malting (10 to 14 to fold). The greatest protein degradation occurs at 50°C but special protein rest is not necessary if well-dissolved malts are used. Medium and high molecular breakdown products arise at 60–70°C and are important for fullness of flavor and foam. These quality criteria as well as carbonation decrease if protein degradation is extended too far. Additionally, risk increases for turbidity in beer. Insufficient protein degradation results in shortage of assimilable nitrogen. Fermentation is heavy and unwished-for side products arise. Proteases may be set free that decrease foam stability.

Cytolysis Breakdown products of hemicelluloses dissolute and increase viscosity during cytolysis. Main breakdown occurs at temperatures below 50°C. Breakdown decreases rapidly with increasing temperature. β-Glucan degradation stops at temperatures in a range between 60°C and 70°C but it is set free by β-glucan-solubiase. Hydrogen bonds of higher ordered β-glucan molecules break during heating and boiling. Hydrogen bonds conjugate to gels if increased shearing forces occur and viscosity of mash increases. Increased viscosity may result in problems at lautern and filtration. Use of well-dissolved malt and minimizing shearing forces avoids these problems. Mostly lipids are insoluble and are removed via spent grist. Lipases split a small part into glycerine and fatty acids. Especially, non-saturated fatty acids result from reactions with oxygen or enzymatic breakdown into carbonyls by lipoxygenase. They decrease flavor stability already at low concentrations. Milling under inert gas and oxygen-deficient handling avoids these processes. Processes are additionally minimized by mashing at temperatures above 60°C and mash pH-value below 5.2. *Polyphenol* dissolution from husks and endosperm increases with increasing mashing duration and temperature. Peroxidases and polyphenoloxidases digest them enzymatically. Oxidation by oxygen occurs, too. Polymerization of polyphenols decreases the antioxidative potential of beer. This includes reduction of flavor stability. The use of high mashing temperatures and intensively kilned malts reduces peroxidase contents in mash and polyphenols originated from malts are saved. *Organic phosphates* are broken down enzymatically by phosphatases. Products are phosphate and primary phosphates. They decrease pH-value and increase buffering capacity. Lowest pH-values and lowest buffering capacity result at mashing temperatures in a range of 62–65°C. These conditions also promote welcome pH-fall during fermentation. *Zinc* content of wort is also fixed during mashing. It is one product from alcohol dehydrogenase. Low mash pH-values, low mashing temperatures (45–50°C), as well as reduced mash liquor favor zinc release. Zinc concentrations in a range between 0.1 and 0.15 mg/l are recommended.

Generally, most mashing processes go on better at low pH-values. So some brewers do "biological mash acidification." This procedure includes fermentation of first wort with malt borne *Lactobacillus amylovorus* or *L. amylolyticus*. Result is a 2% lactic acid which may be added to mash for decreasing pH-value. International brewers add substances including glucoamylase to mash to increase conversion of starch to fermentable sugar. It is heat-resistant, cops off glucose (like maltase), and has also an exo-action (like β-amylase).

Mash is prepared in special mashing containers (mash tun). Addition of much water (3–4 hl/kg malt) accelerates enzymatic reactions. Such "thin mash" is used for pale brews. Dark brews get by with 3–3.5 hl/kg malt. Generally, there are two types of mashing:

1. Infusion mashing indicates only enzymatic digestion at different temperatures and durations (rests).
2. Decoction mashing includes additionally thermal degradation. Part of the mash is removed, boiled, and returned. This procedure is recommended for use of unmalted cereals.

Well-dissolved malt should be mash in at higher temperatures as mentioned earlier. This results in technological and economic advantages. An adequate mashing procedure is the "high-short-mashing-procedure." It includes mash in at 60–63°C. This temperature is kept for 30–45 min. Then mash is heated at 1°C/min to 72°C. Rest at this temperature is retained until iodine normality is reached (Narziss, 1992; Bamforth, 2003; Briggs *et al.*, 2004; Back, 2005a).

Lautering The aim of lautern is separation of liquids (wort) and solids (spent grist). Husks act as a filter during this procedure. At first, liquid drains off (first wort, extract content: 16–20%). Then, residual spent grist is flushed several times with hot water (last runnings, last extract concentration: 0.5–1%). First wort and last runnings represent wort. The volume of last runnings depends on aimed extract concentration. Temperature is important during lautern, because increasing temperature decreases viscosity and lautern is accelerated. However, temperatures above 80°C are unfavorable. Then, α-amylase is destroyed and undissolved starch cannot be saccharified. Wort will not be iodine normal and starch haze will result in beer.

Generally, lautern is processed in a lauter tun or mash filter. Mash has to rest after transfer into the lauter tun to build a grain bed. First wort run off contains a lot of particles, so it is removed into the lauter tun. Then, first wort runs off and water is added continuously or stepwise for last runnings. Polypropylene filter sheets separate wort and spent grist in a mash filter. This procedure is independent of particle size. Extract content in spent grist fixes the end of lautern. Final extract content in spent grist has to be below 0.8% (Narziss, 1992; Kunze, 1999; Birgss *et al.*, 2004).

Wort Boiling After lautern, wort is transferred to a boiling device (kettle). International brewers may add liquid sugar adjuncts like invert, dextrose, corn syrup, etc., in country specific maximum amounts (e.g. United States 2.5%). Aims of wort boiling are:

- water evaporation, adjustment of extract content in cast wort (original gravity),
- evaporation of unwanted flavor substances like DMS,
- formation of color and flavor substances,
- isomerization of hop bitter substances,
- precipitation of coagulated proteins (flocculation),
- wort sterilization,
- enzyme inactivation.

Here, three points are discussed in more detail.

1. Evaporation of *DMS* that gives a cabbage and vegetable-like flavor. Its concentration in all malt beer should be below the taste threshold of 100 μg/l. Transformation of DMS-P into DMS and evaporation of DMS increase with continued wort boiling.
2. Formation of *color and flavor substances.* Wanted melanoidins arise during boiling, which have antioxidative effects. But unwanted Strecker aldehydes are built up too, and these are precursors for stale flavor. The thermal stress

is characterized by thiobarbitur acid value that should be as low as possible.

3. *Flocculation.* Too much protein in beer results in turbidity. Too little protein is bad for foam and full taste. Concentration of coagulated nitrogen is an indicator that should be in a range of 15 and 25 mg/l. These three parameters have to be optimized for each system.

Hop is added during wort boiling. Brewers do this at the beginning or end of boiling or dose hop into the whirlpool. Hop dosage at the beginning of wort boiling serves for bittering and is generally carried out with bitter hop. A second dosage at the end of boiling or into the whirlpool gives a favorable hop dose. Few brewers add hop cones after fermentation (filling hop). Isomerized hop products may be added after fermentation or before filtration by brewers operating outside the German *Reinheitsgebot.*

Natural lactate acid may be added to wort (analogous to biological mash acidification). This is carried out at the end of wort boiling because isomerization and DMS degradation are decreased at low pH-values. Biological wort acidification facilitates protein precipitation and accelerates pH-fall during fermentation. Substances in lactate acid like zinc and vitamins stimulate yeast vitality. Generally, resulting beers are of increased quality. Taste is rounded off, full, and soft. Carbonation is fresh and sparkling. Brews show a high chemical–physical stability as well as high foam and flavor stability.

Commonly, original gravity is in a range between 11% and 12% at the end of boiling. Output of boiling is increased by so-called high gravity brewing. There, original gravity is up to 16%. Adjustment of alcohol content and residual extract takes place subsequently and mostly before filtration by addition of degassed water. It is an internationally applied procedure used mostly in larger breweries.

Formation of technical elements depends on brewers' demands:

- Use as wort tun only – or additionally as mash container, whirlpool, etc.
- Type of heating – base heating, internal or external boiling, etc.
- Hop and sour property dosage – often an additional container is necessary.
- Boiling under atmospheric pressure – above or below.

Stepwise boiling below atmospheric pressure facilitates evaporation of unwanted substances at reduced energy input. Boiling above atmospheric pressure can proceed continuously and accelerates chemical and physical processes.

Hot trub (hop particles and precipitated proteins) has to be removed after boiling. It can aggravate yeast metabolism, clarification of green beer, and filtration. Mostly a whirlpool separates hot trub. Hot trub settles down in the middle by resulting rotation (tea cup effect). The wort has to be cooled down as fast as possible to minimize infection risk. The temperatures aimed at are 5–10°C for bottom fermentation and 15–25°C for top fermentation. Nowadays, heat is exchanged with the temperature of icy water in a stainless steel plate cooler. Proteins precipitate in wort again at temperatures below 60°C. Particles of this "*cold trub*" (0.5–1 μm) are smaller than those of hot trub (0.5–500 μm). It is removed by separation, filtration, or flotation (aeration of wort). Recent studies show that cold trub is advantageous for fermentation in less recycled yeast.

Aeration of wort is necessary for yeast propagation. Oxygen concentration should be 8–9 mg/l. It has to be added excessively because not all oxygen dissolves in wort (Narziss, 1992; Heyse, 2000; Bamforth, 2003; Briggs *et al.*, 2004; Back, 2005a).

Fermentation, Maturation, and Storage Cooled and aerated wort has to be mixed rapidly with yeast (pitching) for reduced bacteria development. A common yeast dosage is 15–20,000,000 cells/ml at good yeast vitality. Dosages in amounts of 30,000,000 cells/ml are recommended for strong ales or high gravity brews. Yeast is aerated continuously after pitching, which additionally secures homogeneous distribution. The fermentation tank may be open or closed. Larger breweries mostly prefer closed tanks. There brewers may regulate fermentation by pressure and CO_2. *Fermentation temperature* is the decisive factor for fermentation: the higher the temperature, the faster the processes, and the higher the side product concentrations. Applied pressure reduces yeast propagation and decreases formation of side products. Movement in the fermentation tank can also be controlled by temperature. Adapted convection secures good contact between wort and yeast and allows sedimentation for clarifying green beer at the end of fermentation. *Final attenuation* fixes the end of fermentation. It describes the amount of fermentable sugars in wort. No fermentable sugars (*residual extract*) should be left in final beer. This would increase infection risk and decrease digestibility. Generally, green beer has residual extract in a range of 6–10%. This secures sufficient formation of CO_2 during maturation. It may be significantly lower if one tank processes or "krausening" are applied. A further important process is development of pH-value. It should decrease from 5.6 to 4.5 during fermentation (pH-fall). Sour milieu inhibits infections in final beer. *Maturation* serves fermentation of the residual extract. Volatile substances like aldehydes and sulfur compounds are removed by CO_2 bubbles (CO_2-wash). Degradation of alpha-aceto-lactate and especially diacetyl takes place. Sedimentation of yeast clarifies the brew. Degradation of diacetyl as far as possible fixes the end of maturation. *Storage* at low temperatures (0°C and lower, beer freezes at approximately −2°C) serves for further clarification and stabilization of beer. It binds CO_2 and rounds off-flavor. Residual, settled yeast should be removed if not wished otherwise. Dead cells release substances during decomposition that influence flavor and stability of beer. Sometimes international brewers use wooden spans for homogeneous distribution and flotation of yeast during fermentation. Extra zinc addition to yeast equalizes potential shortage. Addition of enzymes during maturation and storage serves filtration and colloidal stability of beer in countries other than Germany. In traditional ale production, finings, such as isinglass (the swim bladder of fish) or Irish moss (a seaweed), are placed in the cask to drag down the yeast and clear the beer (Heyse, 2000; Bamforth, 2003; Briggs *et al.*, 2004; Back, 2005a; Narziss, 2005).

Filtration and Stabilization Consumers expect not only immaculate taste but also a clear or sparkling beverage. Often storage alone does not suffice. Artificial *clarification* takes place by filtration or centrifugation. One, or a combination, of three different processes serves artificial clarification:

1. Coarse, dispersed particles settle down by *sedimentation* or centrifugal force during centrifugation. Colloids remain in beer.
2. *Sieving effect* retains all particles bigger than pore size of filter. Trub particles and larger colloids as well as beer spoiling bacteria remain depending on pore size.
3. Particles and also dissolved substances can be removed by *adsorption*. It is based on affinity of substances to filter material.

Grade of filtration and intensity of stabilization depend on demands of shelf life. *Kieselguhr* filtration alone may be sufficient for a shelf life of 2 months. *Stabilization* via PVPP (polyvinylpolypyrrolidon) and/or silica gel is recommended for a shelf life of 6 months and more. Outside Germany, proteins may be hydrolyzed by papain (enzyme from paw paw).

Yeast, bacteria, and colloids are almost completely removed from beer depending on the selected filtration plate. Filtration plates consist of cellulose fibers from different types of wood, *kieselguhr*, perlite, synthetic fibers, and resins that increase stability of filters. Large surfaces serve optimum adsorption of trub substances. PVPP removes polyphenols, silica gel removes proteins. The last one is applied before filtration. PVPP is added between *kieselguhr* and plate filtration. Recently, membrane filtrations have been developed because *kieselguhr* resources will run short and disposal costs will increase. Membranes consist of polyester, nylon, etc. Filtration is based on sieving effect at membrane surfaces and may be used for sterile filtration, if sufficient pore sizes are chosen (Bamforth, 2003; Briggs *et al.*, 2004; Narziss, 2005).

Filling The aim of filling is to conserve beer quality and to give an attractive appearance for consumers. It is the most expensive process in the brewery (costs and labor). Basics that have to be considered during filling are:

- *Filling under pressure.* CO_2 containing beverages release CO_2 if partial pressure of dissolved CO_2 is fallen below.
- *Avoiding air contact.* Low oxygen concentrations in beer (0.01 mg O_2/l) result in decreased flavor and colloidal stability of beer.
- *Axhaustive cleaning.* Cleaning and disinfection inhibit contamination by beer spoiling organisms (Kunze, 1999; Heyse, 2000; Back, 2005a; Narziss, 2005).

Quality Criteria of Beer

Microbial stability

Microbial stability describes the susceptibility of beer to contamination by micro-organisms. Beer has several selective properties:

- anaerobic conditions (CO_2 containing beverage),
- low pH-value (approximately 4.5),
- alcohol content (approximately 5% per volume),
- hop bitter substances and hop oils,
- shortage of easily digestible sugars and amino acids,
- low temperatures during manufacturing process.

Weakening of these properties by, for example, lack of alcohol or decreased tidiness may cause adverse effects. Beer spoiling organisms decrease aroma and taste quality and cause haze and precipitations after a certain adaptation phase. *Saccharomyces diastaticus*, for example, is an "over fermentating" yeast that digests dextrins, too. The resulting beer tastes blank, strangely bitter, and tends to foam over. Contamination by bacteria like *Megasphera cerevisia* causes a sewer-like smell. An increased butterscotch aroma indicates high diacetyl levels that may be due to an infection by *Pediococcus* or *Lactobacillus* bacteria. It is important to note that basically no pathogenic germs grow in beer. Beer can be treated thermally to increase microbial stability. Commonly, a short period of heating before filling or a subsequent pasteurization is applied (Back, 2005a; Back, 2005b; Narziss, 2005).

Flavor stability

The taste and aroma of beer are not stable. An aged impression arises from the loss of positive flavoring substances and development of an aged flavor. The main reason is contamination with oxygen, which is unavoidable in spite of the latest filling systems. International brewers may add sulfites or ascorbic acid to reduce oxygen impact besides oxygen-poor operation. Beer flavor changes within few days after filling and lasts for several years. Aging starts with a "ribes flavor" that turns into a "cardboard flavor." Flavor impression further changes from a bread-like taste to caramel, a honey-like flavor, and finally to a sherry-, or whiskey-like character (Briggs *et al.*, 2004; Back, 2005a; Narziss, 2005).

Colloidal stability

Colloidal stability (turbidity) describes precipitation of protein-tanning agent compounds after filling and aging of beer. Instability depends on oxygen content, temperature (heat), movement, light, and presence of metal ions in beer. There are several methods to increase colloidal stability by removal of proteins or tanning agents (polyphenols, see section "Filtration and stabilization"). Biological acidification, oxygen-poor operation, etc. affects colloidal stability (Heyse, 2000; Briggs *et al.*, 2004; Back, 2005a; Narziss, 2005).

Foam stability

Often consumers expect stable foam on their beer. Foam is the result of the complex collaboration between technology and gastronomy. Selection of malt, mashing above protein rest, reduced boiling intensity, or yeast management influences foam development and stability. International brewers additionally may add adjuncts based on alginates to increase foam stability. Attention in gastronomy should especially be stressed on the tidiness of glasses. Fatty residues (e.g. lipstick) or residues of cleaning and disinfectant solutions decrease foam stability. Lastly, the kind of drawing is decisive for optimum presentation. A white, airy head results from CO_2 that also occurs in the drawing device. Manual pumping is applied on brews with less CO_2 that should not develop a distinct head. Drawing with nitrogen gas imparts a tight, creamy head, and a creamy texture (Briggs *et al.*, 2004; Back, 2005a; Narziss, 2005).

Non-alcoholic beer and other brewing technologies

Worldwide interest in non-alcoholic beer is increasing. Athletes appreciate beer's typical properties, reduced calories, and the isotonic properties of most non-alcoholic beers. Legally fixed maximum alcohol contents differ in countries. Arabic countries demand contents below 0.05% per volume. Germany allows contents below 0.5% per volume. Two procedures especially have been established for manufacturing non-alcoholic beer. On the one hand, thermal removal of alcohol is applied subsequently to brewing conventional beer. On the other hand, "cold contact procedure" involves contact of yeast with wort at 0°C or stopping fermentation before the alcohol limit is reached. Brews, according to the second procedure, differ in composition and sensorial properties because no complete fermentation took place. Beers produced by stopped fermentation may have a sweet wort character. Others often show a blank, untypical sour character. A combination of both procedures increases flavor quality.

It is possible to emphasize certain properties of beer by variations of brewing technology. As brewing technologists, we see a chance to improve the image of beer because health awareness increases continuously. Recently, special technologies were developed, for example, for enrichment of folic acid or xanthohumol in beer. Innovations like this, in addition to publicizing the healthy effects of beer ingredients, may strengthen consumer interest in a tasty and healthy beer (Back, 2005a; Narziss, 2005).

Summary Points

- Manufacturing beer is a complex mixture of technical and (bio-)technological processes.
- Main ingredients of most beers are:
  - water
  - barley
  - hops
  - yeast.
- Commonly, barley and other starch suppliers have to be malted to facilitate starch dissolution. This takes place during:
  - steeping (wetting grains, activation of enzymes)
  - germination
  - kilning (drying grains).
- Brewing itself is subdivided into:
  - mashing (activation of enzymes, dissolution of starch, conversion to sugars) and lautering (removal of solids)
  - boiling (thermal and enzymatic processes, addition of hops)
  - fermentation (conversion of sugars to alcohol), maturation (degradation of undesirable side products), and storage (development and fixation of CO_2)
  - filtration and stabilization (removal of residual yeast, causes of haze, and further unwanted substances for shelf-life).
- Every production step influences the resulting beer.
- Every beer variety has to fulfill quality criteria of:
  - microbial stability (no infections)
  - flavor stability (conservation of the original taste and aroma as long as possible)
  - colloidal stability (no haze)
  - foam stability.

References

Back, W. (ed.) (2005a). *Ausgewählte Kapitel der Brauereitechnologie.* Fachverlag Hans Carl, Nürnberg.

Back, W. (2005b). *Colour Atlas and Handbook of Beverage Biology.* Fachverlag Hans Carl, Nürnberg.

Bamforth, C.W. (2003). *Beer: Tap into the Art and Science of Brewing*, 2nd edn. Oxford University Press, NewYork.

Bamforth, C.W. (2004). *Beer: Health and Nutrition.* Blackwell Science, Oxford.

Briggs, D.E. (1998). *Malts and Maltings.* Blackie, London.

Briggs, D.E., Boulton, C.A., Brookes, P.A. and Stevens, R. (2004). *Brewing: Science and Practice.* Woodhead, Cambridge, UK.

BGBI (1993). *Teil 1 Das vorläufige Biersteuergesetz von 29.7.1993*, pp. 1399–1401.

Heyse, K.-U. (ed.) (2000) *Praxishandbuch der Brauerei*, Behr's Verlag, Hamburg.

Kunze, W. (1999). *Technology Brewing and Malting*, 2nd international edn. VLB, Berlin.

Narziss, L. (1992). *Die Bierbrauerei, Band II: Die Technologie der Würzebereitung*, 7th edn. Enke Verlag, Stuttgart.

Narziss, L. (1999). *Die Bierbrauerei, Band I: Die Technologie der Malzbereitung*, 7th edn. Enke Verlag, Stuttgart.

Narziss, L., Back, W. (2005). *Abriss der Bierbrauerei*, Wiley-VCH, Weinheim.

Piendl, A. (2000). *Physiologische Bedeutung der Eigenschaften des Bieres*. Fachverlag Hans Carl, Nürnberg.

2

Non-lager Beer

Andrea Pavsler and Stefano Buiatti Department of Food Science, University of Udine, Udine, Italy

Abstract

Many thousands of different beer brands are produced worldwide and most of them can be classified into defined beer styles which have developed over the course of time in different countries or regions. Depending on the process used, a first classification can be made according to the fermentation process in top and bottom fermentation beers. Top fermented beers represent only a small percentage of the total beer consumption. Top fermented beers are very common in Britain, Germany, Canada's eastern provinces, United States and, last but not least, Belgium. However, lager (the term generally used for bottom fermented beer) is the dominant style in almost all countries and represents more than 90% of the beer produced worldwide. Until the sixteenth century, ale (the term generally used for top fermentation beers) was the main type of beer in Europe. Traditionally, ales are fermented with the use of top-cropping yeasts which rise to the top of the beer in the head of foam at temperatures between 16°C and 24°C. At these temperatures, the yeast produces significant amounts of esters and other secondary flavor and aromatic products, and the result is often a beer with slightly "fruity" compounds. Typical ales have a sweeter, fuller body than lagers.

Introduction

The birthplace of beer is generally known to be the Middle East and Egypt. The first detailed mention of beer was made more than 5,000 years ago by the Sumerians. By the medieval period, the practice of brewing had spread into Europe, bringing a competitor for wine. Until the sixteenth century, ales (the generic name for beers produced by top fermentation) were the main type of beer in Europe. Historically, in the Middle Ages, the words *Ale* and *Beer* had two different meanings, ale describing a non-hopped malt beverage (also called *spiced ale*) as opposed to hopped beer, introduced to Britain by Flanders workers possibly not very keen about the sweet taste of English beers. In fact, in the sixteenth century (when hops had been used for many centuries in Germany), during the reign of Henry the VIII, hops were still considered a "… *wicked and pernicious weed*" (Bamforth, 2003). Nowadays top fermented beers represent only a small percentage of the total beer consumption. Nevertheless, ales are very common in Britain, Germany, Canada's eastern provinces, United States and Belgium. However, lager beer is the dominant type of beer in almost all countries and represents more than 90% of beer produced worldwide.

Top fermented beer is typically fermented at temperatures between 16°C and 24°C. At these temperatures, yeast produces significant amounts of esters and other secondary flavor and aroma products, and the result is often a beer with slightly "fruity" compounds resembling but not limited to apple, pear, pineapple, banana, plum or prune. Typical ales have a sweeter, fuller body than lagers.

Top Fermented Beer Production

- **Malting is the controlled germination of cereals, followed by a termination of this natural process by the application of heat.**

Malt is a cereal grain, usually barley, that has been germinated for limited period of time, and finally dried. During germination, the endosperm is degraded by enzymes that attack the cell walls, starch granules and the protein matrix. Usually, the malt used to produce ales is more and better modified than malt for lagers.

During kilning when the temperature is increased, destruction of malt enzymes is accelerated, and color and flavor are developed; consequently there are several malt types that can be used to provide appropriate substrates and enzymes to yield a soluble extract or simply as wort coloring agents (specialty malt) (Hough, 1985; Freeman, 1999).

- **Milling and mashing are the most critical operations in the brewing process.**

Milling increases the surface area of the malt and makes the starch more accessible to enzymic attack. An important objective is to keep the malt husk as intact as possible, to have an open filter bed that helps wort separation (Briggs *et al.*, 2004). Mashing is the most critical operation in the brewhouse because it directly determines both

Beer in Health and Disease Prevention
ISBN: 978-0-12-373891-2

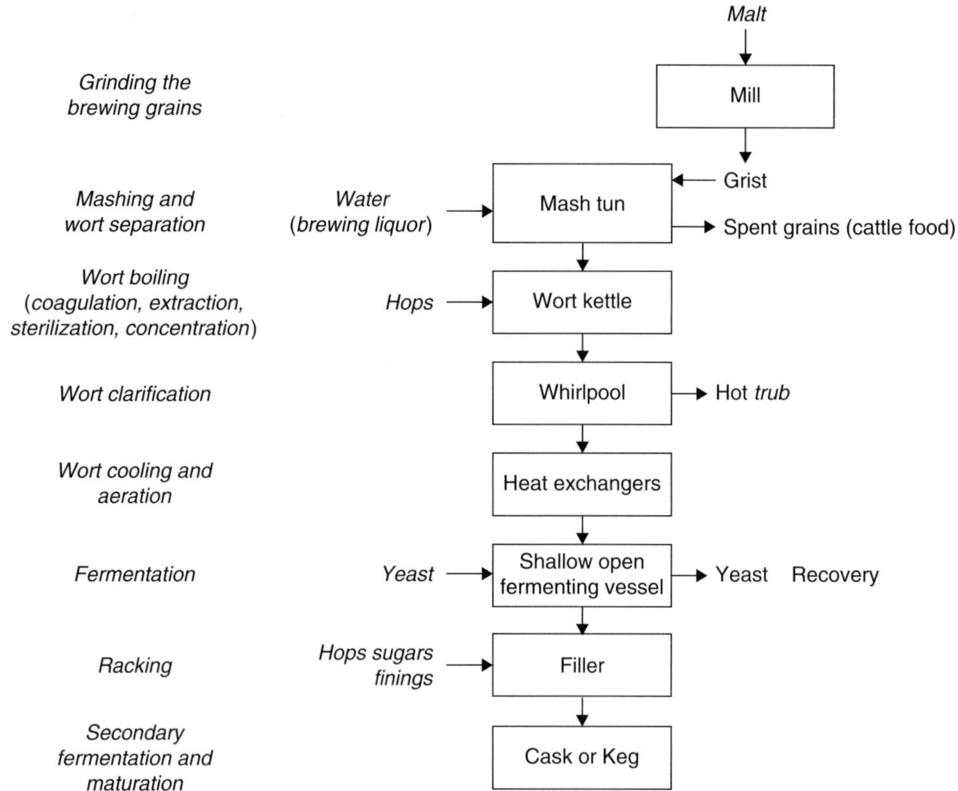

Figure 2.1 The traditional ale brewing process.

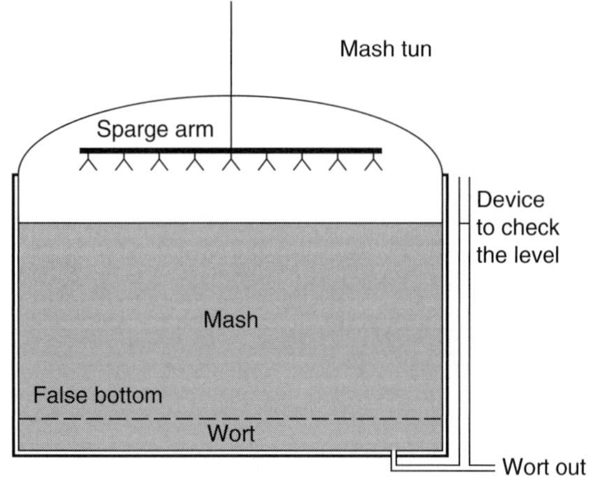

Figure 2.2 Mash tun.

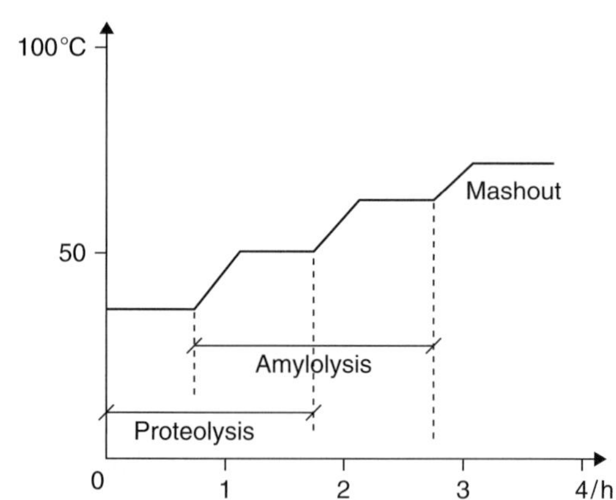

Figure 2.3 Infusion mashing system.

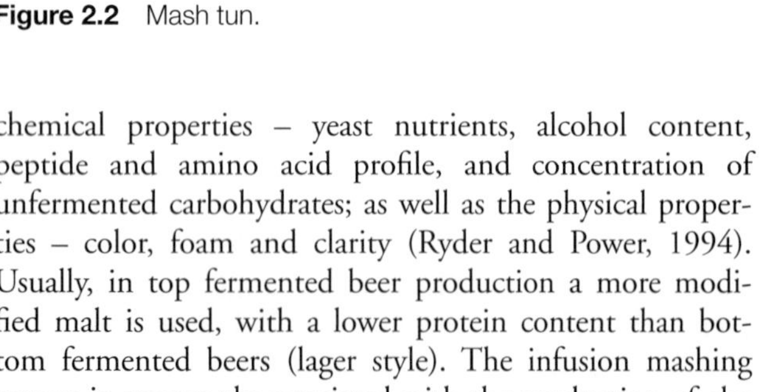

chemical properties – yeast nutrients, alcohol content, peptide and amino acid profile, and concentration of unfermented carbohydrates; as well as the physical properties – color, foam and clarity (Ryder and Power, 1994). Usually, in top fermented beer production a more modified malt is used, with a lower protein content than bottom fermented beers (lager style). The infusion mashing system is commonly associated with the production of ales and stouts (Figure 2.1). It requires a single and unstirred vessel, equipped with a false bottom, called a "mash tun" (Figure 2.2). In this vessel the total mash is always kept together and heated with rests being used at a temperature determined by enzyme properties (Figure 2.3) (Lewis and Young, 1995). The single-step infusion mash is the simplest mash schedule and is used extensively in ale brewing (Figure 2.4). At a mash temperature range of 65–70°C, enzymes in the malt activate and convert complex starches to simple sugar molecules (saccharification rest).

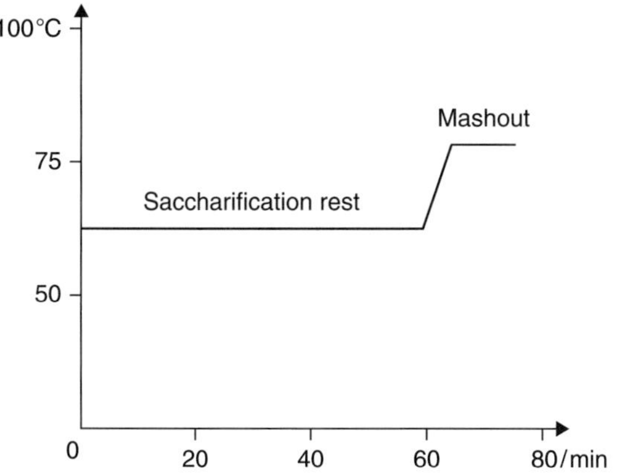

Figure 2.4 Single-step infusion mashing system. A single-step infusion mash is the simplest kind of mash. During the saccharification rest, malt enzymes convert the grain's starch into fermentable sugars.

- **During mashing there is usually no "protein rest" because ale malts present a good modification and degradation of protein.**

Since the malts used to produce ales are better modified with protein (more degraded) there is no "protein rest" (near 50°C) which is typical in a multiple-step infusion. Therefore, a protein rest is used when the endosperm of the malt used is less enzymically degraded and requires more extensive enzymic action (e.g. in lager production) (Briggs *et al.*, 1982; Goldammer, 1999; Briggs *et al.*, 2004).

- **After the mash and before the boil, the wort must be separated from the mash.**

The objectives are to collect as much sugar from the mash as possible while leaving behind as many undesirable compounds as possible, and to make the wort as clear as possible. Filtration is directly run in the mash tun (Figure 2.2) which has a false bottom that allows efficient separation of wort from the spent grain (Lewis and Young, 1995). The sweet wort is transferred to a vessel (boiling kettle) where it is boiled with hops usually for 60–90 min. The boiling process is often associated with the addition of sugars or syrups, and hops or bitter products derived from hops. When hopped wort is clarified, it must be cooled as quickly as possible to fermentation temperatures (16–24°C) through a plate heat exchanger before yeast is pitched (Kunze, 1996). After cooling, it is usual to oxygenate or aerate the wort to provide oxygen for the yeast in the initial stages of fermentation (Briggs *et al.*, 2004).

- **To produce ale, strains of *Saccharomyces cerevisiae* are commonly used in the range of 16–24°C.**

To produce top fermented beers, strains of *Saccharomyces cerevisiae* are commonly used in the range of 16–24°C.

Table 2.1 Flavour compounds associated with yeast metabolism in lager and ale

Class of volatile	*Name*	*Lager (mg/l)*	*Ale (mg/l)*
Higher alcohols	Ethanol	23–25 (g/l)	27–32 (g/l)
	Isopentanol	32–57	47–61
	β-Phenylethanol	25–32	36–53
	n-Propanol	5.0–10	31–48
	Isobutanol	6.0–11	18–33
	2-Methylbutanol	8.0–16	14–19
Esters	Ethyl acetate	8.0–14	14–23
	Isopentylacetate	1.5–2.0	1.4–3.3
Diketone	Diacetyl	0.02–0.08	0.06–0.30
	Pentane-2,3-dione	0.01–0.05	0.01–0.20
Sulfur compounds	Hydrogen sulfide (H_2S)	0.0015–0.008	0.0015–0.008
	Dimethyl sulfide (DMS)	15+ (μg/l)	15+ (μg/l)

Source: Modified from Hough (1994).

The inoculation of wort is called "pitching," and the pitching rate depends on fermentation temperature (pitching rate in ale is lower than lager beer), wort gravity, yeast strain and other variables (Munroe, 1994). As a rule of thumb, the pitching rate is 1×10^6 cells per Plato (°P) per ml of wort (Knudsen, 1999). The pitching rate is very important as it affects both beer flavor and fermentation rate. As shown in Table 2.1, the ester content in ale is higher than in lager beer. It is generally accepted that top fermented beer is more aromatic than bottom fermented beer, both having an identical original gravity. Top fermented beers, with their typically higher fermentation temperatures (16–24°C) and different yeast strains, usually contain more esters and fusel alcohols, and they often have a higher alcohol content (Derdelinckx and Neven, 1996).

Traditionally, ales are fermented with "top yeasts" that rise to the top of the beer in the head of foam. Major differences between ales and lagers do exist in the process conditions, traditional fermentation vessels and methods of yeast recovery. Ale fermentation uses the top-cropping yeast strain *S. cerevisiae*, which is used at higher temperatures than lagers, so the fermentation is faster. It rises to the top of the beer toward the end of the fermentation because the yeast flocs entrap carbon dioxide (CO_2), making them buoyant. The yeast is either removed by suction or by skimming and the fermenter may be the shallow open type (Munroe, 1994). With the development of cylindroconical vessels, the distinction between top and bottom yeasts tends to disappear. With this kind of vessel, brewers may use a bottom-cropping *S. cerevisiae* strain to produce ales. Therefore, the flocculating behavior of yeast is no longer used to exclusively distinguish between strains (Hough, 1985). Ale wort is pitched at about 16°C and fermentation is carried out at 16–24°C. The higher temperature than in lager fermentation causes ale primary fermentation to be completed in much less time (2–3 days) (Briggs *et al.*, 2004).

- **Cask conditioning is the oldest method for maturation and conditioning of ale.**

The oldest method for maturation and conditioning of ale is cask conditioning. At the end of fermentation, which occurs either when the beer has achieved the required present gravity or the gravity has not changed for 24 h (about 2–3 days after fermentation starts), the beer is ready for cooling at 8–10°C to assist in removing any surplus yeast. The beer is then ready for racking into casks, where the maturation or secondary fermentation takes place. To achieve an effective secondary fermentation the beer requires a fermentable residue, and active cell in suspension of about $0.35–2.00 \times 10^6$ cells/ml, so the beer is rarely filtered. This additional carbonation is necessary if primary fermentation takes place in a shallow open-type vessel. To clarify beer, isinglass finings are added to bring the yeast out of suspension. A further addition may be hop products (dry hopping). The benefit with dry hopping is that the brewer can get as much flavor and aroma as possible into the final beer, due to the fact that no volatile oils are boiled off. This addition does not contribute to the bitterness because boiling is necessary to extract and isomerize the bitter resins. After packaging, the beer has to be kept between 12°C and 14°C (Hough, 1985; Carry and Grossman, 2006).

Refermentation of top fermenting beers in bottles is a frequently used process in Belgium. Mature beer is mixed with yeast and fermentable extract and subsequently bottled (Landschoot *et al.*, 2004). Historically, the origin of beer conditioning is related with the transport of beer kegs from brewery to pubs. Due to warm climatic conditions, remaining unfermented sugars in beer were fermented in the kegs. Carbonation gives a refreshing taste, creates foam and causes flavor compounds to escape from the glass (Vanderhaegen *et al.*, 2002).

- **Lambic is a beer produced by spontaneous fermentation.**

Lambic is a very distinctive style of beer brewed only in the Pajottenland region of Belgium (southwest of Brussels). Unlike conventional ales which are fermented by strains of *S. cerevisiae*, lambics are produced by spontaneous fermentation with airborne wild yeast and bacteria. Up to 86 microorganisms have been identified in lambic beer, the most significant ones being *Brettanomyces bruxellensis* and *Brettanomyces lambicus*. The process is generally only possible between October and May, because in summer, there are too many unfavorable organisms in the air that could spoil the beer. Another important feature of lambic is the raw material used to brew it. It is generally made from a grist containing approximately 55% barley malt and 35% unmalted wheat. The temperature of mashing is increased by two or three decoctions and then, the wort is boiled for about 3–6 h, with the addition of aged hop. Hop aging leads to loss of much of its bitterness, but its antiseptic properties are still present. Consequently, lambics often have a strong cheese-like aroma, derived from oxidation of α-acids and β-acids and consequent low-molecular weight acids production (Lewis and Young, 1995). Before it was discovered that hops were a preservative and spice, all types of fruits, herbs and other seasonings were used to flavor the wort of barley and wheat. Cooling and aeration of wort is conducted in the cooling tun at a depth of 20–25 cm where it is exposed to the open air so that fermentation may occur spontaneously (Goldammer, 1999). It is this unusual process which gives the beer its distinctive flavor: dry, vinous and cidery, with a slightly sour aftertaste. The lambic style of beer includes many different sub-categories, such as lambic, gueuze, faro, fruit lambics and Kriek. The most significant ones are described in the section "Beer types."

- **A Trappist beer is a top fermented bottle-conditioned beer, brewed by or under the control of Trappist monks.**

To be called Trappist, the beer must be brewed within the walls of a Trappist abbey, by or under the control of Trappist monks. Trappist beer is therefore not so much a style as an appellation of origin. Trappists, or Order of Cistercians of the Strict Observance (O.C.S.O. or *Ordo Cisterciensis Strictioris Observantiae*), are a contemplative Roman Catholic religious order and their life follows the Rule of St. Benedict written in the sixth century. They originated in the Cistercian monastery of La Trappe, France, in reaction to the relaxation of practices in many Cistercian Monasteries. The Trappists live a life of prayer and penance. Their day is divided between work and prayer. Manual work is preferred over other types of work, and Trappist monasteries generally provide for themselves through the sale of goods produced in the monastery. One of the Rules of St. Benedict states "*You are only really a monk when you live from the work of your hands.*" By this rule, most Trappist monasteries produce goods that are then sold to provide an income for the monastery. The order does not require abstention from alcohol, and the goods produced are beer, cheese, bread and other foodstuffs. The Trappists, like many other religious people, brewed beer to fund their work, and monastery brewhouses existed all over Europe. Among these monastic breweries, the Trappists were certainly the most active brewers. In 1997, eight Trappist abbeys – six from Belgium (Orval, Chimay, Westvleteren, Rochefort, Westmalle and Achel), one from The Netherlands (Koningshoeven) and one from Germany (Mariawald) – founded the International Trappist Association (ITA) to prevent non-Trappist commercial companies from abusing the Trappist name. This private association created a logo that is assigned to goods (cheese, beer, wine and liquors) that respect their precise production criteria. For beers, the rules are the following:

- The beer must be brewed within the walls of a Trappist abbey, by or under control of Trappist monks.
- The brewery, the choices of brewing and the commercial orientations must obviously depend on the monastic community.
- The economic purpose of the brewery must be directed toward assistance and not toward financial profit.

There are currently seven breweries (six in Belgium, one in The Netherlands) that are allowed to have their products bear the Authentic Trappist Product logo. These are Chimay, Orval, Rochefort, Westmalle, Westvleteren and Achel in Belgium and De Koningshoeven in The Netherlands. The brewery De Koningshoeven produces the only Dutch Trappist beer that is able to carry the "Authentic Trappist Product" logo. However, between 1999 and October 2005 their use of the logo was withdrawn. Trappist beers have become quite famous and are considered by many beer critics to be amongst the finest in the world.

Unlike Trappist beers, abbey beers are not made under the control of monks. Officially recognized abbey beers are made under license by a commercial brewery, using the name and recipes of an abbey that has ceased brewing itself. Only a couple of brands, including Val-Dieu and Abbaye d'Aulne, are actually made within the walls of an abbey.

Beer Types

There are many thousands of different beer brands throughout the world, many of which can be classified into defined beer types which have developed over the course of time in a few countries or regions. Depending on the process used, a first classification could be made into top fermentation and bottom fermentation beer types. Table 2.2 gives a breakdown of some principal beer types.

Top fermentation beer types

The sections below contain a list of top fermentation beer types (BJCP, 2004). Beer strength may be defined in several ways; and in order to explain the vital statistics of each style, the content of hop bitter substances (IBU, International Bitterness Units), the color (EBC, European Brewery Convention), the specific gravity of wort before fermentation (OG, original gravity) and post-fermentation (FG, final gravity), and the alcohol content (ABV or alcohol by volume) are used.

Table 2.2 Some principal beer types

Types of beers	*Origin*	*Characteristics*	*Typical range of alcohol (% by vol.)*
Top fermentation			
Standard/ordinary bitter	Britain	Low gravity, low alcohol levels	3.2–3.8
English pale ale	Britain	Dry hop, bitter, estery, malty, low carbonation	4.6–6.2
Mild	Britain	Refreshing, yet flavorful	2.8–4.2
Brown Porter	Britain	English dark ale with restrained roasty characteristics	4.0–5.4
Robust Porter	Britain	Malty dark ale	4.8–6.0
Dry stout	Ireland	Dark, roasty, bitter, creamy ale	4.0–5.0
Sweet stout	Britain	Dark, sweet, full-bodied, slightly roasty ale	4.0–6.0
Kölsch	Germany (Cologne)	Smooth and crisp	4.4–5.2
Lambic	Belgium	Fermented by a variety of Belgian microbiota	5.0–7.0
Rauchbier	Germany	Smoky aroma and flavor and a somewhat dark color	4.8–6.0
Weizen/Weissbier	Germany	Pale, spicy, fruity, refreshing wheat-based ale	4.3–5.6
Bottom fermentation			
German Pilsner (Pils)	Germany	Crisp, clean, refreshing beer	4.4–5.2
Bohemian Pilsener	Czech Republic	Crisp, complex and well-rounded yet refreshing	4.2–5.4
Classic American Pilsner	United States	Rice contributes a crisper, more neutral character	4.5–6.0
Vienna Lager	Austria	Soft, elegant maltiness	4.5–5.7
Oktoberfest/Märzen	Germany	Depth of malt character	4.8–5.7
Dark American Lager	United States	Sweeter version of standard lager	4.2–6.0
Munich Dunkel	Germany	Depth and complexity	4.5–5.6
Schwarzbier (Black Beer)	Germany	Probably a variant of the Munich *Dunkel* style	4.4–5.4
Maibock/Helles Bock	Germany	Pale, strong, malty lager beer	6.3–7.4
Traditional Bock	Germany	Dark, strong, malty lager beer	6.3–7.2
Doppelbock	Germany	Strong and rich lager	7.0–10+
Eisbock	Germany	An extremely strong, full and malty dark lager	9.0–14+

Source: Most of the data in this table is from the BJCP Style Guidelines (2004).

American Ale

American Pale Ale

Overall impression: Refreshing and hoppy, yet with sufficient supporting malt.

History: An American adaptation of English pale ale, reflecting indigenous ingredients (hops, malt, yeast and water). Often lighter in color, cleaner in fermentation by-products and having less caramel flavors than English counterparts.

Comments: There is some overlap in color between American pale ale and American amber ale. The American pale ale will generally be cleaner, have a less caramelly malt profile, less body and often more finishing hops.

Ingredients: Pale ale malt, typically American two-row. American hops, often but not always ones with a citrus character, American ale yeast. Water can vary in sulfate content, but carbonate content should be relatively low. Specialty grains may add character and complexity, but generally make up a relatively small portion of the grist. Grains that add malt flavor and richness, light sweetness, and toasty or bready notes are often used (along with late hops) to differentiate brands.

Vital statistics:	OG: 1.045–1.060 (11.2–14.7°P)
IBUs: 30–45+	FG: 1.010–1.015
EBC: 9.8–27.6	ABV: 4.5–6%

Commercial examples: Sierra Nevada Pale Ale, Stone Pale Ale, Great Lakes Burning River Pale Ale, Full Sail Pale Ale, Three Floyds X-Tra Pale Ale, Anderson Valley Poleeko Gold Pale Ale, Left Hand Brewing Jackman's Pale Ale, Pyramid Pale Ale, Deschutes Mirror Pond.

American Amber Ale

Overall impression: Like an American pale ale with more body, more caramel richness and a balance more toward malt than hops (although hop rates can be significant).

History: Known simply as Red Ales in some regions, these beers were popularized in the hop-loving Northern California and the Pacific Northwest areas before spreading nationwide.

Comments: Can overlap in color with American pale ales. However, American amber ales differ from American pale ales not only by being usually darker in color, but also by having more caramel flavor, more body and usually being balanced more evenly between malt and bitterness. Should not have a strong chocolate or roast character that might suggest an American brown ale (although small amounts are OK).

Ingredients: Pale ale malt, typically American two-row. Medium to dark crystal malts. May also contain specialty grains which add additional character and uniqueness. American hops, often with citrus flavors, are common but others may also be used. Water can vary in sulfate and carbonate content.

Vital statistics:	OG: 1.045–1.060 (11.2–14.7°P)
IBUs: 25–40+	FG: 1.010–1.015
EBC: 19.7–33.5	ABV: 4.5–6%

Commercial examples: Mendocino Red Tail Ale, North Coast Red Seal Ale, St. Rogue Red Ale, Avery Redpoint Ale, Anderson Valley Boont Amber Ale, Bell's Amber, Hoptown Paint the Town Red, McNeill's Firehouse Amber Ale.

American Brown Ale

Overall impression: Can be considered a bigger, maltier, hoppier interpretation of Northern English Brown Ale or a hoppier, less malty Brown Porter, often including the citrus-accented hop presence that is characteristic of American hop varieties.

History/comments: A strongly flavored, hoppy brown beer originated by American homebrewers. Related to American Pale and American Amber Ales, although with more of a caramel and chocolate character, which tends to balance the hop bitterness and finish. Most commercial American Browns are not as aggressive as the original home-brewed versions and some modern craft-brewed examples. India Pale Ale (IPA)-strength brown ales should be entered in the Specialty category.

Ingredients: Well-modified pale malt, either American or Continental, plus crystal and darker malts should complete the malt bill. American hops are typical, but UK or noble hops can also be used. Moderate carbonate water would appropriately balance the dark malt acidity.

Vital statistics:	OG: 1.045–1.060 (11.2–14.7°P)
IBUs: 20–40+	FG: 1.010–1.016
EBC: 35.5–68.9	ABV: 4.3–6.2%

Commercial examples: Brooklyn Brown Ale, Great Lakes Cleveland Brown Ale, Avery Ellie's Brown Ale, Left Hand Deep Cover Brown Ale, Bell's Best Brown, North Coast Acme Brown, Lost Coast Downtown Brown, Big Sky Moose Drool Brown Ale.

English Pale Ale

Standard/Ordinary Bitter

Overall impression: Low gravity, low alcohol levels and low carbonation make this an easy-drinking beer. Some examples can be more malt balanced, but this should not override the overall bitter impression. Drinkability is a critical component of the style; emphasis is still on the bittering hop addition as opposed to the aggressive middle and late hopping seen in American ales.

History: Originally a draft ale served very fresh under no pressure (gravity or hand pump only) at cellar temperatures (i.e. "real ale"). Bitter was created as a draft alternative (i.e. running beer) to country-brewed pale ale around the start of the twentieth century and became widespread once brewers understood how to "Burtonize" their water to successfully brew pale beers and to use crystal malts to add a fullness and roundness of palate.

Ingredients: Pale ale, amber and/or crystal malts may use a touch of black malt for color adjustment. May use sugar adjuncts, corn or wheat. English hops most typical, although American and European varieties are becoming more common (particularly in the paler examples). Characterful English yeast. Often medium sulfate water is used.

Vital statistics:	OG: 1.032–1.040 (8.0–10.0 °P)
IBUs: 25–35	FG: 1.007–1.011
EBC: 7.9–27.6	ABV: 3.2–3.8%

Commercial examples: Boddington's Pub Draught, Fuller's Chiswick Bitter, Oakham Jeffrey Hudson Bitter (JHB), Young's Bitter, Brakspear Bitter, Adnams Bitter.

Extra Special/Strong Bitter (English Pale Ale)
Overall impression: An average-strength to moderately strong English ale. The balance may be fairly even between malt and hops to somewhat bitter. Drinkability is a critical component of the style; emphasis is still on the bittering hop addition as opposed to the aggressive middle and late hopping seen in American ales. A rather broad style that allows for considerable interpretation by the brewer.

History: Strong bitters can be seen as a higher-gravity version of best bitters (although not necessarily "more premium," since best bitters are traditionally the brewer's finest product). Since beer is sold by strength in the United Kingdom, these beers often have some alcohol flavor (perhaps to let the consumer know they are getting their due). In England today, "ESB" is a brand unique to Fullers; in America, the name has been co-opted to describe a malty, bitter, reddish, standard-strength (for the United States) English-type ale. Hopping can be English or a combination of English and American.

Ingredients: Pale ale, amber and/or crystal malts, may use a touch of black malt for color adjustment. May use sugar adjuncts, corn or wheat. English hops most typical, although American and European varieties are becoming more common (particularly in the paler examples). Characterful English yeast. "Burton" versions use medium to high sulfate water.

Vital statistics:	OG: 1.048–1.060+ (11.9–14.7 °P+)
IBUs: 30–50+	FG: 1.010–1.016
EBC: 11.8–35.5	ABV: 4.6–6.2%

Commercial examples: Fullers ESB, Adnams Broadside, Shepherd Neame Bishop's Finger, Samuel Smith's Old Brewery Pale Ale, Bass Ale, Whitbread Pale Ale, Shepherd Neame Spitfire, Marston's Pedigree, Black Sheep Ale, Vintage Henley, Mordue Workie Ticket, Morland Old Speckled Hen, Greene King Abbot Ale, Bateman's XXXB, Gale's Hordean Special Bitter (HSB), Ushers 1824 Particular Ale, Hopback Summer Lightning, Redhook ESB, Great Lakes Moondog Ale, Shipyard Old Thumper, Alaskan ESB, Geary's Pale Ale, Cooperstown Old Slugger.

English Brown Ale

Mild
Overall impression: A light-flavored, malt-accented beer that is readily suited to drinking in quantity. Refreshing, yet flavorful. Some versions may seem like lower gravity Brown Porters.

History: May have evolved as one of the elements of early porters. In modern terms, the name "mild" refers to the relative lack of hop bitterness (i.e. less hoppy than a pale ale, and not so strong). Originally, the "mildness" may have referred to the fact that this beer was young and did not yet have the moderate sourness that aged batches had. Somewhat rare in England, good versions may still be found in the Midlands around Birmingham.

Ingredients: Pale English base malts (often fairly dextrinous), crystal and darker malts should comprise the grist. May use sugar adjuncts. English hop varieties would be most suitable, though their character is muted. Characterful English ale yeast.

Vital statistics:	OG: 1.030–1.038 (7.6–9.5 °P)
IBUs: 10–25	FG: 1.008–1.013
EBC: 23.6–49.2	ABV: 2.8–4.5%

Commercial examples: Moorhouse Black Cat, Highgate Mild, Brain's Dark, Banks's Mild, Coach House Gunpowder Strong Mild, Gale's Festival Mild, Woodforde's Norfolk Nog, Goose Island PMD Mild.

Southern English Brown
Overall impression: A luscious, malt-oriented brown ale, with a caramel, dark fruit complexity of malt flavor. May seem somewhat like a smaller version of a sweet stout or a sweet version of a dark mild.

History: English brown ales are generally split into sub-styles along geographic lines. Southern English (or "London-style") Brown Ales are darker, sweeter and lower gravity than their Northern cousins.

Ingredients: English pale ale malt as a base with a healthy proportion of darker caramel malts and often some roasted malts. Moderate to high carbonate water would appropriately balance the dark malt acidity. English hop varieties are most authentic, although with low flavor and bitterness almost any type could be used.

Vital statistics:	OG: 1.035–1.042 (8.8–10.5 °P)
IBUs: 12–20	FG: 1.011–1.014
EBC: 37.4–68.9	ABV: 2.8–4.2%

Commercial examples: Mann's Brown Ale (bottled, but not available in the United States), Tolly Cobbold Cobnut Nut Brown Ale.

Northern English Brown Ale

Overall impression: Drier and more hop-oriented than Southern English Brown Ale, with a nutty character rather than caramel.

History/comments: English brown ales are generally split into sub-styles along geographic lines.

Ingredients: English mild ale or pale ale malt base with caramel malts. May also have small amounts of darker malts (e.g. chocolate) to provide color and the nutty character. English hop varieties are most authentic. Moderate carbonate water.

Vital statistics:	OG: 1.040–1.052 (10.0–12.9 °P)
IBUs: 20–30	FG: 1.008–1.013
EBC: 23.6–43.3	ABV: 4.2–5.4%

Commercial examples: Newcastle Brown Ale, Samuel Smith's Nut Brown Ale, Tolly Cobbold Cobnut Special Nut Brown Ale, Goose Island Hex Nut Brown Ale.

Porter

Brown Porter

Overall impression: A fairly substantial English dark ale with restrained roasty characteristics.

History: Originating in England, porter evolved from a blend of beers or gyles known as "Entire." A precursor to stout. Said to have been favored by porters and other physical laborers.

Ingredients: English ingredients are most common. May contain several malts, including chocolate and/or other dark roasted malts and caramel-type malts. Historical versions would use a significant amount of brown malt. Usually does not contain large amounts of black patent malt or roasted barley. English hops are most common, but are usually subdued. London- or Dublin-type water (moderate carbonate hardness) is traditional. English or Irish ale yeast, or occasionally lager yeast, is used. May contain a moderate amount of adjuncts (sugars, maize, molasses, treacle, etc.).

Vital statistics:	OG: 1.040–1.052 (10.0–12.9 °P)
IBUs: 18–35	FG: 1.008–1.014
EBC: 39.4–59.1	ABV: 4–5.4%

Commercial examples: Samuel Smith Taddy Porter, Fuller's London Porter, Burton Bridge Burton Porter, Nethergate Old Growler Porter, Nick Stafford's Nightmare Yorkshire Porter, St. Peters Old-Style Porter, Bateman's Salem Porter, Shepherd Neame Original Porter, Flag Porter, Yuengling Porter, Geary's London Style Porter.

Robust Porter

Overall impression: A substantial, malty dark ale with a complex and flavorful roasty character.

History: Stronger, hoppier and/or roastier version of porter designed as either a historical throwback or an American interpretation of the style. Traditional versions will have a more subtle hop character (often English), whereas modern versions may be considerably more aggressive. Both types are equally valid.

Ingredients: May contain several malts, prominently dark roasted malts and grains, which often include black patent malt (chocolate malt and/or roasted barley may also be used in some versions). Hops are used for bittering, flavor and/or aroma, and are frequently UK or US varieties. Water with moderate to high carbonate hardness is typical. Ale yeast can either be clean US versions or characterful English varieties.

Vital statistics:	OG: 1.048–1.065 (11.9–15.9 °P)
IBUs: 25–50+	FG: 1.012–1.016
EBC: 43.3–68.9+	ABV: 4.8–6%

Commercial examples: Anchor Porter, Great Lakes Edmund Fitzgerald Porter, Sierra Nevada Porter, Bell's Porter, Thirsty Dog Old Leghumper, Otter Creek Stovepipe Porter, Portland Haystack Black Porter, Avery New World Porter, Deschutes Black Butte Porter, Redhook Blackhook Porter.

Stout

Dry Stout

Overall impression: A very dark, roasty, bitter, creamy ale.

History: The style evolved from attempts to capitalize on the success of London porters, but originally reflected a fuller, creamier, more "stout" body and strength. When a brewery offered a stout and a porter, the stout was always the stronger beer (it was originally called a "Stout Porter"). Modern versions are brewed from a lower OG and no longer reflect a higher strength than porters.

Ingredients: The dryness comes from the use of roasted unmalted barley in addition to pale malt, moderate to high hop bitterness and good attenuation. Flaked unmalted barley may also be used to add creaminess. A small percentage (perhaps 3%) of soured beer is sometimes added for complexity (generally by Guinness only). Water typically has moderate carbonate hardness, although high levels will not give the classic dry finish.

Vital statistics:	OG: 1.036–1.050 (9.0–12.4 °P)
IBUs: 30–45	FG: 1.007–1.011
EBC: 49.2–78.8+	ABV: 4–5%

Commercial examples: Guinness Draught Stout (also canned), Murphy's Stout, Beamish Stout, O'Hara's Celtic Stout, Dorothy Goodbody's Wholesome Stout, Orkney

Dragonhead Stout, Brooklyn Dry Stout, Old Dominion Stout, Goose Island Dublin Stout, Arbor Brewing Faricy Fest Irish Stout.

Sweet Stout
Overall impression: A very dark, sweet, full-bodied, slightly roasty ale. Often tastes like sweetened espresso.

History: An English style of stout. Historically known as "Milk" or "Cream" stouts, legally this designation is no longer permitted in England (but is acceptable elsewhere). The "milk" name is derived from the use of lactose, or milk sugar, as a sweetener.

Comments: Gravities are low in England, higher in exported and US products. Variations exist in the level of residual sweetness, the intensity of the roast character, and the balance between the two being the variables most subject to interpretation.

Ingredients: The sweetness in most sweet stouts comes from a lower bitterness level than dry stouts and a high percentage of unfermentable dextrins. Lactose, an unfermentable sugar, is frequently added to provide additional residual sweetness. Base of pale malt, and may use roasted barley, black malt, chocolate malt, crystal malt, and adjuncts such as maize or treacle. High carbonate water is common.

Vital statistics:	OG: 1.042–1.056 (10.5–13.8 °P)
IBUs: 25–40	FG: 1.010–1.023
EBC: 59.1–78.8+	ABV: 4–6%

Commercial examples: Mackeson's XXX Stout, Watney's Cream Stout, St. Peter's Cream Stout, Marston's Oyster Stout, Samuel Adams Cream Stout, Left Hand Milk Stout.

India Pale Ale

English IPA
Overall impression: A hoppy, moderately strong pale ale that features characteristics consistent with the use of English malt, hops and yeast. Has less hop character and a more pronounced malt flavor than American versions.

History: Brewed to survive the voyage from England to India. The temperature extremes and rolling of the seas resulted in a highly attenuated beer upon arrival. English pale ales were derived from IPA.

Ingredients: Pale ale malt (well modified and suitable for single-temperature infusion mashing); English hops; English yeast that can give a fruity or sulfury/minerally profile. Refined sugar may be used in some versions. High sulfate and low carbonate water is essential to achieve a pleasant hop bitterness in authentic Burton versions, although not all examples will exhibit the strong sulfate character.

Vital statistics:	OG: 1.050–1.075 (12.4–18.20 °P)
IBUs: 40–60	FG: 1.010–1.018
EBC: 15.8–27.6	ABV: 5–7.5%

Commercial examples: Freeminer Trafalgar IPA, Hampshire Pride of Romsey IPA, Burton Bridge Empire IPA, Samuel Smith's India Ale, Fuller's IPA, King & Barnes IPA, Brooklyn East India Pale Ale, Shipyard Fuggles IPA, Goose Island IPA.

American IPA
Overall impression: A decidedly hoppy and bitter, moderately strong American pale ale.

History: An American version of the historical English style, brewed using American ingredients and attitude.

Ingredients: Pale ale malt (well modified and suitable for single-temperature infusion mashing); American hops; American yeast that can give a clean or slightly fruity profile. Generally all-malt, but mashed at lower temperatures for high attenuation. Water character varies from soft to moderately sulfate.

Vital statistics:	OG: 1.056–1.075 (13.8–18.20 °P)
IBUs: 40–60+	FG: 1.010–1.018
EBC: 11.8–29.5	ABV: 5.5–7.5%

Commercial examples: Stone IPA, Victory Hop Devil, Anderson Valley Hop Ottin', Anchor Liberty Ale, Sierra Nevada Celebration Ale, Three Floyds Alpha King, Harpoon IPA, Bell's Two-Hearted Ale, Avery IPA, Founder's Centennial IPA, Mendocino White Hawk Select IPA.

Imperial IPA
Overall impression: An intensely hoppy, very strong pale ale without the big maltiness and/or deeper malt flavors of an American barleywine. Strongly hopped, but clean, lacking harshness and a tribute to historical IPAs.

History: A recent American innovation reflecting the trend of American craft brewers "pushing the envelope" to satisfy the need of hop aficionados for increasingly intense products. Category may be stretched to cover historical and modern American stock ales that are stronger, hoppier ales without the malt intensity of barleywines. The adjective "Imperial" is arbitrary and simply implies a stronger version of an IPA; "double," "extra," "extreme" or any other variety of adjectives would be equally valid.

Ingredients: Pale ale malt (well modified and suitable for single-temperature infusion mashing); can use a complex variety of hops (English, American, noble). American yeast that can give a clean or slightly fruity profile. Generally all-malt, but mashed at lower temperatures for high attenuation. Water character varies from soft to moderately sulfate.

Vital statistics:	OG: 1.075–1.090+
IBUs: 60–100+	FG: 1.012–1.020 (3.07–5.0 °P)
EBC: 15.8–29.5	ABV: 7.5–10%+

Commercial examples: Dogfish Head 90-min IPA, Rogue I^{2}PA, Stone Ruination IPA, Three Floyd's Dreadnaught, Russian River Pliny the Elder, Moylan's Moylander Double

IPA. Stock ales include examples such as Stone Arrogant Bastard and Mendocino Eye of the Hawk.

German Wheat and Rye Beer

Weizen/Weissbier
Overall impression: A pale, spicy, fruity, refreshing wheat-based ale.

History: A traditional wheat-based ale originating in Southern Germany that is a specialty for summer consumption, but generally produced year round.

Ingredients: By German law, at least 50% of the grist must be malted wheat, although some versions use up to 70%; the remainder is Pilsner malt. A traditional decoction mash gives the appropriate body without cloying sweetness. Weizen ale yeasts produce the typical spicy and fruity character, although extreme fermentation temperatures can affect the balance and produce off-flavors. A small amount of noble hops are used only for bitterness.

Vital statistics:	OG: 1.044–1.052 (11.0–12.9 °P)
IBUs: 8–15	FG: 1.010–1.014
EBC: 3.9–15.8	ABV: 4.3–5.6%

Commercial examples: Schneider Weisse, Paulaner Hefe-Weizen, Hacker-Pschorr Weisse, Franziskaner Hefe-Weisse, Penn Weizen, Capitol Kloster Weizen, Sudwerk Hefeweizen, Brooklyner Weisse, Barrelhouse Hocking Hills HefeWeizen, Sprecher Hefeweizen.

Dunkelweizen
Overall impression: A moderately dark, spicy, fruity, malty, refreshing wheat-based ale. Reflecting the best yeast and wheat character of a Hefeweizen blended with the malty richness of a Munich dunkel.

History: Old-fashioned Bavarian wheat beer was often dark. In the 1950s and 1960s, wheat beers did not have a youthful image, since most older people drank them for their percieved health-giving qualities. Today, the lighter Hefeweizen is more common.

Ingredients: By German law, at least 50% of the grist must be malted wheat, although some versions use up to 70%; the remainder is usually Munich and/or Vienna malt. A traditional decoction mash gives the appropriate body without cloying sweetness. Weizen ale yeasts produce the typical spicy and fruity character, although extreme fermentation temperatures can affect the balance and produce off-flavors. A small amount of noble hops are used only for bitterness.

Vital statistics:	OG: 1.044–1.056 (11.0–13.8 °P)
IBUs: 10–18	FG: 1.010–1.014
EBC: 27.6–45.3	ABV: 4.3–5.6%

Commercial examples: Franziskaner Dunkel Hefe-Weisse, Hacker-Pschorr Weisse Dark, Schneider Dunkel Weiss, Tucher Dunkles Hefe Weizen, Ayinger Ur-Weisse, Brooklyner Dunkel-Weisse.

Belgian and French Ale

Witbier
Overall impression: A refreshing, elegant, tasty, moderate-strength wheat-based ale.

History: A 400-year-old beer style that died out in the 1950s; it was later revived by Pierre Celis at Hoegaarden, and has grown steadily in popularity over time.

Ingredients: About 50% unmalted wheat (traditionally soft white winter wheat) and 50% pale barley malt (usually Pils malt) constitute the grist. In some versions, up to 5–10% raw oats may be used. Spices of freshly ground coriander and Curaçao or sometimes sweet orange peel complement the sweet aroma and are quite characteristic. Other spices (e.g. chamomile, cumin, cinnamon, Grains of Paradise) may be used for complexity but are much less prominent. Ale yeast prone to the production of mild, spicy flavors is very characteristic. In some instances a very limited lactic fermentation, or the actual addition of lactic acid, is done.

Vital statistics:	OG: 1.044–1.052 (11.0–12.9 °P)
IBUs: 10–20	FG: 1.008–1.012
EBC: 3.9–7.9	ABV: 4.5–5.5% (5% is most typical)

Commercial examples: Hoegaarden Wit, Vuuve 5, Blanche de Bruges, Blanche de Bruxelles, Brugs Tarwebier, Sterkens White Ale, Celis White (now made in Michigan), Blanche de Brooklyn, Great Lakes Holy Moses, Unibroue Blanche de Chambly, Blue Moon Belgian White.

Belgian Pale Ale
Overall impression: A fruity, moderately malty, somewhat spicy, easy-drinking, copper-colored ale.

History: Produced by breweries with roots as far back as the mid-1700s, the most well-known examples were perfected after World War II with some influence from Britain, including hops and yeast strains.

Ingredients: Pilsner or pale ale malt contributes the bulk of the grist with Vienna and Munich malts adding color, body and complexity. Candy sugar is not commonly used as high gravity is not desired. Noble hops, Styrian Goldings, East Kent Goldings or Fuggles are commonly used. Yeasts prone to moderate production of phenols are often used but fermentation temperatures should be kept moderate to limit this character.

Vital statistics:	OG: 1.048–1.054 (11.9–13.3 °P)
IBUs: 20–30	FG: 1.010–1.014
EBC: 15.8–27.6	ABV: 4.8–5.5%

Commercial examples: De Koninck, Speciale Palm, Dobble Palm, Ginder Ale, Op-Ale, Vieux-Temps, Brewer's Art

House Pale Ale, Ommegang Rare Vos (unusual in its 6.5% ABV strength).

Saison

Overall impression: A medium to strong ale with a distinctive yellowish-orange color, highly carbonated, well hopped, fruity and dry with a quenching acidity.

History: A seasonal summer style produced in Wallonia, the French-speaking part of Belgium. Originally brewed at the end of the cool season to last through the warmer months before refrigeration was common. It had to be sturdy enough to last for months but not too strong to be quenching and refreshing in the summer. It is now brewed year round in tiny, artisanal breweries whose buildings reflect their origins as farmhouses.

Ingredients: Pilsner malt dominates the grist though a portion of Vienna and/or Munich malt contributes color and complexity. Adjuncts such as candy sugar and honey can also serve to add complexity and thin the body. Hop bitterness and flavor may be more noticeable than in many other Belgian styles. A saison is sometimes dry-hopped. Noble hops, Styrian or East Kent Goldings are commonly used. A wide variety of herbs and spices are generally used to add complexity and uniqueness in the stronger versions. Varying degrees of acidity and/or sourness can be created by the use of gypsum, acidulated malt, a sour mash or *Lactobacillus*. Hard water, common to most of Wallonia, can accentuate the bitterness and dry finish.

Vital statistics:	OG: 1.048–1.080 (11.9–19.3 °P)
IBUs: 25–45	FG: 1.010–1.016
EBC: 9.8–23.6	ABV: 5–8.5%

Commercial examples: Saison Dupont, Foret and Moinette Blonde; Fantome Saison(s); Saison de Pipaix and La Folie; Saison Silly; Saison Regal; Saison Voisin; Lefebvre Saison 1900; Ellezelloise Saison 2000; Brooklyn Saison; Southampton Saison; New Belgium Saison; Pizza Port-Carlsbad Saison.

Belgian Specialty Ale

Overall impression: This category encompasses a wide range of Belgian ales produced by truly artisanal brewers more concerned with creating unique products than in increasing sales.

History: Unique beers of small, independent Belgian breweries that have come to enjoy local popularity but may be far less well-known outside of their own regions. Many have attained "cult status" in the US (and other parts of the world) and now owe a significant portion of their sales to export.

Ingredients: May include herbs and/or spices. May include unusual grains and malts, though the grain character should be apparent if it is a key ingredient. May include adjuncts such as candy sugar and honey. May include Belgian microbiota such as *Brettanomyces* or *Lactobacillus*. Unusual techniques, such as blending, may be used though primarily to arrive at a particular result. The process alone does not make a beer unique to a blind judging panel if the final product does not taste different.

Vital statistics:	OG: varies
IBUs: varies	FG: varies
EBC: varies	ABV: varies

Commercial examples: Orval; De Dolle's Arabier, Oerbier, Boskeun and Still Nacht; La Chouffe, McChouffe, Chouffe Bok and N'ice Chouffe; Ellezelloise Hercule Stout and Quintine Amber; Unibroue Ephemere, Maudite, Don de Dieu, etc.; Minty; Zatte Bie; Caracole Amber, Saxo and Nostradomus; Silenrieu Sara and Joseph; Fantôme Black Ghost and Speciale Noël; St. Fullien Noël; Gouden Carolus Noël; Affligem Nöel; Guldenburg and Pere Noël; De Ranke XX Bitter; Bush (Scaldis); Grottenbier; La Trappe Quadrupel; Weyerbacher QUAD; Bière de Miel; Verboden Vrucht; New Belgium 1554 Black Ale; Cantillon Iris and many more.

Sour Ale

Berliner Weisse

Overall impression: A very pale, sour, refreshing, low-alcohol wheat ale.

History: A regional specialty of Berlin; referred to by Napoleon's troops in 1809 as "the Champagne of the North" due to its lively and elegant character. Only two traditional breweries still produce the product.

Comments: In Germany, it is classified as a *Schankbier* denoting a small beer of starting gravity in the range 7−8 °P. Often served with the addition of a shot of sugar syrups (mit schuss) flavored with raspberry (himbeer) or woodruff (waldmeister) or even mixed with Pils to counter the substantial sourness. Has been described by some as the most purely refreshing beer in the world.

Ingredients: Wheat malt content is typically well under 50% of the grist (generally 30%) with the remainder being Pilsner malt. A symbiotic fermentation with top fermenting yeast and *Lactobacillus delbruckii* provides the sharp sourness, which may be enhanced by blending of beers of different ages during fermentation and by extended cool aging. Low head and carbonation may be incorrectly caused by the yeast's adverse reaction to elevated levels of lactic acid. Hop bitterness is extremely low. A turbid mash is traditional, although some homebrewers use a sour mash.

Vital statistics:	OG: 1.028–1.032 (7.1–8.0 °P)
IBUs: 3–8	FG: 1.004–1.006
EBC: 3.9–5.9	ABV: 2.8–3.6%

Commercial examples: Schultheiss Berliner Weisse, Berliner Kindl Weisse, Nodding Head Berliner Weisse.

Flanders Red Ale

Overall impression: A complex, sour, red wine-like Belgian-style ale.

History: The indigenous beer of West Flanders, typified by the products of the Rodenbach brewery, established in 1820 in West Flanders but reflective of earlier brewing traditions. The beer is aged for up to 2 years, often in huge oaken barrels which contain the resident bacteria necessary to sour the beer. It was once common in Belgium and England to blend old beer with young to balance the sourness and acidity found in aged beer. Although blending of batches for consistency is now common among larger breweries, this type of blending is a fading art.

Comments: Long aging and blending of young and well-aged beer often occurs, adding to the smoothness and complexity, though the aged product is sometimes released as a connoisseur's beer. Known as the Burgundy of Belgium, it is more wine-like than any other beer style. The reddish color is a product of the malt although an extended, less-than-rolling portion of the boil may help add an attractive Burgundy hue. Aging will also darken the beer. The Flanders red is more acetic and the fruity flavors more reminiscent of a red wine than an Oud Bruin.

Ingredients: A base of Vienna and/or Munich malts and a small amount of Special B are used with up to 20% flaked corn or corn grits. Low alpha acid continental or British hops are commonly used (avoid high alpha or distinctive American hops). *Saccharomyces*, *Lactobacillus* and *Brettanomyces* (and acetobacters) contribute to the fermentation and eventual flavor.

Vital statistics:	OG: 1.046–1.054 (11.4–13.3 °P)
IBUs: 15–25	FG: 1.008–1.016
EBC: 19.7–31.5	ABV: 5–5.5%

Commercial examples: Rodenbach Klassiek, Rodenbach Grand Cru, Bellegems Bruin, Duchesse de Bourgogne, New Belgium La Folie, Petrus Oud Bruin, Southampton Publick House Flanders Red Ale, Verhaege Vichtenaar.

Flanders Brown Ale/Oud Bruin

Overall impression: A malty, fruity, aged, somewhat sour Belgian-style brown ale.

History: An "old ale" tradition, indigenous to East Flanders, typified by the products of the Liefman brewery (now owned by Riva), which has roots back to the 1600s. Historically brewed as a "provision beer" that would develop some sourness as it aged. These beers were typically more sour than current commercial examples. Although Flanders red beers are aged in oak, the brown beers are not.

Comments: Long aging and blending of young and aged beer may occur, adding smoothness and complexity and balancing any harsh, sour character. A deeper malt character distinguishes these beers from Flanders red ales. This style was designed to lay down, so examples with a moderate-aged character are considered superior to younger examples. As in fruit lambics, Oud Bruin can be used as a base for fruit-flavored beers such as kriek (cherries) or frambozen (raspberries), although these should be entered in the classic-style fruit beer category. The Oud Bruin is less acetic and maltier than a Flanders red, and the fruity flavors are more malt-oriented.

Ingredients: A base of Pils malt with judicious amounts of crystal malt and a tiny bit of black or roast malt. Low alpha acid continental or British hops are typical (avoid high alpha or distinctive American hops). *Saccharomyces* and *Lactobacillus* (and acetobacters) contribute to the fermentation and eventual flavor. *Lactobacillus* reacts poorly to elevated levels of alcohol. A sour mash or acidulated malt may also be used to develop the sour character without introducing *Lactobacillus*. Water high in carbonates is typical of its home region and will buffer the acidity of darker malts and the lactic sourness. Magnesium in the water accentuates the sourness.

Vital statistics:	OG: 1.043–1.077 (10.7–18.7 °P)
IBUs: 15–25	FG: 1.012–1.016
EBC: 29.6–39.4	ABV: 4–8%

Commercial examples: Liefman's Goudenband, Liefman's Odnar, Liefman's Oud Bruin, Ichtegem Old Brown.

Straight (Unblended) Lambic

Overall impression: Complex, sour/acidic, pale, wheat-based ale fermented by a variety of Belgian microbiota.

History: Spontaneously fermented sour ales from the area in and around Brussels (the Senne Valley) stem from a farmhouse brewing tradition several centuries old. Their numbers are constantly dwindling.

Comments: Straight lambics are single-batch, unblended beers. Since they are unblended, the straight lambic is often a true product of the "house character" of a brewery and will be more variable than a gueuze. They are generally served young (6 months) and on tap as cheap, easy-drinking beers without any filling carbonation. Younger versions tend to be one-dimensionally sour since a complex Brett character often takes upward of a year to develop. An enteric character is often indicative of a lambic that is too young. A noticeable vinegary or cidery character is considered a fault by Belgian brewers. Since the wild yeast and bacteria will ferment ALL sugars, they are bottled only when they have completely fermented. Lambic is served uncarbonated, while gueuze is served effervescent.

Ingredients: Unmalted wheat (30–40%), Pilsner malt and aged (surannes) hops (3 years) are used. The aged hops are used more for preservative effects than bitterness, and makes actual bitterness levels difficult to estimate. Traditionally these beers are spontaneously fermented with naturally occurring yeast and bacteria in predominately oaken barrels. Home- and craft-brewed versions are more typically made with pure cultures of yeast, commonly including

Saccharomyces, *Brettanomyces*, *Pediococcus* and *Lactobacillus*, in an attempt to recreate the effects of the dominant microbiota of Brussels and the surrounding countryside of the Senne River valley. Cultures taken from bottles are sometimes used but there is no simple way of knowing which organisms are still viable.

Vital statistics:	OG: 1.040–1.054 (10.0–13.3 °P)
IBUs: Up to 10	FG: 1.000–1.010
EBC: 5.9–13.8	ABV: 5–6.5%

Commercial examples: The only bottled version readily available is Cantillon Grand Cru Bruocsella of whatever single batch vintage the brewer deems worthy to bottle. De Cam sometimes bottles their very old (5 years) lambic. In and around Brussels there are specialty cafes that often have draft lambics from traditional brewers/blenders such as Boon, De Cam, Cantillon, Drie Fonteinen, Lindemans and Girardin.

Gueuze

Overall impression: Complex, pleasantly sour/acidic, balanced, pale, wheat-based ale fermented by a variety of Belgian microbiota.

History: Spontaneously fermented sour ales from the area in and around Brussels (the Senne Valley) that stem from a farmhouse brewing tradition several centuries old. Their numbers are constantly dwindling and some are untraditionally sweetening their products (post-fermentation) to make them more palatable to a wider audience.

Comments: Gueuze is traditionally produced by mixing 1- to 3-year-old lambic. "Young" lambic contains fermentable sugars whereas old lambic has the characteristic "wild" taste of the Senne River valley. A good gueuze is not the most pungent, but possesses a full and tantalizing bouquet, a sharp aroma and a soft, velvety flavor. Lambic is served uncarbonated, whereas gueuze is served effervescent.

Ingredients: Unmalted wheat (30–40%), Pilsner malt and aged (surannes) hops (3 years) are used. The aged hops are used more for preservative effects than bitterness, and makes actual bitterness levels difficult to estimate. Traditionally these beers are spontaneously fermented with naturally occurring yeast and bacteria in predominately oaken barrels. Home- and craft-brewed versions are more typically made with pure cultures of yeast commonly including *Saccharomyces*, *Brettanomyces*, *Pediococcus* and *Lactobacillus* in an attempt to recreate the effects of the dominant microbiota of Brussels and the surrounding countryside of the Senne River valley. Cultures taken from bottles are sometimes used but there is no simple way of knowing which organisms are still viable.

Vital statistics:	OG: 1.040–1.060 (10.0–14.4 °P)
IBUs: Up to 10	FG: 1.000–1.006
EBC: 5.9–13.8	ABV: 5–8%

Commercial examples: Boon Oude Gueuze, Boon Oude Gueuze Mariage Parfait, De Cam Gueuze, De Cam/Drei Fonteinen Millennium Gueuze, Drie Fonteinen Oud Gueuze, Cantillon Gueuze, Hanssens Gueuze, Lindemans Gueuze Cuvée René, Girardin Gueuze (Black Label), Mort Subite (Unfiltered) Gueuze, Oud Beersel Oude Gueuze.

Fruit Lambic

Overall impression: Complex, fruity, pleasantly sour/acidic, balanced, pale, wheat-based ale fermented by a variety of Belgian microbiota. A lambic with fruit, not just a fruit beer.

History: Spontaneously fermented sour ales from the area in and around Brussels (the Senne Valley) that stem from a farmhouse brewing tradition several centuries old. Their numbers are constantly dwindling and some are untraditionally sweetening their products (post-fermentation) with sugar or sweet fruit to make them more palatable to a wider audience. Fruit was traditionally added to lambic or gueuze, either by the blender or publican, to increase the variety of beers available in local cafes.

Comments: Fruit-based lambics are often produced like gueuze by mixing 1- to 3-year-old lambic. "Young" lambic contains fermentable sugars while old lambic has the characteristic "wild" taste of the Senne River valley. Fruit is commonly added halfway through aging and the yeast and bacteria will ferment all sugars from the fruit. Fruit may also be added to unblended lambic. The most traditional styles of fruit lambics include kriek (cherries), framboise (raspberries) and druivenlambik (Muscat grapes).

Ingredients: Unmalted wheat (30–40%), Pilsner malt and aged (surannes) hops (3 years) are used. The aged hops are used more for preservative effects than bitterness, and makes actual bitterness levels difficult to estimate. Fruits traditionally used include tart cherries (with pits), raspberries or Muscat grapes. More recent examples include peaches, apricots or merlot grapes. Tart or acidic fruit is traditionally used as its purpose is not to sweeten the beer but to add a new dimension. Traditionally these beers are spontaneously fermented with naturally occurring yeast and bacteria in predominately oaken barrels. Home- and craft-brewed versions are more typically made with pure cultures of yeast commonly including *Saccharomyces*, *Brettanomyces*, *Pediococcus* and *Lactobacillus* in an attempt to recreate the effects of the dominant microbiota of Brussels and the surrounding countryside of the Senne River valley. Cultures taken from bottles are sometimes used but there is no simple way of knowing which organisms are still viable.

Vital statistics:	OG: 1.040–1.060 (10.0–14.4 °P)
IBUs: Up to 10	FG: 1.000–1.010
EBC: 5.9–13.8	ABV: 5–7%

Commercial examples: Boon Framboise Marriage Parfait, Boon Kriek Mariage Parfait, Boon Oude Kriek, Cantillon Fou' Foune (apricot), Cantillon Kriek, Cantillon Lou Pepe

Kriek, Cantillon Lou Pepe Framboise, Cantillon Rose de Gambrinus, Cantillon St. Lamvinus (merlot grape), Cantillon Vigneronne (Muscat grape), De Cam Oude Kriek, Drie Fonteinen Kriek, Girardin Kriek, Hanssens Oude Kriek, Oud Beersel Kriek.

The information about the bottom fermentation beer types comes from the 2004 BJCP Style Guidelines, which are Copyright © 2004, Beer Judge Certification Program, Inc. The most current version of the guidelines is found on the BJCP website (http://www.bjcp.org).

References

Bamforth, C. (2003). *Tap into the Art and Science of Brewing.* Oxford University Press, UK.

BJCP Style Guidelines (2004). Beer Judge Certification Program, Inc. (The most current version of the guidelines are found on the BJCP website, http://www.bjcp.org).

Briggs, D.E., Hough, J.S., Stevens, R. and Young, T.W. (1982). *Malting and Brewing Science. I. Malt Sweet Wort.* Chapman and Hall, London. pp. 32–387.

Briggs, D.E., Boulton, C.A., Brookes, P.A. and Stevens, R. (2004). *Brewing Science and Practice.* Woodhead publishing limited and CRC Press, LLC. Boca Raton, USA. pp. 20–542.

Carey, D. and Grossman, K. (2006). In Ockert, K. (ed.), *Fermentation, Cellaring, and Packaging Operations,* pp. 1–134. Masters Brewers Association of the Americas, USA.

Derdelinckx, G. and Neven, H. (1996). *Cerevisia* 21, 41–58.

Freeman, P.L. (1999). Barley and malting. In McCabe, J.T. (ed.), *The Practical Brewer,* pp. 53–98. Master Brewers Association of America, Wauwatosa, WI.

Goldammer, T. (1999). *The Brewers' Handbook – The Complete Book to Brewing Beer.* KVP Publishers, Clifton, VA. pp. 73–104.

Hough, J.S. (1985). *The Biotechnology of Malting and Brewing.* Cambridge, UK. pp. 135–159.

Kunze, W. (1996). *Technology Brewing and Malting,* pp. 303–587. International edn, translated Wainwright, T. VLB, Berlin.

Knudsen, F.B. (1999). Fermentation, principles and practices. In McCabe, J.T. (ed.), *The Practical Brewer,* pp. 235–261. Master Brewers Association of the Americas, Wauwatosa, Wisconsin.

Landschoot, A.V., Vanbeneden, N., Vanderputten, D. and Derdelinckx, G. (2004). *Cerevisia* 29, 140–146.

Lewis, M.J. and Young, T.W. (1995). *Brewing,* pp. 84–251. Chapman and Hall, London.

Munroe, J.H. (1994). Fermentation. In Hardwick, W.A. (ed.), *Handbook of Brewing,* pp. 323–379. Marcel Dekker, New York.

Ryder, D.R. and Power, J. (1994). Miscellaneous ingredients in aid of the process. In Hardwick, W.A. (ed.), *Handbook of Brewing,* pp. 203–245. Marcel Dekker, New York.

Vanderhaegen, B., Coghe, S., Verachtert, H. and Derdelinckx, G. (2002). *Cerevisia* 28, 48–58.

3
Lager Beer

Andrea Pavsler and Stefano Buiatti Department of Food Science, University of Udine, Udine, Italy

Abstract

Beer is one of the world's oldest alcoholic beverages. Brewing industry is a huge global business, consisting of several multinational companies and many thousands of smaller producers ranging from brewpubs to regional breweries. A great many of different types, or style, of beer are brewed across the world. For this reason, it is difficult to generalize on the relationship between beer and relative impact on nutrient intake because the composition of beers will range quite considerably depending on raw materials and how they are produced. Lager represents more than 90% of beer produced worldwide. It is typically brewed at low temperatures (bottom fermentation) in cool conditions using a particular yeast, and then stored (the word "lager" comes from the German *lagern* meaning "to store") in cool conditions to have maturation or improvement of its organoleptic characteristics. Until the sixteenth century ale (top fermentation) was the main type of beer in Europe. So it is only a myth that lager-style products have always been the characteristic beer in Germany. The monks of Bavaria were responsible for an innovation that was to change the face of beer brewing, the "bottom fermentation." The Bavarian monasteries first attempted to store beer for long periods in cool cellar. At lower temperatures, instead of frothing to the top of the fermenting vessel, the yeast sank to the bottom end fermenting more slowly. The Bavarian lager was still different from the widely known modern lager. They remained a fairly conventional dark brown or amber-red color, until 1842, when Joseph Groll mashed his first batch of beer in *Plzeň* (in Czech Republic) and the world's first ever golden colored lager was born.

List of Abbreviations

ABV	Alcohol by volume
CO_2	Carbon dioxide
DMS	Dimethyl sulfide
EBC	European Brewery Convention
FG	Final gravity
H_2S	Hydrogen sulfide
IBU	International Bitterness Units
OG	Original gravity
°P	Plato
PVPP	Polyvinylpolypyrrolidone
SO_2	Sulfur dioxide
SMM	*S*-methyl methionine
VDKs	Vicinal diketones

Introduction

Until the sixteenth century ale (top fermentation) was the main type of beer in Europe. So it is only a myth that lager-style products have always been the characteristic beer in Germany. The monks of Bavaria were responsible for an innovation that was to change the face of beer brewing, the "bottom fermentation." At the time, during summer, fermentation was likely to run out of control and bacteria could spoil the drink. The problem was so great that in Germany in 1533, Prince Maximilian I ordained that anyone wishing to brew between April 23 and September 29 had to obtain special permission. This edict was one of the main driving forces for the development of lager beer type. The Bavarian monasteries first attempted to store beer for long periods in cool cellar. This storage method caused some yeasts to change their character. At lower temperatures, instead of frothing to the top of the fermenting vessel, the yeast sank to the bottom end fermenting more slowly. Actually, the most apparent difference between ales and lagers is that lagers use bottom-fermenting yeast. In 1836, Gabriel Sedlmayr took over the running of the *Spaten* Brewery in Munich and developed the art of producing more stable, bottom-fermented beer through cold storage. The Bavarian lager was still different from the widely known modern lager. They remained a fairly conventional dark brown or amber-red color, until 1842, when Joseph Groll mashed his first batch of beer in *Plzeň* (in Czech Republic) and the world's first ever golden colored lager was born.

The development of the present bottom fermentation beer types did not occur until the end of the nineteenth century. This depended on some circumstances such as the invention of the refrigerating machine by Linde in 1871,

Beer in Health and Disease Prevention
ISBN: 978-0-12-373891-2

Table 3.1 Beverage beer consumption (2004)

Country	*Total consumption (million liters)*
China	286.40
United States	239.74
Germany	95.55
Brazil	84.50
Russia	84.50
Japan	65.49
United Kingdom	59.20
Mexico	54.35
Spain	33.76
Poland	26.70
South Africa	25.30
Canada	21.83
France	20.20
South Korea	18.97
Czech Republic	18.78
Ukraine	17.29
Italy	17.19

Source: Kirin Research Institute of Drinking and Lifestyle (2004).

Table 3.2 *Per capita* consumption of beer and wine

Country	*Beer (l)*	*Wine (l)*
Czech Republic	160.0	15.4
Germany	115.2	18.1
Republic of Ireland	114.0	8.8
Denmark	107.7	29.1
United Kingdom	95.6	17.6
Slovak Republic	93.8	15.2
Belgium	91.5	26.7
Australia	95.0	19.7
New Zealand	84.7	17.0
United States	83.7	7.3
The Netherlands	84.3	18.4
Spain	80.6	35.0
Finland	79.1	8.3
Portugal	61.7	58.0
Canada	67.0	8.9
South Africa	59.5	8.0
Brazil	52.9	1.9
Sweden	57.3	14.6
Japan	57.2	3.3
Norway	49.7	11.0
France	33.0	60.0
Italy	30.3	52.0
Russia	22.5	6.0
China	15.6	0.2

Source: Bamforth (2003) and Assobirra (2006).

the development of mechanical glassblowing to manufacture cheap bottles and the invention of beer filtration in 1878 (Kunze, 1996). Every year more than 1,500 millions of hectoliters (1 hl equals 100 l) are consumed in the world (Table 3.1). Lager beers are by far the most widespread beer type throughout the world. As shown in Table 3.2, beer consumption statistics differ enormously among countries. In most

Table 3.3 Beer production in EU

Countries	*Million liters*
Germany	108.249
Spain	31.600
United Kingdom	56.255
Poland	31.421
Holland	24.560
Czech Republic	19.788
France	16.029
Italy	13.170
Ireland	9.377
Austria	8.818
Denmark	8.704
Finland	4.587

Source: Assobirra (2006).

countries beer is consumed more when compared to wine, but Italy and France drink considerably more wine than beer.

The Czech Republic has the highest *per capita* consumption of beer, over 33 l more than that of their nearest challenger, Germany. Table 3.3 shows that in Europe the first country in beer production is Germany, followed by United Kingdom and Holland (Bamforth, 2003).

Beer Production

- **The first step of brewing process is the milling of malt followed by mashing in which water is added to ground malt.**

In the brewing process, the first step is the milling of the malt (Figure 3.1). The objective is to break up malt and adjuncts to such an extent that the greatest yield of extract is produced in the shortest time in the mashing equipment in use. With most wort separation systems an important objective is to keep malt husk as intact as possible, in order to have an open filter bed that helps wort separation (Briggs *et al.*, 2004).

Ground malt represents a rich source of carbohydrate, degraded protein, various B vitamins, inorganic materials and many enzymes which progressively catalyze the hydrolysis of insoluble polymers (proteins, nucleic acids and carbohydrates) to give soluble products (Hough *et al.*, 1982). The preparation of the malt mash is the most critical operation in the brew house. The malting process will directly determine both chemical properties such as yeast nutrients, alcohol content, peptide and amino acid profile, concentration of unfermented carbohydrates and physical properties such as color, foam and clarity (Ryder and Power, 1994).

There are several methods of mashing to obtain satisfactory wort (an aqueous extract of the malt). In all cases, a mash should be held at a chosen temperature (or at successive different temperatures), for pre-determined times, to allow enzymes to degrade substances. At the end of mashing the sweet or unhopped wort is separated from the undissolved solids,

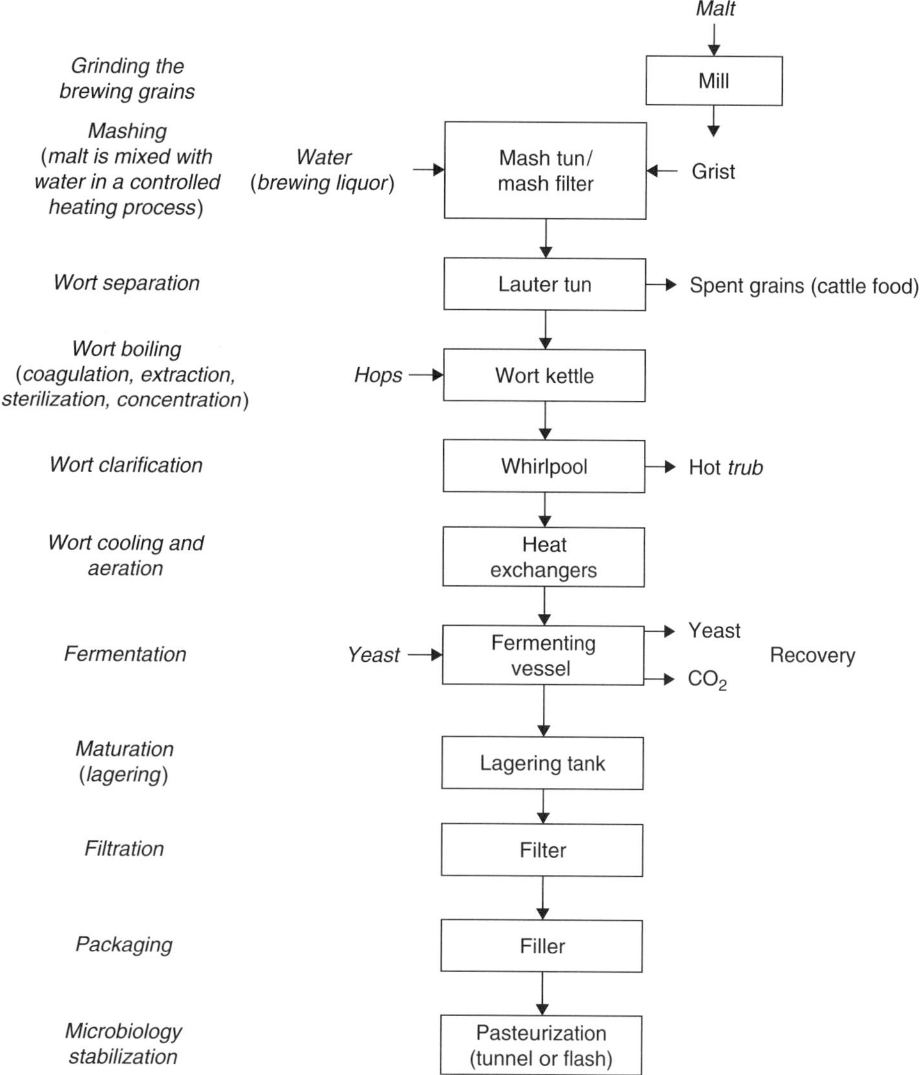

Figure 3.1 The lager brewing process. *Source*: Modified from Buiatti (2004).

the spent grains. The single-step infusion mashing system, commonly associated with the production of ales and stouts, involves the intimate mixing of the ground material, or grist as it is called, with hot water. In brewing, water is commonly known as liquor. The temperature of about 63–65°C is held constant (called "conversion temperature") for a period which may be as short as 30 min or may extend up to 60–90 min. In order to wash virtually all the sweet wort from the undegraded material (the spent grains), further supplies of hot water at say 78–80°C are sprayed over the surface of the mash. The single temperature mashing system is best for the highly modified malt produced in Britain (Briggs *et al.*, 1982), that require only a saccharification rest and no protein rest. Advantages are simplicity of operation and lower capital, energy cost compared to other mashing systems (Goldammer, 1999).

The decoction mashing system is traditional for mainland European lager brewers (Figure 3.2). It differs from infusion mashing in several aspects. The endosperm of the malt used is usually less enzymically degraded and requires more extensive enzymic action in mashing. To aid this, the

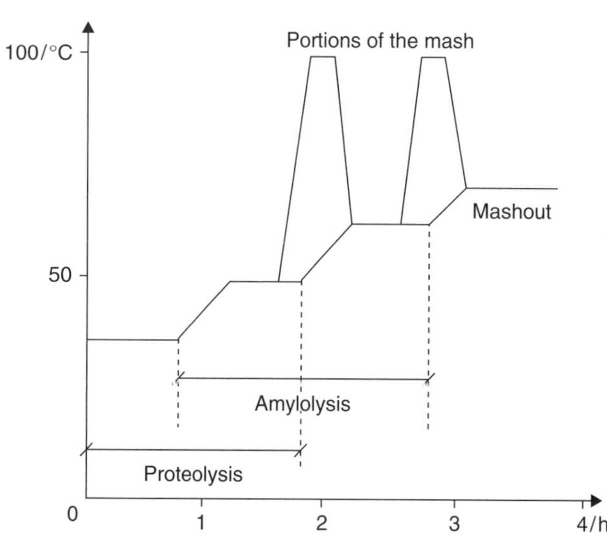

Figure 3.2 A temperature scheme for a typical two-decoction mashing program. Two portions of the mash are boiled separately.

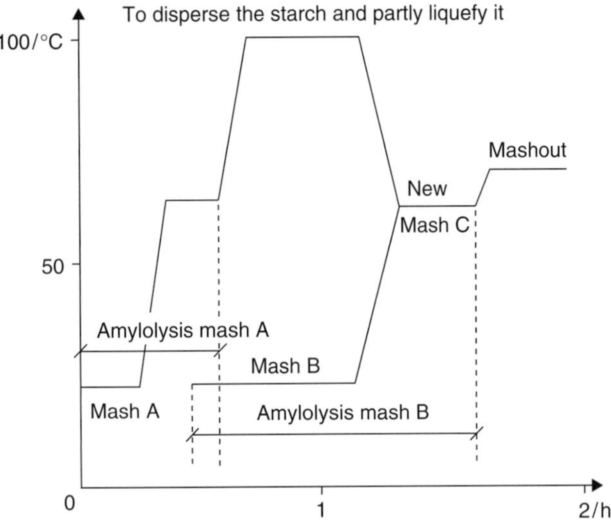

Figure 3.3 Typical temperature schedule of double mash infusion process. A scheme of the temperatures using a cereal cooker. (A) the temperature of the adjuncts/grits mash in the cereal cooker, (B) temperature in the malt mash and in the combined mash during and after mixing and (C) mash obtained mixing mashes A and B.

malt is both ground more finely than in infusion process and mixed with water of lower temperature, at 35–40°C. Extensive proteolysis and solubilization occur. During the conversion a portion of the mash (often one-third) is boiled. On return to the main mash, the temperature rises to about 50°C. Later a further third of the mash is withdrawn and boiled; when it is sent back to the main mash, the temperature increases to about 65°C and hydrolysis of carbohydrates (amylolysis) now occurs rapidly. After a last decoction all enzyme activity ceases (mashout) in the consolidated mash at 75°C.

The double mash infusion system (Figure 3.3), common in North American practice, is a method having features in common with infusion and decoction. This is called double mashing because the mash starts as two separate mashes which are later combined. A cereal cooker for boiling adjuncts and a mash tun for well-modified malts is used. The malt is ground and mixed with water to obtain a mash at 38°C (peptonizing rest). After about 20 min, the temperature is rose to 50°C. Unmalted cereal in the form of maize (corn) or rice grits is mixed with a little malt and/or a preparation of microbial enzymes (if permitted by countries regulations), milled and carefully heated in a cereal cooker to 100°C to disperse the starch and partly liquefy it. The two mashes are then mixed together to achieve about 65–72°C, for about 30–40 min. Upon completion of saccharification, temperature rose to a "mashing out" temperature (75–77°C). The wort is then separated from the grain in a process known as lautering. Additional water may be sprinkled on the grains to extract additional sugars (Briggs *et al.*, 1982; Goldammer, 1999).

- **At the end of mash filtration the wort is boiled, clarified, cooled and aerated.**

The sweet wort is transferred to a vessel, boiling kettle, where it is boiled with hops or hop preparations, usually for 60–90 min in order to arrest further enzymes action, sterilize and concentrate the wort and precipitate some of the proteinaceous material as a coarse coagulum (hot *trub*). The boiling process is often associated with the addition of sugars or syrups, and hops or bitter products derived from hops. Additions may be regulated by weight or by α-acid content, and several additions may be made at different stages of the boil. The bitter resins of the hops are extracted during the boil, and particular attention is paid to levels of humulones (α-acids) and lupulones (β-acids). During wort boiling the humulones are isomerized to isohumulones which are more bitter and water soluble. The hot *trub* and any insoluble material from hop is taken out of the wort by centrifugation or by a whirlpool tank. When hopped wort is clarified, it must be brought down to fermentation temperatures before yeast is added through a plate heat exchanger. Further protein and tannin material tend to come out from solution. This precipitation is called cold break (cold *trub*). During the cooling, it is usual to oxygenate or aerate the wort to provide oxygen for the yeast in the initial stages of fermentation (Briggs *et al.*, 2004).

- **After boiling the cooled and aerated wort is pitched with yeast.**

The yeasts used in breweries are conventionally divided into two main classes, top-fermenting and bottom-fermenting. Beer is also divided into two very broad categories according to which yeast is used, respectively, lager and ale. Lager yeast, known as *Saccharomyces pastorianus* or *Saccharomyces carlsbergensis*, runs the fermentation at cool temperatures (8–15°C), and forms a cloudy mass (flocculates) on the bottom of the vessel (Bamforth, 2003). The beers so produced are called bottom fermented. Lager term therefore refers to the secondary fermentation, maturation and storage which these beers traditionally receive after primary fermentation. To produce ale beers, strains of *Saccharomyces cerevisiae* are commonly used in the temperature range of 16–24°C. The inoculation of wort is called "pitching," and the pitching rate depends on fermentation temperature (so lager and ale are different), wort gravity, yeast strain and other variables (Munroe, 1994). A pitching range of $10–25 \times 10^6$ cells/ml is normally used. As a rule of thumb, the pitching rate is 1×10^6 cells per Plato (°P) per milliliter of wort (Knudsen, 1999). The pitching rate is very important and affects both beer flavor and fermentation rate. Compared to low pitching rates, higher pitching rates will lead to a lower number of cells doubling under fixed oxygen supply. As the pitching rate becomes too low, the oxygen requested to synthesize sterols for new cells is lower and overall growth is lowered.

Poor yeast can also lead to high sulfur dioxide (SO_2) concentrations (Munroe, 1994).

- **The fermentation process starts after 4–6 h, depending on the temperature.**

Lager beers produced by bottom-fermenting yeasts are the most widespread beer types throughout the world (more than 90%). Lager yeast typically undergoes primary fermentation at 8–15°C, followed by a long secondary fermentation between −1°C and +4°C (the "lagering phase"), by having some 1% remaining fermentable extract and also about $1–4 \times 10^6$ cells/ml of yeast in suspension. Now, with modern improved fermentation control, most lager breweries use only short periods of cold storage, typically 1–3 weeks.

- **Lager beer after primary fermentation is stored in cool conditions to have maturation with improvement of its flavor.**

This period causes proteins to coagulate and settle out with the yeast giving improved beer stability. During the maturation, the yeast continues to attack the residual fermentable material, and the carbon dioxide (CO_2) produced is effective in purging any air out of the beer and also much of hydrogen sulfide (H_2S, odor of rotten eggs), sulfur dioxide (SO_2) and dimethyl sulfide (DMS). These are all the results of yeast metabolism, although the majority of DMS comes from *S*-methyl methionine (SMM), an amino acid present in malt, when wort is heated or malt is kilned. In general, for bottom-fermented beers, the technique of maturation must ensure the production of a balanced beer flavor with the minimum concentration of diacetyl (2,3-butanedione). Diacetyl and the related compound 2,3-pentanedione are called vicinal diketones (VDKs). They are generally undesidered contributors to the flavor of lager beers. VDKs are originated by yeast as it synthesizes the amino acids, valine and leucine (Figure 3.4). In this pathway, α-acetolactate is transported out of the cell, where it is non-enzymically converted in diacetyl, compound with a negative buttery flavor. This chemical reaction is accelerated by higher temperature and lower pH. Diacetyl is later converted to 2,3-butanediol by the yeast, compounds having a lower flavor impact (Munroe, 1994). Still another possibility is to add to the lager tank fermenting wort at the *Kräusen* stage (phase in which yeast shows its maximum activity). This addition of fermentable extract at the rate of 5–10% by volume is called "Kräusening" (Hough *et al.*, 1982). The active yeast from the *Kräusen* beer can reduce the diacetyl level in the original beer in shortest time.

- **After fermentation beer is extremely turbid, due to the presence of residual yeast and colloidal haze. The purpose of filtration is to obtain a beer stable for a long time.**

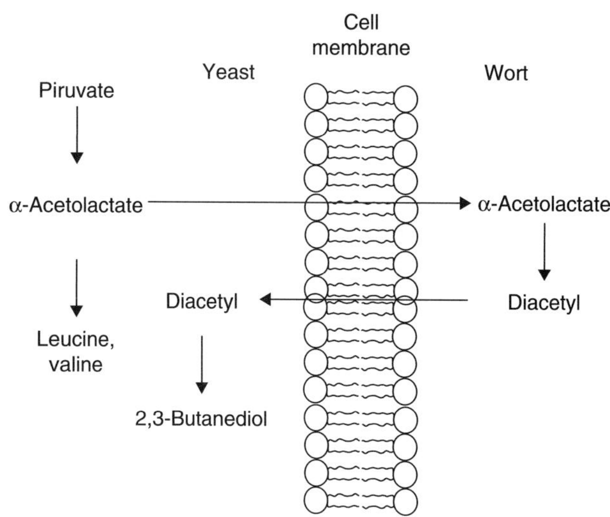

Figure 3.4 Formation of diacetyl and its conversion.

There are various processing techniques for clarification (gravity sedimentation, centrifugation and filtration), but only filtration is able to give the brilliance required in the marketplace. Several chillproofing techniques are employed in order to remove proteins and tannins present in beer which tend to combine together slowly and form colloidal haze. Insoluble polyvinylpolypyrrolidone (PVPP) is, for example, an effective adsorbent of tannins and it is normally added to a tank of pre-filtered beer. Other media used are silica gels and diatomaceous earth (*Kieselguhr*). Silica gels have been successfully used as protein adsorbents, so they cannot combine with polyphenols. *Kieselguhr* selectively removes particles of a certain size and is the filtering coadjutant most commonly used to remove yeast cells. The small diatoms, deposited upon a filter septum, form a rigid and porous filter cake which sieves out the particulate matter in beer. The precoats, made of cellulose and/or *Kieselguhr* of different sizes, would soon become blocked with the suspended particles in the beer, but this is avoided by regular injections of fresh *Kieselguhr* (Patino, 1999).

- **The yeast, besides ethanol and CO_2, produces several by-products that have a great effect on the flavor of beer.**

Fermentation by-products have a great effect on the flavor and aroma of the beer, and the factors which influence their formation are very important to the brewer. As previously described, diacetyl is the most important aroma of not mature beer, and the technique of maturation must ensure the production of a balanced beer flavor with the minimum concentration of diacetyl. Moreover, sulfur compounds (H_2S, SO_2, DMS, see above) have a very strong smell taste. The CO_2 produced during the fermentation is effective in purging any air out of the beer. On the other hand, there are other

Table 3.4 Flavor compounds associated with yeast metabolism in lager and ale

Class of volatile	*Name*	*Lager (mg/l)*	*Ale (mg/l)*
Higher alcohols	Ethanol	23–25 (g/l)	27–32 (g/l)
	2-methylbutanol	8–16	14–19
	Isobutanol	6–11	18–33
	n-Propanol	5–10	31–48
	Isopentanol	32–57	47–61
	B-phenylethanol	25–32	36–53
Esters	Ethylacetate	8–14	14–23
	Isopentylacetate	1.5–2.0	1.4–3.3
Diketones	Diacetyl	0.02–0.08	0.06–0.30
	Pentane-2,3-dione	0.01–0.05	0.01–0.20
Sulfur compounds	Hydrogen sulfide (H_2S)	0.0015–0.008	0.0015–0.008
	Dimethyl sulfide (DMS)	15+ (μg/l)	15+ (μg/l)

Source: Modified from Hough (1985).

flavor compounds such as higher alcohol (or fusel alcohols) and esters that contribute directly to final product aroma.

Most of higher alcohols are formed during primary fermentation. They can be formed from amino acids, from sugars and by other biosynthetic ways (Kunze, 1996). The most important higher alcohols are reported in Table 3.4. The lower temperature fermentations of lagers, limit the production of fusel alcohols (Goldammer, 1999).

Esters, which are produced during fermentation by esterification of fatty acids by ethanol or, in small amounts, by higher alcohols, have long been recognized as important flavor determinants in beers, with many being present at or near their sensory thresholds (Engan, 1981; Kunze, 1996). In general they impart fruity taste to beer. The production of esters is dependent on several factors, such as fermentation temperature, oxygen content, original gravity, pitching rates and yeast strain (Lewis and Bamforth, 2006). As showed in Table 3.4, the ester content in ale is higher than lager beer. It is generally accepted that top-fermented beer is more aromatic than a bottom-fermented beer, both having an identical original gravity (OG). Top-fermented beers, with their typically higher fermentation temperatures (16–24°C) and different yeast strains, usually contain more esters and fusel alcohols, and they often have higher alcohol content (Derdelinckx and Neven, 1996).

- **The microbiological stabilization, through pasteurization or sterile filtration, are the last operations before packaging.**

The term "microbiological stabilization" describes a process whereby spoilage mechanisms, such as bacteria and yeast, are destroyed or removed from the product. These spoilage mechanisms can cause off-flavor and hazing in the final beer and affect the expected shelf-life. Thus, it is important that such contaminants are removed. A traditional method used to destroy the number of microorganisms is pasteurization. The basis of this process is the heating of the beer to a specific temperature for a pre-determined period of time to attain the minimum degree of pasteurization necessary to inactivate beer-spoiling bacteria. The two main pasteurization techniques used are "flash" and "tunnel". Flash pasteurization is used for the continuous treatment of bulk beer prior to filling kegs. It is typically carried out in a plate heat exchanger, with steam as the heat exchange medium. The beer is heated to between 72°C and 74°C and held in this temperature range for 15–30 s.

Tunnel pasteurization, on the other hand, is applied after the bottles and cans have been filled and sealed. The bottles are loaded at one end of the pasteurizer and passed under sprays of hot water as they move along the conveyor. The sprays are arranged so that the bottles are subjected to increasingly hot water until the beer in the bottles reaches the pasteurization temperature of 60°C. The bottles are then cooled gradually with water until they are discharged from the end of the pasteurizer. The temperature changes are made in stages to prevent the bottles from breaking. The heating and cooling of the bottles are performed using various water circulation paths to enable the reuse of the recovered heat. In this way, the energy usage by the tunnel pasteurizer can be kept to a minimum. Although disagreement exists within the brewing community, one criticism leveled against the use of pasteurization is the risk of damaging the flavor of the beer with the heat treatment. An alternative to pasteurization that has been used for many years is sterile filtration. This process has the obvious advantage over pasteurization of eliminating the risk of adversely affecting the beer's flavor characteristics, while at the same time effectively removing the spoilage microorganisms (Scanlon, 2004; Lewis and Bamforth, 2006).

Beer Types

There are many thousands of different beer brands throughout the world, many of which can be classified in defined beer types which have developed in the course of time in a few countries or regions. Depending on the process used, a first classification could be made into top fermentation and bottom fermentation beer types. Table 3.5 gives a breakdown of some principal beer types.

Bottom fermentation beer types

In the text below, there are reported a list of bottom fermentation beer types (BJCP, 2004). Beer strength may be defined in several ways; to explain the vital statistics of each style, it is used to explain the content of hop bitter substances (IBU, International Bitterness Units), the color

Table 3.5 Some principal beer types

Types of beers	*Origin*	*Characteristics*	*Typical range of alcohol (% by vol.)*
Bottom fermentation			
German Pilsner (Pils)	Germany	Crisp, clean, refreshing beer	4.4–5.2
Bohemian Pilsner	Czech Republic	Crisp, complex and well rounded yet refreshing	4.2–5.4
Classic American Pilsner	United States	Rice contributes a crisper, more neutral character	4.5–6.0
Vienna lager	Austria	Soft, elegant maltiness	4.5–5.7
Oktoberfest/Märzen	Germany	Depth of malt character	4.8–5.7
Dark American lager	United States	Sweeter version of standard lager	4.2–6.0
Munich Dunkel	Germany	Depth and complexity	4.5–5.6
Schwarzbier (black beer)	Germany	Probably a variant of the Munich *Dunkel* style	4.4–5.4
Maibock/Helles bock	Germany	Pale, strong, malty lager beer	6.3–7.4
Traditional bock	Germany	Dark, strong, malty lager beer	6.3–7.2
Doppelbock	Germany	Strong and rich lager	7–10+
Eisbock	Germany	An extremely strong, full and malty dark lager	9–14+
Top fermentation			
Standard/ordinary bitter	Britain	Low gravity, low alcohol levels	3.2–3.8
English Pale Ale	Britain	Dry hop, bitter, estery, malty, low carbonation	4.6–6.2
Mild	Britain	Refreshing, yet flavorful	2.8–4.2
Brown Porter	Britain	English dark ale with restrained roasty characteristics	4.0–5.4
Robust Porter	Britain	Malty dark ale	4.8–6.0
Dry Stout	Ireland	Dark, roasty, bitter, creamy ale	4.0–5.0
Sweet Stout	Britain	Dark, sweet, full-bodied, slightly roasty ale	4.0–6.0
Kölsch	Germany (Cologne)	Smooth and crisp	4.4–5.2
Lambic	Belgium	Fermented by a variety of Belgian microbiota	5.0–7.0
Rauchbier	Germany	Smoky aroma and flavor and a somewhat dark color	4.8–6.0
Weizen/Weissbier	Germany	Pale, spicy, fruity, refreshing wheat-based ale	4.3–5.6
Weizenbock	Germany	Strong, malty, fruity, wheat-based ale	6.5–8.0+

Source: Most of the data in this table is from BJCP Style Guidelines (2004).

(EBC, European Brewery Convention), the specific gravity of wort before fermentation (OG, original gravity) and after fermentation (FG, final gravity), and the alcohol content (ABV or alcohol by volume).

Pilsner

German Pilsner (pils)

Aroma: Typically features a light grainy malt character and distinctive flowery or spicy noble hops. Clean, no fruity esters, no diacetyl. May have an initial sulfuric aroma (from water and/or yeast) and a low background note of DMS (from pils malt).

Appearance: Straw to light gold, brilliant to very clear, with a creamy, long-lasting white head.

Flavor: Crisp and bitter, with a dry to medium-dry finish. Moderate to moderately low yet well-attenuated maltiness, although some grainy flavors and slight malt sweetness are acceptable. Hop bitterness dominates taste and continues through the finish and lingers into the aftertaste. Hop flavor can range from low to high but should only be derived from German noble hops. Clean, no fruity esters, no diacetyl.

Mouthfeel: Medium-light body, medium to high carbonation.

Overall impression: Crisp, clean, refreshing beer that prominently features noble German hop bitterness accentuated by sulfates in the water.

History: A copy of Bohemian Pilsner adapted to brewing conditions in Germany.

Comments: Drier and crisper than a Bohemian Pilsner with a bitterness that tends to linger more in the aftertaste due to higher attenuation and higher sulfate water. Lighter in body and color, and with higher carbonation than a Bohemian Pilsner.

Ingredients: Pilsner malt, German hop varieties (especially noble varieties such as Hallertauer, Tettnanger and Spalt for taste and aroma), medium sulfate water, German lager yeast.

Vital statistics:	OG: 1.044–1.050 (11.0–12.4 °P)
IBUs: 25–45	FG: 1.008–1.013
EBC: 3.9–9.8	ABV: 4.4–5.2%

Commercial examples: Bitburger, Warsteiner, König Pilsner, Jever Pils, Holsten Pils, Spaten Pils, Victory Prima Pils, Brooklyn Pilsner.

Bohemian Pilsner

Aroma: Rich with complex malt and a spicy, floral Saaz hop bouquet. Some diacetyl is acceptable, but need not be present. Otherwise clean, with no fruity esters.

Appearance: Very pale gold to deep burnished gold, brilliant to very clear, with a dense, long-lasting, creamy white head.

Flavor: Rich, complex maltiness combined with a pronounced yet soft and rounded bitterness and flavor from Saaz hops. Some diacetyl is acceptable, but need not be present. Bitterness is prominent but never harsh, and does not linger. The aftertaste is balanced between malt and hops. Clean, no fruity esters.

Mouthfeel: Medium-bodied (although diacetyl, if present, may make it seem medium-full), medium carbonation.

Overall impression: Crisp, complex and well rounded yet refreshing.

History: First brewed in 1842, this style was the original clear, light-colored beer.

Comments: Uses Moravian malted barley and a decoction mash for rich, malt character. Saaz hops and low sulfate, low carbonate water provide a distinctively soft, rounded hop profile. Traditional yeast sometimes can provide a background diacetyl note. Dextrins provide additional body, and diacetyl enhances the perception of a fuller palate.

Ingredients: Soft water with low mineral content, Saaz hops, Moravian malted barley, Czech lager yeast.

Vital statistics:	OG: 1.044–1.056 (11.0–13.8 °P)
IBUs: 35–45	FG: 1.013–1.017
EBC: 6.9–11.8	ABV: 4.2–5.4%

Commercial examples: Pilsner Urquell, Budweiser Budvar (Czechvar in the United States), Czech Rebel, Staropramen, Gambrinus Pilsner, Dock Street Bohemian Pilsner.

Classic American Pilsner

Aroma: Low to medium grainy, corn-like or sweet maltiness may be evident (although rice-based beers are more neutral). Medium to moderately high hop aroma, often classic noble hops. Clean lager character, with no fruitiness or diacetyl. Some DMS is acceptable.

Appearance: Yellow to deep gold color. Substantial, long-lasting white head. Bright clarity.

Flavor: Moderate to moderately high maltiness similar in character to the Continental Pilsners but somewhat lighter in intensity due to the use of up to 30% flaked maize (corn) or rice used as an adjunct. Slight grainy, corn-like sweetness from the use of maize with substantial offsetting hop bitterness. Rice-based versions are crisper, drier, and often lack corn-like flavors. Medium to high hop flavor from noble hops (either late addition or first-wort hopped).

Mouthfeel: Medium body and rich, creamy mouthfeel. Medium to high carbonation levels.

Overall impression: A substantial Pilsner that can stand up to the classic European Pilsners, but exhibiting the native American grains and hops available to German brewers who initially brewed it in the United States. Refreshing, but with the underlying malt and hops that stand out when compared to other modern American light lagers. Maize lends a distinctive grainy sweetness.

History: A version of Pilsner brewed in the United States by immigrant German brewers who brought the process and yeast with them when they settled in America. They worked with the ingredients that were native to America to create a unique version of the original Pilsner. This style died out after prohibition but was resurrected as a home-brewed style by advocates of the hobby.

Comments: The classic American Pilsner brewed both pre-prohibition and post-prohibition with some differences. OGs of 1.050–1.060 would have been appropriate for pre-prohibition beers while gravities dropped to 1.044–1.048 after prohibition. Corresponding IBUs dropped from a pre-prohibition level of 30–40 to 25–30 after prohibition.

Ingredients: Six-row barley with 20–30% flaked maize to dilute the excessive protein levels. Native American hops such as Clusters, traditional continental noble hops or modern noble crosses (Ultra, Liberty, Crystal) are also appropriate. Water with a high mineral content can lead to an inappropriate coarseness in flavor and harshness in aftertaste.

Vital statistics:	OG: 1.044–1.060 (11.0–14.7 °P)
IBUs: 25–40	FG: 1.010–1.015
EBC: 5.9–11.8	ABV: 4.5–6%

Commercial examples: Occasional brewpub and microbrewery specials.

European Amber Lager

Vienna lager

Aroma: Moderately rich German malt aroma (of Vienna and/or Munich malt). A light-toasted malt aroma may be present. Similar, though less intense than Oktoberfest. Clean lager character, with no fruity esters or diacetyl. Noble hop aroma may be low to none. Caramel aroma is inappropriate.

Appearance: Light reddish amber to copper color. Bright clarity. Large, off-white, persistent head.

Flavor: Soft, elegant malt complexity is in the forefront, with a firm enough hop bitterness to provide a balanced finish. Some toasted character from the use of Vienna malt. No roasted or caramel flavor. Fairly dry finish, with both malt and hop bitterness present in the aftertaste. Noble hop flavor may be low to none.

Mouthfeel: Medium-light to medium body, with a gentle creaminess. Moderate carbonation. Smooth. Moderately crisp finish. May have a bit of alcohol warming.

Overall impression: Characterized by soft, elegant maltiness that dries out in the finish to avoid becoming sweet.

History: The original amber lager developed by Anton Dreher shortly after the isolation of lager yeast. Nearly extinct in its area of origin, the style continues in Mexico where it was brought by Santiago Graf and other Austrian immigrant brewers in the late 1800s. Regrettably, most modern examples use adjuncts which lessen the rich malt complexity characteristic of the best examples of this style. The style owes much of its character to the method of malting (Vienna malt).

Comments: American versions can be a bit stronger, drier and more bitter, while European versions tend to be sweeter. Many Mexican amber and dark lagers used to be more authentic, but unfortunately are now more like sweet, adjunct-laden American Dark Lagers.

Ingredients: Vienna malt provides a lightly toasty and complex, melanoidin-rich malt profile. As with Oktoberfests, only the finest quality malt should be used, along with continental hops (preferably noble varieties). Moderately hard, carbonate-rich water. Can use some caramel malts and/or darker malts to add color and sweetness, but caramel malts should not add significant aroma and flavor, and dark malts should not provide any roasted character.

Vital statistics:	OG: 1.046–1.052 (11.4–12.9 °P)
IBUs: 18–30	FG: 1.010–1.014
EBC: 11.0–31.5	ABV: 4.5–5.7%

Commercial examples: Great Lakes Eliot Ness (unusual in its 6.2% strength and 35 IBUs), Gösser Dark, Noche Buena, Negra Modelo, Samuel Adams Vienna Style Lager, Old Dominion Aviator Amber Lager, Gordon Biersch Vienna Lager, Capital Wisconsin Amber.

Oktoberfest/Märzen

Aroma: Rich German malt aroma (of Vienna and/or Munich malt). A light- to moderate-toasted malt aroma is often present. Clean lager aroma with no fruity esters or diacetyl. No hop aroma. Caramel aroma is inappropriate.

Appearance: Dark gold to deep orange-red color. Bright clarity, with solid foam stand.

Flavor: Initial malty sweetness, but finish is moderately dry. Distinctive and complex maltiness often includes a toasted aspect. Hop bitterness is moderate, and noble hop flavor is low to none. Balance is toward malt, though the finish is not sweet. Noticeable caramel or roasted flavors are inappropriate. Clean lager character with no diacetyl or fruity esters.

Mouthfeel: Medium body, with a creamy texture and medium carbonation. Smooth. Fully fermented, without a cloying finish.

Overall impression: Smooth, clean and rather rich with a depth of malt character. This is one of the classic malty styles, with a maltiness that is often described as soft, complex and elegant but never cloying.

History: Origin is credited to Gabriel Sedlmayr, based on an adaptation of the Vienna style developed by Anton Dreher around 1840, shortly after lager yeast was first isolated. Typically, brewed in the spring, signaling the end of the traditional brewing season and stored in cold caves or cellars during the warm summer months. Served in autumn amidst traditional celebrations.

Ingredients: Grist varies, although German Vienna malt is often the backbone of the grain bill, with some Munich malt, Pils malt and possibly some crystal malt. All malt should derive from the finest quality two-row barley. Continental hops, especially noble varieties, are most authentic. Somewhat alkaline water (up to 300 ppm) with significant carbonate content is welcome. A decoction mash can help to develop the rich malt profile.

Vital statistics:	OG: 1.050–1.056 (12.4–13.8 °P)
IBUs: 20–28	FG: 1.012–1.016
EBC: 13.8–27.6	ABV: 4.8–5.7%

Commercial examples: Paulaner Oktoberfest, Hacker-Pschorr Original Oktoberfest, Ayinger Oktoberfest-Märzen, Hofbräu Oktoberfest, Spaten Oktoberfest, Eggenberger Märzen, Goose Island Oktoberfest, Capital Oktoberfest, Gordon Biersch Märzen, Samuel Adams Oktoberfest (a bit unusual in its late hopping).

Dark Lager

Dark American lager

Aroma: Little to no malt aroma. Medium-low to no roast and caramel malt aroma. Hop aroma may range from none to light spicy or floral hop presence. Hop aroma may range from none to light, spicy or floral hop presence. Can have low levels of yeast character (green apples, DMS or fruitiness). No diacetyl.

Appearance: Deep amber to dark brown with bright clarity and ruby highlights. Foam stand may not be long lasting, and is usually light tan in color.

Flavor: Moderately crisp with some low to moderate levels of sweetness. Medium-low to no caramel and/or roasted malt flavors (and may include hints of coffee, molasses or cocoa). Hop flavor ranges from none to low levels. Hop bitterness at low to medium levels. No diacetyl. May have a very light fruitiness. Burnt or moderately strong roasted malt flavors are a defect.

Mouthfeel: Light to somewhat medium body. Smooth, although a highly carbonated beer.

Overall impression: A somewhat sweeter version of standard/premium lager with a little more body and flavor.

Comments: A broad range of international lagers that are darker than pale, and not assertively bitter and/or roasted.

Ingredients: Two- or six-row barley, corn or rice as adjuncts. Light use of caramel and darker malts. May use coloring agents.

Vital statistics:	OG: 1.044–1.056 (11.0–13.8 °P)
IBUs: 8–20	FG: 1.008–1.012
EBC: 27.6–43.3	ABV: 4.2–6%

Commercial examples: Dixie Blackened Voodoo, Shiner Bock, San Miguel Dark, Beck's Dark, Saint Pauli Girl Dark, Warsteiner Dunkel, Crystal Diplomat Dark Beer.

Munich Dunkel

Aroma: Rich, Munich malt sweetness, like bread crusts (and sometimes toast.) Hints of chocolate, nuts, caramel and/or toffee are also acceptable. No fruity esters or diacetyl should be detected, but a slight noble hop aroma is acceptable.

Appearance: Deep copper to dark brown, often with a red or garnet tint. Creamy, light to medium tan head. Usually clear, although murky unfiltered versions exist.

Flavor: Dominated by the rich and complex flavor of Munich malt, usually with melanoidins reminiscent of bread crusts. The taste can be moderately sweet, although it should not be overwhelming or cloying. Hints of caramel, chocolate, toast or nuttiness may be present in the background. Burnt or bitter flavors from roasted malts are inappropriate, as are pronounced caramel flavors from crystal malt. Hop bitterness is moderately low but perceptible, with the balance tipped firmly toward maltiness.

Mouthfeel: Medium to medium-full body, providing a firm and dextrinous mouthfeel without being heavy or cloying. Moderate carbonation. May have a light astringency and a slight alcohol warming.

Overall impression: Characterized by depth and complexity of Munich malt and the accompanying melanoidins. Rich Munich flavors, but not as intense as a bock or as roasted as a *Schwarzbier*.

History: The classic brown lager style of Munich which developed as a darker, malt-accented beer in part because of the moderately carbonate water.

Comments: Unfiltered versions from Germany can taste like liquid bread, with a yeasty, earthy richness not found in exported filtered *Dunkels*.

Ingredients: Grist is primarily made up of German Munich malt (up to 100% in some cases) with the remainder German Pilsner malt. Very small amounts of crystal malt can add dextrins and color but should not introduce excessive sweetness. Very slight additions of roasted malts (such as Carafa or chocolate) may be used to improve color but should not add any flavor. Noble German hop varieties and German lager yeast strains should be used. Moderately carbonate water.

Vital statistics:	OG: 1.048–1.056 (11.9–13.8 °P)
IBUs: 18–28	FG: 1.010–1.016
EBC: 27.6–55.1	ABV: 4.5–5.6%

Commercial examples: Ayinger Altbairisch Dunkel, Hacker-Pschorr Alt Munich Dark, Paulaner Alt Münchner Dunkel, Weltenburger Kloster Barock-Dunkel, Penn Dark Lager, Capital Munich Dark, Harpoon Munich-type Dark Beer, Gordon Biersch Dunkels, Dinkel Acker Dark.

Schwarzbier (black beer)

Aroma: Low to moderate malt, with low aromatic sweetness and/or hints of roast malt often apparent. The malt can be clean and neutral or rich and Munich-like, and may have a hint of caramel. The roast can be coffee-like but should never be burnt. A low noble hop aroma is optional. Clean lager yeast character (light sulfur possible) with no fruity esters or diacetyl.

Appearance: Medium to very dark brown in color, often with deep ruby to garnet highlights, yet almost never truly black. Very clear. Large, persistent, tan-colored head.

Flavor: Light to moderate malt flavor, which can have a clean, neutral character to a rich, sweet, Munich-like intensity. Light to moderate roasted malt flavors can give a bitter-chocolate palate that lasts into the finish, but which are never burnt. Medium-low to medium bitterness, which can last till the end. Light to moderate noble hop flavor. Clean lager character with no fruity esters or diacetyl.

Mouthfeel: Medium-light to medium body. Moderate to moderately high carbonation. Smooth. No harshness or astringency, despite the use of dark, roasted malts.

Overall impression: A dark German Lager that balances roasted yet smooth malt flavors with moderate hop bitterness.

History: A regional specialty from southern Thuringen and northern Franconia in Germany, and probably a variant of the Munich Dunkel style.

Comments: In comparison with a Munich Dunkel, usually darker in color, drier on the palate and with a noticeable (but not high) roasted malt edge to balance the malt base. While sometimes called a "black pils," the beer is rarely that dark; do not expect strongly roasted, porter-like flavors.

Ingredients: German Munich malt and Pilsner malts for the base, supplemented by a small amount of roasted malts (such as Carafa) for the dark color and subtle roast flavors. Noble-type German hop varieties and clean German lager yeasts are preferred.

Vital statistics:	OG: 1.046–1.052 (11.4–12.5 °P)
IBUs: 22–32	FG: 1.010–1.016
EBC: 27.6–55.1+	ABV: 4.4–5.4%

Commercial examples: Köstritzer Schwarzbier, Kulmbacher Mönchshof Premium Schwarzbier, Einbecker Schwarzbier, Weeping Radish Black Radish Dark Lager, Sprecher Black Bavarian, Sapporo Black Beer.

Bock

Maibock/Helles bock

Aroma: Moderate to strong malt aroma, often with a lightly toasted quality and low melanoidins. Moderately low to no noble hop aroma, often with a spicy quality. Clean. No diacetyl. Fruity esters should be low to none. Some alcohol may be noticeable. May have a light DMS aroma from pils malt.

Appearance: Deep gold to light amber in color. Lagering should provide good clarity. Large, creamy, persistent, white head.

Flavor: The rich flavor of continental European pale malts dominates (pils malt flavor with some toasty notes and/or melanoidins). Little to no caramelization. May have a light DMS flavor from pils malt. Moderate to no noble hop flavor. May have a low spicy or peppery quality from hops and/or alcohol. Moderate hop bitterness (more so in the balance than in other bocks).

Mouthfeel: Medium-bodied. Moderate to moderately high carbonation. Smooth and clean with no harshness or astringency, despite the increased hop bitterness. Some alcohol warming may be present.

Overall impression: A relatively pale, strong, malty lager beer. Designed to walk a fine line between blandness and too much color. Hop character is generally more apparent than in other bocks.

History: A fairly recent development in comparison to the other members of the bock family. The serving of Maibock is specifically associated with springtime and the month of May.

Comments: Can be thought of as either a pale version of a traditional bock or a Munich Helles brewed to bock strength. While quite malty, this beer typically has less dark and rich malt flavors than a traditional bock. May also be drier, more hopped and more bitter than a traditional bock. The hops compensate for the lower level of melanoidins. There is some dispute whether Helles (pale) Bock and Mai (May) Bock are synonymous.

Ingredients: Base of pils and/or Vienna malt with some Munich malt to add character (although much less than in a traditional bock). No non-malt adjuncts. Noble hops. Soft water preferred so as to avoid harshness. Clean lager yeast. Decoction mash is typical, but boiling is less than in traditional bocks to restrain color development.

Vital statistics:	OG: 1.064–1.072 (15.7–17.5 °P)
IBUs: 23–35+	FG: 1.011–1.018
EBC: 11.8–21.7	ABV: 6.3–7.4%

Commercial examples: Ayinger Maibock, Hacker-Pschorr Hubertus Bock, Einbecker Mai-Urbock, Augustiner Hellerbock, Hofbräu Maibock, Capital Maibock, Victory St. Boisterous, Gordon Biersch Blonde Bock.

Traditional bock

Aroma: Strong malt aroma, often with moderate amounts of rich melanoidins and/or toasty overtones. Virtually no hop aroma. Some alcohol may be noticeable. Clean. No diacetyl. Low to no fruity esters.

Appearance: Light copper to brown color, often with attractive garnet highlights. Lagering should provide good clarity despite the dark color. Large, creamy, persistent, off-white head.

Flavor: Complex maltiness is dominated by the rich flavors of Munich and Vienna malts, which contribute melanoidins and toasty flavors. Some caramel notes may be present from decoction mashing and a long boil. Hop bitterness is generally only high enough to support the malt flavors, allowing a bit of sweetness to linger into the finish. Well attenuated, not cloying. Clean, with no esters or diacetyl. No hop flavor. No roasted or burnt character.

Mouthfeel: Medium to medium-full bodied. Moderate to moderately low carbonation. Some alcohol warmth may be found, but should never be hot. Smooth, without harshness or astringency.

Overall impression: A dark, strong, malty lager beer.

History: Originated in the Northern German city of Einbeck, which was a brewing center and popular exporter in the days of the Hanseatic League (fourteenth to seventeenth centuries). Recreated in Munich starting in the seventeenth century. The name "bock" is based on a corruption of the name "Einbeck" in the Bavarian dialect, and was thus only used after the beer came to Munich. "Bock" also means "billy-goat" in German, and is often used in logos and advertisements.

Comments: Decoction mashing and long boiling plays an important part of flavor development, as it enhances the caramel and melanoidin flavor aspects of the malt. Any fruitiness is due to Munich and other specialty malts, not yeast-derived esters developed during fermentation.

Ingredients: Munich and Vienna malts, rarely a tiny bit of dark roasted malts for color adjustment, never any non-malt adjuncts. Continental European hop varieties are used. Clean lager yeast. Water hardness can vary, although moderately carbonate water is typical of Munich.

Vital statistics:	OG: 1.064–1.072 (15.7–17.5 °P)
IBUs: 20–27	FG: 1.013–1.019
EBC: 27.6–43.3	ABV: 6.3–7.2%

Commercial examples: Einbecker Ur-Bock Dunkel, Aass Bock, Great Lakes Rockefeller Bock.

Doppelbock

Aroma: Very strong maltiness. Darker versions will have significant melanoidins and often some toasty aromas. A light caramel flavor from a long boil is acceptable. Lighter versions will have a strong malt presence with some melanoidins and toasty notes. Virtually no hop aroma, although a light noble hop aroma is acceptable in pale versions. No diacetyl. A very slight chocolate-like aroma may be present in darker versions, but no roasted or burned aromatics should ever be present. Moderate alcohol aroma may be present.

Appearance: Deep gold to dark brown in color. Darker versions often have ruby highlights. Lagering should provide good clarity. Large, creamy, persistent head (color varies with base style: white for pale versions, off-white for dark varieties). Stronger versions might have impaired head retention, and can display noticeable legs.

Flavor: Very rich and malty. Darker versions will have significant melanoidins and often some toasty flavors. Lighter versions will have a strong malt flavor with some melanoidins and toasty notes. A very slight chocolate flavor is optional in darker versions, but should never be perceived as roasty or burnt. Clean lager flavor with no diacetyl. Some fruitiness (prune, plum or grape) is optional in darker versions. Invariably there will be an impression of alcoholic strength, but this should be smooth and warming rather than harsh or burning.

Mouthfeel: Medium-full to full body. Moderate to moderately low carbonation. Very smooth without harshness or astringency.

Overall impression: A very strong and rich lager. A bigger version of either a traditional bock or a helles bock.

History: A Bavarian specialty first brewed in Munich by the monks of St. Francis of Paula. Historical versions were less well attenuated than modern interpretations, with consequently higher sweetness and lower alcohol levels (and hence was considered "liquid bread" by the monks). The term "doppel (double) bock" was coined by Munich consumers. Many doppelbocks have names ending in "-ator," either as a tribute to the prototypical Salvator or to take advantage of the beer's popularity.

Comments: Most versions are dark colored and may display the caramelizing and melanoidin effect of decoction mashing, but excellent pale versions also exist. The pale versions will not have the same richness and darker malt flavors of the dark versions, and may be a bit drier, more hopped and more bitter.

Ingredients: Pils and/or Vienna malt for pale versions (with some Munich), Munich and Vienna malts for darker ones and occasionally a tiny bit of darker color malts (such as Carafa). Noble hops. Water hardness varies from soft to moderately carbonate. Clean lager yeast. Decoction mashing is traditional.

Vital Statistics:	OG: 1.072–1.096+ (17.5–22.9+ °P)
IBUs: 16–26+	FG: 1.016–1.024+
EBC: 11.8–49.2	ABV: 7–10+%

Commercial examples: Paulaner Salvator, Ayinger Celebrator, Spaten Optimator, Tucher Bajuvator, Augustiner Maximator, Weihenstephaner Korbinian, Weltenburger Kloster Asam-Bock, EKU 28, Eggenberg Urbock 23°, Samichlaus, Bell's Consecrator, Moretti La Rossa.

Eisbock

Aroma: Dominated by a balance of rich, intense malt and a definite alcohol presence. No hop aroma. No diacetyl. May have significant fruity esters, particularly those reminiscent of plum, prune or grape. Alcohol aromas should not be harsh or solventy.

Appearance: Deep copper to dark brown in color, often with attractive ruby highlights. Lagering should provide good clarity. Head retention may be impaired by higher-than-average alcohol content and low carbonation. Pronounced legs are often evident.

Flavor: Rich, sweet malt balanced by a significant alcohol presence. The malt can have melanoidins, toasty qualities, some caramel and occasionally a slight chocolate flavor. No hop flavor. Hop bitterness just offsets the malt sweetness enough to avoid a cloying character. No diacetyl. May have significant fruity esters, particularly those reminiscent of plum, prune or grape.

Mouthfeel: Full to very full bodied. Low carbonation. Significant alcohol warmth without sharp hotness. Very smooth without harsh edges from alcohol, bitterness, fusels or other concentrated flavors.

Overall impression: An extremely strong, full and malty dark lager.

History: A traditional Kulmbach specialty brewed by freezing a doppelbock and removing the ice to concentrate the flavor and alcohol content (as well as any defects).

Comments: Eisbocks are not simply stronger doppelbocks; the name refers to the process of freezing and concentrating the beer. Some doppelbocks are stronger than Eisbocks. Extended lagering is often needed post-freezing to smooth the alcohol and enhance the malt and alcohol balance. Any fruitiness is due to Munich and other specialty malts, not yeast-derived esters developed during fermentation.

Ingredients: Same as doppelbock. Commercial eisbocks are generally concentrated anywhere from 7% to 33% (by volume).

Vital statistics:	OG: 1.078–1.120+ (18.9–28.1+°P)
IBUs: 25–35+	FG: 1.020–1.035+
EBC: 35.5–59.1+	ABV: 9–14+%

Commercial examples: Kulmbacher Reichelbräu Eisbock, Eggenberg Urbock Dunkel Eisbock, Niagara Eisbock, Southampton Eisbock.

The information about the bottom fermentation beer types comes from the 2004 BJCP Style Guidelines, which are Copyright © 2004, Beer Judge Certification Program, Inc. The most current version of the guidelines is found on the BJCP website (http://www.bjcp.org).

References

Assobira (2006). Annual report 2006, Roma.

Bamforth, C. (2003). *Beer: Tap into the Art and Science of Brewing*, pp. 1–233. Oxford University Press, New York.

BJCP Style Guidelines (2004). Beer Judge Certification Program, Inc. (The most current version of the guidelines are found on the BJCP website, http://www.bjcp.org).

Briggs, D.E., Hough, J.S., Stevens, R. and Young, T.W. (1982). *Malting and Brewing Science. I. Malt Sweet Wort*, pp. 20–387. Chapman and Hall, London.

Briggs, D.E., Boulton, C.A., Brookes, P.A. and Stevens, R. (2004). *Brewing Science and Practice*, pp. 32–542. Woodhead publishing limited and CRC Press, LLC, Cambridge.

Buiatti, S. (2004). Birra. In Cabras, P. and Martelli, A. (eds), *Chimica degli Alimenti*, pp. 557–597. Piccin Nuova Libraria s.p.a., Padova.

Derdelinckx, G. and Neven, H. (1996). *Cerevisia* 21, 41–58.

Engan, S. (1981). *European Brewery Convection Monograph* 7, 123–134. 189–190.

Goldammer, T. (1999). *The Brewers' Handbook – The Complete Book to Brewing Beer*, pp. 73–104. KVP Publishers, Clifton, VA.

Hough, J.S. (1985). *The Biotechnology of Malting and Brewing.* Cambridge University Press, Cambridge. pp. 114–134.

Hough, J.S., Briggs, D.E., Stevens, R. and Young, T.W. (1982). *Malting and Brewing Science. II. Hopped Wort and Beer*, pp. 389–914. Chapman and Hall, London.

Kirin Research Institute of Drinking and Lifestyle (2004). Beer Consumption in Major Countries in 2004, Report Vol. 29. Kirin Holdings company, Limited, Tokyo.

Knudsen, F.B. (1999). Fermentation, principles and practices. In McCabe, J.T. (ed.), *The Practical Brewer*, pp. 235–261. Master Brewers Association of the Americas, Wauwatosa, WI.

Kunze, W. (1996). In Wainwright, T. (trans.), *Technology Brewing and Malting*, International edition, pp. 323–587. VLB Berlin, Berlin.

Lewis, M.L. and Bamforth, C.W. (2006). *Essays in Brewing Science*, pp. 3–170. Springer Science+Business Media, LLC, New York.

Munroe, J.H. (1994). Fermentation. In Hardwick, W.A. (ed.), *Handbook of Brewing*, pp. 323–379. Marcel Dekker, New York.

Patino, H. (1999). Overview of cellar operations. In McCabe, J.T. (ed.), *The Practical Brewer*, pp. 299–326. Master Brewers Association of America, St. Paul, MN.

Ryder, D.R. and Power, J. (1994). In Hardwick, W.A. (ed.), *Handbook of Brewing*, pp. 203–245. Marcel Dekker, New York.

Scanlon, M. (2004). *Filtration and Separation* 41, 26–27.

4

Traditional and Modern Japanese Beers: Methods of Production and Composition

Masato Kawasaki Research Laboratories for Brewing, Technology Development Department, Production Division, Kirin Brewery Company, Limited, Yokohama, Japan
Shuso Sakuma Quality Assurance Center for Alcoholic Beverages, Quality Assurance Department, Production Division, Kirin Brewery Company, Limited, Yokohama, Japan

Abstract

We can trace the roots of Japanese beer industry to the early Meiji Era (1868–1912), as well as note the significant growth of the industry after the conclusion of World War II. Traditional Japanese beer is a Pilsner-style lager developed during the early Showa Era (1926–1989), relying on hops, and being pasteurized before packaging in bottles. The major difference between traditional Japanese beer and that of Europe is the use of adjuncts. The prevalent modern Japanese beer is a highly fermented beverage, using weakened hops, being fermented in cylindro-conical tanks, and then aged. While characteristically unpasteurized, modern Japanese beer is subjected to membrane filtration before being shipped for consumption. Over the past 10 years or so, techniques related to the use of adjuncts have changed significantly, resulting in the introduction of happo-shu (low-malt beer) with low malt ratios and so-called "New Genre" products containing no malt whatsoever. These products feature a fresher/crisper flavor with low levels of bitterness. However, the industry will continue to develop a wider variety of beer products and techniques to meet the increasingly diverse customer taste preferences.

Introduction

The origin of Japan's beer industry can be traced back to the early Meiji Era (1868–1912). Initially, the Japanese produced both a German-style beer and an English-style beer. However, gradually, well-capitalized manufacturers of German-style beer became prevalent. During this time, the Japanese introduced the use of adjuncts, forming the archetype of traditional and modern Japanese beers. Beer production underwent major growth during the post-war economic boom, including a transition from returnable bottle packaging to cans, and a move away from pasteurization to membrane filtration for "draft" beer. Over the past 20 years, the advent of highly fermented dry beers, the lifting of bans on microbreweries, and the birth of new products called happo-shu and "New Genre" have all significantly changed the structure of the market in Japan. In this chapter, we will introduce the history of the beer business in Japan, changes in manufacturing methods of beer, happo-shu (low-malt beer), and "New Genre" products, and trends in beer composition.

Japanese Beer Production and Consumption Volumes

In 2004, worldwide beer production was approximately 1.5 billion hl. Japan's production volume for that year, including happo-shu, was 66 million hl, helping Japan to reach the No. 7 spot behind China, America, Germany, Brazil, Russia, and Mexico, accounting for 4.3% of the world's beer production volume. Total consumption of beer in Japan was 65.5 million hl, placing Japan in the 6th place worldwide after China, America, Germany, Brazil, and Russia. However, on a per-individual basis, Japanese consumed 51.3 l of beer for that year, placing Japan on the 32nd position among the world's beer-consuming countries (Brewers Association of Japan, 2006). At present, Japan is home to five major beer-manufacturing companies, with approximately 200 small-scale "microbreweries." However, microbrewery production of beer only accounts for about 1% of Japan's total beer production. The main beer product in Japan is a Pilsner-style beverage, but Japan's microbreweries produce a diverse mix of beers, ale, dark ale, Weizen, Kölsch, etc. In 2005, happo-shu, introduced to the market in 1993, accounted for 27% of all beer sales at 17.6 million hl. The year 2005 also saw the introduction of "New Genre" products, that is, a beer-type happo-shu not using malt, representing 16% of all beer sales at 10.1 million hl. Commercial-use beer sales represented 44.7% of the market, while beer for home/private consumption was 55.3%. Four percent of happo-shu was sold for commercial purposes, with 96% consumed at home. The entire amount of "New Genre" product sold during 2005

Beer in Health and Disease Prevention
ISBN: 978-0-12-373891-2

was consumed at home. As for packaging, 27% of Japan's beer sales in 2005 were bottles, 44% cans, and the remaining 29% kegs. About 96% of happo-shu was sold in cans with 4% sold in kegs. All "New Genre" sales were sold in cans (Jozo Sangyo News, 2006). It is apparent that most of the beer for home consumption is purchased in cans.

History of Japanese Beer

In the Edo Period, prior to the opening of Japan to global trade in 1854, the Dutch people were the only westerners allowed to trade with Japan. These foreigners brought beer to the Land of the Rising Sun, which was apparently enjoyed by a certain number of Japanese who were specializing in western learning. When Perry reached Japan in 1853, it is said that, Komin Kawamoto a doctor of western medicine, saw descriptions of beer noted in western texts, and became the first Japanese to attempt to brew beer in Japan (Hashimoto, 1997). Later, in 1868, the Edo Shogunate collapsed, ushering in the advent of Japan as a modern nation. It was in 1870 that the first serious commercial production of beer was engaged. The setting was at Yokohama, and it was William Copeland, a Norwegian-American, who took on the endeavor. As a young man, Copeland studied brewing for 5 years at the foot of a German brewer. Copeland subsequently traveled to Yokohama when he was 30 years of age. There, he observed a plot of land in the Yamate foreigner's residential area of Yokohama that featured a clear water spring. Copeland built a brewery on this location, calling the facility "Spring Valley Brewery." William Copeland's beer was tremendously popular among the foreigners living in Yokohama, and was even known among the local Japanese, who called the product "Amanuma Beer Sake."

Shozaburo Shibutani is said to be the first Japanese to seriously engage in the beer production and sales in the Osaka area beginning in 1872. In 1874, Mitsu Uroko Beer was founded in Kofu. Later, in 1876, the Hokkaido Kaitakushi Sapporo Brewery was established as a government-run enterprise in Hokkaido. The following year, Sapporo Beer was introduced to the Japanese market. In 1887, the Japan Beer Brewery Company was founded, purchasing brewing equipment and malt from Germany. The company brought in brewing specialists from overseas, and introduced Ebisu Beer to Japan in 1890. In connection with government divestment in 1886, the Sapporo Brewery was granted to the Okura Group from the Hokkaido Prefectural Government; the Sapporo Beer Company was later formed in 1888. In 1885, the land and buildings of the Spring Valley Brewery were carried over to the Japan Brewery Company, Limited, and in 1888, the company began selling Kirin Beer. Asahi Beer was introduced to the Japanese market in 1892 by the Osaka Beer Company, Limited, which was established in 1889. At one point in Japan's history, more than 100 different labels of beer were for sale in the market. Most of the smaller beer breweries produced English-style beer without the need to use refrigeration equipment. At that time, the price of one large bottle of beer was very expensive, equivalent to 4,000 yen in today's terms.

At the time, the Japanese government had yet to assess a liquor tax on beer. However, Japanese military expansion precipitated a tax on beer, beginning in 1901. The combination of high-quality German-style beers produced by well-funded manufacturers and the commencement of tax levies on beer forced a wave of bankruptcies among smaller breweries, leaving only the larger producers to continue. In 1906, the Japan Beer Brewery Company merged with the Osaka Beer Company and the Sapporo Beer Company to form the Dai-Nippon Beer Company, Limited, which continued to expand. In 1907, Kirin Brewery was established, taking over the business operations of the Japan Brewery Company, Limited. It was about this point in time that some breweries began to use rice as an adjunct, with the use of such being recognized in the Revised Liquor Tax Law of 1904. World War I broke out in 1914, but Japan experienced an economic boom due to its fortunate geographical location. The war was also a blessing for Japan's beer industry, which used this opportunity to penetrate into the Southeast Asian and Indian markets suffering from interrupted supplies of beer from Europe. Beer prices were not immune to post-war deflation, and while prices could have been considered somewhat geared for the mass market, overall beer consumption did not increase to a great extent. Rather than recovering, beer sales declined even further during the subsequent period of Japanese militarization. The price of a large bottle of beer in 1918 was the equivalent to 1,500 yen in today's prices. Beer consumption volume in 1939 marked the highest levels at 3.1 million hl before World War II, half of which was consumed by the military. World War II broke out in 1939. Beer price controls were instituted at the time, and home consumption of beer was rationed. The Pacific War made it extremely difficult for Japanese breweries to procure barley and hops, leading to decreases in beer production. War-time shortages in 1940 resulted in an increase in the volume of adjuncts used in beer, leading to standards still in use today. In the year following the war, total beer production volume had fallen to one-fourth of pre-war levels. The rationing system was abolished after the war in 1949, and Dai-Nippon Beer was separated into today's Asahi Breweries and Sapporo Breweries under the terms of the Law for the Elimination of Excessive Concentration of Economic Power. Japan had ample access to supplies of raw materials, fuel, and building materials after the outbreak of the Korean War in 1950, and with the abolition of raw material controls in 1952, beer production for 1953 outpaced any production level of pre-war times. After that point, the growth of Japan's beer industry was remarkable, growing approximately 15 times between 1955 and 1975, and reaching nearly 40 million hl of annual production. In 1987, total beer production in Japan exceeded 50 million hl, reaching 60 million hl by 1989, and a record of 71 million hl by 1994. The spread of access to beer throughout Japan due to pre-war rationing system, soldiers, who developed a taste for beer, returning to

Japan from battlefields overseas, and mass production resulting in more accessible beer prices can all be cited as underlying reasons for the rapid increase in beer consumption in Japan (Hashimoto, 2003). The availability of electric refrigerators from around 1960 was another major factor behind the increased beer consumption.

Canned beer, first introduced to Japan in 1958, represented only 16% of beer sales in Japan as of 1985 (Beverage Japan, 1990). By 1995, however, the ratio of canned beer had risen to 45% of the market, even outpacing bottled beer sales (Packpia, 1995). Today, most beer consumption at home is of the canned product (Jozo Sangyo News, 2006). Suntory entered the beer market in 1963, and began selling all of their beer products as membrane-filtered draft beer in 1968 (Sasaki, 1983). In 1989, membrane-filtered bottled/canned draft beer represented 63% of the market (Hashimoto, 1990), and at present, most bottled/canned beer is of the draft variety. The Japanese diet included an increasing preference for meat, and the volume of animal fat consumption increased accordingly. As a result, a lighter option was sought for accompanying dishes and drinks.

In this way, we see that the taste preferences and beer consumption patterns were changing in Japan, and in 1987, a dry beer concept called "karakuchi" was introduced. The "dry" beer featured a smooth sensation at first, with a refreshing aftertaste, and was designed to keep the interest of consumers in their 20s and 30s (Usuba, 1996).

In 1994, government deregulatory policies led to the revision of the Liquor Tax Law, under which annual minimum beer production volume was reduced from 20,000 to 600 hl. This swung the gates to beer production wide open in Japan, with new microbreweries springing up all over the country. According to the National Tax Agency, Japan was home to 232 microbreweries in 2002 (National Tax Agency Japan, 2006). Besides Pilsner-style beer, Japan's microbreweries produce several other types, including ales, dark ales, Weizen, Kölsch, etc.

The strong yen valuation of the 1990s brought a flood of cheap beer from overseas. At that time, domestically produced canned beer was sold for 225 yen, whereas a major supermarket chain was contracting with a Belgian beer maker, offering canned beer for 128 yen retail. Meanwhile, thanks to deregulation, discount liquor stores were popping up all around the country, destroying the foundation of the fixed-price sales system that had been an industry practice for many years. The market-share growth of imported beers in Japan was remarkable, reaching 4.2% in 1994 (Packpia, 1995). To compete with cheap beer imports, the ratio of malt was reduced to 65% to be exempted from high taxation on beer, and the sales of happo-shu (low-malt beer) at a significantly lower price point of 180 yen was initiated. With the Revised Liquor Tax Law in 1994, beer containing more than 66.7% malt was assessed a high tax of 77.7 yen per 350 ml, but happo-shu containing less than 66.7% malt enjoyed a 31% reduction in liquor taxes. The line drawn at 66.7% for malt usage ratio defining beer on one side and happo-shu on the other, with the difference consisting of only a few percent, seemed quite arbitrary. Accordingly, the Revised Liquor Tax Law of 1997 reduced tax rates only on two types of happo-shu, one containing less than 50% malt and the other containing less than 25% malt. Later, the Liquor Tax Law was further revised; at present, most happo-shu contains less than 25% malt. Happo-shu is a cheaper alternative to beer, and has been warmly accepted by consumers as a light, easy to drink option (Hashimoto, 1998).

The 2003 revision of the Liquor Tax Law increased the tax on happo-shu by approximately 10 yen per 350 ml. In response to this change in law, a version of happo-shu without malt was introduced in Japan. This new product has come to be known as "New Genre" in Japan. According to Japanese Liquor Tax Law as of 2006, happo-shu without malt is categorized as "Other Sparkling Spirits," taxed at 28 yen per 350 ml, a lower rate compared to the 46.99 yen levy on happo-shu with less than 25% malt, or the 77 yen assessment on beer using 66.7% or greater malt. Since "New Genre" products do not use malt, they have a fresher/crisper flavor compared to regular happo-shu (Kashiwada and Oono, 2004; Nakamura, 2005) (Table 4.1).

Table 4.1 Beer category definitions and taxes according to Japan's Liquor Tax Law

Category	*Malt ratio (%)*	*Tax (yen/350 ml)*
Beer	≥66.7	77.0
Happo-shu	≥50	77.0
Happo-shu	50>, ≥25	62.3
Happo-shu	25>	46.9
"New Genre"	None	28.0

Note. According to Japanese Liquor Tax Law in 2006, beer is defined as beer made from malt more than 66.7%. The tax for beer is 77 yen/350 ml. Beer made from malt less than 66.7% is defined as Happo-shu (low-malt beer). The tax for Happo-shu that made from malt more than 50% is 77 yen/350 ml. The tax for Happo-shu that made from malt between 25% and 50% is 62.3 yen/350 ml. The tax for Happo-shu that made from malt less than 25% is 46.9 yen/350 ml. Happo-shu not containing malt is categorized as "New Genre." The tax for "New Genre" is 28 yen/350 ml.

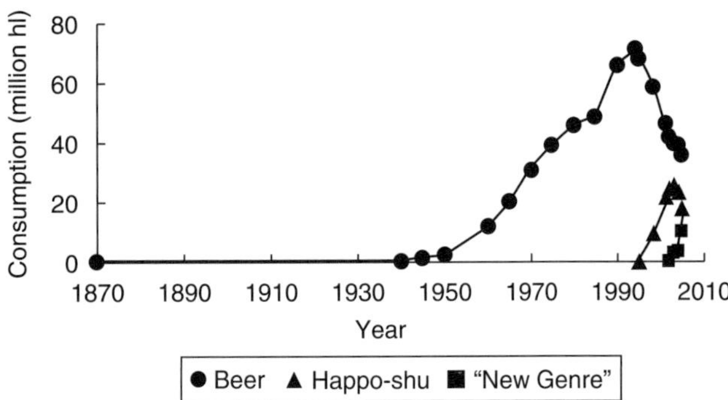

Figure 4.1 Consumption trends for beer, happo-shu, and "New Genre."

Figure 4.1 shows the trend for beer, happo-shu, and "New Genre" consumption in Japan. The increasing consumption of happo-shu has led directly to a decrease in beer consumption, while the introduction of "New Genre" products has eaten into consumption of both beer and happo-shu. Beer consumption in 2005 was 36.2 million hl, while happo-shu consumption was 22.1 million hl, and "New Genre" consumption was 10.1 million hl (Jozo Sangyo News, 2006). Table 4.2 shows the history of beer production in Japan.

The consumption of beer increased rapidly during the post-war economic boom and went up to 71.0 million hl in 1994. Happo-shu was put on sale in 1994. The increasing consumption of happo-shu has led directly to a decrease in beer consumption. "New Genre" that was put on sale in 2004 has eaten into consumption of both beer and happo-shu. Beer consumption in 2005 was 36.2 million hl, while happo-shu consumption was 22.1 million hl, and "New Genre" consumption was 10.1 million hl.

Table 4.2 History of beer production in Japan

Year	*Details*
1853	Beer first brewed in Japan by Komin Kawamoto, a practitioner of western medicine
1870	Norwegian-American William Copeland establishes the Spring Valley Brewery in Yokohama
1876	Government-run Hokkaido Kaitakushi Sapporo Brewery established
1885	Copeland's Spring Valley Brewery taken over by Japan Brewery Company Limited
1887	Japan Beer Brewery Company founded
1887	Sapporo Beer Company (successor of Sapporo Brewery) established
1889	Osaka Beer Company Limited established
1901	Beer tax instituted in conjunction with Japanese military expansion
1904	Revised Beer Tax Law allows addition of rice (up to 30% vs. malt volume)
1906	Dai-Nippon Beer Company Limited established with merger of Japan Beer Brewery Company, Osaka Beer Company, and Sapporo Beer Company
1907	Kirin Brewery established, taking over business of Japan Brewery Company Limited
1940	Allowed adjuncts ratio increased to 50%
1949	Dai-Nippon Beer Company Limited separated into Asahi Breweries and Sapporo Breweries under the Law for the Elimination of Excessive Concentration of Economic Power
1967	First "draft beer" marketed; precision filtered and bottled, rather than pasteurized
1987	"Dry" type beer ("karakuchi") introduced
1994	Revised Liquor Tax Law reduces minimum production from 20,000 to 600 hl; many new microbreweries enter the market
1994	Happo-shu (65% malt) introduced
1995	25% malt happo-shu introduced
2004	Beer-flavored "New Genre" beverages containing 0% malt introduced

Traditional Japanese Beer Production Methods

Traditional Japanese beer is the hops-infused Pilsner-style lager that was created during the early Showa Era (1926–1989). It is a pasteurized, bottled product, but one that uses adjuncts, marking a difference between the Japanese version and the Pilsner-style beer of Europe. The consumption of beer in Japan increased dramatically during the post-war economic boom (1960s through 1970s), and all of Japan's beer manufacturers were busy building new production facilities. Generally speaking, traditional Japanese beer was brewed of malt of 76–82% extract, a Kolbach Index of between 34% and 42%, and a fermentability of between 78% and 85%. Baled hops were used most often with rice, starch, and even corn grits, following the pattern used in America, as adjuncts.

Saccharification was generally achieved through decoction, while wort filtration was conducted via lauter tun or mash filtration. A plate cooler was used for wort cooling. Two- to three-meter tall fermentation tanks made of steel, aluminum, or stainless steel, using either an open or closed type system, were installed inside the fermentation room. The fermentation room itself was cooled. The temperature of the maturation room was kept between 0°C and 2°C, with the room usually located directly beneath the fermentation room. The maturation tanks used were of the horizontal type, similar to the fermentation tanks. To improve haze stability, an exogenous enzyme such as papain was also used. The standard maturation period was 2 months. Beer filtration was performed through a combination of a filter using filter cotton, which is called "Schalenfilter" and a sheet filter using filter paper. Filled and capped bottles were sent through a pasteurizer for low-temperature pasteurization.

Modern Beer Production Methods

Characteristics of Japan's beer production methods

In the modern era, most beer produced in Japan is still of the Pilsner style. The following are particular characteristics of beer produced in Japan. Most of the beer now produced in Japan is not pasteurized, but is rather precisely sterilized under membrane filtration before shipping. This type of beer was first bottled and shipped as "draft beer" in 1967 (Sasaki, 1983), with more manufacturers following suit in 1977. Beginning in 1980, beer not subjected to pasteurization was advertised as "draft beer." In Japan, the sense behind the term "draft" is to imply an image of freshness, which is considered as one factor behind the popularization of the phrase "draft beer." While avoiding pasteurization does preserve the enzymatic activity of invertase and so on, there is no other clearly recognized effect on flavor.

The second characteristic of modern Japanese beer production is the use of adjuncts. Beer produced in 1876 by Japanese technicians holding formal manufacturing licenses from Germany consisted of 100% malt; however, the use of adjuncts was gradually adopted subsequently. In 1904, the Liquor Tax Law recognized the addition of up to 30% rice, and the Revised Liquor Tax Law in 1953 defined the usage of rice, corn, starches, and other adjuncts of up to 50% malt. Presently, regular beer uses rice, corn grits, starch, or other adjuncts; however, the purpose of these ingredients is to adjust the flavor and richness of the beer. Even premium beers in the higher-priced segments consist of both all-malt versions and versions using adjuncts. One could say that adjuncts are an indispensable part of producing a beer product that meets the taste preferences of the Japanese.

A third characteristic of modern Japanese beer is the advent of happo-shu (low-malt beer) and "New Genre" beers. While the category originally emerged in response to needs for a low-cost product, it also developed in response to changing taste preferences amid regulatory restrictions related to malt usage ratios.

Beer

Japan's brewery facilities built before the 1970s underwent wholesale renovations, focusing on scale and automation. The prevailing form of modern beer in Japan is fermented and aged in cylindro-conical tanks, highly fermented, and made of weakened hops. Most modern beer is not pasteurized, but rather subjected to membrane filtration. Most malt used in Japan is imported from overseas, having a Kolbach Index of between 40% and 45%. Malt having a high enzymatic capacity and high fermentability is used to produce beer with a high degree of fermentation (Usuba, 1996). Saccharification is achieved through decoction, as well as infusion for highly fermented wort production. The mashing process incorporates a mechanism to minimize contact with oxygen to improve flavor stability (Kimura and Araki, 2000). Removing air from the water used in the brewing process, and slowly inserting/removing wort from the bottom of the mash vessels ensures that the mixing in of air is kept to a minimum. Lauter tun is the prevalent form of mash separation used in modern beer manufacturing in Japan. During mash separation, the initial liquid produced is the first wort, while the second wort is collected by reintroducing hot water, and then recovering the remaining extract.

Due to the ratio of tannin components seeping out of the husk of the malt is high, the first wort gives rise to a refined, refreshing taste, and a straight-forward drinkability, while second wort imbues beer with a rich, stimulating drinking experience. Normally, first and second worts are blended and fermented; however, some beers are manufactured solely with first wort to produce a light, refreshing flavor. The practice of using hops in both pellet and extract form is increasing; however, there are also cases of hops being used in cone form.

Yeast is selected according to the characteristics of the product in question; however, to produce a beer with a high degree of fermentation, yeast with a strong fermentability is used. Under traditional production methods, fermentation and maturation tanks are installed indoors, but today, outdoor cylindro-conical tanks are prevalent. Some production tanks exceed 5,000 hl in volume. Since refrigeration units are directly wound around the tanks, the temperatures inside the tank can be precisely controlled, and it is even possible to promote the maturation process. This is a process whereby, during the course of maturation, the oxidative decarboxylation of α-acetolactic acid to diacetyl is accelerated through high temperatures, shortening the maturation period. The maturation period varies according to the type of beer in question, but the shortest method takes approximately 2 weeks. High gravity brewing is being tested at the pilot plant level; however, production has not spread to the extent found in the United States and Europe.

After kieselguhr filtration, beer is normally subjected to precise filtration via membrane. Sometimes silica gel and PVPP are added during kieselguhr filtration to remove proteins and polyphenols that cause chill haze. Membrane filtration can produce beer products that can be stored for lengthy periods of time, even without pasteurization.

Happo-shu (low-malt beer)

Under Japan's Liquor Tax Law, alcoholic beverages fermented using malt, hops, and water as raw materials, or alcoholic beverages fermented using malt, hops, water, and barley, rice, corn, kaoliang (type of sorghum), potatoes, starches, and/or sugars in a volume by weight of less than half of that of malt are defined as "beer." Alcoholic beverages other than beer that use malt or barley as a portion of ingredients having effervescent properties are defined as happo-shu (low-malt beer). In 1994, happo-shu was reintroduced to the market. Happo-shu containing 65% malt was first marketed to compete with the low-priced import beer being sold in Japan. In the following year, happo-shu utilizing a malt ratio of less than 25% was brought to the market. At that time, only two companies were producing happo-shu; but later, in 1998 and then in 2001, other manufacturers entered the market, and all four of Japan's major beer producers began selling happo-shu.

The biggest challenge in developing happo-shu is restricted malt ratios. The questions were how to maintain original beer flavor while having a low-malt component, as well as how to compensate in the production process for reduced fermentability caused by lower levels of malt nutrients. With most happo-shu on the market, malted barley comprises less than 25% of the total raw materials, while the treatment of adjuncts, such as rice, corn, or starches is what determines the flavor of the product. To compensate for reduced malt levels, manufacturers use ungerminated barley and/or extract from barley as adjuncts. Manufacturers also use mineral-enriched deep ocean water to ensure that the yeast has enough required nutrients. A reduction in malt composition also results in a reduction in saccharification enzyme activity; however, the addition of liquid sugar as well as starches is frequently used as an adjunct. The production of happo-shu is virtually identical to that of beer, with the exception of malt ratio and the techniques for using adjuncts. The results of the techniques described above have produced a product having a taste equal to beer. Another characteristic of happo-shu is a reduced level of nitrogen in comparison to beer.

"New Genre"

Beer taste preferences in Japan have changed. While beers with rich and deep flavors were once the main characteristic of such beverages in Japan, Japanese tastes have turned to prefer beers with a fresher, crisper flavor profile. In 2004, a beer-flavored beverage using no malt was introduced to the Japanese market (Kashiwada and Oono, 2004). In 2005, three other companies marketed a similar beverage, and these products have come to be known as "New Genre" beers in Japan. With no malt component, liquid sugars are used as a carbon source, which means there is no need for the saccharification process to be conducted, as normally would be the case. Just as with beer production, hops are added and boiled, the liquid is cooled, yeast is added for fermentation, and then the liquid is matured. As malt is not used, the most important issue is to ensure that there is enough nitrogen for yeast propagation. After a process of trial-and-error using different raw materials, manufacturers settled on using pea proteins, soybean proteins, soy peptides, and/or corn. Yeast extract is also used at times to make up for the nitrogen deficiency. Under the current Liquor Tax Law, beverages consisting of spirits added to happo-shu are included in this "New Genre" category.

The lack of malt in "New Genre" beers also affects the color of the product. Most of beer color derives from the malt, and some pigmentation is a by-product of the Maillard Reaction that occurs during the wort boiling process. Since no malt is used for "New Genre" products, caramel coloring is used more often than not to adjust the color of the beverage.

"New Genre" products are noted for a fresh, crisp taste; however, some "New Genre" products are designed specifically for "flavor." One such product is manufactured by adding sugars to peptides/amino acids derived from soy proteins. The mixture is heated, and then the Maillard Reaction imparts a deep flavor, distinct in its richness. Since an amber color is added through the Maillard Reaction, there is no need to add any caramel coloring (Ohta and Sasaki, 2006). Compared to traditional beers, "New Genre" beers were developed with the clear concept of providing a fresh, crisp taste to the consumer. The concept was practically realized by lowering the nitrogen content in the beverage, and reducing the bitterness value (Figures 4.2 and 4.3).

Figure 4.2 shows the total nitrogen levels in Japanese major beer, happo-shu, and "New Genre" brands. Each bar indicates the average value of the major brand of each manufacturer. The levels of total nitrogen in happo-shu and "New Genre" are lower than beer as a result of their low malt ratio.

Figure 4.3 shows the bitterness levels in Japanese major beer, happo-shu, and "New Genre" brands. Each bar indicates

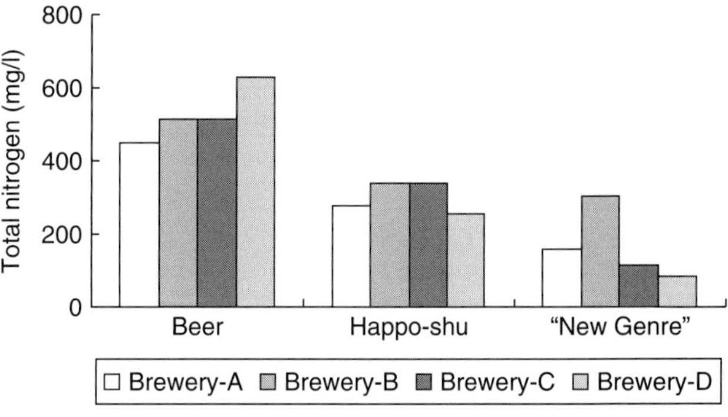

Figure 4.2 Total nitrogen analysis in major beer, happo-shu, and "New Genre" brands (2005).

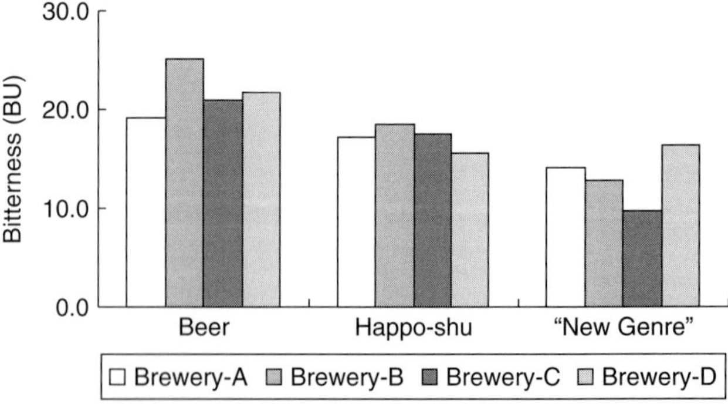

Figure 4.3 Bitterness analysis in major beer, happo-shu, and "New Genre" brands (2005).

the average value of the major brand of each manufacturer. The concept of fresh, crisp taste of "New Genre" was realized by reducing the bitterness level.

Changes in Beer Composition

Table 4.3 shows changes in the main indices used in beer analysis. While the levels of original extract and alcohol concentration have remained almost unchanged, real degree of fermentation have increased, and real extract, total nitrogen, bitterness, and polyphenol levels have decreased. Beers of the Meiji Era were Pilsner-style beers brewed without adjuncts, adopted during a period when beer brewing techniques were brought to Japan from Germany. The beer of that day contained high levels of original extract and nitrogen components, with strong richness and body. With the introduction of low-polyphenol grains, corn or rice, for example as adjuncts replacing a portion of malt, the polyphenol levels in the beer decreased, and the haze problem in the beer improved. At the same time, nitrogen components such as proteins and amino acids also decreased, causing a lightness in the flavor of the beer. The bitterness of different beers can be compared using beverage unit (BU). During the Meiji Era, beer BU was greater than 30; however, consumers reacted negatively to strong bitterness as beer flavors became lighter, resulting in gradually decreasing bitterness in beer through time. The "dry" beers put on market in 1987 used a reduced amount of malt, and increased degree of fermentation, leading to a crisp, very drinkable flavor (Hashimoto, 1998). Happo-shu, for which the malt ratio is less than 25%, uses exogenous enzymes to make up for the lack of malt. Liquid sugar, barley, and other adjuncts are used to generate a more "beer-like" flavor. The low levels of nitrogen in happo-shu result in a light, agreeable flavor, with an elegant, easygoing flavor that matched perfectly to the hint of bitterness. "New Genre" beverages use peas, soybeans, or corn as a nitrogen source (Nakamura, 2005). Most beers derive their color from malt, with pigmentation also created by the Maillard Reaction occurring in the brewing process. To generate a "beer-like" color in "New Genre" products, which use no malt, caramel is added, and the so-called Browning process is utilized to promote the Maillard Reaction by boiling sugar and proteins during the mashing process, as described earlier (Ohta and Sasaki, 2006). The complete lack of malt in "New Genre" beverages results in a fresher, crisper flavor compared to happo-shu.

Beer caloric content depends on the amount of alcohol and extract contained. For example, beer with a 3.2% extract, 5% alcohol content contains approximately 42 kcal per 100 ml. Assuming that the daily caloric requirements of an adult averages to 2,500 kcal, the caloric content of 1 l of beer represents approximately one-sixth of the daily requirement. The harmful effects of alcohol on the human body appear due to excessive consumption particularly for highly concentrated alcoholic beverages, while no ill effects are a concern as related to low-alcohol beverages. Appropriate alcohol consumption enhances the appetite, helps digestive organ and heart function, and aids in recovery from muscle fatigue. In addition, beer contains vitamins B1, B2, B6, niacin, pantothenic acid, biotin, folic acid, and other helpful nutrients, as well as rutin, vital salts such as phosphoric acid, and calcium (Takahashi, 2000). Research into the effects of beer on preventing lifestyle-related diseases have variously reported that xanthohumol, a component in hops, demonstrates anti-cancer activity; that iso-humulones improve insulin resistance and fat metabolism; that iso-xanthohumols help resist bone-density decline; and that polyphenols demonstrate antioxidant properties in living organisms (Kondo, 2004). The reduction in malt and hops content made in response to consumer taste preferences have reduced the efficacy of beer as a healthful food. Purines contained in beer are considered as a cause of gout, and doctors recommend that persons with high levels of uric acid avoid beer altogether. In response, purines-free beers have been developed, warmly received by persons with high levels of uric acid (Fujino and Sakuma, 2006).

Table 4.3 Changes in major beer composition

	Meiji[a]	*Early Showa*[a]	*Dry beer A*[b]	*Happo-shu B*[b]	*"New Genre" C*[b]
Real extract (% Plato)	5.2	3.8	3.2	3.6	3.0
Alcohol (V/V%)	5.1	5.3	5.2	5.5	5.0
Original extract (% Plato)	12.9	11.8	11.2	12.0	10.7
RDF[c] (%)	59.8	67.9	72.4	71.6	73.2
Total nitrogen (mg/l)	697	557	445	334	109
pH	4.3	4.3	4.1	4.0	3.7
Color (EBC units)	7.5	8.4	7.5	7.2	6.9
Bitterness (BU)	35	30	19	19	10
Polyphenol (mg/l)	150	122	140	103	27.3

[a] These beers were reproduced by Kirin Brewery.
[b] Typical product of each category.
[c] RDF: Real degree of fermentation.

Summary Points

- Traditional Japanese beer is a Pilsner-style lager developed during the early Showa Era (1926–1989), relying on hops, and being pasteurized before packaging in bottles. The major difference from that of Europe is the use of adjuncts. Most modern Japanese beer is not pasteurized, but rather subjected to membrane filtration, and then filled in cans.
- Together with the wide-spread adoption of cylindro-conical tanks, beers featuring a high fermentation level and weakened hops have become prevalent over the past 20 years.
- Over the past 10 or so years, happo-shu (using low amounts of malt) and "New Genre" beers (using no malt at all) have been developed to compete against low-cost imported beer.
- Since beer was first produced in Japan, the trend has been increasing real degree of fermentation with lowering bitterness. Happo-shu and "New Genre" beers feature a cleaner, crisper flavor than traditional beer, with less bitterness.

References

Beverage Japan (1990). *Beverage Japan* 13, 42–63.

Brewers Association of Japan (2006). Viewed October 23, <http://www.brewers.or.jp/data/t00-tokei.html>

Fujino, S. and Sakuma, S. (2006). Japanese Patent No. 3730935.

Hashimoto, N. (1990). *New Food Ind.* 32, 18–24.

Hashimoto, N. (1997). *New Food Ind.* 39, 7–11.

Hashimoto, N. (1998). *New Food Ind.* 40, 43–48.

Hashimoto, N. (2003). Sugiyama Chemical and Industrial Laboratory Annual Report 2002, 118–125, Totsuka-ku Yokohama, Japan.

Jozo Sangyo News (2006). *Food and Packaging* 47, 106–111.

Kashiwada, S. and Oono, M. (2004). *Journal of the Brewing Society of Japan* 99, 509–513.

Kimura, T. and Araki, S. (2000). The publication of Japanese Laid-Open Patent Application No. 2000-004866.

Kondo, K. (2004). *Bio Factors* 22, 303–310.

Nakamura, T. (2005). *Seibutsu-kogaku* 83, 494–495.

National Tax Agency Japan (2006). Viewed October 23, <http://www.nta.go.jp/category/sake/10/siori/h16/pdf/07.pdf>

Ohta, Y. and Sasaki, N. (2006). The publication of Japanese Laid-Open Patent Application No. 2006-191910.

Packpia, S. (1995). *Packpia* 39, 70–73, Nippo Co., Ltd., Chiyoda-ku, Tokyo, Japan

Sasaki, E. (1983). *Proceedings of Annual Meeting of Japanese Society for Food Science and Technology* 30, 87–93.

Takahashi, T. (2000). *Journal of the Brewing Society of Japan* 95, 183–192.

Usuba, H. (1996). An Additional Volume of Chemistry 1996, 50–55.

5

Sorghum Beer: Production, Nutritional Value and Impact upon Human Health

Maoura Nanadoum Laboratoire de Recherche sur les Substances Naturelles, Faculté des Sciences Exactes et Appliquées N'Djaména, Tchad

Jacques Pourquie UMR Microbiologie et Génétique Moléculaire, CNRS/INA-PG/INRA, CBAI, Thiverval-Grignon, France

Abstract

In Africa, traditional SMM (sorghum, millet, maize) beers are typically consumed by people who do not have access to sufficient dietary intake. These so-called opaque beers provide their consumers with significant amounts of valuable nutrients (calories, proteins, minerals and vitamins) which they would have difficulty in obtaining from other sources. They are produced in a home-made manner on a very small scale but by numerous individual brewers. They thus support an economic activity which brings cash money to an underpaid part of the population (sorghum growers, firewood collectors and especially women brewers). For example, we discuss bili bili sorghum beer which is produced and consumed in the Republic of Chad. We describe the technical and socioeconomic aspects of its making, and also discuss how the nutritional value of the starting cereal is improved through the different steps of the brewing process. From a risk–benefit point of view, despite their alcoholic content and the very poor sanitary conditions under which they are made, these beverages contribute more to sustain a minimum welfare to their consumers than to add an extra health hazard.

List of Abbreviations

DM	Dry matter
FAO	Food and Agriculture Organization
g	Gram
Mg	Milligram
μg	Microgram
Nd	Not determined
NGO	Non-governmental organization
SMM	Sorghum, millet, maize

Introduction

The history of beer making is as long and as rich as the history of humankind. Many kinds of sorghum or millet beers, known as opaque beers, have been reported across African countries (Table 5.1) (Périsse *et al.*, 1959; Bismuth and Ménage, 1961; Adrien and Jacquot, 1964; Odunfa, 1985; Novellie and De Chaepdrijver, 1986; Haggblade and Holzapfel, 1989; Sanni *et al.*, 1999; Seignobos, 2002). They are produced and sold on village scale markets and in many cities. They form the basis of a significant economic activity, providing both a source of nutrients to undernourished people and an additional income to an otherwise underpaid

Table 5.1 Typical names of traditional African beers

Country	*Local name*	*Malt type*
West Africa		
Benin, Togo, Burkina Faso, Ivory Coast, Mali, Niger	Dam, Tchakpalo, Dolo	Sorghum, millet, Maïs
Ghana, Nigeria	Pito, Burukutu	Sorghum, millet
Central Africa		
Angola	Walwa	Maize
Cameroon	Amgba, Bili bili	Sorghum, millet
Central African Republic	Bili bili	Sorghum, millet
Republic of Chad	Bili bili, Djala, Mbouke	Sorghum, millet
Rwanda	Ikigage	Sorghum
East Africa		
Ethiopia	Bouzza	Sorghum
Kenya	Busaa	Sorghum, millet
Sudan	Merissa, Bili bil	Sorghum
Tanzania	Pombe, Bwalwa	Sorghum, millet
Uganda	Omwenge	Sorghum, millet
South Africa		
Botswana	Bojalwa ja	Sorghum, millet
Lesotho	Yalwa	Sorghum
Republic of South Africa	Utshwala, bjalwa ja, Bogule	Sorghum, maize
Zambia	7-day beer	Sorghum, millet
Zimbabwe	Zezuru	Sorghum, millet

Source: Haggblade and Holzapfel (1989).

Beer in Health and Disease Prevention
ISBN: 978-0-12-373891-2

population. Although this activity is disparaged by non-governmental organizations (NGOs), religious parties and local administrations which consider that the production of sorghum beers is one of the causes of malnutrition, alcoholism, juvenile delinquency and deforestation, its nutritional, economic and social importance cannot be denied (Nanadoum, 2001; Magrin and Mbayhoudel, 2002).

This chapter will focus on the example of the Republic of Chad, where the local traditional beer is called bili bili. We will first give a short overview of the economic and social aspects of bili bili making and consumption. We will then give a technical description of the currently employed process and also discuss the biochemical and microbiological transformations occurring and how these transformations affect the quality of the beer and the health of the consumers.

Sorghum Beer in the Present Chad Society

In ancient times, sorghum beer had a sacred value and its consumption was strictly restricted to social events and work parties. This strong social connotation has progressively vanished; today, sorghum beer production has become a significant economic activity and its consumption is commonplace.

Bili bili beer is obtained by fermentation of malted sorghum and millet. It is an opaque beer which has to be consumed on the very day of its production. It is produced in a home-made manner using a procedure which is roughly similar to that of the production process of European type beers, and the details of which are transmitted orally from generation to generation. It is made exclusively by adult women who individually perform, on a weekly basis, the series of operations which in 2–3 days lead from the sorghum grain to the fermented beer. It demands great physical efforts and the production of each batch is thus limited to an average volume of 150 l.

There are no national statistical figures concerning the total annual production of bili bili, but some studies have been performed on a regional scale in the main cities of the south of Chad (ECOSIT 1, 1998; Ngardiguim and Digali, 2003). They show that around 70% of the local production of sorghum and millet is transformed into bili bili by women brewers who represent 0.5% of the total population. Most important is the flow of cash money which is induced by this transformation; in 2001, it has been estimated that in the town of Moundou (145,000 inhabitants), 840 million CFA Francs ($1.2 million) has been distributed between grain producers and traders, brewers, hirers of taverns and local administration (Magrin and Mbayhoudel, 2002). As a significant part of this money goes to the women brewers who get from this activity an average monthly income of 25,000 CFA ($35), beer production can be regarded as a way to redistribute to women a part of the cotton production income from which they tend to be excluded by the still strongly non-egalitarian structure of the Chad society.

- Bili bili making is a significant source of cash for African women and underpaid people.

Bili bili making

- Sorghum is the fifth largely grown cereal crop in the world. It is a graminaceous annual plant from the Poaceae family. It is well adapted to grow in arid lands and under hot climates; it is much more resistant to drought than any other major cereal. Sorghum and maize have similar nutritional values though sorghum is richer in protein and poorer in lipids.
- Millet is a generic name which encompasses various graminaceous species. Their agronomical and nutritional characteristics are similar to sorghum but their seeds are much smaller.

Bili bili is exclusively prepared by adult women. A survey among 71 of these women brewers (Nanadoum, 2001) has shown that 90% of them use the process which is depicted in Figure 5.1. As shown in this figure, this process encompasses the same basic steps as those of an industrial production (sprouting, malting, mashing and fermentation), but of course these steps are operated under very different conditions.

Sprouting and Malting Great care is taken of the quality of the grain. Seeds which are too old or too young are not used. Although many varieties are available, the most frequently used is djigari, a tannin rich red variety to which small amounts of maize are sometimes added. The kourgho variety, with a lower content of tannins, is considered superior, but its use is limited by its high cost and lesser availability.

Using large earthenware jars, grains are soaked for 10–18 h in water to remove husks and soil impurities, and to reach the optimal moisture content. They are then placed in wooden baskets or porous bags, and washed once or twice before draining. They are then heaped up in a vat until sprouting starts. Sprouting is favored by the rise of temperature inside the heap, caused by endogenous metabolism. During the warm season, this heaping-up step is often omitted.

Grains are then spread on a plastic sheet to form a layer 1–2 in. thickness, and kept covered. Green plantain leaves are still used in some villages in place of plastic sheets. If needed, initial moisture is maintained by spraying with water. Sprouting takes 2–3 days after which germinated grains are heaped up again and set aside overnight. This step results in withering of the plantlets due to the heat evolved within the heap and to an acidification, which is considered as a prerequisite to the correct flavor of the product.

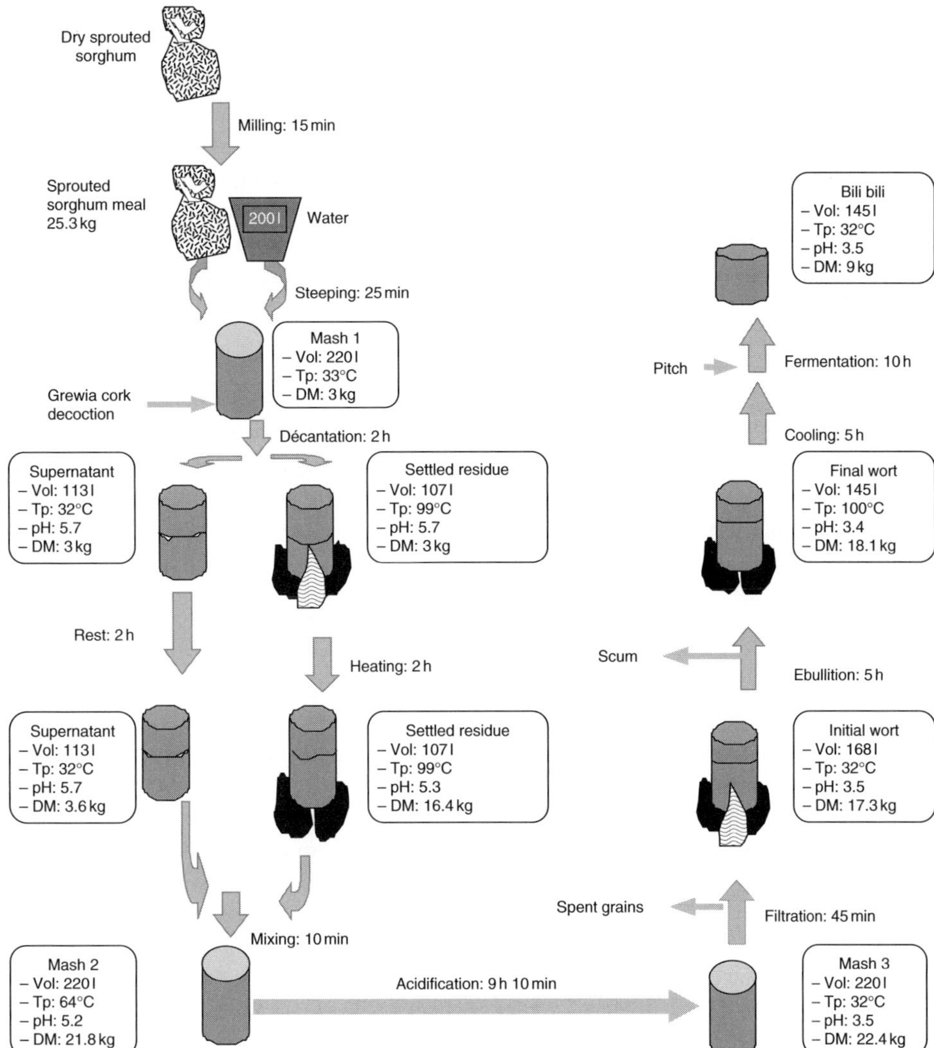

Figure 5.1 Bili bili making. Dry matter (DM) was measured in the liquid phase. *Source*: Nanadoum *et al.* (2005).

Germinated grains are then sun dried. Thin layers of germinated grains are spread over rush mats, corrugated iron or even clean soil, and frequently turned over. They are stored under protection during the night to avoid rehydration. This drying step takes 2–3 days depending on the intensity of sunlight. Due to quality losses during storage, the malting step is always scheduled to allow for an immediate usage of the malt.

Mash Preparation

Milling Once dried, the malt is crushed in a mortar or milled over a millstone to produce a coarse flour. In urban areas, the use of mechanical, gasoline or fuel oil powered hammer mills is becoming more frequent.

Steeping: The steeping step usually starts around 4 p.m. The whole milled malt corresponding to a minimum weight of 35 kg is mixed with 200 l of water in a vessel, either a metal drum or a jar, devoted to this exclusive use, and stirred with a wooden stick. A decoction of *Grewia mollis* bark is often added to promote the sedimentation of insoluble matter and subsequently the filterability of the mash. An opaque mash is obtained which corresponds to the mash obtained in the brewing industry. This mash is left to stand for at least 2 h during which time decantation occurs yielding a supernatant phase and a settled residue. Using a calabash, the supernatant phase is carefully collected from the settled phase and set aside at ambient temperature. This cloudy tea-colored liquid has a slight sour sweet taste.

Cooking of the residue. The settled residue is then cooked over a wood fire. This cooking step is thought to aid the gelatinization of the starch. Depending on the quality of the wood and the thermal conductivity of the vessel, the duration of this cooking step may vary widely around an average of 2 h. While still boiling, the thick mash obtained is poured into the supernatant phase which had been set aside and the temperature of this mix drops to 65–70°C.

Souring – Filtration: This reconstituted mash is thoroughly homogenized and stands overnight in the open air. During this time the temperature falls to 32–40°C, decantation occurs and acidity develops progressively. This acidification is considered to be a critical step of the process and is therefore assessed by frequent tasting. When the brewer considers that it has reached the correct value, she carefully withdraws the supernatant phase with a calabash. More liquid is recovered from the decanted residue using a rudimentary press filter made of a nylon cloth stretched over a bowl and raked with a wooden stick. The semi-solid residue which is obtained is sold as a livestock feed; the liquid which is recovered is mixed with the supernatant phase to constitute the wort. Due to the crude filtration process, an appreciable amount of insoluble material goes into the filtrate and contributes to the typical opaqueness of these beers. In the earlier days, filtration was performed in a woven basket filled with grass in the bottom. Although the obtained filtrate was much clearer, this process was time consuming and has been abandoned.

When the tasted acidity is considered as too strong, the brewer may decide to neutralize it by adding ash or potash, a procedure which results in some degradation of the organoleptic quality of the beer.

Boiling: The wort is boiled in jars or, more and more frequently, metal drums for an average time of 5 h. During this step, a foam, called *ngôph*, is formed on the top. As its nutritive value is high, it is continuously skimmed to be used as an infant gruel. Often, at the end of boiling, brewers drop burning charcoals into the mash, believing that this will "purify" it and clear out bad germs and unpleasant odors. Apart from charcoal, nothing should be added to the mash during its cooking. However, it is suspected that some brewers add bran of penicillary millet or bark of *Kaya senegalensis* to increase the bitterness of the beer.

At the end of this step, the total volume of the mash is reduced to two-thirds of its initial value.

Cooling: To reduce the cooling time, the mash is distributed between small 20 l and 30 l vessels. During this cooling phase, a pitch is prepared by mixing a volume of around 2.5 l of fresh mash with one-tenth volume of a former preparation of beer. This culture is put to stand at ambient temperature.

Fermentation Brewers know by experience that when the fermentation is started at a very high temperature, it takes a longer time to develop. This is probably due to the killing or inactivation of the pitch culture and the replacement by a spontaneous flora which requires some time to become installed.

When they consider that the mash has cooled to the correct temperature, they gather the formerly distributed aliquots in a clean drum and add the pitch which they mix carefully with a calabash reserved for this purpose. Fermentation then takes place at ambient temperature. It is necessary that the fermentation be started in the evening to be able to sell the beer the next morning.

After 2–3 h, the mash becomes effervescent and foam develops, this being considered to be an indication of a good and rapid fermentation. The next morning, at around 5 a.m., the bili bili is covered with a thick head of foam typical of a successful preparation. The beer is then strained and distributed in large aluminum vessels called *tawas* which can be hermetically closed. These *tawas* have replaced earthenware jars. Bili bili is ready to be sold but brewers usually let it rest for two more hours to ensure a good further development of the foam and to afford them with enough time to prepare for the sale. Beer is thus sold from 8 a.m. to 20 p.m. by which time the brewer must clear the market stand. Beer which is left over is distilled at the brewer's home.

As it is the case with many home-made productions, bili bili production associates a precise protocol, transmitted orally from generation to generation, with significant sources of variability resulting from to the variety of operators, raw materials, tools and energy sources, and a complete absence of instrumental and analytical controls. A detailed study (Nanadoum, 2001; Nanadoum *et al.*, 2005) based on a thorough survey of more than 70 brewers and analyses of their intermediate and final products has pinpointed the most invariant features of this process. It has allowed for a chemical and microbiological characterization of the different steps of the transformation of the raw material. Based on this characterization, the specific technological functions of these steps have been identified. We discuss below these main functions.

From germination to malting: This step results in a malt endowed with the required amylolytic properties but also enriched with an abundant lactic flora. Three functions can be assigned to this flora:

1. Lactic acid production lowers the pH to values that are more favorable to amylolytic activities.
2. Supplementary amylolytic activities are produced by the lactic flora as it is usual in many homemade African transformations of starchy foods such as cassava (Daeschel, 1989; Giraud *et al.*, 1991).
3. Amensalistic interactions provide protection against pathogenic or unwanted spoilage flora.

From steeping to sedimentation: As no significant solubilization of the total dry matter is observed, the functions to be assigned to this step are: the preservation of the amylolytic activities and of the lactic flora which would otherwise be impaired by heat, and the decrease in the total volume of material to be submitted to cooking.

Setting aside of the supernatant phase: This standing of the liquid results in a strong acidification the role of which is unclear.

Cooking of the settled phase: This step results in a significant solubilization of the total dry matter mostly due to the gelatinization, dextrinization and hydrolysis of the starch content. Forty-four percent of the dry matter is converted into soluble sugar. By analogy with industrial brewing, it cannot be excluded that other transformations occur, which do not significantly affect the mass balance but are important from both technological and organoleptic points of view (precipitation of proteins, phytates and tannins, hydrolysis of β-glucans, etc.).

Mixing of the supernatant and cooked settled phases: This mixing results in a significant increase of the total concentration in fermentable sugars which amount up to 65% of the total dry weight, probably due to the immediate action of the amylolytic enzymes of the supernatant phase upon the dextrins which have been produced during the cooking step.

Acidification: Due to the continued hydrolysis of dextrins, total fermentable sugar concentration rises to 80% of the total dry weight. An increase in lactic acid concentrations and in counts of lactic acid bacteria suggests that there is development of a vigorous lactic fermentation. The responsible flora probably originates from the flora which developed in the supernatant phase and survived the thermal shock caused by the mixing operation.

Wort cooking: Three main functions have to be assigned to this step:

1. Reduction of the total volume due to water evaporation
2. Precipitation of proteins and tannins
3. Disinfection of the wort

Given the absence of sterile procedures during subsequent stages of production, the main interest of disinfection is probably to free the wort from any bacterial populations which could compete with the intentionally added populations during the fermentation step.

Final fermentation: Both microbiological examinations (parallel development of yeasts and lactic bacteria counts) and analytical assays (parallel productions of lactic acid and ethanol) show that lactic and ethanolic fermentation develop concurrently during this step. The identification and typing of yeast strains isolated from bili bili have shown that these strains belong predominantly to the *Saccharomyces cerevisiae* species, to display a strong interstrain polymorphism and to be accompanied by low numbers of genera and species such as *Kluyveromyces marxianus*, *Candida albidus* and *Debaryomyces hansenii* (Nanadoum *et al.*, 2005).

When compared to European brewing technologies (Table 5.2), bili bili production displays three main differences:

1. The operating procedure and complexity of the mashing step are probably justified by the rudimentary heating technique. And it does not allow for a tight control of the specific temperatures which would be required for the specific needs of gelatinization, dextrinization and hydrolysis of the various components.
2. The presence and activity of an abundant indigenous lactic bacterial flora throughout the process.
3. The shortness of the final fermentation step which is performed under higher-temperature conditions.

Table 5.2 Comparison of traditional African beer with industrial European beers

		Beer		
		Industrial European	*Bili bili from Chad*	*Dolo from Burkina*
Starting materials	Starchy substrate	Barley malt	Sorghum or millet malt	Sorghum malt
	Complement	Other cereal or sugar syrup	None	Millet or maize
Fermentations conditions	Microorganisms	Yeast	Yeast and lactic bacteria	Yeast and lactic bacteria
	Fermentation type	Alcoholic	Lactic and alcoholic	Lactic and alcoholic
	Pitching	Perfectly identified yeast strains	Complex polymicrobial pitch issued from a former fabrication of beer	Complex polymicrobial pitch issued from a former fabrication of beer
	Fermentation time	Several days	10–12h	10–12h
Characteristics	Nutritional value	Limited value	Rich in dry matter and vitamins	Rich in dry matter and vitamins
	Shelf life	Very long after bottling	Less than 24h	2–3 days
Equipments		Highly sophisticated large scale stainless steel equipments, etc.	Rudimentary tools (jars, drums, wood fire, mats, etc.)	Rudimentary tools (jars, drums, wood fire, mats, etc.)

Source: Adapted from Griffon and Hébert (2001).

Characteristics of bili bili sorghum beer

As do many traditional African sorghum beers, bili bili beer displays a number of features which make it distinct from more conventional beers. It is a viscous liquid, slightly cloudy as it has still retained part of the yeast and cellulosic impurities. This is why it is named "opaque beer" in contrast with European beers which are often filtered and pasteurized. Its color varies from brown to golden yellow depending on the sorghum variety which has been used. It is a sparkling and foamy beverage which does not contain any extraneous aromatic compound. This acidic drink (pH 3.5) displays a pronounced sourness associated with fruity overtones.

The alcoholic content is around 4.2% (w/v) but the beer is also rich in soluble sugars (30.4 g/l), soluble protein (10.1 g/l) and lactic acid (12.6 g/l). It is served while still warm during a time period which does not exceed 24 h because of rapid spoilage. It is sold at a price 10 times lower than that of the industrial domestic beer.

Table 5.3 Comparison of sorghum, millet and maize compositions

Constituants	*Sorghum*	*Millet*	*Maize*
Protein (g)	11	10.6	9.5
Lipids (g)	3.2	4.1	4.0
Available sugars (g)	59.3	73.2	66
Dietary fibers (g)	14.5	Nd	0
Calcium (mg)	26	22	16
Phosphorus (mg)	330	286	220
Iron (mg)	10.6	20.7	3.6
Vitamin B1 thiamine (mg)	0.30	0.30	0.33
Vitamin B2 riboflavin (mg)	0.15	0.22	0.10
Vitamin PP (vitamin B3) nicotinamide (mg)	5.3	4.7	3.1
Vitamin B12 (mg)	Nd	Nd	0.4
Vitamin B5 pantothenic acid (mg)	1.2	1.25	0.65

Note: Values expressed for 100 g of grain at 10% moisture. Nd, not determined.

Source: FAO (1974).

Nutritional Value and Impact upon Human Health

In terms of total volume consumed, sorghum beer is the alcoholic beverage most commonly drunk in the Sahel, but it also plays an important role in the nutrition of low-income urban as well as of rural populations. Consumption of the drink begins at teenage, for both men and women. This consumption is frequent since this beverage, which is often called "eat drink," is considered as both nourishing and euphoriant. Thus the question posed by Novellie (1963) "is this beer a food or an alcoholic drink?" is still open.

In the course of our survey in N'djamena (Nanadoum *et al.*, 2006), we noted that the majority of regular consumers were low-salaried civil servants, unemployed people, students and rural people. They appear to be in as good health as are drinkers of the domestic industrial Gala beer which is marketed in Chad. Some consumers stated that they often went for 2 or 3 days drinking sorghum beer as their only source of nutrition. A similar observation was made by Dirar (1993) who noted that 40% of construction workers in Sudan substituted two or three daily meals by consumption of merrissa ("merrissa" is the Arab name for sorghum beer). Platt (1964) also reports that half of the annual consumption of beer in African villages occurs during cooperative works where it constitutes 35% of the caloric intake. According to these statements, sorghum beer can be regarded as an important and safe food.

Nutritional value of the raw material

Cereals such as sorghum, millet or maize which are used for traditional beer production display similar gross chemical compositions (Table 5.3). The digestible form of sugar, mainly as starch, amounts to 65–70% of the total dry weight, corresponding to a caloric value of 3.3–3.8 kcal/g.

Dietary fibers content varies over a large range from 2% to 30% depending on the size of the grain, the proportion of husk being higher in the smallest ones.

Protein content varies between 6% and 18%, but most frequently between 8% and 13%. Despite these somewhat low figures, the protein contribution of these cereals is most important as they make up the major staple diet of numerous populations. The qualitative nutritional value of this protein contribution is rather poor as their content in lysine and tryptophan is low.

Lipids are scarce but of high value due to their richness in polyunsaturated fatty acids.

Mineral content is low and most ions (Fe, Mg, Zn, etc.) are complexed by phytic acid as total calcium is too low to neutralize these acids.

Vitamin C is lacking as well as, except for few species, vitamin A. Group B (except B12) vitamins are present but they are often lost during husking.

Most importantly, digestibility and biological availability of these various nutrients are impaired by the presence of two classes of inhibitors of digestion: phytic acid and tannins.

Nutritional value of the beer

Numerous studies have been devoted to the nutritional interest of African cereal beers (Richards, 1939; Périsse *et al.*, 1959; Novellie, 1963, 1966b; Platt, 1964; Chevassus-Agnes *et al.*, 1976; Van Heerden, 1985; Novellie and De Chaepdrijver, 1986; Van Heerden and Glennie, 1987; Haggblade and Holzapfel, 1989; Dirar, 1993).

The significant dry matter losses due to alcoholic fermentation seem to be balanced by the improvement in protein and amino-acid digestibility, mineral availability and vitamin content (Tables 5.4 and 5.5).

According to Taylor (1983), sprouting increases the digestive availability of essential amino acids tenfold, which is preserved in the subsequent stages of production.

Table 5.4 Evolution of the contents in soluble materials during the production of bili bili

		Production steps			
	Malt	*Mash 1*	*Mash 3*	*Final wort*	*Beer*
Soluble starch	3.8	0.11	0.1	0.43	0.27
Soluble sugar	5.2	10.82	94.41	110.4	30.43
Soluble protein	3.6	12.64	8.14	9.22	10.15
Lactic acid	Nd	3.22	16.27	9.12	12.69
Ethanol	Nd	0	0	0	41.8

Note: The production steps correspond to those in Figure 5.1. Contents are given as % of soluble DM except for malt where they are given as % of total DM. DM, dry matter and Nd not determined.

Source: Adapted from Nanadoum *et al.* (2005).

Table 5.5 Comparison of chemical compositions of sorghum, malted sorghum and amgba, a Cameroonian sorghum beer

	Grain	*Malt*	*Amgba*
Calories	381	380	394
Protein (g)	9.4	9.8	8.7
Lysine (g% proteins)	3.3	3.7	7.2
Lipids (g)	2.8	2.2	0.3
Total sugars (g)	85.6	86.2	86.1
Non-digestible sugars (g)	2.3	3.7	0.3
Ash (g)	2.1	1.7	4.1
Calcium (mg)	11	9.3	20.7
Total phosphorus (mg)	319	327	630
Phytic phosphorus (mg)	166	85	112
Potassium (mg)	391	361	1101
Sodium (mg)	14.5	14.7	26.9
Thiamine (μg)	407*(1)	426*(2)	3441*(3)
Riboflavine (μg)	98	231*(4)	760
Niacin (μg)	4.3	5.3	8

Note: Expressed for 100 g DM.
*Extreme values: (1) 170–545; (2) 168–565; (3) 1693–5241; (4) 169–300. DM, dry matter.

Source: Adapted from Chevassus-Agnès *et al.* (1976).

Sprouting also leads to a decrease in phytic phosphorus which results in a significant increase in ionizable iron and zinc (Malleshi and Desikachar, 1986b; Udayasekhara Rao and Deosthale, 1988).

Phenolic compounds and tannins confer to the grains of brown sorghum a strong astringency which renders them both mold resistant and repellent for birds. But these compounds also impair the nutritional value by sequestering exogenous and endogenous proteins in the form of indigestible complexes (Eggum and Christensen, 1975; Griffiths, 1985; Asquith and Butler, 1986). It has been reported that germination (Osuntogun *et al.*, 1989), cooking (Price *et al.*, 1980) and fermentation (Dhankher and Chauhan, 1987) removed significant amounts of tannins.

Finally, proliferation of lactic acid bacteria and yeasts gives important additional properties to the final product, in relation to increased vitamin content and also probiotic effects.

- Through the improvements in protein and mineral availability and the enrichment in vitamins content, bili bili has a better nutritional value than crude cereal grains.

Hygienic quality and potential hazards

The survey (Nanadoum *et al.*, 2006) conducted among bili bili consumers has stressed the fact that their prevailing complaint was concern about the poor sanitary conditions during beer production: open air operation, incomplete washing, and lack of disinfection. Yet most of them recognize that they never experienced any health problem after having taken bili bili. A small minority stated that they did sometimes suffer from diarrhea, vomiting or headache after having consumed some bad tasting products.

With respect to the mycotoxin hazard, analysis performed in other countries (Okafor, 1966; Lovelace and Nyathi, 1977; Novellie and De Schaepdrijvers, 1986; Odhav and Naicker, 2002; Isaacson, 2005; Nkwe *et al.*, 2005) have shown quite high amounts in maize grains and maize malts but somewhat lower in maize beers. Sorghum malts were found to be weakly contaminated while sorghum beers were devoid of any mycotoxin.

No pathogenic bacteria could be isolated from the bacterial flora of African SMM beers. This is probably due to the strong amensalistic interactions exerted by the lactic flora against pathogenic invaders through the establishment of acidic conditions and bacteriocin excretion.

- Sorghum beers are pathogen- and mycotoxin-free.

Conclusion

Bili bili beer suffers from two important drawbacks:

1. It is prepared under quite poor sanitary conditions.
2. It is an alcoholic drink.

Yet it remains an important and cheap source of calories, digestible proteins, minerals and vitamins. It contributes to sustain the nourishment of a significant part of an urban population, too poor to access other sources of transformed food and for many of them without any means to prepare their own home-made food. This contribution is obtained at an epidemiological cost which is undoubtedly lower than the cost of infectious, parasitic and other diseases which arise in this undernourished population.

It is our opinion that, as long as economic conditions do not improve up to a point where safe and well-balanced food becomes available to the poorest part of the population, bili bili consumption, if moderate, will play a positive role in providing these people with the essential nutrients they could not obtain elsewhere.

Acknowledgment

The authors gratefully acknowledge the helpful assistance of Prof. C. Tinsley in rereading of the text.

References

Adrien, J. and Jacquot, R. (1964). In Vigot Frères (ed.), *Le mil et le sorgho dans l'alimentation humaine*, pp. 99–108. Paris, France.

Asquith, T.N. and Butler, L.C. (1986). *Phytochemistry* 25, 1591–1593.

Bismuth, A. and Ménage, C. (1961). *Sci. Humaine, Série B* 23, 60–118.

Chevassus-Agnes, S., Favier, J.C. and Joseph, A. (1976). *Cah. Nutr. Diététique* 11, 89–104.

Daeschel, M.A. (1989). *Food Technol.* 1, 164–166.

Dhankher, N. and Chauhan, B.M. (1987). *J. Food Sci.* 52, 828–829.

Dirar, H.A. (1993). *African Fermented Food Nutrition.* CAB International University Press, Cambridge, UK. pp. 224–302.

ECOSIT 1 (1998). Project CHD/91/003 "appui à la gestion du développement." (ed. Ministère du Plan et de l'aménagement d territoire/PNUD-DAES), Rapport final, 119 p.

Eggum, B.O. and Christensen, K.D. (1975). *Breeding for Seed Protein Improvement Using Nuclear Techniques.* Agence internationale de l'énergie atomique, pp. 135–143. Vienne, Autriche.

FAO (1970). *Table de composition des aliments à l'usage de l'Afrique.* FAO, Rome, Italie .

Giraud, E., Brauman, A., Keleke, S., Lelong, B. and Raimbault, M. (1991). *Microbiol. Biotechnol.* 36, 379–383.

Griffon, D. and Hébert, J.-P. (2001). *Bière et dolo: Document de cours*, 117 p. Ensia-Siarc, Montpellier.

Griffiths, D.W. (1985). *Exp. Biol. Med.* 199, 504–516.

Haggblade, S. and Holzapfel, W.H. (1989). In Steinkraus, K.H. (ed.), *Industrialization of Fermented Food*, pp.191–283. New York, USA.

Isaacson, C. (2005). *Med. Hypotheses* 64, 658–660.

Lovelace, C.E.A. and Nyathi, C.B. (1977). *J. Sc. Food Agric.* 28, 288–299.

Magrin, G. and Mbayhoudel, K. (2002). *Actes du IVe colloque Méga-Tchad CNRS/Orstom.* Institut Recherche en Développement. Paris, France.

Malleshi, N.G. and Desikachar, H.S.R. (1986b). *J. Inst. Brew.* 92, 174–176.

Nanadoum, M. (2001). Thèse de doctorat en Sciences Agronomiques de l'Institut National Agronomique Paris–Grignon (France), 168 p.

Nanadoum, M., Mbailao, M., Gaillardin, C. and Pourquié, J. (2005). *Afr. J. Biotechnol.* 4, 646–656.

Nanadoum, M., Mbailao, M., Gaillardin, C. and Pourquie, J. (2006). *Afr. Sci.* 2, 69–82.

Ngardiguim, D. and Digali, Z. (2003). Rapport d'étude (ed Initiative Mil Sorgho-Tchad), N'Djaména, Tchad.

Nkwe, D.O., Taylor, J.E. and Siame, B.A. (2005). *Mycopathologia* 160, 177–186.

Novellie, L. (1963). *Food Ind. S. Afr.* 16, 28.

Novellie, L. (1966b). *Food Technol.* 20, 101–102.

Novellie, L. and De Chaepdrijver, P. (1986). *Progr. Ind. Microbiol.* 20, 155–159.

Odhav, B. and Naicker, V. (2002). *Food Addit. Contam.* 19, 55–61.

Odunfa, S.A. (1985). In Wood, B.J.B. (ed.), *Microbiology of Fermented Food*, Vol. 2, pp. 155–191. Amsterdam, The Netherlands.

Okafor, N. (1966). *West Afri. J. Biol. and Appl. Chem.* 9, 4–13.

Osuntogun, B.O., Adewusi, S.R.A., Ogundiwin, J.O. and Nwasike, C.C. (1989). *Cereal Chem.* 66, 87–89.

Périsse, J., Adrian, J., Rerat, A. and Le Berre, S. (1959). *Ann. Nutr. Et Alim.* 13, 1–13.

Platt, B.S. (1964). *Food Technol.* 18, 662–670.

Price, M.L., Hagerman, A.E. and Butler, L.G. (1980). *Nutr. Rep. Int.* 21, 761–767.

Richards, A.I. (1939). *Land, labour and diet in northern Rhodesia:* An economic study of the Bemba tribe. Oxford University Press, London.

Sanni, A.I., Onilude, A.A., Fadahunsi, I.F. and Afolabi, R.O. (1999). *Food Res. Int.* 32, 163–167.

Seignobos, C. (2002). In *Colloque Mega – Tchad.* Paris, France.

Taylor, J.R.N. (1983). *J. Sci. Food Agric.* 34, 885–892.

Udayasekhara, Rao, P. and Deosthale, Y.G. (1988). *Plant Foods Hum. Nutr.* 38, 35–41.

Van Heerden, I.V. (1985). *S. Afr. J. Sci.* 81, 587–589.

Van Heerden, I.V. and Glennie, C.W. (1987). *Nutr. Rep. Int.* 35, 147–155.

6

Production of Alcohol-Free Beer

Luigi Montanari, Ombretta Marconi, Heidi Mayer and Paolo Fantozzi Italian Brewing Research Centre (CERB), University of Perugia, Via San Costanzo, Perugia, Italy

Abstract

With greater interest in health and concern about weight and considering the warnings about alcohol abuse, especially when driving, consumer preference for low-alcohol and alcohol-free beer is increasing, but the definitions of "low-alcohol" and "alcohol-free" beers vary in different countries as well as their composition.

Low-alcohol or any other word or description which implies that the drink being described is low in alcohol may not be applied to any alcoholic drink unless: (a) the drink has an alcoholic strength by volume of not more than 1.2% and (b) the drink is marked or labeled with an indication of its maximum alcoholic strength immediately preceded by the word "not more than."

The most common way to produce non-alcoholic beers is to modify the normal brewing process so that fermentation is limited and almost no ethanol is produced. There are several techniques for determining alcohol concentration by controlling the extent of fermentation. Moreover, beers produced in a traditional way and in different brands can be made alcohol-free by using physical methods to remove the alcohol at the end of the production process.

The biological methods used to produce alcohol-free beers do not usually require special extra plant, but rather a more accurately controlled process to prevent an overproduction of alcohol.

List of Abbreviations

% (v/v) of alcohol	Alcohol concentration % by volume
°C	Celsius degree
°P	Plato degree
ADH	Alcohol dehydrogenase
Ca	Calcium
CCP	Cold contact process
CO_2	Carbon dioxide
DMS	Dimethyl sulfide
EBC	European Brewing Convention
EBU	European Bitterness Unit
EU	European Union
g	Gram
h	Hour
HG	High gravity
hPa	hectopascal
HPLC	High-performance liquid chromatography
IBC	International Bitterness Unit
ml	Milliliter
n.d.	Not detectable
N_2	Nitrogen
NAD	Nicotinamide adenine dinucleotide
NADP	Nicotinamide adenine dinucleotide phosphate
ppb	Parts per billion
ppm	Parts per million
S. ludwigii	*Saccharomycodes ludwigii*
SHG	Super high gravity
wt%	Percent in weight

Introduction

With greater interest in health and concern about weight and considering the warnings about alcohol abuse, especially when driving, consumer preference for low-alcohol and alcohol-free beers is increasing. The definitions of "low-alcohol" and "alcohol-free" vary in different countries (Table 6.1).

The European Union (EU) has no law that refers to "low-alcohol" and "alcohol-free" beers, but each country has its own legislation. In many countries such as Germany, Switzerland, Austria, Finland and Portugal, the ethanol content of alcohol-free beer is restricted to 0.5% (v/v). In Belgian legislation, "alcohol-free" is used for a beer with less than 0.5% (v/v) alcohol and a specific gravity higher than 2.2°P, while the alcohol

Beer in Health and Disease Prevention
ISBN: 978-0-12-373891-2

Table 6.1 Data related to relation to alcohol content and energy in beers from different countries

Country	*Light beer (% v/v alcohol)*[a]	*Low-alcohol beer (% v/v alcohol)*	*Alcohol-free beer (% v/v alcohol)*	*Reference*
Austria	≤3.7	>0.5 and ≤1.9	≤0.5	Codex Alimentarius Austriacus Kapitel B 13, April 1998
Belgium	Gravity ≥1° and ≤4°P[b] 30% energy reduction	>0.5 and ≤1.2 and gravity ≥2.2°P	≤0.5 and gravity ≥2.2°P	Real Decree March 31, 1993
Denmark	<2.8		<0.1	None
Finland	30% less energy content	<2.8	≤0.5	Finnish food legislation
France			≤1.2	Decree n° 92–307 of March 31, 1992
Germany	30% energy reduction	>0.5 and ≤1.2	≤0.5	Nährwert – Kennzeichnungsverordnung, Diät – Verordnung
Italy	>1.2 and ≤3.5 gravity ≥5° and ≤10.5°P[b]		≤1.2 gravity ≥3° and ≤3°P[b]	Law 16 August 1962 n. 1354
The Netherlands	33% less calorific value	>0.1 and ≤1.2	≤0.1	Beer Ordinance 2003, Commodity Board for Beverage
Portugal		>0.5 and ≤1.2	<0.5	Decree n° 1/96 of January 3, 1996
Spain	30% energy reduction	From 1 to 3	<1	Real Decree 53/1999 of 20 January and agreement with Ministry of Health and Consumption dated 1990
Sweden		≥2.25		Alcohol low and agreement with Ombudsman regarding advertising (i.e. self-regulation)
United Kingdom		≤1.2	≤0.05	Statutory Instrument 1996 n° 1499
United States		≤2.5	Absolutely no alcohol is present[c]	

[a] Alcohol concentration % by volume.
[b] 1°P is equal to 1 g of sugar/100 g wort.
[c] non-alcoholic beer <0.5% v/v alcohol.
Source: The Brewers of Europe (2004).

content % (v/v) ranges from 0.5% to 1.2% for low-alcohol beers. Other countries, like Italy and France, consider beer as "alcohol-free" if it has less than 1.2% (v/v) of alcohol and as light beer if it has 1.2–3.5%. (v/v) of alcohol In France, Decree n° 92–307 of March 31, 1992 states that "bier sans alcool" is not a claim but a sales denomination. In Denmark and The Netherlands the term "alcohol-free" may be applied to beer with less than 0.1% (v/v) of alcohol. In the United Kingdom, the Statutory Instrument 1996 n° 1499 established that the term "alcohol-free" may not be applied to any drink from which alcohol has been extracted unless (The Brewers of Europe, 2004):

(a) the drink has an alcoholic strength by volume of not more than 0.05%;
(b) the drink is marked or labeled with an indication of its maximum alcoholic content immediately preceded by the word "not more than" or, if appropriate, with an indication that it contains no alcohol.

Low-alcohol or any other word or description which implies that the drink being described is low in alcohol may not be applied to any alcoholic drink unless:

(a) The drink has an alcoholic strength by volume of not more than 1.2%;
(b) The drink is marked or labeled with an indication of its maximum alcoholic strength immediately preceded by the word "not more than."

"Low-alcohol beer" or "reduced-alcohol beer" is defined by the US Government as a beer with less than 2.5% (v/v) of alcohol. Furthermore, in the United States, "near-beer" or non-alcoholic beer means that it contains less than 0.5% (v/v) of

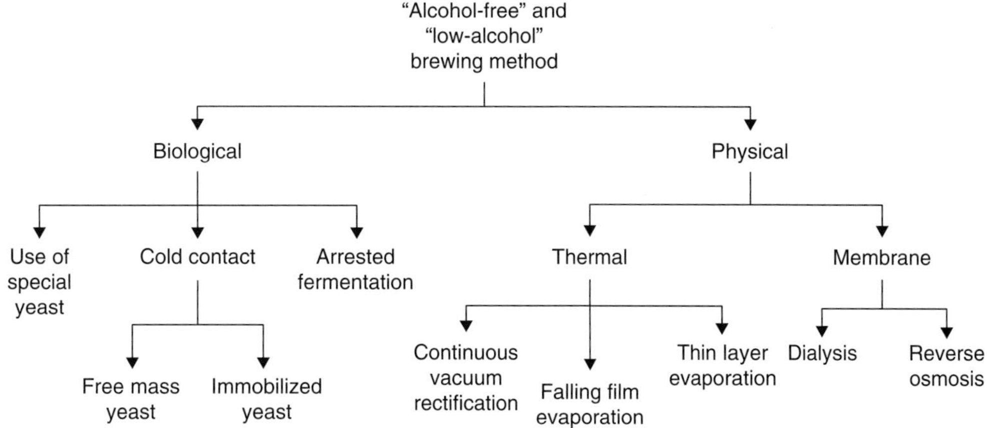

Figure 6.1 The scheme of alcohol-free and low-alcohol beer production methods. Biological and physical processes exist for producing alcohol-free beer. The biological processes include the use of special yeasts, arrested fermentation and CCP. The physical processes include thermal processes and membrane processes.

alcohol by volume, while "alcohol-free" means that there is absolutely no alcohol present (Munroe, 1995), that is to say, below the common analytical detection limit which is 0.05 (v/v) % of alcohol. Islamic countries also demand absolutely no alcohol (Caluwaerts, 1995).

This chapter deals with "alcohol-free" and "low-alcohol" beers production technologies, as well as with their chemical, physical and sensorial characteristics. Over the last few years, several methods, listed below, have been developed for the production of low-alcohol or alcohol-free beer (Scott and Huxtable, 1995) (Figure 6.1).

The biological processes include:

1. use of special yeasts (*S. ludwigii*);
2. arrested fermentation;
3. cold contact process (CCP).

The physical processes include thermal and membrane processes such as:

1. thin-layer evaporation;
2. falling film vacuum evaporation;
3. continuous vacuum rectification;
4. reverse osmosis;
5. dialysis.

Less used processes include pervaporation, freeze concentration, extraction processes, such as extraction with organic solvents and extraction with carbon dioxide, as well as adsorption on special kieselgels or on special adsorbent resins (Von Hodenberg, 1991). An alternative technique for producing beer with a reduced ethanol content is the use of a genetically modified yeast strain that forms less ethanol during complete fermentation of wort sugars (Nevoigt *et al.*, 2002). Technologically, it is possible to produce beer with less than 0.05% (v/v) of alcohol. The alcohol concentration of beer obtained from the different methods is reported in Table 6.2.

Table 6.2 Alcohol-free beers obtained with different production technologies

Brewing method	*% (v/v) alcohol*	*References*
Arrested fermentation and dilution	0.3–1.0	Zasio (1996)
Cold contact	0.36–0.64	Perpete and Collin (1999)
Special yeasts (*S. Ludwigii*)	0.48	Narziss *et al.* (1992)
Continuous vacuum rectification	0.1	Firmenschrift (2004)
Falling film vacuum evaporation	0.4	Zufall and Wackerbauer (2000a)
Reverse osmosis	0.4	Zufall and Wackerbauer (2000b)
Dialysis	0.4	Zufall and Wackerbauer (2000b)

Production Technologies

Biological methods

The most common way to produce non-alcoholic beers is to modify the normal brewing process so that fermentation is limited and almost no ethanol is produced. There are several techniques for determining alcohol concentration by controlling the extent of fermentation. Generally, worts with a low concentration of fermentable carbohydrates are used for all of these techniques. Such worts can be produced by using a high-temperature mash cycle that involves removing and boiling a portion of the mash (the decoction); it is then returned to the main mash to increase the temperature. Briefly, the grist is mashed with hot water at 52°C. The first decoction is performed by removing a part of the mash which is then heated to boiling and then mixed again with the main mash to obtain a temperature of 76°C. This temperature, used for mashing, lautering and sparging, inactivates the amylases (mainly β-amylase) which prevents the formation of normal concentrations of fermentable sugars. The mashing process is dependent on the different biochemical characteristics of the enzymes involved. The enzyme α-amylase is largely responsible for the breakdown of starch into lower-molecular-weight sugars and dextrins. Some of these sugars are fermentable but the dextrins, that are the majority, are not. The other important enzyme is β-amylase that attacks dextrins and soluble starch at the non-reducing chain ends to form fermentable sugar maltose. These enzymes have different thermal stabilities; α-amylase is more stable than β-amylase at high temperatures. These properties can be exploited to control the carbohydrate composition and the fermentability of the final wort (Montanari *et al.*, 2005). In the brewing environment, it is necessary to produce a wort fermentability of about 25–30% to produce a low-alcohol beer (Muller, 2000), whereas a wort fermentability of 80% is needed to obtain pale beers (Kunze, 2004). The different fermentable sugar composition of two worts with 1.040 gravity produced at a mashing temperature of 65°C and 85°C is reported in Table 6.3. The worts had the same total carbohydrate content, but the amount of fermentable sugars found in the wort produced at 85°C was considerably lower than that obtained at 65°C. The fermentable sugar composition was determined using high-performance liquid chromatography (HPLC) (Muller, 1991; Floridi *et al.*, 2001).

A further decrease in the alcohol concentration in the final beer can be obtained by fermenting worts produced by high gravity (HG) (15°P) or super high gravity (SHG) (18°P) (Younis and Stewart, 1999) followed by dilution. Biological processes for alcohol-free beer production include:

1. the use of weakly fermenting yeast strains or of yeast strain mixtures which cannot ferment maltose (Von Hodenberg, 1991);
2. stopped fermentation techniques that halt conventional beer fermentation at a low-alcohol level by suddenly increasing the pressure or lowering the temperature;
3. cold contact process.

Table 6.3 Wort sugars analysis

Sugar	*Low fermentability*	*Normal fermentability*
Glucose	0.17	0.58
Sucrose	0.27	0.38
Maltose	0.38	4.41
Maltoriose	0.14	0.81
Total	0.96	5.96

Note: Two worts (gravity 1.040) were prepared at 65°C (normal fermentability) and at 85°C (low fermentability) and the single fermentable sugars were determined by HPLC (g/100g).
Source: Muller (1991).

Use of Special Yeasts Alcohol-free beer with an alcohol concentration not lower than 0.05% by volume can be obtained with this technique. *Saccharomycodes ludwigii* yeast is closely related to *Saccharomyces uvarum*, but it is capable of fermenting glucose, sucrose and fructose sugars but not maltose, because it does not have invertase and maltase. Considering that *S. ludwigii* attenuates very slowly Narziss *et al.* (1992) obtained an alcohol-free beer by carrying out the fermentation of a wort with 11.5wt% at 20°C, then reduced the temperature to 0°C during the last fermentation day. After a fermentation time of 120h at 20°C *S. ludwigii* had formed 0.68wt% of ethanol. With a dilution to 7.5% of the original gravity, about 0.45% ethanol would have been formed. This yeast has the advantage of being easy to handle – at least during fermentation – and does not require continuous monitoring of the extract reduction.

Stopped Fermentation Methods Stopped fermentation, where the yeast is removed before full attenuation, can be distinguished from limited fermentation, in which yeast metabolism is restrained. The fermentation may be stopped by removing the yeast cells or by rapidly cooling the fermenting wort. This technique requires worts with a low concentration of fermentable carbohydrates. The fermentation step is conducted at low temperatures, about 2–3°C, with a contact time of about 150–200h. During fermentation, the wort is not aerated to prevent yeast reproduction and to lengthen the lag-phase where the yeast consumes and metabolizes, but does not propagate or produce ethanol. The metabolites produced during the lag phase influence beer flavor. These beers are characterized by high level of sulfur compounds which do not completely evaporate during the wort boiling. Dimethyl sulfide (DMS) could therefore be used as an analytical marker. Recent experiments have attempted to strip wort in the presence of carbon dioxide or nitrogen. After cooling the wort to about 20°C, it is stripped under pressure to avoid foam production. This method allows a good quality beer with less than 0.2% of alcohol by volume to be produced, but it requires accurate analytical control. The yeast mass and alcohol content must be checked every 8h. The beers are produced using HG or SHG processes. In the SHG production starting from 18°P, 6°P is obtained after centrifugation at about 0.2–0.3°C and dilution, before or after final filtration, with desalinated water to reach the alcoholic and saccharometric level desired. When producing non-alcoholic beers by means of arrested fermentation, the predominant objective is to reduce the worty flavor impression or limit it from the beginning. When fermentation is arrested at an early stage, the short active phase of the yeasts can contribute to the formation of fermentation by-products that influence the taste of the beer. When producing non-alcoholic beer by using stopped fermentation factors, it is necessary to consider the composition of added malt, the time of dilution, the time and extent of acidification, the fermentation conditions in relation to the yeast type, as well as the fermentation time and temperature (Narziss *et al.*, 1992). The following is an example of a method used to produce a beer with 0.31 wt% of ethanol. A brew was diluted so that the finished wort contained 8% extract, which was then divided into two parts and boiled. One part was fermented with the top fermentation yeast and the other with the bottom fermentation yeast. After a "whirlpool rest," the worts were cooled to 10°C and then to 0°C and then pitched without aeration. Once an attenuation of 10% was reached, the products were filtered, stored and carbonated; after a 3-week storage period, they were bottled. At the fermentation temperatures applied (about 0°C), the top-fermenting yeast took effect rather slowly so that attenuations were considerably lower than for the bottom yeast. The use of top fermentation instead of bottom-yeast fermentation results in the formation of more fermentation by-products such as higher alcohols and esters as well as more diacetyl. When bottom yeasts are used, a higher fermentation temperature is more advantageous despite the short fermentation time and the diacetyl level is reduced if the same temperature is used as that used for top-fermenting yeasts (Table 6.4).

Malt composition influences the final alcohol-free beer obtained with stopped fermentation. Compared to the brew pitched with 100% pale malt, the beers with the special malts clearly contained more beer flavor substances. In particular, pale caramel malt contributed the highest amount of furfural; when a slight excess of caramel malt was added the beer had an unusual color. In conclusion, special malts contribute positive taste characteristics and these beers have a less worty flavor impression than beers produced exclusively with pale malt.

Cold Contact Process In 1983, Schur (1983) proposed a "CCP" combining a long fermentation time with low temperature thus limiting fermentation. During this process, high temperatures (15–20°C) are sometimes combined with short fermentation times (0.5–8 h). However, low temperatures are used (0–5°C), often in combination with longer fermentation times (up to 24 h) (Huige *et al.*, 1990). No ethanol is produced under these conditions, but the yeast exhibit moderate metabolism such as the production of ester and fusel alcohol or carbonyl reduction. During CCP, alcohol-free beers are produced starting from a normal wort cooled to 0–1°C before pitching. In most cases, a high yeast cell concentration is used (>10^8 cells/ml); thus thick yeast slurry is mixed with a HG wort. One disadvantage of this method is that the yeast slurry used for inoculation may have a relatively high ethanol concentration (6.5% v/v) (Schur and Sauer, 1990). Primary metabolism is slow under these conditions, although many biochemical reactions can take place. Carbonyl compounds, suspected of imparting the worty flavor, are partially reduced, while some esters are synthesized. The pH is not as low as usual, so the wort must be acidified either chemically or by immobilized lactic bacteria (Perpete and Collin, 1999).

The CCP is currently applied in two ways:

1. Free mass yeast
2. Immobilized yeast.

CCP with Free Mass Yeast Worts with low concentration of fermentable sugars are stripped at a low temperature and under pressure with CO_2 or N_2 to eliminate the sulfur compounds which were not evaporated during wort boiling. Generally, the yeasts eliminate them during normal

Table 6.4 Influence of yeast type and fermentation temperature on beer composition

Fermentation yeast temperature (°C)	*Bottom 0*	*Bottom 4*	*Bottom 8*	*Bottom 12*	*Top 8*	*Top 12*
Original gravity (wt%)	11.4	7.5	7.5	7.5	7.4	7.4
Ethanol (wt%)	0.27	0.37	0.37	0.42	0.32	0.27
Apparent extract (wt%)	10.5	6.6	6.6	6.3	6.7	6.8
Real extract (wt%)	10.64	6.79	6.79	6.52	6.87	6.94
Attenuation (wt%)	8	12	12	16	9	8
Color (EBC)	8.4	5.6	5.6	5.6	5.6	5.6
pH	5.01	4.87	4.92	4.89	4.87	4.89
Bitter substances (EBC)	25.4	17.5	17.7	17.4	17.7	17.8
DMS (μg/l)	30	22	30	32	35	45
Acetoin (mg/l)	7.0	6.9	6.6	8.2	2.9	2.3
Total diacetyl (mg/l)	0.06	0.09	0.08	0.14	0.51	0.35
2,3-pentadione (mg/l)	0.01	0.03	0.03	0.06	0.08	0.05

wt%: weight percent; DMS: dimethyl sulfide.

Source: Narziss *et al.* (1992).

fermentation, but in CCP yeast metabolism is limited. The use of CO_2 rather than N_2 is preferable because CO_2 is present in the final beer at a concentration of 5/6 g/l. CO_2 prevents spontaneous fermentation. This technique is characterized by a contact time of 50–100 h and stripping with CO_2 at a temperature of 0°C. Stripping improves the contact of yeast with the wort because of convective movements. Using an SHG process, this method produces beer with less than 0.1% alcohol by volume. It is an economical method but requires considerable analytical control; the yeast and alcohol production must be checked every 8 h.

CCP with Immobilized Yeast CCP is currently applied to low-density worts in immobilized yeast reactors. Arrested batch fermentation is a simple operation, but is difficult to control when producing alcohol-free beers. The use of immobilized yeast is currently of great interest to brewers. Fermentation takes a very short time, but the yeast can be used for a long time. A decisive factor is the immobilization of the yeast on a macroporous carrier material (Kunze, 2004). In general, four immobilization technique categories can be distinguished, based on the physical mechanism of cell localization and on the nature of the support mechanisms (Karel *et al.*, 1985; Verbelen *et al.*, 2006):

1. *Attachment to a surface*: The yeast cells are allowed to attach to a solid support. Many different carrier materials are being used. Cellular attachment to the carrier can be induced using linking agents (such as metal oxides, glutaraldehyde or amilosilanes).
2. *Entrapment within a porous matrix*: Two methods of entrapment exist. In the first one, cells are allowed to diffuse into a pre-formed porous matrix. After the cells begin to grow, their mobility is hindered by the presence of other cells and by the matrix, and they are entrapped (Baron and Willaert, 2004). In the second one, the porous matrix is synthesized *in situ* around the cells. Natural and synthetic polymeric hydrogels such as Ca-alginate, *k*-carrageenan, agar, polyurethane, polystyrene and polyvinyl alcohol are being used.
3. *Containment behind a barrier*: This can be attained either by using microporous membrane filters or by entrapping cells in microcapsules. This type of immobilization is most suitable when a cell-free product is required, or when high-molecular-weight products need to be separated from the effluent.
4. *Self-aggregation*: Yeast flocculation is a reversible, asexual and calcium-dependent process in which cells adhere to form flocs consisting of thousands of cells (Bony *et al.*, 1997). Because of their macroscopic size and mass, the yeast flocs settled out rapidly from the fermenting medium, thereby the cells are immobilized naturally. The use of flocculating yeast is simple and cheap.

Immobilization carriers must be inert, cheap, stable, reusable and usually non-toxic, and support a high yeast cell concentration. In brewing, the carriers are usually calcium alginate, carrageenan beads for gel entrapment, DEAE cellulose as an inert support and sintered glass for entrapment in a pre-formed carrier. Other techniques, such as covalent attachment and cell aggregation are mentioned, but not applied. The attachment of yeast cells to suitable carrier materials allows a controlled use of the enzyme potential of the yeast, especially during the exponential and stationary phases of fermentation, and consequently of the formation and removal of fermentation by-products. Currently, only beer maturation and alcohol-free beer production are carried out in commercial-scale immobilized yeast reactors. The main objective during fermentation of alcohol-free beer is to reduce wort carbonyl flavors by yeast, without the formation of alcohol. Traditionally, alcohol-free beer has been produced by arresting fermentation. By keeping the yeast in an optimal steady state condition at low temperature leads to a more complete reduction of wort carbonyl with minimum alcohol formation (Verbelen *et al.*, 2006). In the continuous production of non-alcoholic beer by immobilized yeast at low temperature three aspects are important:

1. The Cultor carrier, a DEAE-cellulose-based granular material, is used in a packed bed reactor, which is operated under down-flow. The yeast cells bind to the rough surface in a monolayer, and the cells are not subject to starvation by substrate limitation. By packing the carrier particles in a bed reactor, and operating under down-flow, a flexible and easily controlled system is obtained.
2. A low temperature (2–4°C) is used. Yeast growth, which could clog the reactor after long production periods, is suppressed and metabolism is limited; however, substrate conversion and product formation are still sufficient. Because of the low temperature, viability remains high over long periods.
3. Anaerobic conditions are maintained, which suppress yeast growth and prevent oxidation of wort lipids that give carbonyl off-flavors.

The combined stress factors thus suppress yeast growth and sugar metabolism, and decrease the risk of contaminants developing in the reactor. In this system, the yeast is made to form a colony on the carrier material. The growth rate in the bioreactor depends on the temperature (Figure 6.2).

S. cerevisiae were grown at very low temperatures, with growth rates of 0.007 and 0.022 h^{-1} at 2°C and 4°C, respectively, in two batch cultures. In a bioreactor, Van Iersel *et al.* (1995) calculated a growth rate of 0.012/h, in agreement with the rates determined in the above-mentioned batch cultures. The temperature and square root of the growth rate are linearly related. In the reactor, combined stress factors,

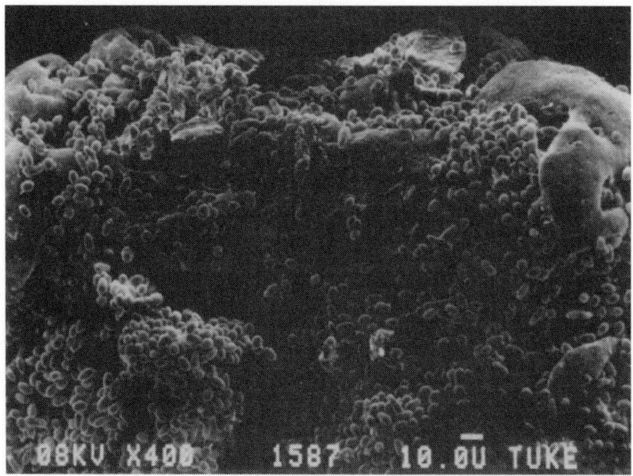

Figure 6.2 Scanning-electron micrograph of yeast cells immobilized on a carrier particle. Bar represents 10 zm^{-1}. In the yeast immobilized system, the yeast forms a colony on the carrier material. The growth rate in the bioreactor depends on the temperature. *Source*: Van Iersel *et al.* (1995).

Table 6.5 Fermentable sugar concentrations (g/100 g) in the wort and in non-alcoholic beer, produced by an immobilized yeast/CCP

Sugars	*In-flowing wort*	*Out-flowing wort*	*Change in concentration*
Glucose	0.58 ± 0.01	0.61 ± 0.02	+0.03
Fructose	0.10 ± 0.10	0.25 ± 0.01	+0.15
Sucrose	0.40 ± 0.02	0.16 ± 0.01	−0.24
Maltose	5.05 ± 0.10	5.00 ± 0.10	−0.05
Maltotriose	0.92 ± 0.03	0.92 ± 0.02	0.00

Source: Van Iersel *et al.* (1995).

such as low temperature (2–4°C) and anaerobic conditions, limit cell metabolism. Growth at low temperatures requires changes in the cell physiology. Inhibition of transport processes might be responsible for the absence of growth. Yeast cells metabolize glucose and reduce numerous wort components to alcohols and esters. Starting from a wort of 12°P which contained approximately 7.05 g/100 g of fermentable sugar, and operating at a temperature of 3°C with a flow rate of 1 m^3/h, a non-alcoholic beer with approximately the same amount of sugars and a concentration of ethanol of less than 0.1% (v/v) was obtained (Table 6.5).

S. cerevisiae takes up glucose more than other sugars. This yeast uses invertase to hydrolyze sucrose in a mixture of various sugars. Due to glucose repression of the maltose and maltotriose transport system, these sugars are not metabolized. At low temperature, regulation of sugar metabolism is apparently centered around glucose which is metabolized preferentially. During fermentation with immobilized yeast at low temperature under anaerobic conditions, yeast cells reduce wort off-flavors and produce beer flavor. The main wort off-flavors are given by aldehydes, such as 2- and 3-methylbutanal, hexanal and heptanal which are reduced to the corresponding alcohols. In addition, aldehydes, formed as intermediates in cell metabolism, are reduced to fusel alcohols (e.g. 1-propanol, isobutanol and isoamyl alcohol). Aldehydes are reduced by alcohol dehydrogenase (ADH). Several ADHs are present in yeast, most of which are dependent on the coenzyme nicotinamide adenine dinucleotide. ADH1 is the main fermentative enzyme and its functioning is essential under anaerobic condition. ADH2 is glucose-repressed, but when cells grow on ethanol, it is the main enzyme that oxidizes ethanol to acetaldehyde. Under physiological conditions, this enzyme uses NADPH primarily. In addition, NAD phosphate (NADP) specific activity increased slightly during alcohol-free beer production. Overall, NADP-specific activity was 3–5 times higher in immobilized cells compared to suspended cells under anaerobic conditions (Van Iersel *et al.*, 2000). The Bavaria Brewery (The Netherlands) uses a packed bed immobilized yeast bioreactor with a production capacity of 150,000 hl of alcohol-free beer per year (Van Dieren, 1995), and according to information from the company, the bioreactor operates for months without problems with no biomass being formed. Further advantages of this method are considered to be:

- better utilization of raw materials;
- no losses;
- no environmental problems;
- very rapid start-up phase.

Physical methods

Beers produced in a traditional way and in different brands can be made alcohol-free by using physical methods to remove the alcohol at the end of the production process. But in comparison with the original beer, there can be a great loss of flavor, body and freshness; this can be mitigated by adding krausen, green beer or fully mature beer up to the permissible alcohol content. While, according to Zufall and Wackerbauer (2000a), beers produced with a manipulated fermentation often have a worty and sweet flavor (Kunze, 2004). Generally, two types of physical processes can be distinguished: thermal and membrane processes. Both require an extra process step with additional costs compared to manipulated fermentation.

Thermal Processes Distillation at atmospheric pressure is the simplest method for making "alcohol-free" and "low-alcohol" beer. The beer is heated to boiling and the volatile substances are separated in the vapor phase and the non-volatile substances are concentrated in the liquid phase. Maintaining a high temperature for a long period degrades the beer quality by increasing the color, caramelizing the naturally occurring sugars and eliminating or damaging the flavor notes. The resulting beer is completely different from the original one; this technology is no longer in use. Nowadays, a vacuum is applied which decreases the boiling temperature and thus reduces the thermal stress on the beer. Most vacuum distillation systems evaporate the beer at temperatures between 30°C and 60°C at pressures of 40–200 hPa absolute (Zufall and Wackerbauer, 2000a). Besides alcohol, other volatile aroma substances like esters and higher alcohols which contribute to a good beer flavor are transferred into the distillate or extracted by vacuum pump. To compensate for these disadvantages, many breweries use a modified brewing technology to produce a more aromatic original beer. Another way to compensate for sensory disadvantages is to blend de-alcoholized beer with a small quantity of original beer or with a beer aroma extract that is recovered from the evaporation plants with rectification columns (Zürcher *et al.*, 2005). The end product of all thermal processes is an alcohol-free beer concentrate to which water and CO_2 must be added.

Continuous Vacuum Rectification A modern, thermal process for gentle removal of alcohol in beer is the SIGMATEC process (API Schmidt-Bretten, 2004). The beer is degassed and then pre-heated in a plate heat exchanger. The beer is fed to the stripping section of a rectifying column. The fluid flows down the column at a temperature between 43°C and 48°C. In counterflow, the product comes in contact with rising vapors which bring about the selective separation of alcohol from the product. The alcohol-free beer is then fed into an evaporator from the bottom of the column. In the evaporator, vapors necessary for the rectification process are produced and then redirected into the column. The completely de-alcoholized product is pumped out of the plant after passing through a cooler. The alcohol-rich vapors pass from the stripping section to the rectification section where they are concentrated. In an aroma recovery unit, aroma components are recovered and redirected into the beer. So, through the de-alcoholization process, the alcohol level can be reduced to less than 0.1%. In trials performed by Zürcher *et al.* (2005) in an industrial vacuum evaporation plant equipped with a rectification column in which very low-alcohol concentrations are achieved, the levels of most of the aroma compounds of the de-alcoholized beer were below the detection limits. The reduction levels were influenced minimally by the temperature of the process (Table 6.6).

The quality of the separation depends on the equilibrium of the vapor and liquid phases as well as on the time that the beer is on the heat exchange surface which is minimized when the liquid layer is reduced. Thin-layer evaporators with gravimetric (falling film evaporator) or mechanically (vacuum rotation evaporator) operated surfaces are mainly used.

Thin-Layer Evaporation An example of a thin-layer evaporator is the Centritherm system (Flavourtech Company). It is a single-effect, centrifugal evaporator that operates under vacuum and uses steam as the heating medium. The heating surface is the underside of a hollow, rotating cone. The full-fermented beer enters the evaporator through a feed tube, and injection nozzles distribute the product to the heating surface. Centrifugal force instantaneously spreads the beer over the entire heating surface in an extremely thin layer (0.1 mm). The beer passes across the heating surface in less than 1 s and collects at the outer edge of the cone and then leaves the evaporator through the stationary paring tube. The product vapor removed from the extract rises through the center of the cone stack and enters an exhaust pipe that transfers it to an external condenser. Steam is supplied to the steam chamber inside each hollow cone through a hollow spindle. As the steam condenses, the condensate is immediately projected to the upper wall of the hollow steam chamber through a channel and is removed from the evaporator by way of a paring tube (Figure 6.3).

The Centritherm evaporator has minimal thermal impact compared to other types of evaporators due to its short delay time and low operating temperatures (35–60°C). The product contacts the heating surface for approximately 1 s. In other evaporation systems contact time is often greater than 30 s. The only negative aspect is the risk of oxygen being introduced into the moving system (Zufall and Wackerbauer, 2000a).

Table 6.6 Aromatic compounds and turbidity of a beer de-alcoholized by vacuum evaporation under different conditions

	Original beer	*De-alcoholized beer (53°C; 150 mbar)*	*De-alcoholized beer (38°C; 60 mbar)*
Ethanol (vol%)	5.3	0.02	0.03
Acetaldehyde (mg/l)	8.7	3.4	2.3
Propanol (mg/l)	23.4	n.d.	n.d.
Ethyl acetate (mg/l)	23.1	n.d.	n.d.
Isobutanol (mg/l)	24.3	n.d.	n.d.
Isoamyl acetate (mg/l)	2.8	n.d.	n.d.
3-methylbutanol (mg/l)	64.1	0.2	0.3
2-methylbutanol (mg/l)	22.4	Traces	0.1
Phenylethanol (mg/l)	35.9	33.6	35.1
Furfuryl alcohol (mg/l)	3.2	2.5	2.8
Diacetyl (mg/l)	0.11	0.08	0.1
DMS (μg/l)	78	n.d.	n.d.
Hexanoic acid (μg/l)	1,024	745	801
Octanoic acid (μg/l)	2,062	1,338	1,590
Decanoic acid (μg/l)	338	107	138
Dodecanoic acid (μg/l)	16.8	10.4	12.8
Ageing compounds (μg/l)	40.2	27	19.2
Turbidity (IBC)	0.3	2.3	1.2

n.d. = not detectable.
Source: Zürcher *et al.* (2005).

Falling Film Evaporator The falling film evaporator is, according to Zufall and Wackerbauer (2000a), the cheapest

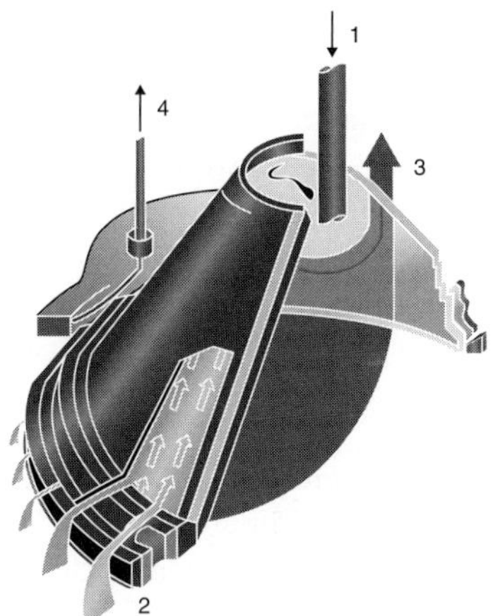

Figure 6.3 Thin-layer evaporator: Centritherm process. The full-fermented beer enters the evaporator through a feed tube and injection nozzles distribute the product to the heating surface. The beer passes across the heating surface in less than 1 s and collects at the outer edge of the cone and then leaves the evaporator through the stationary paring tube. (1) product feed; (2) steam/condensate; (3) vapor to condenser and (4) product concentrate (Centritherm process, Flavourtech., www.ft-tech.net).

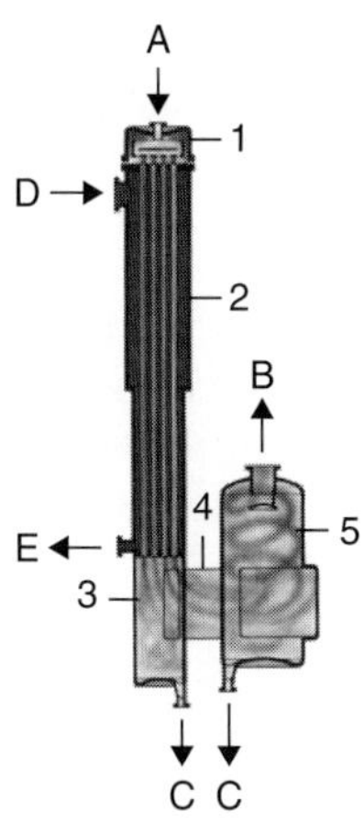

Figure 6.4 Thin-layer evaporator: falling film evaporator. In falling film evaporators, the original beer is pre-heated to boiling. Then even thin film enters the heating tubes through a distribution device in the head of the evaporator, flows downward at boiling temperature and is partially evaporated. The beer therefore has a very short product contact time, generally just a few seconds per pass. The alcohol is removed in a separator connected to the outlet of the evaporator and is finally condensed in a condenser. (1) head, (A) product, (2) calandria, (B) vapor, (3) calandria, lower part, (C) concentrate, (4) mixing channel, (D) heating steam, (5) vapor separator, (E) condensate.

technology that uses thermal processes to produce alcohol-free beer because of its simple construction and great efficiency. Investment and regular operating costs are cheaper than the thin-layer evaporator systems. They are easier to clean and there are no moving parts and no wear. In falling film evaporators the original beer is pre-heated to boiling which occurs at a lower temperature because the whole system is kept under defined vacuum conditions. Even thin film enters the heating tubes through a distribution device in the head of the evaporator, flows downward at boiling temperature and is partially evaporated. This gravity-induced downward movement is augmented by the co-current vapor flow. The beer therefore has a very short product contact time, generally just a few seconds per pass. The contact time is slightly longer than in the thin-layer evaporator. From the beginning to the end of the tube, the layer of the beer becomes thinner because the vapor mass increases while the liquid mass decreases. The alcohol is removed in a separator connected to the outlet of the evaporator and is finally condensed in a condenser (Figure 6.4).

Zufall and Wackerbauer (2000a) examined some parameters and found that conventional analysis does not show important changes, except for the ethanol content. The de-alcoholized beer has only slightly more color and slightly lower concentrations of hop-bittering substances than the original beer. The pH of the de-alcoholized beer is 0.18 higher than that of the original beer which could be due to the loss of volatile organic acids (Table 6.7).

In contrast, the aromatic substances are considerably reduced (Table 6.8).

Table 6.7 Conventional analysis before and after falling film evaporation

	Original beer	*De-alcoholized beer*
Original gravity (wt%)	11.57	4.54
Apparent extract (wt%)	1.96	3.64
Real extract (wt%)	3.75	3.76
Color (EBC)	7.00	7.75
pH	4.52	4.7
Bitter substances (EBC)	31.2	28.7
Total nitrogen (mg/l)	830	830
Coagulable nitrogen (mg/l)	24	24
Polyphenols (mg/l)	107	119
Ethanol (wt%)	4.02	0.40
Ethanol (vol%)	5.04	0.51

Note: The de-alcoholized beer obtained by falling film evaporation does not show important changes with respect to the original beer, except for the ethanol content.

Source: Zufall and Wackerbauer (2000a).

Two- or Three-Stage Falling Film Evaporator The equipment consists of two or three falling film evaporators. According to Zufall and Wackerbauer (2000a), energy can be saved with this kind of plant because the alcohol-containing vapor of the first evaporator is used as heating steam for the second, while the alcohol-containing vapor of the second evaporator is used as heating steam for the third. One disadvantage is the relatively high evaporation temperature of the first evaporator which is necessary to have enough energy for the evaporation in the last falling film evaporator. There is a significant thermal impact on the beer because the temperature of the beer in the first stage is normally about 60°C and 35–40°C in the last one.

Membrane Processes All of the membrane processes have less thermal impact on the beer (Pilipovic and Riverol, 2005). The alcohol is removed with the aid of a semipermeable membrane which separates a full-fermented beer from an alcohol-free liquid; only small molecules like ethanol and water are allowed to pass from the beer to the other liquid. The membranes are placed in modules. Generally, the membranes used are made of cellulose acetate with hollow fiber membranes or the newer spiral-wound membranes. Two types of membrane processes can be distinguished: dialysis and reverse osmosis. These systems are very expensive when alcohol is removed to a content of 0.7% by volume (Zasio, 1996).

Table 6.8 Aromatic substances before and after falling film evaporation

	Original beer	*De-alcoholized beer*
Acetaldehyde (mg/l)	1.5	1.6
n-propanol (mg/l)	7.7	0.6
Isobutanol (mg/l)	9.5	0.4
3-methylbutanol (mg/l)	15.3	0.7
2-methylbutanol (mg/l)	42.4	2.1
Phenylethanol (mg/l)	15.8	11.7
Isoamylacetate (mg/l)	1.0	<0.1
Ethylformiate	<0.1	<0.1
Ethylacetate (mg/l)	13.3	<0.1
Phenylethylacetate (mg/l)	<0.1	<0.1
Total higher aliphatic alcohols	74.9	3.8
Total esters	14.3	<0.1
Ethanol (wt%)	4.02	0.40
Ethanol (vol%)	5.04	0.51

Note: The de-alcoholized beer obtained by falling film evaporation shows a reduction of the aromatic substances with respect to the original beer (de-alcoholized beer was diluted to the original volume).

Source: Zufall and Wackerbauer (2000a).

Dialysis In a dialysis process, the exchange of substances (Bandel *et al.*, 1986) from different liquids through a semipermeable membrane occurs almost exclusively practically only by means of diffusion (Figure 6.5).

The degree of compound exchange is therefore determined by the concentration gradient at the membrane as well as by the contact time between beer and dialysate. The concentration of all the dissolved substances on both sides of the membrane try to come into equilibrium. In this case, the beer passes along a dialysis membrane at a low-pressure differential, while an alcohol-free dialysate liquid simultaneously flows in counter-current along the other side of the membrane. The principle of counter-current flow guarantees a high concentration gradient between the dialysate and the beer in terms of the alcoholic content so that an optimal diffusion can be obtained (Donhauser *et al.*, 1991). The alcohol escapes from the fermented beer through the membrane into the dialysate liquid. However, a portion of the low-molecular-weight components such as higher alcohols also diffuse with the alcohol weakens the taste of the beer. The esters and higher alcohols are almost completely eliminated (Table 6.9) and only 50% of the short-chain fatty acids remain (Table 6.10).

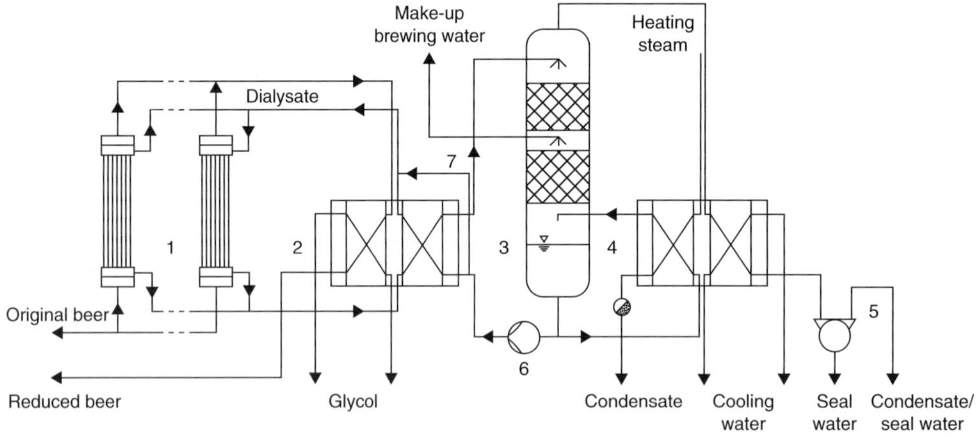

Figure 6.5 Flow diagram of the production of non-alcoholic beer by dialysis. The beer passes along a dialysis membrane at a low-pressure differential, while an alcohol-free dialysate liquid simultaneously flows in counter-current along the other side of the membrane. The alcohol escapes from the fermented beer through the membrane into the dialysate liquid. The alcohol is removed again from the alcohol-enriched dialysate in a rectification column and the dialysate is then pumped back into the module by a dialysate pump. (1) Dialysis membrane module, (2) Plate heat exchanger/low-temperature cooling plant, (3) stripper column, (4) evaporator/condenser, (5) vacuum pump, (6) dialysate pump and (7) temperature control for dialysate infeed. *Source*: Donhauser *et al.* (1991).

This loss of taste components can be prevented if the dialysate liquid has a composition similar to fully fermented beer. For example, alcohol-free beer could be used as the dialysate liquid or the dialysate could be recovered after dialysis, enriched with beer substances and then made alcohol-free in a rectification column and recirculated. On the other hand, substances from the dialysate can also pass into the beer, namely salts (sodium, calcium, nitrate) in the water which are concentrated in the dialysate during rectification and then pass into the beer during dialysis, thus increasing the final values (Donhauser *et al.*, 1991). The beer:dialysate flow ratio determines the amount of ethanol removed. US Patent 4581236 reports a beer:dialysate flow ratio of 1:0.4 that will reduce the alcohol content by 30% lowering the contents of extractive matter by about 10% only with a taste that is fully comparable to the initial beer. By lowering the throughput of beer to 1:1.2 and keeping the amount of dialysate liquid unchanged, a 65% reduction of the alcohol content is obtained, giving a so-called low-alcohol beer. If an alcohol-free beer is desired, the throughput of beer has to be reduced further. The beer: dialysate flow ratio needed is about 1:2.3, but, according to Zufall and Wackerbauer (2000b), with these proportions the efficiency of the plant decreased noticeably and the energy costs for the rectification of the dialysate increased too much. They proposed a mixed production of de-alcoholized beer by manipulated fermentation followed by removal of ethanol by dialysis to less than 0.5% (v/v) of alcohol. The body, freshness and flavor of these beers are of good quality and the production costs are reasonable. The membranes in a dialysis unit are usually hollow fiber membranes and the process fluids flow at high velocity parallel to the membrane surface. The resulting turbulent flow continuously cleans the membrane surface allowing it to be consistently permeated at the highest possible output for any given feed concentration level. The total pressure in the system is generally slightly overpressure, but it has to be increased above the saturation level of the carbon dioxide in the fully fermented beer to keep the carbon dioxide that is still in solution at the membrane surface and to prevent gas formation in the case of carbon dioxide permeating through the membrane. Carbon dioxide may be dissolved in the dialysate liquid in an amount corresponding to the amount of carbon dioxide in the fermented beer which is subjected to analysis (Bandel *et al.*, 1986). In this way, the beer leaves the dialysis plant with the normal content of carbon dioxide. In comparison with reverse osmosis, in the dialysis method there is no concentration for the beer (Zufall and Wackerbauer, 2000b), there is no post-carbonating of the alcohol-free beer, and no need of a high-pressure pump. Therefore, the costs are lower.

Table 6.9 Aromatic substances concentration in beer before and after dialysis

	Original beer	*De-alcoholized beer*
Acetaldehyde (mg/l)	5.4	3.7
n-propanol (mg/l)	9.4	0.5
Isobutanol (mg/l)	7.0	0.3
3-methylbutanol (mg/l)	9.9	0.4
2-methylbutanol (mg/l)	43.6	1.5
Isoamylacetate (mg/l)	2.2	<0.1
Ethylformiate	<0.1	<0.1
Ethyl acetate (mg/l)	12.1	<0.1
Phenylethyl acetate (mg/l)	<0.1	<0.1
Total higher aliphatic alcohols	69.9	2.7
Total esters	14.3	<0.1
Ethanol (wt%)	3.75	0.37
Ethanol (vol%)	4.80	0.47

Source: Zufall and Wackerbauer (2000b).

Table 6.10 Small-chain fatty acids concentration in beer before and after dialysis

	Original beer (mg/l)	*De-alcoholized beer (mg/l)*
i-valeric acid (I-C_5)	1.22	0.49
Valeric acid (C_5)	<0.01	<0.01
Caproic acid (C_6)	1.88	1.02
Caprylic acid (C_8)	4.61	2.55
Capric acid (C_{10})	0.35	0.21
Lauric acid (C_{12})	<0.01	<0.01
Total small-chain fatty acids	8.82	4.27
Ethanol (wt%)	3.75	0.37
Ethanol (vol%)	4.80	0.47

Source: Zufall and Wackerbauer (2000b).

Reverse Osmosis In a reverse osmosis process, the pressure differential of the different liquids is the determining factor for the passage of substances through the membrane and must be substantially higher than the osmotic pressure. An example is the Carlsberg brewery described by Von Hodenberg (1991) (Figure 6.6).

A fully fermented and filtered beer led to the reverse osmosis plant by a feed pump and a valve battery. A pressure of 40 bar is generated by a high-pressure piston pump on the side of the retentate. The beer is passed through a semipermeable membrane, that is a flat cellulose–acetate membrane installed between a spacer and a support plate. During alcohol removal, the beer (concentrate) runs between the membrane and the spacer. The alcohol–water mixture (permeate) goes through the membrane in the direction of the support plate and from there into the void area of the plate; it is then taken away by a hose. One module is made up of 380 membranes. Six modules constitute a unit in a loop. A circulating pump is installed ahead of each loop because the beer must flow past the membrane at a high velocity to avoid that substances such as proteins, α-glucans and β-glucans from being deposited on the membrane and blocking the pores or decreasing the

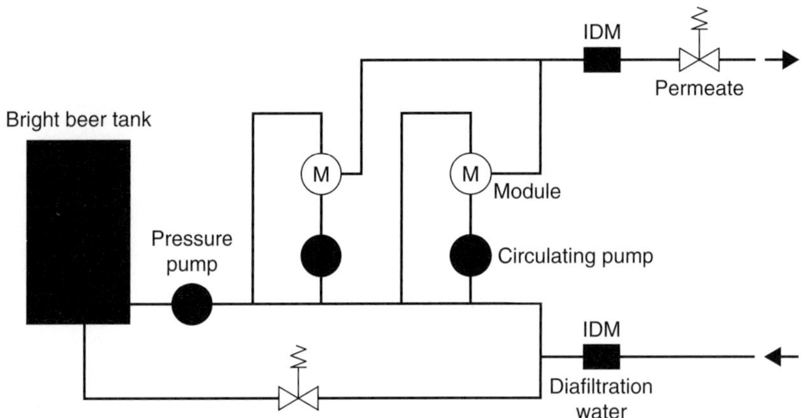

Figure 6.6 Flow diagram of the production of non-alcoholic beer by reverse osmosis. A fully fermented and filtered beer is led to the reverse osmosis plant by a feed pump and a valve battery. The beer is passed through a semi-permeable membrane. During alcohol removal, the beer (concentrate) runs between the membrane and the spacer. The alcohol–water mixture (permeate) goes through the membrane in the direction of the support plate and from there into the void area of the plate. *Source*: Von Hodenberg (1991).

flow capacity during reverse osmosis. Especially, developed cleansers and disinfectants are used to clear the membranes. Cellulose–acetate membranes can only be used in the pH 2–8 range and up to a maximum of 30°C. Careless treatment with excess temperatures or excessive pH leads to a structural change in the membrane and a change in the pores, which makes the membrane unusable. Proven cleansing agents contain β-glucanase and proteinase. Due to the high pressure, the temperature of the beer increases and ice water is used as a cooling medium. Tubular heat exchangers are used in the line downstream of the circulating pump. There are three separate phases: the concentration phase, the diafiltration phase and the make-up phase. During the concentration phase, the permeate (water, alcohol, CO_2 and aromatic substances) is removed from the beer which concentrates the beer and causes an apparent increase in the alcoholic content. At a particular concentration, the beer constituents, for example, the β-glucan gel, reduce the permeability. The following factors are responsible for this: shear forces (arising from the circulating pump), alcoholic content (higher than the original level of the starting beer) and temperature. The lower the temperature during alcohol removal, the more the β-glucan gel that is formed in conjunction with other factors. The concentration phase ends after a defined quantity of permeate is removed which is proportionally replaced by diafiltration water in the diafiltration phase. The diafiltration water has to be sterile, completely de-mineralized and have an oxygen content of less than 0.1 ppm. For storing, only CO_2 may be used as a propellant. Should air be used, oxygen would diffuse into the water by virtue of the partial pressure gradient. The carbon dioxide contained in the beer can also go through the membrane, so there has to be a pressure reducer to maintain a pressure sufficient to prevent carbon dioxide from being released into the permeate. Bubble-free permeate is required to have an accurate measurement of the quantity. This phase continues until the desired alcoholic content in the concentrate has been reached. Following this, during the make-up phase, the concentrate is brought up to the original volume of the starting beer with diafiltration water. Because of reverse osmosis and of the makeup with diafiltration water, little carbon dioxide is present in the beer, therefore carbonation to the required CO_2 level is necessary. According to Pilipovic *et al.* (2005), the reverse osmosis is not economically feasible for the production of beer with an alcohol percentage less than 0.45.

Chemical Composition and Sensorial Properties of Alcohol-Free and Low-Alcohol Beers

Chemical composition

The chemical composition of commercial alcohol-free beers is reported in Table 6.11.

The real beer extract which is usually brewed with an initial gravity of 4.13–7.4°P often remains above 4.11–6.60°P. Comparing alcohol-free beer and lager beer, however, is complex. Alcohol-free beer has no more than 0.1% ethanol but contains dextrins and fermentable sugars. Lager beer usually contains around 5% ethanol, residual dextrins up to 3°P, but no more fermentable sugars if attenuation is complete (Perpete and Collins, 2000; Floridi *et al.*, 2001). The alcohol-free beers have a higher pH than regular beers. The beers obtained using special yeasts have less bitter substances (EBU) than the beer obtained with arrested fermentation and they have a high concentration of DMS.

Table 6.11 Conventional analysis of commercial alcohol-free beers. Minimum, maximum and average values

	Minimum	*Maximum*	*Average*
Original gravity (wt%)	4.13	7.42	6.63
Ethanol (wt%)	0.01	0.54	0.30
Apparent extract (wt%)	4.11	6.43	5.82
Real extract (wt%)	4.11	6.60	6.03
Attenuation (wt%)	0.5	18	12
Color (EBC)	6.6	11.5	8.6
pH	4.25	5.10	4.59
Bitter substances (EBC)	12.1	29.1	22.9
DMS (μg/l)	10	60	28
Acetoin (mg/l)	1.80	9.00	4.70
Total diacetyl (mg/l)	0.04	1.4	0.24
2,3-pentadione (mg/l)	Traces	0.06	0.03

Note: Alcohol-free beer has no more than 0.1% ethanol and attenuation average of 12 wt%. The alcohol-free beers have a higher pH than regular beers with value of 4.59.

Source: Narziss *et al.* (1992).

Sensorial properties

The sensorial properties of an alcohol-free beer are quite different from a full-fermented beer because alcohol is an important flavor contributor. Notwithstanding, alcohol-free beers are of good quality even if they have worty off-flavors and lack the pleasant fruity or ester aroma found in regular beers. Such defects in the process of manipulated fermentation may be due to a fermentation procedure that fails to reduce the chemical compounds responsible for the worty flavor and to produce fusel alcohol and esters. Several carbonyl compounds may contribute to the worty off-flavor, while esters are known to impart the fruity flavor to regular beers. A comparison of the ester and fusel alcohol concentrations of regular and alcohol-free beers shows that alcohol-free beers have little fruity aroma (Perpete and Collin, 1994). The total ester content is below 1 ppm after CCP fermentation (Schur, 1983) (Table 6.12).

S. cerevisiae usually produce high levels of estery flavors. The final level in the end product depends on factors such as high sugar concentrations, temperature increases and low oxygen level. The acetate esters, such as ethyl acetate and isoamyl acetate, are synthesized by alcoholysis of acetyl-coenzyme A (CoA) which is closely linked to the metabolism of lipids. The production of acetate ester is low during the growth phase when lipids are accumulated and is enhanced as the acetyl-CoA increases during the stationary phase. During the production of alcohol-free beer with immobilized *S. cerevisiae* at a temperature of 12°C, the production rate of ethyl acetate is 2–4 times higher compared to rates at 2°C. The beer flavor is strongly affected by the amount of acetalactate because during storage it is converted into a diacetyl that gives a strong off-flavor. At a temperature of 12°C a high level of acetalactate is produced in a short time. An optimal and constant alcohol-free beer profile can be achieved by introducing a regular aerobic period to stimulate yeast growth. Temperature can be used to control the rate of growth and the rate of flavor formation (Van Iersel *et al.*, 1999). Wort carbonyl compounds have long been considered responsible for worty aroma in alcohol-free beer. The main carbonyl compounds present in wort are formed by three different reactions: Maillard reactions between amino acids and sugar, Strecker degradation of amino acids and degradation of lipids (Debourg *et al.*, 1994). During the production of alcohol-free beer, wort aldehydes are reduced by the activity of alcohol dehydrogenases of the yeast (Table 6.13).

Isobutanal, 3- and 2-methylbutanal are reduced by alcohol dehydrogenases and aldehyde dehydrogenase using either NADH or NADPH as cofactors. There is

Table 6.12 Concentration (ppb) of fusel alcohols and esters in a CCP before and after fermentation

Compounds	*Initial concentration*	*Final concentration*
Isobutanol	150	350
Isopentanol	180	380
2-phenylethanol	210	130
Isoamyl acetate	0	70
Ethyl butyrate	0	10
Ethyl caprylate	0	60
Ethyl caprylate	0	75
Isoamyl caproate	0	6
Phenylethylacetate	0	6
Total	540	1,102

Note: The concentration of esters and fusel alcohols in the CCP increases during the fermentation. The total ester level after fermentation is below 1 ppm.

Source: Schur (1983).

Table 6.13 Concentration (ppb) and reduction of carbonyl compounds during a CCP fermentation[a] and immobilized yeast/CCP fermentation[b]

Compounds	*Initial concentration*	*Final concentration*	*% Reduction*
Furfural[a]	480	280	42
Benzaldehyde[a]	12	8	33
Methional[a]	18	8	55
Trans-2 nonenal[a]	12	Traces	99
Pentanal[a]	13	11	15
2-hexenal[a]	5	2	60
2-octenal[a]	2	Traces	99
2-methylbutanal[b]	87.4	19.1	77.9
3-methylbutanal[b]	344	101.2	70
Heptanal[b]	7.6	3.9	49

Note: The concentration of several carbonyl compounds decreases during CCP fermentation and immobilized yeast/CCP fermentation because of their reduction by alcohol dehydrogenases and aldeyde dehydrogenase using either NADH or NADPH as cofactors.

Source: [a]Schur (1983) and [b]Collin *et al.* (1991).

a 77.9% and 70% reduction of 3-methylbutanal and 2-methylbutanal, respectively, but worty flavor imparting compounds remain after fermentation. The worty off-flavor of alcohol-free beers produced by a CCP was attributed to insufficient aldehyde reduction by yeast enzymes due to a limited fermentation. It appears, however, that perception of the aldehydes responsible for the worty flavor is influenced by the medium. In a typical lager beer, ethanol increases aldehyde retention, while in alcohol-free beers, both the absence of ethanol and the higher sugar level could strengthen worty off-flavors (Perpete and Collin, 2000). On the other hand, beers gently de-alcoholized by thermal and membrane processes do not have any off-flavor, except the mild caramel aroma when a thermal process is used. Moreover, they are characterized by the loss of flavor and body. Only an unpleasant sourness was noted in the case of the alcohol-free beer produced by dialysis. Of prime importance is the quality of the original beer (Zürcher *et al.*, 2005). All of the above-mentioned techniques are used and the combination of manipulated fermentation with a process which removes alcohol from a slightly fermented beer can produce very good results.

Technological Evaluation

The biological methods used to produce alcohol-free beers do not usually require an extra plant or process, but rather a more accurate control (Perpete and Collin, 1999). It is extremely important to control the fermentation to prevent an overproduction of alcohol. The use of special yeasts (e.g. *S. Ludwigii*) requires a particular attention to avoid yeast contamination of either the special yeast or the normal brewery yeast. On the other hand, the physical methods require another step in the process which increases the cost for equipment and management (energy and water service). The thermal methods produce an alcohol-free beer with up to 0.05% alcohol by volume, but the colloidal stability of this product is less than the beers made with membrane processes. Furthermore, they have a light caramel flavor due to the thermal impact and a high value of the tiobarbituric acid number. The thermal methods are less selective than membrane methods because they eliminate all of the volatile compounds which can then be recovered by rectification and redirected into the alcohol-free beer. The flavors of beers produced by membrane processes have less body and a low aromatic profile, while the beers obtained by biological methods have a sweet and worty off-flavor.

Summary Points

- There are several different ways to intend "low-alcohol" and "alcohol-free" beers.
- The production of "low-alcohol" and "alcohol-free" beers has different regulation in different countries, therefore the composition of these beers could change from country to country.
- Table 6.1 reports some data related to alcohol content and energy in beers from different countries.
- Over the last few years, biological and physical methods have been developed for the production of low-alcohol or alcohol-free beer.
- The main biological processes include: (1) use of special yeasts (*S. ludwigii*); (2) arrested fermentation and (3) CCP.
- The physical processes include thermal and membrane processes such as: (1) thin-layer evaporation; (2) falling film vacuum evaporation; (3) continuous vacuum rectification; (4) reverse osmosis and (5) dialysis.
- Less used processes include pervaporation, freeze concentration, extraction processes, such as extraction with organic solvents and extraction with carbon dioxide, as well as adsorption on special kieselgels or on special adsorbent resins.
- Alternative techniques for producing beer with a reduced ethanol content include the use of genetically modified yeast strain that forms less ethanol during complete fermentation of worth.
- Technologically, it is possible to produce beer with less than 0.05% (v/v) of alcohol. The alcohol concentration of beer obtained from the different methods is reported in Table 6.2.
- A common chemical composition of commercial alcohol-free beers is reported in Table 6.11.
- The biological methods used to produce alcohol-free beers do not usually require an extra plant or process, but they need a more accurately controlled process. It is extremely important to control the fermentation to prevent an overproduction of alcohol.
- The use of special yeasts (e.g. *S. Ludwigii*) requires a particular attention to avoid yeast contamination of either the special yeast or the normal brewery yeast.
- The physical methods require another step in the process which increases the cost for equipment and management (energy and water service).
- The thermal methods produce an alcohol-free beer with up to 0.05% alcohol by volume, but the colloidal stability of this product is less than the beers made with membrane processes. Furthermore, they have a light caramel flavor due to the thermal impact and have a high level of tiobarbituric acid.
- The thermal methods are less selective than membrane methods because they eliminate all volatile compounds which can then be recovered by rectification and redirected into the alcohol-free beer.
- The flavors of beers produced by membrane processes have less body and a low aromatic profile, while the beers obtained by biological methods have a sweet and worty off-flavor.

Acknowledgments

The authors thank to Eng. Giorgio Zasio and the Italian Beer and Malt Industries Association (ASSOBIRRA) for the help received in collecting and showing several data reported. Moreover, we greatly thank Dr. Giuseppe Ambrosio, Head of the "Department for Development Policy" of "Italian Ministry of Agriculture, Food and Forestry Policies" for his precious help in founding and explaining many specific laws.

References

API Schmidt-Bretten, Entalkoholisierungsanlagen, Firmenschrift Nr. 372, 10/2004.

Bandel, W., Schmitz, F.J., Ostertag, K., Garske, F. and Breidohr, H.G. (1986). US Patent 4581236.

Baron, G.V. and Willaert, R.G. (2004). Cell immobilization in preformed porous matrices. In Nedovic, V. and Willaert, R. (eds), *Fundamentals of Cell Immobilization Biotechnology*, pp. 229–244. Kluwer Academic Publishers, Dordrecht, The Netherlands.

Bony, M., Thines-Sempoux, D., Barre, P. and Blondin, B. (1997). *J. Bacteriol.* 179, 4929–4936.

Caluwaerts, H.J.J. (1995). US Patent 5384135.

Collin, S., Montesinos, M., Meersman, E., Swinkels, W. and Doufour, I.P. (1991). *Proceedings of the 23rd European Brewery Convention Congress*. IRL Press, Oxford, UK, pp. 409–416.

Debourg, A., Layrent, M., Goossens, E., Borremans, E., Van De Winkel, L. and Masschelein, C.A. (1994). *J. Am. Soc. Brew. Chem.* 52, 100–106.

Donhauser, S., Glas, K. and Müller, O. (1991). *Brauwelt International.* 139–144.

Flavoutech. www.ft-tech.net (angulted data 22 October 2006).

Floridi, S., Miniati, E., Montanari, L. and Fantozzi, P. (2001). *Monatsschr. für Brauwiss* 9/10, 209–215.

Huige, N.J., Sanchez, G.W. and Leiding, A.R. (1990). US Patent 4970082.

Karel, S.F., Libicki, S.B. and Robertson, C.R. (1985). *Chem. Eng. Sci.* 40, 1321–1354.

Kunze, W. (2004). *Technology of Brewing and Malting*. VLB, Berlin.

Montanari, L., Floridi, S., Marconi, O., Tironzelli, M. and Fantozzi, P. (2005). *Eur. Food Res. Technol.* 221, 175–179.

Muller, R. (1991). *J. Inst. Brew.* 97, 85–92.

Muller, R. (2000). *J. Inst. Brew.* 97, 85–92; *Enzyme Microb. Technol.* 27, 337–344.

Munroe, J.H. (1995). Fermentation. In: Hardwick, W.A. (ed.), *Handbook of Brewing*, pp. 323–353. Marcel Dekker, New York.

Narziss, L., Miedaner, H., Kern, E. and Leibhard, M. (1992). *Brauwelt Int.* 4, 396–410.

Nevoigt, E., Pilger, R., Mast-Gerlach, E., Schmidt, U., Freihammer, S., Eschenbrenner, M., Garbe, L. and Stahl, Ulf. (2002). *FEMS Yeast Res.* 2, 225–232.

Perpete, P. and Collin, S. (1994). *Proceedings of the VI J. De Clerck Chair, Leuven* 1, 27–33.

Perpete, P. and Collin, S. (1999). *Cerevisia* 1, 27–33.

Perpete, P. and Collin, S. (2000). *Food Chem.* 70, 457–462.

Pilipovic, M.V. and Riverol, C. (2005). *J. Food Eng.* 69, 437–441.

Schur, F. (1983). *Proceedings of the 19th European Brewery Convention Congress*, IRL Press, Oxford, UK, pp. 353–360.

Schur, F. and Sauer, P. (1990). US Patent 4971807.

Scott, J.A. and Huxtable, S.M. (1995). *J. Appl. Symp.* 79, 19–28.

The Brewers of Europe (2004). *Statements in Relation to Alcohol Content and Energy Content.*

Van Dieren, B. (1995). *EBC Symposium "Immobilised Yeast Applications in the Brewery Industry," Monograph XXIV, October 1995.* Verlag Hans Carl Getranke – Fachverlag, pp. 66–76. Espoo, Finland Nürnberg, Germany.

Van Iersel, M.F.M., Meersman, E., Swinkels, W., Abee, T. and Rombouts, F.M. (1995). *J. Ind. Microbiol.* 14, 495–501.

Van Iersel, M.F.M., Van Dieren, B., Rombouts, F.M. and Abee, T. (1999). *Enzyme Microb. Technol.* 24, 407–411.

Van Iersel, M.F.M., Brouwer-Post, E., Rombouts, F.M. and Abee, T. (2000). *Enzyme Microb. Technol.* 26, 602–607.

Verbelen, P.J., de Schutter, D.P., Delvaux, F., Verstrepen, K.J. and Delvaux, F.R. (2006). *Biotechnol. Lett.* 28, 1515–1525.

Von Hodenberg, G.W. (1991). *Brauwelt Int.* 2, 145–149.

Younis, O.S. and Stewart, G.G. (1999). *J. Am. Brew. Chem.* 57, 39–45.

Zasio, G. (1996). *Tecnologie Alimentari.* 2, 114–118.

Zufall, C. and Wackerbauer, K. (2000a). *Monatsschrift f. Brauwiss* 53, 124–137.

Zufall, C. and Wackerbauer, K. (2000b). *Monatsschrift f. Brauwiss* 53, 164–179.

Zürcher, A., Jakob, M. and Back, W. (2005). *Proceedings of the 30th EBC Congress*, Prague, 240–248.

7

Yeast Diversity in the Brewing Industry

Linda Hellborg and Jure Piškur Department of Cell and Organism Biology, Lund University, Lund, Sweden

Abstract

Yeast strains involved in the fermentation greatly influence the beer characteristics. The importance of these unicellular organisms for beer industry is due to their ability to ferment various substrates into ethanol and secondary metabolites. The variation in nature is enormous with over 1,000 different yeast species recognized and many more strains. Taking this into account the possibility of forming even new variants in the laboratory is immense. The best characterized yeast is *Saccharomyces cerevisiae*, and it is also the most common top-fermenting brewer's yeast. The most common bottom-fermenting lager yeast is *Saccharomyces pastorianus*, a hybrid between *Saccharomyces cerevisiae* and *Saccharomyces bayanus* – like yeast. The genomes from these two yeasts and around 20 other yeasts have now been fully sequenced, and a few more are partially done. From these sequences different post-genomics tools have been derived and can now be used, in combination with other genetic and molecular biology tools, to study and manipulate certain yeast traits that are important for beer industry.

List of Abbreviations

ARS	Autonomous replicating sequence
C	Cytosine
DNA	Deoxyribonucleic acid
GMO	Gene modified organisms
G	Guanine
mRNA	Messenger RNA
mtDNA	mitochondrial DNA
NADH	Reduced form of nicotinamide adenine dinucleotide
rDNA	Ribosomal DNA
SHAM	Salicylhydroxamic acid

Introduction

The change from hunters to farmers approximately 10,000 years ago was one of the largest evolutionary steps for mankind and made our lifestyle of today possible. This step included growing cereals and developing two of the oldest food technologies that we still use today, baking and brewing. The brewing technology provided early societies with a nutritious and relatively safe drink that also acted as an intoxicant. The necessary ingredient for both baking and brewing is unicellular yeast. Yeasts are therefore one of the earliest domesticated species (Fay and Benavides, 2005). Chemical tests of ancient pottery jars reveal that a fermented beverage of rice, honey and fruit was made in China 7000 before Christ (BC). This was refined into different beverages fermented from different raw materials and described in the earliest texts from the Shang and Zhou Dynasty, in China 1200–200 BC. Residues from wine have also been found on pottery from Egypt dating back to 3150 BC (Cavalieri *et al.*, 2003; McGovern *et al.*, 2004). Beer was also brewed in Mesopotamia 3000 BC, but not until first century AD in Europe (Corran, 1975).

In the mid-1600 Antoine van Leuwenhoek made the first observation of yeast cells, but the importance of yeast in the food and beverage industries was not realized until 200 years later (1850–1900). Scientists like Louis Pasteur (1822–1895), Hermann Emil Fisher (1852–1919) and Emil Christian Hansen (1842–1909), and their discoveries on yeast have importantly influenced the modern brewing industry (reviewed in Barnett, 2000).

Louis Pasteur, a French chemist and biologist, solved the mysteries of rabies, anthrax, chicken cholera and silkworm diseases, and contributed to the development of the first vaccines. He also discovered that fermentation is caused by microorganisms and thereby contributed a scientific explanation for wine making and brewing of beer. This insight led to the process of pasteurization (as reviewed by Barnett, 2003).

Emil Fischer was a German chemist and the founder of carbohydrate chemistry in the late nineteenth century. His father had a brewery in Dortmund, where young Emil Fischer made his first experiments with beer yeast to ferment different sugars. He as well as Louis Pasteur found that yeast utilized only one of the two optical forms of sugar, and Emil Fischer also discovered that different yeasts fermented different sugars. This led to his famous conclusion about enzyme and corresponding substrate that have to fit like a lock and key to affect each other. He also speculated about differentiation of main keys and special keys referring to enzymes with a broad and narrow substrate range (reviewed in Barnett, 2003).

Beer in Health and Disease Prevention
ISBN: 978-0-12-373891-2

Emil Christian Hansen, a Danish biologist, was employed by the Carlsberg Laboratories in Copenhagen. He discovered a way to isolate and culture a pure yeast strain, and by this method he described a number of new yeast species. He also developed a standardized procedure of using clones from bottom-fermenting yeast in the production of beer. A clone isolated from the Carlsberg brewery called Carlsberg bottom yeast no. 1 gave consistently good beer (Barnett and Lichtenthaler, 2001). *This yeast has become known as Saccharomyces carlsbergensis* but its "true" name is *Saccharomyces pastorianus* (Kurtzman and Robnett, 1998).

Yeast Biodiversity

Yeasts are unicellular fungi (Figure 7.1a) that can be classified into two phylogenetic groups: ascomycetous yeasts and basidiomycetous yeasts. Phylogenetics is derived from Greek *phylon* = tribe, race and *genetikos* = relative to birth, from *genesis* = birth, and is the study of evolutionary relatedness among various groups of organisms. The distinction between the two groups of fungi is not easy if they do not reproduce sexually. In the old days these yeast were called fungi imperfecti. Ascomycetous yeasts produce sexually by forming asci (sing. ascus), sacks where the spores are produced by a simple meios like the bakers yeast (*Saccharomyces cerevisiae*). The Basidiomycetes on the other hand produce basidia (sing. basidium), which are the cells on which sexual spores are produced. There is a great range of variation in morphology of the basidium, the number of spores formed and how the spores are borne on the surface of the basidium (Ingold, 1991). The two phyla separated from each other probably over 1,000 million years ago (Ma) (Heckman *et al.*, 2001). The per cent of the two bases guanine (G) and cytosine (C) in the nuclear deoxyribonucleic acid (DNA) is very different where ascomycetous yeast strains have a gas chromatography (GC) content between 28% and 50% and Basidiomycetes range from 50% to 70% (Price *et al.*, 1978; Kurtzman and Phaff, 1987) (Figure 7.1b).

Today the classification is made by sequence analysis of a region in ribosomal DNA (rDNA). A major advantage of rDNA is that it is present in all living organisms, has a

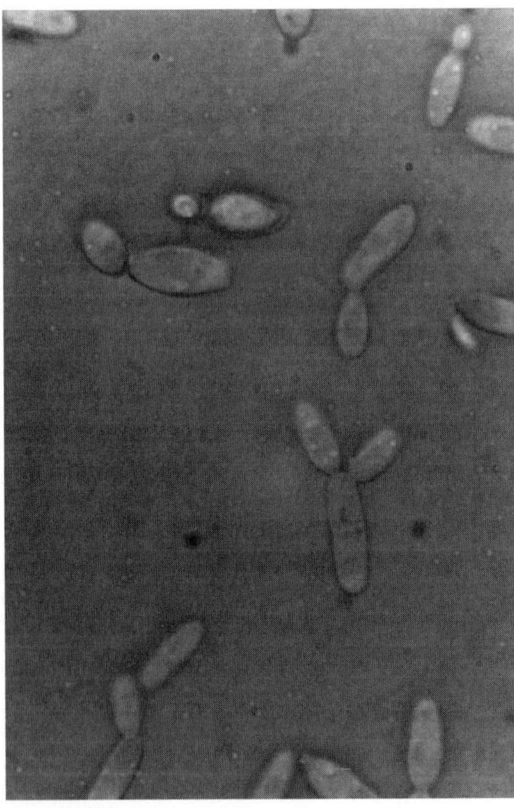

Figure 7.1a Cells from a wine-spoilage yeast *Dekkera bruxellensis*, which is also found in some Belgian beers (kindly provided by A. Merico and C. Compagno).

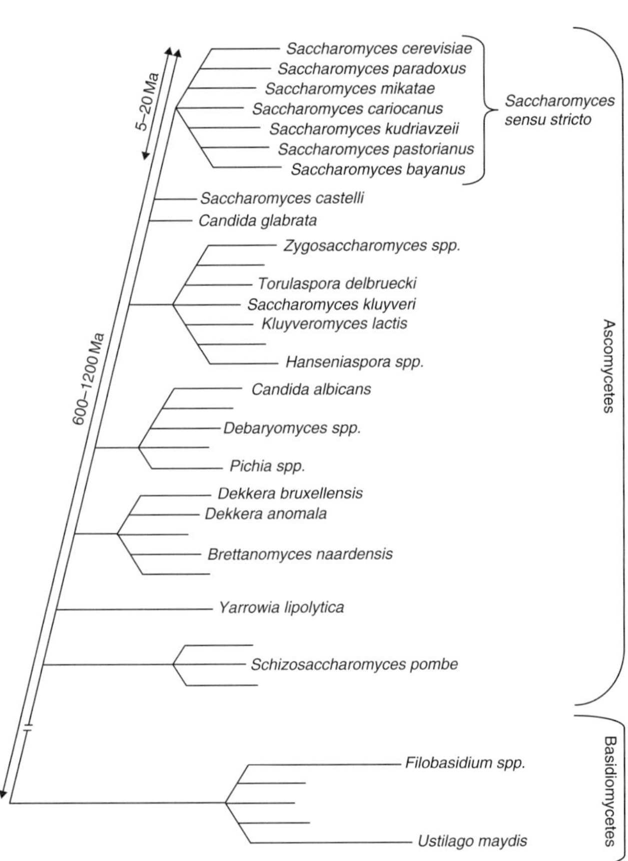

Figure 7.1b A simplified phylogenetic tree of yeast and some other fungi representing the species mentioned in this chapter. The empty branches are a reminder of known species omitted from the figure. The numbers on the vertical branch indicate times of divergence of the species indicated by the arrows. *Source*: Adapted from Kurtzman and Phaff (1987), Heckman *et al.* (2001), Kellis *et al.* (2003), Kurtzman and Robnett (2003), Kurtzman and Fell (2006) and Woolfit *et al.*, 2007.

common evolutionary origin, occurs in multiple copies and is easy to sequence because primer pairs for conserved regions can generally be used for all organisms. It has been suggested that in fungi the intraspecies (within a species) differences are between 0 and 3 bases per 600 nucleotides (0–0.5%) and a strain differing in more than 6 bases (1%) is considered a separate species (Kurtzman and Robnett, 1998; Fell *et al.*, 2000). Intermediate base substitutions are showing the intermediates between subspecies and fully recognized species. Given time these could evolve to a true species level. With this classification system the number of recognized species of fungi has increased and during the last years doubled the number of recognized yeast species. Although more than 1,000 species of ascomycetous yeast and over 30,000 species of basidiomycetous yeast have been described, it is likely that they are just the top of the iceberg constituting less than 1% of the natural flora. This assumption can be inferred from the high frequency of long single-species branches in the phylogenetic tree implying that there are a lot of genera and species missing (Figure 7.1b) (Kurtzman and Fell, 2006).

One of the best studied eukaryotes is *S. cerevisiae.* Its genome together with its closest relatives has been sequenced and form a group of their own called the *Saccharomyces sensu stricto.* They are supposed to have diverged from each other between 5 and 20 Ma (Kellis *et al.*, 2003). In this group three of the most important species for the beer industry are found: *S. cerevisiae*, *S. bayanus* and a hybrid, *S. pastorianus.* In this group, gene transfer and hybridization between different species is possible, resulting in new variants (Marinoni *et al.*, 1999). The progress of classifying old species and the discovery of new ones has led to many changes in the taxonomy, and a considerable number of species has recently been renamed.

Comparative genomics

Comparative genomics is a branch of genetics that is becoming more and more useful and sophisticated thanks to the growing number of DNA sequences from different organisms. By 2006 the complete sequences of more than 400 genomes have become available, and some 1,600 additional genomes are currently being sequenced. The number of sequenced yeast genomes is increasing strongly due to the industrial and scientific importance of this group of organisms and also because of their small genome sizes (Axelson-Fisk and Sunnerhagen, 2006). Within these sequences lie answers to questions on biological features, the evolution of species and their phylogenetic relation to other organisms. The quest for the "Tree of Life" in which all organisms on earth today will find their ancestors and be connected to one another biologically is getting closer. However, it is complicated by the fact that yeast and bacteria can transfer genetic material between very distantly related species, invalidating previous simple assumptions on the inheritance of a gene (Rokas, 2006). These horizontally transferred DNA fragments could be very important, such as the *URA1* gene coding for dihydroorotate dehydrogenase in *S. cerevisiae,* which allows its owner to live almost without oxygen and thereby promote the development into good brewing strains (Nagy *et al.*, 1992; Gojkovic *et al.*, 2004). Genetic material can also be transferred between much more closely related species, as seen in the *Saccharomyces sensu stricto* group, which will be described later.

Large-scale comparisons of genomes (Sunnerhagen and Piskur, 2006 and references cited therein) can also suggest answers to many basic questions about genes, like the number of functional genes in a species, identification of species-specific genes, distribution of genes among functional families, gene density, preservation of gene order, mechanisms of genome reshuffling, the rate of sequence divergence, etc. The sequence of a gene determines also its function, and generally, the more similar the sequences, the more similar are the functions. By comparing an unknown sequence from a gene to already annotated gene sequences, the function can be distinguished. In this way a lot of experimental work is reduced.

In 2006, more than 20 different yeast species had been fully sequenced, and the sequences had been published (Sunnerhagen and Piskur, 2006). Apart from yeast a few other fungi have been sequenced. The first genome to be fully sequenced in 1996 was that of *S. cerevisiae.* In the *Saccharomyces sensu stricto* group, *S. paradoxus*, *S. mikatae*, *S. bayanus* and *S. kudriavzevii* are now also completely sequenced. From the rest of the Ascomycete group we can find the whole genome sequences from *S. castelli*, *Candida albicans*, *Candida glabrata*, *Yarrowia lipolytica*, *Debaryomyces hansenii*, *Kluyveromyces lactis*, *Kluyveromyces waltii*, *Hansenula polymorpha*, *Ashbya gossypii*, *Aspergillus nidulans*, *Giberella zea*, *Magnaporthe grisea*, *Neurospora crassa* and *Schizosaccharomyces pombe.* In Basidiomycetes three genome sequences are currently available, from *Phanerochaete chrysosporium*, *Ustilago maydis* and *Cryptococcus neoformans.* The genome size is between 8.7 Mb in *A. gossypii* and 38.9 Mb in *N. crassa.* The number of genes is correlated with genome size and is found to be between 4,718 in *A. gossypii* and 10,082 in *N. crassa* (reviewed in Axelson-Fisk and Sunnerhagen, 2006). *S. cerevisiae* has a genome size of 12.5 Mb divided into approximately 5,777 genes and intergenic regions (Goffeau *et al.*, 1996). The genome sequences are a strong basis for development of a wide array of tools, including tools for manipulation of the corresponding yeasts.

Comparative genomics is also a very good tool to elucidate evolutionary events, like the whole genome duplication in an ancestor of the *Saccharomyces* clade and the subsequent loss and refinements of pathways leading to the species of today (see Figure 7.2) (Piskur *et al.*, 2006).

Why are they here to serve us?

At the end of the Cretaceous age 140–64 Ma, an excess of different fruits developed, and with them an increased amounts of sugars. These sugars, mostly hexoses (C_6), were used as substrates by many microbes (Friis and Crepet, 1987). The ability of some microorganism to ferment these sugars into ethanol, a two-carbon molecule (C_2), plus carbon dioxide, coupled with a high ethanol tolerance, was probably a winning strategy to inhibit the growth

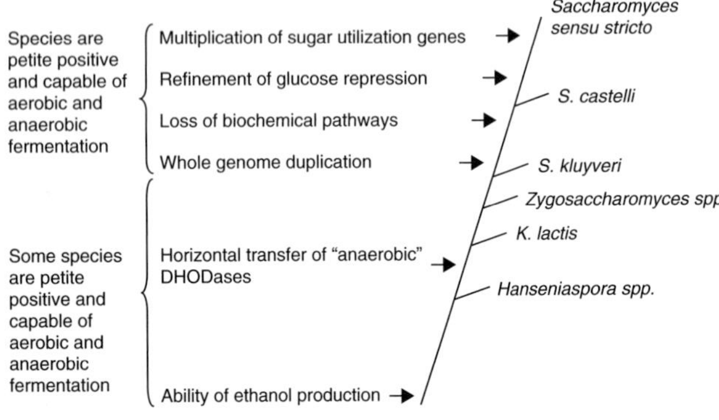

Figure 7.2 Evolutionary tree of important genomic events in Saccharomycetae. *Source*: Modified from Piskur and Langkjaer (2004) and Merico *et al*. (2007).

of competing organisms by high ethanol concentrations (Piskur *et al.*, 2006 and references cited therein). This feature was invented by ancestors of *Saccharomyces* yeasts (see Figure 7.3). However, the degradation of glucose to ethanol instead of a full oxidation to carbon dioxide (CO_2) and water is a very inefficient use of the carbon source. This "peculiarity" is circumvented by a change in the metabolism called the diauxic shift. This strategy involves shifting substrate from glucose to ethanol when the consumption of hexoses has depleted the sugar storage and generated ethanol instead. The accumulated ethanol is now "digested" (the "make-accumulate-consume" strategy) and oxidized into CO_2 (Pronk *et al.*, 1996; Johnston, 1999; Verstrepen *et al.*, 2004).

The ability to produce ethanol in an anaerobic (absence of oxygen) environment is probably a very old trait, originating more than 200 Ma before the yeast lineage (Ascomycetes) diverged. All studied yeasts belonging to Ascomycetes have both the genes responsible for consuming ethanol and also the reverse reaction, production of ethanol in the absence of oxygen. In the presence of oxygen the respiratory pathway can oxidize the sugars to CO_2.

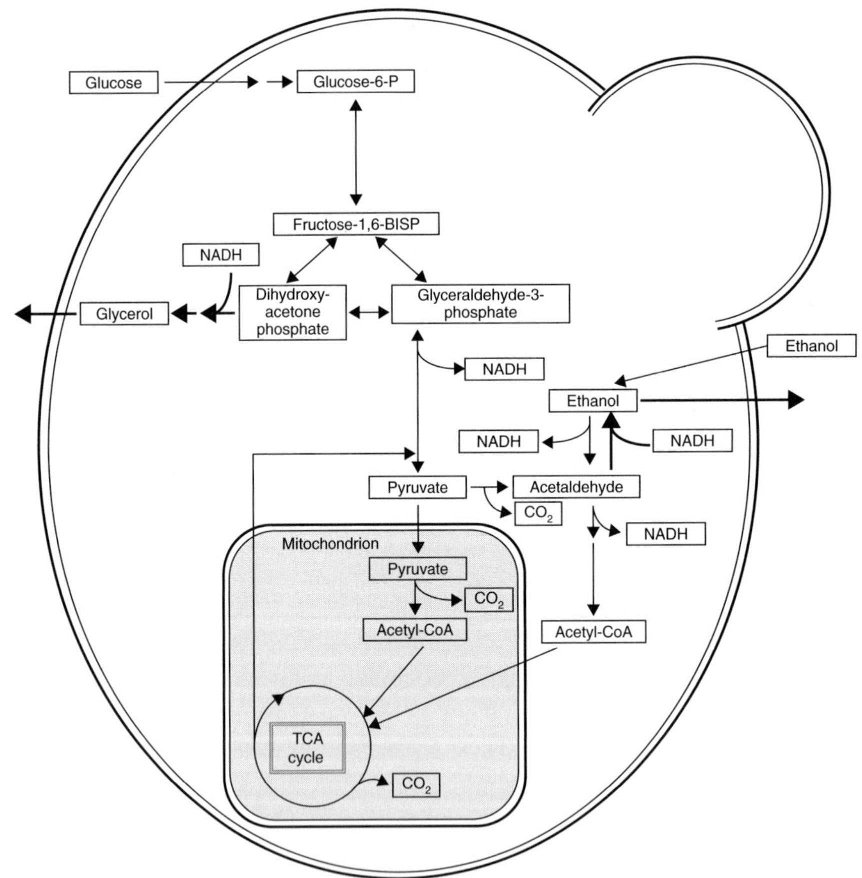

Figure 7.3 Pathways involved in glucose and ethanol assimilation under aerobic conditions, underlining the differences between a Crabtree-negative yeast *Kluyveromyces lactis* (thin arrows), which degrades hexoses directly to CO_2, and a Crabtree-positive yeast, *Saccharomyces cerevisiae* (thin and thick arrows), which can accumulate ethanol. P: phosphate; TCA cycle: tri-carboxylic acid cycle. *Source*: Modified from Piskur *et al.* (2006).

But some yeast lineages, like the *Saccharomyces sensu stricto* group, have developed the ability to suppress the respiratory metabolism in the presence of glucose and oxygen, and can thereby accumulate ethanol even under aerobic conditions. This feature is called the Crabtree effect, and all organisms capable of it are called Crabtree positive (De Deken, 1966).

Species Involved in Brewing

Traditionally ale and lager yeast were differentiated by the ability to ferment melibiose, and whether the yeast was at the top (top fermenting) or the bottom (bottom fermenting) of the fermentation tank after the primary fermentation (see Table 7.1). The lager yeasts produced the extracellular enzyme melibiase (α-galactosidase), which catalyzes the hydrolysis of melibiose into galactose and glucose. The lager yeasts could thereby ferment melibiose, whereas ale strains did not (Tornai-Lehoczki and Dlauchy, 2000; Hornsey, 2004). The ale yeasts used to be all top-fermenting yeasts, where the yeast cells flocculated and floated on the top of the fermentation tank and could easily be removed by carefully scraping them off the surface. These yeasts are mostly closely related to *S. cerevisiae*. The lager brewing yeasts are hybrids between *S. cerevisiae* and other *Saccharomyces* species and usually called *Saccharomyces pastorianus*. They flocculate and sink to the bottom, thereby the name bottom fermenting (Vaughan-Martini and Martini, 1987).

The fermenting temperatures of ales are between 15°C and 23°C, and lager beers has a primary fermentation at 7–12°C and a long second fermentation between 4°C and 7°C. The long second fermentation in lager is the "lagering phase" where the beer clears and mellows resulting in a "crisper" and "cleaner" tasting beer.

The yeast chosen for ale production:

1. ferments more quickly than lager yeasts;
2. converts less sugar to alcohol, which results in a sweeter and fuller body;
3. produces esters, which usually add a fruity taste;
4. produces diacetyl, which provides the beer with a buttery taste.

Table 7.1 Traditional differences in production of lager and ale

	Lager	*Ale*
Yeast species used	*S. pastorianus*	*S. cerevisiae*
Hops used	Yes	No (till seventeenth century)
Ferment meliobiose	Yes	No
Fermenting temperature	4–12°C	14–25°C
Collection of yeast	Bottom	Top
"Taste"	"Clean" beer	Flavor compounds produced

Source: Tornai-Lehoczki and Dlauchy (2000) and Hornsey (2004).

Today 99% of all beer is lager and only 1% is ale, and the brewing yeasts are mainly selected for their uptake capabilities of carbohydrates and other compounds and the conversion of these compounds into alcohol, energy and aroma compounds. Other features that are selected for are the sedimentation characteristics, stress response, vitality and viability. This has led to an almost never-ending search for the ultimate strain, in which certain properties are optimized for different beer characteristics.

Saccharomyces sensu stricto

This group includes *S. bayanus*, *S. cariocanus*, *S. cerevisiae*, *S. kudriavzevii*, *S. mikatae* and *S. paradoxus* (Kurtzman and Robnett, 2003) and are by far the most used in the brewing industry. They have several properties that make them outstanding for industrial use and especially the brewing industry, including fast growth, good ability to produce ethanol and a tolerance for several environmental stresses, such as high ethanol concentration and low oxygen levels (as reviewed by Piskur and Langkjaer, 2004). Within this group, hybridization between two or more species is common, resulting in new sets of genes and new metabolic characteristics (see Figure 7.4a). Rainieri *et al.* (2006) tested different strains isolated from beer and compared the genomes to

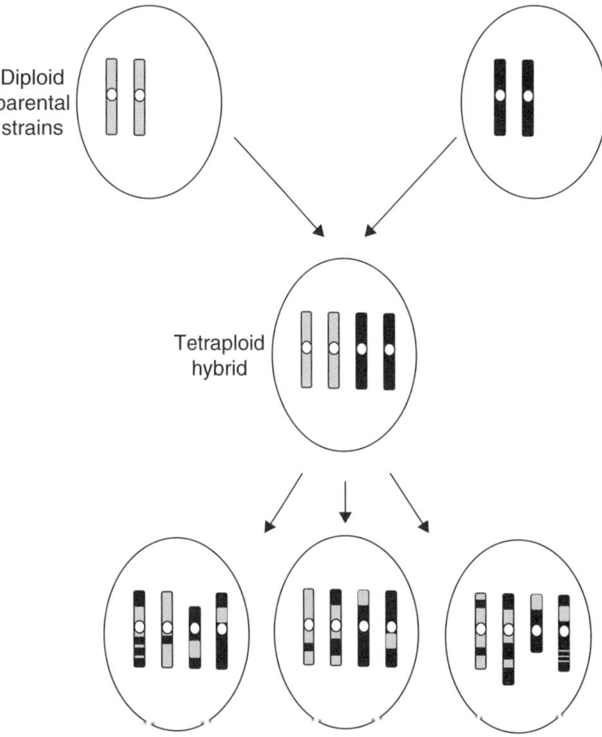

Figure 7.4a Hybridization between two diploid yeast cells forming an allotetraploid progeny and its possible further evolution by genetic events such as homologous recombination, chromosomal translocation, inversion, deletion, duplication and other mutations, making lineages more and more genetically divergent.

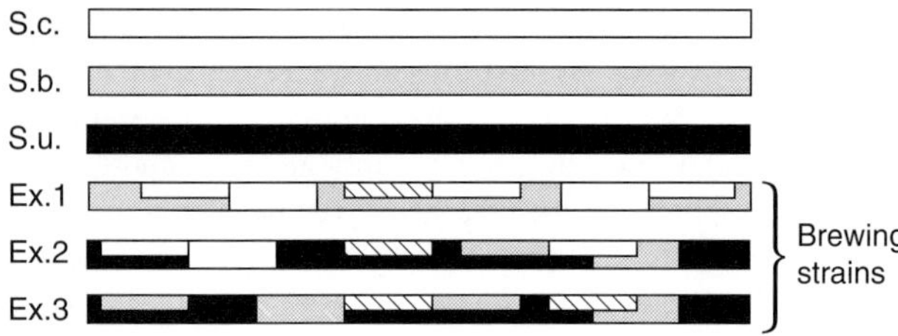

Figure 7.4b Genomes in the polyploid brewing strains, here represented by example 1, 2 and 3. In the brewing strains four different progenitor genomes could be found: *Saccharomyces cerevisae*, S.c. ☐, *Saccharomyces bayanus*, S.b. ▒, *Saccharomyces uvarum*, S.u. ■ and a fourth called "lager" ▧. *Source*: Modified from Rainieri *et al*. (2006).

the well established *S. cerevisiae*, *S. bayanus* and a third, non-hybrid strain derived from an ancestor of *S. bayanus*, called *S. uvarum*. Within the brewery strains, all of these three different genomes could be found in different hybrid compositions, but a diverged fragment could also be detected in some chromosomes not deriving from any of the three non-hybrid strains mentioned above. The authors refer to this fourth ancestor as the "lager" type (see Figure 7.4b). Three different hybrid groups were found, one containing genomic parts from *S. bayanus*/*S. cerevisiae*/lager, another with genes from all four types, and the last one with genetic compositions of *S. bayanus*/*S. uvarum*/lager. The authors also suggest that the hybrids containing *S. cerevisiae* should all be referred as *S. pastorianus* since this is the scientific name for the most common yeast found in lager brewing (see below).

Saccharomyces cerevisiae *S. cerevisiae* is the most common top-fermenting brewery species, but the variation in this species is large. The different strains are carefully tested and chosen for their unique characteristics in the fermentation of a brew made from grain and hops into a specific brand of beer. In this species we also find spoilers, typically producing too much of some flavor compound that is not wanted in the beverages. In a recent study (Douglas *et al*., 2006), different *S. cerevisiae* strains and their effect on the fermentation products from a chemically defined, simulated wort and a hopped ale or stout wort were tested. The choice of strain was found to affect all tested parameters, like foam, filterability and haze characteristics of the final beer.

The search for a better strain is a never-ending task of the yeast engineers, and the number of improvements seems endless. Below are only a few examples breeding efforts on brewery strains of *S. cerevisiae*.

Nevoigt *et al*. (2002) tried to lower the ethanol content in beer to get a healthier and safer (regarding driving and drinking) beverage with the same taste. They over-expressed the gene *GPD1*, which encodes glycerol-3-phosphate dehydrogenase, thereby favoring the production of glycerol at the cost of ethanol production. They managed to increase the glycerol content 5.6 times, and ethanol was decreased by 18% when compared to the wild type. Over-expression of *GPD1* did not affect the consumption of wort sugars and caused only minor changes in the concentration of higher alcohols, esters and fatty acids. However, the concentrations of several other unwanted by-products, particularly acetoin, diacetyl and acetaldehyde, were considerably increased.

β-glucan is a polysaccharide found in the barley cell walls, causing reduced filterability, formation of gels and hazes in the beer, if not broken down by β-glucanase during the grain modification associated by malting. The adverse effects of the presence of β-glucan in the mash from insufficiently modified malt may be remedied by addition of bacterial β-glucanase produced from, for example, *Bacillus subtilis*. In a genetically engineered *S. cerevisiae* strain where the β-glucanase from *Trichoderma reesei* was expressed, the β-glucans were digested very efficiently, resulting in a reduction of beer viscosity. *Trichoderma reesei's* β-glucanase has a lower pH optimum more suited for *S. cerevisiae* than *B. subtilis'* β-glucanase (Penttila *et al*., 1987, 1988; Penttilä *et al*., 1987; Suihko *et al*., 1990, 1991).

Saccharomyces pastorianus In 1883 Emil Christian Hansen isolated a single cell from *Saccharomyces carlsbergensis*, or *S. pastorianus* as it is called today. This was the first time someone generated a pure yeast culture from one single, isolated cell, which was then used as a starter culture in the production of beer. Together with its close relatives it is the most studied lager brewing yeast. The strains are often non-maters, they sporulate poorly and they have very low spore viability. The lager brewing yeast, *S. pastorianus* has a mosaic genome with parts deriving from other members in the *Saccharomyces* group (Kodama *et al*., 2006).

In eukaryotes two different sets of genomes exist, one in the nucleus, and one in an organelle called the mitochondrion (mtDNA). If the cell only contains one set of chromosomes in its nucleus, it is called a haploid cell, and if it contains two sets of chromosomes, the cell is diploid, three sets triploid, four sets tetraploid and so on. The DNA in the nucleus is usually inherited with a haploid set from one parent and a haploid set from the other parent, resulting in a diploid progeny cell. The mtDNA on the other hand is usually only inherited from one parent, but sometimes it can be inherited as a recombinant of that of the two parents.

As initially found for a single linkage group (Nilsson-Tillgren *et al*., 1981), *S. pastorianus* strains are allopolyploid with chromosomes derived from different species (reviewed by Kielland-Brandt *et al*., 1995). The whole genome of a lager brewing yeast has been sequenced recently (Nakao *et al*., 2003; Kodama *et al*., 2006). The hybrid nature of the lager strain has been first proposed on the basis of chromosome III transfer studies (Nilsson-Tillgren *et al*., 1981). Several studies have tried to identify the parental strains of *S. pastorianus* and from DNA–DNA reassociation with members

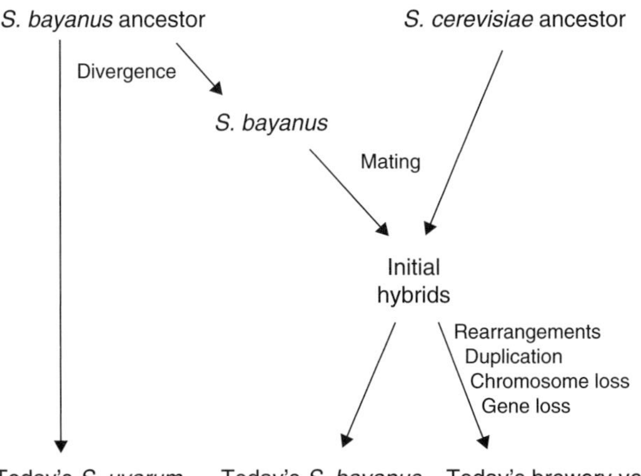

Figure 7.4c Schematic representation of the evolution of the modern brewing strains. *Source*: Modified from Casaregola *et al.* (2001) and Kodama *et al.* (2006).

of the *Saccharomyces sensu stricto* group. Vaughan-Martini and Kurtzman (1985) suggested that lager brewing yeasts are hybrids between *S. cerevisiae* and *S. bayanus.* A competing hypothesis was at the time a hybridization between *S. cerevisiae* and *Saccharomyces monacensis* (now classified as a *S. pastorianus* strain), a brewing yeast also isolated by Emil Christian Hansen in the Carlsberg breweries. The reason for this was that several genes (*HIS4*, *LEU2*, *MET2* and *ACB1*) are represented by two different alleles in *S. carlsbergensis*, one identical to *S. cerevisiae* and the other to *S. monacensis* (Pedersen, 1983, 1986; Hansen & Kielland-Brandt, 1994; Borsting *et al.*, 1997). A comprehensive analysis by Casaregola *et al.* (2001) of the different yeast strains involved in developing the lager brewing strains suggested a complex pedigree where today's *S. bayanus* diverged into two different strains, of which one mated with *S. cerevisiae* and evolved into *S. pastorianus* and the other became today's *S. uvarum* (see Figure 7.4c). However, the nature of the participating parental strains and the offspring is still debated. Today's *S. pastorianus* is composed of two whole sets of genomes, one from an *S. cerevisiae* ancestor and a second from an ancestor of *S. bayanus*. The combination of genomes from *S. bayanus*, *S. cerevisiae*, *S. uvarum* and lager has been rearranged, duplicated and some parts lost, and resulted in the modern allotetraploid genome, *S. pastorianus*. The mitochondrial genome was only inherited from the non-*cerevisiae* part, which in itself is odd because all experiments on mitochondrial hybridization between *S. cerevisiae* and *S. bayanus* have resulted in a daughter cell sharing the nuclear genome between the two parents, but the mtDNA molecule only from the *S. cerevisiae* parent (Marinoni *et al.*, 1999).

Since *S. pastorianus* is an allopolyploid yeast, it is more difficult to genetically engineer it compared to the haploid *S. cerevisiae* laboratory strains. However, it can be done (Hansen & Kielland-Brandt, 1996).

Saccharomyces bayanus An important characteristic of *S. bayanus* is its ability to grow and ferment at low temperature. It can still utilize substrates at 2°C, which is impossible for *S. cerevisiae*. To improve the fermentation capability of *S. cerevisiae* at low temperature, this yeast has been hybridized with *S. bayanus*, resulting in hybrids capable of growing and fermenting at 7°C (Kishimoto, 1994; Sato *et al.*, 2002).

The yeasts within the *S. bayanus* have been subdivided further into two groups (Nguyen and Gaillardin, 1997; Rainieri *et al.*, 1999; Naumov, 2000; Nguyen *et al.*, 2000), *S. bayanus*, which contains a miscellany of various hybrids, and *S. uvarum*, which contains strains of non-hybrid origin, usually isolated from grapes or wine fermentations (Naumov *et al.*, 2000, 2002; Demuyter *et al.*, 2004). *S. uvarum* is the only group found in the above described species in which all strains have equal and consistent characteristics (Giudici *et al.*, 1998; Pulvirenti *et al.*, 2000; Rainieri *et al.*, 2003; Nguyen and Gaillardin, 2005). The *S. bayanus* genome has been sequenced (Kellis *et al.*, 2003), and a lot of studies comparing it to its more famous relative *S. cerevisiae* have been carried out (Beltrao and Serrano, 2005; Hall *et al.*, 2005; Naumova *et al.*, 2005; Romov *et al.*, 2006).

Torulaspora delbrueckii

Torulaspora delbrueckii, Saccharomyces delbrueckii and *Saccharomyces fermentati* are all names for the same species of yeast. This yeast, along with *S. cerevisiae* and *Kluyveromyces lactis*, is used in vinification and brewing. They have the ability to transform a range of monoterpene alcohols using a variety of reactions (King and Dickinson, 2000). Since monoterpenoids are found in hops, they have a strong influence on the aroma quality of the beer (Ribéreau-Gayon *et al.*, 1975; Bauer *et al.*, 1990), so the yeast transformation of these compounds into other compounds is very important for the flavor (see Table 7.2).

In a study by King and Dickinson (2000) the reactions catalyzed by these yeasts led mainly to the formation of linalool and α-terpineol, but the different yeast strains would influence the beer differently. For example, *T. delbrueckii* forms linalool from geraniol, with no citronellol production (see Figure 7.5). Therefore, using *T. delbrueckii* may produce beers with an aroma more like that of the Muscat wines, characterized by a high linalool content. The modifications of the terpenoids may not only alter the type of aroma, but also the intensity. For example, conversion of linalool to α-terpineol may have a negative effect, as its sensory threshold is 4.6 times lower and then the beer would loose some of its aroma. On the other hand, conversion of nerol to linalool would be expected to be beneficial for the floral flavor.

Table 7.2 Properties of monoterpenoids produced by yeast

Compound	*Aroma*	*Systematic name*	*Sensory threshold (μg/l)*
Geraniol	Floral, rose-like, citrus	3,7-Dimethyl-*trans*-2,6-octadien-1-ol	132
Citronellol	Sweet, rose-like citrus	3,7-Dimethyl-6-octen-1-ol	100
Linalool	Floral, fresh, coriander	3,7-Dimethyl-1,6-octadien-3-ol	100
Nerol	Floral, fresh, green	3,7-Dimethyl-*cis*-2,6-octadien-1-ol	400
α-Terpinol	Lilac	1-*p*-Menthen-8-ol	460

Source: Aroma data from Bauer *et al.* (1990) and sensory threshold data (in water) from Ribéreau-Gayon *et al.* (1975).

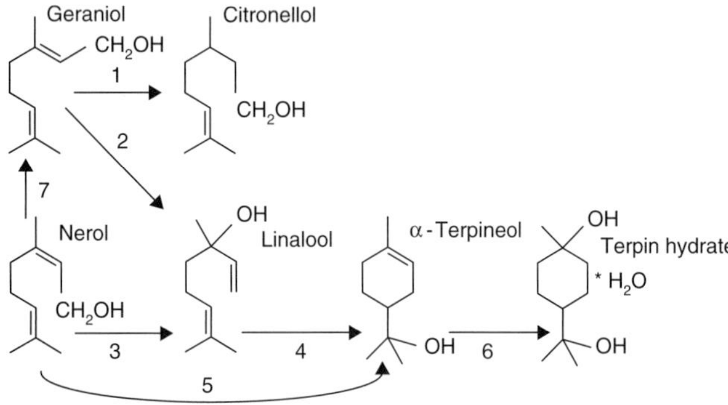
1. Reduction of geraniol to citronellol (except *T. delbrueckii*)
2. Isomerization of geraniol to linalool
3. Isomerization of nerol to linalool
4. Isomerization of linalool to α-terpineol
5. Isomerization of nerol to α-terpineol
6. Hydration of α-terpineol to terpin hydrate
7. Isomerization of nerol to geraniol (except *S. cerevisiae*)
Geraniol
CH_2OH
Citronellol
CH_2OH
Nerol
CH_2OH
OH
Linalool
α-Terpineol
OH
OH
Terpin hydrate
$\cdot H_2O$
OH
1
2
3
4
5
6
7

Figure 7.5 Biotransformations of monoterpenoids catalyzed by *S. cerevisiae*, *T. delbrueckii* and *K. lactis*. *Source*: Modified from King and Dickinson (2000).

Torulaspora delbrueckii has until recently been only poorly studied, but the academic interest in the yeast has increased notably due to its high resistance to several types of stress, including salt and osmotic imbalance. Now genetic tools, such as transformation protocols and knock-out studies, have been developed to study its unique properties (Hernandez-Lopez *et al.*, 2006a,b).

Dekkera/Brettanomyces

Dekkera and *Brettanomyces* are present in spontaneously fermented Belgian lambic and gueuze beer types. They belong to the same genus, where *Dekkera* species are fungi perfecti (reproduce sexually) and *Brettanomyces* species are fungi imperfecti (reproduce asexually). The genus includes the species *D. bruxellensis*, *D. anomala*, *B. naardensis*, *B. custersianus* and *B. nanus* (Walt, 1998). This group is not closely related to *Saccharomyces* (Woolfit *et al.*, 2007), but at least *D. bruxellensis* exhibits a physiology similar to very characteristic features of *S. cerevisiae* and other *Saccharomyces sensu stricto* strains, such as the Crabtree effect, anaerobic growth, the ability to produce respiratory deficient petite mutants, and to produce and tolerate high ethanol concentrations. However, the species is a well-known spoiler of wine and beer, generating off-flavors in the maturation part of the beverage. These off-flavors are often called "brett" flavors and are mainly due to three different compounds produced by *Dekkera/Brettanomyces*:

1. 4-ethylphenol smells like: band-aids, barnyard, horse stable, antiseptic;
2. 4-ethylguaicol smells like: bacon, spice, cloves, smoky;
3. isovaleric acid smells like: sweaty saddle, cheese, rancidity.

Recently 40% of the genome of a *D. bruxellensis* strain has been sequenced and analyzed (Woolfit *et al.*, 2007). Approximately 2,700 genes, among them a lot of transporters and genes involved in nitrogen and lipid metabolism have been identified. A somewhat surprising finding was the presence of a salicylhydroxamic acid (SHAM) sensitive alternative oxidase (*AOX1*). This gene is connected with the ability of an alternative respiration pathway. There are two known responses to glycolytic overflow in the presence of high levels of glucose, namely aerobic fermentation (leading to the formation of ethanol, defining Crabtree-positive yeasts) and alternative respiration (Crabtree-negative yeast). Both pathways reoxidize NADH (reduced form of nicotinamide adenine dinucleotide) that is overproduced from the glycolysis to NAD^+, either by reduction of pyruvate to ethanol (Crabtree positive) or to reduce oxygen to water by alternative oxidase (Crabtree negative). Another alternative that could be used to reoxidize NADH to NAD^+ is to form glycerol from pyruvate (see Figure 7.3). At the moment it is unclear what the function of the *D. bruxellensis*' SHAM pathway is.

Despite the importance of this yeast species as a spoiler of wine not much is known about its physiology, ecology and variation. There are currently no published studies how to genetically manipulate this yeast, even if it may represent a valuable resource of various aromatic compounds.

Other yeasts

The wort in beer production is a rich growth medium for a number of yeast species. Yeasts not deliberately used in the brewery and thus uncontrolled are called wild yeast (Holm and Poulsen, 1888; Priest, 1981). These unwanted organisms can produce substances that will alter the quality and the flavor of the beer even in concentration as low as one wild yeast per 10^5-10^6 of the culture yeast. The wild yeasts are traditionally divided into non-*Saccharomyces* and *Saccharomyces* yeasts (Back, 1987). The non-*Saccharomyces* wild yeasts belong to different genera such as *Brettanomyces*, *Candida*, *Debaryomyces*, *Filobasidium*, *Hanseniaspora*, *Kluyveromyces*, *Pichia*, *Torulaspora* and *Zygosaccharomyces* (Ingledew and Casey, 1982; Campbell and Msongo, 1991; Campbell, 1996). The majority of the *Saccharomyces* wild yeasts belong to *S. cerevisiae*, but other *Saccharomyces* species have also been reported (Lawrence, 1988; Campbell, 1996). The *Saccharomyces* wild yeasts are often regarded as the most hazardous wild yeasts. The diversity of spoilage yeasts means that no general description can be given and no general detection method can be used.

Methods to Increase the Diversity

Nature has provided us with an enormous number of species that can ferment ethanol (Merico *et al.*, 2007). However, additional diversity has been and can be created by employment of genetic and molecular methods (reviewed in Polaina, 2002; Hansen and Piskur, 2004).

Selective breeding

Many beer strains are polyploid (have more than two sets of chromosomes) which makes it very hard to manipulate the genome with only molecular methods. As demonstrated by Gjermansen and Sigsgaard (1981), one may circumvent this problem by sporulating and breeding them under specific conditions (Kielland-Brandt *et al.*, 1995). Yeast lineages can be selected for desired characteristics, sporulated and crossed, thereby producing different strains with different characteristics. However, the sporulation ability can be limited. "Rare mating" is another approach, in which haploid maters are mixed with a population of brewing yeasts; this technique may produce rare hybrids that can be selected. Another approach is fusion of yeast cells after the cell wall has been taken away, producing cells with whole or parts of the genome from both of the fused cells. These mating techniques involve the transfer of many genes or parts of the whole genomes, and the outcome is very unpredictable (reviewed in Hansen and Piskur, 2004).

Hybrids

Hybridization, the genetic combination from two different yeast strains to form a progeny, is relatively easy to carry out in the laboratory. Interspecific hybridization offers almost unlimited variation and has only been poorly explored, and the future outcome can only be speculated upon. Another approach to novel and improved brewing strains is the transfer of limited amounts of genetic material within the *Saccharomyces* yeasts by molecular techniques.

One example of combining two different species to get enhanced brewing yeast has been given by Mukai *et al.* (2001). They took a lysine auxotrophic mutant of sake yeast and fused it with a respiratory deficient mutant of a top-fermenting brewer's yeast. The different mutations in the parents are supposed to complement each other in the fused yeast cells, so only progeny with both parental genomes will survive on a selective medium. The rationale for the fusion rested on the ability of the Sake yeast to produce a fruity flavor and its tolerance to higher concentrations of ethanol (Mukai *et al.*, 1998). The characteristics of the fused hybrid have been intermediate compared to the parents, in both ethanol tolerance and production. The content of isoamyl acetate in the beer brewed using the hybrid increased by 1.5-fold compared to the parental yeast. In addition, the content of acetic acid in the beer decreased significantly. The beer brewed using the hybrid had a strong fruity aroma and a sharp aftertaste compared to the beer brewed by the parental yeast (Mukai *et al.*, 2001).

Molecular techniques

To manipulate and alter the characteristics of yeast, methods have been developed for eliminating the function of a gene (gene deletion or disruption) or insert a new gene from another species, to give the organism a new function. These procedures can rely on homologous recombination where a specific target in the genome can be replaced by a functional gene or disrupted to destroy the function of an existing gene. The transformation of genetic material can also be done by a plasmid (small circular DNA), which usually contains a specific gene, a selection gene and an autonomous replicating sequence (ARS). When the plasmid is introduced into the cell, the ARS enables the plasmid to replicate itself (reviewed in Hansen and Piskur, 2004). There are many variants of these two methods, and of course they can be combined to delete an unwanted gene and replace it with a desired functional one at the same time (Amberg *et al.*, 2005). These methods can also generate novel strains with potentially improved traits for the brewing industry. So far, many recombinant strains have been developed but have only rarely been used in the breweries because of an unfavorable attitude toward gene modified organisms (GMO) in the general public.

Post-genomic methods

The sequenced genomes generated from organisms have been a basis for so-called post-genomic methods developed to find out more about the cell physiology and biochemistry. An example is the DNA microarrays, in which the principle is to hybridize (bind) different messenger RNAs (mRNA) to short sequences of known DNA; the results show different concentrations of the mRNA produced in the cell. These concentration differences are compared against a standard and in this way deviating concentrations of a specific mRNA is recognized. mRNA is the link between DNA and protein, and for those proteins required in the cell at a specific condition, the corresponding mRNA will often be produced in higher amounts. The mRNA signal for a protein can also be completely absent under a certain condition where the protein is not needed (Kumar and Snyder, 2001; Bochner, 2003; Panda *et al.*, 2003; Steinmetz and Davis, 2004). Microarrays detect the expression of the whole genomic set of genes, and not just a single gene.

The mRNA is, as mentioned above, only a link between the instructors (DNA) and the workers (protein), and there is no absolute correlation between the two. Protein microarray technology, on the other hand, has just been introduced, but it has already been successfully applied for the identification, quantification and functional analysis of proteins (reviewed in Poetz *et al.*, 2005). There are a number of different approaches depending on the field of application, but the principle is based on the specific interaction between an antibody and a protein. When attached to each other, a measurable signal, correlated quantitatively with the number of binding pairs, can be detected. These genes can then be manipulated using standard molecular techniques.

Future Trends

The breweries are constantly trying to improve their beers and to find new kinds with other flavors and enhanced characteristics, like foam and color. To do this all components involved in the brewing process are meticulously checked and improved if possible, including the yeast. Yeasts represent a very important part for the final quality of the beer, and not surprisingly there has been lot of research to improve the strains already used and to find new ones. A lot of tools are available to modify the yeast, and a lot of improved strains have been made (reviewed in Dequin, 2001). However, despite the remarkable progress in this field only a limited number of genetically modified brewery strains have been approved officially (Hammond, 1995). An organism is considered a GMO if it has been modified by molecular tools (recombinant DNA technology) described above. It is however not considered a GMO if one uses the selective breeding approach where specific mutations are selected for and crossed with each other or other strains with desirable mutations. The difference at the end is basically precision and the time spent in the laboratory; whereas the recombinant DNA technology is a precise and very fast technique, the breeding process is an often very time-consuming approach. The concern about the GMO is generally due to limited knowledge in the general public about recombinant DNA technology, the benefit for the public and the potential risk of a release into nature. In most beers (not the unfiltered beers) the yeast has been filtered away, so only the product of the yeast will be engulfed and not the yeast itself.

Another way to enhance the beer variability could be to add different yeast strains during the fermentation process to get a specific flavor or degrade a specific substrate. The more we learn about different yeast strains, the more we can use their potentials. An example could be the "brett" flavors produced by *Dekkera/Brettanomyces*, which in small amounts are desired in particular products. If this yeast is added toward the end of fermentation, the amount of volatile phenols (flavors) produced will be less than if it was added from the beginning of fermentation. In this way the taste could be varied enormously.

Summary Points

- Yeasts are essential in beer production.
- There are over 1,000 different yeast species.
- The different yeasts have different characteristics, which can be studied by various approaches.
- Selective breeding and recombinant DNA technology are different ways of modifying yeast and generating more diversity.
- *Saccharomyces sensu stricto* is a group of well-known yeasts and brewing species.
- *Saccharomyces cerevisiae* is the best characterized yeast and the most common top-fermenting species.
- *Saccharomyces pastorianus* is an allopolyploid yeast derived from *S. cerevisiae* and *S. bayanus-like* and the most common bottom-fermenting lager yeast.
- Other important yeasts include *Saccharomyces bayanus, Torulaspora delbrueckii, Dekkera/Brettanomyces* and hybrids.
- Improvements have been developed in different yeast strains using recombinant DNA technology, but because of the resistance toward GMO, they have not been used in the brewing industry.

Acknowledgments

We would like to thank Olof Björnberg, Anders Clausen and Morten Kielland-Brandt for reading and commenting on this chapter.

We are also thankful for the financial support from Carl Tryggers Stiftelse, Futura, Nilsson-Ehle and Sörensen's Foundations.

References

Amberg, D.C., Burke, D.J. and Strathern, J.N. (2005). *Methods in Yeast Genetics: A Cold Spring Harbor Laboratory Course Manual.* Cold Spring Harbor, New York.

Axelson-Fisk, M. and Sunnerhagen, P. (2006). Comparative genomics and gene finding in fungi. In Sunnerhagen, P. and Piskur, J. (eds), *Comparative Genomics Using Fungi as Models*. Springer, New York.

Back, W. (1987). *Brauwelt* 127, 735–737.

Barnett, J.A. (2000). *Yeast* 16, 755–771.

Barnett, J.A. (2003). *Microbiol. Rev.* 149, 557–567.

Barnett, J.A. and Lichtenthaler, F.W. (2001). *Yeast* 18, 363–388.

Bauer, K., Garbe, D. and Surburg, H. (1990). *Common Fragrance and Flavor Materials. Preparation and Uses*. VCH, New York.

Beltrao, P. and Serrano, L. (2005). *PLoS Comput. Biol.* 1, e26.

Bochner, B.R. (2003). *Nat. Rev. Genet.* 4, 309–314.

Borsting, C., Hummel, R., Schultz, E.R., Rose, T.M., Pedersen, M.B., Knudsen, J. and Kristiansen, K. (1997). *Yeast* 13, 1409–1421.

Campbell, I. (1996). Wild yeast in brewing and distilling. In Priest, F.G. and Campbell, I. (eds), *Brewing Microbiology* (2nd edn). Chapman and Hall, London.

Campbell, I. and Msongo, H.S. (1991). *J. Inst. Brew.* 97, 279–282.

Casaregola, S., Nguyen, H.V., Lapathitis, G., Kotyk, A. and Gaillardin, C. (2001). *Int. J. Syst. Evol. Microbiol.* 51, 1607–1618.

Cavalieri, D., Mcgovern, P.E., Hartl, D.L., Mortimer, R. and Polsinelli, M. (2003). *J. Mol. Evol.* 57, S226–S232.

Corran, H.S. (1975). *A History of Brewing*. David and Charles, Newton Abbott, UK.

De Deken, R.H. (1966). *J. Gen. Microbiol.* 44, 149–156.

Demuyter, C., Lollier, M., Legras, J.L. and Le Jeune, C. (2004). *J. Appl. Microbiol.* 97, 1140–1148.

Dequin, S. (2001). *Appl. Microbiol. Biotechnol.* 56, 577–588.

Douglas, P., Meneses, F.J. and Jiranek, V. (2006). *J. Appl. Microbiol.* 100, 58–64.

Fay, J.C. and Benavides, J.A. (2005). *PLoS Genet.* 1, 66–71.

Fell, J.W., Boekhout, T., Fonseca, A., Scorzetti, G. and Statzell-Tallman, A. (2000). *Int. J. Syst. Evol. Microbiol.* 50, 1351–1371.

Friis, E.M. and Crepet, W.L. (1987). *The Origins of Angiosperms and Their Biological Consequences*. Cambridge University Press, Cambridge, UK.

Giudici, P., Caggia, C., Pulvirenti, A. and Rainieri, S. (1998). *J. Appl. Microbiol.* 84, 811–819.

Gjermansen, C. and Sigsgaard, P. (1981). *Carisberg research communications* 46.

Goffeau, A., Barrell, B.G., Bussey, H., Davis, R.W., Dujon, B., Feldmann, H., Galibert, F., Hoheisel, J.D., Jacq, C., Johnston, M., Louis, E.J., Mewes, H.W., Murakami, Y., Philippsen, P., Tettelin, H. and Oliver, S.G. (1996). *Science* 274. 546, 563–567.

Gojkovic, Z., Knecht, W., Zameitat, E., Warneboldt, J., Coutelis, J.B., Pynyaha, Y., Neuveglise, C., Moller, K., Loffler, M. and Piskur, J. (2004). *Mol. Genet. Genomics* 271, 387–393.

Hall, C., Brachat, S. and Dietrich, F.S. (2005). *Eukaryot. Cell* 4, 1102–1115.

Hammond, J.R. (1995). *Yeast* 11, 1613–1627

Hansen, J. and Kielland-Brandt, M.C. (1994). *Gene* 140, 33–40.

Hansen, J. and Kielland-Brandt, M.C. (1996). *J. Biotechnol.* 49, 1–12.

Hansen, J. and Piskur, J. (2004). Fungi in brewing: biodiversity and biotechnology perspectives. In Arora, D.K. (ed.), *Handbook of Fungal Biotechnology*. Marcel Dekker, New York.

Heckman, D.S., Geiser, D.M., Eidell, B.R., Stauffer, R.L., Kardos, N.L. and Hedges, S.B. (2001). *Science* 293, 1129–1133.

Hernandez-Lopez, M.J., Panadero, J., Prieto, J.A. and Randez-Gil, F. (2006a). *Eukaryot. Cell* 5, 469–479.

Hernandez-Lopez, M.J., Randez-Gil, F. and Prieto, J.A. (2006b). *Eukaryot. Cell* 5, 1410–1419.

Holm, J.C. and Poulsen, S.V. (1888). *Compt. Rend. Trav. Lab. Carlsberg* 2, 137–142.

Hornsey, I.S. (2004). *A History of Beer and Brewing*. Royal Society of Chemistry, Cambridge, UK.

Ingledew, W.M. and Casey, G.P. (1982). Media for wild yeast. *Brewers Dig.* 57, 18–22.

Ingold, C.T. (1991). *Mycol. Res.* 95, 618–621.

Johnston, M. (1999). *Trends Genet.* 15, 29–33.

Kellis, M., Patterson, N., Endrizzi, M., Birren, B. and Lander, E.S. (2003). *Nature* 423, 241–254.

Kielland-Brandt, M.C., Nilsson-Tillgren, T., Gjermansen, C., Holmberg, S. and Pedersen, M.B. (1995). Genetics of brewing yeasts. In Rose, A.H., Wheals, E. and Harrison, J.S. (eds), *The Yeasts* (2nd edn). Academic Press, London.

King, A. and Dickinson, R.J. (2000). *Yeast* 16, 499–506.

Kishimoto, M. (1994). *J. Ferment. Bioeng.* 77, 132–135.

Kodama, Y., Kielland-Brandt, M.C. and Hansen, J. (2006). Lager brewing yeast. In Sunnerhagen, P. and Piskur, J. (eds), *Comparative Genomics Using Fungi as a Model*. Springer-Verlag, Heidelberg.

Kumar, A. and Snyder, M. (2001). *Nat. Rev. Genet.* 2, 302–312.

Kurtzman, C.P. and Fell, J.W. (2006). Yeast systematics and phylogeny – implications of molecular identification methods for studies in ecology. In Rosa, C.A. and Peter, G. (eds), *Biodiversity and Ecophysiology of Yeast*. Springer-Verlag, Heidelberg.

Kurtzman, C.P. and Phaff, H.J. (1987). Molecular taxonomy. In Rose Ah, H.J. (ed.), *The Yeasts* (2nd edn). Academic, London.

Kurtzman, C.P. and Robnett, C.J. (1998). *Antonie Van Leeuwenhoek* 73, 331–371.

Kurtzman, C.P. and Robnett, C.J. (2003). *FEMS Yeast Res.* 3, 417–432.

Lawrence, D.R. (1988). Spoilage organisms in beer. In Robinson, R. K. (ed.), *Developments in Food Microbiology*. Elsevier, London.

Marinoni, G., Manuel, M., Petersen, R.F., Hvidtfeldt, J., Sulo, P. and Piskur, J. (1999). *J. Bacteriol.* 181, 6488–6496.

Merico, A., Sulo, P., Piskur, J. and Compagno, C. (2007). *FEBS J* 274, 976–989.

Mcgovern, P.E., Zhang, J.N., Tang, J., Zhang, Z., Hall, G.R., Moreau, R.A., Nunez, A., Butrym, E.D., Richards, M.P., Wang, C., Cheng, G., Zhao, Z. and Wang, C. (2004). *Proc. Natl. Acad. Sci. USA* 101, 17593–17598.

Mukai, N., Okada, A., Suzuki, A. and Takahaski, T. (1998). *J. Brew. Japan* 93, 975–976.

Mukai, N., Nishimori, C., Fujishige, I.W., Mizuno, A., Takahashi, T. and Sato, K. (2001). *J. Biosci. Bioeng.* 91, 482–486.

Nagy, M., Lacroute, F. and Thomas, D. (1992). *Proc. Natl. Acad. Sci. USA* 89, 8966–8970.

Nakao, Y., Kodama, Y., Nakamura, N., Ito, T., Hattori, M., Shiba, T. and Ashikari, T. (2003). Whole genome sequence of a lager brewing yeast. *Proceedings of the 29th European Brewery Convention Congress*, Dublin.

Naumov, G.I. (2000). *Mikrobiologiia* 69, 410–414.

Naumov, G.I., Masneuf, I., Naumova, E.S., Aigle, M. and Dubourdieu, D. (2000). *Res. Microbiol.* 151, 683–691.

Naumov, G.I., Naumova, E.S., Antunovics, Z. and Sipiczki, M. (2002). *Appl. Microbiol. Biotechnol.* 59, 727–730.

Naumova, E.S., Naumov, G.I., Masneuf-Pomarede, I., Aigle, M. and Dubourdieu, D. (2005). *Yeast* 22, 1099–1115.

Nevoigt, E., Pilger, R., Mast-Gerlach, E., Schmidt, U., Freihammer, S., Eschenbrenner, M., Garbe, L. and Stahl, U. (2002). *FEMS Yeast Res.* 2, 225–232.

Nguyen, H.-V. and Gaillardin, C. (1997). *Syst. Appl. Microbiol.* 20, 286–294.

Nguyen, H.V. and Gaillardin, C. (2005). *FEMS Yeast Res.* 5, 471–483.

Nguyen, H.V., Lepingle, A. and Gaillardin, C.A. (2000). *Syst. Appl. Microbiol.* 23, 71–85.

Nilsson-Tillgren, T., Gjermansen, C., Kielland-Brandt, M. C., Petersen, J.G.L. and Holmberg, S. (1981). *Carlsberg Res. Commun.* 46, 65–76.

Panda, S., Sato, T.K., Hampton, G.M. and Hogenesch, J.B. (2003). *Trends Cell Biol.* 13, 151–156.

Pedersen, M.B. (1983). *Carlsberg Res. Commun.* 48, 485–503.

Pedersen, M.B. (1986). *Carlsberg Res. Commun.* 51, 163–183.

Penttila, M.E., Andre, L., Saloheimo, M., Lehtovaara, P. and Knowles, J.K. (1987). *Yeast* 3, 175–185.

Penttila, M.E., Andre, L., Lehtovaara, P., Bailey, M., Teeri, T.T. and Knowles, J.K. (1988). *Gene* 63, 103–112.

Penttilä, M., Suihko, M.L., Lehtinen, U., Nikkola, M. and Knowles, J.K.C. (1987). *Curr. Genet.* 12, 413–420.

Piskur, J. and Langkjaer, R.B. (2004). *Mol. Microbiol.* 53, 381–389.

Piskur, J., Rozpedowska, E., Polakova, S., Merico, A. and Compagno, C. (2006). *Trends Genet.* 22, 183–186.

Poetz, O., Schwenk, J.M., Kramer, S., Stoll, D., Templin, M.F. and Joos, T.O. (2005). *Mech. Age. Dev.* 126, 161–170.

Polaina, J. (2002) Brewer's yeast: genetics and biotechnology. In Khachatourians, G.G. and Arora, D.A. (eds). *Applied Mycology and Biotechnology*. Elsevier Science, Amsterdam, The Netherlands.

Price, C.W., Fuson, G.B. and Phaff, H.J. (1978). *Microbiol. Rev.* 42, 161–193.

Priest, F.G. (1981). Contamination. In *An Introduction to Brewing Science and Technology, Part II*. The Institute of Brewing, London.

Pronk, J.T., Yde Steensma, H. and Van Dijken, J.P. (1996). *Yeast* 12, 1607–1633.

Pulvirenti, A., Nguyen, H., Caggia, C., Giudici, P., Rainieri, S. and Zambonelli, C. (2000). *FEMS Microbiol. Lett.* 192, 191–196.

Rainieri, S., Zambonelli, C., Hallsworth, J.E., Pulvirenti, A. and Giudici, P. (1999). *FEMS Microbiol. Lett.* 177, 177–185.

Rainieri, S., Zambonelli, C. and Kaneko, Y. (2003). *J. Biosci. Bioeng.* 96, 1–9.

Rainieri, S., Kodama, Y., Kaneko, Y., Mikata, K., Nakao, Y. and Ashikari, T. (2006). *Appl. Environ. Microbiol.* 72, 3968–3974.

Ribéreau-Gayon, P., Boidron, J.N. and Terrier, A. (1975). *J. Agric. Food Chem.* 23, 1042–1047.

Rokas, A. (2006). *Science* 313, 1897–1899.

Romov, P.A., Li, F., Lipke, P.N., Epstein, S.L. and Qiu, W.G. (2006). *J. Mol. Evol.* 63, 415–425.

Sato, M., Kishimoto, M., Watari, J. and Takashio, M. (2002). *J. Biosci. Bioeng.* 93, 509–511.

Steinmetz, L.M. and Davis, R.W. (2004). *Nat. Rev. Genet.* 5, 190–201.

Suihko, M.L., Blomqvist, K., Penttila, M., Gisler, R. and Knowles, J. (1990). *J. Biotechnol.* 14, 285–300.

Suihko, M.L., Lehtinen, U., Zurbriggen, B., Vilpoa, A., Knowles, J. and Penttilä, M. (1991). *Appl. Microbiol. Biotechnol.* 35, 781–787.

Sunnerhagen, P. and Piskur, J. (2006). *Comparative Genomics Using Fungi as Models*. Springer, New York.

Tornai-Lehoczki, J. and Dlauchy, D. (2000). *Int. J. Food Microbiol.* 62, 37–45.

Walt, J.P.V. (1998). Dekkera In. *The Yeasts a Taxonomic Study*. Elsevier Science, Amsterdam, The Netherlands.

Vaughan-Martini, A. and Kurtzman, C.P. (1985). *Int. J. Syst. Bacteriol.* 35, 508–511.

Vaughan-Martini, A. and Martini, A. (1987). *Antonie Van Leeuwenhoek* 53, 77–84.

Verstrepen, K.J., Iserentant, D., Malcorps, P., Derdelinckx, G., Van Dijck, P., Winderickx, J., Pretorius, I.S., Thevelein, J.M. and Delvaux, F.R. (2004). *Trends Biotechnol.* 22, 531–537.

Woolfit, M., Rozpedowska, E., Piskur, J. and Wolfe, K.H. (2007). *Eukaryot. Cell* 6, 721–733.

8

The Brewer's Yeast Genome: From Its Origins to Our Current Knowledge

Sandra Rainieri Department of Agricultural Sciences, University of Modena and Reggio Emilia, Reggio Emilia, Italy

Abstract

Brewing yeasts play the fundamental role of converting malt sugars into ethanol, carrying out the alcoholic fermentation that is at the basis of beer manufacturing. Their metabolism is of major importance for establishing the technological and nutritional characteristics of beer, therefore the understanding of their genome is an essential step for optimizing the brewing process, as well as improving the overall beer quality. Many microorganisms and different yeast species can grow and ferment spontaneously in a rich media such as malted barley juice, the fermentation substrate of beer. However, only two types of yeasts have been selected over the years and are currently employed for industrial beer production: ale and lager yeasts.

Ale yeasts are polyploid *Saccharomyces cerevisiae* that differ from *S. cerevisiae* laboratory strains and show a high degree of interspecific polymorphism. Lager yeasts are now considered as part of the *Saccharomyces pastorianus* species, even though their classification has always been controversial. Their genome is very complex and seems to be composed of at least two different genomes: one nearly identical to *S. cerevisiae* and one originating from a non-*S. cerevisiae* yeast, closely related to *Saccharomyces bayanus*. This chapter illustrates the development of the complex taxonomical grouping of ale and lager brewing yeasts; it describes the steps that led to the current knowledge on the characteristics of their genome; and finally it attempts at elucidating the way they possibly originated and developed.

List of Abbreviations

AFLP	Amplified Fragment Length Polymorphism
CBS	Centraal Bureau voor Schimmelcultures, Utrecth, The Netherlands
CHEF	Contour-Clamped Homogeneous Electric Field
FSY1	Gene encoding a specific fructose symporter in *S. bayanus* and *S. pastorianus* yeasts
Lg	Lager-type genome; a portion of the lager brewing strain total genome
NBRC	NITE Biological Resource Center, Department of Biotechnology, National Institute for Technology and Evaluation, Chiba, Japan
PCR	Polymerase chain reaction
RAPD	Random amplified polymorphic DNA
RFLP	Restriction fragment length polymorphism
Sb	*S. bayanus* genome
Sc	*S. cerevisiae* genome
Su	*S. uvarum* genome

Introduction

Beer is the product resulting from the fermentation of the juice extracted from malted barley (the wort), carried out by yeasts. Yeasts play the fundamental role of converting the fermentable sugars of wort into ethanol and CO_2, moreover they release a number of minor fermentation by-products that are critical for defining the general aromatic characteristics of beer.

Far before the existence and the role of yeast was even suspected, its ability of converting sugars into ethanol has been exploited by mankind and has been used for guaranteeing the preservation of foodstuff, providing men with safe and nutritious food supplies. An ancestor of beer was already produced more than 5,000 years ago in Mesopotamia (Corran, 1975); for centuries beer represented a good source of nutrients (such as vitamins, proteins and sugars) and its inebriating effect was probably sought for to overcome years of darkness, famine and fear.

Nowadays, beer is one of the most popular fermented beverages in the world. Two different brewing techniques are currently employed for industrial beer production: (1) lager brewing, the worldwide major technique, contributing to 90% of the global beer production and (2) ale brewing, contributing to a 5% of the total world beer production. The remaining 5% is represented by other minor productions generally manufactured at artisan level (Dufour *et al.*, 2003) that will not be discussed in this chapter.

Beer in Health and Disease Prevention
ISBN: 978-0-12-373891-2

Ale brewing

Ale brewing is probably the earliest technique used for beer manufacturing and the ancestor of beer was most likely produced in this way. Wort is fermented at 20–25°C; yeasts remain in suspension during the fermentation but, toward the end of the process, the cells adhere to the ascending CO_2 bubbles of the foam and are then carried to the surface of the fermenting wort. The fermentation process is completed within a few days and the product is then ready for consumption. In former times, the foam of the best batches used to be manually transferred to start the fermentation of new batches, thus acting as a natural starter.

Currently, ale brewing is used for producing ales and stouts, which are products generally regarded as a specialty beers mainly produced and consumed in United Kingdom and Ireland.

Lager brewing

The lager brewing technique originated in Bavaria (Germany) during the mid-nineteenth century from the practice of storing food into caves, with the scope of preservation. As a matter of fact, the origin of the name "lager" reflects this practice (in German "to store" = "lagern"). In lager brewing, wort is fermented at 8–15°C; the yeasts stay in suspension during the fermentation, but tend to deposit at the bottom of the fermentation vessel once the fermentation has terminated. These deposited yeasts are used again to ferment new batches. After fermentation, lager beer is generally matured at low temperatures for several weeks; during this period, a secondary fermentation occurs, refining the taste and the quality of the product. Lager beer is then filtered and commercialized.

Yeast cultures in brewing

Until the end of the nineteenth century, yeast was not identified as the fermentation agent of wort, and beer was traditionally obtained by the action of a miscellanea of unidentified microorganisms, mainly represented by yeasts and bacteria, that were perpetuated from one batch to the other. It was thanks to the studies of E.C. Hansen from Carlsberg Brewery (Denmark) that yeast cultures could be individually studied. Hansen was the first to apply the pure culture technique (a practice originally elaborated by R. Koch for bacteria) ensuring that isolated cultures were not a mixture of different microorganisms, but individual entities. This allowed Hansen to establish the basis for using selected yeast strains as starter cultures in brewing. Thanks to Hansen's approach, Carlsberg Brewery started the first industrial production of lager beer in 1883 employing a selected starter culture (Polaina, 2002). Figure 8.1 shows an example of cells originating from a pure yeast culture of *S. cerevisiae*.

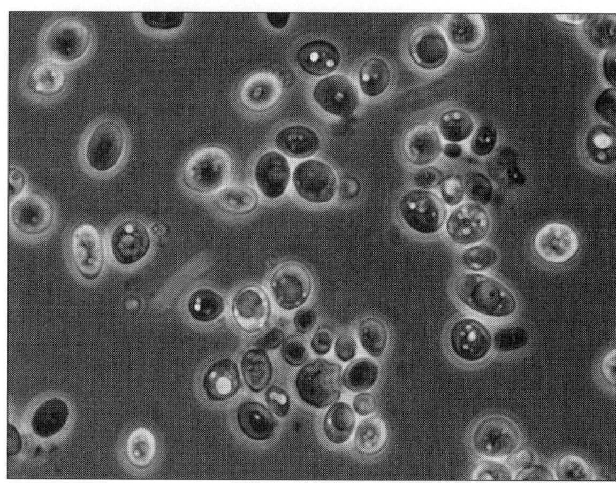

Figure 8.1 Example of brewing yeast cells originating from a pure culture of *S. cerevisiae*. Yeast pure cultures originate from the multiplication of one single cell, therefore all the daughter cells will be genetically identical to the mother cells and identical among them. This pictures has been taken under an optic microscope with a 1,000 times magnification.

It became soon clear that the two brewing techniques, ale and lager, implied the activity of two different types of yeasts. On the basis of the analysis of some phenotypic characteristics, Hansen was the first to define ale brewing yeasts and to distinguish them from lager brewing yeasts (Hansen, 1883). In particular, Hansen named ale yeasts as *S. cerevisiae* and lager yeasts as *Saccharomyces carlsbergensis* (Hansen, 1908).

Ale and lager yeasts are also commonly known as top and bottom fermenting yeasts, respectively. These names reflect the aforementioned property of ale cells to be carried to the top of the fermentation vessel and of lager cells to precipitate to the bottom of the vessel. The difference in this behavior seems to be related to the fact that ale cells have a higher content of surface protein, which makes them highly hydrophobic thus facilitating their adherence to the bubbles of CO_2 (Dengis and Rouxhet, 1997).

Objective of This Chapter

With the exception of some rare cases, such as some traditional Belgian beers (e.g. Lambic beer) that are still fermented with the natural microflora of wort, industrial ales and lagers are currently produced employing specific yeast starter cultures that have been selected to guarantee a product with constant, programmable and desired characteristics. The study of the genome of brewing yeasts is at the basis for the understanding of their metabolic and physiological processes, which are indispensable for the efficient selection and manipulation of industrial strains.

In this light, the objectives of this chapter are: (1) to provide an updated description of the genome of ale and lager yeast and (2) to attempt at tracking the origin of these genomes.

In Table 8.1, some of the technical terms used in this chapter are defined and explained.

Table 8.1 Definitions and explanation of some of the technical terms used through the chapter

Terms used in the text	*Definition*
Allele	One of the alternative forms of a gene that occupies a specific position on a chromosome (genetic locus).
Cloned genes	Genes of interest can be isolated among a population of many different genes. Each isolated gene is then perpetuated through insertion into a vector (plasmid) and insertion of the vector into a host organism (a bacterial cell). The obtained cloned gene can be studied, sequenced, etc.
DNA probes	DNA fragments that are denatured, labeled enzymatically (employing a chemioluminescence detection system) or with radioactivity, and used to detect the presence of a DNA fragment bearing a complementary sequence by Southern hybridization. Probes can be gene fragments or entire genes.
DNA reassociation	Pairing of complementary single-strand DNA to form a double helix. This technique is used as a taxonomic tool to distinguish yeast species and bacterial species and is expressed in percentage.
Flow cytometry analysis	Analysis of biological material by detection of the light-absorbing or fluorescing properties of cells or subcellular fractions such as chromosomes, passing in a narrow stream through a laser beam. Through this measurement it is possible to estimate the ploidy of a yeast.
Genome	All of the hereditary information encoded in the DNA possessed by an organism.
Genomics	Science that studies genes and their function, attempting at understanding the structure of the genome, the gene products, and how, when and why these products are synthesized.
Meiosis	Nuclear division which results in daughter nuclei, each containing half the number of chromosomes of the parent.
Microarray	A device consisting of different DNA probes that are chemically attached to a substrate (e.g. a microchip, a glass slide or a microsphere-sized bead). This device is used to analyze the information contained within an entire genome by hybridization.
PCR and PCR-based techniques (AFLP, PCR–RFLP and RAPD)	Polymerase chain reaction, a technique for selectively replicating and producing a large amount of a specific stretch of DNA *in vitro* starting from a DNA sample. PCR-based techniques: AFLP = following restriction enzyme digestion of DNA, a subset of DNA fragments is selected for PCR amplification and visualization. It is a high sensitive method for detecting polymorphisms in DNA. PCR–RFLP = amplification by PCR of a specific DNA fragment and its subsequent digestion with selected enzymes that produce fragments of different lengths reflecting differences in the DNA nucleotide sequence. RAPD = amplification by PCR of undefined regions of a template DNA. Many fragments are generated from a single reaction and are later separated by agarose or polyacrylamide gel electrophoresis.
Ploidy (includes the terms: haploid, diploid, allopolyploid, aneuploid, polyploid)	Ploidy = number of sets of chromosomes in a cell. Haploid = cells having one set of chromosomes; diploid = cells having two sets of chromosomes; polyploid = cell with more than two chromosome sets; allopolyploid = polyploidy produced by a hybrid between two or more different species therefore possessing two or more different sets of chromosomes; aneuploid = cell having more or fewer of the exact multiple of the haploid number of chromosomes.
Proteomics	The analysis of the expression, locations, functions and interactions of the proteins expressed by the genetic material of an organism.
Southern hybridization	Technique for the detection of specific sequences among DNA fragments. Fragments are separated by gel electrophoresis and then blotted onto a sheet of nitrocellulose for detection with labeled nucleic acid probes.
Starter cultures	Microorganisms selected for their optimal fermentation characteristics and used to initiate and guide a fermentation process.
Type strain	The first strain isolated and characterized of a microbial species. In some cases, it is not the most representative strain of the species but possesses an historical value.

Note: Important biological terms required for the understanding of this chapter are collected here.

Brewing Yeasts Taxonomy and Nomenclature

The taxonomy of the *Saccharomyces sensu stricto* species complex

Ale and lager brewing yeasts belong to the *Saccharomyces sensu stricto* species complex, a grouping originally based on the ability of yeasts to give vigorous alcoholic fermentations (Van der Walt, 1970). The taxonomy of *Saccharomyces sensu stricto* yeasts has always been controversial, particularly at species level. Over the years, this group has undergone many changes that were a consequence of the development of the techniques employed for yeasts classification. At the early stage of yeast taxonomy, the only tests employed to identify yeasts were basically colony and cell morphology, the ability to sporulate and to ferment some carbon sources. With the development of new techniques, the system of yeast classification was progressively enlarged; the number of physiological tests, based on fermentation and assimilation of carbon and nitrogen sources, increased, and some biochemical characteristics

Table 8.2 Changes over the years in the classification of the *Saccharomyces sensu stricto* species complex

Guillermond (1912)	*Lodder and Kreger van Rij (1952)*	*Van der Walt (1970)*	*Yarrow (1984)*	*Vaughan-Martini and Martini (1998)*	*Kurtzman (2003)*
S. cerevisiae	S. cerevisiae	S. cerevisiae	S. cerevisiae	S. cerevisiae	S. cerevisiae
S. ellipsoideus			(17 physiological races)	**S. bayanus**	**S. bayanus**
S. turbidans				**S. pastorianus**	**S. pastorianus**
S. ilicis				S. paradoxus	S. paradoxus
S. vordermanni					S. cariocanus
S. sake					S. kudriavzevii
S. cartilaginosus					S. mikatae
S. batatae					
S. tokyo					
S. yeddo					
S. coreanus	S. coreanus	S. coreanus			
S. willianus	S. willianus				
S. intermedius					
S. validus					
S. carlsbergensis	**S. carlsbergensis**				
S. monacensis	**S. uvarum**	**S. uvarum**			
	S. logos				
	S. bayanus				
S. uvarum	**S. pastorianus**	**S. bayanus**			
S. logos	S. oviformis				
	S. beticus				
S. bayanus					
S. pastorianus					
	S. heterogenicus	**S. heterogenicus**			
	S. globosus	**S. globosus**			
		S. abuliensis			
		S. inusistatus			
		S. aceti			
		S. prostoserdovi			
		S. oleaginosus			
		S. olaceus			
		S. caensis			
		S. diastaticus			
		S. hispaniensis			
		S. norbensis			
		S. cardubensis			
		S. gaditensis			
		S. hispalensis			
	S. chevalieri	S. chevalieri			
	S. fructum				
	S. italicus	S. italicus			
	S. steineri				

Note: Yeast important for the Fermentation Industry belong to the *Saccharomyces sensu stricto* species complex. The classification of these species has undergone numerous changes depending on the classification technique employed. Over the years, species have been created, eliminated and fused, causing confusion among yeast scientists and technologists. In this table are reported the *Saccharomyces sensu stricto* species acknowledged from the first yeast classification of Guillermond (1912) to the currently accepted classification (Kurtzman, 2003). In bold are marked the species involved in the lager brewing yeast genome.

were also being evaluated. With the further development of molecular based techniques, such as nucleotide sequencing and polymerase chain reaction (PCR), yeast grouping has been carried out in an increasingly accurate way. However, depending on the tests employed, yeasts ended up being grouped in different ways and the number of species within the *Saccharomyces sensu stricto* complex changed accordingly (Rainieri *et al.*, 2003). This situation contributed to confuse yeast scientists and technologists. Table 8.2 shows the development of the changes within the *Saccharomyces sensu stricto* yeasts, starting from the first published study on yeast taxonomy to the currently accepted classification.

Saccharomyces bayanus and *Saccharomyces pastorianus* taxonomy

In spite of the sophisticated taxonomic techniques now available and in spite of the importance that some of these species have for the Fermentation Industry, the most recent yeast classification is not yet considered sufficiently accurate. This is especially true for the species *S. bayanus* and *S. pastorianus*, which are the most relevant for the Fermentation Industry as they include wine, brewing and cider strains. Isolates belonging to these two species are very heterogeneous, as they include cultures of hybrid nature, which make difficult their exact taxonomic collocation. Some authors (Nguyen and Gaillardin, 1997; Rainieri *et al.*, 1999; Nguyen *et al.*, 2000) divided the *S. bayanus* species into two groups: (1) *S. bayanus* variety *bayanus*, a group containing the current type strain (CBS 380) and a miscellanea of hybrid strains not generally isolated in natural environments, but preserved in Cultures Collections and (2) *S. bayanus* variety *uvarum*, commonly referred to as *Saccharomyces uvarum*, which contains strains of non-hybrid origin, widespread in nature, especially in the oenological environment (Naumov *et al.*, 2000; Naumov *et al.*, 2002; Demuyter *et al.*, 2004). *S. uvarum* is the only group within the two species that shows homogeneous and consistent genetic and metabolic characteristics (Giudici *et al.*, 1998; Pulvirenti *et al.*, 2000; Nguyen and Gaillardin, 2005) and because of this, a representative of this group has been chosen to be fully sequenced (Kellis *et al.*, 2003). *S. pastorianus* also contains strains of hybrid origin that possess very variable characteristics and are therefore very difficult to group (Yamagishi and Ogata, 1999; Casaregola *et al.*, 2001). Lager brewing strains are currently classified as *S. pastorianus*.

Table 8.3 Grouping of *S. bayanus* and *S. pastorianus* yeasts according to their genome constitution

Genetic line	*Genome*	*Representative strain*	*Species according to current classification*
Pure line 1	*S. uvarum*	CBS[a] 7001	
Pure line 2	*S. bayanus*	NBRC[b] 1948	*S. bayanus*
Hybrid line 1	*S. bayanus* + *S. uvarum* + Lg[c]	CBS 380	
Hybrid line 2	*S. cerevisiae* + *S. bayanus* + Lg	Lager yeasts	*S. pastorianus*
Hybrid line 3	*S. cerevisiae* + *S. bayanus* + *S. uvarum* + Lg	Hybrid wine yeasts	

Notes: *S. bayanus* and *S. pastorianus* are important species for the Fermentation Industry as they include wine, cider and lager brewing strains. In spite of their importance, they have not yet been satisfactorily classified. In fact, they are highly heterogeneous species containing strains of hybrid and non-hybrid nature. A detailed study on the genome constitution of these two species carried out on a high number of strains, highlighted that they can be subdivided into five genetic groups: (a) two pure genetic lines (formed by strains that are not a product of interspecific hybridization) and (b) three hybrid lines (formed by strains that are the product of multiple hybridization). The hybrid lines containing the *S. cerevisiae* genome are currently considered as a part of the *S. pastorianus* species, whereas both pure lines and the hybrid line not containing the *S. cerevisiae* genome are part of the *S. bayanus* species. A representative strain of reference is shown for each group.

[a]CBS (Centraal Bureau voor Schimmelcultures, Utrecth, The Netherlands).

[b]NBRC (NITE Biological Resource Center, Department of Biotechnology, National Institute for Technology and Evaluation, Chiba, Japan).

[c]Lg (Lager type genome, a type of genome recently detected in lager yeast that differs from the *S. bayanus* and *S. uvarum* genomes and is present in various portions of the non-*S. cerevisiae* genome of lager yeasts).

Source: Rainieri *et al.* (2006).

Current developments of brewing yeasts classification

Recently, Rainieri *et al.* (2006) studied the genetic variability of *S. bayanus* and *S. pastorianus* yeasts and concluded that indeed five distinct groups of yeasts contribute to form these two species, namely; (a) two pure genetic lines, represented by: (1) *S. uvarum* and (2) a novel *S. bayanus* non-hybrid group typified by strain NITE Biological Resource Center (NBRC) 1948 and (b) three multiple genetic lines: (1) containing both the *S. bayanus* and the *S. uvarum* genome plus a novel genome referred to as Lager (Lg genome), (2) containing the *S. cerevisiae*, the *S. bayanus* and the Lg genome and (3) containing the *S. cerevisiae*, the *S. bayanus*, the *S. uvarum* and the Lg genome (Rainieri *et al.*, 2006). According to this grouping, lager brewing strains are part of multiple genetic line containing the *S. cerevisiae*, the *S. bayanus* and the Lg genomes. Table 8.3 shows the details of this grouping.

This controversial taxonomic situation has affected differently the two types of brewing yeasts: ale yeasts have been classified by Hansen as *S. cerevisiae* more than one century ago, and still today this grouping has proved to be valid. On the contrary, lager brewing yeasts have been classified in several different ways over the years. Hansen initially classified them as *S. carlsbergensis* (Hansen, 1908); however, in the 1970s this species was not considered valid any longer and lager yeasts were referred to as *S. uvarum* (Van der Walt, 1970). In the following yeasts classification, all *Saccharomyces* species were gathered under the only species *S. cerevisiae*, which was subdivided into 17 physiological races, and lager yeasts became *S. cerevisiae* physiological race *uvarum* (Yarrow, 1984). Since 1998, lager yeasts have been classified as *S. pastorianus* (Vaughan-Martini and Martini, 1998).

Brewing scientists and technologist have generally faced the problem of lager yeast taxonomy in a very practical and sensible way: still today, in fact, in the brewery, lager strains are generally referred to as *S. carlsbergensis*, the original name assigned by Hansen to these cultures.

Characteristics of Ale and Lager Yeasts

Ale yeasts

Phenotypic Characteristics Ale yeasts generally form branched chains of cells, do not ferment melibiose, have an optimal fermentation temperature of 20–25°C and can grow above 37°C (Tornai-Lehoczki and Daluchy, 2000).

One of the distinctive technological traits of ale yeasts is their ability to produce high concentrations of esters, compounds that impart a fruity aroma to beer; ale beers are, in fact, often described as "fruity" (Stewart *et al.*, 1977). Another characteristic that within brewing strains has been detected only in some ale strains, is the ability to decarboxylate phenolic acids producing some compounds considered off-flavors such as 4-vinylguaiacol (McMurrough *et al.*, 1996). This trait is generally negative; however, it is acceptable for some specialty beer such as the German wheat beer (Bamforth, 2000). Table 8.4 summarizes some of the most important phenotypic characteristics and technological features of ale yeasts in comparison to lager yeasts.

Genomic Characteristics All in all, not many studies have been carried out to define the genome of ale yeasts and this is probably due to the fact that ale beers represent a minor production compared to lager beers.

With no doubt, ale strains belong to the *S. cerevisiae* species. Investigations carried out by Pedersen (1986) demonstrated that they are closely related to the *S. cerevisiae* laboratory strain S288C. A number of further studies investigating the entire genome of ale yeasts using the Amplified Fragment Length Polymorphism (AFLP) analysis (Azumi and Goto-Yamamoto, 2001), Random Amplified Polymorphic DNA (RAPD) analysis (Tornai-Lehoczki and Daluchy, 2000), as well as the chromosomal banding pattern obtained by Contour-Clamped Homogeneous Electric Field (CHEF) analysis (Johnston *et al.*, 1989), and more recently the construction of a two-dimensional protein map specific for ale strains (Kobi *et al.*, 2004), have confirmed this association. All these studies have also highlighted a high degree of interspecific heterogeneity in ale yeasts.

In spite of having a genome that is highly similar to *S. cerevisiae* laboratory strains, ale yeasts also show a number of characteristics that make them unique among *Saccharomyces* yeasts. These features have probably evolved as a consequence of adaptation to the fermentation substrate, the fermentation technique, and are also a consequence of the artificial selection carried out by brewers, who would chose and perpetuate only the cultures providing a final product with highly desirable characteristics. While laboratory *S. cerevisiae* strains are mainly haploid or diploid, *S. cerevisiae* ale strains, as the majority of industrial *Saccharomyces* yeasts, are polyploid (Stewart *et al.*, 1977). Moreover, they sporulate very poorly and the rare spores are generally non-viable.

Lager yeasts

Phenotypic Characteristics Among the distinctive physiological characteristics of lager brewing strains are the ability to use melibiose as a carbon source; the ability to ferment well at low temperatures (8–10°C); the inability to grow above 37°C; and the presence of an active system in the cell for fructose transport (Rodrigues de Sousa *et al.*,

Table 8.4 Some of the major characteristics typical of ale and lager yeasts

Ale yeasts	*Lager yeasts*
Species specific characteristics	
S. cerevisiae polyploid strain	*S. pastorianus* allotetraploid strains
Single genome	Multiple genome
Do not ferment the sugar melibiose	Generally ferment the sugar melibiose
Grow above 37°C	Do not grow above 37°C
Absence of fructose transport system	Presence of fructose transport system
Characteristics influencing technological process of brewing	
Ferment well at 25°C	Ferment well at 10°C
Highly hydrophobic cells	Low hydrophobic cells
Slow uptake of maltotriose	Efficient uptake of maltotriose
Characteristics influencing the final product	
Can decarboxilate phenolic acids → off-flavors	Unable to decarboxilate phenolic acids → no off-flavors
High esters production	Low esters production
Low amount sulfite production	High amount sulfite production

Note: Ale and lager yeasts are the agents of alcoholic fermentation in brewing. They belong to two different species, namely *S. cerevisiae* and *S. pastorianus*, and are employed in two different brewing techniques: ale brewing (where fermentation is carried out at 20–25°C) and lager brewing (where fermentation is carried out at 8–10°C). These yeasts show different characteristics; (i) some of these reflect the traits typical of the species, (ii) others are exploited by the technique of production and (iii) others are responsible for the distinctive traits of the beer obtained. Species-specific traits are also used taxonomically to distinguish yeasts at species level, in particular the ability to grow above 37°C, the ability to ferment the sugar melibiose and the presence of an active transport system for fructose. Important characteristics exploited by the different technological use of the two types of yeasts are: the ability to carry out efficient fermentation at the temperature employed in the two different brewing techniques (10°C and 25°C for lager and ale, respectively), the high hydrophobicity of ale cells that make them adhere to the CO_2 particles of the foam and to be carried to the top of the vessel, and the efficient uptake by lager yeasts of maltotriose, which is the most abundant but less efficiently metabolized sugar of wort. Important traits that influence the characteristics of the final product are the inability of lager yeasts, and actually of most brewing yeasts, to decarboxilate phenolic acid, this decarboxilation causes the release of unwanted off-flavors in beer. The effect of this decarboxilation is acceptable in wheat beer. Esters are compounds imparting a fruity aroma in beer; they are specifically produced by ale yeasts that impart to is beer a specific fruity aroma. Sulfites play in beer an antioxidant activity and contribute to flavor stability, lager yeast produce more sulfites than ale, and lager beer are generally regarded as "sulfury" beers.

1995). These features have been used for years to differentiate lager yeasts from other *Saccharomyces* yeasts, including ale strains (Vaughan-Martini and Martini, 1993).

Some of the most important brewing characteristics that are considered typical of lager yeasts are an efficient uptake of maltotriose, and a high production of sulfite. The efficient uptake of maltotriose is a very important trait. Actually, maltotriose is one of the most abundant sugars in wort; however, it has the lowest priority of uptake compared to the other sugars and its slow metabolization is often the cause of reduced fermentation activity. Lager yeasts utilize maltotriose faster compared to ale yeasts (Zheng *et al.*, 1994) and this seem to be due to a difference in the sugar transport system. Ale yeasts possess broad substrate-specificity transporters that could cause competition between the uptake of different sugars, whereas lager strains possess a more specific transport system for sugars (Vidgren *et al.*, 2005). Sulfite plays an antioxidant activity in beer and is also a key compound for beer flavor stability. Lager yeasts produce higher amounts of sulfite compared to ale yeasts and lager beer is often described as a type of beer with a "sulfury aroma" (Stewart *et al.*, 1977), see Table 8.4.

Genomic Characteristics A high number of studies have been carried out over the years to elucidate the genome and the functionality of lager brewing yeasts; these studies have led to interesting findings not only under the technological point of view, but have also set the basis for the development of studies on the evolution of industrial yeasts.

The Multiple Genome of Lager Brewing Strains Many works have supported the hypothesis that the genome of lager brewing yeasts is composed of at least two divergent genomes; a *S. cerevisiae*-type and a non-*S. cerevisiae*-type genome, very likely related to the genome of the *S. bayanus* species. Table 8.5 summarizes some of the most important

Table 8.5 Some of the major strategies employed for elucidating the multiple nature of the lager brewing yeast genome

Strategy	*Genome area*[a]		*Authors*
Sc type gene probe/sequencing	Chr. II	*BAP2*	Kodama *et al.* (2001)
Sc type gene probe/sequencing/PCR–RFLP[b]	Chr. III	*HIS4*; *LEU2*; *MAT*; *HML*; *HMR*; *SUP-RL1*	Nillson-Tillgren *et al.* (1981), Casaregola *et al.* (2001), Pedersen (1985) and Holmberg (1982)
Sc type gene probe/sequencing	Chr. IV	*HO*	Tamai *et al.* (2000)
Sc type gene probe/sequencing/PCR–RFLP	Chr. V	*ILV1*; *CAN1*; *CYC7*; *URA3*; *MXR1*	Nilsson-Tillgren *et al.* (1986), Casaregola *et al.* (2001) and Hansen (1999)
Cloning and sequencing	Chr. VI	*MET10*	Hansen and Kielland-Brandt (1994)
Cloning and sequencing	Chr. VII	*ACB1*	Børsting *et al.* (1997)
Sc type gene probe/sequencing	Chr. X	*ILV3*; *CYC1*	Casey *et al.* (1986a)
Sc type gene probe/sequencing	Chr. XI	*MET14*	Johannesen and Hansen (2002)
Sc type gene probe/sequencing	Chr. XII	*ILV5*; *ILV2*	Petersen *et al.* (1987)
Sc type gene probe/sequencing/PCR–RFLP	Chr. XIV	*MET2*	Hansen and Kielland-Brandt (1994) and Casaregola *et al.* (2001)
Sc type gene probe/sequencing	Chr. XV	*ATF1*	Fuji *et al.* (1996)
Proteome analysis	Entire genome		Jubert *et al.* (2000)
Probes on chromosomes CHEF[c] pattern	Entire genome		Tamai *et al.* (1998) and Yamagishi and Ogata (1999)
DNA reassociation analysis	Entire genome		Vaughan-Martini and Martini (1987)
AFLP[d] analysis	Entire genome		De Barros Lopes *et al.* (2002)
RAPD–PCR[e] analysis	Entire genome		Fernandez-Espinar *et al.* (2003)
Total sequencing of lager strain	Entire genome		Nakao *et al.* (2003)
PCR–RFLP/sequencing	48 genes over 16 chromosomes		Rainieri *et al.* (2006)

Notes: Many studies have confirmed that lager brewing yeast is composed by at least two different genomes; one nearly identical to *S. cerevisiae* and one similar to *S. bayanus*. Most of the approaches taken were based on the Southern hybridization analysis of lager yeast DNA employing DNA probes made with genes isolated from *S. cerevisiae*. A number of genes relevant for the brewing process and located in different chromosomes have been cloned from *S. cerevisiae* and used as probes to detect the presence of complementary DNA fragments in lager yeasts, these complementary fragments have been subsequently characterized by PCR–RFLP or sequencing. In all cases, the genome of lager yeasts showed two types of genes corresponding to the *S. cerevisiae* gene probe; one nearly identical to *S. cerevisiae* and one showing a high similarity to *S. bayanus*. Results confirming this finding have been obtained also by other techniques, such as Southern hybridization of *S. cerevisiae* probes on the chromosomes separated on an agarose gel (CHEF technique), the *S. cerevisiae* genome hybridization to a lager yeasts (DNA reassociation analysis), AFLP and PCR–RFLP analysis on areas covering the entire genome, the detection of all the proteins expressed in comparison with those expressed by *S. cerevisiae* and *S. bayanus* (proteome analysis), until the total nucleotide sequencing of a representative lager yeasts. A brief description of all the techniques mentioned here is given in Table 8.1.

[a] Chromosome location (Chr.) and genes (BAP2, etc.) are indicated for the studies carried out on specific genes.
[b] PCR–RFLP = polymerase chain reaction–restriction fragment length polymorphism.
[c] CHEF = Contour-clamped Homogeneous Electric Field.
[d] AFLP = Amplified Fragment Length Polymorphism.
[e] RAPD–PCR = Random Amplified Polymorphic DNA–PCR.

strategies adopted over the years to investigate lager yeast genome. Most of the approaches taken were based on the Southern hybridization analysis of lager yeast DNA employing DNA probes made with genes isolated from *S. cerevisiae*. A number of genes relevant for the brewing process and located in different chromosomes have been cloned from *S. cerevisiae* and used as probes to detect the presence of complementary DNA fragments in lager yeasts, these complementary fragments have been subsequently characterized by PCR–RFLP (restriction fragment length polymorphism) or sequencing. In all cases, the *S. cerevisiae* probe could detect two types of genes in lager yeasts; one nearly identical to *S. cerevisiae* and one showing a high similarity to *S. bayanus*. Works based on the study of the entire genome using different PCR-based techniques such as RFLP, RAPD, AFLP, corroborated this evidence. In the year 2000, the release of a protein profile specific for lager brewing strains provided further evidence of the co-existence of two types of genomes, as two co-existing protein profiles, one identical to *S. cerevisiae* and one highly similar to *S. bayanus*, were detected (Joubert *et al.*, 2000).

The Chromosomal Set Up of Lager Brewing Yeasts The existence of two divergent genomes in lager brewing yeasts implies also the presence of a multiple chromosomal set made of at least two types of chromosomes: one representing the *S. cerevisiae* genome and the other the non-*S. cerevisiae* genome. Since the 1980s, the co-existence of two types of chromosomes have been investigated at the Carlsberg Laboratories; some pioneer techniques were developed to enable the transfer of individual lager strains chromosomes into laboratory well-defined *S. cerevisiae* strains (Nilsson-Tillgren *et al.*, 1981; Nilsson-Tillgren *et al.*, 1986; Casey *et al.*, 1986b; Petersen *et al.*, 1987; Kielland-Brandt *et al.*, 1995). The study of the meiosis product of such artificial strains enabled these Authors to identify three types of chromosomes in lager brewing strains:

1. Chromosomes that could recombine efficiently with *S. cerevisiae* (homologous chromosomes).
2. Chromosomes that could recombine with difficulty with *S. cerevisiae* (homeologous chromosomes).
3. Chromosomes composed of parts of recombining and not recombining portions (mosaic chromosomes).

The existence of a multiple set of chromosomes has also been demonstrated by studies carried out by Tamai *et al.* (1998) and Yamagishi and Ogata (1999) based on the hybridization of DNA probes on the lager yeasts chromosomes separated by pulsed-field electrophoresis. Both studies confirmed the co-existence of *S. cerevisiae*-type and *S. bayanus*-type chromosomes in lager brewing strains.

In their recent studies, Rainieri *et al.* (2006) investigated the genome composition of several lager brewing strains, by PCR–RFLP or sequencing of 48 genes fragments from three distinct areas of each of the 16 chromosomes corresponding to the *S. cerevisiae* chromosomal set. This investigation, besides confirming the co-existence of the two different genomes (*S. cerevisiae*-type and *S. bayanus*-type), also highlighted the existence of a third type of genome, never detected before, referred to as Lg genome. Table 8.6 shows the genome composition detected with this study for some representative lager strains compared to the genome of *S. bayanus* and *S. uvarum* representative strains.

The Total Genome Sequence of a Representative Lager Yeast One of the most important efforts in elucidating the nature of lager yeasts has been the completion of the total nucleotide sequence of a representative lager brewing strain (Weihenstephan 34/70) carried out at the Institute of Fundamental Research of Suntory Research Center of Osaka (Japan). The details of this sequence have not been made public yet; however, the approach taken and the major implications of this outstanding scientific achievement are described by Nakao *et al.* (2003) and Kodama *et al.* (2006). The sequencing of a lager yeasts has revealed instrumental in: (a) definitely proving the co-existence of at least two genomes in lager yeasts; (b) defining how these two co-existing genomes are organized in the lager yeast; cell: and in (c) characterizing the complex chromosome structure of lager yeasts.

According to the results obtained with this sequencing, the presence of at least two genomes in lager yeasts was confirmed, as well as the existence of three types of chromosomes. Moreover, this investigation highlighted that lager brewing strains contain at least eight mosaic chromosomes and that in chromosomes VIII, X and XI, mosaic chromosomes co-exists with homologous and homeologous chromosomes (Kodama *et al.*, 2006). This complex situation has been confirmed also by competitive comparative genome hybridization of lager yeasts to the *S. cerevisiae* genome (Bond *et al.*, 2004).

Interspecific Diversity of Lager Brewing Strains The comparison of several lager brewing strains by comparative genomic hybridization with a *S. cerevisiae* DNA microarray revealed a very high degree of genetic diversity, and highlighted how the chromosomal set up can vary for lager yeasts at strain level (Kodama *et al.*, 2006). The major degrees of diversity have been detected between ancient lager strains (such as the first lager strains studied by Hansen referred to as *S. pastorianus*-type and *S. carlsbergensis* type strains) and strains currently used at industrial level for lager beer production. In particular, the ancient strains seem to have lost most of the *S. cerevisiae* genome that remains present in modern brewing yeasts. These findings are in agreement with the results of DNA reassociation experiments carried out in the 1980s, showing that the values of reassociation to *S. bayanus* are similar for most lager strains, while the values of reassociation to *S. cerevisiae* can differ greatly and are particularly low for the *S. pastorianus*-type strain (Vaughan-Martini and Martini, 1987).

Table 8.6 Genome composition deduced by PCR–RFLP and sequencing of 48 gene fragments in current lager strains compared to type strains relevant for the lager brewing yeast

	L	*C*	*R*	*L*	*C*	*R*	*L*	*C*	*R*	*L*	*C*	*R*
		Chr. I			*Chr. II*			*Chr. III*			*Chr. IV*	
S. cerevisiae	Sc	Sc	Sc	Sc	Sc	Sc	Sc	Sc	Sc	Sc	Sc	Sc
S. bayanus	Sb	Sb	Sb	Sb = Su	Sb	Sb	Sb	Sb	Sb	Sb	Sb = Su	Sb = Su
S. uvarum	Su	Su	Su	Sb = Su	Su	Su	Su	Su	Su	Su	Sb = Su	Sb = Su
S. pastorianus	Sc + Sb	Sc + Sb	Sc + Sb	Lg	Lg	Sb	Lg	Lg	Lg	Sb	Lg	Lg
S. carlsbergensis	Sc + Sb	Sc + Sb	Sc + Sb	Sc + Lg	Sc + Lg	Sc + Sb	Sc + Lg	Sc + Lg	Sc	Sc + Sb	Sc + Lg	Sc + Lg
Lager strain	Sc + Sb	Sc + Sb	Sc + Sb	Sc + Lg	Sc + Lg	Sc + Sb	Sc + Lg	Sc + Lg	Sc	Sc + Sb	Sc + Lg	Sc + Lg
		Chr. V			*Chr. VI*			*Chr. VII*			*Chr. VIII*	
S. cerevisiae	Sc	Sc	Sc	Sc	Sc	Sc	Sc	Sc	Sc	Sc	Sc	Sc
S. bayanus	Sb	Sb	Sb	Sb	Sb	Sb	Sb	Sb	Sb	Sb	Sb	Sb
S. uvarum	Su	Su	Su	Su	Su	Su	Su	Su	Su	Su	Su	Su
S. pastorianus	Sc + Sb	Sc + Sb	Sb	Lg	Lg	Lg	Sb	Sb	Sb	Sb	Sb	Sb
S. carlsbergensis	Sc + Sb	Sc + Sb	Sc + Sb	Lg	Lg	Lg	Sc + Sb	Sc + Sb	Sc + Sb	Sc + Sb	Sc + Sb	Sb
Lager strain	Sc + Sb	Sc + Sb	Sc + Sb	Sc + Lg	Sc + Lg	Sc + Lg	Sc + Sb	Sc + Sb	Sc + Sb	Sb	Sc + Sb	Sc + Sb
		Chr. IX			*Chr. X*			*Chr. XI*			*Chr. XII*	
S. cerevisiae	Sc	Sc	Sc	Sc	Sc	Sc	Sc	Sc	Sc	Sc	Sc	Sc
S. bayanus	Sb	Sb	Sb	Sb	Sb	Sb	Sb	Sb	Sb	Sb	Sb	Sb
S. uvarum	Su	Su	Su	Su	Su	Su	Su	Su	Su	Su	Su	Su
S. pastorianus	Sb	Sc + Sb	Sc + Sb	Sc + Sb	Sc + Sb	Sc + Sb	Sc + Sb	Sc + Sb	Sc + Sb	Sb	Sb	Sb
S. carlsbergensis	Sc + Sb	Sc + Sb	Sc + Sb	Sc + Sb	Sc + Sb	Sc + Sb	Sb	Sb	Sb	Sb	Sb	Sb
Lager strain	Sc + Sb	Sc + Sb	Sc + Sb	Sc + Sb	Sc + Sb	Sc + Sb	Sc + Sb	Sb	Sb	Sb	Sc + Sb	Sc + Sb
		Chr. XIII			*Chr. XIV*			*Chr. XV*			*Chr. XVI*	
S. cerevisiae	Sc	Sc	Sc	Sc	Sc	Sc	Sc	Sc	Sc	Sc	Sc	Sc
S. bayanus	Sb = Su	Sb	Sb	Sb	Sb = Su	Sb	Sb	Sb	Sb	Sb	Sb	Sb
S. uvarum	Sb = Su	Su	Su	Su	Sb = Su	Su	Su	Su	Su	Su	Su	Su
S. pastorianus	Lg	Lg	Sb	Sc + Lg	Sc + Lg	Sc + Sb	Sb	Sb	Sb	Sb	Lg	Lg
S. carlsbergensis	Lg	Sc + Lg	Sc + Sb	Sc + Lg	Sc + Lg	Sc + Sb	Sc + Sb	Sc + Sb	Sb	Sb	Lg	Lg
Lager strain	Sc + Lg	Sc + Lg	Sc + Sb	Sc + Sb	Sc + Sb	Sc + Sb	Sc + Sb	Sc + Sb	Sc + Sb	Sc + Sb	Sc + Lg	Sc + Lg

Note: PCR–RFLP and sequencing was carried out on the genome of some selected yeasts involved in the genome constitution of lager brewing strains. These include *S. cerevisiae*, *S. bayanus*, *S. uvarum*, ancient representatives of lager brewing strains (*S. pastorianus* and *S. carlsbergensis*) and a representative strain of lager yeasts currently employed in lager brewing production. For each strain, gene fragments located in three different areas for each of the 16 chromosomes corresponding to the *S. cerevisiae* chromosome set (left, center and right area, indicated as L, C and R, respectively), were amplified by PCR and distinguished by RFLP or sequencing. *S. cerevisiae*, *S. bayanus* and *S. uvarum* resulted pure genetic lines (with a single genome) whereas the lager strains tested showed a combination of the genomes of *S. cerevisiae*, *S. bayanus* and of a new genome never detected before and indicated as Lg (lager type genome). The genome of *S. uvarum* was never detected in the lager brewing strains analyzed. In the Table, for each chromosome location it is indicated which type/s of genome was found (Sc = *S. cerevisiae* type genome; Sb = *S. bayanus* type genome; Su = *S. uvarum* type genome; Lg = lager type genome). Chr. = chromosome; L = left telomere of chromosome; C = centromere area; R = right telomere area.

The Ploidy of Lager Brewing Strains In the light of these reports, establishing the exact ploidy of lager strains seems quite an arduous task. Flow cytometry analysis on some ancient lager yeasts (including the type strains of *S. pastorianus*, *S. carlsbergensis*, and *S. monacensis*), showed different ploidy for different strains; the type strains of *S. pastorianus* and *S. monacensis* resulting diploid, and the *S. carlsbergensis*-type strain resulting triploid (Naumova *et al.*, 2005). Bond *et al.* (2004) examined the copy number of *S. cerevisiae*-like genes in two lager yeasts: the detection of two copies in most cases, but also some discrete changes at distinct loci, led these Authors to conclude that lager yeasts should be aneuploid organisms. Considering all the data reported, including the new sequencing data and the latest microarray hybridization results, it seems reasonable to consider lager strains allopolyploid yeasts, with a highly irregular chromosomal set up that is aneuploid for some regions and that is variable for each strain. As a consequence of the allopolyploid and aneuploid nature, lager yeast do not generally show sexual reproduction, therefore they do not sporulate, and this makes very difficult to perform genetic studies, or to set up programs of genetic improvement using traditional genetic techniques.

Aneuploidy, polyploidy, and lack of sporulation are common traits of industrial yeasts, as mentioned already for ale yeasts. This condition, in spite of hampering the development of improvement programs, shows some advantages. The presence of multiple copies of the same gene, in fact, reduces the possible negative effects of mutations that very unlikely will affect all the existing gene copies; polyploid non-sporulating cultures are generally very stable and this feature guarantees that they do not modify their metabolic properties during subsequent use, a practice commonly employed in brewing (Dufour *et al.*, 2003).

The Origin of the Non-*S. cerevisiae*-Type Genome and the Shaping of Lager Brewing Yeast Genome The co-existence of at least two genomes in lager brewing strains has definitely been established; however, it still remains to clarify which is the exact contribution coming from each of these genomes. To achieve this, the understanding of the non-*S. cerevisiae* genome portion of lager yeasts is crucial. In fact, it is likely that the most useful features of lager brewing strains originated from specific traits of this part of the genome. So far, the nature of this portion is not fully clear; a number of studies revealed that it has a high similarity to the *S. bayanus* genome; nevertheless, a representative *S. bayanus* strain contributing to the lager genome has not been identified.

The Interaction Between Wine and Brewing Yeasts Rainieri *et al.* (2006) demonstrated that the only strains that are not the result of inter- or intraspecific hybridizations within the *S. bayanus* species are *S. uvarum* strains and one type of *S. bayanus* typified by strain NBRC 1948. Their work demonstrates that the genome of *S. uvarum* is not directly involved in the genetic composition of lager brewing strains. On the other hand, *S. bayanus* strain NBRC 1948 shares the same PCR–RFLP pattern as lager brewing strains in 67% of the 48 gene fragments that they examined.

S. uvarum is typically found in oenological environments, whereas *S. bayanus* strain NBRC 1948 was originally isolated from a brewing environment. These two groups of strains seem to have evolved from a common ancestor that diverged into two groups probably to become better suited to different nutritional habitats; oenological and brewing, respectively. In support of this hypothesis is the fact that the bottom fermenting brewing technique was originally created in Bavaria (Germany) towards the end of the nineteenth century when beer was cold conditioned in caves and the use of yeast cultures started becoming popular for bottom fermenting beer. The use of caves for preserving food was a common ancient practice. Bavaria has long been a wine producing area, and wines that were made in those days were also traditionally fermented and stored in the same caves were the lager brewing batches were kept. A cold fermenting type of strain was very likely responsible for the fermentation of such wines, as the low temperature inside caves (8–10°C) should have favored the development and activity of *S. uvarum*-like yeasts. Ecological studies on the distribution of *S. uvarum* strains have confirmed, in fact, that these yeasts are associated with low temperature climatic conditions and dominate wine fermentations conducted at low temperatures (Naumov *et al.*, 2000; Naumov *et al.*, 2002; Demuyter *et al.*, 2004). It is therefore very likely that *S. uvarum* strains could have contaminated the brewing batch or that the same type of yeast acted as the fermentation agent of both products (beer and wine) and differentiated at a later stage probably to adapt to the different nutritional habitat of the brewing environment. This hypothesis is sustained by physiological, metabolic, and molecular traits that are common to the *S. uvarum*, *S. bayanus* and *S. pastorianus* yeasts. For example, all these yearts have an optimal temperature for growth that is lower compared to other *Saccharomyces* yeasts and are not able to grow above 37°C. Furthermore, it has recently been proved that only strains belonging to these species have a gene (*FSY1*), which is specifically designed to promote an active transport inside the cell of fructose and consequently to optimize its utilization (Goncalves *et al.*, 2000). Fructose is one of the major sugars of grape juice; however, its concentration is not relevant in wort. The presence of an optimized system for fructose transport in lager brewing strains could simply represent a function inherited from a *S. uvarum*-like wine strain that, in a brewing habitat, gradually lost its role and scope.

The Lg Genome The nature of the non-*S. cerevisiae*-type genome of lager brewing strains is very complex and does not seem to be associated to any specific single strain or any pure genetic line. At least two types of complements seem to be composing this portion; namely, the *S. bayanus* genome and the Lg genome detected for the first time by Rainieri *et al.* (2006). The Lg genome has not yet been attributed to other existing *Saccharomyces* pure genetic lines and so far it has only been detected in association with other genomes; namely *S. cerevisiae*, *S. bayanus* and/or *S. uvarum* (see Table 8.5). In lager brewing strains, the Lg genome was detected exactly in all the cases when RFLP analysis was not sufficient to distinguish the *S. uvarum* from the *S. bayanus* genome and this could indicate that perhaps in lager brewing strains the *S. uvarum* genome (or the ancestral genome that originated both *S. bayanus* and *S. uvarum*) was gradually substituted by or gradually evolved to the Lg genome and therefore there might not be in nature a pure genetic line containing solely Lg genome.

The Hybrid Nature of the Non-S. cerevisiae Portion of Lager Brewing Yeast Genome The aforementioned findings suggest that lager brewing strains could have originated via a multiple hybridization event. De Barros Lopes *et al.* (2002) demonstrated that multiple hybridization events are possible in *Saccharomyces* yeasts. These authors proposed that lager brewing strains originated from a double hybridization event; one occurring between a *S. cerevisiae*- and a *S. bayanus*-like strain to form *S. pastorianus*, and one between this new formed *S. pastorianus* and a *S. cerevisiae* ale strain. A multiple hybridization event followed by chromosomal loss and rearrangements

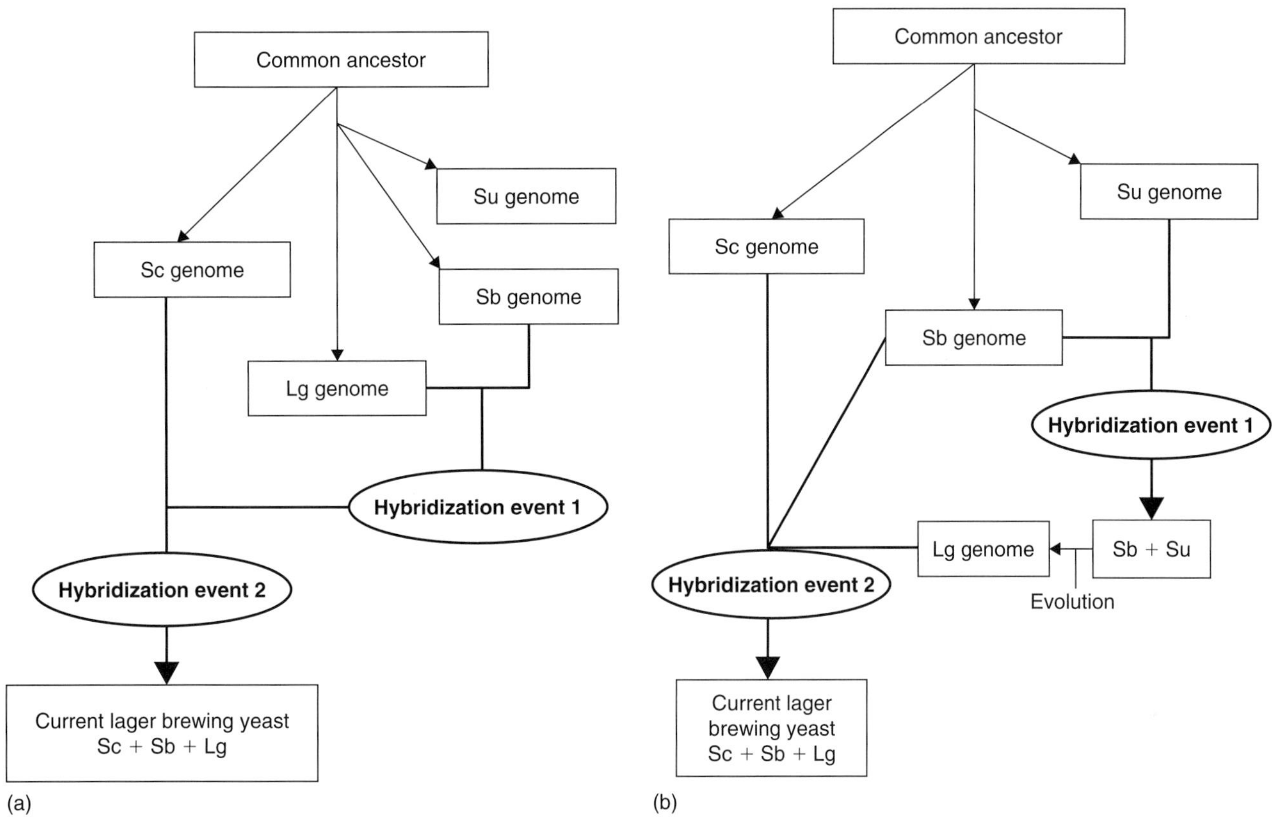

Figure 8.2 Two hypothesis on the origin of lager brewing yeast and on the lager-type genome (Lg genome) formation. Lager brewing yeasts are composed of at least two divergent genomes: one nearly identical to *S. cerevisiae* and one similar to *S. bayanus*. Recently, a new genome has been detected as a further portion of lager brewing genome by Rainieri *et al.* (2006) and was named Lg genome. The two hypothesis described in the figure attempt to establish the origin of lager yeasts and of this newly detected genome. *Saccharomyces* yeasts could have originated from a common ancestor, here only the species related to lager brewing strains are shown; *S. cerevisiae* diversified from *S. bayanus* and *S. uvarum* branched out from *S. bayanus* (or the other way around). (a) Hypothesis 1: The Lg genome evolved independently from the common ancestor of *Saccharomyces* yeasts, it hybridized with *S. bayanus* (first hybridization event) and the result of this mating hybridized a second time with a *S. cerevisiae* strain (second hybridization event). (b) Hypothesis 2: *S. bayanus* hybridized with *S. uvarum* (hybridization event 1) and the result of this hybridization underwent some evolutionary rearrangements that lead to the conversion of the *S. uvarum* genome to the Lg type genome. A second multiple hybridization event occurred between *S. cerevisiae*, the newly formed Lg genome and the *S. bayanus* genome (hybridization event 2) that formed the current lager brewing strains. Sc genome = genome from *S. cerevisiae*; Sb genome = genome from *S. bayanus*; Su genome = genome from *S. uvarum*; Lg genome = newly detected genome referred to as Lager genome or Lg genome. In bold are marked the possible ways to the hybridization events.

is a common mechanism of yeast genome evolution (Wolfe and Shields, 1997) and could also be at the basis of the non-*S. cerevisiae*-type genome in lager yeasts. Figure 8.2 shows two of the possible hypothesis on how current lager strains could have originated and on how the Lg genome portion could have evolved. Assuming that all *Saccharomyces* yeast originate from a common ancestor, Figure 8.2(a) shows hypothesis 1: the Lg genome evolved independently from the common ancestor of *Saccharomyces* yeasts, it hybridized with *S. bayanus* and the result of this mating hybridized a second time with a *S. cerevisiae* strain. Figure 8.2(b) shows hypothesis 2: *S. bayanus* hybridized with *S. uvarum* and the result of this hybridization underwent some evolutionary rearrangements that lead to the conversion of the *S. uvarum* genome to the Lg genome. A second multiple hybridization event occurred between *S. cerevisiae,* the newly formed Lg genome and the *S. bayanus* genome.

The alternative hypothesis of lager yeast being itself the common ancestor that originated the species composing or related to its genome (*S. cerevisiae*, *S. bayanus*, and *S. uvarum*) cannot be excluded.

Conclusions

The study of the origin and the characteristics of industrial yeast genomes is critical for understanding the metabolic properties of cultures guiding the fermentation processes. In brewing, as well as in any other fermented food, this knowledge is at the basis for the development of genetic improvement programs aimed at selecting and constructing yeasts targeted to optimize the brewing process and the overall beer quality. The case of lager brewing strains is particularly challenging and at the same time exciting. These strains represent, in fact, a unique example in yeast genetics, where the genome has evolved through the rearrangement of divergent genomes in a favorable and stable combination particularly suited to the brewing environment. In the light of the most recent scientific achievements, such as the genome sequence of a representative lager yeast, genomics and proteomics represent a great potential that can be exploited not only for the efficient manipulation of industrial yeasts, but also for the counteraction of pathogenic or undesirable cultures.

Summary Points

- Currently two types of beer are produced industrially: ale and lager beer. Lager beer contributes to the 90% of the global beer production, ale beer to the 5%. These two products are obtained by fermentation of malted barley juice (the wort) at 20–25°C and 8–10°C, respectively, by the activity of two types of yeasts named ale and lager yeasts.
- Ale yeasts are classified as *S. cerevisiae*; they differ from lager yeasts for their phenotypic and genomic characteristics. Among the major distinctive traits of these yeasts are the ability to ferment well at 20–25°C and to produce high concentrations of esters, thus imparting to ale beer a typical fruity aroma.
- Lager yeasts are currently classified as *S. pastorianus*, however, their name has changed several times over the years and their taxonomy is still controversial. Lager strains generally cannot grow above 37°C and ferment well at 8–10°C. They commonly produce a higher concentration of sulfites compared to ale yeasts, thus contributing to enhance the flavor stability of lager beer.
- The genome of lager yeasts is very complex and this is probably the cause of their difficult taxonomic collocation as well as their technological properties. The lager yeast genome is a multiple genome, composed by two portions: a *S. cerevisiae* portion and a non-*S. cerevisiae* portion. The latter is composed by two types of genomes: a *S. bayanus*-like genome and a newly discovered genome referred to as Lg genome. So far the Lg genome has not been associated to any existing yeast species; however, it seems genetically related to other cold fermenting *Saccharomyces* yeasts, such as *S. uvarum* wine strains.
- The multiple genome of lager yeasts seems to have originated from a series of hybridization events that involved the hybridization of the *S. cerevisiae* to the non-*S. cerevisiae* genome. The non-*S. cerevisiae* genome seems to be itself the product of hybridization.
- Three types of chromosomes can be detected in lager yeasts, *S. cerevisiae*-type chromosomes, *S. bayanus*-type chromosomes, and mosaic chromosomes between the two. The cells of lager yeasts are allopolyploid, with an irregular chromosomal set up that is aneuploid for some regions and variable for each strain. The total genome sequence of a representative lager brewing strain has recently confirmed the complex nature of the lager yeast genome and elucidated its chromosomes organization.
- The exploitation of these findings in studies of expression analysis, comparative genomics, and structural analysis will provide novel insight into the improvement of brewing production and beer quality as well as in elucidating beer beneficial characteristics.

Acknowledgments

Sandra Rainieri is supported by a fellowship from the Italian Ministry of University and Research under the program "Promoting the mobility of foreign researcher and Italian researcher residing abroad."

References

Azumi, M. and Goto-Yamamoto, N. (2001). *Yeast* 18, 1145–1154.

Bamforth, C.W. (2000). *Chem. Educ.* 5, 102–112.

Bond, U., Neal, C., Donnelly, D. and James, T.C. (2004). *Curr. Genet.* 45, 360–370.

Børsting, C., Hummel, R., Schultz, E.R., Rose, T.M., Pedersen, M.B., Knudsen, J. and Kristiansen, K. (1997). *Yeast* 13, 1409–1421.

Casaregola, S., Nguyen, H.V., Lepathitis, G., Kotyk, A. and Gaillardin, C. (2001). *Int. J. Syst. Evol. Microbiol.* 51, 1607–1618.

Casey, J.P. (1986a). *Carlsberg Res. Commun.* 51, 327–341.

Casey, J.P. (1986b). *Carlsberg Res. Commun.* 51, 343–362.

Corran, H.S. (1975). *A History of Brewing*. David and Charles PLC., Newton Abbot.

De Barros Lopes, M., Bellon, J.R., Shriley, N.J. and Ganter, P.F. (2002). *FEMS Yeast Res.* 1, 323–331.

Demuyter, C., Lollier, M., Legras, J-L. and Le Jeune, C. (2004). *J. Appl. Microbiol.* 97, 1140–1148.

Dengis, P.B. and Rouxhet, P.G. (1997). *Yeast* 13, 931–943.

Dufour, J-P., Verstrepen, K. and Derdelinckx, G. (2003). In Boekhout, T. and Robert, V. (eds), *Yeasts in Food*, pp. 347–388. Beher's Verlag, Hamburg.

Fernandez-Espinar, M.T., Barrio, E. and Querol, A. (2003). . *Yeast* 20, 1213–1226.

Fuji, T., Yoshimoto, H., Nagasawa, N., Bogaki, T., Tamai, Y. and Hamachi, M. (1996). *Yeast* 12, 593–598.

Giudici, P., Caggia, C., Pulvirenti, A. and Rainieri, S. (1998). *J. Appl. Microbiol.* 84, 811–819.

Goncalves, P., Rodrigues de Sousa, H. and Spencer-Martins, I. (2000). *J. Bacteriol.* 182, 5628–5630.

Guillermond, A. (1912). *Les Levures*. Octave Doin et Fils, Paris.

Hansen, E.C. (1883). *Medd. Carlsberg Lab.* 2, 29–86.

Hansen, E.C. (1908). *Compt. Rend. Trav. Lab. Carlsberg* 7, 179–217.

Hansen, J. (1999). *Appl. Environ. Microbiol.* 65, 3915–3919.

Hansen, J. and Kielland-Brandt, M.C. (1994). *Gene* 140, 33–40.

Holmberg, S. (1982). *Carlsberg Res. Commun.* 47, 233–244.

Johannesen, P.F. and Hansen, J. (2002). *FEMS Yeast Res.* 1, 315–322.

Johnston, J.R., Curran, L., Contopopulu, R.C. and Mortimer, R.K. (1989). *7th International Symposium on Yeast*, Perugia, Italy. Wiley and Sons, Chichester, UK, p. S255.

Joubert, R., Brignon, P., Lehmann, C., Monribot, C., Gendre, F. and Boucherie, H. (2000). *Yeast* 16, 511–522.

Kellis, M., Patterson, N., Endrizzi, M., Birren, B. and Lander, E.S. (2003). *Nature* 423, 241–254.

Kielland-Brandt, M.C., Nilsson-Tillgren, T., Gjermansen, C., Holmber, S. and Pedersen, M.B. (1995). In Wheals, A.E., Rose, A.H. and Harrison, J.S. (eds), *The Yeast*, pp. 223–254. Academic Press, London.

Kobi, D., Zugmeyer, S., Potier, S. and Jaquet-Gutfreund, L. (2004). *FEMS Yeast Res.* 5, 213–230.

Kodama, Y., Omura, F. and Ashikari, T. (2001). *Appl. Environ. Microbiol.* 67, 3455–3462.

Kodama, Y., Kielland-Brandt, M.C. and Hansen, J. (2006). In Sunnerhagen, P. and Piškur, J. (eds), *Comparative Genomics Using Fungi as Models*, pp. 145–164. Springer-Verlag, Berlin.

Kurtzman, C. (2003). *FEMS Yeast Res.* 4, 233–245.

Lodder, J. and Kreger van Rij, N.J.W. (1952). *The Yeast: A Taxonomic Study*. North-Holland Publishing Company, Amsterdam.

McMurrough, I., Madigan, D., Donnelly, D., Hurley, J., Doyle, A.M., Hennigan, G., McNulgy, N. and Smyth, M.R. (1996). *J. Inst. Brew.* 102, 327–332.

Nakao, Y., Kodama, Y., Nakamura, N., Ito, T., Hattori, M., Shiba, T. and Ashikari, T. (2003). *Proceedings of the 29th Congress European Brewing Convention*, May, 15–22, Dublin. Fachverlag Hans Carl, Nürnberg, pp. 524–530.

Naumov, G.I., Masneuf, I., Naumova, E.S., Aigle, M. and Dubourdieu, D. (2000). *Res. Microbiol.* 151, 683–691.

Naumov, G.I., Naumova, E.S., Antunovics, Z. and Sipiczki, M. (2002). *Appl. Microbiol. Biotechnol.* 59, 727–730.

Naumova, E.S., Naumov, G.I., Masneuf-Pomarede, I., Aigle, M. and Dubourdieu, D. (2005). *Yeast* 22, 1099–1115.

Nilsson-Tillgren, T., Gjermansen, C., Kielland-Brandt, M. C., Petersen, J.G.L. and Holmberg, S. (1981). *Carlsberg Res. Commun.* 46, 65–76.

Nilsson-Tillgren, T., Gjermansen, C., Holmberg, S., Petersen, J.G.L. and Kielland-Brandt, M.C. (1986). *Carlsberg Res. Commun.* 51, 309–326.

Nguyen, H-V. and Gaillardin, C. (1997). *Syst. Appl. Microbiol.* 20, 286–294.

Nguyen, H-V. and Gaillardin, C. (2005). *FEMS Yeast Res.* 5, 471–483.

Nguyen, H-V., Lepingle, A. and Gaillardin, C. (2000). *Syst. Appl. Microbiol.* 23, 71–85.

Pedersen, M.B. (1985). *Carlsberg Res. Commun.* 50, 263–267.

Pedersen, M.B. (1986). *Carlsberg Res. Commun.* 51, 163–183.

Petersen, J.G.L., Nilsson-Tillgren, T., Kielland-Brandt, M.C., Gjermansen, C. and Holmberg, S. (1987). *Curr. Genet.* 12, 167–174.

Polaina, J. (2002). In Arora, D.K. and Khachatourians, G.G. (eds), *Applied Mycology and Biotechnology*, pp. 1–17. Elsevier, Amsterdam.

Pulvirenti, A., Nguyen, H-V., Caggia, C., Giudici, P., Rainieri, S. and Zambonelli, C. (2000). *FEMS Microbiol. Lett.* 192, 191–196.

Rainieri, S., Zambonelli, C., Hallsworth, J.E., Pulvirenti, A. and Giudici, P. (1999). *FEMS Microbiol. Lett.* 177, 177–185.

Rainieri, S., Zambonelli, C. and Kaneko, Y. (2003). *J. Biosci. Bioeng.* 96, 1–9.

Rainieri, S., Kodama, Y., Kaneko, Y., Mikata, K., Nakao, Y. and Ashikari, T. (2006). *Appl. Environ. Microbiol.* 72, 3968–3974.

Rodrigues de Sousa, H., Madeira-Lopes, A. and Spencer-Martins, I. (1995). *Syst. Appl. Microbiol.* 18, 44–51.

Stewart, G.G., Goring, T.E. and Russell, I. (1977). *J. Am. Soc. Brew. Chem.* 35, 168–178.

Tamai, Y., Momma, T., Yoshimoto, H. and Kaneko, Y. (1998). *Yeast* 14, 923–933.

Tamai, Y., Tanaka, K., Umemoto, N., Tomizuka, K. and Kaneko, Y. (2000). *Yeast* 16, 1335–1343.

Tornai-Lehoczki, J. and Daluchy, D. (2000). *Int. J. Food Microbiol.* 62, 37–45.

Van der Walt, J.P. (1970). In Lodder, J. (ed.), *The Yeast: A Taxonomic Study*, pp. 555–718. North-Holland Publishing Company, Amsterdam.

Vaughan-Martini, A. and Martini, A. (1987). *Antonie van Leeuwenhoek* 53, 77–84.

Vaughan-Martini, A. and Martini, A. (1993). *Syst. Appl. Microbiol.* 16, 113–119.

Vaughan-Martini, A. and Martini, A. (1998). In Kurtzman, C. and Fell, J.W. (eds), *The Yeast: A Taxonomic Study*, pp. 358–371. Elsevier Science, Amsterdam.

Vidgren, V., Ruohonen, L. and Londesborough, J. (2005). *Appl. Environ. Microbiol.* 71, 7846–7857.

Wolfe, K.H. and Shields, D.C. (1997). *Nature* 387, 708–713.

Yamagishi, H. and Ogata, T. (1999). *Syst. Appl. Microbiol.* 22, 341–353.

Yarrow, D. (1984). In Kreger-van Rij, N.J.W. (ed.), *The Yeast: A Taxonomic Study*, pp. 379–393. Elsevier Science Publishers, Amsterdam.

Zheng, X., D'Amore, T., Russell, I. and Stewart, G.G. (1994). *Ind. Microbiol. Biotechnol.* 13, 159–166.

9

Flocculation in *Saccharomyces Cerevisiae*

Eduardo V. Soares Chemical Engineering Department, Superior Institute of Engineering from Porto Polytechnic Institute, Porto, Portugal
IBB-Institute for Biotechnology and Bioengineering, Centre for Biological Engineering, Universidade do Minho, Braga, Portugal

Abstract

Yeast flocculation is a reversible, non-sexual and multivalent process of cell aggregation into multicellular masses, called flocs, with the subsequent rapid removal of flocs from the medium in which they are suspended. Traditionally associated with beer production, flocculation might also be useful in modern biotechnology as a low cost and easy method of cell separation. Flocculation characteristics, namely the degree and the time of onset of flocculation, are of exceptional interest to brewing industry because they can affect beer characteristics.

Flocculent cells have a specific lectin-like protein, which sticks out of the yeast cell wall, recognizes and interacts with the carbohydrates residues of α-mannan (receptors) of adjoining cell walls; calcium ions are required to activate the lectin. Taking into account the sugar sensitiveness and ethanol dependence, four flocculation phenotypes have been described: Flo1 phenotype, NewFlo phenotype, mannose insensitive (MI) phenotype and strains whose flocculation requires the presence of ethanol.

Yeast flocculation is a complex process, influenced by multiple factors, namely: cell surface characteristics, chemical characteristics of the medium, fermentation conditions and the expression of several specific genes such as *FLO1*, *FLO5*, *FLO8* and *Lg-FLO1*.

This work reviews, discusses and updates the current knowledge on yeast flocculation with particular attention to the aspects related with brewing yeasts. The loss and the onset of flocculation in brewing yeasts belonging to NewFlo phenotype are also examined and discussed. Finally, the possibility of flocculation to constitute a long-term survival mechanism or a means of protection against an unfavorable environment is discussed.

List of Abbreviations

$[Ca^{2+}]_f$	Free calcium concentration
Con A	Concanavalin A
CSH	Cell surface hydrophobicity
EDTA	Ethylenediaminetetraacetic acid
GPI	Glycosylphosphatidylinositol
Kbp	Kilobase pair
MI	Mannose insensitive
mnn mutants	Mannan synthesis mutants
NCYC	National Collection of Yeast Culture
PCR	Polymerase chain reaction
S. cerevisiae	*Saccharomyces cerevisiae*
YEPD	Yeast extract, peptone, dextrose
YNB	Yeast nitrogen base

Introduction

Cellular aggregation is a well-known phenomenon in higher organisms and widespread in microbial world, being observed within bacteria, yeasts, filamentous fungi, algae and protozoa (Calleja, 1987). Yeast flocculation has been traditionally used in many fermentation processes, like wine making or in the brewing industry. Nevertheless, this property might also be useful in modern biotechnology, as in the production of heterologous proteins or ethanol in continuous fermentations (Domingues *et al.*, 2000, 2005; Verbelen *et al.*, 2006), since it is a natural, easy, eco-friendly and a low cost method of cell separation from the fermentation broth (Figure 9.1), thus facilitating further downstream processing.

Although flocculation is fundamentally linked with the yeast *Saccharomyces cerevisiae* and particularly with brewing yeast strains, it seems to be a more generalized phenomena, being found in other yeast genera, namely *Candida utilis, Hansenula anomala, Kluyveromyces marxianus, Pichia pastoris, Saccharomycodes ludwigii, Schizosaccharomyces pombe and Zygosaccharomyces* sp. (Stratford, 1992c).

The present contribution concerns almost exclusively to the present knowledge of flocculation in *S. cerevisiae,* with particular attention to the aspects related to its use in brewing industry. Recent reviews of yeast adhesion and yeast flocculation specifically, where complementary viewpoints can be found, were performed by Jin and Speers (1998), Domingues *et al.* (2000), Verstrepen *et al.* (2003) and Verstrepen and

Beer in Health and Disease Prevention
ISBN: 978-0-12-373891-2

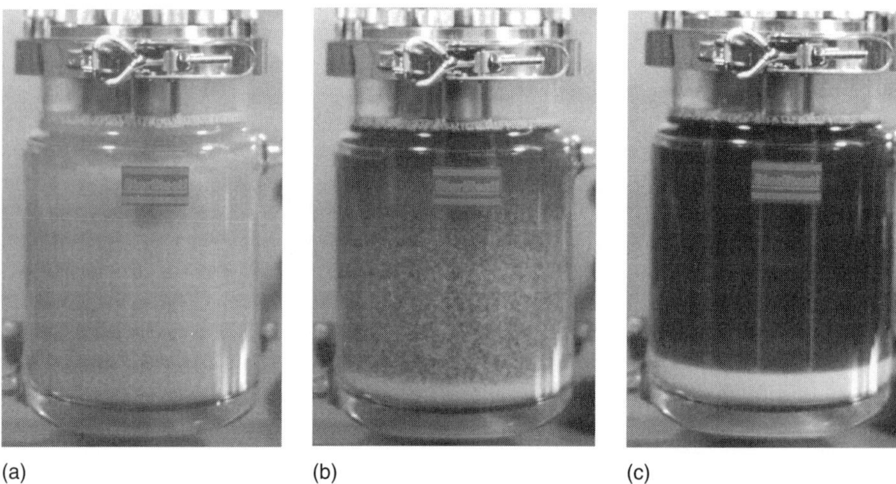

Figure 9.1 Flocculating culture of the ale-brewing yeast strain of *S. cerevisiae* National Collection of Yeast Culture (NCYC) 1195. (a) Culture continuously aerated and stirred; (b) and (c) 30 s and 1 min, after aeration and stirring was stopped, respectively.

Klis (2006). For an earlier work, the reader may consult the reviews by Calleja (1987) and Stratford (1992a, c).

Types of Yeast Aggregation

Cellular aggregation can be defined as a meeting of several units in order to form a large unit called the aggregate. The aggregates formation implicates the cell movement, which is initially as a form of isolated cells, and the establishment of reversible multicellular contacts. The aggregation process should be spontaneous and compatible with the life of the cells (Calleja, 1987). Common examples of yeast aggregation, which should be distinguished from flocculation, are sexual aggregation and chain formation (Table 9.1); however, the last phenomenon does not fulfill the definition of aggregation.

Yeast flocculation can be defined as a reversible, multivalent and non-sexual aggregation of yeast cells into multicellular masses (called flocs) (Figure 9.2), dispersible by ethylenediaminetetraacetic acid (EDTA) or specific sugars, with subsequent fast sedimentation of these flocs from the medium in which they were suspended (Table 9.1) (Stewart, 1975; Calleja, 1987). The word floc derives from the Latin word *floccus*, which means a lock of wool. The cells with the ability to form flocs are called flocculants and look like tufts of wool (Figure 9.1), while the cells not able to form flocs are usually known as powdery.

Although Amory *et al.* (1988) made a distinction between flocculence and flocculation, in the present work, the expressions, flocculation, flocculence, aggregation, adhesion and cell–cell interactions will be used indiscriminately to designate the flocculation phenomenon.

Table 9.1 Different types of *S. cerevisiae* aggregation

	Sexual aggregation	*Chain formation*	*Flocculation*
Type of cells involved	Two	One	One
Mechanism	Protein–protein bonding	Covalent linked	Lectin–carbohydrate bonding
Aggregate dispersion	EDTA and sugar insensitive	Mechanical shear; reaggregation not possible	By EDTA (Ca^{2+} sensitive), sugars or heat

Note: Aggregation can be formed between complementary mating types cells (α and a) after exchange of pheromones, a and α factors, respectively (sexual aggregation), due to a failure of buds to separate from mother cell (chain formation) or within single strains (flocculation).

Yeast Flocculation and Beer Production

The flocculation characteristics of a brewing yeast strain, namely the timing (during the fermentation cycle) of the onset of flocculation as well as the degree of flocculation, are of exceptional commercial interest to the brewing industry because they can determine the extent of attenuation (conversion of sugars into ethanol) of the wort. Ideal brewing yeasts should grow and ferment wort sugars, as free cells, and flocculate after its metabolic role has finished. Classically, ale strains raise to the top of the fermenter, probably due to the affinity for the CO_2 bubbles (top fermentation), while the lager strains settle in the bottom of the fermenter (bottom fermentation) (Stewart and Russell, 1981).

The onset of flocculation marks, as a rule, the end of primary fermentation, limits the wort nutrients to yeast cells and leads to a decrease of the number of cells to secondary fermentation. Early or premature flocculation is one of the common causes of "hung" or "stuck" fermentations giving rise to sweeter and less fermented beers (with low alcohol contents). A delay or a lack of flocculation can cause filtration difficulties and some problems occur for obtaining

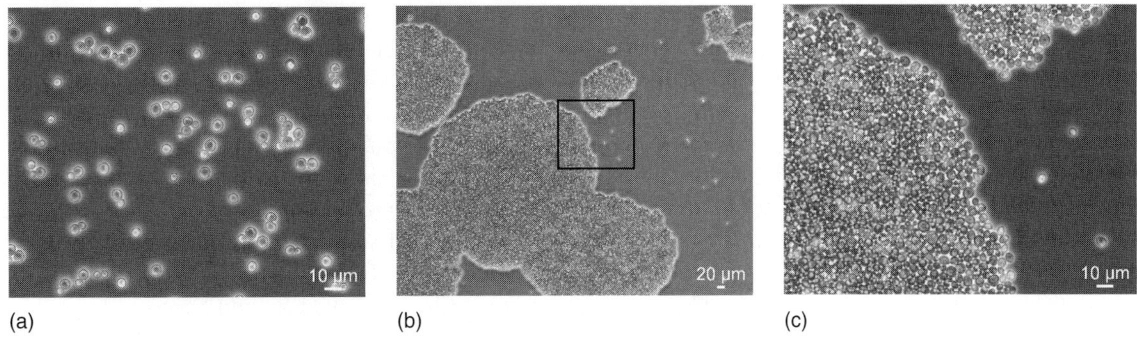

Figure 9.2 Photomicrographs of non-flocculent and flocculent cells of *S. cerevisiae*. (a) Non-flocculent cells of *S. cerevisiae* S646-8D; (b) flocculated cells of the ale-brewing strain of *S. cerevisiae* NCYC 1364; (c) detail of figure (b).

a bright sparkling beer; moreover, the presence of excess yeast in beer during aging can cause off-flavors due to yeast autolysis (Stewart and Russell, 1981).

Measurement of Yeast Flocculation

Sedimentation test

The sedimentation method described by Burns (1937) is the base of most of the flocculation assays reported in the literature. This method has been modified and refined by many authors in order to standardize the steps and turn it quantitative (Helm *et al.*, 1953; Stewart, 1975; Bendiak, 1994; Soares and Mota, 1997; D'Hautcourt and Smart, 1999). Basically, it consists of the separation, by sedimentation, of the flocs from the free cells. After a defined period of settling (usually between 6 and 10 min), free cells remaining in suspension are determined spectrophotometrically (600 nm) without (Bendiak, 1994) or with a previous deflocculation step (Soares and Mota, 1997). The fraction of flocculated cells is calculated by subtracting the fraction remaining in suspension from the total cell count previously determined.

In these tests, cells are removed from the growth medium, washed and then flocculation is promoted, usually, in 150 mmol/l acetate buffer, at pH 4.5, with about 4 mmol/l Ca^{2+} (ASBC, 1996). In order to become more close to fermentation conditions and take into account ethanol–flocculation dependence shown by several yeast strains, some authors proposed the inclusion of 4% ethanol in the buffer solution (Speers and Ritcey, 1995; D'Hautcourt and Smart, 1999).

Other methods of measurement

In the years 1980 and 1990, a more detailed analysis of the influence of the initial cell concentration and agitation in the quantification of yeast flocculation was performed (Miki *et al.*, 1982b; Stratford and Keenan, 1987, 1988; Soares and Mota, 1997). Yeast cells are usually negatively charged leading to its dispersion; mechanical agitation gives enough energy to yeast cells to overcome this repulsion barrier, allowing the establishment of a flocculent bond (Stratford, 1992a). The colloidal aspects of yeast flocculation, particularly concerning to predict the cell–cell interaction energies and the rate at which cells collide and associate, were reviewed by Jin and Speers (1998).

Stratford and co-workers described a standardized method, in which the cell suspension was shaken in Erlenmeyer flasks during several hours (4–6 h) until the equilibrium between the fraction of flocculated and free cells had reached (Stratford and Keenan, 1987; Stratford *et al.*, 1988). A comparative study between Stratford test and a sedimentation test has shown that the results obtained by both methods are not significantly different, having the sedimentation method the advantage of being much faster (Soares and Mota, 1997).

Beyond the tests reported above, other methods were developed based on the dispersion of the flocculated yeast's suspensions by the action of sugars (Eddy, 1955), heat (Taylor and Orton, 1975) or EDTA (Stahl *et al.*, 1983). On-line measurement of yeast flocculation has been attempted by several authors (Van Hamersveld *et al.*, 1993; Mas and Ghommidh, 2001). Recently, a new method was proposed by Jibiki *et al.* (2001) based on polymerase chain reaction (PCR) amplification of the *FLO5* gene.

Physiology of Yeast Flocculation

pH and presence of ions

Changing the pH value of the solution can cause a reversible dispersion of the flocs in a strain-dependent process (Figure 9.3). For several laboratory and industrial strains, flocculation occurs over a broad pH range, 2.5–9.0; conversely, many brewing yeasts only flocculate within a narrow pH range, with an optimum pH value between 3.0 and 5.0 (Figure 9.3) (Stratford, 1996; Soares and Seynaeve, 2000b).

There is a general agreement that Ca^{2+} is the most effective ion in the promotion of flocculation (Miki *et al.*,

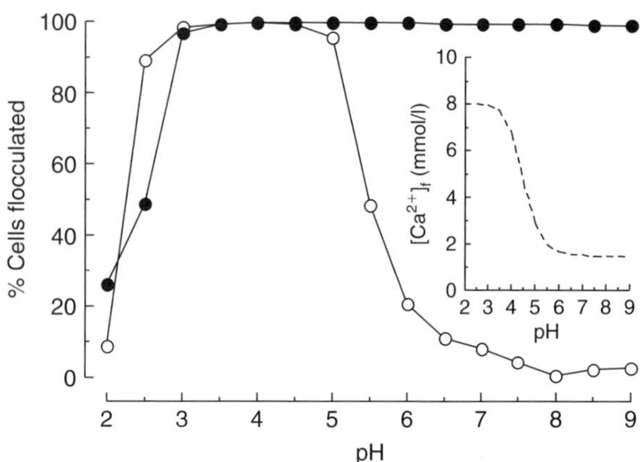

Figure 9.3 Influence of pH on the flocculation. Flocculation of the ale-brewing strains *S. cerevisiae* NCYC 1214 (○) (narrow pH range) and NCYC 1364 (●) (broad pH range). Flocculation was evaluated in standard conditions, in buffer containing Ca^{2+}. Insert: Influence of pH in the free Ca^{2+} concentration ($[Ca^{2+}]_f$). Theoretical calculations of variation of $[Ca^{2+}]_f$ with the pH in the presence of 8 mmol/l of total Ca^{2+} concentration and a ligand (50 mmol/l of succinic acid). *Source*: Reprinted with permission of the editor; from Soares and Seynaeve (2000b).

1982a; Stratford, 1989). For some strains, trace amounts of Ca^{2+} (10^{-5}–10^{-8} mol/l) are sufficient to induce flocculation (Taylor and Orton, 1975), while other strains require a higher amount (5×10^{-4} mol/l) of Ca^{2+} (Soares and Seynaeve, 2000b). More important than the total Ca^{2+} concentration present in the media is the available Ca^{2+} (the free and labile Ca^{2+}); this fraction is the only one which is able to induce the correct conformation of the lectins, and is influenced, among other factors, by the pH, as it can be seen in the insert of Figure 9.3 (Soares and Seynaeve, 2000b). The promotion of flocculation by other ions, such as Rb^+, Cs^+, Fe^{2+},Co^{2+}, Al^{3+} and particularly Mg^{2+} and Mn^{2+} was also reported (Miki *et al.*, 1982a; Nishihara *et al.*, 1982; Sousa *et al.*, 1992).

Ba^{2+}, Sr^{2+}, Pb^{2+} and with less intensity Na^+ inhibit competitively yeast flocculation, probably due to the similarity of their ionic ratio to Ca^{2+} (Nishihara *et al.*, 1982; Gouveia and Soares, 2004); most likely, these cations compete for the same "calcium binding site" of flocculation lectins, being not able to activate the lectin-like component of yeast flocculation.

Ethanol and ionic strength

Flocculation of the majority of brewing strains is not affected by ethanol (Stratford, 1992c); for some strains, where flocculation mechanism is most likely different from the lectin-like model, flocculation increases with ethanol concentration or only occurs in the presence of ethanol (Mill, 1964b; Dengis *et al.*, 1995; Dengis and Rouxhet, 1997). Conversely, a negative effect of ethanol in yeast flocculation was reported (Kamada and Murata, 1984). It has been suggested that the positive effect of ethanol is due to its adsorption at cell surface, which may cause a reduced local dielectric constant, leading to a decrease of cell–cell electrostatic repulsion; alternatively, ethanol can allow the protrusion of polymer chains into the liquid phase, carrying binding sites for non-specific (hydrogen binding) or specific interactions (Amory *et al.*, 1988; Dengis *et al.*, 1995). Ethanol seems to produce a pronounced effect in the promotion of flocculation in yeast strains with a strong surface hydrophobicity (Jin and Speers, 2000).

The increasing of ionic strength seems to have a negative impact on yeast flocculation, both for Flo1 and NewFlo phenotype strains, probably due to modifications in the conformation of flocculation lectins (Kamada and Murata, 1984; Jin and Speers, 2000).

Cell surface charge and hydrophobicity

Factors that facilitate cell–cell contact, namely the increase of cell surface hydrophobicity (CSH) or the decrease of cell surface charge, could play an important role on flocculation. However, no clear relationship between electrical properties and the onset of flocculation was found (Amory *et al.*, 1988; Dengis *et al.*, 1995; Dengis and Rouxhet, 1997).

Although an extensive research about the role of CSH on yeast flocculation has been undertaken, a controversy still exists. For instance, CSH and more recently the presence of 3-hydroxy fatty acids (3-OH oxylipins) on yeast cell wall has been positively correlated with the onset of flocculation (Straver *et al.*, 1993; Jin *et al.*, 2001; Strauss *et al.*, 2005). However, other authors described no significant differences in CSH or surface concentrations of proteins, polysaccharides or hydrocarbons between flocculent and non-flocculent cells at stationary and exponential phases of growth, respectively (Dengis *et al.*, 1995; Dengis and Rouxhet, 1997).

Temperature

Temperature affects a multiplicity of factors complicating the interpretation of its effect on the flocculation process. The lowering of fermentation temperature reduces the level of yeast metabolism and the production of CO_2 with the consequent reduction of turbulence favoring yeast sedimentation. Temperature also acts at surface level, in the cell–cell interactions, promoting a reversible dispersion of the flocs at 50–60°C (Mill, 1964b; Taylor and Orton, 1975). Additionally, the growing temperature seems to have a deep impact on yeast flocculation expression. A brief heat shock (52°C, 5 min) in brewing strains in exponential phase of growth delayed the onset of flocculation; a permanent mild heat stress (incubation at a supra-optimum temperature) impair or delay the triggering of flocculation (Williams *et al.*, 1992; Garsoux *et al.*, 1993; Soares *et al.*,

1994; Claro *et al.*, 2007). Probably, a continuous mild heat stress can act directly on the mitochondrial activity and indirectly on the cell membrane structure, affecting the secretion of flocculation lectins with the consequent reduction of flocculation (Soares *et al.*, 1994).

Sugars and nitrogen source

The floc dispersion effect of sugars is well documented in the literature (Mill, 1964b; Taylor and Orton, 1978). A detailed study of the effect of sugars and their derivatives on the floc dispersion promotion has shown the existence of three flocculent phenotypes: Flo1, NewFlo and mannose insensitive (MI) phenotype (see section "Flocculation phenotypes") (Stratford and Assinder, 1991; Masy *et al.*, 1992). On the other hand, the presence of sugars in the wort or culture medium can provoke a loss or a modification in yeast flocculation ability by affecting the expression of *FLO* genes (see section "The flocculation cycle").

High molecular weight polysaccharides from wort rich in arabinose and xylose have been implicated in premature flocculation (Herrera and Axcell, 1991). These polysaccharides have a higher affinity than sugars present in medium for yeast flocculation lectins inducing premature yeast settling by acting as a bridge between cells (Stratford, 1992a).

Strains grown in worts with high level of assimilable nitrogen or in medium supplemented with basic amino acids or ammonia showed a delay on the onset of flocculation (Mill, 1964a; Baker and Kirsop, 1972). Many ale strains do not flocculate in chemically defined media yeast nitrogen base (YNB) or in rich media yeast extract, peptone, dextrose (YEPD), being only flocculent in wort. It was proposed that these strains require the addition of nitrogen compounds (gelatine, peptones or yeast extract) to YNB in order to flocculate (Stewart, 1975; Beavan *et al.*, 1979). More recent works have shown that the lack of flocculation can be explained by the narrow pH range of flocculation of these strains (see above, effect of pH) plus the limited available Ca^{2+} in solution (Stratford, 1996; Soares and Seynaeve, 2000b). YNB has a small buffer capacity and consequently the pH falls rapidly to near 2.0 during yeast growth. On the other hand, the pH at the end of growth in YEPD (near 5.5–6.0) do not correspond to the pH range where these strains flocculate; in these culture media, flocculation is restored by Ca^{2+} addition and/or by correcting the pH to a suitable value (Soares and Seynaeve, 2000a, b).

Oxygen

The presence/absence of O_2 seems to have a deep effect on yeast flocculation. A moderate aeration produces a benefit effect, while a strong aeration leads to a lack of flocculation (Kida *et al.*, 1989; Soares *et al.*, 1991). On the other hand, the absence of oxygen seems to lead to a reduction of flocculation in laboratory and industrial strains (Miki *et al.*, 1982b; Soares *et al.*, 1991; Straver *et al.*, 1993; Iung *et al.*, 1999). In anaerobic conditions, the integrity and functionality of plasma membrane of *S. cerevisiae* can be affected, influencing the secretion of flocculation lectins and consequently yeast flocculation.

Cell age

It was proposed that flocculation increased with the genealogical age, being the bottom part of the yeast crop constituted by the more flocculent and aged cells (Hough, 1961). Thus, the brewing practice of cell reuse (repitching) leads to the constant selection of the more flocculating cells. Powell *et al.* (2003) have shown that virgin and non-virgin cells are both flocculent, the aged being more flocculent than the younger counterparts. However, the analysis of the distribution of the genealogical age of settled and cells remaining in suspension did not detect any difference (Gyllang and Martinson, 1971).

A more recent and detailed analysis of the different zones of the cone of the fermenter has shown cell populations with an extensive heterogeneity of flocculation, cell size and replicative age (Powell *et al.*, 2004).

Since flocculation of cells with zero genealogical age is not so different from the parent cells, it was suggested that daughter (virgins) and parent (old) cells should be flocculent or non-flocculent, depending on the growth phase (Soares and Mota, 1996). The genealogical distribution throughout the growth was essentially identical comprising 44–54% of daughter cells; in this way, the onset of flocculation observed toward the end of exponential phase of growth can hardly be explained by the genealogical age of the cells (Soares and Mota, 1996).

Genetic Control of Yeast Flocculation

The best known flocculation gene is *FLO1*, which has been cloned and sequenced by different groups (Teunissen *et al.*, 1993a, b; Watari *et al.*, 1994). The *FLO1* is a dominant gene localized at 24 kbp from the right end of chromosome I (Teunissen *et al.*, 1993a) and encodes a cell wall protein involved in flocculation process of *S. cerevisiae* (Watari *et al.*, 1994; Bony *et al.*, 1997). Other *FLO* genes are *FLO2* and *FLO4*, which are in fact alleles of *FLO1*, and the genes *FLO5*, *FLO9* and *FLO10*, which are highly homologous to *FLO1*; thus, the *FLO5* and *FLO9* gene products are 96% and 94% similar to *FLO1* product, respectively, while *FLO10* and *FLO1* gene products are 58% similar (Teunissen and Steensma, 1995). Expression of *FLO1* gene causes flocculation of Flo1 phenotype (Watari *et al.*, 1994). A new *FLO1* homolog, named *Lg-FLO1*, was isolated and it is believed that it encodes to an adhesine responsible for the NewFlo phenotype of brewer's yeasts

(Kobayashi *et al.*, 1998; Sato *et al.*, 2002). The analysis of the N-terminal region of Flo1 protein and Lg-Flo1 protein suggested that threonine 202 in Lg-Flo1 protein interacts with mannose and glucose, while tryptophan 228 and its neighboring amino acids residues in Flo1 protein recognize C-2 hydroxyl group of mannose but do not recognize the C-2 hydroxyl group of glucose (Kobayashi *et al.*, 1998).

It was proposed that *FLO1* gene is transcriptionally regulated by the proteic complex Ssn6–Tup1 that acts as global repressor in a regulatory cascade (Teunissen *et al.*, 1995). It was shown that the Swi–Snf coactivator and Tup1–Ssn6 corepressor control an extensive chromatin domain in which regulation of the *FLO1* gene takes place (Fleming and Pennings, 2001). The *FLO8* gene encodes a transcriptional activator *FLO1*, *FLO11* and *STA1* genes (Kobayashi *et al.*, 1996, 1999). Recently, it was shown that the transcription factor Mss11p, together with the Flo8p, is required for the induction of flocculation, controlled by *FLO1* gene (Bester *et al.*, 2006).

The *FLO11* gene encodes a protein critical for diploid pseudohyphal development and haploid invasive growth (Guo *et al.*, 2000; Lo and Dranginis, 1998). Expression of *FLO11* has been shown to be controlled by several major pathways, including the mitogen-activated protein (MAP) kinase pathway and the protein kinaseA/cAMP pathway (Verstrepen and Klis, 2006).

Besides the dominant genes, recessive/semi-dominant genes *flo3*, *flo6*, *flo7* have been described (Teunissen and Steensma, 1995). Several lines of evidence suggest that the expression of *FLO1* may be inhibited by suppressor genes: *fsu1*, *fsu2* and *fsu3* (Teunissen and Steensma, 1995). Additionally, many mutations give rise to flocculation involving regulatory, mitochondrial or genes implicated in the cell wall biosynthesis; these mutations and their pleiotropic effects were listed and reviewed by Teunissen and Steensma (1995).

Mechanism of Yeast Flocculation

The presence of proteins

The cell wall of *S. cerevisiae* has a layered structure, consisting of an amorphous inner layer and a fibrillar outer layer. The inner layer is mainly composed by β-glucan and chitin, whereas the outer layer consists predominantly of α-mannan associated with proteins (Lesage and Bussey, 2006).

Yeast flocculation is an intrinsic surface phenomenon, as isolated cell walls from flocculent strains are able to flocculate (Nishihara *et al.*, 1982; Sousa *et al.*, 1992). The outer mannoprotein layer of yeast cell wall is involved in the flocculation process because the treatment of flocculent cells with proteases as well as chemical modification of functional groups of amino acids residues, promote the irreversible desaggregation of the flocs (Nishihara *et al.*, 1977, 1982). The addition of a protein synthesis inhibitor (cycloheximide) impairs the onset of flocculation, which clearly shows that flocculation is a protein-dependent process (Baker and Kirsop, 1972; Stratford, 1993).

The Flo1 protein

The open reading frame of *FLO1* gene is composed by 4.6 kbp, which encodes for a protein of 1,537 amino acids (Watari *et al.*, 1994). Flo1 protein contains many repeated sequences, a large number of serine and threonine residues (which provide sites for *O*-glycosylation) and 14 potential *N*-glycosylation sites (Teunissen *et al.*, 1993b; Watari *et al.*, 1994). Flo1 protein is a structural protein localized at yeast cell surface (Bidard *et al.*, 1995; Bony *et al.*, 1997, 1998) and is directly involved in the flocculation process (Bony *et al.*, 1997). The functional analysis of the major repeated sequence showed that the degree of flocculation can be modulated by adjusting the number of repeated sequences in the Flo1 protein (Bidard *et al.*, 1995).

Flo1 protein has a hydrophobic C-terminal region, which likely corresponds to a glycosylphosphatidylinositol (GPI) anchor signal addition (Watari *et al.*, 1994). Deletion of this hydrophobic region prevents cell surface anchorage of the protein, resulting in the loss of flocculation and the release of the protein in the culture medium (Bony *et al.*, 1997).

Prediction of the secondary structure of Flo1 protein shows that it is almost composed by β sheets and coils, being the α-helix found only at N- and C-terminal regions (Watari *et al.*, 1994). As a consequence of *O*-glycosylation of serine and threonine residues, the Flo1 protein would increase the stiffness and adopt an extended conformation, being the N-terminus exposed toward the cell surface (Teunissen *et al.*, 1993b; Watari *et al.*, 1994). The truncated form of Flo1 protein, in which the N-terminal region was deleted, could not develop a flocculent phenotype, although it can be detected in the cell wall (Bony *et al.*, 1997). It was shown that the N-terminal region of Flo1 protein contains the sugar recognition domain (Kobayashi *et al.*, 1998).

The involvement of α-mannan

Reversible inhibition of flocculation by mannose and mannosyl derivatives suggests the involvement of the α-mannan in the flocculation (Taylor and Orton, 1978); in the same line, the blocking or chemical modification of α-mannan also prevents flocculation (Miki *et al.*, 1982a; Nishihara *et al.*, 2000).

Flocculation theories

Calcium Bridge Theory The calcium bridge theory was dominant in 60–70 years and proposed that flocculent cells were linked by calcium bridges formed by the carboxylic groups (Mill, 1964b; Beavan *et al.*, 1979) or the phosphate groups (Lyons and Hough, 1970, 1971) of the cells involved. This theory is unsatisfactory to explain the flocculation inhibition by the action of bivalent ions like Sr^{2+}, Ba^{2+} or Pb^{2+} (Nishihara *et al.*, 1982; Gouveia and Soares, 2004), as well as by sugars (Taylor and Orton, 1978) or concanavalin A (Con A) (Miki *et al.*, 1982a).

Lectin-Like Mechanism The lectin-like theory was formally proposed in the beginning of the 80 years and is the theory that prevailed until now in almost all of its basic concepts.

The term lectin derives from the Latin word *legere*, which means to choose, pick up or select. Lectins are glycoproteins of non-immune origin that bind sugars, often with high specificity (Goldstein *et al.*, 1980). In lectin-like model (Miki *et al.*, 1982a), it was proposed that a specific lectin (only present on flocculent cells) recognize and interact with carbohydrate residues of α-mannans (receptors) of adjoining cells (Figure 9.4). The calcium ion has the role to assure the correct conformation of the lectin (Miki *et al.*, 1982a; Stratford, 1989). The receptors are present both in flocculent and non-flocculent cells (Miki *et al.*, 1982a; Soares *et al.*, 1992), since *S. cerevisiae* cells have mannans on the outer part of cell wall. A detailed analysis of the inhibitory action of sugars and the use of *mnn* mutants and Con A suggests that flocculation receptors of Flo1 and NewFlo phenotype are the non-reducing termini of $\alpha(1\rightarrow3)$-linked mannan side branches, two or three mannopyranose residues in length (Stratford and Assinder, 1991; Stratford, 1992b).

Using atomic force microscopy, adhesion forces of $121 \pm 53\,pN$ were measured; these forces reflect the specific interactions between cell surface flocculation lectins

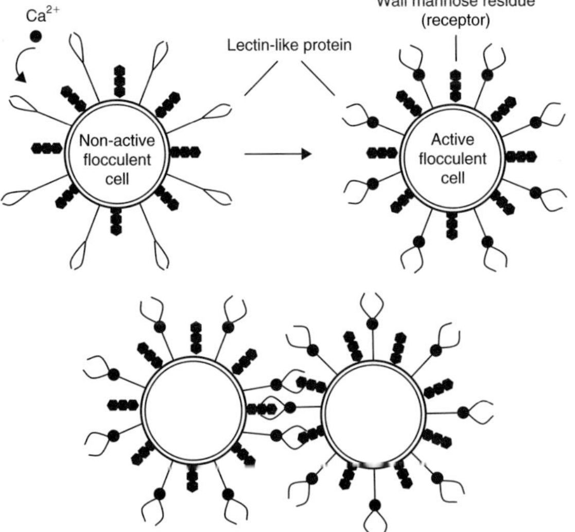

Figure 9.4 Lectin-like model for yeast flocculation. A specific lectin-like protein, previously activated by calcium ions, sticks out of the yeast cell wall, recognizes and interacts selectively with the mannose residues (receptors) of adjoining cells.

and sugar residues (receptors) (Touhami *et al.*, 2003). It was suggested that the specific interactions (lectin-receptor) were stabilized by non-specific interactions: hydrogen bonds and hydrophobic interactions (Amory *et al.*, 1988; Dengis *et al.*, 1995; Jin and Speers, 2000; Jin *et al.*, 2001).

Flocculation phenotypes

Taking into account the flocculation reversible inhibition by sugars, salt and proteases sensitiveness, two main types of flocculent yeast cells were found: Flo1 phenotype, comprises strains where cell–cell interactions are specifically inhibited by mannose and derivatives; NewFlo phenotype, is composed mostly by ale-brewing strains where flocculation is reversibly inhibited by mannose, maltose, glucose and sucrose, but not by galactose (Stratford and Assinder, 1991).These phenotypes also possess different sensitiveness to culture conditions, namely temperature, pH and glucose availability (Soares *et al.*, 1994; Soares and Mota, 1996; Stratford, 1996; Soares and Seynaeve, 2000b).

Later on, two other phenotypes have been described: MI phenotype, composed by strains where flocculation is not inhibited by sugars, including mannose (Masy *et al.*, 1992), and a fourth phenotype, comprising strains whose flocculation occurs in the presence of sufficiently high ethanol concentration (Dengis *et al.*, 1995; Dengis and Rouxhet, 1997). The exact mechanism of aggregation of these strains is far from being understood.

The Flocculation Cycle

Although the Flo1 phenotype flocculation is generally constitutively expressed throughout growth (Figure 9.5a), the majority of brewer yeast strains belong to the NewFlo phenotype and possess cyclic flocculation ability (Stratford and Assinder, 1991; Soares and Mota, 1996). NewFlo strains progressively lose their flocculation in the early period of growth (Figure 9.5b) and become flocculent toward the end of logarithmic phase of growth (Stratford and Carter, 1993; Soares and Mota, 1996; Soares *et al.*, 2004, Sampermans *et al.*, 2005). Flocculation receptors were found in all stages of growth (Stratford, 1993; Soares and Mota, 1996), while Flo 1 protein is not permanently present at the cell surface, increasing at the end of the exponential phase growth (Bony *et al.*, 1998). These facts, together, indicate that the availability of Flo proteins in the cell wall determines the flocculation level.

The loss and triggering of flocculation can be influenced by many and varied factors that can act at different stages. The action of culture medium components on cell–cell interactions and the disappearance/emergence of flocculation lectins on yeast cell surface are two important levels of control of flocculation cycle. On the other hand, the presence of active lectins on yeast cell surface can be controlled at different levels: by transcriptional control of *FLO* genes

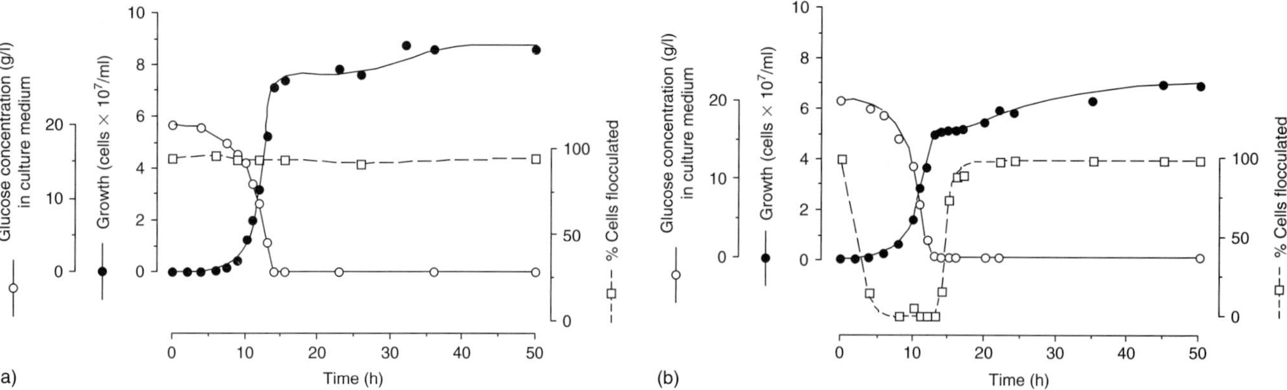

Figure 9.5 Flocculation and glucose utilization during the growth of Flo1 and NewFlo phenotype strains. (a) *S. cerevisiae* NCYC 869 (Flo1 phenotype) flocculates during all phases of growth, being insensitive to the presence of nutrients. (b) *S. cerevisiae* NCYC 1195 (NewFlo phenotype) lose flocculation ability in the early phase of growth, occurring the onset of flocculation at the end of exponential phase. This phenomenon coincides with the attainment of the lowest amount of glucose in the culture medium. Flocculation was evaluated in standard conditions, in buffer containing Ca^{2+}. *Source*: Reprinted with permission of the editor; from Soares and Mota (1996).

or during the secretion process. This means that the regulation of flocculation cycle of *S. cerevisiae* is not a straightforward mechanism.

The loss of flocculation

Fermentable sugars (glucose, maltose and sucrose), present in commercial worts as well as in most culture media, cause the dispersion of flocculated yeasts of NewFlo phenotype. With the fermentation progress, sugars are consumed and their inhibitory effect decreases. Recently, it has been shown that, besides this surface level action, sugars have a central role in the induction of flocculation loss both in starved cells (Soares and Duarte, 2002; Soares and Vroman, 2003) and in growing conditions (Figure 9.5b) (Soares and Mota, 1996; Soares *et al.*, 2004), most likely via the yeast metabolism. The loss of flocculation is an energy-dependent process, influenced by carbon source metabolism, and requires *de novo* protein synthesis by an unknown mechanism; probably, different proteases are involved on the dismantling of flocculation mechanism because the presence of protease inhibitors prevented partially or completely flocculation loss induced by glucose (Soares and Vroman, 2003; Soares *et al.*, 2004).

The onset of flocculation

The pH value, Ca^{2+} availability, residual concentration of sugars or nitrogen and the presence of ethanol are important factors on the controlling of the onset of flocculation. In brewing conditions, the pH of the wort falls from 5.2–5.8 to 4.0–4.4, which seems to be enough to induce flocculation in strains that flocculate in a narrow (3.0–5.0) pH range (Figure 9.3) (Stratford, 1996; Soares and Seynaeve, 2000b). In addition, available Ca^{2+} (the free and labile Ca^{2+}) increases as a consequence of pH decrease (insert of Figure 9.3), which favors the triggering of flocculation (Soares and Seynaeve, 2000a, b).

The onset of flocculation occurs at the end of exponential phase of growth, when a low sugar (Figure 9.5b) and/or nitrogen concentration is reached in the culture media (Smit *et al.*, 1992; Soares and Mota, 1996; Sampermans *et al.*, 2005). The triggering of flocculation is an energetic-dependent process, requiring a residual external carbon source, most likely for the production of energy required for the secretory pathway (Mill, 1964a; Stratford, 1992a; Soares and Mota, 1996); conversely, it does not require an external source of nitrogen (Sampermans *et al.*, 2005). The nutrients shortage combined with the presence of ethanol, which in a small amount has a positive effect on yeast flocculation, may be the signal nutrient that induces the onset of flocculation (Sampermans *et al.*, 2005; Claro *et al.*, 2007).

Nutrients availability or limitations may directly repress or induce, respectively, *FLO* genes in NewFlo phenotype strains (Verstrepen *et al.*, 2003; Verstrepen and Klis, 2006). It was proposed that *FLO1* gene is regulated at the transcriptional level by the proteic complex Ssn6–Tup1 (Teunissen *et al.*, 1995). However, nothing is known about the regulation of the *Lg-FLO1*, which is believed to encode the lectin responsible for the NewFlo phenotype. Although much information has been obtained last year about the flocculation cycle of NewFlo phenotype strains, the upstream sensors as well as the signaling pathway(s) of regulation of NewFlo phenotype flocculation in laboratory and brewing conditions remain unknown.

To Be or Not to Be Flocculent: The Art of Survival?

Why do yeast cells, which suffer from nutrient limitations under flocculating conditions, keep on insisting in separating from the culture medium?

In nature, the majority of biomass is under starving conditions and the multicellular lifestyle of microorganisms appears to be prevalent (Palková and Váchová, 2006). Brewing yeasts belonging to NewFlo phenotype, in the presence of available nutrients, are preferentially under the form of individual cells (Soares *et al.*, 2004). Interestingly, the nutrient shortage, probably combined with the presence of ethanol, induces the triggering of flocculation (Sampermans *et al.*, 2005); thus, the cells aggregated in flocs do not have anything to lose, under a nutritional viewpoint. On contrary, they can cooperate within a multicellular structure (floc) and in this case the union may be the basis of the strength. The autolysis of some cells of the center of the floc will originate compounds that can support the survival of the other cells of the floc. Herker *et al.* (2004) proposed that yeast cells commit altruistic suicide (apoptosis – programed cell death) in order to provide nutrients for the others, probably younger and healthy cells. In this way, flocculation can be seen as a form of making possibly a long-term survival of a cellular community in an unfavorable environment with a limited nutrient supply, as it was suggested by B. F. Johnson (personal communication to Stewart and Russell (1981).

Flocculation can also be seen as a means of protection against a harmful environment (Stratford, 1992c). Brewing yeasts are usually exposed to different detrimental conditions during beer production. In this perspective, flocculation can be a strategy of survival, as the cells outside the floc can offer some protection to external adverse environmental conditions to the cells inside.

Although the question raised above remains without a straight and definitive answer, future work, namely about the regulation of yeast flocculation as well as the impact of stress on the triggering of flocculation, could give a little more light on these conjectures.

Summary Points

- Yeast flocculation is a reversible process of cell aggregation into multicellular masses called flocs.
- Traditionally associated with beer production, flocculation might also be useful in modern biotechnology as a low cost and easy method of cell separation.
- Yeast flocculation is affected by multiple factors, namely pH, Ca^{2+} availability, temperature, sugars and nitrogen sources and dissolved oxygen.
- Brewing flocculent strains have a specific lectin-like protein, which interacts with the sugars (receptors) of adjoining cells; calcium ions are required to activate the lectin.
- Four flocculation phenotypes have been described: Flo1, NewFlo, MI and strains whose flocculation requires the presence of ethanol.
- Several dominant, recessive and suppressor genes have been described. Expression of *FLO1* and *Lg-FLO1* genes causes flocculation of Flo1 or NewFlo phenotype, respectively.
- In brewing NewFlo phenotype strains, sugars induce the loss of flocculation in the early period of growth; the onset of flocculation occurs toward the end of logarithmic phase when low sugar and/or nitrogen concentration is reached in the culture medium.
- Yeast flocculation can constitute a long-term survival mechanism or a means of protection against a harmful environment.

References

Amory, D.E., Rouxhet, P.G. and Dufour, J.P. (1988). *J. Inst. Brew.* 94, 79–84.

ASBC (1996). *J. Am. Soc. Brew. Chem.* 54, 245–248.

Baker, D.A. and Kirsop, B.H. (1972). *J. Inst. Brew.* 78, 454–458.

Beavan, M.J., Belk, D.M., Stewart, G.G. and Rose, A.H. (1979). *Can. J. Microbiol.* 25, 888–895.

Bendiak, D.S. (1994). *J. Am. Soc. Brew. Chem.* 52, 120–122.

Bester, M.C., Pretorius, I.S. and Bauer, F.F. (2006). *Curr. Genet.* 49, 375–383.

Bidard, F., Bony, M., Blondin, B., Dequin, S. and Barre, P. (1995). *Yeast* 11, 809–822.

Bony, M., Thines-Sempoux, D., Barre, P. and Blondin, B. (1997). *J. Bacteriol.* 179, 4929–4936.

Bony, M., Barre, P. and Blondin, B. (1998). *Yeast* 14, 25–35.

Burns, J.A. (1937). *J. Inst. Brew.* 43, 31–43.

Calleja, G.B. (1987). In Rose A.H. and Harrison, J.S. (eds), *The Yeasts*, Vol. 2, 2nd edn, pp. 165, 238. Academic Press, London and New York.

Claro, F.B., Rijsbrack, K. and Soares, E.V. (2007) *J. Appl. Microbiol.* 102, 693–700.

D'Hautcourt, O. and Smart, K.A. (1999). *J. Am. Soc. Brew. Chem.* 57, 123–128.

Dengis, P.B. and Rouxhet, P.G. (1997). *J. Inst. Brew.* 103, 257–261.

Dengis, P.B., Nélissen, L.R. and Rouxhet, P.G. (1995). *Appl. Environ. Microbiol.* 61, 718–728.

Domingues, L., Vicente, A.A., Lima, N. and Teixeira, J.A. (2000). *Biotechnol. Bioprocess. Eng.* 5, 288–305.

Domingues, L., Lima, N. and Teixeira, J.A. (2005). *Process. Biochem.* 40, 1151–1154.

Eddy, A.A. (1955). *J. Inst. Brew.* 61, 313–317.

Fleming, A.B. and Pennings, S. (2001). *EMBO J.* 20, 5219–5231.

Garsoux, G., Haubursin, H., Bilbaut, S. and Dufour, J.P. (1993). *Proc. Eur. Brew. Conv. Congr.* 24, 275–282.

Goldstein, I.J., Hughes, R.C., Monsigny, M., Osawa, T. and Sharon, N. (1980). *Nature* 285, 66.

Gouveia, C. and Soares, E.V. (2004). *J. Inst. Brew.* 110, 141–145.

Guo, B., Styles, C.A., Feng, Q. and Fink, G. (2000). *Proc. Natl. Acad. Sci. USA* 97, 12158–12163.

Gyllang, H. and Martinson, E. (1971). *Proc. Eur. Brew. Conv. Congr.* 13, 265 271.

Helm, E., Nohr, B. and Thorne, R.S.W. (1953). *Wallerstein Lab. Commun.* 16, 315–326.

Herker, E., Jungwirth, H., Lehmann, K.A., Maldener, C., Fröhlich, K.U., Wissing, S., Büttner, S., Fehr, M., Sigrist, S. and Madeo, F. (2004). *J. Cell Biol.* 164, 501–507.

Herrera, V.E. and Axcell, B.C. (1991). *J. Inst. Brew.* 97, 359–366.

Hough, J.S. (1961). *J. Inst. Brew.* 67, 494–495.

Iung, A.R., Coulon, J., Kiss, F., Ekome, J.N., Vallner, J. and Bonaly, R. (1999). *Appl. Environ. Microbiol.* 65, 5398–5402.

Jibiki, M., Ishibiki, T., Yuuki, T. and Kagami, N. (2001). *J. Am. Soc. Brew. Chem.* 59, 107–110.

Jin, Y. and Speers, R.A. (1998). *Food Res. Intern.* 31, 421–440.

Jin, Y. and Speers, R.A. (2000). *J. Am. Soc. Brew. Chem.* 58, 108–116.

Jin, Y., Ritcey, L.L., Speers, R.A. and Dolphin, P.J. (2001). *J. Am. Soc. Brew. Chem.* 59, 1–9.

Kamada, K. and Murata, M. (1984). *Agric. Biol. Chem.* 48, 2423–2433.

Kida, K., Yamadaki, M., Asano, S., Nakata, T. and Sonoda, Y. (1989). *J. Ferment. Bioeng.* 68, 107–111.

Kobayashi, O., Suda, H., Ohtani, T. and Sone, H. (1996). *Mol. Gen. Genet.* 251, 707–715.

Kobayashi, O., Hayashi, N., Kuroki, R. and Sone, H. (1998). *J. Bacteriol.* 180, 6503–6510.

Kobayashi, O., Yoshimoto, H. and Sone, H. (1999). *Curr. Genet.* 36, 256–261.

Lesage, G. and Bussey, H. (2006). *Microbiol. Mol. Biol. Rev.* 70, 317–343.

Lo, W.-S. and Dranginis, A.M. (1998). *Mol. Biol. Cell.* 9, 161–171.

Lyons, T.P. and Hough, J.S. (1970). *J. Inst. Brew.* 76, 564–571.

Lyons, T.P. and Hough, J.S. (1971). *J. Inst. Brew.* 77, 300–305.

Mas, S. and Ghommidh, C. (2001). *Biotechnol. Bioeng.* 76, 91–98.

Masy, C.L., Henquinet, A. and Mestdagh, M.M. (1992). *Can. J. Microbiol.* 38, 1298–1306.

Miki, B.L.A., Poon, N.H., James, A.P. and Seligy, V.L. (1982a). *J. Bacteriol.* 150, 878–889.

Miki, B.L.A., Poon, N.H. and Seligy, V.L. (1982b). *J. Bacteriol.* 150, 890–899.

Mill, P.J. (1964a). *J. Gen. Microbiol.* 35, 53–60.

Mill, P.J. (1964b). *J. Gen. Microbiol.* 35, 61–68.

Nishihara, H., Toraya, T. and Fukui, S. (1977). *Arch. Microbiol.* 115, 19–23.

Nishihara, H., Toraya, T. and Fukui, S. (1982). *Arch. Microbiol.* 131, 112–115.

Nishihara, H., Kio, K. and Imamura, M. (2000). *J. Inst. Brew.* 106, 7–10.

Palková, Z. and Váchová, L. (2006). *FEMS Microbiol. Rev.* 30, 806–824.

Powell, C.D., Quain, D.E. and Smart, K.A. (2003). *FEMS Yeast Res.* 3, 149–157.

Powell, C.D., Quain, D.E. and Smart, K.A. (2004). *J. Am. Soc. Brew. Chem.* 62, 8–17.

Sampermans, S., Mortier, J. and Soares, E.V. (2005). *J. Appl. Microbiol.* 98, 525–531.

Sato, M., Maeba, H., Watari, J. and Takashio, M. (2002). *J. Biosci. Bioeng.* 93, 395–398.

Smit, G., Straver, M.H., Lugtenberg, B.J.J. and Kijne, J.W. (1992). *Appl. Environ. Microbiol.* 58, 3709–3714.

Soares, E.V. and Duarte, A.A. (2002). *Biotechnol. Lett.* 24, 1957–1960.

Soares, E.V. and Mota, M. (1996). *Can. J. Microbiol.* 42, 539–547.

Soares, E.V. and Mota, M. (1997). *J. Inst. Brew.* 103, 93–98.

Soares, E.V. and Seynaeve, J. (2000a). *Biotechnol. Lett.* 22, 859–863.

Soares, E.V. and Seynaeve, J. (2000b). *Biotechnol. Lett.* 22, 1827–1832.

Soares, E.V. and Vroman, A. (2003). *J. Appl. Microbiol.* 95, 325–330.

Soares, E.V., Teixeira, J.A. and Mota, M. (1991). *Biotechnol. Lett.* 13, 207–212.

Soares, E.V., Teixeira, J.A. and Mota, M. (1992). *Can. J. Microbiol.* 38, 969–974.

Soares, E.V., Teixeira, J.A. and Mota, M. (1994). *Can. J. Microbiol.* 40, 851–857.

Soares, E.V., Vroman, A., Mortier, J., Rijsbrack, K. and Mota, M. (2004). *J. Appl. Microbiol.* 96, 1117–1123.

Sousa, M.J., Teixeira, J.A. and Mota, M. (1992). *Biotechnol. Lett.* 14, 213–218.

Speers, R.A. and Ritcey, L.L. (1995). *J. Am. Soc. Brew. Chem.* 53, 174–177.

Stahl, U., Kües, U. and Esser, K. (1983). *Appl. Environ. Microbiol.* 17, 199–202.

Stewart, G.G. (1975). *Brew. Dig.* 50, 42–62.

Stewart, G.G., Russell, I. (1981). In Pollock, J.R.A. (ed.), *Brewing Science*, Vol. 2, pp. 61, 62. Academic Press, London.

Stratford, M. (1989). *Yeast* 5, 487–496.

Stratford, M. (1992a). *Adv. Microb. Physiol.* 33, 1–72.

Stratford, M. (1992b). *Yeast* 8, 635–645.

Stratford, M. (1992c). *Biotechnol. Gen. Eng. Rev.* 10, 283–341.

Stratford, M. (1993). *Yeast* 9, 85–94.

Stratford, M. (1996). *FEMS Microbiol. Lett.* 136, 13–18.

Stratford, M. and Assinder, S. (1991). *Yeast* 7, 559–574.

Stratford, M. and Carter, A.T. (1993). *Yeast* 9, 371–378.

Stratford, M. and Keenan, M.H.J. (1987). *Yeast* 3, 201–206.

Stratford, M. and Keenan, M.H.J. (1988). *Yeast* 4, 107–115.

Stratford, M., Coleman, H.P. and Keenan, M.H.J. (1988). *Yeast* 4, 199–208.

Strauss, C.J., Kock, J.L.F., Van Wyk, P.W.J., Lodolo, E.J., Pohl, C.H. and Botes, P.J. (2005). *J. Inst. Brew.* 111, 304–308.

Straver, M.H., Aar, P.C.V.D., Smit, G. and Kijne, J.W. (1993). *Yeast* 9, 527–532.

Taylor, N.W. and Orton, W.L. (1975). *J. Inst. Brew.* 81, 53–57.

Taylor, N.W. and Orton, W.L. (1978). *J. Inst. Brew.* 84, 113–114.

Teunissen, A.W.R.H. and Steensma, H.Y. (1995). *Yeast* 11, 1001–1013.

Teunissen, A.W.R.H., Van Den Berg, J.A. and Steensma, H.Y. (1993a). *Yeast* 9, 1–10.

Teunissen, A.W.R.H., Holub, E., Van Der Hucht, J., Van Den Berg, J.A. and Steensma, H.Y. (1993b). *Yeast* 9, 423–427.

Teunissen, A.W.R.H., Van Den Berg, J.A. and Steensma, H.Y. (1995). *Yeast* 11, 435–446.

Touhami, A., Hoffmann, B., Vasella, A., Denis, F.A. and Dufrêne, Y.F. (2003). *Microbiology* 149, 2873–2878.

Van Hamersveld, E.H., Van Loosdrecht, M.C.M., Gregory, J. and Luyben, K.C.A.M. (1993). *Biotechnol. Tech.* 7, 651–656.

Verbelen, P.J., De Schutter, D.P., Delvaux, F., Verstrepen, K.J. and Delvaux, F.R. (2006). *Biotechnol. Lett.* 28, 1515–1525.

Verstrepen, K.J. and Klis, F.M. (2006). *Mol. Microbiol.* 60, 5–15.

Verstrepen, K.J., Derdelinckx, G., Verachtert, H. and Delvaux, F.R. (2003). *Appl. Microbiol. Biotechnol.* 61, 197–205.

Watari, J., Takata, Y., Ogawa, M., Sahara, H., Koshino, S., Onnela, M., Airaksinen, U., Jaatinen, R., Penttilä, M. and Keränen, S. (1994). *Yeast* 10, 211–225.

Williams, J.W., Ernandes, J.R. and Stewart, G.G. (1992). *Biotechnol. Tech.* 6, 105–110.

10

Use of Amylolytic Enzymes in Brewing

N.P. Guerra, A. Torrado-Agrasar, C. López-Macías, E. Martínez-Carballo, S. García-Falcón, J. Simal-Gándara and L.M. Pastrana-Castro Nutrition and Bromatology Group, Department of Analytical and Food Chemistry, Food Science and Technology Faculty, Ourense Campus, University of Vigo, Ourense, Spain

Abstract

One of the main problems in the production of fermented alcoholic beverages from amylaceous raw materials is the efficient conversion of starch into fermentable sugars for *Saccharomyces cerevisiae*. α-Amylase, β-amylase, α-glucosidase, and limit dextrinase are the enzymes responsible for the hydrolysis of starch into maltose and glucose in beer elaboration.

Two different strategies are used in traditional brewing: to favor the activity of the endogenous enzymes that are present in the ingredients during the malting and mashing steps (beer in Western countries), or to use amylolytic microorganisms in a previous step to yeast fermentation (koji in Eastern countries). More recently, the development of technologies for the efficient production of enzymes, mainly of microbial origin, has allowed the application of exogenous amylases in beer elaboration to improve classical brewing by compensating enzymatic deficits in poor malts and by reducing the needs of malt for mashing. But, moreover, the addition of exogenous enzymes has also allowed the use of new starchy materials with low amylolytic potential and the preparation of worts with adequate sugars composition to elaborate new kinds of beer with interesting functional properties, as low-caloric and gluten-free beers for celiac people.

The importance of the amylolytic potential of the amylaceous material, the synergic activity of the three main enzymes (α-amylase, β-amylase, and limit dextrinase) involved in starch hydrolysis during mashing, and the need of a correct performance of the malting and mashing steps to maximize the expression and activity of these enzymes and to minimize the losses of enzymatic activity due to the thermal treatments applied during brewing are here described, paying special attention to the use of barley and sorghum as the most used starchy substrates and sources of amylases. Finally, examples of the application of exogenous enzymes in brewing for the use of new starchy materials as chestnut, and for the elaboration of new kinds of functional beers, are also included.

List of Abbreviations

AA	Total amylolytic activity in the mixture
AA_t	Total amylolytic activity (expressed as percentage referred to the initial total activity) for the amylases mixture at time *t* in equation (10.3)
AA_α	α-Amylase activity (expressed as percentage referred to the initial total activity) in equation (10.3)
a and *b*	Pre-exponential parameters in equation (10.3) for each glucoamylase form present in the commercial enzyme.
DP	Diastatic power
E	Total enzyme concentration
EBC	European Brewery Convention
EC	Enzyme Commission
EU	Enzymatic units
FAO	Food and Agricultural Organization of the United Nations
GA3	Gibberellic acid
GRAS	Generally recognized as safe
I	Inhibitor (glucose) concentration in equation (10.2)
ICRISAT	International Crops Research Institute for the Semi-Arid Tropics
IoB	Institute of Brewing
IUBMB	International Union of Biochemistry and Molecular Biology
JECFA	Joint FAO/WHO Expert Committee on Food Additives
ka and *kb*	First order constants in equation (10.3) for each glucoamylase form present in the commercial enzyme
K'_m	Operational Michaelis–Menten constant in equation (10.2)
K'_s	Operational substrate inhibition constant in equation (10.2)

Beer in Health and Disease Prevention
ISBN: 978-0-12-373891-2

K'_{iC}	Operational competitive inhibition constant in equation (10.2)
K'_{iNC}	Operational non-competitive inhibition constant in equation (10.2)
LD	Limit dextrinase
°L	Degrees Lintner
R	Ratio of α-amylase/glucoamylase enzymatic units
S	Substrate concentration in equation (10.2)
S_1, S_2	Synergism terms in equation (10.3)
SABS	South African Bureau of Standards
SDU	Sorghum diastatic units
V	Initial enzymatic reaction rate in equation (10.2)
V'_m	Maximal initial enzymatic reaction rate in equation (10.2)
°WK	Degrees Windisch–Kolbach

Introduction

Brewing is one of the best examples of the important role of enzymes in the elaboration of traditional food and beverages.

Briefly, beer can be defined as the alcoholic beverage elaborated by means of yeast fermentation with *Saccharomyces cerevisiae* of a starch-based material. The most used material is barley, although there are also beers made from wheat, rice, oats, rye, corn, sorghum, potato, cassava root, or agave among others. Hop is added to give bitterness. Adjuncts can also be added as additional sources of fermentable sugars and nutrients for yeast development during the fermentation stage.

Starch is the molecule of sugar storage in plants. It is the main component of cereal grains and tubercles. Starch can be defined as the mixture of two polymers of glucose: amylose – a linear molecule of D-glucose linked by α-1,4-glucosidic bonds; and amylopectin – a branched molecule of α-1,4-glucose residues and α-1,6-glucose bonds at the branching points (Figure 10.1).

The inability of *Saccharomyces* to directly utilize the starch molecule as a carbon source makes necessary the previous hydrolysis of the polymer into smaller sugars, preferably the monomeric (glucose) and dimeric (maltose) molecules. The same happens with the proteins present in starchy materials since they must be hydrolyzed to amino acids to be used by the yeast as nitrogen sources.

According to that, the first steps in beer elaboration are directed to allow the hydrolysis of both starch and proteins; amylases, limit dextrinase (LD), and proteases are the enzymes responsible for it. The fermentability of the wort (Figure 10.2) and the final levels of alcohol and remaining sugars in beer are strongly dependent on the activity of these enzymes.

Amylases, limit dextrinase, and proteases are naturally present in the cereal grains or in the tubercles during germination. Therefore, traditional brewing takes advantage of it stimulating the synthesis and activity of these endogenous enzymes. Still more, the election of barley as the most used material for brewing is not surprising, considering the high content of this cereal in amylases.

Figure 10.2 shows the main stages in beer elaboration, indicating those in which enzymes are implied for a correct brewing.

During the first stage (*steeping*) of barley *malting*, the grains are soaked in water for 1–3 days at 10–15°C to increase the humidity of the cereal. Afterwards, the steeping water is drained away and the grain is spread out to allow germination for 4–7 days with periodical aeration. During this phase proteases and the starch-degrading enzymes are accumulated. At this step proteases also contribute to starch degradation releasing bound β-amylase from starch

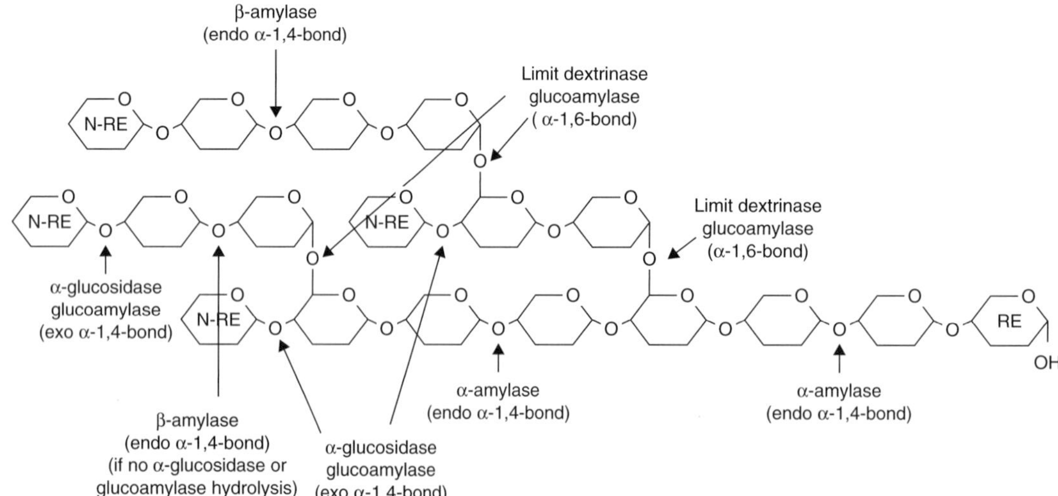

Figure 10.1 Amylopectin structure and hydrolysis points depending on the different enzymes involved in starch hydrolysis. RE, reducing end; N-RE, non-reducing end.

(Loreti *et al.*, 1998) and releasing the inactive limit dextrinase forms from their inhibitors (Longstaff and Bryce, 1993; McCafferty *et al.*, 2004).

Final drying (*kilning*) provides brown coloring and flavor by the Maillard reaction. In the case of malt storage, kilning also allows malt stabilization by stopping the enzymatic reactions and inhibiting an undesirable microbial growth by decreasing the water activity. This malt is still not readily fermentable by *S. cerevisiae.* Since hydrolysis must be continued in the next stage of brewing, kilning is a critical step because an intensive heating treatment can lead to enzymes deactivation.

The next step (*mashing*) is performed to obtain the wort. Mashing starts by milling and mixing the malt with water in ratios between 3:1 and 4:1. Extra carbon and nitrogen sources can be added at this point as adjuncts. Mashing is a critical operation in brewing. Hydrolysis of starch and proteins must be completed at this stage by continuation of the enzymatic hydrolysis, which had started during germination, to allow next the fermentation. This stage ends heating at 75–80°C to inactivate the enzymes, and filtering to eliminate the residual solids. The resulting wort is thus enriched in low molecular weight compounds, mainly maltose, glucose, and amino acids, and also in starch dextrins that were not hydrolyzed by the endogenous amylases. Mashing is the last step for starch and protein hydrolysis.

Before yeast inoculation, hop and adjuncts are added to the filtered wort, which is finally boiled to inactivate residual enzymatic activities, to sterilize the medium, to coagulate proteins, and to give flavor by improving hop extraction and inducing Maillard reactions.

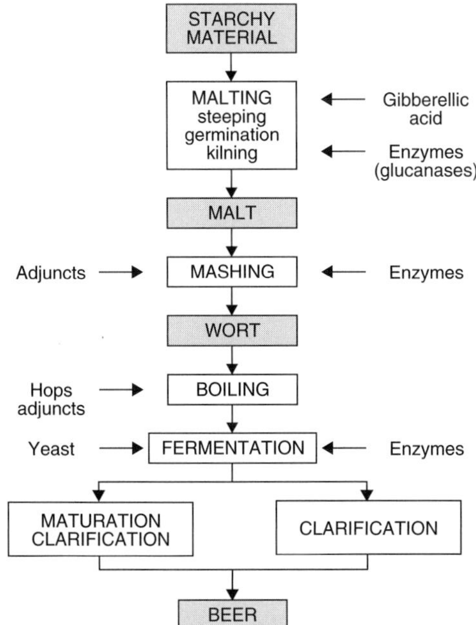

Figure 10.2 Stages in beer elaboration.

Besides the central role of amylases, limit dextrinase, and proteases in wort fermentability and beer composition, there are other enzymes implied in brewing. β-Glucanases are the enzymes responsible for the solubilization and hydrolysis of the β-glucans, which are major components of the cell wall of the starchy endosperm of barley. The synthesis and activity of these enzymes during germination is essential in brewing to improve the extraction of the grain components (mainly starch and proteins). During mashing these enzymes continue the hydrolysis of the solubilized β-glucans, which increase the viscosity of the medium and make difficult the operations of filtering (Georg-Kraemer *et al.*, 2004; Kuusela *et al.*, 2004).

Amylases in Traditional Brewing

The efficient extraction and transformation of starch into fermentable sugars is the critical step in brewing. Hence, amylases and limit dextrinase expression, stability, and performance under the conditions applied by the malting and brewing industries are critical.

The concentration of fermentable and non-fermentable starch-derived sugars in the wort defines the quality of the beer in terms of alcoholic degree and caloric content. The elaboration of high ethanol beers employs worts with high concentrations of fermentable sugars, which can be achieved by addition of adjuncts rich in fermentable sugars and by extensive hydrolysis of the starch coming from malt and adjuncts. On the opposite, low ethanol beers are elaborated by limiting the activity of the enzymes during mashing to reduce the amount of fermentable sugars.

Among the starch-derived sugars, only the monosaccharide (glucose) and the lineal disaccharide (maltose) are readily fermentable by *S. cerevisiae*, while the α-1,6-disaccharide (isomaltose) and the lineal trisaccharide (maltotriose) are only partially consumed (Yoon *et al.*, 2003). The lineal and branched oligosaccharides of higher degree of polymerization are not fermentable for this yeast. Fructose and saccharose, which are not starch sugars but are present in many starchy materials, are also good carbon sources for *S. cerevisiae.* A high degree of hydrolysis of the starch molecule is then necessary to obtain high concentrations of fermentable sugars.

The enzymatic hydrolysis of starch is carried out by the joint action of three amylases (α-amylase, β-amylase, and α-glucosidase) and of limit dextrinase (Table 10.1 and Figure 10.1). α-Amylase (EC 3.2.1.1) is an endo-acting enzyme that rapidly and randomly attacks the α-1,4-glucosidic linkages of starch and related oligosaccharides to produce linear and branched oligosaccharides. The final products of the exhaustive hydrolysis of starch by α-amylase are maltose, glucose, and α-limit dextrins, which contain the α-1,6-glucosidic linkages of the branched molecules of starch. The action of the α-amylase on starch produces a

Table 10.1 Enzymes involved in starch degradation during brewing according to the IUBMB nomenclature

Trivial name	*Systematic name*	*Code number*	*Reaction*	*Substrates*	*Products*
α-Amylase, alpha-amylase, glycogenase, endoamylase, Taka-amylase A	1,4-α-D-glucan glucanohydrolase	EC 3.2.1.1	Random endohydrolysis of 1,4-α-D-glucosidic linkages	Starch, glycogen and related polysaccharides, and oligosaccharides with three or more 1,4-α-linked D-glucose units	α-Oligosaccharides, α-maltose, α-glucose (low amounts), α-limit dextrin
β-Amylase, beta-amylase, saccharogen amylase, glycogenase	1,4-β-D-glucan maltohydrolase	EC 3.2.1.2	Successive hydrolysis of 1,4-α-D-glucosidic linkages to remove β-maltose units from the non-reducing ends of the chains	Starch, glycogen and related polysaccharides, and oligosaccharides	β-maltose, β-limit dextrin
α-Glucosidase, maltase, glucoinvertase, glucosidoinvertase, maltase-glucoamylase, α-glucoside hydrolase, glucosidosucrase, α-Glucopyranosidase	α-D-glucoside glucohydrolase	EC 3.2.1.20	Successive hydrolysis of terminal non-reducing 1,4-linked α-D-glucose residues with release of α-D-glucose	Polysaccharides Oligosaccharides (more rapidly)	α-D-glucose
Glucoamylase, amyloglucosidase, glucose amylase, exo-1,4-α-glucosidase, γ-amylase, acid maltase, γ-1,4-glucan glucohydrolase, lysosomal α-glucosidase	1,4-γ-D-glucan glucohydrolase	EC 3.2.1.3	Successive hydrolysis of terminal non-reducing 1,4-linked α-D-glucose residues with release of β-D-glucose Hydrolysis of terminal 1,6- α-D-glucosidic linkages when the next bond in the sequence is 1,4	Polysaccharides (more rapidly) Oligosaccharides	β-D-glucose
Limit dextrinase, R-enzyme, amylopectin-1,6-glucosidase	Dextrin α-1,6-glucanohydrolase	EC 3.2.1.142	Hydrolysis of 1,6-α-D-glucosidic linkages	α- and β-limit dextrins of amylopectin (complete reaction), amylopectin (incomplete reaction)	Oligosaccharides, maltose (as the smallest sugar released)

fast reduction of the viscosity of the medium. For that reason α-amylase is also called liquefying amylase. β-Amylase (EC 3.2.1.2) is an exo-acting enzyme that cleaves β-maltose from the non-reducing ends of the lineal chains, but does not hydrolyze the α-1,6-glucosidic linkages. Consequently, the final products of starch hydrolysis by β-amylase are β-maltose and β-limit dextrins. α-Glucosidase (EC 3.2.1.20) is also an exo-acting enzyme that cleaves non-reducing α-1,4-linkages liberating glucose. This amylase participates in starch hydrolysis mainly during the early stages of starch degradation in germinating barley seeds (Sun and Henson, 1991). β-Amylase and α-glucosidase are also called saccharifying amylases. Limit dextrinase (EC 3.2.1.142) is an endo-acting enzyme that removes the α-1,6-linkages in α- and β-limit dextrins to allow their further hydrolysis by β-amylase.

The activity of mainly α-amylase, β-amylase, and limit dextrinase is collectively called "diastatic power" (DP). In the brewing industry, DP is a key parameter of malting quality since it is an estimate of the capacity of the malt to degrade starch into fermentable sugars (Delcour and Verschaeve, 1987). Methods for estimating the diastatic activity of malt are generally based on its ability to generate reducing sugars. The main units and criteria used to measure the DP of a malted cereal are:

- Degrees Lintner (°L), defined by the JECFA (the Joint FAO/WHO Expert Committee on Food Additives) and the IoB (Institute of Brewing) as follows: "A malt has a diastatic power of 100°L if 0.1 ml of a clear 5% infusion of the malt, acting on 100 ml of a 2% starch solution at 20°C for 1 h, produces sufficient reducing sugars to reduce completely 5 ml of Fehling's solution." For a complete description of the method see http://www.fao.org/ag/agn/jecfa-additives/specs/Monograph1/Additive-270.pdf. The DP is around 35–40 for standard barley malts, but it can be as high as 100–125 for lager malts, and over 160 for some high-protein North American malts which have far more enzymatic power than they require to hydrolyze the starch from the malt. Therefore, they enable the brewer to use these malts as an amylases source in the case of unmalted starch adjuncts addition (The BREWER Inter-national, 2002, p. 29).
- Degrees Windisch–Kolbach (°WK), used by the EBC (European Brewery Convention), which can be converted to Lintner units as follows:

$$\mathrm{DPL} = \frac{{}^{\circ}\mathrm{WK} + 16}{3.5}$$

- Sorghum diastatic units (SDU), used by the SABS (South African Bureau of Standards) especially for sorghum, and not easily comparable to °L and °WK (EtokAkpan, 2004).

Next, the importance of every stage during brewing to enhance the activity of the enzymes and to obtain an adequate wort for beer elaboration is briefly described.

Malting: Germination and Kilning The first step of germination is critical in the brewing process if no exogenous enzymes are added. At this stage, all the enzymes must be expressed and activated to start the process of starch solubilization and hydrolysis. α-Amylase, α-glucosidase, and bound limit dextrinase are synthesized *de novo* during seed germination, while β-amylase (Ziegler, 1999) and free limit dextrinase are activated by endogenous proteases. In addition to the effect of the genotype on enzymes expression, the main factors that affect both expression and activation of these enzymes during germination are temperature, water/solid ratio, oxygen availability, and concentration of gibberellic acid (GA3) – the hormone that stimulates the synthesis of α-amylase and other hydrolases.

α-Amylase synthesis is synergically improved with the increase in temperature from 20–25°C to 30–35°C and the addition of exogenous GA3 (Singh *et al.*, 1988). β-Amylase, which is synthesized during the development of the grain and accumulated in an inactive starch-bound form, is released from starch and activated by a proteolytic process. Anoxic conditions during germination prevent the production of the endoprotease involved in β-amylase activation. Oxygen deficit also inhibits α-amylase synthesis (Hanson and Jacobsen, 1984; Loreti *et al.*, 1998). Limit dextrinase in barley is partially synthesized following germination (Hardie, 1975) under the influence of GA3 (Lee and Pyler, 1984) and the hydration conditions. Continuous humectation during germination produces higher levels of limit dextrinase than addition of water at the beginning (Pratt *et al.*, 1978; Longstaff and Bryce, 1993; Stenholm, 1997). Nevertheless, limit dextrinase activity is usually low in malted cereals, making up less than 20% of the potential total activity (Longstaff and Bryce, 1991) and leading to high concentrations of non-fermentable limit dextrins. This low activity is due to the major presence of LD as inactive forms of the enzyme bound to endogenous proteinaceous inhibitors (MacGregor *et al.*, 2000). LD activation probably occurs by proteolysis of these inhibitors by endogenous thiol proteases (Longstaff and Bryce, 1993) and/or specific reduction of inhibitors by thioredoxin (Cho *et al.*, 1999). In agreement with it, anaerobically germinated grain, following a period of normal malting, produced grains containing a limit dextrinase activity constituting over 80% of the potential total limit dextrinase activity (McCafferty *et al.*, 2004) due to the application of reducing conditions that could improve the activity of cysteine proteases (McCafferty *et al.*, 2000). In consequence, considering the high levels of limit dextrinase inhibitors usually present in malt, it does not seem suitable to improve the levels of this enzyme in the wort by selecting cereal lines with a high potential for limit dextrinase synthesis. It will be more effective to optimize those malting and mashing conditions that promote the release of free enzyme from the inhibitors-bound enzyme (MacGregor *et al.*, 1999).

In spite of enzymes synthesis and activation during germination, at this stage the starch is attacked only in a small extent because starch in the grain is in a crystalline non-soluble form that shows resistance to the enzymatic hydrolysis. α-Amylase and α-glucosidase are the only enzymes that are able to partially attack native (not boiled) starch (Sun and Henson, 1990). Consequently, the enzymes present in the germinated grain must retain their activity during the heating treatment of kilning to be active in the next step of mashing. Kilning is then a critical operation in brewing because excessive temperatures will lead to dramatic losses of the amylolytic ability of the malt. The thermostability of the synthesized and activated enzymes during germination is also of great importance for correct mashing. It depends on the enzyme, its origin, and even on the variety of the starchy material (Evans *et al.*, 2003). Under a typical kilning regimen, approximately 30% of the β-amylase activity is irreversibly deactivated (Evans *et al.*, 1997). α-Amylase, α-glucosidase, and limit dextrinase are also negatively affected, although the inhibitor-bound forms of this last enzyme are more resistant to thermal degradation (Sissons *et al.*, 1995).

Mashing At this stage starch hydrolysis must be completed to produce wort with an adequate composition of fermentable sugars. The use of malt with high DP will be the first requirement if no exogenous enzymes are added. Nevertheless, some considerations must be made at this respect.

The DP of a malted starchy material depends on the total and relative amounts of enzymes present in the malt. In the case of barley, β-amylase has been significantly correlated to DP (Gibson *et al.*, 1995; Clarke *et al.*, 1998), what is in agreement with the presence of maltose in barley wort as the major fermentable sugar (typically >55%) (Kunze, 1996) and with the presence of β-amylase as the enzyme that contributes in a greater extent to the total amylolytic activity in barley malt. Nevertheless, the levels and composition of fermentable sugars depend on not only the β-amylase but also the synergistic interaction between all the enzymes that are involved in starch degradation in such a way that, for the same content in β-amylase, the differences in α-amylase and limit dextrinase activities will be responsible for the differences in the levels of non-fermentable sugars in the wort (MacGregor *et al.*, 1999). In effect, in spite of the importance of β-amylase to generate maltose, the activity of this enzyme is positively affected by α-amylase, which improves synergically the activity of the β-amylase providing it oligosaccharides of adequate molecular weight for this saccharifying enzyme. On the other hand, limit dextrinase is the only enzyme capable of hydrolyzing α-1,6-linkages. Since high levels of limit dextrins, which can constitute as much as 25% of total carbohydrates, often remain in the wort as non-fermentable sugars (Enevoldsen and Schmidt, 1974), wort fermentability also depends strongly on the activity of the free limit dextrinase (Stenholm and Home, 1999). Nevertheless, this enzyme cannot attack starch granules without the previous action of α-amylase on starch (Maeda *et al.*, 1978). On the other hand, high levels of maltose, produced by the intensive action of β-amylase, can inhibit the activity of the free limit dextrinase during the mashing stage of brewing (MacGregor *et al.*, 2002). In conclusion, optimal starch hydrolysis will require an adequate equilibrium between α- and β-amylases and free limit dextrinase, which reflects the empirical model obtained by MacGregor *et al.* (1999) including the main effects of α- and β-amylases, as well as the interactions between these enzymes and the free limit dextrinase.

The relative ratio and total amounts and activity of each enzyme in malt depends first of all on the genotypic characteristics of the starchy material, the variety, the cultivar, and the malting conditions, as commented before. Nevertheless, the activity of the enzymes during mashing is strongly affected by the conditions of pH, which must be in the range 5–6 – as usual in the wort – by the presence of Ca^{2+} that is necessary for the activity and stability of the α-amylase, and mainly by the temperature and time of operation.

During mashing, temperature must reach at least 60°C to ensure starch gelatinization that makes it adequate for the enzymatic hydrolysis (Slack and Wainwright, 1980). This increase of temperature affects the activity of every enzyme in a different extent depending on their specific activities at each temperature and on their resistant to thermal denaturation, these effects being stronger as the time of operation increases. This way, an adequate amount and ratio of the enzymes could be suboptimal if the conditions of mashing are particularly inadequate for one of them. In general terms, α-amylase is the most resistant enzyme to heat inactivation and an amylase with higher optimal temperature (around 70°C). β-Amylase and limit dextrinase show maximum enzymatic activities at 60–62.5°C (Stenholm and Home, 1999), but while limit dextrinase retains most of its activity at these temperatures, especially under conditions of high gravity mashing (Stenholm, 1997), β-amylase suffers an important inactivation. This is in agreement with the apparent excess of β-amylase needed in malt compared to *in vitro* assays, what could be explained by the need of higher amounts of this enzyme to counterpart the loss of activity due to heat inactivation during mashing (MacGregor *et al.*, 1999). In this sense, there is already some evidence that improving the heat stability of β-amylase may be more beneficial than selecting barleys with higher β-amylase levels to increase the levels of fermentable sugars in the wort (MacGregor *et al.*, 1999).

Mashing can be performed isothermally at approximately 65°C (infusion mash) or by using a ramped temperature profile from approximately 45°C–70°C (temperature programmed mash). The time of operation is usually between 1 and 3 h. According to all that, an accurate selection of the mashing conditions of temperature and time of operation must be carefully done depending on malt and adjuncts composition (if added), and on the cereal enzymes profile, to improve the activity of the enzymes that control the extent of starch hydrolysis (Brandam *et al.*, 2003), according to the desired final characteristics of the beer, and to optimize extraction from malt. This way, when it is necessary to reduce the amount of non-fermentable sugars in the wort to obtain beers with high levels of alcohol or a low-caloric content, different mashing temperature profiles can be assayed to minimize limit dextrinase and β-amylase thermal losses by avoiding long periods of high temperature. On the contrary, in the case of low ethanol beers, low levels of fermentable sugars are needed in the wort and, consequently, mashing at high temperature can be a good strategy to reduce the activity of β-amylase and limit dextrinase.

Consequently with all of it, it is suggested to add, to the conventional malt quality DP criterion, the description of the individual enzymatic activities, mainly for α-amylase, β-amylase, and free limit dextrinase, to make easier to brewers the choice of the kind of malt and the mashing conditions that will allow the elaboration of good quality and special beers (Evans *et al.*, 2003).

Koji

Koji can be considered the substitute of malt in the Eastern World. Koji elaboration consists of the solid-state culture of molds on seeds to produce hydrolytic enzymes, including amylases and proteases. The koji thus obtained can be used as source of enzymes for the hydrolysis of starchy materials as a previous step in the manufacture of a variety of Oriental fermented foods as sake (the traditional alcoholic beverage of Japan made from rice), soy sauce, or sufu (soybean cheese). There are different kinds of koji depending on the material used (mainly rice and soybean, but also barley), the mold inoculated (mainly *Aspergillus oryzae*, but also *Aspergillus flavus* and species belonging to *Zygomycetous* spp.), and the final use of the koji. In all cases the growth of microorganisms is not only a source of enzymes, but also of vitamins and flavors that give the particular organoleptic character to the final food or beverage.

The Role of Amylases in Modern Brewing

Nowadays, the development of the enzyme technology has allowed optimizing the enzymatic steps of brewing to secure an adequate and constant quality of the wort (see at The BREWER International, 2002, p. 17) a "first enzymatic aid kit" to solve different problems that can appear during all the brewing process). In addition to the optimization of temperature and time conditions during the enzymatic steps, the addition of exogenous enzymes, especially thermostable amylases, has been introduced in brewing to compensate enzymatic deficits in case of incomplete germination or in case of materials with low enzyme production. This has allowed the extending of the number of starchy materials suitable for beer elaboration, offering the possibility to use local cultivars for brewing and to elaborate new beers with special tastes and nutritional characteristics, as gluten-free beers for celiac people, made from gluten-free starchy materials with low DP, as sorghum (Maccagnan *et al.*, 1999).

The use of exogenous enzymes has also allowed elaborating beer for diabetics (Curin *et al.*, 1988), or diet (low caloric) beers (Annemueller and Schober, 1999) with a caloric-content reduction between 15% and 50%. Considering that the caloric content in beer can be calculated approximately as (Lewis and Young, 1995)

$$\text{Calories in 10 cl} = 4 \times \%\ (\text{w/v})\ \text{solids} \times 7 \times \%\ (\text{w/v})\ \text{alcohol} \tag{10.1}$$

and considering that in a typical beer residual dextrins account for 75% of the solids, diet beers are elaborated by reducing the remaining non-fermentable dextrins with the addition of exogenous enzymes, mainly glucoamylase.

Substitution of the malting step by addition of all the necessary amylolytic enzymes to avoid the synthesis of β-glucanases during germination is also described as a strategy to elaborate functional beers, mainly from oats or barley, with beneficial coronary effects due to the high content of soluble glucans in these cereals (Triantafylloy, 2000) (Table 10.2).

The most used amylases in beer elaboration are α-amylase, α-glucosidase, and glucoamylase (see Table 10.1), although the use of these two last enzymes can affect negatively the fermentation of mashing worts with high concentrations of maltose since the presence of high concentrations of glucose as a result of the action of these amylases could inhibit maltose consumption in some yeast strains (Stewart *et al.*, 1979; Phaweni *et al.*, 1993). β-Amylase is also added, especially in case of those materials, as sorghum, lacking this enzyme.

The addition of limit dextrinase is not suitable since the inhibitors present in the malt will complex and deactivate part of the added enzyme (Stenholm, 1997). Pullulanase (EC 3.2.1.41) can substitute limit dextrinase in brewing (Enevoldsen, 1970; Odibo and Obi, 1989) since this enzyme is not inhibited as limit dextrinase. However, pullulanase is commonly used in the production of syrup adjuncts, but it is not approved for use in brewing in many countries (MacGregor *et al.*, 1999). Exogenous hydrolysis of α-1,6-linkages can be performed by glucoamylase, which offers the advantage over α-glucosidase of also hydrolyzing α-1,6-glucosidic bonds when the next bond is α-1,4. Care must be taken in the use of thermostable glucoamylases (many

Table 10.2 List of patents including the use of exogenous enzymes in brewing for different purposes

Patent number	*Title*
General brewing; starch sources for brewing	
US2005095315	Process for the production of alcoholic beverages using maltseed
DD99179	Highly fermented beer manufacture with barley processing
ZA9803237	Process for brewing beer
WO2002074895	Improved fermentation process
CN1594525	Method for manufacturing barley extracts for beer production
DE2153151	Starch degradation for the manufacture of ethanol beverages
ZA2003009381	A method of producing a fermentable wort
RU2190012	Method for manufacture of beer Arsenal'noe Temnoe 4
FR2203875	Manufacturing beer
DE2352906	Enzymes in beer wort manufacture
ZA7004735	Brewers' wort for making beer
NL7713669	Brewer's wort
SU379615	Beer
US3066026	Wort treatment with hectorite and enzyme
CN1616636	Preparation of a potato syrup for special use in beer
ZA6900044	Production of beer
WO9805788	Improved process for the production of alcoholic beverages using maltseed
DD109400	Beer wort after substitution of traditional raw materials
JP2004024151	Beer-like alcoholic beverages brewing from wheat starch
Enzymatic preparations	
DE10027915	Methods for isolation from malted grain of enzymes and enzyme mixtures and their application in beer and food production
DE10241647	Preparation of enzymes and culture media components from malted grain for use in beverage and food industries
WO9742839	Enzyme granulate for use in food technology
US6031155	Isolation and characterization of barley endoxylanase gene and products and their use to enhance arabinoxylan degradation in brewing processes
FR2676456	Thermostable variants of *Bacillus amyloliquefaciens* α-amylase and their preparation and use
Special new beers with nutritional benefits	
CN1740301	Method for producing dry beer from oats
WO2000024864	Preparation of wort and beer of high nutritional value, and corresponding products
CN1116652	Method for brewing health beer series not containing carcinogen but containing anticarcinogen
CN1401754	Enzymatic transglycosylation method for producing bifidus factor beer
US4355047	Low-calorie beer
EP949329	Gluten-free beer
CS236212	Method of manufacturing a light beer for diabetics by treating the mash with amylase
US4251630	Preparation of malt high in alpha-1,6-hydrolase
US4666718	Preparation of low calorie beer

commercial fungal glucoamylases) since they can retain some activity even after beer pasteurization, thus increasing the sweetness of the beer in the bottle at the expense of residual dextrins (James and Lee, 1997). Therefore, yeast thermolabile glucoamylases are usually applied.

These enzymes can be added individually or in enzymatic mixtures that generally include other enzymes not directly involved in starch hydrolysis (Souppe and Beudeker, 1998; Annemueller *et al.*, 2001; Annemueller *et al.*, 2004) such as glucanases and xylanases, which contribute to the filterability of the wort (Dale *et al.*, 1990) and to improve starch solubilization through the hydrolysis of cell wall polymers in the case that glucanases are added during the germination step (Grujic, 1998). Proteases are usually added with amylases to increase nitrogen availability for fermentation.

The exogenous enzymes applied in brewing can be of plant origin. Examples are the addition of *Curculigo pilosa* as an exogenous β-amylase source in the traditional elaboration of sorghum beer in West Africa, which additionally offers the advantage of high activity and stability, and the ability to attack raw starch from wheat, corn, potato, and rice (Dicko *et al.*, 1999), the employ of β-amylase from sweet potato for partial replacement of malt in brewing (Jiang *et al.*, 1994), or the use of multienzymatic preparations obtained from malted cereals (Annemueller *et al.*, 2001). Nevertheless, the exogenous enzymes applied in brewing are usually of microbial origin due to the advantages that fermentation offers in comparison to plant enzymes recovery, as higher yields and less time-consuming procedures. Microbial enzymatic preparations containing one or several amylases are obtained from GRAS ("generally recognized as safe") bacteria or fungi in cultures made on starch, as bacterial and fungal α-amylases (Sobral and De Vasconcelos, 1983; Imayasu *et al.*, 1989; Goode *et al.*, 2002; Goode *et al.*, 2003), bacterial β-amylases (Xu *et al.*, 1994), yeast glucoamylases (Lowery *et al.*, 1987), or bacterial pullulanases (Odibo and Obi, 1989).

Several strategies can be applied for exogenous enzyme enrichment. Generally, enzymes are added during mashing to complete the hydrolysis of starch before the enzyme deactivation that takes place during wort pasteurization. But there is also the possibility to include exogenous enzymes during fermentation (Dickscheit *et al.*, 1973; Mizuno *et al.*, 2004) to progressively release glucose and/or maltose, thus avoiding substrate inhibition of the yeast during the elaboration of beers with high ethanol degree.

Finally, there are other possibilities for the use of exogenous enzymes. They include the use of transgenic seeds and recombinant *Saccharomyces* strains, which will express heterologous enzymes during malting in the first case, and during fermentation in the second situation. The modification of barley seeds by inclusion of a fungal thermotolerant endo-1,4-beta-glucanase (EC 3.2.1.4) from microbial origin (*Trichoderma reesei*) to reduce wort viscosity and improve beer filtration (Nuutila *et al.*, 1999) is already reported. The construction of different amylolytic brewing yeasts (*S. cerevisiae* and *S. pastorianus*) by transformation of the wild strains with yeast and fungal α-amylase and glucoamylase genes that allow growth on starch as sole carbon source for the manufacture of low-carbohydrate diet beers (Hollenberg and Strasser, 1990; Liu *et al.*, 2004) is also described. The transformation of laboratory strains of *S. cerevisiae* and brewers' and distillers' yeasts with both genes encoding a glucoamylase from *S. diastaticus* and an α-amylase from *Bacillus amyloliquefaciens*, and the synergistic effect of the co-expression of both genes into the same strain to improve starch assimilation with an efficiency as high as 93% is also reported (Steyn and Pretorius, 1991).

Starchy materials for brewing other than barley

As commented before, adding exogenous enzymes during mashing allows to extent the possibilities of brewing with starchy materials that show low DP and difficulties for correct starch hydrolysis during mashing, whenever the fermentability of the wort and the organoleptic quality of the beer thus elaborated are adequate.

In these cases three strategies can be applied: partial addition of malted cereals as source of enzymes during mashing, addition of exogenous enzymes, mainly during mashing or even during the fermentation step, and use of an amylolytic microorganism that grows on the starchy material in a first stage, producing the amylases needed to hydrolyze in a second stage the starch present in the fresh material.

Addition of malted barley as source of enzymes has the advantage of contributing to color and flavor in the beer if the main starch material gives no enough adequate organoleptic profile to the beer. But even in that case, exogenous enzymes can be added to reinforce the amylolytic ability of barley (Goode *et al.*, 2000; Goode and Arendt, 2003). Addition of exogenous enzymes has the advantage of allowing to regulate the degree of starch hydrolysis needed depending on the type of beer, as well as correcting the levels of assimilable nitrogen and the filterability of the wort if proteases and glucanases are also applied. The possibility of using amylolytic microorganisms constitutes the basis for koji elaboration, as commented before.

Next, two examples of exogenous enzyme applications in beer elaboration with starchy materials other than barley are exposed.

Sorghum Beer A good example of exogenous enzyme application in brewing is the case of sorghum beer elaboration. Sorghum is the world's fifth most important cereal grain and constitutes a strategic natural food resource in areas subject to hot and dry agroecologies, where it is difficult to grow other grains. In fact, 90% of the world's sorghum area lies in the developing countries, mainly in Africa and Asia (FAO and ICRISAT, 1996).

For that reason sorghum has been widely used for several traditional food purposes, including brewing of African beers as burukutu (Faparusi, 1970; Novellie, 1977; Ogundiwin and Tehinse, 1981). Recently, sorghum beer brewing has also developed into a major industry for European-type lager beer elaboration, especially in the case of Nigeria, where barley importations have been restricted since 1988 (EtokAkpan, 2004).

There are several studies about the use of sorghum in brewing (Owuama, 1997; Agu and Palmer, 1998; Jani *et al.*, 1999; Obeta *et al.*, 2000; Okungbowa *et al.*, 2002; Goode and Arendt, 2003; EtokAkpan, 2005). As well as economic reasons, sorghum offers an interesting potential as raw material for brewing due to its high starch content and the absence of gluten, what makes it suitable for the elaboration of gluten-free beers for celiac people. Nevertheless, there are some inherent problems associated with sorghum that must be solved to better compete with barley in the elaboration of European-type beer.

A major disadvantage for the use of malted sorghum in brewing is the usual low DP and amylolytic activity during mashing. Although α-amylase isoenzymes are *de novo* synthesized during sorghum germination, very low (Dufour *et al.*, 1992; Taylor and Robbins, 1993) or even total absence (Uriyo and Eigel, 2000) of β-amylase levels are detected, causing incomplete saccharification of starch and low levels of maltose in comparison to barley wort (Dicko *et al.*, 2006). In addition, the higher gelatinization temperature of sorghum starch with regard to barley increases thermal deactivation of the enzymes (Jani *et al.*, 1999).

Several studies have been developed to improve α- and β-amylase activities in malted sorghum in relation with variety, cultivar, steep regime, steep liquor composition, and kilning temperature (Taylor and Robbins, 1993; Jani *et al.*, 1999; Obeta *et al.*, 2000; Okungbowa *et al.*, 2002). Nevertheless, the best solution to reduce the levels of non-fermentable sugars in sorghum worts is the use of mixtures of malted barley with sorghum during mashing (Goode and Arendt, 2003), or the addition of exogenous enzymes such as α-amylase and amyloglucosidase (Clayton, 1969), β-amylase from potato (Etim and EtokAkpan, 1992), or microbial α-amylases (Goode *et al.*, 2003), to the unmalted sorghum. In this last case it is also reported the convenience of including a percentage of malted sorghum as source of endogenous proteases to avoid the need of adding these enzymes since a poor foam retention has been associated to commercial proteolytic enzymes (Agu and Palmer, 1998).

Chestnut in Brewing Among the above-mentioned seeds used as raw materials for the preparation of fermented drinks, other indigenous crops like chestnut can constitute local alternative sources of starches for industrial purposes (especially sugar and alcohol manufacture) and lead to the conservation of agriculturally marginal lands. In fact, it is already described the elaboration of a new Chinese chestnut beer with beneficial health effects such as anti-cancer, reducing blood sugar, and lowering blood fat activities (Li *et al.*, 2005). Therefore, chestnut is here studied as a source of starch for brewing.

As sorghum, chestnut has no gluten but shows low endogenous amylolytic activity. According to it, chestnut is included in the elaboration of a kind of koji as a prior stage to ethanol fermentation for the elaboration of wine (Iwasaki *et al.*, 2002) or shochu (a Japanese popular distilled light alcoholic drink produced from steamed cereals, mainly rice and barley, but also from sweet potato soba (buckwheat), and chestnut in a lesser extent). Addition of malt (Li *et al.*, 2005) is also reported as a source of exogenous enzymes to complete chestnut starch hydrolysis.

Another strategy for brewing chestnut consists on substituting koji by direct addition of exogenous enzymes. This alternative takes as basis the two-step industrial process for starch hydrolysis. In the first stage simultaneous gelatinization and liquefaction of starch with a high-temperature α-amylase are performed. The maltodextrins thus generated are then saccharified with a glucoamylase in the second stage (Slominska, 1993). Optimal reaction conditions depend on the amylases used, as well as on the starch origin, which affects the composition, viscosity, and degradation resistance of the polysaccharides.

In our laboratory, we have optimized the enzymatic hydrolysis of chestnut starch in solid (chopped) and submerged (aqueous liquid pastes) operation in a single step with an enzymatic mixture of a commercial heat resistant α-amylase (Termamyl 120L(S)) and a glucoamylase (AMG 300L), both purchased by Novo Nordisk A/S Industries (López *et al.*, 2004, 2005, 2006). Some details of these enzymatic processes are next briefly described as an example of practical application and optimization of the addition of exogenous enzymes in brewing of new starchy materials.

The submerged process of hydrolysis was performed at 70°C to reduce purée viscosity. In these conditions total conversion of starch to glucose in a single step was only achieved when an adequate concentration and composition of the enzymatic mixture of α-amylase/glucoamylase was present in the reaction medium (López *et al.*, 2004). Figure 10.3 shows the linear increasing effect of the concentration of the enzymes on chestnut starch solubilization and hydrolysis, being the best the higher value assayed (60 EU/g raw chestnut, corresponding to 10.5 EU/ml), and the second order effect of the ratio of α-amylase/glucoamylase, which implies the existence of an optimum value corresponding to glucoamylase enriched mixtures (α-amylase/glucoamylase ratio of 0.35/0.75 EU). Sugar profile in this hydrolyzate corresponded to glucose (as the only final product of starch hydrolysis) and saccharose (present in chestnut) in concentrations of 70 and 15 g/l respectively.

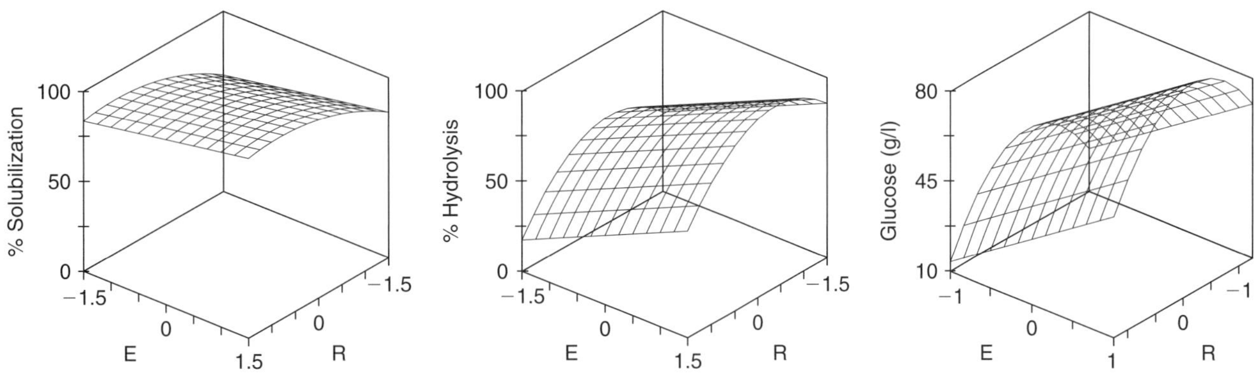

Figure 10.3 Combined effect of the enzyme concentration and the ratio of α-amylase/glucoamylase (in codified values) on the solubilization, hydrolysis, and glucose release from chestnut purée with a mixture of amylases. E, enzyme concentration; R, ratio of α-amylase/glucoamylase in the mixture. Published with permission of the American Chemical Society (Copyright 2004).

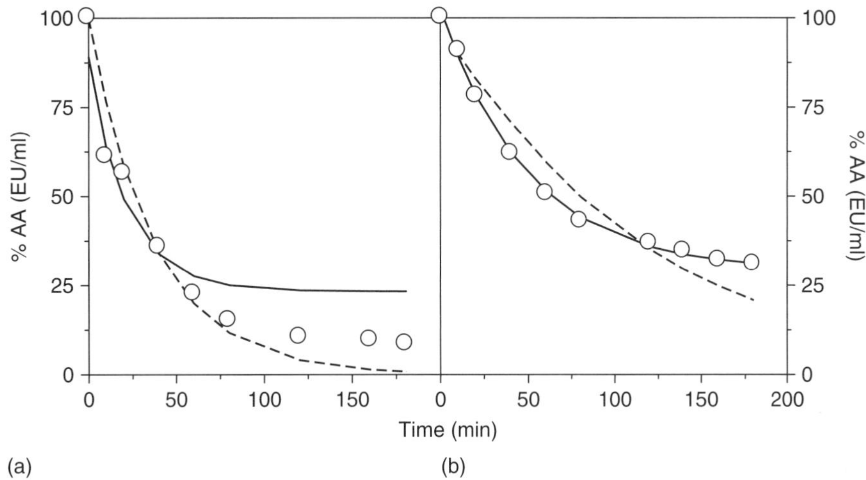

Figure 10.4 Thermal loss of amylolytic activity of a mixture of α-amylase and glucoamylase (respective ratio: 0.35/0.65) at 70°C in (a) 50 mM citric–phosphate buffer pH 4.75 and (b) 225 g/l pH 4.75 buffered chestnut purée. AA, total amylolytic activity expressed as percentages referred to the initial value (1.35 EU/ml). Symbols represent the mean values of two experimental points; dashed and solid lines represent, respectively, the fittings to a first order model and to model (10.3).

Incomplete starch conversion at low enzyme concentrations was attributed to product and substrate inhibition, as well as thermal deactivation (López *et al.*, 2006). In effect, substrate and product inhibition were confirmed and modeled by equation (10.2), this derived from Michaelis–Menten and Briggs–Haldane's models considering simultaneous competitive and non-competitive product inhibition, and substrate inhibition:

$$v = \frac{v'_m S}{\left(K'_m\left(1+\frac{I}{K'_{iC}}\right)+S+K'_S S^2\right)\left(1+\frac{I}{K'_{iNC}}\right)} \qquad (10.2)$$

where v and v'_m are respectively initial and maximal initial reaction rates of the enzyme mixture in chestnut purée, S is the substrate concentration, K'_m and K'_s represent operational Michaelis–Menten and substrate inhibition constants, respectively, I is the inhibitor (glucose) concentration, and K'_{iC} and K'_{iNC} are operational competitive and non-competitive product inhibition constants, respectively.

Anyway, substrate and glucose inhibition was not strong enough to explain the low percentage of hydrolysis reached at low enzyme concentration. Consequently, thermal deactivation of the α-amylase and glucoamylase mixture at low enzyme concentration was also studied in presence and absence of substrate (Figure 10.4), and the losses of amylolytic activity were fitted to model (10.3), based on Aymard and Belarbi's one for an enzymatic mixture (Aymard and Belarbi, 2000), and modified to include a synergistic effect between these two enzymes (López *et al.*, 2006):

$$\begin{aligned} AA_t &= AA_\alpha + ae^{-kat} + be^{-kbt} \\ &\quad + S_1 AA_\alpha(ae^{-kat}) + S_2 AA_\alpha(be^{-kbt}) \end{aligned} \qquad (10.3)$$

where AA_t represents the total amylolytic activity (expressed as percentage referred to the initial total activity) of the mixture at time t, AA_α is the α-amylase activity expressed as percentage, a and b, and ka and kb are, respectively, pre-exponential parameters and first order constants for each glucoamylase form present in the commercial enzyme (Amirul *et al.*, 1996), and S_1 and S_2 are the synergism terms between the α-amylase and each glucoamylase form.

Experimental and modeled data showed a strong decrease of the enzymatic activity in both cases, which reflects the important role of enzyme thermal deactivation as a reason for incomplete starch hydrolysis. Glucoamylase, following a biexponential kinetics pattern, was only responsible for the thermal deactivation of the mixture, while the α-amylase kept 100% of the initial activity at the end of the incubation in these conditions. Therefore, the slightly retarded addition of glucoamylase with regard to α-amylase, to reduce the exposure of this enzyme to high temperatures while taking advantage of the synergic action of both enzymes working together, was finally proposed as an alternative to reduce the need of high concentrations of enzymes, especially of glucoamylase (López *et al.*, 2004).

Two main factors prevent the achievement of high-glucose hydrolyzates from chestnut, they condition the utility of chestnut as an adequate starchy material for use in brewing or as adjunct. They are the low concentration of starch in raw chestnut (around 30%) and the impossibility of working with chestnut purée concentrations higher than 300 g/l due to their viscosity. Therefore, two procedures were developed to increase the glucose levels in chestnut hydrolyzates.

In a way, the elaboration of hydrolyzates in consecutive cycles of submerged one-step hydrolysis of chestnut purée, carried out by using the hydrolyzate obtained in the first cycle – free of solids – to make a new chestnut pureé for the next cycle of hydrolysis, led to a 65% increase of the glucose concentration in the hydrolyzate obtained after three cycles of operation (López *et al.*, 2004) with regard to the simple one-step operation.

On the other hand, solid state hydrolysis, performed with chopped-wet chestnut without free water, also showed the suitability of this mode of operation to increase the levels of glucose in the hydrolyzates obtained after one-step solid state operation and posterior aqueous extraction (López *et al.*, 2005). Applying the same optimal enzyme concentration and α-amylase/glucoamylase ratio defined for the submerged operation, total hydrolysis was achieved operating in solid state at 70°C (López *et al.*, 2005) (Figure 10.5), what led to a 50% increase of the glucose concentration in the hydrolyzate comparing to the submerged process. The assays performed at lower temperatures to check the possibility to develop a process of simultaneous hydrolysis and fermentation showed the inability of the system to achieve total hydrolysis of the chestnut starch (Figure 10.5) as a consequence of mass transfer restrictions (López *et al.*, 2005).

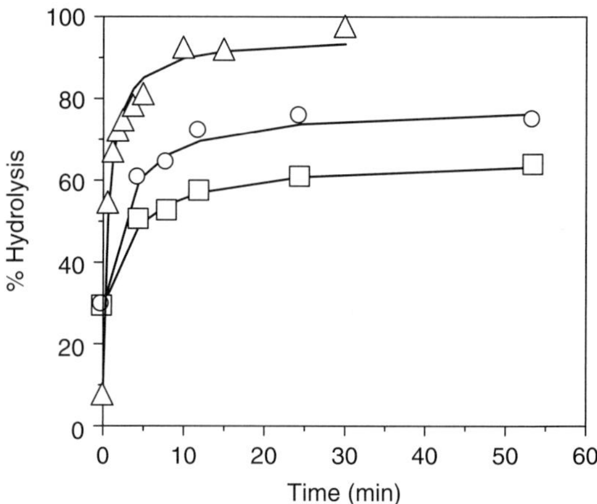

Figure 10.5 Kinetics of the one-step solid-state hydrolysis of chestnut with a mixture of 0.35/0.65 α-amylase/glucoamylase and 60 EU/g of raw chestnut at three temperatures: 70°C (triangles), 30°C (circles) and 17°C (squares). Published with permission of the American Chemical Society (Copyright 2005).

Summary Points

- Enzymes are the underlying responsible for all the biochemical reactions that take part in the elaboration of many foodstuffs. Beer is an example of that.
- Amylases are, together with limit dextrinase and proteases, the main enzymes implicated in brewing. Their action during the stages of malting and mashing allows the degradation of the starch and proteins present in the cereal grain to transform them into yeast assimilable sugars and amino acids.
- The fermentability of the wort and the final levels of alcohol and remaining sugars in beer are strongly dependent on the activity of the starch degrading enzymes (amylases and limit dextrinase). Low levels of enzymes or inadequate conditions of pH, temperature, and time of operation during malting and mashing can lead to low-quality beers.
- The profile of cereal endogenous starch degrading enzymes includes α-amylase, β-amylase, α-glucosidase, and limit dextrinase. It depends mainly on the cereal, although variety, cultivar, and malting conditions also affect the levels of the enzymes synthesized. They are accumulated during the malting step by *de novo* synthesis or by proteolytic transformation into active forms.
- The main amylases in barley and sorghum are β- and α-amylase. The former is the major amylase in barley. It is an exoenzyme that liberates β-maltose from starch, providing a readily fermentable substrate for the yeast. The latter is the major amylase in sorghum. It is an endoenzyme that reduces starch viscosity breaking the starch molecule in lower weight non-directly assimilable oligosaccharides, maltose, and glucose in low amounts. The only action of α-amylase on starch provides low levels of fermentable

sugars. Therefore, this enzyme needs the following action of β-amylase or α-glucosidase as saccharifying amylases.

- Limit dextrinase is the debranching enzyme responsible for the hydrolysis of the α-1,6-linkages in α- and β-limit dextrins resulting from the exhaustive action of α- and β-amylases on starch. The activity of this enzyme during mashing is usually low in malted cereals, making up less than 20% of its potential total activity due to the major presence of limit dextrinase as inactive forms of the enzyme bound to endogenous proteinaceous inhibitors.
- Exogenous amylases (mainly α-amylase, α-glucosidase, and glucoamylase) can be added during the mashing stage to reinforce the action of the endogenous enzymes. This strategy has interesting operational benefits increasing the wort fermentability of poorly modified malts, reducing the need of malt for mashing, and allowing the use of other non-easily maltable starchy sources as chestnut.
- New kinds of beers with interesting nutritional characteristics can be obtained by different strategies related to the role of amylases:
  - Beers with low ethanol content can be obtained by limiting the activity of the endogenous enzymes during mashing to reduce the amount of fermentable sugars in the wort.
  - Beers for diabetics, light or diet beers, which are characterized by low levels of residual sugars in the final product, can be elaborated increasing the extent of starch hydrolysis during mashing by adding amylase-rich multienzyme preparations.
  - Beers for celiac people can be elaborated employing gluten-free starchy sources with low DP (as sorghum) in combination with the addition of exogenous enzymes.

References

Agu, R.C. and Palmer, G.H. (1998). *Bioresource Technol.* 66, 253–261.

Amirul, A.A., Khoo, S.L., Nazalan, M.N., Razip, M.S. and Azizan, M.N. (1996). *Folia Microbiol.* 41, 165–174.

Annemueller, G. and Schober, J. (1999). *Brauwelt* 139, 862–867.

Annemueller, G., Bauch, T., Fischer, W., Schoeber, J.J. and Tiep, H.A. (2001). Patent no. DE10027915.

Annemueller, G., Schoeber, J.J., Manger, H.J. Schauermann, P.S. and Thormann, C. (2004). Patent no. DE10241647.

Aymard, C. and Belarbi, A. (2000). *Enzyme Microb. Technol.* 27, 612–613.

Brandam, C., Meyer, X.M., Proth, J., Strehaiano, P. and Pingaud, H. (2003). *Biochem. Eng. J.* 13, 43–52.

Cho, M.-J., Wong, J.H., Marx, C., Jiang, W., Lemaux, P.G. and Buchanan, B.B. (1999). *Proc. Natl. Acad. Sci. USA* 96, 14641–14646.

Clarke, D., Sissons, M. and Proudlove, M.O. (1998). HGCA Project Report no. 162.

Clayton, D.H. (1969). Patent no. ZA6900044.

Curin, J., Cernohorsky, V. and Faktor, J. (1988). Patent no. CS236212.

Dale, C.J., Young, T.W. and Omole, A.T. (1990). *J. Inst. Brew.* 96, 403–409.

Delcour, J.A. and Verschaeve, S.G. (1987). *J. Inst. Brew.* 93, 296–301.

Dicko, M.H., Searle van Leeuwen, M.J.F., Beldman, G., Ouedraogo, O.G., Hilhorst, R. and Traore, A.S. (1999). *Appl. Microbiol. Biotechnol.* 52, 802–805.

Dicko, M.H., Gruppen, H., Zouzouho, O.C., Traoré, A.S., van Berkel, W.J.H. and Voragen, A.G.J. (2006). *J. Sci. Food Agric.* 86, 953–963.

Dickscheit, R., Glaser, W., Grochowski, S., Raehse, K., Raehse, K., Siebert, N., Beubler, A., Nielebock, C., Ehlies, H. and Dempwolf, M. (1973). Patent no. DD99179.

Dufour, J.P., Melotte, L. and Sebrenik, S. (1992). *J. Am. Soc. Brew. Chem.* 50, 110–119.

Enevoldsen, B.S. (1970). *J. Inst. Brew.* 76, 546–552.

Enevoldsen, B.S. and Schmidt, F. (1974). *J. Inst. Brew.* 80, 520–533.

Etim, M.U. and EtokAkpan, O.U. (1992). *World J. Microbiol. Biotechnol.* 8, 509–511.

EtokAkpan, O.U. (2004). *J. Inst. Brew.* 110, 335–339.

EtokAkpan, O.U. (2005). *Process Biochem.* 40, 2489–2491.

Evans, D.E., Wallace, W., Lance, R.C.M. and MacLeod, L.C. (1997). *J. Cereal Sci.* 26, 241–250.

Evans, E., van Wegen, B., Ma, Y. and Eglinton, J. (2003). *J. Am. Soc. Brew. Chem.* 61, 210–218.

FAO and ICRISAT (1996). *The World Sorghum and Millet Economies. Facts, Trends and Outlook*, pp. 5–27. FAO and ICRISAT, Rome, Italy, and Andhra Pradesh, India.

Faparusi, S.I. (1970). *J. Sci. Food Agr.* 21, 79–81.

Georg-Kraemer, J.E., Caierão, E., Minella, E., Barbosa-Neto, J.F. and Cavalli, S.S. (2004). *J. Inst. Brew.* 110, 303–308.

Gibson, T.S., Solah, V., Glennie Holmes, M.R. and Taylor, H.R. (1995). *J. Inst. Brew.* 101, 277–280.

Goode, D.L. and Arendt, E.K. (2003). *J. Inst. Brew.* 109, 208–217.

Goode, D.L., Halbert, C. and Arendt, E.K. (2000). *VTT Symposium* 207, 321–323.

Goode, D.L., Halbert, C. and Arendt, E.K. (2002). *J. Inst. Brew.* 108, 465–473.

Goode, D.L., Halbert, C. and Arendt, E.K. (2003). *J. Am. Soc. Brew. Chem.* 61, 69–78.

Grujic, O. (1998). *J. Inst. Brew.* 104, 249–253.

Hanson, A.D. and Jacobsen, J.V. (1984). *Plant Physiol.* 75, 566–572.

Hardie, D.G. (1975). *Phytochemistry* 14, 1719–1722.

Hollenberg, C.P. and Strasser, A.W.M. (1990). *Food Biotechnol.* 4, 527–534.

Imayasu, S., Hata, Y., Oishi, K., Kawato, A. and Suginami, K. (1989). *Nippon Nogeikagaku Kaishi* 63, 971–980.

Iwasaki, I., Ichigami, M., Fujiwara, T., Nagatomo, M., Toda, Y. and Takahashi, K. (2002). Patent no. JP2002253209.

James, J.A. and Lee, B.H. (1997). *J. Food Biochem.* 21, 1–52.

Jani, M., Annemüller, G. and Schildbach, R. (1999). *Monatsschrift fuer Brauwissenschaft* 52, 157–162.

Jiang, G.S., Li, Y.N. and Cai, S.J. (1994). *Food Sci. China* 3, 7–11.

Kunze, W. (1996). Wort production. In: Wainwright, T. (ed.), *Technology Brewing and Malting*, pp. 171–316. VLB Berlin, Germany.

Kuusela, P., Hämäläinen, J.J., Reinikainen, P. and Olkku, J. (2004). *J. Inst. Brew.* 110, 309–319.

Lee, W.J. and Pyler, R.E. (1984). *J. Am. Soc. Brew. Chem.* 42, 11–17.

Lewis, M.J. and Young, T.W. (1995). *Brewing*. Chapman and Hall, London. p. 243.

Li, X., Zhang, Z., Wang, X., Zhao, C. and Zhang, H. (2005). *Zhongguo Niangzao* 6, 56–57.

Liu, Z., Zhang, G. and Liu, S. (2004). *J. Biosci. Bioeng.* 98, 414–419.

Longstaff, M.A. and Bryce, J.H. (1991). *Proceedings of the European Brewing Convention Congress*, Lisbon, IRL Press: Oxford, pp. 593–600.

Longstaff, M.A. and Bryce, J.H. (1993). *Plant Physiol.* 101, 881–889.

López, C., Torrado, A., Fuciños, P., Guerra, N.P. and Pastrana, L. (2004). *J. Agric. Food Chem.* 52, 2907–2914.

López, C., Torrado, A., Guerra, N.P. and Pastrana, L. (2005). *J. Agric. Food Chem.* 53, 989–995.

López, C., Torrado, A., Fuciños, P., Guerra, N.P. and Pastrana, L. (2006). *Enzyme Microb. Tech.* 39, 252–258.

Loreti, E., Guglielminetti, L., Yamaguchi, J., Gonzali, S., Alpi, A. and Perata, P. (1998). *J. Plant Physiol.* 152, 44–50.

Lowery, C.E., Duncombe, G.R., Line, W.F. and Chicoye, E. (1987). Patent no. US4666718.

Maccagnan, G., Pat, A., Collavo, F., Ragg, G.L. and Bellini, M.P. (1999). Patent no. EP949329.

Maeda, I., Nikuni, Z., Taniguchi, H. and Nakamura, M. (1978). *Carbohydr. Res.* 61, 309–320.

McCafferty, C.A., Perch-Neilson, N. and Bryce, J.H. (2000). *J. Amer. Soc. Brew. Chem.* 44, 47–50.

McCafferty, C.A., Jenkinson, H.R., Brosnan, J.M. and Bryce, J.H. (2004). *J. Inst. Brew.* 110, 284–296.

MacGregor, A.W., Bazin, S.L., Macri, L.J. and Babb, J.C. (1999). *J. Cereal Sci.* 29, 161–169.

MacGregor, E.A., Bazin, S.L., Ens, E.W., Lahnstein, J., Macri, L.J., Shirley, N.J. and MacGregor, A.W. (2000). *J. Cereal Sci.* 31, 79–90.

MacGregor, A.W., Bazin, S.L. and Schroeder, S.W. (2002). *J. Cereal Sci.* 35, 17–28.

Mizuno, A., Shinoda, N. and Nomura, Y. (2004). *Nippon Jozo Kyokaishi* 99, 873–877.

Novellie, L. (1977). Beverages form sorghum and millets. In Dendy, D.A.V. (ed.), *Proceedings of a Symposium on Sorghum and Millets for Human Food*, pp. 83–103. Tropical Products Institute, London, England.

Nuutila, A.M., Ritala, A., Skadsen, R.W., Mannonen, L. and Kauppinen, V. (1999). *Plant Mol. Biol.* 41, 777–783.

Obeta, J.A.N., Okungbowa, J. and Ezeogu, L.I. (2000). *J. Inst. Brew.* 106, 295–304.

Odibo, F.J.C. and Obi, S.K.C. (1989). *MIRCEN J. Appl. Microbiol. Biotechnol.* 5, 187–192.

Ogundiwin, J.O. and Tehinse, J.F. (1981). *Brew. Distill. Int.* 6, 26–27.

Okungbowa, J., Obeta, J.A.N. and Ezeogu, L.I. (2002). *J. Inst. Brew.* 108, 362–370.

Owuama, C.I. (1997). *World J. Microb. Biotechnol.* 13, 253–260.

Phaweni, M., O'Connor-Cox, E.S.C., Pickerell, A.T.W. and Axcell, B.C. (1993). *J. Am. Soc. Brew. Chem.* 51, 10–15.

Pratt, G.W., Chapple, T.W. and Fahy, M.J. (1978). Patent no. US4251630.

Singh, T., Harinder, K. and Bains, G.S. (1988). *J. Am. Soc. Brew. Chem.* 46, 1–5.

Sissons, M., Taylor, M. and Proudlove, M. (1995). *J. Am. Soc. Brew. Chem.* 53, 104–110.

Slack, P.T. and Wainwright, T. (1980). *J. Inst. Brew.* 86, 74–77.

Slominska, L. (1993). *Starch/Stärke* 45, 88–90.

Sobral, J. and De Vasconcelos, L. (1983). *Cerveza y Malta* 20, 35–40.

Souppe, J. and Beudeker, R.F. (1998). Patent no. WO9805788.

Stenholm, K. (1997). VTT Publication no. 323. VTT, Technical Research Centre of Finland, Espoo, Finland.

Stenholm, K. and Home, S. (1999). *J. Inst. Brew.* 105, 205–210.

Stewart, G.G., Erratt, J., Garrison, I., Goring, T. and Hancock, I. (1979). *Tech. Q. Master Brew. Assoc. Am.* 16, 1–7.

Steyn, A.J. and Pretorius, I.S. (1991). *Gene* 100, 85–93.

Sun, Z. and Henson, C.A. (1990). *Plant Physiol.* 94, 320–327.

Sun, Z. and Henson, C.A. (1991). *Arch. Biochem. Biophys.* 284, 298–305.

Taylor, J.R.N. and Robbins, D.J. (1993). *J. Inst. Brew.* 99, 413–416.

The BREWER International (2002), Vol. 2. http://www.igb.org.uk.

Triantafylloy, O.A. (2000). Patent no. WO2000024864.

Uriyo, M. and Eigel, W.E. (2000). *Process Biochem.* 35, 433–436.

Xu, T., He, B., Zhu, F., Wang, H., Zhang, S., Yang, J., Zheng, Y. and Li, Y. (1994). *Weishengwuxue Tongbao* 21, 336–339.

Yoon, S.-H., Mukerjea, R. and Robyt, J.F. (2003). *Carbohyd. Res.* 338, 1127–1132.

Ziegler, P. (1999). *J. Cereal Sci.* 29, 195–204.

(ii) Beer Drinking

11

Trends of Beer Drinking in Europe

Pedro Marques-Vidal Unidade de Nutrição e Metabolismo, Faculdade de Medicina da Universidade de Lisboa, Lisboa, Portugal

Abstract

The trends in beer drinking in Europe were assessed from the food balance sheets of the Food and Agriculture Organization and the brewers in Europe, together with available national or international studies. In Nordic countries, beer consumption decreased in some countries but increased in others. In Southern European countries, beer consumption tended to increase, whereas in Central European countries beer consumption declined steadily. Finally, in Eastern European countries, no concise pattern could be drawn, although an increase in the consumption was found in most countries studied. Overall, the available data indicate that beer consumption decreases in the Center and North of Europe, while it tends to increase in the Southern and Eastern Europe. The reasons for such changes are multiple, including global market, tax and law enforcement, local supply and trendy fashion.

List of Abbreviations

ESPAD	The European School survey Project on Alcohol and other Drugs
EU	European Union
FAO	Food and Agriculture Organization of the United Nations
USSR	Union of the Soviet Socialist Republics

Introduction

Alcohol drinking can be influenced by several factors at the population level: price policies (Ponicki *et al.*, 1997; Heeb *et al.*, 2003; Kuo *et al.*, 2003), law enforcement (Kubicka *et al.*, 1998; Nordic Council for Alcohol and Drug Research, 2002; Wallin *et al.*, 2005), local availability (Ólafsdóttir, 1998) and fashion (Simpura *et al.*, 1995). Further, assessing the trends in alcohol (and beer) consumption is a relatively challenging task, as there are little longitudinal studies, and the methods used to quantify alcohol consumption do not provide homogeneous results (Giovannucci *et al.*, 1991; Casswell *et al.*, 2002; Koppes *et al.*, 2002). Since earlier trends have already been reported (Leifman, 2000), this chapter will focus mainly on the trends in beer availability as reported in the Food and Agriculture Organization (FAO) food balance sheets (Food and Agriculture Organization, 2006), and by national brewer's associations. The FAO food balance sheets enable the estimation of a per capita supply of different types of foodstuffs for a given period based on the available supply and the population size,[1] but do not take into account the individual imports or home-made alcoholic drinks (Nordlund and Osterberg, 2000; Leifman *et al.*, 2002). Whenever possible, data from national or international studies on the trends of beer drinking will be provided. Regarding adolescents, data from the European School survey Project on Alcohol and other Drugs (ESPAD) study (Hibell *et al.*, 1997, 2004) will be reported; the ESPAD study is a multinational study focusing on alcohol and other drug use among students, encompassing 35 European countries, and provides estimates of the prevalence of adolescents aged 15–16 years who consumed beer at least thrice during 30 days prior to the interview. It should be stressed that the results obtained using the FAO food balance sheets, the per capita consumption as provided by brewer's associations and the data from population studies might differ, as the methodologies are not comparable.

Also, since drinking patterns differ considerably according to geographical region (Sieri *et al.*, 2002), trends will be provided for four regions: Nordic, traditionally spirit-drinking countries; Central, beer-drinking countries, and Southern European, wine-drinking countries (Leifman, 2000); and lastly, the trends in beer consumption will be assessed in the former USSR, Eastern European countries, for which only limited data regarding trends are available.

Results will be expressed in annual per capita consumption (in liters), mean daily beer-related ethanol consumption (in grams of ethanol) and as percentage of overall ethanol consumption. For each country, a linear regression was performed using beer consumption parameters as dependent variable and year as independent variable; this enables to assess

[1] http://www.fao.org/ES/ESS/fbsforte.asp assessed November 26th.

Beer in Health and Disease Prevention
ISBN: 978-0-12-373891-2

Table 11.1 Estimated share of total beer sales consumed in private homes (%)

Country	*2002*	*2003*	*2004*
Austria	65	65	66
Belgium	43	44	45
Denmark	75	–	–
Finland	73	75	75
France	70	72	72
Germany	68	70	–
Greece	35	35	–
Ireland	20	23	–
Italy	59	60	61
Lithuania	–	85	88
Norway	74	73	75
Poland	–	60	60
Portugal	33	34	66
Spain	32	26	–
Sweden	79	79	78
Switzerland	55	57	60
United Kingdom	37	39	40

–: No data.

Source: Adapted from The Brewers of Europe (2006).

whether the beer availability and/or consumption increased, remained stable or decreased during the time period studied.

Nordic Countries

Nordic countries (Denmark, Finland, Iceland, Norway and Sweden) are characterized by high spirit consumption. Beer is also a common beverage, and its alcohol content varies between less than 2.8% (light beer) to nearly 7% (strong beer). Interestingly, although alcoholic beverage sales is a state monopoly, light beer can be found in supermarkets, and changes in sales policies as imposed by European Union (EU) might considerably influence consumption trends (Holder *et al.*, 1995). Most of the beer is consumed in private houses, less than 25% being consumed in restaurants or other premises, and no significant trend was noted (Table 11.1).

Denmark

Denmark is a relatively modest producer of beer in Europe, ranking behind Austria and before Portugal (Table 11.2). Per capita consumption decreased from 128 l per year in 1992 to 85 l in 2004; this decrease being also found for the average daily consumption and the percent of total ethanol consumption as reported by the food balance sheets (Table 11.3). Those findings are in agreement with other authors, and are the result of efforts of some Nordic countries to promote Southern European drinking style, replacing beer and spirits by wine (Gerdes *et al.*, 2002; Nordic Council for Alcohol and Drug Research, 2002). Still, those findings might not apply to all the Danish population, as a recent survey found that alcohol consumption has remained relatively stable in 15–16-year olds for the period 1995–2003 (44% in 1995, 53% in 1999 and 44% in 2003) (Hibell *et al.*, 2004) or even increased in middle-aged and elderly Danes (Bjork *et al.*, 2006).

Finland

Contrary to Denmark, beer consumption in Finland increased in the 1980s (Simpura *et al.*, 1995) and remained stable afterward (Table 11.3). In 1992, the per capita consumption was 88 l per year, with only a slight decrease to 84 l in 2004; similar conclusions can be drawn from the FAO food balance sheet data. Beer represents circa two-thirds of all ethanol consumed, and this figure has remained stable for the period studied (Table 11.3). It should be noted that there is no information available regarding unrecorded beer consumption, such as home-made beer or importing from abroad (Leifman *et al.*, 2002). Also, as in Denmark, total alcohol consumption appears to be increasing among elderly subjects (Sulander *et al.*, 2004), although no information regarding whether this consumption of beer or other types of alcoholic beverages was provided. The prevalence of adolescents who consumed beer three times or more during the last 30 days also increased slightly from 15% in 1995 to 17% in 2003 (Hibell *et al.*, 2004).

Iceland

There is little information regarding the trends in beer consumption for Iceland. A previous study has shown that the consumption of beer increased after the introduction of strong beer in 1989, but leveled off afterward (Ólafsdóttir, 1998). Still, people started shifting from spirits to beer since, and data from the FAO indicate that the consumption of beer increased during 1992–2004: in 1992, beer represented less than 40% of total alcohol consumed, whereas in 2003 it was over 60%. Beer-related ethanol consumption also doubled during that period (Table 11.3), and a slight, non-significant increase in the prevalence of beer drinkers was also noted in the ESPAD study: 17% in 1995 and 1999, 19% in 2003 (Hibell *et al.*, 2004).

Norway

The mean beer-related ethanol consumption increased slightly from 1992 to 2003 (Table 11.3) a trend also observed in the ESPAD study for adolescents (9% in 1995, 17% in 1999, 14% in 2003) (Hibell *et al.*, 2004). Conversely, the share of beer among alcoholic beverages decreased from 70% to 56% (Table 11.3). Those findings indicate that beer consumption is increasing at a lower pace than total alcohol consumption (Strand and Steiro, 2003).

Sweden

As for Denmark, the consumption of beer has been declining in Sweden. Per capita consumption decreased from 64 l in

Table 11.2 Trends in beer production

Year	*Germany*	*United Kingdom*	*Spain*	*The Netherlands*	*France*	*Belgium*	*Italy*	*Ireland*	*Austria*	*Denmark*	*Portugal*	*Finland*	*Greece*	*Sweden*	*Luxembourg*
1992	120158	55887	26082	20659	21297	14259	12161	6633	10014	9775	6893	4576	4010	4973	569
1993	115800	56746	24278	20431	20833	14182	11715	6910	9823	9435	6568	4588	3900	5140	558
1994	118200	58333	25024	22175	20445	14743	12098	7186	10144	9410	6637	4538	4250	5430	561
1995	116900	56800	25313	23118	20634	15046	11990	7402	9662	10058	6928	4726	4005	5309	518
1996	114200	58072	24716	23494	20441	14180	11117	7765	9547	9591	6713	4669	3945	4805	484
1997	114800	59139	24879	24701	19483	14014	11455	8152	9366	9181	6623	4797	3945	4858	481
1998	111500	56652	24991	23988	19807	14105	12193	8478	8830	8075	6784	4787	4012	4568	469
1999	112791	57854	25852	24501	19866	14575	12179	8648	8869	8024	6758	4695	4220	4673	450
2000	110000	55279	26414	25072	18926	14734	12575	8324	8750	7460	6451	4612	4500	4495	418
2001	108500	56802	27702	25232	18866	15039	12782	8712	8588	7233	6554	4631	4454	4449	397
2002	108336	56672	27860	24898	18117	15696	12592	8133	8731	8534	7129	4726	4550	4376	386
2003	105300	58014	30671	25124	18132	15650	13673	8023	8891	8352	7350	4564	4080	4192	390
2004	106190	53800	31600	23828	16800	17409	13170	8142	8670	8550	7440	4617	4150	3788	391

Note: Results expressed in 1.000 hl

Source: Data from The Brewers of Europe (2006).

Table 11.3 Trends in beer consumption in Nordic countries

Year	*1992*	*1993*	*1994*	*1995*	*1996*	*1997*	*1998*	*1999*	*2000*	*2001*	*2002*	*2003*	*2004*	*Trend*
Liters/year														
Denmark	128	126	127	124	121	117	108	105	102	99	97	96	85	Decrease
Finland	88	86	83	80	80	81	79	79	78	80	81	78	84	Stable
Sweden	64	64	67	65	59	62	62	59	56	55	56	55	51	Decrease
Grams of ethanol/day														
Denmark	23.1	23.0	23.4	23.3	23.3	23.1	23.1	23.0	24.8	18.6	18.3	18.1		Decrease
Finland	17.9	17.1	16.6	17.0	15.7	16.0	15.7	15.3	15.5	17.0	16.7	17.1		Stable
Iceland	4.7	4.3	5.2	5.8	6.4	6.9	7.6	8.4	8.9	9.2	9.7	9.9		Increase
Norway	9.7	9.5	9.9	10.0	10.2	10.5	10.3	10.3	10.4	10.2	10.5	10.2		Increase
Sweden	12.0	11.9	12.7	12.3	12.6	12.3	12.1	11.0	11.2	11.0	11.0	10.7		Decrease
% of total ethanol consumption														
Denmark	71	73	73	71	70	68	68	68	67	59	58	56		Decrease
Finland	64	68	72	73	69	73	66	64	62	62	62	65		Stable
Iceland	39	40	45	49	52	54	55	56	58	59	61	62		Increase
Norway	70	70	70	69	68	67	66	65	66	61	60	56		Decrease
Sweden	62	64	68	61	58	59	59	58	64	56	55	55		Decrease

Source: Data from the Food and Agriculture Organization food balance sheets (Food and Agriculture Organization, 2006) and The Brewers of Europe (2006).

1992 to 51l per year in 2004, a trend similar to the percentage of total ethanol (Table 11.3). Again, this trend might be related to the promotion of a Southern European drinking style, replacing beer and spirits by wine (Gerdes *et al.*, 2002; Nordic Council for Alcohol and Drug Research, 2002; Eiben *et al.*, 2004). Still, recent changes regarding alcoholic beverage trading might counter this favorable trend (Berggren and Nystedt, 2006), namely regarding the consumption of strong beer among teenagers (Andersson *et al.*, 2002) and adults (Berg *et al.*, 2005). Interestingly, the ESPAD study showed a relative stabilization in the prevalence of beer drinkers: 19% in 1995, 21% in 1999 and 20% in 2003 (Hibell *et al.*, 2004).

Central European Countries

Central European countries (Austria, Belgium, Germany, Ireland, The Netherlands and the United Kingdom) are traditionally beer-producing and beer-drinking countries. Although Switzerland cannot be considered as a traditional beer-drinking country, it can be considered as a Central European country, and will be analyzed accordingly. It should also be noted that people from Belgium, Ireland and the United Kingdom tend to consume beer mostly outside home, whereas the opposite trend is found for Austrians, Germans and Swiss; still, a slight trend toward a higher home consumption can be noted for all countries (Table 11.1).

Austria

Mirroring the decrease in beer production (Table 11.2), the per capita consumption of beer decreased from 23.3l in 1992 to 22.4l per year in 2004 (Table 11.4). This trend could not be confirmed by the data from the food balance sheets, although the share of total alcohol consumption decreased slightly, indicating a possible shift from beer to other alcoholic beverages (Table 11.5).

Belgium–Luxembourg

Contrary to beer production, which increased in Belgium and decreased in Luxembourg (Table 11.2), the per capita consumption decreased considerably in Belgium from 114l in 1992 to 85l per year in 2004, whereas it remained stable in Luxembourg (Table 11.4). A possible explanation might be the sales of alcoholic beverages to foreign tourists, although a real stability in the consumption of beer cannot be ruled out. Taking both countries together, the average consumption of beer remained stable, as the share of total alcohol consumption (Table 11.5).

Germany

Germany is the biggest beer producer in Europe (Table 11.2) and one of the biggest in the world. Still, the overall production and consumption of beer have been declining steadily. Per capita consumption dropped from 144l in 1992 to 120l in 2004 (Table 11.4), whereas verage beer-derived alcohol consumption also decreased (Table 11.5). Interestingly, the share of beer among total alcohol consumption also decreased from 67% to 61% (Table 11.5), indicating a slight but consistent shift in drinking patterns. Those findings are further confirmed by population studies, which also showed a downward trend in alcohol and beer consumption (Schaeffler *et al.*, 1996;

Table 11.4 Trends in per capita beer consumption in Central European countries (liters/year)

Year	*1992*	*1993*	*1994*	*1995*	*1996*	*1997*	*1998*	*1999*	*2000*	*2001*	*2002*	*2003*	*2004*	*Trend*
Austria	123	117	117	116	114	113	109	109	108	107	109	111	108	Decrease
Belgium	114	107	106	104	102	101	98	100	99	98	96	96	85	Decrease
Germany	144	138	140	138	132	131	127	128	126	123	122	118	120	Decrease
Ireland	123	111	113	113	118	124	124	126	125	125	125	113	108	Stable
Luxembourg	112	104	102	99	95	119	111	110	108	101	99	100	106	Stable
The Netherlands	90	85	86	86	85	86	84	84	83	81	79	79	78	Decrease
United Kingdom	103	104	103	101	102	104	99	99	95	97	101	102	99	Decrease

Source: Adapted from The Brewers of Europe (2006).

Table 11.5 Trends in Central European countries

Year	*1992*	*1993*	*1994*	*1995*	*1996*	*1997*	*1998*	*1999*	*2000*	*2001*	*2002*	*2003*	*Trend*
Grams of ethanol/day													
Austria	23.3	22.1	22.1	21.4	20.1	21.7	21.7	21.9	23.0	21.1	22.4	22.4	Stable
Belgium–Luxembourg	22.0	21.9	20.9	20.9	20.7	23.1	20.1	19.0	23.3	NA	NA	NA	Stable
Germany	27.9	25.1	25.4	25.0	24.0	23.7	23.1	23.3	23.0	23.3	22.1	21.0	Decrease
Ireland	25.0	27.1	27.3	26.7	26.3	26.0	26.6	27.0	26.7	36.9	36.3	36.4	Increase
The Netherlands	17.9	16.7	17.3	17.4	15.7	21.3	21.1	15.0	16.0	15.7	14.7	15.4	Stable
Switzerland	12.9	11.7	11.7	10.9	10.5	10.1	9.8	9.5	9.1	11.1	11.0	10.9	Stable
United Kingdom	20.1	19.6	20.0	19.6	20.0	20.1	19.1	19.3	18.1	19.0	18.6	19.9	Stable
% of total ethanol consumption													
Austria	64	62	62	60	59	60	60	60	56	58	59	57	Decrease
Belgium–Luxembourg	68	68	68	69	68	71	64	67	70	NA	NA	NA	Stable
Germany	67	66	69	70	68	63	64	63	63	63	61	61	Decrease
Ireland	70	71	70	69	67	67	68	69	68	74	73	74	Stable
The Netherlands	69	71	76	76	73	78	74	62	61	62	66	62	Decrease
Switzerland	49	45	48	46	45	43	43	39	38	40	40	42	Decrease
United Kingdom	75	75	74	76	75	74	73	72	72	71	70	72	Decrease

NA, not available.
Source: Data from the Food and Agriculture Organization food balance sheets (Food and Agriculture Organization, 2006).

Bloomfield, 1998). Thus, the available information indicates that the Germans are replacing beer with other alcoholic drinks, mostly with wine.

Ireland

The per capita consumption of beer in Ireland has remained stable between 1992 and 2004, although with a slight decrease in the recent years (Table 11.4). Similar findings were obtained among adolescents aged 15–16 years for the period 1995–2003, with a prevalence of beer consumers between 34% and 36% (Hibell *et al.*, 2004). Still, the overall beer production has increased (Table 11.2), as the average consumption expressed in grams of ethanol (Table 11.5). Conversely, no changes were found regarding the percentage of total alcohol consumption for beer, although a slight increase might be apparent for the period 1996–2003 (Table 11.5). Those findings indicate that beer is the preferred alcoholic beverage in Ireland, accounting for circa three quarters of total alcohol consumed.

The Netherlands

The Netherlands is the fourth biggest beer producer in the former EU, and the production has increased in the beginning of the twenty-first century relative to the beginning of the 1990s (Table 11.2). Still, the per capita consumption has decreased from 90 l in 1992 to 78 l per year in 2004 (Table 11.4), a decrease which was not found regarding beer availability, although the average consumption in the 2000s was lower than in the 1990s; a possible explanation is that the increased production of beer is for exports, thus reducing the actual amount of beer available for local consumption.

The share of total alcohol consumption increased in the beginning of the 1990s to decrease afterward (Table 11.5), thus making the overall trend non-significant. Those findings might indicate temporal changes in drinking patterns, although other reasons cannot be ruled out.

Switzerland

Switzerland is a wine-producing country, and beer consumption remained stable between 1992 and 2003, although a decrease was noted between 1992 and 2000 (Table 11.5). This decrease in beer consumption was also found in population studies (Schmid and Gmel, 1996), and was paralleled by a decrease followed by a slight increase in the share of total alcohol consumption (Table 11.5). This decrease can partly be due to the increased spirit consumption following price changes (Kuo *et al.*, 2003; Mohler-Kuo *et al.*, 2004), with a stable consumption of wine and beer (Heeb *et al.*, 2003).

United Kingdom

In the United Kingdom, most of the beer consumption occurs outside home (Table 11.1), mainly in public bars (McKinney and Coyle, 2005). The per capita consumption has decreased in the 1990s, with a slight recovery in the beginning of the new millennium (Table 11.4). Opposite trends were found for adolescents who consumed beer three or more times during the last 30 days, with an increase from 30% in 1995 to 37% in 1999, followed by a decrease to 31% in 2003 (Hibell *et al.*, 2004). Still, the availability of beer remained rather stable, whereas the share in total alcohol consumption decreased slightly (Table 11.5).

Southern European Countries

Southern European countries (France, Greece, Italy, Portugal and Spain) are usually considered as wine-producing, wine-consuming countries, with a Mediterranean-style diet. Still, in the early 1990s some authors have suggested that alcohol consumption patterns were shifting, with an increased consumption of beer (Pyörälä, 1990; Smart, 1991), but no recent data were available.

France

The production of beer has declined in France, being overcome by Belgium in 2004. This decrease in production has been paralleled by a decrease in consumption from 40.9 l per year in 1992 to 33.7 l in 2004 (Table 11.6) (The Brewers of Europe, 2006). Other sources indicate a 15% decrease in the consumption of beer and cider between 1980 (51.7 l per year) and 1995 (44.2 l per year) (Haut Comité de la Santé Publique, 2000). Indeed, the percentage of French students consuming beer at least thrice during the past 30 days is the lowest when compared to the other countries, and also decreased from 25% in 1999 to 20% in 2003 (Hibell *et al.*, 2004). Conversely, the share of beer has remained relatively stable (Table 11.6), indicating that the decrease in beer consumption might partly be due to the decrease in total alcohol consumption.

Table 11.6 Trends in beer consumption in Southern European countries

Year	*1992*	*1993*	*1994*	*1995*	*1996*	*1997*	*1998*	*1999*	*2000*	*2001*	*2002*	*2003*	*2004*	*Trend*
Liters/year														
France	41	39	39	39	40	37	39	39	36	36	35	36	34	Decrease
Greece	40	42	42	40	39	39	42	43	40	39	39	39	40	Stable
Italy	26	25	26	25	24	25	27	27	28	29	28	30	30	Increase
Portugal	65	64	62	65	62	63	65	64	62	61	59	59	62	Decrease
Spain	71	67	67	67	65	67	66	69	72	75	73	78	81	Increase
Grams of ethanol/day														
France	6.7	6.6	6.6	6.6	6.3	5.7	6.3	6.3	5.5	5.7	5.6	5.7		Decrease
Greece	7.4	7.1	6.9	7.0	7.1	7.4	7.3	6.9	6.7	7.1	7.1	6.3		Stable
Italy	4.4	4.1	4.4	4.3	4.1	4.4	4.7	4.4	5.4	5.1	5.1	5.1		Increase
Portugal	11.9	12.3	12.6	13.0	12.9	12.6	13.4	13.0	12.4	11.9	11.6	11.4		Stable
Spain	12.4	12.4	12.9	13.1	12.9	12.7	12.6	12.7	12.9	12.7	12.9	12.7		Stable
% of total ethanol consumption														
France	23	23	23	23	23	21	23	23	21	23	23	24		Stable
Greece	40	38	42	49	50	43	40	37	34	34	34	33		Decrease
Italy	21	20	21	21	20	22	23	22	26	25	25	26		Increase
Portugal	31	31	31	32	31	31	33	34	32	33	31	30		Stable
Spain	47	48	49	51	49	50	49	49	51	50	51	50		Increase

Source: Data from the Food and Agriculture Organization food balance sheets (Food and Agriculture Organization, 2006) and The Brewers of Europe (2006).

In France, and contrary to Greece, Portugal and Spain, most of beer is consumed in private homes (Table 11.1). Possible explanations include the high consumption of beer by tourists visiting those countries (increased beer consumed in bars, restaurants and other premises) associated with higher weather temperatures, although other reasons related to marketing or drinking patterns cannot be ruled out.

Greece

Greece is usually considered as a minor producer of beer, but in 2004 the Greek production was higher than Sweden (Table 11.2). The per capita consumption has remained stable for 10 years at 40 l per year, half of the EU average, but higher than France or Italy (Table 11.6). This relatively high per capita consumption might partly be due to tourists, as only one-third of beer sales are consumed in private homes (Table 11.1).

Mean consumption remained stable, whereas the share of total alcohol consumption decreased from 40% in 1992 to 33% in 2003 (Table 11.7). A decrease was also found in the ESPAD study for adolescents, from 35% in 1999 to 28% in 2003 (Hibell *et al.*, 2004). Those findings might indicate that, contrary to the other Southern European countries, the Greeks are slowly shifting from beer to other alcoholic beverages, such as wine or spirits.

Italy

Italy has a relatively small production of beer, ranking seventh in front of Ireland, Austria and Denmark. As for France, circa 60% of all beer sales are consumed in private households (Table 11.1). The per capita consumption of beer is the lowest among Europe (29.6 l per year in 2004), with an increase in the recent years (Table 11.6). Those findings are confirmed by the ESPAD reports, where the percentage of male students consuming beer at least thrice during the past 30 days increased from 36% in 1995 to 45% in 2003 (Hibell *et al.*, 1997, 2004); conversely, the authors reported a relative stability of the number of female students consuming beer (21% in 1995 and 22% in 2003), and for the overall sample, no significant trend was observed (Hibell *et al.*, 2004).

Beer consumption shows a seasonal pattern in Italy, being three times higher in summer than in winter (Table 11.7), with no significant change for almost a decade (Associazione degli Industriali della Birra e del Malto, 2002, 2003, 2004, 2005). Those findings might be related to weather temperature, as beer can be consumed as a refreshing beverage, or due to increased number of incoming tourists.

Portugal

The Portuguese production of beer has been increasing regularly since 1992 and, according to the FAO food balance sheets, exceeded wine production in 2003 (Food and Agriculture Organization, 2006). The per capita consumption in 2004 was 61.7 l, the second highest among Southern European countries, although a slight downward trend was noted. Still, no significant evolution was noted using data from the food balance sheets, neither for average consumption nor for the share of total alcohol consumption (Table 11.6). Conversely, individual data from the national health surveys actually showed an increase in beer consumption: in men, beer represented 20% of alcohol consumption in 1995/96 and 22% in 1998/99, the corresponding figures for women being 9% and 35%, respectively (Marques-Vidal and Dias, 2005). Finally, data from the ESPAD report also confirms those trends, with a slight increase in the percentage of male students who consumed beer at least thrice during the past 30 days (25% in 1995 and 27% in 2003); conversely, the percentage of female students reporting a similar consumption decreased slightly

Table 11.7 Monthly consumption of beer in Italy

Month	*1996*	*1997*	*1998*	*1999*	*2000*	*2001*	*2002*	*2003*	*2004*
January	4	4	5	5	5	5	5	5	6
February	5	5	5	5	5	5	6	6	5
March	8	8	7	8	7	7	8	6	7
April	8	8	8	8	7	9	8	8	8
May	10	10	10	10	11	10	11	11	10
June	15	13	13	14	13	12	12	13	12
July	13	14	15	14	13	13	14	14	13
August	11	11	12	11	12	12	10	11	11
September	7	9	8	8	8	7	8	8	8
October	6	7	6	7	7	7	7	7	6
November	6	5	5	6	6	6	6	5	6
December	7	7	6	6	6	6	6	6	7

Note: Results are expressed as percentage of total (yearly) consumption.

Source: Adapted from Associazione degli Industriali della Birra e del Malto (2002, 2003, 2004, 2005).

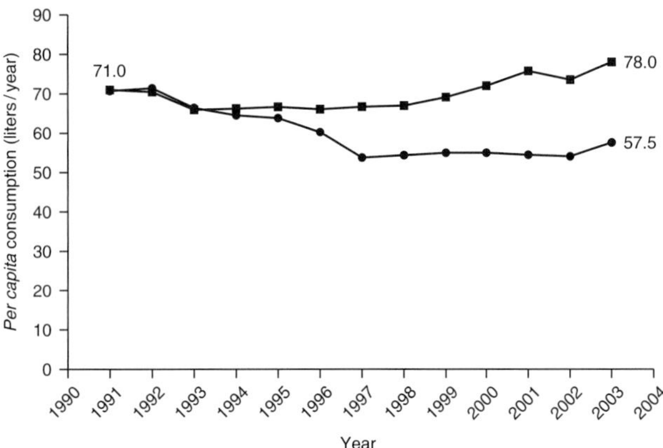

Figure 11.1 Trends in beer consumption in Spain. Squares: overall consumption (Spanish citizens + tourists); circles: Spanish citizens only. *Source*: Adapted from Cerveceros de España (2004).

(12% in 1995 and 10% in 2003), making the overall trend non-significant (Hibell *et al.*, 1997, 2004). Finally, the share of beer sales consumed in private homes increased dramatically between 2003 and 2004 (Table 11.1); those data might indicate that beer is increasingly becoming a popular beverage among households, possibly at the expense of other alcoholic beverages.

Spain

Spain is the third biggest beer producer in the EU and the ninth in the world, ranking in front of Ireland and The Netherlands. Still, the per capita consumption of beer in 2004 was just at the European average (80 l per year, Table 11.6). According to the Spanish Ministry of Agriculture, Fisheries and Food, the per capita consumption of beer in 2003 was 57.5 l, whereas according to the Spanish Beer Producers, this consumption was around 78 l (Cerveceros de España, 2004). Those differences are mainly due to tourists visiting Spain, which account to circa one-third of beer consumption. Indeed, most of the tourists come from traditionally beer-drinking countries such as the United Kingdom and Germany, their per capita consumption is significantly higher than the Spanish. Thus, considering the 1991–2003 period, the consumption of beer has actually declined from 71 to 57.5 l among Spanish citizens, whereas the overall consumption (Spanish citizens + tourists) has slightly increased from 71 to 78 l (80 in 2004 – Figure 11.1). Those findings might also explain the relatively low share of total beer sales consumed in private homes, which decreased between 2002 and 2003 (Table 11.1), possibly indicating that beer is increasingly consumed in bars or other premises open to tourists. Still, data from the food balance sheets suggest that the average consumption of beer-related ethanol has remained stable, and that beer has actually increased its share of total alcohol consumed: since 1999, beer accounts for half of all alcohol consumed in Spain (Table 11.6).

The consumption of beer varies according to region, with a South to North gradient. In 2003, the per capita consumption of beer in the South (Andalucía and Extremadura) was 89 l, whereas the corresponding consumption in the North (Galìcia, Asturias and León) was only 38 l (Cerveceros de España, 2004). Those differences are mainly due to the number of tourists visiting the region and to local weather temperatures, as beer is normally consumed as a refreshing beverage. Indeed, the heat wave that struck Southern Europe in the summer of 2003 is considered as one of the main reasons for the increase in beer consumption between 2002 and 2003. The highest increase was noted in the Northern regions, although it is currently unknown whether this increase was for Spanish citizens or due to the higher number of tourists.

Former USSR and Eastern European Countries

There is little information regarding the trends in the consumption of alcoholic beverages in Eastern European countries. Further, the types of alcohol consumed differ according to country, and it is possible to define spirit-drinking (Russian Federation, Belarus), wine-drinking and beer-drinking (Ukraine) countries (Pomerleau *et al.*, 2005); the prevalence of alcohol drinkers also varies considerably (McKee *et al.*, 2000).

In the Czech Republic, the increase in alcohol consumption following political changes in 1993 (Kubicka *et al.*, 1998) appears to have stabilized, as the mean amount of ethanol and also the share of beer among alcoholic beverages did not show any significant trend (Tables 11.8 and 11.9). Similar findings were obtained in the ESPAD survey: the prevalence of adolescents who consumed beer thrice or more, the previous 30 days increased from 31% in 1995 to 40% in 1999, but remained stable afterward (39% in 2003) (Hibell *et al.*, 2004). Also, no significant trends were found for the period studied for Belarus, Bulgaria and Slovakia (Tables 11.8 and 11.9), although in Slovakia a decrease in alcohol consumption was observed since 1990 (Szantova *et al.*, 1997). Regarding consumption by adolescents, the ESPAD data indicate that the prevalence of subjects who consumed beer thrice or more the previous 30 days increased from 27% in 1999 to 43% in 2003 in Bulgaria, and from 16% in 1995 to 22% in 2003 in Slovakia (Hibell *et al.*, 2004).

Bosnia, Croatia, Estonia, Poland, Romania, the Russian Federation, Serbia–Montenegro and Ukraine showed an increase in beer consumption, both in grams of ethanol and as percentage of all alcoholic beverages, indicating a possible shift of drinking patterns (Tables 11.8 and 11.9).

Table 11.8 Trends in beer consumption in former USSR and Eastern European countries (grams of ethanol/day)

Year	*1992*	*1993*	*1994*	*1995*	*1996*	*1997*	*1998*	*1999*	*2000*	*2001*	*2002*	*2003*	*Trend*
Belarus	5.2	4.1	2.9	2.7	3.3	3.9	4.1	4.2	3.7	3.6	3.4	3.6	Stable
Bosnia	2.6	2.8	3.3	3.3	4.4	7.4	7.3	6.7	5.5	6.0	6.9	7.4	Increase
Bulgaria	10.6	9.6	10.8	9.6	9.5	6.9	8.7	9.5	9.7	9.8	9.6	7.6	Stable
Croatia	10.4	10.2	13.1	13.6	13.5	14.6	14.3	14.8	16.3	16.5	15.9	16.3	Increase
Czech Republic	NA	28.6	30.6	29.9	29.9	30.8	30.8	31.0	30.4	29.9	30.1	30.3	Stable
Estonia	5.5	5.5	6.5	6.9	6.8	8.3	12.2	12.2	12.4	13.4	14.7	14.5	Increase
Hungary	18.0	15.9	16.3	14.4	13.7	13.3	13.3	13.2	13.9	13.9	13.9	14.2	Decrease
Latvia	6.4	3.9	5.0	5.2	5.2	5.8	6.5	8.0	8.0	8.6	9.4	9.0	Increase
Lithuania	6.3	6.5	6.7	6.4	6.5	7.7	8.9	10.5	11.9	12.7	14.9	15.1	Increase
Macedonia	7.6	6.8	6.5	5.7	5.9	5.0	5.9	5.7	5.2	4.7	5.0	5.8	Decrease
Poland	7.3	6.3	7.0	7.5	8.2	9.6	10.4	11.7	12.6	12.6	13.5	14.2	Increase
Romenia	8.3	8.3	8.0	7.5	6.9	6.5	8.5	9.5	10.5	10.4	10.3	11.3	Increase
Russian Federation	3.7	3.4	3.0	3.0	2.9	3.5	4.5	5.8	6.8	8.6	9.4	10.2	Increase
Serbia–Montenegro	7.1	7.2	9.3	10.3	10.2	10.6	11.2	12.5	12.1	10.7	10.5	11.3	Increase
Slovakia	NA	15.5	18.5	16.3	16.6	20.5	16.1	16.4	16.7	16.7	17.7	17.2	Stable
Slovenia	14.9	16.3	17.0	17.1	16.7	15.7	14.5	16.1	12.1	12.4	13.1	12.5	Decrease
Ukraine	4.1	3.4	3.4	2.6	2.3	2.4	2.6	3.2	4.0	4.8	5.5	6.2	Increase

NA: not available.

Source: Data from the Food and Agriculture Organization food balance sheets (Food and Agriculture Organization, 2006).

Table 11.9 Trends in beer consumption in former USSR and Eastern European countries (% of total ethanol)

Year	*1992*	*1993*	*1994*	*1995*	*1996*	*1997*	*1998*	*1999*	*2000*	*2001*	*2002*	*2003*	*Trend*
Belarus	23	18	14	13	14	16	21	21	22	23	22	23	Stable
Bosnia	11	14	17	17	17	23	27	26	23	23	23	31	Increase
Bulgaria	40	36	40	41	46	38	43	46	42	47	45	36	Stable
Croatia	41	40	46	49	49	45	42	50	54	54	51	53	Increase
Czech Republic	NA	78	78	77	73	72	76	75	75	75	75	74	Stable
Estonia	30	28	33	29	41	40	57	57	52	50	49	49	Increase
Hungary	53	49	51	50	47	47	46	47	48	46	45	46	Decrease
Latvia	51	48	42	37	34	35	34	37	37	41	43	39	Stable
Lithuania	61	64	69	42	37	42	54	60	55	54	56	54	Stable
Macedonia	66	67	59	66	57	41	49	56	62	61	74	46	Stable
Poland	45	40	42	45	51	54	56	60	63	65	67	68	Increase
Romenia	41	40	44	40	37	33	49	52	56	49	47	52	Increase
Russian Federation	20	17	19	19	27	32	35	34	39	42	42	43	Increase
Serbia–Montenegro	38	37	41	50	39	41	51	62	58	55	57	49	Increase
Slovakia	NA	60	64	64	59	63	61	62	61	64	68	68	Stable
Slovenia	46	48	54	54	57	57	67	73	42	67	67	67	Increase
Ukraine	31	26	33	29	30	25	29	33	35	43	43	39	Increase

NA: not available.

Source: Data from the Food and Agriculture Organization food balance sheets (Food and Agriculture Organization, 2006).

Those findings are in agreement with the literature, where beer has become the preferred alcoholic beverage among adolescents in the Baltic countries (Zaborskis *et al.*, 2006). Also, the ESPAD study noted an increase in the prevalence of beer drinkers in most countries: Croatia (from 13% in 1995 to 28% in 2003), Estonia (from 12% in 1995 to 25% in 2003), Poland (from 25% in 1995 to 41% in 2003), Romania (from 20% in 1999 to 32% in 2003) and Ukraine (from 12% in 1995 to 34% in 2003), whereas no increasing trend was found for Russia (40% in 1999 and 38% in 2003) (Hibell *et al.*, 2004). Interestingly, for Southern European countries, the consumption of beer in

Estonia is significantly related with weather temperature, being higher in summer (Silm and Ahas, 2005).

In Lithuania, the per capita consumption was 75.51 in 2003 and increased to 81.21 in 2004 (The Brewers of Europe, 2006), in agreement with data from the FAO (Table 11.8), the ESPAD (from 9% in 1995 to 28% in 2003) (Hibell *et al.*, 2004) and previous findings from an urban sample of subjects aged 35–64 years (Tamoshiunas *et al.*, 2005) in adolescents (Grabauskas *et al.*, 2004) and in school-aged children (Sumskas and Zaborskis, 2004). Beer is consumed mostly at home (Table 11.1), and the share of total alcohol from beer remained stable, suggesting an increase in total alcohol consumption (Table 11.9). Conversely, beer has become the most popular alcohol drink in school-aged children (Sumskas and Zaborskis, 2004), indicating that the penetration of beer in the Lithuanian population might differ according to age group. Also, for Latvia, an increase in the average consumption of beer was noted (Table 11.8), although data from the ESPAD showed no significant trend in adolescents (30% of subjects with a consumption ≥ 3 units the previous 30 days in 1999, 32% in 2003); further, no significant change in the share of alcoholic beverages was noted (Table 11.9).

Only three countries registered a decrease in the average consumption of beer: Hungary, Macedonia and Slovenia. In Slovenia, total alcohol consumption decreased significantly (Sesok, 2004); data from the ESPAD study actually showed an increase in the percentage of adolescents consuming beer from 21% in 1995 to 27% in 1999, followed by a decrease to 21% in 2003 (Hibell *et al.*, 2004). The share of beer actually increased, indicating a probable shift in drinking patterns, people preferring beer to other alcoholic beverages (Tables 11.8 and 11.9). The opposite conclusion can be derived for Hungary, where the share of beer tended to decrease, suggesting that beer is being substituted by other alcoholic beverages, although the percentage of adolescents consuming beer increased from 12% in 1999 to 17% in 2003 (Hibell *et al.*, 2004). Finally, data from Macedonia indicate that beer consumption is decreasing but that its share of alcoholic beverages is relatively stable (Tables 11.8 and 11.9).

Conclusion

During the last decade, the consumption of beer showed different trends according to geographical region: mostly a decrease in Nordic and Central European countries, with a concomitant increase in Southern and Eastern European countries. Those trends can be found using data from different sources (FAO, European brewers, ESPAD study), suggesting that beer consumption is slowly coming toward uniformity among European countries, as reported by other authors (Pyorälä, 1990; Gual and Colom, 1997; Walsh, 1997). The reasons for such changes are multiple, such as global marketing, price policies (Ponicki *et al.*, 1997; Heeb *et al.*, 2003; Kuo *et al.*, 2003), law enforcement (Kubicka *et al.*, 1998; Nordic Council for Alcohol and Drug Research, 2002; Wallin *et al.*, 2005) and local availability (Ólafsdóttir, 1998) just to cite a few. Of particular concern is the fact that beer (and alcohol) consumption is increasing among adolescents in a considerable number of European countries, with possible deleterious health consequences in the future.

Summary Points

- The consumption of beer decreased in Nordic and Central European countries, and increased in Southern and Eastern European countries.
- Those trends can also be found for adolescents aged 15–16 years.
- The reasons for those different trends are multiple and include global marketing, price policies, European or local regulations and fashion, and might be different according to country.
- The increase in beer (and total alcohol) consumption in Eastern European countries and in adolescents is of concern.

References

Andersson, B., Hansagi, H., Damstrom Thakker, K. and Hibell, B. (2002). *Drug Alcohol Rev.* 21, 253–260.

Associazione degli Industriali della Birra e del Malto (2002). Annual Report 2002. Rome, Italy. Available at http://www.assobirra.it/annual_report/2002/AnnualReportlast2002%20.pdf.

Associazione degli Industriali della Birra e del Malto (2003). Annual Report 2003. Rome, Italy. Available at http://www.assobirra.it/annual_report/2003/Annual%20Report2003%20.pdf.

Associazione degli Industriali della Birra e del Malto (2004). Annual Report 2004. Rome, Italy. Available at http://www.assobirra.it/annual_report/2004/AnnualReport2004%20.pdf.

Associazione degli Industriali della Birra e del Malto (2005). Assobirra Annual Report 2004. Rome, Italy. Available at http://www.assobirra.it/annual_report/annual_report_2005.htm.

Berg, C.M., Lissner, L., Aires, N., Lappas, G., Toren, K., Wilhelmsen, L., Rosengren, A. and Thelle, D.S. (2005). *Eur. J. Cardiovasc. Prev. Rehab.* 12, 115–125.

Berggren, F. and Nystedt, P. (2006). *Scand. J. Public Health* 34, 304–311.

Bjork, C., Vinther-Larsen, M., Thygesen, L.C., Johansen, D. and Gronbaek, M.N. (2006). *Ugeskr. Laeger* 168, 3317–3321.

Bloomfield, K. (1998). *Eur. Addict. Res.* 4, 163–171.

Casswell, S., Huckle, T. and Pledger, M. (2002). *Alcohol Clin. Exp. Res.* 26, 1561–1567.

Cerveceros de España (2004). Informe económico 2003, datos del sector. In Cerveceros de España (ed.). Available at http://www.cerveceros.org/interior.jsp?url=datos_sector.jsp&franja=datos.

Eiben, G., Andersson, C.S., Rothenberg, E., Sundh, V., Steen, B. and Lissner, L. (2004). *Public Health Nutr.* 7, 637–644.

Food and Agriculture Organization (2006). Food balance sheets. Available at http://faostat.fao.org/site/345/default.aspx (accessed October 2006).

Gerdes, L.U., Bronnum-Hansen, H., Osler, M., Madsen, M., Jorgensen, T. and Schroll, M. (2002). *Public Health* 116, 81–88.

Giovannucci, E., Colditz, G., Stampfer, M.J., Rimm, E.B., Litin, L., Sampson, L. and Willett, W.C. (1991). *Am. J. Epidemiol.* 133, 810–817.

Grabauskas, V., Zaborskis, A., Klumbiene, J., Petkeviciene, J. and Zemaitiene, N. (2004). *Medicina (Kaunas)* 40, 884–890.

Gual, A. and Colom, J. (1997). *Addiction* 92, S21–S31.

Haut Comité de la Santé Publique (2000). Pour une politique nutritionnelle de santé publique en France, Rennes, Editions ENSP.

Heeb, J.L., Gmel, G., Zurbrugg, C., Kuo, M. and Rehm, J. (2003). *Addiction* 98, 1433–1446.

Hibell, B., Andersson, B., Bjarnason, T., Kokkevi, A., Morgan, M. and Narusk, A. (1997). *The 1995 ESPAD Report: Alcohol and Other Drug Use Among Students in 26 European Countries*. The Swedish Council for Information on Alcohol and Other Drugs (CAN), the Pompidou Group at the Council of Europe, Stockholm, Sweden.

Hibell, B., Andersson, B., Bjarnason, T., Ahlström, S., Balakireva, O., Kokkevi, A. and Morgan, M. (2004). *The ESPAD Report: Alcohol and Other Drug Use Among Students in 35 European Countries*. The Swedish Council for Information on Alcohol and Other Drugs, Co-operation Group to Combat Drug Abuse and Illicit Trafficking in Drugs (Pompidou Group) Council of Europe, Stockholm, Sweden.

Holder, H.D., Giesbrecht, N., Horverak, O., Nordlund, S., Norstrom, T., Olsson, O., Osterberg, E. and Skog, O.J. (1995). *Addiction* 90, 1603–1618.

Koppes, L.L., Twisk, J.W., Snel, J. and Kemper, H.C. (2002). *Br. J. Nutr.* 88, 427–435.

Kubicka, L., Csemy, L., Duplinsky, J. and Kozeny, J. (1998). *Addiction* 93, 1219–1230.

Kuo, M., Heeb, J.L., Gmel, G. and Rehm, J. (2003). *Alcohol Clin. Exp. Res.* 27, 720–725.

Leifman, H. (2000). Trends in alcohol consumption in the European Union. *Proceedings of the 26th Alcohol Epidemiology Symposium of the Kettil Bruun Society for Social and Epidemiological Research on Alcohol*, Oslo, Norway.

Leifman, H., Osterberg, E. and Ramstedt, M. (2002). Alcohol in postwar Europe, ECAS II: a discussion of indicators on alcohol consumption and alcohol-related harm. In National Institute of Public Health (ed.). European Comparative Alcohol Study – ECAS, Stockholm, Sweden, 111pp, ISBN 91 7257 167 5.

Marques-Vidal, P. and Dias, C.M. (2005). *Alcohol Clin. Exp. Res.* 29, 89–97.

McKee, M., Pomerleau, J., Robertson, A., Pudule, I., Grinberga, D., Kadziauskiene, K., Abaravicius, A. and Vaask, S. (2000). *J. Epidemiol. Commun. Health* 54, 361–366.

McKinney, A. and Coyle, K. (2005). *Subst. Use Misuse* 40, 573–579.

Mohler-Kuo, M., Rehm, J., Heeb, J.L. and Gmel, G. (2004). *J. Stud. Alcohol* 65, 266–273.

Nordic Council for Alcohol and Drug Research (2002). The effects of Nordic alcohol policies: What happens to drinking and harm when alcohol controls change? In Room, R. (ed.). Nordic Council for Alcohol and Drug Research, Helsinki, Finland. 108pp, ISBN 9515324505. Available at http://www.nad.fi/index.php?lang=en&id=pub/42.

Nordlund, S. and Osterberg, E. (2000). *Addiction* 95, S551–S564.

Ólafsdóttir, H. (1998). *J. Stud. Alcohol* 59, 107–114.

Pomerleau, J., McKee, M., Rose, R., Haerpfer, C.W., Rotman, D. and Tumanov, S. (2005). *Addiction* 100, 1647–1668.

Ponicki, W., Holder, H.D., Gruenewald, P.J. and Romelsjo, A. (1997). *Addiction* 92, 859–870.

Pyorälä, E. (1990). *Br. J. Addict.* 85, 469–477.

Schaeffler, V., Doring, A., Winkler, G. and Keil, U. (1996). *Ann. Nutr. Metab.* 40, 129–136.

Schmid, H. and Gmel, G. (1996). *Schweiz. Med. Wochenschr.* 126, 1099–1106.

Sesok, J. (2004). *Croat. Med. J.* 45, 466–472.

Sieri, S., Agudo, A., Kesse, E., Klipstein-Grobusch, K., San-Jose, B., Welch, A.A., Krogh, V., Luben, R., Allen, N., Overvad, K., Tjonneland, A., Clavel-Chapelon, F., Thiebaut, A., Miller, A.B., Boeing, H., Kolyva, M., Saieva, C., Celentano, E., Ocke, M.C., Peeters, P.H., Brustad, M., Kumle, M., Dorronsoro, M., Fernandez Feito, A., Mattisson, I., Weinehall, L., Riboli, E. and Slimani, N. (2002). *Public Health Nutr.* 5, 1287–1296.

Silm, S. and Ahas, R. (2005). *Int. J. Biometeorol.* 49, 215–223.

Simpura, J., Paakkanen, P. and Mustonen, H. (1995). *Addiction* 90, 673–683.

Smart, R.G. (1991). *World Health Forum* 12, 99–103.

Strand, B.H. and Steiro, A. (2003). *Tidsskr. Nor. Laegeforen.* 123, 2849–2853.

Sulander, T., Helakorpi, S., Rahkonen, O., Nissinen, A. and Uutela, A. (2004). *Prev. Med.* 39, 413–418.

Sumskas, L. and Zaborskis, A. (2004). *Medicina (Kaunas)* 40, 1117–1123.

Szantova, M., Kupcova, V., Bada, V. and Goncalvesova, E. (1997). *Bratisl. Lek. Listy* 98, 12–16.

Tamoshiunas, A., Domarkene, S., Reklaitene, R., Kazlauskaite, M., Buividaite, K., Radishauskas, R. and Benotene, G. (2005). *Ter. Arkh.* 77, 37–41.

The Brewers of Europe (2006). The Brewers of Europe statistics. Available at http://stats.brewersofeurope.org/stats_pages/inhabitants.asp (accessed October 2006).

Wallin, E., Gripenberg, J. and Andreasson, S. (2005). *J. Stud. Alcohol* 66, 806–814.

Walsh, B. (1997). *Addiction* 92, S61–S66.

Zaborskis, A., Sumskas, L., Maser, M. and Pudule, I. (2006). *BMC Public Health* 6, 67.

12

Trends of Beer Drinking: Rest of the World

Qiao Qiao Chen Unidade de Nutrição e Metabolismo, Faculdade de Medicina da Universidade de Lisboa, Lisboa, Portugal
Pedro Marques-Vidal Institut Universitaire de Médecine Sociale et Préventive, Lausanne, Switzerland

Abstract

The trends in beer drinking worldwide were assessed from the food balance sheets of the Food and Agriculture Organization, together with available national or international studies. Overall, the data indicate that beer consumption is decreasing in industrialized countries such as Australia, Canada, Japan, New Zealand and the United States, whereas the opposite trend is observed for developing countries. This increase is particularly strong in Asia, namely in China and Thailand. Conversely, no definite trends were found in other regions such as Latin America or Africa. Although social and religious factors considerably influence alcohol and beer drinking, their effects appear to be lessening in the younger generations, which appear as the major consumers of beer.

List of Abbreviations

FAO Food and Agriculture Organization of the United Nations
USA United States of America

Introduction

In this chapter, it was decided to present only data from countries where alcohol consumption is common in the population. Thus, data from predominantly Muslim countries were not included. Further, while most industrialized countries have reliable data on beer production and consumption, this is not the case for most developing countries, where estimates have to be performed. Thus, some trends should be regarded with caution, as Food and Agriculture Organization of the United Nation (FAO) data do not take into account home-made alcoholic beverages, which are quite common and popular in developing countries (Carlini-Cotrim, 1999; Mohan *et al.*, 2001).

North America

Canada

Canada ranks 12th in beer production worldwide (Brewers Association of Japan, 2004a) but only 19th as regards the per capita consumption of beer (Brewers Association of Japan, 2004b). Overall, the per capita consumption of beer has decreased in the last years from 93 l in 1995 to 88 l in 2005 (Table 12.1), but this decrease was not observed in some provinces such as Québec and Yukon (Table 12.1). It should also be noted that the per capita beer consumption varies considerably between provinces, from less than 80 l per year in Manitoba and Saskatchewan to over 100 l in Newfoundland and 150 l in Yukon (Table 12.1) (The Brewers Association of Canada, 2007b, c). Expressed in percentage of overall ethanol consumption, the importance of beer has also decreased slightly from 85% in 1995 to 80% in 2005 (Table 12.1). Those findings are partly confirmed by the FAO data (Table 12.2), namely as regards the relative importance of beer; conversely, no significant trend was found regarding the amount of beer-derived ethanol consumption (Table 12.2).

The type of beer package also showed differential trends, cans being more frequently purchased, while bottles and draft beer showed a slight decrease (Figure 12.1) (The Brewers Association of Canada, 2007a).

United States of America

The United States were until recently the main producers of beer worldwide, but have been overpowered by China (Brewers Association of Japan, 2004a).

Data from the National Institute on Alcohol Abuse and Alcoholism indicate that the overall consumption of beer has decreased in the recent decades (Figure 12.2) (National Institute on Alcohol Abuse and Alcoholism), a trend also confirmed by the FAO data (Table 12.2) and the USDA

Beer in Health and Disease Prevention
ISBN: 978-0-12-373891-2

Table 12.1 Trends in beer consumption in Canada

Year	*1995*	*1996*	*1997*	*1998*	*1999*	*2000*	*2001*	*2002*	*2003*	*2004*	*2005*
Liters											
Newfoundland	104.7	101.2	99.5	95.7	98.2	102.9	102.2	105.3	100.4	106.7	108.2
Prince Edward Island	81.3	82.9	84.0	81.2	82.8	84.5	84.4	86.4	85.3	86.5	85.9
Nova Scotia	82.1	81.0	80.0	78.7	81.6	83.8	82.9	84.5	83.6	85.5	84.7
New Brunswick	84.0	83.7	80.9	81.5	83.2	86.8	85.6	88.1	85.3	87.0	86.0
Québec	96.9	97.7	97.5	98.2	99.7	100.4	98.1	99.5	98.3	97.8	97.1
Ontario	92.7	92.6	90.3	90.4	87.7	88.6	85.6	85.7	84.8	84.5	83.2
Manitoba	82.4	82.2	81.0	81.8	81.5	80.5	81.0	82.6	81.2	83.3	79.6
Saskatchewan	76.3	77.0	75.9	78.7	80.5	82.0	81.1	84.1	82.9	85.8	79.8
Alberta	93.7	92.0	90.3	94.4	96.9	95.0	93.9	97.4	94.9	96.5	96.8
British Columbia	95.9	93.4	89.4	87.9	87.2	84.1	84.3	83.0	81.9	83.5	82.4
Yukon	154.8	167.4	171.8	166.9	165.4	167.0	168.5	163.8	163.8	161.3	163.5
N.W.T. & Nunavut	96.9	90.5	89.1	86.0	87.5	88.5	88.6	91.5	94.3	96.7	98.4
Canada	93.0	92.6	90.8	91.2	91.0	91.2	89.3	90.2	88.8	89.4	88.2
% of volume consumption											
Newfoundland	90	90	90	89	89	89	88	88	87	87	87
Prince Edward island	87	88	87	86	85	85	84	83	82	82	81
Nova Scotia	86	86	85	85	85	84	83	83	82	82	81
New Brunswick	88	88	88	87	87	86	86	85	84	84	84
Québec	86	86	85	86	85	84	83	82	81	81	80
Ontario	85	85	84	84	83	82	81	80	79	79	79
Manitoba	84	84	84	84	83	83	83	82	82	82	81
Saskatchewan	86	86	85	85	85	85	85	84	84	84	82
Alberta	83	84	83	82	82	82	81	81	81	80	80
British Columbia	80	80	80	80	80	81	80	79	78	78	77
Yukon	84	87	87	86	86	86	86	85	85	85	84
N.W.T. & Nunavut	85	85	84	83	83	82	82	81	82	82	82
Canada	85	85	84	84	83	83	82	81	81	80	80

Source: Data from The Brewers Association of Canada (2007c).

Table 12.2 Trends in beer consumption in North America

Year	*1993*	*1994*	*1995*	*1996*	*1997*	*1998*	*1999*	*2000*	*2001*	*2002*	*2003*	*Trend*
Grams of ethanol/day												
Canada	12.1	12.1	12.3	11.8	11.6	12.0	12.1	11.9	12.2	12.3	10.4	Stable
Mexico	6.7	6.7	6.3	6.5	6.8	6.8	7.1	7.1	7.0	6.5	6.9	Stable
United States	15.2	15.1	14.6	14.6	14.6	14.6	14.6	14.7	14.6	14.7	14.3	Decrease
% of total ethanol consumption												
Canada	68	66	66	67	65	64	63	62	62	62	58	Decrease
Mexico	74	71	78	79	77	78	80	88	92	87	87	Increase
United States	69	69	68	67	67	67	67	67	67	67	67	Decrease

Source: Data from the Food and Agriculture Organization food balance sheets (Food and Agriculture Organization, 2006).

Economic Research Service (Table 12.3) (USDA Economic Research Service Data Sets, 2006). Overall, beer represented between 67% and 54% of all ethanol consumed, and this percentage also tended to decrease in all datasets analyzed. Interestingly, the consumption of beer is not evenly distributed in the United States, representing over 50% of total alcohol consumption in the Midwest and South regions, vs. less than 50% in the Northeast and the West (Table 12.3).

Data from the National Alcohol Surveys showed that the frequency of beer drinkers decreased from 51.5% in 1984 to 45.2% in 1990, but increased slightly to 48% in 1995 (Greenfield *et al.*, 2000); since no consumption data were available, it cannot be assessed whether this slight increase in drinkers was associated with a concomitant increase in individual consumption.

The 2001–2002 National Epidemiologic Survey on Alcohol and Related Conditions provided very interesting data regarding the factors related to beer preference. Overall, beer is the most preferred alcoholic beverage, but considerable gender, ethnicity, education, family income and age differences exist. For instance, 50% of men indicate beer as their preferred alcoholic beverage, vs. 19% of women (National Institute on Alcohol Abuse and Alcoholism, 2006); beer is

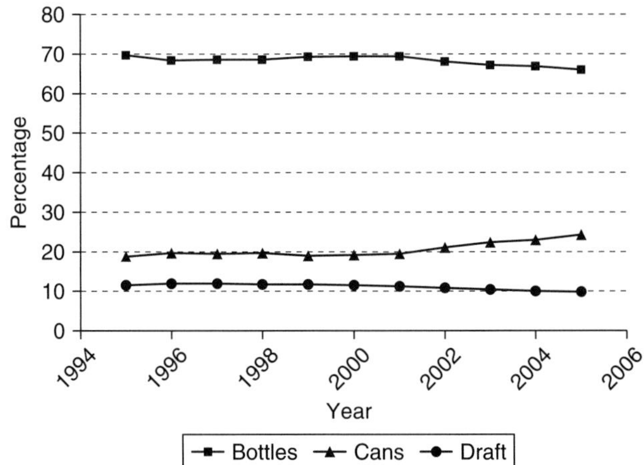

Figure 12.1 Trends in beer consumption by package, Canada. *Source*: Adapted from The Brewers Association of Canada (2007a).

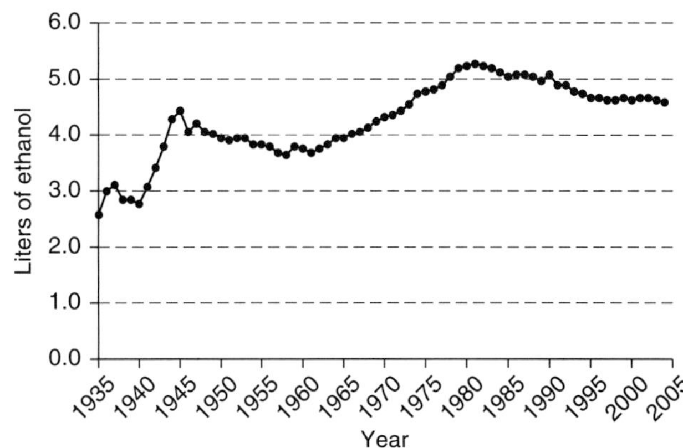

Figure 12.2 *Per capita* beer-derived ethanol consumption in the United States, 1935–2005. *Source*: Data from National Institute on Alcohol Abuse and Alcoholism for subjects aged 14 and older (2006a, b).

Table 12.3 Trends in beer consumption (% of total alcohol consumption) in the United States

Year	*1993*	*1994*	*1995*	*1996*	*1997*	*1998*	*1999*	*2000*	*2001*	*2002*	*2003*	*2004*
Midwest	59.6	60.7	59.9	59.9	59.4	59.8	59.4	59.2	59.2	59.1	57.7	57.7
Northeast	52.6	52.4	52.2	52.2	51.5	52.5	51.0	50.5	51.9	50.9	50.5	49.3
South	60.5	60.6	60.8	60.3	60.4	60.4	60.5	60.2	60.3	59.4	58.3	58.0
West	52.7	51.9	53.5	52.6	52.6	52.9	52.4	51.5	51.7	51.5	50.2	49.4
United States	56.5	57.3	57.2	56.9	57.0	57.0	56.9	56.0	56.4	55.9	55.0	54.3

Source: Data from USDA Economic Research Service Data Sets (2006).

cited by 45% of Hispano or Latino subjects, vs. 37.5% for American Indians/Alaska Natives and 33.8% in Whites (National Institute on Alcohol Abuse and Alcoholism, 2006). Further, over 51% of subjects with 11 years or less of education prefer beer, vs. 33.5% of subjects with 13–15 years and 25.6% of those with 16 years or more of education (National Institute on Alcohol Abuse and Alcoholism, 2006). Among families with less than $20,000 annual income, beer is the preferred beverage for 40.4%, 36.5% for families with incomes between $35,000 and $59,999 and less than 30% for families with an annual income of $60,000 or more (National Institute on Alcohol Abuse and Alcoholism, 2006). Regarding age, 36% of subjects aged 18–24 years report beer as the preferred beverage, vs. 24% of subjects aged over 65 years (National Institute on Alcohol Abuse and Alcoholism, 2006). Finally, 45.5% of current smokers preferred beer, vs. 31.3% for non-smokers, and heavy drinkers reported more frequently preferring beer than light drinkers (National Institute on Alcohol Abuse and Alcoholism, 2006).

Mexico

In 1994, beer was estimated to represent 87% of the Mexican market of alcohol (Medina-Mora *et al.*, 2000) and accounted for 54% of all ethanol consumed (Medina-Mora *et al.*, 1998). Beer is the most frequently consumed alcoholic beverage (78% of drinkers) followed by spirits (72%) (Medina-Mora *et al.*, 2000), although in rural areas it comes second after the traditional *pulque* (Medina-Mora, 1999). Men consume more than women; in men, beer is mainly consumed by high/excessive drinkers, whereas in women it is mainly consumed by low/high drinkers (Medina-Mora *et al.*, 2000). Consumption is irregular and occurs on special occasions such as weekends, paydays and festivities (*fiestas*) (Medina-Mora *et al.*, 2000, 2001) where high amounts can be consumed.

Both beer production and imports have increased considerably; for instance, beer imports increased from only 3041 in 1970 to more than 30 million in 1993 (Medina-Mora, 1999). Although the data from FAO do not support an increase in beer consumption (in absolute ethanol/day), still the relative impact of beer among alcoholic beverages has increased (Table 12.2). It should be noted that those figures do not take into account home-made alcoholic beverages, which might represent as much as 40% of the total volume of ethanol consumed in the country (Medina-Mora, 1999; Medina-Mora *et al.*, 2000).

Central America and the Caribbean

There is little information regarding the trends in beer consumption in Central America and the Caribbean. Data from beer production (Table 12.4) and the FAO (Table 12.5) indicate that the amount of beer-derived alcohol has increased in some countries, namely in Cuba and the Dominican Republic. The highest consumptions are observed for the latter country and Panama, possibly due to a North American influence.

With the exception of Costa Rica and El Salvador, beer accounted for almost half of the ethanol consumption, and increased in Cuba, the Dominican Republic and Nicaragua, whereas it tended to decrease in El Salvador and Panama (Table 12.5).

South America

Argentina

Argentina is traditionally among the countries with the highest per capita wine production, with a relatively low production of beer. Still, in the last decades this balance has shifted, with a considerable increase in the production of beer (Figure 12.3, Tables 12.6 and 12.7) (Camara de la Industria Cervecera y Maltera Argentina, 2007) and a decrease in wine consumption (Munné, 2005). Beer is the preferred alcoholic drink among adolescents, namely boys (Jerez and Coviello, 1998). Although the total amount of beer (expressed in grams of ethanol/day) remained stable in Argentina for period 1993–2003 (Table 12.7), the

Table 12.4 Trends in per capita beer production and consumption in Central America and the Caribbean

	Production					*Consumption*	
Year	*1994*	*1995*	*1996*	*1997*	*1998*	*1997*	*1998*
Costa Rica	38.6	38.4	34.6	31.8	32.4	1.7	1.6
Dominican Republic	32.1	29.4	30.2	29.9	34.6	6.6	7.3
El Salvador	14.7	13.4	12.1	11.6	12.6	2.0	2.0
Guatemala	12.6	15.3	10.7	12.4	13.5	1.1	1.3
Honduras	16.5	15.8	15.5	17.6	18.2	1.9	2.2
Nicaragua	12.9	11.3	11.0	12.0	12.2	1.3	1.4
Panama	51.0	49.7	46.0	49.2	52.3	6.4	6.5

Source: Data expressed in liters/year, from Cerveceros latinoamericanos (2007b).

Table 12.5 Trends in beer consumption in Central America and the Caribbean

Year	*1993*	*1994*	*1995*	*1996*	*1997*	*1998*	*1999*	*2000*	*2001*	*2002*	*2003*	*Trend*
Grams of ethanol/day												
Costa Rica	1.5	1.8	1.7	1.7	1.7	1.7	1.6	1.6	1.7	1.6	1.6	Stable
Cuba	1.8	1.6	1.8	2.0	1.9	2.5	2.6	2.7	2.8	3.0	3.1	Increase
Dominican Republic	4.9	5.6	5.1	5.0	5.7	6.6	7.3	7.9	6.6	7.3	7.5	Increase
El Salvador	2.3	2.2	2.5	2.3	2.2	2.0	2.3	2.2	2.0	2.0	2.3	Stable
Guatemala	1.0	1.0	1.3	1.4	1.3	1.3	1.1	1.4	1.1	1.3	0.9	Stable
Honduras	2.1	1.9	2.0	2.0	2.4	2.2	2.2	2.1	1.9	2.2	2.2	Stable
Nicaragua	1.2	1.1	1.0	0.8	1.0	1.3	1.4	1.3	1.3	1.4	1.7	Increase
Panama	6.6	6.9	6.8	6.4	6.8	7.4	7.3	7.0	6.4	6.5	6.4	Stable
% of total ethanol consumption												
Costa Rica	15	16	16	16	16	16	15	15	15	15	15	Stable
Cuba	38	28	32	37	35	42	39	40	41	44	48	Increase
Dominican Republic	41	44	43	41	45	50	52	49	48	51	51	Increase
El Salvador	54	48	50	51	42	40	40	33	31	30	34	Decrease
Guatemala	31	39	39	40	42	52	51	56	41	40	41	Stable
Honduras	53	54	51	52	57	55	53	50	50	46	50	Stable
Nicaragua	26	25	24	21	24	27	30	29	30	32	42	Increase
Panama	68	67	65	60	61	62	62	61	60	60	59	Decrease

Source: Data from the Food and Agriculture Organization food balance sheets (Food and Agriculture Organization, 2006).

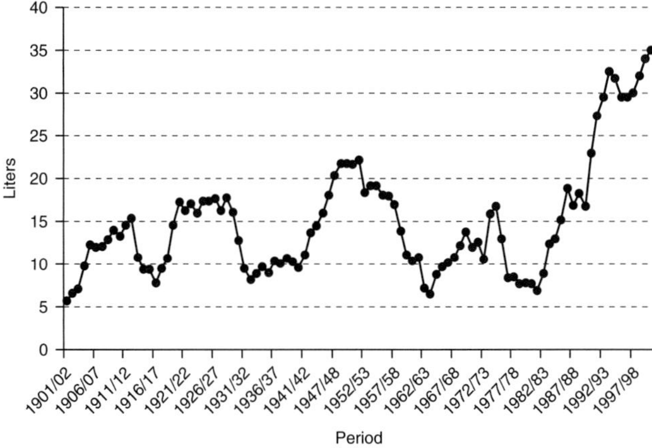

Figure 12.3 Secular trends in beer consumption, Argentina. *Source*: Data from Cerveceros latinoamericanos (2007a).

Table 12.6 Trends in beer production in South America

Year	*1994*	*1995*	*1996*
1,000 hl/year			
Argentina	11,306	10,423	10,287
Bolivia	1,750	1,696	1,705
Brazil	62,500	79,000	80,178
Chile	3,800	4,120	3,929
Colombia	15,875	17,800	16,689
Ecuador	1,947	2,500	2,154
Paraguay	1,750	1,500	1,434
Peru	6,900	8,300	7,664
Uruguay	820	850	780
Venezuela	15,423	16,011	14,993
Per capita (liters/year)			
Argentina	33.4	30.1	29.3
Bolivia	24.2	22.9	22.5
Brazil	40.3	50.7	50.6
Chile	27.0	28.9	27.2
Colombia	43.4	45.9	42.2
Ecuador	17.3	20.8	18.4
Paraguay	37.1	33.5	31.2
Peru	29.8	35.2	32.0
Uruguay	25.9	26.8	24.7
Venezuela	70.9	71.8	67.5

Source: Data from Cerveceros latinoamericanos (2007b).

Table 12.7 Per capita beer consumption (liters/year)

Year	*1997*	*1998*
Argentina	33.2	33.8
Bolivia	18.1	19.8
Chile	27.2	27.4
Colombia	42.1	40.7
Ecuador	19.9	19.7
Paraguay	25.1	26.2
Peru	29.5	27.6
Uruguay	24.9	21.9
Venezuela	81.9	88.0

Source: Data from Cerveceros latinoamericanos (2007b).

percentage of ethanol consumed as beer actually increased, from less than one-quarter to almost one-third (Table 12.8). A possible explanation is the recent economic crisis, which led to considerable changes in drinking patterns, people shifting to lower-quality alcoholic drinks and going less frequently to bars (Munné, 2005), although the long-term effects of this crisis on patterns of alcohol consumption remain to be assessed.

Interestingly, beer consumption in Argentina follows a seasonal pattern (Camara de la Industria Cervecera y Maltera Argentina, 2007), opposite to that observed in Italy (Associazione degli Industriali della Birra e del Malto, 2004) (Table 12.9). Thus, the months of November to January account for one-third of all beer consumed, almost twice the amount of the consumption observed in June to August; the most likely explanation is weather, with increased temperatures during the summer months of the Southern hemisphere.

Brazil

Brazil ranks among the biggest producers of beer worldwide, with an increasing production from 51 millions of hectoliters in 1993 to 80 million in 1999 (Cervesia, 2003) (Table 12.6). The production is unevenly distributed throughout the country, the Southeast region accounting for more than half of the overall brewing capacity (Cervesia, 2003). Beer ranks first in the Brazilian consumption by volume, being second after spirits (*cachaça*) regarding the amount of ethanol consumed (Carlini-Cotrim, 1999).

Beer is the most popular alcoholic drink among adolescents (Pechansky, 1995; Galduróz and Caetano, 2004; Oliveira de Souza *et al.*, 2005) and also in the general population, namely among men, higher educated and non-white subjects (Almeida-Filho *et al.*, 2004). The per capita consumption of beer doubled between 1985 and 1995 (Carlini-Cotrim, 1999), but no significant trend was found afterwards (Table 12.8). In 2003, beer represented slightly more than half of total ethanol consumption (Table 12.8), but this figure should be interpreted with caution as the local, unreported home production of spirits is not considered in the FAO data.

Venezuela

Venezuela is the third biggest producer of beer in South America after Brazil and Colombia (Table 12.6). Still, reported on a per capita basis, Venezuela has the highest per capita production and consumption rates (Cerveceros latinoamericanos, 2007b) (Table 12.7). Those findings are in agreement with data from the FAO (Food and Agriculture Organization, 2006), although the differences between countries are not so stringent. Expressed in grams of ethanol/day, Venezuela has the highest consumptions, comparable to those found in European countries (Table 12.8). Beer

Table 12.8 Trends in beer consumption in South America

Year	*1993*	*1994*	*1995*	*1996*	*1997*	*1998*	*1999*	*2000*	*2001*	*2002*	*2003*	*Trend*
Grams of ethanol/day												
Argentina	4.5	4.8	4.6	4.8	5.2	4.9	4.7	4.6	4.7	4.4	4.7	Stable
Bolivia	2.7	2.7	2.9	2.8	2.9	2.8	3.7	3.7	3.5	3.4	3.3	Increase
Brazil	4.0	4.6	6.0	5.6	5.7	5.6	5.3	5.3	5.5	5.5	5.6	Stable
Chile	3.4	3.1	3.3	3.2	3.3	3.3	3.2	2.8	3.2	3.1	3.5	Stable
Colombia	4.2	3.7	3.9	3.7	3.7	3.6	3.1	2.2	2.6	2.1	2.1	Decrease
Paraguay	7.8	9.2	9.9	9.2	8.7	9.5	9.5	8.8	9.8	8.6	8.6	Stable
Ecuador	2.5	1.5	1.2	1.3	2.5	3.0	2.6	2.2	2.3	2.3	2.3	Stable
Peru	4.2	4.6	4.6	4.3	4.2	3.7	3.4	3.1	3.1	3.2	3.5	Decrease
Uruguay	3.9	4.2	4.3	4.3	4.7	4.6	4.5	3.6	3.7	4.0	3.2	Stable
Venezuela	10.9	10.0	9.9	9.4	10.7	11.5	10.2	10.8	11.6	9.5	9.8	Stable
% of total ethanol consumption												
Argentina	23	26	26	28	29	30	29	30	31	31	32	Increase
Bolivia	55	51	55	56	56	53	60	59	59	59	58	Increase
Brazil	47	49	54	53	52	51	51	51	52	52	53	Stable
Chile	37	33	37	35	39	33	33	28	34	31	34	Stable
Colombia	49	52	50	49	49	53	50	39	44	36	36	Decrease
Ecuador	55	38	36	42	62	65	66	60	60	59	57	Stable
Paraguay	42	48	45	44	44	51	57	64	70	73	67	Increase
Peru	46	49	49	50	50	47	44	42	43	42	42	Decrease
Uruguay	28	30	29	26	29	29	30	27	28	36	29	Stable
Venezuela	59	63	62	62	72	73	67	63	64	58	57	Stable

Source: Data from the Food and Agriculture Organization food balance sheets (Food and Agriculture Organization, 2006).

Table 12.9 Monthly consumption of beer in Argentina

Month	*1989*	*1990*	*1991*	*1992*	*1993*	*1994*	*1995*	*1996*	*1997*	*1998*
January	15	11	11	11	10	10	12	11	12	10
February	12	8	9	10	9	9	9	10	9	8
March	9	4	8	10	10	10	9	9	9	9
April	5	4	7	7	8	7	6	6	7	7
June	4	5	6	5	5	6	6	6	6	6
July	3	4	4	4	4	5	5	5	4	5
August	2	4	5	5	5	5	5	4	5	6
September	4	8	7	7	8	7	6	8	7	7
October	6	9	9	9	9	9	8	7	8	7
November	10	12	10	10	9	9	9	9	9	10
December	13	14	11	10	10	10	11	11	10	10

Source: Data from Camara de la Industria Cervecera y Maltera Argentina (2007).

represents more than half of total ethanol consumption (Table 12.8), but this ratio has remained relatively stable for period 1993–2003. Conversely, beer has replaced other traditional alcoholic drinks such as corn liquor; currently beer is the most frequently consumed alcoholic beverage among the indigenous population (Seale *et al.*, 2002a, b).

Other countries

The production and per capita consumption of beer show wide variations between countries in the other South American countries (Tables 12.6 and 12.7). Expressed in grams of ethanol/day, Paraguay has the second highest consumption, comparable to those found in European countries, whereas the consumption in the other South American countries is much lower. Beer represented more than half of total ethanol consumption in Bolivia and principally Ecuador, where it represented two-thirds of all ethanol consumption (Table 12.8).

Regarding trends, beer consumption (expressed in grams of ethanol) increased in Bolivia, decreased in Colombia and Peru, and remained stable in the other countries. Expressed as percentage of total ethanol consumption, an increase was

Table 12.10 Trends in beer consumption in Asia-Pacific countries

Year	*1993*	*1994*	*1995*	*1996*	*1997*	*1998*	*1999*	*2000*	*2001*	*2002*	*2003*	*Trend*
Grams of ethanol/day												
China	2.0	2.3	2.6	2.7	3.0	3.1	3.3	3.4	3.5	3.6	3.8	Increase
India	0.0	0.1	0.1	0.1	0.1	0.1	0.1	0.1	0.1	0.0	0.0	Stable
Japan	9.5	10.0	9.4	9.4	9.0	8.2	7.8	7.2	6.4	5.6	5.2	Decrease
Malaysia	0.8	0.6	0.6	0.7	0.6	0.6	0.6	0.7	0.8	0.8	0.8	Stable
South Korea	5.7	6.3	6.4	6.2	6.0	5.0	5.2	5.8	6.2	6.3	6.1	Stable
Thailand	1.4	1.7	2.1	2.5	2.8	3.1	3.3	3.6	3.8	3.8	4.7	Increase
Vietnam	0.7	0.9	0.9	1.0	1.0	1.7	1.2	1.3	1.2	1.3	1.5	Increase
Australia	14.1	13.6	13.3	13.0	13.1	12.9	12.9	12.7	12.6	12.4	12.4	Decrease
New Zealand	14.1	14.2	13.5	13.3	12.2	12.4	12.1	11.4	11.6	11.6	11.5	Decrease
% of total ethanol consumption												
China	21	23	21	27	29	35	38	41	34	34	40	Increase
India	3	5	4	5	6	7	6	4	3	3	3	Stable
Japan	42	43	41	41	40	39	37	35	32	28	26	Decrease
Malaysia	80	74	74	81	81	85	73	89	85	79	91	Stable
South Korea	31	34	35	35	34	30	30	35	35	35	33	Stable
Thailand	11	13	13	16	19	20	21	23	24	24	28	Increase
Vietnam	48	56	60	56	48	60	48	48	45	47	49	Stable
Australia	62	60	60	58	60	60	58	58	57	56	57	Decrease
New Zealand	71	74	71	67	64	65	65	62	64	64	64	Decrease

Source: Data from the Food and Agriculture Organization food balance sheets (Food and Agriculture Organization, 2006).

observed in Bolivia and Paraguay, a decrease in Colombia and Peru, while non-significant trends were found for the other countries (Table 12.8). Finally, in Chile, beer is the most popular drink among students, together with spirits (Araneda *et al.*, 1996).

Asia-Pacific Region

The Asia-pacific region is characterized by two main and differential trends: a decreased consumption in Australia and New Zealand, paralleled by a considerable increase in the consumption among emerging Asiatic economies such as China and Thailand.

China

China is the main beer producer worldwide (Brewers Association of Japan, 2004a), and both the amount of beer-derived alcohol and the percentage of total ethanol from beer have increased considerably, almost doubling during the period 1993–2003 (Table 12.10). Beer is the most consumed alcoholic beverage among Chinese adolescents (Li *et al.*, 1996) and the second most consumed among adults (Wei *et al.*, 2001).

India

In India the consumption of beer is very low, representing less than 5% of all ethanol consumption, and no significant trend was noted (Table 12.10). Beer consumption is much lower than country-made liquor or spirits, and might be even lower since there is no good estimation of the amount of illicit, home-produced spirits (Mohan *et al.*, 2001). The very low consumption of beer is probably due to its high price (Gupta *et al.*, 2003), which make this beverage more frequent among middle and upper economic classes and also among the urban youngsters (Saxena, 1999).

Japan

Japan is the sixth biggest beer producer worldwide (Brewers Association of Japan, 2004a) but only the 31st regarding the per capita consumption (Brewers Association of Japan, 2004b). Beer is the most popular alcoholic drink among policemen (Ohno, 1995), male adolescents (Osaki *et al.*, 1999) and adult women (Sobue *et al.*, 2001). Still, beer consumption showed a considerable decrease for period 1993–2003, both in absolute and relative terms (Table 12.10).

Malaysia

In Malaysia, beer and *samsu*, a local distilled alcoholic drink, are the most popular drinks by volume of absolute alcohol (Jernigan and Indran, 1999). Still, the high price of beer precludes its consumption by the lower socio-economic groups of the population (Jernigan and Indran, 1997, 1999). Based on FAO data, the average per capita consumption of beer is very low and has remained constant throughout the period 1993–2003 (Table 12.10). Those figures should be analyzed with caution, since beer and alcohol consumption is unevenly distributed in the population, being almost none among the Muslims and much higher among Chinese (Jernigan and Indran, 1999). Further, and as reported for other countries, the high percentage of alcohol consumed as beer is probably overestimated, since the local, home-based production of spirits cannot be taken into account (Jernigan and Indran, 1999).

Australia

Slightly more than half of all alcohol consumed in Australia is in some form of beer, mostly beer with more than 4.5% alcohol by volume (Chikritzhs *et al.*, 2003), which represents 80% of beer-derived ethanol consumption and an even greater percentage as regards beverage volume (Catalano *et al.*, 2001). Although beer is still considered as the most popular alcoholic drink (Pidd *et al.*, 2006), its consumption has decreased (Drinkwise Australia, 2007), and this decrease is also patent in FAO data, both in absolute and relative terms (Table 12.10). Interestingly, the amount of full strength beer consumed has decreased by 14% while light alcohol beer has increased by 25% over the past one to two decades (Stockwell, 2004), no differences between urban and rural subjects (Dunsire and Baldwin, 1999). Among adolescents, beer consumption is decreasing, being replaced by spirits (King *et al.*, 2005); similar findings among middle-aged women, where beer consumption is lower than consumption of wine or spirits (Young and Powers, 2005). Finally, beer consumption is higher among risky and high-risk drinkers compared to low risk level drinkers (Australian Bureau of Statistics, 2006).

Other countries

In South Korea, beer is a popular alcoholic drink, together with local traditional beverages such as soju and makkolli (Chung, 2004); for period 1993–2003, no significant trends were found regarding the absolute and relative consumption of beer (Table 12.10).

In Thailand and Vietnam, the absolute amount of beer more than doubled during period 1993–2003; in Thailand, the percentage of ethanol consumed as beer increased considerably, whereas no changes were found in Vietnam (Table 12.10).

In Papua New Guinea, locally brewed lager beer is the most popular alcoholic beverage, followed by rum (Marshall, 1999). Men consume more than women, and usually do so in groups. In rural areas consumption is lower and, interestingly, beer is used in exchange ceremonies between kin groups (Marshall, 1999). Finally, in New Zealand, both the total amount as the relative part of beer-derived alcohol decreased (Table 12.10).

Mediterranean Non-European Countries

Only two countries were assessed, Turkey and Israel. In Turkey, the amount of beer-derived ethanol is low and increased only slightly, whereas the percentage of total ethanol from beer showed a steeper increase, from 48% in 1993 to 59% in 2003 (Table 12.11).

In Israel, the amount of beer-derived ethanol remained stable between 1993 and 2003, while the percentage of total ethanol from beer showed a decreased trend, from 56% in 1993 to less than half in 2003 (Table 12.11). A possible explanation might be related to alcoholic beverage preference of Russian emigrants, who tend to prefer spirits and disregard beer; indeed, no difference regarding beer consumption was found between Russian emigrants and other Israeli Jews (Rahav *et al.*, 1999). Finally, among college students, beer and wine were more popular than spirits and consumed in similar frequencies (Isralowitz and Peleg, 1996).

Africa

With the exception of the Seychelles and South Africa, the consumption of beer is very low in African countries.

Table 12.11 Trends in beer consumption in non-European Mediterranean countries

Year	*1993*	*1994*	*1995*	*1996*	*1997*	*1998*	*1999*	*2000*	*2001*	*2002*	*2003*	*Trend*
Grams of ethanol/day												
Israel	2.7	2.3	2.5	2.4	2.6	2.5	2.5	2.5	2.6	2.6	2.5	Stable
Turkey	1.5	1.5	1.6	1.6	1.6	1.7	1.6	1.6	1.8	1.7	1.8	Increase
% of total ethanol consumption												
Israel	56	61	73	65	56	53	54	54	53	50	49	Decrease
Turkey	48	50	51	48	48	49	49	53	56	57	59	Increase

Source: Data from the Food and Agriculture Organization food balance sheets (Food and Agriculture Organization, 2006).

Further, the figures are somewhat hampered by considerable fluctuations, probably due to economical or political changes, and there are few field studies on alcohol consumption. Further, home-made alcoholic beverages are quite common and are not integrated into the national statistics. Thus, the data presented should be interpreted with some caution.

Namibia

In Namibia, 67% of all alcohol is consumed as home-brewed beer and 15% as store-purchased beer (Mustonen *et al.*, 2001). In women, 73% of ethanol consumption comes from home-brewed beer, whereas the corresponding figure in men is 64% (Mustonen *et al.*, 2001); conversely, men tend to consume more store-purchased beer.

Based on FAO data, a considerable increase in the total amount and in the relative importance of beer-derived ethanol consumed was noted till 2002, with a considerable decrease afterwards (Table 12.12). The reasons for such a decrease are not straightforward and might be related to economic or political changes.

Nigeria

In Nigeria, stout beer accounts for 80% and lager beer for 20% of total beer volume sales (Gureje, 1999), and more than 40 brands of locally brewed lager and stout are available (Obot, 2000). Beer is the most common alcoholic beverage, above local traditional beverages made of palm wine: 44% of adults in the middle-belt region and northern part of Nigeria reported consuming beer, vs. 21% for palm wine (Gureje, 1999). Indeed, expressed in volume, beer production is almost double of soft drinks, with a much steeper annual increase (Obot, 2000) (Figure 12.4). Possible reasons for such popularity are the relatively low price of beer, which is also considered a modern and stigma-free alcoholic beverage, and the availability in small-scale, street-corner shops (Gureje, 1999). Still, the consumption of beer and alcohol is unevenly distributed throughout the country, the predominantly Muslim North region being characterized by a very low consumption (Gureje, 1999). According to FAO data, no significant trends were found for both the

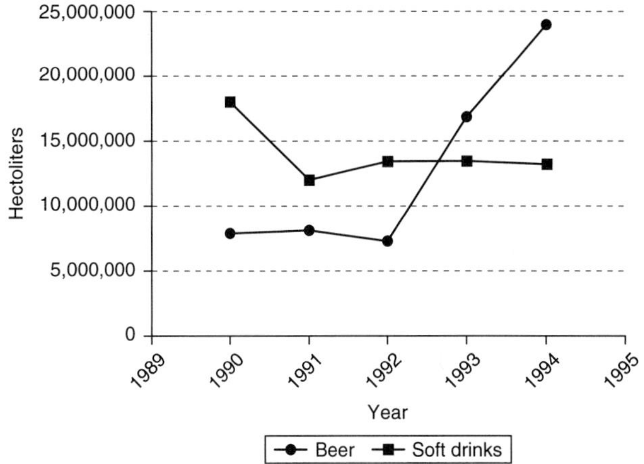

Figure 12.4 Trends in beer and soft drink production, Nigeria. *Source*: Adapted from Obot (2000).

Table 12.12 Trends in beer consumption in Africa

Year	*1993*	*1994*	*1995*	*1996*	*1997*	*1998*	*1999*	*2000*	*2001*	*2002*	*2003*	*Trend*
Grams of ethanol/day												
Angola	1.1	1.2	1.3	1.6	1.9	1.6	1.6	1.7	2.3	3.0	2.8	Increase
Egypt	0.1	0.1	0.1	0.1	0.1	0.1	0.1	0.1	0.2	0.2	0.2	Increase
Mozambique	0.4	0.5	0.7	0.6	0.4	0.6	0.5	0.5	0.5	0.6	0.5	Stable
Namibia	0.0	0.0	0.0	0.0	1.5	0.6	2.6	2.9	6.1	6.2	2.2	Increase
Nigeria	1.6	1.6	1.5	1.5	1.4	1.4	1.7	1.6	1.6	1.9	1.8	Increase
Seychelles	47.5	43.0	41.4	41.2	42.5	47.7	45.3	49.1	49.5	40.7	48.8	Stable
South Africa	8.0	8.3	7.7	8.2	8.7	8.8	9.1	8.0	8.0	9.0	8.7	Stable
Zimbabwe	1.9	4.2	7.0	8.6	7.6	8.7	8.2	8.4	8.8	12.0	14.6	Increase
% of total ethanol consumption												
Angola	36	36	38	42	42	38	43	46	48	55	52	Increase
Egypt	71	71	70	71	69	70	70	75	77	76	76	Increase
Mozambique	51	50	53	53	42	40	32	34	18	25	52	Decrease
Namibia	0	0	0	0	6	4	22	12	28	28	9	Increase
Nigeria	15	15	15	14	12	12	14	13	13	15	15	Stable
Seychelles	78	75	69	72	77	80	77	77	98	73	88	Stable
South Africa	39	39	38	39	40	42	43	41	42	41	38	Stable
Zimbabwe	5.5	9	14	18	13	14	15	15	16	21	25	Increase

Source: Data from the Food and Agriculture Organization food balance sheets (Food and Agriculture Organization, 2006).

overall and the relative amount of beer-derived ethanol consumption (Table 12.12); the relatively low percentage of total ethanol consumed as beer might be related to the low alcohol content of beer relative to the other alcoholic drinks.

Data from the FAO food balance sheets indicate a slight, borderline significant increase in the amount of beer-derived ethanol, whereas no significant trend was found regarding the relative importance of beer among alcoholic beverages (Table 12.12). Based on FAO data, beer accounted for one-sixth (15%) of all ethanol consumed.

Seychelles

Beer is the most frequently consumed alcoholic beverage in the Seychelles: circa 45% of men aged 25–64 years report being regular drinkers (Perdrix *et al.*, 1999; Bovet, 2001). Conversely, beer-derived ethanol consumption is only 31%, the main percentage coming from local distilled beverages such as *baka* (Perdrix *et al.*, 1999). Men consume considerably more than women (17.6 vs. 1.1 ml ethanol/day), and alcoholic beverages are consumed mainly outside home (Perdrix *et al.*, 1999; Bovet, 2001). Beer consumption has been estimated to be 3 million liters for the entire population, although in the year 1994 5.54 million liters of beer were sold (Perdrix *et al.*, 1999; Bovet, 2001). Indeed, FAO data indicate considerable but stable beer consumption (over 45 g of ethanol/day), which accounts for more than 75% of all ethanol consumed (Table 12.12).

South Africa

Two-thirds of the absolute ethanol consumption in South Africa is in the form of malt or sorghum beer, and from 1970 to 1995 the greatest market growth was in malt beer (Parry and Bennetts, 1999). Those figures are not in agreement with the FAO data, which indicates that beer accounts for only 40% of total ethanol consumed (Table 12.12). The most likely explanation is that home-brewed beer production is not considered in the FAO report, thus underestimating the importance of this beverage. Consumers are shifting from sorghum to malt and home-brewed beer, since they contain more alcohol (Parry and Bennetts, 1999). In 1997, malt beer accounted for 44% of the alcoholic beverage market, followed by sorghum beer with 20% (Parry and Bennetts, 1999); this popularity is partly due to the fact that beer prices have been maintained below the inflation rate, making beer more affordable (Parry and Bennetts, 1999). Thus, between 1970 and 1991, the per capita consumption of malt beer increased by over 300, from 13.7 to 58 l per year (Parry and Bennetts, 1999). Based on FAO data, this increase has been contained, since no significant trend was found regarding both absolute and relative ethanol consumption (Table 12.12); again, the unaccounted for home-brewed production might explain part of those differences.

Gender differences regarding the consumption of alcoholic beverages have also been noted, men consuming mainly beer while women consume other alcoholic drinks (Parry and Bennetts, 1999); a similar pattern is also found among teenagers (Madu and Matla, 2003). Interestingly, beer is the preferred alcoholic beverage in men irrespective of race (Parry and Bennetts, 1999).

Zimbabwe

In Zimbabwe, traditional African or opaque beer is the most consumed alcoholic beverage, followed by lager beer (Jernigan, 1999). Consumption is mostly driven by economic forces, people consuming the less expensive beverages, and the industry has kept the price of beer behind the pace of inflation to promote sales (Jernigan, 1999). Indeed, data from the FAO indicate that both the absolute and relative amounts of beer-derived ethanol have increased, beer representing less than one-tenth of all ethanol consumed in 1993 and one-quarter in 2003 (Table 12.12). Women consume very little alcoholic beverages, while the per capita consumption of opaque beer has been estimated to be over 11 l of pure ethanol a year in the 1970s (Jernigan, 1999). Taking into account that in 1995 the beer produced by the country's legal breweries amounted to only 4 l of pure ethanol per capita, the difference between the legal production and the actual per capita consumption is mainly due to illegal, home-brewed beer (Jernigan, 1999).

Other countries

The consumption of beer increased in Angola and Egypt; in Angola it increased from one-third to half of all ethanol consumed (Table 12.12). Conversely, in Mozambique, no trend was found regarding absolute beer consumption, whereas the relative part of beer-derived ethanol consumption showed a slight decreasing trend. Overall, beer accounted for more than half of total ethanol consumption in those three countries (Table 12.12).

Conclusion

The epidemiology of beer drinking worldwide is hampered by the lack of reliable data for most developing countries. The local, home-made and mostly illegal alcoholic beverages (including beer) are difficult to assess and might considerably bias the estimates. Conversely, in industrialized countries, the available data might provide different estimates for the prevalence of beer drinking or the amount of beer consumed; thus, the data source must be properly cited when single estimates are provided.

Still, based on the available information, it can be inferred that the consumption of beer is decreasing in most industrialized countries, while the opposite trend is found in developing countries, namely due to low prices and strong marketing forces. Also in developing countries, traditional and religious beliefs strongly influence beer (and alcohol) consumption. Asia is the continent where the increase in beer consumption is steeper, namely due to China. Finally, in almost all countries, beer consumption is closely linked to male gender and younger age groups.

Summary Points

- Beer accounts for 58–67% of total alcohol consumption in North America; 15–59% in Central America and the Caribbean; 29–58% in South America; 28–91% in Asia-Pacific countries, and 9–88% in selected African countries.
- Beer consumption is increasing in developing countries whereas the opposite trend is observed among industrialized countries.
- This increase is stronger in Asia (China and Thailand) than in other parts of the world.
- This increase is also stronger among younger generations.
- Social and religious factors considerably influence beer consumption, but their effect appears to be lessening.
- In many developing countries, the lack of reliable field studies and the local non-declared production of beer lead to an underestimation of the per capita consumption.

References

Almeida-Filho, N., Lessa, I., Magalhães, L., Araújo, M.J., Aquino, E., Kawachi, I. and James, S.A. (2004). *Revista de Saúde Pública* 38, 45–54.

Araneda, J.M., Repossi, A. and Puente, C. (1996). *Revista Medica de Chile* 124, 377–388.

Associazione degli Industriali della Birra e del Malto (2004). Annual report 2004. Rome, Italy. Available at http://www.assobirra.it/annual_report/2004/AnnualReport2004%20.pdf.

Australian Bureau of Statistics (2006). 4832.0.55.001 – Alcohol consumption in Australia: a snapshot, 2004–05. Canberra, Australia, National Information and Referral Service.

Bovet, P. (2001). Alcohol consumption patterns and association with the CAGE questionnaire and physiological variables in the Seychelles Islands (Indian Ocean). In Department of Mental Health and Substance Dependence (ed.), *Surveys of Drinking Patterns and Problems in Seven Developing Countries*. Geneva, Switzerland, World Health Organization.

Brewers Association of Japan (2004a). Beer consumption around the world. Tokyo, Japan. Available at: http://www.brewers.or.jp/english/10-consupt.html

Brewers Association of Japan (2004b). Beer consumption per capita around the world. Tokyo, Japan. Available at: http://www.brewers.or.jp/english/10-consupt2.html

Camara de la Industria Cervecera y Maltera Argentina (2007). Cerveza. Expendio de cerveza y consumo "per capita." Ejercicio 1901/02 a 2000/2001. Available at: http://www.camaracervecera.com.ar/index.php

Carlini-Cotrim, B. (1999). Country profile on alcohol in Brazil. In Riley, L. and Marshall, M. (eds), *Alcohol and Public Health in 8 Developing Countries*. Social Change and Mental Health, World Health Organization, Geneva, Switzerland.

Catalano, P., Chikritzhs, T., Stockwell, T., Webb, M., Rohlin, C.J. and Dietze, P. (2001). Trends in per capita alcohol consumption in Australia, 1990/91 to 1998/99. In National Drug Research Institute (ed.), *National Alcohol Indicators*. National Drug Research Institute, Curtin University, Perth, WA; Applied Population Research Unit, University of Queensland; Turning Point Alcohol and Drug Centre Inc., Melbourne, Victoria.

Cerveceros latinoamericanos (2007a). Argentina: ventas de cerveza 1987–1997. Available at: http://www.cerveceroslatinoamericanos.com/

Cerveceros latinoamericanos (2007b). Consumo de cerveza per-capita por país (1997–1998). Litros/habitante. Available at: http://www.cerveceroslatinomericanos.com/

Cervesia (2003). O mercado brasileiro de cerveja. Available at: http://www.cervesia.com.br/dados estatisticos.asp

Chikritzhs, T., Catalano, P., Stockwell, T., Donath, S., Ngo, H., Young, D. and Matthews, S. (2003). Australian Alcohol Indicators, 1990–2001. Patterns of Alcohol Use and Related Harms for Australian States and Territories. National Drug Research Institute, Curtin University of Technology, Perth, WA; Turning Point, Alcohol and Drug Centre Inc., Melbourne, Victoria.

Chung, W. (2004). *Alcohol Alcohol.* 39, 39–42.

Drinkwise Australia Alcohol consumption in Australia. Melbourne, Australia, Drinkwise Australia, Ltd.

Dunsire, M. and Baldwin, S. (1999). *Alcohol Alcohol.* 34, 59–64.

Food and Agriculture Organization (2006). Food balance sheets. Available at http://faostat.fao.org/site/345/default.aspx (accessed October 2006).

Galduróz, J.C.F. and Caetano, R. (2004). *Revista Brazileira de Psiquiatria* 26, 3–6.

Greenfield, T.K., Midanik, L.T. and Rogers, J.D. (2000). *Am. J. Pub. Health* 90, 47–52.

Gupta, P.C., Saxena, S., Pednekar, M.S. and Maulik, P.K. (2003). *Alcohol Alcohol.* 38, 327–331.

Gureje, O. (1999). Country profile on alcohol in Nigeria. In Riley, L. and Marshall, M. (eds), *Alcohol and Public Health in 8 Developing Countries*. Social Change and Mental Health, World Health Organization, Geneva, Switzerland.

Isralowitz, R.E. and Peleg, A. (1996). *Drug Alcohol Depend.* 42, 147–153.

Jerez, S.J. and Coviello, A. (1998). *Alcohol* 16, 1–5.

Jernigan, D.H. (1999). Country profile on alcohol in Zimbabwe. In Riley, L. and Marshall, M. (eds), *Alcohol and Public Health in 8 Developing Countries*. Social Change and Mental Health, World Health Organization, Geneva, Switzerland.

Jernigan, D.H. and Indran, S.K. (1997). *Drug Alcohol Rev.* 16, 401–409.

Jernigan, D.H. and Indran, S.K. (1999). Country profile on alcohol in Malaysia. In Riley, L. and Marshall, M. (eds), *Alcohol and Public Health in 8 Developing Countries*. Social Change and Mental Health, World Health Organization, Geneva, Switzerland.

King, E., Taylor, J. and Carroll, T. (2005). *Alcohol Consumption Patterns Among Australian 15–17 year olds from 2000 to 2004.* Department of Health and Ageing, Australian Government, Sydney, Australia.

Li, X., Fang, X., Stanton, B., Feigelman, S. and Dong, Q. (1996). *J. Adolesc. Health* 19, 353–361.

Madu, S.N. and Matla, M.Q. (2003). *J. Adolesc.* 26, 121–136.

Marshall, M. (1999). Country profile on alcohol in Papua New Guinea. In Riley, L. and Marshall, M. (eds), *Alcohol and Public Health in 8 Developing Countries.* Social Change and Mental Health, World Health Organization, Geneva, Switzerland.

Medina-Mora, M.E. (1999). Country profile on alcohol in Mexico. In Riley, L. and Marshall, M. (eds), *Alcohol and Public Health in 8 Developing Countries.* Social Change and Mental Health, World Health Organization, Geneva, Switzerland.

Medina-Mora, M.E., Cravioto, P., Villatoro, J. (1998). El consumo de alcohol en la población urbana de México. *Encuesta nacional de adicciones.* México, Mexico, Secretaría de Salud.

Medina-Mora, M.E., Borges, G. and Villatoro, J. (2000). *J. Subst. Abuse* 12, 183–196.

Medina-Mora, M.E., Villatoro, J., Caraveo, J. and Colmenares, E. (2001). Patterns of alcohol consumption and related problems in Mexico: results from two general population surveys. In Department of Mental Health and Substance Dependence (ed.), *Surveys of Drinking Patterns and Problems in Seven Developing Countries.* World Health Organization, Geneva, Switzerland.

Mohan, D., Chopra, A., Ray, R., Sethi, H. (2001). Alcohol consumption in India: a cross-sectional study. In Department of Mental Health and Substance Dependence (ed.), *Surveys of Drinking Patterns and Problems in Seven Developing Countries.* World Health Organization, Geneva, Switzerland.

Munné, M.I. (2005). *Addiction* 100, 1790–1799.

Mustonen, H., Beukes, L. and Du Preez, V. (2001). Alcohol drinking in Namibia. In Department of Mental Health and Substance Dependence (ed.), *Surveys of Drinking Patterns and Problems in Seven Developing Countries.* World Health Organization, Geneva, Switzerland.

National Institute on Alcohol Abuse and Alcoholism Apparent per capita ethanol consumption for the United States, 1850–2004. (Gallons of ethanol, based on population age 15 and older prior to 1970 and on population age 14 and other thereafter.) National Institutes of Health.

National Institute on Alcohol Abuse and Alcoholism per capita ethanol consumption for States, census regions, and the United States, 1970–2004. (Gallons of ethanol, based on population age 14 and older.) National Institutes of Health. Available at: http://www.niaaa.nih.gov/Resources/DatabaseResources/QuickFacts/AlcoholSales/default.html

National Institute on Alcohol Abuse and Alcoholism (2006). Alcohol use and alcohol use disorders in the United States: main findings from the 2001–2002 National Epidemiologic Survey on Alcohol and Related Conditions (NESARC). Bethesda, USA, National Institutes of Health. Available at: http//niaaa.census.gov/

Obot, I.S. (2000). *J. Subst. Abuse* 12, 169–181.

Ohno, K. (1995). *Arukoru Kenkyuto Yakubutsu Ison* 30, 97–120.

Oliveira de Souza, D.P., Areco, K.N. and da Silveira Filho, D.X. (2005). *Revista de Saúde Pública* 39, 1–8.

Osaki, Y., Minowa, M., Suzuki, K. and Wada, K. (1999). *Nippon Koshu Eisei Zasshi* 46, 883–893.

Parry, C.D.H. and Bennetts, A.L. (1999). Country profile on alcohol in South Africa. In Riley, L. and Marshall, M. (eds), *Alcohol and Public Health in 8 Developing Countries.* Social Change and Mental Health, World Health Organization, Geneva, Switzerland.

Pechansky, F. (1995). *Jornal Brasileiro de Psiquiatria* 44, 231–242.

Perdrix, J., Bovet, P., Larue, D., Yersin, B., Burnand, B. and Paccaud, F. (1999). *Alcohol Alcohol.* 34, 773–785.

Pidd, K., Berry, J.G., Harrison, J.E., Roche, A.M., Driscoll, T.R. and Newson, R.S. (2006). Alcohol and work. Patterns of use, workplace culture and safety. *Injury Research and Statistics,* Australian Institute of Health and Welfare, Adelaide, Australia.

Rahav, G., Hasin, D. and Paykin, A. (1999). *Am. J. Pub. Health* 89, 1212–1216.

Saxena, S. (1999). Country profile on alcohol in India. In Riley, L. and Marshall, M. (eds), *Alcohol and Public Health in 8 Developing Countries.* Social Change and Mental Health, World Health Organization, Geneva, Switzerland.

Seale, J.P., Seale, J.D., Alvarado, M., Vogel, R.L. and Terry, N.E. (2002a). *Alcohol Alcohol.* 37, 198–204.

Seale, J.P., Shellenberger, S., Rodriguez, C., Seale, J.D. and Alvarado, M. (2002b). *Alcohol Alcohol.* 37, 603–608.

Sobue, T., Yamamoto, S. and Watanabe, S. (2001b). *J. Epidemiol.* 11, S44–S56.

Stockwell, T. (2004). *Drug Alcohol Rev.* 23, 377–379.

The Brewers Association of Canada (2007a). Canadian and Imported Beer Sales in HL, Brewers Association of Canada, Ontario, Canada. Available at: http://www.brewers.ca/UserFiles/Documents/pdfs/eng/statistics/asb/2006/Page%2020-06%20Sales% 20by%20Region.pdf

The Brewers Association of Canada (2007b). Per Capita Consumption of Beer, Spirits, and Wine Based on Adult Population, Brewers Association of Canada, Ontario, Canada. Available at: http://www.brewers.ca/UserFiles/Documents/pdfs/eng/statistics/asb/Keystone%20ASB%20(E)%20Final%202006.pdf

The Brewers Association of Canada (2007c). Per Capita Consumption of Beer, Spirits, and Wine Based on Legal Age Population, Brewers Association of Canada, Ontario, Canada. Available at: http://www.brewers.ca/UserFiles/Documents/pdfs/eng/statistics/asb/Keystone%20ASB%20(E)%20Final%202006.pdf

USDA Economic Research Service Data Sets (2006). Food Availability: Custom Queries. USDA Economic Research Service. Available at: http://www.ers.usda.gov/Data/FoodConsumption/FoodAvailQueriable.aspx

Wei, H., Derson, Y., Shuiyan, X. and Lingjiang, X. (2001). Drinking patterns and related problems in a large general population sample in China. In Department of Mental Health and Substance Dependence (ed.), *Surveys of Drinking Patterns and Problems in Seven Developing Countries.* World Health Organization, Geneva, Switzerland.

Young, A. and Powers, J. (2005). *Australian Women and Alcohol Consumption 1996–2003.* Research Centre for Gender and Health, University of Newcastle, Newcastle, Australia.

13

Beer Consumption Patterns in Northern Ireland

Adele Mc Kinney School of Psychology, Life and Health Sciences, University of Ulster, Magee Campus, Derry

Abstract

Alcohol has a long history of use, and due to its ability to promote feelings of joviality it is associated with celebrations. Northern Ireland has a distinct binge drinking culture where excessive amounts of alcohol are consumed at one sitting. The Health Promotion Agency of Northern Ireland (HPA, 2002) revealed that 37% of male drinkers exceeded 21 units per week and 20% of female drinkers exceeded 14 units per week, and this alcohol consumption is concentrated to the weekend. Another characteristic of Northern Irish male drinkers is their preference for beer consumption compared to wine consumption which is more popular in the wider European community. The HPA (2002) observed that the main drink of choice for men is beer (77%). For women the main choice of drink is wine (50%) closely followed by spirits (42%). One further distinctive pattern within Northern Ireland is the high level of abstinence. A Northern Ireland Community Health Study (Blaney and Mc Kenzie, 1978) found that 40% did not drink and of those 37% were life-long abstainers. However this level of abstinence is gradually decreasing. The continuous household survey (NISRA – Northern Ireland Statistics and Research Agency) revealed that the level of abstainers had decreased to 24% in 2002–2003. These drinking patterns are evident in all age groups and all socioeconomic classes of Northern Irish drinkers.

List of Abbreviations

DHSS	Department of Health and Social Services
HPA	Health Promotion Agency of Northern Ireland
HSBC	The Health Behaviour of School Children Survey
NISRA	Northern Ireland Statistics and Research Agency
WHO	World Health Organization

Introduction

To address the topic of "beer consumption patterns" it is important to identify what is meant by patterns. Patterns of beer consumption can relate to where beer is consumed, how much beer is consumed, when beer is consumed and in what environment. Patterns of alcohol consumption may also refer to the differences in beer consumption among different socioeconomic groups, age groups and gender. This chapter aims to address these interpretations of pattern of consumption.

It has been well established that the United Kingdom and in particular Northern Ireland are essentially beer drinking cultures. Another aspect of alcohol consumption in Northern Ireland is the tendency to drink large quantities of alcohol in one sitting, binge drinking. This chapter will compare the drinking patterns in Northern Ireland with other European countries to highlight the binge drinking culture.

Beer is the drink of choice in Northern Ireland especially for males; however, it is important to put the beer drinking into context and describe general drinking habits in Northern Ireland. This chapter will endeavor to describe drinking habits in Northern Ireland in relation to other countries and then focus on the beer drinking culture within the distinctive drinking culture of Northern Ireland.

Alcohol Use/Misuse in Northern Ireland

The classification of problem drinkers is questionable but different research studies have used units of alcohol consumption as a criterion. The recommended weekly intake of alcohol is 14 units for females and 21 units for males. The percentage of females, in Northern Ireland, consuming more than 14 units is reported to have decreased from 12% to 11% between 1987 and 1989, the percentage of males consuming more than 21 units decreased from 33% to 26% during the same period (Sweeney *et al.*, 1990). More recent statistics from NISRA (Northern Ireland Statistics and Research Agency) indicate that this slight decrease in Northern Irish drinking more than the recommended weekly limit has been reversed and 33% of males and

Beer in Health and Disease Prevention
ISBN: 978-0-12-373891-2

11% of females in Northern Ireland consume more than the recommended weekly limit in 2002–2003.

Females consuming more than 35 units per week and males consuming more than 50 units per week are classified as heavy problem drinkers. According to this classification, in 1987 and 1989, only 1% of female drinkers were above the upper risk of 35 units per week (Sweeney *et al.*, 1990). This is in accordance with the figures from "the continuous household survey" and this rate was maintained during the period 1988–1998. However the percentage of females consuming alcohol to a "dangerous" level has increased to 2% in 2002–2003. The percentage of males consuming above the upper risk limit of 50 units per week decreased from 9% in 1987 to 6% in 1989, and this had decreased to 4% in 1989. However there has been a marked increase and the level of "dangerous" drinking in the male population of Northern Ireland from 9% in 2001 to 11% in 2003.

A recent study carried out by the Health Promotion Agency of Northern Ireland (HPA, 2002) confirmed that daily drinking limits are not regularly exceeded by Northern Irish drinkers but that drinking is concentrated. It was observed that 48% of men and 35% of women had a binge drinking session in the previous week. A binge drinking session was defined in this study as 10 units for men and 7 units for women. This study also revealed that 37% of male drinkers and 20% of female drinkers exceeded their weekly sensible drinking limit (21 units for men and 14 units for women) and could be referred to as risk drinkers. These figures are slightly higher than those obtained in the continuous household survey but confirm the fact that an increasing number of people in Northern Ireland are drinking beyond the recommended weekly limits.

Social aspects of alcohol consumption

The media has an influential role in people's lives and has been concerned with the effects of alcohol. One example of an extensively reported problem, associated with alcohol consumption, was the mass media depiction of "lager louts." The heavy drinking was associated with public disorder among young people, especially males (British Medical Association, 1986). Another area of mass media concern is driving while under the influence of alcohol. Driving while under the influence of alcohol is currently the principle cause of road traffic deaths in Northern Ireland and was responsible for 25% of road fatalities in 1996 (DHSS, 1998); this figure has not changed and other dramatic figures related to alcohol consumption include 30% of drowning, 30% of murders, 33% of accidents in the home, 40% of incidents of domestic violence, 44% of theft charges and 88% of criminal damage arrests (HPA, 2002).

The alcohol-related death rate in the United Kingdom increased from 6.9 per 100,000 population in 1991 to 13.0 in 2004, it was also observed that death rates are much higher for males than females and in recent years the gap between the sexes has widened. In 2004 the male death rate was 13.7 deaths per 100,000 while females was 8.5 deaths per 100,000 (NISRA).

A relationship between the type of beverage consumed and the likelihood of driving after the consumption of alcohol has been suggested. Perrine (1970) found that 58% of the Vermont drivers arrested for drink-driving reported daily beer drinking, but only 12% were daily spirit drinkers and 3% reported drinking wine. However the proposed link between beverage choice and drinking-driving may be confounded by the sex and age characteristics of the drinking-driver. Gruenewald *et al.* (2000) investigated the association between beer drinking and driving under the influence. The results failed to establish a relationship between beverage preference and driving while under the influence of alcohol. However the demographic information revealed that the beer drinkers in the sample were from a sub-population of heavy drinking young men with a preference for drinking in bars. Thus they had to travel to and from the place of alcohol consumption.

Cultural variations in beliefs about alcohol effects

The level of social acceptance of alcohol consumption varies between cultures. Within the United Kingdom, Northern Ireland has been associated with a distinctive drinking style. The differences may be due to numerous factors among which are alcohol expectancies. O'Connor (1978) showed that Northern Irish adults expect the consumption of alcohol to reduce anxiety and enhance sociability. In contrast English adults simply view alcohol consumption as a social activity. In a recent qualitative study carried out by the HPA (2002) the participants-perceived benefits of alcohol consumption included reduce stress, increase confidence, strengthens relationships and facilitates meeting new people. The majority of the participants are not aware of any safe drinking guidelines and are shocked to be told that the general definition of binge drinking used in UK studies was 10 and 7 units for men and women respectively. An example of a females' definition of binge drinking was "A binge is when you drink for 3 or 4 days constantly." Another quote from the survey relating to how participants define binge drinking was "If you go for a week or two and drink non-stop." This type of definition was in keeping with the responses from the majority of the sample. The conclusions drawn placed the Irish at greater risk of alcohol-related problems due to the attitudes attached to alcohol consumption. These findings indicate that the change in recommendations by the UK government to update the sensible drinking guidelines from a weekly to a daily limit to discourage saving units for the "weekend binge" Bennett *et al.* (1995) have had little effect in decreasing the pattern of binge drinking for Northern Ireland drinkers.

In Europe it is common for people to consume small amounts of alcohol frequently. In contrast Northern Ireland is associated with a more concentrated drinking style. Marques-Vidal *et al.* (2001) observed that alcohol consumption in France was homogeneous throughout the week with a slight increase at the weekend, this is in contrast to the pattern observed in the Northern Irish drinkers, were 66% of the total drinking occurred on Friday and Saturday. They also observed that the men in the French sample consumed on average 317 ± 249 ml/week compared to Northern Irish men consuming 325 ± 333 ml/week thus Northern Irish men consume more in 2 days than French men consume in 7 days. The second interesting observation is the volume of each type of beverage consumed, wine consumption accounted for 216 ml/week in the French sample but only accounted for 18 ml/week in the Northern Irish sample, spirits accounted for 28 ml/week in the French sample and 91 ml/week in the Northern Irish sample and the beverage of choice in the Northern Irish sample was beer which accounted for 215 ml/week compared to 72 ml/week in the French sample. Thus confirming two facts about the drinking habits in Northern Ireland: (1) there is a tendency to concentrate all drinking to the weekend and (2) the beverage of choice for Northern Irish males in beer.

Drinking habits in Northern Ireland

There have been a few large-scale investigation of drinking habits in Northern Ireland and a distinctive pattern of drinking has emerged. It has been well documented that Northern Ireland has one of the highest levels of abstinence in Europe, with 30% of adults who do not drink at all. However recent research has identified that this abstinence rate is decreasing and that 24% of people are non-drinkers in 2002–2003 (continuous household survey). However within its population of drinkers drinking tends to be less frequent with greater quantities. When considering the identified drinking patterns in Northern Ireland the investigations which look at the consumption of alcohol per capita of population are misleading, due to the high level of abstinence. This causes the consumption within the population as a whole to be artificially deflated. The other factor, which is concealed, is the concentrated drinking. Studies looking at the amount of alcohol consumed per annum fail to identify the tendency, within Northern Ireland, to consume large quantities on few occasions.

Differences within cultures

Differences within cultures as well as between cultures have been identified. A focus of large-scale research has been placed on the examination of drinking practices in terms of user characteristics. Drinking practices have been found to vary according to age, sex, socioeconomic position, income, education, ethnicity, religious affiliation, marital status and urbanization (Cahalan *et al.*, 1969; Dight, 1976; Casswell, 1980). Thus when discussing drinking or beer consumption patterns it is important to take into consideration some of these factors. Recently attention has been directed toward the study of influential factors other than the characteristics of individuals. Situational and contextual variables differ according to demographic variables such as age and sex and have been found to be important determinants of alcohol consumption (Clark, 1977; Harford, 1983). Consequently a complete discussion of beer consumption patterns requires consideration of situational and contextual factors.

Beer Consumption

The Northern Irish have a beer and spirits drinking culture. In Northern Ireland the preferred beer is stout, always ordered by brand name, usually Guinness. Second to Guinness is lager. This is in contrast to England where the beer of choice is real ale, real ale is not popular in Northern Ireland and few bars even stock bitters on tap. The popularity of wine is increasing rapidly, but this trend is not yet evident in the majority of ordinary pubs. In other countries, adults decide when it is time to stop drinking and the public bars are open all night. In Northern Ireland the decision about when to stop drinking is taken out of the punters control and the bars are forced to close at 1.30 with 1/2 h drinking up time.

Drinking Patterns Among the Young People of Northern Ireland

The distinctive drinking patterns associated with Northern Ireland can be identified even at an early age. Three large-scale studies of children in year 8–12 (age 11–19 years) aimed to describe and compare young peoples drinking behavior. The Health Behaviour of School Children Survey (HSBC, 1997) was a cross, a national-research study conducted in collaboration with European Region of the World Health Organization (WHO), data was obtained from a representative sample of 5,607 in 1997, >80% response rate. The Young Persons' Behaviour and Attitudes Surveys (2000 and 2003) were a commissioned work carried out by NISRA. The response rates were 6,297 in 2000 (85%) and 7,223 in 2003 (89%). The results indicate that 41% of young people in the 2003 survey had never taken an alcoholic drink; however, the abstinence rate decreased with increasing age so that only 19% of 16-year olds had never taken an alcoholic drink.

Table 13.1 Choice of drink for those who currently drink

	1997				*2000*			
	All (%)	*Base*	*Boys (%)*	*Girls (%)*	*All (%)*	*Base*	*Boys (%)*	*Girls (%)*
Beer	68	3,823	78	55	60	3,362	74	45
Wine	55	3,509	52	57	49	3,289	46	53
Spirits	50	3,544	49	51	62	3,323	62	62
Cider	51	3,511	55	46	49	3,269	53	44
Alcopops	72	3,748	69	74	81	3,297	78	84

Note: The HPA results for choice of drink for those young people aged 11–19 years who currently drink. The results are presented in percentages for years 1997 and 2000 for each type of alcoholic beverage.
Source: HPA (2004).

Table 13.2 Choice of drink by age group (2000 survey)

	Beer (%)	*Wine (%)*	*Spirits (%)*	*Cider (%)*	*Alcopops (%)*	*Base*
Boys						
Year 8	59	52	39	43	63	181
Year 9	66	49	49	50	72	310
Year 10	65	47	53	52	73	403
Year 11	77	48	68	57	85	482
Year 12	87	39	77	55	84	524
Girls						
Year 8	21	52	21	20	53	121
Year 9	42	50	45	41	75	237
Year 10	45	57	49	49	82	346
Year 11	46	51	67	46	90	444
Year 12	49	55	75	44	93	5,000

Note: The HPA results for choice of drink for those young people aged 11–19 years who currently drink. The results are presented for both boys and girls due to the difference in drink preference. The table presents the percentage of girls and boys in each school year who drink each type of beverage.
Source: HPA (2004).

The HPA conducted secondary analysis on the HSBC (1997) and the Young Persons' Behaviour and Attitudes Surveys (2000, 2003) and revealed that beer was the most popular drink for boys in 1997, but by 2000 it has been overtaken by Alcopops. Alcopops are the main drink of choice for girls in both the 1997 and 2000 survey (see Table 13.1).

However the 2000 survey identified that this drinking preference changes with age (see Table 13.2). For 8-year-old boys who drink, Alcopops (63%) are the most popular; however, when the boys reach year 12 beer becomes the most popular drink (87%). There is a very strong sense of who should drink what in Northern Ireland, working class men can only drink beer or spirits in a pub everything else being effeminate. This could explain the move away from Alcopops when boys reach the age of 18/19 and become aware of the actual trend in drinking style when they can legally drink in a bar.

The percentage of girls choosing beer doubles from 21% in year 8 to 42% in year 9. This increased popularity is maintained and increases slightly to 49% in year 12; however, as can be seen from Table 13.2, the increase in popularity of Alcopops increases by 40% between year 8 and year 12.

Young Adult Drinkers in Northern Ireland

A study carried out by the HPA (2002) collected information on prevalence of drinking from a representative sample of 1,752 individuals aged 18–75 years; 922 individuals also completed a diary of drinking the week prior to the survey, only 7 individuals failed to complete the diary fully; thus the data relating to alcohol consumption in 1 week was based on 915 individuals.

This survey followed previous work and also supported previous findings of a very distinctive drinking pattern in

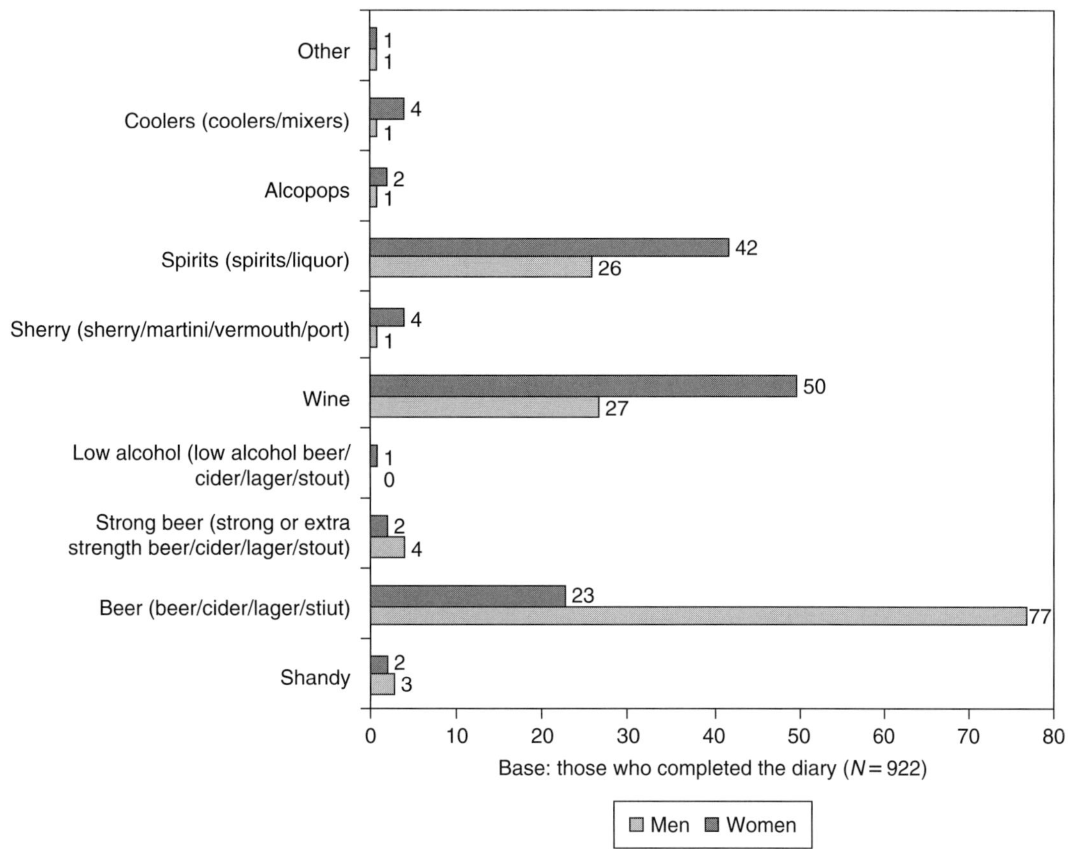

Figure 13.1 Drink of choice analyzed by sex. The graph displays the percentage of men and women who choose each type of alcoholic beverage. *Source*: HPA (2002).

Northern Ireland. One important aspect of drinking patterns is the type of drink consumed. This comprehensive survey confirmed that beer is the drink of choice for men in Northern Ireland. Figure 13.1 presents choice of drink by sex. The main drink of choice for men is beer (77%). For women the main choice of drink is wine (50%) closely followed by spirits (42%).

When investigating drinking patterns other determinants need to be taken into consideration. The HPA (2002) identified some important determinants of choice of drink and subjected their findings to statistical analysis. Table 13.3 illustrates the influence of age group, marital status, socio-economic group, household income, educational status and religious group on the choice of drink. Due to the observed difference in choice of drink between males and females the results were analyzed separately. It was observed that males under 44 years, manual workers, males educated to O level or commercial qualifications, and Catholic males were more likely to choose beer, these differences reached significance. Marital status had no impact on the choice of drinking beer.

The same analysis was performed on the responses from females and revealed that household income was the only factor to significantly influence the female's choice of drinking beer with females in the lower income categories (<£14,999) choosing to drink beer more than the females in the higher income groups (>£15,000) (see Table 13.4).

Another important factor when considering beer drinking patterns is the days of the week that alcohol is consumed. The HPA addressed this issue and revealed that beer was the most popular choice of alcoholic drink for men on each day of the week with a slight increase in popularity on a Saturday and a small decrease in popularity on a Sunday. Table 13.5 illustrates the popularity for males of each type of beverage on each day of the week.

To clarify these results further the HPA ranked the most popular drinks (see Table 13.6) on each day of the week and as expected beer is the most popular each day.

For females it was observed that wine (see Table 13.7) was the most popular choice of drink each day; however, this was closely followed by spirits. Beer was also very popular especially on a Saturday.

To clarify these results further the Health Promotion Agency ranked the most popular drinks (see Table 13.8) on each day of the week and as expected wine was the most popular drink each day with beer being ranked third each day.

Table 13.3 Drink choice for males by respondents' demographic and socioeconomic circumstance

		Beer (%)	Strong beer (%)	Wine (%)	Sherry (%)	Spirits (%)	Alcopop/ coolers (%)	Base
Age group								
	18–29	93	2	13	0	22	2	98
	30–44	83	5	28	1	19	1	167
	45–59	66	4	39	3	31	1	116
	60–75	56	3	27	0	41	0	71
Marital status								
	Single	93	5	9	1	73	2	99
	Married/cohabiting	71	4	35	1	76	1	304
	Separated/divorced	72	0	25	3	66	0	32
	Widowed	82	6	6	0	65	0	17
Socioeconomic group								
	Non-manual	68	2	45	2	25	1	211
	Manual	83	6	13	0	28	1	212
Household income								
	£25,000 or over	66	4	50	2	25	0	142
	£15,000–24,999	81	4	30	2	24	2	105
	£10,000–14,999	76	3	15	0	24	5	62
	Under £10,000	83	4	8	0	32	0	103
Educational status								
	A level/higher education	76	3	37	1	23	1	186
	O level/commercial	84	2	26	2	24	1	134
	No qualifications	70	6	14	1	33	1	132
Religious group								
	Catholic	84	2	21	1	25	2	182
	Protestant	72	6	31	1	27	<1	228

Note: The table illustrates the percentage of male respondents who choose each type of alcoholic beverage. This is presented in terms of age of respondent, their marital status, their socioeconomic group, their household income, their educational status and their religious group.
Source: HPA (2002).

Table 13.4 Drink choice for females by respondents' demographic and socioeconomic circumstance

		Beer (%)	Strong beer (%)	Wine (%)	Sherry (%)	Spirits (%)	Alcopop/ coolers (%)	Base
Age group								
	18–29	35	3	37	1	35	20	92
	30–44	27	2	57	3	37	3	208
	45–59	15	1	53	6	49	3	125
	60–75	4	0	38	13	60	0	45
Marital status								
	Single	34	2	37	2	40	20	85
	Married/cohabiting	20	1	58	4	39	3	310
	Separated/divorced	27	3	36	5	53	3	59
	Widowed	6	0	31	13	63	0	16
Socioeconomic group								
	Non-manual	18	1	61	6	38	5	284
	Manual	29	3	36	2	47	6	160
Household income								
	£25,000 or over	15	1	70	5	33	5	141
	£15,000–24,999	21	4	65	5	40	5	112
	£10,000–14,999	33	1	34	5	44	8	77
	Under £10,000	30	1	24	4	53	8	107
Educational status								
	A level/higher education	19	1	66	5	34	8	166
	O level/commercial	25	4	54	4	39	5	159
	No qualifications	26	1	28	3	55	4	145
Religious group								
	Catholic	27	3	47	1	42	6	216
	Protestant	21	1	51	7	42	5	224

Note: The table illustrates the percentage of female respondents who choose each type of alcoholic beverage. This is presented in terms of age of respondent, their marital status, their socioeconomic group, their household income, their educational status and their religious group.
Source: HPA (2002).

Table 13.5 The choice of drink for male respondents during the week

	Monday (%)	*Tuesday (%)*	*Wednesday (%)*	*Thursday (%)*	*Friday (%)*	*Saturday (%)*	*Sunday (%)*
Shandy	3	2	1	3	2	1	0
Beer	60	54	59	59	67	72	56
Strong beer	4	4	3	5	4	3	4
Low alcohol	0	0	0	0	0	0	0
Wine	18	23	23	21	16	17	36
Sherry	1	2	0	0	1	0	0
Spirits	24	25	24	22	24	23	18
Alcopops	0	0	0	0	<1	<1	<1
Coolers	0	0	0	1	0	<1	<1
Others	1	1	1	2	<1	1	2
Base (*N*)	108	92	118	117	231	342	197

Note: The table illustrates the percentage of male respondents who choose each type of alcoholic beverage on each day of the week.
Source: HPA (2002).

Table 13.6 Drink rating through the week – top three for males

Rank	*Monday*	*Tuesday*	*Wednesday*	*Thursday*	*Friday*	*Saturday*	*Sunday*
1	Beer	Beer	Beer	Beer	Beer	Beer	Beer
2	Spirits	Spirits	Spirits	Spirits	Spirits	Spirits	Wine
3	Wine	Wine	Wine	Wine	Wine	Wine	Spirits

Note: The table illustrates the rank order of drink of choice of alcoholic drink preference for males for each day of the week.
Source: HPA (2002).

Table 13.7 The choice of drink for female respondents during the week

	Monday (%)	*Tuesday (%)*	*Wednesday (%)*	*Thursday (%)*	*Friday (%)*	*Saturday (%)*	*Sunday (%)*
Shandy	1	1	1	2	<1	2	2
Beer	16	15	15	11	19	21	9
Strong beer	0	0	0	1	2	1	1
Low alcohol	0	0	0	0	0	<1	0
Wine	53	53	49	44	39	41	66
Sherry	9	7	10	5	4	2	4
Spirits	28	27	28	39	36	38	27
Alcopops	1	0	1	0	2	2	0
Coolers	3	3	0	8	6	2	0
Others	0	1	0	0	0	<1	<1
Base (*N*)	76	73	72	79	185	326	162

Note: The table illustrates the percentage of female respondents who choose each type of alcoholic beverage on each day of the week.
Source: HPA (2002).

Quantity of Consumption

As identified in previous studies Northern Ireland has a tendency to binge drinking so it is important to investigate the quantity of alcohol consumed at one sitting, when investigating beer consumption patterns. A questionnaire survey carried out in Northern Ireland in 1998 (McKinney and Coyle, 2005) employed an opportunistic sampling technique, aiming to represent students and non-students; 239 questionnaires (39.8% response rate) were returned, 108 (45.2%) from males and 131 (54.8%) from females.

The study employed a short self-report questionnaire (after Knight and Longmore, 1994, p. 97) inquiring about alcohol consumed in the previous month. The focus of this questionnaire was on identifying social drinkers in terms of volume and type of alcohol consumed, days of the week that alcohol is consumed and places where alcohol is consumed. Frequency of drinking, using the previous month as a reference, was assessed using a five-point scale. The five-point scale ranged from consuming alcohol no days in the previous month to 6–7 days per week. This information was obtained for each type of beverage beer, wine and spirits. Respondents also provided information concerning the amount of each alcoholic beverage consumed at one sitting, this ranged from no pints of beer to 8 or more pints, no glasses of wine to 15 or more and no measures of spirits to 15 or more. The question concerning place of alcohol consumption provided four choices in which alcohol is usually consumed: pub or bar, at home or the home of friends or relatives, a club or disco, somewhere else. Using the last week as a reference respondents reported on which day(s) of the week they had consumed alcohol.

Of the alcohol consumers it was revealed that Friday and Saturday are the most popular days for alcohol consumption; 59% of respondents have a drink on Friday and 73.6% have a drink on Saturday. Five-hundred and ninety one drinking events were reported for the total sample within the last month, 54% of all drinking events occur on the weekend, Friday (24%) and Saturday (30%). Thus the prevalence of weekend alcohol consumption is slightly greater than week–day alcohol consumption.

The participants who report beer consumption have the highest volume of consumption on any one occasion. As shown in Table 13.9, 32% of respondents reported the consumption of 7 or more pints (>14 units) of beer at one sitting. The highest percentage of spirit consumers also falls in the highest range, that is, 15% consume 7 or more measures of spirits. The most popular quantity of wine consumption is four glasses accounting for 11% of respondents. However 10% of respondents report wine consumption of two glasses. Thus 21% of the wine drinkers consume four or less glasses of wine at any one sitting. Thus the volume of wine consumed on any one occasion is typically lower than the volume of beer or spirits consumed on any one occasion.

Mixed Drinks

Almost half the sample reports mixing drinks (45%), that is the consumption of, for example, beer, wine and spirits on any one occasion. The most popular mix of drinks is beer and spirits accounting for 17%. A large proportion of people report consuming all three beverage types – beer, wine and spirits 12% (see Table 13.10). The least popular mix of drinks on any one drinking occasion is wine and spirits with only 6%. This is closely followed by the combination of beer and wine (9%). However the highest representation is for the consumption of beer alone (31%). That is beer drinking alone is almost twice as popular as the most popular mix of drinks (beer and spirits).

Table 13.8 Drink rating through the week – top three for females

Rank	*Monday*	*Tuesday*	*Wednesday*	*Thursday*	*Friday*	*Saturday*	*Sunday*
1	Wine	Wine	Wine	Wine	Wine	Wine	Wine
2	Spirits	Spirits	Spirits	Spirits	Spirits	Spirits	Spirits
3	Beer	Beer	Beer	Beer	Beer	Beer	Beer

Note: The table illustrates the rank order of drink of choice of alcoholic drink preference for females for each day of the week.
Source: HPA (2002).

Table 13.9 The number and percentage of participants who consume each volume of each type of beverage

	Beer			*Wine*			*Spirits*	
Pints	*N*	*%*	*Glass*	*N*	*%*	*Measure*	*N*	*%*
0	81	33.9	0	153	64	0	134	56.1
2	18	7.5	2	24	10	2	19	7.9
4	35	14.6	4	26	10.9	4	28	11.7
6	29	12.1	6	18	7.5	6	22	9.2
≥7	76	31.8	≥7	14	5.9	≥7	36	15

Note: The table illustrates the number and percentage respondents who drink each quantity ranging from 0 units to greater than or equal to 7 units of beer, wine and spirits.

Gender

Quantity Independent sample *t*-tests employed to investigate the relationship between gender and alcohol consumption. It was revealed that men consumed significantly (t (237) = 9.689, $p < 0.001$) more beer than women (female mean, 4.32 SD 5.4; male mean, 11.28 SD 5.62) per drinking occasion. And women consumed significantly (t (237) = −4.071, $p < 0.001$) more wine than men (female mean, 2.22 SD 3.10, male mean, 0.7824 SD 2.17) per drinking occasion. No difference in the volume of spirits was observed (t (237) = 0.833, $p > 0.05$). This is shown in Table 13.11.

Table 13.10 The number and percentage of participants who reported consuming each combination of mixed drinks on any drinking occasion

	N	%
Beer	74	31
Wine	26	10.9
Spirits	21	8.8
Beer and wine	16	6.7
Beer and spirits	40	16.7
Wine and spirits	14	5.9
Beer, wine and spirits	29	12.1

Note: It was observed that respondents mix their drinks. The table illustrates the number and percentage of respondents who consume each mix of beer, wine and spirits.

Frequency Independent sample *t*-tests indicated that males drank beer significantly more often than females (t (237) = −7.519, $p < 0.001$) and that females drank wine significantly more often than males (t (237) = 3.950, $p < 0.001$). Table 13.12 shows, 39% of men consume beer 6–7 days a week compared to 11% of women who consume beer daily. No significant difference between genders was revealed for the frequency of consuming spirits (t (237) = 0.240, $p > 0.05$).

Students/Non-students

Investigation into the volume of alcohol consumed revealed no difference in the volume of beer (t (220) = −0.304, $p > 0.05$) and volume of wine (t (209.280) = −1.015, $p > 0.05$)

Table 13.11 The percentage of male and female respondents who consume each volume of each beverage

Quantity Units	*Beer*		*Wine*		*Spirits*	
	Male	*Female*	*Male*	*Female*	*Male*	*Female*
0	14 (13.0)	67 (51.1)	87 (80.6)	66 (50.4)	64 (59.3)	70 (53.4)
2	3 (2.8)	15 (11.5)	9 (8.3)	15 (11.5)	10 (9.3)	9 (6.9)
4	15 (13.9)	20 (15.3)	5 (4.6)	21 (16.0)	10 (9.3)	18 (13.7)
6	15 (13.9)	14 (10.7)	5 (4.6)	13 (9.9)	10 (9.3)	12 (9.2)
≥7	61 (56.5)	15 (11.5)	2 (1.9)	16 (12.3)	14 (12.9)	22 (16.8)

Note: The table illustrates the number and percentage of males and females who drink each quantity (0 to >7 units) of beer, wine and spirits.

Table 13.12 The percentage of people who drink each mix of alcoholic beverage and the place(s) they consume alcohol

	Bar (%)	*Home (%)*	*Club (%)*	*Other (%)*
Beer	24	12	12	4
Wine	4	7	3	0
Spirits	6	4	6	0
Beer and wine	5	3	2	0
Beer and spirits	13	7	7	2
Wine and spirits	5	2	3	1
Beer, wine and spirits	10	5	4	1

Note: It was observed that almost half the sample, mix their drinks on any one drinking occasion. It was also observed that people consume alcohol in more than one place. This illustrates the places people consume alcohol, this is presented in terms of mix of drinks to illustrate that beer is the most popular choice of drink in all locations but especially in a public bar setting.

between students and non-students. However the difference in reported volume of spirits (t (220) = 2.579, $p < 0.05$) indicates that students consume more spirits than non-students. It was also observed that the frequency of drinking spirits was higher for students than non-students (t (220) = 2.14, $p < 0.05$); however, this increased frequency was not observed in beer (t (220) = −0.154, $p > 0.05$) or wine (t (220) = −1.395, $p > 0.05$) drinking.

Place of Alcohol Consumption

It has been shown that respondents tend to mix their drinks with 45% consuming more than one type of alcoholic beverage at any one sitting. It was also observed that respondent consume alcohol in more than one place. They may start drinking in their own home or the home of family or friends, then continue drinking in a pub and even proceed to a club. Table 13.12 illustrates the percentage of people who consume alcohol in either their own home or the home of family or friend, in a public bar in a club or disco or in another place. This is presented in terms of their mix of drink.

It was also observed that participants consume alcohol in more than one place. For example they may start drinking wine in their own home then continue to drink spirits in the public bar. Thus the mixing of drinks could be influenced by the place of alcohol consumption. The present author revealed that the consumption of alcohol in the pub is the most popular single setting accounting for 29% of the respondents; 14% consume alcohol only in the home and 9% consume alcohol only in a club setting; 37% consume alcohol in a pub setting in conjunction with a home setting and/or a club setting. Thus 66% of respondents consume alcohol in a pub. The choice of drink(s) and place of alcohol consumption are presented in Table 13.12. This illustrates that beer is the drink of choice for people who drink in a bar.

Conclusion

This chapter has presented evidence of the very distinctive style of drinking in Northern Ireland. It has highlighted the high, but decreasing abstinence rate. It has also highlighted the prevalence of binge drinking and the preference of beer over other beverages especially for the male alcohol consumers of Northern Ireland.

Summary Points

- 37% of male drinkers and 20% of female drinkers exceeded their weekly sensible drinking limit (21 units for men and 14 units for women) and could be referred to as risk drinkers.
- Northern Irish adults expect the consumption of alcohol to reduce anxiety and enhance sociability.
- There is a high level of abstinence in Northern Ireland approximately 30%.
- There is a high level of abnormal, problem or heavy drinking in Northern Ireland.
- A distinctive style of drinking in which more is consumed on fewer drinking occasions has also been observed.
- Beer was the most popular drink for boys in 1997, but by 2000 it has been overtaken by Alcopops.
- For 8-year-old boys who drink, Alcopops (63%) are the most popular; however, when the boys reach year 12 beer becomes the most popular drink (87%).
- In Northern Ireland the main drink of choice for men is beer (77%). For women the main choice of drink is wine (50%) closely followed by spirits (42%).
- Friday and Saturday are the most popular days for alcohol consumption; 59% of respondents have a drink on Friday and 73.6% have a drink on Saturday.
- The participants who report beer consumption have the highest volume of consumption on any one occasion, 31.8% of respondents reported the consumption of 7 or more pints (>14 units) of beer at one sitting.
- The most popular mix of drinks is beer and spirits.

References

Bennett, *et al.* (1995). *Alcohol and Alcoholism. Sensible Drinking: The Report of an Inter-Departmental Working Group*. Department of Health, London.

Blaney, R. and MacKenzie, G. (1978). A Northern Ireland Community Health Study. Department of Community Medicine, Queen's University, DHSS, Belfast.

British Medical Association (1986). Young People and Alcohol BMA science and education department. *British Medical Association*. BMA. House Tavistock Square, London.

Cahalan, D., Cisin, I. and Crossley, H. (1969). *American Drinking Practices: A National Study of Drinking Behavior and Attitudes.* Rutgers Center of Alcohol Studies, New Brunswick, NJ.

Casswell, S. (1980). 'Drinking by New Zealanders', Results of a National Survey of New Zealanders Aged 15–65 Auckland, Alcoholic Liquor Advisory Council, Wellington and the Alcohol Research Unit, 1–12.

Clark, W.B. (1977). *Contextual and Situational Variables in Drinking Behavior*. University of California, Social research group, Berkeley.

Conger, J.J. (1956). *Q. J. Stud. Alcohol* 17, 296–305.

Dight, S.E. (1976). *Scottish Drinking Habits: A Survey of Scottish Drinking Habits and Attitudes Toward Alcohol.* HMSO, Scottish Home Health Department, London.

Department of Health, Social Services and Public Safety (1998). *The drug strategy for Northern Ireland.* Belfast, UK.

Gruenewald, P.J., Johbson, F.W., Millar, A. and Mitchell, P.R. (2000). *J. Stud. Alcohol* 61, 515–523.

Harbison, J.J.M. and Haire, T. (1982). *Drinking Practices in Northern Ireland*, Belfast: Policy Planning and Research Unit.

Harford, T.C. (1983). *Int. J. Addict.* 18, 825–834.

Health Promotion Agency for Northern Ireland (HPA) (1995). Health Behaviour of School Children in Northern Ireland. A report on the 1994 survey. HPA, Belfast.

Health Promotion Agency for Northern Ireland (HPA) (2001). Health Behaviour of School Children in Northern Ireland. A report on the 1997/1998 survey. HPA, Belfast.

Health Promotion Agency for Northern Ireland (HPA) (2002). *Adult Drinking Patterns in Northern Ireland.* Health Promotion Agency for Northern Ireland, Belfast.

Health Promotion Agency for Northern Ireland (HPA) (2004). Drinking Behaviour Among Young People in Northern Ireland. Secondary analysis of alcohol data from 1997 to 2003. HPA, Belfast.

HSBC (1997). *Health Behaviour in School-aged Children: a WHO Cross-National Study (HSBC) International Report.* WHO Policy Series Health policy for Children and Adolescents Issue 1, WHO Copenhagen and www.hbsc.org.

Knight, R.G. and Longmore, B.E. (1994). *Clinical Neuropsychology of Alcoholism.* East Sussex, UK: Erlbaum.

Lange, J.E., Lauer, E.M. and Voas, B.R. (1999). *Eval. Rev.* 23, 378–398.

Marques-Vidal, P., Arveiler, D., Evans, A. *et al.* (2001). *Hypertension* 28, 1361–1366.

McKinney, A. and Coyle, C. (2005). *Subst. Use Misuse* 40, 573–579.

NISRA, Office for National Statistics, General Register Office for Scotland, Northern Ireland Statistics and Research Agency http://www.nisra.gov.uk.

O'Connor, J. (1978). *The Young Drinkers: A Cross-National Study of Social and Cultural Influences.* Tavistock Publications, Ltd, London.

Perrine, M.W. (1970). *Behav. Res. Highway Saf.* 2, 207–226.

Presley, C.A., Meilman, P.W. and Lyerla, R. (1995). *Alcohol on American College Campuses: Use, Consequences, and Perceptions of the Campus Environment.* The Core Institute Student health Programs, Southern Illinois University at Carbondale, Carbondale, IL.

Steele, C.M. and Josephs, R.A. (1988). *J. Abnorm. Psychol.* 97, 196–205.

Sweeney, K., Gillian, J. & Orr, J. (1990). Drinking habits in Northern Ireland, 1987–1989. Belfast *Policy Planning and research unit Occasional Paper 22, DHSS 1990.*

Tasplin, A.I. (1972). *Proc. Med. Inst. Russia* 110, 160–162.

The Continuous Household Survey (2006). Northern Irelands Statistics and Research Agency http://www.csu.nisra.gov.uk/surveys/survey.asp.

Wechsler, H., Davenport, A., Dowdall, G. *et al.* (1994). *JAMA* 272, 1672–1677.

Wilson, P. (1980). *Drinking in England and Wales: An Enquiry Carried Out on Behalf of the Department of Health and Social Security.* HMSO, London.

14

Beer Consumption in Teenagers in Brazzaville (Congo)

Jean Robert Mabiala Babela, Alphonse Massamba and Senga Prosper Centre Hospitalier et Universitaire, Service de Pediatrie Nourrissons, Brazzaville, Congo
Rajaventhan Srirajaskanthan Department of Nutrition and Dietetics, Kings College, London, UK

Abstract

Brazzaville is the capital of Congo, which is a central African country with a population of around 3 million. Alcohol consumption has been prevalent in the Brazzaville since the colonial period. Beer was introduced to the region during the 1950s. The annual consumption of alcohol is estimated to be 5.21 per person over the age of 15 years, however, a large proportion of the population are teenagers. Following a study done by our group we identified the extent of beer consumption amongst the teenage population. Factors such as non-schooling teenagers and orphans have a higher beer intake than teenagers attending school or teenagers with parents. Furthermore, those who practice religion have a significantly lower prevalence of beer consumption than those who do not. Within 15–19 year old age groups, the consumption of beer is marked and this leads to concerns about long-term health implications. In view of the high incidence of beer consumption, efforts to control drinking patterns amongst teenagers in Brazzaville would be prudent.

List of Abbreviations

CFA Franc	Coopération Financière en Afrique Centrale Franc
WHO	World Health Organization

Introduction

Congo is a central African country, located across the equator covering an area 342,000 km^2; the climate is consistently warm throughout the year. The population is approximately 3 million with 47% of the population being under the age of 18 years (WHO, 2004). There is a high level of urbanization with over 50% of the population living in four main cities: Brazzaville, Point Noire, Dolisie and Nkayi.

The consumption of alcohol in Congo is not a new phenomenon. Initially during the colonial period, the Congolese people consumed alcoholic drinks which were produced by fermentation of cooked cereals, palm wine or fruit juices (Bonnafe, 1988). Following the incursion of the French and Portuguese, wine, liquors and strong drinks were introduced into the region, initially in the costal regions before spreading inland (Vennetier, 1968; Phillis, 1972). Beer was introduced to the region in the 1950s. In 2002, most different types of beverage had become available in Congo, there were two breweries and wine and spirits were openly available.

Alcohol Consumption in Brazzaville

The annual consumption of alcohol is estimated to be 5.21 of alcohol per person over the age of 15 years (CNSEE, 1997). However, as stated earlier a large proportion of the Congalese population are under 15 years of age. Furthermore, in 1994 a survey of the World Health Organization (WHO) about the health of Congolese adolescents revealed that more than a third of 12 year olds from all social backgrounds are involved in the use of lawful drugs (WHO, 1994). The 2004 Global Alcohol report from the WHO showed that 3.9% of drinkers in the Congo are heavy episodic young drinkers. Its consumption is not spread in a homogenous way throughout the different regions of the country. Furthermore, it seems that within a region there are some zones with a high prevalence of youth alcohol consumption. This is associated with social deviation and/or disruption linked to alcohol consumption; one of these areas is Brazzaville, the capital city of Congo. There are a multitude of socio-economic factors that are at the origin of this phenomenon, mainly the repetition of armed conflicts which Brazzaville city was a victim. This chapter analyzes the alcohol consumption, with a specific focus on beer, in teenagers within Brazzaville.

Beer in Health and Disease Prevention
ISBN: 978-0-12-373891-2

Beer Consumption Amongst Teenagers

A study conducted by our research group over a year period from October 2004 looked at the alcohol consumption in teenagers in the seven administrative divisions of Brazzaville (see Figure 14.1). We interviewed 4,315 adolescents from various regions of Brazzaville to give us an accurate representation of drinking habits throughout the entire capital city (Hambleton *et al.*, 1995; Schienger and Dervaux, 2000). All the children and parents gave informed consent prior to interview, and interviews were carried out in the absence of parents. The study group was composed of 2,334 boys and 1,981 girls; the age range was 10–19 years.

Among the 4,315 adolescents questioned, 984 (22.8%) were drinking beer. The prevalence of beer consumption among adolescents in the seven administrative regions varied from 10.2% in Mfilou (a semi-urban area) to 28.3% in Moungali (cosmopolitan area), see Figure 14.1. This prevalence of alcohol consumption is much lower than in European countries, for example, a study by Hibbel *et al.* (1997) showed that the prevalence of alcohol consumption in 16 year olds in Denmark is 50%, Great Britain 39% and 30% in United States. There was no gender difference in the groups that were drinking. Age was a significant variable with regards to beer consumption amongst teenagers. The older the adolescent, the higher the consumption of beer ($p < 0.001$), see Table 14.1. The first contact with beer often occurred by the age of 14 years; 74.1% of children questioned had drunk beer by age of 14 years. This usually occurred in a controlled environment, for example, an anniversary, communion or gathering with peers.

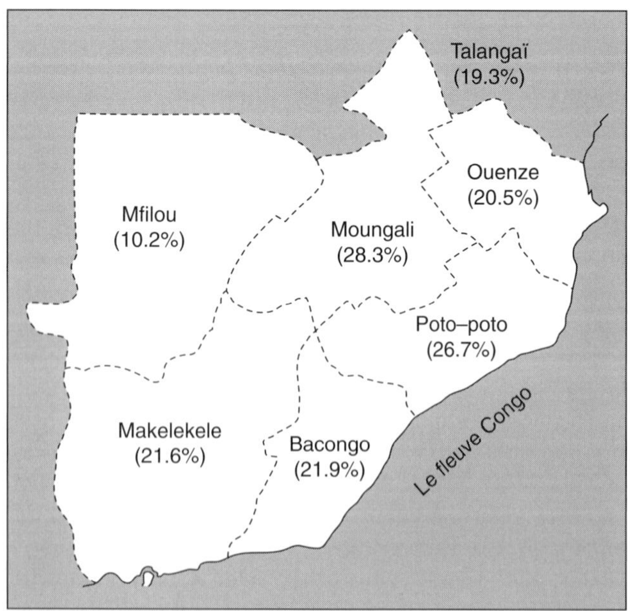

Figure 14.1 Map of Brazzaville showing the seven study sites. The prevalence of beer consumption among teenagers shown in brackets.

There was significantly higher consumption of beer in adolescents that did not attend school than those that did attend school ($p < 0.01$), see Table 14.2. Also, as would be expected there is a significantly higher percentage of children consuming alcohol at secondary school than at primary school ($p < 0.01$).

Table 14.3 indicates the different prevalence found in accordance with the socio-demographic characteristics. The beer consumption frequency among non-schooling adolescents with a weekly or monthly income was higher than that of any other group ($p < 0.05$).

Table 14.1 Prevalence as a function of gender and age

	Sample (N)	*Beer users (n)*	*Prevalence (%)*
Gender			
Male	1,981	582	24.9
Female	2,334	402	20.3
Age			
10–14 years old	2,750	323	11.7
15–19 years old	1,565	661	42.2*

Notes: Shows the number of teenagers questioned and the prevalence of beer drinking within this cohort. There is a significant difference in beer consumption between the 10–14 and 15–10 age groups.

*Significant difference at $p < 0.001$.

Table 14.2 Beer consumption related to school attendance

	Sample (N)	*Beer users (n)*	*Prevalence (%)*
Schooling	3,622	701	19.3
Primary level	1,333	141	10.5
Secondary level	2,289	560	24.4
Non-schooling	693	283	40.8
With pocket money	384	164	42.7
No pocket money	309	119	38.5

Table 14.3 Prevalence as a function of socio-cultural status

	Sample (N)	*Beer users (n)*	*Prevalence (%)*
Religious practice			
Yes	4,168	894	21.4
No	147	90	61.2*
Parental structure			
Living with their parents	2,194	378	17.2
Divorced parents	1,114	259	23.2
Orphaned	1,007	347	34.4**

Notes: A significant difference was illustrated between those who practice religion and those that do not. Orphaned teenagers have a significantly higher prevalence of beer consumption than those with parents.

*Significant difference at $p < 0.05$.

**Significant difference at $p < 0.001$.

There was a significant ($p < 0.001$) relation between abstinence to beer consumption and religious practice, in that those that are religious have a lower rate of consuming beer, see Table 14.3. The consumption of beer was higher among adolescents with one or more parents deceased ($p < 0.001$); whilst children with united families presented a low prevalence 17.2%.

With regard to the types of beer consumption, see Table 14.4, they were variable amongst different groups. Moderate drinkers constituted the majority, whatever the light ale beer is the dominant in the regular consumption (95.4%). In those that use alcohol continually the most commonly used beer was mainly brown ale beer (4.6%). The regular and excessive consumption of beer was most commonly seen amongst boys in comparison to girls ($p < 0.005$). There was also a relation between the mode of consumption and the age.

Regular and excessive drinkers were found in a large number of subjects between 15 and 19 years of age. As for the regular weekly consumption of beer, it approached 100–300 g in 52.7% of cases, with the top volume of consumption of 1,000 g for 1.1% of teenagers. The average intake of beer was different amongst boys (17.4 ± 3.1 g/day) and girls (9.2 ± 0.7 g/day). The univariate analysis revealed that boys drunk more beer than the girls ($p < 0.001$). As for the frequency of becoming drunk, it was more important among boys: 49.2% of them confessed to have been drunk on beer more than twice, against 11.9% of girls. Finally, regular and excessive drinkers were found frequently ($p < 0.01$) amongst non-schooling young people.

Underlying Causes for Teenage Drinking

The consumption of beer increases with age (Arènes *et al.*, 1998; Laure *et al.*, 2001), this pattern is seen in other countries, for example, in Canada from 40% in 12 year olds to 84% in 19 year olds (Adlaf *et al.*, 1999). The growth of prevalence with age is clearly connected to the psychological development stage of adolescents (Bandura, 1980; Damon, 1983).

Some variables can play the role of activator or of moderator in development of beer consumption, four clear variables have been identified, these are: school environment, family background, socio-economic status and way of life (Ferreol, 1999). It has been shown in other countries as well as in Brazzaville that children in primary and secondary school have lower consumption of beer compared to non-schoolers. However, this in part is due to the fact that non-school attenders are usually older. In the Congo, school is compulsory till the age of 15 years. Among non-schooling teenagers, there are multiple reasons for increased beer consumption, first, they usually work and earn an income, thereby, buying beer from their own income. Idleness amongst those without income can also lead to drinking.

A study by Isohanni *et al.* (1994) in Finland noted that the children whose parents are divorced or one of them deceased are more exposed to the consumption of beer and to the drunkenness experience. Our work has shown that the consumption of beer among the adolescents is influenced by those of close persons. It is in fact established that the alcoholism of parents has more impact than the one of the brothers or friends. This is a direct correlation between the ages a child has initial contact with individuals who abuse alcohol and the age at which the child starts consuming beverages. So children exposed to alcoholic parents or relatives at a young age start drinking at an earlier age.

Teenage drinking in Brazzaville follows certain patterns which are gender specific. These patterns pertain to types of beer consumed, frequency and volume of beer consumption and age of commencement of beer drinking (see Figures 14.2 and 14.3). These teenager gender specific patterns have been reported in other studies, for example Harford (1976), Donovan *et al.* (1983), Parquet *et al.* (1986) and Bailly (1999). The reasons for the underlying differences

Table 14.4 Survey of consumption

	Lager beer (%)	*Brown ale beer (%)*	*Imported lager beer (%)*	*Imported brown beer (%)*
Frequency				
Occasional	13.6	43.5	63.7	12.2
Moderate	57.4	35.2	24.1	81.6
Regular	23.9	20.8	11.8	2.3
Abuse	5.1	0.5	0.4	0.9
*Volume**				
<100 g	12.3	30.6	47.4	35.8
100–300 g	70.2	53.2	35.1	52.3
300–500 g	10.5	9.7	12.8	8.6
500–700 g	5.1	5.2	4.8	2.8
>700 g	1.9	1.3	0.9	0.5

Notes: Consumption of imported beer is relatively uncommon especially amongst those with the highest beer consumption. Imported beers are predominately consumed by occasional and moderate drinkers.

*Volume (in gram) of pure alcohol consumed in 1 week.

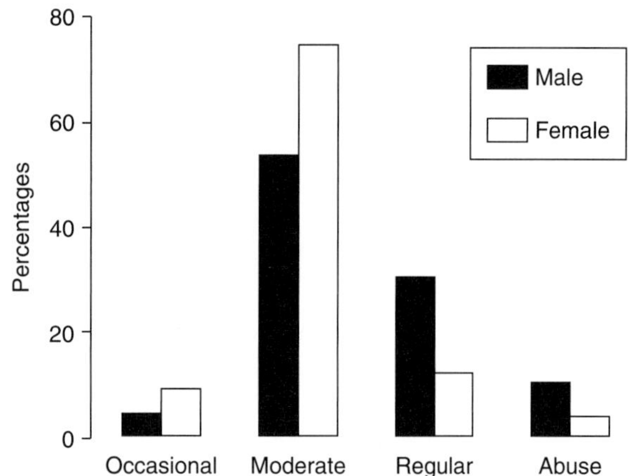

Figure 14.2 Evolution of alcoholic practices shown by gender. A larger percentage of men drink with a regular and heavy frequency than compared to women.

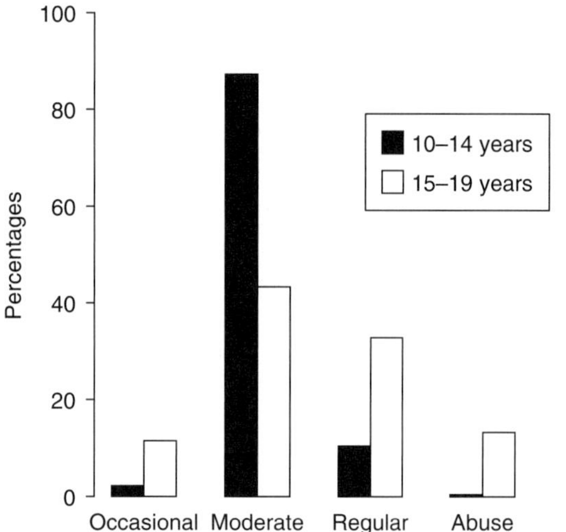

Figure 14.3 Evolution of alcoholic practices separated by age. The majority of 10–14 year olds that drink consume beer on a moderate basis. Heavy intake of beer is almost sorely amongst the 15–19 year old cohort.

between consumption patterns and between the sexes are complex. In part, it is thought to be that from an early age and throughout adolescence, children attain insight into the acceptable behavior and roles of each gender. The figures or role models that provide most of this insight are parents, siblings, peers and institutions. The children then learn to express their interpretation of accepted behavior patterns within society. Beer consumption is a specific type of behavior and different beer consumption practices are accepted for boys and girls. Furthermore, in Congo the social acceptance of the teenagers drinking behavior is almost more important than the legal aspects, since there is an absence of legal law and its enforcement with regards to alcohol consumption (Nsika Nkaya, 1985).

In view of this social system, it is unsurprising that teenagers that have finished school, who are therefore, likely to be older have a higher alcohol intake than those at school. One would expect them to follow different social patterns and in some way follow adult behavior traits. Furthermore, differences seen in regional zones with regard to alcohol consumption would be expected, since they correlate with the socio-demographics and structural characteristics of the region (Sokal and Rohlf, 1969). The region with the highest number of teenage drinkers has the highest population density and the largest number of drink retailers. In addition, the less activities and sport venues available to teenagers have a higher number of regular teenager beer drinkers.

Type of Beer Consumption Amongst Teenagers

As stated earlier light ale beer is the most consumed drink in Brazzaville (Table 14.4); it is also advertised mainly on television. However, there is also a consumption of brown ale and imported beers. This is of some concern because brown ale locally brewed has higher alcohol content than the light ale. The light ale is usually 3–6% alcohol by volume, whilst the brown ale is 6–9% alcohol by volume. The consumption of the stronger beer by adolescents is associated with bad social behavior traits, as well as higher sexual activity and increased rates of delinquency. The price difference between the light beer (500 CFA) and the brown ale (600 CFA) is only 100 CFA, therefore, in teenagers that wish to become drunk, or suffer from alcohol dependence, there is only a relatively small price difference for much stronger beer.

Of some concern is that in 19 year old boys and girls the daily consumption that is being reported at 25.3 ± 2.8 g and 12.1 ± 0.5 g, respectively, is higher than that reported by in the same age group in France (Rigaud *et al.*, 1997). Since France has one of the highest rates of alcohol consumption in the world, it is of concern that within the Congo where medical facilities are not the same, teenagers are consuming large volumes of alcohol. This could potentially lead to high rates of cirrhosis in this group of individuals over the next 10–15 years; unfortunately, they will not have access to the same quality of medical care and support that is available in European countries, with similar rates of alcohol consumption.

Conclusion

The consumption of beer amongst Congolese teenagers is alarming; especially, the high levels being consumed by non-school attending teenagers. If these teenagers continue this level of consumption, a large number will eventually develop medical complications related to alcohol abuse. Government need to address this emerging problem with the adoption of legislative measures to stop teenagers being able to purchase alcohol and also prohibit them from entering drinking premises. In addition, there is a need for education amongst teenagers of the long-term detrimental effects of alcohol.

Summary Points

- Drinking amongst teenagers in Brazzaville increases with age in both boys and girls.
- The behavioral practices of boys and girls differ with regards to consumption of beer.
- There is increased incidence of teenagers drinking in poorer and more urbanized areas, with higher population density.
- In teenagers that do not attend school, the frequency and volume of beer consumption is highest.
- The total weekly consumption of 19 year olds in Brazzaville is comparable to that of Western European countries.
- Efforts to reduce teenage drinking within the Congo need to be implemented to tackle the problem of teenage drinking.

References

Adlaf, E.M., Paglia, A. and Ivis, F. (1999). *Document de recherche du CISM n°5*. Centre de toxicomanie et de Santé, Toronto, Ontario.

Arènes, J., Janvrin, M.P. and Baudier, F. (1998). *Baromètre Santé Jeunes 97/98*. Comité Français d'Education pour la Santé, Vanves.

Bailly, D. (1999). *J. Pediatr. Puériculture* 12, 37–42.

Bandura, A. (1980). *L'apprentissage social*. Mardaga, Paris.

Bonnafe, P. (1988). *Histoire social d'un people congolais*. Orstom Editions, Paris.

Centre National de la Statistique et des Etudes Economiques (1997). La République du Congo en quelques chiffres, 1996. Ministère de l'économie et des Finances, chargé du Plan et de la Prospective, Brazzaville.

Damon, W. (1983). Social and personality development: infancy through adolescence. Norton, New York.

Donovan, J., Jessor, R. and Jessor, L. (1983). *J. Stud. Alcohol* 44, 109–137.

Ferreol, G. (1999). *Adolescence et toxicomanie*. Colin, Paris.

Hambleton, R.K., Swaminathan, H., Algina, J. and Coulson, D. (1995). Criterion-referenced testing and measurement. Review of technical issues and developments. Report of the Annual Meeting of the American Statistical Research Association. American Statistical Research Association, Washington, DC.

Harford, J.C. (1976). *J. Stud. Alcohol* 37, 1747–1750.

Hibbel, B., Anderson, B. and Bjarnasson, T., *et al.* (1997). The 1995 ESPAD Report: the European school survey project on alcohol and other drug–alcohol and other drug use among students in 26 European countries. The Swedish council for information on alcohol and other drugs: CAN – Council of Europe: cooperation group to combat drug abuse and illicit trafficking in drug (Pampidou group).

Isohanni, M. *et al.* (1994). *Soc. Sci. Med.* 38, 715–722.

Laure, P., Lecerf, T. and Le Scanff, C. (2001). *Arch. Pédiatr.* 8, 16–24.

Nsika Nkaya, H. (1985). *Annales de l'Université Marien Ngouabi (Brazzaville) – série Littératures, Langue et Sciences Humaines* 1, 29–43.

Parquet, P.J., Bailly, D., Lejeune, D. and Gignac, C. (1986). *Ann. Pédiatr.* 33, 635–660.

Phillis, M. (1972). *The External Trade of the Lwangu Coast (1576–1870)*. University Press of Oxford, Oxford.

Rigaud, D. *et al.* (1997). *Cah. Nutr. Diet.* 32, 379–384.

Schlienger, J.L. and Dervaux, T. (2000). *Rev. Prat. (Paris)* 50, 209–216.

Sokal, R.F. and Rohlf, S.W. (1969). *Biometry*. Freeman and Co, San Francisco, CA.

Vennetier, P. (1968). *Pointe-Noire et la façade maritime du Congo*. Orstom Editions, Paris.

World Health Organization (1994). *Santé des adolescents au Congo. Analyse de la situation*. Organisation Mondiale de la Santé, Brazzaville.

World Health Organization (2004). Global Alcohol Report.

15

Personality Characteristics Associated with Drinking and Beverage Preference

Colin R. Martin Psychology Group, Faculty of Health, Leeds Metropolitan University, Leeds, UK

Abstract

The study of psychological aspects of alcohol consumption and, in particular, alcohol dependence and problem drinking has produced a vast and broad quantity of research findings over the past 50 years. However, in spite of the breadth of research conducted in this important area of applied psychology, comparatively little research has been conducted into the relationship of personality characteristics and beverage and beer preference. This chapter seeks to highlight some of the significant relationships that have been observed between alcohol beverage choice and selection and personality characteristics and style. Given the relative dearth of robust findings in the area of alcohol beverage choice and psychological factors, the context for this present state of affairs is also explored by highlighting competing and contrasting models of alcohol consumption and abuse in addition to highlighting areas of future research endeavor in this surprisingly under-researched area.

Introduction

This chapter will explore personality attributes associated with drinking behavior and drinking preferences, particularly the characteristics that may influence the main beverage choice of the individual, whether it be beer, wine or spirits. To explore these issues within a coherent psychological context, it is important to establish key factors which have been influential in the development of important personality insights central to the manifestation of drinking behavior and beverage preference. Psychology as a scientific and evidence-based discipline has attempted to determine these pertinent personality characteristics through experimentation and social and clinical observation. The psychological heritage in this area is extensive and complex; however, the milestones encountered in the understanding of drinking behavior from a psychological perspective have also highlighted fundamental omissions in the understanding of personality attributes in certain areas, particularly beverage preferences. There are very good and rationale reasons why this has been the case to date but fortunately, the sophistication of methodological approaches used in this research arena have started to yield valuable and robust insights within the psychological processes and characteristics which influence beverage choice. To understand this fascinating and important story within a coherent and understandable context, the historical perspectives and contemporary approaches to understanding personality antecedents to drinking behavior and beverage preference will be explored. Examination of these factors within this framework will be invaluable in allowing the reader to develop an understanding of not only drinking style and beverage preferences as behavioral end-points, but also an appreciation of the contribution of psychology to separating the normal from the pathological, the hazardous from the hazard-free in the constellation of fundamental personality attributes enmeshed within the complex behavior known as drinking alcohol.

A Psychology of Drinking Behavior

Investigation of the personality and behavioral characteristics of abstinence, normative drinking and pathological drinking has been a key psychological endeavor for clinical researchers for decades (Martin and Bonner, 2005). The historical perspective of psychological study of drinking has, as a modus operandi, the main tenet of psychological science, namely to understand and predict behavior and ultimately to modify it. Unsurprisingly, this enterprise has had as a central focus, a pressing clinical agenda, brought into sharp relief by the huge social, occupational and health consequences of problematic drinking behavior, often encapsulated within the disease concept of "alcoholism" (Jellinek, 1960; Lender, 1979; Piazza and Wise, 1988). The disease model of alcoholism has created a lasting enigma for both the practice of evidence-based medicine and the provision of effective therapeutic intervention. The disease

Beer in Health and Disease Prevention
ISBN: 978-0-12-373891-2

model of alcoholism has also enabled and facilitated psychological science to develop alternative approaches to the disease model of alcoholism that have the identification of personality characteristics which are consistently associated with drinking behavior and preference choice. Prior to proceeding further, it is crucial to reflect on what the disease model of alcoholism is, why it has been needed, how it has endured and how it has facilitated and often driven the development of psychological alternatives to it.

The Disease Model of Alcoholism

The disease model of alcoholism represents a paradox for modern medicine and indeed modern clinical science. The paradox is patently clear within the context of modern medical practice in the area as an evidence-based discipline. The disease model of alcoholism posits that there is a key biological characteristic that distinguishes those people that drink unproblematically and socially, from those that drink hazardously, abusively and ultimately chemically dependent (Jellinek, 1960). Despite the dominance of this model since at least the 1960s, there is absolutely no evidence at all for the notion of a unitary biological antecedent factor that causes the "disease of alcoholism." Jellinek's (1960) model and subsequent developments of it are paradoxical in many respects since the classification system proposed to identify clusters of drinkers includes definable group with critical psychological[1] rather than biological features of presentation (alpha alcoholism) and who could stop if the individual really wanted to! To put this in perspective, the model describes these sub-types in a progressive way leading through the sub-types to increasingly catastrophic drinking. Surprisingly, the focus of this model pays no head to the particular beverage of choice, only that the disease is specific to alcohol. It is readily acknowledged that there are genetic, social, biological and psychological features which may influence the development of problematic drinking (Wallace, 1990; Orford and Velleman, 1991; Zucker *et al.*, 1994); however, in no way could any of these characteristics can be described as having the attributes of a causative biological entity. The consequences of a disease model of alcoholism are highly constrictive to the patient with the "illness" since there is no "cure" to be had, only a lifestyle of abstinence from alcohol, punctuated with periods of "remission" and sadly, "relapse." The disease model does satisfy an agenda of offering treatment to those who have alcohol problems as a disease rather than through choice. Thus the disease model "gives permission" to offer treatment to individuals who would be unlikely to receive medical intervention if their drinking behavior was attributed to their own choice. The focus on the disease model notion

[1]Thus, it could be argued that Jellinek's model was actually a biopsychosocial model rather than a disease model *per se*.

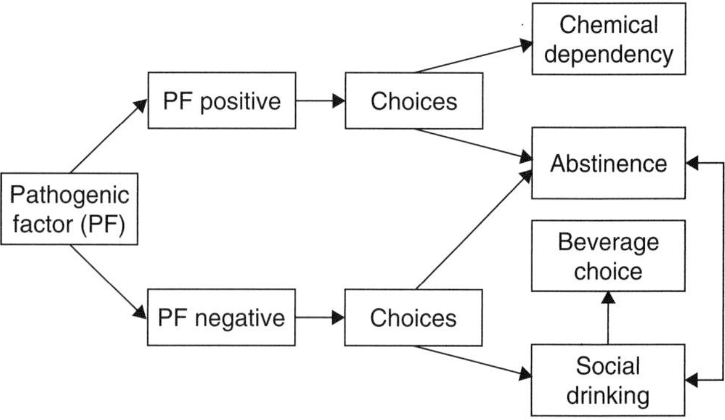

Figure 15.1 The disease model of alcoholism. Only in the case of the individual without the pathogenic factor for alcoholism does beverage choice have any salience.

that alcoholics have no choice or free will in their alcohol pursuits also by implication negates any issues of beverage preference, the goal of the alcoholic being to maintain a significant blood alcohol level. The disease model is described in Figure 15.1.

The medical model of alcoholism is still influential today and a central part of self-help organizations such as Alcoholics Anonymous. The insufficiencies in the evidence for a medical model have led to the development of a number of models of problematic drinking as either a psychodynamic issue or (more commonly) a behavioral problem (Wilson, 1977; Hays, 1985; Vuchinich and Tucker, 1988; Smith and Goldman, 1994; Leonard and Blane, 1999). Contemporary psychological models emphasize that hazardous and chemically dependent drinking is a behavioral problem and that the problem behavior can be modified and extinguished. This psychological perspective on the presentation of problem behavior has facilitated the development of a number of effective psychological interventions for those encountering problematic drinking (Thevos *et al.*, 2000; Ness and Oei, 2005; Kavanagh *et al.*, 2006). Importantly, these psychological interventions may have, as an end-point, a return to controlled responsible drinking, whereby the individual will have a choice over what to drink within firmly proscribed parameters of amount in units. However, even within the most sophisticated psychological models, including those that integrate psychological, personality and biological processes in describing problematic drinking, the issues associated with the choice of beverage is rarely seen. Indeed, the most recent model of psychobiological model of alcohol dependency that includes personality characteristics does not include beverage selection as an integral feature to its overall structure (see Figure 15.2).

Personality Traits and Beverage Choice

The main substantive psychological literature in relation to beverage selection concerns personality traits. The notion

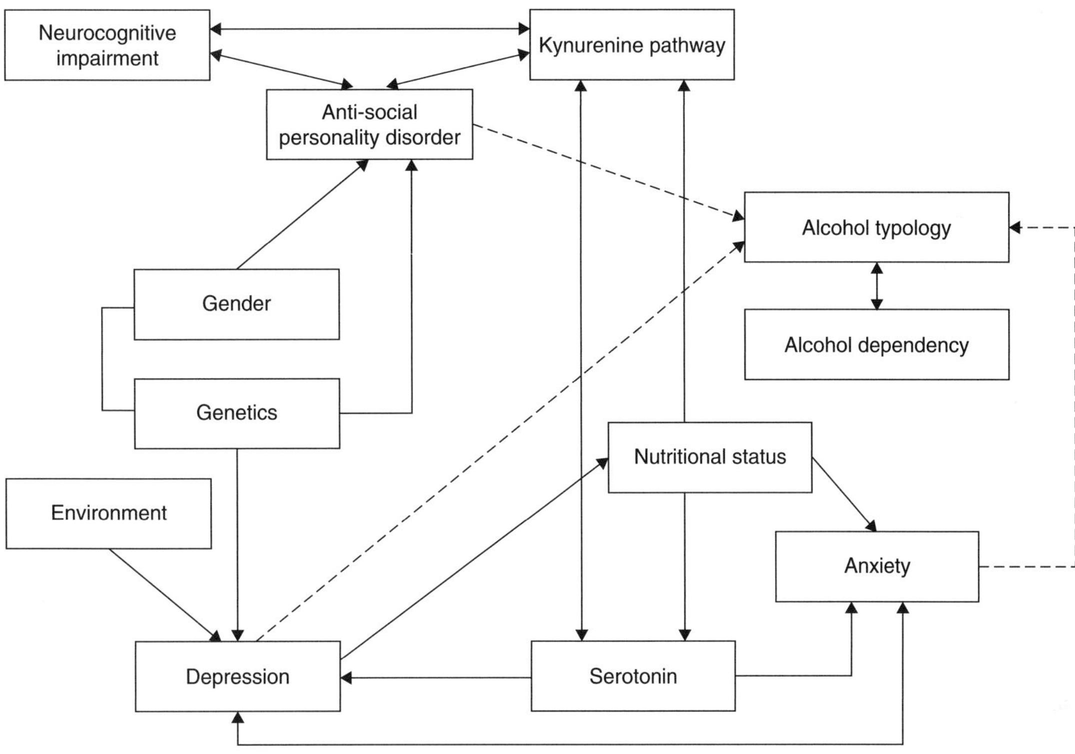

Figure 15.2 Martin and Bonner's (2005) psychobiological model of alcohol dependency. Beverage choice selection is absent within the model, an omission common to psychological models of excessive drinking.

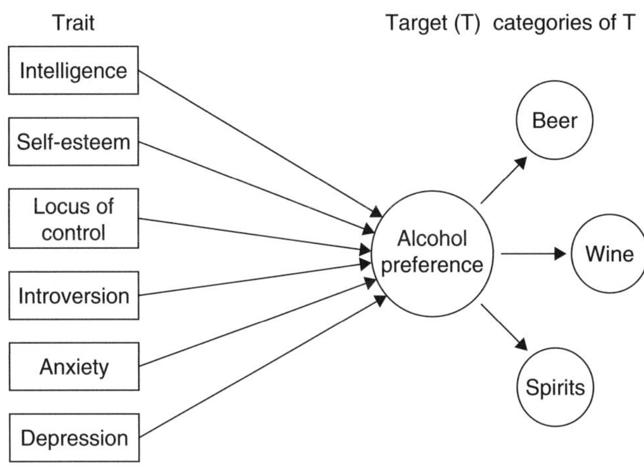

Figure 15.3 A multiple logistic regression predicting beverage preference from personality trait characteristics. The relative contribution of individual traits can be evaluated in terms of their influence on alcohol preference. Cumulative effects of traits can also be evaluated using regression modeling.

of the personality trait is important to psychology because it has a number of key functions. Personality traits do not seek to explain the whole personality, rather they seek to identify key attributes which are stable, measurable, behaviorally influential and predictive. The characteristics of the attributes described are very powerful elements in accounting for behavioral outcomes and also for identifying between groups differences, for example intelligence is a trait personality characteristic and has been found to be predictive of the choice of beer individuals choose to drink (Mortensen *et al.*, 2005). Importantly, though personality traits generally represent uni-dimensional constructs, they can be usefully combined in predictive analysis to determine not only any (statistically) significant predictive value of a personality trait on a target behavior, but also the relative contribution of a personality trait, compared to other personality traits, in predicting a behavioral outcome. The statistical approach taken is multiple linear and multiple logistic regression. To explore which personality traits influenced drinking preference and how important they were to this target behavior, a multiple logistic regression would be used. A hypothetical model of multiple logistic regression model to determine the contribution of personality traits to alcoholic beverage choice is shown in Figure 15.3. Statistical *t*-values and p-values are calculated for each predictor variable (personality traits) in the model. The target variable comprises categorical classifications of beverage preference. Predictor variables are analogs to independent variables and the target variable is analogs to a dependent variable. This approach to modeling is very powerful and has been underutilized in research on alcohol beverage preference to date, though this situation is fortunately changing as the power of this approach becomes increasingly widely recognized.

Personality Characteristics Associated with Alcoholic Beverage Preference

A number of personality characteristics have been identified which discriminate between non-drinkers and drinkers, and drinkers with different beverage preferences. Some of these characteristics cover a number of personality, neurocognitive and neurophysiological domains. Intelligence is a key example of this, certainly, since it is recognized that intelligence does demonstrate the key characteristics of a personality trait including stability, measureability, and is often behaviorally predictive in combination with other personality traits.

Intelligence

Mortensen *et al.* (2005) conducted a large sample study (>1,700) following up men who had been tested for their intelligence quotient (IQ) in early adulthood and the relationship between this and drinking preferences several years later. These researchers found a significant association between IQ and later beverage preference. It was observed that a high IQ was associated with a preference for wine over both beer and spirits. Importantly, IQ was not found to be associated with heavy drinking nor was the IQ advantage of wine drinkers over beer and spirit drinkers associated with socio-economic factors. This important and indeed provocative study has highlighted robust and impressive evidence that beer and spirit drinkers have a lower intelligence than wine drinkers. The findings of this European study were limited by a participant population that was exclusively male; however, extension of this study design to females would be highly desirable to determine how generalizable this finding may be. Intelligence is a key individual differences variable and ultimately mediated by neurophysiological processes and structures. The findings from this study therefore would indicate that preference for beer over wine or vice versa may be potentially "hard-wired" within the brain and involves genetic antecedents.

Contrasting with the findings of Mortensen *et al.* (2005), a study recently conducted in the United States by Paschall and Lipton (2005) revealed that beer drinkers were less educated than wine drinkers. A similar association between beer drinking and lower education was found by McCann *et al.* (2003). These findings may initially seem to support those of Mortensen *et al.* (2005); however, it should be acknowledged that more education is by no means equivalent to more IQ and may be more representative of social opportunity. This distinction also serves to remind that the implications of personality traits are of far greater significance than socio-demographic variables in understanding the intra-personal aspects of beverage preference. Further, the neurophysiological corollaries of personality traits such as intelligence also furnish a pathway between the psychology of beverage preference and the biology of problematic drinking. It has, for example, been observed that beer drinkers are at greater risk of becoming excessive drinkers compared to wine drinkers (Jensen *et al.*, 2002). It would therefore be anticipated that personality variables that have associations between both beverage preference and biological substrates (e.g. intelligence) may be potent and useful markers of broader psychobiological processes. Indeed, this informed conjecture is central to the psychobiological model of alcohol dependency proposed by Martin and Bonner (2005).

Negative evaluation

Negative evaluation, the individuals' perception of how they are seen and evaluated by others, also has many characteristics common to a definition of a personality trait. Certainly, some individuals perceive and fear negative evaluation more than others, therefore negative evaluation represents an enduring individual differences variable. The concept of negative evaluation is also stable across time and conditions, thus confirming the status of the concept as a personality trait. Finally, consistent with personality traits, the fear of negative evaluation will influence behavior. Experimental work has identified a powerful effect of negative evaluation on beer selection specific to females. Corcoran and Segrist (1998) found that in a beverage selection experiment, females with elevated levels of fear of negative evaluation selected beer significantly less often from a selection that included beer among a selection of alcohol-free drinks such as Coke light, tonic water and pineapple juice. This behavioral effect of fear of negative evaluation was not observed in males suggesting an influential gender-specific role of this personality trait in beer selection. Further, research is required in this area to determine the impact of this pervasive trait on actual beer drinking behavior in social settings.

Depression

Depression is often considered within the context of clinical classification for diagnosis, but it should be borne in mind that there is a basal level of depression within the individual which is usually stable over time and a component part of human psychological functioning. Depression then is a personality characteristic and is related to other key psychological domains which also have enduring trait qualities, such as dispositional optimism, dispositional pessimism and anhedonia. Depression is often co-morbid with a diagnosis of alcohol dependency (Martin and Bonner, 2000; Le Fauve *et al.*, 2004; Pettinati, 2004; Lukassen and Beaudet, 2005) and there is consequently a rich ancestry of research exploring the relationship between depression and alcohol dependency. The role of depression on beverage selection is less well explored, however tantalizing insights into the role of depression on beverage selection can be deduced by examination of data from suicide rate studies. This is based on the premise that depression and suicide are associated, since many individuals who chose to end their lives are clearly depressed. Gruenewald *et al.* (1995) in large-scale population study conducted in the United States found that suicide rates were not associated with beer drinking; however, a significant increase in suicides was associated with the purchase and consumption of spirits. This study highlights that it is not ethanol *per se* that impacts on the occurrence and prevalence of suicide, but the form of beverage itself is key. This leads to the very real consideration and possibility of an important association between increased depression and spirit preference compared to beer preference.

Anxiety

Anxiety is a key co-morbid clinical presentation associated with both alcohol dependence and alcohol abuse (Allan, 1995; Martin and Bonner, 2000; Schade *et al.*, 2003; Baigent, 2005). Importantly, anxiety in individuals with alcohol dependency commonly comprises two distinct components. These components are either physiological autonomic manifestations of anxiety symptoms, often exacerbated during withdrawal of alcohol and detoxification, in effect a central nervous system rebound effect. However, a more enduring anxiety component has been observed in individuals with alcohol dependency which represents a relative elevated trait characteristic that is largely independent of the level of alcohol in the bloodstream or the kinetic properties of alcohol metabolism during withdrawal or consumption. This component of anxiety has been associated with relapse as alcohol may be used as a maladaptive attempt at "self-medication" by the individual (Thomas *et al.*, 2003; Tomlinson *et al.*, 2006). Indeed, therapeutic programs aimed at reducing relapse emphasize the importance of anxiety management techniques as integral aspect of treatment. Given the importance and relevance of anxiety to alcohol-related problems, it is surprising to discover a relative dearth of research in the area of anxiety and alcohol preference. However, given the potent effect of alcohol as a central nervous system depressant, the type of beverage, beer, wine, spirits, etc. chosen may actually be immaterial as the goal-seeking behavior of the individual may be primarily geared toward access to ethanol rather than a specific beverage to exploit the potent central nervous system effects of ethanol as a depressant. Clearly, more research is necessary to explore the possible relationships between beverage type and anxiety in selection of a drink of choice and any interaction between alcohol type, anxiety and the problematic compared to non-problematic drinking style.

Motivation

Increasing over recent years within the clinical and health psychology, literature on individual differences factors in relation to health and disease behaviors is a focus on motivational aspects. The role of motivational factors in drinking behavior has been of relevance to the study of psychological aspects of drinking behavior is of particular relevance due to the concept of motivation being key in the treatment of individuals presenting with alcohol abuse and dependency. Motivation to drink has been associated with alcohol preference and as such motivation assumes key status as a behavioral variable of important interest to understanding both normative and problematic decision making in the realm of alcohol consumption. However, before elaborating further, it is of value to reflect that in the points made to beverage preference and anxiety and depression made earlier, motivational factors will inevitably be concurrent with the affective presentation of an individual. Beer and spirit consumption has been shown to be associated with problematic drinking styles compared to other types of alcohol (Clapp and Shillington, 2001). This is an interesting finding, since it immediately raises the issues of preference beyond the constraints of the physiological aspects of the blood alcohol curve, since the profile would be different between beer and spirits as a function of proof volume. However, motivation remains an illusive and multi-factorial construct psychologically, strongly influenced by dispositional, environmental and social factors and as such, robustly implicating motivational factors causally and uni-directionally within an alcohol preference model is likely to remain difficult for some time.

Summary

This chapter has highlighted some of the more interesting and relatively more important psychological dimensions that may have an influence of alcohol beverage and beer choice. A surprising finding is not only how little primary research has been conducted in the psychological arena on alcohol beverage and beer preference characteristics in relation to personality, but also the *relatively* small amount of research conducted compared to a strong body of evidence implicating personality characteristics and individual differences attributes with problem in drinking behavior. Consequently, no firm conclusions can be made regarding personality characteristics and beer preference. Where relationships are found to exist, these seem to represent psychological domains that often lie beyond the bounds of what may be termed exclusively a personality characteristic or attribute, for example in the case of intelligence.

It is enlightening that given the huge industrial base and financial rewards associated with alcohol and beer commercial enterprise, evaluation of personality characteristics which may be associated with beverage choice seems largely ignored and under-researched. In addressing such a vacuum of research and the need and desirability to redress this in the future, the author is minded to comment that such research enterprise should be approached with both investigative zeal and moral responsibility since the relationship between non-problematic alcohol use and alcohol abuse can represent a gray and overlapping area.

A final recommendation is therefore that the issues of personality characteristics and beer preference require further systematic investigation to determine the relationship of these enduring psychological domains to alcoholic choice and beverage selection decision making and further, that such endeavor should be done within the context of a coherent theoretical account and psychological model.

Summary Points

- The relationship between alcohol beverage preference and personality characteristics is currently under-researched.
- A small number of personality characteristics have been found to be associated with beer/alcohol type preference.
- The focus of research into personality characteristics associated with alcohol consumption has largely ignored the issue of alcohol beverage type.
- The clinical/applied bias in research may be responsible for the dearth of research in the area of personality characteristics and alcohol beverage choice.
- There is a pressing need to address through systematic research the absence of robust and replicable findings in the area of personality characteristic and beverage choice.

References

Allan, C.A. (1995). *Alcohol Alcohol.* 30, 141–151.

Baigent, M.F. (2005). *Curr. Opin. Psychiatr.* 18, 223–228.

Clapp, J.D. and Shillington, A.M. (2001). *Am. J. Drug Alcohol Abuse* 27, 301–313.

Corcoran, K.J. and Segrist, D.J. (1998). *Addict. Behav.* 23, 509–515.

Franken, I.H., Muris, P. and Georgieva, I. (2006). *Addict. Behav.* 31, 399–403.

Gruenewald, P.J., Ponicki, W.R. and Mitchell, P.R. (1995). *Addiction* 90, 1063–1075.

Hays, R. (1985). *Br. J. Addict.* 80, 379–384.

Jellinek, E.M. (1960). *The Disease Concept of Alcoholism.* College and University Press, New Haven, CT.

Jensen, M.K., Andersen, A.T., Sorensen, T.I., Becker, U., Thorsen, T. and Gronbaek, M. (2002). *Epidemiology* 13, 127–132.

Kavanagh, D.J., Sitharthan, G., Young, R.M., Sitharthan, T., Saunders, J.B., Shockley, N. and Giannopoulos, V. (2006). *Addiction* 101, 1106–1116.

Le Fauve, C.E., Litten, R.Z., Randall, C.L., Moak, D.H., Salloum, I.M. and Green, A.I. (2004). *Alcohol. Clin. Exp. Res.* 28, 302–312.

Lender, M.E. (1979). *J. Stud. Alcohol* 40, 361–375.

Leonard, K.E. and Blane, H.T. (eds) (1999). *Psychological Theories of Drinking and Alcoholism.* Guilford Press, New York.

Lukassen, J. and Beaudet, M.P. (2005). *Soc. Sci. Med.* 61, 1658–1667.

Martin, C.R. and Bonner, A.B. (2000). *Alcohol Alcohol.* 35, 49–51.

Martin, C.R. and Bonner, A.B. (2005). *Curr. Psychiatr. Rev.* 1, 303–312.

McCann, S.E., Sempos, C., Freudenheim, J.L., Muti, P., Russell, M., Nochajski, T.H., Ram, M., Hovey, K. and Trevisan, M. (2003). *Nutr. Metab. Cardiovasc. Dis.* 13, 2–11.

Mortensen, L.H., Sorensen, T.I. and Gronbaek, M. (2005). *Addiction* 100, 1445–1452.

Ness, M.L. and Oei, T.P. (2005). *Am. J. Addict.* 14, 139–154.

Orford, J. and Velleman, R. (1991). *Br. J. Med. Psychol.* 64, 189–200.

Paschall, M. and Lipton, R.I. (2005). *Drug Alcohol Depend.* 78, 339–344.

Pettinati, H.M. (2004). *Biol. Psychiatr.* 56, 785–792.

Piazza, N.J. and Wise, S.L. (1988). *Int. J. Addict.* 23, 387–397.

Schade, A., Marquenie, L.A., Van Balkom, A.J., De Beurs, E., Van Dyck, R. and Van Den Brink, W. (2003). *Alcohol Alcohol.* 38, 255–262.

Smith, G.T. and Goldman, M.S. (1994). *J. Res. Adolesc.* 4, 229–247.

Thevos, A.K., Roberts, J.S., Thomas, S.E. and Randall, C.L. (2000). *Addict. Behav.* 25, 333–345.

Thomas, S.E., Randall, C.L. and Carrigan, M.H. (2003). *Alcohol. Clin. Exp. Res.* 27, 1937–1943.

Tomlinson, K.L., Tate, S.R., Anderson, K.G., Mccarthy, D.M. and Brown, S.A. (2006). *Addict. Behav.* 31, 461–474.

Vuchinich, R.E. and Tucker, J.A. (1988). *J. Abnorm. Psychol.* 97, 181–195.

Wallace, J. (1990). *West. J. Med.* 152, 502–505.

Wilson, A. (1977). *Addiction* 72, 99–108.

Zucker, R.A., Ellis, D.A. and Fitzgerald, H.E. (1994). *Ann. NY Acad. Sci.* 708, 134–146.

16

Beer and Current Mood State

Ralf Demmel and Jennifer Nicolai Department of Clinical Psychology, University of Münster, Münster, Germany

Abstract

The consumption of beer is closely related to human affect. An individual's current mood state has been shown to act as an internal stimulus eliciting the urge to drink alcohol, thus activating positive outcome expectancies and drinking motives. An individual's beliefs regarding the effects of beer determine his or her labeling of mood states following the consumption of beer. The attribution of the perceived changes in current mood state to the effects of beer strengthens both an individual's alcohol expectancies and his or her drinking motives.

Introduction

An individual's alcohol use is closely related to his or her current mood state. For example, depressed mood may trigger cravings for alcohol in individuals anticipating mood-enhancing effects of alcohol use. Accordingly, high levels of negative affect have been shown to increase the risk for relapse following successful substance abuse treatment (e.g. Hodgins *et al.*, 1995). An individual's current mood state may in turn be the result of his or her previous alcohol use. For example, a low dose of alcohol may produce pleasurable feelings of mild euphoria (e.g. Martin *et al.*, 1993). Thus, changes in current mood state may be either the cause or the consequence of alcohol use.

Researchers in the field of alcohol studies are less intested in the mood effects of specific types of beverages. Administering a mixture of a non-alcoholic beverage and vodka is the standard procedure in alcohol challenge studies (e.g. Croissant *et al.*, 2006). Beer is rarely used as a pharmacological challenge in experimental research. Hence, scientific evidence on the relationship between beer consumption and current mood is limited. In contrast, common beliefs about the mood effects of beer consumption are richly reflected in folklore and art. For example, William Hogarth's famous engraving of Beer Street illustrates eighteenth century beliefs about the positive effects of beer consumption (Figure 16.1). When Hogarth's engraving was first published in 1751, a poem by the Reverend James Townley was included:

Beer, happy product of our Isle
Can sinewy strength impart,
And, wearied with fatigue and toil,
Can cheer each manly heart.
Labor and Art, upheld by thee,
Successfully advance;
We quaff thy balmy juice with glee,
And Water leave to France.
Genius of Health, thy grateful taste
Rivals the cup of Jove,
And warms each English generous breast
With Liberty and Love.

While the appreciation of beer had been echoed in the work of many nineteenth century artists (for a review, see

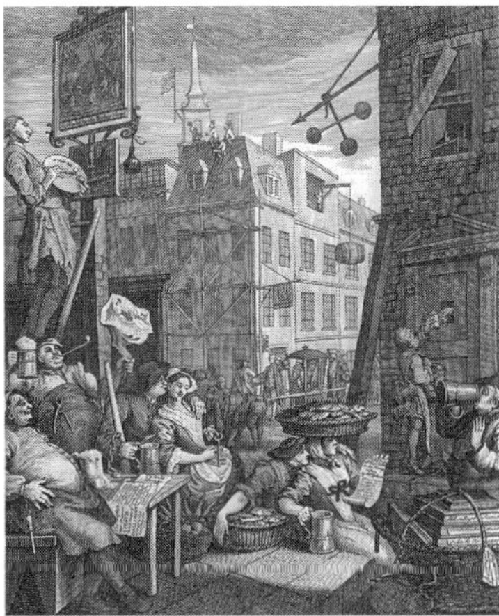

Figure 16.1 William Hogarth, Beer Street.

Beer in Health and Disease Prevention
ISBN: 978-0-12-373891-2

Jung, 1966), empirical research in the second half of the twentieth century started to challenge prevailing beliefs about the psychological effects of alcohol in general and beer in particular. Pharmacological studies proved alcohol to be a sedative rather than a stimulant (for a review, see Fromme and D'Amico, 1999). Psychological studies using the balanced placebo design (Figure 16.2) enabled researchers to separate placebo effects from pharmacological effects (e.g. Gross *et al.*, 2001). Animal studies led to the development of the tension reduction hypothesis stating that individuals use alcohol to gain relief from anxiety and stress, respectively (for a review, see Greeley and Oei, 1999). Recently, psychophysiological studies broadened the focus of alcohol research beyond the relationship between anxiety and alcohol use (for a review, see Lang *et al.*, 1999). To provide a conceptual framework for the interpretation of findings from different lines of research, we suggest a cognitive model of alcohol use taking into account the concepts of cue reactivity, outcome expectancies, drinking motives, and attributional processes (Figure 16.3). Alcohol-related cues such as the smell of beer or an individual's current mood state are assumed to act as stimuli eliciting the urge to drink alcohol. The perception of alcohol cues is likely to activate positive outcome expectancies. The anticipation of positive alcohol effects in turn will motivate the individual to initiate alcohol use. Finally, the model assumes that the attribution of mood enhancement to the effects of alcohol consolidates an individual's alcohol expectancies, thus strengthening his or her drinking motives and making future alcohol use more likely. Before we discuss the model in more detail, we first provide a brief introduction to research on human affect.

		Expected	
		Alcohol	No alcohol
Administered	Alcohol	A	B
	No alcohol	C	D

Figure 16.2 Balanced placebo design.

Current Mood States

Since the 1980s, mood has become a very popular concept in psychology. In contrast to emotions, moods are defined as relatively diffuse and enduring affective states of low intensity. While emotions are assumed to be the consequence of specific circumstances, moods are, by definition, not induced by a salient event. Traditionally, research in the field of human affect has focused on the identification of discrete types of affect, such as anxiety, anger, and joy. However, measures of different types of affect have been shown to be strongly related to each other. For example, individuals feeling sad have been found to report high levels of fear as well (e.g. Watson and Clark, 1992). The non-specificity of affect led many researchers to prefer a dimensional approach to the assessment of affective states. Research based on non-self-report data, for example, the analysis of facial expression, identified two dimensions of affect labelled pleasantness vs. unpleasantness and activation/arousal (Figure 16.4). Findings from studies using self-report questionnaires suggest two independent dimensions of affect often labeled negative and positive. In experimental research so-called mood induction procedures are used for manipulating an individual's current mood state. For example, participants are asked to listen to a piece of serious classical music or to watch a funny movie (for a comprehensive review of research on the assessment of current mood states, see Watson and Clark, 1997). In an early study on the relationship between mood and alcohol consumption social drinkers were randomly assigned to interact with a child confederate trained to enact behaviors characteristic of either well-adjusted or mentally ill children. Interacting with a child confederate exhibiting externalizing behaviors induced negative mood in both males and females. Moreover, male participants anticipating another interaction with the same child consumed more beer during a 20 min

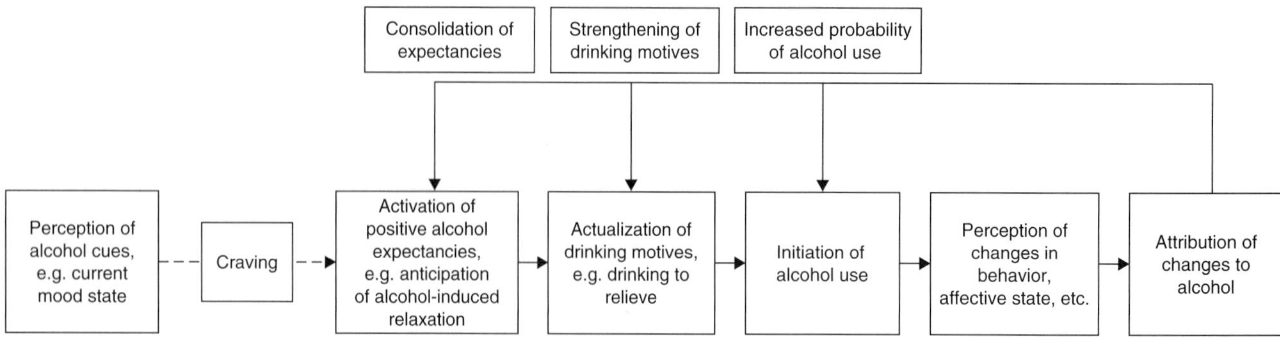

Figure 16.3 Relationship between alcohol use and current mood state.

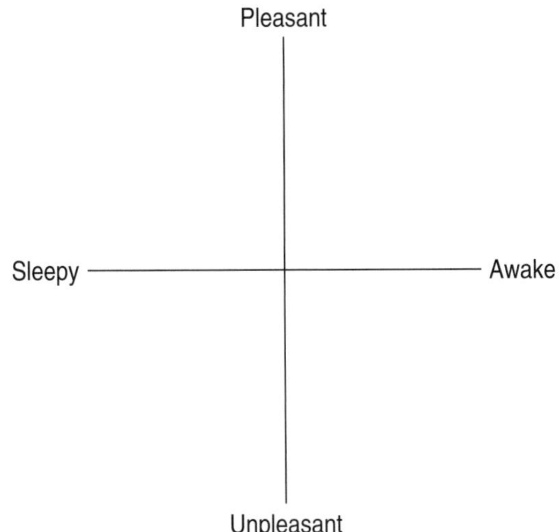

Figure 16.4 The structure of mood.

ad lib drinking period compared to their counterparts anticipating a second encounter with an apparently well-adjusted child (Lang *et al.*, 1989). These findings suggest that negative mood induced by a stressful social interaction may increase beer consumption.

Cue Reactivity

According to learning theory, a previously neutral stimulus becomes capable of eliciting a response from an organism by pairing it several times with either an aversive or a reinforcing stimulus. In other words, due to the repeated association with significant stimuli formerly non-significant stimuli may turn into signals or cues predicting important events, for example the availability of food and beverage. The capability of external alcohol cues, for example the smell and taste of beer, to elicit an appetitive response, that is craving for alcohol, from both non-problem and problem drinkers is well established (for a review, see Carter and Tiffany, 1999). Moreover, an individual's current mood state has been shown to act as an internal stimulus eliciting the urge to drink alcohol (e.g. Willner *et al.*, 1998). Most interestingly, individuals at high risk for alcohol-related disorders have been found to drink more beer following a negative mood induction when compared to low-risk individuals (Randall and Cox, 2001). These findings are in line with research demonstrating an increased sensitivity to the reinforcing effects of alcohol in high-risk individuals (e.g. Finn *et al.*, 1990).

Outcome Expectancies

Cognitive learning theories state that an individual's outcome expectancies determine his or her behavior. For example, the anticipated short-term effects of drinking are assumed to affect both the frequency and the quantity of alcohol use. In accordance with cognitive models of drinking and alcohol dependence, research using self-report questionnaires has consistently shown that alcohol outcome expectancies are related to drinking behavior (e.g. Demmel and Hagen, 2003). Findings from both cross-sectional and longitudinal studies indicate that positive alcohol expectancies enhance the level of alcohol use (for a review, see Jones *et al.*, 2001). Positive alcohol expectancies are beliefs about the reinforcing effects of alcohol such as social and sexual enhancement, tension reduction, and positive affect. In contrast, negative alcohol expectancies include the anticipation of cognitive impairment, physical discomfort, and interpersonal aggression. The strength of alcohol expectancies has been shown to vary with the number of drinks an individual expects to consume within a given time period and his or her current mood state. For example, social drinkers asked to think of how they would feel immediately after drinking four glasses of beer in 60 min anticipate higher levels of alcohol-induced sedation and stimulation than their counterparts expecting to have one glass of beer in 15 min (Demmel *et al.*, 2006). Moreover, those respondents feeling tired and worn out at the time of completing an expectancy questionnaire anticipate higher levels of beer-induced sedation (Demmel *et al.*, 2006). These findings suggest that current mood state may determine the level of beer consumption by altering the strength of outcome expectancies.

Drinking Motives

Drinking motives are assumed to be more proximal antecedents of alcohol use than outcome expectancies. While the term drinking motives refers to an individual's reasons for the initiation of alcohol use, alcohol outcome expectancies are defined as the anticipated short-term effects of alcohol. Drinking motives and alcohol outcome expectancies are – yet conceptually distinct – closely related to each other (for a detailed discussion, see Cox and Klinger, 2004). For example, drinking to cope with negative mood implies that an individual believes alcohol to have mood-altering effects. Findings from longitudinal studies suggest that the desire to regulate both positive and negative affect is the major motivation for alcohol use. While drinking to enhance positive affect seems to be a correlate of externalizing personality traits such as sensation seeking, drinking to cope with negative affect has been found to be related to depressed mood (Cooper *et al.*, 1995).

Attributional Processes

In cognitive psychology, the term attribution is often defined as the causal explanation of an event or an individual's behavior. Moreover, when used synonymously with blame, the term attribution refers to the responsibility for an event, state, or behavior (for a detailed discussion, see Bell-Dolan and Anderson, 1999). Drunkenness has been shown to affect the attribution of responsibility. For example, studies using written acquaintance-rape scenarios revealed that females are considered more responsible for being raped when described as having had a couple of beers (e.g. Cameron and Stritzke, 2003). Findings from experimental studies suggest that attributional processes are also involved in human affect (e.g. Sinclair *et al.*, 1994). For example, an individual's beliefs regarding the effects of beer will determine his or her labeling of mood states following the consumption of beer. Mood states congruent with the anticipated outcomes are likely to be attributed to the effects of beer.

Summary Points

- Moods are relatively diffuse and enduring affective states of low intensity.
- Negative mood induced by a stressful social interaction may increase beer consumption.
- Individuals at high risk for alcohol-related disorders drink more beer following a negative mood induction when compared to low-risk individuals.
- An individual's current mood state may determine the level of beer consumption by altering the strength of his or her outcome expectancies.
- Changes in current mood state congruent with the anticipated outcomes are likely to be attributed to the effects of beer.

References

Bell-Dolan, D. and Anderson, C.A. (1999). Attributional processes: An integration of social and clinical psychology. In Kowalski, R.M. and Leary, M.R. (eds), *The Social Psychology of Emotional and Behavioral Problems: Interfaces of Social and Clinical Psychology*, pp. 37–67. American Psychological Association, Washington, DC.

Cameron, C.A. and Stritzke, W.G.K. (2003). *J. Appl. Soc. Psychol.* 33, 983–1008.

Carter, B.L. and Tiffany, S.T. (1999). *Addiction* 94, 327–340.

Cooper, M.L., Frone, M.R., Russell, M. and Mudar, P. (1995). *J. Pers. Soc. Psychol.* 69, 990–1005.

Cox, W.M. and Klinger, E. (2004). A motivational model of alcohol use: Determinants of use and change. In Cox, W.M. and Klinger, E. (eds), *Handbook of Motivational Counseling: Concepts, Approaches, and Assessment*, pp. 121–138. John Wiley & Sons, Ltd., Chichester.

Croissant, B., Rist, F., Demmel, R. and Olbrich, R. (2006). *Int. J. Psychophysiol.* 61, 253–261.

Demmel, R. and Hagen, J. (2003). *SUCHT* 49, 300–305.

Demmel, R., Nicolai, J. and Gregorzik, S. (2006). *Addict. Behav.* 31, 859–867.

Finn, P.R., Zeitouni, N.C. and Pihl, R.O. (1990). *J. Abnorm. Psychol.* 99, 79–85.

Fromme, K. and D'Amico, E.J. (1999). Neurobiological bases of alcohol's psychological effects. In Leonard, K.E. and Blane, H.T. (eds), *Psychological Theories of Drinking and Alcoholism*, pp. 422–455. The Guilford Press, New York.

Greeley, J. and Oei, T. (1999). Alcohol and tension reduction. In Leonard, K.E. and Blane, H.T. (eds), *Psychological Theories of Drinking and Alcoholism*, pp. 14–53. The Guilford Press, New York.

Gross, A.M., Bennett, T., Sloan, L., Marx, B.P. and Juergens, J. (2001). *Exp. Clin. Psychopharmacol.* 9, 380–388.

Hodgins, D.C., El-Guebaly, N. and Armstrong, S. (1995). *J. Consult. Clin. Psychol.* 63, 400–407.

Jones, B.T., Corbin, W. and Fromme, K. (2001). *Addiction* 96, 57–72.

Jung, H. (1966). *Bier – Kunst und Brauchtum*. Documenta-Verlag, Dortmund.

Lang, A.R., Pelham, W.E., Johnston, C. and Gelernter, S. (1989). *J. Abnorm. Psychol.* 98, 294–299.

Lang, A.R., Patrick, C.J. and Stritzke, W.G.K. (1999). Alcohol and emotional response: A multidimensional-multilevel analysis. In Leonard, K.E. and Blane, H.T. (eds), *Psychological Theories of Drinking and Alcoholism*, pp. 328–371. The Guilford Press, New York.

Martin, C.S., Earleywine, M., Musty, R.E., Perrine, M.W. and Swift, R.M. (1993). *Alcohol Clin. Exp. Res.* 17, 140–146.

Randall, D.M. and Cox, W.M. (2001). *Am. J. Drug Alcohol Abuse* 27, 183–187.

Sinclair, R.C., Hoffman, C., Mark, M.M., Martin, L.L. and Pickering, T.L. (1994). *Psychol. Sci.* 5, 15–19.

Watson, D. and Clark, L.A. (1992). *J. Pers. Soc. Psychol.* 62, 489–505.

Watson, D. and Clark, L.A. (1997). *J. Pers. Assess.* 68, 267–296.

Willner, P., Field, M., Pitts, K. and Reeve, G. (1998). *Behav. Pharmacol.* 9, 631–642.

17

Female Beer Drinking and the Morning After

L. Darren Kruisselbrink and René J.L. Murphy School of Recreation Management and Kinesiology, Acadia University, Wolfville, NS, Canada

Abstract

The goal of this chapter is to review the drinking patterns and hangover effects of beer consumption in women. We first provide an overview of alcohol consumption and the experience of the alcohol hangover. Alcohol is a widely consumed drug. Beer is consumed by both men and women although women typically consume less than men. In North America, per capita consumption of beer has been stable over the past 20 years; total amount of pure alcohol consumed in beer is approximately 4–4.5 l/year. Given that beer contains ~5% alcohol by volume (~17 ml alcohol per 341 ml bottle), this represents the annual consumption of a large quantity of beer. Factors contributing to consumption including consumption rates, locations and social influences are reviewed, as there are some limitations of the methods used to collect these data. There are some differences in alcohol pharmacokinetics between women and men, however when these are controlled, sex does not appear to differentially affect the intoxication or hangover experience. Consumption of alcohol is often associated with negative delayed effects sometimes experienced as hangover symptoms. These delayed or hangover effects are difficult to standardize and have not been widely studied. Although there is little published work on the experience of hangover in women, the few reports that are available indicate that hangover effects on performance do not appear to differ between women and men. Furthermore, there are very few studies on the hangover effects of beer consumption in women. This chapter concludes with a summary of the known effects of beer hangover on physical and psychomotor performance in women, as well as general recommendations for future work.

List of Abbreviations

BAC	Blood alcohol concentration, estimated with an Alco-Sensor IV breathalyzer in grams of alcohol per 100 ml of blood
bpm	Beats per minute
CRT	Choice reaction time
freq.	Frequency
g	Grams
g%	Grams of pure alcohol (1 ml of alcohol weighs 0.79 g) per 100 ml of blood (e.g. in Canada the legal driving limit is set at 0.08 g%)
g/kg	Grams of alcohol per kilogram body weight
HR	Heart rate
kg	Kilograms
l	Liters
min	Minutes
ml/kg	Milliliters of alcohol per kilogram body weight
mmHg	Millimeters of mercury
ms	Milliseconds or 1/1000th of a second
n.s.	Non-significant
POMS	Profile of mood states, a questionnaire measuring negative and positive aspects of mood
RPE	Rating of perceived exertion
SRT	Simple reaction time

"I feel sorry for people who don't drink. When they wake up in the morning, that's as good as they're going to feel all day" (Frank Sinatra).

Hangover is a commonly experienced phenomenon following over zealous consumption of alcohol. Descriptions of the hangover state indicate feeling worse than would be expected if alcohol had not been consumed. The majority of quotations about the alcohol-induced hangover give the impression that it is a male-dominated experience. Perhaps because the temperance movement in the United States in the late 1800s and early 1900s was driven by women, the image of decent women drinking and experiencing hangovers has remained in the background of the North American cultural psyche. Alcohol consumption in twenty-first century North America, however, appears to be an equal opportunity vice, as a trip to many popular bar or lounge will undoubtedly attest. Although women tend to favor wine and spirits over beer, females still consume beer in substantial quantity. All this alcohol consumption suggests the inevitability of the hangover experience that typically follows.

The goal of this chapter is to review the experience and effects of alcohol hangover in females following consumption of beer. To achieve this purpose, we will begin by discussing North American alcohol consumption patterns to

Beer in Health and Disease Prevention
ISBN: 978-0-12-373891-2

provide a general context in which to consider hangover effects. We will also discuss differences in alcohol pharmacokinetics between females and males, as well as the experience and effects of alcohol hangover in females.

Consumption Patterns

Consuming alcohol creates the opportunity to experience a hangover. The alcohol-induced hangover is a commonly experienced phenomenon. In the following section, we outline the prevalence of alcohol consumption primarily in North America, the pros and cons of the methods used to gather these data, the location and frequency of drinking episodes, the average amount consumed per episode and the rate of consumption. Some of these data are provided in summary form in Table 17.1.

Prevalence

Alcohol is widely consumed. In Canada and the United States, various national surveys have reported that the proportion of the population who had consumed alcohol in the previous year ranged from 74% to 80%. Alcohol has been reported as the most used drug, with over 50% of teenagers and higher percentages of college students and adults having consumed alcohol in the past 12 months (Prendergast, 1994; World Health Organization, 2004). In the United States, 49% of adults over 18 years indicated that they were current drinkers (≥12 drinks in the previous year; National Center for Health Statistics, 2006), while in Canada 53% rated themselves as regular drinkers (≥1 drink/month in the previous year; Health Canada, 1999). Across North America, a greater percentage of males than females reported consuming alcohol regularly. Per capita alcohol consumption in both Canada and the United States has remained stable at approximately 8 l of pure alcohol (ethanol) per year since the mid-1990s, but has declined from a peak of over 10 l reported in the mid-1970s (World Health Organization, 2004). In contrast, North American consumption of ethanol in beer has been remarkably stable, totaling approximately 4 l since the early 1960s; recent data indicate that Americans and Canadians consume 3.9 and 4.6 l of ethanol, respectively, in beer (World Health Organization, 2004). The Brewers Association of

Table 17.1 Summary of alcohol consumption data in North America

Item	*Male*	*Female*	*Total*
Percentage of regular drinkers (≥1 drink per month)			
United States 18+ years (National Center for Health Statistics, 2006)	58%	41%	49%
Canada 15+ years (Health Canada 1999; Statistics Canada, 2005)	63–69%	43–51%*	53%
Percentage heavy drinkers (≥5 drinks per occasion ≥12 times per year)			
Canada 20+ years (Statistics Canada, 2004, 2006)	28–30%	10–12%	
Canada 20–34 years (Statistics Canada, 2004, 2006)	40–46%	18–22%	
Estimated mean per capita consumption of absolute alcohol (ethanol) in beer, spirits and wine			
United States (Lakins *et al.*, 2006)			8.4 l
Beer			4.6 l
Spirits			2.6 l
Wine			1.3 l
Canada (World Health Organization, 2004)			8.2 l
Beer			3.9 l
Spirits			2.5 l
Wine			1.7 l
Drinking occasions by location (Single and Wortley, 1993)			
Beer parlor	More freq.	Least freq.	
Lounge/restaurant	Least freq.	More freq.	
Private setting	Most freq.	Most freq.	
Volume consumed by location (Single and Wortley, 1993)			
Beer parlor	–	More	
Lounge/restaurant	–	Less	
Mean drinks per episode (Single and Wortley, 1993)	2–5	1–3	
Consumption rate			
Beer parlor (Single and Wortley, 1993)	~20 min	~30 min	
Lounge (Single and Wortley, 1993)	~30 min	~35 min	
Beer parlor (Kruisselbrink *et al.*, 2006)		30–40 min	

*Statistics Canada (2005) indicates that as of 2003, 55–60% of women aged 15–54 years were regular drinkers.
l = liters; freq. = frequency; min = minutes; ~ = approximately.

Canada estimated that between 1995 and 2005 the per capita consumption of beer was 83–87 l/year (Brewers Association of Canada, 2006). These estimates of drinking prevalence provide a general indication of the extent of alcohol consumption, however, they do not provide any information on the pattern of drinking or the problems that may be associated with drinking (Prendergast, 1994).

Location of drinking episodes

Alcohol consumption has been shown to vary by location. Engs and Hanson (1990), In their review, concluded that males drank most frequently in public places (e.g. ballgame, concert or a dormitory) while females drank most often in restaurants or lounges, nightclubs or bars. Storm and Cutler (1981) interviewed males and females at beer parlors and cocktail lounges, reporting that the number of drinking occasions and number of drinks consumed per occasion varied by sex and location. Specifically, men reported drinking more frequently than women. Women tended to report consuming fewer drinks per occasion in cocktail lounges vs. beer parlors whereas men reported consuming similar amounts in each setting. Compared to males, females were less likely to drink bottled beer in a lounge (16% vs. 4%; Storm and Cutler, 1981).

Drinking in private settings, including parties in private homes, is the location where drinking has been reported to occur most frequently (World Health Organization, 1999). Single and Wortley (1993) also reported that home consumption accounted for the greatest share of alcohol consumption. They concluded that drinking in licensed establishments represented only 25% of the total alcohol consumption.

Amount consumed per episode

Studies by a number of groups (e.g. Plant *et al.*, 1977; Storm and Cutler, 1981) have yielded remarkably similar findings on the number of drinks consumed per episode. On average, females have been reported to consume 1–3 drinks per episode while males typically consume 2–5 drinks per occasion. In the Melbourne Collaborative Cohort Study, Baglietto *et al.* (2006) reported that the majority of women who consumed alcohol tended to drink between 1 and 19 g/day; more men reported consuming alcohol and a greater percentage of those reported drinking larger quantities. By the way of contrast, most patrons observed at drinking establishments consumed a small number of drinks (average: 1.9–3.3 for women and 2.0–4.3 for men; Storm and Cutler, 1981). However, in interviews of men and women drinking in beer parlors and cocktail lounges, they reported consuming an average of 0.9–1.3 additional drinks other than those observed being consumed in the drinking establishment. Furthermore, 35% of women interviewed about their consumption pattern in a beer parlor reported drinking ≥9 drinks that evening while 50% reported drinking ≤4 drinks.

Social context also influences the amount of alcohol consumed. Gerstel (1975, as cited in Storm and Cutler, 1981) has reported that social drinkers are more likely to drink heavily in groups. Rosenbluth *et al.* (1978) also reported that individuals in larger groups drank more than individuals in pairs. Storm and Cutler (1981) observed that females tended to drink in groups of two or more, whereas males were more likely to drink alone in beer parlors. Moreover, they observed that one-third of females drinking in beer parlors in groups of six or more consumed ≥6 beers. Rosenbluth *et al.* (1978) reported that men drank less in the presence of women and women drank more in the presence of men.

The amount of alcohol consumed has also been shown to vary with age. In 2005, 25% of Canadian females and 38% of Canadian males aged 15–19 drank five or more drinks on one occasion, 12 or more times in a year (Statistics Canada, 2006). In the 20–24-year-old demographic, 32% and 55% of females and males, respectively, were heavy drinkers. Conversely, the incidence of heavy drinking in females and males aged 35–64 was in the range of 8–11% and 25–30%, respectively. In women drinking in a beer parlor, there was a significant relationship between age and number of drinks ($r = -0.37$; Storm and Cutler, 1981). Thus, it appears that for young adult women, the consumption of alcohol is a relatively widespread phenomenon.

Rate and duration of consumption

The rate of alcohol consumption observed in women drinking in beer parlors was 29.5 min per drink, whereas it was observed to be 19.7 min for men (Storm and Cutler, 1981). In cocktail lounges, Storm and Cutler (1981) observed the mean rate of consumption in females and males as 35.9 and 31.8 min, respectively. Storm and Cutler also noted that both men and women drank the first beer faster than subsequent ones. Similarly, our direct observations of alcohol consumption rates for female university students in a beer parlor indicated that, on average, women took approximately 30 min to consume the first couple of drinks whereas subsequent drinks were consumed at a rate of approximately 40 min each (reported in Kruisselbrink *et al.*, 2006).

By directly observing patrons drinking, Storm and Cutler (1981) have reported that the average duration of drinking episodes in men and women was ~88 and 106 min, respectively, in beer parlors while the observed duration in a lounge was ~62 min. Since not all drinking occurs in the setting chosen for observation, these data likely do not represent the full duration of the drinking episode.

Data collection methods

Estimates of alcohol consumption patterns have been obtained through direct observation, surveys and through calculations of total sales of alcohol. There are pros and cons to each approach. The benefit of directly observing drinking patterns in naturalistic settings is an accurate tally, however the observed drinking pattern may be unique to the location and setting in which they were recorded, and are not representative of regular consumption patterns. For example, a survey conducted by Storm and Cutler (1981) following observation of drinking patterns in public places revealed that 40% of the respondents had consumed alcohol – sometimes a large volume of alcohol – prior to their arrival at (or after leaving) a public drinking establishment. Population surveys have been used to try to assess alcohol consumption patterns but most have focused on quantity and frequency of drinking and on indicators of problem drinking. These surveys are helpful in defining population tendencies but rarely provide information on location and social context of consumption or other factors like rate of consumption. Rehm *et al.* (1999) have also shown differences in the sensitivity of different methods of assessing alcohol consumption. Alternatively, total sales of alcoholic beverages are good estimates of the total amount of consumption in a region, but they do not provide accurate information on patterns of how, when and by whom alcohol is consumed, and do not take into account the alcohol produced privately or in brew pubs, for example (Brewers Association of Canada, 2006).

Clearly each data collection method provides useful information, however, the conclusions generated using data collected by a specific approach must focus on its strengths and care should be exercised when generalizing, especially when so many potential covariates are often ignored. For instance, it is important to note that alcohol consumption may vary from day to day and from week to week. Occasions of heavy drinking, following which hangovers are much more likely to result, may also account for a disproportionate amount of the total consumption compared to lighter consumption at regular intervals (Storm and Cutler, 1981). All these factors need to be considered and accurately compiled and reported.

Alcohol Pharmacokinetics

Differences in alcohol pharmacokinetics between females and males have the potential to affect the drinking experience of females, which in turn may affect their hangover experience. Research has shown that females have more body fat and less body water per kg of body weight than males. Thus, standardizing the amount of alcohol females and males consume by body weight will produce higher peak blood alcohol concentrations (BACs) in females than males (Goist Jr. and Sutker, 1985; Mumenthaler *et al.*, 1999). Standardizing the amount of alcohol given to females and males by volume of body water eliminates this difference. The available evidence also suggests that females eliminate alcohol faster than males (Lammers *et al.*, 1995).

The phase of menstrual cycle has been reported to alter females' sensitivity to alcohol (e.g. Jones and Jones, 1976). However, in more recent reviews of this literature, Mumenthaler *et al.* (1999) have stated that phase of menstrual cycle is unlikely to affect alcohol pharmacokinetics and performance in females, while Lammers *et al.* (1995) have stated that "for the time being, it cannot be concluded that the human female menstrual cycle has a significant impact on the potency of alcohol" (p. 28).

Although there appear to be some differences in how the female and male body reacts to alcohol, these discrepancies have not produced sex differences in perceived intoxication (Goist Jr. and Sutker, 1985). Nonetheless, some performance differences between females and males have been reported while intoxicated. Jones and Jones (1977) found that short-term memory was affected to a greater degree in intoxicated females than males. Furthermore, Niaura *et al.* (1987) showed that females were slower to recover short-term memory following peak BAC as it returned to zero. Females also showed greater decrements in divided attention than males (Mills and Bisgrove, 1983); however, decrements in psychomotor performance while intoxicated have not been shown to vary according to sex (Mumenthaler *et al.*, 1999).

The Experience of Hangover

Introducing alcohol to the body initiates a number of short-term physiological adaptations including altered neural and endocrine functioning (Lemon, 1993). Hangover is thought to be caused, in part, by re-adaptation processes once alcohol has been fully metabolised and cleared. Hangover symptoms commence with the decline in BAC after drinking has stopped, and peak around the time that it reaches zero (Swift and Davidson, 1998). Following a bout of heavy drinking (1.50–1.75 g/kg ethanol), Anylian *et al.* (1978) have shown that ratings of hangover intensity were greatest (12–16 h) after drinking stopped.

While few would disagree that hangovers exist, generating a precise definition of it has been elusive. In fact, Wiese *et al.* (2000) state that "there is no consensus definition" (p. 897) for hangover. In general terms, Swift and Davidson (1998) state that "a hangover is characterized by the constellation of unpleasant physical and mental symptoms that occur after a bout of heavy alcohol drinking" (p. 55). The result of this lack of consensus in defining hangover is the use of a wide variety of descriptors in various combinations to characterize hangover symptomology. Table 17.2 lists hangover symptoms provided in a pair of recent hangover studies that included a rationale for the symptoms they included, as well as from a number of hangover reviews that included a summary of reported symptoms. While a comprehensive review of hangover symptoms is beyond the scope of this chapter, those gleaned from the literature that was sampled indicate a number of hangover symptoms that appear to be central to the hangover experience; headache, nausea, dry mouth/thirst, fatigue, dizziness/vertigo, tremulous/shakiness, depressed well being and anxiety were reported in >50% of the literature sampled. Other hangover symptoms appear more peripheral to the hangover experience, appearing in <50% of the literature sampled (see Table 17.2).

There appears to be little evidence that hangover severity differs amongst females and males. Verster *et al.* (2003) reported that hangover intensity was greater in females than males; however, sex differences in peak BAC were not

Table 17.2 Summary of hangover symptom descriptors and frequency of use in selected literature

Symptom	*Anylian et al. (1978)*	*Gauvin et al. (1993)*	*Swift and Davidson (1998)*	*Wiese et al. (2000)*	*Slutske et al. (2003)*	*Rohsenow et al. (2006)*	*Kruisselbrink et al. (2006)*	*Symptom frequency*
Headache	X	X	X	X	X	X	X	7
Nausea	X	X	X	X	X	X	X	7
Dry mouth/thirst	X	X	X	X	X	X	X	7
Fatigue	X		X	X	X	X	X	6
Dizziness/vertigo	X	X	X			X	X	5
Tremulous/shakiness		X	X	X	X		X	5
Depressed sense of well being/depression	X		X	X	X			4
Anxious/tense	X	X	X		X			4
Accelerated heart rate		X	X			X		3
Difficulty sleeping		X	X		X			3
Stomach ache/pain			X			X	X	3
Sweating more than usual/feel hot		X	X		X			3
Agitated/irritated			X				X	2
Difficulty concentrating			X		X			2
Loss of appetite				X		X		2
Sensitivity to light and sound			X		X			2
Vomiting			X		X			2
Apathetic/listless/general malaise	X							1
Diarrhea/loose bowels				X				1
Muscle aches			X					1
Postural unsteadiness		X						1
Tinnitus		X						1
Weakness			X					1

X indicates that the symptom was used to describe hangover.

assessed in their study. As ethanol consumption was standardized on the basis of body weight, females may have reached higher peak BACs than males (Goist Jr. and Sutker, 1985). Kruisselbrink *et al.* (2004) allowed females and males to consume alcohol *ad libitum* in the natural setting of their choice. Peak BACs were recorded upon termination of drinking and subjects rated the presence and intensity of eight hangover symptoms approximately 12 h later. Overall, lower mean peak BACs were recorded for females, who also rated their hangover as less severe than males. However, when peak BAC served as a covariate, there was no difference in hangover intensity between females and males (unpublished analysis). Thus, the presence of hangover appears to be independent of sex and more related to the volume of alcohol consumed.

Delayed (Hangover) Effects of Alcohol Consumption

Although a number of studies examining the relationship between hangover and performance have included females as subjects, many of these do not report sex differences. Therefore, we can only assume that the delayed effects of alcohol on performance do not substantially differ between females and males. In general, the extant research is inconsistent in showing decrements in performance with hangover, prompting Lemon (1993) to state, “it must be noted that for nearly every performance difference found in the post-intoxication state, there is at least one other study using the same, or similar, tests which has reported no effect” (p. 309). For example, performance decrements on cognitive and psychomotor tasks such as divided attention, digit-symbol substitution, mental rotation, memory, strategic decision making, simple (SRT) and choice reaction time (CRT), compensatory tracking and fine motor movement have been found by some (Seppälä *et al.*, 1976; Kim *et al.*, 2003; McKinney and Coyle, 2004) but not others (Lemon *et al.*, 1993; Chait and Perry, 1994; Streufert *et al.*, 1995; Rohsenow *et al.*, 2006). Likewise, for longer duration psychomotor tasks such as simulated flying and driving, research indicates both the presence (Yesavage and Leirer, 1986; Yesavage *et al.*, 1994; Petros *et al.*, 2003) and absence (Törnros and Laurell, 1991;

Morrow *et al.*, 1993; Taylor *et al.*, 1996; Petros *et al.*, 2003) of significant decreases in performance. Similarly, some physiological variables (e.g. heart rate (HR), blood pressure and aerobic performance) have been shown to decrease (Karvinen *et al.*, 1962; O'Brien, 1993) whereas others (e.g. grip strength) have not (Karvinen *et al.*, 1962).

One factor that may influence the presence or absence of performance decrements post-intoxication is the peak BAC achieved while drinking. Petros *et al.* (2003) failed to find significant decreases in flight simulator performance following peak BACs of ~0.07 g% in males, but found some differences for the group of men that exceeded 0.10 g%. Similarly, Yesavage and Leirer (1986) and Morrow *et al.* (1993) reported some post-intoxication deficits on flight simulator performance following BACs of >0.10 g%, however Yesavage *et al.* (1994) did not. Törnros and Laurell (1991) also found no differences in post-intoxication driving simulator performance 14–16 h after achieving peak BACs ranging from 0.115–0.247 g%. More recently, despite reporting increases in hangover symptoms and perceived impairment of performance following consumption of beer, Rohsenow *et al.* (2006) reported no post-intoxication effect on ship engine simulator performance in young cadets following heavy drinking (mean peak BAC 0.115 g%). This suggests that peak BAC contributes to, but is not the sole cause of, the obtained results.

In their reviews of the hangover literature, Lemon (1993) and Gauvin *et al.* (1993) both have provided summary tables of the post-intoxication effects of alcohol on performance once BAC had returned to zero. When these data are considered together, the inconsistency in the pattern of results is evident. Table 17.3 is a similarly styled summary table of post-intoxication effects of alcohol on performance conducted since 1993; however, for the purposes of this chapter, we have only included those studies in which females have been included as subjects. Similar to previous patterns of results, an overview of the findings reported in Table 17.3 indicates an inconsistent pattern of results.

The only study to explicitly contrast the psychomotor performance of males and females post-intoxication was conducted by Taylor *et al.* (1996). They found no differences between females and males on flight simulator performance 8 h after drinking terminated. To date, there is no reason to believe that post-intoxication performance differs according to sex; however, this conclusion should be interpreted with caution as it is based on limited data.

The available data also do not provide conclusive evidence that beer hangovers are rated any differently than hangovers induced by other types of alcoholic beverages. Whereas Takala *et al.* (1958) compared a beer hangover to a hangover induced by brandy, no self-rated hangover data were reported. Finally,

Table 17.3 Summary of hangover studies published since 1993 that have included female participants

Study	*Subjects*	*Dose*	*Peak BAC reported*	*Delay*	*Post-intoxication performance results*
Kruisselbrink *et al.* (2006)	12 f	0, 27, 54 and 81 g (in beer)	0, 0.036, 0.070 and 0.106 g%	9 h	↑CRT errors; ↔HR, blood pressure, grip strength, 4 CRT, run to exhaustion
Rohsenow *et al.* (2006)	11 f, 50 m	To reach 0.10 g% (in beer)	0.100 g%	~10 h	↔Ship engine simulation; fell asleep faster, ↑self-rated impairment
Finnigan *et al.* (2005)	35 f, 36 m	*Ad libitum*	Not measured	Next day between 9 a.m. and 1 p.m.	↔Tracking-SRT dual task, ↔probed memory recall
McKinney and Coyle (2004, 2006)	33 f, 15 m	f average of 95 g, m average of 132 g	Not measured	Next day at 9 a.m., 11 a.m., 1 p.m.	↓Free recall 9 and 11 a.m., ↑SRT, ↔5CRT; less sleep, to bed later, fell asleep faster; sleep less satisfying, restful and refreshing; less alert at 11 a.m.
Verster *et al.* (2003)	24 f, 24 m	1.4 g/kg	0.155 g%	~10.5 h	↔Sleep quality; ↓rated alertness; ↔immediate recall, ↓delayed recall, ↔recognition, ↔vigilance
Anderson and Dawson (1999)	8 f, 8 m	*Ad libitum* (>1 g/kg)	Not measured	12–16 h	↓Focused attention, ↓divided attention
Taylor *et al.* (1996)	12 f, 11 m	m 0.8 ml/kg, f 12.5% less ml/kg	f 0.084 g%, m 0.087 g%	8 h	↔Change in flight simulator performance; n.s. gender effect
Chait and Perry (1994)	4 f, 10 m	f 0.5 g/kg, m 0.6 g/kg	0.088 g%	13.5 h	POMS fatigue ↑ in morning; ↔1 leg balancing, ↔digit substitution, ↔divided attention

Note: For subject and dose columns, f = female, m = male; g = grams; g% = grams of alcohol per 100 ml of blood; ml/kg = milliliters of alcohol per kilogram body weight; g/kg = grams of alcohol per kilogram body weight (1 ml of alcohol weighs 0.79 g); ↑ = increase; ↓ = decrease; ↔ = no change; CRT = choice reaction time; SRT = simple reaction time; HR = heart rate; n.s. = non-significant; POMS = profile of mood states, a questionnaire measuring negative and positive aspects of mood.

Source: For summaries of work prior to 1993, see Gauvin *et al.* (1993) and Lemon (1993).

Verster (2006) has recently suggested that beer hangovers are less intense than liquor-induced hangovers, however these data were generated from a survey in which participants were asked to recall post-intoxication experiences caused by beer vs. liquor rather than on more direct and objective state measures taken during the hangover state. Therefore, this finding must be interpreted with caution.

Search and Review of Articles on the Topic

There is a dearth of literature on the delayed effects of beer on physical and psychomotor performances. Moreover, few studies on the delayed effects of alcohol have included females or focused specifically on women. We searched the Web of Science, PsycInfo, PubMed and Google Scholar databases using various combinations of keywords related to alcohol- and beer-induced hangover in females to highlight the number of publications on the topic. The number of results returned from each search is shown in Table 17.4.

Given the dearth of research examining post-intoxication effects of alcohol on various measure of performance in females, the call for more hangover research on females (e.g. Gauvin *et al.*, 1993) and the relatively widespread consumption of beer by females, we investigated the effects of drinking beer on next morning performance in a group of female university students (Kruisselbrink *et al.*, 2006).

Beer-Induced Hangover and Performance in Females

In the only published report specifically assessing the post-intoxication effects of beer in women, Kruisselbrink *et al.* (2006) concluded that there are minimal short-term performance decrements following consumption of up to 6 beers. Kruisselbrink and colleagues reported that consuming moderate quantities of beer altered decision making but had limited effects on short-term physical and physiological variables measured during hangover. Specifically, 12 healthy, non-smoking female university students aged 22 ± 2.8 years completed four testing conditions where they consumed 0 (control), 2, 4 and 6 bottles of beer (341 ml, commercially brewed, 5% alcohol by volume, 13.5 g alcohol/bottle) in a laboratory setting. The rate of consumption was standardized according to typical drinking patterns of female university students in a social setting (30 min/beer for the first 2 bottles; 40 min/beer for subsequent bottles).

Results

In this study, the treatment, ranging from 0 to 6 beers, caused a dose-dependent significant increase in BAC of the female subjects, increasing from 0.000g% in the control (0 beer) to 0.106 g% in the 6 beer condition (see Figure 17.1a). Although the amount of beer consumed was moderate and ingested over time in an ecologically valid manner, it was sufficient to induce some acute deficits in performance as well as some delayed (i.e. hangover) effects 9 h following the end of consumption. For example, in the acute phase (i.e. 15–30 min following the end of consumption), CRT increased as dose increased (Figure 17.1b), indicating a slowing of information processing speed; no differences in movement time emerged with increased dose (Figure 17.1c) which shows that subjects' ability to carry out the simple movement once triggered was unaffected by dose. BAC had returned to 0.000 in all subjects at the time of awakening and post-intoxication testing.

The morning after the control condition (no alcohol consumed), participants' responses on the Post-Intoxication Scale indicated that, for the most part, they experienced the absence of, or mild symptoms typically associated with hangover (77% and 20% of total responses, respectively; Table 17.5). Moreover, the frequency of rating hangover symptoms as mild or severe increased with dose (see Kruisselbrink *et al.*, 2006 for hangover intensity ratings).

Table 17.4 Number of articles identified in commonly used academic databases using various combinations of relevant keywords

	Number of publications returned (as of December 14, 2006)*			
Keywords entered	*ISI Web of Knowledge (Web of Science)*	*PsycInfo*	*PubMed*	*Google Scholar*
Female and alcohol	5,288	10,436	159,695	969,000
Alcohol and hangover	142	128		3,960
Female, alcohol and hangover	8	12	69	1,730
Female and beer	136	223	1,374	49,100
Beer and hangover	7	5	8	1,600
Female, beer and hangover	0	1	4	722

*Note that a large number of articles were not cited in this review because of non-human subjects, outcome measures used or relevance of the topic in the identified publications.

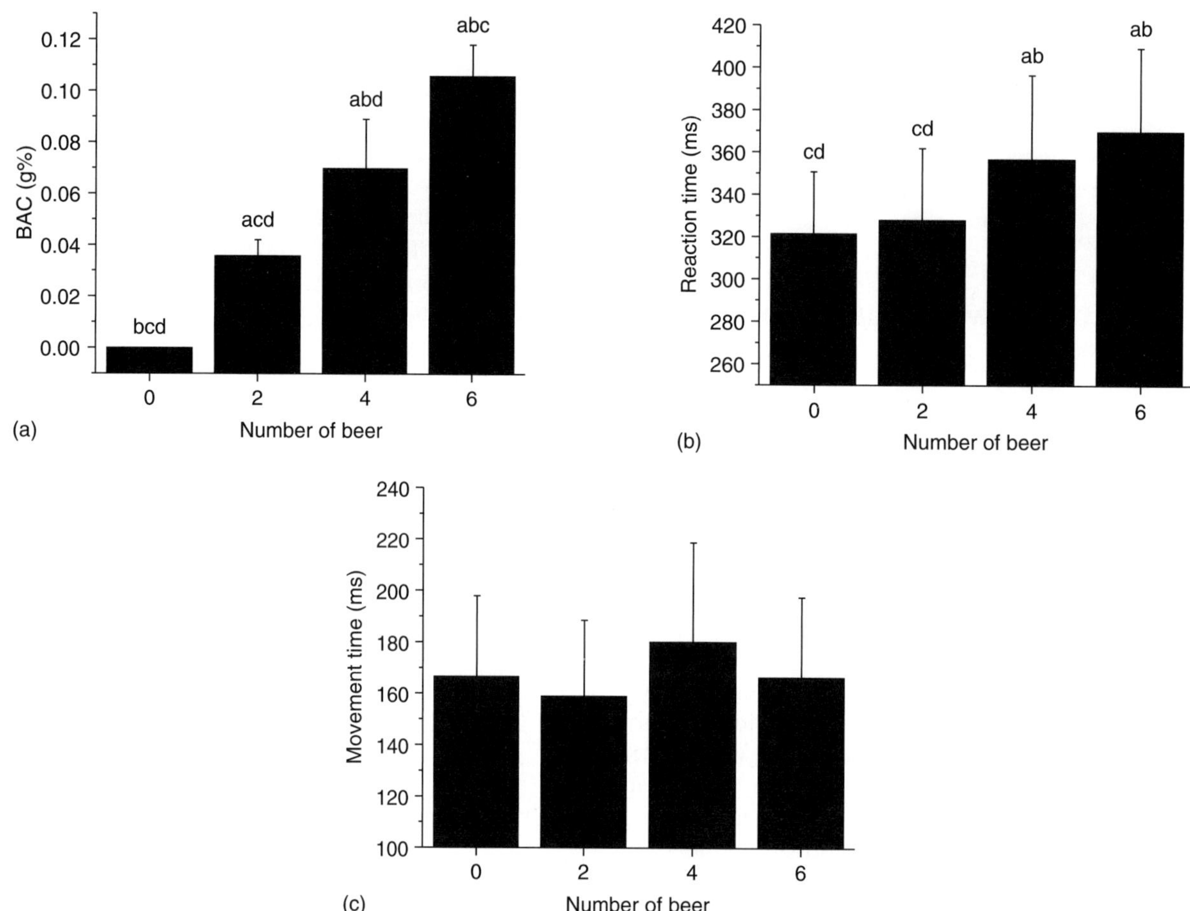

Figure 17.1 Peak mean BAC, four CRT and movement time within the hour following cessation of drinking. BAC = blood alcohol concentration, estimated with an Alco-Sensor IV breathalyzer in grams of alcohol per 100 ml of blood; error bars represent standard deviations; reaction time and movement time were obtained using four stimulus-response alternatives – following a cue, subjects released a central start key and moved up, down, right, left to depress a response key 15 cm away. ms = milliseconds or 1/1000th of a second. Repeated measures ANOVA and Tukey HSD *post hoc* analysis revealed significant differences ($p < 0.05$) between conditions. a, condition significantly different from 0 beer condition; b, condition significantly different from 2 beer condition; c, condition significantly different from 4 beer condition and d, condition significantly different from 6 beer condition.

Table 17.5 Frequency of rating hangover symptoms as absent, mild and severe by females ($n = 12$) the morning after consuming 0, 2, 4 and 6 bottles of beer

	0 beer (0 g alcohol)			*2 beer (27 g alcohol)*			*4 beer (54 g alcohol)*			*6 beer (81 g alcohol)*		
Hangover symptom	*A*	*M*	*S*	*A*	*M*	*S*	*A*	*M*	*S*	*A*	*M*	*S*
Headache	7	5	0	9	3	0	3	8	1	4	7	1
Nausea	12	0	0	8	4	0	10	2	0	6	4	2
Dry mouth/thirsty	7	4	1	3	8	1	2	9	1	0	5	7
Fatigue	3	7	2	4	4	4	3	7	2	1	6	5
Dizziness vertigo	11	1	0	6	6	0	6	6	0	4	5	3
Movement tremors	11	1	0	11	1	0	9	3	0	7	4	1
Upset stomach	12	0	0	9	2	1	12	0	0	6	3	3
Irritable	11	1	0	9	2	1	9	2	1	8	4	0
% of total responses	77	20	3	61	31	7	56	39	5	38	40	23

Note: Each bottle contained 341 ml of beer at 5% alcohol by volume which translates into 13.5 g of alcohol per bottle. Symptoms were rated on a 7 point Likert scale ranging from 0–6. A = absent, symptom given a rating of 0; M = mild, symptom given a rating of 1, 2 or 3; S = severe, symptom given a rating of 4, 5 or 6. Rounding errors are responsible for those conditions in which the % of total responses does not total 100%.

Table 17.6 Physiological and physical hangover effects of beer consumption in females (n = 12) the morning after consuming 0, 2, 4 and 6 bottles of beer

	Resting heart rate (bpm)	*Blood pressure (mmHg)*		*Grip strength (kg)*	*Body weight (kg)*
		Systolic	*Diastolic*		
0 beer (control)	66.8 (6.7)	114.5 (5.2)	73.4 (6.5)	64.8 (14.5)	66.4 (7.1)
2 beer	61.5 (7.1)	115.7 (6.9)	76.0 (10.7)	64.9 (13.1)	66.8 (6.7)
4 beer	63.8 (7.8)	114.3 (5.6)	74.4 (7.7)	65.4 (14.5)	67.0 (7.1)
6 beer	64.4 (11.3)	116.5 (8.3)	75.0 (8.3)	64.0 (13.9)	66.9 (6.9)

Note: bpm = beats per minute; mmHg = millimeters of mercury; kg = kilograms. For each condition, standard deviations are provided in parentheses following the mean value. Heart rate and blood pressure were measured in bed prior to standing. Grip strength is the sum of the better of two trials from each of the dominant and non-dominant hand.

Table 17.7 Hangover effects of beer consumption on physical performance in females (n = 12) the morning after consuming 0, 2, 4 and 6 bottles of beer

	Time to exhaustion (min:sec)	*RPE* (Borg scale)*		*Blood glucose† (mM)*			*Blood lactate† (mM)*		
		Submax	*Max*	*Resting*	*Submax*	*Max*	*Resting*	*Submax*	*Max*
0 beer (control)	12:44 (6:22)	12.7 (2.2)	17.7 (1.2)	4.8 (0.6)	4.6 (1.1)	6.0 (1.7)	1.3 (0.4)	2.7 (1.6)	7.7 (3.8)
2 beer	11:27 (5:39)	13.1 (2.7)	17.1 (1.9)	5.1 (1.5)	4.5 (1.9)	6.1 (1.9)	1.6 (1.7)	2.3 (1.4)	6.4 (2.3)
4 beer	12:53 (6:34)	13.1 (1.6)	17.9 (1.4)	4.9 (0.7)	5.0 (0.8)	6.1 (1.8)	1.5 (0.9)	3.4 (1.4)	8.1 (2.8)
6 beer	11:41 (5:24)	13.6 (2.1)	17.4 (1.4)	4.8 (0.8)	5.2 (1.3)	5.8 (1.5)	1.4 (0.8)	3.2 (1.9)	7.1 (2.2)

Notes: For each condition, standard deviations are provided in parentheses following the mean value. RPE = rating of perceived exertion; min:sec = minutes and seconds; mM = millimoles; submax = the 6 min submaximal portion of the treadmill run during which the treadmill operated at 6 miles per hour at a 0% grade – RPE, glucose and lactate were measured in the last minute; max = the maximal portion of the treadmill run during which the treadmill operated at 6 miles per hour at a 7% grade – RPE, glucose and lactate were measured immediately following termination.

*Dose of beer consumed produced a significant ($p < 0.05$) increase in the ratings of perceived exertion between the 2 and 4 beer conditions during maximal exercise but not during the submaximal run.

†indicates a significant ($p < 0.05$) increase with exercise intensity (from rest to submaximal exercise to maximal exercise).

Post-intoxication resting HR, systolic and diastolic blood pressure and body mass following consumption of 0, 2, 4 or 6 beers in young adult women are presented in Table 17.6. Neither resting HR, resting blood pressure nor body mass was affected by the amount of beer consumed the previous evening.

Physical testing was also performed the morning after consumption. Overall grip strength performance was not affected by dose conditions (Table 17.6) and further analysis demonstrated that grip strength in neither the dominant nor the non-dominant hand was affected by the amount of beer consumed by this group of women (unpublished observation). A submaximal treadmill run and a run to exhaustion were also completed. The effect of dose of beer in the time to exhaustion on the treadmill test the following morning is shown in Table 17.7. There was no statistically significant difference in time to exhaustion with an increasing dose of beer, and the dose of beer did not alter HR in response to exercise in the female subjects the next morning. As expected, there was an increase in HR and perception of effort from submaximal to maximal treadmill exercise regardless of the amount of beer subjects had consumed (Table 17.7). While ratings of perceived effort varied significantly with the dose of beer consumed, the pattern did not follow a dose–response relationship as lower ratings of perceived effort were provided the morning after consuming 6 relative to 4 bottles of beer. As expected, blood glucose and blood lactate increased with exercise intensity but the amount of beer consumed did not alter this anticipated relationship in either variable (Table 17.7).

Psychomotor testing the next morning showed that the mean number of response errors made during CRT testing were greatest following consumption of the highest dose although neither reaction time nor movement time varied significantly with the amount of beer consumed the night before. This finding suggests that the time needed to react to an event does not change when the event is perceived correctly, however at the highest dose the event was misperceived more often (Kruisselbrink *et al.*, 2006).

Conclusions

Overall, this first and only study on the effects of increasing, moderate doses of beer on physical, physiological and psychomotor variables in young female subjects indicates that, despite the moderate dose of beer consumed in a more ecologically valid fashion (i.e. 81 g alcohol in 6 beers over 2 h 40 min for the largest dose), very few performance characteristics were significantly altered. Cardiovascular physiology and aerobic performance, maximal muscle strength and metabolism during a submaximal and maximal run on a treadmill appear to be largely unaffected in healthy young adult women even after reaching BACs of approximately 0.10 g%. A number of variables may have contributed to the null results obtained in this study. These include the amount of beer consumed, age of subjects, tolerance to alcohol, rate of consumption, the laboratory conditions of drinking and sleeping, food consumed, hydration status, the delay between drinking and hangover testing, the relatively short duration of post-intoxication testing and the sensitivity of tests used. Moreover, anecdotally, in the debriefing for the study, a number of participants indicated that their mood likely played a larger role in their ability to perform than the amount of beer consumed the night before. Future studies should attempt to control as many of these variables as possible.

Summary Points

- Approximately 50% of alcohol (ethanol) consumed in North America is in the form of beer.
- To date the available literature shows that there appear to be differences in the consumption of beer by females and males, with females consuming less beer than males.
- The lower volume of body water combined with faster alcohol elimination rates in females will cause females to reach higher peak BACs than males of equal body weight, but they will also likely return to zero faster.
- Any differences in the way the bodies of females and males respond to alcohol appear to have little effect on the experience of drunkenness and hangover, given that females rate perceived intoxication and hangover severity similar to males.
- Physical testing of females has shown no significant impact of hangover on HR, blood pressure, grip strength, metabolism during exercise or running performance even when peak BAC had reached 0.10 g% 9 h previous.
- In the short term, neither physical nor psychomotor performance appears to be greatly compromised in women after consuming up to 6 beers to perform than the amount of beer consumed the night before. No decreases in complex cognitive functioning have been reported; however, the increase in error rates on a CRT test suggests that the delayed effects of alcohol consumption may affect cognitive processing.

Recommendations

- The database of research examining hangover effects of beer consumption is extremely limited. Currently, little is known about whether a beer hangover is rated any differently from hangovers induced by wine or spirits, and if differences do exist, whether they alter performance. In addition to exposing the need for more research into the delayed effects of beer consumption, we also reinforce Gauvin *et al.*'s (1993) recommendation for more hangover research that includes female participants.
- Moreover, we recommend that researchers who include females as research participants in hangover studies provide an analysis of sex differences related to the experience and any effects of hangover, as Taylor *et al.* (1996) did.
- Many of the tasks used in hangover research, with the exception of some flight simulations, are short-duration tasks. Perhaps hangover effects can be overcome in the short term (e.g. 1 h) and emerge to a greater extent when the subject's attention and energy must be sustained over time. We recommend incorporating longer duration tasks into hangover testing batteries.
- We also recommend that researchers continue to search for tests that are sensitive to hangover effects. Perhaps the demands of many of the tests that produce inconsistent results simply do not place sufficient resource demands on hungover subjects.

Acknowledgments

The authors would like to acknowledge Audrey Kruisselbrink for her assistance in preparing tables, as well as Katrina Martin, Michael Megeney and Jonathon Fowles for the many hours spent in the lab collecting data.

References

Anderson, S. and Dawson, J. (1999). *S. Afr. J. Sci.* 95, 145–147.

Anylian, G.H., Dorn, J. and Swerdlow, J. (1978). *S. Afr. Med. J.* 54, 193–198.

Baglietto, L., English, D.R., Hopper, J.L., Powles, J. and Giles, G.G. (2006). *Alcohol Alcohol.* 41, 664–671.

Brewers Association of Canada (2006). Available at http://www.brewers.ca/EN/statistics/asb/page64-05.pdf.

Chait, L.D. and Perry, J.L. (1994). *Psychopharmacology* 115, 340–349.

Engs, R.C. and Hanson, D.J. (1990). *J. Alcohol Drug Educ.* 35, 36–47.

Finnigan, F., Schulze, D., Smallwood, J. and Helander, A. (2005). *Addiction* 100, 1680–1689.

Gauvin, D.V., Cheng, E.Y. and Holloway, F.A. (1993). Biobehavioral correlates. In Galanter, M. (ed.), *Recent Developments in Alcoholism, Volume 11: Ten Years of Progress*, pp. 281–304. Plenum, New York.

Goist Jr., K.C. and Sutker, P.B. (1985). *Pharmacol. Biochem. Behav.* 22, 811–814.

Health Canada (1999). Available at http://www.statcan.ca/english/freepub/82-570-XIE/82-570-XIE1997001.pdf.

Jones, B.M. and Jones, M.K. (1976). *Ann. NY Acad. Sci.* 273, 576–587.

Jones, B.M. and Jones, M.K. (1977). Alcohol and memory impairment in male and female social drinkers. In Birnbaum, I.M. and Parker, E.S. (eds), *Alcohol and Human Memory*, pp. 127–138. Erlbaum, Hillsdale, NJ.

Karvinen, E., Miettinen, M. and Ahlman, K. (1962). *Q. J. Stud. Alcohol* 23, 208–215.

Kim, D.J., Yoon, S.J., Lee, H.P., Choi, B.M. and Go, H.J. (2003). *Int. J. Neurosci.* 113, 581–594.

Kruisselbrink, L.D., Gullick, T., MacDougall, B.D. and Murphy, R.J.L. (2004). *Can. J. Appl. Physiol.* 29, S60.

Kruisselbrink, L.D., Martin, K.L., Megeney, M., Fowles, J.R. and Murphy, R.J.L. (2006). *J. Stud. Alcohol* 67, 416–420.

Lakins, N.E., Williams, G.D. and Hsiao-ye, Y. (2006). Available at http://pubs.niaaa.nih.gov/publications/surveillance78/CONS04.pdf.

Lammers, S.M., Mainzer, D.E. and Breteler, M.H. (1995). *Addiction* 90, 23–30.

Lemon, J. (1993). *Drug Alcohol Rev.* 12, 299–314.

Lemon, J., Chesher, G.B., Fox, A., Greeley, J. and Nabke, C. (1993). *Alcohol. Clin. Exp. Res.* 17, 665–668.

McKinney, A. and Coyle, K. (2004). *Alcohol Alcohol.* 39, 509–513.

McKinney, A. and Coyle, K. (2006). *Alcohol Alcohol.* 41, 54–60.

Mills, K.C. and Bisgrove, E.Z. (1983). *Alcohol. Clin. Exp. Res.* 7, 393–397.

Morrow, D., Yesavage, J., Leirer, V., Dolhert, N., Taylor, J. and Tinklenberg, J. (1993). *Aviat. Space Environ. Med.* 64, 697–705.

Mumenthaler, M.S., Taylor, J.L., O'Hara, R. and Yesavage, J.A. (1999). *Alcohol Res. Health* 23, 55–64.

National Center for Health Statistics (2006). Available at http://www.cdc.gov/nchs/data/series/sr_10/sr10_232.pdf.

Niaura, R.S., Nathan, P.E., Frankenstein, W., Shapiro, A.P. *et al.* (1987). *Addict. Behav.* 12, 345–356.

O'Brien, C.P. (1993). *Sports Med.* 15, 71–77.

Petros, T., Bridewell, J., Jensen, W., Ferraro, F.R., Bates, J., Moulton, P., Turnwell, S., Rawley, D., Howe, T. and Gorder, D. (2003). *Int. J. Aviat. Psychol.* 13, 287–300.

Plant, M.A., Kreitman, N., Miller, T.I. and Duffy, J. (1977). *J. Stud. Alcohol* 38, 867–880.

Prendergast, M.L. (1994). *J. Am. Coll. Health* 43, 99–113.

Rehm, J., Greenfield, T.K., Walsh, G., Xie, X., Robson, L. and Single, E. (1999). *Int. J. Epidemiol.* 28, 219–224.

Rohsenow, D.J., Howland, J., Minsky, S.J. and Arnedt, J.T. (2006). *J. Stud. Alcohol* 67, 406–415.

Rosenbluth, J., Nathan, P.E. and Lawson, D.M. (1978). *Addict. Behav.* 3, 117–121.

Seppälä, T., Leino, T., Linnoila, M., Huttunen, M. and Ylikahri, R. (1976). *Acta Pharmacol. Toxcol.* 38, 209–218.

Single, E. and Wortley, S. (1993). *J. Stud. Alcohol* 54, 590–599.

Slutske, W.S., Piasecki, T.M. and Hunt-Carter, E.E. (2003). *Alcohol. Clin. Exp. Res.* 27, 1442–1450.

Statistics Canada (2004). Available at http://www.statcan.ca/english/freepub/82-221-XIE/2005002/nonmed/behaviours2.htm.

Statistics Canada (2005). Available at http://www.statcan.ca/english/freepub/89-503-XIE/0010589-503-XIE.pdf.

Statistics Canada (2006). Available at http://www.statcan.ca/english/freepub/82-221-XIE/2006001/tables/t015a.pdf.

Storm, T. and Cutler, R.E. (1981). *J. Stud. Alcohol* 42, 972–997.

Streufert, S., Pogash, R., Braig, D., Gingrich, D., Kantner, A., Landis, R., Lonardi, L., Roache, J. and Severs, W. (1995). *Alcohol. Clin. Exp. Res.* 19, 1141–1146.

Swift, R. and Davidson, D. (1998). *Alcohol Health Res. World* 22, 54–60.

Takala, M., Siro, E. and Toivainen, Y. (1958). *Q. J. Stud. Alcohol* 19, 1–29.

Taylor, J.L., Dolhert, N., Friedman, L., Mumenthaler, M. and Yesavage, J.A. (1996). *Aviat. Space Environ. Med.* 67, 407–413.

Törnros, J. and Laurell, H. (1991). *Blutalkohol* 28, 24–30.

Verster, J.C. (2006). *Alcohol. Clin. Exp. Res.* 30, 53A.

Verster, J.C., van Duin, D., Volkerts, E.R., Schreuder, A.H. and Verbaten, M.N. (2003). *Neuropsychopharmacol* 28, 740–746.

Wiese, J.G., Shlipak, M.G. and Browner, W.S. (2000). *Ann. Intern. Med.* 132, 897–902.

World Health Organization (1999). Available at http://www.who.int/substance_abuse/publications/en/GlobalAlcohol_overview.pdf.

World Health Organization (2004). Available at http://www.who.int/substance_abuse/publications/global_status_report_2004_overview.pdf.

Yesavage, J.A. and Leirer, V.O. (1986). *Am. J. Psychiatr.* 143, 1546–1550.

Yesavage, J.A., Dolhert, N. and Taylor, J.L. (1994). *J. Am. Geriatr. Soc.* 42, 577–582.

18

Beer Consumption During Pregnancy

Brittany B. Rayburn and William F. Rayburn Division of Maternal-Fetal Medicine, Department of Obstetrics and Gynecology, School of Medicine, University of New Mexico, Albuquerque, NM, USA

Abstract

Beer is the most commonly chosen and most heavily consumed alcoholic beverage by reproductive-age women. Lower cost, easy access, and a perception by many as being less harmful favors this alcoholic beverage, even after pregnancy awareness. Routine prenatal questioning should focus on beer drinking patterns. Drinking several consecutive beers is a particularly troublesome pattern before and after pregnancy recognition. Some pregnant women, especially heavy drinkers, will continue to drink beer. In addition to abstention-oriented health messages, it is prudent for the obstetrician to educate patients about beverage equivalency and standard drink sizes. Brief interventions and referrals to alcohol treatment programs are urged to reduce exposure and potential harm to the vulnerable fetus. Although evidence is inconclusive about effects from social drinking on fetal growth and neurobehavior development, it is recommended that women limit or preferably cease any alcohol consumption during pregnancy.

Introduction

Maternal alcohol consumption is a leading preventable cause of birth defects and childhood neurobehavior disabilities in the United States (Ebrahim *et al.*, 1998; Centers for Disease Control and Prevention, 2004). Frequent alcohol use during pregnancy has not reduced significantly in the United States during the past 20 years (from 3.9% in 1988 to 3.5% in 1995) (Ebrahim *et al.*, 1998). Adverse fetal outcomes associated with excess alcohol exposure include morphologic, behavioral, cognitive, hormonal, immunologic abnormalities and death (Centers for Disease Control and Prevention, 1995).

Despite the widespread availability of home pregnancy tests, most women are usually unaware that they are pregnant until after the fifth week, once the pregnancy is established and the fetal organs are being formed (Cole *et al.*, 2004). A recent cross-sectional study in 2002, using survey data collected by the United States National Center for Health Statistics, revealed that half of all pregnant women drank alcohol during the 3 months before pregnancy recognition, with one in twenty drinking at moderate-to-heavy levels (National Survey on Drug Use and Health, 2005). In most surveys of women who drank, the number of drinking days decreased considerably once pregnancy was recognized. For example, the survey from the National Center indicated that confirmation of a pregnancy led to a decrease in alcohol use, especially heavy consumption (National Survey on Drug Use and Health, 2005) (Table 18.1).

The type of alcoholic beverage and how it is consumed during pregnancy may affect fetal outcome (Lancaster *et al.*, 1989; Graves and Kaskutas, 2002; Bailey *et al.*, 2004). Beer is consumed often by reproductive-aged women, particularly in a binge pattern (Graves and Kaskutas, 2002; Centers for Disease Control and Prevention, 2004); Bailey *et al.*, 2004). The objective of this chapter is to examine the prevalence of beer consumption before and after pregnancy awareness and to counsel about hazards and therapy.

Table 18.1 Level of consumption of different alcoholic beverages before pregnancy awareness. Beer was consumed more heavily (moderate or heavy) than wine alone ($p < 0.05$) or liquor alone ($p < 0.05$)

	*Level of consumption**		
Beverage	*Light (%)*	*Moderate (%)*	*Heavy (%)*
Beer	5.5	28.8	65.8
Wine alone	25.0	75.0	0
Liquor alone	25.0	15.0	60.0
Wine and liquor combined	25.0	16.7	58.3

*Levels of drink units per drinking day: light (≤2 drinks); moderate (>2, <5 drinks); heavy (≥5 drinks).

Source: Fleming *et al.* (1997) with permission.

Beer in Health and Disease Prevention
ISBN: 978-0-12-373891-2

Beer Preference During Pregnancy

Beverage preference during pregnancy is affected by women's attitudes about the relative safety of different kinds of alcoholic beverages. For example, Graves and Kaskutas (2002) found that more than one-fourth of their surveyed Native American and African-American pregnant patients in 2002 believed that beer and wine were safer than other kinds of alcoholic drinks. In another study, pregnant African-American women who drank beer thought it was safer than other alcoholic beverages (Graves and Kaskutas, 2002). These women thought that reducing their drinking during pregnancy might not prevent birth defects or other harmful fetal effects.

Worldwide, pregnant women appear to prefer beer than other types of alcohol. In a study of 2,913 antepartum gravidas in Cleveland, Ohio, Sokol *et al.* (1981) reported that 57% of the women who reportedly drank while pregnant preferred beer to other forms of alcohol. About 52% of pregnant participants in a study in Sweden reported drinking beer at least once weekly, with one to six bottles or cans per occasion (Halmesmaki *et al.*, 1987). Younger women expressed more tolerant attitudes toward alcohol use and drank more beer on any occasion. Another study in South Africa revealed that women who continued to drink after pregnancy awareness tended to drink beer or to binge (Croxford and Viljoen, 1999).

Beer also appears to be the alcoholic beverage of choice for hazardous pregnant drinkers regardless of ethnicity (Rayburn *et al.*, 2006). Many study populations are predominantly low income, and beer is popular because it is the least expensive alcoholic beverage. These results add to the literature that reported beer products to be the preferred alcoholic beverage in poor or lower income communities. In a 1-year cohort of 872 Swedish nulliparas, Dejin-Karlsson *et al.* (1997) noted that younger women or those with fewer years of education tended to continue drinking alcohol if it was beer. In contrast, we found that more educated women drank wine and in low quantities before pregnancy and negligibly after confirmation of gestation (Rayburn *et al.*, 2006).

Social vs. Heavy Alcohol Consumption

A safe threshold dose for alcohol use in general and for beer in particular during pregnancy has never been established. Women at highest risk to have affected children are those who chronically ingest large quantities and those who engage in binge drinking. For comparison in alcohol consumption, drinks may be converted into standard drink units of 0.5 oz. of ethanol. One unit of alcohol equals approximately 8 g of absolute alcohol which is equivalent to one-half pint of ordinary strength beer, lager or cider or to one-fourth pint of strong beer or lager (Royal College of Obstetricians and Gynecologists, 1996).

Most reproductive-age women consume alcohol at some time. Occasional alcohol consumption is socially acceptable and regarded as normal behavior. This social activity during pregnancy is often discouraged, although its consequences are less clear. Investigations are limited by the often inexact or underreporting of alcohol consumed and by confounding factors, such as other substance use, time of pregnancy awareness, and manner in which alcohol is consumed.

Data are, therefore, inconsistent about the effect of "social drinking" on many pregnancy outcomes such as spontaneous abortion or preterm delivery. There is no conclusive evidence of reduced fetal growth or IQ level with alcohol consumption below 120 g (15 units) per week (Royal College of Obstetricians and Gynecologists, 1996). Social alcohol consumption does have a small negative effect on fetal weight. Separate studies by Mills and Florey reported a 66–83 g deficit in birth weight for an average of two drinks per day (Mills *et al.*, 1984; Florey *et al.*, 1992).

Impairment of intelligence appears to occur at higher levels of alcohol consumption. The best information comes from the Seattle Pregnancy and Health Study as summarized in a 1993 review (Streissguth *et al.*, 1994). That group reported a decrease of five IQ points in children of mothers drinking greater than 250 g of alcohol (>30 units) per week, while 7-year-old children of mothers drinking greater than 165 g (>20 units) per week had a decrease of seven IQ points. Other neurodevelopment impairments included deficits in attention and memory, and difficulties with arithmetic and reading.

Jones *et al.* (1973) were the first to describe "fetal alcohol syndrome" (FAS). Heavy maternal alcohol consumption was associated with the following fetal impacts: (1) growth restriction, (2) central nervous system involvement (neurological abnormalities, development delay, intellectual impairment, head circumference below the third centile, brain malformation), and (3) facial deformities (short palpebral fissures, elongated mid-face, flattened cheek bone). This syndrome is rare with reported incidences of 1.7 per 1,000 and 3.3 per live births in Sweden and France, respectively (Guerri *et al.*, 1999).

Neither fetal alcohol spectral disorders nor fetal alcohol syndrome can be diagnosed prenatally. There is no correlation between alcohol use and ultrasonically detectable facial and intracranial biometrical measurements (Handmaker *et al.*, 2006). Shown in Table 18.2 are prenatal ultrasound findings associated with FAS. While heart defects or cleft lip can be diagnosed sonographically, failure to identify major organ defects does not preclude other alcohol effects.

The syndrome is not seen consistently in infants born to women who are heavy consumers of alcohol. Women ingesting eight or more drinks daily throughout pregnancy have a 30–50% risk of having a child with all features of the alcohol syndrome (Abel, 1999). Susceptibility of fetuses to heavy alcohol exposure is believed to be multifactorial,

Table 18.2 Prenatal ultrasound findings associated with FAS.

- Symmetrical smaller size for gestational age
- Organ defects (heart, kidney, widespread eyes)
- Skeletal and rib abnormalities (small jaw and foot length)
- Vascular abnormalities (single umbilical artery, excess amniotic fluid)

reflecting a complex interplay of genetic factors, social deprivation, nutritional deficiencies, tobacco, and other substance use (Royal College of Obstetricians and Gynecologists, 1996).

Binge Drinking During Pregnancy

Binge drinking, defined as greater than or equal to five drinking units per drinking day, is associated with an increased finding of unplanned pregnancy and continued drinking during pregnancy (Ebrahim *et al.*, 1999). Intermittent fetal exposure to these potentially high levels of alcohol can have important neurologic consequences. Fetuses exposed to binge drinking are at greater risk of cognitive deficits, delinquent behavior at 7 years of age, and IQ scores in the mentally retarded range (Streissguth *et al.*, 1990; Jacobson *et al.*, 1998; Naimi *et al.*, 2003). In addition, maternal consequences of binge drinking include unintentional injuries, exposure to domestic violence, unprotected and unplanned sexual intercourse, spontaneous abortion, and sexually transmitted diseases (Naimi *et al.*, 2003).

This pattern is particularly noteworthy for beer consumption rather than for wine or distilled spirits alone. Binge drinking is common among our hazardous beer drinkers before and after pregnancy recognition. The National Survey on Drug Use and Health reported that 4.1% of pregnant women binge drank during the past month (National Survey on Drug Use and Health, 2005). Ebrahim *et al.* reported that, between 1991 and 1995, binge drinking among pregnant women increased significantly from 0.9% to 3.5% (Figure 18.1), whereas the prevalence changed little for nonpregnant women (11.3% vs. 11.2%) (Lancaster *et al.*, 1989).

Although some studies indicate that fetal injury can result from consuming as little as one to two drinks per day, the effects of binge drinking may have been obscured by computing a daily average alcohol consumption. For example, Jacobson *et al.* (1993) reported that the threshold below which no alcohol-related effects occurred was 0.5 oz. of absolute alcohol per day. Most women with affected children actually drank four to six drinks per occasion, however, which averaged to be lower daily doses. Subsequently, Jacobson *et al.* (1998) found that 80% of functionally impaired infants were born to women who drank more than five drinks per occasion, on several occasions weekly.

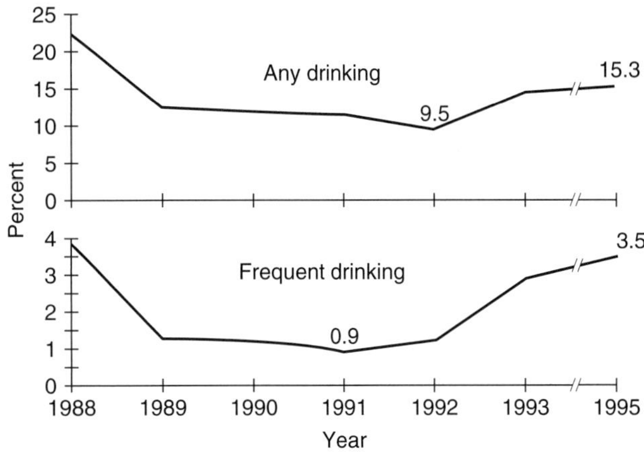

Figure 18.1 Alcohol drinking by pregnant women in the month before the survey, United States, 1988–1995. Percentages were adjusted to the population distribution of pregnant women in 1988. Frequent drinking = binge drinking or at least seven drinks per week. *Source*: Abel (1999) with permission.

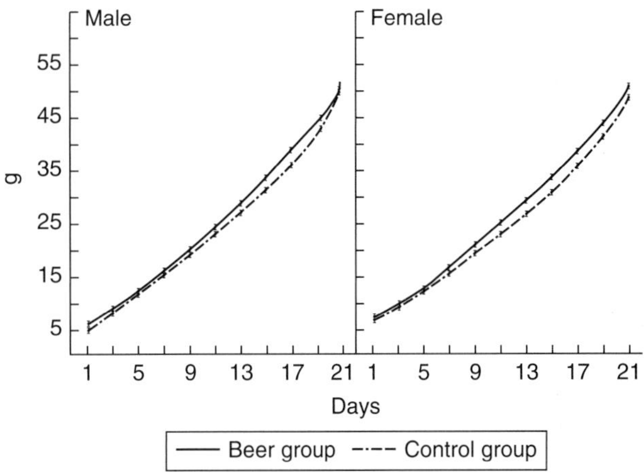

Figure 18.2 Body weights of male and female offspring of control rats and rats which drank beer during gestation. *$p < 0.05$, ANOVA. *Source*: Naimi et al. (2003) with permission.

Limitations with Animal and Human Investigations

We were only able to locate laboratory investigations about beer specifically during pregnancy by Lancaster and his colleagues (Lancaster and Spiegel, 1989, 1992; Lancaster *et al.*, 1989). Their method for voluntary beer drinking by pregnant rats identified subtle consequences of maternal beer drinking. Their findings in rodents suggest beer to be more hazardous to the fetus than other alcoholic beverages. Lancaster observed in gravid rats that beer exposure led to adverse effects on the fetal development. Beer-exposed offspring were less active in the open field than nonexposed offspring and had excess body weight from birth until 21 days of age (Lancaster *et al.*, 1989). As shown in Figure 18.2, gravid rats exposed to beer also had greater weights of their body and specific organs (thymus, spleen, heart, and liver) (Lancaster *et al.*, 1989; Lancaster and Spiegel, 1992).

Limitations of beer investigations in pregnant humans are noteworthy. Study populations may not be representative of all alcohol-exposed pregnancies. Hazardous drinkers often seek late or no prenatal care, and those who sought prenatal care early may not be representative. Many surveys rely on responses by pregnant drinkers to questionnaires to quantitate alcohol consumption. Their self-reported beer consumption is often underestimated (National Survey on Drug Use and Health, 2005).

There is no reliable laboratory technique in screening for long-term alcohol exposure. Alcohol and its metabolites are eliminated rapidly from the body, making them insensitive as biomarkers for chronic intermittent exposure (Bearer, 2001; Cook, 2003). Biological markers of excess alcohol consumption include blood gamma-glutamyl transferase, thiocyanate, and mean corpuscular volume (Bearer, 2001). None is precise, however, and better markers are being developed.

A limitation in counseling would be that it is not possible to focus solely on beer products and their harm to the mother or fetus. Most women drink beer with other alcoholic beverages before and after pregnancy awareness (Rayburn *et al.*, 2006). Furthermore, beer is often consumed with other substances such as cigarettes and marijuana (Rayburn *et al.*, 2006).

In addition to a brief alcohol intervention during initial prenatal care, the obstetrician or other healthcare provider is encouraged to offer a brochure, such as that published by the National Institute on Alcohol Abuse and Alcoholism, about the hazards of drinking during pregnancy. In addition, a list of local substance abuse and mental health treatment agencies, with a referral letter, are encouraged.

Prevention of Beer Drinking During Pregnancy

Prevention involves more than warning people about health hazards of alcohol abuse. It requires screening for early detection of alcohol abuse and providing patient-specific information. One method to screen for beer drinking is to include a prior week's diary of alcohol consumption, including lunchtime and early evening drinking. The T-ACE questionnaire, devised by Sokol *et al.* (1989), can be used to screen either the whole population or those women with growth-impaired fetuses. The survey consists of four questions:

1. **T** How many drinks does it take to make you feel high? (The patient is considered **t**olerant if it takes more than two drinks to her feel high) – 2 points
2. **A** Have people **a**nnoyed you by criticizing your drinking? – 1 point
3. **C** Have you ever felt you ought to **c**ut down your drinking? – 1 point
4. **E** Have you ever had a drink first thing in the morning to steady your nerves or to get rid of a hangover (**e**ye opener)? – 1 point

A total score greater than or equal to two points is considered to be positive and correctly identifies approximately 70% of heavy drinkers during pregnancy.

Very brief physician interventions or trials of advice qualify as prevention or early intervention programs that can be easily offered in medical practice. Randomized trials proved this to be effective in reducing harmful levels of alcohol consumption (Fleming *et al.*, 1997). Individuals should know that their attitudes and behaviors will affect how their children and spouses drink. All should be cautioned that drinking is dangerous in dealing with insomnia and emotional problems.

Counseling During Pregnancy

Therapies can be classified as psychological, behavioral, or sociocultural. Selection is best done on an individualized basis to meet the patient's specific needs. Most programs use a combination of such modalities. The current emphasis is on outpatient care, except for treatment of severe acute withdrawal syndrome. Costly inpatient care remains an option for people who have failed other forms of treatment and who will not deal with the problems so long as they are in environments that maintain destructive drinking.

Alcoholism is associated with special needs that require the therapist to take a more active role than is typical in insight-oriented psychotherapy. One must provide structure, guidance, support, nurturance, and instruction on helping the patient control drinking while working on her underlying conflicts and dysfunctional defense mechanisms. Behavioral–cognitive therapies are based on the notion that alcoholism is a learned behavior that can be extinguished and reshaped. Behavioral therapy is often useful in dealing with problems involving role changes and in motivating behavior change in specific situations. Cognitive therapy attempts to identify the precipitants to abuse and the factors that maintain or perpetuate it.

The primary physician can perform a major service for these patients by understanding available specialized referral resources in one's community and matching them to the patient's needs. Sociocultural treatment emphasizes altering external factors. It includes residential care, halfway houses, and direct social manipulation, such as finding jobs, helping with shelter and money, and removing a person from her family. This is a treatment appropriate for homeless, jobless young people, and severe family problems. Any of these approaches and the community services that follow can be used as adjuncts to other treatments wherever necessary. Alcoholics Anonymous is a community service that provides the critical elements of social support, caring, and structure, which are essential to many patients. Al-Anon and Alateen assist family members of the alcoholic, while Women for Sobriety stresses individual responsibility to boost self-esteem. Employee assistance programs and church organizations can be very helpful when motivation is high.

Drug Therapy During Pregnancy

Specific information about medication to curb beer drinking during pregnancy is unavailable. Drug therapy plays a supportive role in outpatient care, mainly by providing a temporary respite from alcohol consumption to engage in a more comprehensive and durable treatment program (Shaffer and Naranjo, 1998). The duration of therapy is individualized. Treatment should be terminated if the patient fails to keep appointments, resumes drinking, or develops abnormalities in liver function tests or cardiovascular status. Pharmacologic agents are prescribed to reduce the urge to drink, to blunt withdrawal symptoms, and to treat underlying psychiatric problems that may contribute to alcohol abuse. Treatment modalities when nonpregnant have been well summarized (Hanna, 2000).

Aversive therapy is seldom, if ever, used during pregnancy. Disulfiram (Antabuse) is an aversive drug not used during pregnancy. The drug sensitizes the patient to the effects of alcohol by inhibiting hepatic aldehyde-NAD oxidoreductase. Within minutes of taking as little as 1 oz. of alcohol, she can experience an increase in serum acetaldehyde concentration that leads to palpitations, flushing, tachypnea, tachycardia, and shortness of breath. Nausea, vomiting, and headache develop if a greater amount of alcohol is consumed. Symptoms last about 90 min but usually are self-limited. Naltrexone (Trexan), an opioid antagonist that appears to blunt the pleasurable effects of alcohol, is US Food and Drug Administration approved to reduce cravings.

Pharmacologic treatment of underlying psychopathology has been proposed as a means of cutting down on any form of drinking. Anxiolytic agents such as the benzodiazepines have been used with a modicum of short-term (less than 4 weeks) success in patients who drink because of an anxiety disorder. Buspirone has been effective in short trials as a treatment for severely anxious patients, but more work is required to clarify its effectiveness. Selective serotonin reuptake inhibitors may be effective when there is an underlying depression, especially when it is accompanied by neurovegetative symptoms. Lithium has been tried with lesser success.

The acute withdrawal syndrome and its severest manifestations and complications (seizures, hallucinations, and delirium tremens) are best prevented and treated during pregnancy by use of benzodiazepines or barbiturates such as phenobarbital (Hanna, 2000). The Clinical Institute Withdrawal Assessment – Alcohol, revised (CIWA-Ar) is the most validated instrument for objective assessment of withdrawal severity and risk. Women with moderate symptoms (e.g. CIWA-Ar score of 8–15) benefit symptomatically from treatment; those with severe symptoms (scores higher than 15) require pharmacologic therapy, because the risk of seizures is very high. Long-acting benzodiazepines (e.g. lorazepam, diazepam, chlordiazepoxide) appear to be more effective in preventing withdrawal seizures and in achieving a smoother withdrawal with fewer rebound symptoms than the short-acting agents; however, they are more likely to cause sedation. Fixed-dose, loading-dose, and symptom-triggered benzodiazepine regimens are effective when used as intended. Beta-blockers (e.g. atenolol, 50–100 mg/day) can help control adrenergic symptoms and reduce benzodiazepine requirements. Clonidine, a centrally acting inhibitor of noradrenergic activity, is an effective alternative to benzodiazepines in mild to moderate withdrawal syndrome when used in a tapered program. Outpatient administration is appropriate for those with mild symptoms of withdrawal.

Beer and Breastfeeding

Beer is used as a folk remedy to enhance lactation. However, a clinical study by Mennella and Beauchamp (1993) revealed that beer consumption by nursing women altered the sensory qualities of their milk and the short-term behavior of their infants during breastfeeding. The infants consumed significantly less milk shortly after their mothers drank beer. This reduced intake was not due to a decrease in the number of times the babies were fed. Despite this, the mothers believed that their infants had ingested enough milk, reported breast milk letdown while nursing, and felt that enough milk remained in their breasts at the end of most feedings.

Summary Points

- Beer is the most commonly chosen and most heavily consumed alcoholic beverage by reproductive-age women.
- Lower cost, easy access, and a perception by many as being less harmful favors this alcoholic beverage, even after pregnancy awareness.
- Routine prenatal questioning should focus on beer drinking patterns. Inquiring about malt liquor, drink size, and drink numbers is recommended for patients with a positive history of beer consumption.
- Binge drinking is a particularly troublesome pattern when beer is consumed before and after pregnancy recognition.
- In addition to abstention-oriented health messages, it is prudent for the provider to educate patients about beverage equivalency and standard drink sizes.

- Brief interventions and referrals to alcohol treatment programs are urged to reduce harm to the vulnerable fetus.
- Although evidence is inconclusive about effects from social drinking on fetal growth and neurobehavior development, it is recommended that a woman be careful or preferably cease any alcohol consumption during pregnancy.
- Beer consumption by nursing women may affect qualities of milk and short-term behavior of infants during breastfeeding. Decreased milk intake may result.

References

Abel, E.L. (1999). What really causes FAS? *Teratology* 59, 4–6.

Bailey, B.N., Delaney-Black, V., Covington, C., Ager, J., Janisse, J., Hannigan, J. and Sokol, R. (2004). Prenatal exposure to binge drinking and cognitive and behavioral outcomes at age 7 years. *Am. J. Obstet. Gynecol.* 191, 1037–1043.

Bearer, C. (2001). Markers to detect drinking during pregnancy. *Alcohol Res. Health* 25, 210–218.

Centers for Disease Control and Prevention (1995). Update: Trends in fetal alcohol syndrome – United States, 1979–1993. *Morbidity and Mortality Weekly Report* 44, 249–251.

Centers for Disease Control and Prevention (2004). Alcohol consumption among women who are pregnant or who might become pregnant – United States, 2002. *Morbidity and Mortality Weekly Report* 53, 1178–1181.

Cole, L.A., Khanlian, S., Sutton, J., Davies, S. and Rayburn, W. (2004). Accuracy of home pregnancy tests at the time of missed menses. *Am. J. Obstet. Gynecol.* 190, 100–105.

Cook, J.D. (2003). Biochemical markers of alcohol use in pregnant women. *Clin. Biochem.* 36, 9–19.

Croxford, J. and Viljoen, D. (1999). Alcohol consumption by pregnant women in the Western Cape. *South Afr. Med. J.* 89, 962–965.

Dejin-Karlsson, E., Hanson, B.S. and Ostergren, P.O. (1997). Psychological resources and persistent alcohol consumption in early pregnancy: a population study of women in their first pregnancy in Sweden. *Scand. J. Soc. Med.* 25, 280–288.

Ebrahim, S.H., Luman, E.T., Floyd, R.L., Murphy, C.C., Bennett, E.M. and Boyle, C.A. (1998). Alcohol consumption by pregnant women in the United States during 1988–1995. *Obstet. Gynecol.* 92, 187–192.

Ebrahim, S.H, Diekman, S., Floyd, R.L and Decoufle, P. (1999). Comparison of binge drinking among pregnant and non-pregnant women, United States 1991–1995. *Am. J. Obstet. Gynecol.* 180, 1–7.

Fleming, M.F., Barry, K.L., Manwell, L.B. *et al.* (1997). Brief physician advice for problem drinkers: A randomized controlled trial in community-based primary care practices. *J. Am. Med. Assoc.* 277, 1039.

Florey, C. du V., Taylor, D., Bolumar, F., Kaminski, M., Olsen, J., eds. (1992). EUROMAC – A European concerted action: maternal alcohol consumption and its relation to the outcome of pregnancy and child development at 18 months. *Int. J. Epidemiol.* 21, S1–S87.

Graves, K. and Kaskutas, L.A. (2002). Beverage choice among Native American and African American urban women. *Alcohol. Clin. Exp. Res.* 26, 218–222.

Guerri, C., Riley, E. and Stromland, K. (1999). Commentary on the recommendations of the Royal College of Obstetricians and Gynecologists concerning alcohol consumption in pregnancy. *Alcohol Alcoholism* 34, 497–501.

Halmesmaki, E., Raivio, K.O. and Ylikorkala, O. (1987). Patterns of alcohol consumption during pregnancy. *Obstet. Gynecol.* 69, 594–597.

Handmaker, N.S., Rayburn, W.F., Meng, C., Bell, J.B., Rayburn, B.B. and Rappaport, V.J. (2006). Impact of alcohol exposure after pregnancy recognition on ultrasonographic fetal growth measures. *Alcohol. Clin. Exp. Res.* 30, 892–898.

Hanna, E. (2000). Approach to the patient with alcohol abuse. In Goroll, A.H. and Mulley, A.G. (eds), *Primary Care* Medicine: Office *Evaluation and Management of the Adult Patient*, 4th edn, pp. 1174–1178. Lippincott Williams and Wilkins, Philadelphia, PA.

Jacobson, J.L., Jacobson, S.W., Sokol, R.J., Martier, S.S., Ager, J.W. and Kaplan-Estrin, M.G. (1993). Teratogenic effects of alcohol on infant development. *Alcohol Clin. Exp. Res.* 17, 174–183.

Jacobson, J.L., Jacobson, S.W., Sokol, R.J. and Ager, J.W. (1998). Relation of maternal age and pattern of pregnancy drinking to functionally significant cognitive deficit in infancy. *Alcohol. Clin. Exp. Res.* 22, 345–351.

Jones, K.L., Smith, D.W., Ulleland, C.N. and Streissguth, A.P. (1973). Pattern of malformation in offspring of chronic alcoholic mothers. *Lancet* (i), 1267–1271.

Lancaster, F.E. and Spiegel, K.S. (1989a). Voluntary beer drinking by pregnant rats: offspring growth, development, and behavior. *Alcohol* 6, 199–205.

Lancaster, F.E., Raheem, Z.A. and Spiegel, K.S. (1989b). Maternal beer drinking: offspring growth and brain myelination. *Neurotoxicology* 10, 407–415.

Lancaster, F.E. and Spiegel, K.S. (1992). Alcoholic and nonalcoholic beer drinking during gestation: offspring growth and glucose metabolism. *Alcohol* 9, 9–15.

Mennella, J.A. and Beauchamp, G.K. (1993). Beer, breast feeding, and folklore. *Dev. Psychobiol.* 26, 459–466.

Mills, J.L., Graubard, B.I., Harley, E.E., Rhoads, G.G. and Berendes, H.W. (1984). Maternal alcohol consumption and birthweight. How much drinking during pregnancy is safe?. *J. Am. Med. Assoc.* 252, 1875–1879.

Naimi, T., Lipscomb, L., Brewer, R. and Gilbert, B.C. (2003). Binge drinking in the preconception period and the risk of unintended pregnancy: implications for women and their children. *Pediatrics* 111, 1136–1141.

National Survey on Drug Use and Health (2005). Substance use during pregnancy: 2002 and 2003 updates. US Department of Health and Human Services, Rockville, MD. Available at: http://www.oas.samhsa.gov/nhsda/2k2nsduh/2k2sofw.pdf. Retrieved November 23, 2005.

Rayburn, B., Handmaker, N., Meng, C. and Rayburn, W. (2006). Wine consumption among hazardous drinkers during pregnancy. *J. Reprod. Med.* (in press).

Rayburn, W.F., Meng, C., Rayburn, B.B., Proctor, B. and Handmaker, N.S. (2006). Beer consumption among hazardous drinkers during pregnancy. *Obstet. Gynecol.* 107, 355–360.

Royal College of Obstetricians and Gynecologists (RCOG) (1996). Alcohol consumption in pregnancy. *RCOG Guideline No. 9*, November.

Shaffer, A. and Naranjo, C.A. (1998). Recommended drug treatment strategies for the alcoholic patient. *Drugs* 56, 571.

Sokol, R.J., Miller, S.I., Debanne, S., Golden, N., Collins, G., Kaplan, J. and Martier, S. (1981). The Cleveland NIAAA prospective alcohol-in-pregnancy study: the first year. *Neurobehav. Toxicol. Teratol.* 3, 203–209.

Sokol, R.J., Martier, S.S. and Ager, J.W. (1989). The T-ACE questions: practical prenatal detection of risk-drinking. *Am. J. Obstet. Gynecol.* 160, 863–870.

Streissguth, A.P., Barr, H.M. and Sampson, P.D. (1990). Moderate prenatal alcohol exposure: effects on child IQ and learning problems at age 7–12 years. *Alcohol. Clin. Exp. Res.* 14, 662–669.

Streissguth, A.P., Sampson, P.D., Olson, H.C., Bookstein, F.L., Barr, H.M., Scott, M., Feldman, J. and Mirsky, A.F. (1994). Maternal drinking during pregnancy: attention and short-term memory in 14-year-old offspring – a longitudinal prospective study. *Alcohol. Clin. Exp. Res.* 18, 202–218.

19

Beer and Other Alcoholic Beverages: Implications for Dependence, Craving and Relapse

Thomas Hillemacher and Stefan Bleich Department of Psychiatry and Psychotherapy, University Hospital Erlangen, Erlangen, Germany

Abstract

Beer and other types of alcoholic beverages play different roles in alcohol-mediated neurotoxicity, withdrawal symptoms, craving and relapse. This chapter will try to give an overview about pathophysiological mechanisms that are responsible for neurotoxicity and withdrawal symptoms, especially including the role of homocysteine and the glutamatergic system. In this context, differences between beverages and their influence on homocysteine-mediated toxicity are presented. Beer contains higher levels of folate than other alcoholic beverages. It has been found that consumers of beer had nearly consistent serum folate and moderately increased homocysteine levels compared to other patients with alcohol dependence. Also, neurobiological and particularly neuroendocrinological pathways are discussed in the pathogenesis of alcohol craving and relapse. Recently, differences between beverage types have been found to influence alcohol craving during withdrawal. We found that beer consumption was directly associated with the extent of craving, but not consumption of wine or spirits. A possible role of volume regulating mechanism with respect to a dysregulation of the hypothalamic–pituitary–adrenal axis will be discussed as a possible explication for these beverage-dependent differences. This may explain the found association between beer consumption and craving and may help to further understand neurobiological mechanisms of alcohol craving and relapse.

List of Abbreviations

ACTH	Adrenocorticotropic hormone
ANP	Atrial natriuretic peptide
CHD	Coronary heart disease
CRH	Corticotropin releasing hormone
HPA axis	Hypothalamic–pituitary–adrenal axis
ICD	International Classification of Diseases
MRI	Magnetic resonance imaging
MS	Methionine synthase
NF-κB	Natural killer-enhancing factor B
NMDA	*N*-methyl-D-aspartate
NMDAR	*N*-methyl-D-aspartate receptor
OCDS	Obsessive-compulsive drinking scale
PARP	Poly-ADP-ribose polymerase
ROS	Reactive oxygen species

Introduction

Alcohol dependence is, besides nicotine dependence, the clinically most important form of addiction. Lifetime prevalence is estimated in industrialized countries being about 3–6% for alcohol dependence and 4–16% for alcohol misuse. The differentiation between alcohol misuse and alcohol dependence is one first and important step because therapy differs regarding to the diagnosis. Referring to the international classification of diseases (ICD-10), alcohol dependence should be diagnosed if 3 of 6 criteria are positive: craving, loss of control, withdrawal symptoms, increasing tolerance regarding the effects of alcohol, neglect of social activities and interests, and to continue consuming alcohol in spite of damaging sequels. The amount of consumed alcohol or the type of consumed beverage is no criterion for alcohol dependence or misuse.

Excitatory amino acids, such as glutamate, aspartate and homocysteine, have been shown to be increased in patients with chronic alcoholism who underwent alcohol withdrawal. Furthermore, sustained hyperhomocysteinemia occurred in chronic alcoholics with an active drinking pattern. Excitotoxicity can be induced by increased homocysteine levels via rebound activation of *N*-methyl-D-aspartate receptor (NMDAR) mediated glutamatergic neurotransmission upon the removal of ethanol-evoked inhibition. Therefore, hyperhomocysteinemia may be responsible for the higher incidence of complications during alcohol withdrawal (e.g. seizures). In addition, an association between brain atrophy and increased levels of homocysteine in chronic alcoholism was shown. This may have important implications for the

Beer in Health and Disease Prevention
ISBN: 978-0-12-373891-2

pathogenesis of brain atrophy in alcoholics. However, there exist important differences regarding the consumption of different alcoholic beverages, particularly with respect to cardiovascular risks, neurotoxicity, craving and relapse.

Main Text

Homocysteine, alcoholic beverages and cardiovascular risk

Evidence from observational studies suggests that elevated levels of homocysteine are associated with an increased risk of cardiovascular diseases including coronary artery disease, cerebrovascular disease, peripheral vascular disease and venous thrombosis (Nygard *et al.*, 1997). Furthermore, it has been observed that chronic alcoholism is associated with increased homocysteine levels (Bleich *et al.*, 2000a, b, d, 2005; Cravo and Camilo, 2000) and could therefore be responsible for the increased incidence of stroke and myocardial infarction in this group (Bleich and Degner, 2000; Bleich *et al.*, 2000c). The "French paradox" is the lower-than-expected rate of mortality from coronary heart disease (CHD) conferred by mild-to-moderate alcohol consumption in a country where traditional risk factors of CHD (hypertension, hyperlipidemia, smoking, diabetes) are not less prevalent than in other industrialized countries and where the diet is rich in animal saturated fat. Thus, various epidemiological studies suggested that moderate alcohol intake results in a U-shaped curve in which the equivalent of two drinks (20–40 g alcohol per day) of any kind of alcohol, especially red wine consumption, is associated with a decreased incidence of CHD compared with no drinks (St Leger *et al.*, 1979; Renaud and de Lorgeril, 1992; Gronbaek *et al.*, 1995). However, higher doses result in an increased risk of infarction and stroke (Numminen *et al.*, 2000).

As shown in Figure 19.1 and Table 19.1, homocysteine levels are increased in social drinkers with daily alcohol consumption of beer, red wine or spirits (Bleich *et al.*, 2001). The reasons for the significant correlation between blood alcohol concentration on the one hand, and plasma homocysteine on the other, regardless of whether beer, wine or

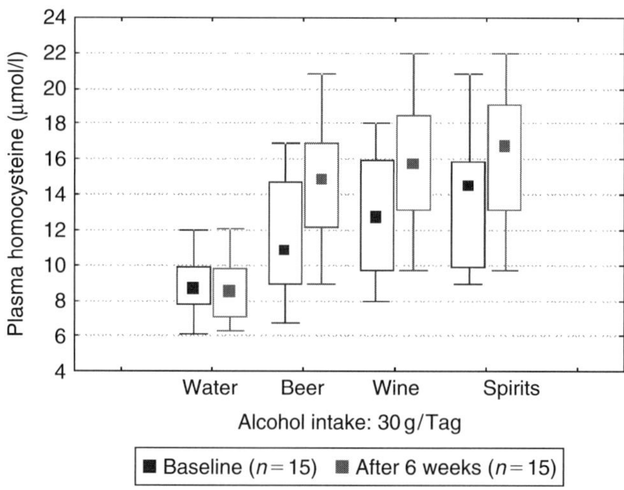

Figure 19.1 Homocysteine levels in dependence of beverage types (see Table 19.1).

Table 19.1 Homocysteine and other laboratory parameters in non-drinking controls and in subjects before and 6 weeks after daily consumption of beer, red wine or spirits

Parameter	*Mineral water*	*Beer*	*Red wine*	*Spirits*
Baseline				
Hcy (μmol/l)	9.06 ± 2.08	11.67 ± 2.17	12.69 ± 1.85	13.80 ± 2.22
Folate (μg/l)	12.3 ± 4.8	9.7 ± 3.3	9.2 ± 3.8	11.3 ± 5.3
B12 (ng/l)	512 ± 198	428 ± 118	612 ± 158	479 ± 87
B6 (μg/l)	11.3 ± 4.2	14.3 ± 6.2	9.9 ± 2.8	10.3 ± 4.1
After 6 weeks				
Hcy (μmol/l)	8.47 ± 1.42	14.58 ± 1.58*	15.61 ± 1.83*	16.25 ± 2.19*
Folate (μg/l)	11.5 ± 3.9	8.9 ± 4.1	7.1 ± 3.9**	9.1 ± 2.3**
B12 (ng/l)	578 ± 112	479 ± 77	543 ± 87	528 ± 115
B6 (μg/l)	9.8 ± 3.1	13.8 ± 4.7	8.4 ± 2.8	9.2 ± 3.9

Notes: Non-drinking individuals (n = 15) consumed mineral water whereas social drinkers (n = 15 per group) daily consumed 30 g alcohol in the form of beer, red wine or spirits over a period of 6 weeks. Homocysteine (Hcy) and vitamin levels (folate, B12, B6) were analyzed at baseline and after 6 weeks, respectively. Scores of folate (normal range: 4–17 μg/l), vitamins B6 (4–20 μg/l) and B12 (170–850 ng/l), and homocysteine (Hcy; 5–15 μmol/l). Homocysteine concentrations were significantly increased in social drinkers, especially in consumers of red wine and spirits (Mann–Whitney *U*-test, $p < 0.01$). The latter alcohol consumers also had significant lower folate levels ($p < 0.02$). Statistical details are summarized in the results section. Significant ($p < 0.02$) changes are marked:

* significant increase;

** significant decrease.

Source: Bleich *et al.* (2001).

spirits had been consumed (Bleich *et al.*, 2000c), are most likely complex ones in alcohol-dependent patients: impairment of remethylation of homocysteine is brought about on account of a dysfunction of methionine synthase (MS), due to an alcohol-induced vitamin deficiency (folic acid and vitamin B12), as well as a direct inhibition of MS due to acetaldehyde (Kenyon *et al.*, 1998), the product of oxidative degradation of alcohol. Regular consumers (daily alcohol intake over a period of 6 weeks) of red wine and spirits had significant lower folate levels when compared with concentrations at baseline (Bleich *et al.*, 2001). In addition, it has been known for many years that ethanol has an effect on folate metabolism, which could not be explained by an alcohol-induced low intake of folate (Sullivan and Herbert, 1964). The etiology of folate deficiency in alcoholism can be ascribed to several causes, such as low dietary intake, poor absorption, decreased hepatic uptake and retention, and increased urinary excretion of folate. Furthermore, beer is a rich source of folate (about 90–120 g/40 g alcohol) and vitamin B6 (about 0.3–0.5 mg/40 g alcohol), whereas red wine and spirits contain negligible amounts of these vitamins, which might explain that the consumers of beer had nearly consistent serum folate and moderately increased homocysteine levels (Bleich *et al.*, 2001). Additionally, abstinent individuals were shown to have significant higher levels of folate which might be explained by the lack of the alcohol-induced folate depletion, as described above.

Mildly elevated plasma homocysteine levels have been associated with an increased risk of CHD (Nygard *et al.*, 1997; Folsom *et al.*, 1998; Refsum *et al.*, 1998). Hence, it has been shown that homocysteine levels increase after 6 weeks consumption of red wine and spirits by 19% and 17%, respectively. The latter increase in homocysteine coincides with an increase of CHD risk of approximately 20% (Verhoef *et al.*, 1998). However, some other effects of alcohol may counteract the effect of homocysteine (Bleich *et al.*, 2000e; Paassilta *et al.*, 1998) and, in addition, other known risk factors for cardiovascular diseases (i.e. hypertension) must be taken into account. Furthermore, elevated plasma homocysteine levels may increase the risk for different types of vascular diseases (i.e. cerebral microangiopathy, brain infarction, peripheral vascular disease) whereby the exact mechanisms are largely unknown (Fassbender *et al.*, 1999).

Homocysteine and alcoholism: implications for neurotoxicity

More recent studies have demonstrated that the plasma homocysteine concentration is not only dependent on the type of alcoholic beverage, but especially on the amount of alcohol consumed and the blood alcohol concentration (Bleich *et al.*, 2000b, d). The degree of the plasma homocysteine levels is strongly determined by the degree of alcoholization. Whereas alcohol-dependent patients only have minimally elevated or already normal homocysteine concentrations a few days after they have stopped drinking, the majority of alcoholized patients have plasma homocysteine levels two to three times higher than the upper normal value of 15 μmol/l (Bleich *et al.*, 2000b, c, e). Course measurements during an alcohol withdrawal treatment show a continuous reduction in plasma homocysteine levels, which return more or less to within the normal range after around 3–7 days (Hultberg *et al.*, 1993; Bleich *et al.*, 2000e). Before withdrawal a remarkable feature is the significant positive correlation between the degree of the plasma homocysteine level and the blood alcohol concentration as well as the significant inverse correlation between homocysteine and the serum folic acid level (Bleich *et al.*, 2000d). The plasma levels of vitamins B12 and B6 are mostly even in the upper normal range and have no effect on the plasma homocysteine concentration (Bleich *et al.*, 2000b, d, e). However, other studies have shown a deficiency of these vitamins (Cravo *et al.*, 1996; Cravo and Camilo, 2000). The interplay of these conditions is important for an understanding of alcoholism-associated hyperhomocysteinemia, since a single intoxication with large amounts of alcohol does not lead to a pathological increase in plasma homocysteine concentrations in healthy subjects (Bleich *et al.*, 2000c).

Several mechanisms of toxic action of homocysteine have been discussed. Homocysteine can act as an agonist at the glutamate binding site of the NMDAR (Lipton *et al.*, 1997) which are expressed in both neurons and astrocytes (Conti *et al.*, 1990). Furthermore, it has been found that astrocytes regulate the expression of NMDAR subtypes which increase neuronal sensitivity to glutamate toxicity (Daniels and Brown, 2001). Thus, homocysteine leads to an enhanced excitatory glutamatergic neurotransmission in different brain areas (Lipton *et al.*, 1997) whereby neuronal damage derives from excessive calcium influx and reactive oxygen generation (Kim and Pae, 1996; Lipton *et al.*, 1997). Homocysteine can induce neuronal apoptosis or apoptotic processes by a mechanism involving DNA damage, poly-ADP-ribose polymerase (PARP), and mitochondrial dysfunction by caspase-3 activation (Kruman II *et al.*, 2000; Anton *et al.*, 2006). Autooxidation of homocysteine is known to generate reactive oxygen species (ROS), whereby the prevention of homocysteine-induced toxicity by catalase, in cell cultures which were coincubated with homocysteine and Cu^{2+}, suggests that hydrogen peroxide acted as a mediator of oxidative injury leading to apoptosis (Huang *et al.*, 2005). In the present study, this mechanism of toxic action seems less probable as the culture media used contained only minimal concentrations of metal ions. Homocysteine also decreases the expression of the antioxidant enzymes glutathione peroxidase and natural killer-enhancing factor B (NF-κB) so that homocysteine could potentially enhance conditions known to cause oxidative stress (Outinen *et al.*, 1998). Like some structurally related excitotoxins homocysteine may competitively inhibit cystine uptake resulting in a decrease in glutathion synthesis and reduced capabilities of blocking oxidative stress (Kato *et al.*, 1992; Meldrum, 1993).

Brain volumetric magnetic resonance imaging (MRI) studies on alcohol-dependent patients show a significant correlation between the degree of plasma homocysteine levels, on the one hand, and the hippocampal volume reduction or global alcoholism-associated brain atrophy, on the other (Bleich *et al.*, 2003; Bleich and Kornhuber, 2003). A new approach to explain the reversibility of "alcohol-induced" brain atrophy observed in many cases may be provided by transient ethanol-associated hyperhomocysteinemia. Accordingly, toxic hyperhomocysteinemia is to be discussed as being causative, but the influence of alcohol regarded as an indirect effect. These investigations are consistent with the observation that patients with hereditary homocystinuria, in addition to mental retardation, remarkably often display cerebral atrophy and suffer from epileptic seizures (Harris *et al.*, 2002). The latter fact is in line with more recent investigations showing that patients with moderate to severe hyperhomocysteinemia significantly more frequently suffer from alcohol withdrawal seizures (Bleich *et al.*, 2000a, 2006; Kurth *et al.*, 2001; Bayerlein *et al.*, 2005).

Craving and relapse in alcoholism

Craving is a well-studied phenomenon in patients with alcoholism (Geerlings and Lesch, 1999) and is known to be associated with a higher risk of relapse in patients suffering from alcohol dependence (Bottlender and Soyka, 2004). The manifestations of craving differ widely while obsession and compulsion have been described by many authors to be the most common characteristics (Modell *et al.*, 1992; Lesch *et al.*, 1997; Tiffany and Conklin, 2000). In fact, craving for alcohol shares many features with obsessive-compulsive disorders. Furthermore, it has much in common with other forms of craving, especially food craving (Pelchat, 2002). Craving is of high importance in treating addictive diseases and must be regarded as an important factor for relapse. Therefore, treatment of craving with psychotherapeutic or pharmacological interventions is of high interest in the therapeutic concept for patients with alcohol dependency. The efficacy of psychotherapeutic and pharmacological anticraving therapy has been described in various studies (Kranzler *et al.*, 1999; Rohsenow and Monti, 1999; Buerger *et al.*, 2002; Flannery *et al.*, 2003). Recently, the COMBINE-Study showed negative findings regarding the efficacy of acamprosate in relapse prevention (Anton *et al.*, 2006). However, the majority of existing studies and meta-analysis show significant effects for both, acamprosate and naltrexone (Kiefer *et al.*, 2003; Mann *et al.*, 2004). New substances like baclofen and topiramate have been studied to treat craving in alcoholism and have shown promising results (Johnson *et al.*, 2003; Addolorato *et al.*, 2006). While pharmacological anticraving therapy seems to be effective it is only one part of the therapeutic concept. An integrative therapeutic concept for relapse prevention should also include psychotherapeutic strategies differentiating in-patients and out-patients treatment, attendance in self-help groups, social activities and a tight connection with the therapist. Only if profiting of all these therapeutic possibilities, a low rate of relapse can be achieved.

The underlying mechanisms of alcohol craving are subject to intense research. Behavioral models intent to explain craving mainly by reinforcement as alcohol improves mood and reduces negative affective states. The mesocorticolimbic dopaminergic neurotransmission most probably is of crucial importance in cue-induced reinforcement (Wise, 1988; Heinz *et al.*, 2003b; Tupala and Tiihonen, 2004; Bowirrat and Oscar-Berman, 2005). Animal-experimental investigations have shown that alcohol directly stimulates dopaminergic neurons (Gessa *et al.*, 1966; Imperato and Di Chiara, 1986; Brodie *et al.*, 1995), while chronic consumption leads to a down-regulation of dopamine receptors. In human beings, reduced dopamine receptor activity has been reported in alcohol-dependent patients (Heinz *et al.*, 1995; Schmidt *et al.*, 2005). During detoxification, a normalization of down-regulated central dopaminergic receptors has been shown in recent studies (Markianos *et al.*, 2000). Furthermore, findings point toward a lower risk of relapse in patients with an increase of dopamine receptor responsivity (Markianos *et al.*, 2001).

Besides the dopaminergic system, recent studies have shown that also various neuroendocrinological conditions are associated with craving in alcoholism (Buerger *et al.*, 2002; Kiefer and Wiedemann, 2004). Many investigations showed that craving is associated with a disturbance of the hypothalamic–pituitary–adrenal (HPA) axis (Buerger *et al.*, 2002; Kiefer and Wiedemann, 2004). Higher craving was found to correlate with lower corticotropin releasing hormone (CRH) in patients suffering from alcohol dependency (Fahlke *et al.*, 1994; Olive *et al.*, 2003). Further studies showed, that also lowered cortisol- and ACTH-(adrenocorticotropic hormone)-serum levels are associated with higher craving and elevated relapse rates (Kiefer *et al.*, 2002; Junghanns *et al.*, 2003). Also changes of the prolactin secretion, possibly as sequel of a disturbed dopaminergic transmission in the tuberoinfundibular circuit, are associated with alcohol craving (Hillemacher *et al.*, 2005b; 2006a).

As described above, craving also shares many neurobiological pathways with food craving and appetite regulation. The peptide leptin, secreted by white adipocytes, is known to play an important role in hypothalamic appetite regulation (Kraus *et al.*, 2001). Kiefer *et al.* showed first evidence for an association between increased plasma concentration of leptin and craving for alcohol in 2001 (Kiefer *et al.*, 2001a, b). Since leptin plasma concentrations were shown to be elevated during chronic alcohol consumption (Nicolas *et al.*, 2001) and normalize during withdrawal and abstinence (Wurst *et al.*, 2003), leptin was discussed as a factor that mediates increased alcohol intake through increased urge to drink. Leptin is known to regulate the HPA axis and to inhibit the cortisol-mediated stress response (Inui, 1999). Also other appetite regulating hormones such as grehlin have been investigated to be associated with alcohol craving without positive findings up to now (Kraus *et al.*, 2005).

Differences regarding alcoholic beverages

The majority of studies on craving and relapse refer to ethanol intake without differentiating the type of consumed beverages. However, recent findings suggest that important differences exist between the different types of alcoholic drinks. So, consumption of low-alcohol drinks such as so-called alcohol free beer was found to be associated with increased craving (Long and Cohen, 1989), which points toward a beverage-dependent effect besides the "pure" ethanol impact. In the study of Willner *et al.* increased craving after exposure to low-alcohol beer was found in male recreational drinkers, which points toward the importance of gender effects in craving (Willner *et al.*, 2003). In female patients, Willner *et al.* found no effect or decreased craving after consumption of low-alcohol beer. In an investigation of our own study group, we demonstrated that craving is not only associated with alcohol intake. Instead, we found that craving for alcohol also depends on the type of alcoholic beverage consumed. In this recent study, we found that beer consumption, in contrast to wine or spirits consumption, is associated with higher alcohol craving (Hillemacher *et al.*, 2005a). The differences between the consumption of different alcoholic drinks with respect to high and low craving (using a median-split division of the OCDS, obsessive-compulsive drinking scale; $N = 198$) are shown in Figure 19.2.

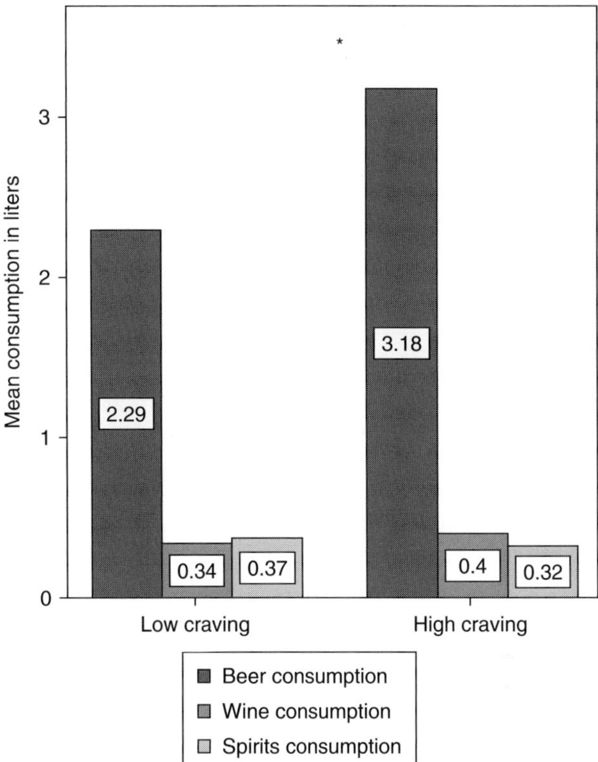

Figure 19.2 Differences regarding alcohol craving and consumption of different beverages. *Significant difference comparing low and high alcohol craving (OCDS median-split division) for beer consumption (Mann–Whitney *U*-test: $Z = -2.8$, $p = 0.004$), not for wine or spirits consumption; OCDS: obsessive-compulsive drinking scale.

The findings of this study are in line with other investigations, observing an association between craving and intake of low-alcohol beer (so-called alcohol free beer) in problem drinkers (Long and Cohen, 1989) and in male recreational drinkers (Willner *et al.*, 2003). These results add evidence to the hypothesis that craving as an important factor for relapse in alcoholism may be a special phenomenon in beer drinkers. Alcoholic patients who prefer wine or spirits may have other risk factors leading toward relapse or may mainly suffer from craving dimensions other than obsession and compulsion (Lesch *et al.*, 1997; Geerlings and Lesch, 1999).

A different motivation for consuming beer may help to explain these findings. In contrast to wine or spirits, beer is often used to quench one's thirst. This may cause an additional reward effect on beer consumption apart from the ethanol impact. Reward effects in alcoholism and craving have been described in recent studies (Heinz *et al.*, 2003a). Also, the similarity between alcohol craving and food craving may help to elucidate our findings (Pelchat, 2002). In this context, the orbito-frontal cortex, which is especially implicated in obsessive-compulsive disorders and alcohol craving (Volkow and Fowler, 2000; Pelchat, 2002), may play an important role. In addition to that, different neurobiological factors such as endogenous opiates that have been described as a factor in food craving and alcohol craving, may contribute to this pathophysiologic model (Buerger *et al.*, 2002; Pelchat, 2002).

One other possible explication of these findings would be associated with the high volume intake in beer drinkers. Especially, beer-drinking patients with alcohol dependence tend to consume high amounts of volume. Therefore, we studied whether the volume intake of alcoholic beverages in general and in comparison to the pure ethanol intake is associated with craving (Hillemacher *et al.*, 2006b). We found that the daily volume intake is significantly associated with craving, independently of the ethanol intake. Of course, these results do not mean that ethanol consumption is not involved in craving but points toward an additional influence of volume intake.

The possible role of volume regulating mechanisms

Changes in volume regulation during alcohol intoxication and withdrawal are well known and have been the focus of various studies (Eisenhofer *et al.*, 1985; Trabert *et al.*, 1992;

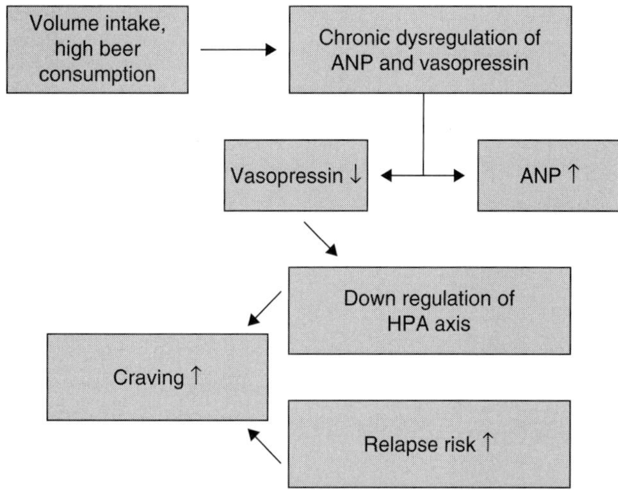

Figure 19.3 Volume regulating mechanisms.

Taivainen *et al.*, 1995; Buerger *et al.*, 2002). Recent investigations have shown that these alterations are persistent after detoxification in long-term abstinent alcoholics (Döring *et al.*, 2003; Jahn *et al.*, 2004). An association between craving and changes in volume regulation has been postulated (van Ree *et al.*, 1994; Döring *et al.*, 2003), but has not been studied in detail until recently.

In numerous studies, neuroendocrinological changes in alcohol dependency have been described (Kiefer and Wiedemann, 2004). We suppose that higher volume intake may lead to higher craving via changes in the vasopressin and atrial natriuretic peptide (ANP) metabolism. In alcohol craving, a role of the vasopressin metabolism and an involvement of the HPA axis has been suggested in different studies (Buerger *et al.*, 2002; Döring *et al.*, 2003; Hillemacher *et al.*, 2005b). The present results suggest that the described findings about the association of beer consumption with craving (Hillemacher *et al.*, 2005a) may be explained by a volume effect, as – evidently – beer consumption is associated with higher volume intake than wine or spirits consumption. This concept has much in common with concepts referring to similarities between alcohol craving and food craving, for example in patients suffering from binge eating disorder. For a schematic illustration of the proposed neurobiological mechanisms see Figure 19.3.

Patients with alcohol dependency can be subtyped not only referring to their consumed beverages but also taking into account other biological and psychosocial factors. In Europe, the Lesch's typology of alcohol dependence is widely used to distinguish different forms of alcohol dependency. The Lesch's typology is a well-established classification taking into account social, mental and somatic factors (Lesch *et al.*, 1990; Lesch and Walter, 1996). The typology differentiates four subtypes: type 1 (model of allergy) is characterized as patients with heavy alcohol detoxifications, who tend to use alcohol to weaken detoxification symptoms. Patients of type 2

Table 19.2 Lesch's typology of alcohol dependence

Lesch Type 1	Severe alcohol withdrawals, alcohol to ease withdrawal symptoms
Lesch Type 2	Alcohol consumption as self-medication in patients with comorbid anxiety disorder
Lesch Type 3	Patients using alcohol to treat an underlying mood disorder
Lesch Type 4	Infantile cerebral damage, behavioral disorders

(model of anxiety or conflict) use alcohol as self-medication because of anxiolytic effects. In patients of Lesch's type 3 an affective disorder is the main characteristic as origin of alcohol abuse (alcohol as an antidepressant). Instead, Type 4 patients (alcohol as adaptation) show pre-morbid cerebral defects, a high social burden and behavioral disorders.

We used the Lesch's typology to analyze whether the described association between volume intake and alcohol craving is more important in a patients subgroup than in other patients. The results show, that this association is of highest importance in Lesch type 2 patients. If proposing a dysregulation of vasopressin and ANP it is notable that ANP has been discussed to have an anxiolytic activity (Wiedemann *et al.*, 2001; Herrmann-Lingen *et al.*, 2003). Animal studies have proposed an involvement of ANP in fear-motivated learning processes (Bidzseranova *et al.*, 1992). Craving and anxiety have many features in common from a psychopathological point of view. Therefore, especially in patients with comorbid anxiety disorder, a dysfunction of volume regulating mechanisms might be important.

Perspectives

Understanding the neurobiological mechanisms is one important step to develop new and more effective therapeutic strategies for treating alcohol withdrawal and dependency. Homocysteine is increasingly regarded as a risk factor for patients to develop alcohol withdrawal seizures and is also already used in some centers as a biological marker to assess the individual seizure risk. Taking into account that high plasma homocysteine levels are helpful in the prediction of alcohol withdrawal seizures, early anticonvulsive therapy could prevent this severe complication. Prospective intervention studies may show whether the incidence of complications of alcohol withdrawal (e.g. withdrawal seizures) or alcoholism-associated damage (e.g. brain atrophy) can be reduced by therapeutic measures with early lowering of elevated homocysteine levels (e.g. folate administration). Supplementation of folate, a cofactor of the homocysteine catabolism, lowers raised homocysteine levels and therefore could be established as a new therapeutic strategy in alcohol withdrawal treatment. The results of various studies highlight the need for further research to prove whether alcoholics benefit from a reduced homocysteine level with respect to both, alcohol-related disorders and alcohol withdrawal symptoms.

Regarding craving and relapse prevention, the described new findings show that relapse and craving not only depend on the amount of consumed ethanol but also differs in dependence of the consumed alcoholic beverages. This leads to new perspectives for research regarding the neurobiology of alcohol craving and may help to consider new therapeutic options in the future. Also, it shows that subtyping patients using specific typologies or just distinguishing different consumption patterns may be important to evaluate the efficacy of pharmacological interventions in future trials.

Summary Points

- Beer and other alcoholic beverages have different effect on the cardiovascular risk factor homocysteine.
- Homocysteine levels on admission may be a useful screening method to identify alcoholic patients at risk for withdrawal seizures.
- Alcohol consumption-associated increase of homocysteine provides new approaches for explaining the damaging consequences of dependent drinking.
- Craving in alcohol dependence differs with respect to the amount of consumed beer, wine or spirits.
- The volume regulating endocrinological system may be one important pathway in the neurobiology of alcohol craving due to a dysregulation of vasopressin and ANP.

References

Addolorato, G., Leggio, L., Agabio, R., Colombo, G. and Gasbarrini, G. (2006). *Int. J. Clin. Pract.* 60, 1003–1008.

Anton, R.F., O'Malley, S.S., Ciraulo, D.A., Cisler, R.A., Couper, D., Donovan, D.M., Gastfriend, D.R., Hosking, J.D., Johnson, B.A., LoCastro, J.S., Longabaugh, R., Mason, B.J., Mattson, M.E., Miller, W.R., Pettinati, H.M., Randall, C.L., Swift, R., Weiss, R.D., Williams, L.D. and Zweben, A. (2006). *JAMA* 295, 2003–2017.

Bayerlein, K., Hillemacher, T., Reulbach, U., Mugele, B., Sperling, W., Kornhuber, J. and Bleich, S. (2005). *Biol. Psychiatr.* 57, 1590–1593.

Bidzseranova, A., Gueron, J., Balaspiri, L. and Telegdy, G. (1992). *Peptides* 13, 957–960.

Bleich, S. and Degner, D. (2000). *Atherosclerosis* 150, 441–442.

Bleich, S. and Kornhuber, J. (2003). *Neurology* 60, 1220. Author reply 1220.

Bleich, S., Degner, D., Bandelow, B., von Ahsen, N., Ruther, E. and Kornhuber, J. (2000a). *Neuroreport* 11, 2749–2752.

Bleich, S., Degner, D., Javaheripour, K., Kurth, C. and Kornhuber, J. (2000b). *J. Neural. Transm. Suppl.* 60, 187–196.

Bleich, S., Degner, D., Kropp, S., Ruther, E. and Kornhuber, J. (2000c). *Lancet* 356, 512.

Bleich, S., Degner, D., Wiltfang, J., Maler, J.M., Niedmann, P., Cohrs, S., Mangholz, A., Porzig, J., Sprung, R., Ruther, E. and Kornhuber, J. (2000d). *Alcohol Alcohol.* 35, 351–354.

Bleich, S., Spilker, K., Kurth, C., Degner, D., Quintela-Schneider, M., Javaheripour, K., Ruther, E., Kornhuber, J. and Wiltfang, J. (2000e). *Neurosci. Lett.* 293, 171–174.

Bleich, S., Bleich, K., Kropp, S., Bittermann, H.J., Degner, D., Sperling, W., Ruther, E. and Kornhuber, J. (2001). *Alcohol Alcohol.* 36, 189–192.

Bleich, S., Bandelow, B., Javaheripour, K., Muller, A., Degner, D., Wilhelm, J., Havemann-Reinecke, U., Sperling, W., Ruther, E. and Kornhuber, J. (2003). *Neurosci. Lett.* 335, 179–182.

Bleich, S., Carl, M., Bayerlein, K., Reulbach, U., Biermann, T., Hillemacher, T., Bönsch, D. and Kornhuber, J. (2005). *Alcohol Clin. Exp. Res.* 29, 334–336.

Bleich, S., Bayerlein, K., Hillemacher, T., Degner, D., Kornhuber, J. and Frieling, H. (2006). *Epilepsia* 47, 934–938.

Bottlender, M. and Soyka, M. (2004). *Alcohol Alcohol* 39, 357–361.

Bowirrat, A. and Oscar-Berman, M. (2005). *Am. J. Med. Genet. B Neuropsychiatr. Genet.* 132, 29–37.

Brodie, M.S., Trifunovic, R.D. and Shefner, S.A. (1995). *J. Pharmacol. Exp. Ther.* 273, 1139–1146.

Buerger, K., Teipel, S.J., Zinkowski, R., Blennow, K., Arai, H., Engel, R., Hofmann-Kiefer, K., McCulloch, C., Ptok, U., Heun, R., Andreasen, N., DeBernardis, J., Kerkman, D., Moeller, H., Davies, P. and Hampel, H. (2002). *Neurology* 59, 627–629.

Conti, A., Monopoli, A., Forlani, A., Ongini, E., Antona, C. and Biglioli, P. (1990). *Eur. J. Pharmacol.* 176, 207–212.

Cravo, M.L. and Camilo, M.E. (2000). *Nutrition* 16, 296–302.

Cravo, M.L., Gloria, L.M., Selhub, J., Nadeau, M.R., Camilo, M.E., Resende, M.P., Cardoso, J.N., Leitao, C.N. and Mira, F.C. (1996). *Am. J. Clin. Nutr.* 63, 220–224.

Daniels, M. and Brown, D.R. (2001). *J. Biol. Chem.* 276, 22446–22452.

Döring, W.K., Herzenstiel, M.N., Krampe, H., Jahn, H., Pralle, L., Sieg, S., Wegerle, E., Poser, W. and Ehrenreich, H. (2003). *Alcohol Clin. Exp. Res.* 27, 849–861.

Eisenhofer, G., Lambie, D.G., Whiteside, E.A. and Johnson, R.H. (1985). *Br. J. Addict.* 80, 195–199.

Fahlke, C., Hard, E., Thomasson, R., Engel, J.A. and Hansen, S. (1994). *Pharmacol. Biochem. Behav.* 48, 977–981.

Fassbender, K., Mielke, O., Bertsch, T., Nafe, B., Froschen, S. and Hennerici, M. (1999). *Lancet* 353, 1586–1587.

Flannery, B.A., Poole, S.A., Gallop, R.J. and Volpicelli, J.R. (2003). *J. Stud. Alcohol.* 64, 120–126.

Folsom, A.R., Nieto, F.J., McGovern, P.G., Tsai, M.Y., Malinow, M.R., Eckfeldt, J.H., Hess, D.L. and Davis, C.E. (1998). *Circulation* 98, 204–210.

Geerlings, P. and Lesch, O.M. (1999). *Alcohol Alcohol* 34, 195–196.

Gessa, G.L., Loddo, B., Schivo, M.L. and Tagliamonte, A. (1966). *Boll. Soc. Ital. Biol. Sper.* 42, 813–815.

Gronbaek, M., Deis, A., Sorensen, T.I., Becker, U., Schnohr, P. and Jensen, G. (1995). *BMJ* 310, 1165–1169.

Harris, B.R., Prendergast, M.A., Gibson, D.A., Rogers, D.T., Blanchard, J.A., Holley, R.C., Fu, M.C., Hart, S.R., Pedigo, N.W. and Littleton, J.M. (2002). *Alcohol Clin. Exp. Res.* 26, 1779–1793.

Heinz, A., Dettling, M., Kuhn, S., Dufeu, P., Gräf, K.J., Kürten, I., Rommelspacher, H. and Schmidt, I.G. (1995). *Alcohol Clin. Exp. Res.* 19, 62–65.

Heinz, A., Lober, S., Georgi, A., Wrase, J., Hermann, D., Rey, E.R., Wellek, S. and Mann, K. (2003a). *Alcohol Alcohol.* 38, 35–39.

Heinz, A., Schäfer, M., Higley, J.D., Krystal, J.H. and Goldman, D. (2003b). *Pharmacopsychiatry* 36, S255–S258.

Herrmann-Lingen, C., Binder, L., Klinge, M., Sander, J., Schenker, W., Beyermann, B., von Lewinski, D. and Pieske, B. (2003). *Psychosom. Med.* 65, 517–522.

Hillemacher, T., Bayerlein, K., Reulbach, U., Sperling, W., Wilhelm, J., Mugele, B., Kraus, T., Bönsch, D., Kornhuber, J. and Bleich, S. (2005a). *Addict. Biol.* 10, 181–186.

Hillemacher, T., Bayerlein, K., Wilhelm, J., Reulbach, U., Frieling, H., Bönsch, D., Kornhuber, J. and Bleich, S. (2005b). *Addict. Biol.* 10, 337–343.

Hillemacher, T., Bayerlein, K., Wilhelm, J., Frieling, H., Sperling, W., Kornhuber, J. and Bleich, S. (2006a). *Neuropsychobiology* 53, 133–136.

Hillemacher, T., Bayerlein, K., Wilhelm, J., Poleo, D., Frieling, H., Ziegenbein, M., Sperling, W., Kornhuber, J. and Bleich, S. (2006b). *Alcohol Alcohol.* 41, 61–65.

Huang, M.C., Chen, C.H., Yu, J.M. and Chen, C.C. (2005). *Addict. Biol.* 10, 289–292.

Hultberg, B., Berglund, M., Andersson, A. and Frank, A. (1993). *Alcohol Clin. Exp. Res.* 17, 687–689.

Imperato, A. and Di Chiara, G. (1986). *J. Pharmacol. Exp. Ther.* 239, 219–228.

Inui, A. (1999). *Trends Neurosci.* 22, 62–67.

Jahn, H., Döring, W.K., Krampe, H., Sieg, S., Werner, C., Poser, W., Brunner, E. and Ehrenreich, H. (2004). *Alcohol Clin. Exp. Res.* 28, 1925–1930.

Johnson, B.A., Ait-Daoud, N., Bowden, C.L., DiClemente, C.C., Roache, J.D., Lawson, K., Javors, M.A. and Ma, J.Z. (2003). *Lancet* 361, 1677–1685.

Junghanns, K., Backhaus, J., Tietz, U., Lange, W., Bernzen, J., Wetterling, T., Rink, L. and Driessen, M. (2003). *Alcohol Alcohol.* 38, 189–193.

Kato, S., Negishi, K., Mawatari, K. and Kuo, C.H. (1992). *Neuroscience* 48, 903–914.

Kenyon, S.H., Nicolaou, A. and Gibbons, W.A. (1998). *Alcohol* 15, 305–309.

Kiefer, F. and Wiedemann, K. (2004). *Addict. Biol.* 9, 205–212.

Kiefer, F., Jahn, H., Jaschinski, M., Holzbach, R., Wolf, K., Naber, D. and Wiedemann, K. (2001a). *Biol. Psychiatr.* 49, 782–787.

Kiefer, F., Jahn, H., Wolf, K., Kampf, P., Knaudt, K. and Wiedemann, K. (2001b). *Alcohol Clin. Exp. Res.* 25, 787–789.

Kiefer, F., Jahn, H., Schick, M. and Wiedemann, K. (2002). *Psychopharmacology (Berl)* 164, 239–240.

Kiefer, F., Jahn, H., Tarnaske, T., Helwig, H., Briken, P., Holzbach, R., Kampf, P., Stracke, R., Baehr, M., Naber, D. and Wiedemann, K. (2003). *Arch. Gen. Psychiatr.* 60, 92–99.

Kim, W.K. and Pae, Y.S. (1996). *Neurosci. Lett.* 216, 117–120.

Kranzler, H.R., Mulgrew, C.L., Modesto-Lowe, V. and Burleson, J.A. (1999). *Alcohol Clin. Exp. Res.* 23, 108–114.

Kraus, T., Haack, M., Schuld, A., Hinze-Selch, D. and Pollmächer, T. (2001). *Neuroendocrinology* 73, 243–247.

Kraus, T., Schanze, A., Groschl, M., Bayerlein, K., Hillemacher, T., Reulbach, U., Kornhuber, J. and Bleich, S. (2005). *Alcohol Clin. Exp. Res.* 29, 2154–2157.

Kruman, II., Culmsee, C., Chan, S.L., Kruman, Y., Guo, Z., Penix, L. and Mattson, M.P. (2000). *J. Neurosci.* 20, 6920–6926.

Kurth, C., Wegerer, V., Degner, D., Sperling, W., Kornhuber, J., Paulus, W. and Bleich, S. (2001). *Neuroreport* 12, 1235–1238.

Lesch, O.M., Benda, N., Gutierrez, K. and Walter, H. (1997). Craving in alcohol dependence: pharmaceutical interventions In Judd, L., Saletu, B. and Filip, V. (eds.), *Basic and Clinical Science of Mental and Addictive Disorders*, pp. 136–147. Karger, Basel.

Lesch, O.M., Kefer, J., Lentner, S., Mader, R., Marx, B., Musalek, M., Nimmerrichter, A., Preinsberger, H., Puchinger, H., Rustembegovic, A. *et al.* (1990). *Psychopathology* 23, 88–96.

Lesch, O.M. and Walter, H. (1996). *Alcohol Alcohol.* 31, 63–67.

Lipton, S.A., Kim, W.K., Choi, Y.B., Kumar, S., D'Emilia, D.M., Rayudu, P.V., Arnelle, D.R. and Stamler, J.S. (1997). *Proc. Natl. Acad. Sci. USA* 94, 5923–5928.

Long, C.G. and Cohen, E.M. (1989). *Br. J. Addict.* 84, 777–783.

Mann, K., Lehert, P. and Morgan, M.Y. (2004). *Alcohol Clin. Exp. Res.* 28, 51–63.

Markianos, M., Moussas, G., Lykouras, L. and Hatzimanolis, J. (2000). *Drug Alcohol Depend.* 57, 261–265.

Markianos, M., Lykouras, L., Moussas, G. and Hatzimanolis, J. (2001). *Drug Alcohol Depend.* 64, 363–365.

Meldrum, B. (1993). *Brain Res. Brain Res. Rev.* 18, 293–314.

Modell, J.G., Glaser, F.B., Cyr, L. and Mountz, J.M. (1992). *Alcohol Clin. Exp. Res.* 16, 272–274.

Nicolas, J.M., Fernandez-Sola, J., Fatjo, F., Casamitjana, R., Bataller, R., Sacanella, E., Tobias, E., Badia, E. and Estruch, R. (2001). *Alcohol Clin. Exp. Res.* 25, 83–88.

Numminen, H., Syrjala, M., Benthin, G., Kaste, M. and Hillbom, M. (2000). *Stroke* 31, 1269–1273.

Nygard, O., Nordrehaug, J.E., Refsum, H., Ueland, P.M., Farstad, M. and Vollset, S.E. (1997). *New Engl. J. Med.* 337, 230–236.

Olive, M.F., Mehmert, K.K., Koenig, H.N., Camarini, R., Kim, J.A., Nannini, M.A., Ou, C.J. and Hodge, C.W. (2003). *Psychopharmacology (Berl)* 165, 181–187.

Outinen, P.A., Sood, S.K., Liaw, P.C., Sarge, K.D., Maeda, N., Hirsh, J., Ribau, J., Podor, T.J., Weitz, J.I. and Austin, R.C. (1998). *Biochem. J.* 332, 213–221.

Paassilta, M., Kervinen, K., Rantala, A.O., Savolainen, M.J., Lilja, M., Reunanen, A. and Kesaniemi, Y.A. (1998). *BMJ* 316, 594–595.

Pelchat, M.L. (2002). *Physiol. Behav.* 76, 347–352.

Refsum, H., Ueland, P.M., Nygard, O. and Vollset, S.E. (1998). *Annu. Rev. Med.* 49, 31–62.

Renaud, S. and de Lorgeril, M. (1992). *Lancet* 339, 1523–1526.

Rohsenow, D.J. and Monti, P.M. (1999). *Alcohol Res. Health.* 23, 225–232.

Schmidt, L.G., Bleich, S., Boening, J., Buehringer, G., Kornhuber, J., Weijers, H.G., Wiesbeck, G.A., Wolfgramm, J. and Havemann-Reinecke, U. (2005). *Alcohol Clin. Exp. Res.* 29, 1282–1287.

St Leger, A.S., Cochrane, A.L. and Moore, F. (1979). *Lancet* 1, 1017–1020.

Sullivan, L.W. and Herbert, V. (1964). *J. Clin. Invest.* 43, 2048–2062.

Taivainen, H., Laitinen, K., Tahtela, R., Kilanmaa, K. and Valimaki, M.J. (1995). *Alcohol Clin. Exp. Res.* 19, 759–762.

Tiffany, S.T. and Conklin, C.A. (2000). *Addiction* 95, S145–S153.

Trabert, W., Caspari, D., Bernhard, P. and Biro, G. (1992). *Acta Psychiatr. Scand.* 85, 376–379.

Tupala, E. and Tiihonen, J. (2004). *Prog. Neuropsychopharmacol. Biol. Psychiatr.* 28, 1221–1247.

van Ree, J.M., Kornet, M. and Goosen, C. (1994). *EXS* 71, 165–174.

Verhoef, P., Stampfer, M.J. and Rimm, E.B. (1998). *Curr. Opin. Lipidol.* 9, 17–22.

Volkow, N.D. and Fowler, J.S. (2000). *Cereb. Cortex.* 10, 318–325.

Wiedemann, K., Jahn, H., Yassouridis, A. and Kellner, M. (2001). *Arch. Gen. Psychiatry.* 58, 371–377.

Willner, E.L., Tow, B., Buhman, K.K., Wilson, M., Sanan, D.A., Rudel, L.L. and Farese Jr., R.V. (2003). *Proc. Natl. Acad. Sci. USA* 100, 1262–1267.

Wise, R.A. (1988). *J. Abnorm. Psychol.* 97, 118–132.

Wurst, F.M., Bechtel, G., Forster, S., Wolfersdorf, M., Huber, P., Scholer, A., Pridzun, L., Alt, A., Seidl, S., Dierkes, J. and Dammann, G. (2003). *Alcohol Alcohol.* 38, 364–368.

(iii) Beer Composition and Properties

20

Beer Composition: An Overview

Stefano Buiatti Department of Food Science, University of Udine, Udine, Italy

Abstract

The word beer comes from the old English *bēor*; but its roots are from late latin *biber* (meaning drink), from *bibere* (to drink) which is the source of English "imbibe" and "beverage" (Encarta World English Dictionary, 1999). Not surprisingly beer is not only the oldest alcoholic beverage but also the most important in terms of amount of volumes produced worldwide. In 2006 nearly 1,700,000,000 hl (one thousand and seven hundred million of hectoliters) of beer were drunk in the world. Hectoliter (hl) is equivalent to 100 l (175.98 UK pints or 211.29 US pints). The amount of wine, the other "historical" alcoholic beverage, produced in the world is about six times smaller (280,000,000 hl). Beers are quite similar in most respects but small differences in their composition can greatly affect both appearance and flavor. Apart from water which normally represents more than 90% of the beer, the only compound present with a concentration greater than 1 g/l are some carbohydrates not fermented by yeast, ethanol, carbon dioxide and glycerol. In spite of this fact beer, is a very complex beverage that contains, besides these compounds, about 800 organic compounds. Many of them have such a low level that only those having a flavor active impact can have a real influence on taste and smell perception. Most chemical compounds in beer were either present in the raw materials (malts, hops and water) or they are by-products of yeast metabolism during the fermentation and are responsible for most of the flavor character that is unique to beer.

List of Abbreviations

ABV	Alcohol by volume
DMS	Dimethyl sulfide
DMSO	Dimethyl-sulfoxide
DP	Degree of polymerization
IBU	International Bitterness Units
kDa	Kilo (thousand) Daltons
MBT	3-methyl-2-butene-1-thiol
SMM	*S*-methyl methionine
VDK	Vicinal diketones

Introduction

Beer is as old as civilization. The origins of beer are lost somewhere in the mists of time but, as one of the world's oldest drinks, it has played an important part in many of the major cultures of the past. It has been known for a long time that Middle East and Egypt were the birthplace of beer and that it can have an important role and contribution to the diet. In the ancient times beer production was strictly related to the baking of bread since they are both made with grain, water and yeast. During 6000 BC in the old cities of Mesopotamia (the area today covered by Iraq) the brewing of beer was well known. Although the great early Middle Eastern civilization did develop brewing to a fine art no one understood how the process of fermentation worked. These beers must have been very different from those we are used today; they probably were thicker, sweeter, lower in alcohol and higher in protein.

Greeks and Romans learned from Egyptians the art of brewing but when wine became the most common drink in the Mediterranean area beer migrated to the north. Throughout the medieval times beer was more than satisfying and warming refreshment, it also provided a safe drink in an age when the purity of water was uncertain and drinks like coffee and tea were unknown. The process of boiling, the antibacterial properties of alcohol and, after they were introduced in fifteenth century, hops kept away the main dangers of infection.

The main constituents of a beer are shown in Table 20.1.

Beer comprises hundreds of different compounds. Some of them are derived from raw materials and pass unchanged through the brewing process, others are produced during the process. Raw materials sources of chemicals in beer are water, malts (and its adjuncts), hops and yeast.

- **Water is quantitatively the main ingredient of beers: it forms more than 90% and often even more than 94% of the final product.**

Not surprisingly its composition is very important and of critical concern to the brewer. Any water that will end

Beer in Health and Disease Prevention
ISBN: 978-0-12-373891-2

Table 20.1 Composition of beer

Substances	*Concentration*	*Number of compounds*	*Source or agent*
Water	90–94%	1	–
Ethanol	3–5% v/v	1	Yeast, malt
Carbohydrates	1–6% w/v	~100	Malt
Carbon dioxide	3.5–4.5 g/l	1	Yeast, malt
Inorganic salts	500–4,000 mg/l	~25	Water, malt
Total nitrogen content	300–1,000 mg/l	~100	Yeast, malt
Organic acids	50–250 mg/l	~200	Yeast, malt
Higher alcohols	100–300 mg/l	80	Yeast, malt
Aldehydes	30–40 mg/l	~50	Yeast, hops
Esters	25–40 mg/l	~150	Yeast, malt, hops
Sulfur compounds	1–10 mg/l	~40	Yeast, malt, hops
Hop derivates	20–60 mg/l	>100	Hops
Vitamin B compounds	5.0–10 mg/l	13	Yeast, malt

Source: Modified from Hardwick (1995).

up in the bottle of beer must be of the highest chemical and microbiological quality. The water must fulfill all legal requirements both chemically and microbiologically as well as satisfy the brewer's standards for clarity, taste, smell and lack of color. Breweries need vast amount of water; for every liter of beer produced, at least five more are required for cleaning, cooling and heating. In some cases brewery might use as much as 20 times more water (Bamforth, 2003).

The mineral content of brewing water has a very large effect on the properties of beer and gives an important contribution to the flavor of the finished product. A wide range of brewing waters ("liquor" is the name given in breweries to the water used for brewing) is employed, giving rise to many classic styles of beers that over the centuries have become very famous. Certain mineral salts were identified in natural water supplies from various locations which produced superior beers of a particular type. Perhaps the best known brewing liquor is that of Burton-on-Trent, a town that became famous for its full flavored and excellent pale ales. This liquor is high in permanent hardness because of the high calcium sulfate (gypsum) content but it also has a lot of temporary hardness due to the high level of bicarbonate. Liquor treatment is the practice of adding or removing mineral salts, to give the brewing liquor properties similar to the most suitable natural supplies. For example, brewers in other parts of the country, with less suitable water supplies, were able to adjust the composition of their supplies to make them the same; the practice became known as Burtonisation. A good water source was a particular key requirement for the earliest breweries. Many of the great brewing towns sprang up around a good liquor supply. At one time most breweries had their own supply which varied little in its mineral content and a liquor treatment could be done to suit the supply. At present, where a brewery is taking its supply from a water authority, water can be taken from several sources which are changed according to the demand of the customers and availability from the sources. Water supplied one day could be quite different in its mineral content the day after; some brewers find this problem so great that they remove all salts from the water and add what they require rather than try to adjust the amounts which are naturally present from day to day. Natural water supplies all contain some salts which are dissolved from the geological strata through which they have to pass. Besides Burton-on-Trent, other towns are famous for their waters: Munich, in Germany, has water poor in sulfates and chloride but contains bicarbonates, which are not very suitable for pale beers but ideal to produce darker, smoother lagers. The carbonates raise the pH during the mashing, producing a wort with a higher dextrin to maltose ratio. The water from Vienna (Austria) is more mineralized than that from Munich. The Bohemian Czech town of Plzen (Pilsen in German), where this famous classic style was first produced in 1842, has very soft water and produces beers renowned for their complex character with a flowery hop aroma and a dry finish. The water of Dortmund (Germany) contains noticeable amounts of both bicarbonate and chloride that aid in the production of full-bodied, malty lagers which are less aromatic than a Pilsner. The principal ions present in most brewing liquors are calcium, magnesium, sodium, potassium, sulfate, chloride, bicarbonate, carbonate and nitrate. Other elements are present but only in small amounts and are known as trace elements. It should be mentioned that brewing materials are also a source of some of these ions; most of the magnesium, potassium and phosphate in wort come from this source (Goldammer, 1999; Warnakulasuriya *et al.*, 2002)

- **Inorganic salts found in beer (Table 20.2) come from brewing water and/or malt and may have positive or negative effect on beer quality depending on their concentration and nature.**

Some ions may be precipitated during the brewing process on the break and others may be absorbed by the yeast; that means the inorganic salts present in beer are very different from those present in the brewing water used. The presence of some minerals (e.g. iron) is avoided by brewers because it can have a negative action as pro-oxidant and so accelerating the beer staling. On the other hand iron has been used as foam stabilizer but its addition to beer is not very common. Trace amounts of many metals are essential for yeast growth whereas larger amounts can be toxic and/or limited by regulations. When specific limit for beer is not indicated the limits for potable beer are usually applied. Beer is cited as being an important dietary source of selenium and the high potassium:sodium ratio (4:1) is consistent with a low sodium diet. Yeast is a source of a

Table 20.2 Inorganic compounds in beer

Inorganic compounds	*Concentration (mg/l)*	*Inorganic compounds*	*Concentration (mg/l)*
Potassium	200–450	Fluoride	0.08–0.71
Sodium	20–350	Hydrogen	0.2–0.3
Calcium	25–120	Iron	0.01–0.3
Magnesium	50–90	Lead	<0.01–0.1
Chloride	120–500	Manganese	0.03–0.2
Sulfate	100–430	Mercury	Negligible
Oxalate	5–30	Nickel	0.03–0.2
Phosphate	170–600	Nitrite	0–2
Nitrate	13–43	Nitrogen	1–14
Aluminum	0.1–2	Oxygen	0.4–4
Arsenic	0.02–0.05	Phosphorus	90–400
Bromine	0.2–0.4	Silica	10.2–22.4
Cadmium	0.03–0.68	Selenium	Negligible
Chromium	<0.04	Tin	0.01–0.02
Cobalt	0.01–0.11	Vanadium	0.03–0.15
Copper	0.01–1.55	Zinc	0.01–1.48

Source: Baxter and Hughes (2001) and Briggs *et al.* (2004).

chromium-containing complex (the so-called glucose tolerance factor) which may play an important role in the regulation of body glucose levels. Iron, tin, lead and zinc were found in beer at higher than minimal concentrations in three-piece tin plate cans that have soldered side seam. Three-piece welded cans are generally welded with a copper-based metal that can cause an increase in copper concentrations in beer. The UK Food Standard Committee recommends a limit for copper in beer of 7.0 mg/kg. In the 1960, cobalt was added to beer as foam enhancer and to prevent gushing but was found to cause heart diseases in heavy drinkers (more than 20 pints/day) and since then no brewer is employing cobalt as foam stabilizer (Hardwick, 1995; Briggs *et al.*, 2004)

- **Beer is mainly rich in magnesium, potassium, sodium and calcium (cations) and chloride, sulfate, nitrate and phosphate (anions).**

Calcium (Ca^{2+})

This ion is by far the most influential mineral in the brewing process because they affect the acidity of the wort; it can react with phosphates in the malt and can form primary, secondary or tertiary phosphates. The secondary phosphate is weakly soluble and the tertiary phosphate is not soluble at all. The more calcium present in the wort the more tertiary phosphate is produced which is accompanied by a release of hydrogen ions making the wort more acidic.

$$3Ca^{2+} + 2(HPO_4)^{2-} \rightarrow 2H^+ + Ca_3(PO_4)_2$$

The lowering of the pH is critical because it provides an ideal environment for α- and β-amylase, proteolytic enzymes. This in turn will increase saccharification and proteolysis, leading to an increase in extract yield and a rise in soluble nitrogen. The lowering of the pH may sufficiently reduce wort viscosity for faster filtration. Moreover, polyphenols (so-called tannins) are extracted to a lesser degree at a lower pH, resulting in less astringent beers with less color. Calcium during wort filtration aids rapid, bright filtration which diminishes the extraction of astringent and coloring substances. During boiling process calcium ions are essential to have a good break formation as it aids in the precipitation of proteins and other substances which might otherwise cause beer haze formation. Calcium enhances yeast flocculation and sedimentation during the primary fermentation and, during maturation, improves clarification, stability and flavor in the final product. Calcium ions initiate the precipitation of oxalate derived from malt which continues to precipitate during the brewing process. When these ions are not sufficient oxalate precipitation might be delayed and, in some cases, causes haze and foam problems in the finished beer. Usually a 4:1 ratio Ca:oxalate is recommended but some brewers advocate 10:1 ratio to prevent haze formation. Too much calcium, however, can lead to an intense precipitation of phosphates causing a wort poor of a vital yeast nutrient. High calcium content also tends to diminish the extraction of hop resins and delay the isomerization of α-acids.

Carbonate $(CO_3)^{2-}$ and Bicarbonate $(HCO_3)^{1-}$

These are not desiderable as they take up hydrogen ions (H^+) from the wort to produce water and carbon dioxide (CO_2). The decrease in acidity (higher pH) is not welcomed. When calcium bicarbonate is present in water producing temporary hardness the detrimental effects of the bicarbonate ions outweigh the beneficial effects of the calcium ions.

$$CaCO_3 \xrightarrow{Ca^{++}} (CO_3)^{2-} \xrightarrow{H^+} (HCO_3)^{1-} \xrightarrow{H^+} H_2O + CO_2$$

Alkalinity is a measure of the buffering capacity of the bicarbonate ions and, to a some extent, the carbonate and hydroxide ions of water. These three ions all react with hydrogen ions to reduce acidity and raise pH. Alkalinity is normally given in mg/l (mg/l) as calcium carbonate ($CaCO_3$) for all three ions. Usually water with more than 100 mg/l of calcium carbonate is considered alkaline and should be treated. Water with less than 100 mg/l of calcium carbonate is considered soft or just slightly alkaline. The pH raise caused by carbonate hardness opposes the pH lowering effect coming from other calcium and magnesium ions present as calcium chloride, calcium sulfate, magnesium chloride and magnesium sulfate. The bicarbonate ion is a very strong buffer and because of that water with a high buffering capacity or alkalinity tends to have a pH very stable, even when bases or acids are added to it (Moll, 1995)

Total water hardness is the measure of the bicarbonate, calcium and magnesium ions present in the water and is measured in two ways: temporary and permanent. Temporary hardness is always strongly alkaline and permanent hardness is only weakly acidic. Total hardness is the combined effect of the two measurements.

The effect of carbonate ions in raising pH can give less fermentable worts due to a higher dextrin/maltose ratio, slow wort filtration and less efficient separation of protein–polyphenol compounds during the hot and cold breaks (indicated with the German word *trub* meaning turbid). Moreover high carbonate concentration can have a negative influence on hop flavor while hop bitterness becomes harsher. Usually carbonate concentration should not exceed 50 mg/l to avoid harsh and bitter flavors. Carbonate in excess of 200 mg/l is acceptable only when a dark roasted malt is used to buffer its excessive acidity.

Magnesium (Mg^{2+})

It has similar properties to calcium ions and also reacts with phosphates in the malt but the phosphates produced are more soluble. Thus fewer hydrogen ions are released and the increase in acidity is therefore less. Magnesium ions are important for the yeast metabolism being required in very small amounts as an enzyme cofactor. Usually, malt and water contain sufficient magnesium to supply the required amount. They can also impart a sour or bitter astringency to the beer in concentration over 15 mg/l.

Sodium (Na^{+})

At low concentration it influences sweetness and smoothness (levels from 70 to 150 mg/l) which is most pleasant when paired with chloride ions than when associated with sulfate ions. Higher concentrations give a salty and unpleasant taste. When sodium sulfate is present in the brewing liquor the combined effect of the ions on the beer is an unpleasant harshness and sour taste; 150 mg/l is considered the upper limit of this salt for brewing water. In some, breweries is preferred adding potassium chloride rather than sodium chloride as potassium is free from the slightly sour flavor given by the sodium ion. However when sodium chloride is added at the correct concentration palate fullness is produced.

Potassium (K^{+})

It has similar properties to sodium ions but does not give beer the sourness that sodium ions do. If chloride ions need adding in a water treatment potassium chloride is therefore often used in preference to sodium chloride. It is required for yeast metabolism and above 10 mg/l inhibits some mash enzymes and makes beers laxative. However, its concentration is rarely high enough to have any effect on beer flavor.

Sulfate $(SO_4)^{2-}$

This ion has a positive effect on starch and protein degradation which favor wort filtration and *trub* sedimentation. It can give a dry, crisp palate to beer and increase the perceived bitterness but if in excess, the final product may have a harsh, salty and laxative character. Light ales bitters and even mild ales benefit from the presence of sulfate in brewing water.

Chloride (Cl^{-})

Calcium and magnesium chloride give sweetness, body, fullness to beers. Sodium chloride (common table salt) adds a certain roundness on the palate and this makes the salt suited for all types of sweet beers (e.g. Scotch Ales) and both dark beers and stouts. Concentrations of sodium chloride above 400 mg/l give to pale beers a pasty flavor and above 500 mg/l chloride has a negative effect on yeast metabolism and leads to poor clarification and a flat taste.

Nitrates $(NO_3)^{1-}$ and Nitrites $(NO_2)^{1-}$

Nitrate in itself is not a problem. The nitrate concentration in beer is usually below the legal limit of 50 mg/l for drinking water and is harmless. However nitrate can be converted to nitrite which is harmful to health. Moreover high nitrite levels may slow the fermentation rate and cause an increase of vicinal diketones (VDK) levels in beer. It has been reported that nitrite can cause gushing when it reacts with amino acids.

Trace Elements

Iron (Fe^{2+})

Iron salts above 0.2 mg/l can have a negative effect slowing the saccharification, resulting in hazy worts and reduced yeast activity. If its concentration is above 0.3 mg/l causes grayish foam and an increase in color and with more than 1 mg/l iron weakens yeast, increases haze problems and oxidation of tannins.

Copper (Cu^{2+})

This ion in concentration as low as 0.1 mg/l has an effect of catalyst of oxidants causing beer haze formation. When its concentration is above 10 mg/l copper becomes toxic to yeast.

Zinc (Zn^{2+})

Zinc has an important role in yeast metabolism and fermentation process with a positive action on protein synthesis and yeast growth. A zinc level between 0.08 and 0.2 mg/l is recommended to have positive effects on fermentation while zinc content above 0.6 mg/l can vice versa affect negatively fermentation and colloidal stability of beer. More than 1 mg/l zinc is toxic to yeast cells and inhibits enzymes. Like iron, zinc can give a metallic taste if present with too high concentrations.

Manganese (Mn^{2+})

Manganese has an important role as enzyme cofactor and a positive action on protein solubilization. This ion can inhibit yeast metabolism and affect negatively colloidal stability of beer. The manganese level should be from 0.1 to 0.2 mg/l in wort and in any case not more than 0.5 mg/l.

- **Malt is the germinated and dried barley and it is the grist component of more than 90% of beer produced in the world.**

The cultivated barley (*Hordeum vulgare*) belongs to the grass family (*Gramineae*). On average to produce 1 hl of beer 15–20 kg of malt are used. This raw material is the primary source of the protein, lipid, carbohydrate, polyphenols compounds present in beers. Most malt components are changed during mashing; protein degradation, for example, to peptones and peptides started during germination goes on in the mash vessel. Even if these composition changes are not really great they are significant and important to obtain a regular fermentation for the yeast growth and for the development and synthesis of flavor compounds that will be formed throughout the brewing process.

- **Substances different from barley malt which provide fermentable carbohydrates in addition to those from malt are known as adjuncts.**

Adjuncts are used to replace malt not only for economic reasons, being usually cheaper than barley malt, but also to modify the flavor. Thus, the resulting beers may have a lighter flavor and a less satiating impact (especially when sugars, as adjuncts, have been added) or an increased flavor depending on the adjunct (e.g. roasted raw barley) added to barley malt. These adjuncts are primarily cereals such as corn (maize), rice, wheat, rye, sorghum used as sources of starch. Also invert sugar (hydrolyzed cane or beet sugar) glucose syrups (derived from maize starch) or other cereal syrups are adjuncts. The starch coming from the cereals, once gelatinized, is hydrolyzed by malt enzymes in the same manner as malt starch. These adjuncts can be used as grits, flakes or torrefied products. Classification and substances which can be legally used vary from country to country and from time to time the lists and amounts permitted adjuncts change.

- **Barley malt and adjuncts are the sources of several constituents present in beer such as, nitrogenous compounds, lipids, carbohydrates and vitamins.**

Nitrogenous compounds: Nitrogenous compounds in beer are in the range of 0.3–1.0 g/l (equivalent to 0.11–0.63% protein multiplying by the conversion factor 6.3) and comprise amino acids, peptides and polypeptides, nucleic acid fragments, amines and heterocyclic compounds. Some strong beers (particularly the not filtered ones) can contain up to nearly 2,000 mg/l of total nitrogen equivalent to 1.26% protein; 80–85% of these nitrogen components are derived from the malt (10–15% are from the yeast). The total nitrogen content multiplied by the factor 6.25 is often expressed as "protein." It is suggested that peptides may contain up to 10 amino acids, polypeptides from 11 to 100 amino acids residues and proteins more than 100 amino acids. However Bamforth suggests that the term protein should be used only for undegraded molecules. On this basis only few proteins are still present in the finished product and most of the nitrogen as polypeptides (Briggs *et al.*, 2004).

During mashing, proteins and peptides in malt are broken down to amino acids thereby continuing the enzymatic degradation started during malting operations. As a consequence the level of nitrogenous compounds that will be available to the yeast later in fermentation is increased. Most of these amino acids will be used by the yeast for its multiplication, apart from proline which is not utilized by yeast in anaerobic conditions and carried out through the beer. The amino compounds found in beer are almost exclusively nitrogenous compounds that were not utilized by the yeast. Some wort amino acids are metabolized by yeast to form higher alcohols (or fusel alcohols) which are important flavor compounds in beer. In fact deamination and transamination reactions carried out by the yeast cell are responsible for the presence of several organic acids, aldehydes, alcohols and esters in beer; most of them are cast-out carbon skeleton of amino acids which were in wort. As already known malt contains different peptides and polypeptides which increase during mashing due to proteolytic enzyme action degrading malt protein and other complex polypeptides to smaller compounds. Some of these smaller units can be metabolized by yeast while the larger, more complex polypeptides, made up of hundreds of amino acids, are still soluble in beer. These compounds can give an important contribution to foam stability and to the mouthfeel of beer. The biggest polypeptides and the undegraded proteins will precipitate and eliminate during the brewing process.

Purines and pyrimidines as well as nucleotides and nucleosides are present in beer as degradation products of nucleic acids which took place during malting and mashing. Their concentration is included between 0.2 and 139 μg/ml and guanosine, uridine and cytosine are the major constituents. Other nitrogenous constituents of beer are choline, tryptophol and nicotinic acid which are a B vitamin, essential for human growth.

Other nitrogenous constituents are the heterocyclic compounds originated mainly from the Maillard reaction which took place during the malt kilning. Above 80°C the reducing sugars and amino acids can react to form a great group of compounds referred generically as Maillard reaction products, which are coloring and with a strong flavor. The intermediate compounds called Amadori rearrangements products will decompose to various chemicals such as 2-acetylfuran and other compound carrying the furan ring. Substitution of nitrogen or sulfur into the furan ring structure results in the formation of pyridines, pyrrolizines, pyrroles, maltoxazines, thiazolines, thiazoles and thiophenes; other heterocyclic compounds are the pyrazines, alkyl-substituted pyrazines, furyl pyrazines and cyclopentapyrazines responsible for a nutty, toffee, green wood, burnt, roasted odors. These compounds have a concentration between 2 and 400 mg/l. Biogenic amines are also present in beer and polyamines that, at low concentrations found in beer, do not have a very significant influence on the flavor of beer. Dimethylamine is the major component of this class; tyramine, obtained from the decarboxylation of tyrosine, has been detected in beer. People under treatment with monoamine oxidase inhibitors (antidepressant) do not have to drink due to the build up of toxic levels of tyramine. Even ethyl carbamate (urethane), which is reported to be carcinogenic, has been detected in many fermented and spirits beverages, but according to Canas *et al.* (1989) could be found only in few beers. Secondary amines, such as dimethylamine, can react with oxides of nitrogen to form carcinogenic *N*-nitrosamines. Some of these compounds have been detected in beers and after several studies it was finally found that the nitrosamines were formed during the direct fired kilning of malts (e.g. as in the German *Rauchmalz*, smoked malt); the oxides of nitrogen (NO_X) react with amines such as hordenine to form nitrosamine. Since then (mid-1970s) the level of these compounds has been strongly reduced and today the level set by the American Food and Drug Administration is not more than 5 μg/l of *N*-nitrosodimethylamine in beer.

Lipids: Lipids in beer come mainly from barley malt and are fatty acids, diglyceraldehydes and triglyceraldehydes. In fact barley contains approximately 3% w/w lipid, present in the living tissues (embryo and aleurone layer) but only very little is still present in the final product making this beverage basically a fat-free food, beers in fact contain trace amounts of lipids. The concentration of the lipids is very low, less than 0.1%, and the yeast metabolism can affect the presence of these compounds and modify them. The effect of lipids is negative for the shelf life of beers and particularly a fatty aldehyde, the *trans*-2-nonenal, is a very flavor potent compound, detectable in beer at less than 1 μg/l. This aldehyde is considered responsible for the cardboard flavor in stale beer. However, most of these compounds are eliminated during the brewing process in different ways, by the spent grain and hot *trub* after the whirlpool and by the filtration at final beer clarification. The concentration of free fatty acids, very low at the beginning of the process, decreases further on during the brewing process. Particularly during fermentation it has been observed that there is an increase in C8 to C10 and a considerable decrease in C12 to C18:3 as consequence of yeast metabolism. The concentration of total fatty acids in finished beers is about 15–30 mg/l and the most abundant are C4–C10 (Bamforth, 2002).

Table 20.3 Unfermented carbohydrates in beer

Carbohydrates	*Concentration (g/l)*
Fructose	0–0.19
Glucose	0.04–1.1
Sucrose	0–3.3[a]
Maltose	0.7–3.0
Maltotriose	0.4–3.4

[a] Higher levels in primed beers.

Source: Baxter and Hughes (2001).

Carbohydrates: Carbohydrates present in beer are showed in Table 20.3.

Obviously most of the sugar in wort is fermented to ethanol by yeast but some carbohydrates are still present at the end of the process and their content is estimated for a range of beer values between about 1.0% and 6.0%. The sugars found in beer range from the simple unit, such as glucose, to molecules having more than 250 glucose units (M_r~45 kDa). In fact the carbohydrates surviving into beer from wort are the non-fermentable dextrins or α-glucans (90%), remnants of enzymatic starch hydrolysis and some polysaccharides compounds (10%) coming from cell walls, in starchy endosperm of barley kernel. In general beers will contain only low levels of fermentable sugars other than those added to sweeten the final product (primings). The dextrins are formed by many glucose units and their number is expressed by the degree of polymerization (DP); the 72.4% of dextrins range from a DP 4 to DP 34 while higher dextrins (DP > 35) are 15.2%. The surviving β-glucans in beer can have a positive influence on beer smoothness and foam retention, however it is important that the concentration of β-glucans in the final beer is not too high because it can cause a "soupy" effect and mouth filling flavor will linger in the mouth and the beer is no longer sharp and fresh.

Carbohydrates are the major components of the residual unfermented solids present in beer which is named "real extract"; it is a measure of the total dissolved solids in beer and consists approximately of 75–80% carbohydrates, mainly dextrins, 6–9% nitrogenous compounds, 4–5% glycerol and

Table 20.4 Vitamin B compounds in beer

Vitamin B compounds	*Concentration (mg/l)*
Aminobenzoic acid	0.01–0.15
Biotin (B_8)	<0.015
Ethyl nicotinoate	<1.5
Folic acid (B_9)	0.04–0.6
Methylbutylnicotinoate	<0.01
Methyl nicotinoate	<0.01
Nicotinic acid, niacin (B_3)	0.3–5
Phenylethylnicotinoate	<0.01
Pyridoxine (B_6)	0.07–1.7
Riboflavin (B_2)	0.02–0.1
Pantothenic acid (B_5)	0.04–2
Thiamin (B_1)	0.08
Cyanocobalamin (B_{12})	<0.03

Source: Modified from Hardwick (1995).

β-glucans, inorganic compounds, phenolic compounds and bitter substances and other compounds which, despite their low concentration, can have an important effect on the sensorial properties and quality of final beer.

Vitamins: Barley and malt are rich sources of several vitamins that, being present in the embryo and aleurone layer, are solubilized into wort during the brewing process. Their importance to the brewing process depends on their content in wort, more than sufficient to ensure a regular yeast performance during fermentation. In particular the B-group vitamins are crucial as growth factor for yeast, especially biotin, inositol and panthotenic acid. This is why beer contains considerably lower levels of these vitamins than does wort.

Some vitamins are present in the malt in bound forms and released during mashing by enzymes. Riboflavin, panthotenic acid and pyridoxine increase during malting, as it happens to ascorbic acid, which is later on completely destroyed by high temperature during kilning. Beer contains (see Table 20.4) small amounts of vitamins of the B-group and for this reason are considered as a valuable source of many of the water-soluble vitamins (particularly folate, riboflavin, panthotenic acid, pyridoxine and niacin). The fat-soluble vitamins do not survive into beer and are lost during the brewing process with insoluble compounds (spent grain, *trub* and yeast). Some beers may contain ascorbic acid (Vitamin C) because it can be added as antioxidant.

- **Yeast is responsible for the fermentation process and has a fundamental impact on the quality of beer. Most breweries use carefully selected strain which are stored and grown to be used within the brewery.**

Yeast (unicellular *fungi*) is the most important microorganism responsible of fermented beverages production. The yeast is used by the brewer several times (usually four to six times) and taken from one fermentation to start the next.

The pitching rates most often used are between 10 and 25 million cells/ml. As a rule of thumb the pitching rate is 1 million viable cells per Plato degree per ml of wort. For example, a 13°P wort would require 13×10^6 cells/ml.

1 Plato degree equates to 1 g sucrose per 100 g water. So, if wort has a specific gravity of 12° Plato, it has the same specific gravity as a 12% solution of sucrose.

Many large and small breweries use several strains of *S. cerevisiae* and/or *S. carlsbergensis* (*S. uvarum*) to produce different beers. The brewer knows very well that the properties of the beer produced depend very much on yeast used. It plays a fundamental role in the synthesis and formation of several compounds found in beers. As yeast grows and metabolizes during fermentation almost all carbohydrates (hexoses, disaccharides and trisaccharides) are converted to ethanol and carbon dioxide. Yeast cell uses some organic carbon skeletons from glycolysis to form new cell substances; there is a combination of these fragments with amino groups from degraded malt proteins to form new amino acids, proteins and nucleic acids. Many other compounds are modified and a lot of yeast-produced compounds in beer are metabolic by-products which are eliminated by the yeast cell. Moreover the yeast enzymes may modify other compounds through reduction, oxidation and esterification reactions forming organic acids, esters and alcohols. The total amount of these compounds expressed as percentage is quite low, less than 1% (not considering ethanol production) but nevertheless they number in the hundreds and they play an important role on the flavor, aroma and final quality of the beer.

- **The properties of the beer depend very much on the yeast used. It produces not only ethanol and carbon dioxide but even other compounds (higher alcohols, organic acids, esters, aldehydes, ketones, sulfur compounds) which play a key role on the sensorial profile of beer.**

Ethyl alcohol (*ethanol*): It is the most important alcohol in beer and its concentration range on average from 30 to 50 g/l (3–5% w/v). However many different beer styles can contain much less (e.g. free alcohol beers and light beers) or much more alcohol (e.g. stronger beers such as Belgian Trappists or Barley wine or German Doppelbocks). It seems that the strongest beer in the world is the American Utopias MM II, brewed in Boston, and with an alcohol content of 25.6% alcohol by volume (ABV). The strength of beer and other alcoholic drinks is expressed in United States as alcohol by weight and in EU as ABV. Since alcohol has a lower specific gravity than beer its concentration expressed "by volume" gives a larger number. The specific gravity of alcohol and beer are respectively and approximately 0.8 and 1 and this means 4% alcohol by weight (w/w) is equal to 5% ABV (v/v). In other words, the percentage of alcohol by weight figure is approximately 20% lower than the ABV figure because alcohol weighs less than its equivalent volume of water (alcohol by weight/0.8 = ABV; ABV × 0.8 = alcohol by weight). Aqueous solutions of ethanol cause a warming sensation in the mouth and, after swallowing, it continues in the throat and into the stomach. Ethanol is a flavor enhancer and also increases sweetness in beer.

Other alcohols: Besides ethanol beer contains several alcohols which are derived mainly from yeast metabolism and from hops and malts (see Table 20.5). Alcohols which are derived by yeast metabolism are formed during fermentation. These compounds, so-called higher alcohols as they have a larger molecular weight, are referred to as fusel oils and in large quantities can cause headaches, hangovers and general discomfort that follow excessive beer consumption. Higher alcohol content is about 60–100 mg/l but concentrations above 100 mg/l can negatively affect the flavor of beer (Lewis and Young, 1995).

Larger amounts of these alcohols are correlated to high alcohol content in the product, whereas beers with low alcohol content contain less higher alcohols and may be considered more agreeable with a better drinkability. These alcohols are produced by the yeast removing amino groups from the amino acids and replacing them with the —OH group of the alcohols; the concentration of amino acids content is therefore very important and plays a fundamental role in fusel oils synthesis. The main higher alcohols present in beer are 3-methylbutanol (isoamylalcohol), 2-methylbutanol (active-amyl alcohol), 2-methylpropanol (isobutyl alcohol), propanol (propyl alcohol) and β-phenylethanol (phenetyl alcohol). Smaller number of primarily phenolic alcohols is derived from the breakdown of malt and hops polyphenols and can contribute to beer texture in the mouth (mouthfeel) and to harshness. Many hop-derived alcohols give a positive flavor. Floral aromas from some of these contribute to the pleasing aroma of beer.

Table 20.5 Some alcohols commonly present in beer

Alcohols	*Concentration (mg/l)*	*Flavor descriptors*
Ethanol	20,000–80,000	Alcoholic, strong
Methanol	0.5–3.0	Alcoholic, solvent
1-Propanol	3–16	Alcoholic
2-Propanol	3–6	Alcoholic
2-Methylbutanol	8–30	Alcoholic, vinous, banana
3-Methylbutanol	30–70	Alcoholic, vinous, banana
2-Phenylethanol	8–35	Roses, bitter, perfumed
1-Octen-3-ol	0.03	Fresh-cut grass, perfume
2-Decanol	0.005	Coconut, aniseed
Glycerol	1,200–2,000	Sweetish, viscous
Tyrosol	3–40	Bitter, chemical

Source: Baxter and Hughes (2001).

Glycerol is an important compound, classified as alcohol, and originated during fermentation as a product of yeast carbohydrate metabolism. The interest for this compound comes from the relationship between carbohydrate level, yields of glycerol and ethanol: the latter decrease in proportion to the amount of carbohydrate used to produce glycerol and other fermentation by-products. Its content in beers is 1.5–3.5 g/l, glycerol plays an important role on the beer taste enhancing smoothness and mouthfeel.

Carbon dioxide: During the fermentation, chemical conversion of fermentable sugars in the wort, approximately equal parts of ethanol and carbon dioxide gas, are formed through the action of yeast. The final product contains 3.5–4.5 g/l (0.35–0.45%) of carbon dioxide but oversaturated beers and bottle conditioned beers may contain as much as 6 g/l but gas will be lost as soon as the container is open and the pressure released. The sensory threshold of carbon dioxide is about 1 g/l so the amount present will have an effect on the flavor of beer. The carbon dioxide is responsible of the extent of foam formation and influences the delivery of volatiles into the headspace of beers.

Organic acids: Most beers range on average in pH from about 4 to 5, so beer is a beverage slightly acidic. Other beers (e.g. Lambic) have a pH much lower, around 3.0. Organic acids and carbonic acid (dissolved CO_2 in beer) are responsible for this acidity. These acids are basically all metabolic by-products or intermediates excreted by yeast cells. The total amount is very low and range from 0.2 to 0.5 g/l (see Table 20.6).

These acids, in concert with carbonic acid which also provides the "tingle" in beer, are responsible for the pleasurable sensation of tartness. The most abundant is the acetic (ethanoic) acid (~30–200 mg/l) followed by lactic and succinic acids (respectively about 60–120 and 20–140 mg/l). In some Belgian "acid" beers (such as lambic and gueuze), however, the amount of lactic and acetic acids can be much higher, even more than 1 g/l for acetic acid and 3 g/l for lactic acid. Most of the acids are of yeast origin or, more precisely, they are yeast waste products. The organic acids are formed mainly from the amino acids present in wort: yeast uses the amino group $—NH_2$, removed from the amino acid, because it needs to synthesize its own proteins releasing the corresponding organic acid formed by this deamination into the beer.

The aliphatic acids with short to middle carbon chain length have distinctive and familiar odors; caprylic and capric acids can be responsible for aromas in beer described as "cheesy" or "goaty" but generally are not at concentrations high enough to negatively affect the beer flavor.

Most of the phenolic acids present in beer are extracted from malt but small amounts can come from hops and adjuncts. Phenolic acids contribute to astringency which is essential to characteristic beer flavor and probably the different chemical structure of these phenolic acids gives variety to this astringency in beer; however when it is too high is not pleasant.

Table 20.6 Important organic acids in beer

Acids	*Concentration (mg/l)*	*Flavor descriptors*
Acetic	30–200	Acid, vinegar
Propanoic	1–5	Acid, vinegar
Butanoic	0.5–1.5	Butter, cheese, sweat
2-Methylpropanoic	0.1–2	Sweet, bitter, sour
Pentanoic	0.03–0.1	Sweat, body odor
2-Methylbutanoic	0.1–0.5	Cheese, old hops, sweat
3-Methylbutanoic	0.1–2	–
Octanoic	2–12	Caprylic, goaty
Lactic	20–80	Acid
Pyruvic	15–150	Acid, salt, forage
Succinic	16–140	–
Phenolic acids		
Caffeic	1–10	Bitter, harsh, sour, diacetyl
Chlorogenic	1–10	Bitter, harsh, bitter–sweet, astringent
Cinnamic	0.5	
p-Courmaric	0.1–0.2	Sour, dry, bitter, astringent, medicinal
Ellagic	1–10	
Ferulic	1.1–6	Bitter–sweet, sour, vanilla, malty
Gallic	1–5	Bitter, harsh, astringent, dry, sour, sweet
Hydroxybenzoic	0.13	Bitter, harsh, astringent, acidic, vinegar
Isochlorogenic	1–10	
Salicylic	0.02–5	
Sinapic	1–10	Bitter, astringent, harsh, sour, dry
Syringic	1–10	Bitter, harsh, astringent, winey, malty
Vanillic	1–10	Harsh, bitter–sweet, sour, astringent, peppery, medicinal

Source: Hardwick (1995) and Baxter and Hughes (2001).

Table 20.7 The most important esters in beer

Esters	*Concentration (mg/l)*	*Flavor descriptors*
Ethyl acetate	10–60	Solvent-like, sweet
Isoamyl aceta te	0.5–5.0	Banana, ester, solvent
Ethyl hexanoate	0.1–0.5	Apple, fruity, sweet
Ethyl octanoate	0.1–1.5	Apple, tropical fruit, sweet
2-Phenylethyl acetate	0.05–2.0	Roses, honey, apple, sweet
Ethyl nicotinate	1.0–1.5	Grainy, perfume

Source: Baxter and Hughes (2001).

Esters: All alcohols and acids present in beer are theoretically capable of esterification reaction, potentially forming almost 4,000 esters. In beers many esters have been detected (60–80 mg/l) but since the main alcohol is ethanol, ethyl acetate is by far the most common ester found; its concentration is larger than expected from the equilibrium constant of the reaction between acetic acid and ethanol (see Table 20.7).

This shows the important role played by the yeast in the biosynthesis of esters. Ethyl esters are the most abundant in beer but the acetates (ethanoate) of the higher alcohols are also important (e.g. isoamylacetate, the so-called "banana" ester) and common as are ethyl esters of long-chain fatty acid (caproic and caprylic). The esters in beer contribute several pleasing fruit-like and floral aromas, however wild yeast such as *Hansenula* and *Pichia* produce high quantities of ethyl acetate that may be considered as off-flavors. Yeast strain can influence both the quantity and type of ester produced in beer and an abnormal increase in ethyl acetate is caused by worts with a high sugar concentration. Although some increase in the concentration of ethyl esters takes place also during the beer shelf life (Fix, 2000).

Aldehydes: Aldehydes are derived from alcohols through dehydrogenation (oxidation) (Rabin and Forget, 1998). They contain the radical —CHO and their content in beer is around 10–20 mg/l (see Table 20.8).

Several of the aldehydes are of the yeast origin and others are the result of Strecker degradation of amino acids during kettle boil and still others appear to be the result of a random decarboxylation of organic acids. Acetaldehyde (ethanal) is the most common aldehyde in beer and is

Table 20.8 Important aldehydes in beer

Aldehydes	*Concentration (mg/l)*	*Flavor descriptors*
Acetaldehyde	2–20	Green, paint
Propanal	0.01–0.3	Green, fruity
Butanal	0.03–0.02	Melon, varnish
trans-2-Butenal	0.003–0.02	Apple, almond
2-Methylpropanal	0.02–0.5	Banana, melon
C_5 Aldehydes	0.01–0.3	Grass, apple, cheese
Hexanal	0.003–0.07	Bitter, vinous
trans-2-Hexenal	0.005–0.01	Bitter, astringent
Heptanal	0.002	Aldehyde, bitter
Octanal	0.001–0.02	Orange peel, bitter
Nonanal	0.001–0.011	Astringent, bitter
trans-2-Nonenal	0.00001–0.002	Cardboard
cis-3-Nonenal	–	Soy bean oil
trans-2-*cis*-6-Nonadienal	–	Cucumber, green
Decanal	0.0–0.003	Bitter, orange peel
Decadienal	–	Oily, deep fried
Furfural	0.01–1.0	Papery, husky
5-Methylfurfural	<0.01	Spicy
5-Hydroxymethylfurfural	0.1–20	Aldehyde, stale

Source: Baxter and Hughes (2001).

excreted into the green beer by yeast during the first 3 days of fermentation and it is responsible for the "green" young beer flavor. In the young beer phase the acetaldehyde content is about 20–40 mg/l and it decreases to 5–15 mg/l in the final product. During fermentation, after the first 3 days when its formation is faster than its reduction, acetaldehyde is reduced to ethanol but it can be oxidized to acetic acid, which is, as mentioned above, the most abundant organic acid in beer.

As beer ages in commercial package, aldehydes may be produced through oxidation of higher alcohols by melanoidins. These aldehydes have a much lower threshold values than the origin alcohols and may be responsible for off-flavors. As mentioned above the cardboard flavor typical of stale beer is probably due to *trans*-2-nonenal. Other aldehydes found in beer are 5-hydroxymethylfurfural, 5-methylfurfural and furfural, compounds formed during wort boiling. The furfural content can increase also during pasteurization and storage at 40°C. Usually its concentration is very low (<15 μg/l) but a level of more than 1,843 μg/l was reported by Bernstein and Laufer (1977).

Ketones: Ketones belong, as aldehydes, to the group of carbonyl compounds. A carbonyl is a radical made up of one atom of carbon and one atom of oxygen connected by a double bond (=C=O). The most important ketones in beer are the diacetyl (butane-2,3-dione) and the related compound pentane-2,3-dione, which are produced from yeast metabolites secreted into beer.

Both diketones are highly aromatic and considered undesiderable in lighter-flavored beer. Diacetyl is the most important beer aroma. Its taste threshold is very low (0.15 mg/l) and above this value it imparts to beer an unclean, sweetish, butterscotch taste, which in high concentration is responsible for the aroma of butter. Since pentane-2,3-dione has a similar effect but with a higher taste threshold (0.9 mg/l) these compounds are often considered together and referred to as VDK because both compounds have adjacent carbonyl group (see Table 20.10). The breakdown of these VDK occurs at the same time to other maturation reactions during the beer conditioning process and for this reason considered as the fundamental criterion to evaluate the state of maturation of a beer. The guideline for the total diacetyl content (expressed as VDK) for a fully matured beer is not more than 0.1 mg/l (see Tables 20.9 and 20.10).

Sulfur compounds: Sulfur compounds may be present in the raw material, primarily in malt but they may also result from the metabolism or from infecting microorganisms (see Table 20.11).

Occasionally hops can have sulfur present as residue from crop treatment. The most common volatile sulfur compounds found in beer are sulfur dioxide (SO_2) and hydrogen sulfide (H_2S) plus a number of organic sulfur mercaptans (thiols) and organic sulfides. The raw materials used in brewing may contain different amounts of sulfur dioxide but most of it disappears during wort boiling and the

Table 20.9 Vicinal diketones in beer

Vicinal diketones	*Concentration (mg/l)*	*Flavor descriptors*
2,3-Butanedione (Diacetyl)	0.01–0.4	Butterscotch
3-Hydroxy-2-Butanone	1–10	Fruity, mouldy, woody
2,3-Butanediol	50–150	Rubber, sweet, warming
2,3-Pentanedione	0.01–0.15	Butterscotch, fruity
3-Hydroxy-2-pentanedione	0.05–0.07	–

Source: Baxter and Hughes (2001).

Table 20.10 Summary of ketones in beer

Ketones	*Concentration (mg/l)*	*Flavor descriptors*
3-Methylbutan-2-one	<0.05	Ketone, sweet
3-Methylpentan-2-one	0.06	–
4-Methylpentan-2-one	<0.013	–
3,3-Dimethylbutan-2-one	–	–
6-Methyl-5-hepten-2-one	0.05	–
Heptan-2-one	0.04–0.11	Varnish, hops
Octan-2-one	0.01	Varnish, walnut
Nonan-2-one	0.03	Ketone, varnish
Decan-2-one	–	Ketone, flowery
Undecan-2-one	–	Ketone, green plant
Oct-1-en-3-one	–	Metallic, mushroom
Octa-1-*cis*,5-dien-3-one	–	Metallic, geraniums

Source: Baxter and Hughes (2001).

Table 20.11 Sulfur compounds in beer

Sulfur compounds	*Concentration (μg/l)*	*Flavor descriptors*
Hydrogen sulfide (H_2S)	1–20	Sulfidic, rotten eggs
Sulfur dioxide (SO_2)	200–20,000	Sulfidic, burnt match
Carbon disulfide	0.01–0.3	–
Methanethiol	0.2–15	Putrefaction, drains
Ethylene sulfide	0.3–2	–
Ethanethiol	0–20	Putrefaction
Propanethiol	0.1–0.2	Putrefaction, rubber
Dimethyl sulfide (DMS)	10–100	Sweetcorn, tin tomatoes
Diethyl sulfide	0.1–1	Cooked vegetables
Dimethyl disulfide	0.1–3	Rotten vegetables
Diethyl disulfide	0–0.01	Garlic, burnt rubber
Dimethyl trisulfide	0.01–0.8	Rotten vegetables, onion
Methyl thioacetate	5–20	Cabbage
Ethyl thioacetate	0–2	Cabbage
Methionol	50–1,300	Raw potatoes
Methional	20–50	Mash potatoes
3-methyl-2-butene-1-thiol (MBT)	0.001–0.1	Skunk

Source: Baxter and Hughes (2001).

sulfur dioxide in beer is mainly formed during fermentation by yeast. The main factors influencing the sulfur dioxide content in beer are the original gravity of worts (sugar concentration) and the type of fermentation and to a lesser extent the yeast strain. Usually top fermented beers have significantly lower sulfur dioxide levels than bottom fermented beers.

Sulfur-containing amino acids taken up by yeast may be further broken down and the excess sulfur is cast off as hydrogen sulfide which may be responsible for the rotten egg off-flavor. Normal beers, when not contaminated and free from infection, contain little, if any, free hydrogen sulfide. The production of this compound is influenced by the yeast strain and its formation runs parallel with the intensity of fermentation process. However hydrogen sulfide is very volatile and it is swept out during fermentation and maturation by the evolving carbon dioxide.

Dimethyl sulfide (DMS) is a by-product of *S*-methyl methionine (SMM) degradation in the brew kettle and has the odor of fresh corn and is not compatible with beer flavor. In general, however the level of DMS in beer is low and present under taste threshold of 50–60 μg/l but according to Bamforth its threshold is around 30 μg/l. Usually DMS concentration in lager beers seems to be considerably higher than in ales because their malts are highly modified at very high temperatures that partly destroy the SMM, the DMS precursor. The lower DMS values in ales could also be explained by the higher enzymatic activity during the infusion mashing (typical in ales production) or may be due to the higher temperatures used in top fermentation, which may give a more efficient carbon dioxide wash out of volatiles during fermentation. Yeast itself cannot remove the DMS but in some cases more may be produced through reduction of dimethyl-sulfoxide (DMSO) by yeast cell.

Mercaptans are thioalcohols, compounds in which the —OH of the alcohol has been replaced by the thiol group —SH. The most important is the 3-methyl-2-butene-1-thiol (MBT) which imparts to beer an unpleasant, skunk-like flavor (described also as sun-struck or light-struck flavor) by exposure to light. This causes the photolysis of the 4-methyl-pentenyl side chain of iso-α-acids (bitter substances of beer) to release an isopentenyl radical which reacts with a thiol radical to form MBT. The threshold of this compound is extraordinary low, in fact it can be detected at level as low as 0.4 parts per trillion (ng/l). The formation and presence of this compound explains why beer is usually packaged in brown or dark green glass bottles which usefully absorb visible light below about 550 nm providing some protection of the product from the photolysis. To prevent this reaction, in beer packaged into ordinary clear glass bottle (e.g. Ice beers), hop extracts are used that have been chemically reduced; the carbonyl group (=C=O) in the side chain of iso-α-acid is reduced by sodium borohydride to a secondary alcohol group.

- **The main reason for using hops is to provide bitterness and characteristic hoppy flavors in beer. Moreover they provide some protection against bacterial spoilage and they are fundamental for good foam formation.**

Hops are a climbing herbaceous perennial vine (*H. lupulus*) member of the *Cannabiniceae* family. The Romans called it *L. salictarius* (*lupus* meaning wolf) because the plant grew wild among the willows like a wolf among sheep (Bamforth, 2003). The female plant yields flowers of soft-leaved pine-like cones (called strobile) which are used for flavoring beer. In brewing process about 200–600 g are required for every hectoliter of beer. Although all hop varieties provide both bitterness and aromas, some are mainly used for their ability to provide bitterness and others specifically to provide hop aromas. Hops contain a range of chemical species but only two of these constituents are fundamental for the brewer: the resins and the essential oils. However hops also contain several phenols which may be important for the flavor of the finished beer.

Resins: Resins may be separated into what are called soft resins (soluble in hexane) and hard resins (not soluble in hexane). The hard resins are mostly oxidized and polymerized form of the substances present in soft resins. The soft resin fraction contains two groups of compounds known as humulones (α-acids) and lupulones (β-acids); they are acidic because they contain a phenolic group able to release a hydrogen ion (H^+). The α-acids are solubilized and extracted during wort boiling when they are oxidatively isomerized to iso-α-acids (iso-humulones), which are the most important bitter compounds in beer. In fact, using fresh, not deteriorated hops, about 70% of the bitterness in beer is obtained as a consequence of this isomerization reaction. The iso-humulones content in beer is about 20–60 mg/l but a number of other substances, including oxidized β-acids, provide the rest of bitterness. The amount of iso-α-acids is measured by the International Bitterness Units (IBU) which are approximately equal to the concentration expressed as mg/l.

Essential oils: Hops may contain 0.5% to as much as 3.0% essential oils and much of the flavor of a beer depends on the aroma compounds added by the hops. Essential oils of hops are a complex mixture of several hundred components and comprise two major fractions: the first belong to the group of hydrocarbons of which terpene hydrocarbons account for about 70% (Wainwright, 1998). The remaining 30% are compounds containing oxygen (oxygenated fraction which is generally more aromatic and less volatile) such as esters, aldehydes, ketones, acids and alcohols (see Table 20.12). The hydrocarbon fraction of most hops contains the monoterpene myrcene and the sesquiterpenes caryophillene and humulene as the most significant component plus a plethora of other chemically related monoterpenes and sesquiterpenes. The hydrocarbons are very volatile and are present only in dry-hopped beers. The pleasant aroma in beer originated from kettle-hoping (the so-called late hop aroma) which probably depends on substances derived from the oxygenated fraction.

The essential oil has influence on both the flavor and aroma of beer although most of the oil added to boiling wort is lost by steam distillation. Some of this loss is desiderable because some of the hop oil components have an unpleasant smell and would make beer undrinkable. In general, however, most of the hops used to impart aroma are added near the end of wort boiling to minimize losses. A process known as "dry hopping" is used when producing cask ales; in this case hops are added to the fermented beer and the oils extracted are retained in the beer.

Phenolic compounds: Beers contain several and different polyphenols which are derived from malt (two-thirds) and hops (one-third). The nomenclature of all these compounds is confusing and terms such as tannins, flavonoids, polyphenols are used, often in a very generic way, to describe a group of compounds chemically complex and different. A schematic classification is given in Table 20.13

The proanthocyanidin are very similar in their chemical structure to the anthocyanidins which are the colored pigments (red and blue) presents in many plants and in the red wine, tea, some fruits and vegetables (e.g. tomatoes). In beer an important percentage of phenolic compounds are present in the monomeric form such as hydroxycinnamic acids (e.g. p-coumaric, ferulic, chlorogenic and caffeic acids) and phenolic acids (e.g. gallic). The most important hydroxycinnamic acid found in beer (0.52–2.36 mg/l) is ferulic acid originated mainly from endosperm cell wall of barley (Pollock, 1981; Baxter and Hughes, 2001):

- **Considering the caloric value of beer generally about two-thirds are originated from alcohol and one-third from the residual carbohydrates and proteins. However beers can differ enormously in their composition, depending on their strength and how they were made.**

Before calculating the calorific value of beers it may be useful to keep in mind that beers produced worldwide can greatly differ in their composition, depending on their alcohol content and how they are brewed. In fact the alcohol content may range from less than 0.05% ABV like in

Table 20.12 Some hop oil-derived compounds found in beers

Compound	*Concentration (μg/l)*[a]
Linalool	1–470
Linalool oxides	Nd–49
Citronellol	1–90
Geraniol	1–90
Geranyl acetate	35
α-Terpineol	1–75
Humulene epoxide I	Nd–125
Humulene epoxide II	1.9–270
α-Eudesmol	1–100
T-Cadinol	Nd–200
Humulenol	1–1,150
Humuladienone	Nd–43
Humulol	Nd–220
Clovanediol	51–677

[a] Nd: not detectable.

Source: Baxter and Hughes (2001).

Table 20.13 Classification of phenolic compounds in beer.

Class	*Group*	*Congeners*	*Concentration*
Monophenols	Phenolic alcohols	Tyrosol	3–40 mg/l
	Phenolic acids	p-coumaric acid, ferulic, vanillic, gallic, caffeic, syringic, sinapic acids, etc.	10–30 mg/l including esters and glycosides, e.g. chlorogenic acid, neochlorogenic acid
	Phenolic amines and amino acids	hordenine, tyramine, *N*-methyltyramine, tyrosamine, tyrosine	10–20 mg/l (3–8 mg/l as tyrosine)
Monomeric polyphenols	Flavonoids catechines (flavan-3-ols)	(+) catechin (+) epicatechin, possibly other isomers	0.5–13 mg/l 1–10 mg/l
	Anthocyanogens (leucoanthocyanins, flavan-3,4-diols)	Leucocyanidin	4–80 mg/l
		Leucopelargonidin	0–5 mg/l
		Leucodelphinidin	1–10 mg/l
	Flavonols	Quercetin, kaempferol, myricetin (occur as glycosides) iso-quercitin, astragalin, rutin	Less than 10 mg/l
Condensed polyphenols		Dimeric catechins	5–8 mg/l
		Trimers	1 mg/l
		Polymers of catechins and anthocyanogens	Uncertain

Source: Modified from Pollock (1981).

no-alcohol beers to more than 10% ABV in some Trappist Belgian beers or may even be exceptionally up to 25.6% ABV like in Utopias MM II, an American top fermented beer. However most beers produced in the world have an alcohol content of 3–6% ABV. The energy values of ethanol (7 kcal/g), protein (4 kcal/g), carbohydrates (3.75 kcal/g) and lipids (9 kcal/g) must be considered to evaluate the calorific value of foodstuffs. Obviously, the beer being a fat-free food, the latter class of compounds will not be considered. There are different formulas to calculate this value, Martin in 1982 suggested one which takes quite precisely into consideration the major beer components and their contribution.

$$\text{Energy value (kcal/100 ml)} = (a \times 7) + (b \times 7) + (c \times 3.75)$$

where a = ethanol as g/100 ml [% (w/v)]
b = protein as g/100 ml [% (w/v)]
c = carbohydrates (as glucose) as g/100 ml [% (w/v)]

The calorific value of most beers is between 20 and 40 kcal/100 ml (80–180 kJ/100 ml). About two-thirds of this energy is originated from alcohol and one-third from the residual carbohydrates and proteins. The light beers generally contain very low amounts of carbohydrates, however they can still have a high energy value if the alcohol content is significant. This may generate some confusion because the term "light" is used to describe beers with low carbohydrate (as in United States) or low alcohol (as in Europe). In the United Kingdom the energy value is calculated according to a formula defined by Food Labelling Regulations:

$$\text{Energy value (kJ/100 ml)} = (\text{ethanol} \times 29) + (\text{carbohydrate} \times 17) + (\text{protein} \times 17)$$

where ethanol, carbohydrate and protein is expressed as above in g/100 ml [% (w/v)] (Baxter and Hughes, 2001).

References

Bamforth, C.W. (2003). *Beer: Tapping into the Art and Science of Brewing.* Insight Books Plenum Publishing Corporation, New York, London. pp. 60–65.

Bamforth, C.W. (2002). *Standards of Brewing.* Brewers Publications, Boulder, CO. pp. 123–136.

Baxter, E.D. and Hughes, P.S. (2001). *Beer: Quality, Safety and Nutritional Aspects, Vol. xiv.* The Royal Society of Chemistry, Cambridge. 138–151.

Bernstein, L. and Laufer, L. (1977). *J. Am. Soc. Brew. Chem.* 35, 21–24.

Briggs, D.E., Boulton, C.A., Brookes, P.A. and Steven, R. (2004). *Brewing Science and Practice.* Woodhead Publishing Limited and CRC Press, Cambridge, UK. pp. 687–705

Canas, B.J., Havery, D.C., Robinson, L.R., Sullivan, M.P., Joe, F.R. and Diachenko, G.W. (1989). *J. Assoc. Off. Analyt. Chem.* 78, 783–792.

Encarta World English Dictionary (1999). p. 162. Bloomsbury Publishing Plc, London, UK.

Fix, G. (2000). *Principles of Brewing Science.* Brewers Publications, Boulder, CO. pp. 106–119.

Goldammer, T. (1999). *The Brewers' Handbook – The Complete Book to Brewing Beer.* KVP Publishers, Clifton, VA. pp. 73–104.

Hardwick, W.A. (1995). *Handbook of Brewing.* Marcel Dekker Inc, New York. pp. 551–586.

Lewis, M.J. and Young, T.W. (1995). *Brewing.* Chapman and Hall, London, UK. pp. 175–190.

Moll, M.M. (1995). *Handbook of Brewing.* Marcel Dekker Inc, New York. pp. 133–156.

Pollock, J.R.A. (1981). *Brewing Science, Vol. 12.* Academic Press, London, UK. pp. 121–157.

Rabin, D. and Forget, C. (1998). *Dictionary of Beer and Brewing.* Brewers Publications, Boulder, CO.

Wainwright, T. (1998). *Basic Brewing Science.* Magic Print Limited, South Africa. pp. 275–294.

Warnakulasuriya, S., Harris, C., Gelbier, S., Keating, J. and Peters, T. (2002). *Clin. Chim. Acta* 320, 1–4.

21

Identification of Taste- and Aroma-Active Components of Beer

Paul Hughes International Centre for Brewing and Distilling, Heriot-Watt University, Riccarton, Edinburgh, UK

Abstract

The flavor of beer is a holistic perception, derived from a complicated interplay between well-defined volatile and non-volatile components. Additionally, the presence of oligo- and polymeric components in beer contributes to flavor attributes, such as body, mouthfeel and fullness. It is assumed here that the challenges for the identification of flavors are driven by research and trouble-shooting needs. Thus, the emphasis for identification of taste- and aroma-active compounds is focused on identification of those species that either have not been observed (at the level seen) before in a given beer or because there is an outstanding requirement to understand the sensory properties of a novel component. Two approaches to the identification of taste- and aroma-active compounds in beer are outlined here. The first approach is based on an initial observation of analytical anomalies in a beer, which are subsequently shown to have unusual flavor properties. The ensuing steps focus on understanding whether the observed analytical observations have a cause-and-effect relationship with the sensory observations. The second approach is based on an initial observation of sensory anomalies and how analysis can be used to try and identify the cause of the flavor.

In this chapter, the analytical techniques used to identify potentially flavor-active materials are described. The possible difficulties that arise in trying to compare sensory and analytical data are indicated, particularly in relation to the experimentation that is normally applied in analytical and sensory sciences.

List of Abbreviations

AED	Atomic emission detector
AEDA	Aroma extract dilution analysis
ECD	Electron capture detector
ELSD	Evaporative light scattering detector
FID	Flame ionization detector
FPD	Flame photometric detector
GC	Gas chromatography
GC–O	Gas chromatography–olfactometry
GC × GC	Two-dimensional gas chromatography
HPLC	High performance liquid chromatography
LC	Liquid chromatography
MIPs	Molecular imprint resins
MS	Mass spectrometry
PCA	Principal component analysis
PFBOA	*O*-(2,3,4,5,6-Pentafluorobenzyl)hydroxylamine
QDA	Quantitative descriptive analysis
SCD	Sievers' chemiluminescence detector
SPE	Solid phase extraction
SPME	Solid phase microextraction
ToF	Time-of-flight
UV	Ultraviolet

Introduction

The term beer is a generic one, encapsulating any beverage, the creation of which requires the fermentation of a sugar source that is ultimately derived from plant material, and flavored with aromatic plants. More specifically, the sugar source is most often malted barley, which can be partially replaced with other sugar sources such as maize, rice and fermentable syrups. The flavoring components are almost always derived, at least in part, from hops or products derived from hops. In 2005, global production volumes of beer exceeded 1,500 million hl (1 hl = 100 l) or around 23 l per capita per year.

It is recognized that the composition of beer is complex, consisting of a mixture of well-defined volatiles, well-defined non-volatiles, and oligo- and polymeric materials, all present in true solution or in a colloidal state in a carbonated, alcoholic matrix. In this chapter, the sources of flavors will be reviewed, which sets the scene for the approaches that are required for the identification of taste- and aroma-active materials in beer. For the purposes of this chapter, flavor-active is considered to be the overarching term for a substance that elicits some form of sensorial response from human subjects, whilst taste-active is restricted to components that elicit a response by direct interaction with the buccal cavity, either in the classical sense (i.e. sweet, salt, sour, bitter, umami) or in terms of body and mouthfeel. Aroma-active

Beer in Health and Disease Prevention
ISBN: 978-0-12-373891-2

substances are those that are perceived by the olfactory epithelium, whether nasally or retro-nasally.

Sources of Beer Flavor

The flavor of beer can be considered to be derived from four sources: raw materials, the impact of the process, in-pack flavor changes and the ingress of taint materials (Table 21.1). The major raw materials are cereals, in particular malted barley, and hops or hop products (see, for instance, Hughes, 2003). Typically, barley is subject to hydration, partial germination, then kilning, which arrests germination but ensures that specific enzyme activities of the grain survive. This process starts to release simple sugars and free amino acids that, under the influence of heat, combine to yield a complex portfolio of Maillard reaction products. The exact nature of these products will depend on the severity of the kilning regime and the water activity in the grain. Thus low-color, so-called lager malts, will tend to yield low levels of color and flavor, whilst specialty malts can make a substantially larger contribution to beer color and flavor. Malted barley replacements tend to make less of a flavor impact, although when cereals such as sorghum are used, the final beer has a quite distinct flavor, due to different flavor-active compounds being developed from the parent grain. Hops and hop products contribute both the characteristic bitterness and hoppy aroma to beer. Whilst the bitter compounds are well-defined (Verzele and De Keukeleire, 1991), the major impact compounds for the expression of hoppy aroma are poorly understood. Some workers, though, have attempted to define the expression of hop aroma in beer, based purely on the analytical levels of specific beer components (Nickerson and van Engel, 1992).

The process of beer production can in itself influence the final flavor of beer. The most important of these process considerations is the fermentation – where yeast is added to the boiled cereal extract or "wort," primarily to affect the biosynthesis of ethanol. Other components are also generated, particularly a series of esters, longer chain alcohols and free fatty acids, the exact concentrations of which are dependent on factors such as the design of the fermenter, the yeast strain used and its state of health, the temperature of fermentation, the spectrum of sugars in the fermentation and the concentration of the sugars themselves (MacDonald *et al.*, 1984). Other processes, such as the time of maturation (principally to reduce the concentration of the highly flavor-active compound diacetyl), the duration and intensity of the wort boil, which precedes fermentation, and the severity of pasteurization all impact on the final flavor of beer. It is clear then that only by close control of beer production throughout the whole process can a brewer reasonably expect to produce beers with consistent flavor quality.

An additional complication is that beer is not a completely stable product in pack. It is prone to oxidative, non-oxidative and light-induced flavor changes. There are two potentially deleterious flavor changes that can occur to a beer in-pack. Firstly, the formation of the highly flavor-active 3-methyl-2-butene-1-thiol (MBT) in beer when exposed to light in green or clear glass can occur in seconds. Reminiscent of the aroma emitted by skunks, it is also described as a key attribute for certain beers that are unprotected from light. Secondly, a range of flavor-active aldehydes, formed either by lipid oxidation or the Strecker degradation of residual amino acids in the beer, can confer flavors described as cardboard, cooked potato and generally an "oxidized" flavor to an aging beer. However, it is considered that flavor deterioration during beer aging extends beyond the portfolio of aldehydes formed and, indeed is, on the basis of the recent publication record, an active area of research (see, for instance, Sanchez *et al.*, 2003).

The final source of flavors in beer, those derived from tainting materials, are generally undesired and can cause substantial difficulty in a production context. Often these compounds have flavor activities below the level of 1 μg/l so that they can be highly elusive in any analytical evaluation. Viable bacteria or wild yeast in the final packaged beer can also cause significant flavor problems during storage. Off-flavors from bacteria generally include diacetyl, short-chain fatty acids, volatile sulfur compounds and acetaldehyde. Fungi, especially wild (i.e. non-brewing) yeast strains, often have the ability to decarboxylate ferulic acid to the highly flavor-active 4-vinylguaiacol, which confers a smoky flavor to beer.

Table 21.1 Sources of flavors in typical beers, with an indication of their flavor descriptors

Flavor source	*Major flavor contributions*
Raw materials	
– Malted barley	– Maillard reaction products, dextrins
– Wheat	– Fullness, mouthfeel
– Hops/hop products	– Bitterness, hoppy aroma
Process-derived	
– Wort boiling	– Evaporation of volatiles (e.g. hoppy, sulfury)
– Fermentation	– Ethanol, CO_2, esters, higher alcohols
– Maturation	– Reduction of diacetyl
Changes in-pack	
– Ageing	– Various esters, dioxolanes
– Oxidation	– Aldehydes
– Light-induced	– 3-Methyl-2-butene-1-thiol, H_2S
– Microbiological	– Various, including sulfurs, fatty acids, 4-vinylguiaicol
Taints	
– Chlorophenols	– Confer a "medicinal" taint
– Chloroanisoles	– Musty, "corked" flavours
– Others (e.g. geosmin, isoborneol)	– Include earthy, musty

Note: Desired flavors are derived by the impact of the beer production process on selected raw materials. Generally, flavor changes during ageing and taints/off-flavors are undesirable.

Approaches to the Detection of Taste- and Aroma-Active Compounds in Beer

The composition of beer has been systematically investigated over the past few decades, particularly since the advent of gas chromatography (GC) and high performance liquid chromatography (HPLC). However, there is still a need to identify flavor activities in beer, either to understand the contributors to product quality or to troubleshoot potential flavor defects. Another reason for attempting to elucidate the chemical composition of beer is to ensure that there are no compounds that pose a health and safety risk to the consumer. (These will not be considered explicitly here, although the approaches outlined below can be applied in this area.) The flavor goals can be addressed in one of two ways, depending on whether a flavor has been flagged up by instrumental analysis (analysis-led) or by a sensory evaluation (sensory-led; Figure 21.1).

It is important to appreciate that whether initial discovery is analysis- or sensory-led, there is still a need to link the two observations together so that a sensory-led discovery is demonstrated to show a cause-and-effect relationship with one or more analytes. Conversely, an analysis-led discovery must be similarly confirmed by sensory evaluation.

There are specific issues with regard to the instrumental analysis and sensory evaluation of beer that need to be considered. A typical beer can be described as an aqueous ethanolic solution (typically 0.5–1.0 M ethanol), containing around 0.1 M carbon dioxide. The liquid medium is acidic (pH 3.8–4.8), and contains dissolved and colloidal, non-volatile components (typically around 40 g/l) and about 0.5 g/l volatiles. Additionally, glycerol may be present at around 1 g/l. The heterogeneity of beer and its propensity both to develop insoluble precipitates and to foam, often make sample handling difficult and can compromise the reliability of certain flavor compound determinations. Perhaps the best example of this is the loss of the bitter iso-α-acids into foam if it is allowed to form, resulting in systematically low bitterness analysis results. Thus, the compositional attributes of beer can provide sampling and analytical challenges. In addition, the quantity of beer consumed in a tasting session should not, of course, unduly overburden tasters.

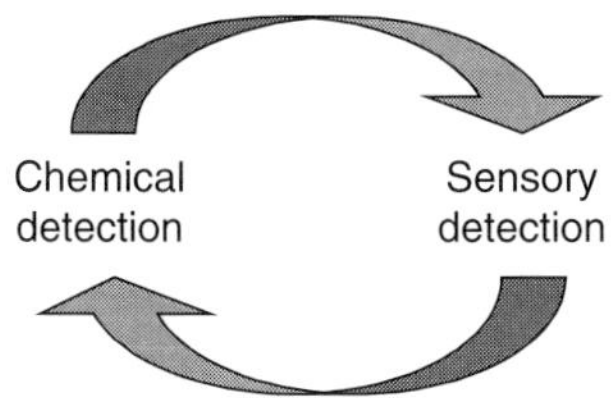

Figure 21.1 Interrelationship between sensory- and flavor-led identification of flavors in beer. The identification of flavor-active components in beer can be driven either by sensory detection, triggering a need to investigate the chemical cause, or by the chemical detection of a compound that requires sensory evaluation.

Analysis-led identification of flavor-active components in beer

The most effective approach for an analysis-led identification of a flavor-active component in beer requires some form of chromatographic technique and the appropriate detection systems (Table 21.2).

Here only HPLC- and GC-based approaches will be considered, although it is recognized that complementary techniques such as capillary electrophoresis and planar chromatography can be useful. The approach for an analysis-led

Table 21.2 Chromatographic detection systems commonly used for the identification of flavor-active components in beer

Chromatography	*Detector*	*Application*
HPLC	UV-visible	Compounds with absorption from 190 to 800 nm
	Fluorescence	Selective for compounds with defined excitation and emission wavelengths
	Refractive index	Universal detector, relying only on the ubiquitous property of refractive index
	Evaporative light scattering	Universal detector: useful for compounds with few analytical "handles," such as sugars
	Mass spectrometry	Almost universal detector; often complex fragmentation patterns with few rules for spectral interpretation
	Electrochemical	Can be used in oxidation or reduction modes as a selective detector
	Chemiluminescence	Highly selective for chemiluminescent compounds
GC	Flame ionization	General purpose: detects carbon
	Electron capture	Sensitive to specific compounds such as halogen- and nitro-containing species and 1,2-diketones
	Atomic emission	Can be set to detect a wide range of elements
	(Pulsed) flame photometric	Used mainly for sulfur-containing compounds
	Sievers' chemiluminescence	Used mainly for sulfur-containing compounds
	Nitrogen phosphorus	Specific for nitrogen- or phosphorus-containing species
	Mass spectrometry	Very common, general-purpose detector
	Olfactometry	Used extensively for flavor volatile research and troubleshooting

Note: Detector selection depends on the specific sensitivities of the analytes of interest and the degree of selectivity required to eliminate or suppress responses from unwanted, interfering, components.

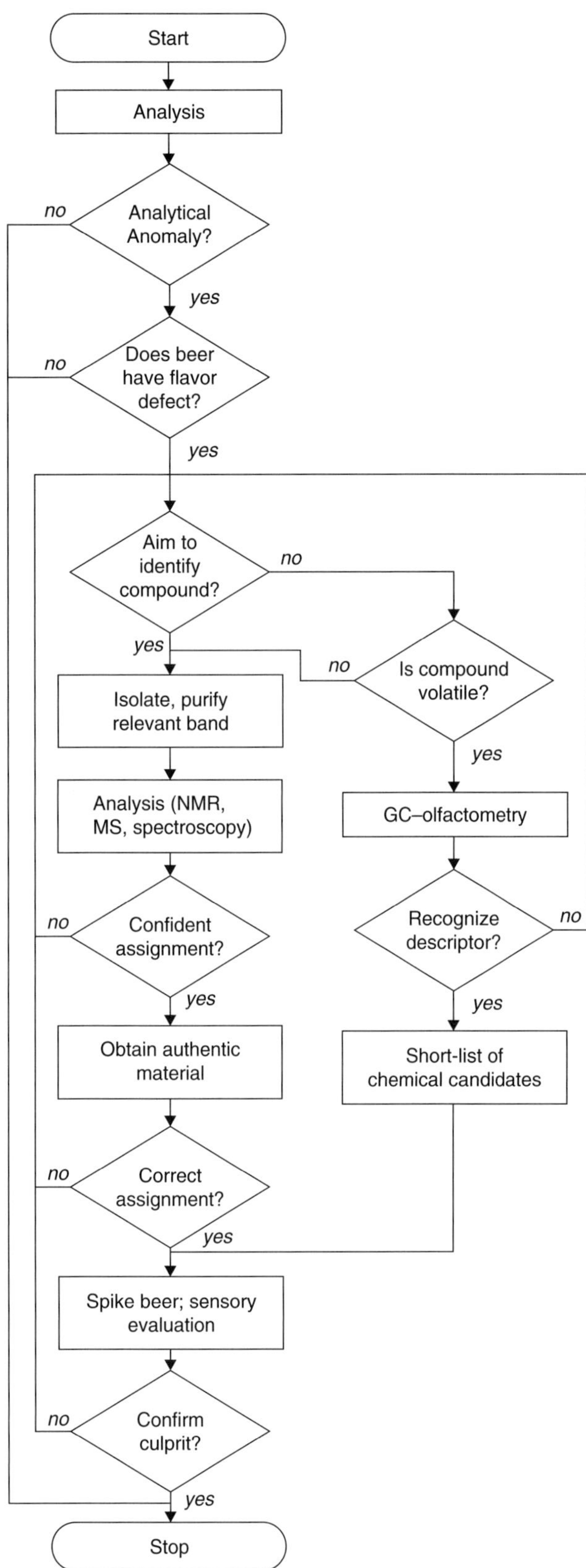

Figure 21.2 Flowchart illustrating the steps and decision-making points for identification of flavor-active compounds in beer, driven by initial analytical observations. Executed processes (represented by rectangular boxes) require decisions to be made (diamond boxes).

identification of a flavor-active compound (Figure 21.2) often presents itself either as an analytical anomaly (i.e. a chromatographic band at unusually elevated levels or, unexpectedly, present at all) or as a result of analytical screening. In both cases, the implication is that the analysis-led approach relies initially on some form of comparison, either between samples or the "expert eye" perceiving an observation outside expectations. Such an approach can, in its simplest form, be a visual comparison of the appropriate chromatograms. The approach can also be more sophisticated, by applying tools such as principal component analysis (PCA) to identify outlying samples from chromatographic data and probing the variables that make up specific principal components.

So, once the analytical anomaly has been observed and confirmed, the next step is to understand whether the subject beer is also presenting with an unexpected or unusual flavor. As mentioned earlier, sensory evaluation is an essential part of beer quality control, so there is a need to check the sensory records. If these records are deemed to be reliable (i.e. trained panelists, possible track-record that proves sensory evaluation credentials) then we reach a point where the subject beer not only shows analytical anomaly, but also has a specific sensory characteristic flagged up during a routine tasting session.

This correlation does not mean that there is a cause-and-effect relationship, so there is now a need to demonstrate this. There are two approaches to understanding whether or not the anomaly is flavor-active or not. Firstly, the analyst can focus on identification of the chemical entity and use existing knowledge to understand its flavor impact. This can be subsequently confirmed by adding back the authentic material into a beer with a more typical analytical profile, and subsequent sensory evaluation. This is often straightforward when there are high-quality mass spectrometric library hits, although this is only likely to be useful for gas chromatography–mass spectrometry (GC–MS), as identification of unknown compounds by liquid chromatography–mass spectrometry (LC–MS) remains problematic.

However, it is not essential that the chemical identity is known. Here there is a requirement to evaluate the flavor attributes *in situ*, by applying techniques such as GC–olfactometry (GC–O), or by isolation, purification and adding this material back into a "clean" beer. (Currently, there is no non-volatile alternative to GC–O, although there have been some advances made in this area (Frank *et al.*, 2003).) It is asserted here that, in most cases, it is highly desirable to know the chemical identity of a potentially flavor-active compound as:

- It provides a clue as to its origin and will often suggest approaches for elimination or control.
- In most cases, it obviates the need to go through a laborious process of isolation and purification, as chemical

compound, once its identity is known, can be acquired either by purchase from existing catalogs or by custom synthesis.

There are, however, several potential problems associated with this approach. Firstly, the suspect compound may not be considered to be suitable for human consumption. Even if it is, isolation techniques may well involve hazardous materials (e.g. preparative HPLC often requires methanol- or acetonitrile-based mobile phases), and chemical synthesis can suffer from the same limitations. It is clear then that rigorous purity appraisal is essential before submitting "spiked" beers for sensory evaluation. A further complication is the possible chemical lability of the suspect compound. Oxidation-, heat- and light-instability can make isolation and purification difficult, and also encourage the wrong conclusions to be made. Again, knowledge of the chemical structure of the suspect compound can help the flavor chemist appraise any potential difficulties here.

Sensory-led identification of flavor-active components in beer

Most if not all beers produced globally are evaluated by some form of sensory experiment prior to release on to the market. The rationale is straightforward here: the chemical complexity of beer precludes complete analysis, so that whilst the costs associated with reliable sensory evaluation are high, sensory testing allows beer to be evaluated in a fashion similar to that performed by the consumer. Most beer sensory testing relies on some form of flavor profiling, where the beer is assessed on aroma and taste and the assessor is asked to score each of a number of flavor descriptors. Often most of these descriptors are negative terms, so that scoring such terms not only indicates a flavor problem, but also suggests where the flavor problem might lie. Indeed, many flavor-negative terms on a flavor profile are chemically oriented, examples including butyric, metallic, diacetyl and sulfury.

The approach that can be applied for instance to the chemical characterization of an off-flavor (Figure 21.3) requires the problem product to be submitted for analysis. The descriptors scored by the flavor assessors can provide some clue as to where the problem might lie and facilitate analytical detection. For instance, if a product is scoring high on sulfury, initial analysis should logically focus on sulfur volatile determination, which in turn requires specific detection systems (Table 21.2) to enable detection of the potential problem. Again, it is highly desirable to have a typical example of the same brand available for comparison, particularly if the analyses required are not routinely performed and there is little experience in the interpretation of these data. Comparative brands should be of a similar age to the problem beer, to help prevent changes in flavor during aging confounding the flavor evaluation.

Experimental Techniques

Till now, the discussion has in the main used terms such as "instrumental analysis" and "sensory evaluation" as catch-all categories, with some reference to specific techniques. However, both disciplines require rigor and expertise in their application if they are to yield reliable data. The steps taken to derive data from instrumental analysis of unknown compounds in a beer matrix indicate three distinct stages: sample preparation, analysis and data interpretation.

Sample preparation

As mentioned earlier, the composition of beer presents several challenges for the flavor chemist, not least of which is the presence of carbon dioxide and, in some cases, nitrogen gas. The analysis of volatile compounds has been successfully carried out on beers by first applying a wide range of techniques (Table 21.3). For volatile compounds the simplest approach, in principle, is by direct injection of beer. However, this is undesirable due to the solid content of beer, which will have a rapid and deleterious effect on column performance. For non-volatile components, though, direct injection onto an HPLC can often prove straightforward and reliable. Thus the hop-derived iso-α-acids and sugars can be analyzed by initial direct injection. However, it is essential to ensure that the beer is sufficiently degassed to ensure that gas bubbles are not introduced into the HPLC pump. Typically degassing achieved by careful pouring of the beer onto glass beads and leaving for a period of hours.

A commonly used analytical technique for the quantification of higher esters and higher alcohols is to perform direct headspace injection onto the GC, with subsequent flame ionization detector (FID) detection (Strating, 1988). The concentration ranges of these components ranges from less than 1 mg/l for heavier esters such as ethyl octanoate to 80 mg/l for 2- and 3-methylbutanol. The active purging of beer to sweep volatiles onto the GC has been a common approach for the evaluation of the highly flavor-active sulfur volatiles. Whilst detection systems for sulfur analysis tend to be highly selective due to their low concentration (quantification is required from around 0.2 μg/l for methanethiol to 30 μg/l for ethyl thioacetate), this purge-and-trap approach successfully suppresses matrix effects. This is critical for optimal performance of all sulfur detectors with two, the AED and the SCD, being particularly sensitive.

Extraction techniques are perhaps the most traditional of sample preparation methods. Liquid–liquid extraction is rarely used today, although extraction of acidified beer with 2,2,4-trimethylpentane (isooctane) can be used for preparation of an iso-α-acid sample for HPLC analysis. More commonly, solid phase extraction (SPE) can be used both for polyphenol (Lee, 2000) and iso-α-acid analysis (Donley, 1992). The application of SPE can extend to the use of immunoaffinity SPE cartridges. These are most often

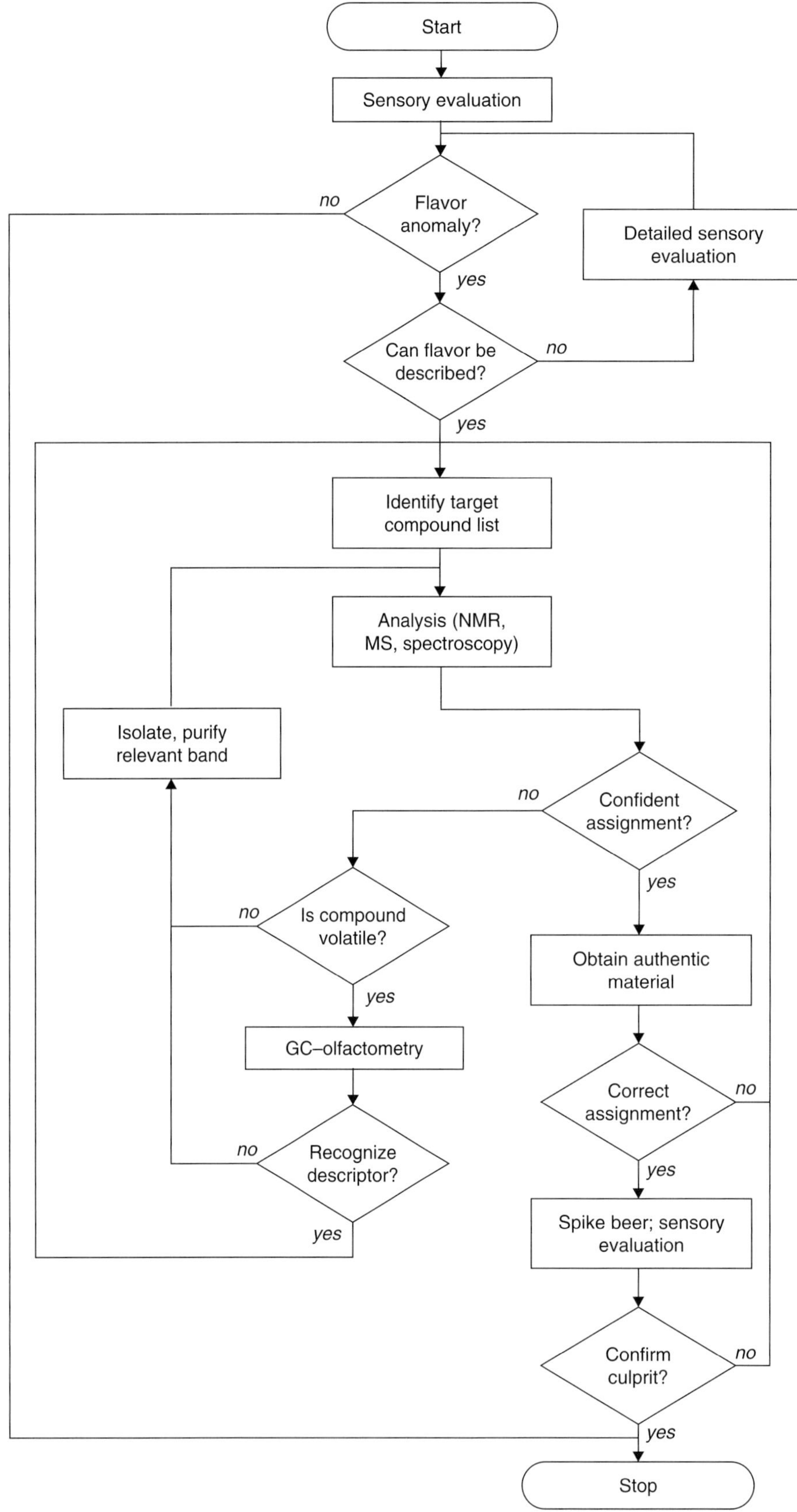

Figure 21.3 Flowchart illustrating the steps and decision-making points for identification of flavor-active compounds in beer, driven by initial sensory observations. Executed processes (represented by rectangular boxes) require decisions to be made (diamond boxes).

Table 21.3 Sample preparation methodologies for beer flavor analysis

Sample preparation method	*GC?*	*HPLC?*	*Examples*	*References*
Direct injection	×	✓	Sugars	Analytica-EBC (1998)
			Hop acids	Buckee (1985)
Headspace	✓	×	Esters, alcohols	Strating (1988)
Purge-and-trap	✓	×	Sulfur volatiles	Walker (1991)
Solid phase extraction (SPE)	✓	✓	Polyphenols	Lee (2000)
Solvent extraction	✓	✓	Hop volatiles	Wu *et al.* (1999); Harayama *et al.* (1994)
SPME*	✓	×	Sulfur volatiles	Hill and Apostolescu, (1999)
On fiber-derivatization SPME	✓	×	Aldehydes	Vesely *et al.* (2003)

*Solid phase microextraction. The aim of any sample preparation is to prepare the analytes of interest in a compatible format for the analysis of choice. Additionally, there may be a requirement to concentrate analytes and/or suppress background interferents.

used for environmental contaminants, such as mycotoxins, rather than flavor components. Recently, Sellergren *et al.* (2004) indicated that molecular imprint resins (MIPs) could be usefully prepared to selectively scavenge specific analytes from beer. However, to date, there do not appear to be any commercial applications of either immunoaffinity cartridges or MIPs for beer flavor analysis.

Since the 1990s there has been a surge of interest in the application of solid phase microextraction (SPME). Here, a fiber, coated internally with one of a range of phases, is introduced to the beer sample, either in its headspace or by immersion into the beer liquid. The volatile analytes partition into the fiber coating, which are then subsequently desorbed in the hot injector of the GC. Automation of this adsorption–desorption cycle has done much to improve the reproducibility of this technique. This technique has been further modified, by pre-adsorption of a derivatizing agent onto the fiber prior to its introduction to the beer sample. The best example of this is the adsorption of the aldehyde derivatizing agent *O*-(2,3,4,5,6-pentafluorobenzyl)hydroxylamine (PFBOA) onto the fiber (Vesely *et al.*, 2003). Aldehydes, when subsequently adsorbed, react with the derivatizing agent and, as the derivatives themselves are appreciably volatile, they can be desorbed and measured by GC analysis.

Separation systems

Detailed consideration of chromatographic separation systems is beyond the scope of this chapter (for additional information, see, for instance, Nollet, 2000). However, the understanding of whether or not a compound has sufficient volatility and thermal stability is essential if some form of gas chromatographic analysis is to be performed. For GC analysis, the thermal program and choice of column chemistry are the key decisions to be made, although for particularly difficult separations, some advantages can be gained by judicious selection of carrier gas (either hydrogen, helium or nitrogen) and optimization of linear gas velocities. Similarly, HPLC columns can, to a first approximation, be categorized into normal- and reverse-phase. The former is a highly polar silica-based stationary phase, and is used in conjunction with organic solvents. In contrast, reverse phase consists of an organic substance grafted onto silica (usually C_{18} alkyl groups), effectively reversing the polarity of silica. Mobile phases often consist of water in conjunction with polar organic solvents (most commonly methanol, acetonitrile, tetrahydrofuran and ethanol). Additionally, buffers can be used to adjust the pH of the aqueous phase, and ion-pairing agents can be used to mask any molecular charges on the analytes. This is important as such charges often cause tailing of peaks and a loss of resolving power of the analysis.

In some circumstances, it is important to achieve separation of optically active substances. This is most often addressed by using chiral stationary phases, which are available for both HPLC and GC separations. These phases are commonly based on cyclodextrins, and have been used, for instance, in the HPLC analysis of hop-derived bitter compounds (Ting and Goldstein, 1996).

Recently, there has been increasing application of the so-called GC × GC separation approach. Here, specific bands from a GC column are transferred on to a second column (see Bertsch, 1999, 2000; Phillips and Beens, 1999). This second column provides further opportunity for band resolution. This technique has shown that certain mixtures are exceedingly complex. This has been used successfully for the identification of off-flavors in beer (Sakuma *et al.*, 2000).

Detection systems

Chromatographic detection systems can be conveniently classified according to whether they are "universal," selective or based on mass detection. The term universal indicates that the analyte in question merely needs to exist above its detection limit to enable detection. For GC analysis, the best-known universal detector is the FID, which is universal in the sense that it detects molecules based on their ability to burn to give carbon. It is clear then that there is little selectivity here, apart from the exclusion of a rare few volatile molecules that lack carbon atoms (for beer, this includes sulfur dioxide, hydrogen sulfide and carbonyl sulfide). The detector that best epitomizes universal detection in the HPLC domain is the so-called ELSD (evaporative light scattering detector). Detection relies on the substances of interest possessing an ability to scatter light after the mobile phase has been evaporated, a property common to all sufficiently non-volatile components.

There is a range of selective detection systems available for both HPLC and GC. Selective implies that the molecules of interest possess physicochemical properties that are not universal. For HPLC, the most common is the UV-visible detector, either in a single wavelength or diode array configuration. The latter can collect complete spectra of chromatographic bands. The analytes of interest must, of course, exhibit absorption bands between around 190 and 800 nm, with a sufficiently high molar absorption coefficient so that it can be detected at the concentrations at which it is likely to be present. The higher the absorption wavelength, the more selective the detection is likely to be. Thus, at 254 nm, a common single wavelength detection setting, many compounds absorb. In beer, this includes a whole array of proteins, polyphenols, aromatic amino acids and the iso-α-acids. At longer wavelengths, the absorbing chromophore needs to be longer. Thus at 500 nm, riboflavin can be detected, although its concentration in beer (typically 0.2–0.3 mg/l) is too low for reliable quantification.

An alternative selective HPLC detection can be based on fluorescence. Here, both the excitation and detection wavelengths can be set, enhancing selectivity. Certain polyphenols, and beer flavin derivatives, can be observed readily by fluorescence detection. In some instances, electrochemical detection can be applied with good effect. In particular, in oxidative mode, it can be used to detect polyphenols and phenolic acids. Whilst electrochemical detection can also be used in reductive mode, in practice, it is highly challenging to exclude atmospheric oxygen sufficiently to allow sensitive detection in this mode. The ESA CoulArray, which can use up to 16 electrodes in series, has found application, again predominantly for polyphenols and phenolic acids (Rehova *et al.*, 2004).

There is a range of selective GC detectors available. One of the most common is the electron capture detector (ECD). It can detect species that are able to accept electrons, which in practice is most commonly nitrated or halogenated derivatizing agents, which are used to assign an analytical handle of sufficient sensitivity to molecules of interest. An example of this, the use of PFBOA to derivatize aldehydes, is mentioned above. The ECD can also detect diacetyl, and is the method of choice for many brewing laboratories. Selective detection is an essential prerequisite for sensitive and reliable sulfur volatile analysis. Traditionally, the flame photometric detector (FPD) had been used to good effect here, allowing quantification of short-chain thiols, di- and trisulfides, and thioesters. One disadvantage of the FPD is its non-linear response curve, which is close to quadratic. This was effectively solved with the advent of the pulsed FPD (Hill and Apostolescu, 1999), which has typical calibration plots that are more linear. More recently, the Sievers chemiluminescence detector (SCD) has become more commonplace in the brewing laboratories of several of the larger companies. This is highly sensitive detector, although it can be challenging to run consistently. The atomic emission detector (AED) can, in principle, be set up to detect a wide range of chemical elements, including sulfur. However, there are few applications of this detector in the context of beer flavor. For certain heterocycles, the nitrogen phosphorus detector (NPD) has been used, its selectivity being derived from its high level of discrimination for nitrogen and phosphorus atoms (Herent *et al.*, 1997).

Without doubt, the development of cost-effective mass spectrometric detectors has enabled the flavor chemist to derive mass data from individual chromatographic bands (for a review, see Fay *et al.*, 2001). This is far more developed in the GC arena, with substantial collections of library mass spectra and sophisticated software routines available for comparing unknown spectra with known compounds. This, together with catalogs of retention indices, substantially simplifies the flavor chemist's job. Most commonly, the mass detection for the GC is based on ion trap or quadrupole technology. Both determine unit masses, so that no definitive molecular formula information can be derived directly from such mass spectra. Recently, the wider availability of time-of-flight (ToF) mass spectrometric detectors has given the flavor chemist the opportunity to obtain accurate mass data. This is extremely useful, for instance, when attempting to identify unknown compounds, as, with careful calibration, the resolving power of the ToF detector is sufficient to generate a short list of molecular formula possibilities.

Mass spectrometric HPLC detectors are also available in various configurations. However, unlike the situation for GC, there are no substantial libraries of liquid chromatography–mass spectrometry (LC–MS) spectra and, indeed, the rules for interpretation of LC–MS spectra are, as yet, poorly defined. Thus identification of unknown compounds is often far more problematic. The quadrupole and triple quadrupole detectors are useful alternatives for selective HPLC detectors and can be used to determine a wide range of analytes in one chromatographic run. The ToF and quadrupole-ToF (QToF) detectors again allow for accurate mass determination, which is invaluable in any attempt to identify unknown compounds.

GC–olfactometry

The application of GC–O deserves special mention here as it arguably spans the instrumental and sensory interface.

This is intuitively appealing; after all, it focuses detection closely on the property of interest – its olfactory behavior. The use of the human nose as a GC detection system, often in parallel with more conventional detectors, has been increasingly employed with examples of applications including: the identification of aroma-active taints from plastics (Bravo *et al.*, 1992; Marin *et al.*, 1992), aroma thresholds of enantiomeric forms of octalactone derivatives (Abbott *et al.*, 1995), the assessment of lobster meat extracts for their aroma properties (Cadwallader *et al.*, 1995), assessment of virgin olive oil aroma (Morales *et al.*, 1995) and the aroma properties of wines (Ferreira *et al.*, 1995).

GC–O has also been applied to the aroma properties of hops. In two papers, Sanchez *et al.* (1992a, b) describe the sensory properties of hop oil oxygenated compounds and beers brewed with the three different hop varieties compared with unhopped beer. In each case the data was collected using a method called Osme (da Silva *et al.*, 1994). This is based on a time-intensity (TI) device connected to a PC and allows the evaluation of the odor activity of compounds eluting from a GC both qualitatively (by use of descriptors) and quantitatively (by use of intensity ratings). Alternative methods are CharmAnalysis™ and a similar method known as aroma extraction and dilution analysis (AEDA). Both methods are based on the GC–O analysis of serial dilutions of a sample. In CharmAnalysis™, volatiles are extracted from the sample with solvents and separated by GC. The presence or absence of odor in the effluent as a function of time is recorded by the subject using a PC. The data has a value of "zero" (i.e. cannot be detected) or "one" (can be perceived) at every time during the run. A serial dilution of the sample is continued until no odor is detected at all. Combining these results produces a chromatogram-like response called a charm chromatogram (Acree *et al.*, 1984).

Abbott *et al.* (1993) compared AEDA and Charm Analysis for the characterization of beer extracts isolated by SPE. Whilst the authors could not advocate one method over the other, they advised caution if only one approach is employed. Indeed, Marin *et al.* (1988) pointed out that there were significant differences between assessors carrying out CharmAnalysis. When applying GC–O, it is important to relate band elution times to standard retention indices. In this way, small changes in GC parameters (temperature, gas flow rates, *etc.*) can be compensated for. Such indices are generally only dependent on the nature of the stationary phase (Farkas *et al.*, 1994).

It is apparent that these techniques measure different aspects of aroma detection. It can be argued that the use of Osme is more subjective, relying on real-time intensity evaluations. This is known to be problematic (Dijksterhuis and van den Broek, 1995). However, CharmAnalysis is more time consuming, requiring the determination of several "sniffograms" (one for each sniffer employed) to enable a charm chromatogram to be evaluated. In this case, sensory fatigue becomes a pertinent issue. In addition, sniff ports are invariably located near a heat source. Although they are now designed to produce humidified air to the sniffer, care is required with the ergonomic design of sniff-ports to minimize heat drying the assessor's eyes. Nevertheless, it is undeniable that GC–O offers a route to the evaluation of the sensory characteristics of complex mixtures of volatile compounds, allowing the derivation of both descriptive and intensity parameters.

Whilst there is a need for this type of analytic approach, it should be remembered that work with extracts must be substantiated in whole beer. It is now recognized that a number of macromolecules, whilst not necessarily being flavor-active in themselves, influence the release of aroma compounds from complex matrices (Harrison and Hills, 1997). An extension of this complexity is to consider the dynamics of aroma release in the buccal cavity. This latter approach, though, is challenging (Taylor and Linforth, 1994).

Sensory evaluation

The options available for the sensory evaluation of beers depend on the question posed by the experimentalist. The circumstances in which sensory data will be required are diverse and include the following:

- Ensuring acceptability of an established product prior to its release to the market.
- Ensuring that any (minor) process change, such as new season malt or modification of stabilization treatments, do not affect the flavor attributes of a brand.
- To define the sensory attributes of unfamiliar brands (e.g. new own brands, competitor brands).
- Troubleshooting possible flavor defects.
- Comparison of brand performance, either within the company or at a consumer level.

Each of the above circumstances requires different skills of the taster and different questionnaires to be posed by the sensory analyst. Whilst it is outside the scope of this chapter to review sensory analysis methods in detail (for more information see Meilgaard *et al.*, 1999), it is worthwhile to consider the types of methods that can be applied.

Perhaps the simplest test is to ask the taster to compare two or more products. Typically, three glasses of beer are presented, one of which is different from the other two (a so-called triangle taste test). The taster is simply asked to identify the odd one out. Typically, 24 or more tasters are required to perform such a test, but testing for statistical significance is straightforward and unambiguous. If one of the beers is a control (e.g. a product known to be acceptable for the market), such a test can be used to pass a beer for sale. Alternatively, it can be used to confirm that minor changes in production have not had a significant impact on the flavor qualities of the brand.

For more major process changes, such as brewing an existing brand in a different brewery, it is likely that a period of flavor-matching will be required due to differences in brewery design and operation. A triangle test, at least at the outset, will often show significant differences, and there is a clear need to understand how the beer is performing differently from the flavor benchmark. One approach is to invoke some form of magnitude estimation for a range of flavor descriptors. Here a trained panel of tasters is asked to judge the intensity of a range of taste and aroma descriptors. Depending on the methods of training, tasters will score the various descriptors, either numerically or by marking off on a line scale. The descriptors will often be of both positive attributes (e.g. estery, fruity, bitter, malty) and negative attributes (e.g. diacetyl, butyric, sour), although it is important to remember that some negatives for one brand are acceptable at controlled levels in another. The outcome is a flavor profile, and often around 8–10 tasters will make their judgments independently, and the resulting data processed in an attempt to establish whether the test has identified possible flavor attributes that affect the overall flavor quality. These in turn can give hints as to how the process can be adjusted to bring it in line with the existing flavor benchmark.

Flavor profiling finds other applications too, such as developing flavor benchmarks for new brands, trouble-shooting off-flavors, and comparison between brands to develop a product map. There are occasions though when the scope of a flavor profile is not sufficiently broad to capture the attributes of all the brands being studied. In this case, there may be a requirement to generate new descriptors. Here, procedures such as quantitative descriptive analysis (QDA) can be useful. Here, a group of experienced tasters evaluate a range of beers and record their own flavor impressions and descriptions. After several sessions of this vocabulary generation, the tasters, under the leadership of the sensory analyst, agree a subset of descriptors. Often tasters then train to use these in scaling exercises before the modified profile is applied. QDA finds application in areas such as defining new products and concepts and for capturing brand data for a broad range of products.

Consumer sensory data is often important to brewing companies. Unlike trained sensory panels, consumers require more commonly known flavor descriptors, which can be defined, for instance, in a QDA environment. Tools such as preference mapping (MacFie and Hedderley, 1993; Greenhoff and MacFie, 1994) can be helpful in mapping analytical data and expert sensory data onto consumer sensory data. This can often highlight consumer segments and also indicate what it is about specific products that drives this segmentation.

The management and control of sensory panels and deriving relevant and reliable information from them represents a significant challenge. In particular, as discussed below, the structure of sensory panel data is such that common approaches to data analysis can be flawed.

The Challenges of Relating Sensory and Analytical Data

Earlier, it was indicated that, to identify flavor-active substances in beer, there is a necessity to relate some flavor property with a chemical identification. There are several challenges here that need to be overcome if this relationship is to be firmly established (Table 21.4). Firstly, analysis, as the term implies, requires some form of resolution of a complex composition into simpler parts. Here, analysis is used to resolve chemical mixtures into a number of bands. The ultimate aim is to have an unambiguous chemical identification of the band or bands of interest. This suggests a promise of being able to recreate the flavor effects of identified bands by adding authentic material back to the beer. However, this is often a difficult task. At its simplest, it requires rigorously pure authentic materials to be used for additions, as there are several examples of apparent flavor compounds actually containing low levels of a much more potently flavor-active substance.

One such example is that of oct-1-en-3-ol, endowed with flavor descriptors such as mushroom and metallic. In fact, these flavor characteristics are actually due to the presence of small quantities of its oxidation product, oct-1-en-3-one. Here we encounter the sheer scale of the sensory dynamic range, in comparison with that for analysis. Estimates of the flavor thresholds of oct-1-en-3-ol and oct-1-en-3-one are 1,000 ng/l (Buttery *et al.*, 1988) and 5 ng/l (Buttery *et al.*, 1990), respectively, different by more than three orders of magnitude. Thus the flavor characteristics of oct-1-en-3-ol at 99.5% pure, containing 0.5% oct-1-en-3-one, will be dominated by the trace of the latter compound. However, analytical scrutiny of the former would not necessarily reveal this impurity, as it may be present in too low a relative concentration to be routinely detected if the oct-1-en-3-ol is submitted for chromatographic analysis.

An additional difficulty is that flavor descriptions can often be concentration dependent. This is a particular problem with off-flavors, as they can be present over a vast range

Table 21.4 A comparison of sensory and analytical data attributes

Instrumental analysis	*Sensory evaluation*
Simplify: eliminate matrix	Holistic: full matrix
Sequential measurements	Virtually instantaneous assessment
All components considered singly	All components can interact
Aim is to measure concentration	Aim is to determine sensory activity
Instrumentation can be calibrated	Time-consuming to "calibrate" tasters
Output: hard numbers	Output: subjective values

Note: Chemical components do not map singly or exclusively on to specific flavor descriptors, although for certain flavors and off-flavors, there is an approximate one-to-one mapping.

of concentrations. Furthermore, the dose–response relationship between flavor component and human judgment of intensity is well-known to be non-linear, so that the application of conventional statistics (which often rely on assumptions of normality) is flawed. However, applying linearized scales for sensory magnitude estimation, such as the Linear Magnitude Scale developed by Green *et al.* (1993, 1996), can improve the chances of success in relating sensory judgments with analytical concentrations or activities.

In short, relating sensory evaluation to analytical data is often challenging. It requires high-quality data from both perspectives and a consideration of the structure of both data sets to ensure that subsequent data analyses do not fatally contravene the assumptions of the data analysis methods employed.

Future Perspectives: Detection of Non-sensory Components of Physiological Significance

The presence of compounds in beer with potential physiological effects has been discussed elsewhere in this book. The approaches described here can, in principle, be used to assess whether specific components are physiologically active (analysis-led) or whether some form of biological activity can be traced to specific beer components (assay-led). Thus, the observation of some form of biological activity can be probed using the analytical approach outlined above. Similarly, the observation in beer of compounds with known or purported biological activity can be evaluated in the appropriate biological assay. Some of the deficiencies mentioned above in relation to the inclusion compared with the control of the matrix may also be important here; biological activity could be a synergistic expression of more than one compound, so that isolation of single components may mean that the most exhaustive search is doomed to failure.

Conclusions

The identification of taste- and aroma-active components in beer has occupied brewing scientists for more than a century. The major chemical contributors to beer flavor have been mapped on to flavor descriptors. Thus the most substantial contributors to bitterness, estery, sulfury, and a myriad of off-flavors are known. The challenge today is to complete this mapping exercise, in the knowledge that flavors, even of quite disparate origin, can interact both synergistically and antagonistically so that flavor expression is specific to a given beer. The role of the relatively abundant non-volatile fraction, particularly in terms of how they impact on the flavor release and flavor intensity of volatile beer components, has been studied in other systems, and also from a theoretical standpoint. The fact that dextrins have been shown to affect the partitioning behavior of volatiles into the headspace of solutions indicates that this could be a possible expression of the impact of the beer matrix on flavor perception.

Summary Points

- Beer is a complicated mixture of well-defined volatile and non-volatile components, together with a range of oligo- and polymeric substances. These are either truly solvated or in the colloidal state, in a carbonated, acidic matrix (pH 3.8–4.8) of aqueous ethanol (typically 0.5–1.0 M).
- The flavor components of beer can be considered to originate from its raw materials (most commonly malted barley and hops/hop products), the impact of the process (particularly boiling and fermentation) and changes to the beer during its shelf-life. Additionally, unwanted taints can be found in clearly defective beers.
- The motivation for identification of taste- and aroma-active compounds in beer is either to troubleshoot problems or to understand specific flavor expression. In the case of the former and the need is to eliminate the problem, in the case of the latter the need is to apply the appropriate control to ensure product quality and consistency.
- Analysis-led identification of flavor-active components relies on applying chromatographic techniques to spot analytical anomalies, either by comparison with data from other beers, or the experience of the flavor chemist.
- Sensory-led identification of flavor-active components relies on sensory evaluation reliably flagging up flavor issues, which the flavor chemist attempts to identify cause-and-effect relationships with beer components.
- The rigorous proof of the flavor impact of a specific compound requires obtaining authentic material, either by isolation and purification from source, or by (custom) synthesis. Before using any such materials in a sensory evaluation experiment, all efforts must be made to ensure its purity and its safety.
- Instrumental analysis often requires some form of sample preparation to eliminate or control the matrix of the analyte, such that subsequent analytical methodology, almost always based on chromatography, can be applied to reliably detect, identify and/or measure target components.
- Relating sensory and analytical data can be problematic for several reasons, so that attempting to map one or more compounds to a specific flavor attribute can often meet with failure in all but the simplest cases.
- This correlation problem can be addressed, at least in part, by simple mathematical transformation of magnitude estimation data or by applying techniques such as the Labeled Magnitude Scale (LMS) which improves the linearity of sensory data.
- Ultimately, the ability of the flavor chemist to allow for the matrix effects in any sensory evaluation, which are

controlled or eliminated in the analytical experiment, will enhance his/her chances of success.

- The approaches indicated here can in principle be used to relate analytical data to other functional detection systems beyond sensory evaluation. One example is the appraisal of biological activities through specific functional assays.

References

Abbott, N., Puech, J.-L., Bayonove, C. and Baumes, R. (1995). *Am. J. Enol. Vitic.* 46, 292–294.

Abbott, N., Etievant, P., Issanchou, S. and Langlois, D. (1993). *J. Agric. Food Chem.* 41, 1698–1703.

Acree, T.E., Barnard, J. and Cunningham, D.G. (1984). *Food Chem.* 14, 273–286.

Analytica-EBC Methods (1998). *Method 9.27, European Brewery Convention.* Verlag, Nurnberg.

Bertsch, W. (1999). *J. High Resolut. Chromatogr.* 22, 647–665.

Bertsch, W. (2000). *J. High Resolut. Chromatogr.* 23, 167–181.

Bravo, A., Hotchkiss, J.H. and Acree, T.E. (1992). *J. Agric. Food Chem.* 40, 1881–1885.

Buckee, G. (1985). *J. Inst. Brew.* 91, 143–147.

Buttery, R.G., Teranishi, R., Flath, R.C. and Ling, L.C. (1990). *J. Agric. Food Chem.* 38, 792–795.

Buttery, R.G., Turnbaugh, J.G. and Ling, L.C. (1988). *J. Agric. Food Chem.* 36, 1006–1009.

Cadwallader, K.R., Tan, Q., Chen, F. and Meyers, S.P. (1995). *J. Agric. Food Chem.* 43, 2432–2437.

Dijksterhuis, G. and van den Broek, E. (1995). *J. Sensory Stud.* 10, 149–161.

Donley, J.R. (1992). *J. Am. Soc. Brew. Chem.* 50, 89–90.

Farkas, P., Quere, J., Maarse, H. and Kovac, M. (1994). In Maarse, H. and van der Heij, D.G. (eds), *Trends in Flavour Research*, pp. 145–149. Amsterdam, Elsevier.

Fay, F.B., Yeretzian, C. and Blank, I. (2001). *Chimia* 55, 429–434.

Ferreira, V., Fernàndez, P., Gracia, J.P. and Cacho, J.F. (1995). *J. Sci. Food Agric.* 69, 299–310.

Frank, O., Jezussek, M. and Hofmann, T. (2003). *J. Agric. Food Chem.* 51, 2693–2699.

Green, B.G., Dalton, P., Cowart, B., Shaffer, G., Rankin, K. and Higgins, J. (1996). *Chem. Senses* 21, 323–334.

Green, B.G., Shaffer, G.S. and Gilmore, M.M. (1993). *Chem. Senses* 18, 683–702.

Greenhoff, K. and MacFie, H.J.H. (1994). In MacFie, H.J.H. and Thomson, D.M.H. (eds), *Measurement of Food Preferences*, pp. 137–166. London, Blackie.

Harayama, K., Hayase, F. and Kato, H. (1994). *Biosci. Biotechnol. Biochem.* 58, 2246–2247.

Harrison, M. and Hills, B.P. (1997). *J. Agric. Food Chem.* 45, 1883–1890.

Herent, M.-F., Vanthournhout, C., Gijs, L. and Collin, S. (1997). *Proceedings of the European Brewery Convention Congress*, Maastricht, Canes, pp. 167–174.

Hill, P.G. and Apostolescu, L. (1999). *Proceedings of the European Brewery Convention Congress*, Cones, pp. 87–93.

Hughes, P. (2003). In Caballero, B., Trugo, L. and Finglas, P. (eds), *Encyclopedia of Food Sciences and Nutrition*, 2nd edn. pp. 422–429. Amsterdam, Elsevier.

Lee, H.S. (2000). In Nollet, L.M.L. (ed.), *Food Analysis by HPLC.* Marcel Dekker Inc, Basel.

MacDonald, J., Reeve, P.T.V., Ruddlesden, J.D. and White, F.H. (1984). Industrial fermentations. In Bushell, M.E. (ed.), *Progress in Industrial Micro-biology*, Vol. 19, pp. 47–198. Elsevier, Amsterdam.

MacFie, H.J.H. and Hedderley, D. (1993). *Food Qual. Pref.* 4, 41–49.

Marin, A.B., Acree, T.E., Hotchkiss, J.H. and Nagy, S. (1992). *J. Agric. Food Chem.* 40, 650–654.

Marin, A.B., Acree, T.E. and Barnard, J. (1988). *Chem. Senses* 13, 435–444.

Meilgaard, M.C., Civille, G.V. and Carr, B.T. (1999). *Sensory Evaluation Techniques*, 3rd edn. CRC Press, Boca Raton, FL.

Morales, M.T., Alonso, M.V., Rios, J.J. and Aparicio, R. (1995). *J. Agric. Food Chem.* 43, 2925–2931.

Nickerson, G.B. and van Engel, E.L. (1992). *J. Am. Soc. Brew. Chem.* 50, 77–81.

Nollet, L.M.L. (ed.) (2000). *Food Analysis by HPLC*, 2nd edn. Marcel Dekker, Inc, Basel.

Phillips, J.B. and Beens, J. (1999). *J. Chromatogr. A* 856, 331–347.

Rehova, L., Skerikova, V. and Jandera, P. (2004). *J. Sep. Sci.* 27, 1345–1359.

Sakuma, S., Amano, H. and Ohkochi, M. (2000). *J. Am. Soc. Brew. Chem.* 58, 26–29.

Sanchez, B., Reverol, L., Galindo-Castro, I., Bravo, A., Rangel-Aldao, R. and Ramirez, J. (2003). *Tech. Q. Master Brew. Assoc. Am.* 40, 204–221.

Sanchez, N.B., Lederer, C.L., Nickerson, G.B., Libbey, L.M. and McDaniel, M.R. (1992a). Food science and human nutrition. *Dev. Food Sci.* 29, 371–402.

Sanchez, N.B., Lederer, C.L., Nickerson, G.B., Libbey, L.M. and McDaniel, M.R. (1992b). Food science and human nutrition. *Dev. Food Sci.* 29, 403–426.

Sellergren, B., Manesiotis, P. and Hall, A.J. (2004). Patent WO 2004/067578.

da Silva, M.A.A.P., Lundahl, D.S. and McDaniel, M.R. (1994). In Maarse,, H. and van der Heij, D.G. (eds), *Trends in Flavour Research*, pp. 191–209. Elsevier, Amsterdam.

Strating, J. (1988). In Linskens, H.F. and Jackson, J.F. (eds), *Beer Analysis, Modern Methods of Plant Analysis*, Vol. 7, pp. 254–263. Springer-Verlag, London.

Taylor, A.J. and Linforth, R.S.T. (1994). In Maarse, H. and van der Heij, D.G. (eds), *Trends in Flavour Research*, pp. 3–14. Elsevier, Amsterdam.

Ting, P.L. and Goldstein, H. (1996). *J. Am. Soc. Brew. Chem.* 52, 103–109.

Verzele, M. and De Keukeleire, D. (1991). Developments on food science. In *Chemistry and Analysis of Hop and Beer Bitter Acids*, Vol. 27. Elsevier, Amsterdam.

Vesely, P., Lusk, L., Basarova, G., Seabrooks, J. and Ryder, D. (2003). *J. Agric. Food Chem.* 51, 6941–6944.

Walker, M.D. (1991). *Proceedings of the European Brewery Convention Congress*, Lisbon, pp. 521–528.

Wu, Z., Buiatti, S. and Hughes, P.S. (1999). *Proceedings of the European Brewery Convention Congress*, Canes, pp. 79–86.

22

Hop Essential Oil: Analysis, Chemical Composition and Odor Characteristics

Graham Eyres and Jean-Pierre Dufour Department of Food Science, University of Otago, Dunedin, New Zealand

Abstract

The essential oil of hops (*Humulus lupulus* L.) imparts odor and aroma characteristics to beer. Hops can influence beer aroma in terms of floral, spicy, herbal, woody and fruity characters. There are a large number of hop varieties commercially available with distinct odor characteristics, which can be attributed to the different composition of their essential oils. This composition is complex, potentially containing up to 1,000 compounds from a wide range of chemical classes. Fresh essential oil is dominated by terpene hydrocarbons, predominantly myrcene, α-humulene and β-caryophyllene. The composition varies depending on: intrinsic and extrinsic factors during growth, processing conditions, and the extraction method used to isolate the essential oil. In addition, oxidation and hydrolysis reactions occurring during storage alter the composition and further increase the chemical complexity.

Despite more than 50 years of research, not all character-impact odorants in hop essential oil have been identified. Due to its abundance, myrcene is important for the odor of fresh hop essential oil. Linalool and geraniol have been determined to be important odorants contributing to the floral character of hop essential oil and beer. Other compounds such as β-ionone, β-damascenone, geranial, neral, *trans*-4,5-epoxy-(*E*)-2-decenal, 1,3(*E*),5(*Z*)-undecatriene, 1,3(*E*),5(*Z*),9-undecatetrene, ethyl 2-methylpropanoate, methyl 2-methylbutanoate, propyl 2-methylbutanoate, (*Z*)-1,5-octadien-3-one, nonanal and isovaleric acid have been implicated as potent odorants in hop essential oil.

Hoppy aroma in beer is still not completely understood due to the physical, biochemical and chemical changes that occur during brewing and fermentation. Hop-derived odorants identified in beer but not present in hop essential oil include citronellol, γ-nonalactone, humuladienone, geranyl acetate and ethyl cinnamate. Oxidation and hydrolysis products of sesquiterpenes (e.g. humulene epoxides) have commonly been associated with "noble" hop characters in beer; however, the importance of these compounds remains controversial. The complexity of hop aroma in beer has led to increasing trends to add fractionated hop oils with specific odor characteristics to beer post-fermentation.

List of Abbreviations

AU	Aroma Units
^{1}D	First column
^{2}D	Second column
DMS	Dimethyl sulfide
DMTS	Dimethyl trisulfide
FID	Flame ionization detector
GC × GC	Comprehensive two-dimensional gas chromatography
GC–O	Gas chromatography–olfactometry
HACP	Hop aroma component profile
HPLC	High performance liquid chromatography
MDGC	Multidimensional gas chromatography
MS	Mass spectrometry
SDE	Simultaneous distillation extraction
SPE	Solid-phase extraction
Syn.	Synonym
TOFMS	Time-of-flight mass spectrometry

Introduction

Hops (*Humulus lupulus* L.) are added to beer to impart bitterness, odor and aroma. Both hop resins and essential oil are found in the lupulin glands of the female flower cone. The essential oil is comprised of the components that are volatile in steam, usually isolated by distillation (Lawrence, 2002). The iso-α-acids originating from hop resins are predominantly responsible for bitterness, whereas a number of compounds in the essential oil are responsible for imparting hoppy odor and aroma to beer. Essential oil makes up between 0.5% and 3% of the gross composition of the

Beer in Health and Disease Prevention
ISBN: 978-0-12-373891-2

dried hop cone, varying between varieties (Benitez *et al.*, 1997; Briggs *et al.*, 2004).

Hops are typically added to wort during the boil (kettle hopping) to extract the bitterness and allow the chemical isomerization of the α-acids to the more bitter iso-α-acids. To minimize evaporation of essential oil and retain aroma compounds, premium aroma hops are added at the end of boiling (late hopping) or even to the whirlpool (Benitez *et al.*, 1997; Fritsch and Schieberle, 2003).

There are a large number of hop varieties commercially available with varying α-acids contents, essential oil levels and odor profiles (Benitez *et al.*, 1997; Briggs *et al.*, 2004). It is well known that different hop varieties produce beers with distinct aroma characteristics. Differences in the odor profiles between hop varieties can be attributed to the composition of their essential oil (Gardner, 1994). Brewers often use several varieties in a single beer to achieve the desired balance of bitterness, odor and aroma. This is usually based on α-acids content (which does not directly contribute to aroma), past experience, and trial and error. Varieties of hops are typically classified into bitter varieties with high α-acids, aroma varieties with desirable odor characteristics and dual purpose varieties that meet both criteria.

The terms odor, aroma and flavor are often used synonymously, but in this chapter a distinction will be made between them. Odor and aroma both result from a perception of volatile compounds at the olfactory epithelium in the nose. *Odor* can be defined as an orthonasal perception, where volatiles are breathed in directly through the nose. In comparison, *aroma* is a retronasal perception, where volatiles reach the olfactory epithelium via the mouth during consumption (Acree, 1993; Blank, 2002). Finally, *flavor* is a complex and integrated perception consisting of odor, aroma, taste, texture or mouthfeel, and any other trigeminal sensations such as irritation, cooling or heat (Lawless and Heymann, 1998).

This chapter discusses the chemical composition of hop essential oil and the factors that influence its composition. Methods of extraction, methods of analysis and the fractionation of essential oil are also considered. The odor characteristics of hop essential oil and the current understanding of the compounds responsible are presented with an inference to hop aroma in beer.

Variation and Changes in Composition

Much like other plant essential oils, the composition of hop oil depends on a number of intrinsic and extrinsic factors during growth. The most important of these are genetic differences where the composition varies markedly between hops of different varieties. Minor genetic variation may also occur between hops of the same variety from different growing regions. Hops are typically grown without male plants to reduce the amount of seeds, but this may reduce yields (kg/ha) (Benitez *et al.*, 1997). However, seedless hops typically produce more essential oil (Briggs *et al.*, 2004). An alternative method is the production of seedless triploid varieties, which have three sets of chromosomes instead of the normal two (diploid), and produce normal harvest yields (Beatson *et al.*, 2003).

Geographical location, climate and agronomical factors also affect the oil composition, potentially creating different profiles for hop samples with the same genetic material. Good yields depend on adequate soil nutrients and nitrogen levels, thus fertilizer is typically applied (Benitez *et al.*, 1997). Variation also occurs between harvest years due to different climatic conditions such as rainfall, temperature and sunshine. Irrigation is also required in arid conditions to ensure a good yield of hops and α-acids." As the flower cone develops, not only does the amount of essential oil increase but the proportions of compounds change. For example, oxygenated compounds are synthesized first, followed by sesquiterpenes (predominantly α-humulene (**1**) (Figure 22.1) and β-caryophyllene (**2**)), and the monoterpenes (primarily myrcene (**3**)) are produced last as the flowers ripen (Briggs *et al.*, 2004). Therefore, the harvest time will impact upon the composition of the essential oil and myrcene concentration can be used as a measure of hop ripeness. However, the humulene:caryophyllene ratio remains constant and is a varietal characteristic.

Infection from viruses and diseases, such as downy mildew, powdery mildew and verticillium wilt, and attack from pests, such as the damson hop aphid, the red spider mite and the two-spotted spider mite, can also change the composition and yield of essential oil as the plant becomes stressed (Benitez *et al.*, 1997; Hysert *et al.*, 1998). This has implications on the quality of the hops and the consistency of the oil composition. These pests and diseases are controlled by selective breeding for natural resistance, application of pesticides and fungicides (Briggs *et al.*, 2004), or alternatively via biological control using predatory mites (Barber *et al.*, 2003).

The composition of the essential oil changes during post-harvest processing, storage and transport. Compounds are partially lost through evaporation to varying degrees depending on their volatility. Furthermore, the composition of the essential oil continues to change due to oxidative degradation. The degree of change during storage depends on: the extent of physical damage to the lupulin glands withstood during harvesting, baling and kiln drying; the processing and packaging method; and the subsequent storage temperature. Larger bale sizes and density increase the damage to the lupulin glands (Forster, 2001). Baled hop cones waiting processing are often stored at ambient temperature, which allows significant changes to occur. It is recommended that temperatures during kiln drying do not exceed 60°C to prevent major losses of essential oil and oxidative degradation (Forster, 2001).

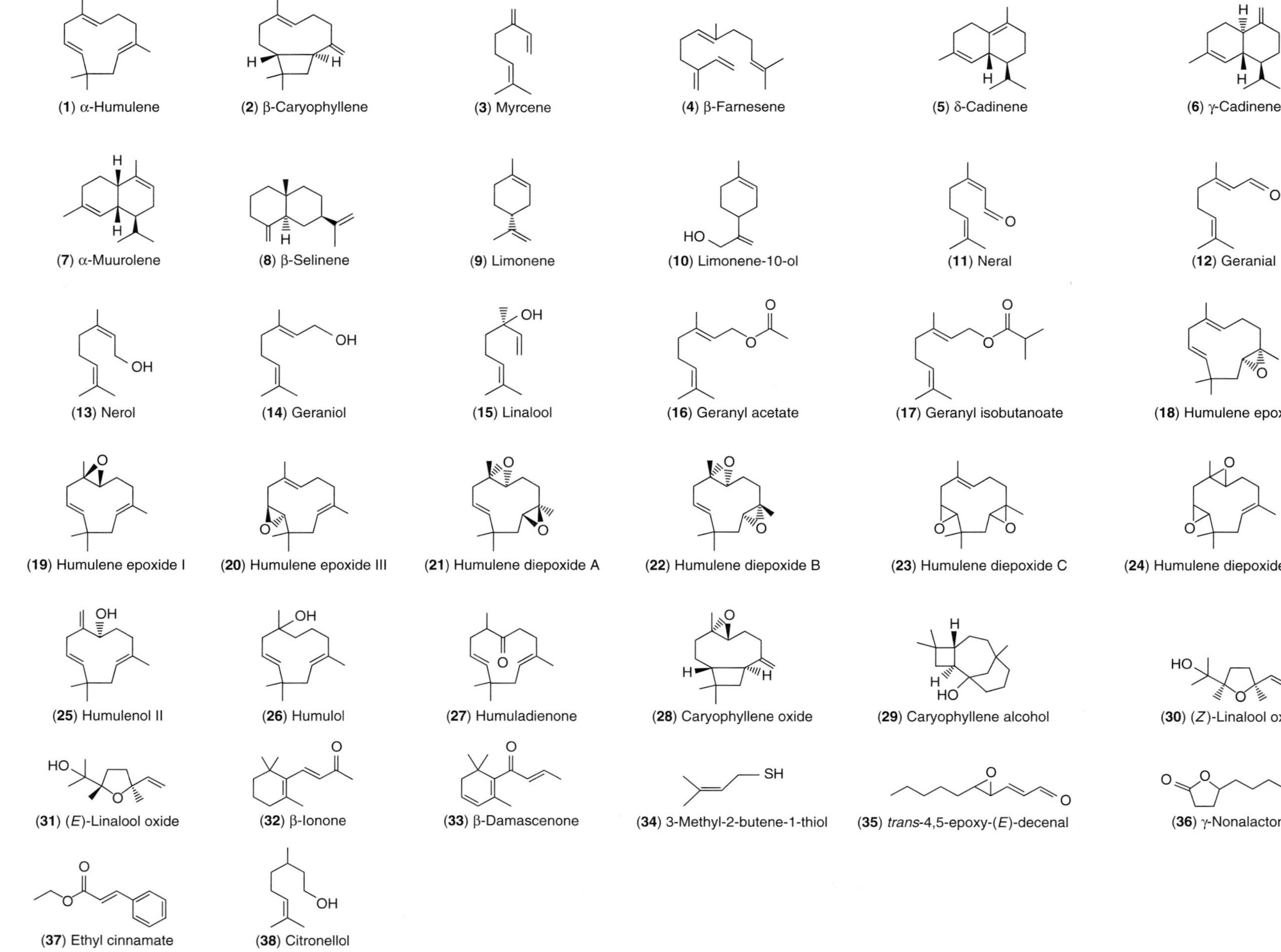

Figure 22.1 Chemical structures of major compounds and potential odorants in hop essential oil and beer.

Whole hops are the most susceptible to oxidation during storage, with significant losses of resins and essential oil occurring. Between 50% and 70% of the essential oil can be lost during 6 months storage at 20°C, mainly due to loss of myrcene (Beatson *et al.*, 2003). Therefore, hop bales should ideally be stored at refrigeration temperatures (0–5°C) (Forster, 2001).

During pelletization, hops are exposed to temperatures up to 65°C due to friction in the pelleting die, which causes the resins and essential oil that are released from the crushed lupulin glands to be susceptible to rapid oxidation. The EBC Manual of Good Practice for Hops and Hop Products (Benitez *et al.*, 1997) advocates a maximum pelleting temperature of 55°C followed by immediate cooling and vacuum packaging under an inert atmosphere (CO_2 or N_2). Packaged pellets should ideally be stored at refrigeration temperatures, but where this is impractical, keeping the temperature below 15°C should be sufficient to maintain freshness and quality (Benitez *et al.*, 1997; Forster, 2001). Extracts of resins and essential oil (see section "Methods of Extraction") are considerably more stable than pellets or whole hops, and therefore a maximum storage temperature of 20°C is acceptable (Forster, 2001).

Essential oil composition also depends on the method of isolation, as different techniques vary in their selectivity for different compound classes. This will be discussed further below (see section "Methods of Extraction").

Analysis and Characterization of Hop Essential Oil

The first characteristic of interest for a hop variety is the percentage yield of essential oil from the dried hop cones. This is determined by measuring the volume of oil recovered from steam distillation of dried hop cones and expressed in ml/g (Analytica-EBC, 2005; ASBC Methods of Analysis, 2006). The ratio of oil to α-acids is also important as brewers will primarily add hops to the kettle based on the content of α-acids to achieve a desired bitterness. Subsequently, the variable volume of essential oil added concurrently with the resins will impact upon the consistency of hop aroma in beer.

Routine analysis to determine the composition of hop essential oil is performed by gas chromatography with either flame ionization detection (GC–FID) or mass spectrometry (GC–MS). The hop essential oil is usually isolated prior to analysis (see section "Methods of Extraction"), although headspace analysis of hop cones or pellets is also performed. Headspace analysis can be achieved by either static or dynamic sampling, and the volatiles may also be concentrated by trapping on adsorbents. A convenient and popular technique for rapid characterization of hop volatiles is solid-phase microextraction (Kenny *et al.*, 2000; Steinhaus *et al.*, 2003).

Common criteria used to characterize a hop variety are the ratios of various sesquiterpene hydrocarbons, the most important being the humulene:caryophyllene ratio. A high humulene:caryophyllene ratio is typically associated with European aroma hops (Deinzer and Yang, 1994). The ratio of these sesquiterpenes is characteristic of a variety, independent of ripeness or storage, and have therefore been used to discriminate between varieties (Kralj *et al.*, 1991; Moir, 1994). However, while these ratios may be useful markers, they cannot be used to predict or explain differences in odor characteristics between varieties.

Consistent bitterness is achieved in beer by hop addition based on α-acids content. However, controlling hop aroma is more difficult as there is no single compound to measure to determine hopping rate. Addition based on total essential oil is not satisfactory due to variable composition, varietal differences and changes during storage. To address this, Foster and Nickerson (1985) proposed the "hoppiness potential" concept to control hopping rates based on the quantitative analysis of 24 compounds per gram of α-acids. This concept was further developed by Nickerson and Van Engel (1992) who refined the list of compounds and renamed it the "hop aroma component profile" (HACP) (Table 22.1). The compounds were classified into three categories: humulene and caryophyllene oxidation products; floral–estery compounds and citrus–piney compounds. These authors defined Aroma Units (AU) as the quantitative sum of the 22 HACP compounds per gram of hops (nl/g). HACP has subsequently been commonly used as a criterion for characterizing the essential oil of different hop varieties. It was envisaged that the compounds comprising HACP would evolve as new odorants were identified and their impact on beer aroma

Table 22.1 Classification of compounds comprising the hop aroma component profile[a]

Oxidation products[b]	*Floral–estery compounds*	*Citrus–piney compounds*
Humulene epoxide I (**18**)	Geraniol (**14**)	δ-Cadinene (**5**)
Humulene epoxide II (**19**)	Linalool (**15**)	γ-Cadinene (**6**)
Humulene epoxide III (**20**)	Geranyl acetate (**16**)	α-Muurolene (**7**)
Humulene diepoxide A (**21**)	Geranyl isobutanoate (**17**)	β-Selinene (**8**)
Humulene diepoxide B (**22**)		Limonene (**9**)
Humulene diepoxide C (**23**)		Limonene-10-ol (**10**)
Humulenol II (**25**)		Citral (neral + geranial)[c]
Humulol (**26**)		Nerol (**13**)
Caryophyllene oxide (**28**)		
Caryophyllene alcohol (**29**)		

[a] Adapted from Nickerson and van Engel (1992). Numbers in parentheses refer to the chemical structure depicted in Figure 22.1.
[b] Oxidation products of humulene and caryophyllene.
[c] Citral is a mixture of the two isomers – neral (**11**) and geranial (**12**).

elucidated. This has not really eventuated and an updated review of HACP is required for its potential to be realized.

The problem with analysis of hop essential oil using conventional GC is that the maximum number of compounds that can be resolved on a single 50 m column is limited to only 260 peaks (Bartle, 2002). In addition, peaks are neither evenly nor randomly distributed in a chromatogram because compounds demonstrate related chemical properties (Marriott, 2002). Because the number of compounds present in hop oil exceeds this peak capacity, severe co-elution occurs in conventional GC. This makes identification and quantification of compounds challenging, particularly for trace odorants co-eluting with larger odor inactive peaks. A solution is to use GC–MS in single ion monitoring (SIM) mode to quantify known compounds by a unique mass. This may be performed in conjunction with stable isotope dilution assay, which uses the deuterated target compound as an internal standard (Blank *et al.*, 1999; Steinhaus *et al.*, 2003). However, identification of unknown compounds remains difficult, particularly for trace odorants.

A potential solution to improve resolution is multidimensional gas chromatography (MDGC), which uses two columns with different stationary phases to create two independent separations. Compounds that co-elute on a first column may be resolved on a second column. For example, two compounds with similar boiling points that co-elute on a non-polar column may be resolved on a polar second column if they differ in their polarity. Traditional MDGC (Figure 22.2a) uses either a mechanical or pneumatic valve (V) to selectively transfer discrete regions, known as "heart-cuts," from the first column (^{1}D) to a second column (^{2}D) (Marriott, 2002). Regions that are not heart-cut to the ^{2}D column are diverted to FID 1, which monitors the separation on the ^{1}D column. The second detector is often another FID, but a mass selective detector may also be used to identify the compounds eluting from the ^{2}D column. The limitation of the heart-cut technique is that there must be sufficient time between sequential heart-cuts to prevent compounds from the two separate cuts overlapping on the ^{2}D column. Therefore, only a certain number of regions can be transferred and only a portion of the sample can be separated in two dimensions.

Another technique known as comprehensive two-dimensional gas chromatography (GC × GC) separates the *entire* sample in two dimensions in a single analysis. This is achieved using two columns connected in series with a cryogenic modulator (M) at the interface (Figure 22.2b). The modulator sequentially traps and pulses zones from the first column to the second column (e.g. every 5 s) creating two independent separation dimensions based on different compound properties. A short (0.5–2 m), narrow diameter (0.1 mm) and thin-film (0.1 μm) ^{2}D column is typically used to create a fast, efficient separation in the second dimension so that peaks from sequential pulses do not overlap (wraparound). GC × GC results are typically converted to a matrix and plotted as a contour plot analogous to a topographical map (Figure 22.3b). Retention time on the ^{2}D column is plotted against retention time on the ^{1}D column with detector signal plotted on the *z*-axis with shaded or colored contour levels used to denote peak height and compound abundance.

The greater peak capacity, resolution and sensitivity of GC × GC provide superior analyses compared with conventional GC analysis. Figure 22.3a presents a section of a single column separation of a sample of Cascade hop essential oil and exhibits considerable co-elution in the complex region of oxygenated sesquiterpenoid compounds. Figure 22.3b demonstrates the superior resolution obtained using GC × GC and illustrates the complexity of the region.

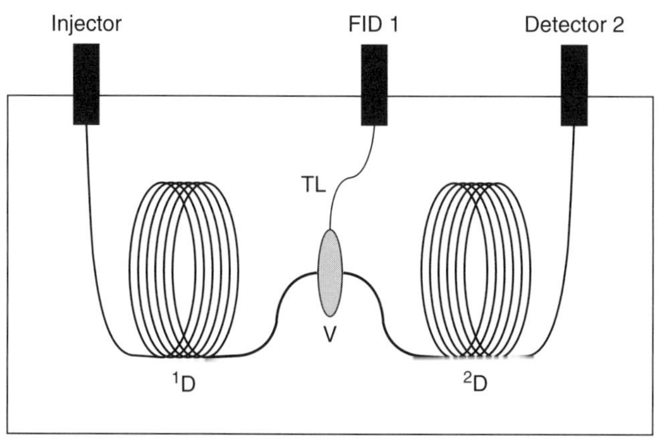

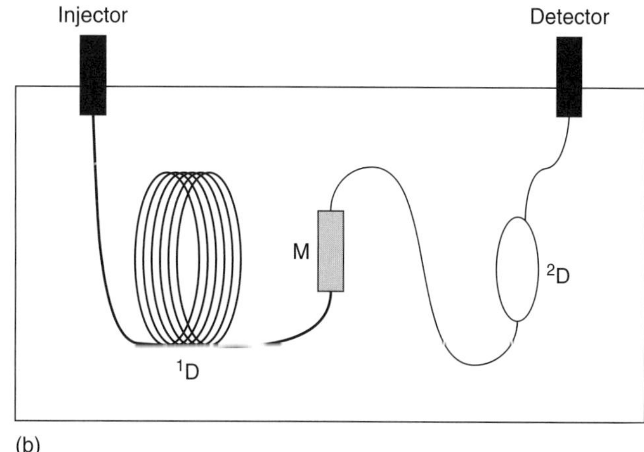

Figure 22.2 Schematic diagrams of (a) a traditional heart-cut MDGC system and (b) a comprehensive GC × GC system. ^{1}D, first column; ^{2}D, second column; V, valve; TL, transfer line to FID 1; M, cryogenic modulator. Detector 2 in the MDGC system could either be a FID or a mass selective detector. The detector in the GC × GC system could either be a FID or a TOFMS.

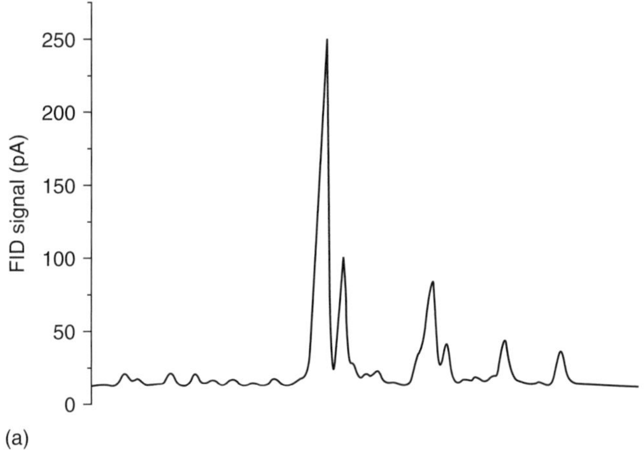

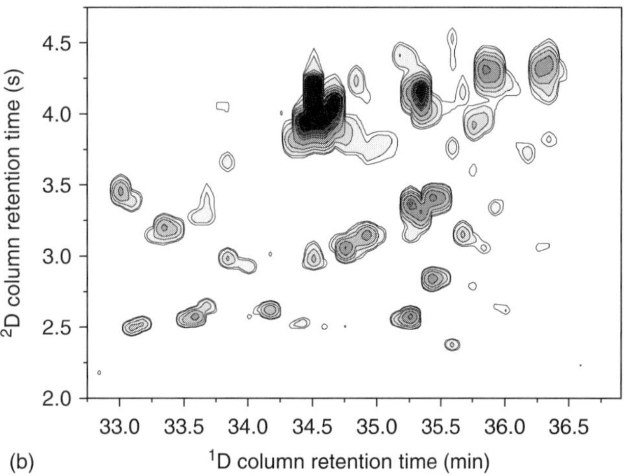

Figure 22.3 Separation of the oxygenated sesquiterpenoid region of Cascade hop essential oil sample using (a) conventional GC–FID and (b) GC × GC–FID. Note the severe co-elution of compounds for conventional GC and the superior resolution achieved using GC × GC. For the GC × GC plot, retention time on the ^{2}D column (polar) (*y*-axis) is plotted against retention time on the ^{1}D column (non-polar) (*x*-axis). Detector signal is plotted in the *z*-axis with abundance indicated by the contour levels and increasing shading.

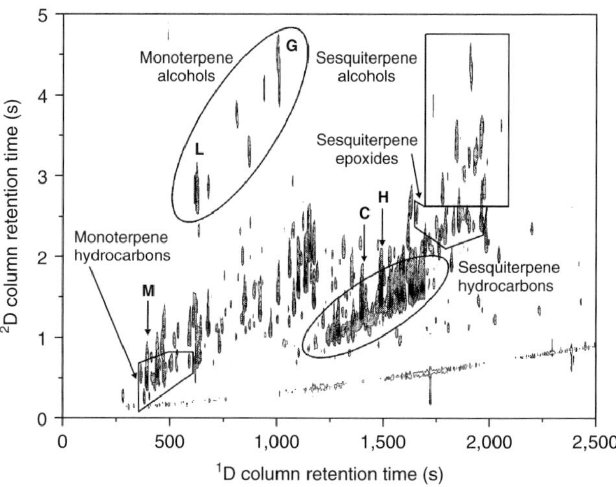

Figure 22.4 Contour plot of GC × GC separation of Target hop essential oil. Outlined regions correspond to regions where classes of terpenoid compounds elute. M, myrcene; C, β-caryophyllene; H, α-humulene; L, linalool; G, geraniol.

Combining GC × GC to time-of-flight mass spectrometry (TOFMS) results in a very powerful identification tool (Roberts *et al.*, 2004).

Another advantage of GC × GC is that it generates a structured chromatogram which aids peak identification. Different compound classes elute in specific regions and clusters of the chromatogram depending on their interaction with the two stationary phases. For example, using a polar ^{2}D column, early eluting hydrocarbons are at the bottom of the GC × GC plot whereas alcohols are at the top (Figure 22.4). In addition, homologous series of compounds form linear or logarithmic relationships in the separation plane which helps to discriminate between isomeric compounds (Roberts *et al.*, 2004; Eyres *et al.*, 2005) (Figure 22.5).

At present, these multidimensional techniques are generally used for research purposes rather than routine analysis, but their potential for the discovery of new compounds is immense. For more information on the development and operation of GC × GC and TOFMS the reader is directed toward two comprehensive reviews (Phillips and Beens, 1999; Marriott, 2002).

Composition of Hop Essential Oil

The composition of hop essential oil is complex. Nijssen *et al.* (1996) compiled a comprehensive list of 425 compounds reported in hop essential from 75 references. During the last decade, a further 60 compounds have been identified and reported bringing the total to 485 (Roberts *et al.*, 2004). However, recent research suggests that up to 1,000 compounds may actually be present (Roberts *et al.*, 2004). This leaves great scope for further identification and discovery of important odor active compounds. Hop essential oil contains a wide range of aliphatic, aromatic and terpenoid compound classes. Figure 22.4 presents a GC × GC separation of a sample of Target hop essential oil demonstrating the complexity of the chemical composition.

Terpenoid compounds

Figure 22.4 shows the main classes of terpenoid compounds present in hop essential oil, namely monoterpene hydrocarbons, monoterpene alcohols, sesquiterpene hydrocarbons, sesquiterpene epoxides and sesquiterpene alcohols. The composition of fresh hop essential oil is dominated by terpene hydrocarbons, primarily the monoterpene

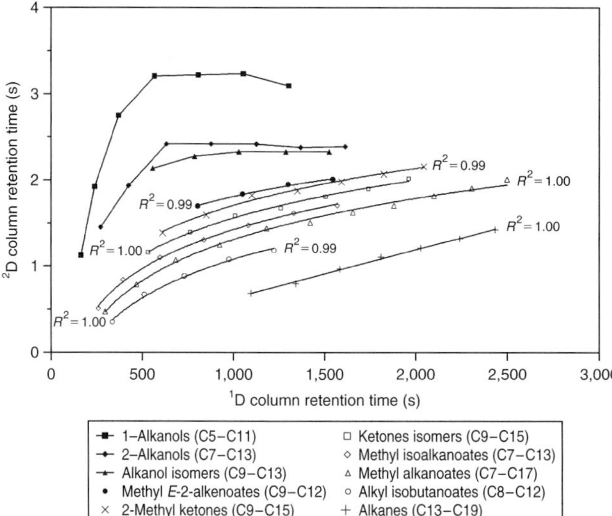

Figure 22.5 Homologous series of compounds identified in a GC × GC separation of Target hop essential oil. The apex of each peak is plotted with ^{2}D retention time (*y*-axis) plotted against ^{1}D retention time (*x*-axis). The trendline for the alkane series was fitted using a linear function. Ester and ketone series were fitted with a logarithmic function. Trendlines could not be fitted to the alcohol series. The numbers in parentheses in the key refer to the range of total number of carbons in each series.

myrcene (**3**) and sesquiterpenes α-humulene (**1**), β-caryophyllene (**2**) and β-farnesene (**4**). Other monoterpenes include α- and β-pinene, sabinene, δ-3-carene, camphene, *p*-cymene, (*Z*)- and (*E*)-β-ocimene, α- and γ-terpinene, α-terpinolene and limonene (**9**). There is a bewildering array of over 40 acyclic, monocyclic, bicyclic and tricyclic sesquiterpene hydrocarbons including (*Z*)- and (*E*)-α-bergomotene, cadinenes (e.g. **5**, **6**), muurolenes (e.g. **7**), selinenes (e.g. **8**), ylangenes, copaenes, germacrenes, selinadienes and many others (Moir, 2000). Sesquiterpenoids are notoriously difficult to resolve and identify because they have the same molecular formulae and therefore interact with column stationary phases in the same manner and exhibit very similar mass spectra.

Autoxidation and subsequent hydrolysis and rearrangement of sesquiterpene hydrocarbons lead to a large number of reaction products that increase during storage of hops (Deinzer and Yang, 1994). These include the epoxides, with the most abundant being humulene epoxide II (**19**) and caryophyllene oxide (**28**). Humulene epoxides I (**18**) and III (**20**) are typically present at lower levels. However, humulene epoxide I is more resistant to hydrolysis than humulene epoxide II and III, and therefore persists during storage and is found at greater concentrations in beer (Deinzer and Yang, 1994). Further oxidation results in the formation of five humulene diepoxide isomers (A–E) (**21–24**), although humulene diepoxide A (**21**) predominates in hop oil and beer (Deinzer and Yang, 1994). Sesquiterpene epoxides and diepoxides undergo further hydrolysis and rearrangements to form various ketones and alcohols (see below).

Monoterpene alcohols are generally biosynthetic products related to the biosynthesis of myrcene. These include geraniol (**14**) and linalool (**15**), which are particularly important as floral odorants in hop essential oil. Other monoterpene alcohols present are nerol (**13**), α-terpineol, borneol, fenchol, myrtenol and limonene-10-ol (**10**). Sesquiterpene alcohols are typically oxidation degradation products and among many others include humulenol II (**25**), humulol (**26**), caryophyllene alcohol (syn. caryolan-1-ol) (**29**), caryophyllenol, nerolidol, farnesol isomers, cadinol isomers and eudesmol isomers. Biosynthetic alcohols tend to decrease during storage, whereas oxidation-derived alcohols tend to increase (Moir, 1994).

The monoterpene aldehydes neral (**11**) and geranial (**12**) have been identified in freshly distilled hop essential oil but these compounds will be rapidly reduced to their corresponding alcohols during storage or fermentation (Sanchez *et al.*, 1992a). The terpenoid ketones β-ionone (**32**) and β-damascenone (**33**) are found at trace levels in hop essential oil resulting from the degradation of β-carotene (Sell, 2003). The ketones humulenone and humuladienone (**27**) result from the oxidation reactions of humulene.

A number of esters of the terpene alcohols are also present including methyl geranate, methyl nerolate, geranyl propanoate, neryl propanoate, geranyl isobutanoate (**17**), neryl isobutanoate, geranyl acetate (**16**), neryl acetate and linalyl acetate.

Oxygen heterocyclic compounds in hop essential oil include (*Z*)- and (*E*)-linalool oxide (**30, 31**), rose oxide and cyclic ethers such as hop ether and karahana ether (Moir, 1994).

Non-terpenoid compounds

The composition of hop essential oil includes many homologous series of aliphatic compounds (Figure 22.5). Aliphatic hydrocarbons are present at low levels and are represented by a series of linear alkanes, a number of branched alkanes and several trace alkenes. Hop essential oil contains a number of isomeric series of straight chain and branched ketones. The foremost series is the methyl ketones with the most abundant compound being 2-undecanone (syn. methyl nonyl ketone). Levels of aldehydes are generally low in hop essential oil and are mainly lost during kiln drying. Aldehydes identified include linear alkanals (e.g. nonanal), *E*-2-hexenal, *Z*-3-hexenal, *E*-2-nonenal, benzaldehyde and phenylacetaldehyde (Nijssen *et al.*, 1996).

Hop essential oil is rich in a large variety of aliphatic esters. Many exist as homologous series including: linear methyl alkanoates (e.g. methyl decanoate); branched methyl alkanoates such as methyl 2-methyl-alkanoates and the methyl isoalkanoates (e.g. methyl 6-methyl-heptanoate); unsaturated methyl alkenoates (e.g. methyl *E*-2-decenoate); alkyl propanoates (e.g. pentyl propanoate); alkyl isobutanoates (e.g. hexyl 2-methyl-propanoate) and unsaturated alkenyl acetates with unconfirmed stereochemistry (e.g. octenyl acetate). Important esters that do not exist in homologous series include methyl *Z*-4-decenoate, 2-methylpropyl 2-methyl-propanoate (syn. 2-methylpropyl isobutanoate), 2-methylbutyl 2-methyl-propanoate (syn. 2-methylbutyl isobutanoate), 3-methylbutyl 3-methylbutanoate (syn. isoamyl isovalerate) and 2-methylbutyl 3-methyl-butanoate (syn. 2-methylbutyl isovalerate). The homologous series of straight chain methyl esters most likely originate from fatty acid biosynthesis, whereas the branched chain esters (e.g. 2-methylbutyl isobutanoate) are derived from amino acid biosynthesis (Briggs *et al.*, 2004).

Alcohols are represented by straight chain alcohols, such as 1- and 2-alkanols, and branched chain alcohols, such as 2-methyl-3-buten-2-ol, which is formed by cleavage of the isoprenyl side chains of the α- and β-acids (Briggs *et al.*, 2004). Acids are also present in hop essential oil and are usually associated with aged hops as degradation products of the α- and β-acids. Cleavage of the acyl side chains yields 3-methylbutanoic acid (syn. isovaleric acid) from humulone and lupulone, 2-methylbutanoic acid from adhumulone and adlupulone, and 2-methylpropanoic acid (syn. isobutyric acid) from cohumulone and colupulone. These acids are responsible for the cheesy aroma of aged hops (Benitez *et al.*, 1997; Briggs *et al.*, 2004). Photo-oxidation of the ring structure of the α- and β-acids also produces 4-methyl-3-pentenoic acid. Other acids include decanoic acid and *Z*-4-decenoic acid. The degree of acids found in essential oil also varies depending on the sample preparation and extraction or distillation method used to isolate the oil.

Sulfur compounds

Lermusieau and Collin (2003) recently reviewed the occurrence and origins of sulfur compounds in hops and beer. Sulfur compounds are present at trace levels but can have very low odor thresholds and so impact upon the odor of essential oil and beer (Lermusieau *et al.*, 2001). Methyl thioesters have been commonly identified in hop essential oil and Lermusieau and Collin (2003) assert that these are not artifacts of steam distillation because they are also present in cold solvent extracts. The authors suggested a possible biosynthetic pathway from methionine degradation. The concentration of thioesters depends on variety and local growing conditions, and increase considerably upon kiln drying, independent of sulfur dioxide (SO_2) application.

Other sulfur containing compounds include thiophenes, sulfur adducts of myrcene and humulene, and episulfides of sesquiterpenes. These compounds result from reactions with elemental sulfur either applied in the field to control powdery mildew (Briggs *et al.*, 2004) or from burning sulfur during kilning (Benitez *et al.*, 1997). In the presence of light or heat, sesquiterpenes react with the residual elemental sulfur to generate episulfides. These compounds have the same structure as the corresponding epoxides except oxygen is substituted by sulfur. A number of sulfur adducts of myrcene and humulene also form due to reaction with elemental sulfur. These compounds are also formed during steam distillation as a result of the high temperature applied, and can be thought of as artifacts of sample preparation. In contrast, vacuum distillation and CO_2 extracts have much lower levels of sulfur compounds (Briggs *et al.*, 2004). However, these compounds could also form in the kettle during boiling and be introduced into the beer, particularly upon late hopping where limited evaporation occurs (Lermusieau and Collin, 2003).

Dimethyl sulfide (DMS) is also generated during steam distillation and wort boiling by thermal degradation of *S*-methylcysteine sulfoxide. The levels of DMS and polysulfides (e.g. dimethyl trisulfide, DMTS) also increase with levels of elemental sulfur and when kilning is performed without SO_2. These sulfide compounds have characteristic cooked vegetable, onion, rubbery and sulfury odors that may impact on beer aroma. The compound responsible for the skunky aroma of lightstruck beer, 3-methyl-2-butene-1-thiol (**34**), has also been found in hop pellets being derived from the isoprenyl side chains of α- and β-acids (Lermusieau *et al.*, 2001).

Odor Characteristics of Hop Essential Oil

Although there maybe several hundred compounds present in hop essential oil, only a certain number will be present at a concentration above their detection threshold and contribute to the odor of the oil (Guadagni *et al.*, 1966; Buttery, 1999). Compounds that are responsible for, or significantly contribute to, a sample's distinctive odor profile are known as *character-impact odorants*.

Instrumental analysis of character-impact odorants

The characterization of essential oils is usually based on chemical composition determined by GC–MS or GC–FID. However, odor detection thresholds of volatile compounds can differ by many orders of magnitude (e.g. parts per trillion up to odorless compounds) (Buttery, 1999). The relationship between concentration and odor intensity may also vary considerably between compounds. Therefore, the response of a chemical detector is not representative of odor activity. For example, the most abundant compound in a chromatogram may not be the most important odorant (Eyres *et al.*, 2005). Consequently, the impact of

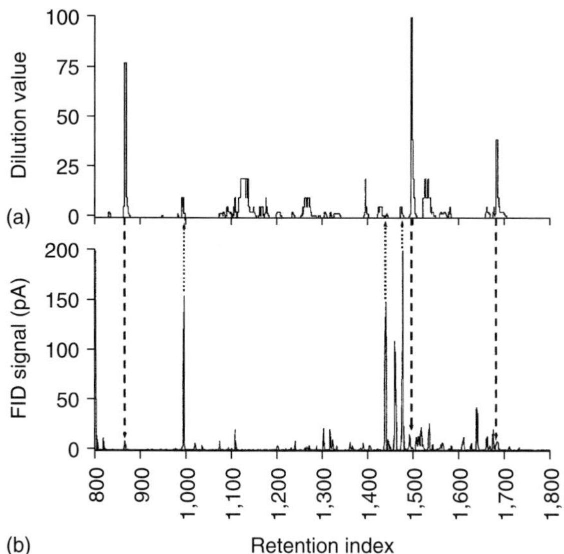

Figure 22.6 Comparison of (a) the GC–O "aromagram" with (b) the FID chromatogram for Saaz hop essential oil. Retention index (*x*-axis) is plotted against (a) dilution value for GC–O and (b) FID signal. Peak areas in the GC–O aromagram are proportional to odor potency.

a compound on the odor of a sample must be evaluated using human assessors. A valuable tool for identifying character-impact odorants is gas chromatography–olfactometry (GC–O), where human "sniffers" are used to detect and evaluate the odor of compounds as they elute from a GC separation (Delahunty *et al.*, 2006). Figure 22.6 demonstrates that the odor profile generated by GC–O is rather different than the FID chromatogram for a hop essential oil sample. Several odor peaks correspond to major FID peaks but conversely, other important odorants do not correspond to any noteworthy FID peaks, only being present at trace concentrations. The advantage of GC–O is that it specifically measures odor activity and can therefore be used to locate character-impact odorants. Once odorants have been identified and their odor activity confirmed, their concentrations can be routinely measured using a conventional detector.

There are a number of issues that should be taken into account when interpreting GC–O data. Various GC–O methodologies use different properties to rate odorant importance, including odor potency by dilution analysis (concentration/threshold; synonymous to odor activity values or odor units), detection frequency of a panel and direct odor intensity (Delahunty *et al.*, 2006). Two methods may produce different results because the relationship between concentration and odor intensity differs considerably between compounds (Petersen *et al.*, 2003). The objective of GC–O is to assess the odor activity of compounds individually without co-elution. This allows identification of the odorants that are potentially important but does not take into account possible interactions that occur in the mixture such as synergistic, antagonistic (suppression) or additive effects (Delahunty *et al.*, 2006). For these reasons, assessment of hops using sensory evaluation is indispensable.

Sensory evaluation of odor characteristics

There have been relatively few sensory evaluations of raw hop cones or essential oils. Sanchez *et al.* (1992b) used a descriptive sensory panel and GC–O to evaluate oxygenated fractions of three hop varieties. Stucky and McDaniel (1997) used free-choice profiling to discriminate 15 varieties, and correlated the sensory results with the concentration of 21 compounds. Myrcene and linalool demonstrated a strong association with the combined sensory characters of fruity, floral, pine and sage in principal components analysis (PCA).

Odorants identified in hop essential oil

The odor characteristics of compounds that are potential odorants in hop essential oil and beer are summarized in Table 22.2. At harvest, the most potent odorant in green hops is *Z*-3-hexenal (green, cut grass), but this is mostly lost during kiln drying (Steinhaus and Schieberle, 2000). This odorant is common in plants and herbs as a secondary metabolite of linoleic acid. Myrcene is typically the most abundant compound in fresh hop essential oil. Its odor threshold in water has been determined to range between 13 and 36 ppb (Guadagni *et al.*, 1966; Ahmed *et al.*, 1978; Masanetz and Grosch, 1998), and so is expected to exert a large impact on the odor profile of the essential oil. This has been supported in studies using GC–O (Steinhaus and Schieberle, 2000). It has odor descriptors of resinous, herbaceous, balsamic and geranium-like (Masanetz and Grosch, 1998; Steinhaus and Schieberle, 2000).

Odorants that contribute to floral characteristics of hop essential oil include linalool (floral – citrusy), geraniol (floral – rose, geranium) and β-ionone (floral – violet). The importance of linalool in hop essential oil has been confirmed by various authors using GC–O (Sanchez *et al.*, 1992b; Steinhaus and Schieberle, 2000; Lermusieau *et al.*, 2001). Geraniol has been determined to be a potent odorant in hop essential oil (Peacock and Deinzer, 1981; Lam *et al.*, 1986; Eyres *et al.*, 2006) but was not deemed important by Sanchez *et al.* (1992b) because only one of four assessors detected it during GC–O. It was also not detected by Steinhaus and Schieberle (2000). These results could be influenced by varietal differences (Peacock *et al.*, 1981) or the age of the hops, as geraniol concentration increases during storage. The monoterpene aldehydes geranial and neral have also been implicated for the floral odor of essential oil (Nickerson and Van Engel, 1992). Sanchez *et al.* (1992b) reported that neral contributed a citrus-spicy odor during GC–O analysis. However, these compounds

Table 22.2 Odor characteristics of hop-derived compounds that potentially contribute to the odor of the essential oil and beer

Compound[a]	*Odor descriptors*	*References*[b]
α-Humulene (**1**)	Balsamic	1
β-Caryophyllene (**2**)	Cloves, turpentine	2
Myrcene (**3**)	Resinous, herbaceous, balsamic, geranium-like	1, 2
Z-3-hexenal	Green, cut grass, leafy	1, 2
Neral (**11**)	Citrus, spicy, lemon	2, 3
Geranial (**12**)	Citrus, lemon	2
Nerol (**13**)	Floral – rose	2
Geraniol (**14**)	Floral – rose, geranium	2, 4
Linalool (**15**)	Floral – citrus, coriander seed	2, 4
Geranyl acetate (**16**)	Floral – lavender, perfumed pine	2, 5
Geranyl isobutanoate (**17**)	Floral – rose	2
Humulene epoxide I (**18**)	Hay-like	6
Humulene epoxide II (**19**)	Moldy, cedar	6, 7
Humulene epoxide III (**20**)	Cedar	7
Humulene epoxides I, II, III	Musty, floral, spicy	3
Humulene diepoxide A, B (**21**, **22**)	No odor	3
Humulenol II (**25**)	Sage-brush, pineapple	6, 7
Humulol (**26**)	Hay-like	6
Humuladienone[c] (**27**)	Flowery, fresh	5
Caryophyllene oxide (**28**)	Musty, floral, spicy, cedar	3, 7
β-Ionone (**32**)	Floral – violet	2, 4
β-Damascenone (**33**)	Cooked apple, tobacco, prunes	3, 4
3-Methyl-2-butene-1-thiol (**34**)	Sulfurous, skunky, mercaptan	2
Dimethyl disulfide	Cheesy, glue	5
Dimethyl trisulfide	Onion, soup	2, 5
trans-4,5-epoxy-(*E*)-2-decenal (**35**)	Metallic	1
γ-Nonalactone[c] (**36**)	Coconut, fruity, sweet	2, 5
Ethyl cinnamate[c] (**37**)	Cinnamon-like, honey-like strawberry, sweet	2, 5
Citronellol[c] (**38**)	Floral – rose, fruity, apple, citrus	2, 8
Isovaleric acid	Rancid, sweaty, cheesy	2, 4
Ethyl 2-methylpropanoate	Sweet, fruity	1, 2
Methyl 2-methylbutanoate	Sweet, fruity, apple-like	1, 2
Propyl 2-methylbutanoate	Sweet, fruity	1
1,3(*E*),5(*Z*)-undecatriene	Fresh, balsamic	1
1,3(*E*),5(*Z*),9-undecatetrene	Fresh, balsamic	1
(*Z*)-1,5-octadien-3-one	Geranium-like	1
Nonanal	Citrus, soapy, fatty	1, 2

[a] Numbers in parentheses refer to the chemical structure depicted in Figure 22.1.
[b] References: 1: Steinhaus and Schieberle (2000); 2: Burdock (2002); 3: Sanchez *et al*. (1992b); 4: Eyres *et al*. (2006); 5: Lermusieau *et al*. (2001); 6: Fukuoka and Kowaka (1983); 7: Deinzer and Yang (1994); 8: Sanchez *et al*. (1992a).
[c] Hop-derived compounds in beer not found in hop essential oil.

will be rapidly reduced to their corresponding alcohols during storage (Briggs *et al.*, 2004).

β-ionone and β-damascenone (cooked apple) have previously been suggested to be important odorants due to their low odor thresholds (Tressl *et al.*, 1978), which range between 0.008–0.17 ppb and 0.002–0.009 ppb in water, respectively (Plotto *et al.*, 2006). Their importance as odorants has also been supported by various GC–O investigations for β-ionone (Eyres *et al.*, 2006) and β-damascenone (Sanchez *et al.*, 1992b; Lermusieau *et al.*, 2001; Murakami *et al.*, 2003), respectively. However, it is estimated that approximately 1/3 of the population have a specific anosmia for β-ionone and therefore cannot detect it (Brenna *et al.*, 2002; Plotto *et al.*, 2006). Recent research indicates that β-damascenone may also be partially affected by anosmia (Plotto *et al.*, 2006) and that it has low odor intensity even at high concentrations above threshold (Petersen *et al.*, 2003). Therefore, the overall impact of these two compounds is still unconfirmed.

Steinhaus and Schieberle (2000) found *trans*-4,5-epoxy-(*E*)-2-decenal (**35**), a fatty acid oxidation product with a metallic odor, to be the most potent odorant in an extract of dried hop cones using GC–O. However, it was not present in a headspace sample and has not been reported in hops since, so its importance is still unverified. The same study also identified 1,3(*E*),5(*Z*)-undecatriene and 1,3(*E*),5(*Z*),9-undecatetrene as important odorants in both the extract and headspace samples contributing a fresh, balsamic odor. Other potent odorants identified were ethyl 2-methylpropanoate (sweet, fruity), methyl 2-methylbutanoate (sweet, fruity), propyl 2-methylbutanoate (sweet, fruity), (*Z*)-1,5-octadien-3-one (geranium-like), nonanal (citrus, soapy), and 2- and 3-methylbutanoic (isovaleric) acid (cheesy).

A panel of four assessors used the terms musty, floral and spicy to describe the odors perceived during GC–O for humulene epoxide I, II and III and caryophyllene oxide in oxygenated fractions of hop oil (Sanchez *et al.*, 1992b). This was confirmed using a synthesized mixture of the three humulene epoxides. In contrast, no odors were detected for humulene diepoxide A or B, even for a synthesized sample at high concentration. Steinhaus and Schieberle (2000) did not detect any humulene oxidation products by GC–O, but the oil may have been too fresh for oxidation to have occurred. Deinzer and Yang (1994) reported that almost all humulene and caryophyllene oxidation products exhibited cedar-like aromas during sensory evaluations. Fukuoka and Kowaka (1983) evaluated the aroma of several synthesized oxidation products. Humulene epoxide I and humulol had a hay-like odor, humulene epoxide II had a moldy odor and humulenol II had a sage-brush odor. The authors concluded that these compounds were not responsible for the odor of a concentrated high performance liquid chromatography (HPLC) fraction exhibiting a strong herbal, spicy character. The two herbal odorants actually responsible were not identified, but were reported to have an oxygenated sesquiterpenoid structure ($C_{15}H_{24}O$ and $C_{15}H_{26}O$). One of these compounds was also found in a sample of commercial Japanese beer.

Guadagni *et al.* (1966) and Tressl *et al.* (1978) suggested that hop ether, karahana ether, methyl-4-decenoate and methyl thiohexanoate were important odorants based on their odor activity values (concentration/threshold). The detection threshold and the odor impact of the two ethers in beer were re-evaluated by Lam and Deinzer (1986) who determined that neither compound was a major contributor to hop aroma.

Hop Aroma in Beer

Because all of the compounds responsible for hop aroma in beer have not been completely identified, sensory evaluation is still the method of choice for product development and quality control of beer. It is well established that the hoppy aroma in beer is due to the perception of complex mixtures of volatiles rather than single compounds. Hop aroma in beer is usually complex, and accurately describing the specific characteristics can be challenging. In addition, it is often difficult to differentiate hop-derived aroma from aroma compounds produced during fermentation. Hops can impact on beer aroma in terms of floral, spicy, herbal, woody and fruity (particularly citrus and tropical fruit) characters. However, the official beer flavor wheel does not adequately reflect this complexity of hop aroma, only using "hoppy" as a specific first-tier term (Meilgaard *et al.*, 1979). This is subdivided into three second-tier terms which are "kettle hop," "dry hop" and "hop oil." Use of the term "noble hop aroma" is common in the literature and is usually associated with traditional aroma hop varieties from Europe such as Hallertauer mittelfrüh, Hallertauer Hersbrucker, Saaz, Spalter and Tettnanger (Sanchez *et al.*, 1992b; Deinzer and Yang, 1994). However, the actual aroma description of this character is poorly defined, but is often described as herbal or spicy (Sanchez *et al.*, 1992b).

Physical, chemical and biochemical changes that occur during wort production and fermentation complicate the analysis of hop-derived compounds in beer. Thereby, not all compounds present in hop essential oil are found in kettle-hopped beer, and conversely not all hop-derived compounds in beer are found in hop essential oil itself. Hydrocarbons are not typically detected in beer except when dry hopping is used. Conversely, oxygenated compounds are much more likely to dissolve into wort and survive the boiling and fermentation processes.

Correlating sensory characteristics of hopped beer with instrumental composition may elucidate associations to aid understanding of hop aroma in beer. For example, Peppard *et al.* (1989) used multivariate statistics to correlate sensory characteristics for beer brewed with 8 different hop varieties with the concentration of 36 hop-derived compounds. Linalool oxide, and to a lesser extent caryophyllene alcohol and humulol, were correlated with "European hop aroma." A large number of compounds were associated with the spicy character including spiroacetal, dihydrospiroacetal, humulene epoxide I, humulenol II and humulene diepoxides. However, a good correlation does not prove a cause and effect relationship, so the impact of the compounds reported must still be directly confirmed (Peppard *et al.*, 1989).

Peacock *et al.* (1981) concluded that geraniol and linalool were responsible for most of the floral aroma in a beer brewed with Cascade hops. Geranyl isobutanoate was present below threshold, but could be hydrolyzed by yeast to yield free geraniol and contribute to the aroma. Linalool in particular has been implicated as being important in overall hoppy aroma and the noble hop aroma in beer (Steinhaus and Schieberle, 2000; Steinhaus *et al.*, 2003; Fritsch *et al.*, 2005). These compounds would be expected to produce a floral hop aroma in beer when added post-fermentation but are also expected to survive fermentation (Irwin, 1989).

There is also a difference in sensory threshold and odor character between linalool enantiomers. In hop essential oil, 92–95% of linalool is present as the more active (*R*)-enantiomer, which has an odor threshold approximately 80 times lower than (*S*)-linalool (Kaltner *et al.*, 2003; Steinhaus *et al.*, 2003). It has been shown that interconversion between the enantiomers occurs during wort boiling so that (*S*)-linalool may actually constitute 30% in beer, potentially decreasing the overall odor impact of linalool

(Fritsch and Schieberle, 2003). The extent of this conversion appears to be dependent on the wort pH (Marriott *et al.*, 2006).

Lermusieau *et al.* (2001) assessed amberlite resin (XAD-2) extracts of beer using GC–O. The authors compared the odorants present in unhopped beer with those in two beers late-hopped with Saaz and Challenger, respectively. Potent hop odorants were linalool, β-damascenone, dimethyl disulfide (cheesy, glue), DMTS (onion, soup) and an unidentified spicy, hoppy odorant eluting with a retention index of 810 on an apolar stationary phase. Hop-derived odorants that were detected in hopped beer but not in steam distilled hop essential oil were γ-nonalactone (fruity, sweet) (**36**), humuladienone (flowery, fresh), geranyl acetate (perfumed pine) and ethyl cinnamate (strawberry, sweet) (**37**). Sanchez *et al.* (1992a, 1992b) reported 9-methyl-2-decanone (musty, vinyl, rancid) as a possible odorant in hop oil and beer extracts.

Citronellol (floral – citrus, fruity, apple) (**38**) has also been identified as a hop-derived compound in beer by GC–MS and GC–O and is implicated in contributing to hop aroma (Lam *et al.*, 1986; Sanchez *et al.*, 1992a). It has been shown that citronellol can be transformed from geraniol by yeast during fermentation (King and Dickinson, 2000, 2003). It has also been suggested that it is formed by reduction of geranial and neral by yeast (Lam *et al.*, 1986; Sanchez *et al.*, 1992a).

β-damascenone has been identified as a potent odorant in beer by various authors (Schieberle, 1991; Sanchez *et al.*, 1992a; Lermusieau *et al.*, 2001; Chevance *et al.*, 2002; Fritsch *et al.*, 2005). Its concentration has been shown to increase during wort boiling (Kishimoto *et al.*, 2005), decrease during fermentation due to reduction or adsorption by yeast, and then increase again upon storage (Chevance *et al.*, 2002). β-damascenone is likely to contribute to the odor of beer because of its low threshold. However, its sensory impact on overall beer flavor still needs to be confirmed using sensory evaluation to assess its odor intensity and interaction with other aroma compounds. It should also be noted that β-damascenone only partially originates from hops, also being present in unhopped wort and beer (Lermusieau *et al.*, 2001; Chevance *et al.*, 2002; Fritsch and Schieberle, 2003).

Oxidation and hydrolysis products of sesquiterpenes have been associated with the noble and spicy hop characters in beer (Peacock and Deinzer, 1981; Lam *et al.*, 1986; Deinzer and Yang, 1994; Goiris *et al.*, 2002). Good correlations between increasing concentrations of humulene epoxides and these hop characters have been demonstrated (Kowaka *et al.*, 1983; Peppard *et al.*, 1989). As a result, so-called noble hop varieties are often purposefully stored prior to brewing to increase the levels of oxygenated compounds (Deinzer and Yang, 1994; Briggs *et al.*, 2004). However, a good correlation does not prove a cause and effect relationship (Peppard *et al.*, 1989), and the importance of these oxidation compounds for imparting hoppy aroma remains controversial (Fukuoka and Kowaka, 1983; Irwin, 1989; Goiris *et al.*, 2002). The compounds so far identified have exhibited concentrations below their detection thresholds and their aroma characteristics do not correspond to the desired spicy or noble hop aroma (Deinzer and Yang, 1994).

Yang *et al.* (1993) found that a hydrolysis reaction mixture from humulene epoxide I and II contributed a cedar, lime, spicy character to beer, but with a relatively high sensory threshold of 2.3 ppm. This concentration was exceeded in pilot beers, but not in any commercial brands tested. In the study by Sanchez *et al.* (1992a), only one out of four assessors detected the odors associated with humulene oxidation products in beer extracts using GC–O, despite being detected in hop oil and identified in the beer extracts by GC–MS. It was concluded that the compounds were not present at high enough concentration. This may indicate that humulene epoxides may contribute to hop aroma but are not essential to it (Deinzer and Yang, 1994).

Goiris *et al.* (2002) found that adding 20 ppb of an oxygenated sesquiterpene fraction isolated by supercritical CO_2 extraction and solid-phase extraction (SPE) to a bland pilot beer produced a desirable spicy or herbal aroma reminiscent of noble hop aroma. The authors concluded that this was due to unidentified compounds present in this fraction, associated with humulene oxidation products.

There is growing evidence for the release of glycosidically bound hop aroma compounds during wort boiling, fermentation or ageing (Goldstein *et al.*, 1999; Chevance *et al.*, 2002; Fritsch *et al.*, 2005; Kishimoto *et al.*, 2005). Examples that are implicated in hop aroma are geraniol, linalool and β-damascenone. These glycosidically bound compounds are not isolated with the essential oil but may affect hop aroma in kettle-hopped beer as they are released by acid catalyzed hydrolysis during boiling (Chevance *et al.*, 2002).

Methods of Extraction

One should distinguish between methods used to isolate hop essential oils for analysis or for the manufacture of commercial products. The simplest method for isolation of essential oil is either steam distillation or hydro-distillation. A method solely used for analytical sample preparation are many adaptations of the Likens–Nickerson simultaneous steam distillation-solvent extraction (SDE) (Likens and Nickerson, 1964). Distillation methods involve the application of heat and therefore there is the possibility to produce artifacts by thermal degradation. Composition will differ depending on whether the distillation is performed at atmospheric or reduced pressure due to the temperature that is applied (Briggs *et al.*, 2004). Steam distillation at atmospheric pressure is known to cause a number of degradative changes so that the odor of the resultant oil is not representative of the original sample (Moyler, 1993; Gardner, 1994). As a result, early attempts at using these oils for dry hopping were unsuccessful (Gardner, 1994).

Solvent extraction is another method of obtaining hop volatiles, although according to Lawrence (2002) these extracts cannot strictly be called essential oils and are more accurately described as "volatile concentrates." However, for all intents and purposes the final result is very similar – an isolated volatile oil. Various solvents have been used commercially including hexane, ethanol, methanol, trichloroethylene and methylene chloride (Gardner, 1993). However, only hexane and ethanol are still in use and even these are in decline (Briggs *et al.*, 2004). These solvent extracts are known to decrease the yield and alter the composition and odor characteristics of hop essential oil due to the loss of volatile compounds during evaporation of the solvent (Gardner, 1993; Benitez *et al.*, 1997). The most volatile compounds, which are responsible for top notes in the odor profile, are most severely affected. There are also safety and regulation concerns regarding solvent residues remaining in the extracts.

Currently the method of choice to extract hop essential oil is extraction using liquid or supercritical CO_2. Liquid CO_2 extraction is typically carried out at 5–15°C and 60–65 bar whereas supercritical CO_2 requires greater temperature (40–60°C) and pressure (200–250 bar) (Benitez *et al.*, 1997). Composition of the two extracts is likely to be extremely similar, except that supercritical CO_2 extracts contain more hard resins, polar bitter substances and pigments (e.g. chlorophyll), the latter giving a dark green color to supercritical extracts (Gardner, 1993; Benitez *et al.*, 1997). The extraction efficiency and flexibility of supercritical CO_2 are greater, because the solvent properties can be altered by varying the temperature and pressure. In comparison, the properties of liquid CO_2 can only be altered by small changes in temperature (Gardner, 1993; Benitez *et al.*, 1997). The impact on trace odor compounds has not been thoroughly investigated, with liquid CO_2 extraction theoretically giving a milder extraction and a more representative extract (Moyler, 1993). In practice, liquid CO_2 is used when the extract is further processed for essential oil and aroma products due to its greater selectivity and lower temperature (Gardner, 1993).

Oil enriched extracts (~26 ml oil per 100 g extract) may be produced using either partial extraction with liquid CO_2 or by two-step fractionation using supercritical CO_2, where the resins are initially precipitated by reducing the pressure to 100–120 bar before recovering the essential oil in an evaporator (Benitez *et al.*, 1997). However, it is more practical to make a total extract comprising both hop resins and essential oils and isolate the essential oil using molecular distillation under high vacuum (1.33×10^{-6} bar) (Gardner, 1994; Benitez *et al.*, 1997; Briggs *et al.*, 2004). For essential oils, the great advantage of CO_2 extraction is that the aroma compounds are obtained quantitatively without the creation of artifacts. Therefore, the odor profile is much more representative of the original sample than steam distillation or other solvent extraction methods (Moyler, 1993; Gardner, 1994). Separating the essential oil from the resins allows hop aroma and bitterness to be controlled independently in the brewing process (Gardner, 1993).

Essential Oil Fractionation

Hop essential oils are often fractionated by physical and chemical properties in an attempt to improve the resolution of compounds for the chemical analysis of hop essential oils. Historically, hop essential oils were separated into a hydrocarbon fraction and an oxygenated fraction by elution from a silica gel column with light petroleum and ether, respectively. More recently, pre-analytical fractionation has been achieved by HPLC (Fukuoka and Kowaka, 1983; Deinzer and Yang, 1994) and SPE (Irwin, 1989; Goiris *et al.*, 2002).

A great deal of research has been invested into developing commercially fractionated hop oil products with specific aroma qualities that may be added either pre- or post-fermentation (Haley and Peppard, 1983; Westwood and Daoud, 1985; Westwood, 1987; Gardner, 1994; Marriott, 2001; Goiris *et al.*, 2002). Isolated hop oil was originally dosed into wort and beer as aqueous emulsions or entrained in a liquid CO_2 stream (Westwood, 1987). However, post-fermentation products must be soluble in beer to prevent problems with haze. A soluble Dry Hop Essence was subsequently developed by removing the insoluble monoterpene and sesquiterpene hydrocarbons by liquid–liquid extraction (Westwood and Daoud, 1985; Marriott, 2001).

Further fractionation by functional groups using a combination of fractional distillation and column chromatography gave rise to four Late Hop Essences with specific aroma characteristics (Westwood and Daoud, 1985; Gardner, 1994; Marriott, 2001). These fractions became known as: the Spicy fraction, rich in monoterpene and sesquiterpene alcohols; the Floral fraction, containing ketones, epoxides and esters; the Ester fraction, predominantly made up of branched and straight chain fatty acid methyl esters; and the Citrusy fraction, composed of a mixture of terpene alcohols, short chain aliphatic alcohols and ketones (Marriott, 2001). Post-fermentation products are currently sold as Pure Hop Aroma and also now include Herbal (herbaceous, green, vetivert odor) and Sylvan (woody, earthy, resinous, pine odor) fractions (Marriott and Parker, 2004). They are supplied dissolved in food grade ethanol and are used at typical dose rates of 50–100 ppb (Marriott, 2001). The impact on hop aroma in beer will greatly depend on interactions with the aroma compounds present in the base beer and must therefore be evaluated in each case (Gardner, 1994; Marriott and Parker, 2004). Hop fractions obtained from different hop varieties also retain distinct aroma profiles due to differences in their chemical composition (Gardner,

1994; Marriott, 2001). Post-fermentation products allow great flexibility in new product development and allow the introduction of specific hop aroma without the changes that occur during wort boiling and fermentation (Marriott, 2001).

Concluding Remarks

Despite more than 50 years of research, the compounds responsible for important odorants in hop essential oil and hop aroma in beer are still not completely understood (Moir, 2000). More research is required to identify character-impact odorants in hop essential oil, determine their sensory impact on beer aroma and ascertain their fate during the brewing process. Identification of important odorants will allow hop breeders to select for varieties containing these compounds. In addition, knowledge of the important odorants for "hoppy" aroma in beer will allow for better quality control and development of new products. The authors contend that MDGC techniques in combination with GC–O are essential to improve our understanding of hop aroma in beer. The impact of identified character-impact odorants must then be confirmed using sensory evaluation.

Summary Points

- Hop essential oil is a complex mixture of volatile compounds from a wide range of compound classes.
- Differences in odor characteristics of hop varieties can be attributed to differences in the composition of the essential oil.
- The composition of the essential oil varies considerably with genetics, geographical location, growth conditions, infection from diseases and attack from pests. The composition alters during storage increasing the complexity due to oxidation, hydrolysis and rearrangements.
- Composition also depends on how the essential oil is isolated prior to analysis.
- Routine analysis of composition is performed by conventional GC but multidimensional techniques using two columns are often required to resolve and identify co-eluting compounds.
- The odor of hop essential oil and hop aroma in beer is due to a complex mixture of contributing volatile compounds.
- Not all character-impact odorants in hops have been identified and hoppy aroma in beer is still not completely understood.
- Hop aroma in beer is complex and complicated by physical, biochemical and chemical changes occurring during brewing and fermentation. This has led to increasing trends to add fractionated hop oils with specific odor characteristics to beer post-fermentation.

References

Acree, T.E. (1993). Bioassays for flavour. In Acree, T.E. and Teranishi, R. (eds.), *Flavor Science: Sensible Principles and Techniques*, pp. 1–22. American Chemical Society, Washington, DC.

Ahmed, E.M., Dennison, R.A., Dougherty, R.H. and Shaw, P.E. (1978). *J. Agric. Food Chem.* 26, 187–191.

American Society of Brewing Chemists (ASBC) (2006). *Methods of Analysis, Hops-13 Total Essential Oil in Hops and Hop Pellets by Steam Distillation.* American Society of Brewing Chemists, St. Paul, MN, USA.

Barber, A., Campbell, C.A.M., Crane, H., Lilley, R. and Tregidga, E. (2003). *Biocontrol Sci. Technol.* 13, 275–284.

Bartle, K.D. (2002). Introduction. In Mondello, L., Lewis, A.C. and Bartle, K.D. (eds), *Multidimensional Chromatography*, pp. 3–16. John Wiley and Sons, Chichester, England.

Beatson, R.A., Ansell, K.A. and Graham, L.T. (2003). *MBAA Tech. Q.* 40, 7–10.

Benitez, J.L., Forster, A., De Keukeleire, D., Moir, M., Sharpe, F.R., Verhagen, L.C. and Westwood, K.T. (1997). *EBC Manual of Good Practice: Hops and Hop Products.* Getränke-Fachverlag Hans Carl, Nürnberg, Germany.

Blank, I. (2002). Gas chromatography-olfactometry in food aroma analysis. In Marsili, R. (ed.), *Flavor, Fragrance and Odor Analysis*, pp. 297–331. Marcel Dekker, Inc, New York.

Blank, I., Milo, C., Lin, J. and Fay, L.B. (1999). Quantification of aroma-impact components by isotope dilution assay – recent developments. In Teranishi, R., Wick, E.L. and Hornstein, I. (eds), *Flavor Chemistry: 30 Years of Progress*, pp. 63–74. Kluwer Academic/Plenum Publishers, New York.

Brenna, E., Fuganti, C., Serra, S. and Kraft, P. (2002). *Eur. J. Org. Chem.* 6, 967–978.

Briggs, D.E., Boulton, C.A., Brookes, P.A. and Stevens, R. (2004). *Brewing Science and Practice.* Woodhead Publishing Limited, Cambridge, UK.

Burdock, G.A. (2002). *Fenaroli's Handbook of Flavor Ingredients*, 4th edn. CRC Press, Boca Raton, FL.

Buttery, R.G. (1999). Flavor chemistry and odor thresholds. In Teranishi, R., Wick, E.L. and Hornstein, I. (eds), *Flavor Chemistry: 30 Years of Progress*, pp. 353–365. Kluwer Academic/Plenum Publishers, New York.

Chevance, F., Guyot-Declerck, C., Dupont, J. and Collin, S. (2002). *J. Agric. Food Chem.* 50, 3818–3821.

Deinzer, M. and Yang, X. (1994). *EBC Monograph XXII: Symposium on Hops, Zoeterwoude, The Netherlands.* Verlag Hans Carl, Nürnberg, Germany, pp. 181–197.

Delahunty, C.M., Eyres, G. and Dufour, J.-P. (2006). *J. Sep. Sci.* 29, 2107–2125.

European Brewery Convention (2005). *Analytica-EBC, 7.10 Hop Oil Content of Hops and Hop Products.* Fachverlag Hans Carl, Nürnberg, Germany.

Eyres, G., Dufour, J.-P., Hallifax, G., Sotheeswaran, S. and Marriott, P.J. (2005). *J. Sep. Sci.* 28, 1061–1074.

Eyres, G., Dufour, J.-P. and Marriott, P.J. (2006). *Proceedings of the Institute of Brewing and Distilling Convention – Asia Pacific Section (CD-ROM).* Hobart, Australia. March 19–24.

Forster, A. (2001). *Proceedings of the 48th International Hop Growers Congress.* Canterbury, England. August 6–10.

Foster, R.T. and Nickerson, G.B. (1985). *J. Am. Soc. Brew. Chem.* 43, 127–135.

Fritsch, H. and Schieberle, P. (2003). *Proceedings of the 29th EBC Congress, Dublin (CD-ROM).* Fachverlag Hans Carl, Nürnberg, Germany.

Fritsch, H., Kaltner, D., Steiner, S.H., Schieberle, P. and Back, W. (2005). *Brauwelt Int.* 23, 22–23.

Fukuoka, Y. and Kowaka, M. (1983). *Rep. Res. Lab. Kirin Brew. Co.* 26, 31–36.

Gardner, D. (1993). Commercial scale extraction of alpha-acids and hop oils with compressed CO_2. In King, M. and Bott, T. (eds), *Extraction of Natural Products Using Near Critical Solvents*, pp. 84–100. Blackie, Glasgow, UK.

Gardner, D. (1994). *EBC Monograph XXII: Symposium on Hops, Zoeterwoude, The Netherlands.* Verlag Hans Carl, Nürnberg, Germany, pp. 114–126.

Goiris, K., De Ridder, M., De Rouck, G., Boeykens, A., Van Opstaele, F., Aerts, G., De Cooman, L. and De Keukeleire, D. (2002). *J. Inst. Brew.* 108, 86–93.

Goldstein, H., Ting, P., Navarro, A. and Ryder, D. (1999). *European Brewery Convention. Proceedings of the – 27th Congress Cannes, France.* IRL Press Ltd., Oxford, England, pp. 53–62

Guadagni, D.G., Buttery, R.G. and Harris, J. (1966). *J. Sci. Food Agric.* 17, 142–144.

Haley, J. and Peppard, T.L. (1983). *J. Inst. Brew.* 89, 87–91.

Hysert, D., Probasco, G., Forster, A. and Schmidt, R. (1998). *The 64th Annual Meeting of the American Society of Brewing Chemists.* Boston, MA, June 20–24.

Irwin, A.J. (1989). *J. Inst. Brew.* 95, 185–194.

Kaltner, D., Steinhaus, M., Mitter, W., Biendl, M. and Schieberle, P. (2003). *Monatsschr. Brauwiss.* 56, 192–196.

Kenny, S., Barber, L., Hill, P., Pruneda, T., Smith, R., Tinginys, A. and Murphey, J. (2000). *J. Am. Soc. Brew. Chem.* 58, 180–183.

King, A.J. and Dickinson, J.R. (2000). *Yeast* 16, 499–506.

King, A.J. and Dickinson, J.R. (2003). *FEMS Yeast Res.* 3, 53–62.

Kishimoto, T., Wanikawa, A., Kagami, N. and Kawatsura, K. (2005). *J. Agric. Food Chem.* 53, 4701–4707.

Kowaka, K., Fukuoka, Y., Kawasaki, H. and Asano, K. (1983). *European Brewery Convention. Proceedings of the 19th Congress, London.* IRL Press Ltd, Oxford, England. pp. 71–78

Kralj, D., Zupanec, J., Vasilj, D., Kralj, S. and Psenicnik, J. (1991). *J. Inst. Brew.* 97, 197–206.

Lam, K.C. and Deinzer, M.L. (1986). *J. Am. Soc. Brew. Chem.* 44, 69–72.

Lam, K.C., Foster, R.T. and Deinzer, M.L. (1986). *J. Agric. Food Chem.* 34, 763–770.

Lawless, H.T. and Heymann, H. (1998). *Sensory Evaluation of Food: Principles and Practices.* Chapman and Hall, New York.

Lawrence, B.M. (2002). Commercial essential oils: truths and consequences. In Swift, K.A.D. (ed.), *Advances in Flavours and Fragrances. From the Sensation to the Synthesis* Special Publication 277, pp. 57–83. Royal Society of Chemistry, Cambridge, UK.

Lermusieau, G. and Collin, S. (2003). *J. Am. Soc. Brew. Chem.* 61, 109–113.

Lermusieau, G., Bulens, M. and Collin, S. (2001). *J. Agric. Food Chem.* 49, 3867–3874.

Likens, S.T. and Nickerson, G.B. (1964). *Proc. Am. Soc. Brew. Chem.*, 22, 5–13.

Marriott, P.J. (2002). Orthogonal GC–GC. In Mondello, L., Lewis, A.C. and Bartle, K.D. (eds), *Multidimensional Chromatography*, pp. 77–108. John Wiley and Sons Ltd, Chichester, England.

Marriott, R. (2001). *EBC Monograph 31: European Brewery Convention Symposium – Flavour and Flavour Stability, Nancy, France (CD-ROM).* Fachverlag Hans Carl, Nürnberg, Germany, pp. 1–6.

Marriott, R. and Parker, D. (2004). *Book of Abstracts – World Brewing Congress, San Diego, CA, USA, 24–28 July*, p. 60.

Marriott, R., Birkby, J. and Parker, D. (2006). *Proceedings of the Institute of Brewing and Distilling Convention – Asia Pacific Section (CD-Rom).* Hobart, Australia. March 19–24.

Masanetz, C. and Grosch, W. (1998). *Flav. Fragr. J.* 13, 115–124.

Meilgaard, M.C., Dalgliesh, C.E. and Clapperton, J.F. (1979). *J. Inst. Brew.* 85, 38–42.

Moir, M. (1994). *EBC Monograph XXII: Symposium on Hops, Zoeterwoude, The Netherlands.* Verlag Hans Carl, Nürnberg, Germany, pp. 165–180.

Moir, M. (2000). *J. Am. Soc. Brew. Chem.* 58, 131–146.

Moyler, D.A. (1993). *Flav. Fragr. J.* 8, 235–247.

Murakami, A.A., Goldstein, H., Navarro, A., Seabrooks, J.R. and Ryder, D.S. (2003). *J. Am. Soc. Brew. Chem.* 61, 23–32.

Nickerson, G.B. and Van Engel, E.L. (1992). *J. Am. Soc. Brew. Chem.* 50, 77–81.

Nijssen, L., Vissher, C., Maarse, H., Willemsens, L. and Boelens, M. (1996). *Volatile Compounds in Food: Qualitative and Quantitative Data*, 7th edn. TNO Nutrition and Food Research Institute, Zeist, The Netherlands.

Peacock, V.E. and Deinzer, M.L. (1981). *J. Am. Soc. Brew. Chem.* 39, 136–141.

Peacock, V.E., Deinzer, M.L., Likens, S.T., Nickerson, G.B. and McGill, L.A. (1981). *J. Agric. Food Chem.* 29, 1265–1269.

Peppard, T.L., Ramus, S.A., Witt, C.A. and Siebert, K.J. (1989). *J. Am. Soc. Brew. Chem.* 47, 18–26.

Petersen, M.A., Ivanova, D., Møller, P. and Bredie, W.L.P. (2003). Validity of ranking criteria in gas chromatography – olfactometry methods. In Le Quéré, J.L. and Étiévant, P.X. (eds), *Flavour Research at the Dawn of the Twenty-First Century*, pp. 494–499. Lavoisier, Paris, France.

Phillips, J.B. and Beens, J. (1999). *J. Chromatogr. A* 856, 331–347.

Plotto, A., Barnes, K.W. and Goodner, K.L. (2006). *J. Food Sci.* 71, S401–S406.

Roberts, M.T., Dufour, J.-P. and Lewis, A.C. (2004). *J. Sep. Sci.* 27, 473–478.

Sanchez, N.B., Lederer, C.L., Nickerson, G.B., Libbey, L.M. and McDaniel, M.R. (1992a). Sensory and analytical evaluation of beers brewed with three varieties of hops and an unhopped beer. In Charalambous, G. (ed.), *Food Science and Human Nutrition* Developments in Food Science 29. Elsevier Science, Amsterdam, The Netherlands, pp. 403–426.

Sanchez, N.B., Lederer, C.L., Nickerson, G.B., Libbey, L.M. and McDaniel, M.R. (1992b). Sensory and analytical evaluation of hop oil oxygenated fractions. In Charalambous, G. (ed.), *Food Science and Human Nutrition* Developments in Food Science 29. Elsevier Science, Amsterdam, The Netherlands, pp. 371–402.

Schieberle, P. (1991). *Z. Lebensm. Unters. Forsch.* 193, 558–565.

Sell, C.S. (2003). *A Fragrant Introduction to Terpenoid Chemistry.* The Royal Society of Chemistry, Cambridge, UK.

Steinhaus, M. and Schieberle, P. (2000). *J. Agric. Food Chem.* 48, 1776–1783.

Steinhaus, M., Fritsch, H.T. and Schieberle, P. (2003). *J. Agric. Food Chem.* 51, 7100–7105.

Stucky, G.J. and McDaniel, M.R. (1997). *J. Am. Soc. Brew. Chem.* 55, 65–72.

Tressl, R., Friese, L., Fendesack, F. and Koppler, H. (1978). *J. Agric. Food Chem.* 26, 1422–1426.

Westwood, K.T. (1987). *EBC Monograph XIII: Symposium on Hops, Freising/Weihenstephan, Fe. Rep. of Germany.* Verlag Hans Carl, Nürnberg, Germany, pp. 243–253.

Westwood, K.T. and Daoud, I.S. (1985). *European Brewery Convention. Proceedings of the 20th Congress, Helsinki.* IRL Press Ltd, Oxford, England. pp. 579–586.

Yang, X., Lederer, C., McDaniel, M. and Deinzer, M. (1993). *J. Agric. Food Chem.* 41, 1300–1304.

23

Ethanol Content of Beer Sold in the United States: Variation Over Time, Across States and by Individual Drinks

William C. Kerr Alcohol Research Group, Emeryville, CA, USA

Abstract

Research studies estimating the average alcohol content of beer sold in the United States indicate that beer strength has generally declined over time from around 5% alcohol by volume (% ABV) in the 1950s to a low of 4.5% ABV in 2005. This decline is mainly attributed to the growth in popularity of light beer, with a market share of over 50% in 2005, and to growth in lower alcohol content brands in other categories, particularly Mexican beers among the imported beers. Differences in the popularity of beer types by state also result in varying estimates of average % ABV by state. Some states in recent years have a market share for light beer of over 60%, while others are below 40% and consume more imported and super premium beers. The particularly strong beer types, malt liquor and ice beer, also show substantial variation in market share across states. Individual beer drinks in the United States have been found to be more consistent and to have less alcohol on average than wine or spirits drinks but also to vary by size and alcohol content, especially when served in bars and restaurants. For example, a 16 oz. beer with a strength 7.3% ABV contains nearly two US standard drinks of alcohol. The research presented highlights the importance of obtaining information on drink size and brand or alcohol content in understanding survey response to questions regarding the number of beer drinks consumed and of taking estimates of mean beer % ABV into account when evaluating trends in alcohol consumption or modeling relationships between alcohol consumption from beer and health or other outcomes.

List of Abbreviations

% ABV	Percentage alcohol by volume
AEDS	Alcohol Epidemiologic Data System
NAS	National Alcohol Survey
NIAAA	National Institute on Alcohol Abuse and Alcoholism
USA	The United States of America

Introduction

Individual's beer drinks

The alcohol content of individual drinks of beer and the mean alcohol content of beer sold in the United States in a given year are important factors in the accuracy and interpretation of epidemiologic research regarding the effects of beer on health and other outcomes. Beer is the most popular alcoholic beverage in the United States, comprising 59.4% of the ethanol consumed in 2002 (Kerr *et al.*, 2006a). In their respective analyses and consumption decisions, researchers and, in many cases, consumers typically assume that all beer drinks contain roughly the same amount of ethanol. However, the detailed description of the US beer market presented here indicates considerable variation in the ethanol content of the beer drinks available at any given time. This variation has important implications for both consumer decision-making and survey assessment of consumer behavior. The essential dimensions of beer drink ethanol content variation are straightforward: the liquid volume of beer in the container or glass and the alcohol (ethanol) content by volume (% ABV) of that beer. Yet it is difficult for consumers to gauge the size and strength of the beer they drink and even harder for them to translate these into the often vaguely described "standard drink" in terms of which they are expected to report for many surveys. In the United States a standard drink of beer is most often defined as 12 oz. at 5% ABV, containing 0.6 oz. (14 g) of alcohol. This difficulty may be reflected in the inability of general population surveys to account for all of the beer (and similarly wine and spirits) sold (Rogers and Greenfield, 2000). Further, systematic differences in the ethanol content of beer drinks across individuals could lead to differential under- and over-estimates of their consumption, confounding the modeling of the determinants of and outcomes related to beer consumption.

Beer in Health and Disease Prevention
ISBN: 978-0-12-373891-2

Aggregate beer sales

Similarly, aggregate analyses of trends and cross-state differences in per capita consumption of beer, wine, spirits and total alcohol, and the estimation of population-level relationships between alcohol consumption measures and outcome measures require accurate estimates of the mean % ABV for each beverage, year and geographic unit. Only recently have empirically based estimates of mean % ABV become available for the United States and for specific states (Kerr *et al.*, 2006a). For beer, as suggested in guidelines published by the World Health Organization (2000), these estimates are based on information on producer-reported brand % ABV, national brand-level sales, national and state beer type sales and measures of malt and other ingredients per barrel for earlier years. Estimates for wine and spirits mean % ABV are based on similar types of information and also utilize different types of information for some years (Kerr *et al.*, 2006a, b). These estimates were found to differ from the *ad hoc* estimates, which were originally developed by the Rutgers Center for Alcohol Studies (Efron *et al.*, 1974) and are currently used by the Alcohol Epidemiologic Data System (AEDS) (Lakins *et al.*, 2004). The empirically based estimates described in Kerr *et al.* (2006a) indicate that beer had more alcohol in all years and wine and spirits less alcohol in most years than the AEDS estimates had assumed. Mean % ABV estimates for beer, wine and spirits were also found to vary across states (Kerr *et al.*, 2004; 2006a, b), a factor not considered in any previous analyses of US state-level relationships between alcohol measures and outcomes.

This chapter presents a variety of information on the alcohol content of the beer sold in the United States and beer drinks consumed by US drinkers. This information has been collected and organized as part of two ongoing research programs at the Alcohol Research Group in Emeryville, California. One focused on estimating per capita consumption of alcohol for use in modeling relationships between alcohol intake and potentially alcohol-related mortality outcomes in the US states and a second focused on estimates of the amount of alcohol contained in individual drinks of beer, wine and spirits consumed in the United States and the key sources of variation in these amounts to better understand and estimate self-reported alcohol intake in surveys. Both of the projects are supported by grants from the National Institute on Alcohol Abuse and Alcoholism (NIAAA).

US Beer Types and Brand % ABV

Beer sold in the United States is generally divided into seven types by sources that monitor and track beer industry statistics: premium, popular, light, super premium (including craft, microbrew and flavored malt beverages), imported, ice and malt liquor (Adams Beverage Group, 2006). The popularity of these types varies by state (as discussed below) and has changed considerably over time as seen in Figure 23.1.

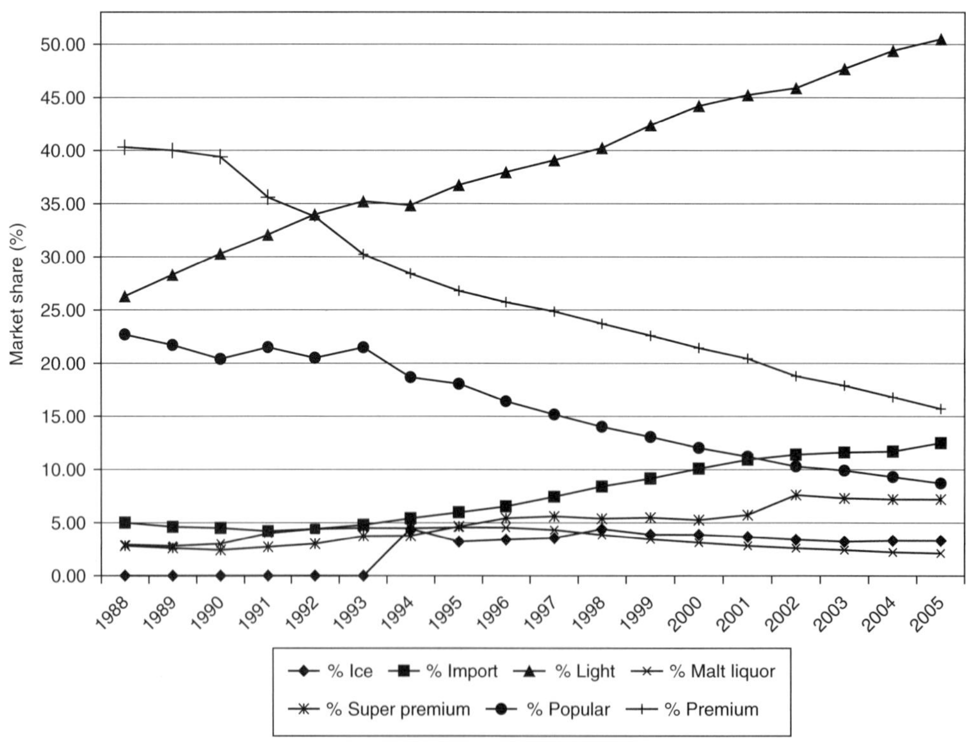

Figure 23.1 US market shares of industry beer types as a percentage of beer sold. Each line represents the percentage of overall beer sales accounted for by each type of beer in each year from 1988 to 2005.

Statistics on the market share of beer types presented here come from all issues of the Beer Handbook (Jobson Publishing Corporation, 1994, 1995; Adams/Jobson Publishing Corporation, 1996; Adams Business Media, 1997, 1998, 1999, 2000; Adams Business Research, 2001; Adams Beverage Group, 2002, 2003, 2004, 2005, 2006).

Light beer

Light beer has by far the largest market share of any category comprising over 50% of the beer sold in 2005. Light beer is generally defined as beer with at least 20% fewer calories than the regular version of the same brand. In practice this also means less alcohol since most beer calories come from the alcohol so the major light beers have 4.2% ABV. The market share of light beer in the United States has risen annually since its invention in the late 1960s. Its market share has doubled since1988 (see Figure 23.1).

Premium beer

Much of the rise in market share for light beer has been at the expense of the premium beer category, which declined from 40% of the market in 1988 to only 15.7% in 2005. Premium beer is considered to be the regular US beer and includes brands from the largest US breweries such as Budweiser, Coors and Miller Genuine Draft. These beers are generally 5% ABV although they have all changed over time. Most recently Miller Genuine Draft reduced its % ABV to 4.7%, returning to its pre-1995 level. In 1995 Coors was 4.6% ABV and Budweiser was 4.8% ABV. These shifts by major brands over time highlight the difficulty of tracking the alcohol content of beer for both researchers and consumers as these changes are not usually announced and, in some cases, do not appear on the label.

Popular beer

Popular beer has also lost popularity over time and now makes up less than 10% of the market. This category consists of lower priced brands from major breweries and some historically regional brands. Many of these brands have been consolidated by Pabst Brewing. These include Old Milwaukee, Schlitz, Rainer and Pabst Blue Ribbon. The alcohol content of popular beers varies widely with some as low as 4.3% such as Milwaukee's Best, others around 4.6% such as Busch or 4.7% like Miller High Life, while others are as high as 5% ABV including Pabst Blue Ribbon. The % ABV of popular beer brands has changed over time as well, for example Busch was 4.9% ABV in the late 1990s and is now 4.6% ABV (Table 23.1).

Imported beer

Imported beer has grown substantially in recent years and now constitutes 12.5% of the beer market. Much of this growth is due to the popularity of Mexican beers which now make up 5 of the top 10 imported brands. As with domestic beers, the lighter brands have grown most in popularity resulting in a lower mean % ABV for this category over time. While a few 5% ABV brands such as Heineken and Labatt Blue are still among the most popular, most have lower % ABVs. The leading imported brand is Corona Extra (4.6%) and other Mexican brands are 4.4% ABV. In addition some imported light brands like Corona Light (4.1%) and Amstel Light (3.5% ABV) have become popular. Guiness Stout at 4.2% ABV has always had an alcohol content similar to light beers.

Super premium beer

The super premium category, which includes craft beers, microbreweries and in recent years flavored malt beverages,

Table 23.1 2005 alcohol content and market share of top beer brands

Brand	*% ABV*	*Market share (%)*	*Cumulative market share (%)*
Bud Light	4.2	19	19
Budweiser	5.0	13	32
Miller Lite	4.2	9	40
Coors Light	4.2	8	48
Natural Light	4.2	4	53
Corona Extra	4.6	4	56
Busch	4.6	3	59
Busch Light	4.1	3	62
Miller High Life	4.7	2	65
Heineken	5.0	2	67
Miller Genuine Draft	4.7	2	69
Michelob Ultra	4.2	2	70
Keystone Light	4.2	1	72
Natural Ice	5.9	1	73
Budweiser Select	4.3	1	74
Milwaukee's Best	4.3	1	75
Milwaukee's Best Light	4.2	1	76
Michelob Light	4.3	1	77
Icehouse	5.5	1	78
Yuengling Traditional Lager	4.4	1	78
Milwaukee's Best Ice	5.9	1	79
Pabst Blue Ribbon	5.0	1	80
Coors	5.0	1	80
Old Milwaukee	4.6	1	81
Tecate	4.4	1	81
Modelo Especial	4.4	1	82
Labatt Bluo	5.0	0	82
Smirnoff Twisted V	5.0	0	83
Colt 45	6.1	0	83
King Cobra	6.0	0	84
Mean % ABV of top brands	4.5	84	84

Note: Producer reported % ABV and estimated market share from the Adams Beer Handbook 2006 for leading brands in 2005.

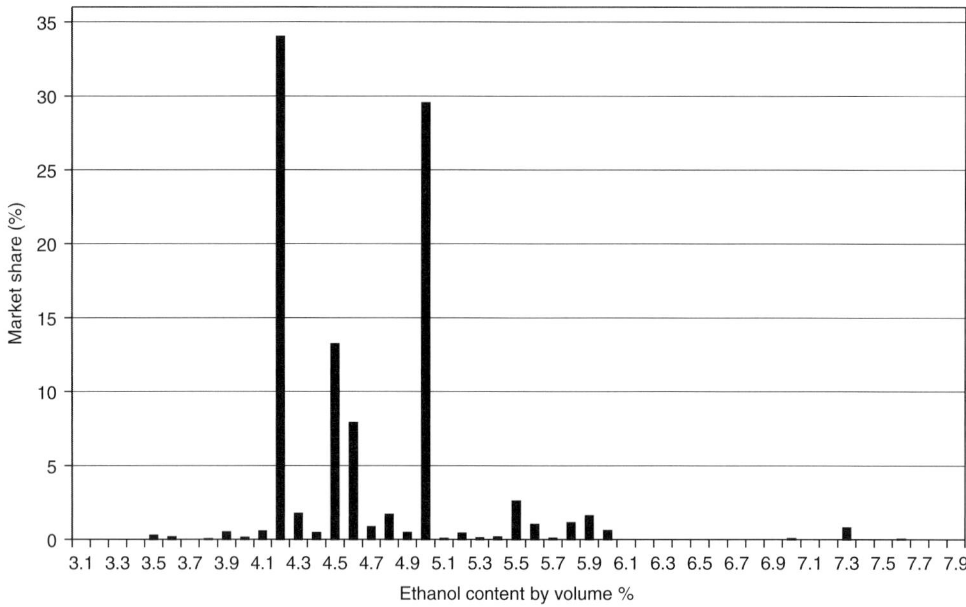

Figure 23.2 Beer ethanol content distribution for 2000. Bars represent the percentage of beer sold among major brands that had the labeled percentage ethanol content by volume in the year 2000.

has also grown over time and is now over 7% of the beer market. While the Michelob brand led this category for many years, the top brand is now Yuengling Lager, which is lower in alcohol than most beers in this category at 4.4% ABV. Many beers in this category have higher alcohol contents such as Sierra Nevada Pale Ale (5.6%) and some are as high as 7% or 8% ABV. The category includes a very large number of low production beers and is thus difficult to form a complete picture of it in terms of the % ABV distribution.

Ice beer

Ice beer is a type of beer that has been clarified by forming small ice crystals and then removing them. This process also removes some of the water, increasing the alcohol content such that these beers are typically 5.5–5.9% ABV. As seen in Figure 23.1, this category was introduced in 1994 and has maintained a small share of the market since. This category is a mix of low cost high alcohol beers with 5.9% ABV such as Natural Ice, Milwaukee's Best Ice and Keystone Ice that compete with malt liquors in offering the most alcohol for the dollar among beers and 5.5% ABV brands including Icehouse and Bud Ice that are priced like premium beers. The stronger, lower priced brands have gained a larger share of this category in recent years, possibly through some consumers switching from the declining malt liquor category.

Malt liquor beer

Malt liquor is generally lower priced, higher alcohol content beer that is often sold in larger containers such as 16 or 40 oz. Malt liquor consumption peaked in the mid-1990s at nearly 5% of the beer market and has since declined to only 2.1% in 2005. This category covers a range of % ABVs from Mickey's at 5.6% ABV to King Cobra and Colt 45 at 5.9% to Olde English 800 or St. Ides at 7.3% ABV or more. Malt liquor % ABV appears to be more complicated than other beers because versions with very different strengths have been sold in different parts of the country. Some brands have sold 5.9% ABV versions in the Eastern United States due to certain states that do not allow higher % ABVs while selling much stronger versions in the Western states. Brand % ABVs also change over time as with other beer types.

Distribution of beer alcohol contents

The beer ethanol content distribution for major beer brands in 2000 is shown in Figure 23.2. This illustrates the concentration of % ABVs at 4.2%, 5% and between these in that year with much smaller market shares for beers with higher or lower % ABVs. By 2005 there has been a further shift toward lower % ABV beer as can be seen in Table 23.1. These beers represent 84% of the beer market and have an average % ABV of 4.5. While this estimate is based on less detail than those presented in Kerr *et al.* (2004), it indicates that the average % ABV of beer has likely fallen since 2001 due to the increasing market share of light beers and lower % ABV imports like Corona and reduced % ABVs for major brands such as Busch and Miller beers. Considering the strong trend in this direction it can be expected that even further declines in the mean % ABV of beers in the United States will occur in the future.

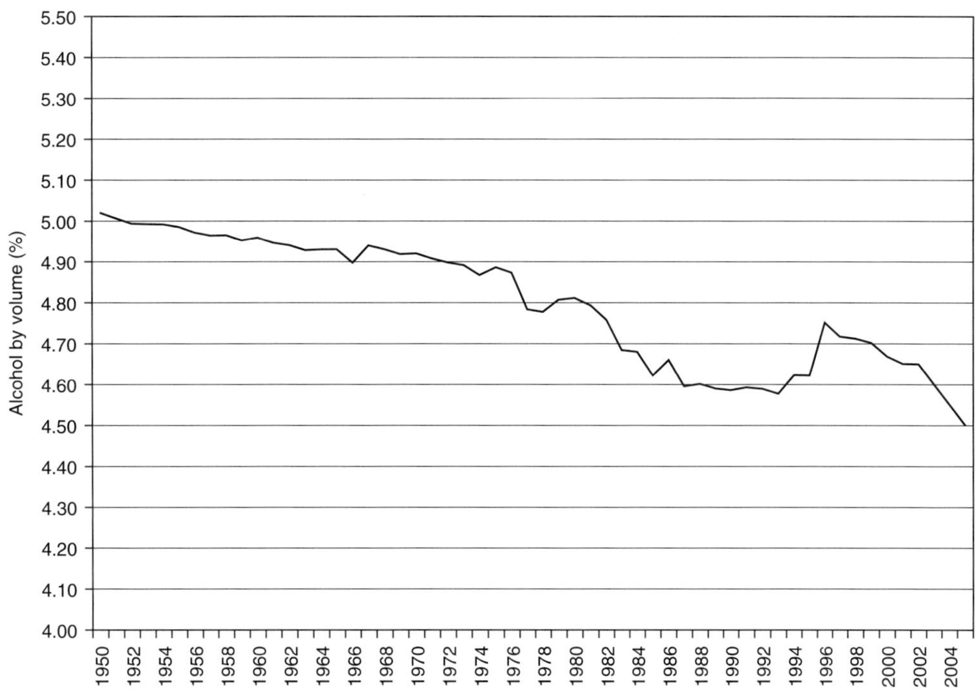

Figure 23.3 Estimated mean % ABV of beer in the United States. The line shows the estimated mean % ABV for all beer sold in the United States in each year from 1950 through 2005.

Time Trends in % ABV and Beer Consumption

Estimates of the mean % ABV of beer sold in the United States (Figure 23.3) indicate a generally declining trend over the past 50 years from about 5% ABV in the early 1950s to 4.5% ABV in 2005. One exception to this was a rise in the late 1990s, which was mainly due to the increase % ABV of certain brands (Kerr *et al.*, 2004). As noted above, the major factor in this shift has been the relentless rise in the popularity of light beer.

The importance of the changing alcohol content of beer can bee seen in Figure 23.4 where trends in the liters of beer sold and the ethanol contained in that beer are charted. While both are seen to peak around 1980, at the same time as overall alcohol consumption, the ethanol consumed in the form of beer has declined proportionally more than beer sales. For purposes of estimating the relationship between alcohol consumption from beer and health outcomes, it is the ethanol, rather than the beer, that would be relevant. This has increased from a low of about 4 l per capita aged 15 years and older in the late 1950s and early 1960s to a high of about 5.5 l per capita around 1980 and has subsequently fallen to below 5 l from the early 1990s.

In comparison to wine and spirits, beer has been the largest source of alcohol for the US population since the end of prohibition. As seen in Figure 23.5, the proportion of US alcohol intake from beer declined from over 55% in the early 1950s to below 50% around 1970. During that time spirits rose in popularity from 35% of the alcohol sold to nearly 42%. With the decline of spirits popularity since the mid-1970s, beer's share of US alcohol intake has risen to over 60% by the mid-1990s. Wine has never comprised more than 15% of the alcohol sold in the United States but has risen from about 10% through 1970 to nearly 15%. Spirits have also seen a small increase in recent years resulting in a small decline in beer's share of US alcohol intake. However, beer remains by far the main source of alcohol for the US population.

State Differences in % ABV and Type Shares

The mean % ABV of beer sold has been found to vary across states in the United States in addition to changing over time as discussed above (Kerr *et al.*, 2004). Estimates of state mean % ABV utilize each state's market shares of the seven beer types along with estimates of the mean % ABV by beer type calculated using national sales of major brands. These estimates are presented in Table 23.2 for selected years for states sorted by the 2001 % ABV estimate. While it would be preferable to utilize brand-level sales by state to calculate these means, this information has not yet been found, although producers or wholesalers are likely to have these data due to the separate licensing and

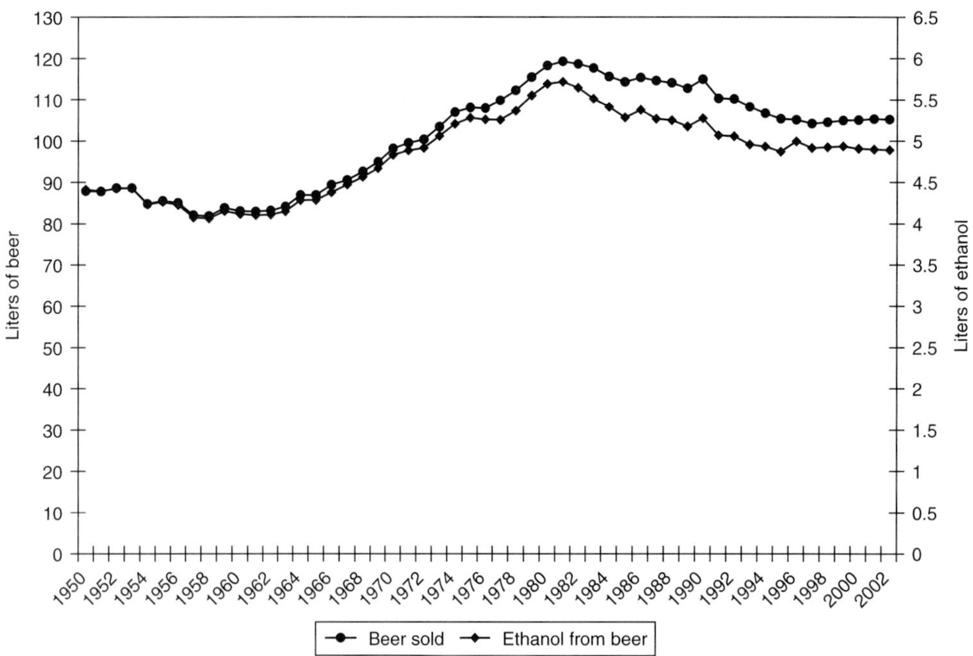

Figure 23.4 Per capita (15+) liters of beer and ethanol from beer for the United States Line with circles shows the amount of beer sold in liters on the left axis and the line with diamonds show the amount of ethanol sold as beer in liters on the right axis for each year.

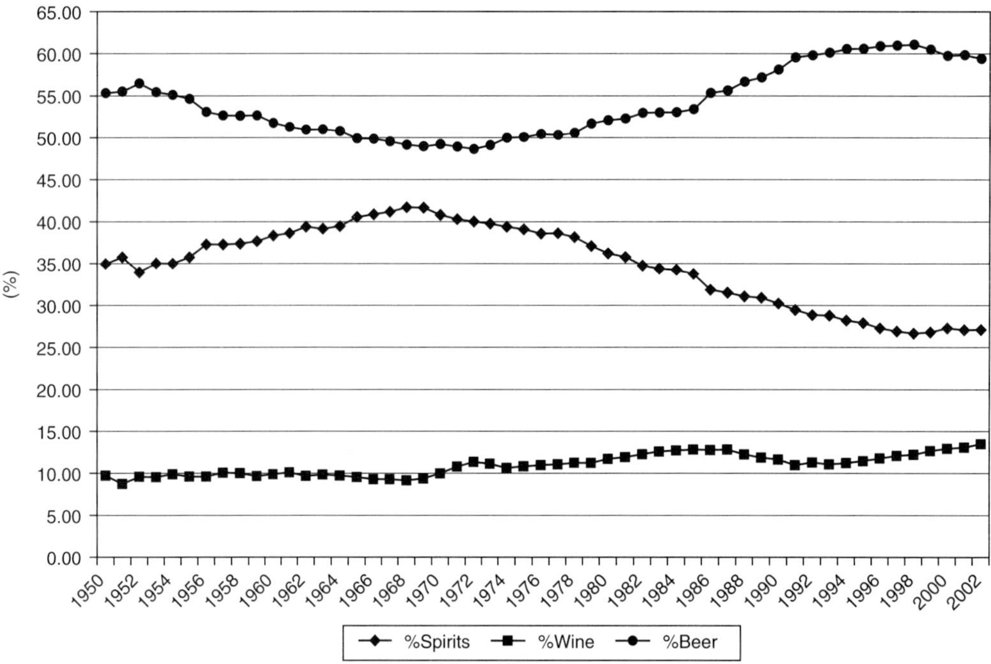

Figure 23.5 Proportion of total ethanol from beer, wine and spirits in the United States over time. Each line represents the percentage of total ethanol consumed in the United States from each beverage type with circles for beer, diamonds for spirits and squares for wine.

tax requirements of each state. State means are found to differ by about 0.25% ABV from the highest to lowest in later years with somewhat less variation seen in earlier years. The main source of this variation is in the share of light beer relative to the share of imported and super premium beer across states. The states with higher mean % ABV such as New York and New Jersey have particularly high shares of imported beer in 2005 at over 20% and super premium beer, about 9%, as well as ice beer and malt liquor, over 8% combined in New York compared to 5.4% nationally

Table 23.2 Estimated mean % ABV of beer in selected years by state (sorted by 2001 estimate)

State	*1993 (%)*	*1995 (%)*	*1997 (%)*	*1999 (%)*	*2001 (%)*
New York	4.59	4.66	4.82	4.81	4.74
New Jersey	4.59	4.66	4.79	4.77	4.72
District of Columbia	4.57	4.62	4.76	4.73	4.72
Maryland	4.57	4.60	4.79	4.76	4.71
Washington	4.72	4.77	4.78	4.76	4.71
North Carolina	4.56	4.60	4.80	4.77	4.71
Mississippi	4.60	4.63	4.79	4.75	4.70
Virginia	4.57	4.61	4.78	4.75	4.70
Alaska	4.64	4.72	4.74	4.74	4.70
Georgia	4.57	4.61	4.76	4.74	4.69
South Carolina	4.55	4.58	4.78	4.73	4.69
Florida	4.57	4.61	4.76	4.74	4.69
Michigan	4.61	4.65	4.75	4.73	4.69
Kentucky	4.57	4.60	4.75	4.74	4.68
Oregon	4.71	4.74	4.76	4.75	4.68
Vermont	4.56	4.63	4.72	4.73	4.68
Illinois	4.63	4.70	4.73	4.72	4.67
Ohio	4.60	4.63	4.74	4.72	4.67
Delaware	4.58	4.62	4.73	4.72	4.66
Maine	4.56	4.61	4.72	4.72	4.66
Connecticut	4.56	4.63	4.71	4.70	4.66
Massachusetts	4.55	4.62	4.72	4.71	4.66
Tennessee	4.57	4.60	4.73	4.71	4.66
Montana	4.68	4.72	4.72	4.71	4.65
Rhode Island	4.56	4.62	4.70	4.69	4.65
Minnesota	4.64	4.67	4.71	4.70	4.65
California	4.56	4.62	4.71	4.69	4.65
Arkansas	4.56	4.59	4.71	4.70	4.65
Pennsylvania	4.58	4.64	4.72	4.72	4.65
Indiana	4.59	4.62	4.70	4.70	4.65
Missouri	4.57	4.60	4.72	4.70	4.65
Alabama	4.53	4.57	4.70	4.69	4.65
Nebraska	4.58	4.60	4.70	4.69	4.65
New Hampshire	4.54	4.58	4.69	4.69	4.64
Louisiana	4.55	4.58	4.71	4.68	4.64
Nevada	4.52	4.58	4.68	4.67	4.63
Wyoming	4.53	4.56	4.68	4.67	4.62
Wisconsin	4.66	4.71	4.68	4.68	4.62
Colorado	4.52	4.56	4.68	4.68	4.62
Arizona	4.54	4.58	4.67	4.67	4.61
West Virginia	4.56	4.58	4.67	4.65	4.61
New Mexico	4.51	4.54	4.66	4.65	4.61
Hawaii	4.53	4.58	4.66	4.64	4.61
Kansas	4.51	4.54	4.65	4.64	4.60
North Dakota	4.60	4.62	4.66	4.65	4.60
Idaho	4.57	4.62	4.66	4.65	4.60
South Dakota	4.57	4.58	4.66	4.65	4.59
Utah	4.51	4.56	4.67	4.64	4.59
Oklahoma	4.47	4.54	4.64	4.63	4.59
Texas	4.53	4.57	4.59	4.57	4.52
Iowa	4.62	4.64	4.53	4.53	4.48
USA	4.58	4.62	4.72	4.70	4.65

(Adams Beverage Group, 2006). Conversely these states have low share of light beer at around 40% of the market while states like Texas and especially Iowa have very high shares of light beer. In 2005, nearly 70% of the beer sold in Iowa was light beer and a number of other states including Texas, Louisiana, Kansas, Oklahoma and South Dakota had around a 60% share of light beer (Adams Beverage Group, 2006). As both light beer and the imported and super premium categories show increasing trends in market share, the differences in mean % ABV across states may also be expanding over time highlighting the importance of considering these differences in research studies utilizing cross-state variation in beer consumption.

Alcohol Content of Beer Drinks

Containers

In 2000, 51% of beer sold in the United States was packaged in cans, 40% was in bottles and 9% was on draft (Beer Institute, 2001). States differ in these percentages with 15% of sales or more in the form of draft beer in Iowa, Minnesota, New Jersey, Oregon, Pennsylvania, Washington and Wisconsin, while 5% or less of sales were in the form of draft beer in Alabama, Arkansas, Georgia, Louisiana, Mississippi, New Mexico, North Carolina, Oklahoma, South Carolina, Tennessee and Texas (Beer Institute, 2001). Including sales of both draft and cans and bottles, 24.9% of beer in 2000 was sold for on-premise consumption while 75.1% was sold for off-premise consumption (Adams Beverage Group, 2002). Less information is available on the size of the cans and bottles sold but figures are available from 1992. In that year about 90% of the volume of beer sold in both bottles and cans of beer were 12 oz., not including malt liquor (about 5% of the packaged market), which typically is sold in larger containers. About 6.4% of beer sold was in 16 oz. cans and about 1.4% was sold in 32 oz. bottles with the small remainder being of unknown size (Beer Institute, 1998). While it is clear that 12 oz. containers make up a large majority of total beer sales, roughly 82%, other sizes and draft beer could account for significant drink size differences if larger-sized containers, or various-sized glasses of draft, are reported as a single drink.

Brand % ABV

As shown in Table 23.1 and discussed in the section about beer types, the % ABV of different brands varies widely. Figure 23.2 shows that while most of the beer sold is between 4.2% and 5% ABV, a wide variety of strengths are available. The importance of a beer's % ABV and container size in determining the number of 0.6 ethanol ounce (14 g) standard drinks consumed for a given number of beer drinks is shown in Figure 23.3. When beer is 3.6% ABV even six 12 oz. drinks do not add up to five drinks, the typical threshold used to determine heavy drinking occasions. For 4.2% or 4.6% beers, six 12 oz. drinks must be consumed to reach five standard drinks. For stronger beer or larger sizes, fewer drinks will be required. For beer above 7% ABV only four 12 oz. drinks and only three 16 oz. drinks are needed to reach five standard drinks. These conversions to standard drinks clearly illustrate the importance of considering size and % ABV in determining an individual's alcohol intake (Table 23.3).

Table 23.3 The effect of beer drink size and % ABV on the number of standard (0.6 oz. of ethanol) drinks consumed when drinking one to six drinks

	Number of drinks					
% ABV	*1*	*2*	*3*	*4*	*5*	*6*
12 oz.						
3.6	0.72	1.44	2.16	2.88	3.6	4.32
4.2	0.84	1.68	2.52	3.36	4.2	5.04
4.6	0.92	1.84	2.76	3.68	4.6	5.52
5.0	1	2	3	4	5	6
5.6	1.12	2.24	3.36	4.48	5.6	6.72
5.9	1.18	2.36	3.54	4.72	5.9	7.08
7.3	1.46	2.92	4.38	5.84	7.3	8.76
7.7	1.54	3.08	4.62	6.16	7.7	9.24
16 oz.						
3.6	0.96	1.92	2.88	3.84	4.80	5.76
4.2	1.12	2.24	3.36	4.48	5.60	6.72
4.6	1.23	2.45	3.68	4.91	6.13	7.36
5.0	1.33	2.67	4.00	5.33	6.67	8.00
5.6	1.49	2.99	4.48	5.97	7.47	8.96
5.9	1.57	3.15	4.72	6.29	7.87	9.44
7.3	1.95	3.89	5.84	7.79	9.73	11.68
7.7	2.05	4.11	6.16	8.21	10.27	12.32

Note: Each cell represents the number of US standard drinks (14 g of ethanol) that would be consumed for a given number of actual drinks and a given % ABV for two common drink sizes 12 and 16 oz.

Measured drinks

More detailed information on the size and strength of beer drinks consumed in the United States is available for individuals surveyed in the 2000 National Alcohol Survey (NAS) Methodological Follow-up Study, a national sample of 323 individuals conducted in the winter of 2003–2004 (Kerr *et al.*, 2005) and the 2003 San Francisco Bay Area Pilot Study of drink ethanol content measurement where 24 individuals reported on beer drink size and brand in consumed in bars or restaurants. Variation in both glass and container size and in brand ethanol content were found to influence drink ethanol content. Figure 23.6 shows the distribution of beer drink ethanol content for home drinks from the 2000 NAS Follow-up Study. Home beer drinks were found to average 0.56 oz. of ethanol with large numbers reporting either 0.5 oz., the amount in 12 oz. of light beer, or 0.6 oz., the amount in 12 oz. of regular 5% ABV beer. The ethanol content of beers served in restaurants and bars reported in the 2003 Bay Area Pilot Study are more varied and are, on average, larger than those of beer consumed at home in that study or in the 2000 NAS Follow-up Study. Beer served at bars and restaurants averaged 0.69 oz. of ethanol with a substantial proportion of drinks being larger than 0.7 oz. of ethanol, as seen in Figure 23.7. In this sample, the beer drinks served at restaurants and bars tended to be larger, 21.5% larger on average, than those served at

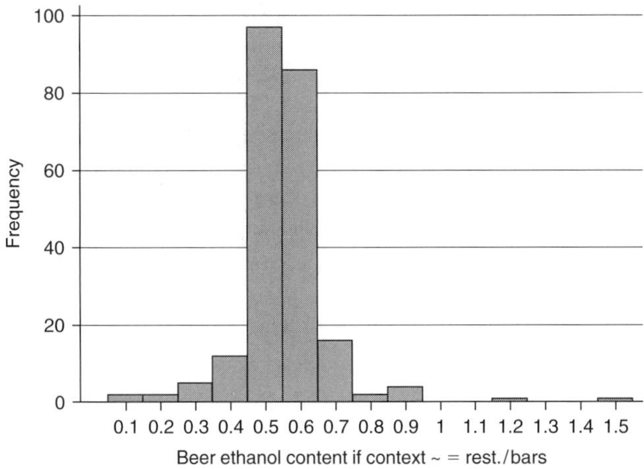

Figure 23.6 Distribution of beer ethanol content in measured home drinks from the 2000 NAS Methodological Follow-up Study. Histogram shows the number of respondents in the 2000 NAS Methodological Follow-up Study reporting home drink ethanol content in 0.1 oz. groupings between 0.05 and 1.55 oz. of ethanol per drink.

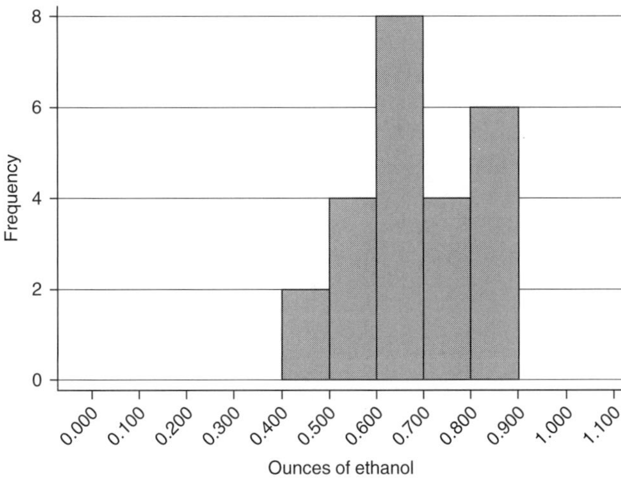

Figure 23.7 Ethanol content of beer drinks at restaurants and bars in Pilot Study. Histogram shows the number of respondents in the 2003 Bay Area Pilot Study reporting drink ethanol content in 0.1 oz. groupings between 0.4 and 0.9 oz. of ethanol per drink.

home. Most (38 of 43) home drinks were reported to be consumed from 12 oz. cans, bottles or glasses while bar and restaurant drinks included thirteen 16 oz., two 14 oz. and three 24 oz. glasses compared to only six 12 oz. drinks. The results of this pilot study clearly indicate the importance of both size and ethanol concentration in determining the amount of alcohol in one drink of beer. The home drinks measured in the larger study indicate that for these drinks the brand % ABV is the main varying factor in this context and both studies together indicate that context of drinking may be an important determinant of beer drink alcohol content.

Limitations and Measurement Issues

The results reported here do not represent the final word on the alcohol content of beer sold or the alcohol content of beer drinks in the United States. Considerable extrapolation from available data was required to achieve the mean beer % ABV estimates. This is especially true for years prior to 1988 and for state-level estimates. More detailed information could certainly alter these estimates if it was to become available. These estimates also utilize producer provided brand % ABV in most cases and the accuracy in these is not known. Further studies where samples are directly measured may indicate that there is a degree of error or even systematic bias in these reports. Also, as mentioned above, the use of type averages rather than state-specific brand sales reduces the accuracy of the estimates presented.

Research on the alcohol content of beer drinks by US consumers is at a very early stage. Our national estimates of home beer drinks have shown that these drinks are less varied and contain, on average, less alcohol than wine or spirits drinks but larger samples are need to confirm these results and explore potential sources of variation. The pilot study results also indicate that beer drinks in bars, at least in one part of the United States, tend to be larger and to contain more alcohol than drinks consumed at home. Future research to directly measure the alcohol content of drinks consumed in bars and restaurants across the United States is needed to fully understand the dimensions of this important issue.

Concluding Remarks

Considering the wide range of beer choices available to American beer drinkers and the changes over time in the brand % ABV and market share, it is particularly important for both survey and aggregate-level analyses to consider the details of beer size and strength to the extent possible. Unlike some countries where almost complete brand-level sales information is available, for example Sweden, Norway and some Canadian provinces, in most countries, including the United States, this information is more difficult and time consuming to obtain. Often, as in the figures presented in this chapter, a variety of information sources that are less than perfect can be used to generate the best possible estimates while still leaving considerable room for improvement. The assessment of individual's beer drink ethanol content is important for surveys and other types of individual-level research. It is now clear that not all drinks contain the same amount of alcohol, particularly across beverage types but also within them. Therefore, beer drinks should be assessed separately from wine and spirits drinks and information on the size and brand or type of beer should be collected where possible.

The importance of accurate ethanol measurement is probably most keen in studies of health and medical outcomes.

In these studies an individual's self-reported number of drinks, often from relatively simplistic question formats, is converted into a number of grams per day variable that gives the appearance of precision. These variables are then used to estimate relationships and risk thresholds in terms of grams of alcohol, which are then extrapolated to populations and used to form drinking guidelines and recommendations. In fact, almost none of the literature regarding alcohol's relationship with health outcomes is based on detailed measures of drink alcohol content and very little of it includes assessment of drinking patterns (Rehm *et al.*, 2006), another dimension likely to be essential in most of these relationships. Hopefully this overview of the US beer market and individual beer drinks will encourage researchers and consumers of research finding to consider these important dimensions in the conduct and interpretation of future studies.

Summary Points

- The mean % ABV of beer sold in the United States has generally declined since 1950 from around 5% to a low of 4.5% in 2005.
- The popularity of beer types, as represented by US market share, has changed over time with light beer increasing to over 50% of the market in 2005 and popular and premium beer types declining. Imported beer has also grown substantially since the early 1990s.
- The alcohol content of major beer brands sold in the United States ranges from 3.5 to over 8% ABV. However, most beers are between 4.2% ABV, the typical strength of light beer, and 5% ABV, the typical strength of regular beer.
- Beer is the most commonly consumed form of alcohol in the United States, representing around 60% of all alcohol since 1990.
- The estimated mean alcohol content of beer differs by US state with the lowest % ABVs found in states with large market shares for light beer and the highest % ABVs seen in states with the highest shares of imported and super premium beers and lower shares of light beer.
- Individual's drinks of beer in the United States are more consistent and lower on average in terms of alcohol content than wine or spirits drinks since most beer is consumed from 12 oz. bottles or cans.

References

Adams Beverage Group (2002). *Adams Beer Handbook*. Adams Beverage Group, Norwalk, CT.

Adams Beverage Group (2003). *Adams Beer Handbook*. Adams Beverage Group, Norwalk, CT.

Adams Beverage Group (2004). *Adams Beer Handbook 2004*. Adams Beverage Group, Norwalk, CT.

Adams Beverage Group (2005). *Adams Beer Handbook 2005*. Adams Beverage Group, Norwalk, CT.

Adams Beverage Group (2006). *Adams Beer Handbook 2006*. Adams Beverage Group, Norwalk, CT.

Adams Business Media (1997). *Adams Beer Handbook*. Adams Business Media, New York.

Adams Business Media (1998). *Adams Beer Handbook*. Adams Business Media, New York.

Adams Business Media (1999). *Adams Beer Handbook*. Adams Business Media, New York.

Adams Business Media (2000). *Adams Beer Handbook*. Adams Business Media, New York.

Adams Business Research (2001). *Adams Beer Handbook*. Adams Business Media, Norwalk, CT.

Adams/Jobson Publishing Corporation (1996). *Adams/Jobson's Beer Handbook 1996*. Adams/Jobson Publishing Corporation, New York.

Beer Institute (1998). *Brewers Almanac 1998*. Beer Institute, Washington, DC.

Beer Institute (2001). *Brewers Almanac 2001*. Beer Institute, Washington, DC.

Efron, E., Keller, M. and Gurioli, C. (1974). *Statistics on Consumption of Alcohol and on Alcoholism*. Journal of Studies on Alcohol, Inc., New Brunswick, NJ.

Jobson Publishing Corporation (1994). *Jobson's Beer Handbook 1994*. Jobson Publishing Corporation, New York.

Jobson Publishing Corporation (1995). *Jobson's Beer Handbook 1995*. Jobson Publishing Corporation, New York.

Kerr, W.C., Brown, S. and Greenfield, T.K. (2004). *Alcohol. Clin. Exp. Res.* 28, 1524–1532.

Kerr, W.C., Greenfield, T.K., Tujague, J. and Brown, S. (2005). *Alcohol. Clin. Exp. Res.* 29, 2015–2021.

Kerr, W.C., Greenfield, T.K. and Tujague, J. (2006a). *Alcohol. Clin. Exp. Res.* 30, 1583–1591.

Kerr, W.C., Greenfield, T.K., Tujague, J. and Brown, S. (2006b). *Alcohol. Clin. Exp. Res.* 30, 516–522.

Lakins, N.E., Williams, G.D., Yi, H.-y. and Smothers, B.A. (2004). *National Institute on Alcohol Abuse and Alcoholism*. National Institutes of Health, Rockville, MD.

Rehm, J., Greenfield, T.K. and Kerr, W.C. (2006). *Contem. Drug Probl.* 33, 205–235.

Rogers, J.D. and Greenfield, T.K. (2000). *Contemp. Drug Probl.* 27, 367–381.

World Health Organization (2000). World Health Organization, Department of Mental Health and Substance Dependence, Noncommunicable Diseases and Mental Health Cluster, Copenhagen, Denmark.

24

Soluble Proteins of Beer

Marion Didier and Bakan Bénédicte INRA Unité Biopolymères, Interactions, Assemblages, Nantes cedex, France

Abstract

Soluble beer proteins are heat-stable proteins from malted barley. These proteins are mainly composed of proteins that would be involved in the defense of barley against microbial pathogens as a serpin-like cysteine protease inhibitor (protein Z) and lipid transfer proteins (LTPs). These proteins are essential for the formation of beer foam. To become surface active these barley proteins undergo a structural maturation including glycation through Maillard reaction on malting and unfolding on heating during the brewing process. In the case of LTP1, another modification involves an acylation by a product of the activity of two enzymes from barley embryo (i.e. lipoxygenase and allene oxide synthase) on polyunsaturated fatty acids. These structural modifications increase the amphiphilic character of the proteins and their spreading behavior at the gas–liquid interfaces. Finally, minor beer proteins, weakly soluble in water, barley storage proteins (i.e. hordeins) are responsible for the haze formation of freshly fermented beer.

List of Abbreviations

9-LOX	9-Lipoxygenase
AOS	Allene oxide synthase
FFA	Free fatty acids
RCL	Reactive center loop
LTP	Lipid transfer protein

Introduction

Beer contains 0.5–1 g/l proteins with molecular mass from 5 to 100 kDa (Sorensen and Ottesen, 1978). The major beer proteins are involved in haze formation and foam stability, two significant criteria that define the quality of a beer for the consumer. Actually, other plant raw products such as maize grits or wheat malt can be added in the brewing process, but most of the data available on beer proteins have been obtained starting from barley malt, the major plant source of beer.

Beer Concentrate Heat-Stable Barley Albumins

Beer proteins have been characterized after fractionation using different chromatographic procedure including ion exchange, size exclusion and hydrophobic interaction chromatographies. Recently, using the current strategy of proteomic, two-dimensional electrophoresis coupled with mass spectrometry, an overall view of beer proteins was provided (Figure 24.1). Most data converge with the presence of two main proteins in beer: protein Z and lipid transfer proteins (LTPs). Protein Z is a protein with a molecular mass of 45 kDa protein. The second major beer protein, LTP, is composed by two proteins, LTP1 (about 9 kDa) and LTP2

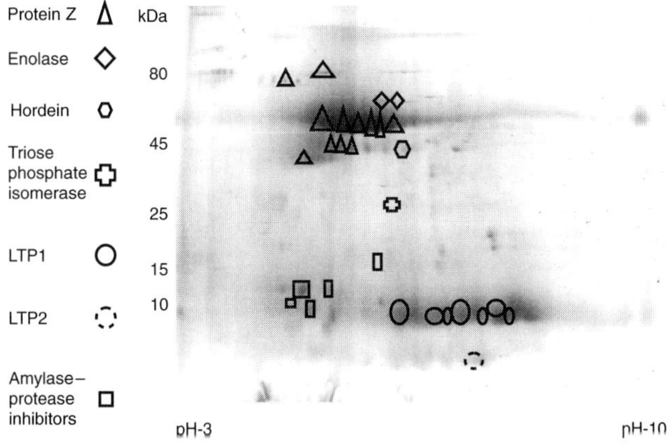

Figure 24.1 Two-dimensional electrophoresis of beer proteins (pH 3–10). The protein spots were identified by mass spectrometry after trypsin cleavage. *Source*: Perrocheau *et al.* (2005).

Beer in Health and Disease Prevention
ISBN: 978-0-12-373891-2

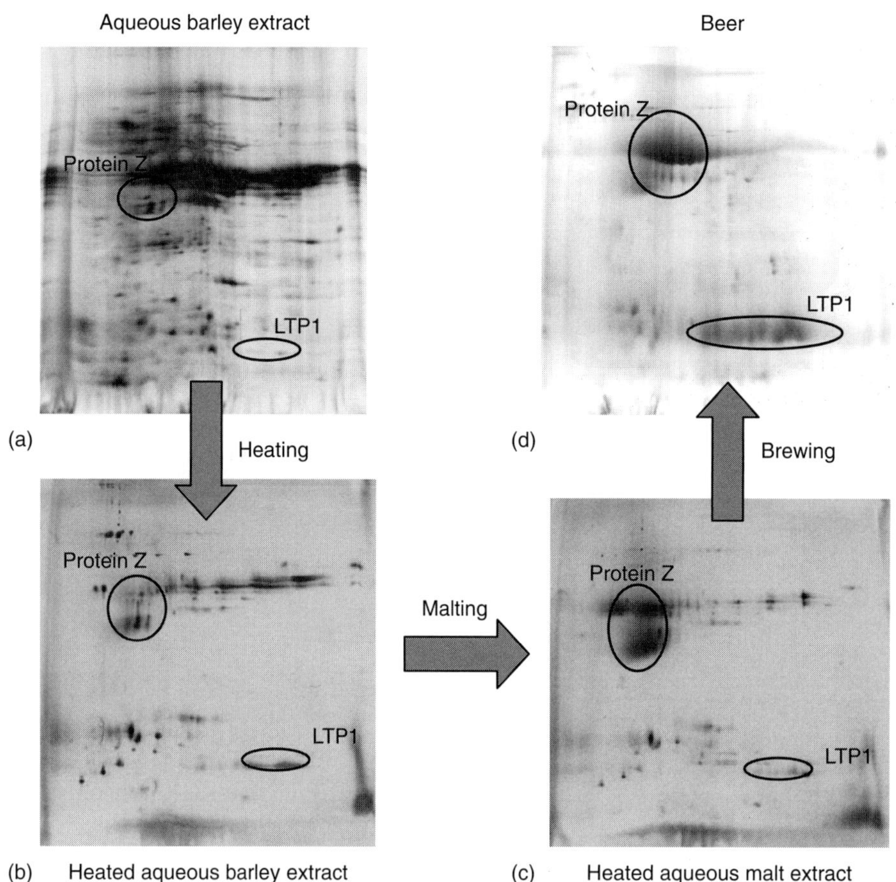

Figure 24.2 Two-dimensional electrophoresis of soluble proteins from barley, before (a) and after (b) boiling, malt after boiling (c) and beer (d).

(about 7 kDa). LTP1 is the most abundant protein of this family. Other minor proteins have been highlighted as protease and amylase–protease inhibitors, barwin and storage proteins (i.e. hordeins). Yeast proteins were also identified in beer such as enolase and triose phosphate isomerase, enzymes that play a major role in the metabolism of yeast cells (Perrocheau *et al.*, 2005). Except hordeins, most of the identified proteins are soluble proteins (i.e. albumins) as expected from the aqueous extraction of malted barley. However, not all soluble proteins of barley are recovered in beer. Actually, it was shown that only heat-stable soluble proteins were present in agreement with the boiling procedure of the brewing process (Figure 24.2). Comparing heated malt extract and beer more hordeins are extracted from malt. Most of these proteins precipitate during the maturation of beer in part by forming large aggregates with phenolic compounds from hop and malt. These complexes are responsible for the haze formation in beer (see below).

Protein Z belongs to the serpin superfamily of serine protease inhibitors and are composed by protein Z4 and protein Z7 that share about 75% sequence identity (Østergaard *et al.*, 2000) and are encoded by chromosomes 4 and 7 (Hejgaard and Kaersgaard, 1983). These soluble and lysine-rich proteins (>5% lysine) are abundant in the starchy endosperm of monocots where they account for about 5% of barley albumins. Although there are different consensus glycosylation sites in protein Z, no glycosylation was observed on the proteins purified from barley seeds. However, this protein is glycated in beer (Curioni *et al.*, 1995). Glycation of protein Z is due to Maillard reaction that occurs on malting. The Maillard reaction is a reaction between the amine group of lysine and reducing sugar (glucose and maltose) (Figure 24.3) that occurs on during the kilning step of the malting process (Jégou *et al.*, 2001). Protein Z irreversibly inhibits chymotrypsin and other non-plant proteases but are not inhibitory for endogenous protease, including cysteine proteinase that degrades storage protein on germination. It was suggested that protein Z, by inhibiting exogenous protease, could play a role in the defense of plant against their predators (fungi, insects, etc.) (Østergaard *et al.*, 2000). Recently, it was shown in *Arabidopsis thaliana* that serpin is a suicide inhibitor of a cysteine protease, metacaspase9 (Vercammen *et al.*, 2006). Plant metacaspases are involved in signaling of cell death. The normal development of barley endosperm, that is, as in other cereals, lead in fine to its death. Cereal serpin could play a role in the control of endosperm cell death in preventing premature apoptosis of this storage compartment of

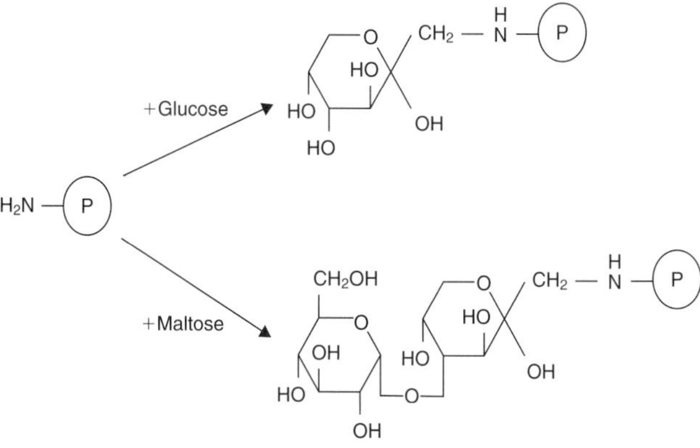

Figure 24.3 Schematic glycation of proteins in the Maillard reaction.

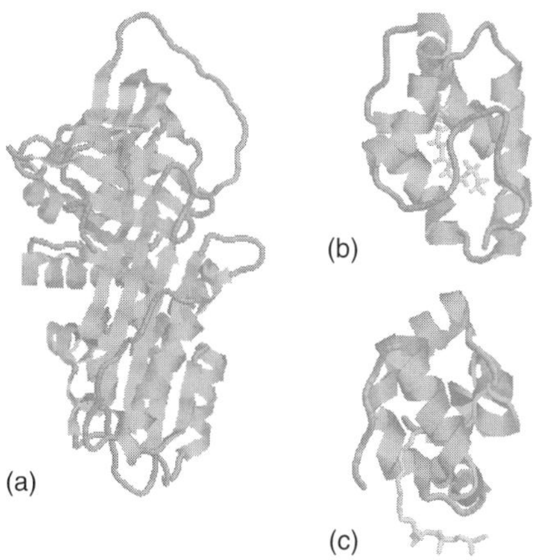

Figure 24.4 Structure of the main beer proteins. (a) Protein Z (the structure of the prototypical serpin α1-antitrypsin is presented with the RCL, up, pdb code 1QLP; Elliott *et al.*, 2000). (b) Barley LTP1 complexed with a fatty acid (1BE2; Lerche and Poulsen, 1998). (c) Wheat LTP2 complexed with lysophosphatidylglycerol (1TUK; Pons *et al.*, 2003).

the grain. This protein could participate in the mechanisms determining the final protein content of the grain, a key factor that determines the quality of malt for the brewers. The structure of plant serpins has not yet been determined but by analogy with animal serpins, it can be suggested that they are composed of nine helices and three β-sheets (Figure 24.4a). They are composed by a loop of about 20 amino acid residue, that is, the reactive center loop (RCL) that is flexible and contains a sequence complementary to the active site of its target protease (Huntington, 2006). Serpins display high metastability especially with respect to the RCL. This loop, exposed in the native protein, is fully incorporated in a β-sheet for the irreversible high-energy state. The serpin with the RCL incorporated in the β-sheet denatures at temperature above 100°C while the native protein denatures at about 60°C (Kaslik *et al.*, 1997). This unique behavior of serpins could explain the concentration of protein Z in beer. However, no data are available on the folded state of protein Z in beer.

LTPs (i.e. LTP1 and LTP2) are ubiquitous plant lipid binding proteins. They form a multigenic family where the expression of the different proteins is spatially and temporally regulated. This is well illustrated for wheat seeds where the nine LTPs are expressed at the different stages of the developing grain. The major LTP1 and LTP2 of barley and wheat seeds are expressed in the aleurone cells at the last stage of grain development (Boutrot *et al.*, 2005). These helical proteins are stabilized by four disulfide bonds. Within the protein, there is a large hydrophobic cavity or a tunnel that is the lipid binding site (Figure 24.4b and c). These proteins are capable of binding all sorts of lipids and hydrophobic molecules. Lipid binding generally involved non-covalent bonds between lipids and the protein (Douliez *et al.*, 2000). However, it has been recently shown that the barley LTP1 is also capable to bind covalently oxygenated fatty acid derivatives (i.e. oxidation products of polyunsaturated fatty acids) also called oxylipins (Bakan *et al.*, 2006; Perrocheau *et al.*, 2006). A specific site has been highlighted for these oxylipins (see below). The biological role of LTPs is still unknown but most data converge for a role of these proteins in the defense signaling of plants against microbial pathogens (Douliez *et al.*, 2000). Some LTPs are capable to inhibit fungal growth by permeabilizing the membranes of the pathogens (Blein *et al.*, 2002). These proteins could also inhibit protease and especially barley endoproteases (Jones, 2005). LTPs are also ubiquitous plant food allergens and the corresponding beer proteins have been described in rare patients as a major allergen (Asero *et al.*, 2001; Marion *et al.*, 2004). These proteins are highly stable to heat treatments and only long boiling procedure or heating in presence of reducing agent allow their denaturation (Van Nierop *et al.*, 2004; Perrocheau *et al.*, 2006). As for protein Z these proteins are not glycosylated in barley seeds but are glycated in beer. The glycation of LTPs occurs on the last step of kilning through Maillard reaction when the hydration of the green malt decreases and kilning temperature increases (Jégou *et al.*, 2001). In beer, most of the LTP1 is unfolded and some to all disulfide bonds are broken (Jégou *et al.*, 2000). Interestingly, some rearrangement of disulfide bonds can occur and a chimeric protein associating LTP1 and LTP2 have been observed in beer (Jégou *et al.*, 2000).

Structural Maturation of Proteins and Development of Beer Foam

Formation and stability of head foam strongly determine the perception of the quality of beer by the consumer (Bamforth, 1985; Evans and Sheehan, 2002). Proteins are essential in the foaming properties of a beer in forming a visco-elastic film around gas bubbles (Maeda *et al.*, 1991;

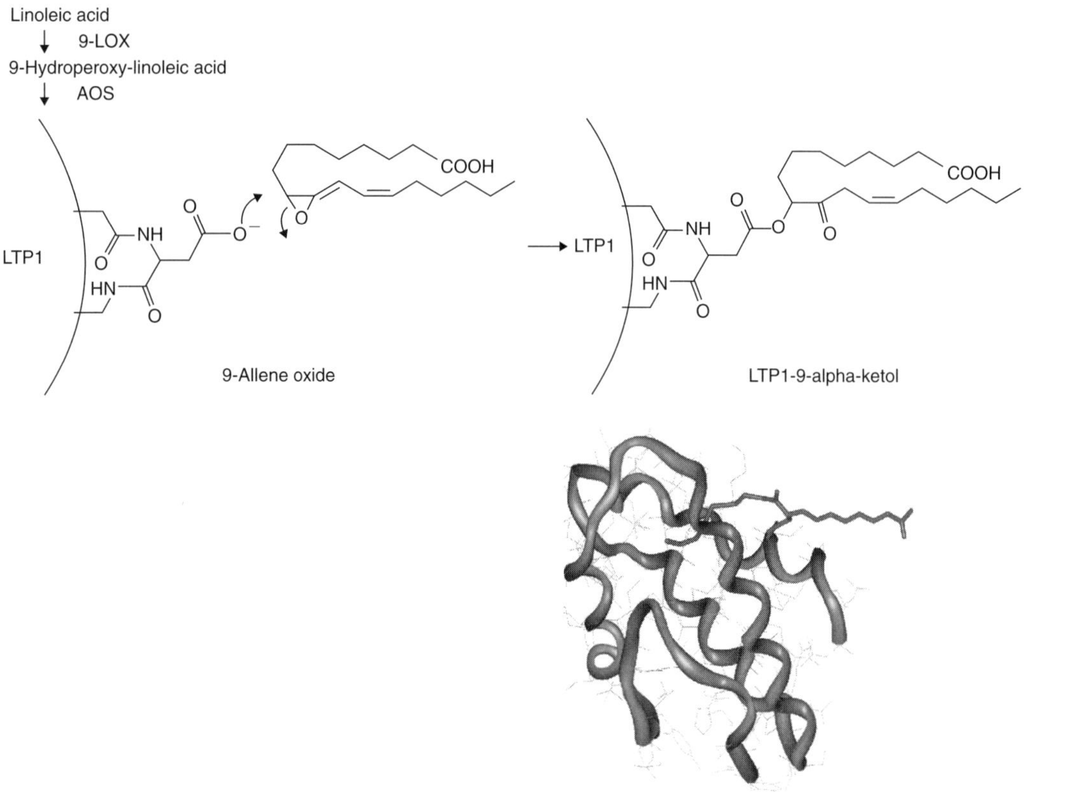

Figure 24.5 Biochemical mechanism of the adduction of barley LTP1 with 9-hydroxy-10-oxo-12(Z)-octadecenoic acid (alpha-ketol).

Sorensen *et al.*, 1993; Wilde *et al.*, 2003). Other components can influence the formation and stability of beer foam. For example, ethanol improves foam formation but decreases its stability (Brierley *et al.*, 1996; Evans and Sheehan, 2002). Hop acids increase foam stability in forming complexes with protein at the gas–liquid interface (Smith *et al.*, 1998; Evans and Sheehan, 2002). Lipids are the main foam-negative substance of beer. These hydrophobic and/or amphiphilic molecules adsorb rapidly at the interface and destabilize the protein film by displacing protein and decreasing protein–protein interactions. This leads to the rupture and coalescence of foam bubbles (Wilde *et al.*, 2003).

The malting and brewing process transforms the barley albumins into foaming proteins. The mechanism involved in these structural maturation has been recently delineated, especially for one of the major beer proteins, LTP1. Actually, the barley LTP1 does not form any foam while the corresponding beer protein display good foaming properties (Bech *et al.*, 1995; Marion *et al.*, 2001). In beer, LTP1 is a mixture of glycated proteins displaying different unfolding state (Jégou *et al.*, 2000). Glycation occurs on kilning during the malting process while unfolding occurs on brewing (Jégou *et al.*, 2001; Van Nierop *et al.*, 2004). Heat-induced unfolding of LTP1 is strengthened by the reduction of disulfide bonds of the protein during the extraction of malt (Perrocheau *et al.*, 2006). The disulfide bond reducing mechanism of malt has not been identified yet, but it should involve the thioredoxin and/or glutathione oxido-reducing pathways (Marx *et al.*, 2003). The other important modification is the acylation of LTP1. This acylation is catalyzed by two enzymes from the embryo, a 9-lipoxygenase (9-LOX) and an allene oxide synthase (AOS). 9-LOX generates a 9-hydroperoxide from linoleic acid, the major polyunsaturated free fatty acids (FFAs) from cereal seeds while the AOS transforms the hydroperoxide in the corresponding allene oxide. The electrophilic attack of the unstable allene oxide by an acidic side chain of the protein (Asp7) leads to the covalent binding of an alpha-ketol to LTP1 (Figure 24.5). This acylation has been observed in beer for the glycated LTP1 (Jégou *et al.*, 2000). Up to two alpha-ketol can be covalently bound to the barley LTP1 (Jégou *et al.*, 2001; Perrocheau *et al.*, 2006). Finally, glycation and acylation increase the amphiphilic character of the protein while unfolding improves spreading of the protein at the air–water interface allowing a better anchoring in the interface through the acyl adducts and formation of protein–protein interaction in the film surrounding gas bubbles (Figure 24.6). Lipids and especially FFAs are detrimental to the formation and stability of beer foam (Wilde *et al.*, 2003). Trapping of the major barley FFA (i.e. linoleic acid) by LTP1 through

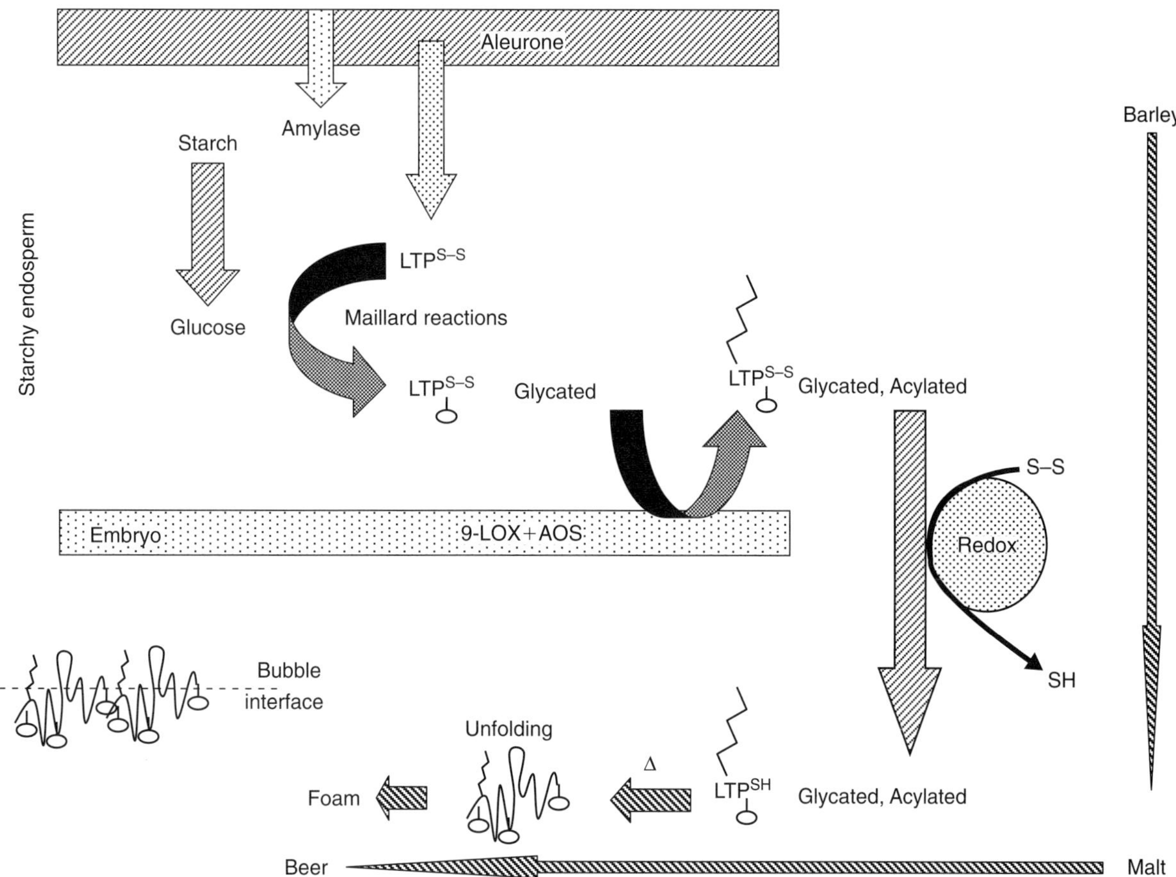

Figure 24.6 Structural maturation of LTP1 from a non-foaming protein to a foaming protein during the malting and brewing processes. During germination of barley, amylase secreted by the aleurone cells into the starchy albumen provides glucose and maltose (starch hydrolysis) necessary for glycation of the LTP1 during the kilning step of malting. During germination of barley or extraction of malt, LTP1 or glycated LTP1 from the aleurone cells is acylated by the enzyme complex from the embryo (i.e LOX and AOS). On mashing the non-reduced $LTP^{S\text{–}S}$ is reduced to LTP^{SH} by a redox system from malt. The disulfide bond reduction and boiling promote protein unfolding during brewing. The glycated, acylated and unfolded beer LTP1 displays higher foaming properties than the corresponding non-modified protein from barley.

the combined activity of LOX and AOS should limit the accumulation of the foam-destabilizing FFAs. This mechanism could act synergistically with the non-covalent lipid binding (Cooper *et al.*, 2002) to protect beer against lipid-induced foam destabilization. Finally, it should be emphasized that the quality of beer foam is not due to a unique protein but to complex associations between the different beer proteins and between proteins and other components (phenolic compounds, hop acids, minerals, etc.) as well as to the technological process (i.e. malting and brewing) that induce different structural modifications essential to generate pro-foaming entities.

Over-foaming can produce on opening packages. This phenomenon called gushing is one of the major source of economical losses for the brewers. Primary gushing is caused by factors from malt or other cereal raw material entering in the brewing process. Secondary gushing is due to the presence of aggregates and particles related to technological impurities or to haze. Primary gushing is closely related to *Fusarium* contamination of malt and is assumed to be due to surface active proteins that form a highly stable film around gas bubbles. Most studies converge for a role of small proteins of fungi (i.e. hydrophobins). These fungal proteins with four disulfide bonds are highly stable. They can survive to heating on brewing and only small quantities of these proteins can induce gushing (Linder *et al.*, 2005). These proteins display an amphiphilic character that allow rapid adsorption at the gas–water interface to form stable and ordered aggregated protein films with unique elasticity (Szilvay *et al.*, 2007). As suggested by Hippeli and Elsner (2002), the modified forms of LTPs (i.e. glycated and acylated proteins) could also be involved in gushing. These proteins share structural characteristics with the gushing factor isolated from wort (Kitabatake, 1978). Although these proteins are essential to the foaming properties of beer, they could induce gushing above a threshold concentration. Since synthesis of most LTPs is induced on pathogen attack (Douliez *et al.*, 2000; Blein *et al.*, 2002), higher level of

LTPs could be produced in response to the fungal infection of barley. The role of LTPs in gushing, alone or in interaction with fungal hydrophobins, has not been highlighted yet, but has to be investigated in the perspective of improving the quality of beer foam by increasing LTP content either through barley breeding or by genetic modifications.

Proteins and Beer Haze

Brilliance or brightness (i.e. absence of a haze or sediment) is considered as a significant parameter for the acceptance of beer by most consumers. Haze is generally formed on cold conditioning of freshly fermented beer and can be due to multiple materials as yeast cells and colloidal particles of organic or mineral origin (Bamforth, 1999). Much research has been conducted to characterize the haze-forming materials in beer as well as in other beverages by analyzing the chemical composition of the sediment (Siebert, 1999). Significantly, haze-forming molecules are mainly composed of polypeptides derived from the storage proline-rich proteins of barley endosperm (i.e. hordeins) and polyphenols from malted barley and hops. Another protein, the barley trypsin inhibitor, that is not a proline-rich proteins in regard to hordeins, also seems to play a role in the formation of beer haze (Robinson *et al.*, 2007). Although carbohydrates are present in high amount in the sediment, it was shown that they are not involved in haze formation but co-aggregate with haze particles (Siebert, 1999). Haze is mainly due to the formation of protein and polyphenol aggregates on cold conditioning. The polyphenol–protein complex grows to sufficient size to result in turbidity and finally can form large particles that can sediment.

Conclusion

As illustrated here for two important factors of the quality of beers (i.e. foams and haze) proteins are essential components. Until now, individual protein components have been identified as the major actor of these properties. Their technological role involves structural maturation that is under the control of both physiological and technological processes. Today, there is also evidence that the role of proteins on the quality of beer involves molecular and macromolecular interactions. These interactions have been poorly studied and it will be essential in the future to devise a beer interactome strategy to delineate the precise role of these interactions on the foaming and haze-forming properties of beer. These studies will allow to improve the quality of beer through barley breeding and technological processes. Finally, it is worthy to note that beer concentrates on plant allergens and especially the ubiquitous plant LTP allergen. The low prevalence of allergy to beer can be related to the structural modification that occurs on malting and brewing. Actually, chemical modifications and unfolding should improve the sensitivity of this putative beer allergen to proteases of the digestive tract (Marion *et al.*, 2004).

References

Asero, R., Mistrello, G., Roncarolo, D., Amato, S. and van Ree, R. (2001). *Ann. Allergy Asthma Immunol.* 87, 65–67.

Bakan, B., Hamberg, M., Perrocheau, L., Maume, D., Rogniaux, H., Tranquet, O., Rondeau, C., Blein, J.-P., Ponchet, M. and Marion, D. (2006). *J. Biol. Chem.* 281, 38981–38988.

Bamforth, C.W. (1985). *J. Inst. Brew.* 91, 370–383.

Bamforth, C.W. (1999). *J. Am. Soc. Brew. Chem.* 57, 81–90.

Bech, L.M., Vaag, P., Heinemann, B. and Breddam, K. (1995). *Proceedings of the European Brewery Convention Congress, Brussels.* IRL Press, Oxford, UK. pp. 561–568.

Blein, J.-P., Coutos-Thévenot, P., Marion, D. and Ponchet, M. (2002). *Trend. Plant Sci.* 7, 293–296.

Boutrot, F., Guirao, A., Alary, R., Joudrier, P. and Gautier, M.F. (2005). *Biochim. Biophys. Acta* 1730, 114–125.

Brierley, E.R., Wilde, P.J., Onishi, A., Highes, P.J. and Clark, D.C. (1996). *J. Sci. Food Agric.* 70, 531–537.

Cooper, D.J., Husband, F.A., Mills, E.N.C. and Wilde, P.J. (2002). *J. Agric. Food Chem.* 50, 7645–7650.

Curioni, A., Pressi, G., Furegon, L. and Peruffo, A.D.B. (1995). *J. Agric. Food Chem.* 43, 2620–2626.

Douliez, J.-P., Michon, T., Elmorjani, K. and Marion, D. (2000). *J. Cereal Sci.* 32, 1–20.

Elliott, P.R., Pei, X.Y., Dafforn, T.R. and Lomas, D.A. (2000). *Protein Sci.* 9, 1274–1281.

Evans, D.E. and Sheehan, M.C. (2002). *J. Am. Soc. Brew. Chem.* 60, 47–57.

Hejgaard, J. and Kaersgaard, P. (1983). *J. Inst. Brew.* 89, 402–410.

Hippeli, S. and Elsner, E.F. (2002). *Z. Naturforsch.* 57c, 1–8.

Huntington, J.A. (2006). *Trend. Biochem. Sci.* 31, 427–435.

Jégou, S., Douliez, J.-P., Molle, D., Boivin, P. and Marion, D. (2000). *J. Agric. Food Chem.* 48, 5023–5029.

Jégou, S., Douliez, J.-P., Molle, D., Boivin, P. and Marion, D. (2001). *J. Agric. Food Chem.* 49, 4942–4949.

Jones, B.L. (2005). *J. Cereal Sci.* 42, 271–280.

Kaslik, G., Kardos, J., Szabo, E., Szilagyi, L., Zavodszky, P., Westler, W.M., Markley, J.L. and Graf, L. (1997). *Biochemistry* 36, 5455–5464.

Kitabatake, K. (1978). *Bull. Brew. Sci.* 24, 21–32.

Lerche, M.H. and Poulsen, F.M. (1998). *Protein Sci.* 7, 2490–2498.

Linder, M.B., Szilvay, G.R., Nakari-Setälä, T. and Penttilä, M. (2005). *FEMS Microbiol. Rev.* 29, 877–896.

Maeda, K., Yokoi, S., Kamada, K. and Kamimura, M. (1991). *J. Am. Soc. Brew. Chem.* 49, 14–18.

Marion, D., Jégou, S., Douliez, J.-P., Gaborit, T. and Boivin, P. (2001). *Proc. Eur. Brew. Conv.* 28, 67–74.

Marion, D., Douliez, J.-P., Gautier, M.-F. and Elmorjani, K. (2004). Plant lipid transfer proteins: Relationships between allerginicity and structural, biological and technological properties. In Mills, E.N.C. and Shewry, P.W. (eds), *Plant Food Allergens*, pp. 57–69. Blackwell Publishing, Oxford, UK.

Marx, C., Wong, J.H. and Buchanan, B.B. (2003). *Planta* 216, 454–460.

Østergaard, H., Rasmussen, S.K., Roberts, T.H. and Hejgaard, J. (2000). *J. Biol. Chem.* 275, 33272–33279.

Perrocheau, L., Rogniaux, H., Boivin, P. and Marion, D. (2005). *Proteomics* 5, 2849–2858.

Perrocheau, L., Bakan, B., Boivin, P. and Marion, D. (2006). *J. Agric. Food Chem.* 54, 3108–3113.

Pons, J.L., de Lamotte, F., Gautier, M.F. and Delsuc, M.A. (2003). *J. Biol. Chem.* 278, 14249–14256.

Robinson, L.H., Juttner, J., Milligan, A., Lahnstein, J., Ellington, J.K. and Evans, D.E. (2007). *J. Cereal Sci.* 45, 343–352.

Siebert, K.J. (1999). *J. Agric. Food Chem.* 47, 353–362.

Smith, R.J., Davidson, D. and Wilson, R.J.H. (1998). *J. Am. Soc. Brew. Chem.* 56, 52–57.

Sorensen, S.B. and Ottesen, M. (1978). *Carlsberg Res. Commun.* 43, 133–144.

Sorensen, S.B., Bech, L.M., Muldbjerg, M., Beenfeldt, T. and Breddam, K. (1993). *Tech. Q. Master Brew. Assoc. Am.* 30, 136–145.

Szilvay, G.R., Paananen, A., Laurikainen, K., Vuorimaa, E., Lemmetyinen, H., Peltonen, J. and Linder, M.B. (2007). *Biochemistry* 46, 2345–2354.

Van Nierop, S.N., Evans, D.E., Axcell, B.C., Cantrell, I.C. and Rautenbach, M. (2004). *J. Agric. Food Chem.* 52, 3120–3129.

Vercammen, D., Belenghi, B., Van de Cotte, B., Beunens, T., Gavigan, J.-A., De Rycke, R., Brackenier, A., Inzé, D., Harris, J.L. and Van Breugesem, F. (2006). *J. Mol. Biol.* 364, 625–636.

Wilde, P.J., Husband, F.A., Cooper, D., Ridout, M.J. and Mills, E.N.C. (2003). *J. Am. Soc. Brew. Chem.* 60, 31–36.

25
Amino Acids in Beer

Marta Fontana Department of Agriculture and Environmental Sciences, University of Udine, Udine, Italy
Stefano Buiatti Department of Food Science, University of Udine, Udine, Italy

Abstract

Nitrogenous compounds are considered very important in beer playing a key role in determining the quality and stability of the finished product. They include amino acids, peptides, polypeptides, proteins, nucleic acids and their degradation products. These compounds affect flavor, foam stability, haze formation, color, yeast nutrition and biological stability. The nitrogenous compounds in beer are derived mainly from barley malt and its adjuncts. Moreover the brewing process may have an important role in determining complex profile of nitrogenous compounds present in the final beer. The content of nitrogen compounds in barley depends on variety and on environmental condition in cultivation. During malting the storage proteins are degraded to amino acids and other peptides. These amino acids are important in wort to promote a good fermentation and the yeast budding. During fermentation amino acids are used in different ways by yeasts and may have many effects on the final quality of beer: in particular the amino nitrogen content influences the flavor profile of beer. The amino acids present in final beer could influence negatively the stability of product promoting haze formation. Nitrogen compounds may also play an important role influencing the foam quality and stability.

List of Abbrevations

kDa	Kilodaltons
PVPP	Polyvinylpolypyrrolidone
LPT1	Lipid transfer protein 1
EBC	European Brewery Convention

Introduction

Quality and stability are the most important qualities of alcoholic beverages, particularly in beer. Different and complex compounds are responsible for these properties. About 800 constituents have been characterized in beer and very important are macromolecules such as proteins, nucleic acids, polysaccharides and lipids (Briggs *et al.*, 2004). Several authors considered that the most important substances present in beer are alcohol and proteins. These proteins in beer are present at 0.3–1.0 g/l of total nitrogen, equivalent to 0.11–0.63% of protein (Hough *et al.*, 1982). If there is general agreement on the fact that hydrolysis of proteins produces polypeptides, peptides and amino acids, there is discordance about the classification of the same proteins. Some authors classify proteins by their function, others by molecular size. Only few proteins survive into beer and most of the nitrogen is present as polypeptides. The simpler nitrogen constituents of beer comprise mainly α-amino acids and the estimation of the latter has been the subject of several researches (Charalambous, 1981), therefore, the study of amino acids is frequently associated to the study of proteins. Proteins and their derivatives play a key role in determining beer quality and stability; they are in fact responsible for yeast nutrition and performance, influence malt color, foam formation, permanent haze and may affect the flavor. Amino acids in beer are originated mostly from malt and in particular, content and composition of proteins and amino acids depend on raw materials and on technological process of brewing.

Nitrogenous Compounds

The content of nitrogenous compounds is often reported as the protein content. The factor 6.25 is used to convert total nitrogen to total protein because, on average, proteins contain 16% nitrogen. But not many proteic substances contain nitrogen and the protein value obtained in this way could be too high. Thus, it is sometimes utilized the factor 5.7. Amino acids are the principal building blocks of proteins. They are incorporated into proteins by transfer

Beer in Health and Disease Prevention
ISBN: 978-0-12-373891-2

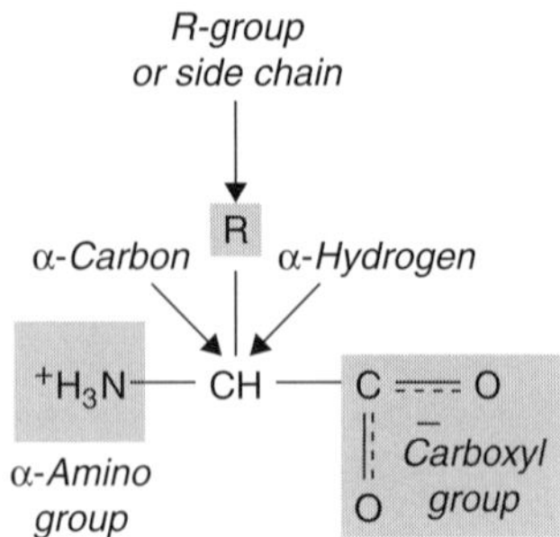

Figure 25.1 Basic structure of an amino acid.

Table 25.1 The amino acids are grouped according to the characteristics of the side chains

Side chains	*Amino acids*
Aliphatic	Alanine, glycine, isoleucine, leucine, proline, valine
Aromatic	Phenylalanine, tryptophan, tyrosine
Acidic	Aspartic acid, glutamic acid
Basic	Arginine, histidine, lysine
Hydroxylic	Serine, threonine
Sulfur-containing	Cysteine, methionine
Amidic (containing amide group)	Asparagines, glutamine

RNA according to the genetic code while messenger RNA is being decoded by ribosomes. During and after the final assembly of a protein, the amino acid content dictates the spatial and biochemical properties of the protein. The amino acids in peptides and proteins (excluding proline) consist of a carboxylic acid (—COOH) and an amino (—NH_2) functional group attached to the same tetrahedral carbon atom. This carbon is the α-carbon (Figure 25.1).

All amino acids found in proteins have this basic structure, differing only in the structure of the R-group or the side chain. The amino acids are grouped according to the characteristics of the side chains (Table 25.1).

Amino Acids in Barley

Production of high-quality malt depends on a number of factors. One of the most important parameters is the nitrogen content in malting barley. The nitrogenous components in barley change with the variety, the growing season, the soil and the amount of fertilizer and topography of the field (Bertholdsson, 1999; Agu and Palmer, 2003). In particular, variation in quality is caused by a complex set of interacting factors during the growth of the crop (De Ruiter and Haslemore, 1996). For example, high availability of nitrogen and stress situation (drought or heat in association with drought) may increase the protein level above the limit for malting barley. In fact, it is very important that barley used to produce malt has a grain protein concentration (GPC) lower than 11.5% (Bertholdsson, 1999); higher protein in barley is undesirable because of reduced potential fermentable extract which decreases the amount of beer that can be made from barley's malt. Nevertheless higher nitrogen barleys are likely to produce extracts that are rich in soluble nitrogen, free amino nitrogen (FAN) and peptide nitrogen. In contrast, lower nitrogen barleys are likely to produce extracts that are rich in carbohydrates. While some researchers and maltsters believe that barleys containing higher nitrogen levels would produce higher enzyme levels, other authors seem to disagree with this concept (Agu, 2003). Many studies have evaluated the content of proteins and their fractions in barley and beer but only few works have considered the evaluation of amino acids content. Table 25.2 shows the content of amino acids (%) in grain protein of barley.

Instead, it is usually accepted to classify barley proteins, and generally cereal proteins, with their solubility characteristics in different solvents. By classifying barley proteins with solvents, four different fractions can be obtained. Proteins soluble in salt solution are albumins and globulins which include enzymes. The protein material, which is insoluble in salt solution but soluble in warm alcohol, is prolamine (called hordein in barley). Finally, protein material insoluble in warm alcohol is glutelin (Hough, 1994). In Table 25.3 the protein composition of barley is reported.

Hordein is the major storage protein in the endosperm. It is a complex mixture of proteins that can be separated using sodium dodecyl sulfate and polyacrylamide gel electrophoresis (SDS-PAGE) into four groups with different molecular weight: A (<25 kDa), B (35–46 kDa), C (59–72 kDa) and D (90–105 kDa) (Palmer, 1989). Fraction A has low molecular weight, with bands frequently indistinct and variable for distinguishing barley varieties (Baxter and Wainwright, 1979). Shewry (1992) has reported a fractioning of hordein using SDS-PAGE and two-dimensional analyses (isoelectrofocusing IEF/SDS-PAGE): these polypeptides are classified into two main sub-fractions: B and C and at least two minor sub-fractions: D and γ. These groups are also called, on the basis of their amino acid content, sulfur poor (C hordein), sulfur rich (B and γ hordein) and high molecular weight prolamins (D hordein). The amino acids composition of B, C, D and γ fractions have been reported in Table 25.4.

Hordeins are characterized by having high levels of amino acids proline and glutamine. The levels of tryptophan and threonine are low and level of lysine is reported to be limited (Bewley and Black, 1994). The B and D hordeins fractions are reported to contain sulfur (cystine) bridges (Field *et al.*, 1983). Howard *et al.* (1996) have suggested that the amount of fraction D hordein in grain should be an accurate guide to malting quality than the use of total protein alone. The amino acid composition of the total protein fraction present in grains is strongly influenced by hordein (Bewley and Black, 1994) but the proportion of the different hordein

Table 25.2 Amino acids present in barley proteins

Amino acid	*(%)*
Alanine	3.8
Arginine	4.6
Aspartic acid	6.0
Cystine	1.1
Glutamic acid	26.8
Glycine	3.6
Histidine	2.1
Isoleucine	3.7
Leucine	6.7
Lysine	3.4
Methionine	1.2
Phenylalanine	5.9
Proline	12.6
Serine	4.3
Threonine	3.4
Tryptophan	–
Tyrosine	2.8
Valine	4.8

Source: Modified from Bewley and Black (1994).

Table 25.3 Approximate percent protein composition of barley

Protein composition	*(%)*
Albumin	13
Globulin	12
Prolamin (Hordein)	52
Glutelin	23

Source: Modified from Bewley and Black (1994).

Table 25.4 Amino acid composition (mol%) of the groups of hordein polypepties

	Groups of hordein			
Amino acid	*B*	*C*	*D*	γ
Aspartic acid	1.4	1.0	1.3	2.9
Threonine	2.1	1.0	8.1	3.1
Serine	4.7	4.6	9.7	5.5
Glutamic acid	35.4	41.2	29.6	32.4
Proline	20.6	30.6	11.6	16.5
Glycine	1.5	0.3	15.7	5.9
Alanine	2.2	0.7	2.5	2.6
Cysteine	2.5	0	1.5	2.7
Valine	5.6	1.0	4.5	3.7
Methionine	0.6	0.2	0.2	1.2
Isoleucine	4.1	2.6	0.7	2.9
Leucine	7.0	3.6	3.3	8.6
Tyrosine	2.5	2.3	3.9	1.7
Phenylalanine	4.8	8.8	1.4	4.7
Histidine	2.1	1.1	3.4	2.0
Lysine	0.5	0.2	1.1	1.6
Arginine	2.4	0.8	1.5	2.0

Note: Hordein is a complex mixture of protein that can be classified and separated into two major groups (B and C hordeins) and into two minor groups (D and γ hordeins) which vary in their molecular weight, isoelectric point and amino acid composition.

Source: Shewry (1992).

fractions present in mature grain are affected by growth conditions, particularly nitrogen nutrition. Glutelin is a storage protein present in the aleurone layer and globulin is the storage protein of embryo but it represents only a small proportion of the total reserve protein of the whole grain. Albumins and globulins, which include many enzymes, are not seriously deficient in specific amino acids. They contain a higher level in lysine and methionine than hordein (Briggs, 1998). However, Kunze (1999) has reported that globulin does not completely precipitate during boiling of wort and can promote haze in beer, whereas albumins precipitate completely when wort is boiled. Unmalted adjuncts such as rice or corn for all practical purposes do not contain proteins that are soluble in wort. Thus, their use will directly dilute the protein content of wort (Fix, 2000).

Amino Acids in Brewing Process

During malting, the storage proteins of barley, mainly in the endosperm, are hydrolyzed by proteases into polypeptides, peptides and amino acids. During this step there is some utilization of amino acids (other loss of protein will occur during mashing due to precipitation), but for the most part, the protein content of malt is similar to that of the barley from which the malt was made. There is some continuation of protein breakdown in the mash, but the extent is greatly influenced by the mashing program used (Fix, 2000). The amino acids present in wort are necessary to promote yeast multiplication and a good fermentation. The presence of FAN, peptides and polypeptides also influences yeast growth, the foam and haze properties of derived beer (Agu and Palmer, 1999). The value of 150–175 mg/l of α-amino nitrogen is optimal to maintain a healthy yeast and maximum fermentation.

- **During fermentation amino acids are used in different ways by yeasts.**

Wort amino acids represent the major source of assimilable nitrogen for brewing yeast. Yeast metabolizes each one of them in a different way largely independent of the conditions of fermentation. On the basis of yeast assimilation, amino acids have been categorized into four groups. In Table 25.5 the order of absorption of amino acids from brewer's wort by yeast is illustrated.

Group A amino acids are absorbed rapidly, in the first step of fermentation (about 20 h). Amino acids of group B are utilized more slowly, and group C amino acids are taken up only after the complete removal of group A amino acids in wort. Group D consists only in proline, in fact yeast uses proline more slowly under anaerobic condition. Proline has no free amino group and therefore cannot take part directly in transamination reactions that often cause the formation of flavor-producing beer compounds. If proline is present in final beer it supports the instability of product. The order of amino acid assimilation is not affected by the concentration of specific amino acids but appears to involve the nature and specificities of amino acids permeases. The process of uptake of amino acids by yeast appears very complex. It is often convenient to consider individual aspects of metabolism in terms of biochemical pathways. In fermentation, amino acids present in wort are preferentially taken up and utilized to supply nitrogen to the cell and yeasts are considered to incorporate up to 50% of wort amino acids directly into protein. Of these, approximately one-third are excreted back into wort, but this proportion can be higher in adverse conditions. Under normal conditions, 33.5% of the wort amino acids are consumed during the fermentation, while 16.5% of the wort amino acids are assimilated, only to be excreted back into the fermenting wort (Fix, 2000). As seen before, yeasts take up amino acids in a definite order. The amino nitrogen is used as a nutrient, while the carbon skeleton is sent to the oxo-acid pool in the yeast cell for further processing. As a general rule, amino acids are not treated separately, but rather in pairs. The Strickland reaction is a major mechanism whereby one amino acid donates hydrogen atoms and the second acid acts as an acceptor.

Table 25.5 Classification of wort amino acids according to their consumption rate by yeast

Group A	*Group B*	*Group C*	*Group D*
Fast absorption	*Intermediate absorption*	*Slow absorption*	*Little or no absorption*
Glutamic acid	Valine	Glycine	Proline
Aspartic acid	Methionine	Phenylalanine	
Asparagine	Leucine	Tyrosine	
Glutamine	Isoleucine	Tryptophan	
Serine	Histidine	Alanine	
Threonine			
Lysine			
Arginine			

In Figure 25.2, amino nitrogen and carbon skeletons (oxo-acids) are shown.

When amino acids enter the cell their amino groups are removed by a transaminase system and their carbon skeletons assimilated. Transaminase catalyze readily reversible reactions dependent on the presence of cofactors. The oxo-acids, derived from the carbon skeleton of the amino acid present in wort or from carbohydrate metabolism, enter the cell's metabolic pools. The synthesis of amino acids by the yeast cell then proceeds and, in the latter instance, *ex novo* synthesis of amino acids is said to occur and the penultimate reaction is usually transamination (Hough *et al.*, 1982). Yeast-synthesized amino acids, including lysine, histidine, arginine and leucine, are extremely critical because their carbon skeletons are derived entirely from exogenous wort amino acids with no carbon contribution from sugar catabolism. Low levels of lysine, histidine, arginine and leucine can cause important changes in yeast-induced metabolism of nitrogen, lowering the final quality of beer (Meilgaard, 1976). Amino acids such as proline, threonine and methionine are essential because they are generally produced by yeast until late in the fermentation and valine, glycine and tyrosine are critical because late they serve as the major sources of yeast carbon skeletons. Jones and Pierce (1969) have reported that concentration in wort of amino acids isoleucine, valine, phenylalanine, glycine, alanine, tyrosine, lysine, histidine, arginine and leucine are considered important and changes in the concentration of amino acids in wort will influence nitrogen metabolism.

- **Free amino acids are very important on influencing flavor development in beer.**

Many factors may influence the beer flavor but, in general, aromatic profile of beer is determinated by yeast and by their ability to grow and to metabolize the nitrogenous constituents of wort. The amino nitrogen content influences the flavor profile of beer mainly via higher alcohol and ester formation. In this metabolism, the amino group of amino acids may be transferred to an enzyme (transaminase) and the remaining carbon skeleton excreted or used to regenerate adenine dinucleotide phosphate (NAD^+). The oxo-acid produced by transamination is decarboxylated to give carbon dioxide and an aldehyde. The aldehyde

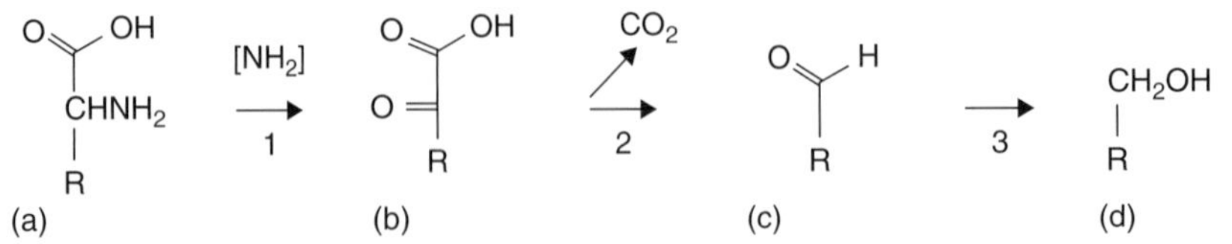

Figure 25.2 Formation of higher alcohols, aldehydes and oxo-acids from amino acids. (generalized pathway: R any amino acid chain) a = amino acid; b = oxo-acid; c = aldehyde; d = alcohol [NH_2] indicates group transferred to transaminase enzyme CO_2 = carbon dioxide Enzyme involved: 1 = transaminase; 2 = decarboxylase; 3 = dehydrogenase.

is then reduced to an alcohol, called higher alcohol. These substances have higher boiling points than ethanol and are potently aromatic. A variety of alcohols are produced during yeast metabolism and in Table 25.6 the amino acids level present in wort and flavors compound obtained during their catabolism are reported.

A similar correlation was found between the wort amino acid content and the formation of higher alcohols, ester and carbonyl compounds in the resulting beer by Äyräpää (1971). In their work, Vesely *et al.* (2004) have reported the use of single amino acids by yeast during two different fermentation temperatures: 10°C and 15°C. The effect of the fermentation temperature on the yeast causes different use of single amino acids with different aromatic profiles in beer. The higher the temperature, the more significant the amino acid level decrease during fermentation, and the higher rate of yeast growth. At the end of a fermentation carried out at 15°C, 90% of amino acids are metabolized, except for glycine and proline. It is well known that glycine is one of the last amino acids utilized by yeast and proline is not a substrate of yeast metabolism. At 10°C fermentation, utilization of amino acids by the yeast was slightly lower, particularly for alanine, glycine, histidine and tyrosine. Limited nitrogen concentration may alter the time course of flavor precursor production and therefore change the flavor of the final beer (Dufour and Devreux, 1986). The compounds responsible are mainly butane-2,3-dione (diacetyl) and pentane-2,3-dione, by-products of valine, leucine and isoleucine amino acids (Almeida *et al.*, 2004). If valine is deficient in wort, yeast synthesizes it by a pathway involving α-acetolactate as an intermediate. Accumulation and oxidation of acetolactate produce diacetyl that causes flavor defects (Pollock, 1988). Sulfur compounds also influence the flavor and aroma of beer. They can derive from organic sulfur compounds in wort, such as the amino acids methionine and cysteine and peptides and proteins that contain sulfur. Wainwright (1971) has reported that the wort's content of the sulfur-containing amino acid methionine greatly influences the production of volatile sulfur compounds by yeast: a methionine-poor wort leads to higher sulfur dioxide and hydrogen sulfide levels in beer.

- **The color of final beer depends on malt used and products of Maillard reaction originated from amino acids and sugar.**

During kilning, malting and boiling of wort various complex compounds are generated, mainly melanoidines. These compounds are the products of Maillard reaction, partly responsible of the color of beer, and obtained through a reaction between amino acids and sugar. Charalambous (1981) has reported that the most important browning reaction is believed to take place between the amino acid proline and maltose to 3-hydroxy-2-metyl-4-pyrone (maltol). The level of proline in wort can thus affect color development in beer.

Amino Acids in Final Beer

Only about 30% of nitrogen compounds in barley are present in the final beer. As previously reported, beers contain only low levels of amino acids, since during fermentation amino acids are assimilated for yeast growth (Briggs *et al.*, 2004); in particular the content of proline is quantitatively higher if compared to other amino acids. In beer, nitrogenous compounds comprise denatured proteins, denatured nucleic acid, amino acids, amides, amines and heterocyclic compounds. Beers from all malt wort contain 32.6–44.7 mg/l α-amino nitrogen equivalent to 8.2% of the total nitrogen and beers brewed from a grist containing 22.8% of wheat flour contained 21.3–26.7 mg/l α-amino nitrogen, 5.8% of the total nitrogen (Hough *et al.*, 1982). Table 25.7 has reported the content of amino acids found in different beers.

Table 25.6 Compounds originated by amino acid catabolism in anaerobic environment

Amino acid	*α-Keto acid*	*Aldehydes*	*Alcohols*	*Carboxylic acids*	*Others*
Asparagine	Oxaloacetate	–	–	Malate	Diacetyl, acetoine
Isoleucine	α-Keto-β-methylvaleate	2-Methylbutanal	2-Methylbutanol	2-Methylbutanoic acid	
Leucine	α-Keto-iso-caproate	3-Methylbutanal	3-Methylbutanol	3-Methylbutanoic acid	
Methionine	α-Keto-butyrate	3-Methylthiopropanal	3-Methylthiopropanol	3-Methylthiopropionic acid	Methenethiol
Phenylanine	Phenyl pyruvate	Phenylacetaldehyde	Phenylethanol	Phenylacetic acid	
Tryptophane	Indole pyruvate	Indole-3-acetaldehyde	Tryptophol	Indol-3-acetic acid	Skatole
Tyrosine	*p*-OH-phenyl puruvate	*p*-OH-phenylacetaldehyde	*p*-OH-phenyl-ethanol	*p*-OH-phenylacetic acid	*p*-Cresol
Valine	α-Keto-isovalerate	2-Methylpropanal	2-Methylpropanol	2-Methylpropanoic acid	

Source: Ardö (2006).

Table 25.7 Amino acid composition of different kinds of beers

			After Hough et al.[a]									
Amino acid	*After Derby*[a] *(mg/l)*	*After Hardwick*[a] *(mg/l)*	*India pale ale (mg/l)*	*Draft bitter (mg/l)*	*Stout (mg/l)*	*After Drawer*[b] *European (German) (mg/l)*	*After Chen*[b] *Canadian (mg/l)*	*Indian pale ale*[c] *(mg α-amino N/L)*	*Brown ale*[c] *(mg α-amino N/l)*	*Draft bitter*[c] *(mg α-amino N/l)*	*Mild ale*[c] *(mg α-amino N/l)*	*Stout*[c] *(mg α-amino N/l)*
Alpha alanine						28.2–206.1	65–175					
Beta alanine						0.6–2.7						
Alanine	14.5–21.6	10–130		2.7					0.19	0.43		0.2
Ammonia								1.07	0.92	1.88	1.36	1.7
Arginine	2.0–9.4	9–110		1.1		24.6–292.6	165–185			0.18		
Asparagine						1.0–15.7						
Aspartic acid	4.5–20.6	6–45		1	1.25	16.7–82.4	48–68		0.04	0.16	0.4	0.2
Citrullin						1.1–8.1						
Cysteine	Traces	0–11				7.7–21.4	94–130					
Cystine		1–6				2.5–7.8						
Gamma aminobutyric acid						30.4–78	124–163					
Glutamic acid	1.2–6.6	9–50		0.9		17.3–76.3	70–97		0.04	0.14	0.2	
Glutamine						5.8–17.5						
Glycine	8.1–11.5	9–45		0.5		10.8–50.9	59–68	0.21	0.01	0.08	0.19	
Histidine	5.9–20.4	9–50				16.1–46.3	14–18	0.14				
Hydroxyproline						3.2–7.8	25–34					
Isoleucine	2.1–6.6	5–40		0.06	2.5	11.6–75.0	40–65			0.01		0.4
Leucine	2.0–10.9	3–60		0.19	2.5	23.5–159.1	57–89			0.03		0.4
Lysine	0.2–4.4	5–60	2.6	3.1	1.25	16.4–47.1	77–80	0.42	0.31	0.50	0.32	0.4
Methionine	1.4–2.7	0–10		1.5		5.0–9.6	29–36			0.24		
Ornithin						0–7.1	51–63					
Phenylalanine	3.1–32.4	5–99		3.1		9.5–38.0	56–76		0.04	0.49	0.07	
Proline	151–169	~400	177	178	2.38	242.2–761.9	45–46	28.25	13.32	28.53	22.05	39.05
Pyroglutamic acid						5.1–13.8						
Sarcosine						1.9–4.9						
Serine	5.3	2–12		0.9	1.25	9.3–29.6	59–63			0.15	0.05	0.2
Threonine	3.7–4.6	0–10		4.1	1.25	7.1–18.6	67–116			0.66		0.2
Tryptophan	8.6	1–12	11.1	12.9	3.1	4.5–19.9	48–61	1.77	1.62	2.06	1.62	0.8
Tyrosine	14.7–28.4	9–80		2.2		13.9–96.2	38–65		0.50	0.35	0.07	
Valine	2.9–17.8	5–80		0.19		21.6–149.6	159–169			0.03		0.5
Total amino acids						574.6–2284.5	1882–2192					

Source: Modified from [a]Bamforth (2004), [b]Charalambous (1981), [c]Briggs *et al.* (2004).

The level of protein in beer is low but it has very important effect on the quality of beer. Many studies on the characterization of proteins in beer are associated to studies of the quality aspect, often associated to foam and haze stability. In fact, these two aspects, foam and haze stability, are of critical importance to brewers (Evans *et al.*, 2003).

- **Nitrogenous compounds can combine with polyphenols to form complex responsible of haze in beer.**

One of the most common quality defects found by the consumers in beer is cloudiness or haze, which can negatively effect the shelf-life of the product and its acceptability. Many consumers think that it is caused by a microbial contamination, but beers are biologically safe after the pasteurization treatment which destroys microbial contamination. In fact it is important to distinguish the two different kinds of haze in beer: biological haze and non-biological (or colloidal) haze. Microbiological haze is caused by infections that involve bacterial or yeast and can be avoided with a sterile filtration and pasteurization. The presence of colloidal or non-biological haze can appear in bright beer and it can be caused by several types of substances. The most important non-biological haze is chill (or permanent) haze. Chill haze starts to develop at low temperature (0–4°C) with particle size between 0.1 and 1.0 μm, but it disappears when the beer is returned to 20°C. On the contrary, permanent haze is present in beer even at 20°C with particle between 1 and 10 μm (Bamforth, 1999). Chill haze is an important problem with lager beers which are served at lower temperatures than ales. The appearance of haze is a visual clue of the reduced flavor stability of beer since the haze and flavor stability is both directly influenced by oxidation processes during storage (Robinson *et al.*, 2004). Several chemical species can enter into such insoluble complexes. However the most common chill hazes found in beer are originated by interactions between proteins and polyphenols. These compounds form weak, temperature-sensitive hydrogen bonds that are broken as the beer's temperature increases. The other form of haze is permanent and is characterized by strong bonds of covalent type in which constituent atoms share the available electrons to achieve a more stable energy state. Typical protein–polyphenol haze consisted of about 50% protein, 25% polyphenol and the remaining 25% from polysaccharides and metals. The 0.1% of the total nitrogen in beer is sufficient to produce protein–polyphenol haze (McMurrough *et al.*, 1999). A quantity as 2 mg/l of protein can produce a haze of 1 EBC (Chapman, 1993), equivalent to 69 FTU (formazin turbidity units). Haze-active proteins isolated from beer have been found to be derived primarily from residues of the barley proteins group, the hordeins. These protein fragments consist of several different molecular weights and are relatively rich in proline. This description matches the characteristics of the nitrogen-terminal sequence repeats of the hordeins that are rich in glutamine (which comprise 30 mol% of hordein) and proline (20 mol%), which are produced by proteolytic modification during malting and

Table 25.8 Chemical composition of four different fractions from haze-forming proteins and in hordein and albumin plus globulin from malt

	Haze-forming proteins				*Malt*	
	I	*II*	*III*	*IV*	*Hordein*	*Albumin and globulin*
Protein content (%)	69	76	65	75		
Amino acid Composition of Protein (mol%)						
Alanine	6.1	3.1	7.4	8.6	2.1	8.6
Arginine	4.2	1.4	3.6	3.4	1.3	4.3
Aspartic acid	6.6	3.0	8.5	6.6	1.2	9.3
Cysteine	1.2	0.9	1.9	–	0.6	1.5
Glutamic acid	12.1	20.9	14.3	14.2	29.1	9.6
Glycine	9.3	4.7	9.2	7.5	1.8	8.7
Histidine	2.3	0.6	2.7	3.4	0.9	1.7
Isoleucine	2.2	2.3	2.8	3.4	2.8	3.2
Leucine	3.3	2.3	5.3	8.3	4.7	6.5
Lysine	3.9	1.3	2.5	3.3	0.3	3.6
Methionine	0.7	0.5	1.1	–	0.6	1.7
Phenylalanine	1.2	2.6	1.5	4.1	4.4	2.7
Proline	5.5	19.9	10.3	8.7	18.2	7.3
Serine	4.6	3.4	5.9	7.5	3.3	6.0
Threonine	0.4	2.0	4.1	3.9	1.4	3.5
Tyrosine	1.6	2.0	1.7	1.1	1.6	2.7
Valine	3.6	2.2	5.5	6.4	3.1	6.4

Note: Four fractions responsible for haze are isolated in beer and they are called haze-forming proteins I, II, III and IV. Their molecular weights were estimated to be 1–10 kDa (fraction I); 19 kDa (fraction II); 16 kDa (fraction III); 40 kDa (fraction IV).

Source: Modified from Asano et al. (1982)

mashing (Robinson *et al.*, 2004). Properties and compositions of haze-forming proteins have been studied by Asano *et al.* (1982). They used a procedure to isolate and fractionate four different fractions of haze-forming proteins in beer. The amino acids composition of these four fractions and hordein, albumin, globulin present in malt is shown in Table 25.8.

They concluded that haze-forming proteins derived from hordein were rich in proline, and derived from polypeptides albumin and that globulin may also react with polyphenols to form haze. Proline is the amino acid that has a specific affinity for polyphenols. The force of attraction between polyphenols and proteins is mainly described as hydrogen and hydrophobic bonding involving hydrophobic amino acids such as proline but also tryptophan, phenylalanine, tyrosine, isoleucine and valine. Hough *et al.* (1982) have reported that the main amino acids present in haze are proline, glutamic acid, arginine and aspartic acid. It is extensively accepted that protein with high levels of amino acid proline and polyphenols with higher degree of polymerization are most likely to form haze (Siebert *et al.*, 1996). Many researchers have studied influences of proline amino acid in beer stability. This imino acid, not metabolized during fermentation, is the principal amino acid present in the finished product. Gorinstein *et al.* (1999) have studied protein, proline and lysine contents of beer during brewing process. They emphasized that maximum proline content corresponds to the fermentation and storage stages while in the final product the content of proline decreases remaining significantly higher than in wort. In all cases, final filtration decreases the level of amino acids. Polypeptides which contain low level or no proline produce little or no haze (Briggs *et al.*, 2004). Protein and polyphenol complexes cross-link together by weak interactions such as hydrogen bonds and hydrophobic interactions; alcohol, pH, free amino acids, and metal content may influence protein–polyphenol haze formation as well. The amount of alcohol in the beer will change the hydrophobic bonding between the proteins and the polyphenols due to the lesser polarity of ethanol than water. Siebert *et al.* (1996), in a model system, have studied the effect of pH on haze formation and concluded that there was decreased haze formation at a lower pH value with a maximum haze formation at pH 4.2. Asano *et al.* (1982) have described the chemical combination between protein and polyphenols. The pyrrolidine rings of proline forming proteins have unfolded molecular structures that facilitate the entry of polyphenols into them. Furthermore, the pyrrolidine ring of proline cannot form intramolecular and intermolecular hydrogen bonds with oxygen atoms of peptide bonds and, consequently, these free oxygen atoms readily form hydrogen bonds with hydroxyl groups of polyphenols. Moreover proline also participates in hydrophobic bonding between the haze-forming proteins and polyphenols. These two mechanisms of combination between the haze-forming proteins and polyphenols were probably responsible for chill haze formation of beer. Siebert *et al.* (1996) have investigated the mechanism of protein–polyphenol interaction and they proposed a model where only a fixed number of sites in the protein (primarily proline containing proteins) serve as attachment point for polyphenols. In protein–polyphenol complexes, the polyphenolic compounds act as a bridge between adjacent protein molecules. A diagram of a model for protein–polyphenol interactions is shown in Figure 25.3.

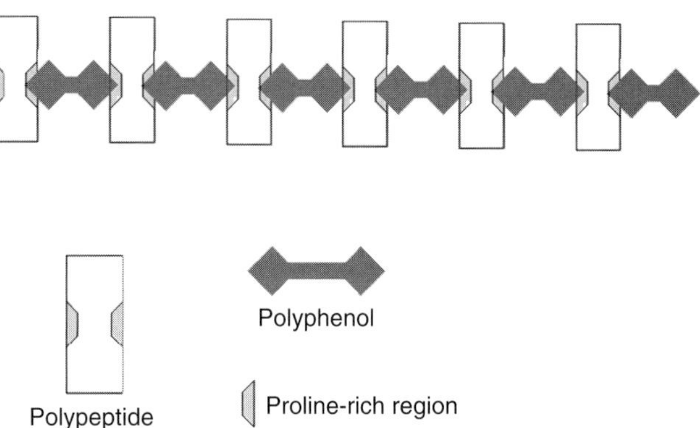

Figure 25.3 Model for protein–polyphenol interaction causing haze. *Source*: Modified from Siebert and Lynn (1998).

The model assumes that polyphenol has a fixed number of binding ends (two or more) and each protein also has a fixed number of polyphenol binding sites (two or more). If the number of polyphenol ends is equal to the number of protein binding sites, the largest network of protein and polyphenols should be produced thereby creating the largest amount of haze. If the amount of protein is in excess relatively to the polyphenols, as it usually happens in beer, then each polyphenol molecule can bridge two protein molecules, making it unlikely that an extended network of bridges would be formed between the protein and polyphenol molecules. If the number of polyphenol molecules significantly exceeds the number of haze-active protein molecules, all of the haze-active protein binding sites would likely be bound to polyphenols making it unlikely that an extended network of bridges between haze-active protein and polyphenol molecules would be created (Siebert *et al.*, 1996). The fixed number of binding sites on haze-active protein is considered to be accessible prolines, which are attachment sites for the polyphenols (Siebert and Lynn, 1998). More haze results from the same amount of protein and polyphenol when their ratio is more nearly even; later on use of compounds that reduce some haze-active protein could result in an initial increase in haze (Siebert and Lynn, 1997). Stabilization treatments are necessary to improve the colloidal stability and to extend the shelf-life of beer. Bamforth (1999) reported three different strategies: protein removal, polyphenol removal or remove a proportion of each. Many different substances can be used to improve the stability of beer and to remove polyphenols polyvinylpolypyrrolidone (PVPP) is commonly used. Its chemical structure, in comparison with polyproline structure, is reported in Figure 25.4.

A fraction of polyproline A fraction of PVPP

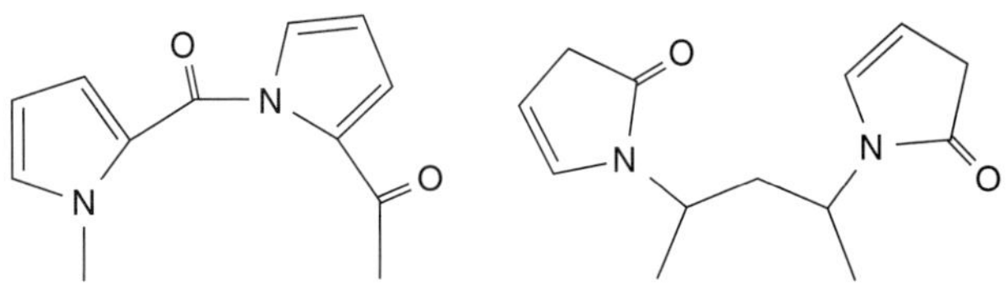

Figure 25.4 Comparison of partial structures of polyproline and PVPP. *Source*: Modified from Siebert and Lynn (1998).

Siebert and Lynn (1998) have showed that the structure of PVPP strongly resembles the structure of polyproline and that it binds polyphenols in the same way proteins rich in proline bind with polyphenols. Both substances have five-membered, saturated, nitrogen-containing rings and amide bond with no other functional groups. Proteins have not to be eliminated completely because they are associated with important characteristics of beer such as the head-forming properties and the development of a full palatability (Hough *et al.*, 1982). It is not clearly established if the haze-forming and foam-forming proteins are different. Hough *et al.* (1982) have reported that two proteins, which reacted with barley antibodies, were present in both foam and haze. It is important to use coadjuvants that are able to remove constituents of haze without reducing foam stability, flavor and taste. Papain was one of the first stabilizers used in brewing. It is a proteolytic enzyme; it hydrolyzes peptides but it reduces the foam quality (Bamforth, 1999). Also tannic acid and bentonite, used as a specific precipitant of haze-active proteins, can damage foam in beer. It is most common to use silica gels that bind to proline residue in the protein with minimal negative effects on the protein fraction involved in beer foam-active quality (Siebert and Lynn, 1998). Lopez and Edens (2005) have proposed alternatives to the traditional stabilization compounds. A proline-specific protease in wort that can hydrolyze proteins rich in proline has been used, yielding a peptide fraction that is unable to form a haze without negative effect on foam stability. Evans *et al.* (2003) have proposed a different approach; since haze activity is dependent on the distribution of proline in the hordein, they have studied immunological methods that can predict the potential of malt samples to produce beer with superior foam and haze stability.

- **The quality and stability of foam are influenced by proteins in beer and by their complex with other substances.**

According to Omrod (1994) volume and quality of beer foam are generally considered by consumers as a major factor in beer quality. Foams are colloids composed of gas bubbles dispersed through a liquid. The stability of the beer foam is related to the stability of the bubbles and anything that disrupts the bubbles will result in unstable foam. Compounds that influence foam stability and quality include proteins, bittering substances of hops, metal ions, polysaccharides and melanoidins. The foam is richer than the beer in such substances as specific proteins and hop components, particularly iso-α-acids. Beer proteins are considered the major foaming agents and variations in foaming behavior are due to interaction of the protein with other substances (Hough *et al.*, 1982). Other components foam-negatives, such as lipids, are also important in determining the overall head-forming characteristics of a particular beer. Beer proteins form complex with iso-α-acids and metal ions. These strongly hydrophobic complexes are known to enhance foam stability and adhesion. During foam formation, amphipathic proteins surrounding the bubbles interact with hydrophobic region, forming a stable "bridge" between the hydrophobic gas bubbles and the aqueous beer; these are then cross-linked by hop bitter acids and metal ions, forming a semirigid structure (Dickie *et al.*, 2001). Ryder *et al.* (1991) have reported the chemical interaction and colloidal aspect present in beer foam. Formation of foam requires the presence of surfactants in solution and one property of proteins, or polypeptides, and iso-α-acids present in beer, is to be surfactants. In fact only few proteins are surface active to some degree and tend to form foams: the incorporation of both hydrophilic and hydrophobic amino acid gives proteins their amphipathic properties. The principal components of beer that stabilizes foam are proteins derived from barley (Bamforth, 1985) but they undergo considerable modification during malting, mashing and brewing. Several researchers have reported that proteins present in beer foam are greater than 10 kDa (Siebert and Knudson, 1989). Other studies have considered that beer proteins with a molecular weight between 5–10 and 100 kDa (termed as high molecular weight fraction – HMW) have a positive effect on beer foam quality and compounds with a molecular weight below 10 kDa (termed as low molecular weight fraction – LMW) have a negative effect on foam and the ratio of these two fractions, rather than their absolute amounts, is very important (Sharpe *et al.*, 1981; Omrod, 1994). Protein associated with beer foam formation and stability are protein Z, lipid transfer protein 1 (LPT1), hordein and glutelin fragments (Siebert and Knudson, 1989). Protein Z and LPT1 are considered the predominant proteins in beer (Leisegang and Stahl, 2005). Protein Z is a 40 kDa protein derived from barley albumin which has been related to beer foam stability (Bamforth *et al.*, 1993). Protein Z with 50–200 mg/l (Leisegang and Stahl, 2005) is partially homologous to serine protease inhibitors and these inhibitory properties might be the reason why protein Z is not degraded by proteolytic enzymes during malting and mashing. Protein Z can be resolved into two isoforms: Z4 (80%) and Z7 (20%) (Briggs *et al.*, 2004). Protein LPT1 has a rate of 50–90 mg/l and is concentrated in beer foam

(Leisegang and Stahl, 2005). LPT1 is a 9.6 kDa protein and it has been suggested that it is important in beer foam formation. It is made up of 91 amino acid residues including eight cysteines that are probably present in the beer protein in the oxidized form as four cystines (Lusk *et al.*, 1995). Leisegang and Stahl (2005) have evaluated the degradation of LTP1 by protease A. This is an enzyme primarily released by autolysis from dead yeast cell and the degradation of LPT1 may have a negative influence on beer foam stability. Kapp and Bamforth (2002) have established that albumin and hordein fractions from barley are capable of foaming and that the foam stability of the albumin fraction is greater than that of the hordein fraction. Evans *et al.* (2003) have described that malt derived, foam positive proteins, including protein Z4, LPT1 and some members of the hordein storage protein family, interact principally with isomerized hop acids to stabilize foam. Several research groups have studied the influence of polymeric amino acids on beer foam. Amino acids and their concentrations in the main beer protein may vary from beer to beer depending on the type of malt and adjuncts used in brewing. Wheat contain more foam stability proteins than the equivalent proteins from barley; adjuncts based on corn, rice and sugars provide no foaming material and their use, therefore, dilutes foam potential (Lewis and Bamforth, 2006). Asano and Hashimoto (1980) have studied amino acids composition of foaming proteins. They isolated three different molecular weight fractions of foaming proteins: higher, medium and lower with molecular weights from 90 to 100 kDa, 40 kDa and 15 kDa. The result of analysis is reported in Table 25.9.

The amino acid composition of these three fractions were similar to that of barley albumin or globulin. Lysine occurred more frequently in higher and medium molecular weight fractions than in lower fraction; cysteine and methionine were not present in the third fraction. ε-Amino groups of lysine residue in foaming proteins combine electrostatically with acidic groups of iso-α-acids molecules derived from hops (Asano and Hashimoto, 1976). Because higher and medium molecular weight fractions have the higher content of lysine, these fractions must combine preferentially with iso-α-acids and this complex increases the foaming of beer. Asano *et al.* (1982) also provided data for malt hordein and malt albumin plus globulin; amino acid composition shows that beer haze-forming protein is derived from malt hordein and the beer foam-active protein originates from the malt albumins and globulins. Siebert and Knudson (1989) have proposed a Coomassie blue dye binding assay to determine high molecular weight protein (over 5 kDa) in beer. The dye-binding procedure responds strongly to basic and aromatic amino acids, mainly present in foam-active proteins. Yokoi *et al.* (1994) have studied the hydrophobic beer proteins and their function in beer foam; they have fractioned beer proteins and analyzed the amino acid composition of these fractions. They reported that proteins in beer have a different hydrophobicity; proteins rich of hydrophobic amino acids form strongly complex with iso-α-acids and are concentrated in beer foam and play an important role in foam stability.

Table 25.9 Amino acid composition of "foaming proteins"

	Beer foam		
	Higher	*Medium*	*Lower*
Protein content (%)	21	75	65
Amino acid composition of protein (mol%)			
Alanine	6.7	8.6	7.4
Arginine	5.7	3.4	3.6
Aspartic acid	5.6	6.6	8.5
Cysteine	–	–	1.9
Glutamic acid	9.0	14.2	14.3
Glycine	6.1	7.5	9.2
Histidine	3.4	3.4	2.7
Isoleucine	2.4	3.4	2.8
Leucine	5.7	8.3	5.3
Lysine	3.6	3.3	2.5
Methionine	–	–	1.1
Phenylalanine	2.2	4.1	1.5
Proline	3.9	8.7	10.3
Serine	6.9	7.5	5.9
Threonine	3.6	3.9	4.1
Tyreonine	0.9	1.1	1.7
Valine	4.1	6.4	5.5

Note: Three different molecular weight fractions of foaming proteins are isolated in beer: Higher, Medium and Lower with molecular weights from 90 to 100 kDa, 40 kDa and 15 kDa.

Source: Modified from Asano and Hashimoto (1980).

- **Amino acids are precursors of formation of biogenic amines.**

Biogenic amines can be found in beer, in fact brewing process fulfills the three factors that govern the formation of amines. Free precursors of amino acid are available; microorganisms with amino acid decarboxylating activity can occur and favorable conditions for the growth of microorganisms can be found. Biogenic amines formation is attributed to thermal amino acid decarboxylation and possibly to enzymatic activity in malt. Only few studies are available on the relationship between precursor of amino acids and formation of their corresponding amines. Ardö (2006) has reported a research about amino acid catabolism and Table 25.10 shows the amines produced from decarboxylation of amino acids.

Izquierdo-Pulido *et al.* (2000) have investigated the influence of a precursors amino acid on tyramine formation during beer fermentation. They concluded that it is difficult to establish a direct relation between tyramine and tyrosine. Probably more attention should be paid to keep under control the bacteria contamination than the amount of free tyrosine present in wort.

Table 25.10 Biogenic amines originated from corresponding amino acids

Amino acid	*Biogenic amine*
Tyrosine	Tyramine
Histidine	Histamine
Ornithine	Putrescine
Lysine	Cadaverine
Tryptophane	Tryptamine
Phenylalanine	Phenylethylamine

Source: Modified from Ardö (2006).

- **Amino acids can influence the sensory quality of beer.**

Aroma profile in beer is depending on many different compounds, responsible of different sensations. According to Hough (1994) some amino acids are involved in taste perception; it has been reported that L-alanine and L-tryptophan are respectively associated to sweet and bitter sensation.

- **Amino acids in excess are responsible of biological stability in beer.**

Above all, the beer's biological stability is related to resistance to *Lactobacillus* infection. When present in excess, the amino acids in beer can promote infections by acting as nitrogen sources for spoilage microorganism (Bamforth, 2004).

References

Agu, R.C. (2003). *J. Inst. Brew.* 109, 106–109.

Agu, R.C. and Palmer, G.H. (1999). *Process Biochem.* 35, 497–502.

Agu, R.C. and Palmer, G.H. (2003). *J. Inst. Brew.* 109, 110–113.

Almeida, R.B., Almeida e Silva, J.B., Lima, U.A., Assis, A.N. and Silva, D.P. (2004). *Cerevisia* 29, 147–154.

Ardö, Y. (2006). *Biotech. Adv.* 24, 238–242.

Asano, K. and Hashimoto, N. (1976). *Rep. Res. Lab. Kirin Brew. Co.* 19, 9–16.

Asano, K. and Hashimoto, N. (1980). *J. Am. Soc. Brew. Chem.* 4, 129–137.

Asano, K., Shinagawa, K. and Hashimoto, N. (1982). *J. Am. Soc. Brew. Chem.* 40, 147–154.

Äyräpää, T. (1971). *J. Inst. Brew.* 77, 266.

Bamforth, C.W. (1985). *J. Inst. Brew.* 91, 370–383.

Bamforth, C.W. (1999). *J. Am. Soc. Brew. Chem.* 57, 81–90.

Bamforth, C.W. (2004). *Health and Nutrition.* Blackwell, New Delhi, India. pp. 81, 105.

Bamforth, C.W., Canteranne, E., Chandley, P. and Onishi, A. (1993). *Proceedings of the EBC Congress*, Oslo, Norway, p. 331.

Baxter, E.D. and Wainwright, T. (1979). *J. Am. Soc. Brew. Chem.* 1, 8–12.

Bertholdsson, N.O. (1999). *Eur. J. Agron.* 10, 1–8.

Bewley, J.D. and Black, M. (1994). *Seeds. Physiology of Development and Germination.* Plenum Press, New York, USA. pp. 18–20.

Briggs, D.E. (1998). *Malts and Malting.* Blackie Academic and Professional, London, UK. pp. 169–175.

Briggs, D.E., Boulton, C.A., Brookes, P.A. and Stevens, R. (2004). *Brewing Science and Practice.* Woodhead Publishing Limited and CRC Press, Cambridge, UK. pp. 701–705

Chapman, L. (1993). *J. Inst. Brew.* 99, 49–56.

Charalambous, G. (1981). In Pollock, J.R.A. (ed.), *Brewing Science*, Vol. 2, pp. 203–207. Academic Press London, UK.

De Ruiter, J.M. and Haslemore, R.M. (1996). *New Zeal. J. Crop Hort.* 24, 77–87.

Dickie, K.H., Cann, C., Norman, E.C., Bamforth, C.W. and Muller, R.E. (2001). *J. Am. Soc. Brew. Chem.* 59, 17–23.

Dufour, J.P. and Devreux, A. (1986). *Proc. EBC Congr. Monog.* 11, 227–249.

Evans, D.E., Robinson, L.H., Sheehan, M.C., Hill, A., Skerritt, J.S. and Barr, A.R. (2003). *J. Am. Soc. Brew. Chem.* 61, 55–62.

Field, J.M., Shewry, P.R. and Miflin, B.J. (1983). *J. Sci. Food Agric.* 34, 367–369.

Fix, G. (2000). *Principles of Brewing Science.* Brewers Publications, CO, USA. pp. 99–100.

Gorinstein, S., Zemser, M., Vargas-Albores, F., Ochoa, J.-L., Paredes-Lopez, O., Scheler, C., Salnikow, J., Martin-Belloso, O. and Trakhtenberg, S. (1999). *Food Chem.* 67, 71–78.

Hough, J.S. (1994). Malt – a package of enzymes and food substances (Chapter 3), pp. 25–26; Post fermentation treatments (Chapter 9), p. 155. *The Biotechnology of Malting and Brewing.* pp. 25–26, 155. University Press, Cambridge, UK.

Hough, J.S., Briggs, D.E., Stevens, R. and Young, T.M. (1982). *Malting and Brewing Science.* Chapman and Hall University Press, Cambridge, UK. Vol. 2, pp. 458, 799.

Howard, K.A., Gayler, K.R., Eaglest, H.A. and Halloran, G.M. (1996). *J. Cereal Sci.* 24, 47–53.

Izquierdo-Pulido, M., Mariné-Font, A. and Vidal-Carou, M.C. (2000). *Food Chem.* 70, 329–332.

Jones, M. and Pierce, J.S. (1969). *Proceedings of the EBC Congress*, Interlaken, Switzerland, pp. 151–160.

Kapp, G.R. and Bamforth, C.W. (2002). *J. Sci. Food Agric.* 82, 1276–1281.

Kunze, W. (1999). *Technology Brewing and Malting*, International Edition. Verlagsabteilung, Berlin, Germany. p. 33.

Leisegang, R. and Stahl, U. (2005). *J. Inst. Brew.* 112, 112–117.

Lewis, M.J. and Bamforth, C.W. (2006). *Essays in Brewing Science.* Springer, CA, USA. pp. 39–40.

Lopez, M. and Edens, L. (2005). *J. Agric. Food Chem.* 53, 7944–7949.

Lusk, L.T., Goldstein, H. and Ryder, D. (1995). *J. Am. Soc. Brew. Chem.* 53, 93–103.

McMurrough, I., Madigan, D., Kelly, R.I. and O'Rourke, T. (1999). *Food Tech.* 53, 58–62.

Meilgaard, M.C. (1976). *MBAA Tech. Q.* 13, 78–90.

Omrod, I.H.L. (1994). *Symposium EBC "Malting Technology."* Andernach, Germany. pp. 137–146.

Palmer, G.H. (1989). Cereal in malting and brewing. In Palmer, G.H. (ed.), *Cereal Science and Technology*, pp. 71–134. University Press, Aberdeen, UK.

Pollock, J.R.A. (1988). *Ferment* 1, 31–32.

Robinson, L.H., Evans, D.E., Kaukovirta-Norja, A., Vilpola, A. and Aldred, P. (2004). *MBAA Tech. Q.* 41, 353–362.

Ryder, D.S., Power, J., Foley, T. and Hsu, W.-P. (1991). *Proceedings of the 3rd Scientific and Technical Convention of Institute of Brewing*, Zimbabwe. pp. 104–112.

Sharpe, F.R., Jacques, D., Rowsell, A.G. and Whitear, A.L. (1981). *Proceedings of the EBC Congress*, Copenaghen, Denmark, pp. 607–614.

Shewry, P.R. (1992). Barley seed storage proteins – structure, synthesis, and deposition. In Mengel, K. and Pilbeam, D.J. (eds), *Nitrogen Metabolism of Plants*, pp. 201–208. Clarendon Press, Oxford, UK.

Siebert, K.J. and Knudson, E.J. (1989). *MBAA Tech. Q.* 26, 139–146.

Siebert, K.J. and Lynn, P.Y. (1997). *J. Am. Soc. Brew. Chem.* 55, 73–78.

Siebert, K.J. and Lynn, P.Y. (1998). *J. Am. Soc. Brew. Chem.* 56, 24–31.

Siebert, K.J., Carrasco, A. and Lynn, P.Y. (1996). *J. Agric. Food Chem.* 44, 1997–2005.

Vesely, P., Duncombe, D., Lusk, L., Basarova, G., Seabrooks, J. and Ryder, D. (2004). *MBAA Tech. Q.* 41, 282–292.

Wainwright, T. (1971). *Proceedings of the EBC Congress*, Estoril, Portugal, p. 437.

Yokoi, S., Yamashita, K., Kunitake, N. and Koshino, S. (1994). *J. Am. Soc. Brew. Chem.* 52, 123–126.

26

Purines in Beer

Tetsuya Yamamoto and Yuji Moriwaki Division of Endocrinology and Metabolism, Department of Internal Medicine, Hyogo College of Medicine, Hyogo, Japan

Abstract

As compared with other alcoholic beverages, beer contains considerable amounts of purines, which high-performance liquid chromatography has shown to consist of purine nucleosides and bases. According to that analysis, the nucleoside guanosine was most abundant, as compared with other types of purines. Purine ingestion causes an increased production of uric acid, leading to an increase in the serum concentration of urate. According to the results of a study on nucleic acid ingestion, the serum concentration of urate was increased to a greater degree in patients with hyperuricemia or gout than in normal subjects. In addition, the serum concentration of urate was increased by ingestion of nucleotides (adenosine monophosphate (AMP), guanosine monophosphate, and inosine monophosphate (IMP)) and purine bases (adenine, hypoxanthine, xanthine) in all three subject groups, while it was shown that hypoxanthine, AMP, and IMP had greater hyperuricemic effects on patients with gout than those with hyperuricemia and the normal subjects. The effects of guanosine (the most plentiful purine in beer) on the serum urate levels were not examined in previous human studies. However, since it was found that guanosine was more readily absorbed than other nucleosides, nucleotides, or bases and rapidly converted to uric acid via guanine and xanthine in animals, it is suggested that its ingestion may increase the serum concentration of urate. Since purines in beer have a clinical effect on serum urate and augment hyperuricemic effect in patients with gout, it is important for those patients to refrain from consuming large amounts of beer that contains considerable amounts of purines.

List of Abbreviations

ADP	Adenosine diphosphate
AMP	Adenosine monophosphate
ATP	Adenosine triphosphate
GMP	Guanosine monophosphate
HPLC	High-performance liquid chromatography
IMP	Inosine monophosphate
S-AMP	Adenylosuccinic acid
SDS	Sodium dodecyl sulfate
XMP	Xanthosine monophosphate

Introduction

A purine is a heterocyclic aromatic organic compound that consists of a pyrimidine ring fused to an imidazole ring (Figure 26.1), and the term purines refers to substituted purines and their tautomers. Many purine bases including hypoxanthine, xanthine, adenine, guanine, and uric acid are present in the body. Deoxynucleic acid contains two of the bases, adenine, and guanine. Therefore, purines are known to play an important role in animals, bacteria, fungi, viruses, and plants, as well as in other organisms. Beer is produced from malt by fermentation with yeast fungus, and since malt contains considerable amounts of purines, beer also contains high levels of purines. In the human body, most ingested purines are metabolized to the end-product uric acid (Figure 26.2) (Clifford *et al.*, 1976). Therefore, ingestion of large amounts of purines causes an increased production of uric acid, leading to hyperuricemia. Continued hyperuricemia causes gouty attack, tophus, and

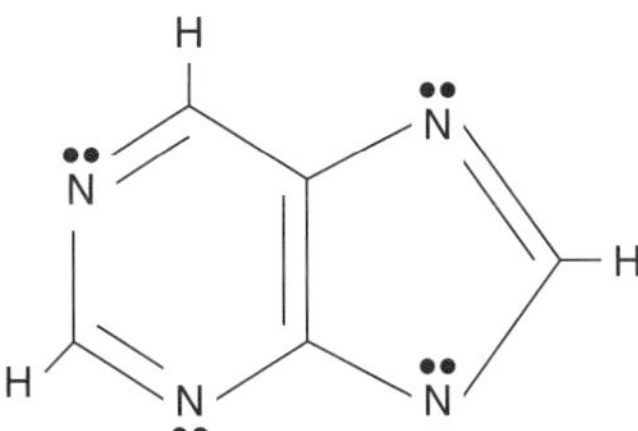

Figure 26.1 Purine ($C_5H_4N_4$). A purine is a heterocyclic aromatic organic compound that consists of a pyrimidine ring fused to an imidazole ring.

Figure 26.2 Uric acid. In the human body, most ingested purines are metabolized to the end-product uric acid.

Beer in Health and Disease Prevention
ISBN: 978-0-12-373891-2

gouty kidneys; therefore, it is important for individuals at risk to restrict the intake of large amounts of purines as well as reduce other factors that contribute to hyperuricemia, such as obesity and vigorous exercise (Yamashita *et al.*, 1986; Takahashi *et al.*, 1997; Yamamoto *et al.*, 1997). Beer contains greater amounts of purines than other alcoholic beverages as shown in Table 51.2 of this book in the article entitled "Relationship between exercise and beer ingestion in regard to metabolism" (Chapter 51 of this book) and may contribute to hyperuricemia to a greater degree than other alcoholic beverages. Therefore, it is important to obtain data regarding the contents and effects of purines in beer and other beverages.

Analysis of Purines in Beer

Purines in beer consist of nucleosides and bases, the majority of which are derived from the malt contained in beer, and it is important to use a reliable method to measure these nucleosides and bases in beer easily and accurately. In several studies (Yamamoto *et al.*, 2002, 2004a; Cortacero-Ramirez *et al.*, 2004a, b), purines in beer were analyzed using a high-performance liquid chromatography (HPLC) technique, which is known to be rapid and easy, and able to determine the amounts of purines in aqueous solution accurately. In our previous study (Yamamoto *et al.*, 2002, 2004b), the concentrations of hypoxanthine, xanthine, inosine, adenosine, guanosine, deoxyinosine, deoxyguanosine, and deoxyadenosine in beer were determined by reversed-phase HPLC, with the mobile phase of 20 mM/l phosphate buffer (pH 2.2), the flow rate of 1 ml/min, and the detection wavelength of 254 nm, using a Wakosil 5C18-200 (Wako Pure Chemicals Industries, Osaka, Japan). In addition, the concentrations of adenine, guanine, and deoxyuridine in beer were determined by another HPLC method. In brief, the chromatograph consisted of two CCPM pumps (Tosoh, Tokyo, Japan), a SC-8020 system controller (Tosoh, Tokyo, Japan), two spectrophotometric detectors (UV-8010 and UV-8020) (Tosoh, Tokyo, Japan), and a VC-8020 column switching valve (Tosoh, Tokyo, Japan). The chromatographic columns were a Wakosil 5C18-200 (4.6 × 250 mm) (Wako Pure Chemicals Industries, Osaka, Japan) as the first column and a NAVI C18-5 (4.6 × 250 mm) (Wako Pure Chemicals Industries, Osaka, Japan) as the second column. In the first column, the mobile phase was 20 mM KH_2PO_4 (pH 4.70) and in the second column, the mobile phase was 20 mM KH_2PO_4 (pH 2.20). The flow rate was 1 ml/min and the detection wavelength was 254 nm. Using two methods, the purine nucleosides and bases in Japanese regular beer (Kirin Brewery, Yokohama, Japan) were determined, with the results shown in Table 26.1.

Another method termed the capillary electrophoretic method, which uses micellar electrophoretic capillary chromatography, has also been reported (Cortacero-Ramirez, 2004a) and shown to have high resolving power, high separation efficiency, high sensitivity, and unique selectivity. The advantages of this method include a low consumption of solvents and less rigorous requirements for sample cleanup, as compared with traditional HPLC. The system comprises a 0–30 kV high-voltage built-in power supply and is equipped with a diode array detector. In their study, the mobile phase was 25 mM $Na_2B_4O_7$ adjusted to pH 10.5 and 110 mM sodium dodecyl sulfate, with detection wavelengths of 210 and 270 mM while the separation voltage was 14 kV at a constant temperature of 25°C. All of the capillaries had an inner diameter of 75 mm, a total length of 50 cm, and an effective separation length of 50 cm. The concentrations of purines in each of seven different kinds of beer determined by this method are shown in Table 26.2. Further, in another study (Cortacero-Ramirez, 2004b), using the same method, the concentrations of purines in different kinds of beers were determined (Table 26.3). However, the methods are not sufficient to determine the quantities of purines in beer, as only guanosine, adenosine, adenine, and xanthine were detected in contrast to the large variety present in beer.

Table 26.1 Concentrations of purine nucleosides and bases, and uridine and its metabolites in Japanese beer (μmol/l)

Hypoxanthine	17.5 ± 1.5
Xanthine	58.5 ± 3.6
Guanine	42.4 ± 3.6
Adenine	17.2 ± 2.3
Uric acid	ND
Uracil	17.6 ± 1.5
Inosine	20.3 ± 2.5
Guanosine	174 ± 16.1
Adenosine	42.1 ± 7.9
Uridine	210.6 ± 27.2
2'-Deoxyguanosine	ND
2'-Deoxyadenosine	19.4 ± 3.7
2'-Deoxyinosine	ND
2'-Deoxyuridine	7.9 ± 2.1

Note: Values are expressed as mean ± SD. Beer contains various purines.

Purines in Beer and Other Beverages

British beer, home-brewed beer, and lager beer each contain many different types of purines, such as adenine, hypoxanthine, adenosine, and guanosine (Table 26.4) (Gibson *et al.*, 1984). Japanese beer contains greater amounts of purines than other types of beer, including purine nucleosides (inosine, guanosine, adenosine, and deoxyadenosine) and purine bases (hypoxanthine, xanthine, guanine, and adenine), with guanosine being the most abundant (Table 26.1). Guanosine is more quickly absorbed and rapidly converted to uric acid via guanine and xanthine in animals (Figure 26.3), and thus it may increase the serum concentration of uric acid (Potter *et al.*, 1980). In Japan, low malt liquor (happo-shu) and purine-free happo-shu have been developed (Yamamoto *et al.*, 2004), and have a taste that is similar to beer. Happo-shu contains 249.4 μmol/l

Table 26.2 Analysis of different types of beer samples

	Concentration (mg/l)						
Analytes	*Extra*	*Classic I*	*Classic II*	*Special*	*Special black*	*Light*	*Non-alcoholic*
Adenosine	n.q.	n.q.	8.3 ± 1.0	7.1 ± 0.9	n.q.	21.3 ± 1.9	12.3 ± 1.4
Adenine	1.6 ± 0.2	3.0 ± 0.4	n.d.	n.d.	n.d.	1.9 ± 0.4	n.d.

Note: n.d. not detected; n.q. not quantified. Values are expressed as mean ± SD. Different types of beer contain small amounts of adenine.

Table 26.3 Analysis of different types of beer

	Concentration (mg/l)						
Analytes	*Belgian origin*	*Abbey beer*	*Red malt beer*	*Trapense beer*	*Double malt beer*	*Extra lager beer*	*Wheat beer*
Adenosine	11.8 ± 2.0	7.3 ± 1.6	8.7 ± 1.5	14.0 ± 3.8	15.3 ± 2.2	4.8 ± 0.2	9.6 ± 1.9
Adenine	n.d.	n.d.	n.d.	n.d.	n.d.	n.d.	n.q.
Guanosine	78.2 ± 1.2	87.4 ± 7.7	97.5 ± 3.9	71.3 ± 4.3	96.8 ± 4.9	38.1 ± 1.0	51.2 ± 7.5
Xanthine	94.0 ± 5.1	95.9 ± 3.6	116.6 ± 5.5	77.6 ± 6.0	99.0 ± 6.7	34.7 ± 1.1	35.3 ± 5.9

Note: n.d. not detected; n.q. not quantified. Values are expressed as mean ± SD. Different types of beer contain considerable amounts of purines including guanosine and xanthine.

Table 26.4 Purine bases and nucleosides in different types of beer

	Adenine	*Hypoxanthine*	*Xanthine*	*Adenosine*	*Guanosine*	*Total purines*
British beer	1.2	0.6	3.3	3.5	13.6	22.2
(Range)	(0.4–3.0)	(0–2.5)	(2.6–3.8)	(0–6.0)	(10–17.3)	(20.3–27.5)
Home-brewed beer	0.7	1.2	0.2	0	1.8	3.9
Guinness	0	0	5.5	7.7	10.6	23.8
Lager beer	4.3	3.0	3.5	0	6.9	17.7

Note: Values are expressed in mg purine nitrogen/l. British beer, Guinness, and Lager beer contain considerable amounts of purines.

of purines, indicating that it contains lower amounts of malt and purine (Table 26.5) as compared with Japanese regular beer that contains 391.4 μmol/l of purines (Table 26.1). However, happo-shu still contains a considerable amount of purines, especially guanosine (Table 26.5). On the other hand, purine-free happo-shu contains the same amounts of malt and very low levels of purines (13.2 μmol/l), as compared with regular happo-shu (249.4 μmol/l). Purine-free happo-shu was recently developed for individuals who were concerned about increases in urate serum concentration. However, ingestion of large amounts of purine-free happo-shu causes an ethanol-induced increase in that concentration.

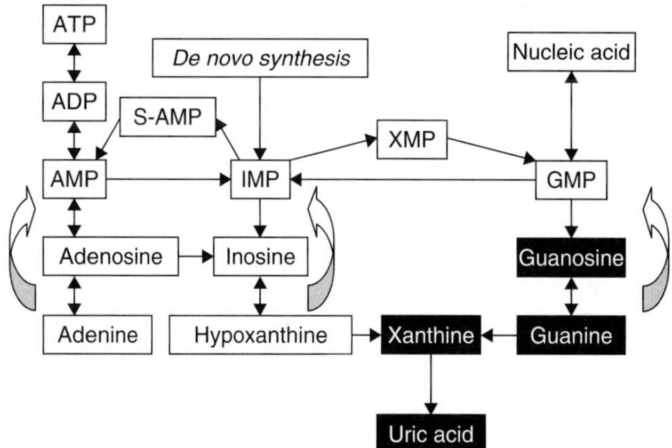

Figure 26.3 Guanosine degradation. Words in white indicate pathway of guanosine degradation.

Comparison of Purines Between Beer and Other Beverages

Wine contains 1.6 mg/l of purines and sake contains 4.6 mg/l of purines expressed contains mg purine nitrogen/l, while whisky, brandy, and shouchu (a traditional Japanese distilled sprits, which has a high ethanol concentration at about 20–40% spirit), each a type of distilled liquor, contain 0.5, 1.6, and 0.1 mg/l (Table 51.2 in the article entitled "Relationship between exercise and beer ingestion in regard to metabolism", Chapter 51 of this book). As compared with beer and happo-shu, these alcoholic beverages contain lower amounts of purines, suggesting that the serum concentration of urate may not be increased if they are not ingested in large amounts.

Table 26.5 Concentrations of purine and pyrimidine nucleosides and bases in regular and purine-free happo-shu (μmol/l)

	Regular happo-shu	*Purine-free happo-shu*
Adenosine	30.9 ± 1.0	0.3 ± 0.1
Deoxyadenosine	5.5 ± 0.5	Nd
Guanosine	162.6 ± 4.1	12.1 ± 1.8
Deoxyguanosine	Nd	Nd
Inosine	9.6 ± 1.5	Nd
Deoxyinosine	Nd	Nd
Xanthine	32.5 ± 1.1	0.8 ± 0.1
Hypoxanthine	1.4 ± 0.1	Nd
Adenine	4.4 ± 0.1	Nd
Guanine	2.5 ± 0.2	Nd
Uric acid	Nd	Nd
Uridine	113.2 ± 5.7	20.8 ± 1.3
Deoxyuridine	3.8 ± 0.2	Nd
Thymidine	42.8 ± 1.7	4.6 ± 0.1
Cytidine	80.4 ± 4.3	7.6 ± 0.3
Deoxycytidine	Nd	Nd
Uracil	17.0 ± 0.9	1.2 ± 0.1
Thymine	Nd	Nd
Cytosine	Nd	Nd

Note: Nd denotes not detected. Values are shown as the mean ± SE. Happo-shu is a low malt liquor, which has a taste that is similar to beer and it contains lower amounts of purine.

Effects of Purines on the Serum Concentration and Urinary Excretion of Uric Acid

Since beer contains many kinds of purines, it is important to investigate the hyperuricemic effects of each. Previous studies (Griebsch and Zollner, 1974; Clifford *et al.*, 1976) have demonstrated that intake of nucleic acid increased the serum concentration and urinary excretion of uric acid. Further, those studies also showed relationships among nucleic acid (RNA) and serum and urinary uric acid levels (Table 26.6) (Clifford *et al.*, 1976). According to those findings, nucleic acid intake was positively correlated to serum concentration and urinary excretion of uric acid, and the increase in the serum concentration of urate following the same amounts of RNA intake was greater in patients with hyperuricemia than in normal control subjects, while the increase in urinary excretion of uric acid was not different between the two groups. In addition, it was reported that the intake of 2 g of RNA per day increased the serum concentration of uric acid by 1.13–1.80 mg/100 ml and the urinary excretion of uric acid by 226–328 mg in 24 h in normal subjects. In patients with gout or hyperuricemia who ingested 2 g of RNA per day, the serum concentration of urate was 1.5-fold greater than that in normal subjects. Although the mechanism by which RNA increased the serum concentration of uric acid to greater levels in the patients was not elucidated, it may have been ascribable to various unknown deficiencies of purine metabolism in individuals with gout. In addition to nucleic acid, the effects of adenine, guanine, hypoxanthine, xanthine, adenosine monophosphate (AMP), guanosine monophosphate (GMP), and inosine monophosphate (IMP) on the serum concentration and urinary excretion of uric acid were investigated in normal subjects, patients with hyperuricemia, and patients with gout (Tables 26.7 and 26.8) (Clifford *et al.*, 1976). Each of those purines (0.1 mmol/kg body weight), except guanine, increased the serum concentration of urate, while each, except for guanine and xanthine, also increased the urinary excretion of uric acid. These findings indicate that many types of purines have hyperuricemic effects. In that study, hypoxanthine, GMP, AMP, and IMP had greater hyperuricemic effects than xanthine and guanine in the control subjects. In the hyper-uricemic patients, hypoxanthine, GMP, AMP, IMP, and adenine had greater hyperuricemic effects than guanine, while AMP, hypoxanthine, GMP, IMP, and adenine had greater hyperuricemic effects than xanthine and guanine in the patients with gout. In addition, hypoxanthine, AMP, and IMP had greater hyperuricemic effect in the patients with gout than in those with hyperuricemia and the control subjects. Each of the examined purines, except for xanthine, guanine, and adenine, increased the urinary uric acid/creatinine ratio in all of the groups. On the other hand, adenine increased the urinary uric acid/creatinine ratio in the control subjects and patients with hyperuricemia, but not in the patients with gout, while neither xanthine nor guanine had effects on the urinary uric acid/creatinine ratio in any of the groups. The differences in effects of the hypoxanthine, AMP, IMP, xanthine, and guanine on the serum concentration and urinary excretion of uric acid may be ascribable to differences in absorption, utilization, and degradation of each purine, as well as differences among the three groups. Nevertheless, these findings suggest that most purines in beer contribute to hyperuricemia in normal subjects and gouty attack in patients. On the other hand, the influence of guanosine toward the increase in the serum concentration of urate in humans has not been studied, even though it is the most abundant purine in beer. However, since guanosine is more readily absorbed than other nucleosides, nucleotides, or bases and rapidly converted to uric acid via guanine and xanthine in animals (Potter *et al.*, 1980), it is suggested that its ingestion may increase the serum concentration of uric acid.

Effects of Purines in Beer and Happo-shu, on Plasma Concentration of Urate

The ingestion of beer is known to increase the plasma concentration of urate. In a previous study (Gibson *et al.*, 1984), 41% of the subjects with gout consumed more than 60 g of ethanol daily and the intake of purine nitrogen, half of which was derived from beer, was higher in those with gout who consumed more than 60 g of ethanol daily. Those results suggested that purines in beer have a clinical effect on serum urate and augment the hyperuricemic effect following its

Table 26.6 Regression equations describing the relationship among dietary RNA intake and serum and urinary uric acid levels in human adults

	Regression equation of diet RNA g/day (X) on	
Type of subjects	*Serum urate mg/100 ml (Y)*	*Urinary uric acid mg/day (Y)*
Normal	$Y = 4.84 + (0.65)(\text{g RNA})$	$Y = 367.8 + (147.2)(\text{g RNA})$
Normal	$Y = 5.05 + (0.56)(\text{g RNA})$	$Y = 645.0 + (163.6)(\text{g RNA})$
Normal	$Y = 3.25 + (0.9)(\text{g RNA})$	$Y = 377.0 + (113)(\text{g RNA})$
Hyperuricemic	$Y = 4.4 + (1.46)(\text{g RNA})$	$Y = 286.0 + (120)(\text{g RNA})$

Note: Dietary RNA intake increases serum and urinary uric acid levels.

Table 26.7 Effects of ingestion of oral purines (0.1 mmol/kg body weight) on serum urate concentrations in normal, hyperuricemic, and gouty subjects

	Subjects		
	Normal	*Hyperuricemic*	*Gouty*
Fasting serum urate (mg/dl)	63 ± 0.5	8.5 ± 0.2	8.3 ± 0.7
Changes in serum			
Urate due to			
Adenine	+1.8 ± 0.3	1.6 ± 0.1	2.0 ± 0.2
Guanine	−0.2 ± 0.1	+0.1 ± 0.2	+0.2 ± 0.3
Hypoxanthine	+2.4 ± 0.2	+2.8 ± 0.2	+4.1 ± 0.4
Xanthine	+0.7 ± 0.1	–	+0.7 ± 0.1
AMP	+2.2 ± 0.3	+1.9 ± 0.1	+4.2 ± 0.4
GMP	+2.3 ± 0.6	+2.2 ± 0.2	+3.3 ± 0.2
IMP	+1.5 ± 0.1	+1.7 ± 0.2	+3.2 ± 0.3

Note: Values are shown as mean + SE. – denotes "not determined." Changes in serum uric acid were determined by subtracting the fasting value from the highest subsequent value after purine intake and are expressed as mg/100 ml. All purines except guanine significantly elevated serum urate levels above fasting values ($p < 0.05$).

Table 26.8 Effects of ingestion of oral purines (0.1 mmol/kg body weight) on urine uric acid/creatinine ratio

	Subjects		
	Normal[a]	*Hyperuricemic*[b]	*Gouty*[a]
Before test purines	0.39 ± 0.03	0.40 ± 0.04	0.34 ± 0.04
After administering			
Adenine	0.46 ± 0.02[c]	0.53 ± 0.02[c]	0.40 ± 0.02
Guanine	0.35 ± 0.02	0.50 ± 0.06	0.34 ± 0.03
Hypoxanthine	0.55 ± 0.07[c]	0.58 ± 0.08[c]	0.68 ± 0.09[c]
Xanthine	0.40 ± 0.04	–	0.38 ± 0.03
AMP	0.51 ± 0.04[c]	0.54 ± 0.04[c]	0.58 ± 0.06[c]
GMP	0.47 ± 0.01[c]	0.64 ± 0.04[c]	0.51 ± 0.01[c]
IMP	0.47 ± 0.06[c]	0.54 ± 0.06[c]	0.57 ± 0.04[c]

Note: Values are shown as mean ± SE.

[a] Based on complete 24-h urine collections.

[b] Based on spot urine samples.

[c] Greater than the ratio before loading ($p < 0.05$). All purines except guanine and xanthine increased urine uric acid/creatinine ratio.

ingestion in gout patients. In our recent study (Yamamoto *et al.*, 2002), we found that regular beer (10 ml/kg body weight) increased the plasma concentration of urate by 30 μmol/l, while freeze-dried beer (0.34 g/kg body weight) also increased that by 20 μmol/l. Since 10 ml of regular beer contains 0.34 g of content when freeze-dried, the amount of purines in freeze-dried beer are the same as those in regular beer. These results indicate that the contents of beer contribute to an increase in urate in blood (Figure 51.7). Accordingly, beer may cause a greater increase in the plasma concentration of urate than

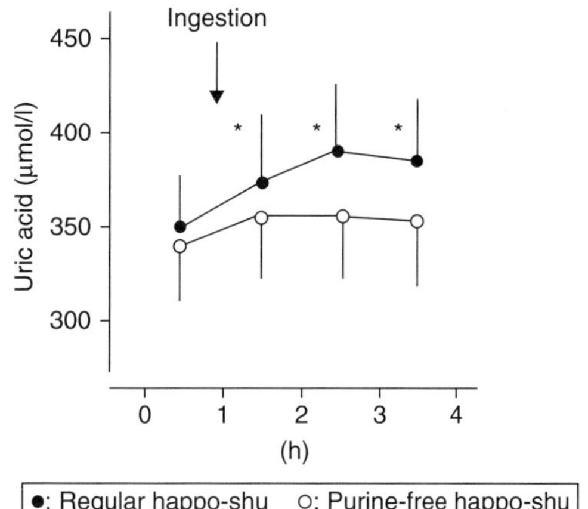

Figure 26.4 Effects of regular and purine-free happo-shu on plasma concentration of urate. *denotes $p < 0.05$, as compared with the reference value before ingestion. Happo-shu is a low malt liquor, which has a taste that is similar to beer and it contains lower amounts of purine. Purine-free happo-shu contains the same amounts of malt and very low levels of purines.

other alcoholic beverages. This result strongly suggested that the purines in beer are the cause of an increase in plasma concentration of urate. In another study (Yamamoto *et al.*, 2004), ingestion of purine-free happo-shu (10 ml/kg body weight) did not increase the plasma concentration of urate, whereas regular happo-shu (10 ml/kg body weight) did, which confirmed our earlier speculation that purines in beer cause an increase in the plasma concentration of urate (Figure 26.4).

Effects of Beer and Other Alcoholic Beverages on Serum Urate Levels

Recently, a prospective study related to nutrition found that subjects who drank 40 ml of distilled liquor (whisky and brandy) had their serum concentration of urate increased by 0.29 mg/dl (Choi *et al.*, 2004). Since distilled liquor rarely contains purines, this finding indicates that the ethanol content increased the level of serum urate. However, the increase in urate caused by distilled liquor is less than that caused by beer ingestion, even when the ingested ethanol volume is not different. Thus, it is considered important for individuals at risk to refrain from drinking large amounts of beer to prevent the development of gout. That prospective study also found that ingestion of 4 oz. of wine per day decreased the serum concentration of uric acid by 0.04 mg/dl, while another study showed that drinking not more than 236 ml (less than 22.0 g ethanol) of wine per day did not increase the risk of gout. Therefore, it was speculated that the components present in wine which were not related to alcohol, such as polyphenol, may prevent ethanol from increasing serum urate, as well as cause a decrease in uric acid production and/or increase urinary uric acid excretion. On the other hand, another report (Abu-Amsha *et al.*, 2001) indicated that ingestion of red wine (5 ml/kg body weight) rapidly increased the serum concentration of urate, while four glasses of red wine each day for 12 weeks increased the serum concentration of urate by 9%, as compared with an 8% increase caused by ingestion of regular spirits containing the same volume of ethanol. Together, these findings suggest that the effect of red wine on serum urate is not significantly different from that of regular spirits.

Summary points

- Beer contains greater amounts of purines than other alcoholic beverages.
- Beer purines consist of purine nucleosides and purine bases, with guanosine being the most abundant.
- Purines in beer augment the hyperuricemic effect following its ingestion.
- It is considered important for individuals at risk to refrain from drinking large amounts of beer to prevent the development of gout.

References

Abu-Amsha Caccetta, R., Burke, V., Mori, T.A., Beilin, L.J., Puddey, I.B. and Croft, K.D. (2001). *Free Radic. Biol. Med.* 30, 636–642.

Choi, H.K., Atkinson, K., Karlson, E.W., Willett, W. and Curhan, G. (1976). *Lancet* 363, 1277–1281.

Clifford, A.J., Rumallo, J.A., Young, V.R. and Scrimshow, N.S. (1976). *J. Nutr.* 106, 428–450.

Cortacero-Ramirez, S., Segura-Carretero, A., Cruces-Blanco, C., Hernainz-Bermudez de Castro, M. and Fernandez-Gutierrez, A. (2004a). *Electrophoresis* 25, 1867–1871.

Cortacero-Ramirez, S., Segura-Carretero, A., Cruces-Blanco, C., Romero-Romero, M.L. and Fernandez-Gutierrez, A. (2004b). *Anal. Bioanal. Chem.* 380, 831–837.

Gibson, T., Rodgers, A.V., Simmonds, H.A. and Toseland, P. (1984). *Br. J. Rheumatol.* 23, 203–209.

Griebsch, A. and Zollner, N. (1974). *Adv. Exp. Med. Biol.* 41, 443–449.

Potter, C.F., Cadenhead, A., Simmonds, H.A. and Cameron, J.S. (1980). *Adv. Exp. Med. Biol.* 122A, 203–208.

Takahashi, S., Yamamoto, T., Tsutsumi, Z., Moriwaki, Y., Yamakita, J. and Higashino, K. (1997). *Metabolism* 46, 1162–1165.

Yamamoto, T., Moriwaki, Y., Takahashi, S., Tsutsumi, Z., Yamakita, J. and Higashino, K. (1997). *Metabolism* 46, 1339–1342.

Yamamoto, T., Moriwaki, Y., Takahashi, S., Tsutsumi, Z., Ka, T., Fukuchi, M. and Hada, T. (2002). *Metabolism* 51, 1317–1323.

Yamamoto, T., Moriwaki, Y., Ka, T., Inokuchi, T., Takahashi, S., Tsutsumi, Z., Fukuchi, M. and Hada, T. (2004). *Horm. Metab. Res.* 36, 231–237.

Yamashita, S., Matsuzawa, Y., Tokunaga, K., Fujioka, S. and Tarui, S. (1986). *Int. J. Obes.* 10, 255–264.

27
Beer Carbohydrates

Isabel M.P.L.V.O. Ferreira REQUIMTE, Serviço de Bromatologia, Faculdade de Farmácia, Universidade do Porto, Porto, Portugal

Abstract

Cereals provide the carbohydrates for beer production. Barley that has been malted is the most usual cereal used. However, other cereals, including wheat, rice, maize, oats, sorghum and sugar syrups, may also be used. During malting all enzymes necessary for total degradation of starch are synthesized and/or activated, together with enzymes that contribute to the hydrolysis of β-glucans and in less extension arabinoxylans. Important transformations occur during mashing, namely, starch is converted into maltose and dextrins. Carbohydrates form 90% of the wort extract, 64–77% of which is usually fermentable by yeast to produce ethanol and carbon dioxide.

Carbohydrate levels in beer range from 3 to 61 g/l. Specific data concerning the beer carbohydrate contents reported by different authors are presented. Different contents of total and fermentable sugars are reported according to beer type. Lagers are in general more fully fermented than ales. Total carbohydrate content of lager and ale beers range between 10–30 and 15–60 g/l, respectively. Lagers also contain less residual carbohydrates than ales, 1–7 g/l and 5–10 g/l, respectively. New brewing styles include fully attenuated low carbohydrate beers that contain less carbohydrate amounts (4–9 g/l) because dextrins have been more or less completely digested and fermented. In general, non-alcohol beers produced by short fermentation present higher level of fermentable sugars (about 55 g/l).

List of Abbreviations

α-L-Ara	α-L-Arabinofuranosyl units
β-D-Glc	β-D-Glucopyranosyl units
β-D-Xyl	β-D-Xylopyranosil units
HPLC	High performance liquid chromatography
TCA	Tricarboxylic acid cycle
t_R	Retention time

Introduction

Beer is a fermented beverage made from malted grains (usually barley), hops, yeast and water. It has a complex composition, containing a vast number of compounds widely ranging in nature and in concentration level. In addition to water and ethanol, major beer components are carbohydrates comprising fermentable sugars as well as glucose oligosaccharides and arabinoxylans (Brandolini *et al.*, 1995; De Keukeleire, 2000; Duarte *et al.*, 2003).

The source of carbohydrates in beer is starch-rich cereals, mainly malted barley, but other cereals including wheat, rice, maize, oats, sorghum and sugar syrups may also be used. The brewing process converts the malt starch to soluble sugars and then uses yeast to ferment these to alcohol. Fermentation takes place at 7–13°C for lagers (using bottom-fermenting yeast, *Saccharomyces carsbergensis*) or 16–18°C for ales (using top-fermenting yeast *Saccharomyces cerevisiae*) (Fix, 1989; Bamforth, 1998; Hughes and Baxter, 2001; Pelter and MaQuade, 2005).

Beers of the lager type include different styles, namely, Bock, Dortmunder, Munchner, Pilsener and Vienna (Marzen). All too often the term lager is used synonymously with Pilsener, the classic style originated in mid-nineteenth century, in the Pilsen city brewhouse. Beers of ale type include a variety of styles such as, Porter, Stout, Salsons, Alt, Light ale, Pale ale, Bitters and Barley wines (Caballero *et al.*, 2003). New brewing styles are introduced, such as those involved in the production of light, dry and low alcohol beers. Here, aspects related to beer carbohydrates, origin and concentration in lager and ale beers will be described. For clarity, brewing specific vocabulary is introduced in Table 27.1.

Origin of Beer Carbohydrates

Beer preparation involves incubating and extracting malt and sometimes other starchy materials and/or enzymes with warm water. After filtration the solution is boiled with hops or hop preparation and the cooled liquid is fermented by added yeast. Cereals provide the carbohydrates and amino acids for the yeast to grow, generate ethanol and carbon dioxide, and produce key flavors in the final beer. Thus, three polysaccharides, starch, pentosan (arabinoxylan) and β-glucan together with saccharose, are the primary source of carbohydrates in beer.

Beer in Health and Disease Prevention
ISBN: 978-0-12-373891-2

Table 27.1 Definitions of common malting and brewing terms

Term	*Definition*
Adjunct	Any source of fermentable extract other than malted barley used in the mash tun, for example, cereal grits or sugar syrup
Aleurone	Layer of living cells in the mature barley kernels, which surround the starchy endosperm
Boiling	Operation that follow lautering. Wort sterilization. Hop is added. Yeast is added to the cooled product to begin fermentation
Fermentation	Metabolization of wort constituents into ethanol and other fermentation products to produce beer
Germination	The sprouting of the barley seed to form new roots and shoots
Lautering	Filtration of mash assisted by insoluble husk material that creates a filter bed
Malt milling	Process carried out in the brewery to reduce the size of the malt particles
Malting	Partial germination to convert barley into malt, followed by quickly drying before the plant develops. Technologically, it is divided into three stages, steeping, germination and kilning
Mashing	Process in which milled malt is mixed with water to form the "mash," which is heated under controlled conditions between 40 and 70 K°C (1–2 h). Important transformations are carried out, namely, proteins are hydrolyzed and amino acids are released, starch is converted into maltose and dextrins
Primings	Sugar added after the primary fermentation to provide additional fermentable extract for secondary fermentation
Sorghum	A small-grained cereal grown in Africa and southern United States
Wort	The liquid obtained after lautering. Sweet wort contains high level of fermentable sugars. Bitter wort or hopped wort is obtained after addition of hop
Yeast	A single-celled microorganism which, in the absence of oxygen, can use glucose as a respiratory substrate and convert it to ethanol.

Table 27.2 Summary of the enzymes necessary for degradation of malt carbohydrates synthesized and/or activated during malting

Type	*Enzyme*	*Substract*	*Function*
Amylases	α-Amylase	Starch	Breakdown of α(1,4) glucosyllinkages
	β-Amylase	Starch and malto-oligosaccharides	Cleave the penultimate α(1,4) glucosyllinkages from non-reducing end
	Limit dextrinase	Amylopectin and branched dextrins	Cleave α(1,6) glucosyllinkages
	α-Glucosidases	Oligosaccharides and maltose	An exoenzyme that releases glucose
Carbohydrases	Endo-β-glucanases	β-Glucan	Releases β-D-glucopyrano-syl oligosaccharides
	Exo-β-glucanases	Oligosaccharides released by endo-β-glucanases	Produce glucose from β-glucan oligosshacarides
	Endo-β-xylanases	Arabinoxylans	Cleave β-1,4 xylan linkages
	β-Xylopyranosidases	Arabinoxylans	Breakdown xylan polymers
	α-L-Arabinofuranosidase	Arabinoxylans	Release α-L-arabinofura-nosyl units from pentosans
Carboxipeptidases	β-Glucan solubilase	β-Glucan	Degrades ester linkages between proteins and β-glucan, releases β-glucan

Source: Adapted from Hughes and Baxter (2001), Caballero *et al.* (2003) and Eliasson (2006).

Malt

Barley that has been malted is the most usual cereal used in beer production. It has an appropriate level of protein (8–12% dry weight), low level of lipids, develops high levels of amylolytic enzymes during germination and it has a husk (the outer case of the barley grain) that creates a filter bed and assists in the separation of insoluble material from the extract.

Barley grain germination is initiated by the uptake of water. The grain is hydrated or steeped by immersion in water. Germination occurs in a cool, moist atmosphere with occasional turning, and involves partial development of the embrion, activating several endogenous enzymatic systems. Hydrolytic enzymes are secreted from the aleurone and the scutellar epithelium and migrate into the starchy endosperm. Thus, during malting all enzymes necessary for total degradation of starch are synthesized and/or activated (Table 27.2). Some enzymes also contribute to the hydrolysis of β-glucans and hordeins (water insoluble proteins), which would otherwise restrict access of enzymes to the starch granules.

...4) – β-D-Glc (1,3) – β-D-Glc (1,4) – β-D-Glc (1,4) – β-D-Glc (1,4) – β-D-Glc (1,4) – β-D-Glc (1,3) –

↑ ↑

Figure 27.1 Structure of barley β-glucan. β-D-Glc, β-D-glucopyranosyl units; (1,3), β-1,3 linkages (about 30%); (1,4), β-1,4 linkages (about 70%). ↑ Examples of sites of hydrolysis by endo-β-glucanases.

Germination is allowed to proceed over around 5 days to obtain green malt, which is stopped during the kilning phase by forced flow of hot air. Hydrolases produced during malting are partially inactivated during this process and the malt is suitable for the milling process, which precedes brewing.

During mashing the crushed malt, named grist, is mixed with hot water in the mash tun and the whole mash is held at around 65°C for about 1 h. This temperature is chosen as it is the temperature at which malt (i.e. barley) starch will gelatinize – making it more susceptible to enzyme attack.

Adjuncts

Other cereals, both malted and unmalted, including wheat, rice, maize, oats and sorghum, are used as adjuncts for certain beers. Adjuncts come in a variety of forms, for example grits that are fragments of starchy endosperm from cereal grains. If they are used directly in the brewery they must be cooked or flaked (the grain is heated at 85°C and passed through feed rolls to flaking rolls).

To use in the brewery, all grits must be cooked to disrupt them and gelatinize the starch. Because the starch is already gelatinized the flakes do not need cooking and can be added directly to the mash. Like barley starch, wheat starch also gelatizes at 65°C. Rice and maize starches gelatinize at higher temperatures, so if either of these cereals is used as an adjunct, it must be pre-cooked in a separate vessel (known as a cereal cooker) before being added to the mash (Hughes and Baxter, 2001; Briggs *et al.*, 2004; Urias-Lugo and Saldivar, 2005).

Syrups of sucrose and its hydrolysis product, inverted sugar, are used by some brewers during beer production, produced either from sugar cane or from sugar beet, the range of products is large.

Adjuncts are used to reduce the quantity of malt used, since malt is more expensive than these products, and so the use of adjuncts in relatively large amounts (20–30%) significantly reduces the cost of brewing process. Good quality malt presents amylolytic activity surplus to requirements. Thus, an adjunct's starch is hydrolyzed during mashing by enzymes from the malt, not only to provide a less expensive source of sugars, but also to change the character of the wort. For example, small quantities of wheat are often used in ales to enhance the beer foam, while unmalted rice and maize grits may be used to improve the flavor stability of light-flavored lagers. In a few countries the use of adjuncts is forbidden. In Germany, the *Reinheitsgebot* stipulates that beer may be made only with water, malt, hops and yeast (Hughes and Baxter, 2001; Caballero *et al.*, 2003; Urias-Lugo and Saldivar, 2005).

Degradation of cell-wall polymers

The major component of the endosperm of barley cell walls are β-glucans, which are linear polymers composed of β-D-glucopyranosyl residues linked with a mixture of β-1,3 (about 30%) and β-1,4 (about 70%) linkages (Figure 27.1). About 90% of the 4-linked residues occur in groups of two or three residues, separated by (1,3) linkages. Breakdown of the endosperm cell walls initiates from the scutellum and advances more or less uniformly through the grain. The extent to which β-glucans are degraded during malting depends on the moisture content of the steeped grain, on the amount of cell-wall-degrading enzymes, and on the structure of the cell walls. Endo-β-glucanases are enzymes that hydrolyze high molecular weight β-glucans and produce tri and tetrasaccharides. Exo-β-glucanases produce glucose from β-glucan or oligosacchacarides. β-Glucan solubilase are carboxipeptidases that degrade ester linkages between proteins and β-glucan (see Table 27.2) (Eliasson, 2006).

Incomplete breakdown of the β-glucan linkage can cause several problems during brewing, namely, decrease rates of wort separation and beer filtration, formation of hazes and precipitates in the final beer.

Arabinoxylans consist of a linear xylan backbone of β-1,4 linked to D-xylopyranosil residues to which α-L-arabinofuranosyl units are attached mostly as single substitutes. These pentosans are side-chain branched heteroglycans built from pentose sugars, arabinose and xylose (Figure 27.2). Several enzymes are involved in the hydrolytic breakdown of barley arabinoxylans, namely, endo-β-xylanases, β-xylopyranosidases, α-L-arabinofuranosidase (see Table 27.2). However, whereas β-glucans are degraded extensively during malting, pentosans are not and remain in malt (Beldman *et al.*, 1988).

Starch Degradation

Cereal starch consists of approximately 75% amylopectin and 25% amylase. Although built up from the same glucopyranose units, they differ in the type of glycosidic linkages and require different enzymes for their degradation. Amylopectin is a very large, branched molecule (the molecular weight has been estimated at several million,

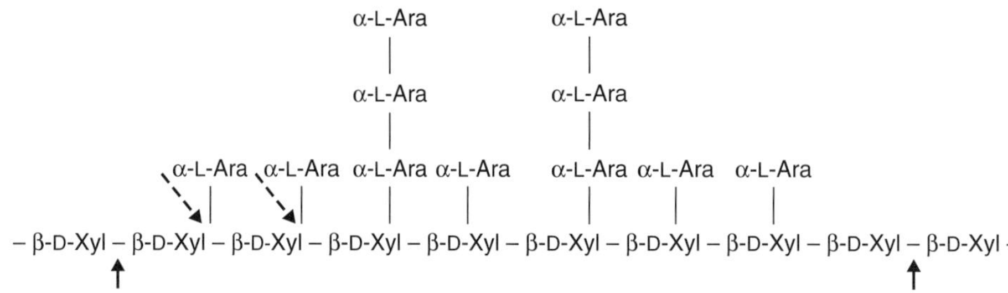

Figure 27.2 Structure of barley arabinoxylans. α-L-Ara, α-L-arabinofuranosyl units; β-D-Xyl, β-D-xylopyranosil units. ↑ Examples of sites of hydrolysis by endo-β-xilanases. ↘ Examples of sites of hydrolysis by α-L-arabinofuranosidase.

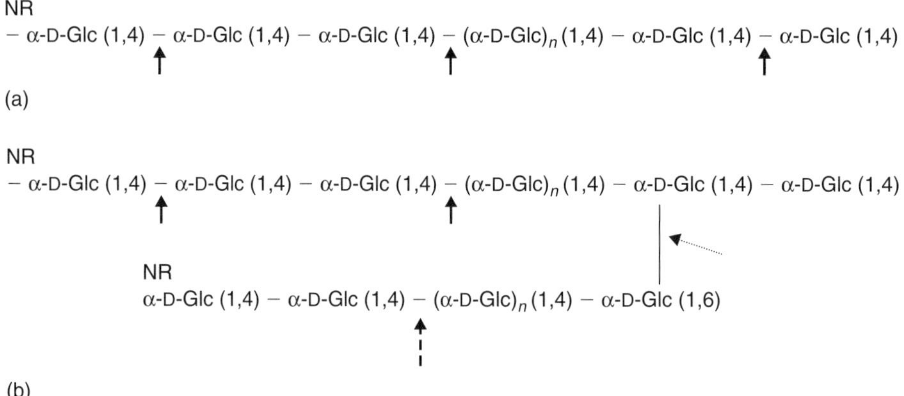

Figure 27.3 Structure of amylose and amylopectine. (a) Amylose and (b) amylopectine. α-D-Glc: α-D-glucopyranosyl units; (1,4), α-1,4 linkages; (1,6), α-1,6 linkages. ↑ Examples of sites of hydrolysis by α-amylases. ⇡ Examples of sites of hydrolysis by β-amylases. ← Examples of sites of hydrolysis by limit dextrinase.

10^6–10^8 Da) made up of glucose units linked by α-1,4 bonds (which give linear chains) and α-1,6 bonds (which give branch points). On average, each branch is made up of around 25 glucose units. Amylose, on the other hand, is a linear molecule made up of up to 2,000–5,000 glucose units linked by α-1,4 bonds only (Figure 27.3(a) and (b)).

During malting starch is only partially degraded (15–18%). It is during mashing that the malt amylolytic enzymes break down the starch into fermentable sugars. Both α- and β-amylase can hydrolyze α-1,4 bonds. α-Amylase hydrolyze intact starch granule, degrade amylose to oligosaccharides, maltose and glucose. It also attacks lengths of α-1,4 chains between branch points of amylopectin, releasing smaller, branched dextrins with long straight side-chains. These provide more substances for β-amylase action. β-Amylase attacks from the outer reducing ends of the amylopectin and amylase molecules, releasing free maltose (two glucose units), but stopping when it reaches an α-1,6 bond. α- and β-Amylases acting together reduce amylose to maltose, maltotriose and glucose, however, amylopectin gives rise to small branched dextrins which cannot be further broken down during mashing.

Limit dextrinase hydrolyzes α-1,6 linkages in amylopectin or in branched dextrins. It requires at least one α-1,4-glicosidic linkage on either side of the α-1,6 linkage. However, this enzyme is inhibited by a heat-stable protein present in barley. α-Glucosidase converts maltose and other small dextrins to glucose (Hughes and Baxter, 2001; Caballero *et al.*, 2003; Pelter and MaQuade, 2005).

Wort Carbohydrates

Carbohydrates form 90% of the wort extract, 64–77% of which is usually fermentable by yeast. Its composition will depend on the make-up grist and the mashing conditions. However, the most important sugars and dextrins in wort are made of glucose, which also occurs free and d-glicopyranosyl units joined by α(1,4) linkages or α(1,6) linkages for dextrins. Maltose and maltotriose are the major sugars in brewer's wort, but other carbohydrates are present, some of them detected in tiny amounts (Table 27.3). Maltose usually accounts for 50–60% of the fermentable sugar in wort (Briggs *et al.*, 2004). Carbohydrate

Table 27.3 Major and minor wort saccharides

Major wort saccharides	*Content (g/l)*	*Minor wort saccharides*	*Content (mg/l)*
Fructose + glucose	9–12	Xilose	15
Maltose	56–59	Arabinose	14
Saccharose	4–5	Ribose	2
Maltotriose	14–17	Isomaltose	Traces
Maltotetraose	6–7	Panose	Traces
Dextrins + glucans + pentosans	22–26	Isopanose	Traces
		Nigerose	Traces
		Maltulose	Traces

Source: Adapted from Briggs *et al.* (2004).

fermentability of the wort is determined by the evaluation of "fermentable sugars" and "dextrins" and the results are presented as fermentable carbohydrates as a percentage of the total carbohydrates.

The carbohydrates undergo some changes during wort boiling which include browning reactions that take place between reducing sugars and the primary amines. These reactions consist of condensation reactions between simple sugars, such as glucose with primary amines to give aldosylamines. These unstable compounds can undergo Amadori rearrangement to form ketosamines, which condense with another aldose molecule to form diketosamines that can undergo further condensation reactions with additional amines (Hughes and Baxter, 2001). All these reactions are complex and not completely understood, however, they occur in very low extension. Whole hops and pellets only contribute to 0.15% of the total carbohydrates in hopped wort, thus, the carbohydrate composition of hopped wort is very similar to that of sweet wort.

Beer Carbohydrates

Brewing yeast strains (ale and lager strains) are capable of utilizing saccharose, glucose, fructose, maltose and maltotriose in this order, whereas the higher oligomers remain in solution. Consequently, the total carbohydrates in beer include residual fermentable sugars and a variable amount of higher dextrins, most of which contain two or more branches (Uchida *et al.*, 1991; Shanta-Kumara *et al.*, 1995; Clement *et al.*, 1992; Castellari *et al.*, 2001). Nevertheless, trace amounts of other carbohydrates have been detected in beer including the monosaccharides; D-ribose, L-arabinose, D-xilose, D-mannose and D-galactose, the positional isomers of α and β-glucobioses and the trisaccharides panose and isopanose and β-linked materials are derived from the β-glucan and arabinoxylan present in barley (Vinogradov and Bock, 1998; Duarte *et al.*, 2003; Briggs *et al.*, 2004; Bamforth, 2005). Table 27.4 summarizes monosaccharides, disaccharides, trisaccharides and oligosaccharides identified in several types of beers. The total carbohydrates remaining

Table 27.4 Monosaccharides, disaccharides, trisaccharides and oligosaccharides identified in beer

Monossaccharides	*Disaccharides*	*Trisaccharides*	*Oligosaccharides*
L-Arabinose	Cellobiose	Maltotriose	4-α-Isomaltosyl-D-maltose
Fructose	Isomaltose	Isopanose	Maltotetraose
Glucose	Maltose	Panose	Maltopentose
D-Galactose	Saccharose	Xylotriose	Maltohexose
D-Manose	Kojibiose	Cellotriose	Maltoheptose
Pentose	Xylobiose	Raffinose	Malto-octose
D-Ribose	Trehalose	Gentianose	Maltononanose
D-Xylose	Melibiose	Isokestose	Stachyose
	Turanose	Kestose	
	Maltulose	Melizitose	

Source: Adapted from Gey *et al.* (1996), Vinogradov and Bock (1998), Floridi *et al.* (2001), Duarte *et al.* (2003), Briggs *et al.* (2004), Bamforth (2005), Ramirez *et al.* (2005), Bruggink *et al.* (2005).

Table 27.5 Carbohydrate content of beers reported by different authors

	Carbohydrate (g/l)		
Beer type	*Total*	*Sugars (including maltotriose)*	*Dextrins*
Beer mean values[a]	2.8–61	1.3–22	7–39
Pilsener[b]	30	3.65	24
Lagers[c]	10–30	1–7	10–20
Ales and stouts[c]	15–60	5–10	10–40
Primed beers[c]	20–70	13–36	10–40
"Lite" beers[c]	2–9	1–6	1–3

Source: Adapted from [a] Buckee and Hargitt (1977), [b] Caballero *et al.* (2003), [c] Hughes and Baxter (2001).

in beer can be estimated spectrophotometrically with anthrone in 85% sulfuric acid (Analytica-EBC, 1998) for a range of beers values between 2.8–61 g/l as glucose were found. However, in general, carbohydrate levels range from 20 to 30 g/l. Table 27.5 presents more specific data concerning the beer carbohydrate contents reported by different authors.

Beer fermentable sugars

Alcoholic fermentation of wort sugars to ethanol and carbon dioxide is conducted by yeasts predominantly under anaerobic conditions, however, oxygen is required by brewing yeasts in the initial stages of wort fermentation for the biosynthesis of membrane sterols and fatty acids. Thus, yeast, when under anaerobic conditions (which means that air exposure is to be kept to a minimum), converts glucose to pyruvic acid via the glycolysis pathways, then go one step farther, converting pyruvic acid into ethanol, a C-2 compound (see Figure 27.4). Once most of the available sugars are fermented, metabolism slows down. The freshly produced or "green" beer is held for a period of maturation or secondary fermentation. During this process the flavor of the mature beer is improved. Sometimes "priming" sugar or a small amount of wort is added to boost yeast metabolism and the "maturation," "conditioning" or "lagering" process (Briggs *et al.*, 2004).

Fermentable sugars directly contribute to the sweetness of beer. These can arise either from the malt if they have survived fermentation/or else they have been added as "primings" to stimulate secondary fermentation to bring the beer up to specified carbon dioxide levels. The carbohydrates with more than four glycosyl units possess little sweetness. However, they can be beneficial to the perception of beer in that they contribute to body or mouthfeel (Corradini *et al.*, 1997; Ferreira *et al.*, 2005).

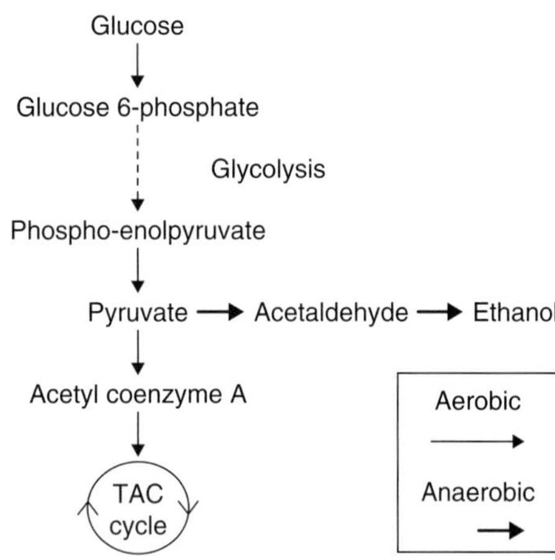

Figure 27.4 Conversion of glucose to ethanol in yeast. *Glycolysis* – the sequence of reactions that converts glucose into pyruvate with the concomitant production of a relatively small amount of adenosine triphosphate (ATP). *Anerobic* (in the absence of oxygen) – pathway for organisms that can ferment sugars and produce the alcohol found in beer. *Aerobic* (in the presence of oxygen) – pathway for pyruvate degradation by the tricarboxylic acid cycle (TCA) or cycle Krebs to produce larger amounts of ATP.

Different contents of fermentable sugars are reported according to beer type (Tables 27.6 and 27.7). Lagers are in general more fully fermented (attenuated) than ales and contain less residual carbohydrates. During fermentation the yeast absorbs and ferments first all the glucose and then maltose. Some lager yeasts can also utilize maltotriose (Thomas *et al.*, 2000).

Fructose, glucose, maltose and maltotriose contents of beers from 10 different countries, including Belgium, Brazil, Czech Republic, Denmark, Germany, Holland, Ireland, Portugal, Spain and UK, were evaluated by high performance liquid chromatography (HPLC)/light scattering (Ferreira *et al.*, 2005; Nogueira *et al.*, 2005). The results obtained in this work (Table 27.8) are in good agreement with others from literature that were reported previously.

Table 27.7 Order of magnitude composition of a pilsner beer

Sugar	*According to Caballero et al. (2003)*	*According to Nogueira et al. (2005)*
Fructose	0.15	Not detected*
Glucose	0.03	Not detected*
Maltose	1.5	0.35
Maltotriose	2.0	1.32
Maltotetraose	Not described	2.95

Source: Adapted from literature. *Detection limit: 0.005 g/l for fructose, 0.008 g/l for glucose.

Table 27.8 Mean values of sugars of 22 beer samples produced in ten different countries

Sugar	*Lager*	*Ale*
Fructose	Not detected	Not detected
Glucose	Not detected	Not detected
Maltose	0.05 ± 0.10	Not detected
Maltotriose	1.25 ± 0.71	2.51 ± 0.40
Maltotetraose	3.45 ± 1.31	7.11 ± 1.91

Source: Values obtained using the HPLC methodology validated by Nogueira *et al.* (2005), $n = 18$ for lagers and $n = 4$ for ales. The detection limit values were 0.005 g/l for fructose, 0.008 g/l for glucose and 0.01 g/l for maltose, maltotriose and maltotetraose.

Table 27.6 Typical levels of sugar content in beer shown as g/l

Sugar	*Range found in beer according to Buckee and Hargitt (1977)*	*Range found in beer according to Hughes and Baxter (2001)*	*Range found in lager beer according to Briggs et al. (2004)*	*Range found in ale beer according to Briggs et al. (2004)*
Fructose	0–5.5	0–0.19	0–1.8	0–0.1
Glucose	0–8	0.04–1.1	0–4.9	0–8
Maltose	0–2	0.7–3.0	0–2.5	0–7
Maltotriose	0.13–7.4	0.4–3.4	0–3.3	0.8–17
Maltotetraose	Not described	Not described	0–2.0	0.4–4

Source: Adapted from cited literature.

Dextrins, pentosans and β-glucan

Dextrins, derived from partial degradation of starch, are not fermentable, thus, when branched dextrins are present in brewer's wort, they will be found in the final beer (Jodelet *et al.*, 1998). Beer dextrins impart body and contribute to calorific value because dextrins are readily hydrolyzed by pancreatic amylase. The branched dextrins are broken down slowly by the oligo-1,6-glucosidase which is found in the mucosal cells lining the intestine.

Pentosan and β-glucan depolymerized to some degree remain partially in beer, where they can cause undesired precipitation and filtration problems.

Carbohydrate Contents in New Brewing Styles

Brewers intent on marketing new brewing styles to answer specific demands of consumers, namely, low carbohydrates beers and low alcohol beers. The enormous incidence of excess body weight in several countries stimulates the interest in these new products, together with the presence of healthy carbohydrates, such as, soluble fiber and prebiotic molecules that it contains and which are derived from the β-glucan and arabinoxylans.

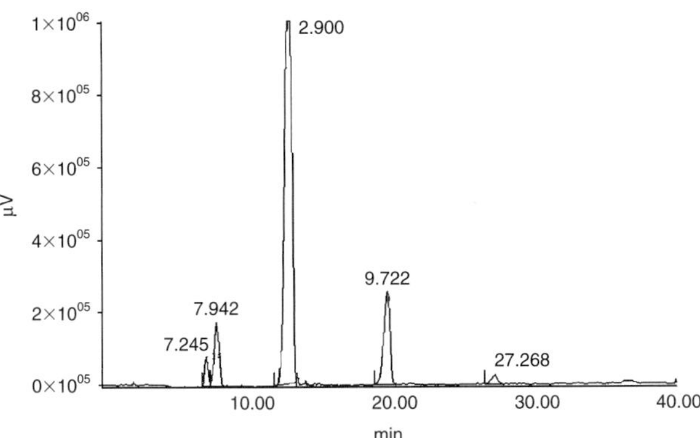

Figure 27.5 Typical chromatogram for separation of five carbohydrates in an alcohol free beer sample. Fructose (t_R = 7.245 min), glucose (t_R = 7.942 min), maltose (t_R = 12.900 min), maltotriose (t_R = 19.722 min), maltotetraose (t_R = 27.268 min). Analyses performed by HPLC with an amine-bonded silica column, acetonitrile–water as eluent, and a light scattering detector.

Table 27.9 Fructose, glucose, maltose, maltotriose and maltotetraose composition of non-alcohol beers.

Sugar	*According to Nogueira et al. (2005)*	*Evaluated in seven brands using the methodology validated by Nogueira* et al. *(2005)*
Fructose	2.57	2.46 ± 0.13
Glucose	4.56	5.60 ± 1.53
Maltose	38.5	44.13 ± 12.14
Maltotriose	8.14	10.89 ± 2.89
Maltotetraose	1.39	2.39 ± 1.03

Source: Values collected from literature, together with results from seven brands from Brazil, Portugal and Spain.

Low carbohydrate beers

Fully attenuated low carbohydrate beers with carbohydrate contents of 4–9 g/l were originally brewed for diabetic patiens, but are now generally available (Briggs *et al.*, 2004; Bamforth, 2005). The low carbohydrate beers contain less carbohydrate because dextrins have been more or less completely digested and fermented by a combination of techniques. For example, special yeasts, known as "highly attenuating yeasts," may be used enabling digestion of a wide range of dextrins. Another possibility is the use of lightly kilned malts, which contain higher levels of debranching enzyme (Hughes and Baxter, 2001).

Non-alcohol beers

Non-alcohol beers can be produced by restricting the ability of yeasts to ferment wort. Figure 27.5 shows the typical chromatographic profile for fructose, glucose, maltose, maltotriose and maltotetraose of a free alcohol beer sample obtained by this process. These samples suffered short fermentation, thus, great part of fructose, maltose, maltotriose and maltotetraose remained in beer (Table 27.9).

Fructose, glucose, maltose and maltotriose contents of beers from three different countries, including Brazil, Portugal and Spain, were evaluated by HPLC/light scattering (Nogueira *et al.*, 2005; Ferreira *et al.*, 2005). The results obtained in this work are also presented in Table 27.8. Low alcohol beers were poorly fermented and contained higher amounts of fermentable carbohydrate. However, another process to obtain non-alcohol beer is removing the alcohol from a full-strength brew by techniques such as vacuum distillation or reverse osmosis. These techniques are more expensive.

Summary Points

- Major beer components are water, ethanol and carbohydrates comprising fermentable sugars (i.e. fructose, glucose, maltose and maltotriose) as well as glucose oligosaccharides and arabinoxylans.
- Barley that has been malted is the most usual cereal used in brewing. However, other cereals, including wheat, rice, maize, oats, sorghum and sugar syrups may also be used.
- During malting all enzymes necessary for total degradation of starch are synthesized and/or activated, together with enzymes that contribute to the hydrolysis of β-glucans and in less extension arabinoxylans.
- Important transformations occur during mashing, namely, starch is converted into maltose and dextrins. Carbohydrates form 90% of the wort extract, 64–77% of

which is usually fermentable by yeast to produce ethanol and carbon dioxide.

- Total carbohydrates in beer include residual fermentable sugars and a variable amount of higher dextrins, most of which contain two or more branches.
- Different contents of fermentable sugars are reported according to beer type. Lagers are in general more fully fermented than ales and contain less residual carbohydrates.
- Brewers intent on marketing new brewing styles to answer specific demands of consumers, namely, low carbohydrates beers and low alcohol beers.

References

Analytica-EBC (1998). *European Brewery Convention*, 5th edn, pp. 57–78. Verlag Hans Carl Getränke, Fachverlag, Nürnberg.

Bamforth, C.W. (2005). *J. Inst. Brew,* 111, 259–264.

Beldman, G., Voragen, A.G.J., Rombouts, F.M., Searle-van, Leeuwen, M.F. and Pilnik, W. (1988). *Biotechnol. Bioeng.* 31, 160–169.

Brandolini, V., Menziani, E., Mazzotta, D., Cabras, P., Tosi, B. and Lodi, G. (1995). *J. Food Comp. and Anal.* 8, 336–343.

Briggs, D.E., Boulton, C.A., Brookes, P.A. and Roger, S. (2004). *Brewing: Science and Practice*, pp. 1–290. Woodhead Publishing Limited and CRC Press, Cambridge and Boca Raton, FL.

Bruggink, C., Maurer, R., Herrmann, H., Cavalli, S. and Hoefler, F. (2005). *J. Chromatogr. A* 1085, 104–109.

Buckee, G.K. and Hargitt, R. (1977). *J. Inst. Brew.* 83, 275–278.

Caballero, B., Trugo, L.C. and Finglas, P.M. (2003). *Encyclopedia of Food Sciences and Nutrition*, pp. 418–451 and Vol 6, pp. 3671–3685. Academic Press Inc., San Diego, CA. Vol 1.

Castellari, M., Sartini, E., Spinabelli, U., Riponi, C. and Galassi, S. (2001). *J. Chromatogr. Sci.* 39, 235–238.

Clement, A., Young, D. and Brechet, C. (1992). *J. Liq. Chromatogr.* 15, 805–817.

Corradini, C., Canali, G. and Nicoletti, I. (1997). *Sem. Food Anal.* 2, 99–111.

De Keukeleire, D. (2000). *Quim. Nova* 23, 108–112.

Duarte, I.F., Godejohann, M., Braumann, U., Spraul, M. and Gil, A.M. (2003). *J. Agric. Food Chem.* 51, 4847–4853.

Eliasson, A.C. (2006). *Carbohydrates in Food,* 2nd edn, pp. 129–209. CRC Press, London and New York.

Ferreira, I.M.P.L.V.O., Jorge, K., Nogueira, L.C., Silva, F. and Trugo, L.C. (2005). *J. Agric. Food Chem.* 53, 4976–4981.

Fix, G. (1989). *Principles of Brewing Science*, pp. 22–108. Brewers Publications, Boulder, CA.

Floridi, S., Miniati, E., Montanari, L. and Fantozzi, P. (2001). *Monatsschrift fur Brauwissenschaft* 54, 209–215.

Gey, M.H., Unger, K.K. and Battermann, G. (1996). *Fresenius J. Anal. Chem.* 356, 339–343.

Hughes, P.S. and Baxter, E.D. (2001). *Beer: Quality, Safety and Nutritional Aspects*, pp. 1–13 and 98–105. Royal Society of Chemistry, Cambridge.

Jodelet, A., Rigby, N.M. and Colquhoum, I.J. (1998). *Carbohydr. Res.* 312, 139–151.

Nogueira, L.C., Silva, F., Ferreira, I.M.P.L.V.O. and Trugo, L.C. (2005). *J. Chromatogr. A* 1065, 207–210.

Pelter, M.W. and MaQuade, J. (2005). *J Chem. Educ.* 82, 1811–1812.

Ramirez, S.C., Carretero, A.S., Blanco, C.C., Castro, M.F.B. and Gutierrez, A.F. (2005). *J. Sci. Food Agric.* 85, 517–521.

Shanta-Kumara, H.M.C., Iserentant, D. and Verachtert, H. (1995). Cerevisia. *Belgian J. Brew. Biotechnol.* 20, 47–53.

Thomas, B.R., Brandley, B.K. and Rodriguez, R.L. (2000). *J. Am. Soc. Brew. Chem.* 58, 124–127.

Uchida, M., Nakatani, K., Ono, M. and Nagami, K. (1991). *J. Am. Soc. Brew. Chem.* 49, 665–673.

Urias-Lugo, D.A. and Saldivar, S.O.S. (2005). *J. Am. Soc. Brew. Chem.* 63, 63–68.

Vinogradov, E. and Bock, K. (1998). *Carbohydr. Res.* 309, 57–64.

28

Dietary Fiber in Beer: Content, Composition, Colonic Fermentability, and Contribution to the Diet

I. Goñi Unidad Asociada Nutrición y Salud Gastrointestinal (UCM-CSIC), Dpt. Nutrición I, Facultad de Farmacia, Ciudad Universitaria, Madrid, Spain
M.E. Díaz-Rubio and F. Saura-Calixto Dpt. Metabolismo y Nutrición (CSIC), Ciudad Universitaria, Madrid, Spain

Abstract

Most reports on carbohydrates in beer deal with sensory and technological properties, but a nutritional approach indicates that dietary fiber (DF) is a quantitatively important beer constituent, composed mainly of indigestible carbohydrates. DF is usually determined exclusively in plant foods probably because the official methods of analysis are not applicable to beverages. Consequently, international food composition tables report zero DF content in beer and other beverages. A specific method to determine DF in beer is reported. DF content in beer is around 2 g/l, the largest constituents being arabinoxylans and β-glucans. Beer DF is highly fermented by colonic bacteria, similarly to healthy soluble DF-like psyllium and β-glucans.

The consumption of beer (150 ml person/day) in Spain accounts for 1.6% and 5% of the total DF and soluble DF intake of the diet, respectively.

DF occurs in beer as a complex with appreciable amounts of indigestible carbohydrates (88–91%), polyphenolic compounds (4.2–2.9%) and indigestible protein (7.7–5.9%).

Further research on the physicochemical structure and biological properties of beer DF is needed to elucidate its nutritional significance.

List of Abbreviations

DF	Dietary Fiber
SDF	Soluble Dietary Fiber
SCFAs	Short Chain Fatty Acids
IDF	Insoluble Dietary Fiber
PP	Polyphenols
WHO/FAO	World Health Organization/Food and Agriculture Organization

Introduction

Nowadays, the importance of dietary fiber (DF) in nutrition and health is well defined. Numerous clinical and epidemiological studies have addressed the role of DF in intestinal health, prevention of cardiovascular disease, colon cancer, obesity and diabetes.

The knowledge of the consumption of DF in the diet is important for a proper nutritional evaluation. DF is determined exclusively in plant foods, and it is generally assumed that drinks, including beer, do not contain DF. Consequently, the presence of DF in common dietary beverages is ignored in nutritional studies and in reports of DF intakes in diets. However, drinks are quantitatively important items in any diet and they may contain measurable amounts of soluble dietary fiber (SDF). Here we focus on DF in beer, the most widely consumed drink in many western countries.

This chapter deals with the content, composition and colonic fermentability of DF in beer, and the analytical methodology used to determine this beer constituent. The contribution of beer to DF intake in the diet is also addressed.

First, the concept and main properties of DF are briefly described for readers who are not familiar with this topic. In this respect, there is comprehensive information available on the carbohydrate composition of beer, which is associated with its sensory and technological properties. The second point adopts a nutritional approach, dividing these beer constituents into two groups: indigestible and digestible. Non-digestible polysaccharides are the major constituents of DF.

Official methods for analysis of DF were developed for plant foods and cannot be applied to beverages, and hence the third point of this chapter presents a specific procedure to determine DF in beer. The DF content and composition in different types of beer, which were determined using a specific procedure to determine DF in beer, is presented in the third point.

Fermentation in the large intestine is an essential property of DF. The degree of colonic fermentation of beer DF is described in point four, including the extent of fermentation and the production of short chain fatty acids (SCFAs).

The dietary significance of DF in a specific food or beverage depends on its contribution in the context of a whole

Beer in Health and Disease Prevention
ISBN: 978-0-12-373891-2

diet. This aspect is addressed in point five, where intake and sources of DF in the Spanish diet, including beverages, are presented.

The traditional concept of DF based on indigestible non-starch polysaccharides and lignin is changing. There is agreement among nutritionists to extend the concept of DF to include other non-digestible plant food constituents. Following this line, the last point of the chapter reports the presence of significant amounts of polyphenolic compounds and protein associated with DF in beer.

Dietary Fiber

Plant foods and beverages contain a wide variety of carbohydrates that supply a large part of the energy in human diet and have different metabolic functions relating to fat synthesis, protein sparing, connective tissue, detoxification, cell recognition and others.

Classification of carbohydrates can be based on chemical composition and/or nutritional properties. From a nutritional point of view, there are two main groups of carbohydrates: digestible ones in the small intestine, or glycemic carbohydrates, and non-digestible ones which are partially fermentable in the large intestine (WHO/FAO, 1999).

Digestible carbohydrates are hydrolyzed by digestive enzymes and metabolized after enzymatic hydrolysis. monosaccharides such as glucose and fructose, low-molecular-weight saccharides like sucrose, lactose and maltose, and polysaccharides with α bonds like starch are the main dietary digestible carbohydrates. Indigestible polysaccharides are neither hydrolyzed nor absorbed in the small intestine and become available in the large intestine as fermentable substrates for the colonic microflora. Cellulose, β-glucans, pentosans, arabinoxylans, galactomannans and other β-polysaccharides are the major constituents of DF. Table 28.1 summarizes the definition and main constituents of DF.

DF is one of the most talked-about food constituents in connection with health promotion and disease prevention.

Table 28.1 Definition and main constituents of DF

<table>
<tr><td rowspan="2">Dietary fiber:
Plant food and drinks constituents resistant to digestion and absorption in the small intestine</td><td>Insoluble dietary fiber:
Non-water soluble at 100°C and pH = 6–7</td><td>Main constituents:
Cellulose, lignin, insoluble hemicelluloses</td></tr>
<tr><td>Soluble dietary fiber:
Water soluble at 100°C and pH = 6–7</td><td>β-Glucans, arabinoxylans, gums, pectins, oligosaccharides, soluble hemicelluloses</td></tr>
</table>

Note: DF improves gastrointestinal health. DF constituents are fermented in the large intestine providing energy to maintain the intestinal bacteria.

The definition of DF, besides specifying the constituents, describes their physiological and metabolic significance (Cho and Dreher, 2001; McCleary and Prosky, 2001). DF consists of the indigestible parts of plants that are resistant to digestion and absorption in the human small intestine. DF includes non-starch polysaccharides, lignin and other non-digestible carbohydrates. These DF components are neither degraded nor absorbed during their passage through the upper part of the gastrointestinal tract, and they can exert nutritionally important effects by slowing down gastric emptying and affecting nutrient assimilation in the small intestine. When non-digestible compounds pass into the large intestine, they can be degraded by bacterial enzymes and their degradation products can be fermented to produce SCFAs as well as gases and water.

Also, DF includes many components that are categorized by whether or not they are soluble in the human digestive system. Insoluble dietary fiber (IDF) includes cellulose and other polysaccharides along with non-carbohydrate compounds such as lignin and cutin and other cell wall constituents. SDF includes pectins, β-glucans, arabinoxylans, galactomannans and other indigestible polysaccharides and saccharides.

Both SDF and IDF are present in all plant foods, with varying degrees of each depending on a plant's characteristics. Insolubility refers to lack of solubility in water, but it also implies passive water-attracting properties that help to increase bulk soften stools and shorten transit time through the intestinal tract. Solubility indicates a fiber source that will readily dissolve in water and form viscous solutions. Soluble fibers delay gastric emptying, slow glucose absorption, enhance immune functions and lower serum cholesterol levels. These terms proved very useful in the initial understanding of the physiological properties of DF, allowing a simple division into those which principally affected glucose and lipid absorption from the small intestine, SDF, and those which were slowly and incompletely fermented and had more pronounced effects on bowel habit, IDF.

The soluble fraction is mainly contained in fruits, vegetables and legumes and is associated with colonic degradation and high fermentability, while insoluble fiber is thought to affect primarily the function of the large bowel and is predominant in cereals and legumes. Insoluble fiber consists mainly of cell wall components such as cellulose, lignin and hemicellulose.

DF is an essential nutrient in human nutrition. Dietary guidelines from the WHO and many national government health bodies recommend an increase in the daily intake of DF, which is especially low in the current diets of western countries. One important aspect of epidemiological and nutritional studies is estimation of the intake of DF in populations and specific diets.

All solid plant foods contain both IDF and SDF, while only beverages can be expected to contain SDF. Nevertheless, international food composition tables report zero DF content in most drinks, including beer.

The literature contains little information on DF in beer because studies on non-digestible carbohydrates in beer have mainly dealt with organoleptic and technological aspects but not with nutrition and health. A second reason for the absence of values of fiber in beer may be the fact that the official methods for determining DF in foodstuffs are not applicable to beverages.

However, measurable amounts of non-digestible polysaccharides may be solubilized during processes for the making of beer – a drink derived from fiber-rich plant foods – and so we may expect DF to be a common constituent of it.

Carbohydrates and DF in Beer

The composition of beer includes 3.3–4.4 g of carbohydrates per 100 ml, consisting of dextrins as the major constituent along with monosaccharides, oligosaccharides and pentosans. Table 28.2 lists the carbohydrates reported in beer.

Dextrins are saccharide polymers linked primarily by α-(1–4)-D-glucose units and can have different properties and molecular compositions depending on starch and how it is digested. Properties include hygroscopicity, fermentability, viscosity, stability, gelation, solubility and bioavailability. Barley starch contains both linear α-(1 → 4) amylose and branched α-(1 → 6) amylopectin, which are released from starch gelatinized by heating in mashing process. Enzyme hydrolysis with α-amylase efficiently hydrolyzes the α-(1 → 4) linkages but not the α-(1 → 6) linkages, leaving behind a small amount of high-molecular-mass residues. On the other hand, hydrolysis with a α-(1 → 6) specific enzyme (pullulanase) will render a higher proportion of linear α-(1 → 4) oligosaccharides, which are more susceptible to retrogradation and gelling.

The saccharides containing fewer than four glucose units that remain in beer after fermentation include glucose, fructose, maltose, sucrose and maltotriose. Glucose and fructose are the main monosaccharides. The main disaccharides are maltose and sucrose; much of the sucrose emanates from malt itself, while the maltose present is produced in the mash tun (Cortacero-Ramírez *et al.*, 2003).

Table 28.2 Carbohydrates in beer

Digestible carbohydrates	*Non-digestible carbohydrates*
Dextrins	β-Glucans
Maltotriose	Arabinoxylans
Sucrose, maltose	Cellobiose
Fructose, glucose	Laminaribiose
Minor Carbohydrates: Arabinose, galactose, ribose, xylose, isomaltose, panose, isopanose, kojibiose, nigerose, maltulose, maltotetraose	

Note: Major (digestible and non-digestible) and minor carbohydrates reported in beer. Major digestible carbohydrates provide caloric value; non-digestible carbohydrates are the beer DF constituents.

Arabinoxylans and β-glucans are the main non-starch polysaccharides. Arabinoxylans are composed of a complex backbone of D-xylopyranosyl residues linked by β-(1–4) glycosidic bonds and have been reported to constitute 3–11% of the barley kernel. β-Glucans are linear homopolysaccharides. They are the major components of the barley cell walls (Holtekjolen *et al.*, 2006) and are partially degraded by endogenous enzymes during germination of barley, but a part remains in the beer.

Fermentable sugars directly contribute to the sweetness of beer, whereas carbohydrates with more than four glycosyl units contribute to body or mouthfeel. β-Glucans and arabinoxylans are responsible for viscosity (Jian Lu and Yin Li, 2006; Yin Li *et al.*, 2005), rate of filtration or haze formation in beer. β-Glucan and arabinoxylans form viscous solutions and can contribute to extraction problems in the brewing industry (Voragen *et al.*, 1987; Viëtor and Voragen, 1993; Schwarz and Han, 1995). Paul *et al.*'s (2002) research and Sadosky *et al.* (2002) reported that the effects of arabinoxylans on viscosity and filterability were at least as important as the effects of β-glucan. Stewart *et al.* (1998) found that pilot-brewed beer viscosity and membrane filter ability were correlated with arabinoxylan content, whereas β-glucan was correlated only with viscosity. β-glucan may increase the viscosity of beer by forming gels, consisting primarily of high-molecular-weight β-glucan molecules.

It is clear, as it is summarized above, that carbohydrates in beer are usually studied in relation to sensory or technological properties, but a nutritional approach is also appropriate for these compounds.

A major part of beer carbohydrates, as Table 28.2 indicates, are digestible and are responsible for the caloric value of beer. However, an appreciable amount passes to the large intestine, where it may be fermented by the colonic microflora to produce a variety of substances which are metabolized. These indigestible carbohydrates – β-glucan and arabinoxylans – are the largest constituents of DF in beer; there may also be amounts of other compounds such as cellobiose, laminaribiose and some indigestible chains derived from starch.

The concept of beer non-digestible carbohydrates as DF is a relatively new one and there is a shortage of physicochemical or biological data on this fraction. We need to know more about the composition and physiological and nutritional properties of beer DF.

Content and Composition of DF in Beer

A specific method developed to determine DF in beverages was used. This procedure includes four steps: concentration, enzymatic treatments, dialysis and determination of DF (Saura-Calixto *et al.*, 2002; Diaz-Rubio and Saura-Calixto, 2006).

SDF contents of the lager and dark beers most widely consumed in Spain are shown in Table 28.3.

Table 28.3 SDF content in beer

Beer		*Alcohol (%v/v)*	*Soluble dietary fiber (g/l)*[a]
Águila Amstel®	Lager	5	1.98 ± 0.11
Mahou Clásica®	Lager	4.8	1.87 ± 0.07
Bock Damm®	Dark	5.4	1.91 ± 0.09
Voll Damm®	Lager	7.2	2.02 ± 0.01
Buckler®	Lager	<1	1.12 ± 0.05
San Miguel 0.0®	Lager	0	1.64 ± 0.05

Notes: SDF in most common beer in Spain (trade mark, alcohol content).

[a] Each value is the mean ± standard deviation (*n* = 3).

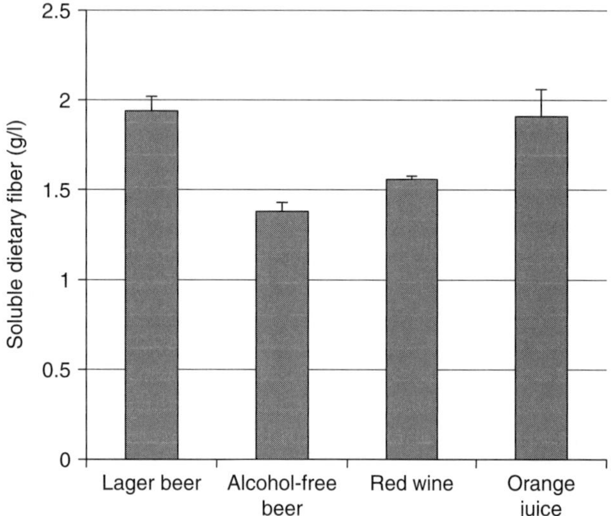

Figure 28.1 SDF in drinks. SDF content in common dietary drinks, determined by enzymatic-dialysis procedure. Data are mean ± standard deviation of three determinations.

Lager and dark beers contain similar amounts of SDF (1.87–2.02 g/l), while the content is lower in low alcohol or alcohol-free beer (1.12–1.64 g/l), presumably due to differences in the brewing procedure (mashing, malting and dealcoholizing). These may be considered reference values for beer, although higher DF contents may be found in other types of beer, depending on the cereals used and the brewing procedure.

SDF is a quantitatively important constituent of beer and is present in larger quantities than vitamins, minerals, PP and others. Probably only water, alcohol and dextrins are present in larger quantities than DF.

Note that in comparison with other common beverages (Figure 28.1) the amount of SDF in beer is higher than in wine and similar to orange juice.

The DF contents of beverages and vegetable foods differ quantitatively and qualitatively. There is naturally less DF in beverages than in solid vegetable foods – DF is expressed in g/l in beverages and in g/100 g in plant foods. On the other hand, vegetables contain both insoluble and soluble fiber, while only soluble fiber is found in beverages. Table 28.4 shows the DF contents of various different items.

Table 28.4 DF content in foods

	Dietary fiber[a] *(g/100 g edible portion)*		
	Soluble	*Insoluble*	*Total*
Oatmeal, medium ground	3.7	2.9	6.6
Rice, white	–	0.5	0.5
Bananas	0.7	0.4	1.1
Apples	0.6	1.0	1.6
Oranges	1.4	0.7	2.1
Corn Meal	0.3	1.4	1.7
Wheat bran	3.8	32.2	36.0
Brussels sprouts	3.0	2.6	5.6
Lettuce, round, raw	0.6	0.6	1.2
Walnuts	1.5	2.0	3.5
Tomatoes	0.4	0.7	1.1
Carrots	1.4	1.0	2.4
Beer[b,c]	0.20	0	0.20
Orange juice[b,c]	0.19	0	0.19
Red wine[b,c]	0.16	0	0.16

Notes: Soluble, insoluble and total DF content in beer and other beverages and foods. Total dietary fiber = SDF + IDF.

[a] Solid foods values from Food Standards Agency (2002).
[b] DF in beverages expressed as g/100 ml.
[c] Values from Saura-Calixto *et al.* (2002).

Table 28.5 Monomers forming soluble DF in beer[a, b]

	Dark	*Lager*	*Alcohol-free*
Xylose	40.1 ± 0.6	34.0 ± 0.7	30.6 ± 0.6
Arabinose	30.1 ± 0.4	24.5 ± 0.4	21.8 ± 0.4
Glucose	17.7 ± 0.5	30.5 ± 0.5	38.7 ± 0.7
Manose	6.9 ± 0.1	6.6 ± 0.1	4.8 ± 0.1
Galactose	5.2 ± 0.1	4.4 ± 0.1	4.1 ± 0.2

Notes: Monomers (monosaccharides) percentage composition of SDF (polymer). Beer soluble DF is a macromolecule make up of different monosaccharides.

[a] Expressed as percentage in neutral sugars.
[b] Each value is the mean ± standard deviation (*n* = 3).

The contribution of beer to the SDF intake in a common diet may be significant; a moderate daily consumption of 250 ml of beer contributes to 0.5 g of SDF, which is equivalent to eating 125 g of tomatoes, 166 g of Brussels sprouts or 83 g of apples.

Table 28.5 shows the monomers forming SDF polysaccharides in beers. Xylose (30.6–40.1%), arabinose (21.8–30.1%) and glucose (17.7–38.8%) were the major constituents in all the different beers, indicating that arabinoxylans and β-glucans are the main polysaccharides in SDF (Figure 28.2).

The high glucose content is mainly derived from β-glucans, but the presence of minor amounts of resistant starch

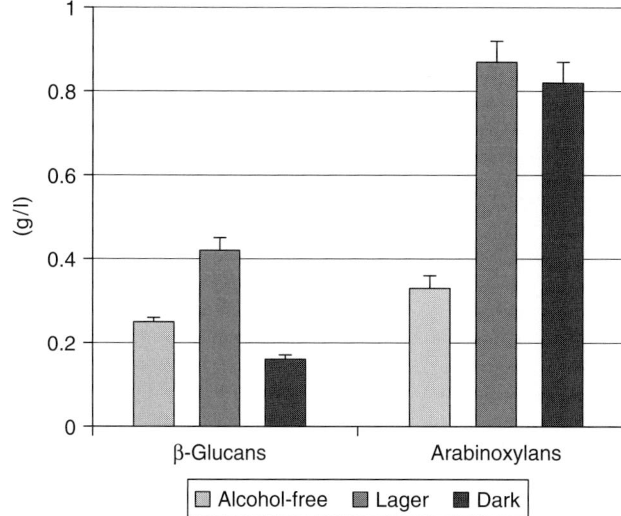

Figure 28.2 β-Glucans and arabinoxylans (arabinose + xylose) in beer. Major polysaccharides constituents of DF in beer. β-Glucans are formed by glucose units and arabinoxylans are formed by arabinose and xylose. Glucose, arabinose and xylose were determined by gas–liquid chromatography. Data are mean ± standard deviation of three determinations.

chains (amylose and amylopectin) cannot be ruled out. The low proportion of galactose and mannose suggests that galactomannans are minor fiber constituents.

In malting and brewing, sizeable proportions of the β-glucan and pentosan survive as oligosaccharides or di-saccharides such as cellobiose and laminaribiose. These saccharides are not detected by the DF analytical method and they cannot therefore be ruled out as minor constituents of the indigestible carbohydrate fraction. In any case, the contribution of these oligosaccharides to the potential pre-biotic properties of beer is surely nutritionally irrelevant given their negligible concentrations.

Fermentability of Beer DF

DF reaches the colon intact, where it may be totally fermented, partially fermented, or remain unfermented. Colonic fermentation consists in the interaction between the non-digestible dietary components and the intestinal ecosystem, involving the metabolism of non-digestible compounds by the bacteria and the effects of DF on the composition, ecology and metabolic activity of the microbiota. The extent to which these processes occur depends on the chemical structure and physical properties of the fiber components, and they can have positive effects on health and well-being (Edwards, 1995).

When the indigestible compounds are fermented, they are metabolized to hydrogen, methane, carbon dioxide and SCFAs, principally acetic, propionic and butyric acids. These SCFAs are absorbed and further metabolized in the colonocytes, the liver cells, or the peripheral tissues (Cummings and Macfarlane, 1991; Macfarlane and Macfarlane, 1993). Fibers also contribute to fecal bulking in a number of ways. They can do so directly via their own mass and/or via the mass of the water they attract. They can also influence fecal bulking indirectly in that they are fermented by colonic microflora; this stimulates their growth and results in increased microbial biomass.

The major end-products of fermentation are the SCFAs which acidify the proximal colon and bulk the stool. Acidity is one of the major factors determining the composition of bacterial population. Water is removed from the colon by osmotic equilibration with the mucosal blood.

The major SCFA metabolites are absorbed from the colon and contribute to the energy balance of the host. Butyrate from the colonic lumen has been shown to be the major source of energy supply to the colonic mucosal cells and is known to be a potent trophic agent. It may therefore be implicated in the prevention of colorectal cancer and in the maintenance of epithelial mucosa. Propionate is cleared by the liver and may modulate hepatic carbohydrate and lipid metabolism. Acetate largely escapes colonic and hepatic metabolism and serves primarily as fuel for peripheral tissues. Acetate and propionate have been associated with hypocholesterolemic effects (Mathers and Sakata, 2003).

Fermentation products can favor colonization resistance by increasing the numbers and variety of bacteria. SCFA fermentation end-products are likely to be major factors in increasing colonization resistance and aiding recovery.

The increase of certain types of bacteria (Lactobacillus, Bifidobacterium) or the decrease of others (Clostridium, Bacteroids, etc.) by DF or specific DF constituents is known as the pre-biotic effect.

Soluble fibers are usually more extensively fermented than insolubles, and hence beverage DF can be expected to be highly fermentable. In fact, beer DF is extensively degraded by colonic bacteria. Ninety-nine percent of DF components are fermented, the bulk of them being converted to SCFAs.

The fermentability (Table 28.6) and high propionic acid production of beer DF (molar ratio: acetic, 61: propionic, 30: butyric, 9) is consistent with the high fermentability of β-glucans (Berggren *et al.*, 1993).

Fermentability and propionic production are comparable to that of psyllium (38%) but significantly higher than other soluble fibers such as citric pectins (7%) or inulin (19%). Psyllium and β-glucan are both recognized as healthy fibers, for which health claims have been accepted by Food and Drug Administration (FDA).

Contribution of Beer to DF Intake in the Diet

The intake of DF should range between 30–35 g/day or 10–13 g/1,000 kcal according to dietary guidelines from international health organizations. A balanced DF composition is also recommended (SDF/total DF ratio: 1/3).

Table 28.6 Fermentability and SCFAs production in beer and some DF

		Molar proportions		
	Fermentability[a]	*Acetic*	*Propionic*	*Butyric*
Beer[b]	85.5	61	30	9
Lactulose[b]	100	81	12	7
β-Gucans[b]	100	67	15	15
Arabinogalactans[b]	65	68	24	8
Guar Gum[b]	71	52	34	14
Arabic Gum[b]	77	66	21	13
Citric pectins[b]	93	90	7	3
Psyllium[b]	27	48	38	14
Inulin[b]	97	72	19	8
Oligofructose[b]	88	78	14	8
Wheat bran[c]	25	61	13	26
Oat[c]	57	59	19	22
Soy[c]	58	62	20	18

Notes: Degree of colonic fermentation and intestinal production of SCFAs (acetic, propionic and butyric) of different DF.

[a] Percentage of fermentability with respect to lactulose.
[b] SDF materials.
[c] Materials containing both, SDF and IDF.

However, the usual intake in developed countries is only about half of that level.

The European nutrition and health report (Elmadfa and Weichselbaum, 2005) indicates DF intakes ranging from 16 to 21 g/person/day in the European Union. Note that beverages are not included in the reports on DF intake.

There are significant differences in DF quality due to considerable regional differences in food sources. Northern European countries obtain 58% of DF (range: 54–64) from cereals, while Mediterranean countries such as France, Italy and Spain obtain only 42% (range: 36–49). Intake of vegetables, fruits and legumes varies reciprocally, with low intakes in Northern Europe and much higher intakes around the Mediterranean. Some of the postulated benefits of diets rich in fruits and vegetables might then be attributable to the intake of fiber. This suggests differences in composition and properties of DF. Fruits, vegetables and legumes possess a higher proportion of SDF than cereals. The fiber intake in the Spanish diet was recently determined (Table 28.7), including an estimation of the contribution of beverages.

The Spanish population consumes around 19 g/day of DF in which 33% is soluble fiber (Saura-Calixto and Goñi, 2004). The contribution of plant foods to the total DF intake is shown in Figure 28.3. Fruits, vegetables and legumes account for 53%, cereals for 43% and beverages for around 3%. The average beer consumption in Spain is 150 g per capita per day, which would contain 0.3 g of SDF.

The contribution of beverages is estimated at 11% of SDF intake, the largest part of that (5%) coming from beer (Figure 28.4). The average per capita beer consumption in the European Union is around 202 g/day, accounting for some 0.4 g of SDF. A moderate consumption of 500 ml of beer per day could imply an intake of 1 g of SDF.

Table 28.7 DF intake in the Spanish diet

	Daily consumption[a] *(g/p/d)*	*Dietary fiber*[a] *(g/p/d)*	
		Soluble	*Insoluble*
Cereals	231.2	1.95	5.33
Vegetables	311.2	1.90	2.79
Legumes	12.9	0.23	0.52
Fruits	264.4	2.09	2.96
Nuts	7.9	0.13	0.45
Beverages[b]	292	0.54	0
Total	1074	6.84	12.05
Total Dietary Fiber (SDF + IDF) = 18.89			

Notes: Main sources of DF in the Spanish diet. Major items in each group: cereals (white bread, rice), vegetables (potatoes, tomatoes), legumes (beans, chickpeas, lentils), fruits (oranges, bananas) and nuts (peanuts, almonds). Beverages include beer, wine and orange juice.

[a] Values from Saura-Calixto and Goñi (2004).
[b] Beer, wine and juices (ml).

Are Polysaccharides the Only Constituent of DF in Beer?

DF was first defined as non-starch polysaccharides and lignin which are resistant to hydrolysis by the digestive enzymes of man (Trowell *et al.*, 1976). On the basis of this definition, an analytical methodology was developed to determine DF in foods and a large number of clinical and epidemiological studies established were performed.

However, our knowledge has grown since DF was first defined, and the general tendency among nutritionists nowadays is to extend the concept of DF to include other compounds of proven resistance to the action of digestive

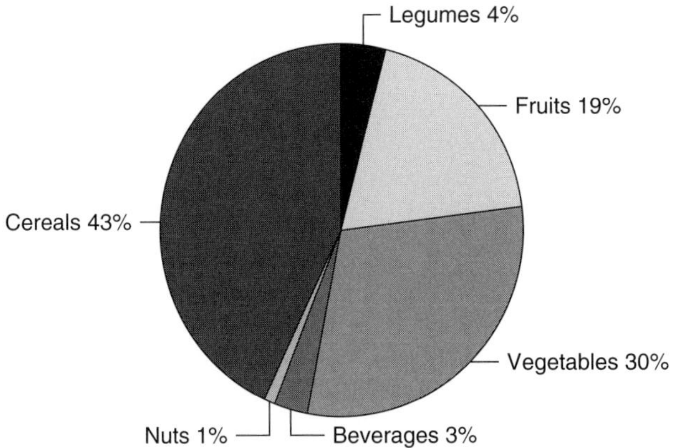

Figure 28.3 Contribution of plant foods to the total DF intake in the Spanish diet (year 2000). Contribution of beverages and vegetable foods to the total DF intake in the Spanish diet (year 2000) (Saura-Calixto and Goñi, 2004). Major items in each group: cereals (white bread, rice), vegetables (potatoes, tomatoes), legumes (beans, chickpeas, lentils), fruits (oranges, bananas) and nuts (peanuts, almonds). Beverages include beer, wine and orange juice.

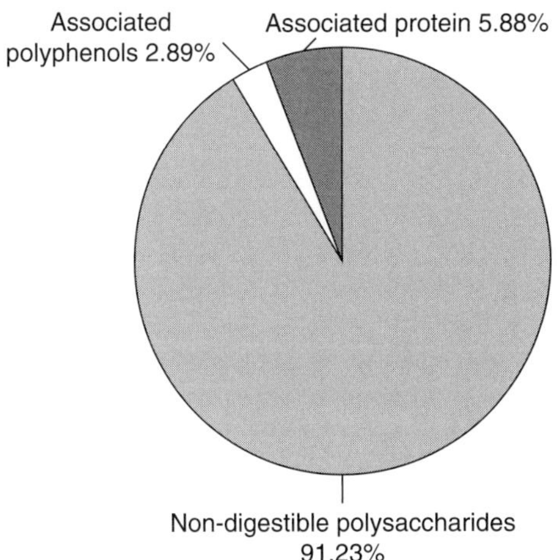

Figure 28.4 DF complex in lager beer DF in beer is made up of non-digestible polysaccharides (β-glucans and arabinoxylans) along with PP compounds and indigestible protein.

enzymes, such as resistant starch, indigestible saccharides or oligosaccharides, indigestible protein and certain PP (Saura-Calixto *et al.*, 2000; Nelson, 2002). These compounds may also be constituents of beer DF.

Resistant starch is a part of dietary starch that is not digested in the human gut and is largely fermented by the colonic bacteria (Asp *et al.*, 1996). Resistant starch is a major component of DF in solid starchy foods such as cereals and legumes, but we may only expect to find minor or negligible amounts in beer DF, made up of indigestible amylose and amylopectin chains. Insoluble saccharides like cellobiose and laminaribiose have also been reported in beer, but at very low concentrations. The presence of resistant starch and indigestible saccharides is therefore nutritionally irrelevant, and only β-glucans and arabinoxylans can be considered significant beer DF constituents.

Proteins from meat and fish are fully digestible, but part of the protein in plant foods remain indigestible after the action of digestive enzymes. Indigestible or resistant protein is a typical constituent of DF in vegetable foods (Goñi *et al.*, 2002).

In the analytical procedure used to determine DF in beer, digestible protein is hydrolyzed to amino acids or peptides by pepsin treatment, but part remains in the dialysis retentate as indigestible protein.

PP and protein content were determined in both beer and the retentates (just after dialysis) which contain the non-digestible polysaccharides solution (Table 28.8). The protein content determined in lager beer (with-alcohol and alcohol-free) was 1.7–1.5%, while a significant amount around 1.3–0.9% of beer protein was found in the SDF solution of the dialysis retentate. Hence, about 76–60% of the beer protein appears to be resistant protein (Table 28.8).

The presence of polyphenolic compounds associated with DF is a characteristic feature of PP-rich plant foods. The presence of PP in both insoluble and soluble DF of grapes and other vegetable materials has been reported by the authors elsewhere (Bravo *et al.*, 1994; Saura-Calixto and Bravo, 2001). Beer contains appreciable amounts of PP. Beer PP are single molecules or oligomers with a molecular weight (MW) considerably below the cut-off (12 kDa) of the dialysis membrane used in our experiment, and they therefore had to be dialyzed. However, appreciable

Table 28.8 Protein and phenolic compounds associated with non-digestible polysaccharides in beer

	Lager[a]		*Free-alcohol*[a]	
	Polyphenols[b] *(mg/l)*	*Protein (mg/l)*	*Polyphenols*[b] *(mg/l)*	*Protein (mg/l)*
Original beer	312.15 ± 2.8	172 ± 3	299 ± 1.4	147 ± 2
Dialysis retentants	66.02 ± 2.2	134 ± 1	52.12 ± 1.34	95 ± 3

Notes: Polyphenols and protein found in original beer (before any treatment) and in dialysis retentants obtained after enzyme treatment and dialysis. Dialysis retentants contain DF and associated compounds.

[a] Each value is the mean ± standard deviation (n = 3).

[b] Expressed as gallic acid.

amounts of total PP remained in the dialysis retentates after enzymatic treatment (Table 28.8). This suggests that the phenolics quantified in the retentates are associated with macromolecules of molecular weights greater than 12 kDa.

Indigestible polysaccharides or DF and protein are the chief beer macromolecules that can bind PP. Polysaccharides and protein undegraded by the enzymes used in the analytical procedure, which constituted the DF, remained in the dialysis retentate and emerged as the chief target for PP bonding.

It has been shown that proteins with high proline content have a high affinity for binding PP. The proteins in beer that are able to bind PP have been shown to originate in barley hordein. Hordein is a prolamin and prolamin is a proline-rich protein (containing approximately 20 mol% proline). Gliadin, or wheat prolamin, is also rich in proline (15 mol%) and exhibits an affinity for binding PP (Siebert, 2006).

Our experiment showed the presence of significant amounts of PP and protein along with DF in the dialysis retentates. We conclude that beer contains a DF complex (DF plus indigestible protein and associated PP) at concentrations of about 1.2–2.3 g/l. We would note particularly that this complex contained from 17% to 21% of the total phenolics in beer and about 75–65% of the protein.

DF complex will not be bioavailable in the human upper intestine and are therefore not susceptible of absorption through the intestinal mucose. Complex may be expected to reach the colon, where the polysaccharides will be extensively fermented as described above, and this could favor fermentation of the associated PP. These PP, and the products of their degradation, may contribute to an antioxidant environment in the colon and may also be absorbed and metabolized.

To sum up, beer contains a considerable amount of DF complex made up of polysaccharides, protein and PP. The objective of this study was simply to show that beer contains DF. The presence of DF in beer should be neither overestimated nor underestimated for purposes of nutrition and health. Further studies on the composition, physicochemical and biological properties of this complex are needed to elucidate its nutritional significance.

Summary Points

- International food composition tables report no DF in beer. However, DF is a quantitatively important constituent of beer.
- Lager and dark beer contain around 2 g of DF/l. Arabinoxylans and β-glucans are the major constituents of beer DF.
- Beer DF presents high colonic fermentability, similar to β-glucans and psyllium, two recognized healthy fibers.
- The contribution of beer (150 ml person/day) to the intake of DF in the Spanish diet is estimated at 1.5% and 5% of total DF and SDF, respectively. A higher contribution may be expected in other European countries where beer consumption is greater.
- DF occurs in beer as a complex (2.3 g/l) made up of indigestible carbohydrates, polyphenolic compounds and indigestible protein.
- The biological and nutritional significance of DF in beer remains to be elucidated.

References

Asp, N-G., Van Amelsvoort, J.M.M. and Hautvast, J.G.A.J. (1996). *Nutr. Res. Rev.* 9, 1–31.

Berggren, A.M., Björck, I.M.E. and Nyman, M. (1993). *J. Sci. Food Agric.* 63, 397–406.

Bravo, L., Abia, R. and Saura-Calixto, F. (1994). *J Agric. Food Chem.* 42, 1481–1487.

Cho, S.S. and Dreher M.L. (eds) (2001). *Handbook of Dietary Fiber*. Marcel Dekker: New York.

Cortacero-Ramírez, S., Hernainz-Bermudez de Castro, M., Segura- Carretero, A., Cruces-Blanco, C. and Fernández-Gutierrez, A.L. (2003). *Trends Anal. Chem.* 22, 440–455.

Cummings, J.H. and Macfarlane, G.T. (1991). *J. Appl. Bacteriol.* 70, 443–459.

Diaz-Rubio, M.E. and Saura-Calixto, F. (2006). *Am. J. Enol. Vitic.* 57(1), 69–72.

Edwards, C.A. (1995). Dietary fibre, fermentation and the colon. In Cherbut, C., Barry, J.L., Lairon, D. and Durand, M. (eds), *Dietary Fibre. Mechanisms of Action in Human Physiology and Metabolism*, pp. 51–60. John Libbey Eurotext, Paris.

Elmadfa, I. and Weichselbaum, E. (eds) (2005). European nutrition and health report 2004. *Forum of Nutrition*, Vol. 58, Karger. Austria.

Food Standards Agency (2002). *McCance and Widdowson's. The Composition of Foods*, 5th edn. Royal Society of Chemistry, Cambridge.

Goñi, I., Gudiel-Urbano, M. and Saura-Calixto, F. (2002). *J. Sci. Food Agric.* 82, 1850–1854.

Holtekjolen, A.K., Uhlen, A.K., Brathen, E., Sahlstrm, S. and Knutsen, S.H. (2006). *Food Chem.* 94, 348–358.

Lu, Jian. and Li, Yin. (2006). *Food Chem.* 98, 164–170.

Macfarlane, G.T. and Macfarlane, S. (1993). *Proc. Nutr. Soc.* 52, 367–373.

McCleary, B.V. and Prosky, L. (eds) (2001). *Advanced Dietar Fiber Technology*. Blackwell Science, Malden, MA.

Mathers, J.C. and Sakoite, T. (2003). *Proc. Nutr. Soc.* 62(1), 67–115.

Nelson, A.M. (2002). Defining high fiber ingredient terminology. In Nelson, A.M. (ed.), *High Fiber Ingredients*, pp. 1–28. Eagan Press, St. Paul, MN.

Paul, S., Paul, B.S. and Richard, D.H. (2002). *J. Am. Soc. Brew. Chem.* 60, 153–162.

Sadosky, P., Schwarz, P.B. and Horsely, R.D. (2002). *J. Am. Soc. Brew. Chem.* 60, 153–162.

Saura-Calixto, F., García-Alonso, A., Goñi, I. and Bravo, L. (2000). *J. Agric. Food Chem.* 48, 3342–3347.

Saura-Calixto, F. and Goñi, I. (2004). *Eur. J. Clin. Nutr.* 58, 1078–1082.

Saura-Calixto, F. and Bravo, L. (2001). In Cho, S.S. and Dreher, M.L. (eds), *Handbook of Dietary Fiber*, pp. 415–433. Marcel Dekker, New York.

Saura-Calixto, F., Goñi, I., Martín Albarrán, C. and Pulido, R. (2002). In Cerveza y Salud Ied., *Fibra dietética en la cerveza:*

Contenido, composición y evaluación nutricional, Madrid, http://www.cervezaysalud.com. Centro de Información Cerveza y Salud, Madrid.

Schwarz, P.B. and Han, Jee-Yup. (1995). *J. Am. Soc. Brew. Chem.* 53, 157–159.

Siebert, K.J. (2006). *LWT-Food Sci. & Technol.*, 39, 987–994.

Stewart, D.C., Hawthorne, D. and Evans, D.E. (1998). *J. Inst. Brew.* 104, 321–326.

Trowell, H.C., Southgate, D.A.T., Wolever, T.M.S., Leeds, A.R., Gassull, M.A. and Jenkins, D.J.A. (1976). *Lancet* 1, 967.

Viëtor, R.J., Voragen, A.G.J. and Angelino, S.A.G.F. (1993). *J. Inst. Brew.* 99, 243–248.

Voragen, A.G.J., Schols, H.A., Marius, J., Rombouts, F.M. and Angelino, S.A.G.F.J. (1987). *J. Inst. Brew.* 93, 202–208.

World Health Organization/Food and Agriculture Organization (WHO/FAO) (1999). Carbohydrates in human nutrition. *WHO Technical Report Series*, World Health Organization/Food and Agriculture Organization, Rome.

Li, Yin, Lu, Jian, Gu, Guoxian, Shi, Zhongping and Mao, Zhonggui (2005). *Food Chem.* 93, 33–38.

29
Beer and Arabinoxylan

Glen P. Fox Plant Science – Wheat, Barley & Oats, Toowoomba, Qld, Australia

Abstract

Arabinoxylans are non-starch polysaccharides (NSP) and are found in a number of tissues, primarily in the cell wall of the aleurone layers and the endosperm. Arabinoxylans are comprised of a mixed linkage between arabinose and xylose. The arabinoxylan structure is degraded, in conjunction with β-glucan, by enzymes during the malting process to facilitate a trouble-free breakdown of the main endosperm contents (protein and starch). Low temperature mashing (<50°C) continues the breakdown of these NSP. However, arabinoxylans have been attributed to contribute to filtration problem during brewing and haze formation in beer. There is variation with a grain type as well as between grain types used for brewing, with barley having a high arabinoxylan content compared to sorghum with a low content. Further research is required to gain a more detailed understanding of the genetic control of arabinoxylan as well as the enzyme systems that degrade this NSP to ensure trouble-free brewing and consistent beer quality. Improvements in filtration technology could increase pressure on barley breeders and maltsters breeders to produce low level arabinoxylan barley and malt which could impact on other quality parameters.

Arabinoxylans are polysaccharides that exist in the cell walls of tissues of grains. These polymers have been reported to be a major positive component of dietary fiber. However, intact arabinoxylans can have a negative impact of malt and beer quality. Arabinoxylans are one of many chemical and biochemical components from grains that are enzymically degraded and solubilized during malting, mashing and boiling to produce beer. To produce trouble-free brewing, a number of grain and malt attributes must meet tight specifications. While the levels of hot water extract, free amino nitrogen and wort β-glucan (BG) can be prescribed to make brewing as trouble free as possible and produce a consistent quality and flavor, one particular group of carbohydrates is generally ignored. This group of carbohydrates is called non-starch polysaccharides (NSP). These important NSPs consist of two main polysaccharides that include β-glucan and arabinoxylan. If these are not degraded during malting and mashing then significant brewing problems can arise.

Arabinoxylans are found in the cell walls of a number of tissues in cereals, including husk (Höije *et al.*, 2006), aleurone (Bacic and Stone, 1981; Rhodes and Stone, 2002) and endosperm cell walls (Henry, 1986). However, there has been more interest in the endosperm cell walls composition in barley (*Hordeum vulgare*), wheat (*Triticum aestivum*) and sorghum (*Sorghum bicolor*) which are the most common cereals used for producing beer. Arabinoxylan also is found in other cereals used as brewing adjuncts such as maize (*Zea mays*) and rice which can also impact on beer production. In addition, arabinoxylan also exits in the minor grains such as buckwheat (*Fagopyrum esculentum*), finger millet (*Eleusine coracana*) (Rao and Muralikrishna, 2004) and pearled millet (*Pennisetum typhoideum*) which are used in producing gluten-free beer.

Arabinoxylan is located in the cell walls of the outer layers of the grains as well as in the endosperm cell wall. There is considerable variation in arabinoxylan content as well as the levels of arabinose and xylose between species. There are differences between cereal species as well as within a species and the portion of arabinoxylan in the endosperm compared to the whole grain (Henry, 1986). Most of the arabinoxylan in grain is in the outlet layers of the grain with a 70/20% arabinoxylan/β-glucan mixture. However, in the endosperm cell walls the reverse proportions exist with only around 20% arabinoxylan (Fincher, 1992).

The Structure of Arabinoxylan

Arabinoxylan has a linear backbone structure of β-D-xylopyranosyl residues linked by β-(1→4)-glycosidic bonds, other monosaccharides such as L-arabinofuranose attached as branches by β-(1→2) or β-(1→3)-linkages

Beer in Health and Disease Prevention
ISBN: 978-0-12-373891-2

(Luchsinger, 1967; Bacic and Stone, 1981; Henry, 1988a; Vietor *et al.*, 1991). Typically, L-arabinofuranose or other side chains are carried on the main chain as non-reducing end groups. Ferulic acid is esterified to some arabinofuranosyl chains. However, there is variation in the esterification of ferulic acid depending on the species and tissue.

Bamforth and Kanauchi (2001) reported a stylized structural model for barley cell wall (Figure 29.1). It was hypothesized that there was a layer of xylose, partially covering the β-glucan. The xylose had arabinose linked in addition to ferulic and acetic acid. This structure provides a rigid backbone to the cell wall but it was not impenetrable to enzymic attack which is critical to allow the movement of protein and starch degrading enzymes and the resultant products during germination (Figure 29.2)

Arabinoxylan can be extracted in either water or alkali solutions (Medcalf *et al.*, 1968; Izydorczyk *et al.*, 1998a, b), with water extractable arabinoxylan able to form viscous solutions (Medcalf *et al.*, 1968). Ferulic acid dimers play a major role in crosslinking in gel formations (Dervilly-Pinel *et al.*, 2001). The negative aspects of gel formation on beer quality will be described later. Cyran *et al.* (2002) concluded that there was more water soluble arabinoxylan present in a barley malt as well as a greater portion of high molecular weight arabinoxylan.

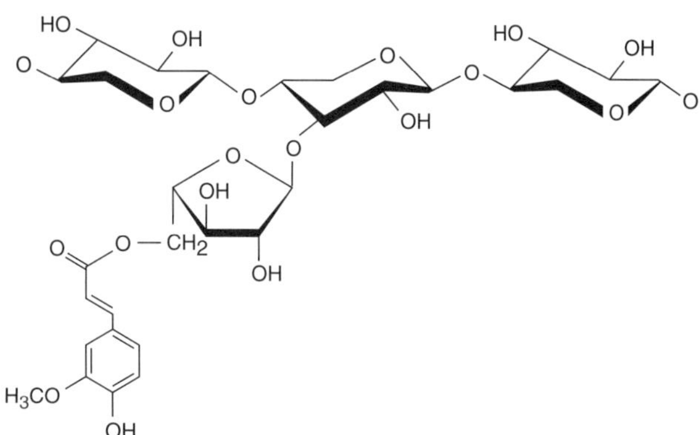

Figure 29.1 Structure of arabinoxylan. *Source*: Fincher and Stone (1986).

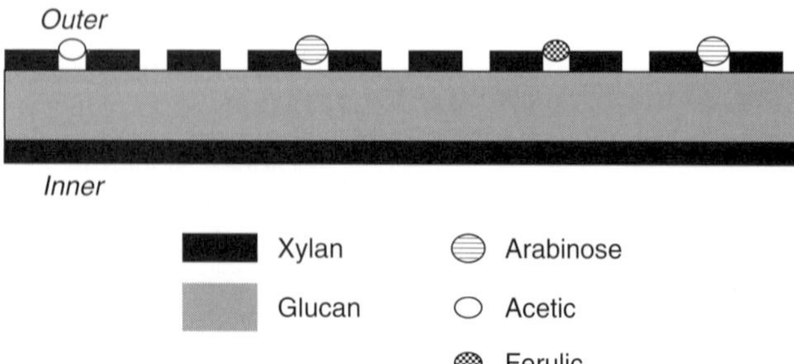

Figure 29.2 Theoretical model of the structure of arabinoxylan in endosperm cell walls. *Source*: Bamforth and Kanauchi (2001).

Arabinoxylan in the Endosperm Cell Wall

As mentioned above arabinoxylan has been detected at around 20% in the endosperm cell walls (Fincher, 1992). There is variation in the level of endosperm arabinoxylan between species as well as within a species (Henry, 1986, 1987). A hypothetical structure for barley is shown in Figure 29.1. While arabinoxylan is the minor partner to β-glucan, like β-glucan, the level can seriously effect the processing of wort in the beer production. The degradation of the cell wall is critical to the efficiency of the malting process. Enzymic attack on the arabinoxylan substrate releases smaller oligosaccharides and simple sugars. In addition, ferulic acid is hydrolyzed from the arabinofuranose side chain. For the degradation of arabinoxylan, a number of enzymes are involved. In recent years, numerous studies have provided more detail on the chromosomal location, gene expression, enzyme functionality and substrate specificity (details provided below).

Arabinoxylan in the Husk and Aleurone Layers

As mentioned previously, a significant amount of the total arabinoxylan is present in the husk and outer layers of barley and other grains where there is approximately 70% arabinoxylan and only 20% β-glucan. Not only is the content of arabinoxylan different but also the structure and the ratio of arabinose to xylose. In barley, the husk and aleurone, the ratio of arabinose:xylose is lower in barley than in wheat. The difference between the arabinose to xylose ratio is also dependant on the genotype, growing environments and extraction solution (Henry, 1988b). These differences can also be measured in the malt (Han and Schwarz, 1996), wort (Debyser *et al.*, 1997) and beer samples (Han, 2000).

Genetic and Environmental Variation

Like most endosperm structures, the cell walls and components within the cell walls are influenced by the growing environment. Arabinoxylan has been detected in the developing endosperm tissue as early as 7 day after anthesis (Wilson *et al.*, 2006). The final arabinoxylan content has been shown by many researchers to be influenced by genotype and environment. In addition, there are differences between species used in brewing. For the purpose of this chapter, the results will describe arabinoxylan from endosperm cell walls only, which is a critical phase in malting and brewing performance.

The variation is quite considerable between species which is influenced partly whether the grain has a husk. The dominant grain used in brewing is barley and the range has been shown to be between 3% and greater than 10%. Henry

(1986) reported significant genetic and environmental effects on a range of malting and non-malting commercial varieties. This study was comprehensive in the number of genotypes and environments used. However, more expansive studies by Lehtonen and Aikasalo (1987), Mikyska *et al.* (2002) and Holtekjølen *et al.* (2006) also showed similar genetic and environmental effects. Lehtonen and Aikasalo (1987) reported differences in pentosan content between barley types (two- vs. six-rowed), varieties and sites with over one hundred varieties tested over three locations.

However, the most difference was between two- and six-rowed barleys. Six-rowed barleys generally have a higher husk content and reduced endosperm. Mikyska *et al.* (2002) reported on the arabinoxylan content in eight varieties grown at four locations in Czechoslovakia. There was significant variation between genotypes as well as locations. In addition, there were correlations between arabinoxylan and malt traits such as hot water extract, friability and viscosity. While Holtekjølen *et al.* (2006) tested 39 barley varieties from a number of countries of origin (Europe and Canada) and found statistically significant variation between cultivars with a hulless variety having the lowest amount, although similar in levels to that reported by Trogh *et al.* (2004). Han (2000) tested two varieties, with one sourced from different locations showed non-significant differences in arabinoxylan content. This was also in the resultant malt and beer samples with around 40–60% loss in arabinoxylan from barley to malt and almost greater than 90% loss from barley to beer.

Variation was identified in water soluble, insoluble and total arabinoxylan between three European hulless barley cultivars (Trogh *et al.*, 2004) with one variety grown at two locations. There were differences between the three varieties and slight difference between the varieties grown at two locations. While Debyser *et al.* (1997) tested the malts of six barley varieties with only slight differences between them.

In regards to wheat, Finnie *et al.* (2006) described the genetic and environmental variation in arabinoxylan in a wide range of wheat varieties. These varieties were not used in brewing but the results highlighted the differences that can be obtained in wheat which can be used as a primary raw ingredient or as an adjunct.

Sorghum has been extensively around the world for brewing either as a raw material or as an adjunct. While detailed analysis has been carried out on most quality attributes usually measured in assessing the suitability for malting and brewing (i.e. protein, amylases, etc.). There has been little reported on the variation of arabinoxylans between varieties of sorghum. Single varieties of sorghum, wheat and pearled millet were assessed for hemicellulose content, with variation between the three species in the arabinose, xylose and arabinose/xylose ratios (Nandini and Salimath, 2001a). Nandini and Salimath (2001b) assessed the structural features of a single sorghum variety.

A less common ingredient used in brewing has been triticale. Triticale is a hybrid species derived from a genetic fusion of wheat and rye. Glatthar *et al.* (2005) found variation in the water soluble and insoluble arabinoxylan content between triticale and wheat varieties grown over multiple years. The triticales were much higher in total, soluble and insoluble arabinoxylan than the wheats tested but had values similar to a commercial barley malt.

Two other grains used in brewing a speciality beer, that is gluten free, are pearled millet and buckwheat. Both of these cereals contain arabinoxylan although there is very limited data on variation between varieties.

Effects in Malting

Many thousand of years ago, the people living in Mesopotamia were the first to "brew" beer, although the process was a little dissimilar to modern brewing practices. These ancient brewers did germinate barley but they had no knowledge of the complex biochemical reactions that convert the endosperm components into food for the growing germ as well important factors having a positive influence on the quality of beer.

The process of malting has had volumes written about it. In simple terms, malting is a four stage process where firstly, grain is steeping in water, which triggers germination. The second stage is germination where the sprouted grain is allowed to germinate, with controlled air flow, temperature and turning of the grain. During this phase, a significant number of the biochemical systems start to work on the insoluble endosperm structures. The third stage is where the grain is dried, again under controlled conditions, where temperature and air flow ensure the malt is finished in the best possible quality. The final stage is malt storage where it is critical for the malt to be maintained in optimal quality. Also, this is where malt is blended to meet brewers' specifications. It is absolutely critical to maintain ideal storage conditions once blending is completed.

The steeping, germinating and kilning processes all impact on the expression and optimal functionality of enzymes that will work to produce the products to be utilized, initially for the growing embryo, but also for the yeast during fermentation. Key enzymes including (1→4)-β-endoxylanases, β-D-xylosidases, α-L-arabinofuranosidases and esterases, involved in degrading the arabinoxylan structure are synthesized during steeping and germination. These enzymes are synthesized in the aleurone layer, stimulated by the presence of gibberellic acid (Taiz and Honigman, 1976; Dashek and Chrispeels, 1977), and move into the endosperm to commence working on the arabinoxylan substrate. Although it is shown that the major (1→4)–β-endoxylanase was synthesized only after day 4 of germination and increased until 15 days in one barley variety (Casper *et al.*, 2001). This supports previous data that suggested the endoxylanase is bound in the aleurone layer cell walls until complete breakdown before it migrates to the endosperm (Fincher, 1989; Slade *et al.*, 1989)

The breakdown of the endosperm cell walls is critical for the successful modification on the two other key endosperm components, the protein matrix and the starch granules. Chandra *et al.* (1999) have shown the effect on the rate of breakdown of β-glucan has an impact on modification regardless of whether a lager or ale malt was produced from three barley varieties. Incomplete breakdown of the cell walls leaves residual β-glucan and arabinoxylan which impacts on brewing efficiency and beer quality (see below). Sungurtas *et al.* (2004) identified differences between four varieties in the expression of three important enzymes, namely (1→4)-β-endoxylanases, β-D-xylosidases and α-L-arabinofuranosidases. There were differences in the rate of expression and total amount of enzymes. The varieties that had the higher levels of the main enzyme (1→4)-β-endoxylanase did not show the highest levels of arabinoxylan content in a hot water extract.

During germination, the cell wall degrading enzymes act on the appropriate substrates, producing smaller, more soluble molecules. While there is a decrease in total arabinoxylan content, there is little change in the amount of the two sugars, namely arabinose and xylose. Kilning effectively suspends the action of the enzymes. However, the high temperature (>60°C up to 85°C) during the later stages of kilning reduces the activity of the enzymes.

These enzymes are temperature sensitive and while they could continue to act on the arabinoxylan substrates, high temperature (infusion) mashing will render the enzymes inactive almost immediately. Li *et al.* (2004) demonstrated the effect of different mashing temperatures and mash stand times on xylanase activity and arabinoxylan content. They developed a model to predict the xylanase activity, arabinoxylan content in wort using laboratory and commercial mashes. For those breweries that mash-in using a lower temperature (<50°C), the breakdown of the arabinoxylan will continue until the temperature increases thereby denaturing the enzymes. Hence, it is important that all the arabinoxylan (and β-glucan) is degraded during the malting process. Although complete degradation of both NSPs is always possible, Cyran *et al.* (2002) showed that there was an increased level of arabinoxylan than β-glucan in malt and there was also a high portion of molecular weight arabinoxylan residues.

Impacts on Brewing

The final quality of beer is influenced by a number of inputs and processes during production. These inputs and processes would include:

- the quality of the primary cereal ingredient (barley, wheat or sorghum);
- the malting quality (ale or lager malts);
- the mashing process (decoction vs. high temperature infusion);
- the adjunct and processing of the adjunct.

The effect of the primary cereal ingredient is twofold, with the level of arabinoxylan as well as the expression of enzymes that degrade it. As mentioned previously, there were genetic and environmental effects on the level of arabinoxylan in barley, wheat, sorghum and a range of other grains (Henry, 1986; Lehtonen and Aikasalo, 1987; Han, 2000; Nandini and Salimath, 2001a, b; Mikyska *et al.*, 2002; Trogh *et al.*, 2004; Glatthar *et al.*, 2005; Holtekjølen *et al.*, 2006; Finnie *et al.*, 2006). Also the malting process impacts on the breakdown of the endosperm cell walls and the degradation of the β-glucan and arabinoxylan.

The differences in malt styles, that is ale or lager malts, and hence, level of endosperm modification, is controlled by the malting process. While the quality of the raw material could impact on the malting performance, the process itself will control the final malt quality. Although the difference in beer style (ale vs. lager) is controlled by the brewing process, the malt itself plays a role. Brewers will set malt specifications for the maltster to produce a malt style that complements the brewing process. Lager malts generally have a lower Kolbach Index (KI) which could therefore have slightly high levels of cell wall material intact, including arabinoxylan. A number of studies have shown significant correlations between arabinoxylan and the KI, suggesting that if there was reduced protein modification there was a higher level of arabinoxylan. A high level of arabinoxylan indicates incomplete endosperm cell wall breakdown (Stewart *et al.*, 1998; Evans *et al.*, 1999). Conversely, ale malts with a higher KI would have greater degradation of the cell walls.

While lager malts may be lower in KI compared to ale malts, the malt could still produce excellent beer with no processing problems. Also, ale malts, with a high level of protein breakdown, could still have a high level of intact cell wall material but produce beer within specifications and causing no brewhouse problems. However, where malts were under-modified, and there are high levels of arabinoxylans then there may be processing problems with low rates of wort separation, high wort viscosity (Li *et al.*, 2004, 2005), beer viscosity, decrease of beer microfiltration rate (Stewart *et al.*, 1998; Stewart *et al.*, 1999), haze formation in the brewery (Coote and Kirsop, 1976) and foam instability (Evans *et al.*, 1999). Furthermore, incomplete degradation of endosperm cell walls reduces the yield of extract which can be derived during mashing.

A number of these studies have identified two important but different effects of arabinoxylan. Firstly, the level of arabinoxylan impacted on wort separation, viscosity (Li *et al.*, 2004, 2005) and haze formation (Coote and Kirsop,

1976). Secondly, the molecular weight of the arabinoxylan residues was shown to affect beer viscosity, filtration rate (Stewart *et al.*, 1998, 2000) and foam stability (Evans *et al.*, 1999). Although there were a small number of samples used in the studies the results clearly indicated that negative effects of undegraded arabinoxylan on beer quality and processing efficiency.

These studies used combinations of commercial malts, pilot scale brewing as well as commercial brewing samples of barley malt. However, similar problem have been shown in wheat malts and beer with high molecular arabinoxylan effect quality and processing (Cleemput *et al.*, 1993; Schwarz and Han, 1995). However, there are few reports of solubilization of arabinoxylans in mashing with grist containing wheat and wheat malt (Lu and Li, 2006). Historically, reduced beer filtration efficiency has been mainly attributed to β-glucan. Sadosky *et al.* (2002) reported that the concentration and molecular weight of arabinoxylan had a negative effect on beer viscosity and filterability. These effects were at least as important as the effects of β-glucan.

There are a number of quality attributes that contribute to the production of beer and well as the visual acceptability of the beer, these include viscosity, haze, filterability and foam retention. Arabinoxylan has been shown to impact on all of these four traits and importantly, it is both the concentration as well as the molecular size of the arabinoxylan residues that influence the quality.

Adjuncts

Most brewers around the world use adjuncts to impact particular characteristics to the final beer quality. Liquid adjunct brewers would use products such as corn syrup or cane sugar (sucrose from sugar cane). The function of liquid adjuncts would be to contribute additional fermentable sugars for fermentation. There would be little non-fermentable sugar present, that is oligo- or polysaccharides from either starch or NSP.

Solid adjunct brewers on the other hand would use either unprocessed or processed (malted or steamed flaked) grains. These grains would include rice, corn, barley or sorghum depending on the flavor target of the brewer. The use of an adjunct cooker would assist in the gelatinization of the starch prior to the addition into the mash. However, the presence of NSP in the form of β-glucan and arabinoxylans could impact on beer processing and quality.

Enzymic Degradation During Malting

As mentioned previously, the action of enzymes on the cell walls and in particular arabinoxylan is critical to producing malt that will cause minimal to no problems during brewing. A number of enzymes are involved in this process (Preece and MacDougall, 1958). These particular enzymes are required to degrade arabinoxylan during germination, which, in conjunction with the breakdown of the major endosperm cell wall component, β-glucan, will allow a more efficient modification of the endosperm.

The endo- and exo-enzymes work synergistically to:

- remove the arabinose side chains;
- attack the xylan backbone;
- cleave individual xyloses and arabinoses from the backbone and side chains;
- cleave ferulic acid.

The natural process of germination induces the development of enzymes. This process is common for all grains. The function and activity of the cell wall degrading enzymes are of particular importance to those grains used in brewing.

Over the years many reports have documented the various enzymes and the roles in degrading the arabinoxylan component as well as describing effects of germination with and between species. It would appear that (1→4)-β-endoxylanase is the main enzyme that cleaves internal bonds of the xylan backbone. There are a number of isoforms of the enzyme and there is variation due to variety (Slade *et al.*, 1989; Debyser *et al.*, 1997; Autio *et al.*, 2001) and species (Autio *et al.*, 2001; Simpson *et al.*, 2003; Grant *et al.*, 2003). (1→4)-β-endoxylanase is synthesized during germination (Preece and MacDougall, 1958) and stimulated by the action of gibberellic acid (Taiz and Honigman, 1976; Dashek and Chrispeels, 1977).

Another critical enzyme is arabinofuranohydrolase and is suggested to act first to remove the arabinosyl side chains. Several reports also describe the differences between barley varieties, species and the effect of germination (Taiz and Honigman, 1976; Autio *et al.*, 2001; Grant *et al.*, 2003). Further Ferré *et al.* (2000) identified an arabinoxylan arabinofuranohydrolase from germinated barley and suggested that this enzyme hydrolyzed arabinose from singly or doubly substituted xylose.

Two other enzymes that play a minor but still important role in breaking down the arabinoxylan structure have been described in recent research. These enzymes are xylanopyranosidase and esterase. The xylanopyranosidase is an exo-enzyme cleaving xylose from the xylan backbone. Grant and Briggs (2002) identified the presence of this enzyme in various wheat tissues. Further, Grant *et al.* (2003) showed the development of two isoforms of β-xylopyranosidase in germinating wheat. Both isoforms increased in total activity during in 7 days of germination.

Finally, esterases hydrolyze the esterified bonds between the non-reducing end arabinose and ferulic acid. Sancho *et al.* (1999) identified the presence of an esterase in barley and followed the activity during germination. The level of the enzyme decreased from the level in barley significantly from day 2 to day 6 of germination. Ward and Bamforth

(2002) also identified esterases in two varieties of barley and malt with a difference between the varieties. Also there were differences in the thermostability between the enzymes suggesting that some of the enzymes could survive malting and mashing. Further, the distribution of the enzymes between the husk/aleurone layer and endosperm indicated that some of the esterases where tissue specific and synthesized during germination. Finally, one particular esterase was involved in cell wall breakdown. Sancho *et al.* (2001) esterases cleaved ferulic acid bound to arabinose in spent brewers grain.

Conclusions

The research carried over the last 20 years has improved understanding of structure of arabinoxylan and its location in tissues. Also there is better understanding of enzymes involved in the breakdown of arabinoxylan, the aleurone and endosperm cell wall, both functionally as well as structurally. Arabinoxylan plays a positive role in dietary fiber when it is in its native state. However, when undegraded arabinoxylan has serious negative impact on malt and brewing quality and it has been suggested that arabinoxylan may impact more on brewing than β-glucan. Like most of the grain endosperm components arabinoxylan must undergo enzymic breakdown so as to ensure trouble-free brewing and beer quality.

For many years, there have been national and international discussions on the relevance of some of the malt specifications in relation to brewhouse performance and beer quality. One of the traits that should be routinely measured in arabinoxylan content and like its cell wall counterpart, the molecular weight of the final arabinoxylan residues is equally as important.

Future research into the genetic variability in the expression of arabinoxylan, the genes and translated proteins responsible for its breakdown during malting and brewing, and changes in brewing practices will herald arabinoxylan to be an equal partner to β-glucan and its importance in brewing.

Summary Points

- Arabinoxylans are NSP.
- They are found in the cell wall of the aleurone layers (75%) and the endosperm (25%).
- Arabinoxylans are degraded by enzymes during the malting process to facilitate continued breakdown of the endosperm contents (protein and starch).
- Low temperature mashing (<50°C) continues the breakdown of these NSP.
- Arabinoxylans contribute to filtration and haze problems in beer.
- Further research is required to gain a more detailed understanding of the genetic control of arabinoxylan as well as the enzyme systems that degrade this NSP to ensure trouble-free brewing and beer production.
- Improvements in filtration technology could increase pressure on barley breeders and maltsters breeders to produce low level arabinoxylan barley and malt which could impact on other quality parameters.

References

Autio, K., Simonen, T., Suortti, T., Salmenkallio-Martilla, M., Lassila, K. and Wilhelmson, A. (2001). Structural and enzymic changes in germinated barley and rye. *J. Inst. Brew.* 107, 19–25.

Bacic, A. and Stone, B.A. (1981). Organisation and chemistry of aleurone cell wall components from wheat and barley. *Aust. J. Plant Physiol.* 8, 475–495.

Bamforth, C.W. and Kanauchi, M. (2001). A simple model for the cell wall of starchy endosperm in barley. *J. Inst. Brew.* 107, 235–240.

Caspers, M.P.M., Lok, F., Sinjorgo, K.M.C., van Zeijl, M.J., Nielsen, K.A. and Cameron-Mills, V. (2001). Synthesis, processing and export of cytoplasmic endo-ß-1,4-xylanase from barley aleurone during germination. *Plant J.* 26, 191–204.

Chandra, G.S., Proudlove, M.O. and Baxter, E.D. (1999). The structure of barley endosperm – an important determinant of malt modification. *J. Sci. Food Agri.* 79, 37–46.

Cleemput, G., Roels, S.P., Vanoort, M., Grobet, P.J. and Delcour, J.A. (1993). Heterogenity in the structure of water-soluble arabinoxylans in European wheat flours of viable bread making quality. *Cereal Chem.* 70, 324–329.

Coote, N. and Kirsop, B.H. (1976). A haze consisting largely of pentosan. *J. Inst. Brew.* 82, 34.

Cyran, M., Izydorczyk, M.S. and Macgregor, A.W. (2002). Structural characteristics of water-extractable nonstarch polysaccharides from barley malt. *Cereal Chem.* 79, 359–366.

Dashek, W.V. and Chrispeels, M.J. (1977). Gibberellic-acid-induced synthesis and release of cell wall degrading endoxylanase by isolated aleurone layers of barley. *Planta* 134, 251–256.

Debyser, W., Derdelinckx, G. and Delcour, J.A. (1997). Arabinoxylan and arabinoxylan hydrolysing activities in barley malts and worts derived from them. *J. Cereal Sci.* 26, 67–74.

Dervilly-Pinel, G., Saulnier, R.L., Andersson, R. and Åman, P. (2001). Water-extractable arabinoxylans from pearled flours of wheat, barley, rye and triticale. Evidence for the presence of ferulic acid dimmers and their involvement in gel formation. *J. Cereal Sci.* 34, 207–214.

Evans, D.E., Sheehan, M.C. and Stewart, D.C. (1999). The impact of malt derived proteins on beer foam quality. II. The influence of malt foam-positive proteins and non-starch polysaccharides on beer foam quality. *J. Inst. Brew.* 105, 171–178.

Ferré, H., Broberg, A., Duus, J.ø. and Thomsen, K.K. (2000). A novel type of arabinoxylan arabinofuranohydrolase isolated from germinated barley. *Eur. J. Biochem.* 267, 6633–6641.

Fincher, G.B. (1989). Molecular and cellular biology associated with endosperm mobilization in germinating cereal grains. *Annu. Rev. Plant Physiol. Plant Mol. Biol.* 40, 305–346.

Fincher, G.B. (1992). Cell wall metabolism in barley. In Shewry, P.R. (ed.), *Barley: Genetics, Biochemistry, Molecular Biology and Biotechnology*, pp. 413–437. CAB International, Wallingford, UK.

Fincher, G.B. and Stone, B. (1986). Cell walls and their components in cereal grain technology. In Pomeranz, Y. (ed.), *Advances in Cereal Science and Technology V8*, pp. 207–295. American Association of Cereal Chemistry, St Paul, MN.

Finnie, S.M., Bettge, A.D. and Morris, C.F. (2006). Influence of cultivar and environment on water soluble and insoluble arabinoxylans in soft wheat. *Cereal Chem.* 83, 617–623.

Glatthar, J., Heinisch, J.J. and Senn, T. (2005). Unmalted triticale cultivars as brewing adjuncts: effects of enzyme activities and composition on beer wort quality. *J. Sci. Food Agri.* 85, 647–654.

Grant, M.M. and Briggs, D.E. (2002). The histochemical location of arabinoxylan and xylanopyranosidase in germinating wheat grains. *J. Inst. Brew.* 108, 478–480.

Grant, M.M., Briggs, D.E., Fitchett, C.S., Stimson, E. and Deery, M.J. (2003). Purification of an arabinofuranosidase and two β-xylopyranosidases from germinating wheat. *J. Inst. Brew.* 109, 8–15.

Han, J.Y. (2000). Structural characteristics of arabinoxylan in barley, malt, and beer. *Food Chem.* 70, 131–138.

Han, J.Y. and Schwarz, P.B. (1996). Arabinoxylan composition in barley, malt, and beer. *J. Am. Soc. Brew. Chem.* 54, 216–220.

Henry, R.J. (1986). Genetic and environmental variation in the pentosan and β-glucan content of barley and their relationship to malt quality. *J. Cereal Sci.* 4, 269–277.

Henry, R.J. (1988a). Changes in β-glucan and other carbohydrate components of barley during malting. *J. Sci. Food Agri.* 42, 333–341.

Henry, R.J. (1988b). The carbohydrates of barley grains – a review. *J. Inst. Brew.* 94, 71–78.

Höije, A., Sandström, C., Roubroeks, J., Andersson, R., Gohil, S. and Gatenholm, P. (2006). Evidence of the presence of 2-O-ß-D-xylopyranosyl-α-L-arabinofuranose side chains in barley husk arabinoxylan. *Carbohydr. Res.* 341, 2959–2966.

Holtekjølen, A.K., Uhlen, A.K., Bråthen, E., Sahlstrøm, S. and Knutsen, S.H. (2006). Contents of starch and non-starch polysaccharides in barley varieties of different origin. *Food Chem.* 93, 348–358.

Izydorczyk, M.S., Macri, L.J. and MacGregor, A.W. (1998a). Structure and physicochemical properties of barley non-starch polysaccharides – I. Water-extractable β-glucans and arabinoxylans. *Carbohydr. Polymer.* 35, 249–258.

Izydorczyk, M.S., Macri, L.J. and MacGregor, A.W. (1998b). Structure and physicochemical properties of barley non-starch polysaccharides – II. Alkali-extractable β-glucans and arabinoxylans. *Carbohydr. Polymer.* 35, 259–269.

Lehtonen, M. and Aikasalo, R. (1987). Pentosans in barley varieties. *Cereal Chem.* 64, 133–134.

Li, Y., Lu, J., Gu, G., Shi, Z. and Mao, Z. (2004). Studies on water-extractable arabinoxylans during malting and brewing. *Food Chem.* 93, 33–38.

Li, Y., Lu, J., Gu, G., Shi, Z. and Mao, Z. (2005). Studies on water-extractable arabinoxylans during malting and brewing. *Food Chem.* 93, 33–38.

Lu, J. and Li, Y. (2006). Effects of arabinoxylan solubilization on wort viscosity and filtration when mashing with grist containing wheat and wheat malt. *Food Chem.* 98, 164–170.

Luchsinger, W.W. (1967). The role of barley and malt gums in brewing. *Brewers Digest.* 42, 56–63.

Medcalf, D.G., D'Appolonia, B.L. and Gilles, K.A. (1968). Comparison of chemical composition and properties between hard red spring and durum wheat endosperm pentosans. *Cereal Chem.* 45, 539–549.

Mikyska, A., Prokes, J., Haskova, D., Havlova, P. and Polednikova, M. (2002). Influence of the species and cultivation area on the pentosan and β-glucan content in barley, malt and wort. *Monschr. Brauwiss.* 55, 88–95.

Nandini, C.D. and Salimath, P.V. (2001a). Carbohydrate composition of wheat, wheat bran, sorghum and bajra with good chapatti/roti (Indian flat bread) making quality. *Food Chem.* 73, 197–203.

Nandini, C.D. and Salimath, P.V. (2001b). Structural features of arabinoxylans from sorghum having good roti-making quality. *Food Chem.* 74, 417–422.

Preece, I.A. and MacDougall, M. (1958). Enzymic degradation of cereal hemicelluloses. II. Pattern of pentosan degradation. *J. Inst. Brew.* 64, 489–500.

Rao, M. and Muralikrishna, G. (2004). Structural analysis of arabinoxylans from native and malted finger millet (*Eleusine coracana*). *Carbohydr. Res.* 339, 2457–2463.

Rhodes, D.I. and Stone, B.A. (2002). Proteins in walls of wheat aleurone cells. *J. Cereal Sci.* 36, 83–101.

Sadosky, P., Schwartz, P.B. and Horsley, R.D. (2002). Effect of arabinoxylan, β-glucans and dextrins on the viscosity and membrane filterability of a beer model solution. *J. Am. Soc. Brew. Chem.* 60, 153–162.

Sancho, A.I., Faulds, C.B., Bartolome, B. and Williamson, G. (1999). Characterisation of feruloyl esterase activity in barley. *J. Sci. Food Agri.* 79, 447–449.

Sancho, A.I., Bartolomé, B., Gómez-Cordové, C., Williamson, G. and Faulds, C.B. (2001). Release of ferulic acid from cereal residues by barley enzymatic extracts. *J. Cereal Sci.* 34, 173–179.

Schwarz, P.B. and Han, J.Y. (1995). Arabinoxylan content of commercial beers. *J. Am. Soc. Brew. Chem.* 53, 157–159.

Simpson, D.J., Fincher, G.B., Huang, A.H.C. and Cameron-Mills, V. (2003). Structure and function of cereal and related higher plant (1→4)-β-xylan endohydrolases. *J. Cereal Sci.* 37, 111–127.

Slade, A.M., Høj, P.B., Morrice, N.A. and Fincher, G.B. (1989). Purification and characterisation of three (1→4)-ß-D-xylan endohydrolases from germinating barley. *Eur. J. Biochem.* 185, 533–539.

Stewart, D., Freeman, G. and Evans, E. (2000). Development and assessment of a small-scale wort filtration test for the prediction of beer filtration efficiency. *J. Inst. Brew.* 106, 361–366.

Stewart, D.C., Hawthorne, D. and Evans, D.E. (1998). Cold sterile filtration: a small scale filtration tests and investigation of membrane plugging. *J. Inst. Brew.* 104, 321–326.

Sungurtas, J., Swanston, J.S., Davies, H.V. and McDougall, G.J. (2004). Xylan-degrading enzymes and arabinoxylans solubilisation in barley cultivars of differing malting quality. *J. Cereal Sci.* 39, 273–281.

Taiz, L. and Honigman, W.A. (1976). Production of cell wall hydrolysing enzymes from barley aleurone layer in response to gibberellic acid. *Plant Physiol.* 58, 380–386.

Trogh, I., Courtin, C.M. and Declour, J.A. (2004). Isolation and characterization of water-soluble arabinoxylan from hull-less barley flours. *Cereal Chem.* 81, 576–581.

Viëtor, R.J., Angelino, S.A.G.F. and Voragen, A.G.J. (1991). Arabinoxylans in barley, malt and wort. *Proc. Cong. Eur. Brew. Con.* 23, 139–146.

Ward, R.E. and Bamforth, C.W. (2002). Esterases in barley and malt. *Cereal Chem.* 79, 681–686.

Wilson, S.M., Burton, R.A., Doblin, M.S., Stone, B.A., Newbigin, E.J., Fincher, G.R. and Bacic, A. (2006). Temporal and spatial appearance of wall polysaccharides during cellularization of barley (*Hordeum vulgare*) endosperm. *Planta* 224, 655–667.

30

Histamine in Beer

Susanne Diel, Maria Herwald, Hannelore Borck and Friedhelm Diel
Institut für Umwelt und Gesundheit (IUG) and University of Applied Sciences, FB:Oe, Biochemistry, Fulda, Germany

Abstract

Histamine is the major mediator in inflammation and allergy. Furthermore, histamine is a product of microbial metabolism especially during fermentation and spoiling of food. In this paper histamine is determined in beverages like beer before and after mechanical and chemical cleaning of tap installation in selected German bars and restaurants. After a couple of weeks without cleaning storage devices, tubes and taps, histamine increases up to 35 mg/l in a beer sample on-draft. However, this contamination can be significantly reduced after mechanical (35%) and after combined mechanical/chemical cleaning (93%), respectively. Beside histamine other biogenic amines, especially tyramine, are produced and must also be taken into account in the health risk assessment. Brewing, brewery location and hygienicity are most important factors for the *Enterobacteriaceae*, *Lactobacillae*, *Pediococcus* and *Staphylococcus* spp. derived biogenic contaminations. The specific mammalian histamine responses are also discussed. Special focus is laid on histamine-activated G protein coupled receptors (GPCR), the signal transduction induced by the gastro/intestinal (H2R) and the "new" lymphocyte (H4R) histamine receptor. It can be suggested that beer consumption is better than wine related to the prevalence of allergic reactions. Specific "beer allergies" are very rare, and only a few articles are published on this matter in the international literature.

List of Abbreviations

AC	Adenylyl cyclase
ALDH	Aldehyde dehydrogenase
AVE	Allergie-Verein in Europa
cAMP	Cyclic AMP
CREB	cAMP-response element-binding protein
DAG	Diacylglycerol
DAO	Diamino-oxidase
ELISA	Enzyme-linked immuno sorbent assay
GPCR	G protein coupled receptor
Gut	Intestinum
HDC	L-histidine decarboxylase
HIS	Histamine
HPLC	High performance liquid chromatography
HR	Histamine receptor
IgE	Immunoglobulin E
InsP3	Inositol triphosphate
JAK	Janus kinase
LTP	Lipid transfer protein
MAO	Monoamino-oxidase
MAPK	Mitogen-activated protein kinase
MC	Mast cells
MMC	Mucosal mast cells
NFkB	Nuclear factor kappa B
OPD	Ortho-phthaldialdehyde
PIP2	Phospho-inositol-diphosphate
PKA	Protein kinase A
PKC	Protein kinase C
PLA2	Phospholipase A2
PLC	Phospholipase C
p.o.	Oral
PTX	Pertussis toxin
RIA	Radioimmunoassay
STAT	Signal transducer and activator of transcription

Introduction

Beer is one of the most popular beverages all over the world. It mainly contains substances derived from malt, hops and brewer's yeast. For the production of special beers, other cereals (e.g. wheat, rice or corn) and enzymes may be added. Malt is obtained from germinated and heated or roasted barley. Hops (*Humulus lupulus*) belong to the cannabinaceae family. It provides the characteristic bitterness and aroma of beer and prevents bacterial contamination. For the fermentation process, the yeast-species *Saccharomyces cerevisiae* and *S. carlsbergensis* are used.

Furthermore, the consumption of beer can provide histamine and other biogenic amines and aids in the release

Beer in Health and Disease Prevention
ISBN: 978-0-12-373891-2

of histamine in the gastric intestinal tissue (gut). As histamine shares the same aldehyde dehydrogenase (ALDH) for its metabolism, increased alcohol from beer can also prevent the breakdown of histamine. This leads to allergy-like reactions including most notable hay fever symptoms like, for example, nasal disorders and flushing of the skin. Combined neuronal responses of alcohol and biogenic amines like migraine and headache are concentration dependent and are related to the individual precondition.

The main responses of histamine can be defined to cause vasodilatation with specific effects to the neuro-immune system. Toxicity thresholds in human subjects are assumed to be in the range 10–100 mg p.o. and are closely related to the individual histamine sensitivity (Beutling, 1996a).

As we could show in recent work histamine obtains only poor sensory characteristics, and the average threshold value of "taste" is difficult to specify even in normal tap water (Rohn *et al.*, 2005). However, as histamine is an important mediator in inflammation and influences the exocrine and paracrine processes in the gastric mucosa, cell regulation in the gut and circulating blood is of special interest (Diel and Szabo, 1986; Wackes *et al.*, 2006).

The aim of the present study is to assess whether histamine can be tasted and measured in commercially available beer. Furthermore, it shall be elucidated in how far hygienic handling can suppress histamine concentration in beer on draft. For a better understanding the biosynthesis of histamine and the mechanistic understanding in health responses shall give the frame of this contribution.

Metabolism of Histamine

As it is shown in Figure 30.1 histamine is synthesized by decarboxylation of histidine. Pyridoxal-5-phosphate-dependent l-histidine decarboxylase (HDC EC **4**.1.1.22) is a widespread ubiquitous enzyme and this is the main pathway for the production of histamine. However, degradation can occur in different pathways: amino-oxidases (unspecific monoamino-oxidase – MAO EC **1**.4.3.4, diamino-oxidase – DAO EC **1**.4.3.6), *O*-and *N*-methylation – methyl-transferases (EC **2**.1.1.8), histidase (L-histidine/-ammonialyase EC **4**.3.1.3) and more or less specific *N*-acetyltransferases as well as hydrolases may participate at the histamine degradation.

The cleavage of L-amino acids (histidine in case of histamine) from proteins is precondition for the production of histamine and other biogenic amines. Furthermore, the amino acid–COOH group must be activated and may not be bound to salt or may not be associated or "deactivated" by other molecular-binding sites. Interestingly, the coenzyme for decarboxylases is ATP-dependent and the lack of Vitamine B6 inhibits the carboxylases in *Enterococcus faecalis* (Beutling, 1996b).

The decarboxylation of other amino acids for the biosynthesis of biogenic amines is analog to the histamine synthesis: lysine is the progenitor for cadaverine, arginine for agmatine, tyrosine for tyramine, ornithine for putrescine, respectively. All these biogenic amines can be toxic for mammals in a concentration-related manner. Biogenic amines are produced by symbiotic bacteria, after resorption through the colon mucosal tissue, entering the blood vessels. Beside histamine, tyramine is reported to be the most important biogenic factor in beer (for review Beutling, 1996b).

Analyses of Histamine in Beer

Determination of histamine in biological samples is not so easy and values in the literature are contradictionary. The most sensitive way to measure histamine is fluorimetry or mass spectrography after high performance liquid chromatography (HPLC). Immunological tests like radioimmunoassay (RIA) and enzyme-linked immuno sorbent assay (ELISA) are not sufficiently specific related to the relative small molecular weight and poor epitopal character of the molecular structure. Best efficacy can be elucidated using the post-column derivatization with ortho-phthalaldehyde (OPD) (Diel, 2001).

Ten test samples were purchased from supermarkets and beer on draft from typical German bars.

Types of beer and alcohol concentration were documented from the label. Sugar was estimated refractometrically.

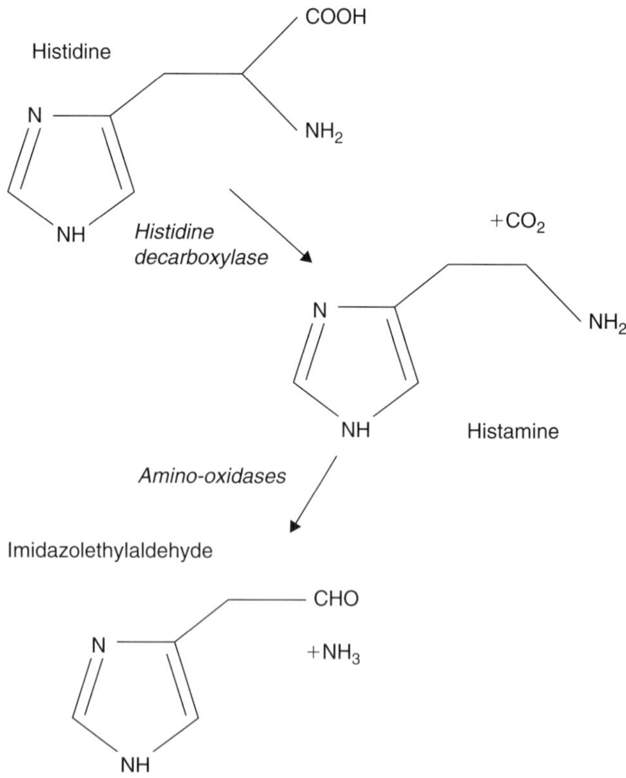

Figure 30.1 The main histamine metabolism. Histamine is synthesized by histidine-decarboxylase (HDC) and degraded by amino-oxidases (MAO and DAO). Methylation and acetylation of histamine are not shown here.

Immediately after opening the bottles, freshly drawn beer was tested using standardized sensitivity assessment methods by 10 instructed assessors – trained according to German DIN 10961/ISO 6658. Triangle test was performed according to DIN ISO 4120 as a double blind method (Bodmer *et al.*, 1999). The reference test samples were diluted in normal tap water (0–5 μM Histamine-HCl; Janssen, Belgium). Specific sensory statistic software FIZZ was used (Rohn *et al.*, 2005). Histamine and other biogenic amines in beer samples like tyramine, cadaverine and putrescine were measured fluorimetrically after HPLC and thin-layer chromatography (data not shown here) (Shore *et al.*, 1959; Busch-Stockfisch, 2002).

Sensory Thresholds

Ten instructed assessors indicated a mean sensory threshold for reference histamine 2.5 ± 1.5 μM (SDM, $n = 10$) in normal tap water. However, the triangle test resulted that only one of the test persons recognized the histamine reference as the right one.

Sensitivity criteria such as pharyngeal irritation, tingling tongue and swelling of mucosal tissues in the mouth were defined to be characteristic for the "specific taste" of the biogenic amines. No positive correlation was found between histamine/biogenic amine concentration in beer and the sensory sensation ($R = 0.6$; ranking of intensity of biogenic amines in seven lager beer samples – data not shown here).

Histamine Concentrations

Histamine concentrations in the international literature

Main methods for the determination of histamine in beverages are RIA, ELISA and fluorimetry after HPLC. Best specificity and validity can be revealed using the OPD-coupled fluorimetric post-column detection as it is mentioned above (Diel *et al.*, 1981).

Related to the method which is used the variety of published histamine concentrations in beer differ depending on origin, brewery and type of beer. Microbial contamination and the hygienic control must also be taken into consideration.

Since six decades histamine is determined in beer. The most important biogenic amines producing bacteria are *Enterobacteriaceae*, *Lactobacillus casei*, *Lactobacillus lindneri*, *Lactobacillus coryniformis*, *Pediococcus inopinatus*, *Lactobacillus brevis* and *Pediococcus cerevisiae* (Koch, 1986).

Histamine concentrations in beer are published in, for example, Scandinavia 2.6–15 mg/l (Granerus *et al.*, 1969), France 0.3–20 mg/l (Zappavigna *et al.*, 1974; Vidal-Carou *et al.*, 1989) and Germany 0.44–35.2 mg/l (Wackes *et al.*, 2006), respectively.

In a review of Beutling (1996b) it is shown that histamine in alcohol-free beer is relatively low (0.04–0.18 mg/l), whereas beer with high contents of basic wort contain relatively high values (approx. 10 mg/l).

It is suggested that the influences of brewing processes and fermentation are crucial on the distinct formation of histamine and other biogenic amines in beer (Romero *et al.*, 2003).

Histamine measured in the Fulda lab

The mean histamine concentration in beer from 10 typical German restaurants, as it is determined in the Fulda lab, ranges 0.49 mg/l (0.44–0.55 mg/l) in the bottled and 10.3 mg/l (range 0.5–35.2 mg/l) in the drawn lager beer, respectively (Table 30.1; Figure 30.1). Although black beer "Schwarzer Hahn" shows a particularly soft taste, the histamine level is pretty high (35.2 mg/l). It must be considered that in this case histamine measurements are performed 2 hours after drawing (Table 30.1).

Table 30.1 Histamine and other compounds in eight selected beer bottled samples

Type of beer	*HIS[a] (HPLC) (mg/l)*	*Sugar[b] (%)*	*Protein[b] (%)*	*Alcohol[c] (Vol. %)*	*Remarks*
Schwarzbier (K.)	0.41	5.2	0.41	4.8	
Kristallweizen 5.3%	0.45	5.2	0.29	5.3	
Ur-Weisse dunkel 5.3%	0.48	5.5	0.34	5.3	
Hefeweizen naturtrüb 5.3%	0.56	5.75	0.35	5.3	
Antoniusweizen	0.54	5.75	0.37	5.3	
Wiesenmühlenbier	0.68	5.75	0.44	4.9	
Pils (hell)	4.83	6.0	0.31	4.9	
Schwarzer Hahn	35.16	5.4	0.32	4.9	2 h after opening

[a] Post-column OPD-fluorimetry after HPLC.
[b] Sugar and protein measurements using a routine photometric test.
[c] Alcohol as indicated on the label.

Table 30.2 Biogenic amines in beer

	Mr (g/mol)	Origin
Group 1		*Exclusively raw material*
Putrescine	88.1	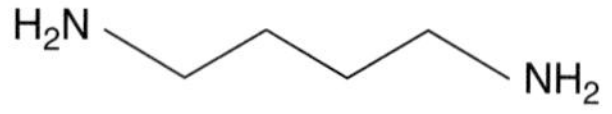
Spermine	202	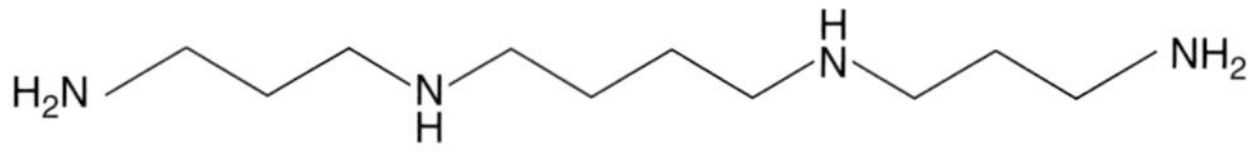
Spermidine	145.5	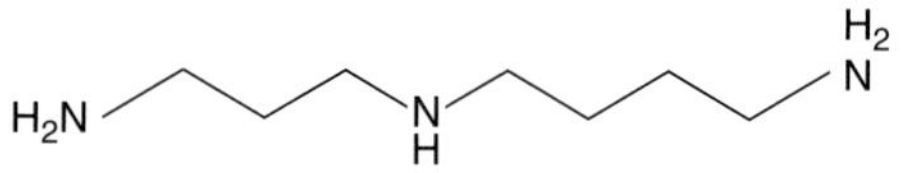
Group 2		*Raw material and processing*
Histamine	111.2	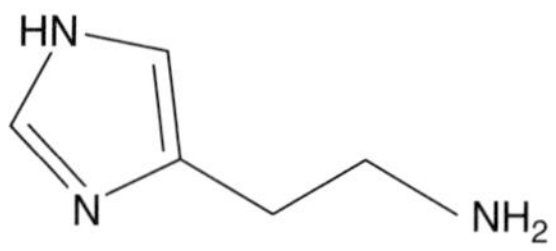
β-Phenylalanine	121.2	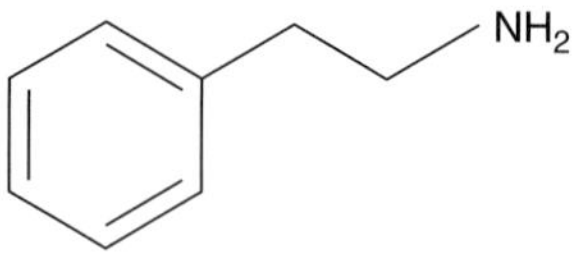
Cadaverine	102.2	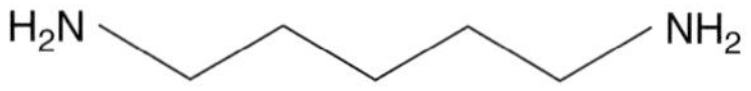
Agmatine	130	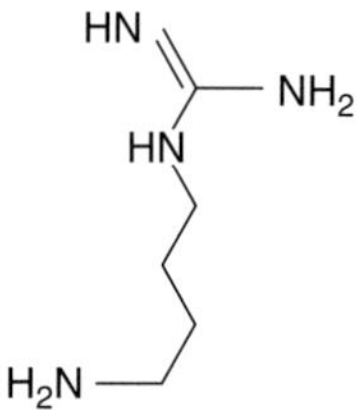
Group 3		*Exclusively processing*
Tyramine	137	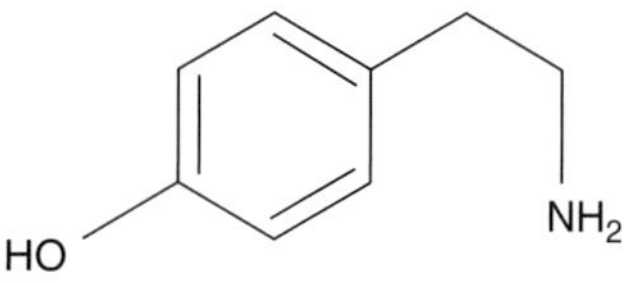
Tryptamine		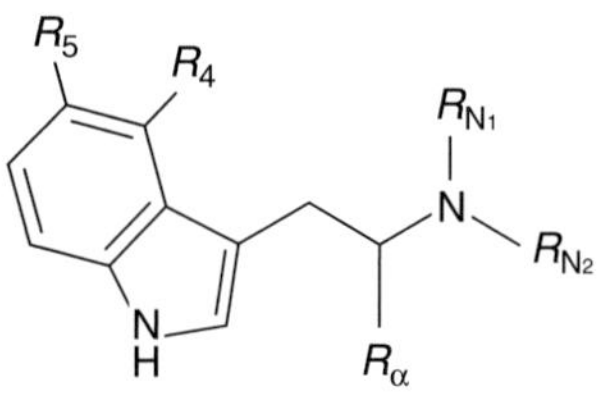

Source: Modified from Beutling (1996b).

In a 15-year-old beer sample the histamine peak is suppressed, however the other biogenic amines seem to dominate the HPLC profile (data not shown).

It can be concluded that only the beer on draft reveals high histamine values (up to 33 mg/l). The sensory characteristics do not correlate to the measured histamine concentrations, using the standardized sensitivity assessment.

Other Biogenic Amines

Biogenic amines are produced predominantly by *Lactobacillae* and *Staphylococcae.* Yeast and other additives are contaminated during the breeding process. Furthermore, storekeeping and drawing lead to additional microbial activity. Tyramine is the most important biogenic factor beside histamine as it is stated already in the introduction. It can be produced rapidly (4 mg/l/day), up to maximal concentrations approx. 45 mg/l (Izquierdo-Pulido *et al.*, 1994). Other biogenic amines are specifically associated to ingredients like malt (spermidine, putrescine, spermine, agmatine, tyramine, tryptamine, cadaverine, phenylalanine …) and hop (spermidine, spermine, phenylalanine, tyramine, putrescine, agmatine …). Related to its origin, biogenic amines in beer can be selected into three groups (Table 30.2).

Hygienic Aspects

In recent work beer on draft samples from distinct city restaurants in central Germany have been examined. Hygienic criteria like organoleptic assessment as well as pH, carbohydrate and protein are measured and compared to the histamine concentrations. The examinations take place before and after mechanical and/or chemical cleaning.

In Figure 30.2a, a typical HPLC graph is shown before cleaning the tap and the beer storage devices. In Figure 30.2b the beer "peak" is significantly suppressed after mechanical cleaning, and in Figure 30.2c it can be demonstrated that after mechanical and additionally chemical cleaning no more histamine contamination can be detected in the drawn beer samples. The results – including also other similar studies – are summarized in Table 30.3.

From the presented results it can be suggested that color and smell of the drawn samples are not varying after the cleaning of the bar equipment. However, there are significant differences of the histamine content before and after cleaning. And it is also of certain importance how the cleaning was performed.

In the present work beer on draft samples from six different Fulda city restaurants are examined. A correlation is found between the histamine contents relevant for health and the present hygienic conditions which depend on several factors as it is shown in Figure 30.3.

From the data of this study it can be concluded that:

1. The hygienic criteria – organoleptic, pH, sugar and protein values do not show significant differences.

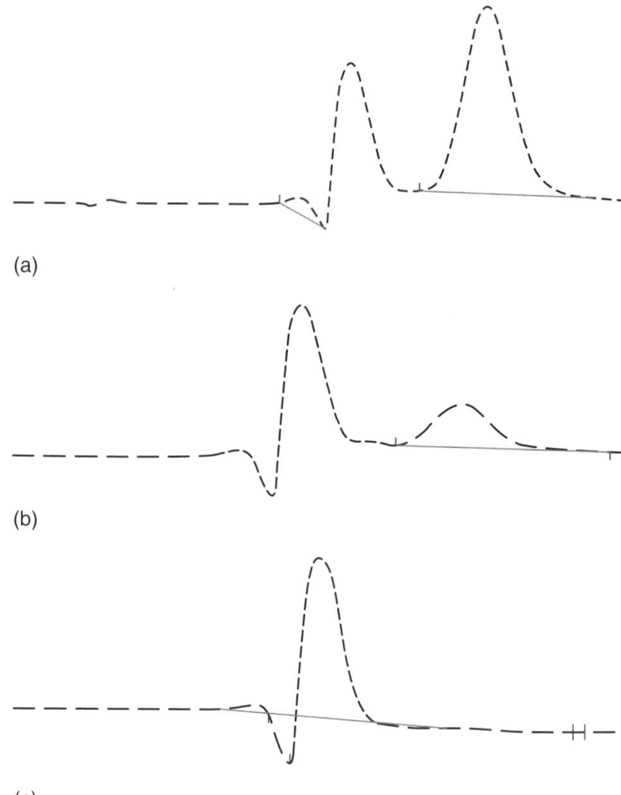

Figure 30.2 Typical ion-exchange HPLC fluorimetry profile of one selected beer sample "Schwarzer Hahn" on draught: (a) before cleaning (last cleaning was 4 weeks ago), (b) after mechanically cleaning, (c) mechanically and chemically cleaning of the tubes and tap devices. For analyses beer samples were treated with perchloric acid and were separated in oxalate/tartrate elutant (0.75/0.5 g/l): 1 ml/min; post-column OPD-derivatization, fluorescence (340/455 nm). The histamine peak is indicated by the arrow.

2. Before and after the cleaning of the tap installation weak sensory differences in taste are ascertained. However, after HPLC the fluorimetric determination of histamine (detection limit 3.8 ng/ml) shows before mechanical cleaning 4.84–31.94 ng/ml, 3.94–6.13 ng/ml after mechanical cleaning, in case of the combined chemical and mechanical cleaning before 2.63–5.5 ng/ml and after 4.06–4.46 ng/ml, respectively.
3. In spite of few data and the fact that the ascertained histamine is concentrated in the allowed range it can be suggested – and this is in particular true for people with elevated histamine sensitivity – that consumption of "unhygienic" beer can induce an increase of health risk.

Histamine Responses and Histamine Receptors

Histamine is a small molecular messenger that regulates a wide variety of physiological responses. Signal transduction is induced via G protein coupled receptors (GPCR)

Table 30.3 Histamine in selected German beer samples before and after mechanical and combined mechanical–chemical cleaning of the tap installations

Selected beer No	*Type of cleaning*	*Histamine before cleaning* (ng/ml)*	*Histamine after cleaning* (ng/ml)*	*Histamine reduction (%)*
1	Mechanical	31,943	6,129	81
2	Mechanical	6,560	5,537	16
3	Mechanical	4,843	3,940	18
4	Chemical–mechanical	5,499	406	93
5	Chemical–mechanical	739	406	45
6	Chemical–mechanical	526	446	15

*Beer samples are examined fluorimetrically 10 min after drawing.

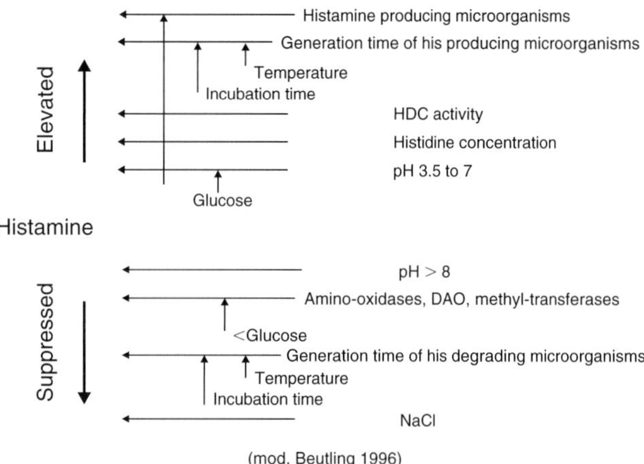

Figure 30.3 Criteria for the microbial histamine contamination. *Source*: Modified from Beutling (1996c).

(Bakker and Leurs, 2005). It acts as a neurotransmitter in the central nervous system (CNS) and also as a major inflammatory factor with certain immune-regulatory potency (Hill *et al.*, 1997). Histamine exerts distinct effects by binding to histamine receptors which is classified on the basis of pharmacological studies influencing gene expression of four histamine subtypes all of which belonging to the superfamily of GPCR.

After the first description of histamine receptors the observation that not all "anti-histamines" can modulate the effects of histamine led Ash and Schild (1966) hypothesize the existence of at least two distinct receptor subtypes antagonizing the responses of histamine on heart and stomach.

Specific H2-receptor (H2R) antagonists are developed in the sixteenths and those are proved to be very useful in gastric ulcer therapy.

Identification of the presynaptic H3R by Arrang *et al.* (1983) gives rise to a new field of interest. For example, sleep/wakefulness, cardiovascular control, nutrition habits like appetite and hormonal secretion are strongly associated to the responses of histamine in mammalian cerebral areas and brain functions.

The identification of a new histamine receptor H4R has possibly been related to genomic database studies. H4R is the target in the regulation of immune function and can be the gate for histamine induced signal transduction of the janus kinase/signal transduction and activation of transcription (JAK/STAT) downstream in human lymphocytes (Oda *et al.*, 2000; Horr *et al.*, 2006).

The four histamine receptors shall be characterized in the following brief summaries. This is for the better theoretical understanding of possible histamine responses derived from exogenous histamine – from beverages like beer. In this context it must be considered that the mammalian mediator cells like mast cells (MC), mucosal mast cells (MMC) and circulating basophilic granulocytes can secrete histamine which can be pathogenic in case of allergy diseases. (*Note*: histamine sensitivity of mammals has nothing to do with constitutively increased precondition for receiving an allergic disease = atopy. This issue – with special focus on "beer allergy" – is discussed in the last chapter.) The H4R is of special interest, because that can be the main histamine receptor of lymphocytes in the human immune system (Schneider *et al.*, 2002). Nevertheless exogenous histamine from beverages must reach those receptor targets once incorporated after drinking beer and penetrating through the intestinal tissues.

H1R

As H1R is involved in many of the allergic symptoms, anti-histaminica against this receptor are developed and widely spread in the western hemisphere (Woosley, 1996). Contractions in airway smooth muscle are histamine induced via H1R mediated Gq/11 stimulation of the inositol phospholipid signaling system. Production of inositol-1,4,5-triphosphate (IP3) and 1,2-diacylglycerol (DAG) as well as activation of protein kinase C (PKC) take place and modulate Ca^{2+} connected to the activation of phospholipase D by monomeric GTP-binding. This can also stimulate phospholipase A2 (PLA2) resulting in arachidonic acid release. Involving immune functions H1R can induce the mitogen-activated protein kinases (MAPK/K) pathway and the transcription factor NFκB.

H2R

H2R is especially known for its role in the gastric regulation and must be considered to be also a first target for histamine and ingredients in beer. An important key for the understanding of ulcer and gastroesophageal reflux diseases can be addressed to this receptor (Bakker and Leurs, 2005).

Activation of H2R transduces Gi-modulated adenylyl cyclase (AC) activity and subsequent regulation of cyclic AMP (cAMP) in the cell (Diel *et al.*, 2006). Downstream activation of protein kinase A and the cAMP-responsive element-binding transcription factor (CREB) modulate the gene transcription. Other signal transduction mechanisms including Ca^{2+} transport are induced by H2R ligand interaction.

H3R

This receptor is located at the CNS and can be associated to a manifold brain derived disorders, including diabetes and obesity, attention deficit hyperactivity disorder (ADHD), Alzheimer's disease, epilepsy, Parkinson and Schizophrenia (Bakker and Leurs, 2005).

Furthermore myocardial ischemia, gastric acid-related and inflammatory diseases are associated centrally via regulatory responses of H3R.

Signal transduction by Gi-subunit predominantly results in an inhibition of AC. Na^{+}/K^{+} exchange is inhibited and activation of efflux (ATPase-activity) decreases the intracellular Ca^{2+} concentration, and in a complex neuronal signal transduction via H3R, for example, glycogen synthase activity 3β (GSK3β) is inhibited (for review Bakker and Leurs, 2005).

H4R

The fourth histamine receptor H4R shares a big part with the H3R derived protein subunits, nevertheless obtains a relatively high affinity for histamine. The expression profile is most abundant in leukocytes including eosinophils, dendritic cells and tonsil B-cells, as well as cells from the bone marrow and spleen (Liu *et al.*, 2001). This receptor may also be relevant in the signal transduction of STAT1 downstream phosphorylation- and histamine-modulated STAT1/STAT6 interaction at the DNA in human lymphocytes (Horr *et al.*, 2006). Furthermore leukotriene B4 production and neutrophil recruitment, chemotaxis and cytoskeletal changes of eosinophils are activated by histamine via H4R (Ling *et al.*, 2004). MC activation (autocrine histamine release!) and B-lymphocyte interleukin-16 (IL-16) secretion are also described. H4R is also expressed in parts of the brain and lung and can indirectly be relevant for the assessment of histamine in beverages with focus on the immune system (for review Bakker and Leurs, 2005).

As it is shown in Figure 30.4 similarly to the H3R, the H4R couples to members of the Gi-family thus inhibiting

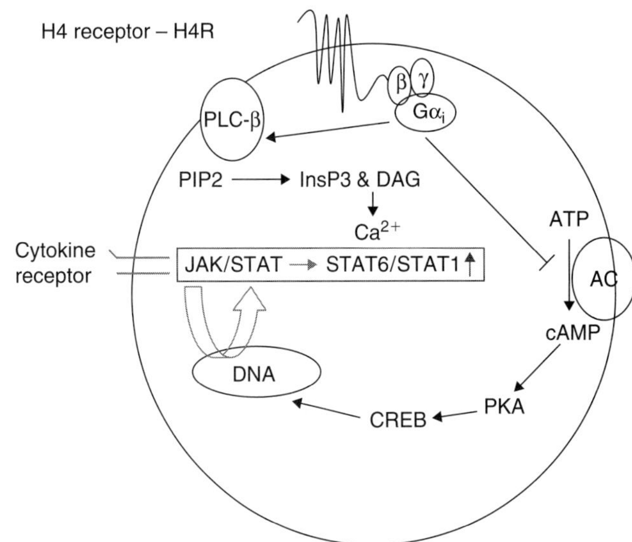

Figure 30.4 Histamine receptor H4R major signaling pathways. *Source*: Modified from Bakker, and Leurs (2005). H4R activates G proteins which inhibit the adenylyl cyclase (AC) resulting in turn a reduced cAMP, protein kinase A (PKA) and CREB-modulated transcription. Ca^{2+} is activated through phospholipase C (PLC) by Gβγ via inositol triphosphate (InsP3) and diacylglycerol (DAG). The janus kinase/signal transduction and activator of transcription (JAK/STAT) pathway provides crosstalk upon the histamine induced STAT6/STAT1 balance. This is constitutively upregulated in atopy (gray).

the AC – CREB pathway. The H4R-mediated Ca^{2+} signaling is induced through a PTX-sensitive (PTX = pertussis toxin) activation of phospholipase C (PLC). Furthermore, the JAK/STAT-downstream activation can induce an intracellular crosstalk to the MAPK/K as well as G protein signal transduction system/pathways in human T-lymphocytes (Michel *et al.*, 2008).

In conclusion the four described histamine receptors have quite different physiological roles and it is still unclear in how far exogenous histamine – particular from beverages like alcohols and beers – succeeds in interacting with H1R–H4R targets. It appears that the constitutive activity of H2R and H3R is more relevant than H1R and H4R, respectively. Nevertheless, H4R shows more constitutive selectivity and specificity concerning the immune responses.

Beer and Allergy

Alcoholic beverages – like beer – obtain a dual effect resulting histamine induced allergic symptoms: a direct one from histamine as a natural ingredient (exogenous), and an indirect one derived from the histamine release after, for example, beer allergenic MC degranulation ("anaphylaxis" – endogenous). As it is shown in Figure 30.5 exogenous and endogenous histamine affect the "immuno-/allergological cycle" in mammals.

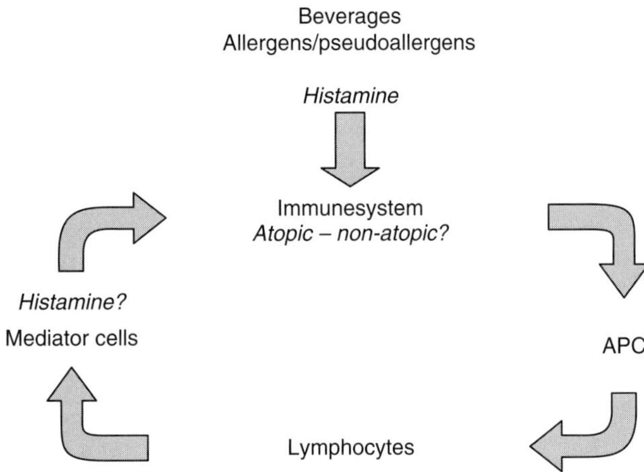

Figure 30.5 The exogenous and endogenous influences of histamine on the "immuno-/allergological" cyclic regulation. APC: antigen/allergen presenting cells.

In general, alcoholic drinks are capable of triggering a wide range of allergic and allergy-like responses, including rhinitis, itching, facial swelling, headache, cough and asthma. Wine is clearly the most frequent reported elicitor for adverse responses. Despite the worldwide and abundant consumption of beer, allergic reactions following beer ingestion are uncommon. One of the first reports was in 1980 (Van Ketel, 1980). Van Ketel described two patients with acute reactions after drinking beer. In scratch tests both persons exhibited positive results to malt. In 1986, Jover *et al.* studied 12 patients with immediate hypersensitivity to beer. They had positive scratch tests to beer, malt, brewer's yeast and rice. Nine of them were also positive to hops. As oral challenge tests with raw rice and yeast powder yielded negative results in these patients, malt was considered the main causative antigen of beer allergy. Fernández-Anaya *et al.* (1999) examined three patients who suffered anaphylactic reactions after consuming beer. The patients experienced a range of symptoms including a tingling sensation in the face, lip or tongue angioedema, chest tightness, coughing, fainting and generalized urticaria. The research team prepared an extract from barley-made beer and performed skin prick testing. The 3 patients had positive skin prick test results, while 20 control patients had negative test responses. Anaphylaxis – with the consequence of immunoglobulin E (IgE)-mediated histamine release – is a severe allergic reaction that affects multiple systems in the body. Symptoms can include severe headache, nausea and vomiting, sneezing and coughing, abdominal cramps, diarrhea, hives, swelling of the lips, tongue and throat, itching all over the body, and anxiety. The most dangerous symptoms include breathing difficulties, a drop in blood pressure and shock. This study indicates that barley-made beer is a potential culprit of severe anaphylaxis and barley-sensitive patients should be questioned about beer tolerance.

As well as the just described data, the majority of studies concerning allergic reactions to beer basically implicate malt to precipitate the observed symptoms. (Gutgesell and Fuchs, 1995; Vidal and González-Quintela, 1995; Santucci *et al.*, 1996; Bonadonna *et al.*, 1999; Curioni *et al.*, 1999) The first identification of allergens in malt and barley was achieved by Figueredo and co-workers in clinical and immunological studies carried out in a patient in whom anaphylaxis developed after drinking beer (Figueredo *et al.*, 1999). Via immunoblotting assays they demonstrated a 38-kDa IgE-binding component in precipitated beer proteins. Interestingly, more and stronger IgE-binding bands were identified in malt than in barley itself. The authors suggest the enzymes that are needed during the germination process to turn starches into brewing sugar as a possible explanation for the enhanced allergenicity of the malted grain. In an ensuing work based on immunoblotting assays and skin prick tests two main barley proteins, that could survive the malting and brewing process, were isolated and characterized as beer allergens (García-Casado *et al.*, 2001). With apparent molecular weights of 9 kDa (lipid transfer protein 1, LTP1) and 45 kDa (barley protein Z_4) these two allergens had in fact previously been identified as the major components of the proteinaceous material present in beer (Curioni *et al.*, 1995).

Besides the barley malt, beer contains other ingredients, including wheat, hops or yeast, which may cause an allergic reaction. They also have been investigated as elicitors of observed allergic symptoms.

Wheat

In 2004, the unusual case of severe anaphylaxis following the ingestion of wheat beer was reported (Herzinger *et al.*, 2004). The patient tolerated lager beer well, but experienced angioedema, generalized urticaria and unconsciousness after ingesting wheat beer. Skin prick tests were positive for wheat flour, but negative for baker's yeast, hops and a brand of lager beer. Specific IgE antibodies to wheat were found in blood serum of the patient. Immunoblot analysis revealed that patient's IgE was bound to a protein of approximately 35 kDa in wheat extract.

Hops

Pradalier *et al.* (2002) reported on a patient who presented four times with systemic urticaria, arthralgias and fever treated successfully with corticosteroids. Wild hop was finally proved to be the causal factor. Hop dermatitis in hop workers population is the most widely described clinical manifestation. Rhinitis, conjunctivitis and asthma are rare as well as contact urticaria.

Yeast

All alcoholic drinks depend on specific yeast metabolism to produce alcohol – obtaining the well-known health risk.

However, in contrast to popular believing, yeast in alcoholic beverages causing allergy is very rare. No allergenic difference has been observed between baker's yeast and brewer's yeast.

Ethanol

As little as 1 ml of pure alcohol (equivalent to 10 ml of wine or a mouthful of beer) is enough to provoke severe rashes, difficulty breathing, stomach cramps or collapse, a condition known as anaphylaxis. Given that the body constantly produces small amounts of alcohol itself, the reason that such reactions occur is poorly understood, but closely associated to gastric histamine release (Diel *et al.*, 1981). Allergy examinations using alcohol are usually negative, but sometimes positive to breakdown products of ethanol such as acetaldehyde or acetic acid. For example, a comprehensive allergological approach in a patient exhibiting hypersensitivity reactions toward beverages and medication containing alcohol led to the observation that the ethanol metabolite acetic acid yielded positive prick test results in concentrations not eliciting reactions in healthy and atopic controls (Boehncke and Gall, 1996). Finally, alcohol can sometimes act as a "co-factor," increasing the likelihood of anaphylaxis from other causes as stated initially.

In a summarizing conclusion it can be stated that different to the declaration of food additives, there is no legal requirement for beer makers to list the ingredients of their product on the can or bottle. However, beer can contain a number of ingredients other than the basic malted grain, hops, water and yeast, as, for example, health risk relevant histamine and biogenic amines.

Organic beers (bio-beer) have a growing consumer base as breweries must conform to stringent standards, anecdotally there appears to be lessened allergic reactions to this type of beer.

Summary Points

- Histamine in beer is a product of microbial metabolism. It is synthesized by decarboxylation of histidine and is mainly be metabolized by amino-oxidases and methyltransferases.
- Histamine concentration is measured fluorimetrically after HPLC separation and ranges 0.4 mg/ml in bottled beer up to 35 mg/l in beer on-draft from typical German bars.
- The sensory threshold of histamine in tap water: 2.5 ± 1.5 μM (SDM, $n = 10$).
- Other biogenic amines are also relevant and specifically associated to ingredients like malt (spermidine, putrescine, spermine, agmatine, tyramine ...) and hop (spermidine, spermine, phenylalanine, tyramine, putrescine ...).
- In a pilot study it could be shown that mechanically cleaning of the tap and the storage devices reduces histamine concentrations up to 35% and combined mechanical and chemical hygienic prevention even 93%, respectively.
- Brewing and brewery location are most important factors for the *Enterobacteriaceae*, *Lactobacillae*, *Pediococcus* and *Staphylococcus* spp. derived biogenic contaminations.
- Specific mammalian histamine responses are discussed and special focus is laid on histamine-activated GPCR, the signal transduction induced by the gastro/intestinal (H2R) and the "new" lymphocyte (H4R) histamine receptor.
- It can be suggested that beer consumption is better than wine related to the prevalence of allergic reactions. Specific "beer allergies" are very rare and only a few articles are published on this matter in the international literature.

Acknowledgments

Beer samples were received from Wiesenmühle brewery (Fulda). The authors thank Inna Michel and Cathleen Krieg for their skillful assistance. The project was supported by funds of the AVE e.V.

References

Arrang, J.M., Garbarg, N. and Schwartz, J.C. (1983). *Nature* 302, 385–390.

Ash, A.S. and Schild, H.O. (1966). *Br. J. Pharmacol.* 27, 427–439.

Bakker, R.A. and Leurs, R. (2005). In Seifert, R. and Wieland, T. (eds) *G Protein Coupled Receptors*, pp. 195–222. Wiley VCH.

Beutling, D.M. (1996a). In Beutling, D.M. (ed.), *Biogene Amine in der Ernährung*, Kapitel 6 pp. 234–247, Springer, Berlin-Heidelberg.

Beutling, D.M. (1996b). In Beutling, D.M. (ed.), *Biogene Amine in der Ernährung*, Kapitel 4 pp. 167–201, Springer, Berlin-Heidelberg.

Beutling, D.M. (1996c). In Beutling, D.M. (ed.), *Biogene Amine in der Ernährung*, Kapitel 3 pp. 59–103–201, Springer, Berlin-Heidelberg.

Bodmer, S., Imark, C. and Kneubühl, M. (1999). *Inflamm. Res.* 48, 296–300.

Boehncke, W.H. and Gall, H. (1996). *Clin. Exp. Allergy* 26, 1089–1091.

Bonadonna, P., Crivellaro, M., Dama, A., Senna, G.E., Mistrello, G. and Passalacqua, G. (1999). *J. Investig. Allergol. Clin. Immunol.* 9, 268–270.

Busch-Stockfisch, M. (2002). *Praxishandbuch Sensorik* (Grundwerk 08/02), pp. 24–32, Behrs's, Hamburg.

Curioni, A., Pressi, G., Furegon, L. and Peruffo, A. (1995). *J. Agric. Food Chem.* 43, 2620–2626.

Curioni, A., Santucci, B., Cristaudo, A., Canistraci, C., Pietravalle, M., Simonato, B. and Giannattasio, M. (1999). *Clin. Exp. Allergy* 29, 407–413.

Diel, F. (2001). *Med. Immunol.* 3, 21–25.
Diel, F. and Szabo, S. (1986). *Regul. Pept.* 13, 235–243.
Diel, F., Neidhart, B. and Opreé, W. (1981). *Int. Arch. Occup. Environ. Health* 48, 369–373.
Diel, S., Klass, K., Wittig, B. and Kleuss, C. (2006). *J. Biol. Chem.* 281, 288–294.
Fernández-Anaya, S., Crespo, J.F., Rodríguez, J.R., Daroca, P., Carmona, E., Herraez, L. and López-Rubio, A. (1999). *J. Allergy Clin. Immunol.* 103, 959–960.
Figueredo, E., Quirce, S., del Amo, A., Cuesta, J., Arrieta, I., Lahoz, C. and Sastre, J. (1999). *Allergy* 54, 630–634.
García-Casado, G., Crespo, J.F., Rodriguez, J. and Salcedo, G. (2001). *J. Allergy Clin. Immunol.* 108, 647–649.
Granerus, S., Svensson, S.E. and Wetterquist, M. (1969). *Lancet* i, 1320.
Gutgesell, C. and Fuchs, T. (1995). *Contact Dermatitis* 33, 436–437.
Herzinger, T., Kick, G., Ludolph-Hauser, D. and Przybilla, B. (2004). *Ann. Allergy Asthma Immunol.* 92, 673–675.
Hill, S.J., Ganellin, C.R., Timmerman, H., Schwartz, J.C., Shankley, N.P., Young, J.M., Schunack, W., Levi, R. and Haas, H.L. (1997). *Pharmacol. Rev.* 49, 253–278.
Horr, B., Borck, H., Thurmond, R., Grösch, C. and Diel, F. (2006). *Int. Immunopharmacol.* 6, 1577–1585.
Michel, I., Borck, H., McElligott, S., Krieg, C. and Diel, F. (2008). *Inflamm. Res.* (in press).
Izquierdo-Pulido, M.L., Mariné-Font, A. and Vidal-Carou, M.C. (1994). *J. Food Sci.* 59, 1104–1107.
Koch, J. (1986). In Koch, J. (ed.), *Handbuch der Lebensmitteltechnologie. Getränkebeurteilung 74*, pp. 377–395. Ulmer, Stuttgart.
Ling, P., Ngo, K., Nguyen, S., Thurmond, R., Edwards, J.P., Karlsson, L. and Fung-Leun, W.P. (2004). *Br. J. Pharmacol.* 142, 161–171.
Liu, C., Wilson, S.J., Kuei, C. and Lovenberg, T.W. (2001). *J. Pharmacol. Exp. Ther.* 299, 121–130.
Oda, T., Morikawa, N., Saito, Y., Masuho, Y. and Matsumoto, S. (2000). *J. Biol. Chem.* 275, 36781–36786.
Pradalier, A., Campinos, C. and Trinh, C. (2002). *Allergie et Immunolgie* 34, 330–332.
Rohn, L., Page, L., Borck, H. and Diel, F. (2005). *Inflamm. Res.* 54, 66–67.
Romero, R., Bagur, M.G., Sanchez-Vinas, M. and Gazquez, D. (2003). *Anal. Bioanal. Chem.* 376, 162–167.
Santucci, B., Cristaudo, A., Cannistraci, C., Curioni, A., Furegon, L. and Giannattasio, M. (1996). *Contact Dermatitis* 34, 368.
Schneider, E., Rolli-Dekinderen, M., Arock, M. and Dy, M. (2002). *Trends Immunol.* 23, 255–263.
Shore, P., Burkhalter, A. and Cohn, C. (1959). *J. Pharmacol. Exp. Ther.* 127, 109–114.
Van Ketel, W.G. (1980). *Contact Dermatitis* 6, 297–298.
Vidal, C. and González-Quintela, A. (1995). *Ann. Allergy Asthma Immunol.* 75, 121–124.
Vidal-Carou, M.C., Izquierdo-Pulida, M.L. and Mariné-Font, A. (1989). *J. Assoc. Anal. Chem.* 72, 412–415.
Wackes, C., Herwald, M., Borck, H., Diel, E., Page, L., Horr, B., Rohn, L. and Diel, F. (2006). *Inflamm. Res.* 55, 67–68.
Woosley, R.L. (1996). *Ann. Rev. Pharmacol. Toxicol.* 36, 233–252.
Zappavigna, R., Brambati, E. and Cerutti, E. (1974). *Riv. Vitic. Enol.* 27, 3–12.

31

Terpenoids in Beer

J. Richard Dickinson Cardiff School of Biosciences, Cardiff University, Cardiff, UK

Abstract

Terpenoids are all derived from the intermediary metabolite isopentyl pyrophosphate. Terpenoids in beer derive mainly from hops. They impart important organoleptic properties to beer. Some are metabolized by yeast during fermentation to other terpenoid compounds. Yeast's ergosterol biosynthetic pathway also comprises intermediates that can potentially serve as precursors to important terpenoids such as farnesol, geraniol and linalool. Attempts to manipulate this pathway for enhanced terpenoid production are now proving successful. One terpenoid in particular (farnesol) has attracted particular attention since it has been demonstrated to have a wide spectrum of desirable properties including: anti-tumour, antioxidative, antifungal and antibacterial effects. Farnesol has been shown to act synergistically at low levels with other compounds/cellular components in some experimental systems. For prevention of oxidative stress or carcinogenesis and tumor development, the required doses of farnesol or geraniol could never be provided by the consumption of beer. However, the farnesol obtained by beer drinking could play a very useful part in antibacterial and some antifungal therapies. A possible role for farnesol in prevention of Parkinsonism warrants further investigation.

Introduction

Terpenoids are all derived from isopentyl pyrophosphate (Figure 31.1). They occur widely in nature and include monoterpenoids (C_{10} comprised of two isopentyl units), sesquiterpenoids (C_{15} comprised of three isopentyl units), diterpenoids (C_{20} four isopentyl units), triterpenoids (C_{30} six isopentyl units), carotenoids, sterols, phytols and quinones. Monoterpenoids and sesquiterpenoids have strong sensory qualities and are highly valued for their flavors and fragrances. They are found in the essential oils of plants (Bauer *et al.*, 1990). Those terpenoids which are important in beers are shown in Figure 31.2 along with their aromas. From perusing Figure 31.2 it is clear that different isomers of a particular terpenoid can have varying

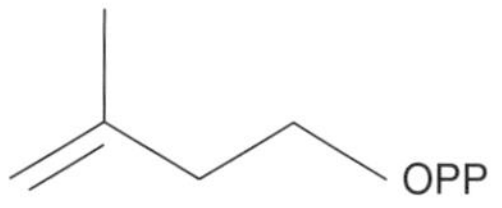

OPP

Figure 31.1 *Isopentyl pyrophosphate: the basic building block of terpenoids.* For simplicity the molecule has been drawn as a line structure in which individual carbon atoms are omitted.

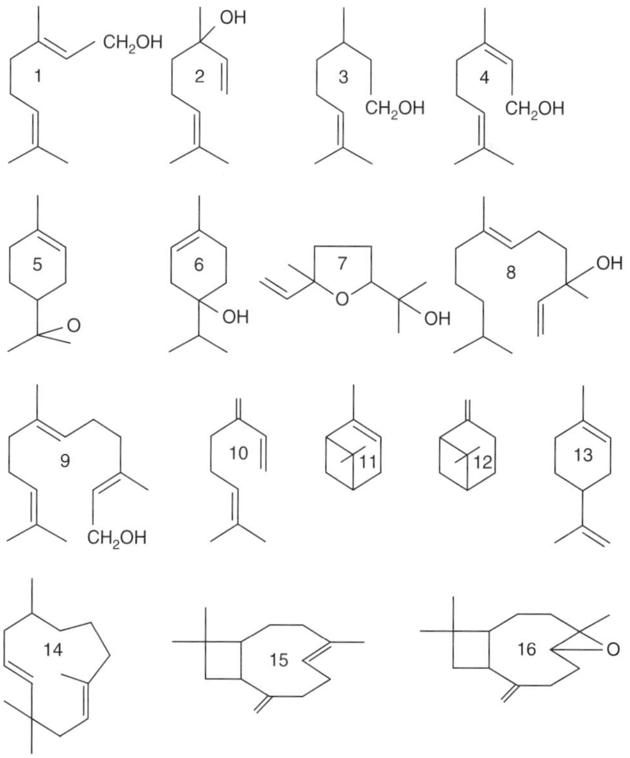

Figure 31.2 *The structures of terpenoids present in beers and their aromas.* 1: geraniol (floral, rose-like, citrus); 2: linalool (floral, fresh, coriander); 3: citronellol (sweet, rose-like, citrus); 4: nerol (floral, fresh, green); 5: α-terpineol (lilac); 6: terpinen-4-ol (spicy, medicinal); 7: linalool oxide (herbaceous, medicinal); 8: nerolidol (floral); 9: farnesol (floral); 10: β-myrcene (medicinal); 11: α-pinene (pine); 12: β-pinene (pine); 13: limonene (sweet, spicy, citrus); 14: α-humulene (medicinal); 15: β-caryophyllene (herbaceous); 16: β-caryophyllene oxide (spicy). The aromas assigned to each compound are as described by Bauer *et al.* (1990). This figure was re-drawn from King and Dickinson (2003) with permission.

Beer in Health and Disease Prevention
ISBN: 978-0-12-373891-2

aromas. For example, geraniol (structure "1" in Figure 31.2) is ascribed a rose-like "citrus" odor, whereas the *cis* isomer, nerol (structure "4"), has a fresh, "green" odor (Bauer *et al.*, 1990). The use of hops (*Humulus lupulus*) in beer making is detailed elsewhere in this volume. Suffice to say, that the essential oil of hops is extremely complex comprising over 200 constituents including terpenoids (Sharpe and Laws, 1981). It is well-known, especially among beer drinkers, that hops impart bitterness and aroma. In past times, hops were also used as preservatives of fermenting worts and finished beers. This notion is disputed by some but it should be recalled that until the advent of municipal water treatment and chlorination, beer was drunk daily by the whole population because it was safer than the water that was available. Undoubtedly, the fact that the water used in beer making was heated (in the wort-boiling step) played a part in its increased potability. However, until relatively recently in terms of the history of brewing, beers were generally brewed to a much lower alcohol content. Hence, a preservative effect is credible. It is appropriate that a twenty-first century appreciation of the health benefits of beers should appraise the contribution of terpenoids.

Terpenoids in Beers

Analysis of the levels of hop-derived terpenoids in beers is not entirely straightforward. Usually, extraction into a solvent (Cocito *et al.*, 1995) is followed by concentration and then detection and quantitation by gas chromatography – mass spectrometry (GCMS). Recently, a new extraction method known as "stir bar-sorptive extraction" (SBSE) has been developed. This is based on the partition coefficient between poly(dimethylsiloxane) and water. A magnetic stirrer bar is coated with poly(dimethylsiloxane) and immersed in the beverage for about 2 h after which it is washed, dried and thermally desorbed into a GCMS. It has been shown to be very suitable for analysis of beers with low-intensity hop aromas such as those from Japan (Kishimoto *et al.*, 2005). One fact is agreed by all: the majority of hop oil is lost during wort boiling. Consequently, (as pointed out by Sharpe and Laws, 1981) brewers have devised a number of strategies to ensure that their products have an appropriate hoppy character. These include late addition of hops to the wort-boiling kettle; restricted evaporation during wort boiling; addition of hops, hop pellets, powdered hops or hop oil at later stages (e.g. during conditioning or prior to final filtration).

The concentrations of the different terpenoids present in finished beer is not the same as in fresh wort. Several different processes occur during fermentation and maturation. The more volatile components simply evaporate. Some adsorb to the various external and internal components of yeast cells and others are metabolized by the yeast. Despite the great differences in beer types, tastes and aromas, the concentrations of many of the terpenoids in beer when actually consumed are surprisingly similar. (The reader is reminded that terpinoids are not the sole flavor and aroma compounds present.) Typical ranges are shown in Table 31.1. From the literature, linalool and α-terpineol display the greatest concentration ranges between beers. The farnesol concentration is frequently below the limit of detection.

Table 31.1 The range of concentrations of some terpenoids found in beers

Compound	*Concentration range (μg/l)*
β-Caryophyllene	0.0–0.2
Citronellol	3.0–22.1
Farnesol	0.0–0.1
Geraniol	2.2–6.1
α-Humulene	0.0–0.2
Linalool	0.0–21.9
β-Myrcene	0.0–0.5
α-Terpineol	0.0–45.0

Note: The table shows the lowest and highest concentration of each compound reported in beers from around the world over the last 40 years.

King and Dickinson (2003) showed that ale and lager yeasts transform the monoterpene alcohols geraniol and linalool during fermentation. In both cases, citronellol was the most abundant product from geraniol. Smaller amounts of linalool, nerol and α-terpineol were also formed. In addition, lager yeast also produced acetate esters of geraniol and citronellol. Linalool was metabolized into α-terpineol, geraniol and nerol. We have little knowledge of the enzymes involved in these transformations (and the genes which encode them). Such a lack of knowledge has not prevented the exploitation of yeast for regio-selective biotransformations in other areas, but the biochemical mind is left unsatisfied. However, one such enzyme activity has been identified. This is an activity which is capable of de-phosphorylating farnesyl pyrophosphate to farnesol, geranyl pyrophosphate to geraniol and geranylgeranyl pyrophosphate to geranylgeraniol (Song, 2006). The activity was assigned to yeast's Pho8p. Geranyl pyrophosphate, farnesyl pyrophosphate and geranylgeranyl pyrophosphate are all intermediates in yeast's sterol biosynthetic pathway which culminates in the end product ergosterol (Figure 31.3) and where the gene products are all well characterized.

Ergosterol is an essential membrane component in yeast and the ergosterol biosynthetic pathway has received considerable attention over the years from researchers eager to modify the pathway to allow enhanced production of specific terpenoids. The reason for wanting to do this is that most terpenoids are currently produced by chemical and/or physical extraction from plant materials or by chemical modification of another terpenoid. Using a yeast culture (with appropriately modified metabolism) to synthesize high levels of a specific terpenoid is an attractive commercial proposition. "Spent" Brewer's yeast which is available in huge quantities worldwide (which commands at best a low

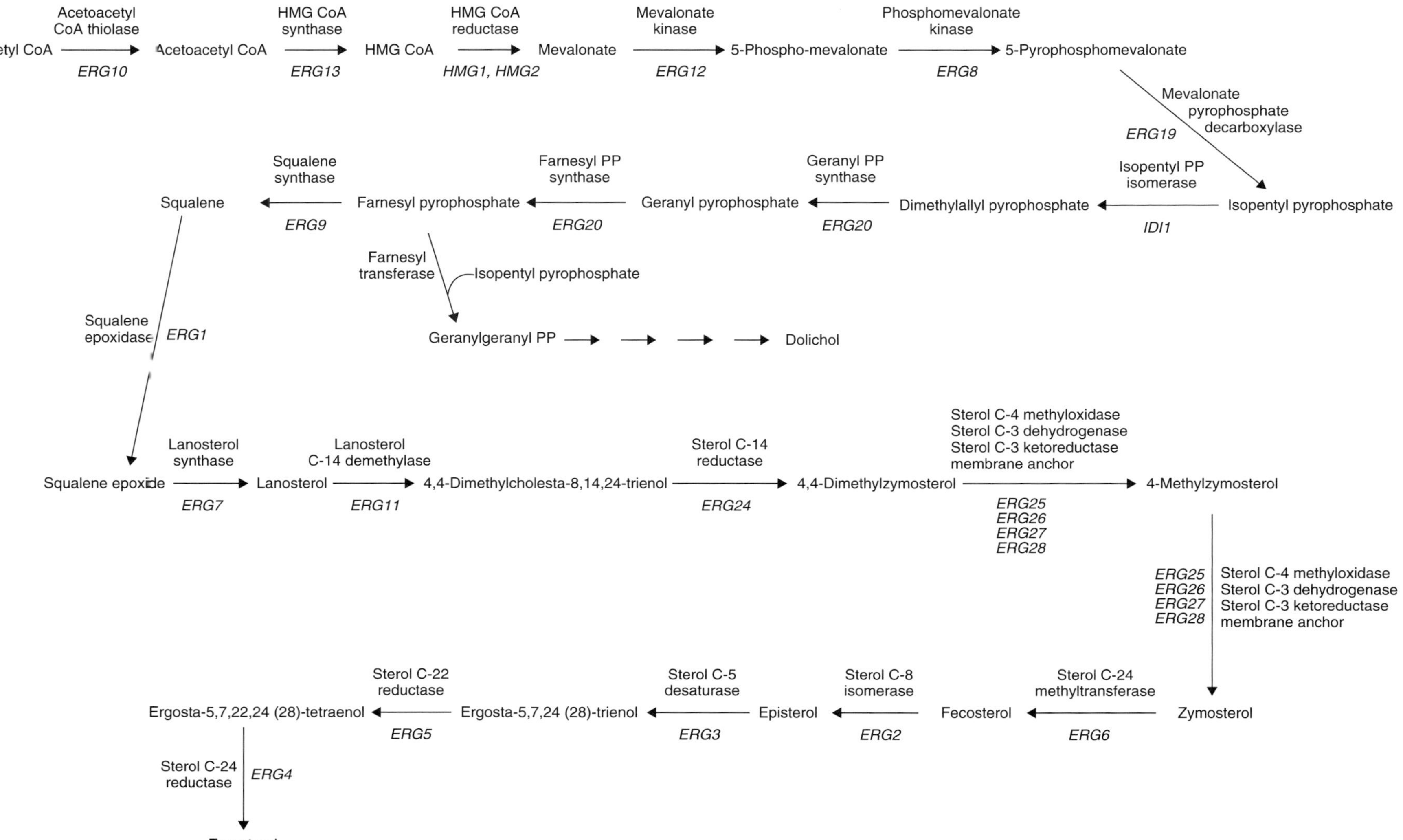

Figure 31.3 *The ergosterol biosynthetic pathway in yeast.* The diagram shows the complete biosynthetic pathway from acetyl CoA to ergosterol. The name of the third intermediate in the pathway (3-hydroxy-3-methyl-glutaryl-CoA) has been shortened to its usual abbreviation "HMG-CoA". Also shown in abbreviated form is the important branch point from farnesyl pyrophosphate via geranylgeranyl pyrophosphate to dolichol. Enzyme names are given (mainly above arrows). The genes which encode each enzyme are denoted by the approved acronym in italics (mainly below arrows).

price for use in products such as "Marmite" or animal feed, and at worst costs the brewer money for disposal) could enjoy a very profitable "second life" in terpenoid production. At present, however, given brewers' apparent universal refusal to use genetically modified strains, this seems an unlikely prospect. Nevertheless, yeast-produced terpenoids, using strains designed solely for this purpose, must arrive in the near future.

Manipulation of Metabolism

Mutants affected in the ergosterol synthesis pathway provided the first step toward the goal of yeast-produced terpenoids. For example, a mutation in the *ERG20* gene which encodes farnesyl pyrophosphate synthase results in excretion of geraniol and linalool but not farnesol (Chambon *et al.*, 1990, 1991). Some attempts to use mutants affected in the ergosterol pathway have been thwarted by its in-built regulation. The early stages are particularly tightly regulated. For example, the first enzyme, acetoacetyl CoA thiolase is subject to feedback regulation by ergosterol acting through translation (Dimster-Denk and Rine, 1996). The two isoenzymes of HMG CoA reductase (encoded by *HMG1* and *HMG2*) are differentially regulated. HMG1p is most abundant during aerobiosis whilst HMG2p is the abundant form under anaerobiosis (Bard and Downing, 1981). Hence, attempts to manipulate the pathway by either genetic or physiological conditions must take account of this situation. Both isoenzymes, but especially HMG1p, are subject to feedback inhibition by ergosterol (Kawaguchi, 1970; Casey *et al.*, 1991). HMG CoA reductase activity is also affected by fatty acid levels. In particular, palmitoleic acid positively regulates HMG1p, whilst oleic acid inhibits HMG2p (Casey *et al.*, 1992). The stabilities of these two crucial enzymes also vary: HMG1p is very stable but HMG2p is prone to rapid degradation during anaerobiosis (Hampton and Rine, 1994). It has been postulated that the two isoenzymes of HMG CoA reductase evolved to allow yeast to control metabolic flux under anaerobic conditions (Hampton *et al.*, 1996). Under aerobic growth, the majority of mevalonate will be converted to ergosterol (and its esters.) These molecules can all be accommodated safely within the yeast cell. During anaerobiosis, sterol production is not possible (because the squalene epoxidase step requires molecular oxygen). Hence ergosterol levels cannot be used to regulate the pathway. However, the yeast cell still requires several compounds that are derived from mevalonate (albeit at reduced rates). These are toxic if allowed to accumulate significantly. Thus, the ability to degrade HMG2p during anaerobiosis is important if these mevalonate-derived materials start to accumulate. It should also be noted that the activity of mevalonate kinase is inhibited by high levels of farnesyl pyrophosphate (Chambon *et al.*, 1991). All this might lead the faint-hearted to conclude that manipulation of the pathway to yield substantially greater metabolic flux into, for example, farnesol or geraniol is bound to fail because of the array of compensatory regulatory mechanisms.

The expression of heterologous (i.e. deriving from sources other than yeast) activities in yeast may be one way around the problem of complex and tight regulation of its own ergosterol pathway. A very recent study (Oswald *et al.*, 2007) described the expression of "geraniol synthase" (an enzyme converting geranyl pyrophosphate to geraniol) from *Ocimum basilicum* (sweet basil) in laboratory strains of *Saccharomyces cerevisiae* which resulted in the excretion of significant quantities (approximately 500 μg/l) of geraniol and linalool into the growth medium. These authors concluded that this shows that wild-type yeast strains contain sufficient levels of available geranyl pyrophosphate for conversion by appropriate enzymes. They contend that it is the absence (non expression?) of the enzymes, not a lack of geranyl pyrophosphate, that explains the normal lack of monoterpenoid alcohols. Oswald *et al.* (2007) also reported a further increase in geraniol synthesis when expressing the plant enzyme in yeast mutants defective in farnesyl pyrophosphate synthase. Not surprisingly, expression of the plant protein also affected yeast's ergosterol pathway. In one strain the level of ergosterol fell about 30% but in another strain (with a different genetic background) there was little change. This clearly shows that we have much more to learn about the metabolic consequences of different genetic backgrounds but it also shows there is considerable scope for further work. This could include the use of other heterologous enzymes, different genetic backgrounds and eventually, fine tuning of industrial production strains and operating processes all of which can be reasonably expected to yield further significant improvements upon the initial "proof of principle."

The Biological Effects of Terpenoids

Besides their involvement in flavors and fragrances, a huge variety of effects have been ascribed to individual terpenoids and to essential oils which contain mixtures of terpenoids and other bioactive chemicals. These include antibacterial, antifungal, insecticidal, medicinal and wound-healing effects. Much of this knowledge pre-dates modern science and medicine and forms the basis of folklore remedies and cures. Nevertheless, many modern enquiries focussing on a single pure terpenoid serve to substantiate the old knowledge. In these modern enquiries one compound is pre-eminent: farnesol. The following subsections of this chapter detail a few of the effects which have recently been ascribed to this remarkable molecule.

Antibacterial effects

The position of *Staphylococcus aureus* as a major pathogen is well-known. The general public has become aware of

"MRSA," even if unable to specify that the acronym stands for "methicillin resistant *S. aureus*." The organism causes infections of the bloodstream and forms biofilms on host tissues and indwelling medical devices (catheters, pacemakers, etc.). Its resistance to antibiotics is almost always greater when growing as a biofilm than in planktonic (freely suspended) form. Thus, it was interesting to read that farnesol has been shown to inhibit biofilm formation in both methicillin resistant and susceptible strains (Jabra-Rizk *et al.*, 2006). Although high concentrations of farnesol (150 nM) were required to reverse resistance to antimicrobial compounds, it was found to enhance the effectiveness of all of the antibiotics to which both types of organism were partly susceptible. Furthermore, farnesol acted synergistically with gentamicin and at 100 nM (22 ng/ml) reduced bacterial growth by 2 log units. These results indicate that farnesol could be used as an adjuvant (i.e. to increase the efficacy) to current antibiotics.

Antifungal effects

Candida albicans is a fungus which can exist in yeast, pseudohyphal and hyphal forms. It is a normal part of the human microflora and in most individuals causes no problem throughout life. However, there are a variety of situations in which infections by this organism can become at least troublesome and at worst deadly. These include the after-effects of antibacterial treatment in which *C. albicans* flourishes in the absence of bacterial competitors, hormonal fluctuations in women, immune suppression (e.g. as a result of HIV infection or treatment with immune suppressing drugs following a transplant) or post-operative systemic infection. It is the third most common cause of nosocomial (hospital acquired) infections. Systemic infection carries a 50% risk of death. The yeast to hyphal transition is widely believed to form a key part of the virulence of *Candida*. The yeast form facilitates dispersal and the hyphal form facilitates penetration of cells and tissues. *C. albicans* produces farnesol to regulate the yeast to hyphal transition (Ramage *et al.*, 2002) and the formation of biofilm (Hornby *et al.*, 2003). Candidiasis is currently treated with antifungal agents such as polyene antibiotics, flucocytosine and azoles. The range of antifungal drugs is clearly limited, some have undesirable side effects and/or counter-indications and resistances are emerging. *In vitro* studies have shown that farnesol not only reduced the growth of *C. albicans*, but also exerted synergistic effects with human gingival tissue (i.e. when *C. albicans*, farnesol and gingival cells were present together, there was much greater inhibition of the yeast to hyphal transition than when farnesol was applied to *Candida* alone) (Saidi *et al.*, 2006.) Farnesol concentrations as low as 10 μM were effective. The approach was not without problems, because farnesol caused some damage to gingival cells. However, as no drug treatment is without side effects, further study of the use of farnesol (possibly as an adjuvant at lower dose) is warranted.

Prevention of carcinogenesis and tumor progression

Rats fed farnesol in their diets for eight consecutive weeks subsequently showed fewer hepatocyte nodules in their livers than geraniol-fed animals compared to controls which received only corn (maize) oil. Compared to the control animals, those consuming either farnesol or geraniol also showed reduced preneoplastic lesion cell proliferation and DNA damage (Ong *et al.*, 2006). Consequently, Ong *et al.* (2006) conclude that both farnesol and geraniol are promising chemopreventative agents against hepatocarcinogenesis. The rats were fed the terpenoids at 25 mg/100 g body weight. If the same dosage were required in a human weighing 75 kg, this would require a terpenoid intake of 18.75 g. Using an upper range for the geraniol concentration in beer of 5 μg/l (see Table 31.1), this would require the consumption of 3,750,000 l of beer! Whilst the health benefits of farnesol and/or geraniol may be undeniable, it is quite obvious that intake at these levels will not come from beer (even if its terpenoid concentrations were to be raised 1,000-fold as seems feasible from the work of Oswald *et al.* (2007)).

Prevention of oxidative stress

Excess iron brings about organ dysfunction in mammals. A principle cause of this is oxidative damage to cells. When rats were given farnesol for 7 days before intoxication with iron, they were able to reverse a wide range of the biochemical processes in their kidneys (markers of oxidative damage) which usually occur. Markers of tumor progression were also reduced in a dose-dependent fashion (Jahangir *et al.*, 2006). Once again, the doses were impossibly huge if one were to attempt to supply the farnesol as beer.

Selective inhibition of monoamine oxidase B in the brain

Inhibition of monoamine oxidase B in the brain protects against the induction of Parkinsonism by a range of chemicals. Farnesol has been demonstrated to selectively inhibit monoamine oxidase B of rat brain (Khalil *et al.*, 2006). Farnesol did not inhibit human placental monoamine oxidase A nor beef liver monoamine oxidase B. Assuming that farnesol can cross the blood–brain barrier, this would indicate that low levels of farnesol may have a beneficial effect in prevention of onset of this debilitating neurological disorder.

Are the Terpenoids in Beers Good for Us?

The recent experiments detailed all point to farnesol and geraniol having beneficial effects for human health and disease prevention. However, as noted above, it is clear that for prevention of oxidative stress or carcinogenesis and tumor development, the doses required are at pharmaceutical levels and could never be provided by the daily consumption of a few glasses of beer. However, it seems reasonable to conclude that farnesol obtained by beer drinking could play a very useful part in antibacterial and some antifungal therapies because the synergism demonstrated (with other antibiotics or even tissues) requires much lower amounts of this terpenoid. The work by Saidi *et al.* (2006) found that regular doses of farnesol every 2 h was particularly effective against oral candidiasis. This would fit well with the regular taking of an antibiotic. Of course, since the medical profession's routine advice is that alcoholic drinks must not be consumed whilst on a course of antibiotics, either the advice must change when farnesol is an adjuvant or the patient must drink alcohol-free beer! With regard to farnesol's selective inhibition of rat brain monoamine oxidase B, it would be very interesting to know if this finding can be replicated in human brain. If as seems likely, it is, then a detailed evaluation of the rates of Parkinsonism amongst beer drinkers and non-beer drinkers could prove illuminating.

In the United Kingdom and elsewhere, a number of food items are required by law to contain supplements. Well-known examples include lysine in flours and vitamins A, B_6, B_{12}, D, E and folic acid in margarines and vegetable oil-based spreads. One is tempted to wonder if we ever see the time when beers are required to contain statutory levels of selected terpenoids. If this ever happens the flavor and aroma of many beers would suffer some extreme changes.

Summary Points

- Terpenoids in beer derive mainly from hops.
- They impart important organoleptic properties to beer.
- Some are metabolized by yeast during fermentation to other terpenoid compounds.
- Yeast's ergosterol biosynthetic pathway comprises intermediates that can potentially serve as precursors to important terpenoids such as farnesol, geraniol and linalool.
- One terpenoid in particular (farnesol) has attracted particular attention since it has been demonstrated to have a wide spectrum of desirable properties including: anti-tumor, anti-oxidative, antifungal and antibacterial effects.
- Farnesol has been shown to act synergistically at low levels with other compounds/cellular components in some systems.
- For prevention of oxidative stress or carcinogenesis and tumor development, the required doses of farnesol or geraniol could never be provided by the consumption of beer.
- The farnesol obtained by beer drinking could play a very useful part in antibacterial and some antifungal therapies.
- A possible role for farnesol in prevention of Parkinsonism requires further investigation.

References

Bard, M. and Downing, J.F. (1981). *J. Gen. Microbiol.* 125, 415–420.

Bauer, K., Garbe, D. and Surburg, H. (1990). *Common Fragrance and Flavor Materials: Preparation and Uses*, 2nd edn. VCH Publishers, New York.

Casey, W.M., Burgess, J.P. and Parks, L.W. (1991). *Biochim. Biophys. Acta* 1081, 279–284.

Casey, W.M., Keesler, G.A. and Parks, L.W. (1992). *J. Bacteriol.* 174, 7284–7288.

Chambon, C., Ladeveze, V., Oulmouden, A., Servouse, M. and Karst, F. (1990). *Curr. Genet.* 18, 16–41.

Chambon, C., Ladeveze, V., Servouse, M., Blanchard, L., Javelot, C., Vladescu, B. and Karst, F. (1991). *Lipids* 26, 633–636.

Cocito, C., Gaetano, G. and Delfini, C. (1995). *Food Chem.* 52, 311–320.

Dimster-Denk, D. and Rine, J. (1996). *Mol. Cell Biol.* 16, 3341–3344.

Hampton, R.Y. and Rine, J. (1994). *J. Cell Biol.* 125, 299–312.

Hampton, R., Dimster-Denk, D. and Rine, J. (1996). *Trend. Biochem. Sci.* 21, 140–145.

Hornby, J.M., Jensen, E.C. and Nickerson, K.W. (2003). *Antimicrob. Agent. Chemother.* 47, 2366–2369.

Jabra-Rizk, M.A., Meiller, T.F., James, C.E. and Shirtliff, M.E. (2006). *Antimicrob. Agent. Chemother.* 50, 1463–1469.

Jahangir, T., Khan, T.H., Prasad, L. and Sultana, S. (2006). *Hum. Exp. Toxicol.* 25, 235–242.

Kawaguchi, A. (1970). *Proc. Natl. Acad. Sci. USA* 88, 6038–6042.

Khalil, A.A., Davies, B. and Castagnoli, N. (2006). *Bioorg. Med. Chem.* 14, 3392–3398.

King, A.J. and Dickinson, J.R. (2003). *FEMS Yeast Res.* 3, 53–62.

Kishimoto, T., Wanikawa, A., Kagami, N. and Kawatsura, K. (2005). *J. Agric. Food Chem.* 53, 4701–4707.

Ong, T.P., Heidor, R., de Conti, A., Dagli, M.L.Z. and Moreno, F.S. (2006). *Carcinogenesis* 27, 1194–1203.

Oswald, M., Fischer, M., Dirninger, N. and Karst, F. (2007). *FEMS Yeast Res.* DOI: 10.1111/j.1567-1364.2006.00172.x.

Ramage, G., Saville, S.P., Wickes, B.L. and Lopez-Ribot, J.L. (2002). *Appl. Environ. Microbiol.* 68, 5459–5463.

Saidi, S., Luitaud, C. and Rouabhia, M. (2006). *Yeast* 23, 673–687.

Sharpe, F.R. and Laws, D.R.J. (1981). *J. Inst. Brew.* 87, 96–107.

Song, L.S. (2006). *App. Biochem. Biotechnol.* 128, 149–157.

32

Proanthocyanidins in Hops

Hui-Jing Li and Max L. Deinzer Department of Chemistry, Oregon State University, Corvallis, OR, USA

Abstract

Liquid chromatography–tandem mass spectrometry (LC/MS^n) coupled with various two-dimensional NMR methods are among the most practical approaches for analyzing proanthocyanidins from hops. Using these and other analytical approaches, it has been shown that hops contain a preponderance of polymeric material, including proanthocyanidins which are dominant, but small quantities of prodelphinidins and propelargonidins are also present. The flavanoids (+) catechin and proanthocyanidin B3 are the most representative followed by B1, B4 and C2. The relative proportions of the various proanthocyanidins vary greatly depending on the variety and climatic conditions as shown by differences in the proanthocyanidins in the same cultivar from different geographic regions. Proanthocyanidins have received a considerable amount of attention in the brewing industry because of their tendency to complex with proteins and contribute to non-biological haze formation, but they stabilize the organoleptic properties and color, and contribute to the astringency and bitterness, which are desirable attributes. Recent studies also show that these compounds, which are classic antioxidants, may also have significant beneficial health effects. Numerous proanthocyanidins including catechin, prodelphinidin B3, procyanidin B3 and epicatechin are present in beer.

List of Abbreviations

APCI	Atmospheric pressure chemical ionization
BFF	Benzofuran-forming fission
C	Catechin
DP	Degree of polymerization
EC	Epicatechin
(E)C	(epi)catechin
(E)GC	(epi)gallocatechin
GC	Gallocatechin
GPC	Gel permeation chromatography
HPLC	High-performance liquid chromatography
HRF	Heterocyclic ring fission
LC/ESI-MS^n	Liquid chromatography/electrospray ionization multistage tandem mass spectrometry
mDP	Mean degree of polymerization
MS	Mass spectrometry
NMR	Nuclear magnetic resonance
PAs	Proanthocyanidins
PC	Procyanidins
PD	Prodelphinidins
PP	Propelargonidins
PVPP	Polyvinylpolypyrrolidone
QM	Quinone methide fission
RDA	Retro-Diels–Alder fission
TLC	Thin layer chromatography

Introduction

Beer is the most widely consumed beverage in the world. Of all the herbs that have been used in beer, only the hop (*Humulus lupulus* L., Cannabinaceae) plant has gained widespread acceptance and is regarded as an essential raw material in the brewing industry (Moir, 2000). Hops are perennial plants grown on trellises, and different varieties are derived from breeding programs. The hop plant is dioecious and cultivated in most temperate zones of the world for its female inflorescences, which are commonly referred to as hop cones or simply hops. The female flower clusters are partly covered with lupulin glands, while male flowers have only a few glands in the crease of their anthers and on their sepals. The resin secreted by these glands contains bitter acids, essential oils and flavonoids (flavonol glycosides, prenylflavonoids and proanthocyanidins) (Stevens *et al.*, 2000). Hops or hop products account for the bitter taste and the flavor of beer. In addition, hops have a favorable influence on the stability of beer foam and contribute to the microbiological stability of beer. Different hop cultivars are traditionally classified into three groups, that is, aroma (noble) hops (e.g. cv. Saaz, Hallertau, Hersbruck, Cascade, Mt Hood), high α-bitter hops (e.g. cv. Northern Brewer, Wye Target, Nugget) and intermediate α-bitter hops (e.g. cv. Kent, Cluster, Brewers Gold). Modern brewing technology allows for the post-fermentation introduction of a variety of hops or hop preparations to adjust bitterness levels and to control formability. Brews may benefit from proper selection of particular hop

Beer in Health and Disease Prevention
ISBN: 978-0-12-373891-2

varieties that add subtle tastes and flavors. Therefore, it is important to know the nature of the hop constituents in different varieties. Among various hop constituents, hop proanthocyanidins have attracted increasing attention, and have been considered as the most reactive of hop polyphenols.

Proanthocyanidins, better known as condensed tannins, are flavan-3-ol oligomers and polymers that give anthocyanidins upon acid-mediated oxidative depolymerization reactions. Proanthocyanidins are widely distributed throughout the plant kingdom, and are present as the second most abundant class of natural phenolic compounds after lignin. There is a growing body of evidence linking these compounds with plant defense mechanisms, organoleptic characteristics and stabilizing effects of pigments in plants (Stevens *et al.*, 2002; Merghem *et al.*, 2004; Callemien *et al.*, 2005; Jerkovic *et al.*, 2005; Maatta-Riihinen *et al.*, 2005; Zhou *et al.*, 2005). Proanthocyanidins exhibit general toxicity toward fungi, yeast and bacteria. They account for astringent properties of many commonly consumed fruits and their beverage products presumably because of interactions with salivary proteins that might contribute to astringency. They also exhibit a wide range of biological activities through their action as antioxidants that lead to protection against cardiovascular disease, immune disorders and neurodegenerative diseases.

Proanthocyanidins or oligomeric proanthocyanidins, names that are often used interchangeably, consist of sequences of phenolic compounds built from single monomer units called afzelechin, epiafzelechin, catechin, epicatechin, gallocatechin and epigallocatechin (Figure 32.1). Although usage of the word "oligomeric" varies somewhat, dimers, trimers and up to heptamers are generally referred to as oligomeric ($n = 2$–7, Figure 32.1), while larger chains are referred to as polymeric or as tannins ($n = 8$–24, Figure 32.1). These flavan-3-ol monomer units are sometimes esterified with gallic acid to form 3-*O*-gallates. Proanthocyanidins can be divided into A-type and B-type proanthocyanidins. The latter are flavan-3-ol oligomers and polymers linked mainly through C4→C8 and sometimes C4→C6 bonds. When an additional ether linkage is formed between C2→O→C7, the compounds are called (C4→C8 or C4→C6) A-type proanthocyanidins. These compounds are also classified as procyanidins, propelargonidins and prodelphinidins. The proanthocyanidins consisting exclusively of (epi)catechin are designated procyanidins. Those containing (epi)afzelechin or (epi)gallocatechin subunits are named propelargonidins or prodelphinidins, respectively. These compounds are mostly heterogeneous in their constituent units and co-exist with procyanidins. Proanthocyanidin structures (Figure 32.1) vary depending on their stereochemistry and the hydroxylation pattern of the flavan-3-ol starter and extension units, the position and stereochemistry of the linkage to the lower unit, the degree of oligomerization, and the presence or absence of modifications such as esterification of the 3-hydroxyl group. The building blocks of most proanthocyanidins are the flavan-3-ols of (+)-catechin and (−)-epicatechin with 2,3-*cis*-stereochemistry of (−)-epicatechin and the 2,3-*trans*-stereochemistry of (+)-catechin.

Up to 30% of the proanthocyanidins present in beer are derived from hops; the rest are derived from the malt.

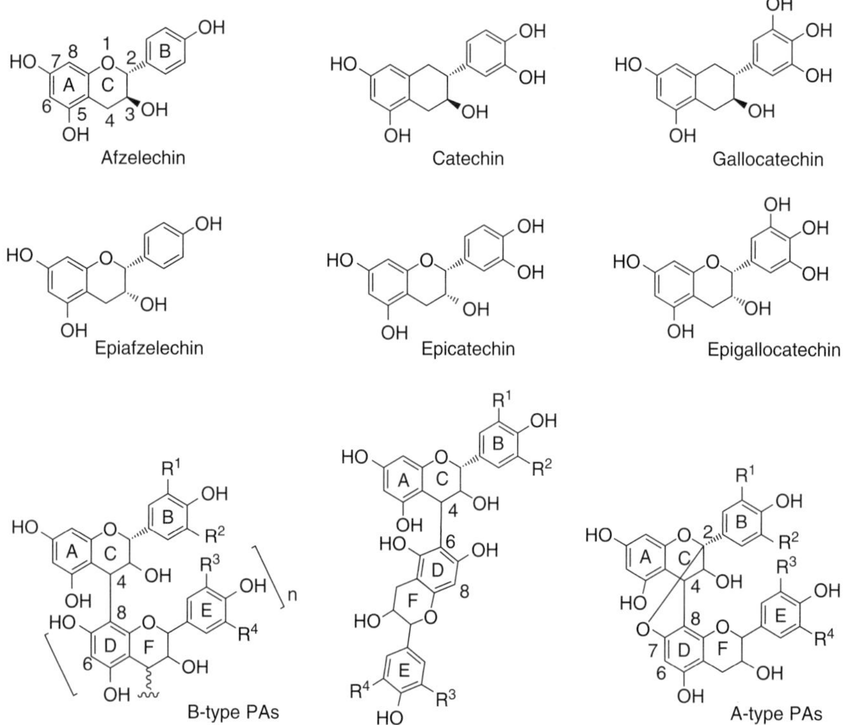

Figure 32.1 Flavanol units of proanthocyanidins (PAs) in hop cones; n: degree of polymerization; A–F: ring labels.

The estimated amount of total hop proanthocyanidins ranges from 0.5% to 5% on a dry weight basis, depending on the variety, geographic origin, freshness and harvesting procedure (Stevens *et al.*, 2002; Callemien *et al.*, 2005). The effects of hop proanthocyanidins in beer depend on their affinity for the proteins that is largely determined by their chemical structures. Therefore, knowing something about the composition and distribution of proanthocyanidins in different hops has become increasingly important. The discussion in this chapter concerns proanthocyanidin composition and their distribution in different hop varieties.

Proanthocyanidin Composition in Hops

Proanthocyanidin compounds in hop samples can be resolved at the preparative scale by a number of chromatographic procedures including such stationary phases as Sephadex G25, Sephadex LH-20 and Toyopearl TSK HW 40 (Ricardo Da Silva *et al.*, 1991; Stevens *et al.*, 2002). A reliable and efficient strategy for the isolation and purification of hop proanthocyanidins involves extraction of the hops with aqueous acetone followed by the removal of the solvent. The resulting extracts are washed with hexane to remove nonpolar material, then with dichloromethane to remove pigments, flavonoids and lipids followed by column chromatography to separate and collect proanthocyanidins and monomeric flavan-3-ols (Taylor *et al.*, 2003).

Previous investigators elucidated the structures of hop proanthocyanidins by combinations of gel permeation chromatography (GPC), high-performance liquid chromatography (HPLC), nuclear magnetic resonance (NMR), acid-catalyzed degradation and mass spectrometry (MS). The mean degree of polymerization (mDP) of crude Willamette hops (Oregon, 2000) proanthocyanidins was shown to be 7.8, with heptamers being the largest oligomers visible in the mass spectra. Seven proanthocyanidins from Saazer hops were elucidated by MS, NMR and chemical degradation, and another 10 were isolated and identified by liquid chromatography–atmospheric pressure chemical ionization tandem MS (HPLC/APCI-MS/MS), and acid-catalyzed degradation in the presence of phloroglucinol, or by partial or complete acid-catalyzed degradation and reaction with benzyl mercaptan followed by desulfurization. Finally, a systematic study was performed on Oregon-Willamette female hop varieties by electrospray ionization multistage tandem MS (ESI-MS^n) through which a total of 25 proanthocyanidins were identified. A new protocol to reliably sequence proanthocyanidin oligomers as described below emerged from these studies.

Molecular weight distribution of proanthocyanidin mixtures

Proanthocyanidins can differ in degree of polymerization (DP), subunit composition and type of linkage between subunits (Porter, 1988). As oligomer size increases, the possible number of isomers increases as well, making chromatographic resolution into pure compounds increasingly difficult. Hop proanthocyanidin mixtures were characterized by acid catalysis, GPC and by MS to give a profile of the molecular weight distribution. Although the individual fractions still were mixtures, a better picture of size distribution is revealed than could be gained from analysis of the whole hop cones.

The mass spectra are usually dominated by the monomers and lower-molecular-weight oligomers, even though chemical methods indicate that large proanthocyanidins are present in appreciable quantities. As demonstrated by Taylor *et al.* (2003), MS methods may not reflect the DP of proanthocyanidins but only the relative ease of ionization or transmission of the ions. A series of solvent mixtures (Table 32.1) was used to rinse the crude proanthocyanidin extracts, which were pooled into eight fractions. The sub-unit composition and DP of the "total" sample and the eight pooled samples were analyzed by acid catalysis in the presence of excess phloroglucinol (Table 32.2).

The proanthocyanidins in Willamette hops are a complex mixture with a large molecular weight range. Catechin is the main terminal unit, and epicatechin is the major extension unit. Prodelphinidin epigallocatechin comprises 25% of the extension unit. In chromatograms of the acid cleaved products, a minor peak (~5 mol%) was observed that is believed to be a prodelphinidin extension unit, and is likely a gallocatechin–phloroglucinol.

The average sample retention times correlate with the molecular weights of the samples. Proanthocyanidins elute later from Sephadex LH-20 because of their greater hydrodynamic volumes. In fact, a comparison of the average molecular weights of the samples determined by compositional and mDP information from acid catalysis (Table 32.2) with their respective chromatographic retention times indicates that these properties are strongly correlated ($R^2 = 0.996$).

Structure identification of individual proanthocyanidins in different hops

The major hop proanthocyanidins, catechin (Stevens *et al.*, 2002), epicatechin (Stevens *et al.*, 2002),

Table 32.1 Solvent mixtures for column chromatographic separation of proanthocyanidine extracts*

	Volume (ml)	*Acetone (vol.%)*	*Methanol (vol. %)*	*Water (vol.%)*
A	800	0	60	40
B	800	0	75	25
C	000	0	90	10
D	600	10	80	10
E	600	20	65	15
F	600	30	40	30
G	800	60	0	40

*Proanthocyanidine extracts obtained with 70% acetone from whole hops (Taylor *et al.*, 2003).

Table 32.2 Results of acid catalysis of hop proanthocyanidin pooled fractions*

Sample	*Sample weight*[a] *(g)*	*mDp by acid catalysis*	*mol% epicatechin in terminal units*	*Overall cis/trans molar ratio*[b]	*Tri-OH/di-OH molar ratio*[c]	*Mass yield of acid catalysis*[d] *(%)*
Total	1.940	7.8	12.5	3.08	0.28	60.6
1	0.042	1.8	19.7	0.80	0.06	12.0
2	0.152	2.3	18.6	0.60	0.06	41.0
3	0.193	3.8	12.9	1.39	0.13	45.6
4	0.186	5.4	12.2	2.04	0.16	61.0
5	0.226	7.6	12.0	2.89	0.21	58.9
6	0.229	10.2	12.0	3.69	0.25	61.6
7	0.242	13.4	12.1	4.50	0.30	61.7
8	0.451	22.2	11.7	6.46	0.44	64.7

[a] Recovered from column = 1.721 g or 88.7%.
[b] 2,3-*cis* to 2.3-*trans* units = (epicatechin + epigallocatechin)/(catechin).
[c] Ratio = (epigallocatechin)/(catechin + epicatechin).
[d] % = 100 × (calculated mass of all subunits)/(measured mass of sample analyzed).
*Taylor, *et al.* (2003).

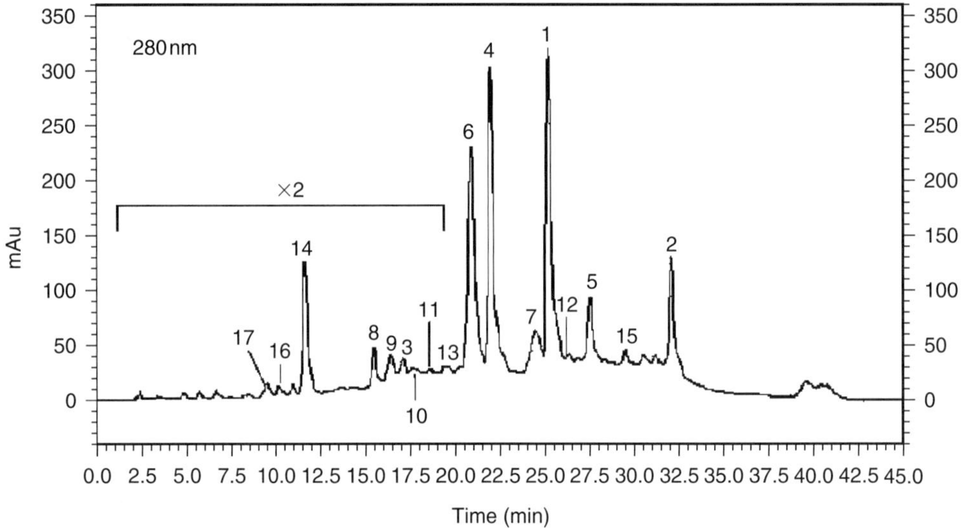

Figure 32.2 HPLC chromatogram of Oregon-Willamette hop proanthocyanidins. HPLC separations were performed on a 250 mm × 4.6 mm Synergi 4 μm Hydro-RP-80A column with a linear gradient of 5–50% methanol in 1% aqueous formic acid over a 50 min period at 0.8 ml/min. Eluting peaks were monitored at 280 nm (Li and Deinzer, 2006).

epicatechin-(4β→8)-catechin (procyanidin B1) (McMurrough, 1981), epicatechin-(4β→8)-epicatechin (procyanidin B2) (McMurrough, 1981; Moll *et al.*, 1984), catechin-(4α→8)-catechin (procyanidin B3) (McMurrough, 1981; Moll *et al.*, 1984), catechin-(4α→8)-epicatechin (procyanidin B4) (McMurrough, 1981; Moll *et al.*, 1984) and epicatechin-(4β→8)-catechin-(4α→8)-catechin (Stevens *et al.*, 2002), were identified early on by several research groups using NMR, HPLC, MS and chemical degradation. But it was difficult to elucidate the structures of minor hop proanthocyanidins by NMR because of both the low amounts available and the multiplicity and broadening associated with rotational and conformational isomerism that often complicates the interpretation of the spectra. Systematic chemical degradation coupled with HPLC and MS technologies was a strategy that helped in the identification of some minor amounts of proanthocyanidins in hops.

Structural Identification of Isolated Hop Proanthocyanidins A liquid chromatogram of a hop extract containing proanthocyanidins (Figure 32.2) shows the large difference in relative amounts of the individual constituents, but some are sufficiently resolved so that, compounds **8**, **9**, **3**, **10**, **11** and **13** could be isolated in pure form by preparative HPLC and identified by systematic chemical degradation, and analysis by HPLC/APCI-MS/MS and HPLC/ESI-MS/MS. Flavan-3-ol monomers were identified by comparison of the LC–MS spectra with authentic samples. Thus compounds **1** ($[M + H]^+$, *m/z* 291), **2** ($[M + H]^+$, *m/z* 291) and **3** ($[M + H]^+$, *m/z* 307) were identified as catechin, epicatechin and gallocatechin, respectively (Figures 32.1 and 32.2). The other 14 proanthocyanidins shown in the chromatogram could be partially characterized by their retention times, molecular ions and molecular fragments, but the confirmation of their identities was achieved by acid-catalyzed

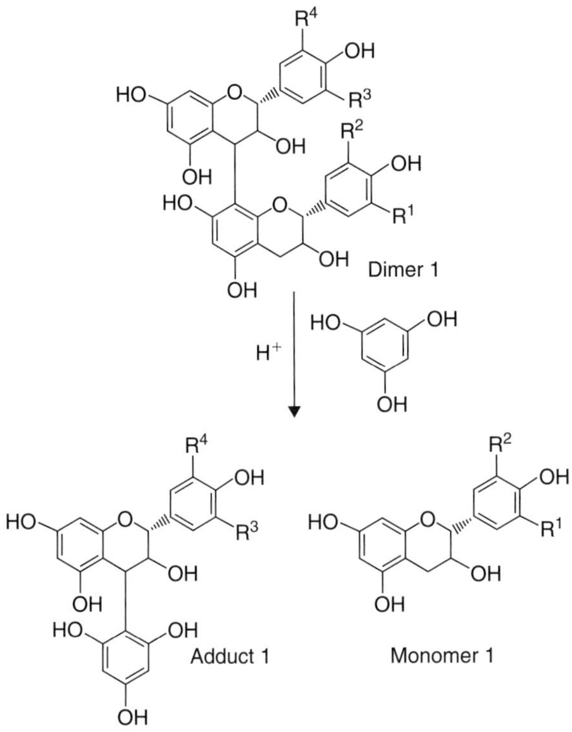

Figure 32.3 Degradation of proanthocyanidins in the presence of phloroglucinol.

degradation in the presence of phloroglucinol, or benzyl mercaptan, through which adducts with known structures were produced.

Acid-Catalyzed Degradation of Proanthocyanidins in the Presence of Phloroglucinol Interflavonoid C—C linkage bonds of hop proanthocyanidins are easy to cleave in mild acidic solution, which makes it relatively straightforward to determine the subunit compositions. Acid-catalyzed degradation with phloroglucinol present reacts to form an adduct (Kennedy *et al.*, 2001) whose identities have been established. Hop proanthocyanidin dimers (dimer 1), for example, can be degraded (Figure 32.3) to release the terminal subunits (i.e. the flavan-3-ol monomers (monomer 1) and in turn the extension subunits. The mechanism involves intermediate C4 carbocations that are trapped by phloroglucinol to generate the analyzable adducts (adduct 1). The authentic samples epicatechin-(4β→2)-phloroglucinol and epigallocatechin-(4β→2)-phloroglucinol can be obtained from grape seeds and the authentic sample of gallocatechin-(4α→2)-phloroglucinol from blackcurrant leaves (Ribes nigrum "Raven") (Foo and Porter, 1981). The authentic sample of catechin-(4α→2)-phloroglucinol can be prepared from commercial (+)-Taxifolin (Kennedy and Jones, 2001). The flavan-3-ol monomers (monomer 1) and phloroglucinol adducts (adduct 1) when compared to authentic samples by HPLC–APCI-MS/MS or HPLC–ESI-MS/MS served to identify the precursors. Phloroglucinol is a popular trapping nucleophile, but benzyl mercaptan can also be used to trap the intermediate carbocations.

To illustrate compound **8** showed a molecular ion with m/z 595 $[M + H]^+$, indicating that it was a proanthocyanidin dimer. After acid-catalyzed degradation and reaction with phloroglucinol, gallocatechin-(4α→2)-phloroglucinol and catechin were obtained, which confirmed that **8** was gallocatechin–catechin. The identity could of course be further confirmed as gallocatechin-(4α→8)-catechin by comparing the data with the authentic sample (Sun *et al.*, 1987; Goupy *et al.*, 1999). Using this procedure hop proanthocyanidin dimer structural identifications were made for **4** (epicatechin-(4β→8)-catechin, procyanidin B1), **5** (epicatechin-(4β→8)-epicatechin, procyanidin B2), **6** (catechin-(4α→8)-catechin, procyanidin B3), **7** (catechin-(4α→8)-epicatechin, procyanidin B4), **8** (gallocatechin-(4α→8)-catechin), **9** (gallocatechin-(4α→6)-catechin), **10** (catechin-(4α→8)-gallocatechin), **11** (catechin-(4α→6)-gallocatechin) and **12** (afzelechin-(4α→8)-catechin) (Figure 32.4).

Acid-Catalyzed Degradation of Hop Proanthocyanidins in the Presence of Benzyl Mercaptan Since no authentic samples of afzelechin-(4α→2)-phloroglucinol and epiafzelechin-(4β→2)-phloroglucinol were available, these prodelphinidin dimers could not be identified by acid-catalyzed adduct formation with phloroglucinol. Instead benzyl mercaptan (Kennedy *et al.*, 2000) was used to trap the acid generated carbocation. Benzyl mercaptan adducts of afzelechin-(4α→2)-benzyl sulfide adduct and epiafzelechin-(4β→2)-benzyl sulfide adduct are desulfurized by hydrogen with Raney nickel to give afzelechin and epiafzelechin, respectively, and their authentic samples can be prepared according to published procedures. Although benzyl mercaptan has an obnoxious odor, the chemical degradation with it can be an efficient method for structural elucidation of proanthocyanidins. For example, compound **12** (Figure 32.5) showed a molecular ion with m/z 563 $[M + H]^+$, indicating that it was a prodelphinidin dimer. After acid-catalyzed degradation and reaction with benzyl mercaptan, compound **12** released catechin and the benzyl mercaptan sulfide adduct of (epi)afzelechin that was desulfurized by hydrogen with Raney nickel catalyst to give afzelechin. Compound **12** was characterized as afzelechin–catechin, and was tentatively identified as afzelechin-(4α→8)-catechin by comparing the data with the authentic sample.

Partial Acid-Catalyzed Degradation of Proanthocyanidins in the Presence of Benzyl Mercaptan Proanthocyanidin trimers are best elucidated by acid-catalyzed degradation in the presence of benzyl mercaptan, which finally releases the terminal subunits, and the benzyl mercaptan adducts of the upper and central subunits (Ricardo Da Silva, 1991; Hsu, 1985; Foo, 1989). The benzyl mercaptan (sulfide) adducts can then be desulfurized by hydrogen and Raney nickel catalyst to give the upper and central subunits as monomers. Partial

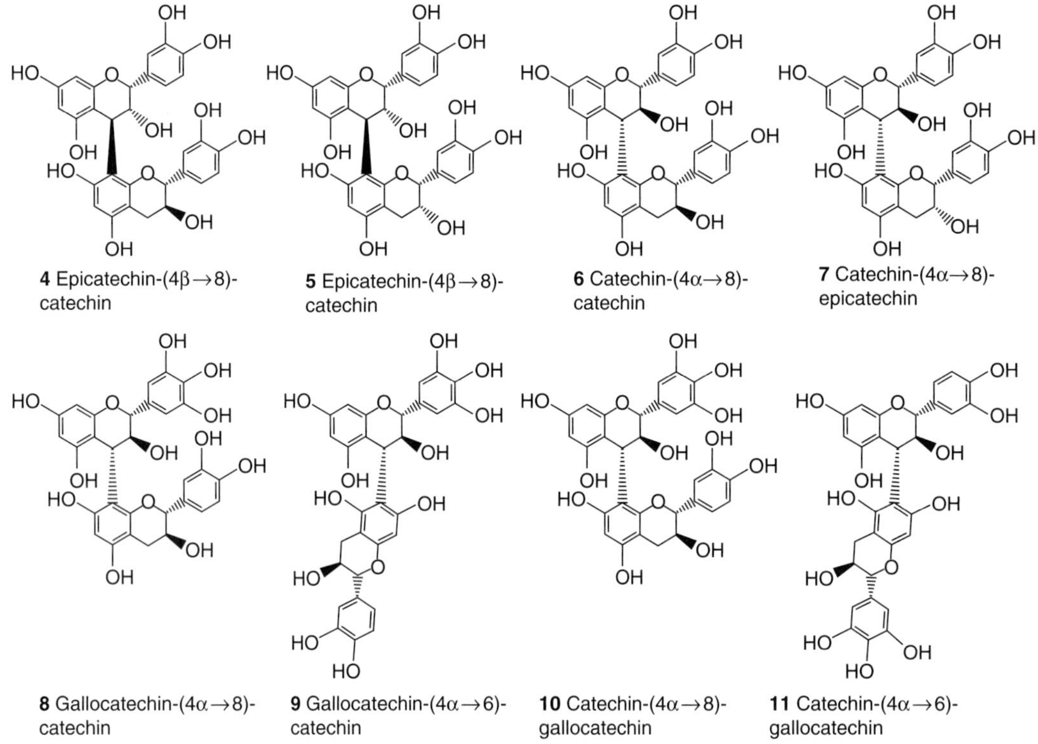

4 Epicatechin-(4β→8)-catechin

5 Epicatechin-(4β→8)-catechin

6 Catechin-(4α→8)-catechin

7 Catechin-(4α→8)-epicatechin

8 Gallocatechin-(4α→8)-catechin

9 Gallocatechin-(4α→6)-catechin

10 Catechin-(4α→8)-gallocatechin

11 Catechin-(4α→6)-gallocatechin

Figure 32.4 Structures of proanthocyanidin dimers isolated from hops.

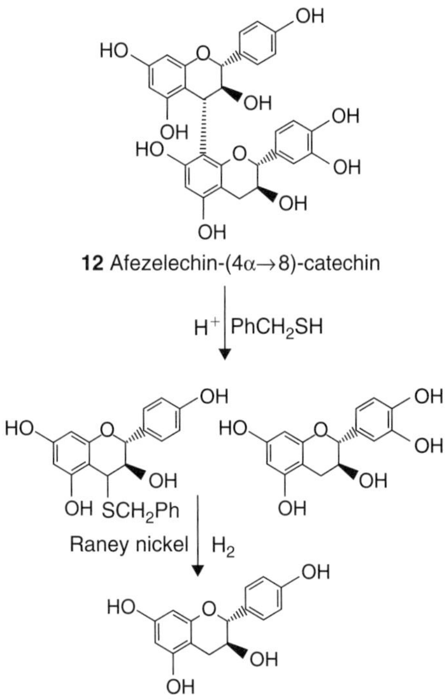

12 Afezelechin-(4α→8)-catechin

H^+ | $PhCH_2SH$

SCH_2Ph

Raney nickel | H_2

Figure 32.5 Degradation of proanthocyanidins in the presence of benzyl mercaptan followed by reduction of sulfide linkage.

acid-catalyzed degradation in the presence of benzyl mercaptan (Figure 32.6) combined with desulfurization allows for controlled chemical reactions yielding a mixture of the central-terminal subunits (dimer 1), terminal subunits (monomer 1) and the benzyl mercaptan adducts of the upper-central and upper subunits which are then analyzed. The benzyl sulfide adducts can be desulfurized to give the upper-central subunits (dimer 2) and upper subunits (monomer 2) that are analyzed. Thus, the structures of the proanthocyanidin trimers (trimer 1, Figure 32.6) are determined from the structures of the upper-central subunits (dimer 2) and central-terminal subunits (dimer 1).

The trimers in the hop extract were identified using this general procedure. Compound **13** (Figures 32.2 and 32.7) showed a molecular ion with m/z 867 $[M + H]^+$, indicat-ing that it was a proanthocyanidin trimer. After partial acid-catalyzed degradation and adduction with benzyl mercaptan, compound **13** yielded its central-terminal subunit ($[M + H]^+$, m/z 579) which identified it as catechin-(4α→8)-catechin and the benzyl mercaptan adduct of the upper-central subunit ($[M + H]^+$, m/z 701) that was desulfurized to give the corresponding upper-central subunit catechin-(4α→8)-catechin. Catechin-(4α→8)-catechin can be confirmed by co-chromatography with the authentic sample, that is, dimer **6**. Thus compound **13** was identified as catechin-(4α→8)-catechin-(4α→8)-catechin. Using the same method (Figure 32.7), the structures of **14** (epicatechin-(4β→8)-catechin-(4α→8)-catechin), **15** (epicatechin-(4β→8)-epicatechin-(4β→8)-catechin), **16** (catechin-(4α→8)-gallocatechin-(4α→8)-catechin) and **17** (gallocatechin-(4α→8)-gallocatechin-(4α→8)-catechin) were established.

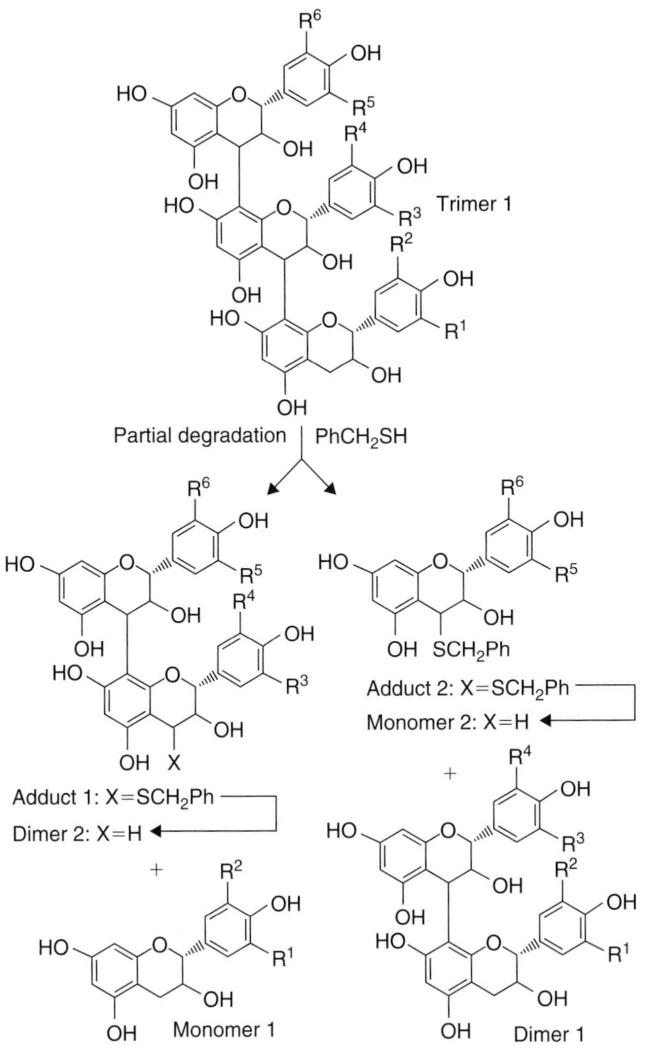

Figure 32.6 Partial degradation of proanthocyanidins in the presence of benzyl mercaptan followed by reduction of sulfide linkage.

Sequencing of Hop Proanthocyanidins by Tandem MS

A general method for establishing the presence of proanthocyanidins in malt, hops and potential beer utilized liquid chromatography-mass spectrometry (LC/MS) (Whittle *et al.*, 1999). The approach is particularly important for hop proanthocyanidins where as noted above the amounts of the individual constituents vary over a very broad range and require the capacity for rapid analysis of small amounts of sample that can be accomplished only by MS. Thus, Li and Deinzer have successfully used ESI-MS^n to reliably identify and sequence hop proanthocyanidins via a systematic analysis of their retro-Diels–Alder (RDA) fission, heterocyclic ring (HRF) fission, benzofuran-forming (BFF) fission, and (QM) fission (Li and Deinzer, 2007). Twenty-five* proanthocyanidins isolated from hops ranging from monomers to hexamers have been sequenced and identified by this approach. All of the fragmentation mechanisms were proposed based on data obtained by ESI-MS^n. These indirect analytical protocols have expanded the possible analytical approaches for sequencing proanthocyanidins in hops and other plants that contain only trace levels of these compounds.

Catechin was used as a representative compound for the off-line HPLC and ESI-MS^n studies to establish the fundamentals of the mass spectral fragmentation pathways for flavan-3-ol monomers, proanthocyanidin oligomers and polymers (Figures 32.2 and 32.8 and Scheme 32.1). Through an examination of complementary fragmentation patterns, the following five general fission rules were postulated: (Rule 1) Fragmentation of the single C-ring by HRF fission cannot undergo further RDA fission and vice versa, fragmentation of this C-ring by RDA fission cannot undergo additional HRF fission. (Rule 2) A ring fragmented by BFF fission cannot undergo HRF fission, and vice versa the product produced by HRF fission cannot fragment further by BFF fission. (Rule 3) A neutral loss of 126 Da always occurs through HRF_C fission (Rule 4) Neutral losses through RDA fissions from (epi)afzelechin, (epi)catechin and (epi)gallocatechin units are 136, 152 and 168 Da, respectively. (Rule 5) Neutral losses through BFF fission of these three compounds respectively are 106, 122 and 138 Da, and neutral losses of H_2O/BFF fission are respectively 124, 140 and 156 Da. Rules 1–5 can be applied to provide an efficient and reliable sequencing protocol for proanthocyanidin dimers, timers and oligomers.

The five rules were applied to analyze proanthocyanidin oligomers. To illustrate the process Compound **4** (Figure 32.2), a dimer, that showed a molecular ion with m/z 563 $[M + H]^+$, is used to illustrate the interpretation of the fragmentation processes. The simplest fragmentation (Figure 32.9a–c) involves a well-known QM fission. Fragment ions with m/z 273 and 291 are formed, thereby identifying the upper and terminal units (Scheme 32.2), and the compound is (epi)afzelechin–(epi)catechin. The abundance of the two characteristic ions were somewhat lower than for the other product ions. The identity, however, can be confirmed by the other general fission rules. Fission of **4** cannot proceed via RDA_C fission and then HRF_C fission (Rule 1), nor can HRF_C fission take place after RDA_C fission (Rule 1), but RDA_F/HRF_C fission can proceed. Neutral loss of a 126 Da fragment by HRF_C fission (Rule 3) following RDA_F fragmentation (Rule 4) yields the ion with m/z 285 (411 – 126 Da). The formation of this ion indicates that the one with m/z 411 (563 – 152 Da) was formed via RDA_F fission (Rule 4), from which it follows that the terminal unit of compound **4** was (epi)catechin (Rule 4). This is confirmed by further H_2O/BFF_C fission (Rule 5) and the upper unit was, therefore, (epi)afzelechin (Figure 32.9b and Scheme 32.2). The ions formed by HRF_C/RDA_F fission give the same result.

*Since the preparation of this chapter, a total of forty-four A- and B-type proanthocyanidins have been identified in hops.

Neutral loss of 126 Da (ion with *m/z* 437, Figure 32.9a and Scheme 32.2) indicating that HRF fission of the C-ring had taken place (Rule 3), hence the ion with 285 (437 – 152) was formed by RDA_F fission (Figure 32.9c), indicating that the terminal unit of compound **4** was (epi)catechin (Rule 4). In addition, a single ring fragmentation by HRF (in this case HRF_C) cannot undergo further BFF_C fission (Rule 2), but $HRF_C/BFF_F/H_2O$ fission (Figure 32.9c and Scheme 32.2)

Figure 32.7 Structures of proanthocyanidin trimers isolated from hops.

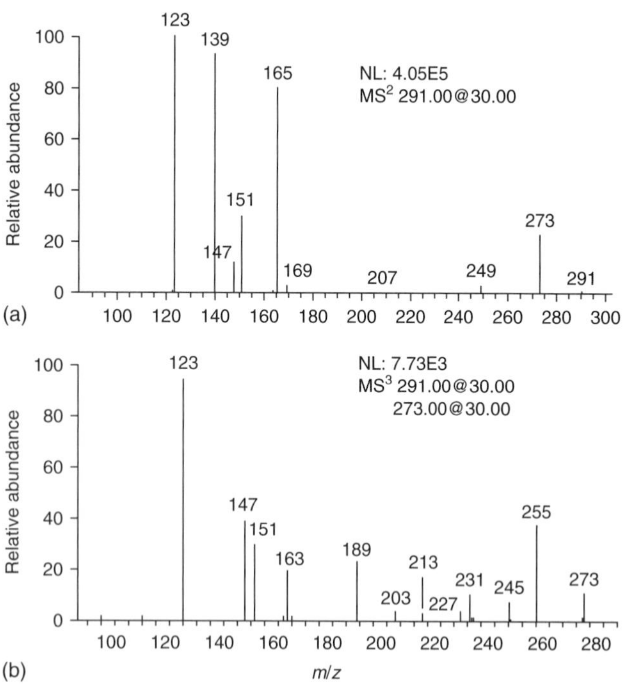

Figure 32.8 Positive ion ESI tandem mass spectra of proanthocyanidin monomer catechin (a) MS^2 of $(M + H)^+$ ion (*m/z* 291) and (b) MS^3 spectrum of ion with *m/z* 273 (Li and Deinzer, 2007).

Scheme 32.1 Fragmentation pathways of the monomer catechin: **RDA**, **HRF**, **BFF** and loss of water (H_2O).

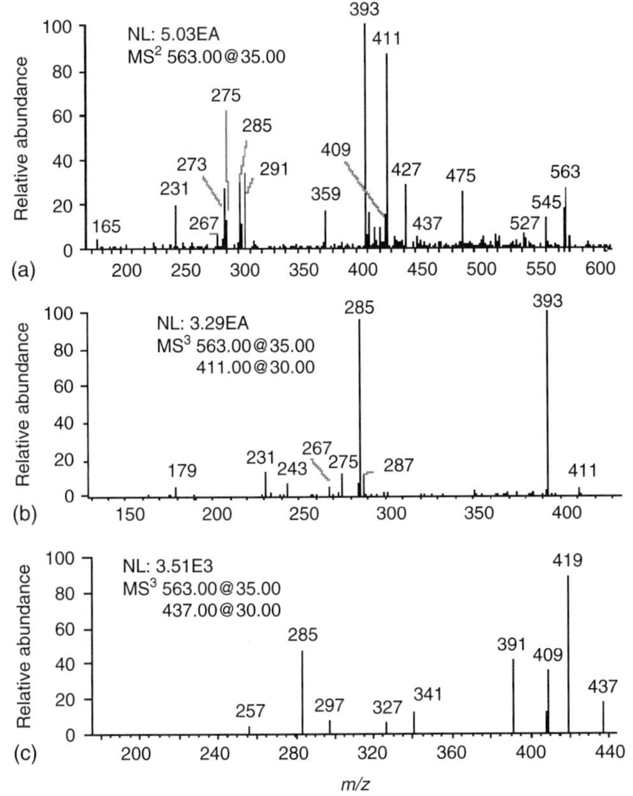

Figure 32.9 Positive ion ESI tandem mass spectra of B-type dimer **4** (a) MS^2 of $(M + H)^+$ (*m/z* 563), (b) MS^3 of *m/z* 411 ion and (c) MS^3 of *m/z* 437 ion (Li and Deinzer, 2007).

can take place to yield the ion with *m/z* 297 (437 – 140 Da) which further confirms the identity of the terminal unit of compound **4** as (epi)catechin (Rule 5). The upper unit also had to be (epi)afzelechin. Finally, the fragment ion with *m/z* 165 ($[M + H - HRF_F$ (398 Da)$]^+$) was formed from HRF_F fission and further serves to confirm that the upper unit of 4 was (epi)afzelechin.

The sequences of 7 B-type dimers (compounds **4–10**) were deduced from the product ions formed via QM fission, RDA_F/HRF_C, $HRF_C/H_2O/BFF_F$ fission and HRF_C/RDA_F fission (Table 32.3). Since the signals of the characteristic ions (low mass) of dimers **4–10** formed by QM fission generally were quite weak or not even present (Table 32.3), HRF, BFF and RDA fragmentation pathways by the indirect MS protocols played a key role in determining their sequences.

The rules for structural elucidation of flavan-3-ol monomers and proanthocyanidin dimers by ESI tandem mass spectral analysis are straightforward and logical as the dimers are generally simple and well-known structures. But the larger the oligomers the more complicated the interpretation becomes and having several different fragmentation routes available makes sequencing these compounds more secure. The rules combined with the general QM fission were used to sequence the B-type trimers **13–17**. All of the above proanthocyanidin monomers and oligomers were successfully sequenced in the mixtures from 13 different hops extracts (Li and Deinzer, 2006). In addition, eight larger proanthocyanidin tetramers, pentamers and hexamers in the extracts present

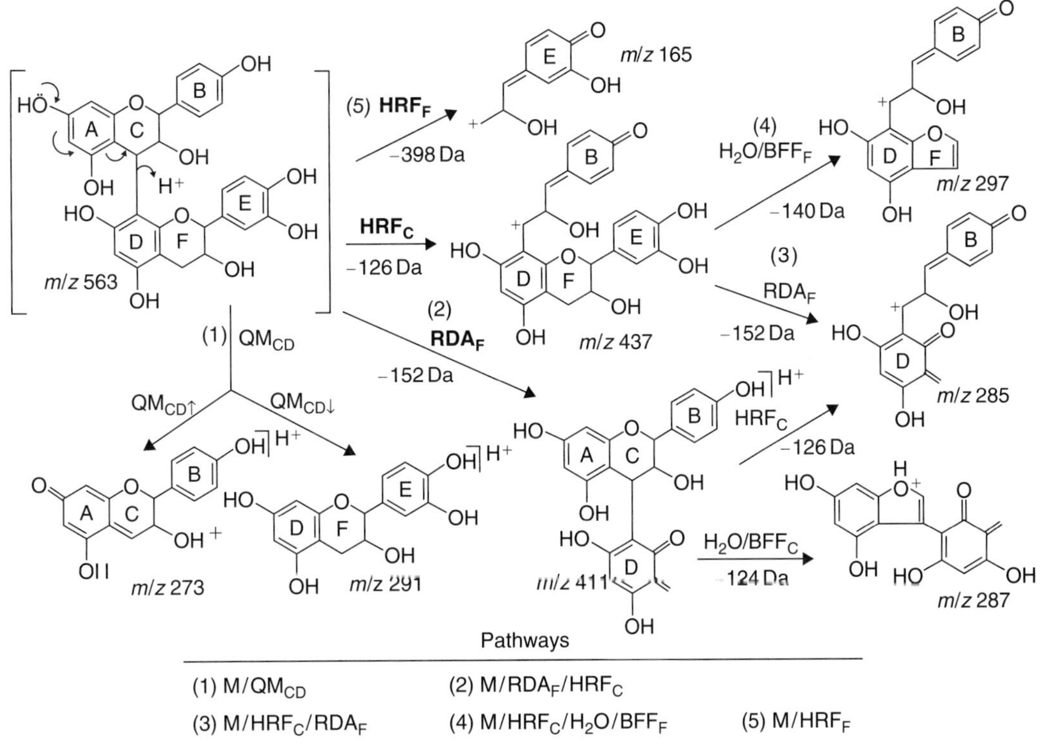

Scheme 32.2 Five characteristic fragmentation pathways of B-type dimer **4**: **RDA**, **HRF**, **BFF**, **QM** fission and loss of water molecule.

Table 32.3 Positive ion ESI tandem mass data (*m/z*), retention time (T_R) and sequences of B-type dimers 4–12

								HRF_C		RDA_F
Compound	T_R *(min)*	$[MH]^+$	$QM_{CD\uparrow}$	$QM_{CD\downarrow}$	HRF_C	RDA_C	RDA_F	RDA_F	H_2O/BFF_F	HRF_C
4 (E)C-(4,8)-(E)C	20.99	579	289	–	453(126)	427(152)	427(152)	301(152)	313(140)	301(126)
5 (E)C-(4,8)-(E)C	22.06	579	–	291	453(126)	427(152)	427(152)	301(152)	313(140)	301(126)
6 (E)C-(4,8)-(E)C	24.58	579	–	291	453(126)	427(152)	427(152)	301(152)	313(140)	301(126)
7 (E)C-(4,8)-(E)C	27.66	579	289	–	453(126)	427(152)	427(152)	301(152)	313(140)	301(126)
8 (E)GC-(4,8)-(E)C	15.55	595	305	–	469(126)	427(168)	443(152)	317(152)	329(140)	317(126)
9 (E)GC-(4,6)-(E)C	16.50	595	–	–	469(126)	427(168)	443(152)	317(152)	329(140)	317(126)
10 (E)C-(4,8)-(E)GC	17.74	595	289	307	469(126)	443(152)	427(168)	301(168)	313(156)	301(126)
11(E)C-(4,6)-(E) GC	18.74	595	289	–	469(126)	443(152)	427(168)	301(168)	313(156)	301(126)
12 (E)Afz-(4,8)-(E)C	26.48	563	273	291	437(126)	427(136)	411(152)	285(152)	297(140)	285(126)

Note: (*m/z*) was omitted. Neutral losses are shown in the parentheses. (E)Afz, (E)C and (E)GC are abbreviations for (epi)afzelechin, (epi)catechin and (epi)gallocatechin. The symbol (E) indicates there are two possibilities: "afzelechin or epiafzelechin, catechin or epicatechin, gallocatechin or epigallocatechin" (Li and Deinzer, 2007).

Table 32.4 Positive ion ESI tandem mass diagnostic ions (*m/z*) and sequences of B-type hop proanthocyanidin oligomers **18–25**

Compound	*Subunit sequences*	$[M + H^+]$	*Diagnostic ions*
18	(E)C-(E)C-(E)C-(E)C	1155	867, 865, 579
19	(E)C-(E)C-(E)GC-(E)C	1171	883, 881, 595
20	(E)C-(E)GC-(E)GC-(E)C	1187	899, 897, 595
21	(E)GC-(E)GC-(E)GC-(E)C	1203	913, 899, 595
22	(E)C-(E)C-(E)C-(E)C-(E)C	1443	1155, 1153, 867, 579
23	(E)C-(E)GC-(E)C-(E)C-(E)C	1459	1171, 1169, 867, 579
24	(E)C-(E)GC-(E)GC-(E)C-(E)C	1475	1187, 1185, 883, 579
25	(E)C-(E)C-(E)C-(E)C-(E)C-(E)C	1731	1441, 1143, 1155, 867, 579

Note: *m/z* was omitted. (E)C and (E)GC are abbreviations for (epi)catechin and (epi)gallocatechin. The symbol (E) indicates there are two possibilities: "catechin or epicatechin, gallocatechin or epigallocatechin" (Li and Deinzer, 2007).

in very small amounts were also sequenced by a systematic analysis starting with QM fission (Table 32.4). Generally however, other diagnostic ions were required either for confirmatory evidence or because QM fission products were not observable in the spectra. The diagnostic ions arising from the other fragmentation pathways always yielded sufficient information to allow sequencing and structural elucidation of the oligomers.

A survey of 13 samples of German and US hop varieties was conducted by isolating individual proanthocyanidins via HPLC, followed by acid degradation and analysis of the acid hydrolysates by ESI-MS (Li and Deinzer, 2006). The chromatograms for the varieties analyzed were qualitatively very similar, that is, peaks were seen at similar retention times for the largest peaks thereby allowing the identification of the largest peaks by comparison with authentic samples. Furthermore, 25 proanthocyanidins were present in all 13 hops, which included Willamette hop cones (Oregon, Idaho, and Washington, USA), Vanguard pellet (USA), Palisade pellet (USA), Tettnang-Hallertauer pellet (Germany), Hallertauer-Hallertauer pellet (Germany), North American Hallertauer pellet (USA), Zeus pellet (USA), Cascade pellet (USA), Saaz 36 pellet (USA), Saaz 72 pellet (USA) and Glacier pellet (USA).

In summary, the structures of hop proanthocyanidins can be elucidated by combinations of GPC, HPLC, NMR, acid-catalyzed degradation and MS. Gas chromatographic analysis generally gives a better representation of the size distribution but for elucidating proanthocyanidins, individual fractions are best analyzed by LC-MS. NMR resonance can be useful for structure analysis, but signal multiplicities, broadening associated with rotational and conformational isomerism and low sample amounts often complicate the interpretations. Acid-catalyzed degradation in the presence of a nuclophile with which the intermediate can react can be very useful for identifying proanthocyanidins provided a sufficient amount of sample is available. Tandem mass spectrometry coupled with liquid chromatography (LC/MS^2) is a new and very powerful method for sequencing proanthocyanidin oligomers because of its capacity for reliably analyzing small sample amounts. Once the sequences are known, NMR spectroscopy can be used to determine the relative stereochemistry of the 2,3-positions (2,3-*cis* vs. 2,3-*trans*) and 3,4-positions (3,4-*cis* vs. 3,4-*trans*) on the C-ring, F-ring and I-ring, as well as to establish the proanthocyanidin interflavan linkages (4→6 vs. 4→8). Thus, LC/MS^2 coupled with various two-dimensional NMR methods are among the most practical approaches for analyzing proanthocyanidins not only from hops, but from any natural product.

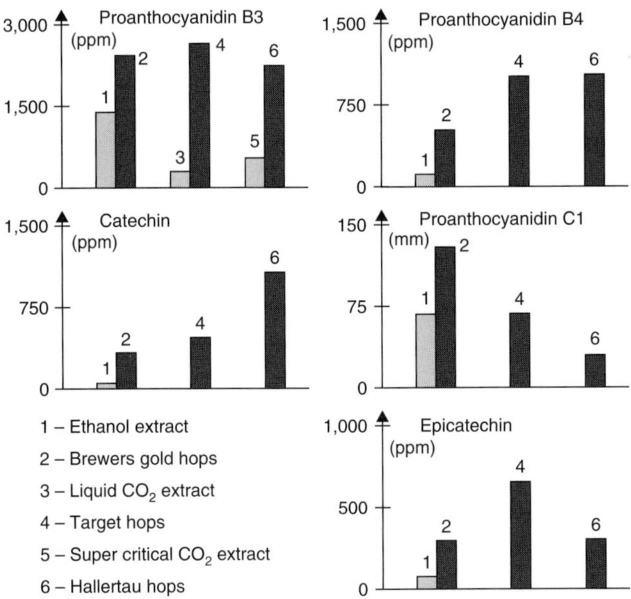

Figure 32.10 Concentrations of polyphenols in hops and hop products (Mollet *et al.*, 1984).

Table 32.5 Flavanoids in hops (mg/g)

Varieties	*(+)-Catechin (mg/g)*	*Procyanidin B3 (mg/g)*	*Procyanidin C2 (mg/g)*
Alsace record	0.8	0.4	0.3
Hallertau	1.1	0.6	0.4
Saaz	2.8	1.5	0.9
Tettnang	1.5	0.8	0.5

Note: mg/g stand for individual proanthocyanidin per gram of hop cone weight (Jerumanis, 1985).

Proanthocyanidin Content of Hops and Beer

The composition of low molecular proanthocyanidins in different hop varieties

McMurrough (1981) reported that hops contained a preponderance of polymeric material. In Challenger hops the relative amounts of the dimers B1, B2, B3 and B4 present were 3:0.5:10:5. Cyanidin and delphinidin were also detected in whole hops with ratios that varied widely, as, for example, 1.2 in Northern Brewer and 6.2 in Talisman. Five flavanols, tentatively identified as trimers, were resolved by HPLC and measured but collectively they amounted to only 0.07 mg/g in hops. The B-series procyanidin dimers amounted to 0.17 mg/g in hops. Whereas the contents of (−)-epicatechin and (+)-catechin were 0.19 and 0.26 mg/g, respectively, in Challenger hops.

Moll *et al.* (1984) reported the identification and concentrations of certain phenolic substances including prodelphinidin, proanthocyanidins B3 and B4, catechin and epicatechin in hops, hop extracts, pellets and finished beer (Figure 32.10). These studies showed that (i) extracts of hops made using liquid or supercritical carbon dioxide contain only proanthocyanidin B3 in low concentration; (ii) hop extracts made with ethanol contain all the known polyphenols, but in view of the small amounts of extracts used when hopping, the quantity of polyphenols introduced into the beer is negligible; (iii) cone hops and pellets contain higher concentrations of proanthocyanidin B3, B4, catechin, epicatechin and the trimer C1; (iv) The relative proportions of the various proanthocyanidins vary greatly depending on the hop variety.

Jerumanis (1985) described an HPLC method for the quantitative analysis of flavanoids in hops. The flavanoids (+) catechin and proanthocyanidin B3 were the most representative followed by procyanidin C2 (Table 32.5). The values found for these three major components in Saaz hops totaled about 5 mg/g.

Forster *et al.* (2002) have undertaken a comparison study of 11 hop varieties harvested in 1997 and 1998 in an effort to determine whether the relative amounts of certain components can be used to identify the hop variety. Some clear differences were evident, but it appears not to be possible to make a variety of identification by means of any single indicator substance such as the level of proanthocyanidin. The relative amounts of several constituents have to be considered. Low-molecular-weight polyphenols may help to differentiate hop varieties. Additionally, the influence of the growing region has been investigated by studying two hop samples of a single variety from the United States and the Hallertau region in Germany. Clear differences were found in the composition of proanthocyanidins between the two growing regions. Generally, the Hallertauer hops showed higher contents of catechin, and procyanidins, B1, B2 and B3 in both Perle and Nugget hops (Table 32.6). The considerable climatic differences between the two regions apparently have a significant influence on proanthocyanidin content in hops.

Li and Deinzer (2006) also studied the relative amounts of individual proanthocyanidins discussed above in 13 different hop varieties to determine whether the composition of proanthocyanidin oligomers had any value in hop variety identification. The mole percent (mol%) composition of proanthocyanidins was based on a comparison of peak integrations at 280 nm. The detector response of proanthocyanidin dimers and trimers was estimated using molar absorption coefficients relative to the monomers. Molar absorptivities of three representative compounds were: monomer (catechin, ε_{280}: 3975); dimer (procyanidin B1, ε_{280}: 6725) and trimer (epicatechin-(4β→8)-epicatechin-(4β→8)-catechin, ε_{280}: 11,360), giving a relative molar response ratio of monomers:dimers:trimers of 1:1.69:2.86. The same 17 hop proanthocyanidin oligomers (Table 32.7) were found in all varieties consisting mostly of three flavan-3-ol monomers, nine proanthocyanidin dimers and five proanthocyanidin

Table 32.6 Proanthocyanidins in Nugget and Perle hops (mg/g)

		1996		*1997*		*1998*	
Compound	*Variety*	*Hallertau*	*USA*	*Hallertau*	*USA*	*Hallertau*	*USA*
Catechin	Nugget	0.73–0.92	0.46–0.53	0.72–0.84	0.54–0.63	0.60–0.81	0.51–0.68
	Perle	0.65–0.78	0.57–0.71	0.82–0.94	0.56–0.80	0.97–0.12	0.40–0.82
Procyanidin B1	Nugget	0.55–0.71	0.32–0.41	0.46–0.55	0.33–0.41	0.32–0.40	0.27–0.34
	Perle	0.45–0.54	0.41–0.54	0.49–0.56	0.32–0.48	0.45–0.55	0.23–0.40
Procyanidin B2	Nugget	0.66–0.76	0.30–0.38	0.48–0.58	0.31–0.40	0.42–0.58	0.27–0.38
Procyanidin B3	Nugget	0.62–0.75	0.33–0.39	0.45–0.50	0.26–0.31	0.29–0.36	0.18–0.23
	Perle	0.64–0.70	0.46–0.53	0.51–0.58	0.40–0.48	0.41–0.50	0.19–0.30

Note: mg/g stand for individual proanthocyanidin per gram of hop cone weight (Forester *et al*., 2002).

Table 32.7 Proanthocyanidin profiles of the 13 different hops

	$1^{\#}$													
Compound	$1a^{\#}$	$1b^{\#}$	$1c^{\#}$	$2^{\#}$	$3^{\#}$	$4^{\#}$	$5^{\#}$	$6^{\#}$	$7^{\#}$	$8^{\#}$	$9^{\#}$	$10^{\#}$	$11^{\#}$	*Average*
1	21.7	16.5	7.7	12.8	14.7	29.5	11.4	17.4	13.2	23.6	32.1	17.7	9.8	17.6
2	20.8	22.7	8.7	12.0	18.3	19.0	17.5	13.8	14.5	12.8	5.5	10.4	15.3	14.7
3	2.5	1.7	3.2	1.6	1.2	1.9	1.8	2.2	2.9	2.2	2.0	4.2	2.2	2.3
4	12.2	13.51	20.7	18.3	14.2	12.0	11.5	10.7	20.0	12.0	19.5	11.3	16.1	14.8
5	8.2	12.0	13.1	5.4	8.7	6.3	4.0	2.2	5.3	7.7	6.6	5.7	8.0	7.2
6	12.8	11.3	18.9	24.7	14.8	6.5	22.7	19.8	15.2	14.9	11.7	4.7	20.2	15.2
7	5.4	6.1	10.0	12.1	18.0	6.0	15.2	20.7	6.8	11.3	4.8	23.4	20.3	12.3
8	1.7	1.2	0.9	1.0	1.3	4.4	1.8	2.1	2.6	1.7	4.5	2.2	1.1	2.0
9	2.2	1.9	3.0	1.0	0.9	2.4	2.7	2.0	4.0	1.7	1.4	2.8	1.0	2.1
10	2.1	1.8	1.0	0.8	0.4	0.7	1.3	1.7	2.3	0.9	0.8	1.9	0.5	1.2
11	2.1	0.9	2.5	1.5	0.2	1.0	1.7	3.0	2.1	0.9	1.2	7.5	0.3	1.9
12	2.1	4.4	4.3	3.7	0.6	3.1	2.5	0.8	0.7	1.0	2.3	0.7	0.6	2.1
13	1.2	0.9	1.6	0.8	0.7	1.1	1.4	1.7	1.9	1.5	1.8	2.8	1.0	1.4
14	2.3	2.6	1.2	0.9	2.2	2.5	0.5	0.4	2.1	2.7	1.4	1.3	0.6	1.6
15	2.2	1.9	2.6	3.1	3.7	3.2	3.7	1.0	5.9	4.8	3.8	3.0	3.0	3.2
16	0.3	0.2	0.3	0.1	0.1	0.2	0.1	0.1	0.3	0.3	0.2	0.1	0.04	0.2
17	0.4	0.2	0.4	0.02	0.1	0.2	0.2	0.2	0.2	0.2	0.1	0.1	0.04	0.2

Note: Abundance (mol%) of the total hops proanthocyanidins determined by HPLC (Procedure 1) at 280nm, mol% is based on oligomeric proanthocyanidin mixtures. **1**$^{\#}$ (Willamette) [**1a**$^{\#}$ (Oregon-Willamette), **1b**$^{\#}$ (Idaho-Willamette) and **1c**$^{\#}$ (Washington-Willamette)], **2**$^{\#}$ (Vanguard), **3**$^{\#}$ (Palisade), **4**$^{\#}$ (Tettnang-Hallertauer), **5**$^{\#}$ (Hallertauer-Hallertauer), **6**$^{\#}$ (Zeus), **7**$^{\#}$ (Idaho-Hallertauer), **8**$^{\#}$ (Cascade), **9**$^{\#}$ (Saaz 36), **10**$^{\#}$ (Saaz 72) and **11**$^{\#}$ (Glacier) (Li and Deinzer, 2006).

trimers, but the concentrations of these individual compounds were significantly different (Figure 32.2).

On average the flavan-3-ol monomers, catechin (**1**, 17.6%), epicatechin (**2**, 14.7%), procyanidin B1 (**4**, 14.8%), procyanidin B2 (**5**, 7.2%), procyanidin B3 (**6**, 15.2%) and procyanidin B4 (**7**, 12.3%) together with the newly identified procyanidin trimer epicatechin-(4β→8)-epicatechin-(4β→8)-catechin (**15**, 3.2%) were the major proanthocyanidins present, with the other 10 proanthocyanidin oligomers amounting to a total of 15.0% (Table 32.7). On the whole, proanthocyanidins (87.5%) were dominant in all samples, but small quantities of prodelphinidins (9.8%) and propelargonidin (2.7%) were also present (Table 32.7).

Saaz 36 and Tettnang-Hallertauer hops had the highest content of catechin, that is, 32.1% and 29.5%, respectively, but the Washington-Willamette and Glacier hop proanthocyanidin oligomers showed exactly the opposite, as the levels were 7.7% and 9.8%, respectively (Table 32.7). With regard to proanthocyanidin dimers, procyanidin B3 (**6**, 15.2%) and procyanidin B1 (**4**, 14.8%) were dominant, followed by procyanidin B4 (**7**, 12.3%) and procyanidin B2 (**5**, 7.2%). The procyanidin B3 content in Vanguard, Hallertauer-Hallertauer and Glacier hop proanthocyanidin oligomers was 24.7%, 22.7% and 20.2%, respectively, but Saaz 72 hop proanthocyanidin oligomers contained only 4.7% procyanidin B3 (Table 32.7). Prodelphinidin dimers (compounds **8**–**11**) and the propelargonidin dimer (afzelechin-(4α→8)-catechin, **12**) were generally present in hop proanthocyanidin oligomers. Tettnanger-Hallertauer and Saaz 36 hop proanthocyanidin oligomers contained gallocatechin-(4α→8)-catechin (**8**) at 4.4% and 4.5%, respectively. Saaz 72 hop proanthocyanidin oligomers contained 7.5% catechin-(4α→6)-gallocatechin (**11**), and the compound **12** content in Idaho-Willamette and Washington-Willamette hop proanthocyanidin oligomers

Table 32.8 Determination of proanthocyanidin content of a number of hop cultivars

Cultivar	*Proanthocyanidins (mg/g)*
Yeoman	12
Target	39
Northern brewer	31
Fuggle	29
Saaz	51

Note: mg/g stand for the whole proanthocyanidins per gram of hop cone weight (Neve, 1992).

was 4.4% and 4.3%, respectively (Table 32.7). Proanthocyanidin trimers included epicatechin-(4β→8)-epicatechin-(4β→8)-catechin (**15**, 3.2%), C2 (**13**, 1.4%) and epicatechin-(4β→8)-catechin-(4α→8)-catechin (**14**, 1.6%). Idaho-Hallertauer and Cascade hop proanthocyanidin oligomers contained compound **15** at 5.9% and 4.8% levels, respectively, but Zeus hop proanthocyanidin oligomers contained only 1.0%. Catechin-(4α→8)-gallocatechin-(4α→8)-catechin (**16**, 0.2%) and gallocatechin-(4α→8)-gallocatechin-(4α→8)-catechin (**17**, 0.2%) were very limited in hop proanthocyanidin oligomers (Table 32.7).

Differences in relative amounts of compounds **1**, **5** and **7** in Saaz 36 and Saaz 72 hop proanthocyanidin oligomers (Table 32.7) were also observed. The two hops were supposedly genetically identical, and they were grown in the same location in Idaho. These clones were established many years apart, and it had been observed that clone selections from varieties established long ago in a given locality might be different. Anecdotally, they were reported to have different brewing characteristics as well. Willamette hops (Oregon, Idaho and Washington) and Hallertauer hops (Germany-Tettnang, Germany-Hallertauer and Idaho) were selected to study the effect of geographic origin on their proanthocyanidin profiles (Table 32.7). Most hop constituents were found to be affected by geographic origin. For example, the relative percentage of compound **1** in Willamette hop proanthocyanidin oligomers, from Oregon, Idaho and Washington, was 21.7%, 16.5%, and 7.7%, respectively (Table 32.7). The relative percentages of compound **6** in Hallertauer hop proanthocyanidin oligomers from Tettnang (Germany, 2004), Hallertauer (Germany, 2004) and Idaho (2004) were 6.5%, 22.7% and 15.2%, respectively (Table 32.7). As in the previous studies by Forester *et al.* (2002), these results indicate that the proanthocyanidin profiles of hops are affected by geographic origin.

Recent barley breeding work by Carlsberg has resulted in the development of cultivars that are free of proanthocyanidins. Brewing with malt from these barleys produces beers with a considerably longer shelf life and if this type of malt were used exclusively, the proanthocyanidin content and hop variety used would likely have a significant impact on beer flavor and overall quality. Determinations of the amounts proanthocyanidins in various hop cultivars made by the Carlsberg brewery (Neve, 1992) showed significant differences (Table 32.8).

In conclusion hops contained a preponderance of polymeric material. The relative proportions of the various proanthocyanidins vary greatly depending on the hop variety. Climatic differences between the different regions apparently have a significant impact on proanthocyanidin content. On the whole, proanthocyanidins were dominant in hops, but small quantities of prodelphinidins and propelargonidin were also present. The flavanoids (+) catechin and proanthocyanidin B3 were the most representative followed B1, B4 and C2.

Proanthocyanidins in beer

Beers are known to contain a wide variety of polyphenols, which originate from the brewing raw materials, that is, barley and hops (Madigan *et al.*, 1994). Polyphenols can protect food such as fats from being spoiled by oxygen which otherwise would affect the taste. They are also active in trapping free radicals in the human body thus exerting an anticarcinogenic effect. Beers contain complex mixtures of polyphenols ranging from 150 to 330 mg/L. The most reactive of the polyphenols are the proanthocyanidins. It is estimated that about 70–80% of the proanthocyanidins in beer are derived from barley, and about 20–30% originate from the hops. The proanthocyanidins from hops are structurally very similar to those found in barley, the main difference being the higher proportion of gallocatechin units in the oligomers derived from barley.

It is generally agreed that polyphenols and more particularly proanthocyanidins are major contributors to the formation of non-biological haze in beer. The haze formed on storage of beer has been shown to consist of polyphenols and proteinaceous material. The protein–polyphenol complexes that are formed are insoluble in beer thus causing beer to appear cloudy. The formation of non-biological hazes in beer can be reduced by the addition of silica gel to reduce the protein content, or polyvinylpolypyrrolidone (PVPP) to reduce the polyphenols during filtration. The use of specially cultivated varieties of barley free of proanthocyanidins such as Caminant or pure-resin hop extracts that are free of polyphenols reduces or eliminates haze formation, but the reduction of proanthocyanidins can affect the final flavor of beer.

Numerous studies have shown that proanthocyanidins are present in beer. Thus, Eastmond (1974) found catechin and procyanidin B3 (catechin-(4α→8)-catechin) in beer by chromatographic methods. Dadic and Belleau (1976) reported procyanidin B3 and procyanidin B4 (catechin-(4α→8)-epicatechin) in beer and confirmed their presence by ^{1}H NMR experiments. Vancraenenbroeck *et al.* (1977) found procyanidin B1 (epicatechin-(4β→8)-catechin), procyanidin B2 (epicatechin-(4β→8)-epicatechin), procyanidin B3 and procyanidin B4, and Jerumanis (1979) found procyanidin B2 and procyanidin B4 in beer by chromatographic means. Kirby and Wheeler (1980) found certain beers contain procyanidin B3 and prodelphinidin B3 (gallocatechin-(4α→8)-catechin) by chromatographic means. Jan and Geert (1984) found procyanidin B3, prodelphinidin B3 and prodelphinidin B9 (epigallocatechin-(4β→8)-catechin) in Pilsner beers by ^{1}H NMR, MS and circular dichroism of their methyl ether diacetates.

Using direct-injection HPLC with electrochemical detection, McMurrough *et al.* (1992) found that lager beers contain catechin, procyanidin B3 and prodelphinidin B3. McMurrough and Baert (1994) developed a method for the measurement of simple flavanols in beer by direct-injection HPLC using dual-electrode electrochemical detection. These investigators used this method successfully to measure small amounts of monomeric and dimeric flavanols in commercial beer. The method offered greatly improved sensitivity and selectivity compared to the ultraviolet detection method used previously. In addition to catechin, epicatechin, prodelphinidin B3 and procyanidin B3, small amounts of three trimer proanthocyanidins T1, T2, T3 and T4 (B4) were also tentatively identified in a typical lager beer. Treatment with PVPP markedly decreased the amounts of total polyphenols and individual PAs in lagered beer, but no decrease in epicatechin was evident (Table 32.9).

Madigan *et al.* (1994) developed an HPLC method using dual-channel electrochemical detection for the determination of proanthocyanidins, and found catechin, epicatechin, prodelphinidin B3 and procyanidin B3 in lager beers. The beer that was taken from the storage vessel (unstabilized) and from cans (stabilized) showed marked differences in flavanol content (Table 32.10). The treatment of beer with PVPP results in a near total reduction in the amount of dimers present, and a significant reduction in monomer content.

Using HPLC/ESI-MS and HPLC/EI-MS to analyze proanthocyanidins in beer, Nigel *et al.* (1999) found proanthocyanidins including catechin, epicatechin, (epi)gallocatechin, (epi)catechin-(epi)catechin, (epi)catechin-(epi)gallocatechin, (epi)gallocatechin-(epi)catechin, (epi)

Table 32.9 Polyphenol composition of commercial lager storage beer and stabilized beer[a]

Analysis	*Storage beer (mg/l)*	*Stabilized beer (mg/l)*
Total polyphenols	260	143
Total flavanols	27	12
(+)-Catechin	2.8	1.6
(−)-Epicatechin	1.0	1.0
Prodelphinidin B3	2.7	0.5
Procyanidin B3	2.1	0.7

Notes: Analysis by HPLC.

[a] Stabilized by PVPP treatment (40g/hl). Stabilized means that, to reduce non-biological hazes, the beer was treated by PVPP to reduce the polyphenols during filtration (McMurrough and Baert, 1994).

Table 32.10 Polyphenolic compounds in beer[a]

Sample	*Concentration (mg/l)* Prodelphinidin B3	Procyanidin B3	Catechin	Epicatechin
Unstabilized lager	3.3	3.1	4.2	1.1
Stabilized lager	0.5	0.3	2.7	0.6

Note: Analysis by HPLC.
[a]Stabilized means that, to reduce non-biological hazes, the beer was treated by PVPP to reduce the polyphenols during filtration (Madigan *et al.*, 1994).

Table 32.12 Effect of stabilized beer with 50g/hl PVPP on the concentration of proanthocyanidins and catechins[a]

Flavanol	*Flavanol concentration (mg/l)* Unstabilized lager	Stabilized lager	Decrease (%)
(+)-Catechin	4.3	1.7	60
(−)-Epicatechin	1.3	0.9	31
Total monomers	5.6	2.6	54
D1 (prodelphinidin B3)	2.5	1.1	56
D2 (procyanidin B3)	1.7	0.7	59
Total dimers	4.2	1.8	57
T1 (prodelphinidin trimer)	0.7	0.4	43
T2 (prodelphinidin trimer)	0.1	0.1	0
T3 (prodelphinidin trimer)	0.3	0.2	33
T4 (procyanidin trimer)	0.5	0.3	40
Total trimers	1.6	1.0	38
Total flavanols measurable by HPLC	11.5	5.5	52

[a] McMurrough and Madigan (1996).

Table 32.11 Concentration of proanthocyanidins in beer[a,b]

Food	*Monomers*	*Dimers*	*Trimers*	*4–6mers*	*7–10mers*	*>10mers*	*Total proanthocyanidins*	*Type*
				mg/l (beverages)				
Beer	4 ± 0	11 ± 1	3 ± 0	4 ± 0	ND	ND	23 ± 2	PC, PD

[a] Values are means S ± D, *n* = 4–8.
[b] Monomers, dimers and trimers are listed separately. Tetramers through hexamers are pooled as 4–6mers. Polymers with DP > 10 are quantified collectively and listed as >10mers. Abbreviations and symbols: ND, not detected. The PP, PC and PD are propelargonidins, procyanidins and prodelphinidins, respectively (Gu *et al.*, 2004).

gallocatechin-(epi)gallocatechin, (epi)catechin-(epi)catechin-(epi)catechin, (epi)catechin-(epi)gallocatechin-(epi)catechin, (epi)gallocatechin-(epi)catechin-(epi)catechin, (epi)gallocatechin-(epi)gallocatechin-(epi)catechin and (epi)gallocatechin-(epi)gallocatechin-(epi)gallocatechin in beer.

An optimized normal-phase HPLC–MS fluorescent detection method (Gu, 2004) was used to estimate the concentrations of proanthocyanidins in common foods and beverages (Table 32.11). With this technique, tetramers through hexamers were first found in beer with concentrations of 4 mg/l. Significant reduction in proanthocyanidins in beer is effected by treatment with 50 g/hl PVPP (Table 32.12).

In summary, numerous studies have shown proanthocyanidins present in hops and malt (barley) are easily extracted from these raw materials into the beer during brewing because of their high solubility. Proanthocyanidin monomers, dimers and trimers have been reported to be present in beer with total amounts generally present around 20 mg/l. Catechin and prodelphinidin B3 are the most representative proanthocyanidins followed by procyanidin B3 and epicatechin. In view of their high aqueous solubilities, it remains to be seen whether larger oligomers may also be present in beers. Proanthocyanidins have received a considerable amount of attention in the brewing industry because they stabilize the organoleptic properties and color, and contribute to the astringency and bitterness, all of which are desirable attributes. Non-biological haze is produced as a result of the protein–polyphenol complexes that are formed on storage of beer. Although the potential for haze formation can be reduced by removing protein or proanthocyanidins or both, marked changes in the balance of these components can negatively affect the quality and flavor of beer as well as the possible health benefits that are associated with the presence of these antioxidants. Future research may show how the beneficial properties of proanthocyanidins may be retained through judicious selection of certain polyphenol components and/or grains with soluble proteins that exhibit a lower tendency for complexation or aggregation.

Summary Points

- Tandem mass spectrometry coupled with liquid chromatography (LC/MS^2) is a new and powerful method for sequencing proanthocyanidin oligomers because of its capacity for reliably analyzing small sample amounts. Once the sequences are known, NMR spectroscopy can be used to determine the relative stereochemistry and the proanthocyanidin interflavan linkages.
- Twenty-five* proanthocyanidins have been structurally identified in hops, and the relative proportions of the various proanthocyanidins have been found to vary greatly depending on the hop variety and climatic differences. Proanthocyanidins were dominant in hops, but small quantities of prodelphinidins and one propelargonidin were also present. The flavanoids (+) catechin and proanthocyanidin B3 were most representative followed B1, B4 and C2.
- Proanthocyanidin monomers, dimers and trimers have been reported to be present in beer with total amounts generally present around 20 mg/l. Catechin and prodelphinidin B3 are the most representative proanthocyanidins followed by procyanidin B3 and epicatechin.
- Proanthocyanidins have received a considerable amount of attention in the brewing industry because they stabilize the organoleptic properties and color, and contribute to the astringency and bitterness of beer, all of which are desirable attributes.
- Although the potential for haze formation can be reduced by removing protein or proanthocyanidins or both, marked changes in the balance of these components can negatively affect the quality and flavor of beer as well as the possible health benefits that are associated with the presence of these antioxidants.

*Since the preparation of this chapter, a total of forty-four A- and B-type proanthocyanidins have been identified in hops.

References

Callemien, D., Jerkovic, V., Rozenberg, R. and Collin, S. (2005). *J. Agric. Food Chem.* 53, 424–429.

Dadic, M. and Belleau, G. (1976). *J. Am. Soc. Brew. Chem.* 34, 154–158.

Eastmond, R. (1974). *J. Inst. Brew.* 80, 188–192.

Foo, L.Y. and Karchesy, J.J. (1989). *Phytochemistry* 28, 1743–1747.

Foo, L.Y. and Porter, L.J. (1981). *J. Sci. Food Agric.* 32, 711–716.

Forster, A., Beck, B., Schmidt, R., Jansen, C. and Mellenthin, A. (2002). *Monatsschrift fuer Brauwissenschaft* 55, 98–108.

Goupy, P., Hugues, M., Boivin, P. and Amiot, M.J. (1999). *J. Sci. Food Agric.* 79, 1625–1634.

Gu, L.W., Kelm, M.A., Hammerstone, J.F., Beecher, G., Holden, J., Haytowitz, D., Gebhardt, S. and Prior, R.L. (2004). *J. Nutr.*, 613–617.

Hsu, F.-L., Nonaka, G. and Nishioka, I. (1985). *Chem. Pharm. Bull.* 33, 3142–3152.

Jerkovic, V., Callemien, D. and Collin, S. (2005). *J. Agric. Food Chem.* 53, 4202–4206.

Jerumanis, J. (1979). *European Brewery Convention, Proceedings of the 17th Congress*, 309–319.

Jerumanis, J. (1985). *J. Inst. Brew.* 91, 250–252.

Kennedy, J.A. and Jones, G.P. (2001). *J. Agric. Food Chem.* 49, 1740–1746.

Kennedy, J.A., Matthews, M.A. and Waterhouse, A.L. (2000). *Phytochemistry* 55, 77–85.

Kirby, W. and Wheeler, R.E. (1980). *J. Inst. Brew.* 86, 15–17.

Li, H.J. and Deinzer, M.L. (2006). *J. Agric. Food Chem.* 54, 4048–4056.

Li, H.J. and Deinzer, M.L. (2007). *Anal. Chem.* 79, 1739–1748.

Maatta-Riihinen, K.R., Kahkonen, M.P., Torronen, A.R. and Heinonen, I.M. (2005). *J. Agric. Food Chem.* 53, 8485–8491.

McMurrough, I. (1981). *J. Chromatogr.* 218, 683–693.

McMurrough, I. and Baert, T. (1994). *J. Inst. Brew.* 100, 409–416.

McMurrough, I., Kelly, R. and Byrne, J. (1992). *J. Am. Soc. Brew. Chem.*, 67–76.

McMurrough, I., Madigan, D. (1996). *J. Agric. Food Chem.* 44, 1731–1735.

Medigan, D., McMurrough, I. and Smyth, M.R. (1994). *Analyst.* 119, 863–868.

Merghem, R., Jay, M., Brun, N. and Voirin, B. (2004). *Phytochem. Anal.* 15, 95–99.

Moir, M. (2000). *J. Am. Soc. Brew. Chem.* 58, 131–146.

Moll, M., Fonknechten, G., Carnielo, M. and Flayeux, R. (1984). *MBAA Tech. Q.* 21, 79–87.

Neve, R.A. (1992). *Hops*, pp. 43–45 Chapman and Hall, London, UK.

Porter, L.J. (1988). In Harborne, J.B. (ed.), *The Flavonoids Tail*, pp. 21–62. Chapman and Hall, London, UK.

Ricardo Da Silva, J.M., Rigaud, J., Cheynier, V., Cheminat, A. and Moutounet, M. (1991). *Phytochemistry* 30, 1259–1264.

Stevens, J.F., Taylor, A.W., Nickerson, G.B., Ivancic, M., Henderson, M.C., Haunold, A. and Deinzer, M.L. (2000). *Phytochemistry* 53, 759–775.

Stevens, J.F., Miranda, C.L., Wolthers, K.R., Schimerlik, M., Deinzer, M.L. and Buhler, D.R. (2002). *J. Agric. Food Chem.* 50, 3435–3443.

Sun, D., Herbert, W. and Foo, L.Y. (1987). *Phytochemistry* 26, 1825–1829.

Taylor, A.W., Barofsky, E., Kennedy, J.A. and Deinzer, M.L. (2003). *J. Agric. Food Chem.* 51, 4101–4110.

Vancraenenbroeck, R., Gorissen, H. and Lontie, R. (1977). European Brewery Convention, *Proceedings of the 16th Congress*, Amsterdam, p. 429.

Whittle, N., Eldridge, H. and Bartley, J. (1999). *J. Inst. Brew.* 105, 89–99.

Zhou, Z.H., Zhang, Y.J., Xu, M. and Yang, C.R. (2005). *J. Agric. Food Chem.* 53, 8614–8617.

33

Metals in Beer

Pawel Pohl Division of Analytical Chemistry, Faculty of Chemistry, Wroclaw University of Technology, Wroclaw, Poland

Abstract

Major, minor and trace metals are important in the fermentation processes since they supply the appropriate growth environment for yeasts and have the influence on their metabolism due to the co-factoring of different enzymes. The presence of the transition metals like copper and iron in their non-complexed forms is a real concern since these metals affect the conditioning and aging of beer by catalyzing the reactions in which the reactive oxygen species are formed. The resulted reactive oxygen species, especially free radicals, are likely to oxidize variety of the organic compounds present in beer which substantially contributes to the foaming quality and the flavor stability of beer. In view of the brewing technology and beer processing, the knowledge regarding the functions of metals and their different speciation forms in brewing liquors and beer is of special significance to the brewers. In the products of final quality, the metals can have a certain nutritional importance to the consumers, however, the effect on the human organism depends on the type of the metal species present in beer since many low and high molecular mass organic species likely bind the metal ions and form the complexes of different stability and availability. This chapter reviews the role of the metals in beer and the processes involved in beer production. The attention is paid to the endogenous and exogenous sources of metals in beer, the nutritional aspects of metals, their bioavailability and partitioning in beer, as well as the roles in brewing and the fermentation performance, and the effect on final quality and taste.

List of Abbreviations

Ag	Silver
Al	Aluminum
ANN	Artificial neural networks
ANOVA	Analysis of variance
Ba	Barium
Ca	Calcium
Cd	Cadmium
Co	Cobalt
Cr	Chromium
Cs	Cesium
Cu	Copper
Da	Dalton, mass unit used for large molecules
Fe	Iron
Ga	Gallium
H_2O_2	Hydrogen peroxide
Hg	Mercury
K	Potassium
LDA	Linear discriminant analysis
Mg	Magnesium
Mn	Manganese
Mo	Molybdenium
Na	Sodium
Ni	Nickel
O_2^-	Superoxide anion
$OH^•$	Hydroxyl radical
$OOH^•$	Perhydroxyl radical
PCA	Principal component analysis
Pb	Lead
pH	Reverse logarithmic representation of relative hydrogen proton (H^+) concentration
Rb	Rubidium
Sr	Strontium
Zn	Zinc
V	Vanadium

Introduction

Sources of metals in beer

Beer is the product of yeast alcoholic fermentation of the extracts of malted cereals, usually barley malts, with or without the starchy material, and to which hops are added. All these natural components used for brewing, that is water, cereals, barleys and yeasts, are the main endogenous sources of metals in beer. Apparently, the mineral composition of

Beer in Health and Disease Prevention
ISBN: 978-0-12-373891-2

beer usually reflects the composition of the ingredients and refers to the brewing processes carried out. In consequence, the content of the metals is rather variable and depends on the quality of the substrates taken, the type of beer brewed and the country of origin of beer (Hardwick, 1995; Moll, 1995; Goldammer, 1999; Baxter and Hughes, 2001; Briggs *et al.*, 2004).

Metals found in beer may originate also from many other adjunctive substances added during the brewing to control the fermentation and the maturation processes taken place in beer. Another exogenous source of metals in beer can be the contamination from different components of the brewery equipment, for example pipes, fluid lines, vessels and tanks, in which beer is fermented, conditioned, filtrated, carbonated and packed, as well as the containers, for example kegs, casks, cans, in which the product of the final quality achieved is kept during the storage and transport. In this case, moderately acidic brewing liquors and beer (pH 4.2 on average) can contribute to a large extent to the ingestion of the metal ions, especially in aluminum cans, kegs and casks (Sharpe and Williams, 1995; Vela *et al.*, 1998; Wyrzykowska *et al.*, 2001). The deterioration of beer can liners and the interaction of the beverage with the containers usually lead to the increase in the concentrations of metals such as Al, Co, Cr, Cu, Fe or Ni, which migrate to the beer components. In the case of Al, it can be presumed that the longer the length of beer storage, the higher concentrations of the metals are found in beer. Moreover, the higher the temperature of storage, the more rapid the rate of can corrosion takes place, regardless of its coating, and the higher the accumulation of the metals in beer occurs (Vela *et al.*, 1998).

Metals in Beer

Total metal content

The major metals of beer are calcium (4–140 mg/l), potassium (20–1,100 mg/l), sodium (1–230 mg/l) and magnesium (20–270 mg/l). At level of minor and trace metals in beer are aluminum (0.005–2.2 mg/l), barium (0.01–0.07 mg/l), cadmium (up to 0.7 mg/l), cobalt (up to 0.0008 mg/l), chromium (up to 0.02 mg/l), copper (0.008–0.8 mg/l), iron (0.02–1.6 mg/l), manganese (0.03–0.8 mg/l), nickel (up to 0.3 mg/l), lead (0.0008–0.03 mg/l), strontium (0.1–0.7 mg/l) and zinc (0.001–1.5 mg/l). Ranges of the concentrations of major, minor and trace metals determined in beers of different country of origin are given respectively in Table 33.1 (Ca, K, Na, Mg), Table 33.2 (Al, Cd, Cu, Fe, Mn, Ni, Sr, Zn) and Table 33.3 (Ba, Co, Cr, Hg, Pb).

With respect to the nutritional value of metals to human and according to relatively high contents of some of them in beer, it is accepted that moderate and reasonable consumption of beer can be to some extent a valuable source of recommended daily dietary intakes of metals. However, it should be noted as well that although the information on the total metal content is advantageous in the estimation of the metal nutrient uptake source, the bioavailability of metals from beer to humans and its absorbability crucially depends on the speciation forms in which they are present in beer (Sharpe and Williams, 1995; Svendsen and Lund, 2000; Pohl and Prusisz, 2007). For example, it has been indicated that aluminum, whose excessive intake is linked with Alzheimer's disease, is predominantly present in beer in the form of citrate and phosphate complexes and that only a small portion

Table 33.1 The concentrations (in mg/l) of major metals in beers of different country of origin

Metal	*Beer*	*Concentration*	*Reference*
Ca	British	40.0–140	Bellido-Milla *et al.* (2000); Alcazar *et al.* (2002); Briggs *et al.* (2004)
	Dutch	42.2–69.8	Bellido-Milla *et al.* (2000); Alcazar *et al.* (2002)
	German	3.80–108	Bellido-Milla *et al.* (2000); Alcazar *et al.* (2002); Briggs *et al.* (2004)
	Spanish	29.0–86.2	Bellido-Milla *et al.* (2000); Alcazar *et al.* (2002)
	Others	16.5–111	Bellido-Milla *et al.* (2000); Alcazar *et al.* (2002)
K	British	135–1100	Bellido-Milla *et al.* (2000); Alcazar *et al.* (2002); Briggs *et al.* (2004)
	Dutch	124–648	Bellido-Milla *et al.* (2000); Alcazar *et al.* (2002)
	German	46.7–833	Bellido-Milla *et al.* (2000); Alcazar *et al.* (2002); Briggs *et al.* (2004)
	Spain	22.9–496	Bellido-Milla *et al.* (2000); Alcazar *et al.* (2002)
	Others	17.5–442	Bellido-Milla *et al.* (2000); Alcazar *et al.* (2002)
Mg	British	60.0–200	Bellido-Milla *et al.* (2000); Alcazar *et al.* (2002); Briggs *et al.* (2004)
	Dutch	55.5–265	Bellido-Milla *et al.* (2000); Alcazar *et al.* (2002)
	German	23.7–266	Bellido-Milla *et al.* (2000); Alcazar *et al.* (2002); Briggs *et al.* (2004)
	Spain	42.0–110	Bellido-Milla *et al.* (2000); Alcazar *et al.* (2002)
	Others	50.0–112	Bellido-Milla *et al.* (2000); Alcazar *et al.* (2002); Pohl and Prusisz (2004)
Na	British	21.9–230	Bellido-Milla *et al.* (2000); Alcazar *et al.* (2002); Briggs *et al.* (2004)
	Dutch	10.4–47.6	Bellido-Milla *et al.* (2000); Alcazar *et al.* (2002)
	German	1.19–120	Bellido-Milla *et al.* (2000); Alcazar *et al.* (2002); Briggs *et al.* (2004)
	Spanish	3.95–103	Bellido-Milla *et al.* (2000); Alcazar *et al.* (2002)
	Others	4.13–66.4	Bellido-Milla *et al.* (2000); Alcazar *et al.* (2002)

of the total Al found in beer is transported through the wall of the gut. Therefore, beer plays a minor part in the bioavailable uptake of Al from the diet (Sharpe and Williams, 1995).

The assessment of the total metal composition of beer, including the determination of major, minor and trace metals, is of particular interest and notice to the brewers and the consumers since, in dependence of the concentration and type, they might be essential or toxic in the human body and they can also have an influence on the brewing process and the quality of beer in view of the flavor stability or the formation of haze (Bellido-Milla *et al.*, 2000; Svendsen and Lund, 2000; Wyrzykowska *et al.*, 2001; Alcazar *et al.*, 2002; Vinas *et al.*, 2002; Bellido-Milla *et al.*, 2004; Pohl and Prusisz, 2004; Asfaw and Wibetoe, 2005; Nascentes *et al.*, 2005; Llobat-Estelles *et al.*, 2006; Onate-Jaen *et al.*, 2006; Pohl and Prusisz, 2007). For example, some metals may be harmful above a certain concentration (Al, Cd, Hg, Pb), some of them are regarded to affect the quality of foam and

Table 33.2 The concentrations (in mg/l) of minor metals in beers of different country of origin

Metal	*Beer*	*Concentration*	*Reference*
Al	Dutch	0.08–0.18	Alcazar *et al.* (2002)
	German	0.05–1.24	Alcazar *et al.* (2002); Briggs *et al.* (2004)
	Spanish	0.05–2.2	Alcazar *et al.* (2002); Vinas *et al.* (2002)
	Others	0.005–6.50	Sharpe and Williams (1995); Vela *et al.* (1998); Alcazar *et al.* (2002); Pohl and Prusisz (2004)
Cd	German	0.0002–0.020	Briggs *et al.* (2004)
	Spanish	0.031–0.40	Briggs *et al.* (2004)
	Others	0.095–0.68	Briggs *et al.* (2004)
Cu	British	0.008–0.80	Bellido-Milla *et al.* (2000); Briggs *et al.* (2004); Asfaw and Wibetoe (2005)
	Dutch	0.032–0.068	Bellido-Milla *et al.* (2000); Asfaw and Wibetoe (2005); Llobat-Estelles *et al.* (2006)
	German	0.019–0.80	Bellido-Milla *et al.* (2000); Briggs *et al.* (2004); Asfaw and Wibetoe (2005); Llobat-Estelles *et al.* (2006)
	Norwegian	0.029–0.050	Svendsen and Lund (2000); Asfaw and Wibetoe (2005)
	Polish	0.029–0.15	Matusiewicz and Kopras (1997); Wyrzykowska *et al.* (2001); Pohl and Prusisz (2004)
	Spanish	0.024–0.080	Bellido-Milla *et al.* (2000); Alcazar *et al.* (2002); Vinas *et al.* (2002); Bellido-Milla *et al.* (2004); Briggs *et al.* (2004)
	Others	0.022–0.16	Bellido-Milla *et al.* (2000); Asfaw and Wibetoe (2005); Nascentes *et al.* (2005)
Fe	British	0.067–0.50	Bellido-Milla *et al.* (2000); Alcazar *et al.* (2002); Briggs *et al.* (2004); Asfaw and Wibetoe (2005)
	Dutch	0.064–0.43	Bellido-Milla *et al.* (2000); Alcazar *et al.* (2002); Asfaw and Wibetoe (2005)
	German	0.040–1.55	Bellido-Milla *et al.* (2000); Alcazar *et al.* (2002); Briggs *et al.* (2004); Asfaw and Wibetoe (2005)
	Norwegian	0.036–0.093	Svendsen and Lund (2000); Asfaw and Wibetoe (2005)
	Polish	0.015–0.53	Matusiewicz and Kopras (1997); Wyrzykowska *et al.* (2001); Pohl and Prusisz (2004)
	Spanish	0.096–0.92	Bellido-Milla *et al.* (2000); Alcazar *et al.* (2002); Bellido-Milla *et al.* (2004)
	Others	0.041–1.06	Bellido-Milla *et al.* (2000); Alcazar *et al.* (2002); Asfaw and Wibetoe (2005)
Mn	British	0.033–0.18	Bellido-Milla *et al.* (2000); Alcazar *et al.* (2002); Asfaw and Wibetoe (2005)
	Dutch	0.047–0.30	Bellido-Milla *et al.* (2000); Alcazar *et al.* (2002); Asfaw and Wibetoe (2005)
	German	0.040–0.51	Bellido-Milla *et al.* (2000); Alcazar *et al.* (2002); Briggs *et al.* (2004); Asfaw and Wibetoe (2005)
	Norwegian	0.046–0.78	Svendsen and Lund (2000); Asfaw and Wibetoe (2005)
	Polish	0.053–0.47	Matusiewicz and Kopras (1997); Wyrzykowska *et al.* (2001); Pohl and Prusisz (2004); Pohl and Prusisz (2007)
	Others	0.032–0.36	Bellido-Milla *et al.* (2000); Alcazar *et al.* (2002); Asfaw and Wibetoe (2005); Nascentes *et al.* (2005)
	Spanish	0.031–0.25	Bellido-Milla *et al.* (2000); Alcazar *et al.* (2002); Bellido-Milla *et al.* (2004)
Ni		up to 0.26	Briggs *et al.* (2004)
Sr	Dutch	0.23–0.41	Alcazar *et al.* (2002)
	German	0.14–0.30	Alcazar *et al.* (2002)
	Spain	0.13–0.74	Alcazar *et al.* (2002)
	Others	0.13–0.39	Alcazar *et al.* (2002)
Zn	Dutch	0.013–0.064	Bellido-Milla *et al.* (2000); Alcazar *et al.* (2002)
	German	0.013–1.48	Bellido-Milla *et al.* (2000); Alcazar *et al.* (2002); Briggs *et al.* (2004)
	Polish	0.004-0.12	Matusiewicz and Kopras (1997); Wyrzykowska *et al.* (2001); Pohl and Prusisz (2007)
	Spain	0.001–0.98	Bellido-Milla *et al.* (2000); Alcazar *et al.* (2002)
	Others	0.007–0.28	Wagner *et al.* (1991); Bellido-Milla *et al.* (2000); Alcazar *et al.* (2002); Nascentes *et al.* (2005)

Table 33.3 The concentrations (in mg/l) of trace metals in beers of different country of origin

Metal	*Beer*	*Concentration*	*Reference*
Ba	Dutch	0.020–0.032	Alcazar *et al.* (2002)
	German	0.034–0.049	Alcazar *et al.* (2002)
	Spanish	0.014–0.033	Alcazar *et al.* (2002)
	Others	0.016–0.068	Alcazar *et al.* (2002)
Co		up to 0.0008	Briggs *et al.* (2004)
Cr		up to 0.022	Briggs *et al.* (2004)
Hg		up to 0.26	Briggs *et al.* (2004)
Pb	German	0.003–0.024	Briggs *et al.* (2004)
	Spanish	0.001–0.006	Briggs *et al.* (2004)
	Others	0.0008–0.033	Briggs *et al.* (2004); Nascentes *et al.* (2005)

flavor (Cu, Fe, Mn), others are essential and have advantageous effect on human health (Fe, Zn).

With regard to different health and/or disease implications of metals, their nutritional value as well as the impact on the quality and sensory properties of beer, the total allowed content claims of the metals in beer are precisely regulated (Baxter and Hughes, 2001; Briggs *et al.*, 2004).

Chemometric differentiation and classification of beer

The information regarding the total contents of metals in beer, typically originated from the natural raw products used for its manufacturing, that is water, cereals, hops and yeasts, the brew processing, further treatment, storage and finally aging in the containers, is documented to be a valuable parameter used for the differentiation and the classification of beer (Bellido-Milla *et al.*, 2000; Wyrzykowska *et al.*, 2001; Alcazar *et al.*, 2002).

For the purpose of the chemometric classification of beer, different pattern recognition techniques are applied to the data matrix referred to the mineral contents found through the analysis of relatively high number of different beer brands. Hence, the principal component analysis (PCA) is used as a result of visualization technique, while the linear discriminant analysis (LDA) and the artificial neural networks (ANN) are the supervised learning methods applied to find adequate classification rules.

This chemometric approach along with the complete information on the mineral composition including the total concentrations of number of metals (Ag, Al, Ba, Ca, Cd, Co, Cr, Cu, Fe, Ga, Hg, K, Mg, Mn, Na, Ni, Pb, Rb, Sr, V, Zn) has been shown to be a very suitable tool for the differentiation and the classification of beer samples in relation to the type, origin and container of beer or the kind of raw material from which beer was brewed. Among others, the concentrations of metals such as Mn, Mg and K have appeared to be the most important variables for such kind of beer classification (Alcazar *et al.*, 2002).

Furthermore, the PCA indicates that a certain degree of association exists between some metals as they tend to group together, that is Cs and Hg, Cd and Co; Cr and Cs; Fe and Zn; or Mn and V (Wyrzykowska *et al.*, 2001). These metal cluster correlations established can be explained bearing in mind two main sources of metal intake in beer, that is the endogenous source associated with raw materials used for the brewing and the exogenous source originated from the contamination taking place during the production and storage of beer.

In addition, the analysis of variance (ANOVA) between the groups is also recognized as a valuable statistical method which can be used for the characterization of beers of different type, country of origin and container as well as for the control of the quality of the final product achieved with respect to its taste and flavor stability (Bellido-Milla *et al.*, 2000). For example, on the basis of the analysis of 25 different beer samples and the determination of seven metals (Al, Ca, Cu, Fe, Mg, Mn, Zn), it has been found that the concentrations of Cu and Fe in canned beers are commonly higher than those found in bottled beers. The notable differences in the contents of Ca, Cu, Fe, Mg, Mn and Na are observed as well among lager, stout, wheat and ale beers which demonstrates that the metals intake is differentiated according to the type of beer and the distinctive technology of its production.

Metal–Organic Matter Associations in Beer

Although the studies devoted to the characterization, the quality control and the estimation of the nutritional value of beers in relation to their total mineral composition are obviously valuable, it should be accentuated that the effect of metals present in beers on their stability and wholesomeness does not depend on their concentrations but foremost on the type of metal species resulted from binding the metals by different low and high molecular organic compounds present in beer and the equilibrium existing between the complexed and the non-complexed metal ions (Pohl and Prusisz, 2007).

Beer contains various classes of natural compounds, including polyphenolics, proteins, amino acids or other organic species, that have a capacity of binding the metals through the donor nitrogen, oxygen and sulfur atoms. Therefore, the metals can be present in beer as non-complexed cations as well as in the form of complexes of different stability and, in a consequence, of different bioavailability and toxicity to the human organisms (Montanari *et al.*, 1999; Gorinstein *et al.*, 2000; Cortacero-Ramirez *et al.*, 2003; Nardini and Ghiselli, 2004; Khatib *et al.*, 2006).

Due to the crucial role of Cu^+ and Fe^{2+} ions in the activation of molecular oxygen and further oxidation of the organic compounds responsible for stability and flavor of beer, the investigations of possible associations of these metals with different endogenous ligands existing in beer are of special interest and significance in terms of the brewing technology and processing (Irwin *et al.*, 1991; Mochaba *et al.*, 1996; Andersen and Skibsted, 1998; Montanari *et al.*, 1999; Blanco *et al.*, 2003; Morales *et al.*, 2005). Apparently, iron and copper are bound by amino acids, polyphenols and melanoids being the products of the last stage of the Maillard reaction and form their very stable complexes. Emphasized complexing reactions are recognized to take place mainly during the storage of beer. Hence, they strictly determine the type of the aging characteristics of beer and its final aroma and taste, as the capture of metal ions and the associations with chelating organic compounds is one of the important anti-oxidative approaches decreasing the formation and the activity of the reactive oxygen species (Bamforth, 1999a; Blanco *et al.*, 2003; Vanderhaegen *et al.*, 2006).

Conversely, the non-complexed copper and iron ions may have a negative effect on beer quality considering their contribution to the deterioration and the changes in stability occurred with aging.

The partitioning of other metals such as manganese or zinc is less explored. The ability of Mn^{2+} ions to form complexes with organic compounds is considered to be rather low (Onate-Jaen *et al.*, 2006). Although the involvement of the divalent cations of that metal in the radical generation and the oxidative staling reactions has not been reported, the chemical properties of manganese tend to the conclusion that its effect on beer colloidal and flavor instability may be possible. The non-complexed manganese ions may enhance the action of copper and iron in catalyzing the staling reactions, however, relatively low concentration of Mn in beer compared to those determined for Cu and Fe may mask this effect (Mochaba *et al.*, 1996).

For the reasons mentioned above, for better elucidation and understanding of the functions of metals in the processes related to the flavor stability, changes during the maturation, taste and odor of beers as well as their health implications and nutritional value referred to the consumption of that alcoholic beverage, it is essential to study the speciation or fractionation of metals in beer.

Metal fractionation pattern in beer

Very few research works have been dedicated so far to the partitioning of metals in beer and the assessment of the pattern of possible metal groupings in terms of the bioavailability of different metal forms.

The charge of Cu, Fe and Mn species in bottled beer (Ringnes Pilsner, Norway) has been established by means of the cation and anion exchange cartridges and off-line measurements by means of the electrothermal atomic absorption spectrometry (Svendsen and Lund, 2000). Analyzing the effluents obtained after separate passing of the aliquots of the untreated beer through the ion exchange cartridges, it has been found that Mn is present in the studied beer in the form of positively charged species (over 94% of the total content) presumably being simple Mn^{2+} cations. On the contrary, Fe has been determined to be entirely present as negatively charged species which indicates the presence of the species of Fe bound to different organic compounds. Finally, in case of Cu, both positively and negatively charged species (34% and 72%, respectively) have been found supposing the existence of different complexes of this metal.

The spiking of the beer sample with free metal cations (Cu^{2+}, Fe^{3+}, Mn^{2+}), followed then by the ion exchange experiments and the evaluation of the metal recoveries, has indicated that beer contains free ligands that readily bind Cu and Fe forming their negatively charged complexes. In contrast to that, added Mn^{2+} has been completely recovered as positive ions.

In addition, in the cited work by Svendsen and Lund (2000), the size exclusion chromatography was subjected to the untreated beer sample for the assessment of possible metal associations with ligands of different molecular weight ranges. The chromatograms, constructed on the basis of the metal quantities found in the column effluents, point out that Mn is present entirely in beer in the non-complexed forms, presumably as Mn^{2+}. In case of the remaining metals under consideration, that is Cu and Fe, the retention volumes of the eluted species (peaks) lead to the conclusion that these metals are likely to be present in beer as negatively charged species bound to organic molecules of the molecular weight of 4–12 and 4–9 kDa, respectively in case of Cu and Fe, and relating to different polyphenolics compounds.

A strong cation exchanger Dowex 50Wx4 has been applied by Pohl and Prusisz (2004) to evaluate the amount of broadly meant cationic fraction of Cd, Co, Cu, Ni and Zn in canned beer (Warka Full Light, Poland). The content of the metals under discussion in that operationally defined fraction was determined by passing the untreated beer sample through the column, followed by their recovery carried out by the acid digestion of the resin beads with adsorbed analytes. It was presumed that this fraction is of the highest bioavailability to the human organisms *via* gastrointestinal system and comprises free cations, stable cationic complexes with small molecular mass, non-volatile acids, including pyruvic acid, malic acid, lactic acid, citric acid, oxalic acid and labile metal species which dissociate the resin badly giving a donation to the cations. In case of Al, Co, Cr and Cu, the quantity of the cationic fraction in relation to the total metal contents was varied from 6% for Cu to 11% for Co. For Mn, Ni and Zn it was ranged from 23% to 28%.

Recently, a tandem column protocol, based on the retention of distinct metals species on a hydrophobic Amberlite XAD7 adsorbent, followed by a strong cation exchanger Dowex 50Wx4, has been developed for the operational fractionation of Mn and Zn, in various Polish canned and bottled beers (Pohl and Prusisz, 2007). The scheme of this fractionation manifold using two different sorption mechanisms to the metal species classification is given in Figure 33.1.

The distinct compounds of Mn and Zn, that is the fraction of the hydrophobic metal species and the fraction of the cationic metal species, were sorbed respectively on solid phase of the Amberlite XAD7 adsorbing resin and the strong cation exchanger Dowex 50Wx4 connected in a series. The metal contents in the respective metal species fractions were measured by means of the flame atomic absorption spectrometry method in the eluates obtained by the subsequent solvent elution. The residual metal fraction was determined on the basis of the metal amount found in the effluents resulted from passing the beer aliquots through the column system.

The procedure proposed by Pohl and Prusisz (2007) has enabled the assessment of the distribution of Mn and Zn among defined chemical species classes, that is the hydrophobic, high molecular weight species of the metal complexes with the polyphenolic and flavonoid compounds, the sum of the free metal cations and the stable cationic metal complexes with the low molecular weight species (mostly amino acids, organic acids being of primary origin (citric, malic) or the secondary products of alcoholic fermentation (pyruvic, lactic, ketoglutaric, succinic, citramalic, fumaric)) and finally the residual metal species, possibly being the anionic and neutral metal associations either with low molecular mass ligands. The distribution of both metals among the fractions distinguished in some Polish bottled and canned beers is exemplified in Figure 33.2.

The case of Mn is of special significance. In comparison to the previous results devoted to the speciation of Mn and reported by Svendsen and Lund (2000), it has been established that possible chemical forms and associations of that metal are more differentiated as it was expected before. In conformity to the former findings, it appears that the predominant class of Mn species is the cationic fraction; the concentrations of Mn in that class of the species vary from less than 60 to over 100% of the total metal concentration. In addition, it was found that there is a considerable donation of the residual metal fraction (from 22% to 42%) to the total content of manganese in the analyzed beers. Manganese has also been determined to be present in the form of the complexes with polyphenolic substances (up to 8% of the total metal concentration).

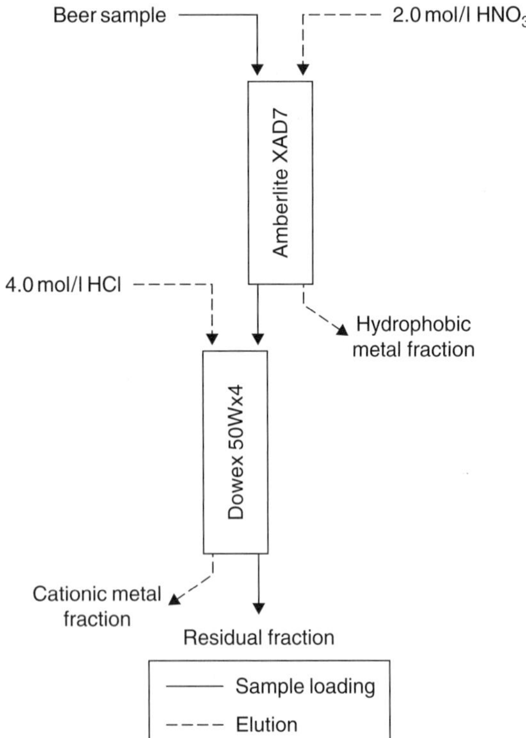

Figure 33.1 Tandem column fractionation protocol used for the classification of Mn and Zn groupings in beer. *Source*: Adapted from Pohl and Prusisz (2007).

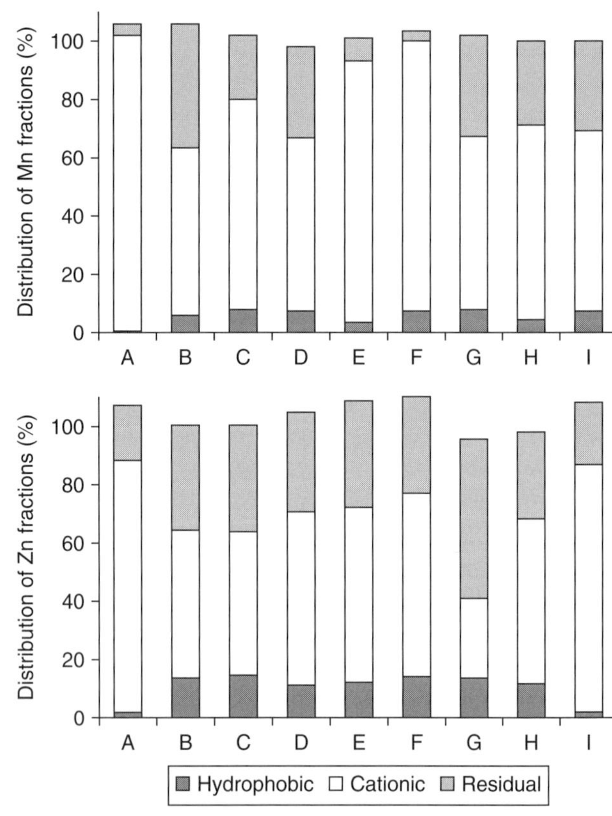

Figure 33.2 The fractionation patterns of Mn and Zn in beer. The distribution of the hydrophobic, the cationic and the residual metal fractions in Polish canned (A, Piast; B, Tyskie; C, Ksiaz; D, Zywiec; E, Karpackie; F, Perla) and bottled beers (G, Mocne dobre; H, Zywe; I, Ksiazece). *Source*: Adapted from Pohl and Prusisz (2007).

It should be noted that, the metal groupings distinguished through the fractionation protocol devised by Pohl and Prusisz (2007) are operationally defined and relate to the sorption behavior of Mn and Zn species toward the adsorbent and the cation exchanger applied; however, with respect to the total content analysis, the information retrieved on the abundance of different metal fractions in analyzed beers yields useful knowledge about metal bioavailability, beverage safety, authenticity and nutrition. Bearing in mind the possible associations of metals with natural organic substances present in beer (Montanari *et al.*, 1999; Cortacero-Ramirez *et al.*, 2003; Khatib *et al.*, 2006), the hydrophobic fraction can be regarded as hardly bioavailable to the humans while the sum of the cationic and the residual metal fractions, accounting respectively for over 92% and 85% of the total manganese and zinc in beers analyzed, can be assumed to be highly absorbable.

Metals in Brewing

Besides the nutrition value of metals of beer in response to their potential relationship and contribution to the daily diary nutrition requirements in diet, they are very important and influential in the brewing processes, especially in terms of proper growth and metabolism of yeasts. In case these last, they are essential co-factors for numerous fermentative enzymes, necessary components of transport systems fulfilling a charge-balancing or structural roles. Typically, the concentrations of metals, for example Ca^{2+}, Co^{2+}, Cu^{2+}, Fe^{3+}, K^{+}, Mo^{2+}, Mn^{2+}, Mg^{2+}, Ni^{2+} and Zn^{2+}, required for the appropriate growth of yeasts are relatively small. At high concentrations, the mentioned metals are usually toxic or exert a salt stress on the yeasts (e.g. Na^{+}) (Briggs *et al.*, 2004).

For that purpose, the metal metabolism of yeast is of special interest to brewers considering the improvement of yields, the enhancement of the fermentative capacity, and finally, the preservation of the consistency of the product quality (Walker *et al.*, 1996; Chandrasena *et al.*, 1997). Usually, the metal ion composition of brewing liquors changes significantly depending on the raw materials used and the conditions of brewing process applied and hence, it should be controlled. However, it should be emphasized that the uptake of the metal ions required by the yeast cells relies on the concentration of the particular ions in the growth environment and on to a great degree to their bioavailability. The latter one depends on both the solubility and the properties of different ion-complexing ligands originated from raw materials used. The most bioavailable are the free metal ions, but the chelating and adsorbing constituents present in wort and other brewing liquors regulate their availability by formation of the complexes of different stability. This reduction of free metal ions' bioavailability (e.g. Ca^{2+}, Mg^{2+}, Zn^{2+}) has a detrimental effect on the yeast growth kinetics and the fermentation performance (Walker *et al.*, 1996; Chandrasena *et al.*, 1997).

The detailed account to the role of particular major, minor and trace metals in the yeast metabolism and the fermentative and sensory performance of beer is given below (Hardwick, 1995; Moll, 1995; Walker *et al.*, 1996; Chandrasena *et al.*, 1997; Goldammer, 1999; Baxter and Hughes, 2001; Briggs *et al.*, 2004).

Role of major metals

Calcium Calcium ions (Ca^{2+}) are regarded as the most significant metal ions in brewing processes; they have several important functions in the metabolism of yeasts and their fermentation action. By the reaction with phosphate, phytate, peptides, proteins and other mash and wort components, the calcium ions involve the release of the hydrogen ions. It results in useful reduction of the mash and wort pH, which is critical for the stabilization of the fermentation enzymes, including α-amylase, β-amylase and other proteolytic enzymes. Their sufficiency is also important in the oxalate precipitation and in the governing of the yeast cells flocculation. Accordingly, the content of the Ca^{2+} ions in the brewing liquors should not exceed a certain concentration (100 mg/l on average) since it would lead to the substantial removal of the phosphate from the wort. In consequence, under conditions of serious deficiency of the phosphate ions, the yeasts would have an inadequate nutrition supply required for their adequate growth.

The effect of the calcium concentration on flavor of beer is rather minor, however, the content of that metal is recommended to be in the range from 20 to 150 mg/l.

Magnesium Magnesium ions (Mg^{2+}) behave similarly as calcium ions but since magnesium salts are more soluble, their effect on the lowering of the mash and wort pH is rather less pronounced. The presence of the magnesium ions is very important and beneficial to the yeast growth and the fermentative metabolism through the stimulation of cell division cycle progression and the co-factoring of more than 300 enzymes, including hexokinases, phosphofructokinase, phosphoglycerate kinase, pyruvate kinase and enolase in glycolysis. The growth demand for the Mg^{2+} ions by yeast cells is very high and cannot be replaced by the other metal ions. In fact, the Ca^{2+} ions may act antagonistically toward Mg^{2+} ions in many biochemical and physiological functions of the yeasts. The magnesium ions may also exert a protective effect on yeast cells from disadvantageous effects caused by ethanol, high temperature and osmotic pressure.

The upper limit of magnesium in beer is proposed to be of 30 mg/l. Much greater concentrations than that usually contribute to a sour or bitter flavor of beer.

Sodium Sodium ions (Na^{+}) have rather no special chemical influence. It is recognized that at higher concentrations, that is above 150 mg/l, which is proposed to be the maximum

Na concentration limit in beer, sodium ions are responsible for sour and salty flavors of beer. Usually, the levels of sodium changing in the range from 75 to 150 mg/l contribute to a round smoothness and accentuate a proper sweetness of beer.

Potassium Like sodium ions, potassium ions (K^+) present at concentrations above 10 mg/l can have different laxative effects and impart a salty taste of beer. They are required for yeast growth since their transport through membrane cells maintains the charge homeostasis. It is also involved in the osmoregulation and in the regulation of divalent cation and phosphate uptake into the yeast cells.

Role of minor metals

Iron Iron can occur in brewing liquors and beer as simple ions (Fe^{2+}, Fe^{3+}) or in the form of complexes with different organic compounds. Being present in too much amounts (above 1 mg/l), iron ions can convey metallic and harsh tastes to beer, as well as dark colors due to associations with phenolic substances from the malt and hops. Negative action of high concentrations of iron ions results also in the hampering of yeast activity, the prevention of complete saccharification and finally the production of haze in beer.

Hence, the concentration of Fe in wort and beer is usually recommended to be lower than 0.1 mg/l. Iron ions also exert a catalytic action in the oxidation processes occurring in beer and are responsible for aerobic aging and flavor stability during storage.

Copper Copper ions (Cu^{2+}), similarly as iron ions, (Fe^{2+}/Fe^{3+}) contribute to the quality of beer and the flavor enhancement due to their oxidation/reduction catalysis action. At too high concentrations, they are toxic and mutagenic to yeasts that accumulate them as well as cause the irreversible beer haze. Usually, brewing liquors should contain less than 0.1 mg/l of Cu.

Manganese Manganese ions (Mn^{2+}, Mn^{4+}) present at trace levels (0.05–0.2 mg/l) in brewing liquors are needed for proper growth of yeasts. Their other role is to attribute the solubilization of proteins and the support of proper enzymatic action. Like copper and iron, manganese ions are supposed to be oxidation/reduction catalysts and have adverse effect on flavor and beer colloidal stability owing to the role in the formation of the reactive oxygen containing species. In appreciable amounts, manganese ions can impart an unpleasant beer taste.

Zinc Zinc ions (Zn^{2+}) are essential micronutrient to the growth and metabolism of yeasts and protein synthesis. They are directly involved in ethanol production as co-factors of the essential enzymes such as alcohol and aldehyde dehydrogenases. At too much high concentration they cause damage to yeasts and affect fermentation. On the other hand, its deficiency leads to impaired fermentation progress. The recommended range of zinc amount in brewing liquors is from 0.15 to 0.5 mg/l.

Beer aging and haze formation

It has been evidenced that in the presence of Fe^{2+} and Cu^+ ions, stable molecules of oxygen dissolved in beer capture the electrons and form the superoxide anions (O_2^-). The resulted metal cations (Fe^{3+}, Cu^{2+}) can be reduced again to the respective lower oxidation state forms (Fe^{2+}, Cu^+ cations) by pro-oxidant molecules, for example some polyphenols. (Bamforth *et al.*, 1993; Uchida and Ono, 1996; Andersen and Skibsted, 1998; Kaneda *et al.*, 1999; Vanderhaegen *et al.*, 2006). By further protonation, the superoxide anions form the perhydroxyl radicals ($OOH^•$) that have much higher oxidative activity. Other reaction is the reduction of O_2^- anions by Fe^{2+} and/or Cu^{2+} cations to peroxide anions (O_2^{2-}), which can be easily protonated in beer to hydrogen peroxide (H_2O_2). Hydroxyl radicals ($OH^•$) that are intensely reactive can be then produced from the resulted H_2O_2 or O_2^- by metal ions induced Fenton and Haber–Weiss reactions, which are given in Figure 33.3.

The resulted reactive oxygen species (O_2^-, $OOH^•$, H_2O_2, $OH^•$) are crucial to beer staling as they react with all classes of organic compounds in beer, that is polyphenols, isohumulones, alcohols, amino acids, fatty acids, iso-α-acids, α-acids and β-acids, leading to permanent changes in the sensory profile of beer and determining the flavor stability of beer. The rate and level of the reactive oxygen species formation is related to the concentration of iron and copper ions (Fe^{2+}/Fe^{3+}, Cu^+/Cu^{2+}), therefore its concentration is of special significance, should be minimized and controlled during the brewing process.

It is established as well that the polyphenols contribute to these beer aging reactions. Some of them are pro-oxidants that are capable of transferring the electrons to metal ions and reducing Fe^{3+} and Cu^{2+}, respectively, to Fe^{2+} and Cu^+ what indirectly stimulates the activation of oxygen in beer. In this process, they may itself become the radicals that react further with other constituents of beer or decompose producing various off-flavors. On the other hand, polyphenols act as anti-oxidants by capture of the iron ions and formation of their stable complexes. Apart from the polyphenols, such components of brewing liquors and beer as amino acids, phytic acid and melanoidins have the ability to sequestrate the metal ions to promote the formation of active oxygen radical species (Vanderhaegen *et al.*, 2006).

It has been also found that the free metal ions can be responsible for the protein–polyphenol haze (chill haze) formed by cross-linkage of proteins by low molecular weight polyphenols (Siebert *et al.*, 1996; McMorrough *et al.*, 1999). In this case, metal effect on the protein–polyphenol haze formation can be presumably attributed to their catalytic action on the polymerization of the polyphenols.

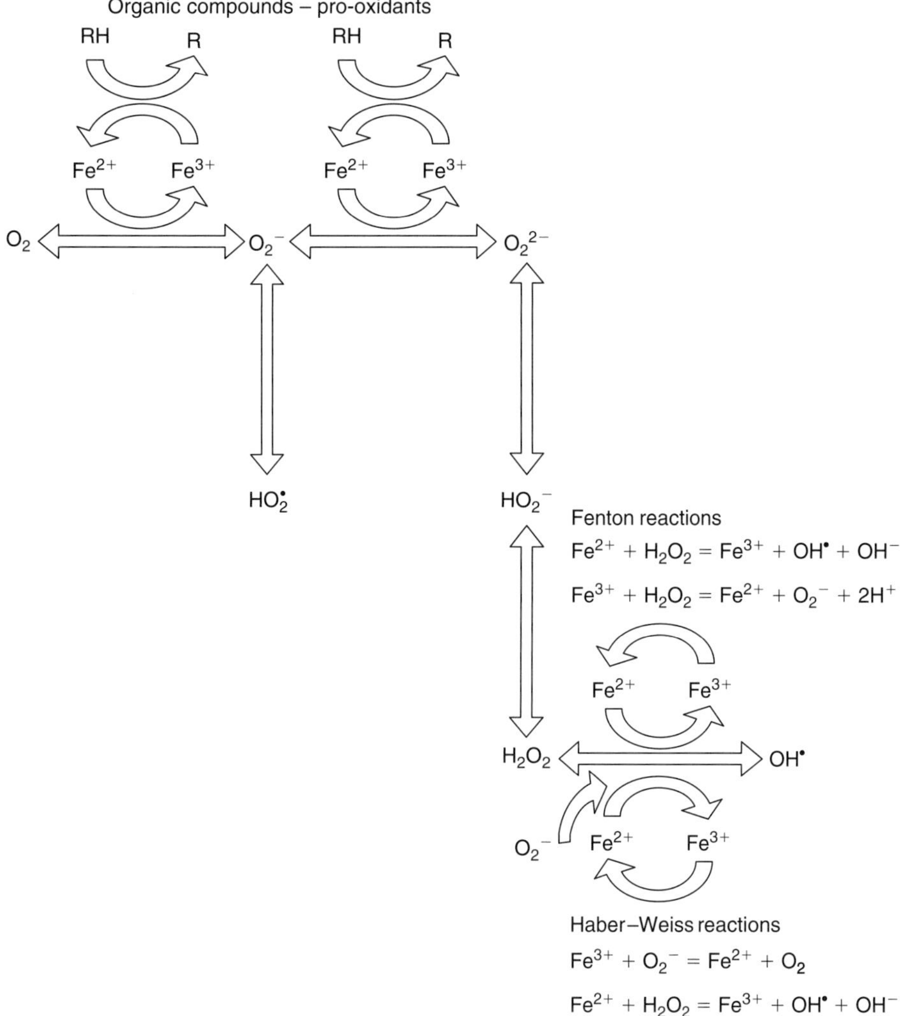

Figure 33.3 The reactions leading to the formation of the reactive oxygen species in stored beer. *Source*: Adapted from Kaneda *et al.* (1999).

The polyphenols, however, are likely to undergo polymerization. When they interact with proteins after this process, they form a "permanent haze" of particle size between 1 and 10 μm. It should also be that the polymerization of the polyphenols is promoted by their oxidation. Therefore, the reactive oxygen species formed in the reactions activated and catalyzed by iron and copper ions (Fenton and Haber–Weiss metal-catalyzed reactions) are responsible for haze formation owing to the efficiency with which they oxidize the polyphenols in beer (Kaneda *et al.*, 1990; Kaneda *et al.* 1992; Bamforth, 1999b).

Summary Points

- The knowledge regarding the content and type of metals in beer is imperative to the beer brewers and the consumers since metal ions determine the quality of beer in terms of the course of the processes involved in brewing, conditioning and storage of beer as well as imply the profound effect on the human health and well-being.
- There is a worldwide awareness of the importance of the controlling of metal composition at various steps of brewing to ensure the excellent quality of beer.
- On account of the nutritious value and critical role of metals in beer performance and final quality, the analysis of beer composition in reference to the total contents of major, minor and trace metals is of particular interest and significance.
- Along with the chemometric methods of data analysis and interpretation, the determination of metals in beer enables its characterization and authentication according to type, origin or packaging what is very useful in beer labeling and fraud tracing.
- It should be expected that the development of new analytical tools and methods linking chromatographic and electrophoretic separation techniques with sensitive

spectrometric method of detection in terms of speciation and fractionation analysis would help in the systematic elucidation of the mechanistic roles of these metals for which metabolic functions in beer processing and implications on beer quality, flavor and taste stability are not yet clearly established.

- On the other hand, the identification and the quantification of ultimate physicochemical forms of major, minor and trace found metals in beer would be determinative in the evaluation of their actual bioavailability or toxicity to human organisms.

References

Alcazar, A., Pablos, F., Martin, M.J. and Gonzalez, A.G. (2002). *Talanta* 57, 45–52.

Andersen, M.L. and Skibsted, L.H. (1998). *J. Agric. Food Chem.* 46, 1272–1275.

Asfaw, A. and Wibetoe, G. (2005). *Microchimica. Acta* 152, 61–68.

Bamforth, C.W. (1999a). *Brauwelt Int.* 17, 98–110.

Bamforth, C.W. (1999b). *J. Am. Soc. Brew. Chem.* 57, 81–90.

Bamforth, C.W., Muller, R.E. and Walker, M.D. (1993). *J. Am. Soc. Brew. Chem.* 51, 79–88.

Baxter, E.D. and Hughes, P.S. (2001). *Beer: Quality, Safety and Nutritional Aspects.* Royal Society of Chemistry, Cambridge, UK.

Bellido-Milla, D., Moreno-Perez, J.M. and Hernandez-Artiga, M.P. (2000). *Spectrochim. Acta Part B* 55, 855–864.

Bellido-Milla, D., Onate-Jaen, A., Palacios-Santander, J.M., Palacios-Tejero, D. and Hernandez-Artiga, M.P. (2004). *Microchim. Acta* 144, 183–190.

Blanco, C.A., Caballero, I., Rojas, A., Gomez, M. and Alvarez, J. (2003). *Food Chem.* 81, 561–568.

Briggs, D.E., Boulton, C.A., Brookes, P.A. and Stevens, R. (2004). *Brewing Science and Practice.* Woodhead Publishing Ltd., Cambridge, UK.

Chandrasena, G., Walker, G.M. and Staines, H.J. (1997). *J. Am. Soc. Brew. Chem.* 55, 24–29.

Cortacero-Ramirez, S., Hernainz-Bermudez de Castro, M., Segura-Carretero, A., Cruces-Blanco, C. and Fernandez-Gutierrez, A. (2003). *Trac-Trends Anal. Chem.* 22, 440–455.

Goldammer, T. (1999). *The Brewer's Handbook.* KUP Publishers, Clifon, Virgina.

Gorinstein, S., Caspi, A., Zemster, M. and Trakhtenberg, S. (2000). *Nutr. Res.* 20, 131–139.

Hardwick, W.A. (1995). The properties of beer. In Hardwick, W.A. (ed.), *Handbook of Brewing,* pp. 551–586. Marcel Dekker, New York.

Irwin, A.J., Barker, R.L. and Pipasts, P. (1991). *J. Am. Soc. Brew. Chem.* 49, 140–149.

Kaneda, H., Kano, Y., Osawa, T., Kawakishi, S. and Kamimura, M. (1990). *J. Agric. Food Chem.* 38, 1909–1912.

Kaneda, H., Kano, Y., Koshino, S. and Ohyanishiguchi, H. (1992). *J. Agric. Food Chem.* 40, 2102–2107.

Kaneda, H., Kobayashi, M., Takashio, M., Tamaki, T. and Shinotsuka, K. (1999). *Tech. Q. Master Brew. Assoc. Am.* 36, 41–47.

Khatib, A., Wilson, E.G., Kim, H.K., Lefeber, A.W.M., Erkelens, C., Choi, Y.H. and Verpoorte, R. (2006). *Anal. Chim. Acta* 559, 264–270.

Llobat-Estelles, M., Mauri-Aucejo, A.R. and Marin-Saez, R. (2006). *Talanta* 68, 1640–1647.

Matusiewicz, H. and Kopras, M. (1997). *J. Anal. Atom. Spectrom.* 12, 1287–1291.

McMorrough, I., Madigan, D., Kelly, R.J. and O'Rourke, T. (1999). *Food Technol.* 53, 58–62.

Mochaba, F., O'Connor-Cox, E.S.C. and Axcell, B.C. (1996). *J. Am. Soc. Brew. Chem.* 54, 164–171.

Moll, M.M. (1995). Water. In Hardwick, W.A. (ed.), *Handbook of Brewing,* pp. 133–156. Marcel Dekker, New York.

Montanari, L., Perretti, G., Natella, F., Guidi, A. and Fantozzi, P. (1999). *LWT-Food Sci. Technol.* 32, 535–539.

Morales, F.J., Fernandez-Fraguas, C. and Jimenez-Perez, S. (2005). *Food Chem.* 90, 821–827.

Nardini, M. and Ghiselli, A. (2004). *Food Chem.* 84, 137–143.

Nascentes, C.C., Kamogawa, M.Y., Fernandes, K.G., Arruda, M.A.Z., Nogueira, A.R.A. and Nobrega, J.A. (2005). *Spectrochim. Acta Part B* 60, 749–753.

Onate-Jaen, A., Bellido-Milla, D. and Hernandez-Artiga, M.P. (2006). *Food Chem.* 97, 361–369.

Pohl, P. and Prusisz, B. (2004). *Anal. Chim. Acta* 502, 83–90.

Pohl, P. and Prusisz, B. (2007). *Talanta* 7l71, 1616–1623.

Sharpe, F.R. and Williams, D.R. (1995). *J. Am. Soc. Brew. Chem.* 53, 85–92.

Siebert, K., Carrasco, A. and Lynn, P. (1996). *J. Agric. Food Chem.* 44, 1997–2005.

Svendsen, R. and Lund, W. (2000). *Analyst* 125, 1933–1937.

Uchida, M. and Ono, M. (1996). *J. Am. Soc. Brew. Chem.* 54, 198–204.

Wagner, H.P., Dalglish, K. and McGarrity, M.J. (1991). *J. Am. Soc. Brew. Chem.* 48, 28–30.

Walker, G.M., Birch, R.M., Chandrasena, G. and Maynard, A.I. (1996). *J. Am. Soc. Brew. Chem.* 54, 13–18.

Wyrzykowska, B., Szymczyk, K., Ichichashi, H., Falandysz, J., Skwarzec, B. and Yamasaki, S. (2001). *J. Agric. Food Chem.* 49, 3425–3431.

Vanderhaegen, B., Neven, H., Verachtert, H. and Derdelinckx, G. (2006). *Food Chem.* 95, 357–381.

Vela, M.M., Toma, R.B., Reiboldt, W. and Pierri, A. (1998). *Food Chem.* 63, 235–239.

Vinas, P., Aguinaga, N., Lopez-Garcia, I. and Hernandez-Cordoba, M. (2002). *J. AOAC Int.* 85, 736–743.

34

Minerals in Beer

Luigi Montanari, Heidi Mayer, Ombretta Marconi and Paolo Fantozzi Italian Brewing Research Centre (CERB), University of Perugia, Via San Costanzo, Perugia, Italy

Abstract

The principal ions in beer are the cations – calcium, magnesium, sodium, and potassium – and the anions – sulfate, nitrate, phosphate, chlorides, and silicate. The minor ions are iron, copper, zinc and manganese. Cereals, water, hops and adjuncts are the main sources of the minerals present in beer, while in yeast, industrial processing and the containers contribute to a lesser extent. The mineral content of the brewing water is particularly important for the brewing process and hence for the quality and flavor of the final beer. In beer most of the minerals originate from the barley. About 75% derives from the malt, while the remaining 25% originates from the water. The mineral composition of the malt depends on the variety, place where it was grown, atmospheric condition, growing techniques, harvesting, storage, and malting system. Hops contribute a negligible amount of the minerals in beer because of the small quantities used (200 g to produce 100 l beer). However hops make a notable contribution of nitrate to the beer wort. In many countries a part of the malt can be substituted with other cereals like maize grits and rice. These cereal matrices normally contain fewer minerals than malt and so the metal level is less than an all-malt wort. The large amount of minerals from the raw materials decreases during the brewing process due to some minerals being removed through precipitations.

List of Abbreviations

°dH	German degree
ATP	Adenosine triphosphate
Ca	Calcium
Cl	Chloride
Cu	Copper
Fe	Iron
K	Potassium
Mg	Magnesium
Mn	Manganese
Na	Sodium
ppm	Parts per million
Zn	Zinc

Introduction

There is a well-balanced amount of minerals contained in beer. Being relatively high in potassium and low in sodium it is an ideal drink to include in diets for hypertensive patients (De Stefano and Montanari, 1996). It is low in calcium and rich in magnesium which may help protect against gall stone and kidney stone formation. These minerals have nutritional importance and also contribute to the flavor of the beer as non-volatile taste-active compounds. Schoenberger *et al.* (2002) showed that all taste qualities (sweet, salty, bitter, and sour) come from the minerals of the beer. Their concentration varies with the raw materials used and with the production process (Table 34.1).

The principal ions are the cations – calcium, magnesium, sodium, and potassium – and the anions – sulfate, nitrate, phosphate, chlorides, and silicate. The minor ions are iron, copper, zinc, and manganese. The level of toxic metals is limited by law. Cereals, water, hops, and adjuncts are the main sources of the minerals present in beer, while in yeast, industrial processing and the containers contribute to a lesser extent.

Calcium

Ca^{2+} ions that derive principally from the brewing water react with malt constituents such as phosphates and proteins during mashing to lower the pH. Most processes in beer production proceed better or faster the more acidic the pH (Kunze, 2004). Wort produced from liquor containing no calcium has a pH on the order of 5.8–6.0, compared to values in the range of 5.3–5.5 for worts produced from treated brewing liquor. For example the Ca^{2+} of neutral calcium sulfate reacts in the mash with the alkaline dipotassium hydrogen phosphate from the malt, forming insoluble

Beer in Health and Disease Prevention
ISBN: 978-0-12-373891-2

Table 34.1 Mineral composition of beer

Inorganic substances	*Amount in beer (mg/l)*	*Recommended daily intake (mg/day)*	*Physiological effects in humans*
Phosphates	300–400	1,250–1,500	Important constituent of bones and teeth; responsible for energy storage and transmission
Sulfate	150–200	–	No important effect
Nitrate	10–80		Nitrate can be converted to nitrite which is harmful to health. The amount of nitrate in beer is usually below the legal limit of 50 mg/l for drinking water and is harmless
Chloride	150–200	2,500	–
Potassium	500–600	2,500	Good for prophylaxis against heart attack; a high potassium content is diuretic
Sodium	30–32	550	Low sodium content desirable
Calcium	35–40	800–1,000	Can prevent heart diseases
Magnesium	100–110	300–350	Lowers the cholesterol level, beneficial effect on cardiac activity

Note: The type and the quantity of the main inorganic substances in the beer and their physiological effects in humans.
Source: Kunze, 2004.

calcium phosphate. Potassium dihydrogen phosphate is acidic and consequently the pH of the solution is lowered.

$$\underset{\text{Calcium sulfate}}{3CaSO_4} + \underset{\text{Dipotassium hydrogen phosphate}}{4K_2HPO_4} \rightarrow$$

$$\underset{\text{Calcium phosphate}}{Ca_3(PO_4)_2\downarrow} + \underset{\text{Potassium dihydrogen phosphate}}{2KH_2PO_4} + \underset{\text{Potassium sulfate}}{3K_2SO_4}$$

It thus has a positive effect on the activity of β-amylase and thus of wort fermentability and extract because the optimum pH for β-amylase activity is about 5.2–5.6. Furthermore, it has a beneficial effect on the precipitation of wort proteins, during both mashing and boiling.

$$\text{Protein} + Ca^{2+} \rightarrow \text{Ca proteinate}\downarrow + 2\,H_3O^+$$

The hydrogen ions released further reduce the pH which encourages further precipitation of proteins, increasing the colloidal stability of the beer. Calcium ions protect the enzyme α-amylase from inhibition by heat. Moreover they eliminate excess oxalate. Calcium oxalate normally separates from beer during fermentation and storage and is the major constituent (50–65%) of the beer stone which forms on the inner surface of fermentation and storage tanks. For this reason various authors recommend having 250 ppm calcium sulfate in the wort (Moll, 1987, 1995). A method commonly used by brewers to have a sufficient amount of calcium, and consequently to decrease the oxalate content in beer, is to add gypsum (calcium sulfate dihydrate) during brewing either to the brewing water at the mashing stage or during wort boiling. The dissolved calcium ions can combine with anionic oxalate to produce an almost totally insoluble calcium oxalate precipitate, which may be removed by settling, centrifugation, or filtration before packaging the product (Madigan and McMurrough, 1994). Thus during ageing, clarification, stability and flavor of the finished beer are improved. Calcium ions are also important for the flocculation of yeast because they activate the protein component essential for floc-forming ability (Nishihara *et al.*, 1994). Flocculation requires at least two types of molecules on the yeast surface: mannan (a type of carbohydrate) and flocculins (sugar-binding proteins). The flocculins bind the mannans on the surface of the neighboring cells in the presence of calcium ions (Dengis *et al.*, 1995; Touhami *et al.*, 2003). Calcium also extracts fine bittering principles of the hops and reduces wort color.

Magnesium

Magnesium ions react like calcium ions, but since magnesium salts are much more soluble, the effect on wort pH is not as great. Magnesium is most important for its benefit to yeast metabolism during fermentation. It is an essential element of the brewing liquor because it is required by yeast as a co-factor for the production of enzymes that are indispensable for the fermentation process. Yeast cells have a very high demand for magnesium that cannot be met by other metal ions. In fact, calcium ions act antagonistically toward magnesium in many biochemical and physiological functions of yeast through inhibitory competitive binding mechanisms. Yeast cells actively take up Mg^{2+}, but exclude Ca^{2+} and so Mg^{2+} functions intracellularly, while Ca^{2+} acts mainly extracellularly influencing yeast flocculation. Mg^{2+} also stabilizes biological membranes and is known to protect yeast cells from stress caused by ethanol, temperature, and osmotic pressure (Walker *et al.*, 1996).

Sodium

Normally, sodium comes from the water supply and brewing ingredients. The level of sodium in malt depends on the levels in the processing water at the malt house (Rehberger and Luther, 1995). Sodium ions are not involved in chemical reactions with other components but pass unchanged into the beer (Kunze, 2004); they contribute to the perceived flavor of the beer by enhancing its sweetness. Sodium levels from 75 to 150 ppm give a round smoothness and accentuated sweetness, which is more pleasant when paired with chloride ions than when associated with sulfate ions. In the presence of sulfate, sodium creates an unpleasant harshness, so the more sulfate there is in the water, the less sodium there should be (and vice versa) (Goldammer, 2000). If the sodium levels exceed 150 ppm, it could indicate contamination by a cleaning solution.

Potassium

Like sodium, potassium can create a "salty" flavor effect. Potassium is required for yeast growth, and like magnesium, is a yeast co-factor that is required at trace levels for satisfactory fermentation. Potassium is particularly necessary for the metabolism of carbohydrates and supports all enzymatic reactions which proceed with ATP. It is more acceptable than sodium from a flavor point of view, giving a salty taste without sour notes. A large amount of potassium (500–600 mg/l) is particularly interesting for the nutritional importance of beer. Due to an osmotic effect, a high potassium content promotes the elimination of sodium and chlorides and therefore helps body dehydration and demineralization (De Stefano and Montanari, 1996). It remains in the final product and accounts for 30% of the recommended daily amount, considering 1 l of medium alcoholic beer as an acceptable daily intake.

Silicon

Beer is a rich source of dietary silicon which is readily absorbed by the body. This silicon comes from two natural sources – water and barley (The Brewer of Europe, 2004). In the form of silicate, it is soluble as a colloid and can be detected in all beer hazes (Kunze, 2004).

Phosphate

Phosphates occur in the structures of many compounds in barley grains (e.g. in phytin, nucleic acids, coenzymes, proteins, etc.). They are released from these compounds in reactions occurring during malting and brewing. Most of the phosphates are bound in phytin that is salts of the organic acid myoinositol hexakis – (dihydrogen phosphate). Phytin is hydrolyzed in the mash tun releasing inorganic phosphate and the B vitamin, myoinosital (deLange, 2004). The amount of phosphate in malt is as much as 1% of its weight (as P_2O_3) according to Briggs *et al.* (1981). The term phosphate refers to compounds that involve the ions of phosphoric acid. Phosphates react with calcium and magnesium as reported earlier. The presence of phosphate is extremely important for fermentation. Phosphorus is required for the formation of ATP, the formation of the phospholipid double membrane around the yeast cell and buffering against pH shift. A deficiency of phosphates causes fermentation problems and reduction in cell growth (Kunze, 2004).

Sulfate

Sulfates positively affect protein and starch degradation, which favors mash filtration and trub sedimentation. However, if the levels are too high, it may result in poor hop utilization (bitterness will not easily be extracted). Sulfates can lend a dry, crisp palate to the finished beer, but if used in excess, the finished beer will have a harsh, salty, and laxative character. The composition of the beer type or beer brand plays an important role in the taste threshold value (TTV). The TTV of $CaSO_4$ in a German lager is 430.5 mg/l, while in wheat beer it is 114.04 mg/l (Schoenberger *et al.*, 2002). Sulfate is absorbed by yeast cells during fermentation (Kunze, 2004).

Chloride

Chloride gives a mellow and full palate. It limits yeast flocculation and improves clarification and colloidal stability.

Nitrate

Nitrate has no effect on beer flavor. It can be reduced to nitrite during the brewing process. Nitrite is a yeast toxin that causes poor multiplication and weak fermentation. Levels as low as 20 mg nitrate/l are dangerous for the yeast (Kunze, 2004).

Zinc

Zinc is found in trace amounts in wort. It is of great physiological importance for protein synthesis and yeast cell growth and thus for fermentation. If zinc is deficient, yeast growth is retarded, fermentation proceeds slowly and there is incomplete reduction of diacetyl. During the brewing process a higher zinc content can be favored by low pH, low mashing temperature, and a grist:liquor ratio of 1:2.5 (Kunze, 2004). However, only about 20% of the zinc in the malt goes into solution on mashing and the zinc content decreases further during mashing. If zinc levels of 0.10–0.15 mg/l are not maintained, the above-mentioned fermentation difficulties may occur because zinc is bound by a number of enzymes, like alcohol, dehydrogenase, and regulatory proteins (Bromber *et al.*, 1997; Kunze, 2004). To compensate for zinc deficiency, zinc chloride, or zinc

Table 34.2 Classic beer styles and the mineral profile of the water of the city where they were developed

Water composition	*Munich beer*	*Pilsner beer*	*Dortmund beer*	*Vienna beer*
Total dissolved solids (mg/l)	284.0	51.2	1,110.0	947.8
Calcium (Ca^{2+}) (mg/l)	75.7	7.0	262.0	162.5
Magnesium (Mg^{2+}) (mg/l)	18.1	0.7	23.0	68.0
SO_4^{2-} (mg/l)	9.0	5.2	289.5	216.5
NO_3^- (mg/l)	Traces	Traces	Traces	Traces
Cl^- (mg/l)	2.0	5.0	107.0	39.0
Total hardness (°dH)[a]	14.8	1.6	41.3	38.5
Non-carbonate hardness (°dH)[a]	0.6	0.3	24.5	7.6
Carbonate hardness (°dH)[a]	14.2	1.3	16.8	30.9

Notes: The mineral content of the brewing water is particularly important for the brewing process. Brewing cities with a characteristic water composition have developed their own style of beer.

[a]dH = German degree.

Source: Schormüller (1968).

sulfate can be added to the wort, but this is not permitted in all countries. Zinc is present in beer at a concentration of 0.02–4.5 ppm.

Sources of Minerals

Most of the minerals in beer derive from the raw materials: brewing water, malt, hops, and adjuncts.

Brewing water

The mineral content of the brewing water is particularly important for the brewing process, and hence for the quality and flavor of the final beer. In the course of time, brewing cities with a characteristic water composition have developed their own styles of beer which are now produced throughout the world, associating the name of the original city with a certain style of beer. For this reason modern brewers add minerals and other natural elements to water or eliminate them by boiling or filtration so that the water used in the brewing process always produces beer with the same flavor and enables brewers to produce identical-tasting beer at different brewing locations throughout the world (Table 34.2).

For example, the Pilsen region of the Czech Republic was the birthplace of the Pilsner style beer which is a crisp, clear golden beer with a very clean hoppy taste. The water of Pilsen is very soft, free of most minerals, and very low in bicarbonates, which allows the proper mash pH to be reached with only base malts. The lack of sulfate provides a mellow hop bitterness. Dortmund Export, a pale lager beer, derives its name from Dortmund, a city in Germany. It has less hop character than a Pilsner, with a more assertive malt character due to higher levels of all minerals. The water of Vienna in Austria is similar to that of Dortmund, but lacks the level of calcium to balance the carbonates, and also lacks sodium and chloride for flavor. So, Vienna malt is used to balance the mash to produce Vienna lager (Frank, 1969; Goldammer, 2000). It is cured at slightly higher temperatures than Pilsner malt. Consequently Vienna malt gives a golden colored beer with increased body. Dark beers require brewing waters rich in carbonate and bicarbonate ions. These ions have a pH-increasing effect which opposes the pH-lowering effect of the dark malts and the other calcium and magnesium ions, present in calcium chloride, calcium sulfate, magnesium chloride, and magnesium sulfate. The calcium, magnesium, and sodium bicarbonates of the brewing water decrease the acidity of the wort in the following order: Ca > Mg > Na. An example of increasing the pH during mashing is the reaction of the acidic potassium dihydrogen phosphate with calcium bicarbonate:

$$\underset{\text{Potassium dihydrogen phosphate}}{2KH_2PO_4} + \underset{\text{Calcium bicarbonate}}{Ca(HCO_3)_2} \rightarrow$$

$$\underset{\text{Calcium hydrogen phosphate}}{CaHPO_4} + \underset{\text{Dipotassium hydrogen phosphate}}{K_2HPO_4} + \underset{\text{Water}}{2H_2O} + \underset{\text{Carbon dioxide}}{2CO_2}$$

Alkaline dipotassium hydrogen phosphate is formed from acidic potassium dihydrogen phosphate (Kunze, 2004).

Malt

In beer most of the minerals originate from the barley. About 75% derives from the malt, while the remaining 25% originates from the water. The minerals include about 35% phosphates (expressed as phosphorous (5)-oxide P_2O_3), about 25% silicates (expressed as silicon dioxide, SiO_2), and about 20% potassium salts (expressed as potassium oxide, K_2O) (Table 34.3).

The mineral composition of the malt depends on the variety, place where it was grown, atmospheric conditions, growing techniques and harvest, storage and malting systems. The malting technique is particularly important.

Table 34.3 Minerals in malt (mg/kg dry matter)

Minerals	*Reference 1*[a]	*Reference 2*[b]	*Reference 3*[c]
K^+		3,530	3,618
PO_4^{3-}	6,329		
Mg^{2+}	1,155	1,370	1,421
Ca^{2+}	479	730	824
Na^+		28.2	25.0
Cl^-	830		
SO_4^{2-}	300		
SiO_2	5,260		

Notes: The quantity of different minerals in malt from different authors.

[a] Kolbach and Rinke (1963).
[b] Holzmann (1975).
[c] Mändl *et al.* (1972).

A short-germinated and undermodified malt has a different grist composition in husks, grits, and flour than a longer-germinated and overmodified malt. In a cereal grain, mineral elements are transferred from the storage tissues to the developing seedling. Minerals are more concentrated in the germ than in the central section, whereas the distal section has an intermediate amount. Rootlets and shoots contain substantially more potassium, phosphorus, iron, zinc, manganese, and copper than kilned malt. Calcium is transported to rootlets but not to shoots, and is more uniformly distributed throughout the kernel than magnesium. High-protein fractions are substantially richer in minerals than low-protein fractions. In differently modified malts, the development of rootlets and acrospires and the extent of metal transport from the central and distal section to the germ end are variable. It can thus be expected that the mineral concentrations in worts derived from such malts will vary. The metal distribution is also highly dependent on protein modification. Consequently, the brewer must carefully plan both malt modification and mashing conditions to achieve a desired mineral level in the wort (Holzman and Piendl, 1976).

Hops

Hops contribute a negligible amount of most minerals in beer because of the small quantities used (200 g to produce 100 l beer). However hops make a notable contribution of nitrate to the beer wort. Approximately 5–30 mg of nitrate/l of wort comes from raw hops or type-90 pellets, depending on beer bitterness and hop variety. A reduction of some 60% can be achieved by using type-45 pellets, the reduction is about 90–95% when using pure ethanol resin extracts, and complete elimination is possible, by using a CO_2 extract (Forster, 1989). New hop products, like potassium salts of the dehydro iso-alpha-acids, are now available that can be added at the end of fermentation to produce a light resistant beer in clear glass bottles, which contribute to the potassium content of the beer. Similarly, the potassium salts of iso-alpha-acids are used to replace bittering hops for utilization or economic reasons and to adjust bitterness in beers that were underhopped in the kettle.

Table 34.4 Minerals in adjuncts

Minerals	*Maize grits (mg/kg)*	*Rice (mg/kg)*
Ca^{2+}	24 ± 8	460 ± 26
K^+	894 ± 93	940 ± 79
Mg^{2+}	270 ± 22	494 ± 25
Na^+	16 ± 7	97 ± 20
PO_4^{2-}	605 ± 15	1,360 ± 25
SiO_2	7.5 ± 1	13.3 ± 8
Zn^{2+}	5.7 ± 0.5	15 ± 1.5

Note: The concentration of the minerals in substitutes of malt.
Source: Moll and Moll (1993).

Adjuncts

In many countries a part of the malt can be substituted with other cereals like maize grits or rice. These cereal matrices normally contain fewer minerals than malt and so the metal level is less than of all-malt wort. Adjunct worts are less buffered, so there is a lower pH during fermentation (Holzman and Piendl, 1976) (Table 34.4).

Influence of the Brewing Process on the Mineral Content of the Beer

The large amount of minerals from the raw materials decreases during mashing due to the formation of insoluble phosphates (e.g. with calcium and magnesium), the formation of salts with the acidic groups of proteins, and the mechanical adsorption on spent grains and trub. The insoluble material precipitates out and thus does not get into the wort. The brewhouse yield of minerals is about 100% for potassium and sodium, 95% for chloride, 84% for sulfuric acid, and 63% for phosphoric acid. More than 50% of the other minerals are lost, and the loss of trace elements is particularly high. The precipitation of nitrogenous compounds at high temperatures removes sequestering agents from the wort leading to a significant loss of minerals. An important parameter that influences the mineral content is the mash concentration. Dilution of the mash concentration leads to a higher solubility of potassium, sodium, calcium, magnesium, manganese, and zinc. Increasing mashing time increases potassium, magnesium, and copper levels and decreases sodium, calcium, iron, manganese, and zinc levels. Wort boiling diminishes the mineral concentration due to metals binding to the precipitated material. With the addition of hops, minerals are also added (Holzman and Piendl, 1976) (Table 34.5).

During fermentation yeast requires minerals, particularly phosphorous and sulfur, as well as a number of metal ions

Table 34.5 Mineral contribution of raw material to the wort (mg/l)

	K^+	Na^+	Ca^{2+}	Mg^{2+}	Cu^{2+}	Fe^{2+}	Mn^{2+}	Zn^{2+}
Malt	556	6	100	184	1.1	6.1	2.1	3.7
Brewing water	3	17	75	21	Traces	0.4	0.04	Traces
Hop	66	Traces	25	9	1.2	0.6	0.3	0.3
Total	627	23	200	214	2.3	7.1	2.4	4.0
Wort 12% *P*	630	24	33	100	0.11	0.05	0.14	0.10
Loss	0	0	83	53	95	99	94	97

Note: The contribution of the different raw materials to the wort minerals and the loss in percent of them after wort boiling during the brewing process due to the formation of insoluble phosphates (e.g. with calcium and magnesium), the formation of salts with the acidic groups of proteins, and the mechanical adsorption on spent grains and trub.

Source: Moll and Moll (1993).

in small amounts. This and other subsequent production steps, like filtration or centrifugation of the final beer, further decrease the mineral content of the beer, bringing it to its desired balanced value.

Summary Points

- There is a well-balanced amount of minerals contained in beer. The principal ions are the cations – calcium, magnesium, sodium, and potassium – with the anions – sulfate, nitrate, phosphate, chlorides, and silicate. The minor ions are iron, copper, zinc, and manganese.
- Ca^{2+} ions derive principally from the brewing water. During mashing they react with malt constituents like phosphates and proteins lowering the pH.
- Magnesium is most important for yeast metabolism during fermentation because it is required by yeast as a co-factor for the production of enzymes that are indispensable for the fermentation process.
- Sodium has its origins in the water supply and brewing ingredients. The level of sodium in malt depends on the levels in the process water at the malt house.
- Potassium is a yeast co-factor and is required at trace levels for satisfactory fermentation and for the metabolism of carbohydrates.
- Phosphates occur in the structures of many compounds in the barley corns (e.g. in phytin, nucleic acids, coenzymes, proteins, etc.). They are released from these compounds in reactions that occur during malting and in the brewery.
- Sulfates positively affect protein and starch degradation, which favors mash filtration and trub sedimentation.
- Zinc is found in trace amounts in wort. It is of great physiological importance for protein synthesis and for yeast cell growth and thus for fermentation.
- The mineral content of the brewing water is particularly important for the brewing process and hence for the quality and flavor of the final beer.
- About 75% of the mineral content derives from the malt, while the remaining 25% originates from the water. The minerals include about 35% phosphates (expressed as phosphorous (5)-oxide P_2O_3), about 25% silicates (expressed as silicon dioxide, SiO_2), and about 20% potassium salts (expressed as potassium oxide, K_2O).
- The mineral composition of the malt depends on the variety, place where it was grown, the atmospheric conditions, growing techniques and harvest, storage and malting systems.
- Hops contribute a negligible amount of the minerals in beer because of the small quantities used (200 g to produce 100 l beer).
- The large amount of minerals from the raw materials decreases during the brewing process due to some minerals being removed through precipitation.
- The brewhouse yield of minerals is about 100% for potassium and sodium, 95% for chloride, 84% for sulfuric acid, and 63% for phosphoric acid. More than 50% of the other minerals are lost, and the loss of trace elements is particularly high.

Acknowledgments

The authors thank Eng. Giorgio Zasio and the Italian Beer and Malt Industries Association (ASSOBIRRA) for the help received in collecting and showing several data reported.

References

Briggs, D.E., Hough, J.S., Stevens, R. and Young, T.W. (1981). *Malting and Brewing Science*, Vol. 1, 2nd edn, pp. 90–91. Chapman & Hall, St Edmundsbury Press, Ltd., Suffolk, UK.

Bromberg, S.K., Bower, P.A., Duncombe, G.R., Fehring, J., Gerber, L. and Tata, M. (1997). *J. Am. Soc. Brew. Chem.* 55, 123–128.

De Stefano, A. and Montanari, L. (1996). *Alcologia* 8, 43–45.

DeLange, A.J. (2004). *Cerevisiae* 29, 188–198.

Dengis, P.B., Nélissen, L.R. and Rouxhet, P.G. (1995). *Appl. Environ. Microbiol.* 61, 718–728.

Forster, A. (1989). Technical publication, www.barthhaasgroup.com (consulted 05/12/2006).

Frank, W.H. (1969). In Acker, L., Bergner, K.G., Diemair, W., Heimann, W., Kiermeier, F., Schormüller, J. and Souci, S.W.

(eds), *Handbugh der Lebensmittelchemie*, Vol. 8/1, pp. 831–833. Springer-Verlag, Berlin, Germany.

Goldammer, T. (2000) *The Brewer's Handbook*, p. 105. Apex Publishers, USA.

Holzmann, A. (1975). *Thesis Technique*. University of Munich, Munich, Germany.

Holzmann, A. and Piendl, A. (1976). *ASBC J.* 35, 1–8.

Kolbach, P. and Rinke, W. (1963). *Monatsschrift fuer Brauerei* 16, 11–16.

Kunze, W. (2004). *Technology of Brewing and Malting*. VLB Berlin, Berlin, Germany.

Madigan, D. and McMurrough, I. (1994). *J. Am. Brew. Chem.* 52, 134–137.

Mändl, B. (1972). *Brauwelt* 115, 1565–1568.

Moll, M.M. (1987). Colloidal stability of beer. In Pollock, J.R.A. (ed.), *Brewing Science*, pp. 2–293. Academic Press, New York, USA.

Moll, M.M. (1995). Water. In Hardwick, W.A. (ed.), *Handbook of Brewing*, pp. 133–156. Marcel Dekker, New York, USA.

Moll, M. and Moll, N. (1993). *Brauerei und Getraenke-Rundschau* 104, 29–36.

Nishihara, H., Fujita, T., Yokoi, N. and Takao, M. (1994). *J. Inst. Brew.* 100, 427–430.

Rehberger, A.J. and Luther, G.E. (1995). In Hardwick, W.A. (ed.), *Handbook of Brewing*, pp. 318–321. Marcel Dekker, New York, USA.

Schoenberger, C., Krottenthaler, M. and Back, W. (2002). *MBAA Tech. Q.* 39, 210–217.

The Brewer of Europe (2004). In Janet Witheridge (ed.), *The Benefits of Moderate Beer Consumption*, 3rd edn, Brewers of Europe, Brussels (www.brewersofeurope.org).

Touhami, A., Hoffmann, B., Vasella, A., Denis, F.A. and Dufrêne, Y.F. (2003). *Microbiology* 149, 2873–2878.

Walker, G.M., Birch, R.M., Chandrasena, G. and Maynard, A.I. (1996). *J. Am. Soc. Brew. Chem.* 54, 13–18.

35

Silicon in Beer: Origin and Concentration

Caroline Walker and Gary Freeman BRI, Lyttel Hall, Nutfield, Surrey, UK
Ravin Jugdaohsingh MRC Human Nutrition Research, Elsie Widdowson Laboratory, Cambridge, UK
Gastrointestinal Laboratory, The Rayne Institute (King's College London), St. Thomas' Hospital, London, UK
Department of Nutrition, King's College London, London, UK
Jonathan J. Powell MRC Human Nutrition Research, Elsie Widdowson Laboratory, Cambridge, UK

Abstract

There is increasing support for an important biological role of the trace element, silicon, in the optimal health of connective tissue, especially bone. Beer contains high levels of dietary silicon, in the well absorbed and biologically active form of orthosilicic acid [$Si(OH)_4$]. It is widely accepted that barley, especially following malting and maceration, provides the major source of silicon within beer. However, how the different aspects of the brewing process then influence the final beer–silicon concentration is not known. Here we describe the findings of two previously unreported studies. First, we confirm that beer contains a high level (typically around 20 mg/l) of silicon. Secondly, from a pilot brewing trial, we show that barley is the major source of silicon in beer. Two different malts (malted barley) had distinctly different silicon concentrations, presumably because silicon levels of barley vary genetically. Silicon levels of the final product also depended on mashing and rinsing (sparging) conditions during the brewing process while filtration was also shown to affect (reduce) silicon levels of the beer, probably due to adsorption of orthosilicic acid onto material that is trapped by or that comprises the filter. Silicon levels of the water used for brewing are likely to have a small additional influence on the final beer–silicon levels, but in this particular work were negligible.

List of Abbreviations

FV	Fermenter vessel
KG	Kieselguhr
PG	Present gravity
PVPP	Polyvinylpolypyrollidone
RO	Reverse osmosis
XE5/XE200	Filtration sheets employed consecutively in filtration operation

Introduction

Silicon is an ubiquitous environmental element that is second only to oxygen in terms of elemental makeup of the earth's crust. Nonetheless, the role of silicon in human biology and health remains enigmatic although there is increasing support for an important biological role of this trace element, when delivered in its orthosilicic acid form [$Si(OH)_4$], in the optimal health of connective tissue, especially bone, skin and blood vessels. Interested readers are referred to a recent review by Sripanyakorn *et al.* (2005) as well as to the Chapter 80 in this book. Indeed, this latter chapter is relevant because of the realization that beer is a potentially rich dietary source of silicon in a form that can be well absorbed by humans into the bloodstream (Sripanyakorn *et al.*, 2004).

Although the source water in the brewing process is likely to contribute to the final beer–silicon content, it is widely accepted that barley, especially following malting and maceration, provides the major source of silicon within beer. However, how the different aspects of the brewing process influence the final beer–silicon concentration is not known. This chapter briefly presents the typical levels of silicon that are found within beers and then reports on an investigation into the unit operations within the brewing process by sampling the process streams at appropriate points for silicon analysis. Thus information has been gained on the inputs, losses and fractionation of silicon in the process. This work was undertaken by two of the authors (Walker and Freeman) at the pilot brewery of BRI and samples then analyzed as previously reported (Sripanyakorn *et al.*, 2004) by Jugdaohsingh and Powell at St. Thomas' Hospital. For solid or slurry samples, prior acid-assisted microwave digestion was undertaken.

Beer in Health and Disease Prevention
ISBN: 978-0-12-373891-2

The Silicon Content of Alcoholic Beverages

We previously reported a mean (±SD) concentration of 19.2 ± 6.6 mg Si/l beer from the analysis of 76 different beers (range: 9–39.4 mg/l; Sripanyakorn *et al.*, 2004). Silicon concentration was not dependent on geographic origin, type of beer, alcohol content or the type of storage and packaging (Sripanyakorn *et al.*, 2004). In contrast, levels of silicon in wines are more varied and although they can be as high as some beers in a recent small analysis (Powell *et al.*, 2005), actual intakes of silicon in terms of servings are at least fivefold lower: 0.62–2.89 mg Si/serving wine (one glass or 125 ml) compared with 3.8–16.3 mg Si/serving for beers (300–574 ml) (Powell *et al.*, 2005). Moreover, it is not clear what the chemical form of silicon is in wine as it may be added as a colloidal, insoluble form during fining (post-vinification). Such an addition is less common in beer, and therefore the silicon is usually only present as soluble orthosilicic acid (Sripanyakorn *et al.*, 2004). Silicon levels in liquors/spirits are much lower being 1.3 ± 0.04 mg/l (Jugdaohsingh *et al.*, 2004) and intake from these beverages are completely unimportant in terms of dietary silicon exposure. Table 35.1 shows analytical results for a small series of previously unreported beer, wine and spirit samples that were analyzed in a single batch with individual sample-based standards. These data emphasize the dominant role of beer in its potential to provide dietary silicon amongst the alcoholic beverages, especially given the likelihood that it is drunk in larger volumetric quantities.

Table 35.1 The silicon content of beers, wines and spirits

	Silicon (mg/l)		
Alcoholic beverages	*Mean*	*Range*	*N*
Beers			
Can lager	20.7	15.4–26.4	4
Can bitter	14.5	9.59–20.1	4
Draft lager	21.5	11.7–39.4	6
Draft bitter/mild	21.0	13.5–30.1	11
Ciders	3.70	2.72–5.53	3
Wines (2 white; 1 red)	7.67	6.61–9.24	3
Spirits	1.26	0.56–2.06	12
Ports/sherry		14.15–19.59	2

Note: Silicon concentrations of different beers available in London (UK) in shops and/or pubs and, for comparison, silicon levels in spirits and wines are also shown. Silicon concentrations were determined by inductively coupled plasma optical emission spectrometry, from sample-based standards. *N* = number of samples analyzed.

Changes in Silicon Content Through the Brewing Process

A pilot study was undertaken to investigate how the different aspects of the brewing process influences the final beer–silicon concentration. The process employed in the pilot brew (Figure 35.1) was typical of commercial brewing processes. Brewing water was tap water that had been through the process of reverse osmosis (RO). The malted barley was milled (ground). Barley varieties were "Pearl" as the standard brewing malt (87.5% by mass of the grist) and crystal malt, which is highly flavored (12.5%). This was then mixed with the hot brewing water (3 kg water to 1 kg malt) and maintained at 64°C for 60 min in a process known as mashing. The separation of liquid from spent grains, or "run-off," involved raising the temperature to 78°C and draining the liquid (sweet wort). The spent grains were then rinsed with water at 78°C (sparging), until the bulked sweet wort volume was 86 l. Yeast (351 wet grams of *Saccharomyces cerevisiae strain NCYC 1681*) was then added and wort fermented for 6 days at 18°C. A 3-day maturation period at 13°C was employed, followed by cold maturation at 3°C for 1 day. Subsequently the settled yeast was removed, followed by cold storage for a minimum of 7 days at 0°C. The beer sample was divided into two, and one sample was filtered through XE5/XE200 filter sheets and bottled. The other sample was filtered through kieselguhr at a dosage rate of 1 g/l. Samples of the bottled beer were processed separately through stabilizers, silica hydrogel (0.8 g/l) and polyvinylpolypyrollidone (PVPP) (0.5 g/l).

Samples collected at the different stages of the brewing process were analyzed by inductively coupled plasma optical emission spectrometry as previously described (Sripanyakorn *et al.*, 2004). Solid or slurry samples were prior digested by acid-assisted microwave digestion.

The brewing process, and the points at which samples were taken for analysis, are shown in Figure 35.1 while the analytical results, and any specific observations (comment) on the sample at the time of analysis, are given in Table 35.2.

Silicon ingress to the process from treated brewing water (liquor) was insignificant in these trials (Table 35.1). However, it should be noted that some water supplies have significant silicon content and the possibility should be considered that this passes *pro rata* through to the finished product. Regardless of the starting liquor silicon content, barley malt is an obvious major source of silicon in beer. Greater than 80% of silicon is in the cereal husks and absolute silicon levels vary between different varieties of barley, which appears to be at least partly genetically determined (Ma *et al.*, 2003). This would translate into different silicon contents of the chosen malts (i.e. malted barley) used for brewing. For example, in this work (Table 35.2), standard ale malt contained 0.28 mg Si/g malt while crystal malt (a darker, toffee-tasting malt) contained 0.45 mg Si/g malt.

Next we considered how silicon from the malted barley passed into solution and into the final product itself (beer). While the initial stirring of the malt in hot water, released

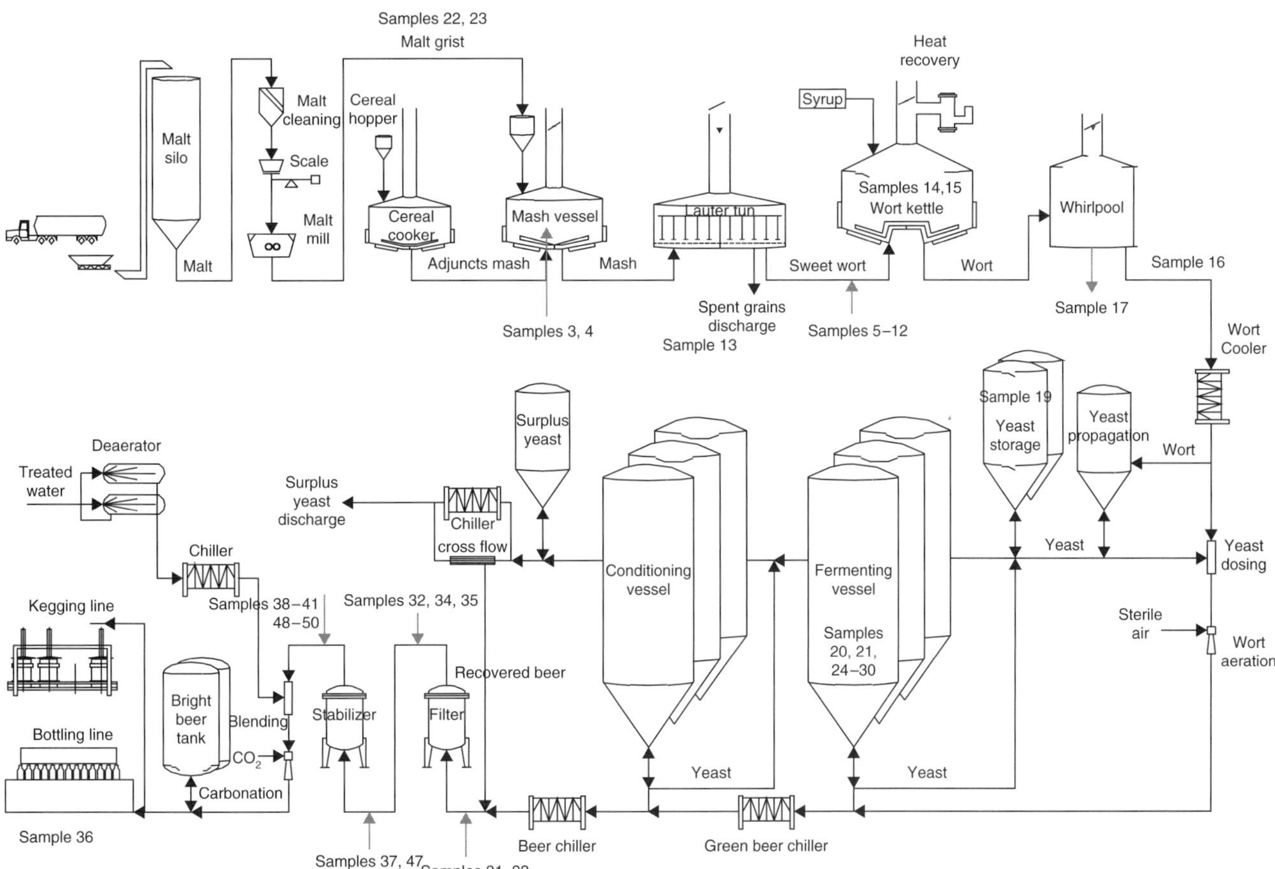

Figure 35.1 The brewing process and samples taken for analysis. Schematic of the brewing process used and the identification of the points at which sampling were undertaken (i.e. sample numbers) for silicon analysis as reported in Table 35.2.

approximately 10 mg Si/l, the first few rinses with very hot water released a further 10–60%, which, with continued rinsing, rapidly fell away as the washed husks were exhausted in terms of dissolvable sugar and silicon (Figure 35.2).

Thus, it is clear that not only does the brewing process release silicon from the malted barley into solution but the rinsing process, that brewers use to recover sugar from the leftover husks, also results in increasing the silicon content of the beer.

Nonetheless, in this work only 19% of the silicon in the malted barley was recovered into the beer. Fermentation had no effect on the silicon content of the beer (Figure 35.3), so the remaining silicon was left in the husks. It would be interesting to see how brewing techniques that grind the husks more finely could further affect how much silicon is released into the final product (presumably increased due to an increase in surface area of the husks). Interestingly, filtration reduced the beer–silicon content by one-third (Figure 35.3), in spite of the fact that orthosilicic acid ($Si(OH)_4$), which is the form of silicon almost exclusively present in beer, is too small to be retained directly as a consequence of filtration. However, there is a possibility of the adsorption of silicon directly onto the filtration mat or indirectly onto material (e.g. yeast cells) trapped by the filtration mat. It should be noted that some brewers also use silicon-containing filters but we found no loss of silicon from these into the beer.

Many brands of beer are treated with process aids (materials that are employed in the brewing process that come into contact with the product, but have no function in the final product). These include kieselguhr (filtration aid, samples 33–35 in Table 35.2) and colloidal stabilizers such as silica hydrogel (samples 37–41) and PVPP (samples 47–50). The effect of these materials was measured on a laboratory pressure filter (a "Walton" filter). There was some evidence of adsorptive loss onto the PVPP but not the kieselguhr or silica hydrogel.

In summary, the silicon content of the beer in this work was at the low end of that found in commercial samples, and this was only a single pilot study, but certain conclusions can still be drawn with confidence. The data clearly show that macerated barley is the predominant source of silicon in beer and that aspects of the brewing process including choice of malt, extent of grinding, maceration and rinsing, as well as filtration could impact upon silicon levels of the final product. These factors will vary between breweries causing the wide range of silicon content seen in commercial beers and explaining why geographical variation and the style/type of beer are not significant factors in determining beer–silicon content.

Table 35.2 Silicon content of samples at the different points of the pilot brewing process

Sample	*Description*	*Comments*	*Si concentration (mg/l)*	*μg Si/g of sample*
1	Water post-RO		0.046	
2	Water post-burtonisation		0.060	
3	Mash at 5 min			27.248
4	Mash end 1 h			17.194
5	Sweet wort at 2 l run-off	PG = 75.27, pH = 5.26	10.034	
6	Sweet wort at 12 l run-off	PG = 71.07, pH = 5.24	9.831	
7	Sweet wort at 24 l run-off	PG = 68.94, pH = 5.21	11.413	
8	Sweet wort at 36 l run-off	PG = 58.38, pH = 5.20	16.170	
9	Sweet wort at 48 l run-off	PG = 35.55, pH = 5.20	13.034	
10	Sweet wort at 60 l run-off	PG = 19.82, pH = 5.22	10.475	
11	Sweet wort at 72 l run-off	PG = 10.90, pH = 5.22	7.661	
12	Sweet wort at 84 l run-off	PG = 6.65, pH = 5.25	6.646	
13	Spent grains			305.850
14	Start boil (less than 5 min) after hop extract and syrup addition		9.500	
15	Boil end (55 min of 1 h boil)			7.366
16	Whirlpool stand end (30 min)			7.401
17	Trub ex-whirlpool	Very wet: volume about 4.5 l		7.740
18	Wort receiver after cutting	PG in FV = 38.4		5.037
19	Pitching yeast			87.873
20	Fermentation day 2	PG = 27.6	11.954	
21	Fermentation day 3	PG = 22.2	13.037	
22	Pale ale malt	BuhlerMiag milled 0.2 mm		279.441
23	Crystal malt	BuhlerMiag milled 0.2 mm		448.656
24	Fermentation day 4	PG = 19.0	12.048	
25	Fermentation day 5	PG = 14.4	12.080	
26	Fermentation day 6	PG = 9.9	11.692	
27	Fermentation day 7	Warm rest 13°C	11.813	
28	Fermentation day 8	Warm rest 13°C	12.175	
29	Fermentation day 9	Warm rest 13°C	12.026	
30	Fermentation day 10	Warm rest 13°C	12.241	
31	Pre-filter XE5/XE200	No PVPP	14.599	
32	Post-filter XE5/XE200	No PVPP	9.120	
33	Pre-KG filter		12.132	
34	Early run KG filtrate	Dilution possible	6.356	
35	KG filtrate bulked		9.720	
36	Bottled beer	Pasteurized		
37	Pre-silica gel	Should be as 36	12.119	
38	Silica gel treated early run	Dilution possible	6.865	
39	Silica gel mid-run		11.162	
40	Silica gel late run		12.369	
41	Silica gel treated bulked		10.338	
42	Walton filter control initial feed		11.903	
43	Control "filtrate" early run		11.075	
44	Control "filtrate" late run		11.939	
45	Control "filtrate" bulked		11.898	
46	Control feed end		12.311	
47	Pre-PVPP start		11.968	
48	Post-PVPP start		1.078	
49	Post-PVPP end		7.399	
50	Post-PVPP bulked		5.046	

Note: Silicon concentration of samples taken at different points of the pilot brewing process (see Figure 35.1 for a schematic representation of the brewing process and points where the samples were collected). Collected samples were analyzed by inductively coupled plasma optical emission spectrometry as previously described (Sripanyakorn *et al.*, 2004). Solid or slurry samples were prior digested by acid-assisted microwave digestion. Specific observations or measurements made on the sample during the brewing process are tabulated under comments. FV: fermenter vessel. KG: Kieselguhr, a filtration aid. PG: present gravity, measured in saccharin, equivalent to density (at 20°C, kg/m^3) × 1,000. PVPP: polyvinylpolypyrollidone, a colloidal stabilization agent. XE5, XE200: filtration sheets employed consecutively in filtration operation.

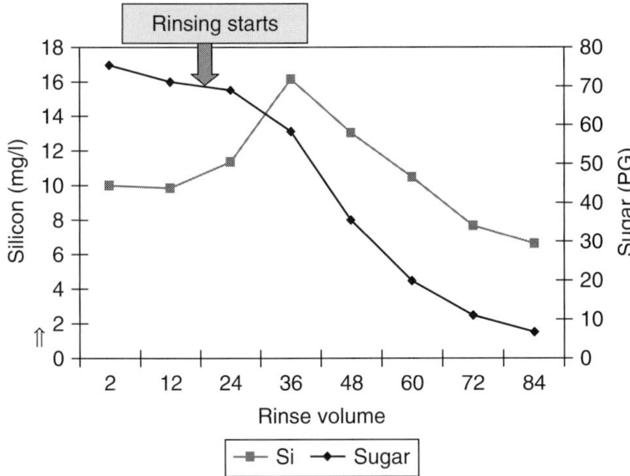

Figure 35.2 Release of silicon and sugars from the malt during rinsing. Silicon (Si) levels (mg/l) in solution as malted barley is stirred and rinsed with separate volumes of hot water. Sugar levels are also shown based on present gravity (PG; equivalent to density (at 20°C, kg/m^3) × 1,000). The individual rinses are combined with the liquor (sweet wort) collected prior to rinsing and the pooled sample then fermented.

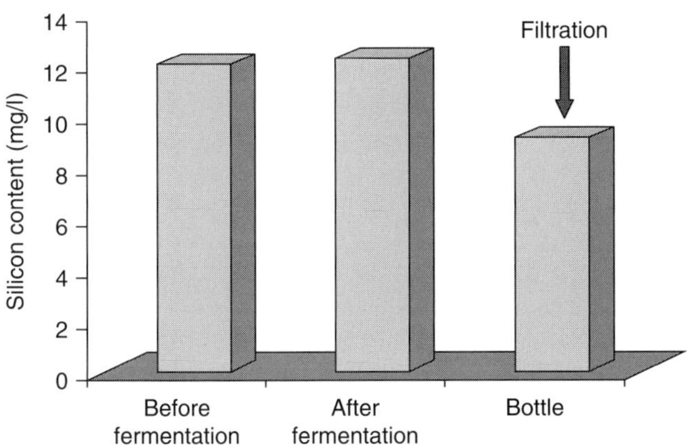

Figure 35.3 The effects of fermentation and filtration on silicon content of the beer. Silicon content (mg/l) of beer before fermentation, after fermentation and following filtration through XE5/XE200 filter sheets where a loss in soluble silicon is observed.

Summary Points

- Beer contains a high level (typically around 20 mg/l) of soluble and absorbable dietary silicon.
- Barley is the major source of silicon in beer.
- Silicon levels of barley vary genetically and thus different malts (malted barley) have varying silicon contents.
- Silicon levels of the final product also depend on mashing and rinsing conditions during the brewing process.
- Filtration may also affect (reduce) silicon levels of the beer due to adsorption onto material that is trapped by or comprises the filter.
- The process aid PVPP, which is employed as a colloidal stabilizer in some brands of beers, may remove some silicon by adsorption but further confirmatory trials should be performed.
- Silicon levels of the water used for brewing are likely to have a small additional influence on the final beer–silicon levels.

Acknowledgments

The work was funded by the Institute and Guild of Brewers in the United Kingdom (now termed the Institute of Brewing and Distilling) and we are grateful for their support as well as the British Beer and Pub Association for their guidance. We also acknowledge Hazel Elliot for assistance with the analysis and other aspects of the studies.

References

Jugdaohsingh, R., Tucker, K.L., Qiao, N., Cupples, L.A., Kiel, D.P. and Powell, J.J. (2004). *J. Bone Miner. Res.* 19, 297–307.

Ma, J.F., Higashitani, A., Sato, K. and Takeda, K. (2003). *Plant Soil.* 249, 383–387.

Powell, J.J., McNaughton, S.A., Jugdaohsingh, R., Anderson, S., Dear, J., Khot, F., Mowatt, L., Gleason, K.L., Sykes, M., Thompson, R.P.H., Bolton-Smith, C. and Hodson, M.J. (2005). *Br. J. Nutr.* 94, 804–812.

Sripanyakorn, S., Jugdaohsingh, R., Elliott, H., Walker, C., Mehta, P., Shoukru, S., Thompson, R.P.H. and Powell, J.J. (2004). *Br. J. Nutr.* 91, 403–409.

Sripanyakorn, S., Jugdaohsingh, R., Thompson, R.P.H. and Powell, J.J. (2005). *Br. Nutr. Found. Nutr. Bull.* 30, 222–230.

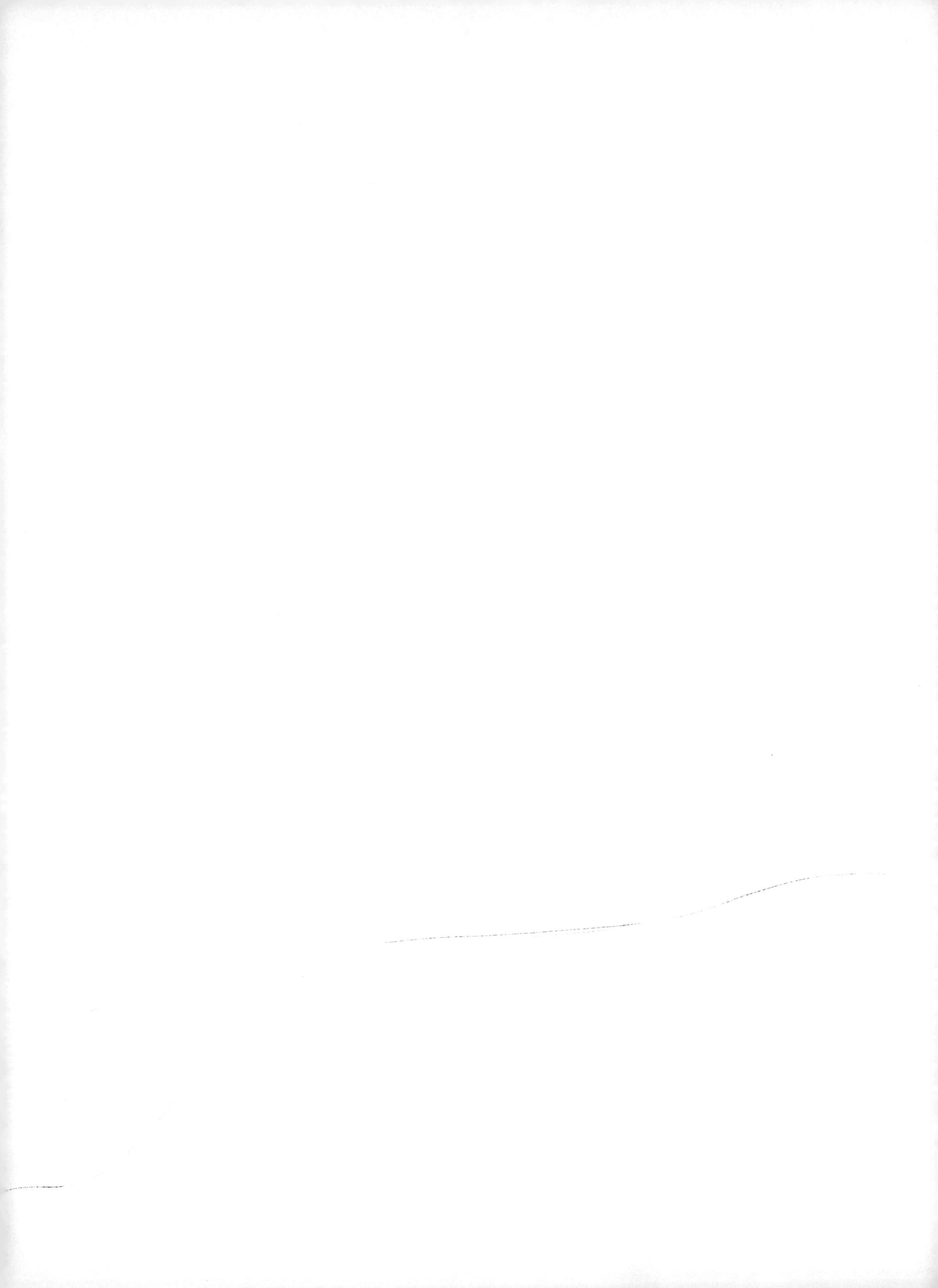

(iv) Beer Stability and Spoilage

36

The Chemistry of Aging Beer

D.P. De Schutter, D. Saison, F. Delvaux, G. Derdelinckx and F.R. Delvaux Department of Microbial and Molecular Systems, Centre for Malting and Brewing Science, Catholic University of Leuven, Belgium

Abstract

Packaged beer is a closed system that continuously will be submitted to alterations by chemical reactions. These alterations will lead to perceivable changes in flavor, foam and colloidal stabilities. In this chapter, the underlying mechanisms of the reactions leading to aging of beer are discussed. Radical reactions, often initiated by reactive oxygen species, have an important contribution to beer staling and form a continuous thread to the stability of beer. Oxidation of unsaturated fatty acids and Maillard reactions leads to hundreds of different compounds. Furthermore degradation of hop bitter acids and carotenoids, oxidation of polyphenols, hydrolysis of glycosides and esters or synthesis of esters, acetalization of aldehydes will all contribute to the aging of beer. When using antioxidants, attention has to be paid to the slower reacting oxygen species such as H_2O_2, rather than the most reactive species as the hydroxyl radical.

List of Abbreviations

1-DH	1-Deoxy-2,3-hexodiulose
3-DH	3-Deoxy-2-hexosulose
$^3RF^{\bullet}$	Riboflavin radical
HMF	Hydroxymethylfurfural
MBT	3-Methyl-2-butene-1-thiol
PVPP	Polyvinylpolypyrrolidone

Introduction

Every living creature alters its environment due to the continuous exchange of metabolites. A closed system will be highly influenced by this metabolism and will evolve to a state of thermodynamic non-equilibrium, far from the minimal Gibbs free energy. When this living entity is removed, a myriad of chemical reactions will slowly lead toward the chemical equilibrium of the system. This principle also counts for beer fermentation. Yeast in concentrations of 60 up to 120 million cells/ml will convert wort sugars into alcohol and CO_2, while producing secondary metabolites and converting components already present in the fermenting wort. Some of these compounds are present above their flavor threshold, while others are precursors of potent compounds arising during beer aging, altering the quality of the beer. When yeast is removed from beer before packaging, exogenous enzymes will still be present, influencing the chemical composition of the beer by enzymatic reactions. When finally the beer is pasteurized, the reactions will have a pure chemical origin, ultimately leading to the minimal enthalpy and maximal entropy. Some of these alterations will remain unnoticed, but others will lead to significant changes in beer flavor, haze and foam stability. While microbiological and colloidal stabilities are largely under control, flavor stability still remains a major concern to the brewer in the twenty-first century. More precisely it is the flavor instability or flavor deterioration that upsets a brewer. If the consumer cannot identify the flavor perception of the tasted beer with the expectation of that particular fresh brand, the beer will be called aged. However, the consumer will not necessarily have less appreciation for the aged beer, as flavor perception is a very personal sensation. Nevertheless flavor stability remains the engine of beer-aging research. At first, with the discovery of (E)-2-nonenal (Palamand and Hardwick, 1969; Jamieson and Van Gheluwe, 1970), the primary focus was set on the oxidation of lipids. At present, it is clear that not only lipid oxidation is responsible for beer deterioration, as other reactions such as radical chain reactions, Maillard reactions, degradation reactions of polyphenols and hop bitter acids also play an important role. This chapter intends to obtain insight in the extreme complexity of beer-aging reactions, focussing on the reaction mechanisms and the chemical nature of compounds, rather than the flavor appreciation that is crucial to brewers.

Chemical Changes During Beer Aging

Pure chemically, beer has to be considered as a water–ethanol solution (ethanol content 3–12 vol.%) with a pH between 4 and 4.5 and several hundreds, or thousands of

Beer in Health and Disease Prevention
ISBN: 978-0-12-373891-2

different compounds. The nature of these compounds can vary from very small volatiles as methanethiol to high-molecular, non-volatile proteins, polyphenols and melanoidins. As these compounds are not in chemical equilibrium, formation and degradation processes will take place during beer storage. Each reaction rate is determined by its reaction rate constant, its activation energy and the initial concentration of substrates, and largely depends on the storage temperature (the storage temperature has to be kept as low as possible) and the initial concentration of the reagents. Therefore, every different kind of beer will age in a typical way, determined by the raw materials, production parameters, packaging techniques and storage conditions. An important staling agent is oxygen, which is present in low levels in beer bottles. Although modern equipment allows not more than 20–50 ppb (μg/l) oxygen in the bottled beer, it is impossible to have the headspace entirely oxygen-free. In this section, first the role of oxygen on radical formation will be discussed, followed by two main chemical reaction pathways: lipid oxidation and Maillard reactions. Then individual beer staling reactions will be considered and finally some antioxidants and pro-oxidants will be highlighted.

Formation of reactive oxygen species

Oxygen in its ground state ($^3O_2$) is relatively non-reactive; it seems thus unlikely that oxygen immediately attacks beer constituents after beer is bottled. However, by energy, light or catalytic activity, activated forms of oxygen can be generated (reactive oxygen species), like singlet oxygen ($^1O_2$), superoxide ($O_2^{\bullet-}$), hydroperoxyl radical ($^{\bullet}OOH$), hydroxyl radical ($^{\bullet}OH$) and hydrogen peroxide (H_2O_2). Reactive oxygen species, as the name indicates, have a strong activity which allows them to react with different kinds of components (Halliwell and Gutteridge, 1984; Bamforth and Parsons, 1985). Recently a general generation pathway (Figure 36.1) of reactive oxygen species in beer has been proposed (Kaneda *et al.*, 1999). First, $O_2^{\bullet-}$ will be produced from O_2 during storage of beer. This reaction will be catalyzed by the oxidation of Fe^{2+} ions or Cu^+ ions to Fe^{3+} and Cu^{2+}, both present in beer in trace amounts. The pKa value of $O_2^{\bullet-}/^{\bullet}OOH$ is 4.7–4.9, the $^{\bullet}OOH$ radical being the most reactive species. Thus the low pH value of beer slightly favors the formation of $^{\bullet}OOH$, unless $O_2^{\bullet-}$ is further reduced to O_2^{2-}. Due to the high pKa values of O_2^{2-}/HO_2^- and HO_2^-/H_2O_2, predominantly H_2O_2 will be formed in beer. It is believed that the formation of hydrogen peroxide is a consequence of mixed function oxidation systems, which involve oxygen in its ground state, Fe^{3+} and Cu^{2+}, but also require electron donors, like ethanol (Chapon and Chapon, 1979), ascorbic acid (Brezova *et al.*, 2002), polyphenols, isohumulones and melanoidins (Irwin *et al.*, 1991; Morales, 2005). Next, $^{\bullet}OH$ is produced by metal-catalyzed reactions such as the Fenton reaction and the Haber–Weiss reaction.

There seems to occur a so-called lag-time in beer before the $^{\bullet}OH$ radical is formed during storage. In that period endogenous antioxidants in beer consume the $O_2^{\bullet-}$, O_2^{2-} and H_2O_2 produced during the coupled oxidation reactions, before the $^{\bullet}OH$ radical can be formed (Uchida *et al.*, 1996). It was reported that an antagonistic action of pro-oxidants,

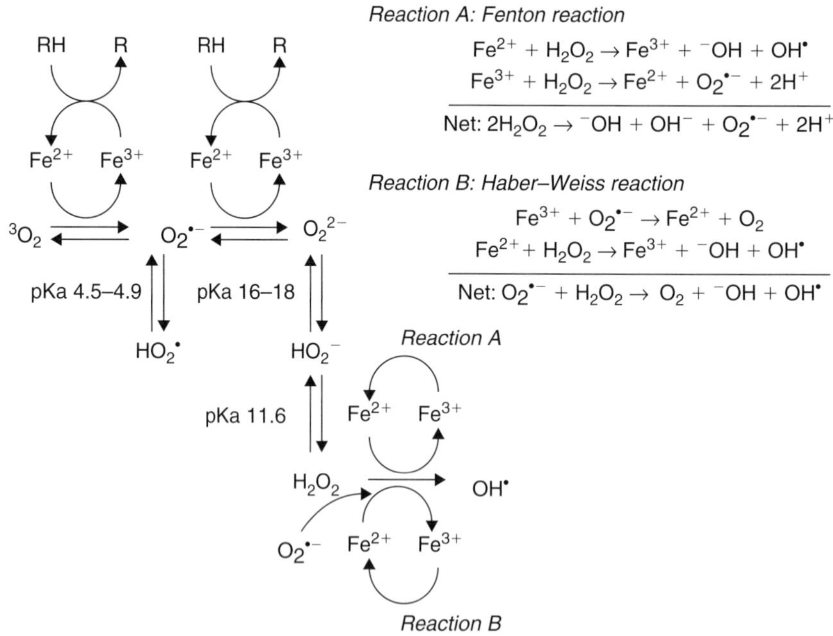

Figure 36.1 Creation of reactive oxygen species (Reprinted from Vanderhaegen *et al.*, 2006, Copyright (2006), with permission from Elsevier). Stable $^3O_2$ will be converted to O_2- and $O_2^{2}-$ by mixed function oxidation systems. Hydrogen peroxide in combination with Fe^{21} or Cu^1 will generate the $OH^{\bullet}$ via the Fenton reaction or the Haber–Weiss reaction.

like iron and Maillard reaction products, shortens the lag-time (Uchida and Ono, 2000). Pro-oxidants are defined as compounds that are known to be able to produce H_2O_2 (like cysteine or sulfhydryl group containing proteins), or are known to be able to reduce metal ions to the oxidation states that are active for the Fenton reactions with peroxides as mentioned before (Brezova *et al.*, 2002).

Antioxidants are defined as compounds able to quench peroxides (like sulfite), or able to inactivate trace amounts of metals that otherwise may generate hydroxyl or alkoxyl radicals from the peroxides (Andersen *et al.*, 2000). After depletion of these antioxidants, $^{\bullet}OH$ radicals will accumulate and can cause damage to beer components. The $^{\bullet}OH$ radical displays a high reactivity toward several beer compounds such as ethanol, sugars, isohumulones, polyphenols, alcohols, fatty acids, etc. This can initiate a series of reactions responsible for the production of carbonyl and phenolic radicals and ultimately lead to staling compounds in beer. This lack of specificity of the $^{\bullet}OH$ radical makes it almost impossible to quench this radical intermediate in beer by adding antioxidants that would react specifically with this radical. Hydrogen peroxide and organic hydroperoxides are the only reactive oxygen species that are stable enough to be trapped efficiently by antioxidants which are normally present in micro-molecular concentrations (Andersen *et al.*, 2000). Because of the high reactivity of ethanol, being the most abundant compound in beer, this compound will be the primary reactant of $^{\bullet}OH$ radical, resulting in the $EtO^{\bullet}$ radical. This radical will bind oxygen, resulting in acetaldehyde and the hydroperoxyl radical (Figure 36.2). The latter can be reduced to hydrogen peroxide, which can react again with metal ions to continue the radical chain reactions (Andersen and Skibsted, 1998). As it is impossible to know all of the variables necessary to prevent oxidative deterioration by reactive oxygen species, minimization of radical formation will be the best strategy. This can be accomplished by keeping the level of O_2 as low as possible, by lowering the temperature, and by introducing chain breakers or quenchers, generally referred to as antioxidants (Bamforth, 2001).

Oxidation of unsaturated fatty acids

Since the identification of (E)-2-nonenal as the volatile which is presumed to be responsible for the cardboard flavor of aged beer (Jamieson and Van Gheluwe, 1970, Palamand and Hardwick, 1969), this powerful odorant was embraced by all beer researchers as the principal cause of beer deterioration. These findings directed the beer-staling research toward the formation of (E)-2-nonenal by the oxidation of unsaturated fatty acids (Drost *et al.*, 1971; Stenroos *et al.*, 1976; Dale *et al.*, 1977; Tressl *et al.*, 1979).

There are two pathways to the oxidation of unsaturated fatty acids: enzymatic oxidation (Drost *et al.*, 1971) and autoxidation (Lindsay, 1973). Enzymatic oxidation occurs during mashing. Due to the activity of both lipase and lipoxygenase, present in malt, linoleic and linolenic acid hydroperoxides are formed (Kobayashi *et al.*, 1993). The limitation of oxygen ingress and a mashing-in temperature at 65°C can decrease the production of hydroxy fatty acids during mashing (Kobayashi *et al.*, 2000b). Nevertheless, the levels of dihydroxyoctadecenoic acid and trihydroxyoctadecenoic acid in commercial beer vary between 0.6–1.6 ppm and 6–15 ppm, respectively (Kobayashi *et al.*, 2000a).

During the boiling process, the enzymes are inactivated due to the high temperature in the wort kettle. As the presence of oxygen cannot completely be excluded, reactive oxygen species are formed due to heat addition to wort. These reactive oxygen species attack susceptible double bonds of oleic, linoleic and linolenic acid, resulting in predominantly 9- and 13-hydroperoxides. Further breakdown of these hydroperoxides leads to the formation of (E)-2-nonenal and other aldehydes. As reduction of these compounds by yeast occurs during fermentation and maturation, it seems evident that yeast exerts a high influence on the overall flavor stability of beer (Wackerbauer *et al.*, 2003).

Despite all the beer-aging models, actual lipid oxidation neither does not seem to occur in bottled beer at normal storage temperatures, nor can nonenol oxidation account for the presence of (E)-2-nonenal (Lermusieau *et al.*, 1999). The total amount of (E)-2-nonenal in aged beer originates from autoxidation during wort boiling (Noël *et al.*, 1999), and enzymatic action during mashing (Liegeois *et al.*, 2002). During mashing and wort boiling, (E)-2-nonenal

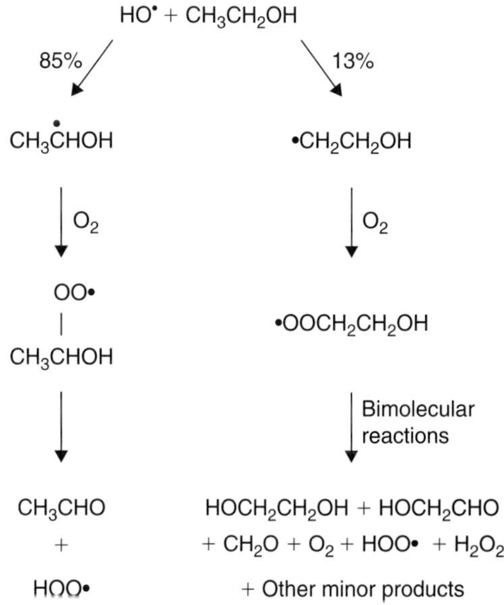

Figure 36.2 Radical reaction of OH with ethanol (Reprinted from Andersen and Skibsted, 1998, with permission from the American Chemical Society). Ethanol is the most abundant molecule in beer and the non-selective $^{\bullet}OH$-radical will quickly react predominantly with ethanol. Preferentially, this will lead to acetaldehyde and the perhydroxyl radical, which after reduction to H_2O_2 can regenerate $^{\bullet}OH$ via the Fenton or Haber–Weiss oxidation pathway.

can form an imine adduct with amino acids and proteins through the formation of Schiff's base. Hence the compound is protected from reduction to nonenol by yeast (Noël and Collin, 1995). During beer aging, (E)-2-nonenal can again gradually be released by acid hydrolysis of (E)-2-nonenal-adducts at beer pH (Lermusieau *et al.*, 1999).

Measures were taken to prevent or to limit oxygen ingress in the brewhouse, which will lead to a decreased oxidation of unsaturated fatty acids, but oxygen cannot completely be excluded during wort production and wort treatment in practical brewing (Drost *et al.*, 1990).

The Maillard reaction

The Maillard reaction predominantly occurs during wort production due to the high temperatures, but some of the reactions will continue during beer storage, even at low temperature.

Initial Reaction Initiated by the reaction of a reducing sugar and an amino-compound, the Maillard reactions develop as a highly complex labyrinth of pathways, which are at present not yet fully elucidated. The complexity of the Maillard reactions was first visualized 40 years after its discovery in a complex scheme of reactions and products (Hodge, 1953). The non-enzymatic browning reactions are ubiquitous in all processed food products; hence they will occur during the production of wort (Tressl, 1979) and continue during beer storage (Bravo *et al.*, 2002).

After mashing, the fermentable sugar content of wort consists of 10% glucose, 60–70% maltose (2 glucose-units linked together in an α-1,4 glycosidic linkage) and 20–30% maltotriose (3 units). Due to the high sugar level and the presence of amino compounds, the Maillard reaction will easily and rapidly occur during wort boiling. An overview of the Maillard reaction involving monomer formation is depicted in Figure 36.3.

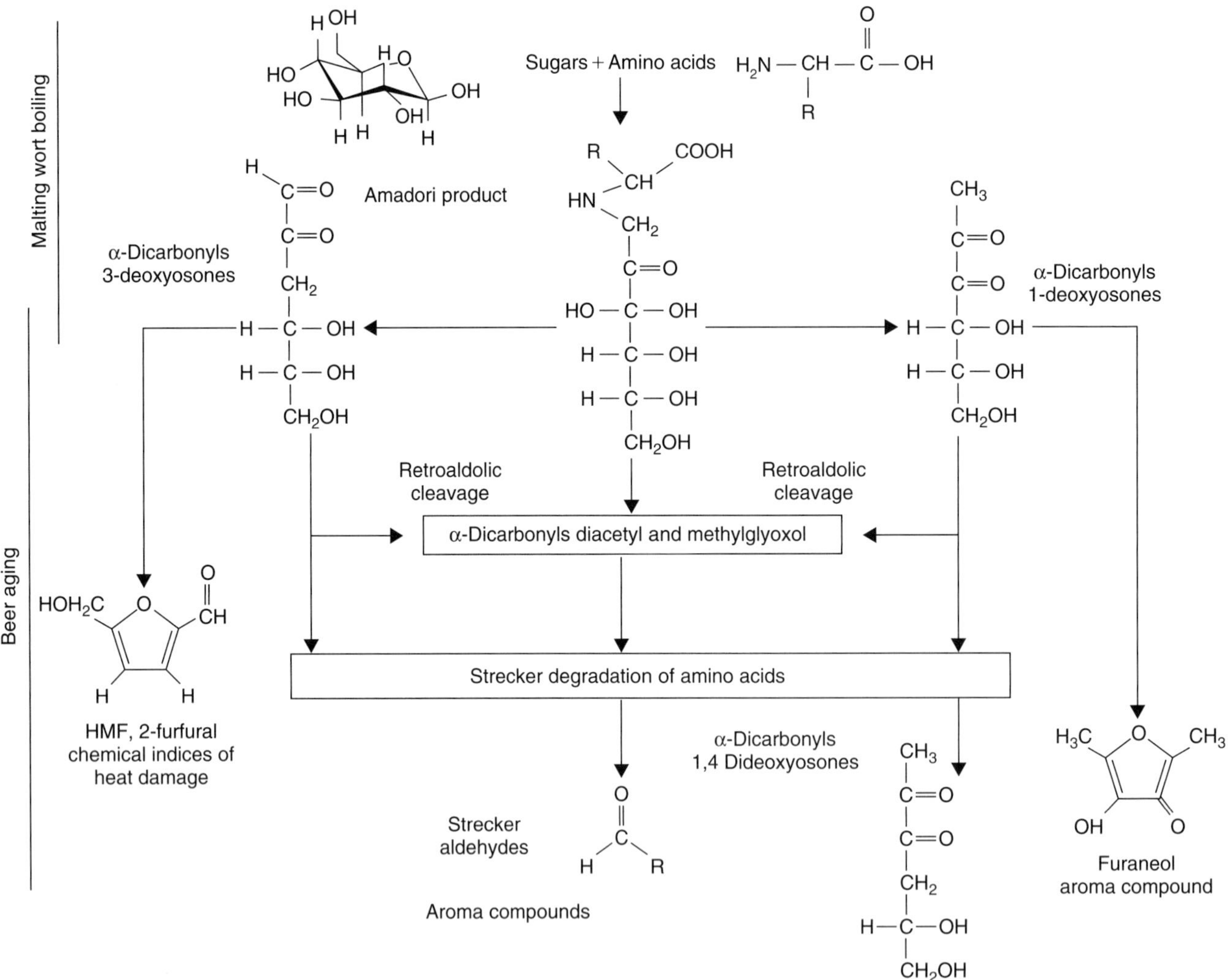

Figure 36.3 The Maillard reaction (Bravo *et al.*, 2002). The reaction of a reducing sugar and an amino acid leads to the formation of the Amadori product. After enolization, 1- and 3-deoxy dicarbonyl compounds can be formed, leading to the synthesis of furanones and furan compounds, respectively. Retro-aldolic cleavage of the dicarbonyl compounds or Strecker degradation give rise to other dicarbonyl compounds or Strecker aldehydes, respectively.

Quantitatively, 5-hydroxymethylfurfural (HMF, originating from hexose sugars) and furfural (from pentose sugars) are the most important Maillard monomers in wort. The reaction is initiated with the formation of a Schiff's base between the carbonyl group of the reducing sugar and an amino-compound (which acts as a nucleophile), resulting in an imine. This undergoes an Amadori-rearrangement to 1-amino-1-deoxyketose (Yaylayan and Huyghues-Despointes, 1994). This Amadori product is subjected to enolization and subsequent release of the amino group; 2,3-enolization resulting in the formation of 1-deoxy-2,3-hexodiulose (1-DH) or 1,2-enolization in the formation of 3-deoxy-2-hexosulose (3-DH) (Hirsch *et al.*, 1995). At wort and beer pH, the latter reaction is favored, so quantitatively more 3-DH is formed. After subsequent dehydrations, finally HMF or furfural can be formed, while 1-DH predominantly generates furanones like furaneol.

The monomeric compounds are not the end products of the Maillard reaction. After further reactions (condensation, cyclization, dehydration, isomerization, . . .), highly colored melanoidins are produced. Notwithstanding several models of melanoidin structures have been proposed so far, the majority of melanoidins is still lying in mysterious obscurity (Tressl *et al.*, 1998; Cammerer *et al.*, 2002; Adams *et al.*, 2003). Although melanoidins are known to act as antioxidants, some reports also indicate a prooxidant activity (Hashimoto, 1972). There are various mechanisms by which Maillard reaction products may act as antioxidants (Ames, 2001): oxygen scavengers, reactive oxygen scavengers (Morales, 2005), reducing agents and metal chelating agents (Wijewickreme *et al.*, 1997). A strong correlation between malt color (and therefore beer color) and antioxidative activity is established. According to Coghe *et al.* (2003), at least two types of Maillard reaction related antioxidants are present in wort: redox-reducing antioxidants and radical scavenging antioxidants. Redox-reducing antioxidants develop linearly with malt color (accounting for the observed correlation between malt color and antioxidative activity). Fast-acting antiradical antioxidants however, seem to be associated with low-colored malts. No correlation has been found between browning intensity and efficiency for scavenging oxygen radicals in solution (Morales, 2005).

Glucose accounts for only 10% of the reducing sugars available in wort, while the concentration of maltose is about 60–70% of the fermentable sugars. Maltose, maltotriose and other malto-oligosaccharides are reducing sugars as well and can also react with amino compounds, yielding α-dicarbonyl compounds via a peeling-off mechanism, proposed by Hollnagel and Kroh (2000). In the case of maltose (Figure 36.4), a β-elimination of D-glucose occurs, resulting in 1-amino-1,4-dideoxysone. The addition of a water molecule and subsequent retro-Claisen condensation yields formic acid and 3-deoxypentosulose, the latter being a precursor of furfuryl alcohol (Vanderhaegen *et al.*, 2004). Furfural, after reduction by yeast, and furfuryl alcohol are precursors of 2-furfuryl ethyl ether, a well-known beer staling compound with a solvent-like flavor and harsh taste (Harayama *et al.*, 1995; Vanderhaegen *et al.*, 2004).

In the following sections, the importance of α-dicarbonyl compounds, the Strecker degradation and aldol condensation will be discussed.

Alpha-Dicarbonyl Compounds Although the Maillard reaction is significantly accelerated at elevated temperatures like wort boiling, the reaction still occurs during beer storage at room temperature. The formation of 10 different α-dicarbonyl compounds was observed during beer storage: glyoxal, methylglyoxal (formed by a retro-aldolic cleavage of 1-DH or 3-DH) according to Weenen (1998), 2,3-butanedione, pyruvate, pentanedione, 1,4-dideoxypentosulose (Strecker degradation product of 1-deoxy-2,3-pentodiulose), 1,4-dideoxyhexosulose (Strecker degradation product of 1-DH), 1-DH and 3-DH (Bravo *et al.*, 2002). The accumulation of these compounds indicates that the Strecker degradation, retro-aldolic cleavage and the degradation of Amadori-compounds still take place during beer aging at moderate temperatures. Due to the central role of α-dicarbonyl compounds in the proceeding of the Maillard reactions, blocking these intermediates could prevent typical aging compounds to develop. The use of α-dicarbonyl trapping reagents like aminoguanidine, also used in diabetes research (Edelstein and Brownlee, 1992), can block these intermediates and inhibit the dicarbonyl-mediated beer aging. When adding aminoguanidine to dicarbonyl compounds, it reacts irreversibly and rapidly to a permanent 3-aminotriazine, as depicted in Figure 36.5 (Hirsch *et al.*, 1992), which prevents any further reaction with the dicarbonyl moiety (Bravo *et al.*, 2001; Rangel-Aldao *et al.*, 2001a). It has been observed that the addition of 2 mM aminoguanidine to fresh beer retards the formation of HMF during storage and moreover, it has a positive effect on the flavor stability during natural aging (Rangel-Aldao *et al.*, 2001b).

Strecker Reaction In the 1970s it was found that an increased formation of 2-methylpropanal and 3-methylbutanal occurred in beer when valine and leucine were added, respectively (Blockmans *et al.*, 1975). This was explained by the Strecker reaction between amino acids and α-dicarbonyl compounds. The reaction of phenylalanine with methylglyoxal is shown in Figure 36.6 as an example. The Strecker degradation involves a transamination, followed by a decarboxylation and hydrolysis, resulting in an aldehyde with one carbon atom less than the amino acid, and an α-aminoketone (Hofmann *et al.*, 2000). Although the Strecker aldehydes (acetaldehyde (Ala), 2-methylpropanal (Val), 2-methylbutanal (Ile), 3-methylbutanal (Leu), methional (Met), phenylacetaldehyde (Phe) and benzaldehyde (Phe)) increase significantly during beer aging, the individual compounds rarely exceed their flavor threshold (Thum *et al.*, 1995). However, they are frequently monitored to get insight in overall quality parameters, brewing

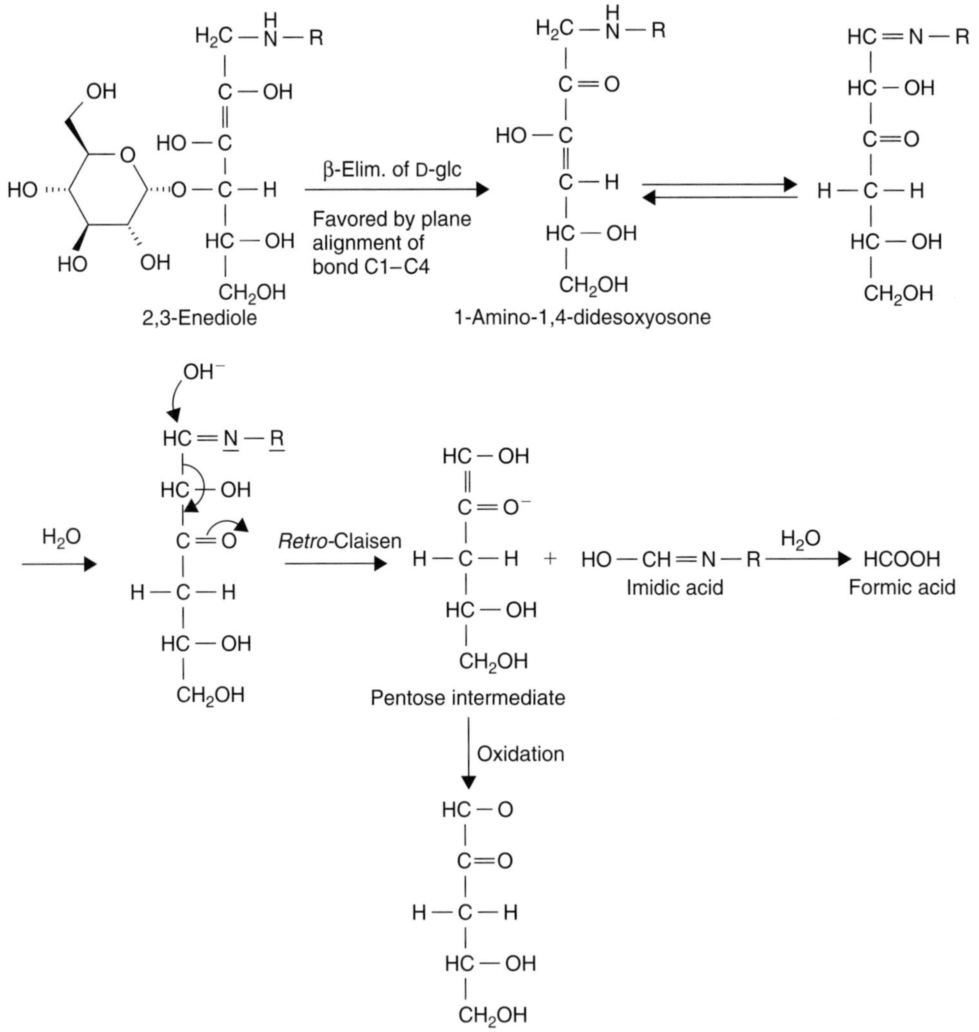

Figure 36.4 Formation of 3-deoxypentosulose from maltose (Reprinted from Hollnagel and Kroh, 2002, with permission of the American Chemical Society). After β-elimination of glucose, a 1-amino-1,4-didesoxyosone is produced, that after water addition and a retro-Claisen reaction leads to formic acid and a C-5 dicarbonyl compound.

technology and storage conditions (Methner *et al.*, 2003). Beside Strecker aldehydes, also α-aminoketones are formed in this reaction, which can further react with other aminoketones to alkylpyrazines, after subsequent cyclization and dehydration (Tressl, 1979). These alkylpyrazines are often characterized by a nutty, roasted flavor.

Recently a Strecker-type degradation of amino acids by oxidation products of unsaturated fatty acids, the 4,5-epoxy-2-alkenals, was observed by Hidalgo and Zamora (2004). Later, the proposed reaction mechanism was extended to hydroxyalkenals as well (Hidalgo *et al.*, 2005). The authors suggested a reaction mechanism, shown in Figure 36.7, where in the first step an imine is formed, followed by a decarboxylation and hydrolysis, yielding a Strecker aldehyde and an alkyl-pyridine. As the reaction proceeds evenly at 37°C and 60°C, the results suggest that heating is not required for this reaction to occur. Moreover, these Strecker-like reactions lead to pyrrole compounds, able to polymerize to brown pigmented melanoidin-like structures (Zamora *et al.*, 2000; Hidalgo *et al.*, 2003). Based on these observations, a merged reaction pathway between the Maillard reaction and lipid oxidation was proposed (Zamora and Hidalgo, 2005).

Aldol Condensation Hashimoto and Kuroiwa (1975) suggested that an aldol condensation in beer is possible under mild conditions during storage. They observed an aldol condensation between acetaldehyde and heptanal, after 20 days of incubation at 50°C, in the presence of proline (which is always present in beer, as it is not metabolized by yeast under normal fermentation conditions). In this reaction amino acids can act as catalysts by the formation of an imine intermediate. This pathway can convert compounds with a medium flavor threshold into compounds with a very low flavor threshold. The proposed reaction mechanism is shown in Figure 36.8.

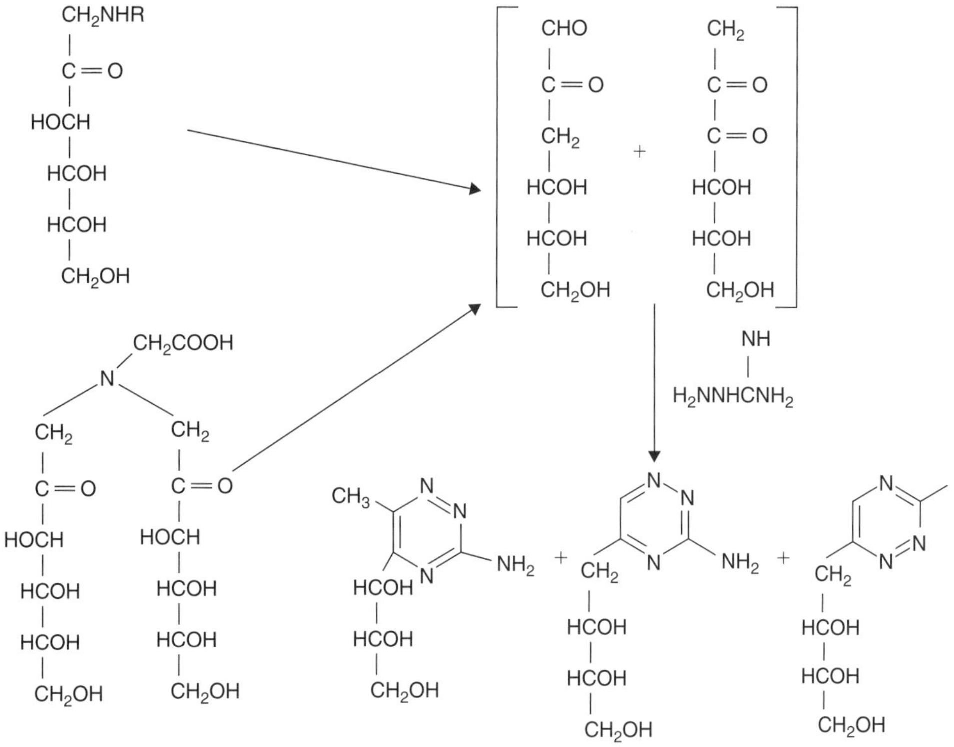

Figure 36.5 Formation of aminotriazine adducts after reaction of aminoguanidine with 1-DH and 3-DH (Reprinted from Hirsch *et al.*, 1995, with permission of Elsevier). Amadori compounds will react to either 1-DH or 3-DH. These dicarbonyl intermediates can be trapped by the reactive guanyl-group of aminoguanidine, which leads to the irreversible formation of triazines.

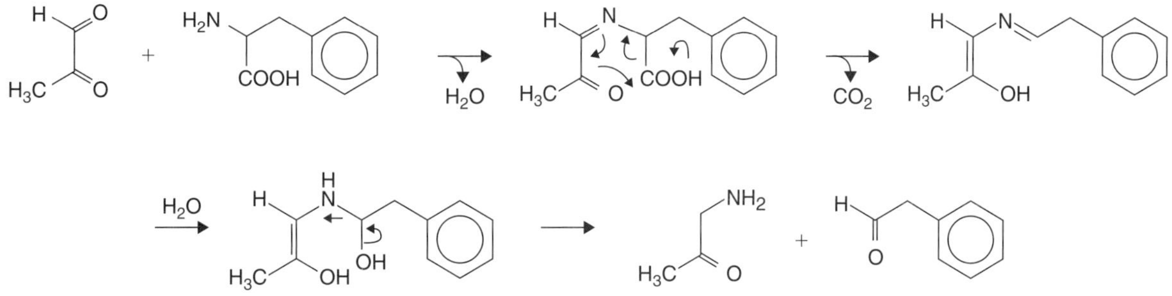

Figure 36.6 Strecker degradation of phenylalanine by methylglyoxal (Reprinted from Hofmann *et al.*, 2000, with permission from the American Chemical Society). After condensation of the α-dicarbonyl compound and the amino acid to an imine intermediate, decarboxylation occurs. Water addition to the intermediate releases the aminoketone and phenylacetaldehyde.

Degradation of Hop Bitter Acids Hop bitter acids (α-acids, β-acids and iso-α-acids) also undergo oxidative degradation during beer storage, resulting in alkanones, alkenals and alkadienals of varying lengths and structures (Hashimoto and Eshima, 1977). Particularly isohumulones are very susceptible to oxidative degradation due to the double bond and the carbonyl group of the isohexenoyl side chain. This oxidation of bitter acids is accompanied by a decrease in beer bitterness (Hashimoto and Eshima, 1979). More recently, it was demonstrated that the gradual decrease of beer bitterness intensity is largely due to the instability of *trans*-iso-α-acids. It was suggested that the ratio of *trans*/*cis*-iso-α-acids offers a reliable criterion to evaluate bitterness deterioration as a function of time (De Cooman *et al.*, 2000). The difference between *cis*- and *trans*-iso-α-acids is depicted in Figure 36.9. Oxidation of α-acids and iso-α-acids leads to complex polycyclic structures by intramolecular reactions, mostly dehydrations. Presumably, as long as functional groups remain in the oxidized bitter substances, oxidation will continue to proceed. Hop β-acids are highly unstable due to the highly susceptible unsaturated side chains and undergo autoxidation which starts already during hop storage. During the brewing process, β-acids will be oxidized almost completely (De Keukeleire, 1981a, b). To overcome the oxidative deterioration of hop bitter compounds, reduced isomerized

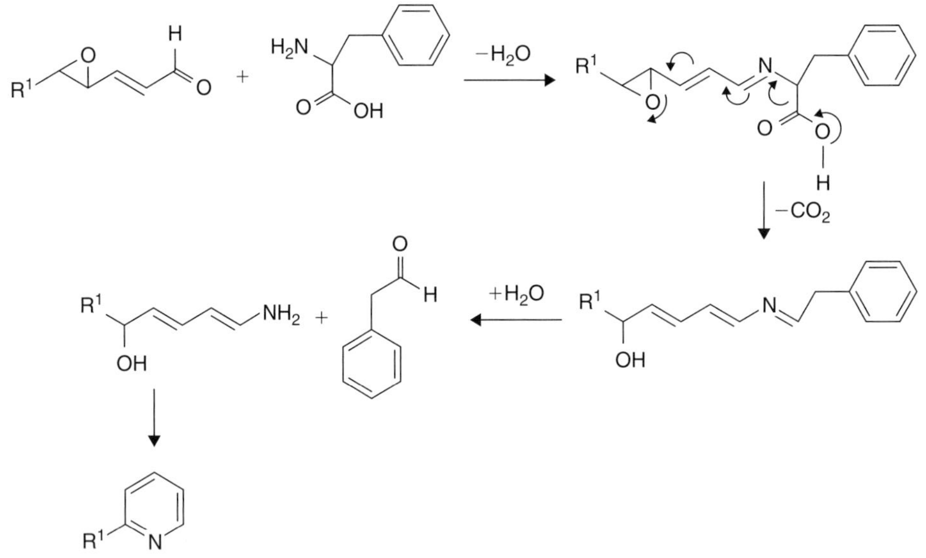

Figure 36.7 Strecker-type degradation of phenylalanine by a 4,5-epoxy-2-alkenal (Reprinted from Hidalgo and Zamora, 2004, with permission of the American Chemical Society). After the condensation of a 4,5-epoxy-2-alkenal and an amino acid to an imine, decarboxylation occurs. Subsequent hydrolysis of the imine compound releases the Strecker aldehyde and the unsaturated amine, which can further react to an alkylpyridine.

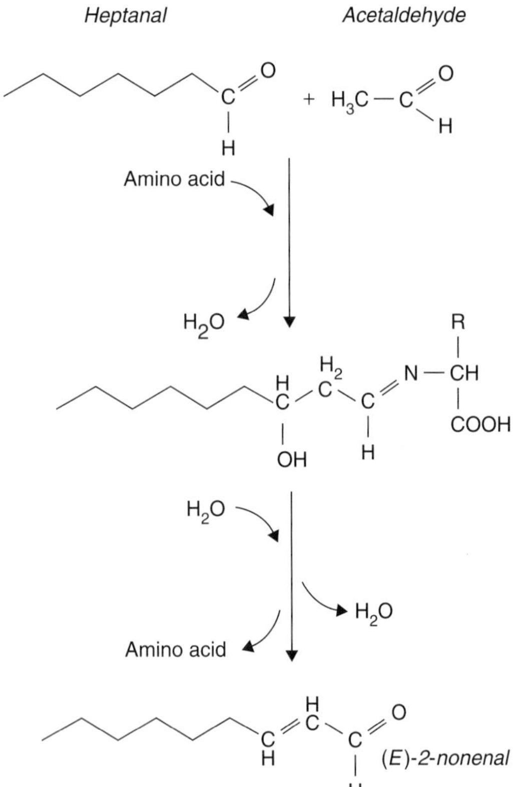

Figure 36.8 Aldol condensation of heptanal and acetaldehyde (Hashimoto and Kuroiwa, 1975). Aldehydes can react via an aldol condensation to unsaturated aldehydes. Amino acids function as catalysts by the formation of an imine intermediate to accelerate the reaction. After hydrolysis of the imine intermediate, the amino acid is recovered and the unsaturated aldehyde is released.

hop extracts are frequently used. Tetrahydroiso-α-acids are extremely resistant to oxidative deterioration and promote foam stability and bitterness consistency, while the light-stable dihydroiso-α-acids do not appear to be stable at all during storage (De Cooman *et al.*, 2001).

A well-known isohumulone degradation compound is 3-methyl-2-butene-1-thiol (MBT), responsible for the light-struck or skunky flavor in beer exposed to visible light. The light-struck flavor compound is characterized by an extreme low flavor threshold, 7 ng/l (Irwin *et al.*, 1993). As isohumulones do not absorb light in the visible region, MBT production has to be triggered by a photo-sensitizer, like riboflavin. There exists a correlation between MBT formation and the riboflavin concentration in beer (Sakuma *et al.*, 1991). Riboflavin, present in beer in concentrations of 0.2–1.3 mg/l, absorbs visible light and can be excited to its triplet state ($^3RF^\bullet$), followed by an electron transfer from iso-α-acids to $^3RF^\bullet$ (Goldsmith *et al.*, 2005). This leads to the formation of the 2-methyl-2-butene radical, which reacts to MBT with H_2S (Huvaere *et al.*, 2005). The initiation of the radical reaction is depicted in Figure 36.10. As this reaction can occur in the absence of oxygen, it can have a major impact on beer quality. Therefore, it is better to store beer in darkness and the use of brown beer bottles is preferred over green or white bottles.

Oxidation of Polyphenols Degradation of polyphenols may affect not only the bitter quality and astringency of beer, but also the beer color (Dadic, 1974). Upon oxidation or acid catalysis, polymerization reactions lead to complex polyphenols of high molecular weight. Possibly, the

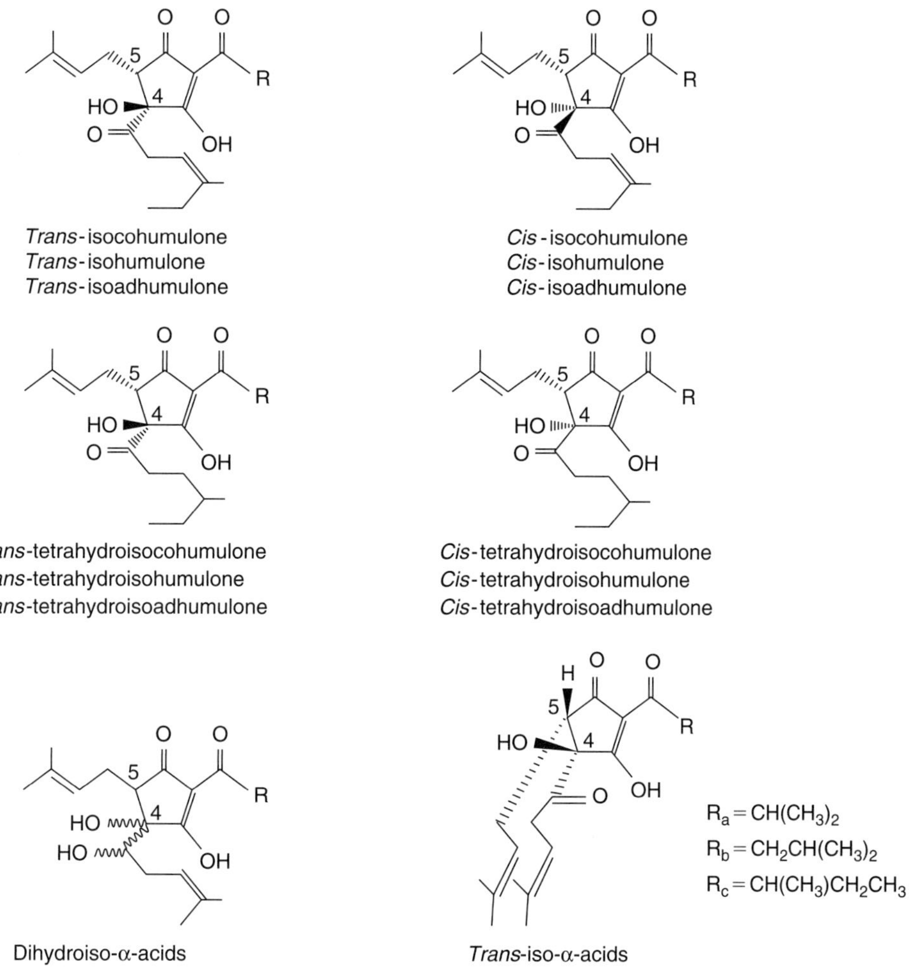

Trans-isocohumulone
Trans-isohumulone
Trans-isoadhumulone

Cis-isocohumulone
Cis-isohumulone
Cis-isoadhumulone

Trans-tetrahydroisocohumulone
Trans-tetrahydroisohumulone
Trans-tetrahydroisoadhumulone

Cis-tetrahydroisocohumulone
Cis-tetrahydroisohumulone
Cis-tetrahydroisoadhumulone

$R_a = CH(CH_3)_2$
$R_b = CH_2CH(CH_3)_2$
$R_c = CH(CH_3)CH_2CH_3$

Dihydroiso-α-acids

Trans-iso-α-acids

Figure 36.9 Reduced and non-reduced *cis*- and *trans*-iso-α-acids (De Cooman *et al.*, 2001). After reduction to dihydro- or tetrahydro-iso-α-acids, the susceptible carbonyl function and unsaturated bonds of the iso-α-acids are transformed in a hydroxyl function and saturated bonds, respectively. The distinction between cohumulone, humulone and adhumulone is made by the composition of the side chain (R).

initiation of the polymerization reactions starts with the oxidation to quinone or semi-quinone radicals, which then further interact with other phenolic compounds (Gardner and McGuinness, 1977). During beer storage, the complex phenolic polymers, called tannoids, as well as oxidized monomeric phenols interact with proteins to form insoluble complexes and hazes, finally leading to colloidal instability.

Treatment of beer with recommended dosages of polyvinylpolypyrrolidone (PVPP) extends effectively the colloidal stability of beer without compromising flavor stability. Although partial removal of flavanoid polyphenols reduces the endogenous-reducing capacity, the resulting beers do not seem to be more susceptible to oxidative flavor damage (McMurrough *et al.*, 1996).

Carotenoid Degradation or Hydrolysis of Glycosides The most important member of the norisoprenoids in beer, β-damascenone, can be found in malt extract (Farley and Nursten, 1980), hops (Tressl *et al.*, 1978a, b), beer (Lermusieau *et al.*, 2001) and wine (Genovese *et al.*, 2005). This compound is characterized by a very low flavor threshold in water (20–90 ng/l) and can be found in naturally aged beer in a concentration up to 210 μg/l. Concerning the mechanism of formation of β-damascenone, acid hydrolysis might explain the increase of β-damascenone during beer aging (Chevance *et al.*, 2002). The hypothesis of acid hydrolysis is supported by the observed increase in β-damascenone concentration when lowering the beer pH (Gijs *et al.*, 2002). Potential precursors include the allene triols and acetylene diols arising from the degradation of neoxanthin (shown in Figure 36.11). Degradation of neoxanthin leads first to the Grasshopper ketone. Reduction of the Grasshopper ketone, followed by acid hydrolysis, ultimately leads to β-damascenone.

It was also found that β-glucosidase treatment of beer leads to an increase in the β-damascenone concentration, due to the hydrolysis of glycosylated β-damascenone precursors (Chevance *et al.*, 2002). Through degradation of

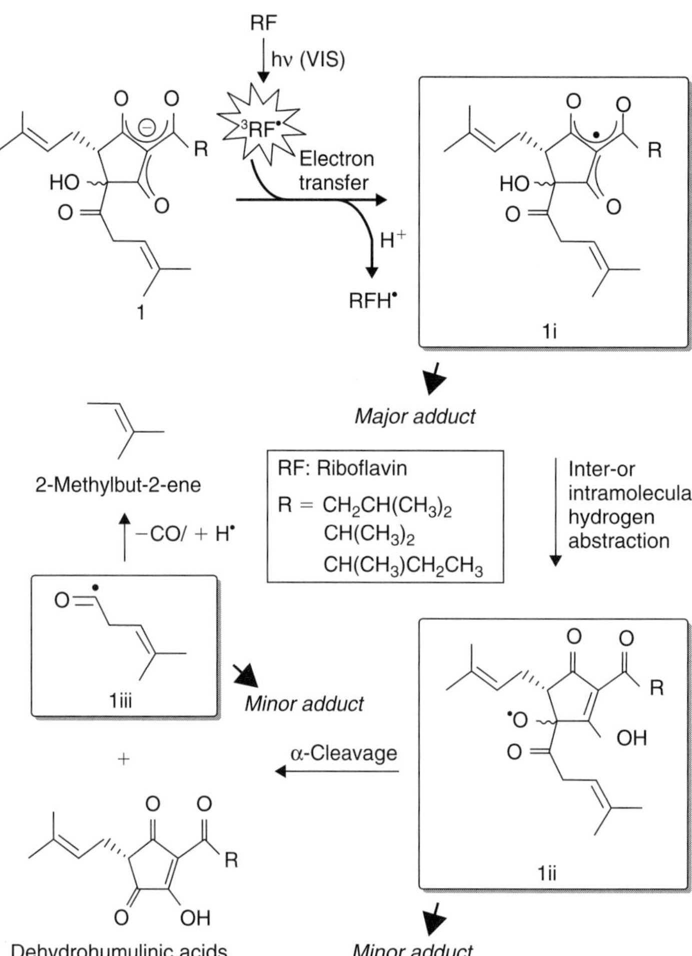

Figure 36.10 Reaction of triplet riboflavin with isohumulones (Reprinted from Huvaere *et al.*, 2005, with permission from the American Chemical Society). Excited riboflavin will extract an electron from bitter acids. This initiates intramolecular reactions, ultimately leading to the formation of the 2-methyl-2-butene radical. After reaction with H_2S, MBT is formed.

carotenoids or hydrolysis of glycosides, other important compounds, contributing to beer aging, might also be released.

Acetalization of Aldehydes A condensation reaction between 2,3-butanediol (concentration up to 280 mg/l in beer) and an aldehyde like acetaldehyde, isobutanal, 3-methylbutanal and 2-methylbutanal, leads to cyclic acetals as 2,4,5-trimethyl-1,3-dioxolane, 2-isopropyl-4,5-dimethyl-1,3-dioxolane, 2-isobutyl-4,5-dimethyl-1,3-dioxolane and 2-secondary butyl-4,5-dimethyl-1,3-dioxolane, respectively (Peppard and Halsey, 1982). The equilibrium between 2,4,5-trimethyl-1,3-dioxolane, acetaldehyde and 2,3-butanediol is reached rapidly in beer. Consequently, during beer aging, the concentration of 2,4,5-trimethyl-1,3-dioxolane will increase similarly to the increase of acetaldehyde (Vanderhaegen *et al.*, 2003).

Synthesis and Hydrolysis of Esters During beer aging, esters formed above their chemical equilibrium will hydrolyze at a characteristic rate. Acetate esters of higher alcohols will hydrolyze more rapidly than the corresponding ethyl esters, independent of the alcohol content of the beverage (Ramey and Ough, 1980). Isoamyl acetate is found to be hydrolyzed both chemically and enzymatically. The enzymatic hydrolysis depends greatly on pH, storage temperature and fermentation/maturation conditions and is performed by esterases released after cell-lysis during fermentation/maturation and bottle conditioning (for beers refermented in the bottle, a typical habit for Belgian specialty beers). The greatest decrease in positive fruity esters is observed in beers refermented in the bottle and in non-pasteurized beers. After pasteurization, the enzymatic hydrolysis is eliminated during beer aging (Neven *et al.*, 1997).

In contrast to hydrolysis, the esterification of ethanol with organic acids also occurs during beer aging. In fresh beer, the concentration of these ethyl esters is relatively low and well under the equilibrium concentration. It is therefore most likely that they were almost not formed by yeast during fermentation (Vanderhaegen *et al.*, 2003).

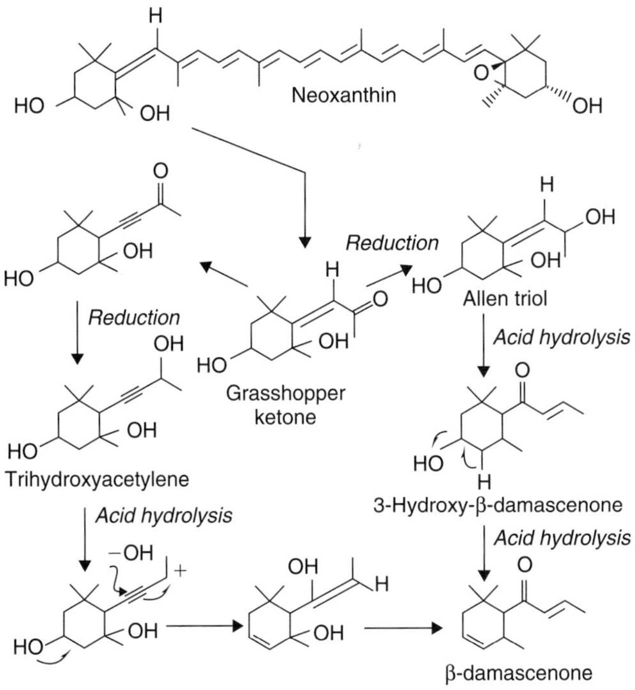

Figure 36.11 Formation of β-damascenone from neoxanthin (Reprinted from Chevance *et al.*, 2002, with permission from the American Chemical Society). Degradation of neoxanthin leads to the formation of the Grasshopper ketone, which after reduction and subsequent acid hydrolysis, gives rise to β-damascenone.

The precursor acids are found to be originating partly from hop, by oxidation of hop bitter acids to, for example, isovalerate and 2-methylbutyrate. After the conversion with ethanol to ethyl esters, these compounds impart a winey, brandy-like flavor to beer (Williams and Wagner, 1978, 1979). Precursors of ethyl ester formation can also be delivered by the Strecker degradation, which can also give rise to organic acids (Hofmann *et al.*, 2000). In addition to the hop acids and the Strecker acids, acids originating from yeast metabolism are present in beer, which may explain the increased concentration of diethyl succinate, ethyl pyruvate, ethyl lactate, ethyl nicotinate and ethyl phenylacetate in aged beer (Vanderhaegen *et al.*, 2003).

Antioxidants and Reducing Agents vs. Pro-oxidants A broad definition of an antioxidant is: a substance that, when present at low concentrations compared with those of an oxidizable substrate, significantly delays or prevents oxidation of that substrate (Halliwell and Gutteridge, 1989). However, the way antioxidants can exert their antioxidant activity differs among compounds. Moreover, most of the presumed antioxidants can have pro-oxidant capabilities as well, for example, ascorbic acid (Brezova *et al.*, 2002), sulfhydryl compounds, chelating agents, polyphenols, Maillard-reaction products (Bamforth, 2001). Maillard-reaction products as melanoidins are known to scavenge free and active oxygen, act as reducing agents and chelate metals (Ames, 2001). However, there have been reports of pro-oxidant activity as well (Hashimoto, 1972).

Phenolic compounds, like (+)-catechin, quercetin, 4-vinylguaiacol and rutin are known to quench superoxide radicals and to inhibit lipid peroxidation. Recently however, it was stated that at beer pH, the scavenging activity of the polyphenols and phenolic acids is very low comparing to sulfite (Nakamura *et al.*, 2003). Other phenolic compounds, as ferulic acid, often demonstrate poor quenching abilities but good peroxidation inhibition. However, some antioxidants can have pro-oxidant properties as well, like (+)-catechin in low concentrations (Walters *et al.*, 1997a). In beer (+)-catechin and ferulic acid also seem to specifically decrease the rate of the *cis*-isohumulone degradation, but they can exert a negative influence on beer colloidal (catechin) or flavor (ferulic acid, after conversion to 4-vinylguaiacol) properties (Walters *et al.*, 1997b).

Sulfite is a very potent inhibitor of flavor deterioration. It is naturally formed by yeast and is frequently used in the food industry. Sulfite stabilizes the flavor in two ways, as antioxidant and as carbonyl scavenger in aldehyde-bisulfite adducts.

Concerning the formation of reactive oxygen species, sulfite is found to be the only compound that is able to effectively retard the formation of radicals in beer during storage. Hydrogen peroxide and organic hydroperoxides are the only reactive oxygen species that are stable enough to be trapped efficiently by antioxidants which normally only are present in micromolecular concentrations (Andersen *et al.*, 2000). Moreover, sulfite reacts with H_2O_2 in an acid-base catalyzed reaction that does not involve radical intermediates. This action prevents the radicals to be produced via the Fenton and Haber–Weiss reactions (Hoffmann and Edwards, 1975).

Sulfite is known to form adducts to staling aldehydes. The strength of the aldehyde bisulfite complexes decreases with increasing chain length and the presence of double bonds. Based on these observations, a staling mechanism was proposed. When the concentration of acetaldehyde rises during beer storage, sulfite will be transferred from staling aldehydes to acetaldehyde, thereby releasing the staling aldehydes (Nyborg *et al.*, 1999).

Kaneda *et al.* (1996) observed the bisulfite adduct of acetaldehyde and other aldehydes, and concluded that the interaction between nonenal and bisulfite was too weak to form stable adducts during beer fermentation. Dufour *et al.* (1999) on the other hand, observed a permanent irreversible sulfite adduct to the double bond of unsaturated aldehydes. The stability of such adducts makes the mechanism of release of unsaturated aldehydes during beer aging relatively improbable. In Figure 36.12 different possible bisulfite adducts are shown. The sulfite addition to the carbonyl group is reversible, but the addition to the carbonyl double bond is irreversible and highly stable.

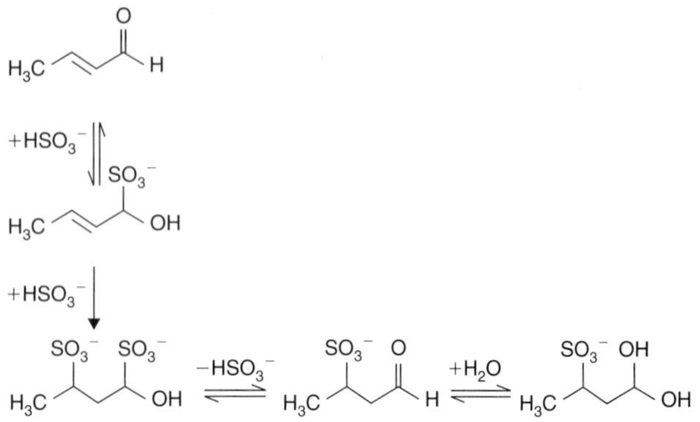

Figure 36.12 Proposed mechanism of bisulfite addition to (E)-2-nonenal (Dufour *et al.*, 1999). The addition of sulfite to the carbonyl group of (E)-2-nonenal is reversible. This is in contrast with the definitive addition of sulfite to the double bond of (E)-2-nonenal.

It is also believed that sulfite stabilizes intermediates of the Maillard reaction by forming adducts. For example, glyceraldehyde forms a stable hydroxysulfonate adduct, which renders this aldehyde non-reactive in processed food (Keller *et al.*, 1999). In conclusion, it can be stated that sulfite stabilizes the flavor as an antioxidant because of the good radical scavenging characteristics rather than its capacity to bind carbonyls (Kaneda *et al.*, 1994). Concerning the formation of reactive oxygen species, sulfite is found to be the only compound that is able to effectively retard the formation of radicals in beer during storage. Moreover, sulfite reacts with H_2O_2 in an acid-base catalyzed reaction that does not involve radical intermediates. This action prevents the radicals to be produced via the Fenton and Haber–Weiss reactions (Hoffmann and Edwards, 1975).

Yeast itself is also a very potent antioxidative creature. *Saccharomyces cerevisiae* is able to reduce a variety of carbonyls and seems to play a very important role in the reduction of beer staling compounds and their precursors (Shimizu *et al.*, 2002).

Conclusion

It is obvious that the knowledge of beer aging is far from complete, given the myriad of reactions that exert an influence on the composition and freshness of beer. Most of the reactions cannot be avoided, but they can at least be minimized. Therefore, excessive heat addition during wort production should be avoided, beer should be bottled with a minimum of oxygen and it should be stored at low temperatures and in the dark.

Summary Points

- Beer changes continuously toward its chemical equilibrium.
- Beer aging will lead to flavor deterioration and colloidal instability.
- Activated forms of oxygen play an important role in beer aging, initiating radical reactions.
- Trace metals function as catalysts during radical formation.
- Lipid oxidation leads to the formation of aldehydes.
- The Maillard reaction pathway is highly complicated and exerts a major influence on beer staling by dicarbonyl compounds and Strecker reactions.
- Degradation of hop bitter acids decreases bitterness but also creates flavor compounds.
- Oxidized polyphenols will form complexes with proteins and cause colloidal haze.
- Certain esters, present above their equilibrium and responsible for the fresh flavor will be hydrolyzed, while other esters will be synthesized chemically.
- Carotenoid degradation and hydrolysis of glycosides lead to the release of potent flavor compounds.
- Most of the used antioxidants are also known to exhibit pro-oxidant behavior in certain circumstances.
- Antioxidants should trap hydrogen peroxide or organic peroxides to efficiently protect beer from aging reactions.

References

Adams, A., Tehrani, K.A., Kersiene, M., Venskutonis, R. and DeKimpe, N. (2003). *J. Agric. Food Chem.* 51, 4338–4343.

Ames, J.M. (2001). *Cerevisia* 26, 210–216.

Andersen, H.A. and Skibsted, L.H. (1998). *J. Agric. Food Chem.* 46, 1272–1275.

Andersen, M.L., Outtrup, H. and Skibsted, L.H. (2000). *J. Agric. Food Chem.* 48, 3106–3111.

Bamforth, C.W. (2001). *Cerevisia* 26, 149–154.

Bamforth, C.W. and Parsons, R. (1985). *J. Am. Soc. Brew. Chem.* 43, 197–202.

Blockmans, C., Devreux, A. and Masschelein, C.A. (1975). *Proceedings of the European Brewing Convention Congress*, pp. 699–714. Elsevier, Nice.

Bravo, A., Scherer, E., Madrid, J., Herrera, J., Virtanen, H. and Rangel-Aldao, R. (2001). *EBC Monograph*, Vol. 31, Nancy.

Bravo, A., Sanchez, B., Scherer, E., Herrera, J. and Rangel-Aldao, R. (2002). *Tech. Q. Master Brew. Assoc. Am.* 39, 13–23.

Brezova, V., Polovka, M. and Stasko, A. (2002). *Spectrochim. Acta Part A* 58, 1279–1291.

Cammerer, B., Jalyschkov, V. and Kroh, L.W. (2002). *Int. Congr. Ser.* 1245, 269–273.

Chapon, L. and Chapon, S. (1979). *J. Am. Soc. Brew. Chem.* 37, 96–104.

Chevance, F., Guyot-Declerck, C., Dupont, J. and Collin, S. (2002). *J. Agric. Food Chem.* 50, 3818–3821.

Coghe, S., Vanderhaegen, B., Pelgrims, B., Basteyns, A.-V. and Delvaux, F.R. (2003). *J. Am. Soc. Brew. Chem.* 61, 125–132.

Dadic, M. (1974). *Tech. Q. Master Brew. Assoc. Am.* 11, 140–145.

Dale, A.R., Pollock, J.R.A., Moll, M. and That, V. (1977). *J. Inst. Brew.* 83, 88–91.

De Cooman, L., Aerts, G., Overmeire, H. and De Keukeleire, D. (2000). *J. Inst. Brew.* 106, 169–178.

De Cooman, L., Aerts, G., Witters, A., De Ridder, M., Boeykens, A., Goiris, K. and De Keukeleire, D. (2001).

Proceedings of the European Brewing Convention Congress, Vol. 28 Budapest, pp. 566–575.
De Keukeleire, D. (1981a). *Cerevisia*, 73–80.
De Keukeleire, D. (1981b). *Cerevisia*, 187–193.
Drost, B.W., van Eerde, P., Hoekstra, S.F. and Strating, J. (1971). *Proceedings of the European Brewing Convention Congress*, Vol. 13, Elsevier, Estoril, pp. 451–458.
Drost, B.W., van den Berg, R., Freijee, F.J.M., van der Velde, E.G. and Hollemans, M. (1990). *J. Am. Soc. Brew. Chem.* 48, 124–131.
Dufour, J.P., Leus, M., Baxter, A.J. and Hayman, A.R. (1999). *J. Am. Soc. Brew. Chem.* 57, 138–144.
Edelstein, D. and Brownlee, M. (1992). *Diabetologia* 35, 96–97.
Farley, D.R. and Nursten, H.E. (1980). *J. Sci. Food Agric.* 31.
Gardner, R.J. and McGuinness, J.D. (1977). *Tech. Q. Master Brew. Assoc. Am.* 14, 250–260.
Genovese, A., Dimaggio, R., Lisanti, M.T., Piombino, P. and Moio, L. (2005). *Annali Di Chimica* 95, 383–394.
Gijs, L., Chevance, F., Jerkovic, V. and Collin, S. (2002). *J. Agric. Food Chem.* 50, 5612–5616.
Goldsmith, M.R., Rogers, P., Cabral, N.M., Ghiggino, K.P. and Roddick, F.A. (2005). *J. Am. Soc. Brew. Chem.* 63, 177–184.
Halliwell, B. and Gutteridge, J.M.C. (1984). *Biochem. J.* 219, 1–14.
Halliwell, B. and Gutteridge, J.M.C. (1989). *Free Radicals in Biology and Medicine*. Clarendon Press, Oxford.
Harayama, K., Hayase, F. and Kato, H. (1995). *Biosci. Biotech. Biochem.* 59, 1144–1146.
Hashimoto, N. (1972). *J. Inst. Brew.* 78, 43–51.
Hashimoto, N. and Eshima, T. (1977). *J. Am. Soc. Brew. Chem.* 35, 145–150.
Hashimoto, N. and Eshima, T. (1979). *J. Inst. Brew.* 85, 136–140.
Hashimoto, N. and Kuroiwa, Y. (1975). *J. Am. Soc. Brew. Chem.* 33, 104–111.
Hidalgo, F.J. and Zamora, R. (2004). *J. Agric. Food Chem.* 52, 7126–7131.
Hidalgo, F.J., Nogales, F. and Zamora, R. (2003). *J. Agric. Food Chem.* 51, 5703–5708.
Hidalgo, F.J., Gallardo, E. and Zamora, R. (2005). *J. Agric. Food Chem.* 53, 10254–10259.
Hirsch, J., Petrakova, E. and Feather, M.S. (1992). *Carbohydr. Res.* 232, 125–130.
Hirsch, J., Mossine, V.V. and Feather, M.S. (1995). *Carbohydr. Res.* 273, 171–177.
Hodge, J.E. (1953). *J. Agric. Food Chem.* 1953, 928–943.
Hoffmann, M.R. and Edwards, J.O. (1975). *J. Phys. Chem.* 79, 2096–2098.
Hofmann, T., Munch, P. and Schieberle, P. (2000). *J. Agric. Food Chem.* 48, 434–440.
Hollnagel, A. and Kroh, L.W. (2000). *J. Agric. Food Chem.* 48, 6219–6226.
Hollnagel, A. and Kroh, L.W. (2002). *J. Agric. Food Chem.* 50, 1659–1664.
Huvaere, K., Andersen, M.L., Skibsted, L.H., Heyerick, A. and De Keukeleire, D. (2005). *J. Agric. Food Chem.* 53, 1489–1494.
Irwin, A.J., Barker, R.L. and Pipasts, P. (1991). *J. Am. Soc. Brew. Chem.* 49, 140–149.
Irwin, A.J., Bordeleau, L. and Barker, R.L. (1993). *J. Am. Soc. Brew. Chem.* 51, 1–3.
Jamieson, A.M. and Van Gheluwe, J.E.A. (1970). *Proc. Am. Soc. Brew. Chem.* 28, 192–197.
Kaneda, H., Osawa, T., Kawakishi, S., Munekata, M. and Koshino, S. (1994). *J. Agric. Food Chem.* 42, 2428–2432.
Kaneda, H., Takashio, M., Osawa, T., Kawakishi, S. and Tamaki, T. (1996). *J. Am. Soc. Brew. Chem.* 54, 115–120.
Kaneda, H., Kobayashi, N., Takashio, M., Tamaki, T. and Shinotsuka, K. (1999). *Tech. Q. Master Brew. Assoc. Am.* 36, 41–47.
Keller, C., Wedzicha, B.L., Leong, L.P. and Berger, J. (1999). *Food Chem.* 66, 495–501.
Kobayashi, N., Kaneda, H., Kano, Y. and Koshino, S. (1993). *J. Ferment. Bioeng.* 76, 371–375.
Kobayashi, N., Kaneda, H., Kuroda, H., Kobayashi, M., Kurihara, T., Watari, J. and Shinotsuka, K. (2000a). *J. Inst. Brew.* 106, 107–110.
Kobayashi, N., Kaneda, H., Kuroda, H., Watari, J., Kurihara, T. and Shinotsuka, K. (2000b). *J. Biosci. Bioeng.* 90, 69–73.
Lermusieau, G., Noel, S., Liegeois, C. and Collin, S. (1999). *J. Am. Soc. Brew. Chem.* 57, 29–33.
Lermusieau, G., Bulens, M. and Collin, S. (2001). *J. Agric. Food Chem.* 49, 3867–3874.
Liegeois, C., Meurens, N., Badot, C. and Collin, S. (2002). *J. Agric. Food Chem.* 50, 7634–7638.
Lindsay, R.C. (1973). *Tech. Q. Master Brew. Assoc. Am.* 10, 16–19.
McMurrough, I., Madigan, D., Kelly, R.J. and Smyth, M.R. (1996). *J. Am. Soc. Brew. Chem.* 54, 141–148.
Methner, F.J., Fritsch, H. and Stephan, A. (2003). *Proceedings of the European Brewing Convention Congress*, Dublin, pp. 732–739.
Morales, F.J. (2005). *Anal. Chim. Acta* 534, 171–176.
Nakamura, Y., Franz, O. and Back, W. (2003). *Proceedings of the European Brewing Convention Congress*, Vol. 65 Dublin, pp. 612–620.
Neven, H., Delvaux, F. and Derdelinckx, G. (1997). *Tech. Q. Master Brew. Assoc. Am.* 34, 115–118.
Noël, S. and Collin, S. (1995). *Proceedings of the European Brewing Convention Congress*, Brussels, pp. 483–490.
Noël, S., Liegeois, C., Lermusieau, G., Bodart, E., Badot, C. and Collin, S. (1999). *J. Agric. Food Chem.* 47, 4323–4326.
Nyborg, M., Outtrup, H. and Dreyer, T. (1999). *J. Am. Soc. Brew. Chem.* 57, 24–28.
Palamand, S.R. and Hardwick, W.A. (1969). *Tech. Q. Master Brew. Assoc. Am.* 6, 117–128.
Peppard, T.L. and Halsey, S.A. (1982). *J. Inst. Brew.* 88, 309–312.
Ramey, D.D. and Ough, C.S. (1980). *J. Agric. Food Chem.* 28, 928–934.
Rangel-Aldao, R., Bravo, A., Galindo-Castro, I., Sanchez, B., Herrera, J., Penttilä, M., Vehkomäki, M.-L., Vidgren, V., Virtanen, H. and Home, S. (2001a). *EBC Monograph 31*, Nancy.
Rangel-Aldao, R., Bravo, A., Galindo-Castro, I., Sanchez, B., Reverol, L., Scherer, E., Madrid, J., Ramirez, J.L., Herrera, J., Penttilä, M., Vehkomäki, M.-L., Vidgren, V., Virtanen, H., & Home, S. (2001b). *Proceedings of the European Brewing Convention Congress* Budapest.
Sakuma, S., Rikimaru, Y., Kobayashi, K. and Kowaka, M. (1991). *J. Am. Soc. Brew. Chem.* 49, 162–165.
Shimizu, C., Ohno, M., Araki, S., Furusho, S., Watari, J. and Takashio, M. (2002). *J. Am. Soc. Brew. Chem.* 60, 122–129.

Stenroos, L., Wang, P., Siebert, K. and Meilgaard, M. (1976). *Tech. Q. Master Brew. Assoc. Am.* 13, 227–232.

Thum, B., Miedaner, H., Narziss, L. and Back, W. (1995). *Proceedings of the European Brewing Convention Congress,* Brussels.

Tressl, R. (1979). *Monatsschr. Brauwiss.* 32, 240–248.

Tressl, R., Friese, L., Fendesack, F. and Koppler, H. (1978a). *J. Agric. Food Chem.* 26, 1422–1426.

Tressl, R., Friese, L., Fendesack, F. and Koppler, H. (1978b). *J. Agric. Food Chem.* 26, 1426–1430.

Tressl, R., Bahri, D. and Silwar, R. (1979). *Proceedings of the European Brewing Convention Congress*, Vol. 17, Berlin, pp. 27–41.

Tressl, R., Wondrak, G.T., Garbe, L.-A., Kruger, R.-P. and Rewicki, D. (1998). *J. Agric. Food Chem.* 46, 1765–1776.

Uchida, M. and Ono, M. (2000). *J. Am. Soc. Brew. Chem.* 58, 30–37.

Uchida, M., Suga, S. and Ono, M. (1996). *J. Am. Soc. Brew. Chem.* 54, 205–211.

Vanderhaegen, B., Neven, H., Coghe, S., Verstrepen, K.J., Verachtert, H. and Derdelinckx, G. (2003). *J. Agric. Food Chem.* 51, 6782–6790.

Vanderhaegen, B., Neven, H., Verstrepen, K.J., Delvaux, F.R., Verachtert, H. and Derdelinckx, G. (2004). *J. Agric. Food Chem.* 52, 6755–6764.

Vanderhaegen, B., Neven, H., Verachtert, H. and Derdelinckx, G. (2006). *Food Chem.* 95, 357–381.

Wackerbauer, K., Meyna, S. and Marre, S. (2003). *Monatsschr. Brauwiss.* 56, 174–178.

Walters, M.T., Heasman, A.P. and Hughes, P.S. (1997a). *J. Am. Soc. Brew. Chem.* 55, 83–89.

Walters, M.T., Heasman, A.P. and Hughes, P.S. (1997b). *J. Am. Soc. Brew. Chem.* 55, 91–98.

Weenen, H. (1998). *Food Chem.* 62, 393–401.

Wijewickreme, A.N., Kitts, D.D. and Durance, T.D. (1997). *J. Agric. Food Chem.* 45, 4577–4583.

Williams, R.S. and Wagner, H.P. (1978). *J. Am. Soc. Brew. Chem.* 36, 27–31.

Williams, R.S. and Wagner, H.P. (1979). *J. Am. Soc. Brew. Chem.* 37, 13–19.

Yaylayan, V.A. and Huyghues-Despointes, A. (1994). *Crit. Rev. Food Sci. Nutr.* 34, 321–369.

Zamora, R. and Hidalgo, F.J. (2005). *Crit. Rev. Food Sci. Nutr.* 45, 49–59.

Zamora, R., Alaiz, M. and Hidalgo, F.J. (2000). *J. Agric. Food Chem.* 48, 3152–3158.

37

Trans-2-nonenal During Model Mashing

José da Cruz Francisco and Estera Szwajcer Dey Pure and Applied Biochemistry, Lund University, Lund, Sweden

Abstract

A study on *trans*-2-nonenal (T2N) production during laboratory mashing of barley malt reveals that during the mashing-in step of kilned malt, an elevated amount of T2N (up to 14 ppb) is produced, and at the mashing-off step, a rapid decrease takes place. The decrease of T2N level observed is independent of the presence of spent grains. At moderate temperature, spent grains have a stabilizing effect on T2N levels. The decreased amount of T2N during mashing-off can be quantitatively determined in a potential test. Reduced levels of T2N have also been observed when the mashing-in liquor was acidified to pH 5.3, or by using coarse ground malt or by making a thicker mash. Increased amounts of T2N have been found in the extracts carried out at 5°C. No correlation between lipoxygenase activity in kilned malt and the corresponding soluble T2N during wort production was found in the study.

List of Abbreviations

GC–MS	Gas chromatography–mass spectrometry
HCB	Hexachlorobenzene
LOX	Lipoxygenase
NICI	Negative ion chemical ionization
PFBHA	*O*-(2,3,4,5,6-pentafluorobenzyl)amine
ppb	Parts per billion
RSD	Relative standard deviation
T2N	*Trans*-2-nonenal

Introduction

Beer off-flavor depends on the production of volatile aldehydes from lipid oxidation during malting, kilning, mashing and wort boiling processes. During beer production, stepwise enzymatic degradation of lipids and fatty acids continues and can lead to the formation of stale flavor substances such as *trans*-2-nonenal (T2N) (Drost *et al.*, 1990). Plants degrade linoleic acid through the action of lipoxygenases (LOX) pathway enzymes, generating T2N and other derivatives of which some are involved in plant defence, gene regulation and plant to plant signaling (Feussner and Waternack, 2002; Hambraeus and Nyberg, 2005).

By enzymatic oxidation of linoleic acid or trilinolein, 9-hydroperoxylinoleic acid is formed by the enzyme LOX-1. T2N is then produced from 9-hydroperoxylinoleic acid by the secondary plant enzyme hydroperoxide lyase (Van Aarle, 1993). It is asserted that flavor stability of beer is inversely related to LOX activity during the early stages of mashing (Martel *et al.*, 1991). The formation of T2N may also occur both during malting and during wort production. Tressl *et al.* (1979) has reported an amount of T2N as high as 200–400 ppb in the final malt. During mashing-in, enhanced amounts of 9-hydroperoxylinoleic acid are produced (Walker *et al.*, 1996); however, it is not elucidated to which degree this compound is converted to T2N by hydroperoxide lyase, or trihydroxy octadecanoic acid by LOX or to ketols produced by dehydrase. Baur *et al.* (1977) have found elevated amounts of trihydroxy fatty acids in beer and after isolation it was established that trihydroxy fatty acids have a bitter taste. T2N is also generated during wort boiling in non-enzymatic process (Noeel *et al.*, 1999). Keeping beer at 38°C for only a few days suffices to increase the concentration of T2N above the threshold (Drost *et al.*, 1990) but exactly how this is formed in the beer remains elusive.

This chapter presents a case study of the changes occurring in soluble T2N and corresponding variations in LOX activity during model laboratory mashing. The experimental design used is described in detail. The methods used for the identification of T2N, its potential determination, the LOX extraction and its activity are simply mentioned to guide the reader for possible repetition.

Experimental Design

For the case studies presented in this chapter, malt is milled to particle size of 1 mm (fine milling). Fifty grams of malt flour is mashed-in with 450 ml of distilled water at 37°C.

Beer in Health and Disease Prevention
ISBN: 978-0-12-373891-2

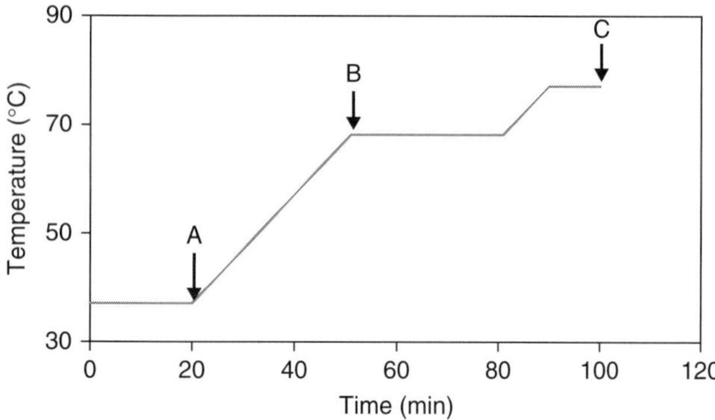

Figure 37.1 Temperature profile and sampling points under standard mashing conditions. Samples are collected at the points marked with arrows and capital letters.

The standard mashing program has three steps (Figure 37.1) with mashing-in at 37°C for 20 min, saccharification at 68°C for 30 min and mashing-off at 77°C for 10 min. Between each step the temperature is raised at 1°C/min.

Samples are collected after mashing-in (point A), at the start of saccharification (point B) and at the end of mashing-off (point C). The entire contents of one mashing beaker is used for each sampling. The sample from each mashing steps is filtered immediately on a folded filter paper. The filtrate is collected in a measuring glass immersed in an ice bath. Collection of filtrate is stopped when 150 ml has been collected. To prevent enzymatic lipid oxidation, pH must be decreased from 6.0 to about 4.0 by the addition of 0.55 ml 8.5% phosphoric acid. The wort (filtrate) is analyzed for T2N after acidification. One part of the wort is analyzed directly and another part is kept at −20°C for the determination of T2N potential.

Monitoring the Mashing Process

Prior to analysis for T2N and T2N potential determination, cleaning up of wort (filtrate) is necessary. For this purpose a solid phase extraction C_{18} column (1 g/6 ml, EC) conditioned with 6 ml of methanol and washed with 6 ml of Milli Q water is recommended. Five milliliters of filtrate is supplemented with 0.8 ml methanol and 4.8 ml of Milli Q water and mixed well. The mixture is then passed through the column. For the described case the column was washed with 6 ml of 30% methanol followed by 3 ml of 70% methanol. T2N was eluted with 6 ml of 90% methanol. T2N present in the eluate from the cleaning is derivatized with 0.5 ml *O*-(2,3,4,5,6-pentafluorobenzyl)amine (PFBHA) solution (0.2 g PFBHA in 50 ml Milli Q water) for 2 h, at room temperature. Fifty microliters sulfuric acid 9 M are added to terminate the reaction. Then T2N is extracted with 2 ml *n*-hexane using a whirl-mixer (minimum 30 s). The *n*-hexane phase is dried with sodium sulfate and quantitatively transferred to a clean test tube and concentrated to less than 0.5 ml under a gentle stream of nitrogen at no more than 40°C. Internal standard hexachlorobenzene for instance is added to the sample and made up to a volume 0.5 ml with hexane and transferred for analysis with gas chromatography–mass spectrometry (GC–MS).

For GC, the interface temperature, the ion source temperature at and the injection temperature are usually kept at 260°C, 190°C and 230°C, respectively. The GC oven temperature is kept at 40°C for 2 min and run at the following temperature gradients: 40–120°C at 25°C/min, 120–240°C at 10°C/min, 240–260°C at 30°C/min held for 15 min.

The mass spectrometer is operated in full scan mode: *m*/*z* 282–317. The acquisition time is 18 min scanning in negative ion chemical ionization mode; *m*/*z* 315 and 285 were used as characteristic ions for T2N. For the case study, *m*/*z* 285 was the quantification ion, *m*/*z* 284 and 286 were used as characteristic ions for the internal standard, and the sum of both ions were used for quantification. For T2N potentialdetermination, the acidified extract/wort (pH 4.0) is boiled for 2 h before measurements as described by Drost *et al.* (1990).

Procedure

The analysis for LOX activity is preceded by the enzyme extraction.

Five grams of malt are milled for 2 min in a water cooled analytical mill. One gram of flour is stirred for 30 min at 5°C with 10 ml of 0.1 M phosphoric buffer, pH 6.0. The suspension is centrifuged for 10 min at 5,500 rpm, and the supernatant used as an enzyme extract. When LOX activity is assayed in filtrates from mashes, the filtrate is used directly as an enzyme extract.

The enzyme assay is then performed by adding 25 μl of freshly prepared enzyme extract to a mixture of 50 μl linoleic acid (25 mM in 1% Tween 20) and 925 μl phosphate buffer (0.1 M, pH 6.0). Afterwards, LOX activity is determined spectrophotometrically by measuring the initial increase at Ab 234 nm indicating the formation of conjugated diene of linoleic acid hydroperoxide with extinction coefficient = 25,000/$M^{-1}cm^{-1}$ at room temperature in a 1 ml quartz cuvette against a blank. One unit of LOX activity is defined as the amount of activity that produces 1 μmol of conjugated diene of linoleic acid hydroperoxide in 1 min at room temperature.

Laboratory Model Mashing Study

During beer production, stepwise enzymatic degradation of lipids and fatty acids continues and can lead to the formation of stale flavor substances such as T2N (Drost *et al.*, 1990). T2N is also generated during wort boiling in a non-enzymatic

Table 37.1 *Trans*-2-nonenal in samples collected at points A, B and C during laboratory mashing

Sampling point/time	*Trans-2-nonenal in wort (ppb)*						
	1 day	*2 days*	*3 days*	*4 days*	*Mean*	*SD*	*RSD (%)*
A	15.1 14.3	13.8 13.3	13.7 13.9	13.2 13.3	13.8	±0.6	4.35
B	4.8 4.8	4.4 3.9	5.1 4.7	4.9 5.0	4.7	±0.4	8.51
C	3.7 3.1	3.7 2.9	3.9 3.9	3.9 3.9	3.6	±0.4	11.1

SD = standard deviation; RSD = relative standard deviation.

Table 37.2 *Trans*-2-nonenal found at points A, B and C in spiked and unspiked filtrates incubated according to the normal mashing program

Sampling point	*Trans-2-nonenal (ppb)*		
	Un-spiked sample	*Spiked sample*	*Difference (ppb)*
Before incubation	15	26	11
A	7	11	4
B	3	5	2
C	2	3	1

process (Noeel *et al.*, 1999). One of the crucial steps in generation of T2N during brewing is the mashing process.

Following the design and the analytical procedures described above, the reproducibility of the T2N analysis (including mashing and sampling) was investigated. Duplicates of Alexis malt mashing were performed on four different days. Samples were collected at points A, B and C; see Figure 37.1.

As displayed in Table 37.1, the T2N values from different batches of wort were reproducible. At all sampling points, the standard deviation was (±)4–6%. However, the coefficient of variations (RSD) for sampling points A, B and C showed increasing values: 4.35%, 8.51% and 11.1%, respectively. The dispersion of the variations increased while the absolute values decreased.

The role of spent grains in reduction of soluble T2N during mashing

A relatively large amount of soluble T2N, approximately 14 ppb, was found after mashing-in (point A). A rapid drop in T2N was observed as the temperature was increased to 68°C (point B). At this point, almost 65% of the T2N found at point A had disappeared. A further decrease was observed after saccharification and mashing-off (point C). The reduction of soluble T2N may be due to a chemical or an enzymatic reaction. Alternatively, T2N may adsorb to the insoluble spent grain particles and thus be removed during filtration. To investigate the role of spent grains, an extract free of spent grains and with a relatively high level of T2N was made by mashing Alexis malt and filtering the mash after mashing-in (point A). A part of this filtrate was spiked with 11 ppb T2N. The two filtrates, spiked and unspiked, were then re-incubated according to the mashing program shown in Figure 37.1. Samples were collected at points A, B and C, and the results are shown in Table 37.2.

Fifteen parts per billion (15 ppb) of T2N was found in the original filtrate free of spent grains made after mashing-in (point A). When this filtrate was re-incubated at 37°C for 20 min, the level of soluble T2N decreased by about 50% to 7 ppb. In the samples collected at points B and C, the level of soluble T2N decreased further to 3 and 2 ppb, respectively, levels somewhat lower than those found in mashing with spent grains present (Table 37.1). In the extracts spiked with 11 ppb, the exogenous T2N disappears just like the endogenous T2N. At points A, B and C, the levels of soluble T2N are only slightly higher in the spiked extract than in the original one. These observations suggest that the reduction in T2N observed during normal mashing was not due to adsorption of spent grain particles. One of the theories is that T2N-adducts are created between the aldehyde and the amino groups of peptides and protein present in wort (Liegeois *et al.*, 1999). Laboratory made adducts between T2N and myoglobin, at pH 7 and 37°C, are water-soluble, non-volatile and flavorless substances (Dey *et al.*, 2005).

T2N potential during mashing

The level of free T2N in fresh beer is below 0.05 ppb, however, during storage the level of free T2N increases. This is explained by the release of the so-called imine-protected T2N at a lower pH during aging (Collin *et al.*, 1999). Drost *et al.* (1990) have introduced the "T2N potential" concept in final pitching wort. This potential is believed to reflect the flavor stability of the resulting beer and is determined by measuring T2N in wort acidified to pH 4.0 (beer pH) and boiled for 2 h. The "T2N potential" during mashing was investigated by analyzing samples from a standard mashing (one of the mashings performed on day 3 in the reproducible experiments, Table 37.1). The results are shown in Table 37.3.

In boiled samples, the concentration of T2N reaches approximately the same level as found after mashing-in in fresh un-boiled samples. These results (Table 37.3) indicate that the reduction of T2N during mashing may be due to a chemical "masking" occurring at elevated temperatures and pH 6.0.

Effect of pH during mashing-in

It has been claimed that the T2N potential in wort is correlated to LOX activity in malt (Drost *et al.*, 1990; De Buck *et al.*, 1997). The activity of LOX-1 was optimal at about pH 6.3 and was markedly reduced at lower pH (Doderer *et al.*, 1992). Earlier, it has been reported that mashing at a lower pH reduces the T2N potential in final wort due to reduced LOX activity during mashing-in.

To see the effect of pH on T2N levels after mashing-in, the mashing-in liquor was acidified with phosphoric acid prior to addition of malt flour. Samples are taken after mashing-in (point A) and pH, T2N and T2N potential are measured in the filtrates. The results are shown in Table 37.4.

The level of free T2N and the T2N potential decrease when pH decreases during mashing-in. When pH was reduced from 6.0 to 4.8, 70% less of T2N was found. This supports the hypothesis that a reduced LOX activity due to low pH during mashing-in leads to reduced levels of T2N in wort.

Effect of temperature

Apart from low pH, LOX activity may also be low due to a low reaction temperature. Thus, at 5°C, LOX activity was expected to be very low, however, the available soluble oxygen at this temperature was higher than at 37°C. The enzyme may also be inactivated by high temperature, and it is known that LOX gets inactivated immediately at temperatures above 60°C. To investigate the effect of temperature, experiments with "mashing-in" at temperatures of 5°C, 37°C and 60°C were carried out. T2N and dissolved LOX activity were followed in filtrates made at fixed time intervals up to 1 h of incubation. The results from this experiment are shown in Table 37.5.

After 5 min incubation at 5°C, 6 ppb T2N was found in the extract, and after 30 min it increased to a steady level of 17 ppb. At 37°C the level of T2N was almost constant at 12 ppb, while at 60°C the level of T2N decreased from 5 ppb after 5 min to 2 ppb after 60 min. T2N potential was measured after 20 min of mashing-in on samples that were at 5°C, 37°C and 60°C, and it was found to be 15, 11 and 20 ppb, respectively. At 5°C, the level of LOX activity was practically constant throughout the extraction period (0.22–0.25 U/ml), at 37°C (after 20 min) it was 0.66 U/ml and at 60°C, no activity was detected. The stability of the LOX already present at temperature higher than 37°C decreases the activity of these enzymes. LOX-1, which survives kilning, is the key enzyme in the pathway leading to T2N in plants

Table 37.3 *Trans*-2-nonenal and *trans*-2-nonenal potential in filtrates from a laboratory mashing

	Trans-2-nonenal (T2N) in filtrates (ppb)	
Sampling point	*Free (T2N)*	*Potential (T2N)*
A	14	11
B	5	18
C	4	16

Table 37.4 *Trans*-2-nonenal and *trans*-2-nonenal potential in filtered samples after incubation at 37°C for 20 min. Mashing-in liquor was acidified with addition of phosphoric acid before addition of malt

Added ml 8.5% phosphoric acid	*pH*	*Trans-2-nonenal (ppb)*	
		Free	*Potential*
0	6.0	13	11
0.45	5.7	13	5
0.9	5.3	9	4
1.2	5.1	7	4
1.6	4.9	5	3
1.8	4.8	4	3

Table 37.5 *Trans*-2-nonenal in filtrates made after mashing-in at 5°C, 37°C and 60°C

	Time of mashing-in (min)					
	5	*10*	*20*	*30*	*40*	*60*
Free trans-2-nonenal in filtrate (ppb)						
Incubation at 5°C	6	9	13	17	17	17
Incubation at 37°C	11	13	12	12	12	13
Incubation at 60°C	5	3	3	3	2	2

(Drost *et al.*, 1990; Van Aarle, 1993; De Buck *et al.*, 1997). LOX-1 has a pH optimum at about 6.3, and at lower pH the activity is markedly reduced (Drost *et al.*, 1990; Yang *et al.*, 1993). It is puzzling that in the "T2N potential test", mashing-in made at 60°C generates as high a level of T2N as the mashing-in at ambient temperature, in spite of the fact that no LOX activity was present.

Effect of malt-to-water ratio and malt particle size

The level of T2N in wort may not only be a result of enzymatic production during mashing. It may also depend on the level of T2N already present in kilned malt. During malting and kilning, T2N may be produced by the same type of reaction as during mashing. It was not clear to which extent T2N was produced during malting, and there was no knowledge about the solubility of T2N from malt during mashing. To investigate a possible effect of solubility of T2N from malt, experiments were performed with different malt-to-water ratios and with different malt particle sizes. The effect of malt-to-water ratio was investigated by incubating 10–50 g of Alexis malt in 450 ml of 37°C water for 20 min. T2N and LOX activity was measured in the filtrates. The results are shown in Table 37.6. The amount of soluble T2N after mashing-in was almost independent of the ratio between malt and water.

Five times more malt results in only 1.6 times more T2N. In contrast, LOX activity increases almost proportionally to the amount of malt.

Table 37.6 *Trans*-2-nonenal in filtrates made after mashing-in (37°C) with different ratios between malt and water

Amount of malt (g)	*Ratio (malt:water)*	*Trans-2-nonenal (ppb)*	*LOX activity (U/ml)*
10	1:45	9	0.026
20	1:23	10	0.044
30	1:15	13	0.066
40	1:11	14	0.080
50	1:9	14	0.077

Note: In all extractions, 450 ml water was used.

Table 37.7 *Trans*-2-nonenal and *trans*-2-nonenal potential after mashing-in and after mashing-off with fine, middle or coarse ground malt

	Trans-2-nonenal (ppb)			
	Mashing-in		*Mashing-off*	
Grinding	*Free*	*Potential*	*Free*	*Potential*
Fine	11	11	3	13
Middle	10	8	2	8
Coarse	4	5	1	5

The role of malt particle size was investigated using Alexis malt milled on a mill, with settings of 0.1, 0.7 and 1.3 mm between the disks giving fine, middle or coarse grindings. T2N and T2N potential are measured after mashing-in (point A) and at mashing-off (point C). Results are shown in Table 37.7.

The amount of T2N in filtrates decreased with increasing malt particle size, both after mashing-in and after mashing-off. There was almost no difference between the level of T2N and T2N potential in filtrates made after mashing-in with malt of the same grinding. The level of T2N at mashing-off was much lower than after mashing-in, but the T2N potential after mashing-off corresponds well to the levels found after mashing-in.

Comparison of LOX activity and T2N in kilned malt

It has been claimed that kilned malt with a high level of LOX(s) produces an enhanced level of T2N potential in wort (Drost *et al.*, 1990; De Buck *et al.*, 1997). To investigate this claim, extracts of seven different kilned malts were assayed for LOX activity. T2N was determined in filtrates made from the same malts after mashing-in. The results are shown in Table 37.8.

No correlation was found between LOX in malt extracts and T2N found after mashing-in in this set of malts. On the other hand, the non-correlation between LOX activity of malt and T2N produced has been previously observed by Kuroda *et al.* (2002), a fact that was considered to depend on peroxidase-like activity (Kuroda *et al.*, 2003).

As shown in this study, it was difficult to clarify whether the level of T2N in wort depends mainly on LOX activity during mashing or on solubility of T2N already present in kilned malt. Most of the research in this area has focused on the role of LOX during mashing, whereas there was very limited knowledge of the impact of the T2N accumulated during the malting process. According to our findings, this part of the process from barley to wort may be just as important as the mashing process for flavor stability in beer.

Table 37.8 LOX activity in seven malts and corresponding T2N found after mashing-in

Malt	*LOX* (U/g of malt)*	*T2N after mashing-in (ppb)*
1	3.6	14
2	6.5	2
3	2.4	26
4	8.4	16
5	3.6	27
6	3.6	19
7	3.8	43

* Extracted at 5°C as described in Procedure.

Summary Points

- At 5°C T2N could already be released and present as free T2N.
- T2N potential correlates with the free T2N extracted at 5°C, after 30 min of incubation.
- Spent grains are not arresting the T2N.
- Endogenous and spiked T2N is arrested by components present in the wort during temperature increases.
- LOX activity was not correlating with the free T2N.
- The ratio between malt and water has no effect on the amount of free T2N, it correlates with the extracted LOX activity.

References

Baur, C., Grosch, W., Wieser, H. and Jugel, H. (1977). *Z. Lebensm Unters Forsh.* 164, 171–176.

Collin, S., Liegeois, C., Noeel, S. and Lermusieau, G. (1999). *Proceedings of the 27th European Brewery Convention Congress*, pp. 113–122.

De Buck, A., Aerts, G., Bonte, S., Dupire, S. and Van den Eynde, E. (1997). *Proc. Eur. Brew. Convention* 26, 333–340.

Dey, E.S., Staniszewska, M., Pasciak, M., Konopacka, M., Rogolinski, J., Gamian, A. and Danielsson, B. (2005). *Polish J. Microb.* 54, 47–52.

Doderer, A., Kokkelink, I., Van der Veen, S., Valk, B.E., Schram, A.W., Douma, A.C., Heineken, T.B. and Zoeterwoude, N. (1992). *Biochim. Biophys. Acta* 1120, 97–104.

Drost, B.W., Van den Berg, R., Freijee, F.J.M., Van der Velde, E.G. and M. Hollemans, M. (1990). *J. Am. Soc. Brewing Chem.* 48, 124–131.

Feussner, I. and Waternack, C. (2002). *Annu. Rev. Plant. Biol.* 53, 275–297.

Hambraeus, G. and Nyberg, N. (2005). *J. Agric. Food Chem.* 53.

Kuroda, H., Kobayashi, N., Kuneda, H., Watari, J. and Takashio, M. (2002). *J. Biosci. Bioeng.* 93, 73–77.

Kuroda, H., Furusho, S., Maeba, H. and Takashio, M. (2003). *Biosci. Biotech. Biochem.* 67, 691–697.

Liegeois, C., Noel, S., Lermusieau, G. and Collin, S. (1999). *Cerevisia* 24, 21–27.

Martel, C., Kohl, S. and Boivin, P. (1991). *Proc. Eur. Brew. Convention Cong.* 23, 425–432.

Noeel, S., Liegeois, C., Lermusieau, G., Bodart, E., Badot, C. (1999). *J. Agric. Food Chem.* 47, 4323–4326.

Tressl, R., Bahri, D. and Silwar, R. (1979). *Proc. Eur. Brew. Convention Cong.* 17, 27–41.

Van Aarle, P.G.M. (1993). Purification and Characterization of Lipoxygenase from Ungerminated Barley, CIP-Gerens Koninjke, University of Urecht, Hague.

Walker, M.D., Hughes, P.S. and Simpson, W.J. (1996). *J. Sci. Food Agric.* 70, 341–346.

Yang, G., Schwarz, P.B. and Vick, B.A. (1993). *Cereal Chem.* 70, 589–595.

38

E-2-nonenal and β-Damascenone in Beer

José Rodrigues and Paulo Almeida Department of Chemistry, Faculty of Science, University of Porto, Porto, Portugal

Abstract

One of the main concerns among brewers is to maintain the organoleptic stability of stored beer. This objective has prompted a series of scientific studies, which have given a better knowledge of all the brewing procedures. Nowadays, the brewers have a better comprehension of the beer-ageing phenomenon and the know-how to increase the organoleptic stability of packaged beers.

E-2-nonenal (also called *trans*-2-nonenal), a compound with an extremely low taste threshold (0.1 μg/l), is widely recognized as the major cause for the development of the typical unpleasant cardboard flavor in aged beers. Recently, an increase of β-damascenone concentration during beer ageing was discovered. These two compounds were proposed as analytical markers for beer-ageing characterization. However, at the levels found in beer, there is no evidence that *E*-2-nonenal and β-damascenone could have effects, adverse or beneficial, on human health. In this chapter, the formation and the determination of these two carbonyl compounds in beer are reviewed.

List of Abbreviations

GC/MS	Gas chromatography/mass spectrometry
HPLC/UV	High-performance liquid chromatography/ ultraviolet detection
LC/MS	Liquid chromatography/mass spectrometry
NMR	Nuclear magnetic resonance
ppb	Parts per billion
SBSE	Stir bar sorptive extraction
SPME	Solid-phase microextraction
UV	Ultraviolet

Introduction

Chemically, the changes in flavor that develop in packaged beers are very hard to define since they occur progressively during storage and are due to a combination of the effects of many flavor components (Vanderhaegen *et al.*, 2006).

Lustig (1996) lists 10 substances as the principal determinants of staling: 2-methylbutanal, 2-furaldehyde, 5-methyl-2-furaldehyde, benzaldehyde, 2-phenylethanal, diethylsuccinate, ethylphenylacetate, 2-acetyl furan, 2-propionyl furan and γ-nonalactone. Compounds such as 2-furaldehyde are generally held to be good markers of oxidation in beer without themselves being present in sufficient quantity to be detectable. Others in this category include acetaldehyde, 5-hydroxymethylfurfural, γ-hexalactone, 3-methylbutanal and the ethyl ester of nicotinic acid and 2-furfurylethyl ether and furfuryl acetate (Bamforth, 1999). It has long been known that the excellent relationship between furanic aldehydes (2-furaldehyde and 5-hydroxymethylfurfural) and the degree of organoleptic deterioration of beer is induced by heat. The impact of oxygen on the development of furanic aldehydes in aged beer is disputable (Madigan *et al.*, 1998), but agreement exists regarding the importance of acetaldehyde, which is the main carbonyl component of beer, as a good indicator of the oxygen levels in the bottle.

The disappearance of the stale off-flavor after addition of carbonyl scavengers to beer, such as aminoguanidine (Bravo *et al.*, 2002), confirms the volatile carbonyl compounds as ones mainly responsible for the beer taste instability. However, the myriad of flavor notes changing during staling are due to a much broader range of chemical entities. Organoleptic-active volatile aldehydes, especially those having 7–10 carbon atoms and very low thresholds, are considered to be the most important. In Table 38.1, some saturated and unsaturated aldehydes that have been detected in beer along with their flavor and threshold level in beer are indicated. Only three of the substances listed – *E*-2-nonenal (also called trans-2-nonenal), (2*E*,6*E*)-nonadienal and (2*E*,4*E*)-decadienal – are present in aged beer in concentrations higher than their flavor thresholds. However, it is known that mixtures of carbonyls can cumulatively cause a perceived flavor.

Of all these aldehydes, *E*-2-nonenal is most frequently cited as the cause of an unpleasant cardboard flavor in beer. A concentration increase of this compound during beer

Beer in Health and Disease Prevention
ISBN: 978-0-12-373891-2

Table 38.1 Typical flavor notes, sensory threshold value and typical concentration of aldehydes in aged beer

Aldehydes	*Typical flavor notes*	*Threshold value (ppb)*	*Concentration in aged beer (ppb)*
Alkanals			
Pentanal	Grassy	500	6
Hexanal	Vinous, bitter	300	4
Heptanal	Vinous, bitter	50	2
Octanal	Vinous, bitter	40	1.7
Nonanal	Astringent	15	4
Decanal	Bitter	5	1
Alkenals			
E-2-hexenal	Astringent	500	1
E-2-Octenal	Bitter, stale	0.3	0.14
E-2-nonenal	Paper, cardboard	0.1	0.16–0.48
E-2-decenal		1.0	0.1
Alkadienals			
(2*E*, 4*E*)-nonadienal	Rancid	0.05	–
(2*E*, 6*E*)-nonadienal	Cucumber	0.5	0.7
(2*E*, 4*E*)-decadienal	Oily, rancid	0.3	0.8

Source: Data from Huige (1993).

ageing has been reported, eventually exceeding its flavor threshold (Jamieson and van Gheluwe, 1970; Wang and Siebert, 1974; Drost *et al.*, 1990).

Recently, an increase of the concentration of another carbonyl compound, β-damascenone, has been found in aged beer. As with *E*-2-nonenal, β-damascenone has also attracted particular attention in the overall context of flavor instability due to its potential use for the characterization of beer ageing (Gijs *et al.*, 2002).

E-2-Nonenal

Since the first manifestation of the term "cardboard flavor" in 1954, by Burger *et al.* (1954), the search to understand the reasons for its development and to identify the compounds responsible for this off-flavor is a main topic in brewing research. Twelve years later, Hashimoto (1966) found a relationship between the development of an oxidized flavor in beer and the level of volatile carbonyl compounds. Jamieson and van Gheluwe in 1970, using GC/MS, were the first to identify *E*-2-nonenal as the compound responsible for the cardboard off-flavor produced in beer when submitted to artificial ageing at elevated temperature and low pH values. Wang and Siebert (1974) demonstrated, 4 years later, that the rise in concentration of *E*-2-nonenal induced by artificial ageing (6 days at 38 °C) causes a perceptible change in beer flavor, from fresh to stale, large enough to account for the papery/cardboard taste sensation, without requiring the synergistic participation of other compounds. The flavor threshold of *E*-2-nonenal, which was reported to be between 0.1 μg/l (Meilgaard, 1975) and 0.03 μg/l in beer (Meilgaard, 1993), is unusually low compared with other aldehydes found in beer.

Drost *et al.* (1990) submitted a packaged beer to natural ageing over 6 months and found, at the end of that time, a *E*-2-nonenal concentration between 0.1 and 0.22 μg/l (Figure 38.1). They suggested that the main mechanism contributing to the generation of *E*-2-nonenal in beer is both the enzymatic and nonenzymatic oxidation of lipids and oxidized free fatty acids.

Recently a study regarding the cytotoxicity of *E*-2-nonenal has been published (Dey *et al.*, 2005). The authors studied the cytotoxicity of unbonded and bonded *E*-2-nonenal and concluded that both forms are cytotoxic at concentration of 95–125 and 200 μg/ml, respectively. However, these levels of *E*-2-nonenal are absolutely impossible to attain only by the ingestion of beer.

The strong dependency with the analytical methodology used should be taken into consideration when comparing the values reported in the literature. Because of the unusual trace level of *E*-2-nonenal in beer, measurement of this compound requires a rather sensitive analytical method. Additionally, since a significant fraction of *E*-2-nonenal in wort and beer is linked to amino acids (Noël and Collin, 1995; Lermusieau *et al.*, 1999) and sulfite (Nyborg *et al.*, 1999; Dufour *et al.*, 1999), a rigorous control of the pH during the sample preparation is required. Most analytical procedures involve a preliminary concentration step followed by a derivatization step. Carbonyl compounds have been isolated from beer by liquid–liquid extraction (Wang and Siebert, 1974), vacuum distillation (Currie *et al.*, 1990), steam distillation (Santos *et al.*, 2003), low-pressure distillation followed by purge and trap (P&T) with Tenax TA (Harayama *et al.*, 1994), and solid-phase extraction (Verhagen *et al.*, 1987; Santos *et al.*, 2003). Solid-phase microextraction (SPME) and stir bar sorptive extraction (SBSE) followed by thermal desorption GC–MS analysis

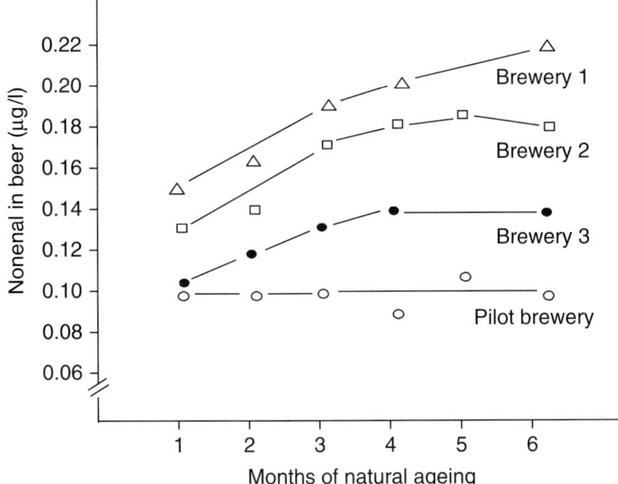

Figure 38.1 Increase of *E*-2-nonenal concentration over 6 months in beers from four different breweries (after Drost *et al.*, 1990).

are methods recently developed for the determination of *E*-2-nonenal in beer (Ochiai *et al.*, 2003; Vesely *et al.*, 2003). In high-performance liquid chromatography (HPLC) with ultraviolet (UV) detection, it is possible to directly determine *E*-2-nonenal (Currie *et al.*, 1990; Santos *et al.*, 2003); however, for a more general determination of aldehydes, a derivatizing procedure can be used. 2,4-Dinitrophenylhydrazine is the most widely used derivatizing agent for aldehydes (Currie *et al.*, 1990), but dansylhydrazine (Verhagen *et al.*, 1987) and dabsylhydrazine (Wu and Lin, 1995) have also been used because of their high sensitivity. These aldehydes derivatives are then separated and estimated by HPLC/UV. Determination of derivatized *E*-2-nonenal by GC/MS was recently reported (Ochiai *et al.*, 2003; Vesely *et al.*, 2003).

The Nonenal Potential Concept

Drost *et al.* (1990) developed a fast and easy method to predict beer flavor stability, assuming the formation of *E*-2-nonenal as one of the main causes of beer staling. The method allows the determination of the so-called nonenal potential of wort. It is defined as the potential of wort to release *E*-2-nonenal under beer conditions and by using a forced ageing procedure. To establish these beerlike conditions, the pH of the wort is adjusted to 4.0 (approximately the beer pH). This solution is then heated at 100°C in a closed tube under an argon atmosphere for 120 min, and the released *E*-2-nonenal is determined. The described heating procedure should simulate a staling process in a closed, almost oxygen-free, beer bottle.

The interactions of *E*-2-nonenal with other groups of substances, such as sulfite (Dufour *et al.*, 1999; Nyborg *et al.*, 1999) and amino acids (Noël and Collin, 1995; Lermusieau *et al.*, 1999), account for the essential control of the pH during this experiment. Furthermore, Wang and Siebert (1974) discovered a strong dependence of the formation of this aldehyde on the pH level: a 400-fold increase in the *E*-2-nonenal concentration in a superacid environment compared to the usual pH of beer conditions was found.

According to some authors (Drost *et al.*, 1990; Lermusieau *et al.*, 1999; Ueda *et al.*, 2001), there is a good correlation between the measured nonenal potential in wort and the results of an overall quality rating of the beer produced. Using this assay, very successful malt selections and malting methods for improving flavor stability of beer have been developed (Fournier *et al.*, 2001). However, the biochemical background of the formation of *E*-2-nonenal during mashing is not completely understood (Kuroda *et al.*, 2005). Some authors argued that the nonenal potential in wort is not a good indicator for the later flavor stability of the produced beers (van Waesberghe, 2002; Wackerbauer and Meyna, 2002).

Formation and Chemical Equilibrium of *E*-2-Nonenal

The earlier theories for aldehydes formation in staled beer only consider their *de novo* synthesis in beer. Although it cannot be disputed that aldehydes are produced by reactions taking place in beer, the extensive research involving *E*-2-nonenal over the past few years reveals that 2-alkenals participate in various chemical equilibria. Consequently, flavor staling could be the result of equilibrium shifting in favor of free aldehydes from compounds that are formed during the malting and mashing processes (Geois *et al.*, 2002). The first evidence for the existence of 3-hydroxy alkanals in malt and wort was provided by Barker *et al.* (1983), who detected 3-hydroxybutanal and 3-hydroxynonanal, formed from aldol condensation of shorter chain aldehydes or by hydration of unsaturated aldehydes. It has been suggested that hydration plays an integral role in the key equilibrium that determines the stability of the α,β-unsaturated aldehyde (Barker *et al.*, 1983).

Isolation and identification of *Z*-3-hexenal and *Z*-3-nonenal in beer extracts led Barker *et al.* (1989) to suggest that these *Z*-3-alkenals, directly derived from the oxidative degradation of linoleic and linolenic acids, would be direct sources of the corresponding *E*-2-alkenals via isomerization induced by heat and under acidic conditions. Results of this investigation suggested that some of the *Z*-3-nonenal, produced by linoleic acid oxidation of barley lipids during malt kilning and wort production, survived from wort into beer, where its ultimate isomerization was likely to be retarded by not only low storage temperatures but also by the formation of sulfite complexes. The flavor imparted by *Z*-3-nonenal is not a cardboard flavor but a soybean-oil-like flavor, and its flavor threshold in beer was determined to be 0.5 μg/l (Sakuma and Kowaka, 1994). The isomerization ratio from *Z*-3-nonenal to *E*-2-nonenal was shown, by Sakuma and Kowaka (1994), to be approximately 20% after 1 day of storage of beer at 5 °C. Sulfite, produced by yeast during fermentation or added before bottling, readily forms adducts with carbonyl compounds, rendering them nonvolatile and flavor-inactive (Nyborg *et al.*, 1999). In addition, the interaction of sulfite with carbonyl compounds was recently demonstrated by voltammetry (Guido *et al.*, 2003). Development of the cardboard flavor in aged beer is strongly retarded when such beers are supplemented with sulfite. Nordlöv and Winell (1983) found that most of the *E*-2-nonenal is bound as a taste-inactive sulfite adduct as long as the level of total SO_2 in aged beer exceeds 2 mg/l, although they do not verify the existence of such adducts. Nyborg *et al.* (1999) demonstrated that flavor-active *E*-2-nonenal disappeared from beer on addition of sulfite species, suggesting the formation of flavor-inactive adducts. They confirmed the adduct formation between *E*-2-nonenal and sulfite, in aqueous solution at beer pH, indirectly by ^1H NMR spectroscopy and directly by LC/MS. The mechanism of the addition reaction proceeds in a two-step process, to initially give a carbonyl adduct and ultimately yield a disulfonate as the thermodynamic product (Dufour *et al.*, 1999).

Another kind of complex was suggested to be the major degradation product of *E*-2-nonenal during mashing and boiling. Approximately 90% of *E*-2-nonenal was retained by an amino acid mixture after 15 min at 36 °C, by forming Schiff bases (Noël and Collin, 1995). The resulting imine, created during mashing and boiling, would protect *E*-2-nonenal from the reducing activity of yeast releasing it at lower pH during beer storage (Lermusieau *et al.*, 1999). Addition of amino acids to beers should therefore delay alkenal release.

The equilibrium proposed above shows various alternative routes for the fate of *E*-2-nonenal and other α,β-unsaturated aldehydes throughout the malting and the brewing process (Figure 38.2). It has been postulated that these reactions equilibriums are interconnected and that volatile carbonyls may be slowly released from their nonvolatile complexes through equilibrium shifts. These shifts may be caused by some perturbation, such as the oxidative loss of sulfite, the decrease in pH or the increase in storage temperature.

Recently, a detailed discussion of reaction mechanisms leading to the formation of aldehydes, particularly of *E*-2-nonenal, in beer was published (Vanderhaegen *et al.*, 2006).

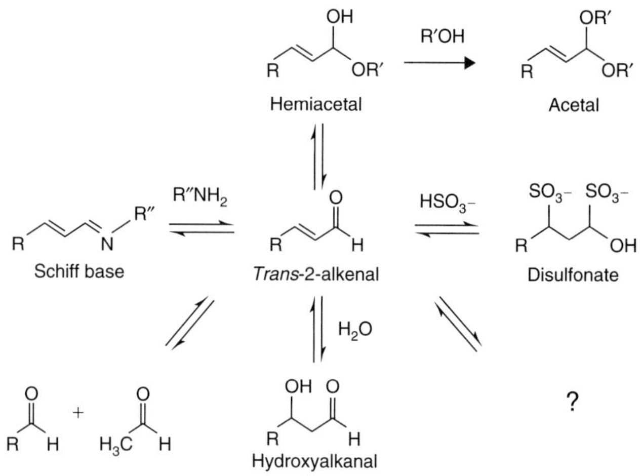

Figure 38.2 Potential equilibrium of α,β-unsaturated aldehydes in beer (after Dufour *et al.*, 1999).

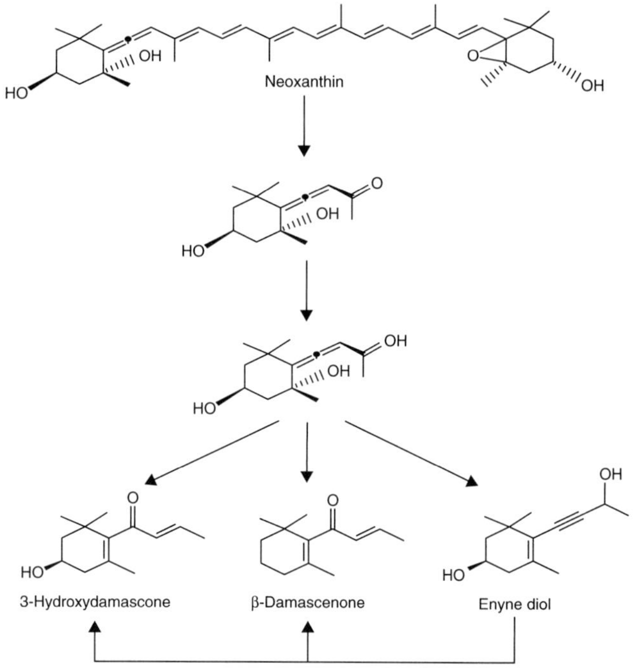

Figure 38.3 Hypothetical pathways for the formation of β-damascenone from neoxanthin (adapted from Puglisi *et al.*, 2001).

β-Damascenone

β-Damascenone, a terpenic ketone (8*E*-megastigma-3,5,8-trien-7-one, Figure 38.3) first identified in Bulgarian rose oil (Demole *et al.*, 1970) and later found in the essential oils of other natural materials, is a highly odoriferous compound important in the creation of modern fragrances (Lee *et al.*, 1991). As it is characterized by a very low odor threshold in water (0.02–0.09 ng/g) (Buttery *et al.*, 1990), β-damascenone was considered to be a significant flavor in many alcoholic beverages such as whiskey, brandy, rum, wine and beer (Masuda and Nishimura, 1980). β-Damascenone has been identified as a key odor in a variety of fruits, vegetables and derived products, including wine where it imparts a pleasant "stewed apple," "fruity" and honeylike character.

Additionally, β-damascenone has been included among the five most important flavor-active compounds in young red wines (Ferreira *et al.*, 2000) and has been identified as the compound with the highest odor activity in Bavarian pale lager beer (Fritsch and Schieberle, 2005).

Fickert and Schieberle (1998) had already identified β-damascenone as an odor-active volatile compound in an extract from barley malt, but only recently an increase in the use of β-damascenone concentration during an artificial ageing of a variety of commercial Belgian beers (Chevance *et al.*, 2002) and top-fermented beers (Vanderhaegen *et al.*, 2003) has been reported. Moreover, β-damascenone was identified as the cause for the most intense aroma in a 6-month-old beer sample (Murakami *et al.*, 2000).

The origin of β-damascenone in beer and its relationship with beer ageing are two topics of great importance that have not yet been clarified. Kotseridis *et al.* (1999) showed that the levels of β-damascenone of wine almost double by heat treatment. Recent studies have indicated that β-damascenone in wine results from the hydrolytic breakdown of complex grape-derived secondary metabolites formed from carotenoids such as neoxanthin (Skouroumounis and Sefton, 2000).

Although the investigation of the mechanisms for the formation of β-damascenone in beer is just beginning, it is believed that it can be formed by acid-catalyzed conversion of the glycoconjugated forms of the allenic triol and derived from enzymatic transformations of the carotenoid neoxanthin (Figure 38.3) present in the basic ingredients of beer (Puglisi *et al.*, 2001). Chevance *et al.* (2002) suggest that the increase in β-damascenone during beer ageing could also be partially explained by acid-catalyzed hydrolysis of glycosides present in fresh beer. A remarkable amount of β-damascenone was formed after acidic hydrolysis of the hop glycoside of 3-hydroxy-β-damascone (Figure 38.4). This glycoside was also found in unhopped beer, suggesting that hop is not the only source for β-damascenone (Biendl *et al.*, 2003).

β-Damascenone is already present at a high level in the initial wort, but it is extensively removed after 7 days of fermentation at 20 °C, after reduction and/or adsorption by yeast (Chevance *et al.*, 2002). Beer pH seems to have a crucial role on the β-damascenone level, with higher concentrations of this compound observed for aged beers having lower pH (Gijs *et al.*, 2002). Air in the headspace of the bottles seems to have no influence on the β-damascenone content of a 6-month-old beer stored at 40 °C (Vanderhaegen *et al.*, 2003).

Clear evidences exist nowadays regarding the relevance of β-damascenone as one of the most important carbonyl compounds contributing to the odor variation observed during beer ageing. It has been recognized by some authors that β-damascenone seems at least as important as *E*-2-nonenal in the flavor of aged beer (Gijs *et al.*, 2002).

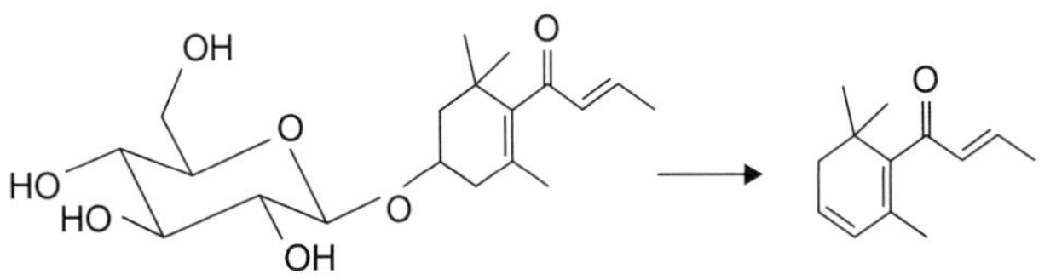

OH, HO, HO, O, O, OH, O, O

β-d-glycoside of 3-hydroxy-β-damascone → β-damascenone

Figure 38.4 Liberation of β-damascenone after acidic hydrolysis of glycosides in hops.

Determination of *E*-2-Nonenal and β-Damascenone in Beer

Most of the methods for the assessment of *E*-2-nonenal in beer are laborious and time-consuming, requiring strong acidic conditions to obtain derivatives, which may change the carbonyl compounds of interest or induce equilibrium shifts. Recently a new analytical method for the simultaneous determination of *E*-2-nonenal and β-damascenone in beer by reversed-phase liquid chromatography with UV detection was developed by Santos *et al.* (2003). The proposed method is fast and easy to implement with no need for derivatization. The method is believed to be more sensitive than the gas chromatographic-mass spectrometric method, provided that potential interferences were effectively removed. The experimental procedure used for the extraction, separation and determination is described in detail elsewhere (Santos *et al.*, 2003). The major advantages of the proposed methodology, when compared to other existing methods, are fastness and simplicity whereas the major drawback is the possibility of some conversion of precursors into *E*-2-nonenal during the steam distillation step used in the extraction of the volatile compounds.

Effect of storage on the concentration of *E*-2-nonenal and β-damascenone found in beer

Using the afore-mentioned methodology, Santos *et al.* (2003) monitored *E*-2-nonenal and β-damascenone in beer during an extended storage time at different conditions. They used two different lots of beer that were stored in the following conditions: 4 weeks at 4 °C, 4 and 12 weeks at 20 °C in the dark (naturally aged beers) and 7 days at 37 °C in the dark (artificially aged beers). As it can be deduced by observing data in Table 38.2, a strong correlation between the storage conditions and the concentrations of *E*-2-nonenal and β-damascenone was verified. No variation was found in the concentrations of *E*-2-nonenal and β-damascenone for beers stored at 4 °C, although the concentration of both compounds increases for beers stored at higher temperatures. It is noteworthy that the concentration of *E*-2-nonenal after 12 weeks of natural ageing exceeds its flavor threshold in beer (roughly 0.1 μg/l). High storage temperatures led to the formation/liberation of β-damascenone, resulting

Table 38.2 Concentration of *E*-2-nonenal and β-damascenone (confidence limits for four determinations) found in beer (Lot A and B) after different storage conditions

Lot	*Fresh beer*	*4°C 12 weeks*	*20°C 4 weeks*	*20°C 12 weeks*	*37°C 1 week*
	E-2-nonenal (μg/l)				
A	0.06 ± 0.01	0.07 ± 0.01	0.08 ± 0.01	0.13 ± 0.03	0.16 ± 0.04
B	0.07 ± 0.01	0.07 ± 0.01	0.09 ± 0.01	0.18 ± 0.04	0.20 ± 0.05
	β-Damascenone (μg/l)				
A	1.8 ± 0.2	1.6 ± 0.2	2.3 ± 0.2	2.6 ± 0.3	2.9 ± 0.3
B	1.8 ± 0.2	1.8 ± 0.2	2.2 ± 0.2	2.6 ± 0.3	2.8 ± 0.3

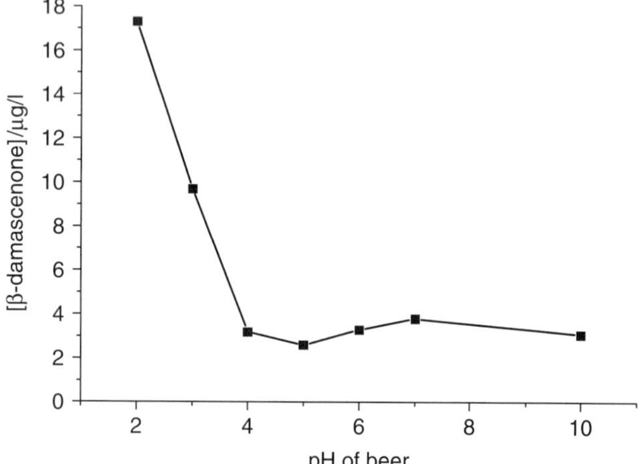

Figure 38.5 Effect of pH on the concentration of β-damascenone found in beer.

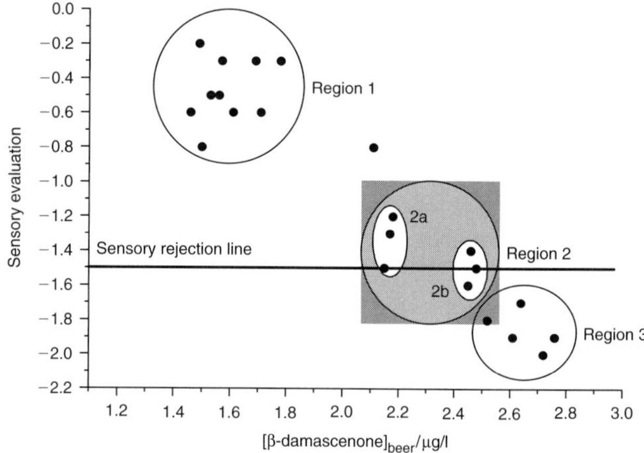

Figure 38.6 Relationship between sensory evaluation and β-damascenone concentration found in beers.

in an increase of the concentration of this compound during beer ageing. Although the mechanisms responsible for this behavior have not been completely elucidated yet, the acidic hydrolysis of glycosides has been described in the literature as the most likely hypothesis (Skouroumounis and Sefton, 2000; Chevance *et al.*, 2002).

Santos *et al.* (2003) have also studied the effect of beer pH, after a pH adjustment, on the concentration of *E*-2-nonenal and β-damascenone, showing that both compounds have a comparable behavior regarding the influence of pH. The results obtained confirm that the formation/liberation of β-damascenone from its precursors is much higher at lower pH values (Figure 38.5), thus supporting the hypothesis that an acidic hydrolysis is responsible for the development of β-damascenone in beer. These results are in agreement with those obtained by Gijs *et al.* (2002).

β-Damascenone as an analytical marker of organoleptic deterioration of beer

Guido *et al.* (2003) have made a specific study to evaluate the possible correlation between the β-damascenone content in beer and the development of off-flavors during beer ageing, with the aid of a sensory panel. β-Damascenone was determined in several beers stored for a long period of time under different conditions and, simultaneously, the sensory changes were followed regularly by an expert evaluation panel. This panel consisted of eight trained tasters who were asked to comment on general quality (discrimination test) as well as to describe the flavor profile according to a special form (description test). All beers were tested at 4°C and evaluated for the degree of staling on a 5-point scale defined as: (+1) no sign of oxidation, (0) very slight oxidation symptoms (−1) slight oxidation symptoms, (−2) enough level of oxidation to reject the beer and (−3) very strong level of deterioration by oxidation. The sensory classification of each beer consisted in the mean value of the scores provided by all the tasters, with an adopted sensory rejection limit of −1.5. The organoleptic state of a beer with a sensory rating lower than −1.5 is considered not satisfactory, implying the rejection of the product by the panel.

As it can be seen in Figure 38.6, a good correlation was found between the concentration of β-damascenone in beer and the sensory evaluation, with higher concentrations of β-damascenone corresponding to lower values of the sensory evaluation. A more detailed inspection of Figure 38.6 allows the identification of three different regions. Region 1 includes beers analyzed immediately after bottling and stored at 4°C for 4 and 12 weeks; these beers obtained the highest score in the sensory evaluation tests and contained the lower concentrations of β-damascenone. Region 2 is formed by beers stored at 20°C; beers stored during 12 weeks (subregion 2b) were given a slightly worse sensory evaluation than beers stored during 4 weeks only (subregion 2a), approaching the sensory rejection line; this decrease in the sensory evaluation was accompanied by an increase in the concentrations of β-damascenone. Finally, all the beers of region 3 (stored at 37°C for 1 week) were considered not satisfactory by the sensory panel, and this worse evaluation was correlated with higher contents of β-damascenone.

The observed correlation between the β-damascenone content and the storage temperature of beers shows that this can be used as a good analytical marker of beer ageing induced by heat. Additionally, the obtained results suggest that β-damascenone can also be used as an analytical marker of the organoleptic state of beer. Obviously, this does not imply that β-damascenone has a direct impact on the organoleptic degradation that beer suffers during ageing, or that the off-flavors perceived by the sensory panel are a direct consequence of the increase in concentration of β-damascenone.

Summary Points

- The knowledge of the mechanisms of beer ageing could help to develop strategies to improve brewing technology and to produce beer with increased flavor stability.
- *E*-2-nonenal has been recognized as the compound responsible for the characteristic cardboard off-flavor, an organoleptic problem that arises during beer storage. Therefore, the study of *E*-2-nonenal and its formation mechanisms is a main topic of research on beer ageing.
- There is strong evidence that the mechanism for development of *E*-2-nonenal in beer begin with the formation of precursors from enzymatic and non-enzymatic lipid oxidation, mainly from linoleic acid, during malting and mashing. These precursors (recognized as nonenal potential) are incorporated into the beer and slowly converted to *E*-2-nonenal during beer storage.
- β-Damascenone, a carotenoid-derived compound, can directly affect beer flavor during ageing, generating a pleasant "stewed apple," "fruity" and honey-like character.
- Both *E*-2-nonenal and β-damascenone have a similar increasing behavior through extended storage of beer. β-Damascenone can advantageously be used as a chemical indicator of beer ageing instead of *E*-2-nonenal, because its analytical determination is easier. The evolution of β-damascenone and *E*-2-nonenal concentrations in beer during storage correlates well with expert sensory panel taste scores.
- There is no evidence that *E*-2-nonenal and β-damascenone could have effects, adverse or beneficial, on human health, at the levels found in beer.

References

Bamforth, C.W. (1999). *Brauwelt Int.* 2, 98–110.

Barker, R.L., Gracey, D.E., Irwin, A.J., Pipasts, P. and Leiska, E.J. (1983). *Inst. Brew.* 89, 411–415.

Barker, R.L., Pipasts, P. and Gracey, D.E. (1989). *J. Am. Soc. Brew. Chem.* 47, 9–14.

Biendl, M., Kollmannsberger, H. and Nitz, S. (2003). *Proc. Congr. Eur. Brew. Conv.* 252–257.

Bravo, A., Sánchez, B., Scherer, E., Herrera, J. and Rangel-Aldao, R. (2002). *Master Brew. Assoc. Am. Tech. Q.* 39, 13–23.

Burger, M., Glenister, P.R. and Becker, K. (1954). *Proc. Am. Soc. Brew. Chem.* 12, 98–107.

Buttery, R.G., Teranishi, R., Ling, L.C. and Turnbaugh, J.G. (1990). *J. Agr. Food Chem.* 38, 336–340.

Chevance, F., Guyot-Declerck, C., Dupont, J. and Collin, S. (2002). *J. Agric. Food Chem.* 50, 3818–3821.

Currie, B.R., Kulandal, J., FitzRoy, M.D., Hawthorne, D.B. and Kavanagh, T.E. (1990). *Proc. Conv. Inst. Brew.* (Aust. & NZ Sect.), 117–125.

Demole, E., Enggist, P., Säuberli, U., Stoll, M. and Kovats, E. (1970). *Helv. Chim. Acta* 53, 541–551.

Dey, E.S., Staniszewska, M., Pasciak, M., Konopacka, M., Rogolinski, J., Gamian, A. and Danielsson, B. (2005). *Polish J. Microbiol.* 54, 47–52.

Drost, B.W., van der Berg, R., Freijee, F.J., van der Velde, E.G. and Hollemans, M. (1990). *J. Am. Soc. Brew. Chem.* 48, 124–131.

Dufour, J.-P., Leus, M., Baxter, A.J. and Hayman, A.R. (1999). *J. Am. Soc. Brew. Chem.* 57, 138–144.

Ferreira, V., López, R. and Cacho, J.F. (2000). *J. Sci. Food Agr.* 80, 1659–1667.

Fickert, B. and Schieberle, P. (1998). *Nahrung* 42, 371–375.

Fournier, R., Dumoulin, M. and Boivin, P. (2001). European Brewery Convention, *Proceedings of the 28th Congress*, Budapest, CD-ROM.

Fritsch, H.T. and Schieberle, P. (2005). *J. Agric. Food Chem.* 53, 7544–7551.

Geois, C.L., Meurens, N., Badot, C. and Collin, S. (2002). *J. Agric. Food Chem.* 50, 7634–7638.

Gijs, L., Chevance, F., Jerkovic, V. and Collin, S. (2002). *J. Agric. Food Chem.* 50, 5612–5616.

Guido, L.F., Fortunato, N.A., Rodrigues, J.A. and Barros, A.A. (2003). *J. Agr. Food. Chem.* 51, 3911–3915.

Harayama, K., Hayase, F. and Kato, H. (1994). *Biosci. Biotechnol. Biochem.* 58, 1595–1598.

Hashimoto, N. (1966). *Rept. Res. Lab. Kirin Brewery Co., Ltd.*, 9, 1–10.

Huige, N.J. (1993). Progress in beer oxidation. In *Beer and Wine Production – Analysis, Characterization and Technological Advances*" (Ed. Barry H. Gump), p. 64–97, ACS Symposium series, 536. American Chemical Society, Washington, DC.

Jamieson, A.M. and van Gheluwe, J.E. (1970). *Proc. Am. Soc. Brew. Chem.*, 28, 192–197.

Kotseridis, Y., Baumes, R. and Skouroumounis, G. (1999). *J. Chromatogr. A* 849, 245–254.

Kuroda, H., Kojima, H., Kaneda, H. and Takashio, M. (2005). *Biosci. Biotechnol. Biochem.* 69, 1661–1668.

Lee, W.Y., Jang, S.Y., Lee, J.-G. and Chae, W.K. (1991). *Bull. Korean Chem. Soc.* 12, 31–35.

Lermusieau, G., Noël, S., Liégeois, C. and Collin, S. (1999). *J. Am. Soc. Brew. Chem.* 57, 29–33.
Lustig, S. (1996). *Proc. Barley, Malt Wort Symp.* (C & SA Sect.), 59–75.
Madigan, D., Perez, A. and Clements, M. (1998). *J. Am. Soc. Brew. Chem.* 56, 146–151.
Masuda, M. and Nishimura, K. (1980). *J. Food Sci.* 45, 396–397.
Meilgaard, M.C. (1975). *Master Brew. Assoc. Am. Tech. Q.* 12, 107–117.
Meilgaard, M.C. (1993). *Food Qual. Pref.* 4, 153–167.
Murakami, A.A., Goldstein, H., Navarro, A., Seabrooks, J.R. and Ryder, D.S. (2000). *J. Am. Soc. Brew. Chem.* 61, 23–32.
Noël, S. and Collin, S. (1995). *Proc. Congr. Eur. Brew. Conv.* 483–490.
Nordlöv, H. and Winell, B. (1983). *Proc. Congr. Eur. Brew. Conv.* 271–278.
Nyborg, M., Outtrup, H. and Dreyer, T. (1999). *J. Am. Soc. Brew. Chem.* 57, 24–28.
Ochiai, N., Sasamoto, K., Daishima, S., Heiden, A.C. and Hoffmann, A. (2003). *J. Chromatogr. A.* 986, 101–110.
Puglisi, C.J., Elsey, G.M., Prager, R.H., Skouroumounis, G.K. and Sefton, M.A. (2001). *Tetrahedron Lett.* 42, 6937–6939.
Sakuma, S. and Kowaka, M. (1994). *J. Am. Soc. Brew. Chem.* 52, 37–41.
Santos, J.R., Carneiro, J.R., Guido, L.F., Almeida, P.J., Rodrigues, J.A. and Barros, A.A. (2003). *J. Chromatogr. A.* 985, 395–402.
Skouroumounis, G.K. and Sefton, M.A. (2000). *J. Agric. Food Chem.* 48, 2033–2039.
Ueda, T., Sasaki, K., Inomoto, K., Kono, K., Kagami, N., Shibata, K. and Eto, M. (2001). *Proc. Congr. Eur. Brew. Conv.* 885–889.
Van Waesberghe, J.W. (2002). *Brauwelt Int.* 6, 375–378.
Vanderhaegen, B., Neven, H., Coghe, S., Verstrepen, K.J., Verachtert, H. and Derdelinckx, G. (2003). *J. Agric. Food Chem.* 51, 6782–6790.
Vanderhaegen, B., Neven, H., Verachtert, H. and Derdelinckx, G. (2006). *Food Chem.* 95, 357–381.
Verhagen, L.C., Strating, J. and Tjaden, U.R. (1987). *J. Chromatogr.* 393, 85–96.
Vesely, P., Lusk, L., Basarova, G., Seabrooks, J. and Ryder, D. (2003). *J. Agric. Food Chem.* 51, 6941–6944.
Wackerbauer, K. and Meyna, S. (2002). *Proc. 4th technical meeting (Oporto), Brewing Science group, Eur. Brew. Conv.*, 170–181.
Wang, P.S. and Siebert, K.J. (1974). *Master Brew. Assoc. Am. Tech. Q.* 11, 110–117.
Wu, H.-Y. and Lin, J.-K. (1995). *Anal. Chem.* 67, 1603–1612.

39

Pathogens in Beer

Garry Menz, Peter Aldred and Frank Vriesekoop School of Science and Engineering, Institute of Food and Crop Science, University of Ballarat, Ballarat, Australia

Abstract

Pathogenic (disease-causing) microorganisms cannot survive in beer due to the presence of various inhibitory factors/hurdles. The major intrinsic hurdles that a pathogen must overcome to survive in a beer are the presence of ethanol produced by yeasts during fermentation (up to 10% (v/v), typically 3.5–5.0% (v/v)), hop (*Humulus lupulus*) bittering compounds (approx. 17–55 parts per million *iso*-α-acids), low pH (approx. 3.9–4.4), carbon dioxide (approx. 0.5% (w/w)), low oxygen (<0.1 ppm), and the lack of nutritive substances. Ethanol and hops interfere with essential cell membrane functions, the low pH hinders enzyme activity, the lack of nutrients and oxygen starves many potential pathogens, whilst elevated dissolved carbon dioxide lowers the pH, inhibits enzymes, affects cell membranes, and creates an anaerobic environment. In addition to these intrinsic factors, many stages of the brewing process reduce the potential for contamination, such as mashing, wort boiling, pasteurization, filtration, aseptic packaging and cold storage. Various studies have shown that the survivability of pathogens such as *Escherichia coli*, *Salmonella* Typhimurium, and *Vibrio cholerae* in most beers is very poor. However, beers without, or with, reduced levels of one or more of these antimicrobial "hurdles" are more prone to the survival and/or growth of pathogenic organisms. Examples are low-alcohol and unpasteurized beer, for which special attention must be paid to ensure their safety.

List of Abbreviations

°C	Degrees Celsius
<	Less than
Approx.	Approximately
B.	*Bacillus*
CFU	Colony forming units
CFU/ml	Colony forming units per milliliter
Cl.	*Clostridium*
CO_2	Carbon dioxide
DNA	Deoxyribonucleic acid
E.	*Escherichia*
h	hour(s)
IPA	India Pale Ale
L.	*Listeria*
Lact.	*Lactobacillus*
ml	Milliliter
min	minutes
O_2	Oxygen
ppm	Parts per million
RNA	Ribonucleic acid
Salm.	*Salmonella*
Sh.	*Shigella*
Staph.	*Staphylococcus*
SO_2	Sulfur dioxide
spp.	Species
V.	*Vibrio*
v/v	Volume per volume
w/w	Weight per weight
WWI	World War I
WWII	World War II
Y.	*Yersinia*

Introduction

Beer is considered to be an intrinsically safe beverage, resistant to microbial contamination. This is mainly due to a number of inhibitory factors (hurdles), which when combined inhibit the growth and survival of pathogenic (disease-causing) microorganisms. The presence of ethanol (up to 10% (v/v), typically 3.5–5.0% (v/v)), hop (*Humulus lupulus*) bittering compounds (approx. 17–55 ppm *iso*-α-acids), low pH (approx. 3.9–4.4), elevated dissolved carbon dioxide (approx. 0.5% (w/w)), low oxygen (<0.1 ppm), and the lack of nutritive substances protect beer from many potential pathogens. In addition to these intrinsic factors, many stages of the brewing process reduce the potential for contamination, such as mashing, wort boiling, pasteurization, filtration, aseptic packaging, and cold storage. This chapter reviews the occurrence and survivability of pathogens in beer, and discusses the antimicrobial hurdles that ensure the microbial safety of beer.

Beer in Health and Disease Prevention
ISBN: 978-0-12-373891-2

Pathogens in Beer

Reports of pathogens in beer and associated products

It is widely recognized that pathogens cannot grow or survive in beer, due to the presence of various intrinsic and extrinsic antimicrobial hurdles. However, there have been several reports of pathogens occurring in beer-like products (Table 39.1). These beer-like products differ from traditional European-style beers, as they either lack one or more of the antimicrobial hurdles typical of beer, or the hurdles are present at a reduced level.

Pseudomonas spp. and *Escherichia* spp. were reported as beer spoilers during World War I and II in "weak" beers, such as those with a pH above 5.0 or with short lagering time (Chevalier, 1946, as cited in Rainbow, 1981). The pathogens *Bacillus cereus, Escherichia coli, Proteus vulgaris, Salmonella* Typhimurium, *Shigella sonnei*, and *Staphylococcus aureus* were detected in boza (a traditional Belgian ale-type product made from millet, with an alcohol content of approx. 1%) (Enikova *et al.*, 1985). This product lacked many of the antimicrobial hurdles that usually protect beer, as boza typically has a low ethanol content (<1%) and is not hopped. However, an investigation into brewing equipment hygiene has yielded coliforms and *Aeromonas* spp. (Nishikawa *et al.*, 1979), although *Aeromonas* spp. is yet to be reported in beer.

Traditional African beers have the potential to support the growth of pathogens, as they typically lack or have lower levels of some of the antimicrobial hurdles that usually offer protection to beer. For example, high levels of coliforms (indicative of the presence of potential pathogens such as *E. coli*, *Salmonella* spp., and *Shigella* spp.) have been detected in Orubisi (Table 39.1), a traditional Tanzanian banana and sorghum beer with a low alcohol content (2.2% ethanol (v/v)) (Shayo *et al.*, 2000). Further, *Bacillus* spp. have been reported in a South African sorghum beer with a lowered ethanol content (<3% ethanol (v/v)) (Pattison *et al.*, 1998).

Although pathogens may not have been detected in beer itself, beer dispensing equipment may be a potential reservoir for pathogenic microorganisms. Schindler and Metz (1990) detected coliforms on beer mugs and tankards, which were suspected to be due to unsatisfactory cleaning. In a later study Taschan (1996) collected 62 samples of beer from German inns, finding that 5% contained *E. coli*, 45% were positive for coliforms, and 70% contained spoilage microorganisms. Comparative studies of bottled beer suggested that the source of contamination was the inn's dispensing equipment. In addition to beer dispensing systems, Storgårds (2000) proposed cross-contamination with food as a potential source of coliforms in beer.

The survival of pathogens in beer

Bacteria Although no pathogenic bacteria have been isolated from beer, several researchers have investigated the survivability of selected pathogenic bacteria in beer. Beer without or with lower levels of one or more of the antimicrobial hurdles will be more susceptible to the growth of bacteria. For example, the potential foodborne pathogens *E. coli*, *Salm.* Typhimurium, *Pseudomonas aeruginosa*, *Shigella flexneri*, *Klebsiella pneumoniae*, *Yersinia enterocolitica*, and *Enterococcus faecium* were capable of growing in an alcohol-free beer (0.5% (v/v) ethanol), although they were destroyed by pasteurization and could not grow in a full strength beer (5% (v/v) ethanol) (L'Anthoën and Ingledew, 1996). Unlike most beers, this alcohol-free beer was nutrient-rich, containing elevated levels of maltose, maltotriose, glucose, and fructose, which supported the bacteria. According to Schmidt (1990), most reduced alcohol beers have a higher pH, are weakly hopped, and contain residual

Table 39.1 Reports of pathogens in beer-like products

Product	*Brief description*	*Major inhibitory factors*	*Pathogen survival*	*References*
Boza	Fermented low-alcohol millet ale	<1% ethanol (v/v), lactic acid	Pathogens detected: *Bacillus cereus, Escherichia coli, Proteus vulgaris, Salmonella* Typhimurium, *Shigella sonnei, Staphylococcus aureus*	Enikova *et al.* (1985)
"Weak beer"	Weak beer produced during WWI and WWII with high pH (>5.0) and/or short lagering time	As for beer, although an increased pH	*Escherichia, Pseudomonas*	Chevalier, as cited in Rainbow (1981)
Orubisi	Traditional Tanzanian banana and sorghum beer, spontaneous alcoholic and lactic fermentation	2.2% ethanol (v/v), pH 3.7, lactic acid	High levels of coliforms indicate presence of the pathogens: *Escherichia coli, Salmonella, Shigella*	Shayo *et al.* (2000)
Sorghum beer	Lactic and alcoholic fermentation South African	<3% ethanol (v/v), pH 3.1, lactic acid	*Bacillus* spp. detected, pathogenicity unreported	Pattison *et al.* (1998)

nutrients, leaving them susceptible to undesirable microbial growth. In these beers, several of the protective hurdles are at reduced levels, thus a secondary treatment such as pasteurization is necessary to ensure their safety.

The survival of the enteric pathogens *E. coli*, *Salm.* Typhimurium, and *Sh. sonnei* in beer was briefly studied by Sheth *et al.* (1988). A single beer was inoculated with 2×10^6 colony forming units (CFU) per ml, and incubated at 36°C. Survival of the pathogens was poor, although small numbers (approx. 5 CFU/ml) could be detected after 48 h. Similar results have been obtained by other workers, such as Zikes (1903) who reported that *Salm.* Typhimurium survived for less than 15 min in beer. Furthermore, Bendová and Kurzová (1968) reported that *Sh. flexneri* and *Salm.* Typhimurium were capable of limited survival in wort and beer maintained at 4°C for 7 days, although no growth was observed. In this study, survival was higher in wort than in beer, highlighting the importance of ethanol and the lack of available nutrients on the antimicrobial properties of beer.

Using various inoculum levels (100–800 CFU/ml), Bunker (1955) investigated the survival of several pathogens in four different beers. The greatest resistance was shown by *E. coli*, which survived up to 3 days, whilst *Salm.* Typhimurium, *Sh. sonnei*, and *Staph. aureus* survived 24 h, and *Corynebacterium diphtheriae* and *Streptococcus haemolyticus* remained viable for up to 1 and 3 h, respectively.

Early work by Lentz (1903) and Sachs-Müke (1908) investigated the survivability of *Salmonella* Typhi in beer. Lentz (1903) showed that the bacterium causing typhoid fever had low viability in beer, and could not be detected after 48 h, whereas Sachs-Müke (1908) reported that *Salm.* Typhi and *Salmonella* Paratyphi remained culturable for 2–5 days. Additional studies by Hompesch (1949) found that *Salm.* Typhi and *Salm.* Paratyphi could survive in beer for up to 5 and 10 days, respectively. Using an unrealistic inoculation level (two million CFU/ml), *Salm.* Typhi remained viable for 55 days, and *Salm.* Paratyphi survived for 63 days (Hompesch, 1949). The viability of *Salm.* Typhi on the rubber seals of swing-top bottles was also studied by Sachs-Müke (1908), who found that the bacteria survived on the rubber seals after 10 days, but could not be isolated out of beer from the same bottles. The author suggested that the bad habit of the working class drinking beer from the bottle (rather than from a glass) could lead to the transmission of typhoid fever.

The survival of the waterborne bacteria *Vibrio cholerae* in beer has been investigated by several authors. Pick (1893, as cited in Zikes, 1903) and Zikes (1903) reported that this pathogen survived for less than 10 min in beer. Other studies have shown that *V. cholerae* could survive for 24 h in a Thai beer (Felsenfeld, 1965), and remained viable for more than 1 h but less than 24 h in another study by Weyl (1892, as cited in Zikes, 1903). Zikes (1903) investigated the factors that influence the survival of *V. cholerae* in beer, by inoculating the bacteria into both fresh and sterilized beer (the sterilization process removed the majority of CO_2 and ethanol). It was concluded that the low survivability of *V. cholerae* in beer is primarily due to the CO_2 and ethanol content (rather than the pH and hops), with the low storage temperature having only a limited influence on survivability.

In a study by Dogel' *et al.* (1984), pathogenic *Yersinia* spp. were found to be resistant to alcohol, surviving for more than 30 min in 3% ethanol. Based on this alcohol tolerance, the authors suggested that beer and other low-alcohol beverages may be involved in the transmission of yersiniosis and pseudotuberculosis. However, the combined effect of the other antimicrobial hurdles in beer (such as hops, low pH and CO_2) was not evaluated.

Protozoa By volume, the major component of beer is water, which is known to be a vehicle for the transmission of various diseases. The majority of brewing water (liquor) is treated and then boiled for at least 45 min during the kettle boil, eliminating the potential for contamination. However, high gravity dilution liquor and water added during filtration are potential sources of pathogenic waterborne protozoa, such as *Cryptosporidium* and *Giardia* (Kuhn and Owades, 1985; Baxter, 1999). Survival of these protozoa was studied by Friedman *et al.* (1997) and Kuhn and Owades (1985). Beer (5% (v/v) ethanol, pH 4.3) was unable to be a host for *Giardia* (Kuhn and Owades, 1985), and Friedman *et al.* (1997) reported that after 24 h in beer at 4°C and 22°C, less than 20% of *Cryptosporidium parvum* oocysts were viable. The reduction in viability was predominantly due to the carbonation and the low pH of the beer.

Opportunistic pathogens

Opportunistic pathogens affect only high-risk subgroups of the population, such as the immunocompromised, and are usually related to an underlying disease (Tauxe, 2002). There have been various reports of species previously associated with the brewing process acting as opportunistic pathogens (Table 39.2). However, these brewery microorganisms generally do not survive into finished beer, and pathogenic strains are yet to be isolated from beer (van Vuuren and Priest, 2003).

Toxins

Despite pathogens being unable to survive in most beers, fungal toxins from contaminated raw materials (such as malt) can prevail and be detected in packaged beer (Scott, 1996). Selected studies reporting on the occurrence of fungal toxins (aflatoxins, deoxynivalenol, ochratoxin A, and zearalenone) in beer are summarized in Table 39.3. Despite aflatoxin levels in beer generally being low (Odhav and Naicker, 2002; Mably *et al.*, 2005), their presence in the food chain must be

Table 39.2 Opportunistic pathogens previously associated with brewing

Opportunistic/emerging pathogen	*Effect on humans*	*Brewing association*	*Reference(s)*[a]
Citrobacter freundii[b]	Diarrhoea	Wort spoiler	Farmer *et al.* (1985)
Enterobacter agglomerans[b]	Endogenous nosocomial infection	Wort spoiler	Sanders and Sanders (1997)
Hafnia alvei[c]	Diarrhoea	Wort spoiler	Ridell *et al.* (1994)
Pediococcus acidilactici[b]	Septicaemia	Malt and mashing	Heinz *et al.* (2000)
Saccharomyces cerevisiae[b]	Invasive infection	Fermentative yeast	Enache-Angoulvant and Hennequin (2005), Murphy and Kavanagh (1999)

[a] Reference to status as an opportunistic pathogen.
[b] Opportunistic pathogen.
[c] Emerging pathogen.

Table 39.3 Selected studies investigating the occurrence of mycotoxins in beer

Toxin(s)	*Country/region*	*Beer type*	*References*
Aflatoxins	Canada	Commercial	Mably *et al.* (2005)
Aflatoxins	South Africa	Commercial, home-brew	Odhav and Naicker (2002)
Deoxynivalenol	Europe	Commercial	Papadopoulou-Bouraoui *et al.* (2004)
Deoxynivalenol	United States	Pilot brew	Schwarz *et al.* (1995)
Ochratoxin A	United States	Pilot brew	Baxter *et al.* (2001), Chu *et al.* (1975)
Zearalenone	Africa	Traditional	Nkwe *et al.* (2005)

minimized as they are considered to be hepatotoxic, carcinogenic, immunosuppressive, and antinutritional (Williams *et al.*, 2004). Other toxins can exhibit similar effects, as deoxynivalenol is immunosuppressive, ochratoxin A is nephrotoxic, teratogenic, immunotoxic, and possibly carcinogenic, fumonisins cause equine leukoencephalomalacia, pulmonary edema in swine, hepatotoxicity, nephrotoxicity, and are carcinogenic, whereas zearalenone has been reported to be genotoxic and a cause of infertility in livestock (Murphy *et al.*, 2006).

In addition to the heat treatments applied during beer production, the presence of brewing yeast minimizes the prevalence of toxins. A significant proportion of the aflatoxins can be mopped up by the yeast during the fermentation (Chu *et al.*, 1975; Scott *et al.*, 1995). The attenuation of the toxicity potentially caused by the aflatoxins is facilitated by yeast cell wall material (Huwig *et al.*, 2001; Ringot *et al.*, 2005), and more specifically due to manno-oligosaccharides associated with the yeast cell wall (Stanley *et al.*, 1993; Baptista *et al.*, 2004). However, while the cell wall mannans are actively involved in the biosorption of aflatoxins, active yeast cells have a greater effect in reducing toxicity symptoms compared to manno-oligosaccharides alone (Baptista *et al.*, 2004). This might be due to the fact that active yeast cells have a greater nutritional value by providing vitamins that could aid in the body's ability to rectify the damage done by aflatoxins.

The other class of microbial toxins that may be of concern is the Gram-negative bacterial endotoxins. However, these were undetectable in packaged beer, albeit in a limited study, by di Luzio and Friedmann (1973).

The Antimicrobial Hurdles of Beer

The microbial safety and stability, the sensory and nutritional quality, and the economic potential of many foods are maintained using a combination of preservative factors (hurdles), termed hurdle technology (Leistner, 2000). By employing numerous hurdles at reduced levels, rather than a single hurdle at an intense level, a product can be produced with more desirable organoleptic properties. A good example of the applied use of hurdle technology in beers is the India Pale Ales (IPAs). During the late 1700s, ales bound for British troops in India spoiled very quickly during the long sea journey (Edgerton, 2005). British brewers needed to increase the stability of their beers, and by the early 1800s this was achieved by brewing beer with higher levels of hops and ethanol (Edgerton, 2005).

Beer contains an array of antimicrobial hurdles that, under most circumstances, prevent the growth of pathogenic microorganisms. Figure 39.1 depicts many of the typical hurdles that ensure the safety of beer, namely boiling in the kettle, the presence of hops, ethanol, carbon dioxide (CO_2), the low pH, and the lack of available nutrients and oxygen (O_2).

Beer is more susceptible to undesirable microbial growth when one or more of these hurdles are absent or at a reduced level. For example, Vaughan *et al.* (2005) noted that beers with elevated pH levels, low ethanol, low CO_2, and those with added sugar (increased nutrients) are more prone to spoilage. According to the work of Fernandez and Simpson (1995), levels of nitrogen (free amino and total soluble), amino acids, maltotriose, beer pH and color significantly

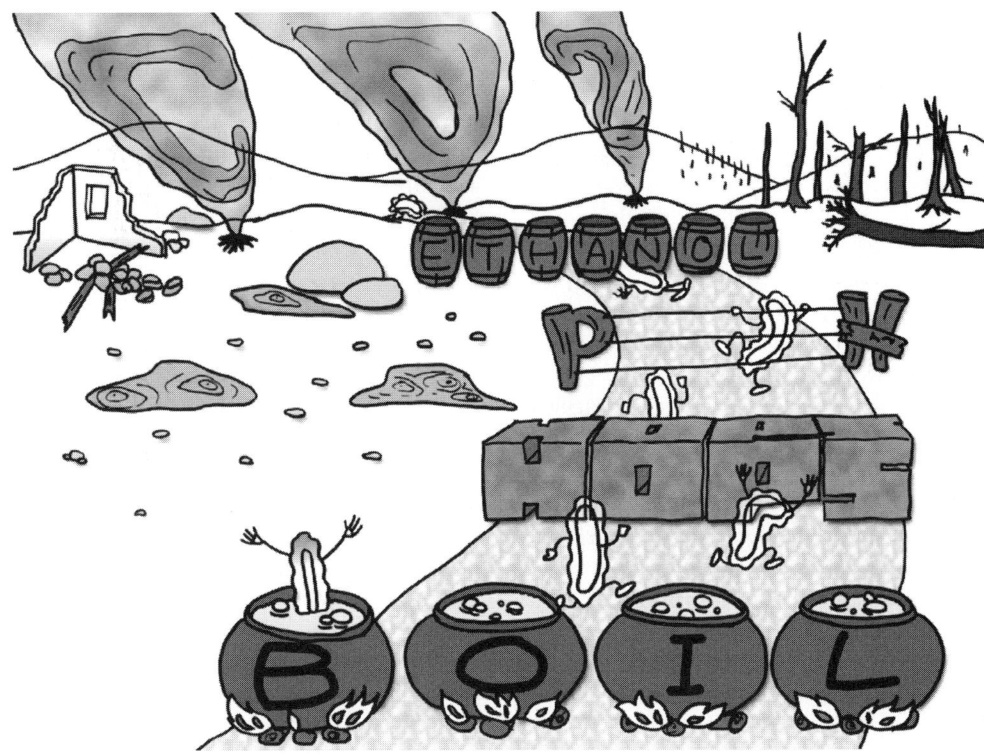

Figure 39.1 Pathogens cannot survive in beer due to the antimicrobial "hurdles," including the kettle boil, hop bitter acids, low pH, ethanol, carbon dioxide (CO_2), and the lack of nutrients and oxygen (depicted by the wasteland). Artwork by Ms. Peggy Hsu.

Table 39.4 Primary targets and mode of inhibition of both the intrinsic and extrinsic (processing) antipathogenic hurdles of beer

Antipathogenic hurdles	*Primary targets*	*Mode of inhibition*
Intrinsic hurdles		
Ethanol	All pathogens	Inhibits cell membrane functions
Low pH	All pathogens	Affects enzymes and permeases (nutrient utilization), enhances inhibitory effects of hops
Hops	Gram-positive bacteria	Inhibits cell membrane functions
Carbon dioxide	Aerobic pathogens	Creates anaerobic conditions, lowers pH, inhibits enzymes, effects cell membrane
Low oxygen levels	Aerobic pathogens, Gram-negative bacteria	Creates anaerobic conditions
Lack of nutrients	All pathogens	Starves cells
Sulphur dioxide*	Gram-negative bacteria	Affects various metabolic systems
Processing hurdles		
Mashing	Gram-negative bacteria	Causes thermal destruction of cells
Kettle boil	All pathogens	Causes thermal destruction of cells
Pasteurization*	All pathogens	Causes thermal destruction of cells
Filtration*	All pathogens	Removes cells by physical size exclusion
Bottle conditioning*	Aerobic pathogens	Creates anaerobic conditions

*Not applicable to all beers.

affected the resistance of beers to spoilage by lactic acid bacteria (non-pathogenic). Unlike the similar study by Dolezil and Kirsop (1980), the cultures were adapted to grow in beer prior to inoculation, providing more reliable results.

Table 39.4 summarizes the primary targets and mode of inhibition of many of the antipathogenic hurdles of beer, which are discussed in more detail below. Although these hurdles are considered in reference to preventing the survival and growth of pathogens, it is important to note that these principles can also be applied to reducing the incidence of beer spoilage bacteria.

Ethanol

The conversion of carbohydrates to ethanol (0.5–10% (v/v), typically 3.5–5.0%) by yeasts during the fermentation of beer provides one of the major hurdles to the growth of pathogens. The antimicrobial properties of ethanol in beer have been recognized for some time, with the prominent brewing microbiologist Shimwell (1935) noting that beers with a higher ethanol content were more resistant to spoilage by *Saccharobacillus pastorianus* (now *Lactobacillus brevis*) than those of lower ethanol content. It can be assumed that the same applies for pathogens.

Mode of Inhibition Ethanol inhibits cell membrane functions (Casey and Ingledew, 1986), and inactivates bacteria by inducing cell membrane leakage (Eaton *et al.*, 1982). At concentrations typical of beer (3.0–4.9% (v/v)), ethanol has been shown to effect the peptidoglycan assembly of some strains of *E. coli* (Ingram and Vreeland, 1980). Like penicillin, ethanol inhibits the transpeptidase reaction, resulting in the production of uncrosslinked peptidoglycan, leading to lysis of the weakened cell wall after 3–4 h (Ingram and Vreeland, 1980). As a result of damage to the cell membrane by ethanol, morphology and a range of cell functions may be affected. These include cell division (filament formation), glycolytic enzymes, membrane permeability, solute uptake/ion pumping systems, and the synthesis of peptidoglycan, DNA, RNA, protein, fatty acids, and phospholipids (Kalathenos and Russel, 2003). Interference with cell division and elongation due to ethanol have also been observed, for example in *E. coli* (Fried and Novick, 1973) and *Clostridium botulinum* (Daifas *et al.*, 2003). Exposure to 5% (v/v) ethanol increased the permeability of the cell membrane of the pathogen *Listeria monocytogenes*, which heightened the sensitivity of the cell to low pH by allowing an increased passage of protons into the cytoplasm, leaving the cell unable to maintain pH homeostasis (Barker and Park, 2001).

At concentrations typical of beer, ethanol exerts only a limited effect on enzyme activity. Few of the glycolytic enzymes studied by Scopes (1989) showed any substantial changes in activity at ethanol concentrations up to 5.8% (v/v), and membrane-bound enzymes in *E. coli* were reported to be relatively insensitive to inhibition by ethanol (NADH oxidase, d-lactate oxidase, and ATPase were inhibited by less than 10% by the presence of 3.9% (v/v) ethanol) (Eaton *et al.*, 1982). A dose-dependent inhibition of lactose permease by ethanol was reported by Ingram *et al.* (1980).

Effect on Pathogens The growth of pathogenic bacteria is mitigated by the presence of ethanol at levels typical of beer, as the growth of *L. monocytogenes* was almost completely inhibited by 6.3% (v/v) ethanol in tryptic soy broth supplemented with yeast extract, whilst only slight growth inhibition was observed at lower concentrations (3.2% (v/v)) (Oh and Marshall, 1993). The maximum ethanol concentrations (v/v) at which growth could occur was determined to be 2.8% for *Salmonella* Enteritidis, 4.9% for *Staph. aureus*, and 4.1% for *B. cereus* (Lanciotti *et al.*, 2001). The effect of ethanol on the survival of four foodborne pathogens (*L. monocytogenes, Salm.* Typhimurium, *Staph. aureus*, and *E. coli* O157:H7) in tryptic soy broth after 24 h was determined by Ahn and Shin (1999). Complete inhibition was obtained with 7% (v/v) ethanol (only present in strong beers), however typical ethanol levels of beer would also provide strong protection against these pathogens, as the inhibition rate was greater than 75% for 5% (v/v) ethanol, and more than 40% for 3% (v/v) ethanol. All ethanol levels (>0% (v/v)) increased the lag phase for the growth of *Cl. botulinum*, whilst 6.9% (v/v) would completely inhibit the growth of this pathogen in trypticase peptone glucose yeast extract broth (Daifas *et al.*, 2003).

The consumption of alcoholic beverages has been reported to enhance a person's resistance to infection by pathogens. Intake of alcohol during or after consumption of contaminated food may protect against *Salmonella* spp. (Bellido-Blasco *et al.*, 2002), and consumption of beverages with >10% alcohol provided a protective effect against Hepatitis A from oysters (Desenclos *et al.*, 1992). Furthermore, moderate alcohol consumption suppresses *Helicobacter pylori* infection (Brenner *et al.*, 1997; Brenner *et al.*, 2001; Murray *et al.*, 2002).

Low pH

A second hurdle common to all beers which prevents the growth of pathogens is a low pH (pH range 3.4–4.8). The importance of a low pH on the stability of beer has been recognized for some time by researchers such as Shimwell (1935), who noted that beer with a lower pH showed increased resistance to spoilage by *Saccharobacillus pastorianus* (now *Lact. brevis*). In addition to its direct action, the low pH of beer exhibits a synergistic effect with the antimicrobial properties of hop compounds, as hops exhibit increased antibacterial activity at lower pH values (Fernbach and Stoleru, 1924; Shimwell, 1937). Simpson and Hammond (1991) reported that a decrease in the pH of 0.2 can increase hop antibacterial activity by up to 50%.

Mode of Inhibition Low pH values disrupt the plasma membrane, cause the destruction of enzyme systems, and reduce nutrient uptake, leading to metabolic exhaustion. For example, Neal (1965) reported that low pH values (4.0) impacted on alcohol dehydrogenase, aldolase, and pyruvate decarboxylase. Microorganisms attempt to maintain a steady, close to neutral intracellular pH, in spite of the pH of the external environment (Beales, 2004). The ability of a cell to maintain a desired internal pH is limited and varies between strains, being primarily driven by the controlled movement of cations across the membrane (Beales, 2004). When the mechanisms of passive and active pH homeostasis are overwhelmed, starvation ensues, leading to cell death.

Effect on Pathogens Figure 39.2 plots the minimum growth pH for many foodborne bacterial pathogens against the typical pH range of beer. The pH values are for growth, not survival, as sufficient comparable data is not available in the literature. The cited minimum pH values are under

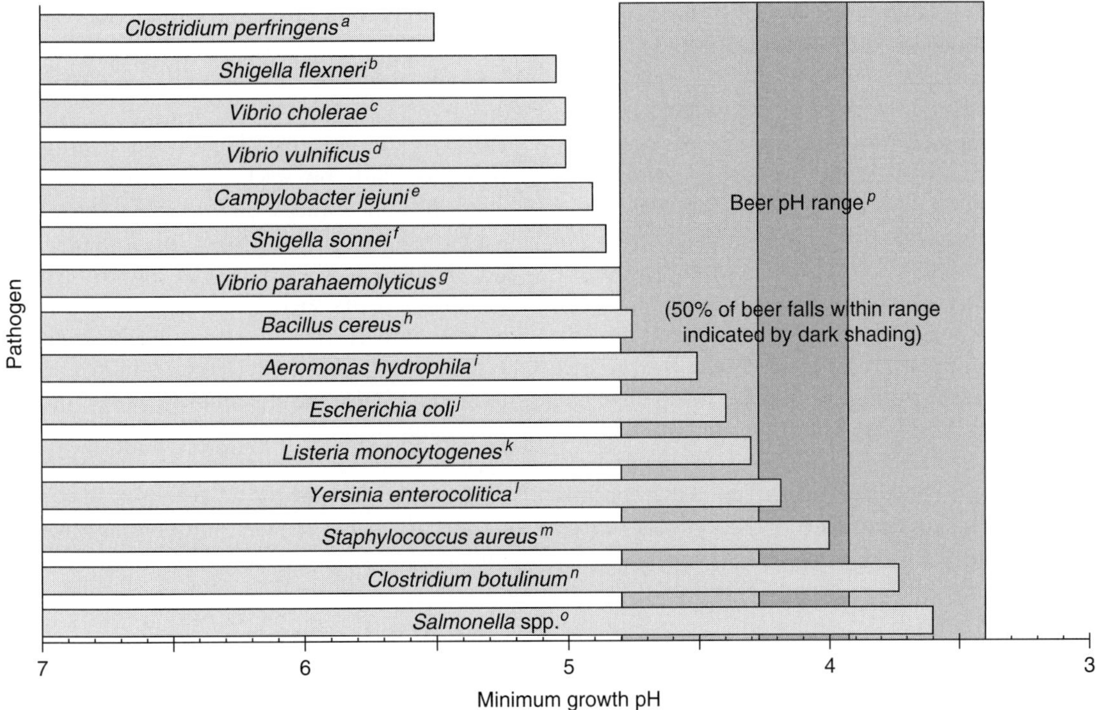

Figure 39.2 Minimum growth pH of pathogens under optimal conditions, compared to the typical pH range of beer. [a]Labbe and Duncan (1974); [b]Fehlhaber (1981); [c]International Commission on Microbiological Specifications for Foods (ICMSF) (1996a); [d]ICMSF (1996b); [e]Doyle and Roman (1981); [f]Fehlhaber (1981); [g]Beuchat (1973); [h]Lanciotti *et al.* (2001); [i]Palumbo *et al.* (1985); [j]ICMSF (1996c); [k]Farber *et al.* (1989); [l]Brocklehurst and Lund (1990); [m]Genigeorgis *et al.* (1971); [n]Wong *et al.* (1988); [o]Růžičková (1996); [p]Range excluding outliers, from analysis of 444 beers of various styles (van Leeuwen, 2006).

optimal conditions for each organism, which is not the case for beer, as it contains other inhibitory factors.

Many pathogens are unable to grow at typical beer pH levels, and only *Y. enterocolitica*, *Staph. aureus*, *Cl. botulinum*, and *Salmonella* spp. have been reported to grow at the pH levels of the majority of beers (Figure 39.1). Even though these pathogens can grow at these low pH values, other hurdles in beer (such as ethanol, hops, and CO_2) provide extra barriers to growth.

Hops

Hops are primarily added to beer to impart a characteristic bitterness and aroma, although their antimicrobial properties have long been recognized. For example, during the late 1700s IPAs were developed with increased levels of hops and alcohols to resist the growth of undesirable microorganisms during extended seaborne transportation (Edgerton, 2005).

Hop compounds can be divided into two fractions; the total resins, and the essential oils. Of most significance are the total resins, which include the α-acids (humulone and its congeners) and β-acids (lupulone and its congeners). The α-acids are isomerized during wort boiling to the more soluble iso-α-acids, which impart bitterness and antimicrobial properties to the beer. Early reports of these chemical changes were documented by Hayduck (1888). Although the β-acids show increased antimicrobial action (Walker and Parker, 1937), they have low solubility in wort (Sakamoto and Konings, 2003), and are therefore of little significance in the resistance of beer to pathogens. Hop aroma is provided to the beer from the essential oils.

Mode of Inhibition The undissociated forms of hop and hop-derived compounds are antimicrobial, whereas their ionized forms have negligible activity (Simpson, 1993b). Hop compounds (lupulone, humulone, isohumulone, and humulinic acid) have been shown to induce leakage of the cell membrane of *Bacillus subtilis* (Teuber and Schmalreck, 1973). This breakdown of the cell membrane led to inhibition of the active transport of sugars and amino acids across the membrane, thus respiration and the synthesis of protein, DNA, and RNA were interrupted. Further studies determined that hop bitter acids act as mobile-carrier ionophores and cause complete dissipation of the transmembrane pH gradient of sensitive cells (Simpson, 1993b). The reduction in intracellular pH leads to inhibition of nutrient transport, and ultimately starvation of the cell (Simpson, 1993a).

Effect on Pathogens With the exception of some resistant strains of lactic acid bacteria, hop compounds exhibit antibacterial activity against Gram-positive bacteria, but not against Gram-negatives (Shimwell, 1937). Hop compounds have been shown to inhibit the growth of the Gram-positive pathogens *L. monocytogenes* (Larson *et al.*, 1996) and *Staph. aureus* (Schmalreck *et al.*, 1975; Haas and Barsoumian, 1994; Sağdiç *et al.*, 2003). For example, *L. monocytogenes* was inhibited by more than 60% in the presence of typical hop levels (30 ppm α-acids) in tryptic soy broth (Larson *et al.*, 1996). In contrast, Gram-negative bacteria are resistant or only affected at higher concentrations, such as the pathogens *E. coli* (Sağdiç *et al.*, 2003), *Salm.* Typhimurium (Schmalreck *et al.*, 1975), *Serratia marcescens* (Schmalreck *et al.*, 1975), and *Y. enterocolitica* (Sağdiç *et al.*, 2003). Gram-negative bacteria are resistant to hop compounds due to the presence of phospholipids in their outer membrane, as lupulone and humulone are inactivated by serum phosphatides (Sacks and Humphreys, 1951). Like the hop acids, hop essential oils exhibited antimicrobial activity against the Gram-positive pathogen *Staph. aureus*, and had only negligible effects on the Gram-negative bacterium (*E. coli*) (Langezaal *et al.*, 1992).

Dissolved gasses

The presence of carbon dioxide (CO_2) and the lack of oxygen (O_2) enhance the microbial resistance of beer. CO_2 is produced during the primary fermentation of beer, and the beer is further carbonated by the direct addition of CO_2 or via secondary fermentation, to give final dissolved CO_2 concentrations of approximately 0.5%. Carbonation and modern bottling techniques limit the amount of dissolved O_2 available for growth in the bottled product. In addition to improving the chemical stability of the beer, decreased O_2 levels reduce the potential for the growth of many pathogenic microorganisms (Schmidt, 1990).

Mode of Inhibition CO_2 inhibits pathogens by a variety of mechanisms; CO_2 creates an anaerobic environment to exclude the growth of aerobic pathogens, causes a lowering of the pH (see section "Low pH"), influences carboxylation and decarboxylation reactions, and exerts a direct inhibitory effect on growth.

The exact mechanism of CO_2 inhibition is not yet clear (Dixon and Kell, 1989), although it has been shown that the inhibitory effects of CO_2 are not solely due to the lowered pH (Coyne, 1933) or displacement of O_2 with CO_2 (King Jr. and Nagel, 1967; Daniels *et al.*, 1985), but rather there is a direct effect of CO_2 (King Jr. and Nagel, 1967; King and Mabbitt, 1982). CO_2 has been shown to inhibit certain enzymes including isocitrate dehydrogenase, malate dehydrogenase, aconitase, succinate dehydrogenase, succinyl-CoA synthetase, fumarase, and formate dehydrogenase (Swanson and Ogg, 1969; Gill and Tan, 1979), and the antimicrobial activity of CO_2 may also be due to adverse affects on the permeability of the cell membrane, as ion uptake is reduced as CO_2 interacts with the membrane lipids (Sears and Eisenberg, 1961). Complementary to the action of hops, CO_2 shows greater inhibition of Gram-negative bacteria than of Gram-postitives, although significant increases in lag phases have been observed for both types of bacteria (Martin *et al.*, 2003).

Effect on Pathogens Hammond *et al.* (1999) reported that beers with low levels of dissolved CO_2 are at a heightened risk of undesirable microbial growth. This study supported the work of Šavel and Prokopová (1980), who documented that a decrease in the dissolved CO_2 level of beer reduced its shelf life (changes in CO_2 levels showed a larger impact than variations in dissolved O_2) (Šavel and Prokopová, 1980). Dissolved CO_2 in raw milk is inhibitory to bacteria (King and Mabbitt, 1982), increasing the lag phase and the generation time of microbes (Daniels *et al.*, 1985). More recent studies have demonstrated the effect of CO_2 on the growth of *B. cereus*, *Enterococcus faecalis*, *E. coli*, *L. monocytogenes*, and *Pseudomonas fluorescens* in milk (Loss and Hotchkiss, 2002; Martin *et al.*, 2003).

Lack of nutrients

The concentrations of nutritive substances available for the growth of pathogenic microorganisms in beer, such as carbohydrates and amino acids, are very low in most beers as the majority of these compounds have been metabolized by the yeast during fermentation (Sakamoto and Konings, 2003). Thus, well-attenuated beers (those with minimal residual nutrients) are the least prone to microbial spoilage (Rainbow, 1971). The effect of a lack of nutrients on the resistance of lager beers to undesirable microbial growth was studied by Fernandez and Simpson (1995). Increased levels of free amino nitrogen, total soluble nitrogen, amino acids, and maltotriose were correlated with an increased incidence of bacterial growth (Fernandez and Simpson, 1995).

Sulfur dioxide

Typically, sulfur dioxide (SO_2) levels in beer range from <1 to 30 mg/l (Ilett, 1995). Sulfur dioxide may be present as a by-product of yeast metabolism, added indirectly through raw materials and processing aids preserved with sulfur dioxide, or added directly (Ilett, 1995). The addition of SO_2 is limited by law to varying amounts in different countries. In beer, sulfur dioxide acts as an antioxidant, reacts with carbonyl compounds to mask stale flavors, and shows antimicrobial action, primarily toward Gram-negative bacteria (Ilett, 1995). However, the antimicrobial action of SO_2 in beers is weak, as most of the SO_2 is bound at typical beer pH levels, therefore it is only a minor hurdle to the growth of pathogens (Hough *et al.*, 1982).

An exact site of action for sulfur dioxide cannot be clearly established, rather it is considered to affect many metabolic systems (Gould and Russel, 2003). These systems include intermediary metabolism (enzymes, cofactors, prosthetic groups), energy production (enzymes, electron carriers, cofactors), protein biosynthesis (proteins, enzymes, nucleic acids), DNA replication (enzymes, nucleic acids), and membranes (proteins, lipids) (Gould and Russel, 2003).

Additional hurdles

In addition to the chief hurdles detailed above, there are a number of other compounds that may increase the antimicrobial nature of beer. Hammond (1999) demonstrated the antimicrobial effects of phytic and ferulic acid on *Lactobacillus* spp., although at much higher levels than typically found in beer. Various specialty beers are brewed with the addition of known antimicrobial compounds such as honey and various spices, which would slightly reduce the products susceptibility. At levels approximately 100 times higher than those found in beer, diacetyl has been shown to inhibit *Salm.* Typhimurium (Archer *et al.*, 1996).

Processing hurdles

As discussed above, beer contains several antimicrobial hurdles to prevent the growth or survival of pathogens. In addition to these, various processing steps add further barriers. Some of the first physical barriers are the use of treated water and the heat applied during mashing. Gram-negative bacteria, yeasts, and molds are rapidly killed in the mash, however lactic acid bacteria and spore forming bacilli are able to survive the mashing process (O'Sullivan *et al.*, 1999). During the kettle boil, the wort is boiled for at least 45 min, destroying vegetative cells and their spores. The majority of craft and microbreweries carbonate their products by bottle conditioning (secondary fermentation), and there is evidence that bottle conditioning reduces a beer's susceptibility to microbial attack, as the fermenting yeast reduces the O_2 content in the bottle headspace by approximately one-third (Derdelinckx *et al.*, 1992). Dolezil and Kirsop (1980) reported that bottle conditioning appeared to be a factor in the production of resistant beer. Many breweries employ post-fermentation treatments such as filtration (physical exclusion), pasteurization (heat treatment), and cold storage to further protect the microbial stability of their beers. However, many small breweries (such as brewpubs and microbreweries) produce unpasteurized and unfiltered beer, thus extra care should be taken to ensure that the intrinsic hurdles are adequate, and that hygiene and sanitation regimes are well maintained.

Conclusion

Beer is rightly considered to be a microbiologically safe product. Various studies have shown that pathogens exhibit poor survival in beer, thus it is unlikely to be a vehicle for the transmission of pathogens. This fermented beverage is protected by an array of intrinsic hurdles, including the presence of ethanol, carbon dioxide, sulfur dioxide, and hops, and the low pH, oxygen, and nutrient levels. Further, extrinsic processing factors provide enhanced protection, including the kettle boil, filtration, pasteurization, and cold storage. However, those beers with reduced levels of these hurdles are more susceptible, such as low-alcohol and unpasteurized beers. In such instances, special attention should be paid to maintaining adequate levels of the other hurdles (such as the pH and ethanol levels), or new hurdles may need to be implemented, such as pasteurization or filtration.

Summary Points

- Pathogenic (disease-causing) bacteria, such as *E. coli* and *Salmonella*, show poor survival in beer.
- The majority of beers are protected against pathogens by antimicrobial "hurdles" (inhibitory factors), including the:
  - Low pH
  - Ethanol content
  - Presence of hops
  - High carbon dioxide content
  - Low oxygen content
  - Lack of nutrients
- Several processing steps also protect beer
  - Mashing
  - Kettle boil
  - Filtration (only for some beers)
  - Pasteurization (only for some beers)
  - Aseptic packaging (only for some beers)
  - Bottle conditioning (only for some beers)
- Beers without, or with, reduced levels of one or more of these antimicrobial "hurdles" are more prone to the survival and/or growth of pathogenic organisms. Such beers include low-alcohol and unpasteurized beers, thus special care needs to be taken to ensure their safety.

Acknowledgments

The authors wish to acknowledge the support of Ms. Sue Taylor from the University of Ballarat for her assistance in locating several hard to find resources. We are grateful to Ms. Peggy Hsu for providing the artwork for Figure 39.1.

References

Ahn, Y.-S. and Shin, D.-H. (1999). *Korean J. Food Sci. Technol.* 31, 1315–1323.

Archer, M.H., Dillon, V.M., Campbell-Platt, G. and Owens, J.D. (1996). *Food Contr.* 7, 63–67.

Baptista, A.S., Horri, J., Calori-Domingues, M.A., Micotti da Gloria, E., Salgado, J.M. and Vizioli, M.R. (2004). *World J. Microbiol. Biotechnol.* 20, 475–481.

Barker, C. and Park, S.F. (2001). *Appl. Enviorn. Microbiol.* 67, 1594–1600.

Baxter, E.D., Slaiding, I.R. and Kelly, B. (2001). *J. Am. Soc. Brew. Chem.* 59, 98–100.

Baxter, D. (1999). *Ferment* 12, 13–18.

Beales, N. (2004). *Compr. Rev. Food Sci. Food Saf.* 3, 1–20.

Bellido-Blasco, J.B., Arnedo-Pena, A., Cordero-Cutillas, E., Canós-Cabedo, M., Herrero-Carot, C. and Safont-Adsuara, L. (2002). *Epidemiology* 13, 228–230.

Bendová, O. and Kurzová, V. (1968). *Kvas. Prům.* 14, 223–234.

Beuchat, L.R. (1973). *Appl. Microbiol.* 25, 844–846.

Brenner, H., Rothenbacher, D., Bode, G. and Adler, G. (1997). *Br. Med. J.* 315, 1489–1492.

Brenner, H., Bode, G., Hoffmeister, A., Koenig, W. and Rothenbacher, D. (2001). *Epidemiology* 12, 209–214.

Brocklehurst, T.F. and Lund, B.M. (1990). *J. Appl. Bacteriol.* 69, 390–397.

Bunker, H.J. (1955). *Proc. Eur. Brew. Conv.* 5, 330–341.

Casey, G.P. and Ingledew, W.M. (1986). *Crit. Rev. Microbiol.* 13, 219–280.

Chu, F.S., Chang, C.C., Ashoor, S.H. and Prentice, N. (1975). *Appl. Microbiol.* 29, 313–316.

Coyne, F.P. (1933). *Proc. R. Soc. Lond. B.* 113, 196–217.

Daifas, D.P., Smith, J.P., Blanchfield, B., Cadieux, B., Sanders, G. and Austin, J.W. (2003). *J. Food Protect.* 66, 610–617.

Daniels, J.A., Krishnamurthi, R. and Rizvi, S.S.H. (1985). *J. Food Protect.* 48, 532–537.

Derdelinckx, G., Vanderhasselt, B., Maudoux, M. and Dufour, J.P. (1992). *Brauwelt Int.* 10, 156–164.

Desenclos, J.-C.A., Klontz, K.C., Wilder, M.H. and Gunn, R.A. (1992). *Epidemiology* 3, 371–374.

di Luzio, N.R. and Friedmann, T.J. (1973). *Nature* 244, 49–51.

Dixon, N.M. and Kell, D.B. (1989). *J. Appl. Bacteriol.* 67, 109–136.

Dogel', L.Z., Dunaev, V.I. and Yushchenko, G.V. (1984). *Gig. Sanit.* 9, 33–34.

Dolezil, L. and Kirsop, B.H. (1980). *J. Inst. Brew.* 86, 122–124.

Doyle, M.P. and Roman, D.J. (1981). *J. Food Protect.* 44, 596–601.

Eaton, L.C., Tedder, T.F. and Ingram, L.O. (1982). *Subst. Alcohol Actions Misuse* 3, 77–87.

Edgerton, J. (2005). *J. Am. Soc. Brew. Chem.* 63, 28–30.

Enache-Angoulvant, A. and Hennequin, C. (2005). *Clin. Infect. Dis.* 41, 1559–1568.

Enikova, R., Kozareva, M., Ivanova, T. and Yangiozova, Z. (1985). *Khranitelnopromishlena Nauka* 1, 73–81.

Farber, J.M., Sanders, G.W., Dunfield, S. and Prescott, R. (1989). *Lett. Appl. Microbiol.* 9, 181–183.

Farmer, J.J.I., Davis, B.R., Hickman-Brenner, W., McWhorter, A., Huntley-Carter, G.P., Asbury, M.A., Riddle, C., Wathen-Grady, H.G., Elias, C., Fanning, G.R., Steigerwalt, A.G., O'Hara, C.M., Morris, G.K., Smith, P.B. and Brenner, D.J. (1985). *J. Clin. Microbiol.* 21, 46–76.

Fehlhaber, K. (1981). *Arch. Exp. Veterinarmed.* 35, 955–964.

Felsenfeld, O. (1965). *Bull. World Health Organ.* 33, 725–734.

Fernandez, J.L. and Simpson, W.J. (1995). *J. Appl. Bacteriol.* 78, 419–425.

Fernbach, A. and Stoleru, I. (1924). *Ann. Brasserie Distillerie* 23, 1–2.

Fried, V.A. and Novick, A. (1973). *J. Bacteriol.* 114, 239–248.

Friedman, D.E., Patten, K.A., Rose, J.B. and Barney, M.C. (1997). *J. Food Saf.* 17, 125–132.

Genigeorgis, C., Foda, M.S., Mantis, A. and Sadler, W.W. (1971). *Appl. Microbiol.* 21, 862–866.

Gill, C.O. and Tan, K.H. (1979). *Appl. Enviorn. Microbiol.* 38, 237–240.

Gould, G.W. and Russel, N.J. (2003). Sulfite. In Russel, N.J. and Gould, G.W. (eds), *Food Preservatives*, 2nd edn, pp. 85–101. Kluwer Academic, New York.

Haas, G.J. and Barsoumian, R. (1994). *J. Food Protect.* 57, 59–61.

Hammond, J., Brennan, M. and Price, A. (1999). *J. Inst. Brew.* 105, 113–120.

Hayduck, F. (1888). *Wochenschr. Brauerei* 5, 937.

Heinz, M., von Wintzingerode, F., Moter, A., Halle, E., Lohbrunner, H., Kaisers, U., Neuhaus, P. and Halle, E. (2000). *Eur. J. Clin. Microbiol.* 19, 946–948.

Hompesch, H. (1949). *Brauwissenchaft* 2, 17.

Hough, J.S., Briggs, D.E., Stevens, R. and Young, T.W. (1982). *Malting and Brewing Science. Vol. 2: Hopped Wort and Beer*, pp. 741–775. Chapman and Hall, London.

Huwig, A., Friemund, S., Kappeli, O. and Dutler, H. (2001). *Toxicol. Lett.* 122, 179–188.

Ilett, D.R. (1995). *MBAA Tech. Q.* 32, 213–221.

Ingram, L.O. and Vreeland, N.S. (1980). *J. Bacteriol.* 144, 481–488.

Ingram, L.O., Dickens, B.F. and Buttke, T.M. (1980). *Adv. Exp. Med. Biol.* 126, 299–337.

ICMSF (International Commission on Microbiological Specifications for Foods) (1996a). *Vibrio cholerae.* In Roberts, T.A., Baird-Parker, A.C. and Tompkin, R.B. (eds.), *Microorganisms in Foods 5: Microbiological specifications of food pathogens*, pp. 414–425. Blackie Academic and Professional, London.

ICMSF (1996b). *Vibrio vulnificus.* In Roberts, T.A., Baird-Parker, A.C. and Tompkin, R.B. (eds.), *Microorganisms in Foods 5: Microbiological specifications of food pathogens*, pp. 436–439. Blackie Academic and Professional, London.

ICMSF (1996c). Intestinally pathogenic *Escherichia coli.* In Roberts, T.A., Baird-Parker, A.C. and Tompkin, R.B. (eds.), *Microorganisms in Foods 5: Microbiological Specifications of Food Pathogens*, pp. 126–140. Blackie Academic and Professional, London.

Kalathenos, P. and Russel, N.J. (2003). Ethanol as a food preservative. In Russel, N.J. and Gould, G.W. (eds), *Food Preservatives*, 2nd edn, pp. 196–217. Kluwer Academic, New York.

King Jr., A.D. and Nagel, C.W. (1967). *J. Food Sci.* 32, 575–579.

King, J.S. and Mabbitt, L.A. (1982). *J. Dairy Res.* 49, 439–447.

Kuhn, O. and Owades, J.L. (1985). *Brewers Dig.* 60, 18.

L'Anthoën, N.C. and Ingledew, W.M. (1996). *J. Am. Soc. Brew. Chem.* 54, 32–36.

Labbe, R.G. and Duncan, C.L. (1974). *Can. J. Microbiol.* 20, 1493–1501.

Lanciotti, R., Sinigaglia, M., Gardini, F., Vannini, L. and Guerzoni, M.E. (2001). *Food Microbiol.* 18, 659–668.

Langezaal, C.R., Chandra, A. and Scheffer, J.J.C. (1992). *Pharm Weekbl [Sci]* 14, 353–356.

Larson, A.E., Yu, R.R.Y., Lee, O.A., Price, S.B., Haas, G.J. and Johnson, E.A. (1996). *Int. J. Food Microbiol.* 33, 195–207.

Leistner, L. (2000). *Int. J. Food Microbiol.* 55, 181–186.

Lentz, K. (1903). *Klin. Jahrb.* 11, 315–320.

Loss, C.R. and Hotchkiss, J.H. (2002). *J. Food Protect.* 65, 1924–1929.
Mably, M., Mankotia, M., Cavlovic, P., Tam, J., Wong, L., Pantazopoulos, P., Calway, P. and Scott, P.M. (2005). *Food Addit. Contam.* 22, 1252–1257.
Martin, J.D., Werner, B.G. and Hotchkiss, J.H. (2003). *J. Dairy Sci.* 86, 1932–1940.
Murphy, A. and Kavanagh, K. (1999). *Enzyme Microb. Tech.* 25, 551–557.
Murphy, P.A., Hendrich, S., Landgren, C. and Bryant, C.M. (2006). *J. Food Sci.* 71, R51–R65.
Murray, L.J., Lane, A.J., Harvey, I.M., Donovan, J.L., Nair, P. and Harvey, R.F. (2002). *Am. J. Gastroenterol.* 97, 2750–2755.
Neal, A.L., Weinstock, J.O. and Lampen, J.O. (1965). *J. Bacteriol.* 90, 126–131.
Nishikawa, N., Kohgo, M. and Karakawa, T. (1979). *Bull. Brew Sci.* 25, 13–16.
Nkwe, D.O., Taylor, J.E. and Siame, B.A. (2005). *Mycopathologia* 160, 117–186.
O'Sullivan, T.F., Walsh, Y., O'Mahony, A., Fitzgerald, G.F. and van Sinderen, D. (1999). *J. Inst. Brew.* 105, 55–61.
Odhav, B. and Naicker, V. (2002). *Food Addit. Contam.* 19, 55–61.
Oh, D.-H. and Marshall, D.L. (1993). *Int. J. Food Microbiol.* 20, 239–246.
Palumbo, S.A., Morgan, D.R. and Buchanan, R.L. (1985). *J. Food Sci.* 50, 1417–1421.
Papadopoulou-Bouraoui, A., Vrabcheva, T., Valzacchi, S., Stroka, J. and Anklam, E. (2004). *Food Addit. Contam.* 21, 607–617.
Pattison, T.-L., Geornaras, I. and von Holy, A. (1998). *Int. J. Food Microbiol.* 43, 115–122.
Rainbow, C. (1971). *Process Biochem.* 31, 15–17.
Rainbow, C. (1981). Beer spoilage microorganisms. In Pollock, J.R.A. (ed.), *Brewing Science*, pp. 491–550. Academic Press, London.
Ridell, J., Siitonen, A., Paulin, L., Mattila, L., Korkeala, H. and Albert, M.J. (1994). *J. Clin. Microbiol.* 32, 2335–2337.
Ringot, D., Lerzy, B., Bonhoure, J.P., Auclair, E., Oriol, E. and Larondelle, Y. (2005). *Process Biochem.* 40, 3008–3016.
Růžičková, V. (1996). *Vet. Med.-Czech.* 41, 25–31.
Sachs-Müke, O. (1908). *Klin. Jahrb.* 11, 351–353.
Sacks, L.E. and Humphreys, E.M. (1951). *Proc. Soc. Exp. Biol. Med.* 76, 234–238.
Sağdiç, O., Karahan, A.G., Özcan, M. and Özkan, G. (2003). *Food Sci. Tech. Int.* 9, 353–358.
Sakamoto, K. and Konings, W.N. (2003). *Int. J. Food Microbiol.* 89, 105–124.
Sanders Jr., W.E. and Sanders, C.C. (1997). *Clin. Microbiol. Rev.* 10, 220–241.
Šavel, J. and Prokopová, M. (1980). *Kvas. Prům.* 26, 124–126.
Schindler, P.R.G. and Metz, H. (1990). *Öff. Gesundh.-Wes.* 52, 592–597.
Schmalreck, A.F., Teuber, M., Reininger, W. and Hartl, A. (1975). *Can. J. Microbiol.* 21, 205–212.
Schmidt, H.-J. (1990). *Brauwelt* 130, 11–14.
Schwarz, P.B., Casper, H.H. and Beattie, S. (1995). *J. Am. Soc. Brew. Chem.* 53, 121–127.
Scopes, R.K. (1989). Effects of ethanol on glycolytic enzymes. In van Uden, N. (ed), *Alcohol Toxicity in Yeast and Bacteria*, pp. 89–109. CRC Press, Boca Raton, Florida.
Scott, P.M. (1996). *J. AOAC Int.* 79, 875–882.
Scott, P.M., Kanhere, S.R., Lawrence, G.A., Daley, E.F. and Farber, J.M. (1995). *Food Addit. Contam.* 12, 31–40.
Sears, D.F. and Eisenberg, R.M. (1961). *J. Gen. Physiol.* 44, 869–887.
Shayo, N.B., Kamala, A., Gidamis, A.B. and Nnko, S.A.M. (2000). *Int. J. Food Sci. Nutr.* 51, 395–402.
Sheth, N.K., Wisniewski, T.R. and Franson, T.R. (1988). *Am. J. Gastroenterol.* 83, 658–660.
Shimwell, J.L. (1935). *J. Inst. Brew.* 41, 245–258.
Shimwell, J.L. (1937). *J. Inst. Brew.* 43, 111–118.
Simpson, W.J. (1993a). *J. Inst. Brew.* 99, 405–411.
Simpson, W.J. (1993b). *J. Gen. Microbiol.* 139, 1041–1045.
Simpson, W.J. and Hammond, J.R.M. (1991). *Proc. Eur. Brew. Conv.* 23, 185–193.
Stanley, V.G., Ojo, R., Woldesenbet, S., Hutchinson, D.H. and Kubena, L.F. (1993). *Poult. Sci.* 72, 1867–1872.
Storgårds, E. (2000). *Process Hygiene Control in Beer Production and Dispensing*. Technical Research Centre of Finland. University of Helsinki.
Swanson, D.H. and Ogg, J.E. (1969). *Biochem. Biophys. Res. Commun.* 36, 567–575.
Taschan, H. (1996). *Brauwelt* 136, 1014–1106.
Tauxe, R.V. (2002). *Int. J. Food Microbiol.* 78, 31–41.
Teuber, M. and Schmalreck, A.F. (1973). *Arch. Microbiol.* 94, 159–171.
van Leeuwen, T. (2006). A comparison of the chemical analysis of beers and judges' scores from the 2004 Australian International Beer Awards. Honours Thesis. University of Ballarat.
van Vuuren, H.J.J. and Priest, F.G. (2003). Gram-negative brewery bacteria. In Priest, F.G. and Campbell, I. (eds), *Brewing Microbiology*, 3rd edn, pp. Kluwer Academic, New York.
Vaughan, A., O'Sullivan, T. and van Sinderen, D. (2005). *J. Inst. Brew.* 111, 355–371.
Walker, T.K. and Parker, A. (1937). *J. Inst. Brew.* 43, 17–30.
Williams, J.H., Phillips, T.D., Jolly, P.E., Stiles, J.K., Jolly, C.M. and Aggarwal, D. (2004). *Am. J. Clin. Nutr.* 80, 1106–1122.
Wong, D.M., Young-Perkins, K.E. and Merson, R.L. (1988). *Appl. Enviorn. Microbiol.* 54, 1446–1450.
Zikes, H. (1903). *Mitt d. österreich. Versuchsstation f. Brauerei u.* Mälzerei, Wien, Heft 11, 20–49.

40

Fate of Pesticide Residues During Brewing

Simón Navarro and Nuria Vela Department of Agricultural Chemistry, Geology and Pedology, School of Chemistry, University of Murcia, Campus Universitario de Espinardo, Murcia, Spain

Abstract

This chapter emphasizes the influence of the different phases of beer-making and the removal of pesticide residues. The effect of their presence on beer quality and health impact is also assessed. With this aim, based on the current data an overview of the behavior and fate of agrochemical residues during the brewing stages (malting, mashing, boiling, fermentation, and stabilization of the beer) is presented. The methodology for analysis of pesticide residues and their metabolites in raw materials, wort, and beer and the main aspects of the food safety and policy in the European Union (EU) are summarized. Depending on the stage involved and the physical–chemical properties (mainly K_{OW} [as $\log P$] value, water solubility, vapor pressure and Henry's law constant) of the residue in the raw materials, differences in the final fate of the residues are observed. As a general rule, the malsters should devote special attention to the residues of hydrophobic pesticides with $K_{OW} > 2$ because they can remain on the malt. On the contrary, brewers should control residues of hydrophilic pesticides with $K_{OW} < 4$ because they can be carried over into beer. Thus, the monitoring and surveillance of pesticide residues with K_{OW} ranging from 2 to 4 (most of them) during the brewing process is essential to get a "healthy drink." Additionally, the influence of pesticide residues on flavor, sugar content, acidity, color or total polyphenol, and flavonoid contents has been pointed out. Therefore, the knowledge of the behavior of pesticide residues must be intended to (i) provide information on the transfers of residues from barley to malt, wort, and beer to calculate concentration or reduction factors during each process; (ii) achieve a realistic estimate of the dietary intake of pesticide residues; (iii) propose maximum residue limits (MRLs) for residues in beer when necessary; and (iv) avoid alterations in the beer quality.

List of Abbreviations

ASE	Accelerated solvent extraction
CAC	Codex Alimentarius Commission
CCP	Control critical point
CEC	Commission of the European Communities
CI	Chemical ionization
CID	Collision-induced dissociation
DMG	Danish Malting Group
EBDC	Ethylene bisdithiocarbamate
ECD	Electron capture detection
EFSA	European Food Safety Authority
ESD	Element-selective detector
ETU	Ethylenethiourea
EU	European Union
FAO	Food and Agriculture Organization
GAP	Good agricultural practices
GC	Gas chromatography
GC/MS	Gas chromatography/mass spectrometry
GLP	Good laboratory practice
HACCP	Hazard analysis critical control point
HPLC	High performance liquid chromatography
IARC	International Agency for Research on Cancer
IPM	Integrated pest management
LC	Liquid chromatography
LC/MS	Liquid chromatography/mass spectrometry
MAE	Microwave-assisted extraction
MRL	Maximum residue limit
MRM	Multiresidue method
MSD	Mass spectrometric detection
MSPD	Matrix solid-phase extraction
NPD	Nitrogen phosphorus detection
OHA	Hydroxy atrazine
OHT	Hydroxy terbuthylazine
OTA	Ochratoxin A
PBDC	Propylene bisdithiocarbamate
PLE	Pressurized liquid extraction
PTU	Propylenethiourea
QA	Quality assurance
QC	Quality control
RAC	Raw agricultural commodity
SBI	Sterol biosynthesis-inhibiting
SFE	Supercritical fluid extraction
SPE	Solid-phase extraction
SPME	Solid-phase microextraction
UNIDO	United Nations Industrial Development Organization
WHO	World Health Organization
WTO	World Trade Organization

Beer in Health and Disease Prevention
ISBN: 978-0-12-373891-2

Introduction

For years there has been a great deal of publicity highlighting the health benefits of a moderate consumption of beer. The influence of beer on health is related to the absence of negative attributes and the presence of positive attributes. Beer, a wholesome beverage that has been a staple part of our diet for many thousands of years, contains a number of components such as antioxidants, which can be beneficial to health. Furthermore, the nutritive aspects of beer include its low sugar content and significant amount of vitamins and minerals (Sendra and Carbonell, 1998; Baxter and Hughes, 2001). One of the most important factors contributing to the public perception of beer as a "healthy drink" has been the accumulation of studies showing that moderate drinkers have lower death rates from all causes, especially from cardiovascular-related diseases, than either non-drinkers or heavy drinkers (Fagrell *et al.*, 1999). The quality of raw materials (barley, hops, water, and yeasts) has a decisive influence on the quality of the final product (Kunze, 2004). Knowledge of the properties of the raw materials and their effects on the process and the product provides the basis for their handling and processing. Therefore, it is important to assess the pollution load of barley and how pesticide residue evolves during the malting process. The ingredients used for brewing must not be allowed to act as a transmitter of unacceptable pollutants that are a risk for the beer consumer and animals.

Barley pests

Because of their high content of starch and storage proteins, barley grains represent an attractive source of nutrients for insects and microbial pathogens. The vulnerability of the grain to insect and pathogen attack is expected to increase during germination, when amino acids, fermentable carbohydrates, nitrogenous bases, and other degradation products of reserve polymers accumulate in the starchy endosperm (Fincher and Stone, 1993). Good weed control is essential to the crop to make efficient use of moisture and to prevent weed seeds from contaminating the harvest. Furthermore a range of head, root, leaf, and stem diseases may affect barley, depending on climate, environment, and farm history. Some of the more common diseases include crown rot, rust, smut, root rot, net blotch, and nematode infection. Finally, armyworms, cutworms, or mites cause important damage to cereals in some areas (Theaker *et al.*, 1989; Domínguez, 2004). Additionally, barley with a moisture content of about 14% may be attacked by fungi during storage especially by *Aspergillus* and *Penicillium* spp. These genera produce secondary metabolites such as ochratoxin A (OTA); it has been shown to be teratogenic and immunosuppressive. The International Agency for Research on Cancer (IARC) lists OTA as possibly carcinogenic to humans, group 2B (IARC, 1993). Some of these metabolites cause gushing, a very severe quality defect, where the beer spontaneously gushes from a bottle on opening. It is therefore important that malting barley is stored under conditions that prevent fungal growth (DMG, 1999).

Use of pesticides on barley

For the reasons mentioned earlier, pesticides are widely used in different combinations at many stages of cultivation and also during postharvest storage. From the past decades there has been, in the developed countries, an increasing concern over possible dangers to human health and/or the environment resulting from the excessive or inappropriate use of chemical pesticides. At present, good agricultural practices (GAP) are formally recognized in the international regulatory framework for reducing risks associated with the use of pesticides, taking into account public and occupational health, environmental, and safety considerations. The International Code of Conduct on the Distribution and Use of Pesticides (the worldwide guidance document on pesticide management for all public and private entities engaged in, or associated with, the distribution and use of pesticides adopted for the first time in 1985 by the Twenty-fifth Session of the FAO Conference) focuses on risk reduction, protection of human health and the environment, and support for sustainable agricultural development by using pesticides in an effective manner and applying integrated pest management (IPM) strategies (FAO, 2002).

The environmental and health impact of pesticides is being reduced through the implementation of a number of concrete programs on pesticide management, such as residue analysis, product standards setting and methods to analyze them, prevention of accumulation of obsolete stocks of pesticides and means to dispose them, and exchange of information on national actions taken to control pesticides.

Presence of pesticide residues in raw materials

The problem is that traces of these pesticides may remain in the beer produced from the treated ingredients, although the residues may also come from the soil itself and the water used; a problem that affects the brewing industry in several countries. During the first step (malting), some residues of pesticides having $\log K_{OW} > 2$ (as $\log P$) would remain on malt as indicated by some authors (Miyake *et al.*, 2002). After mashing and boiling, the pesticides on the malt can pass into the wort in different proportions, depending on the process used, although it should be noted that the removal of material in the form of trub and spent grains tends to reduce the level of pesticides, which are often relatively insoluble in water (Hack *et al.*, 1997; Miyake *et al.*, 1999; Navarro *et al.*, 2005a, 2006). Finally, if pesticide residues, especially some fungicides, are present in the brewer wort, they may cause organoleptic alterations to the finished beer and have toxic effects on the consumer (Jones *et al.*, 1988; Navarro *et al.*, 2007a).

Analysis of Pesticide Residues in Raw Materials and Beer

The widespread use of pesticides in cereals and hops had led to the presence of pesticide residues in beer. Public concern over pesticide residues in malt beverages and beers has been increasing such that it has become a significant food safety issue. Routine analyses of the composition of the raw materials used in the malting and brewing processes aim to assist quality control (QC). Validation protocols are essential for the analyst to provide the proper documentation of analytical results required to meet the QA/QC criteria of GLP/GMP and of various regulation agencies such as the Codex Alimentarius Commission (CAC) (Sherma, 1999). Additional analyses are performed to detect trace amounts of undesirable compounds such as pesticides to confirm that they are not present in the raw materials used in production. For this, multiresidue methods (MRMs) are needed to reliably and rapidly detect and quantitate as many pesticides as possible in the most cost-effective manner (Ghosh *et al.*, 2005).

Traditional batch liquid–liquid solvent extraction in a separatory funnel, Soxhlet extraction, or ultrasonic solvent extraction methods have been progressively substituted by more modern sample preparation methods in the past years (Sherma, 1999). These include general solid-phase extraction (SPE), polymeric reversed-phase (RP)SPE, disk format SPE, automated SPE, matrix solid-phase dispersion (MSPD), solid-phase microextraction (SPME), membrane filtration, solvent extraction flow injection, miniaturized liquid–liquid extraction, accelerated solvent extraction (ASE) or pressurized liquid extraction (PLE), microwave-assisted extraction (MAE), and water or supercritical fluid extraction (SFE). Methods and instruments for modern extraction methods have been reviewed (Jordan, 1998).

Residues in extracts are most commonly separated by gas chromatography (GC) or high performance liquid chromatography (HPLC) using ultraviolet (UV) absorbance, nitrogen phosphorus detection (NPD), or electron capture detection (ECD). However, although these element-selective detectors (ESDs) provide low ppb detection limits and are easy to operate, the data do not provide sufficient information to confirm a compound's presence with confidence. Owing to the universal nature of mass spectrometric detection (MSD), a mass spectrometer provides additional information and increases confidence in the assignment of compound identity (Meng, 2001). GC/MS has features to enhance specificity, such as chemical ionization (CI), selective ion monitoring (SIM), or MS/MS. Even with SIM, where multiple ions are monitored (MIM), the matrix may contain similar ions at the same retention time, so more stringent selectivity must be invoked to remove the matrix ions from the mass spectrum, which eliminates false positives and raises concentration values from matrix interferences. MS/MS does just that by ejecting all except the ion of interest out of the group. Then, a collision-induced dissociation (CID) energy is applied to fragment the ion into a very unique product ion spectrum (Butler and Conoley, 2005). However, although many established MRMs for analysis of food samples have used GC, some water-soluble pesticides that may be very important in beverages such as wine or beer are not suitable for analysis or their recoveries are very low. For these water-soluble pesticides, there are many analytical methods using liquid chromatography (LC). Recently, MS was found to be superior to other LC detectors, in particular, tandem mass spectrometry (MS/MS) was found to be far superior to any other method because of its high selectivity and sensitivity with the advantage of unequivocal analyte identification due to the ion selection of two mass analyzers. Also, as a single analytical procedure is desirable to screen beverage samples, the LC–MS/MS method allows the quantitation of many pesticides in beer without any sample preparation other than centrifugation. Many analytical methods using these techniques have been proposed in recent years for analysis of pesticide residues in cereals, malt, hops, and beer (Williams *et al.*, 1994; Hack *et al.*, 1996; Tadeo *et al.*, 2000; Hengel and Shibamoto, 2002; Wong *et al.*, 2004; Trösken *et al.*, 2005; Omote *et al.*, 2006; Vela *et al.*, 2007).

Food Safety and Policy in the European Union

The agro-food sector is of major importance for the European economy as a whole. The food and drink industry is a leading industrial sector in the European Union (EU), with an annual production worth almost €600 billion, or about 15% of total manufacturing output. An international comparison shows the EU as the world's largest producer of food and drink products. Production of beer worldwide was forecast to increase to an annual growth rate of 2.3% through 2005 to a volume of about 153 billion liters. Concretely, about 34% of the world beer production in 2004 (530 million Hl) was manufactured in Europe – Germany, Great Britain, and Spain being the main producers of the EU (Barth-Haas Group, 2005).

The contamination of food by chemical hazards is a worldwide public health concern and is a leading cause of trade problems internationally. Contamination may occur through environmental pollution, as in the case of toxic metals, polychlorinated biphenyls (PCBs), and dioxins, or through the intentional use of chemicals such as pesticides, animal drugs, and other agrochemicals. Food additives and contaminants resulting from food manufacturing and processing can also adversely affect health. The EU's food policy is based on high food safety standards, which serve to protect and promote the health of the consumer. Regulation (EC) No. 396/2005 on maximum residue levels of pesticides in or on food and feed of plant and animal origin emphasizes the importance of carrying out further work to develop a methodology to take into account cumulative and synergistic effects of pesticides on human health. The EU food safety policy must be based on a comprehensive, integrated approach. This means throughout the food chain ("farm to table"), across all food sectors, between the Member States, at the EU external frontier and within the EU, in international and EU decision-making fore, and at all stages of the policy-making cycle. The pillars of food safety contained in the White Paper (scientific advice, data collection and analysis, regulatory and control aspects, as well as consumer information) must form a seamless whole to achieve this integrated approach (CEC, 2000).

HACCP system in the food industry

The hazard analysis critical control point (HACCP) system is a relatively new approach to the prevention and control of foodborne diseases. The HACCP system identifies specific hazards and preventative measures for their control to ensure the safety of food. HACCP is a tool to assess hazards and establish control systems that focus on preventative measures rather than relying mainly on end-products testing. Table 40.1 summarizes the seven HACCP principles.

For many years public health and food control authorities worldwide, as well as international organizations such as Food and Agriculture Organization (FAO), World Health Organization (WHO), and United Nations Industrial Development Organization (UNIDO) have promoted the application of the HACCP system. FAO/WHO CAC adopted at its 20th Session (1993), the Guidelines for the Application of the HACCP System (CAC/GL 18-1993). This session emphasized that the work of Codex has increased in importance with the establishment of the World Trade Organization (WTO) and the WTO Agreement on the Application of Sanitary and Phytosanitary Measures coming into force. According to this Agreement; Codex standards; guidelines and recommendations relating to food additives, veterinary drug and pesticide residues, contaminants; methods of analysis and sampling; and codes and guidelines of hygienic practice have been recognized as the reference for international food safety requirements, and thus as a benchmark for national requirements.

The Food Hygiene Directive (93/43/EEC) obliges food businesses in the EU to implement systems that are based on the principles of HACCP. Although non-EU suppliers of food products do not legally have to comply directly with the EU directive on food hygiene, they are affected by the Euhygiene rules. It was clearly confirmed that food businesses in Europe, implementing systems to ensure that hazards are identified and controls are in place, have become increasingly selective in dealing with their (foreign) suppliers and request a strict application of HACCP in the request countries of origin of imported products. In some cases, they have even set out additional hygienic requirements for their suppliers regarding specific product(s).

Food businesses in Europe and other industrialized countries, applying systems to assure food safety, will not buy any raw material if they think that, even after sorting and processing, it could make food unfit for human consumption. Any raw material or processed food product that is only suspected or known to be infected or contaminated with parasites or foreign substances will not be accepted.

Therefore, it is important to carry out a HACCP plan (a document describing the activities developed in accordance with the principles of HACCP to ensure control of hazards, which are significant for food safety in the product under consideration and its intended use) in order to reveal the weaknesses of the production line of beer and to suggest the critical limits in compliance with legislation and the corresponding preventive and corrective measures (Kourtis and Arvanitoyannis, 2001).

Table 40.1 Principles of the hazard analysis critical control point (HACCP) system

1. Conduct a hazard analysis. Steps in the process where significant hazards can occur including preventive measures.
2. Identify the critical control points (CCPs) in the process.
3. Establish critical points for preventive measures associated with each identified CCP.
4. Establish CCP monitoring requirements and procedures for using the results of monitoring to adjust the process and maintain control.
5. Establish corrective actions to be taken when monitoring indicates that there is a deviation from an established critical limit.
6. Establish effective record-keeping procedures that document the HACCP system.
7. Establish procedures for verification that the HACCP system is working correctly.

Effects of Brewing on the Pesticide Residues

Depending on the type of process involved and the chemical nature of the residue in the raw agricultural commodity (RAC), differences in the nature of the residue in the processed commodities and the RAC may have to be determined. Once the nature of the residues formed during processing has been clarified and active ingredients and relevant metabolites to be analyzed have been identified, processing studies are conducted with RACs that normally undergo processing in the home or under commercial conditions. The process may be physical or may involve the use of heat or chemicals (Timme and Waltz-Tylla, 2003). These types of processing are intended to (i) provide information on the transfer of residues from RACs to the processed product, in order to calculate reduction/concentration factors; (ii) enable a more realistic estimate to be made of the dietary intake of pesticide residues; and (iii) establish MRLs for residues in processed products when necessary. Figure 40.1 summarizes the principal steps of the brewing process. More detailed descriptions can be found in Eaton (2006).

Dissipation of pesticide residues during storage of barley, malt, and spent grains

When appropriate application methods of agrochemicals are not followed, pesticide residues on barley can be above the maximum residue limits (MRLs) established by the governments of each country, and the time for pesticide dissipation is also high. Desmarchelier *et al.* (1980) reported the losses of several pesticides (bioresmethrin, carbaryl, fenitrothion, *d*-fenothrin, methacrifos, and pirimiphos-methyl) from barley after storage and malting finding losses of 58–100%. Other authors show that after pesticide application using some insecticides (phentoate, fenitrothion, and ethiofencarb) and fungicides (triflumizole, mepromil, propiconazole, and triadimefon), common in barley cultivation, more than 80% of residues of phentoate and fenitrothion (organophosphorus insecticides) remained after 2 months of grain storage at room temperature, whereas the loss of other pesticides ranged from 28% to 85%, and metabolites of triadimefon (triadimenol) and triflumizole (TF-6-1) increased slightly (Miyake *et al.*, 2002). Several models (Timme and Frehse, 1980; Timme *et al.*, 1986; Morton *et al.*, 2001) are used to describe the decay of pesticides in different matrices. Probably, the most commonly used model to describe loss of grain protectants is the following equation, where R_t is the residue at time t, R_0 the residue at time zero, and K the rate constant (Desmarchelier, 1977, 1978).

$$\ln R_t = \ln R_0 - Kt$$

Navarro *et al.* (2007b) found a good linear correlation ($r \geq 0.95$) between $\ln R_t$ and time when they studied the dissipation of several pesticides over 3 months of malt storage at 20 ± 2°C. Additionally, a perfect correlation ($r > 0.99$) between the analytical and theoretical concentration calculated (R_0) at 0 days was observed, which indicates that the model is valid. According to the calculated values for the rate constant (K), the following dissipation rate was observed: myclobutanil > propiconazole > fenitrothion > trifluralin > pendimethalin > malathion > nuarimol with half-lives ranging from 244 to 1,533 days.

A moist by-product from the brewing industry, made up of spent grains, is widely fed to ruminant animals used as a buffer or as a forage or concentrate replacer. Therefore, although the nutritional potential of the spent grains for animals has been demonstrated, it is important to ascertain the pollution load of the same and how any pesticide residues evolve during storage.

To know the dissipation rate of pesticide residues in the spent grains, Navarro *et al.* (2005a, 2006) studied their disappearance during storage (3 months). In all cases, there was a good linear correlation ($r > 0.96$) between residue level and time. The necessary times to reach their respective MRLs in barley were 408, 515, 958, 711, 719, and 934 days for nuarimol, myclobutanil, propiconazole, fenitrothion, trifluralin, and pendimethalin, respectively, which indicates a high persistence level and minimum degradation for all compounds, especially for propiconazole. In the case of malathion, the initial residue was below its MRL.

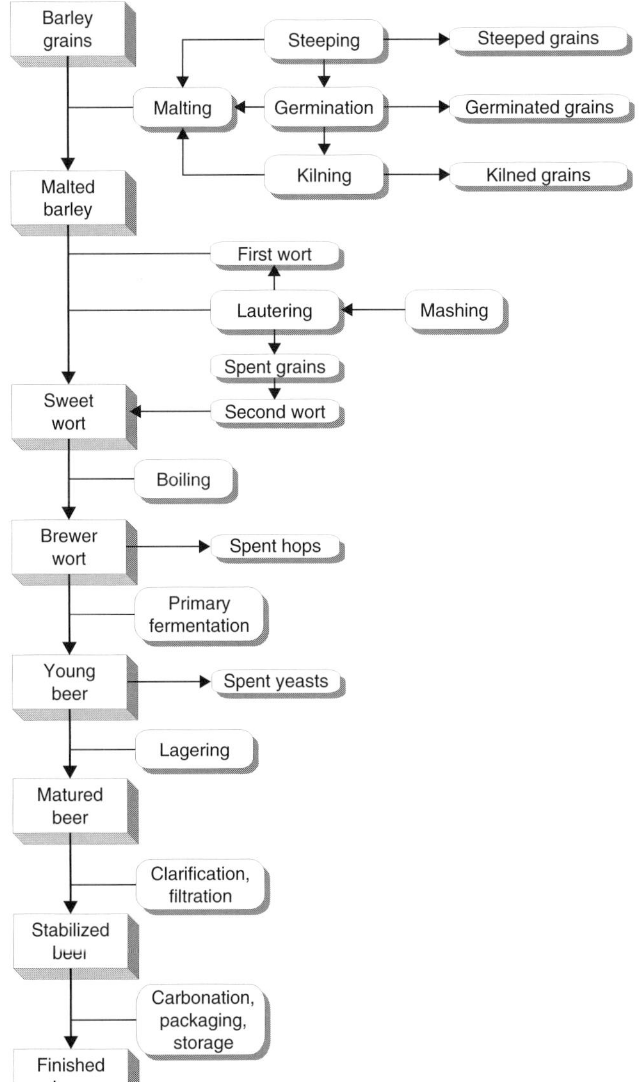

Figure 40.1 Scheme illustrating the principal stages of the brewing process.

Decline of pesticide residues from barley to malt (malting)

Common malting operations involve four basic stages: barley intake, drying and storage, steeping, germination

Table 40.2 Carryover of some pesticide residues after each stage of malting

Pesticides	*Log* P_{OW}*	*Stage*			*References*
		Steeping	*Germination*	*Kilning*	
Ethiofencarb	2.04	3	1	5	Miyake *et al.* (2002)
Mepronil	3.66	24	6	30	
Phentoate	3.69	27	4	18	
Triadimefon	3.11	24	5	30	
Triadimenol	3.08	36	13	47	
Triflumizole	4.36		11	9	
Propiconazole	3.65	50	10	55	Miyake *et al.* (2002)
		55	43	30	Navarro *et al.* (2007b)
Fenitrothion	3.43	52	31	13	Navarro *et al.* (2007b)
Malathion	2.75	45	20	14	
Myclobutanil	2.94	59	42	36	
Nuarimol	3.18	64	57	51	
Pendimethalin	5.18	85	67	49	
Trifluralin	3.07	80	65	50	

*Tomlin (2003).

and kilning (Bamforth and Barclay, 1993). The process commences with the steeping of barley in water to achieve a moisture level sufficient to activate metabolism in the embryonic and aleurone tissues, leading in turn to the development of hydrolytic enzymes. Germination is generally targeted to generate the maximum available extractable material by promoting endosperm modification through the development, distribution, and action of enzymes. Finally, after a period of germination sufficient to achieve even modification, the "green malt" is kilned to arrest germination and stabilize the malt by lowering moisture levels, typically to less than 5%.

Table 40.2 shows some bibliographical data relative to pesticide decline during malting. Although in general terms steeping reduces residue levels significantly, the carryovers for dinitroaniline herbicides (pendimethalin and trifluralin) vary from 80% to 85% in steeped grains. Both are hydrophobic pesticides because of their high log P_{OW} (>5) and low solubility (0.2–0.3 mg/l). In consequence, a low proportion of their residues (10–15%) are removed with the steeping water. Regarding the organophosphorus pesticides, 55% of malathion (log $P_{OW} = 2.7$) is removed from the barley grains after steeping whereas 48% of fenitrothion residues (log $P_{OW} = 3.5$) are removed in this stage (Navarro *et al.*, 2007b). Other published data show carryover of 43% for fenitrothion after steeping process whereas other organophosphorus insecticide such as phentoate remains in lower proportion (27%) as indicated by Miyake *et al.* (2002). On the contrary, other insecticide of the same family as pirimiphos-methyl remains in high proportion (90%) after steeping (Collins and Armitage, 2006). Some fungicides such as nuarimol (pyrimidine), myclobutanil, and propiconazole (triazole) are removed from the barley grains (after steeping) in proportions ranging from 30% to

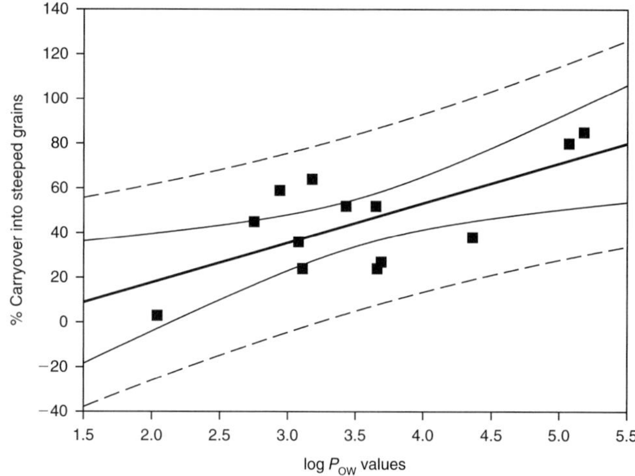

Figure 40.2 Correlation between carryover of some pesticides after steeping and their logP_{OW} values according to the data shown in Table 40.1 (solid line is 95% confidence interval and dash line 95% prediction interval).

41%, this is expected bearing in mind their respective coefficients between *n*-octanol and water (P_{OW} values). Miyake *et al.* (2002) found higher percentages of elimination for some azole fungicides, specifically 50%, 62%, and 76% for propiconazole, triflumizole, and triadimefon, respectively. These data are supported by the relationship between amounts removed after steeping and log P_{OW} of the pesticides used in this study, as can be seen in Figure 40.2. The carryover of hydrophilic pesticides (low log P_{OW}) such us malathion is lower, whereas carryovers of hydrophobic pesticides (pendimethalin and trifluralin) are higher. Miyake *et al.* (1999) suggest that brewers should pay attention to

Table 40.3 Carryover of some pesticide residues after mashing and boiling

Pesticide	Log P_{OW}[a]	Sweet wort	Spent grains	Brewer wort	Spent hops	References
Atrazine	2.5	45	55	42	20	Hack *et al.* (1997)
Terbutylazine	3.2	12	80	7	40	
Triadimenol	3.1	36	ND[b]	ND	ND	Miyake and Tajima (2003)
Captafol	3.8	BDL	3	BDL	BDL	Miyake *et al.* (1999)
Chlorpyrifos	4.7	17	3	4	32	
Deltamethrin	4.6	BDL	45	3	37	
Diclofuanid	3.7	10	10	BDL[c]	BDL	
Dichlorvos	1.9	8	BDL	BDL	BDL	
Dicofol	4.3	BDL	70	18	60	
Fenobucarb	2.8	35	30	64	1	
Fenvalerate	5.0	BDL	50	3	7	
Flucythrinate	6.2	BDL	60	BDL	10	
Glyphosate	−3.2	97	3	95	2	
Oxamyl	0.4	1	BDL	20	BDL	
Parathion-methyl	3.0	1	BDL	10	3	
Permethrin	6.1	BDL	70	BDL	50	
Pirimicarb	1.7	84	14	50	3	
Pirimiphos-methyl	4.2	2	68	6	12	
a-BHC	4.0	8	54	30	15	
Malathion	2.7	20	35	15	5	Miyake *et al.* (1999)
		7	40	4	ND	Navarro *et al.* (2006)
Myclobutanil	2.9	9	38	8	ND	
Nuarimol	3.2	6	26	6	ND	Navarro *et al.* (2005a)
Propiconazole	3.6	4	42	4	ND	
Fenitrothion	3.4	4	30	3	ND	
Pemdimethalin	5.2	1	21	1	ND	Navarro *et al.* (2006)
Trifluralin	5.1	1	17	1	ND	

[a] Tomlin (2003).
[b] Not determined.
[c] Below detection limit.

the residues of hydrophilic pesticides on malt with P_{OW} values <4 because they can be carried over into beer; the steeping stage of the malting process being of special interest. The same authors (Miyake *et al.*, 2002) showed that pesticides with $\log P_{OW} > 2$ can remain on malt. Therefore, the control of pesticides with P_{OW} values ranging from 2 to 4 must be very important for maltster and brewers.

Removal and transference of pesticide residues from malt to sweet wort (mashing)

As a general rule, about 200 g of grains are used to produce 1 litre of wort at 12° Brix, although this amount varies according to whether a higher or lower alcoholic content is desired. Any residues present in the grain, even if completely transferred to the beer, should, therefore, undergo dilution by a factor of 5 although $\log P_{OW}$ values of pesticides should be kept in mind (Miyake *et al.*, 1999). Taking into account the low solubility of most pesticide residues in water and their tendency to be easily adsorbed on the suspended matter, as in wine making, the presence of residues in beer should be very low (Farris *et al.*, 1992).

The carryovers of residues for several pesticides after mashing are shown in Table 40.3. During mashing, the soluble substances (sugars, amino acids, and peptides) produced in malting and mashing are extracted into the liquid fraction (sweet wort), which is then separated from the residual solid particles (spent grains). According to Navarro *et al.* (2005a), at the end of the mashing phase, the remaining percentages are below 10% of the amount recorded in malt; propiconazole showing the greatest decrease (to 4%). On the contrary, the retained amounts on spent grain is relatively high (38%, 42%, and 26% for myclobutanil, propiconazole, and nuarimol, respectively, all the compounds having $K_{OW} > 2$) (Figure 40.3). Similar behavior was observed for atrazine and terbuthylazine during mashing, when 70% and 90%, respectively, were adsorbed on spent grain (Hack *et al.*, 1997). In a general way, adsorption affinity depends on the polarity of the compounds: the more polar the pesticide, the lower the adsorbed amount (Hengel and Shibamoto, 2002). It is necessary to bear in mind that maceration of the malt and adjuncts produces a great quantity of suspended matter, which could adsorb the pesticide residues and, if the recorded levels allow it, the spent grains could be used as animal feeds, implying

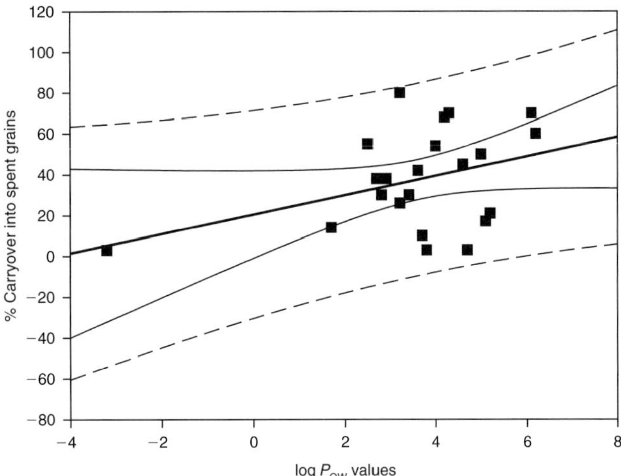

Figure 40.3 Correlation between carryover of some pesticides after mashing and their logP_{OW} values according to the data shown in Table 40.3 (solid line is 95% confidence interval and dash line 95% prediction interval).

a commercial use of this by-product. As shown in Table 40.3, the amounts remaining of dinitroaniline herbicides practically disappear after mashing (<1% of the initial amount in sweet wort), whereas the remaining percentages of fenitrothion and malathion in the sweet wort are greater (4.2% and 6.6%, respectively). On the contrary, the retained amounts on spent grain were relatively high (22%, 17%, 30%, and 40% for pendimethalin, trifluralin, fenitrothion, and malathion, respectively). Other pesticides such as glyphosate (organophosphorus) and pirimicarb (carbamate) were found in sweet wort in proportions higher than 80%. On the contrary, no residues of pyrethroid compounds (fenvalerate, deltamethrin, permethrin, and flucythrinate) were obtained from sweet wort; they were recovered from the spent grains. In the case of oxamyl, dichlorvos, parathion-methyl, chlorpyrifos, dichlofuanid, and captafol, pronounced losses were observed, possibly due to thermal degradation, evaporation, or chemical reactions with some wort components during the mashing process (Miyake *et al.*, 1999).

Removal and transference of pesticide residues from sweet wort to brewer wort (boiling)

Table 40.3 shows the carryovers of several pesticides in brewer wort and spent hops. As can be seen, a very small decrease (<10%) has been observed in the residual content after the wort had been boiled for myclobutanil, nuarimol, and penconazole residues, which points to the stability of the three compounds at temperatures higher than 100°C (Navarro *et al.*, 2005a). The carryovers of pendimethalin and trifluralin recorded from the brewer wort were lower than 30% of their content in sweet wort after wort boiling. With regard to the fall of organophosphorus compounds at this time, the levels of fenitrothion and malathion were 83% and 65%, respectively, of the content in wort after mashing (Navarro *et al.*, 2006). Other authors (Miyake *et al.*, 1999) show that the percentages of residues for glyphosate, fenobucarb, and pirimicarb into the cold wort were prominently high showing a great stability at temperatures above 100°C, whereas dicofol and pyrethroid insecticides were mainly recorded in the spent hops, and dichlorvos, dichlofuanid, and captafol completely disappear, probably due to the higher temperature of the boiling process in this case. However, the sum of residues for oxamyl, parathion-methyl, and chlorpyrifos in cold wort and spent hops was slightly higher than that of the mashing process. Authors assumed this behavior on the basis that these pesticides can react with some components or proteins in the sweet wort but not in the cold wort.

The fate of pesticide residues from hop to wort during boiling has also been studied. Some researchers have demonstrated that no pesticides added to the hops were detected in the young beer after wort boiling (Miyake *et al.*, 1999). Other work carried out by Navarro *et al.* (2005b) shows that residues of malathion, methidathion, and fenamiphos were below their detection limits in the young beer after addition of spiked hop pellets (2 μg/g) to the boiling wort, whereas 1 μg/l was recorded for fenarimol. In most of the cases, the absence of pesticide residues is due to their losses during boiling and the high dilution of hops. Other studies carried out with field-treated hops with several pesticides show that residues of tebuconazole, *Z*- and *E*-dimethomorph were lower than 31% of the amount expected, bearing in mind these were only the diluted residues. Subsequent analysis showed that 84–109% of pesticide residues (chlofenapyr, quinoxyfen, pyridaben tebuconazole, fenarimol, and both *Z*- and *E*-dimethomorph) remain on the spent hops (Hengel and Shibamoto, 2002), which is explained by the highly lipophilic components of hops such as waxes and resins. In Europe, processing studies on hops are only required when residues are higher than 5 mg/kg of dried cones because of the high dilution factor – around 250 (Timme and Waltz-Tylla, 2003).

Evolution of pesticide residues during fermentation

With regard to the influence of the fermentative process on the elimination of pesticide residues (Table 40.4), a significant reduction has been observed for propiconazole residues (47% of the content recorded in brewer wort) but much less for other fungicides such as myclobutanil and nuarimol (around 20%) (Navarro *et al.*, 2005a). However, no residues of dinitroaniline herbicides were found in young beer fermented with bottom-yeasts, although there was a significant reduction in the cases of organophosphorus insecticides fenitrothion and malathion (58% and 71% of the content recorded in brewer wort) (Navarro *et al.*, 2006). Other fermentation studies showed that top-fermenting yeasts (*Saccharomyces cerevisiae*) had a much greater ability

Table 40.4 Carryover of some pesticide residues after fermentation

Pesticide	*Log* P_{OW}[a]	*Young beer*[b]	*Spent yeast*	*References*
Atrazine	2.5	95 (76)	ND[c]	Hack *et al.* (1997)
Terbutylazine	3.2	100 (50)	ND	
Chlorfenapyr	4.8	BDL	34	
Quinoxyfen	4.7	BDL	62	
Tebuconazole	3.7	55	58	
Fenarimol	3.7	41	48	Hengel and Shibamoto (2002)
Pyridaben	6.4	BDL	43	
Z-dimethomorph	2.7	70	22	
E-dimethomorph	2.6	75	23	
Triadimenol	3.1	43	ND	Miyake and Tajima (2003)
Captafol	3.8	BDL[d]	BDL	Miyake *et al.* (1999)
Chlorpyrifos	4.7	12	16	
Deltamethrin	4.6	BDL	15	
Diclofuanid	3.7	17		
Dichlorvos	1.9	65	BDL	
Dicofol	4.3	BDL	10	
Fenobucarb	2.8	94	BDL	
Fenvalerate	5.0	BDL	11	
Flucythrinate	6.2	BDL	2	
Glyphosate	−3.2	110	BDL	
Oxamyl	0.4	30	BDL	
Parathion-methyl	3.0	60	4	
Permethrin	6.1	BDL	11	
Pirimicarb	1.7	50	BDL	
Pirimiphos-methyl	4.2	40	6	
α-BHC	4.0	110	30	
Malathion	2.7	58	2	Miyake *et al.* (1999)
		20	ND	Navarro *et al.* (2006)
Myclobutanil	2.9	78	ND	
Nuarimol	3.2	82	ND	Navarro *et al.* (2005a)
Propiconazole	3.6	52	ND	
Fenitrothion	3.4	35	ND	
Pemdimethalin	5.2	BDL	ND	Navarro *et al.* (2006)
Trifluralin	5.1	BDL	ND	

[a] Tomlin (2003).
[b] Values in parenthesis for atrazine and terbuthylazine are using top-yeasts.
[c] Not determined.
[d] Below detection limit.

to convert triazine herbicide residues into their hydroxylated products than bottom-fermenting yeasts (*Saccharomyces carlsbergensis*) (Hack *et al.*, 1997). For Miyake *et al.* (1999), no significant reduction was observed during the fermentation process for some group of pesticides. Other pesticides such as chlofenapyr, quinoxyfen, and pyridaben show a dramatic drop after addition to the pitching wort, being below detection limit after fermentation, whereas tebuconazole, fenarimol, and both *Z*- and *E*-dimethomorph had relatively high residue recoveries; their carryover, at the end of the fermentation, ranging from 41% to 75% (Hengel and Shibamoto, 2002). These results suggest that there is a relationship between K_{OW} and the amount of pesticides found in the young beer and the trub as can be seen in Figure 40.4. The losses during fermentation may be attributed to biotic metabolism of the yeast and abiotic degradation from the anaerobic environment created by fermentation (Cabras *et al.*, 1995). Also, according to the Henry's law constants (the tendency of a compound to volatilize from aqueous solution to air), those pesticides with high vapor pressure and low solubility in water may escape into the atmosphere (Mackay *et al.*, 1979). This process is also favoredby the constant evolution of CO_2 during the first few days of the fermentation.

Decrease of pesticide residues during maturation phase (lagering), filtration, and beer storage

No important decrease on the residual levels has been observed in any case after maturation and filtration. Nuarimol decreased its concentration (by 10%) with regard to the young beer. However, fenitrothion and malathion decrease their contents with regard to the young beer by

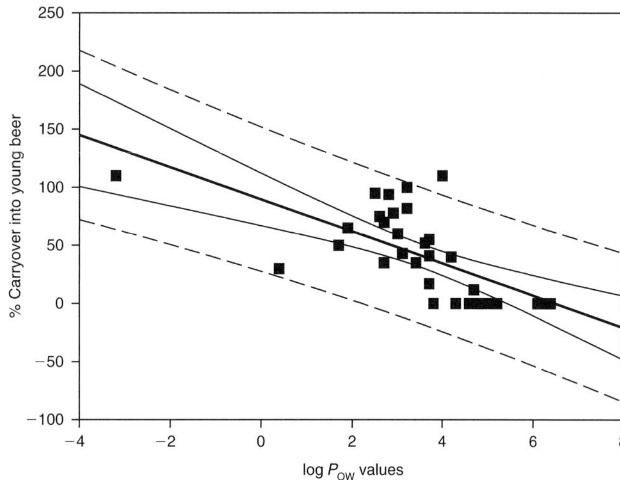

Figure 40.4 Correlation between carryover of some pesticides after fermentation and their $\log P_{OW}$ values according to the data shown in Table 40.4 (solid line is 95% confidence interval and dash line 95% prediction interval).

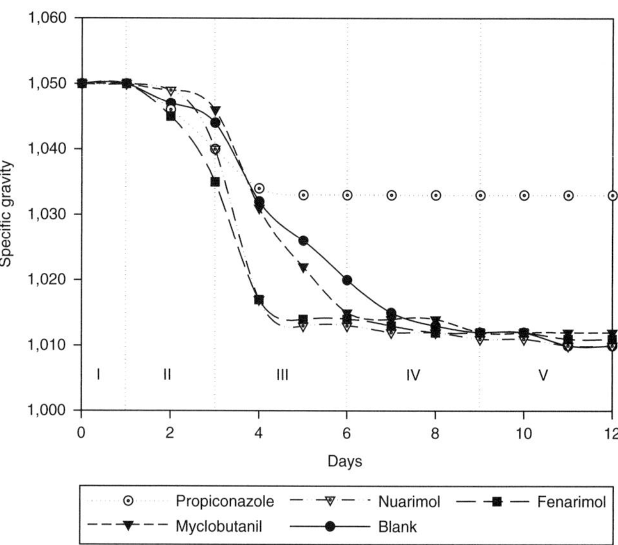

Figure 40.5 Evolution of specific gravity (n = 3) vs. time during fermentation phases (I: initial, II: low krausen, III: high krausen, IV: krausen collapsing, and V: collapsed foam) for blank and treated samples. *Source*: Navarro et al. (2007a).

33% and 37%, respectively (Navarro *et al.*, 2005a; Navarro *et al.*, 2006). Hack *et al.* (1997) did not find loss of triazines after filtration. Finally, after the storage period (3 months), the concentrations of myclobutanil and fenitrothion fall sharply (50% and 75%, respectively), whereas the decrease observed for nuarimol and myclobutanil, being lower than 25% of the amount in the finished beer is less pronounced, and malathion residues are below detection limits.

Influence of Pesticide Residues on the Beer Quality

During fermentation, yeast metabolizes sugars into energy, alcohol, carbon dioxide, secondary by-products, and more yeast. Those fermentation by-products have a considerable effect on the taste, aroma, and other characteristics of the beer. Beer flavor is a very complex subject. More than 800 compounds have been identified that contribute to the characteristic flavor of beer. Some pollutants, such as pesticides, can alter the normal fermentative process, being able to cause in certain cases sluggish and even stuck fermentation, although it will depend to a great extent on the initial concentrations in the malted barley, physical–chemical characteristics of each product, and beer-making procedure. In consequence, the organoleptic properties of the beer should be modified as in other fermented beverages such as wine (Cabras *et al.*, 1987; Navarro, 2000).

Flavor assessment is very important in quality control of beer. One of the most important tools is the sensory analysis by a panel of well-trained tasters. In some cases, the harsh astringent flavor observed in some beer samples was found to be due to products (metabolites) derived from pesticides present in the raw materials. Thus, residues of up to 5 mg/kg of carbaryl were found on treated barley and up to 41 μg/l of carbaryl-derived 1-naphtol were found in beer. Removal of up to 90% of the carbaryl and all of the 1-naphtol occurred during malting. Some tasters were able to consistently identify beer containing 20 μg/l of 1-naphtol (Jones *et al.*, 1988).

According to Navarro *et al.* (2007a), a marked influence of some pesticides in the fermentation rate has been observed (see Figure 40.5 where the evolution of specific gravity with time is shown for blank and treated samples). As can be seen, from the fourth day onward, the fermentation prematurely ceases (stuck fermentation; i.e., the premature termination of fermentation before all fermentable sugars have been metabolized) in the samples with propiconazole residues compared with the blank. No significant differences in the evolution of specific gravity has been found for samples fermented with myclobutanil residues whereas for samples treated with fenarimol and nuarimol residues the fermentative kinetic is quicker, from 2 to 6 days, probably due to the rapid assimilation of nitrogen by the yeasts. The four compounds are sterol biosynthesis-inhibiting (SBIs) fungicides. They inhibit the cytochrome P_{450} monooxygenase, which catalyzes the oxidative C_{14} demethylation of 24-methylenedyhydrolanosterol in the biosynthesis pathway, and are a widely applied class of antifungal agents because of their broad therapeutic window, wide spectrum of activity, and low toxicity (Koller, 1988). Some authors suggest that the complex nitrogen composition of the medium may create conditions resembling those responsible for inducing sluggish/stuck fermentation (Batistote *et al.*, 2006).

The sugars in wort are not all fermented in the same proportion. Figure 40.6 shows the evolution of fermentable

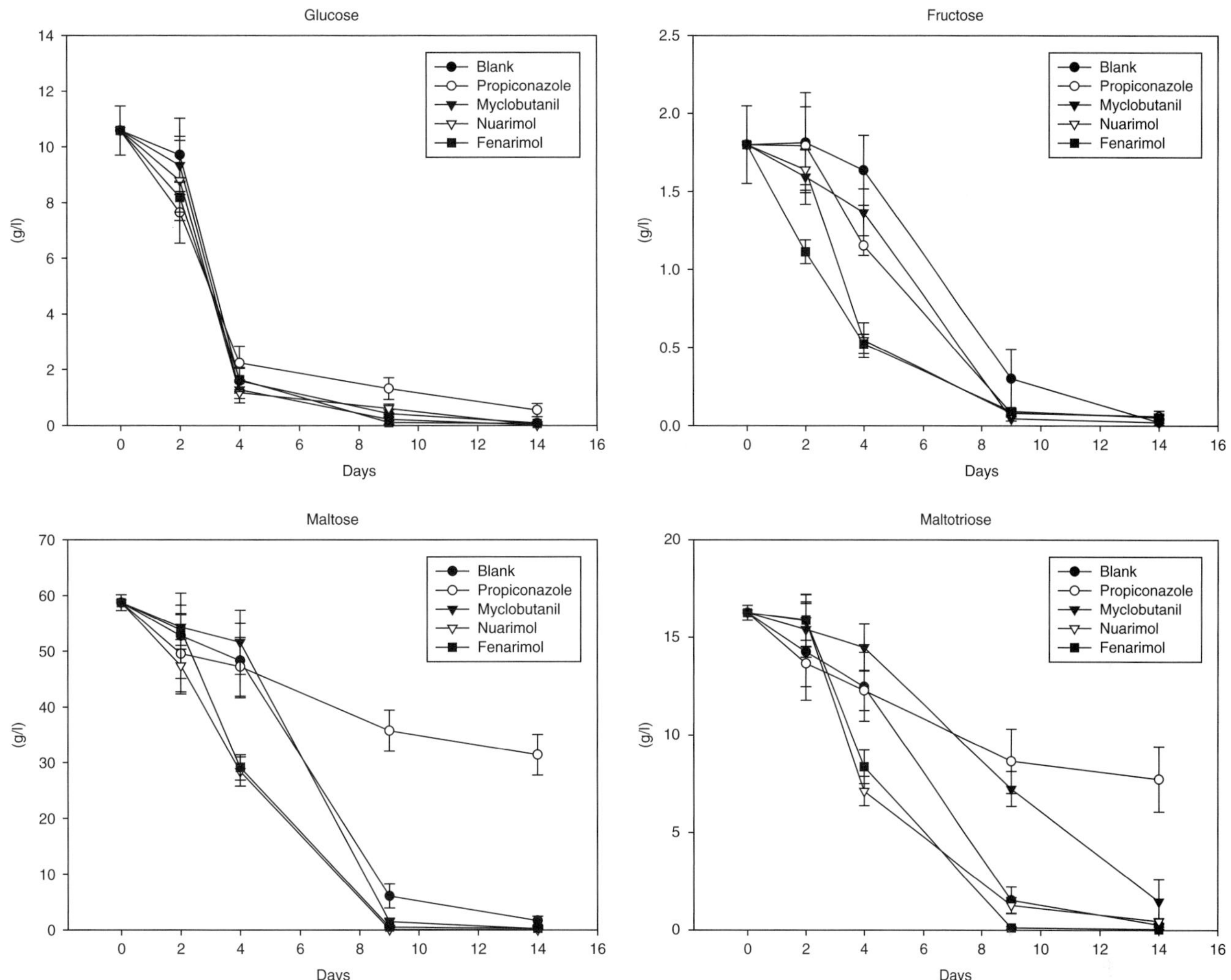

Figure 40.6 Change in glucose, fructose, maltose, and maltotriose content ($n = 3$) vs. time during fermentation for blank and samples treated with fungicides (error bars are 95% confidence intervals). *Source*: Navarro *et al.* (2007a).

carbohydrates during fermentation according to Navarro *et al.* (2007a). Since yeast has to hydrolyze sugar polymers before it can use them, it always attacks hexoses first. For this reason, the yeasts assimilate a greater proportion of glucose during the first 96h. No significant differences were observed between the blank sample and those treated with myclobutanil, nuarimol, and fenarimol residues whereas in the case of propiconazole, a delay in the glucose consumption was observed after 4 days. Sucrose was easily fermented by yeast in all cases because the enzyme that decomposes it, invertase, is located in the cell wall and sucrose is therefore treated as a start of fermentation sugar by the yeast. No significant differences were observed between the blank and the other samples although assimilation of this sugar was to some extent slower in the blank sample during the first 48h. Fructose assimilation follows a different behavior among glucose and sucrose. Samples with nuarimol and fenarimol (pyrim-idine fungicides) residues reduced this sugar quicker than those with propiconazole and myclobutanil (triazole fungicides) residues. The slowest assimilation corresponds to the blank sample. In all cases, the highest reduction occurs from 24 to 216h. Maltose exhibits similar behavior although the biggest consumption takes place between 96 and 216h, during the main fermentation. It is important to remark that after the fourth day the consumption of this sugar decreased drastically by the yeasts in the sample with propiconazole residues with logical bearing in mind that fermentation was stopped at this time. Finally, maltotriose is the last sugar assimilated by the yeasts. No significant differences were observed when comparing the behavior of the blank sample and those with residues of nuarimol and fenarimol. However, triazole fungicides, especially propiconazole, have a marked influence on the assimilation of this sugar by the yeasts.

The effect of some pesticide residues on the pH and color of the beer has also been observed (Navarro *et al.*, 2007a).

Thus, the pH values at the end of the fermentation were 4.1 for the blank sample and 3.0, 3.7, 3.8, and 3.9 for those containing residues of propiconazole, myclobutanil, fenarimol, and nuarimol, respectively. In this case also, the presence of propiconazole alters the final quality of the beer. pH values below 4.0 cause an acidic beer taste and must be avoided, in particular, acidification by microbial infections during fermentation. Therefore, maturation should be completely excluded. Regarding color, at the beginning of the process 5.35 EBC units were recorded. Although a slight increase after 2 days of fermentation can be observed in all cases, color of the beer falls about 1–1.5 EBC units during fermentation. This is possibly due to the decoloration of some substances caused by the drop in pH, and absorption of highly colored compounds in the yeast cells or precipitation in the vessel bottom (Kunze, 2004).

As a result of a decrease in pH during fermentation or adsorption on the yeast cells, a number of colloidally dissolved bitter substances and polyphenols can precipitate as surface active compounds on the CO_2 bubbles in the foam head (Kunze, 2004). As a consequence of their low solubility at a pH below 5 and temperatures lower than 10°C, the α-acids are not isomerized during the boiling of the wort precipitate. For this reason, in the study carried out by Navarro *et al.* (2007a), the values of bitterness are below detection limits in all cases. Regarding the total polyphenol and flavonoid contents found after fermentation, significant differences have been observed between the samples containing residues of triazole fungicides and the others, especially in the case of propiconazole due to the stuck fermentation after 4 days of beginning.

In other cases such as carbaryl residues during brewing its metabolization to 1-naphtol confers, above 20 μg/l, a characteristic harsh astringent flavor to the beer (Jones *et al.*, 1988).

Bearing in mind the aforementioned laser, if the pitching wort contains SBIs, especially triazole compounds, it is important to use fining agents such as activated charcoal, bentonite, or polyvinylpolypyrrolidon (PVPP) to eliminate or at least reduce their concentration in the wort since they can alter the quality of the beer. Some results obtained by Pérez *et al.* (2006) confirm that the use of activated charcoal reduce considerably the level of these compounds in the wort. Specifically, more than 80% and 70% of myclobutanil and propiconazole residues, respectively, can be removed.

Toxicological Risk of Pesticide Residues on Beer

In some cases, pesticide metabolites produced during the brewing phases have the same or more toxicity than their parent compounds and they can persist during fermentation. Agrochemical metabolites are generally water-soluble because most of them have hydroxyl or amine groups. This is the case of triadimenol and TF-6-1, metabolites of triadimefon and triflumizole, respectively. Both have been found in beer (Miyake and Tajima, 2003). Similar behavior has been observed for triazine compounds such as atrazine and terbuthylazine. Hydroxy analogs (OHA and OHT) were mainly detected in top-fermented beers. Monitoring of these herbicides, mainly in the brewing water, is essential because like atrazine these polar degradation products are classified as possible human carcinogens (Hack *et al.*, 1997).

The ethylene bisdithiocarbamate (EBDC) or propylene bisdithiocarbamate (PBDC) fungicides are often used to illustrate the formation of toxicologically relevant metabolites during processing procedures. The conversion of EBDCs and PBDCs into ethylenethiourea (ETU) and propylenethiourea (PTU) is particularly favored by high pH and heat (Timme and Waltz-Tylla, 2003) although the formation of ETU by thermal degradation in aqueous medium can be greatly reduced by the addition of copper sulfate by the formation of a stable cupric EBDC complex (Lesage, 1980). A study carried out with hops treated with radiolabeled EBDCs showed that parent fungicides (maneb/propineb) are mainly changed to ETU/PTU. ETU and PTU are EBDC and PBDC degradation products with carcinogenic effects (Nitz *et al.*, 1984). Therefore, studies to characterize the behavior of pesticide residues during brewing are necessary to perform a more realistic dietary risk assessment.

Summary Points

- Introduction
  - Barley pests
  - Use of pesticides on barley
  - Presence of pesticide residues in raw materials
- Analysis of pesticide residues in raw materials and beer
- Food Safety and Policy in the EU
  - HACCP system in the food industry
- Effects of brewing on the pesticide residues
  - Dissipation of pesticide residues during storage of barley, malt, and spent grains
  - Decline of pesticide residues from barley to malt (malting)
  - Removal and transference of pesticide residues from malt to sweet wort (mashing)
  - Evolution of pesticide residues during fermentation
  - Decrease of pesticide residues during maturation phase (lagering), filtration, and beer storage
- Influence of Pesticide Residues on the beer quality
- Toxicological risk of pesticide residues on beer

References

Bamforth, CW, Barclay, AHP. (1993). Malting technology and the uses of malt. In MacGregor, A.W., Bhatty, S.R. (eds), Barley: Chemistry and technology. St Paul, MN: American Association of Cereal Chemists, Inc., pp. 297–354.

Barth-Haas Group (2005). World Beer Production 2003/2004. Available from: http://www.barthhaasgroup.com/cmsdk/content/ bhg/news/report2/keydata.pdf (accessed October 1, 2006).

Batistote, M., da Cruz, S.H. and Ernandes, J.R. (2006). *J. Inst. Brew.* 112, 84–91.

Baxter, E.D. and Hughes, P.S. (2001). *Beer: Quality, Safety and Nutritional Aspects.* Royal Society of Chemistry, Cambridge, UK.

Butler, J. and Conoley, M. (2005). *Application Note 10017.* Thermo Electron Corporation, USA.

Cabras, P., Meloni, M. and Pirisi, F.M. (1987). *Rev. Environ. Contam. Toxicol.* 99, 83–117.

Cabras, P., Garau, L., Angioni, A., Farris, G., Budroni, M. and Apanedda, L. (1995). *Appl. Microbiol. Biotechnol.* 43, 370–373.

Collins, D, Armitage, D. (2006). Residue and efficacy decline during storage and malting. QualiGrain. Available: http://www.bordeaux.inra.fr/QualiGrain/result-ir.html (Accessed on September, 20 2006).

Commission of the European Communities (CEC) (2000). *White Paper on Food Safety.* Brussels.

Danish Malting Group (1999). Malting Process. Available from: http://www.crc.dk/flab/malting.htm (accessed September 22, 2006).

Desmarchelier, J.M., Goldring, M. and Horgan, R. (1980). *J. Pestic. Sci.* 5, 5539–5545.

Desmarchelier, J.M. (1977). *Aust. J. Exp. Agric.* 17, 818–825.

Desmarchelier, J.M. (1978). *Pestic. Sci.* 9, 33–38.

Domínguez, F. (2004). *Plagas y enfermedades de las plantas cultivadas*, 9ª Edición. Mundi-Prensa, Madrid.

Eaton, B. (2006). An overview of brewing. In Priest, F.G. and Stewart, G.G. (eds), *Handbook of Brewing*, 2nd edn, pp. 77–90. Taylor & Francis, Boca Raton, FL.

Fagrell, B., de Faire, U., Bonday, S., Criqui, M., Gaziano, M., Jackson, R., Klatsky, A., Salonen, J. and Shaper, A.G. (1999). *J. Int. Med.* 246, 331–340.

Food and Agriculture Organization (FAO) (2002). *International Code of Conduct on the Distribution and Use of Pesticides (revised version).* Rome.

Farris, G.A., Cabras, P. and Spanedda, L. (1992). *Ital. J. Food Sci.* 3, 149–169.

Fincher, G.B. and Stone, B.A. (1993). Physiology and biochemistry of germination in barley. In MacGregor, A.W. and Bhatty, S.R. (eds), *Barley: Chemistry and Technology*, pp. 247–295. American Association of Cereal Chemists, Inc, St. Paul, MN.

Ghosh, D., Alder, L., Churchill, M., Gehhardt, W., Genin, E., and Klein, J. (2005). *Application Note 323.* Thermo Electron Corporation, USA.

Hack, M., Nitz, S. and Parlar, H. (1996). *Adv. Food Sci. (CMTL)* 18, 40–45.

Hack, M., Nitz, S. and Parlar, H. (1997). *J. Agric. Food Chem.* 45, 1375–1380.

Hengel, M.J. and Shibamoto, T. (2002). *J. Agric. Food Chem.* 50, 3412–3418.

International Agency for Research on Cancer (IARC) (1993). *Monographs on the Evaluation of Carcinogenic Risks to Humans*, Vol. 56, pp. 489–521. IARC, Lyon, France.

Jones, R.D., Kavanagh, T.E. and Clarke, B.J. (1988). *J. Am. Soc. Brew. Chem.* 46, 43–50.

Jordan, J.R. (1998). *Inside Lab. Manag.* 2, 23–24.

Koller, W. (1988). Sterol demethylation inhibitors: Mechanism of action and resistance. In Delp, C.J. (ed.), *Fungicide Resistance in North America*, pp. 79–88. APS Press, St. Paul, MN.

Kourtis, L.K. and Arvanitoyannis, I.S. (2001). *Food Rev. Int.* 17, 1–44.

Kunze, W. (2004). *Technology of Brewing and Malting*, 3rd International English Edition. The Research and Teaching Institute for Brewing in Berlin (VLB). VLB's Publishing Department, Berlin.

Lesage, S. (1980). *J. Agric. Food Chem.* 28, 787–790.

Mackay, D., Shiu, W. and Sutherland, R. (1979). *Environ. Sci. Technol.*, 13, 333–337.

Meng, C.K. (2001). *Application Note.* Agilent Technologies, USA.

Miyake, Y. and Tajima, R. (2003). *J. Am. Soc. Brew. Chem.* 61, 33–36.

Miyake, Y., Koji, K., Matsuki, H., Tajima, R., Ono, M. and Mine, T. (1999). *J. Am. Soc. Brew. Chem.* 57, 46–54.

Miyake, Y., Hashimoto, K., Matsuki, H., Ono, M. and Tajima, R. (2002). *J. Am. Soc. Brew. Chem.* 69, 110–115.

Morton, R., Bryan, J.G., Desmarchelier, J.M., Dilli, S., Haddad, P.R. and Sharp, G.J. (2001). *J. Stored Prod. Res.* 37, 277–285.

Navarro, S. (2000). Pesticide residues in enology. In Mohan R.M. (ed.), *Research Advances In Agricultural and Food Chemistry*, Vol. 1, pp. 101–112. Global Research Network, Kerala, India.

Navarro, S., Pérez, G., Vela, N., Mena, L. and Navarro, G. (2005a). *J. Agric. Food Chem.* 53, 8572–8579.

Navarro, S., Pérez, G., Mena, L., Navarro, G., Vela, N. and Valverde, P. (2005b). *Cerveza y Malta* 166, 26–30.

Navarro, S., Pérez, G., Navarro, G., Mena, L. and Vela, N. (2006). *J. Food Prot.* 69, 1699–1706.

Navarro, S., Pérez, G., Navarro, G., Mena, L. and Vela, N. (2007a). *J. Agric. Food Chem.* (submitted for publication) 55, 1295–1300.

Navarro, S., Pérez, G., Navarro, G. and Vela, N. (2007b). *Food Addit. Contam.* 24, 851–859.

Nitz, S., Moza, P.N., Kokabi, J., Freitag, D., Behechti, A. and Korte, F. (1984). *J. Agric. Food Chem.* 32, 600–603.

Omote, M., Harayama, K., Sasaki, T., Mochizuki, N. and Yamashita, H. (2006). *J. Am. Soc. Brew. Chem.* 64, 139–150.

Pérez, G., Mena, L., Navarro, G., Vela, N. and Navarro, S. (2006). *Book of Abstracts of 6th European Pesticide Residue Workshop*, Corfu, Greece, pp. 229.

Sendra, J.M. and Carbonell, J.V. (1998). *Evaluación de las propiedades nutritivas, funcionales y sanitarias de la cerveza, en comparación con otras bebidas.* Centro de Información Cerveza y Salud, Madrid.

Sherma, J. (1999). *J. AOAC Int.* 82, 561–574.

Tadeo, J.L., Sánchez-Brunete, C., Pérez, R.A. and Fernández, M.D. (2000). *J. Chromatogr. A* 882, 175–191.

Theaker, P.D., Clarke, B.J., Currie, B.R. and Gough, A.J. (1989). *Tech. Q. Master Brew. Assoc. Am.* 26, 152–160.

Timme, G. and Frehse, H. (1980). *Planzenschutz Nachr Bayer* 33, 47–60.

Timme, G., Frehse, H. and Laska, V. (1986). *II. Planzenschutz Nachr Bayer* 39, 187–203.

Timme, G. and Waltz-Tylla, B. (2003). In Hamilton, D. and Crossley, S. (eds), *Pesticide Residues in Food and Drinking Water: Human Exposure and Risks*, pp. 121–148. Effects of food preparation and processing on pesticide residues in commodities of plant origin. John Wiley & Sons, Ltd, West Sussex, UK.

Tomlin, C.D.S. (ed.) (2003). *The Pesticide Manual*, 13th edn. British Crop Protection Council, Hampshire.

Trösken, E.R., Bittner, N. and Völkel, W. (2005). *J. Chromatogr. A* 1083, 113–119.

Vela, N., Pérez, G., Navarro, G. and Navarro, S. (2007). *J. AOAC Int.* 90, 544–549.

Williams, C., Eastoe, B., Slaiding, I. and Walker, M. (1994). *Food Addit. Contam.* 11, 615–619.

Wong, J.W., Webster, M.G., Bezabeh, D.Z., Hengel, M.J., Ngim, K.K., Krynitsky, A.J. and Ebeler, S. (2004). *J. Agric. Food Chem.* 52, 6361–6372.

Part II

General Effects on Metabolism and Body Systems

(i) General Metabolism and Organ Systems

41

Ethanol in Beer: Production, Absorption and Metabolism

Rajkumar Rajendram Nutritional Sciences Research Division, School of Life Sciences, King's College London, London, UK
Departments of General Medicine and Intensive Care, John Radcliffe Hospital, Oxford, UK
Victor R. Preedy Nutritional Sciences Research Division, School of Life Sciences, King's College London, London, UK

Abstract

Beer is brewed using malted grain (usually barley), water, hops and yeast. The fermentation of malted barley during the brewing process generates ethanol. After caffeine, ethanol is the most commonly used recreational drug worldwide and drinking beer is a very popular way of ingesting ethanol. Although non-alcoholic beers exist, the ethanol content of beer usually varies between 3% and 9% alcohol by volume. However, the concentration of ethanol in some specialist brews can be significantly higher. When beer is consumed, ethanol is absorbed from the gastrointestinal tract and rapidly distributed around the body in the blood before entering tissues. Some ethanol is metabolized to acetaldehyde in the stomach and liver before reaching the systemic circulation (first-pass metabolism). The average rate of oxidation of ethanol to acetaldehyde is approximately 15 mg/dl blood/hour. Acetaldehyde is highly toxic and binds cellular constituents generating harmful acetaldehyde adducts. Acetaldehyde is further oxidized to acetate. The metabolism of acetate and its significance in the effects of ethanol are less well understood.

In one study, consumption of 5 units of alcohol (40 g ethanol) as 1,000 ml of beer with an evening meal resulted in a mean blood ethanol concentration (BEC) of 6.8 mmol/l after 1 h and just below 2 mmol/l after 3 h. However, the relationship between BEC and the effects of ethanol is complex and varies between individuals and also with drinking habits. Many effects correlate with the peak BEC or peak ethanol concentrations within organs during a drinking session. Other effects are due to products of metabolism and the total dose of ethanol ingested over a period of time. The effects of gender, the ethanol content of the beverage consumed and the coincident consumption of food on the absorption, distribution and metabolism of ethanol are reviewed.

List of Abbreviations

ABV	Percentage content of alcohol by volume
ABW	Percentage content of alcohol by weight
ADH	Alcohol dehydrogenase
ALDH	Aldehyde dehydrogenase
AUC	Area under the blood ethanol concentration curve
AUC_{ip}	Area under the blood ethanol concentration curve after intraperitoneal administration of ethanol
AUC_{iv}	Area under the blood ethanol concentration curve after intravenous administration of ethanol
AUC_{oral}	Area under the blood ethanol concentration curve after oral administration of ethanol
BEC	Blood ethanol concentration
CYP2E1	Cytochrome P4502E1
C_2H_5	Carbonyl group of ethanol
FPM	First-pass metabolism
GABA	Gamma aminobutyric acid
GI	Gastrointestinal
GIT	Gastrointestinal tract
GSH	Glutathione
H_2O_2	Hydrogen peroxide
i.v.	Intravenous
*K*m	Half-maximal activity
MEOS	Microsomal ethanol oxidizing system
mRNA	Messenger ribonucleic acid
NAD^+	Nicotinamide adenine dinucleotide to NADH
NADH	Reduced form of nicotinamide adenine dinucleotide
NDMA	*N*-methy-d-aspartate
OH	Hydroxyl group
SD	Standard deviation

Introduction

Beer is a fermented alcoholic beverage which is brewed using malted grain (usually barley), water, hops and yeast. Ethanol is one of the most commonly used recreational

Beer in Health and Disease Prevention
ISBN: 978-0-12-373891-2

Table 41.1 The unit system of ethanol content of alcoholic beverages

Beverage containing ethanol	*Units of ethanol*
Half-pint of beer (284 ml)	1
Pint of beer (568 ml)	2
One glass of wine (125 ml)	1
Bottle of wine (750 ml)	6
One measure of spirits (e.g. whisky)	1
Bottle of spirits (e.g. whisky; 750 ml)	36

Note: The above table outlines the average amount of ethanol in units in some alcoholic beverages. The unit system is a convenient way of quantifying consumption of ethanol and is a helpful means to give practical advice. However, there are several confounding factors. The ethanol content of various brands of alcoholic beverage varies considerably (Table 41.4) and the alcohol consumed in homes bear little resemblance to standard measures.

Table 41.2 The geographical variation in the amount of ethanol in one unit

Country	*One unit of alcohol (g)*	*ml ethanol*
UK	8	10
Australia	10	12.7
Canada	13.5	17.1
USA	14	17.7
Japan	19.75	25

drugs worldwide and drinking beer is one of the most popular ways of ingesting ethanol. Beer has been brewed for thousands of years and gained popularity in Europe during the Middle Ages when clean water was often difficult to find. Where sanitation was poor, beer was often safer to drink than water because of its ethanol content.

In the United Kingdom, a standard alcoholic drink or unit of alcohol (Table 41.1) contains 8 g of ethanol. The UK Department of Health (1995) and Royal College of Physicians, Psychiatrists and General Practitioners (1995) have recommended sensible limits for ethanol intake based on units of alcohol. However, the amount of ethanol in one unit varies around the world (Table 41.2) which causes confusion and prevents international comparisons. Unless otherwise specified all references to units of alcohol in this chapter are based on the UK definitions of standard alcoholic drinks (Table 41.3).

Despite these guidelines, ethanol intake varies significantly between individual drinkers. Many drinkers enjoy the pleasant psycho-pharmacological effects of the ethanol in beer. However, some experience adverse reactions due to genetic variation of enzymes that metabolize ethanol and the consumption of excessive amounts of ethanol undoubtedly affects every organ in the body.

Many of the effects of the ethanol intake correlate with the concentration of ethanol in the blood (blood ethanol

Table 41.3 Guidelines for the consumption of alcohol

	Women (units)		*Men (units)*	
	Weekly[a]	*Daily*[b]	*Weekly*[a]	*Daily*[b]
Harmful	>35	≥1–2[c]	>50	
Hazardous	15–35	≥3	22–50	≥4
Low risk	0–14	2–3	0–21	3–4

Notes: Guidelines on the consumption of alcohol are designed to reduce harm (Royal College of Physicians, Royal College of Psychiatrists, Royal College of General Practitioners, 1995; Department of Health, 1995). Whilst the Department of Health recommendations are concerned with daily consumption, the Royal Colleges' guidelines are for weekly consumption rates.

[a] Recommendations of the Royal College of Physicians, Royal College of Psychiatrists and Royal College of General Practitioners (UK).
[b] Recommendations of the Department of Health (UK).
[c] When pregnant or about to become pregnant consumption of more than 1–2 units of alcohol, 1–2 times per week is harmful.

concentration (BEC)). It is therefore important to understand those factors that influence the BEC achieved from a dose of ethanol (i.e. drinking beer). However, the concentration of ethanol in each type of beer and therefore the dose of ethanol from a pint varies significantly between brews.

In most countries the concentration of ethanol in beer is expressed as a percentage of alcohol by volume (ABV). However, in the United States the legal standard requires the concentration of ethanol in beer to be expressed as a percentage of alcohol by weight (ABW). To approximate ABW from ABV, one needs to multiply ABV by 0.8. To determine ABV, ABW should be multiplied by 1.25. Thus, a beer which is 5% ABV is approximately 4% ABW. To avoid confusion all further references to strength of alcoholic beverages in this chapter will be in terms of ABV.

The strength of beer as ABV typically ranges from 3% to 8%, although some specialist beers can have higher concentrations (Table 41.4). Although low- and non-alcoholic beers are available, the interest in these is minimal. The factors which affect the ethanol content of a beer are described below.

Brewing Beer

The principles of brewing beer have been described by Goldammer (2000) and elsewhere in this book and are only briefly outlined here. All beers are brewed using a process that requires grain, usually barley, which has been malted (allowed to germinate). Germination generates enzymes such as amylase, which are used to convert the starch in the grain into sugars such as maltose (Goldammer, 2000).

The malt is dried in a kiln before being crushed and mixed with hot water in a vat called a "mash tun" where it is "mashed." During mashing, the enzymes within the

Table 41.4 Ethanol content of selected beers

Brewery	*Beer*	*ABV (%)*
Anheuser-Busch	Budweiser Bud Light	4.2
Anheuser-Busch	Budweiser Bud Ice	5.5
Anheuser-Busch	O'Doul's Amber NA	0.5
Carlsberg	Carls Porter	7.8
Chimay	Grand Reserve 1997	9
Clausthaler	Clausthaler	0.9
Carlton & United Breweries	Foster's Lager	5
Guinness	Draught Guinness	4.1
Guinness	Foreign Extra Stout	7.5
Guinness	Special Export Stout	8
Heineken	Export	5
In Bev	Stella Artois	5.2
Shepherd Neame	Spitfire	4.7
Whitbread	Gold Label Barley Wine	10

Note: The above table demonstrates the variability in alcohol content of different beers. ABV: percentage alcohol by volume.

Source: Data from the Oxford bottled beer database (2006) and Realbeer.com (2006).

malt break down the starches of the grain into the sugars required for fermentation (Goldammer, 2000). Mashing usually takes 1–2 h, and time spent at different temperatures (mash rests) activates various enzymes depending on the type of malt and the yeast being used (Goldammer, 2000). These enzymes convert starches to shorter chain carbohydrates such as dextrins and maltotriose. These can be further broken down to sugars such as maltose and glucose which are fermentable.

A mash rest at 40°C activates beta-glucanase, which breaks down beta-glucans, which facilitates the production of sugars later in the process (Goldammer, 2000). A mash rest temperature between 65°C and 71°C is used to convert the starches to fermentable sugars (Goldammer, 2000). A mash rest with a temperature at the lower end of the range results in the production of more low-order sugars. These are easier to ferment and this results in beer with higher ethanol content. Higher temperatures result in the production of higher-order sugars which are more difficult to ferment. This results in a sweet tasting beer with less ethanol. The mash temperature may then be raised to deactivate the enzymes (mashout; Goldammer, 2000). Additional water may then be sprinkled on the grain to extract additional sugars (sparging; Goldammer, 2000).

After mashing, the produced liquid is strained from the grains. The liquid (wort) is moved into a large tank where it is boiled with hops and sometimes other ingredients such as herbs or sugars (Goldammer, 2000). This deactivates enzymes, precipitates proteins and concentrates and sterilizes the wort. The hopped wort is then settled and clarified before being cooled.

The wort is moved into fermentation vessels where yeast is added (Goldammer, 2000). Initially, the concentration of

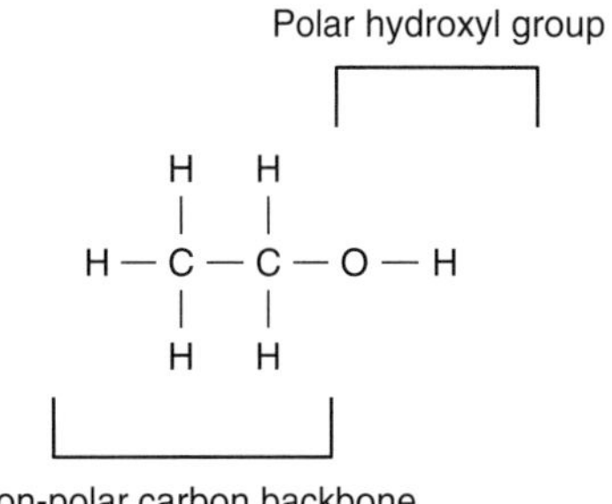

Figure 41.1 The chemical structure of ethanol. *Source*: Adapted from Rajendram *et al.* (2005) with permission from Elsevier.

sugars is high and sugars such as glucose enter the yeast by simple net diffusion, facilitated (carrier-mediated) diffusion or active transport (Pretorius, 2000). Each glucose molecule is broken down by glycolysis into two pyruvate molecules (three carbon sugars; Pretorius, 2000). The pyruvate molecules are then converted into carbon dioxide and ethanol by the yeast (Pretorius, 2000).

After 1–3 weeks, the fresh beer is run off into conditioning tanks (Goldammer, 2000). Conditioning may take several months, after which the beer may be filtered to remove yeast and any other particles. The beer is then ready for serving or packaging (Goldammer, 2000).

Types of yeast used to brew beer

Many different species of yeast are used to make beer, but there are two main types: ale yeasts and lager yeasts (Goldammer, 2000). Ale yeasts rise near to the surface of the beer during fermentation (top fermenting e.g. *Saccharomyces cerevisiae*), and typically prefer temperatures ranging from 10°C to 25°C (Goldammer, 2000). Lager yeasts sink to the bottom of the beer (bottom fermenting e.g. *Saccharomyces uvarum*) and ferment more slowly, preferring colder temperatures, around 7–15°C (Goldammer, 2000).

There are no significant differences between ale and lager yeasts with respect to ethanol tolerance. Ales are generally around 4–5% ethanol while lagers generally contain 4.5–5.2% ethanol. Beer yeast generally cannot tolerate an environment with greater than about 10–11% ethanol (Wyeast Laboratories, 2006) and as the ethanol concentration in the environment rises the efficiency of fermentation declines. However, some specialist brews have higher concentrations of ethanol and are brewed with specific types of yeast which are able to tolerate these levels of ethanol.

The Physical Properties of Ethanol

Ethanol (Figure 41.1) is highly soluble in water due to its polar hydroxyl (OH) group. The non-polar (C_2H_5) group enables ethanol to dissolve lipids and thereby disrupt

Table 41.5 Approximate ethanol concentrations in the GI tract and in the blood following oral ethanol administration (0.8 g/kg)

Site	*Ethanol concentration (g/dl)*
Stomach	7–8
Proximal jejunum	1–5
Ileum	0.1–0.2
Blood (15–120 min after dosage)	0.1–0.2

Note: Ethanol appears in the blood as quickly as 5 min after ingestion and is rapidly distributed around the body. A dose of 0.8 g ethanol/kg body weight (56 g ethanol (7 units) consumed by a 70 kg male) should result in a blood ethanol concentration of 100–200 mg/dl between 15 and 120 min after dosage. Highest concentrations occur after 30–90 min.

Source: Halsted *et al.* (1973); Rajendram *et al.* (2005).

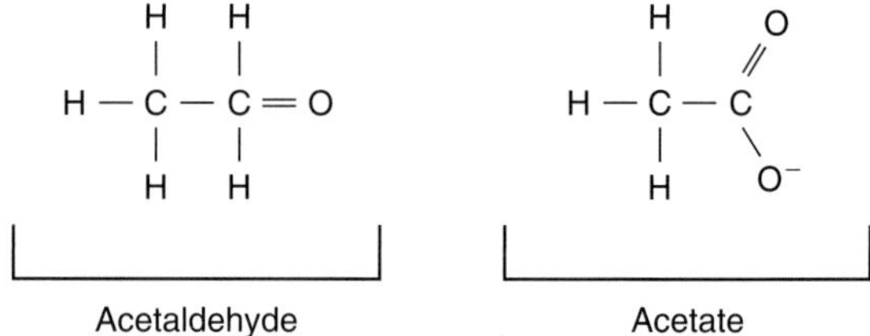

Figure 41.2 The chemical structure of acetaldehyde and acetate. Acetaldehyde and acetate are the products of ethanol metabolism. Their structures are shown above. *Source*: Adapted from Rajendram *et al.* (2005) with permission from Elsevier.

biological membranes. Ethanol crosses cell membranes easily by passive diffusion as it is a relatively uncharged molecule.

Absorption and Distribution of Ethanol in Beer

The basic principles of ethanol absorption from the gastrointestinal (GI) tract, and subsequent distribution are well understood. Alcoholic beverages such as beer pass down the esophagus, into the stomach. Ethanol continues down the GI tract until absorbed (Halsted, 1973; Rajendram *et al.*, 2005). The ethanol concentration therefore decreases down the GI tract. There is also a concentration gradient of ethanol from the lumen to the blood. The concentration of ethanol in plasma is much lower than that in the lumen of the upper small intestine (Table 41.5; Halsted, 1973; Rajendram *et al.*, 2005). Ethanol diffuses passively across the cell membranes of the mucosal surface into the submucosal space and then the submucosal capillaries (Kalant, 2004).

Although absorption is fastest in the duodenum and jejunum, uptake of ethanol occurs across all of the GI mucosa. The rate of gastric emptying is the main determinant of absorption as most ethanol is absorbed after leaving the stomach through the pylorus (Kalant, 2004).

However, concentrations of ethanol within the ileal lumen are not significantly different from BEC (Bode and Bode, 2003). This suggests that ethanol enters the ileum and colon from the blood and any luminal sequelae of ethanol ingestion occur mainly in the upper small intestine.

Ethanol diffuses into tissues from the blood stream through the walls of capillaries. Ethanol concentration equilibrates between blood and the extracellular fluid within a single pass. The time taken for equilibration between blood water and total tissue water can vary from minutes up to an hour or more, depending on the cross-sectional area of the capillary bed and tissue blood flow (Kalant, 2004). Ethanol enters most tissues but its solubility in bone and fat is negligible. Therefore, in the post-absorption phase, the volume of distribution of ethanol reflects total body water. Total body water is highly correlated with fat-free mass and lean body mass. Thus, for a given dose of ethanol, BEC will reflect lean body mass.

Metabolism of Ethanol

The average rate of oxidation of ethanol is approximately 15 mg/dl blood/hour (Fisher *et al.*, 1987). However, many factors influence this rate and there is considerable individual variation.

Absorbed ethanol is initially oxidized to acetaldehyde (Figure 41.2) by one of the three pathways (Figure 41.3):

1. Alcohol dehydrogenase (ADH) – cystosol.
2. Microsomal ethanol oxidizing system (MEOS) – endoplasmic reticulum.
3. Catalase – peroxisomes.

Alcohol dehydrogenase

ADH couples oxidation of ethanol to reduction of nicotinamide adenine dinucleotide (NAD^+) to NADH. ADH also has a wide range of other substrates and functions, including dehydrogenation of steroids and oxidation of fatty acids (Kalant, 2004).

ADH isoenzymes

ADH is a zinc metalloprotein with five classes of isoenzymes that arise from the association of eight different subunits into dimers (Table 41.6; Kwo and Crabb, 2002). A genetic model accounts for these five classes of ADH as products of five gene loci (ADH1-5; Bosron *et al.*, 1993). *Km* is the concentration of substrate that results in half-maximal velocity. Class 1 isoenzymes generally require a low concentration of ethanol to achieve "half-maximal activity" (low *Km*) whilst Class 2 isoenzymes have a relatively high *Km*. Class 3 ADH has a low affinity for ethanol and does not participate in the oxidation of ethanol in the liver (Lieber, 2005). Class 4 ADH

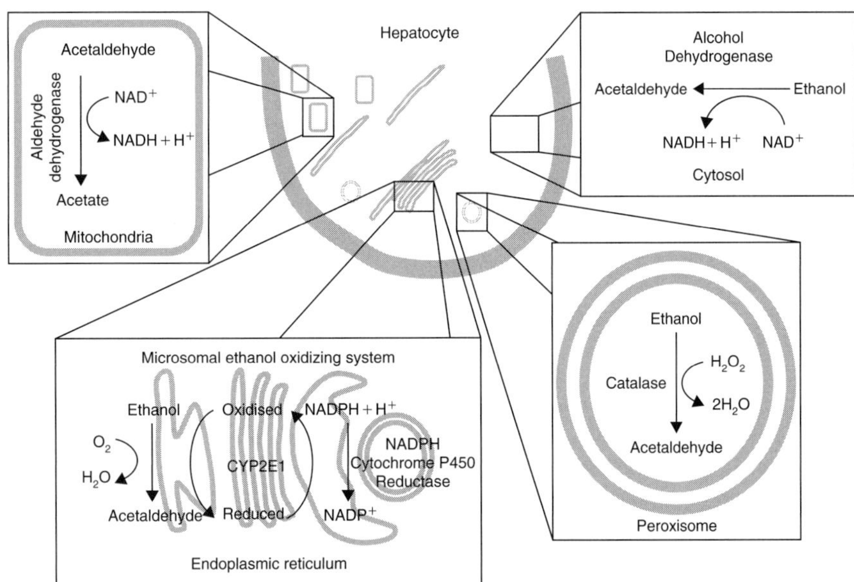

Figure 41.3 Pathways of ethanol metabolism. This figure illustrates the metabolism of ethanol to acetaldehyde and then to acetate. *Source*: Adapted from Rajendram *et al.* (2005) with permission from Elsevier.

Table 41.6 Alcohol dehydrogenase (ADH) isoenzymes

Class	*Subunit*	*Location*	*Km (mmol/l)*[a]	V_{max}
Class 1				
ADH1	α	Liver	4	54
ADH2	β	Liver, lung	0.05–34	
ADH3	γ	Liver, stomach	0.6–1.0	
Class 2				
ADH4	π	Liver, cornea	34	40
Class 3				
ADH5	χ	Most tissues	1,000	
Class 4				
ADH7	σ	Stomach, oesophagus, other mucosae	40	1,510
	μ		20	
Class 5				
ADH6	–	Liver, stomach	30	

[a] *Km* supplied is for ethanol – ADH also oxidizes other substrates.

Source: Adapted from Kwo and Crabb (2002) with permission from the Taylor & Francis Group.

is found in the human stomach (Yin *et al.*, 1990; Moreno and Pares, 1991; Stone *et al.*, 1993) and Class 5 has been reported in liver and stomach (Yasunami *et al.*, 1991). Whilst the majority of ethanol metabolism occurs in the liver, gastric ADH is responsible for some of the oxidation of ethanol.

Catalase

Peroxisomal catalase which requires the presence of hydrogen peroxide (H_2O_2) is of little significance in the metabolism of ethanol (Lieber, 2005). Metabolism of ethanol by ADH inhibits catalase activity as H_2O_2 production is inhibited by the reducing equivalents produced by ADH (Lieber, 2005).

Microsomal ethanol oxidizing system

Chronic administration of ethanol with nutritionally adequate diets increases clearance of ethanol from the blood. This phenomenon could not be adequately explained until 1968 when the MEOS was identified and characterized (Lieber and DeCarli, 1968, 1970). The MEOS has a higher *Km* for ethanol (8–10 mmol/l) than ADH (0.2–2.0 mmol/l) so at low BEC, ADH is more important. However, unlike

Table 41.7 Aldehyde dehydrogenase (ALDH) isoenzymes

Class	*Structure*	*Location*	*Km (μmol/l)[a]*
Class 1			
ALDH1	α4	*Cytosolic*	
		Several tissues: highest in liver	30
Class 2			
ALDH2	α4	*Mitochondrial*	
		Present in all tissues except red blood cells	1
		Liver > kidney > muscle > heart	

Notes: This table describes the properties of the ALDH isoenzymes. *Km* is the concentration of substrate that leads to half-maximal velocity. Although there are several isoenzymes of ALDH the most important are ALDH1 (cytosolic) and ALDH2 (mitochondrial).

[a]*Km* supplied is for acetaldehyde – ALDH also oxidizes other substrates.

Source: Adapted from Kwo and Crabb (2002) with permission from the Taylor & Francis Group.

the other pathways, MEOS is highly inducible by chronic ethanol consumption. The key enzyme of the MEOS is cytochrome P4502E1 (CYP2E1). Chronic ethanol use is associated with a 4–10-fold increase of CYP2E1 due to increases in mRNA levels and rate of translation.

Acetaldehyde metabolism

Acetaldehyde is highly toxic but is rapidly converted to acetate. This conversion is catalyzed by aldehyde dehydrogenase (ALDH) and is accompanied by reduction of NAD^+ (Figure 41.3). There are several isoenzymes of ALDH (Table 41.7; Kwo and Crabb, 2002). The most important are ALDH1 (cytosolic) and ALDH2 (mitochondrial). The presence of ALDH in tissues may reduce the toxic effects of acetaldehyde and thereby ethanol.

In alcoholics the oxidation of ethanol is increased by induction of MEOS. However, the capacity of mitochondria to oxidize acetaldehyde is reduced. In man, hepatic acetaldehyde therefore increases with chronic ethanol consumption (Di Padova *et al.*, 1987). A significant increase of acetaldehyde in hepatic venous blood reflects the high tissue level.

Metabolism of acetate

Acetaldehyde is converted to acetate by ALDH. However, the ultimate fate of acetate is not well understood. Some important principles of acetate metabolism have been elucidated and reviewed by Cornier (2004). Three important points are summarized here:

1. Most of the ethanol absorbed from the GI tract is metabolized in the liver and results in the production and release of acetate. Acetate can be metabolized in the brain and readily crosses the blood–brain barrier. Cardiac and skeletal muscles are also important in the metabolism of acetate.
2. The conversion of acetate to acetyl-CoA is catalyzed by acetyl-CoA synthetase. This reaction requires adenosine triphosphate and results in the production of adenosine monophosphate. 5'nucleosidase catalyses the production of adenosine from adenosine monophosphate.
3. The acetyl-CoA generated from acetate may be used to generate adenosine triphosphate via the Kreb's cycle. Acetyl-CoA may be converted to glycerol, glycogen and lipid particularly, in the fed state. However, this only accounts for a small fraction of absorbed ethanol. The neurotransmitter acetylcholine is produced from acetyl-CoA in cholinergic neurons.

In view of these findings, future investigations of acetate metabolism should consider the effects on skeletal and cardiac muscle and the brain.

Blood Ethanol Concentration

In one study, consumption of 5 units of alcohol (40 g ethanol) with an evening meal (500 ml of beer 1 h before eating and 500 ml beer during the meal) generated mean BECs of 6.8 mmol/l (31 mg/dl) 1 h after the meal and 1.95 mmol/l (9 mg/dl) 3 h after the meal (Hendriks *et al.*, 1994). However, the relationship between BEC and the effects of ethanol is complex and varies between individuals and also with drinking habits. In another study, a 73 kg Japanese male heavy drinker consumed 16 ml of beer per kg body weight (1,168 ml) over 20 min at noon without food. The effect of this on his BEC over the next 6 h is shown in Figure 41.4. For comparative purposes urinary ethanol concentration is also shown in Figure 41.4. However, as with BEC, a number of variables affect the urinary-blood partition (Kroke and Dierkes, 2005).

Many effects correlate with the peak BEC or peak ethanol concentrations within organs during a drinking session. Other effects are due to products of metabolism and the total dose of ethanol ingested over a period of time. These factors are linked as the ethanol concentration during a drinking session may determine which pathways of ethanol metabolism predominate.

The factors which increase the probability of higher maximum ethanol concentrations for any given level of consumption are therefore clinically relevant.

Factors affecting BEC

Gender Differences in BEC When given the same dose of ethanol per kilogram of body weight women achieve higher peak BEC than men (Marshall *et al.*, 1983; Smith *et al.*, 1993). The volume of distribution of ethanol reflects total body water (Marshall *et al.*, 1983). It is therefore not

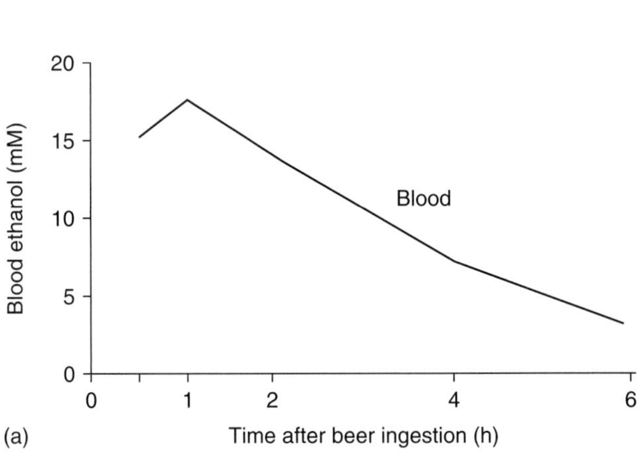

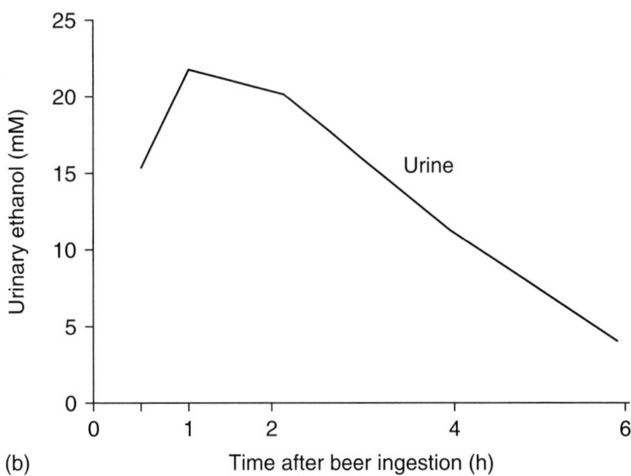

Figure 41.4 Blood and urinary ethanol concentrations after drinking beer. A 73 kg Japanese male consumed 16 ml of beer per kg body weight (1,168 ml) over 20 min at noon without food. The ethanol content of the beer was not provided. (a) Blood and (b) urine were collected at 30 min, 1, 2, 4 and 6 h after beer consumption. It is important to note that the shape of the BEC curve will depend on several factors, including the amount of ethanol consumed, co-ingestion of food and its type, gender, ethnic origins (e.g. if an ALDH2 polymorphism was present) and previous drinking history. See main text for other variables. The data for this figure was derived from a Japanese man classified as a heavy drinker but was a non-flusher (i.e. he had a functional ALDH2*1 genotype rather than a non-functional ALDH2*2 genotype). For comparative purposes urinary ethanol is displayed (b). In general, the ratio of urine to BEC is reported to be about 1:3 but in this study it is about 1:1. However, as with BEC levels, several variables affect the urinary-blood partition (Kroke and Dierkes, 2005). *Source*: Adapted from Tsukamoto *et al.* (1989) with permission from Oxford University Press and the Medical Council on Alcoholism.

surprising that the BEC is higher in women given that the bodies of women contain a greater proportion of fat. Furthermore, when ethanol dosing is based on total body water (TBW) rather than body weight, these sex differences in BEC disappear (Goist Jr. and Sutker, 1985; Savoie *et al.*, 1988). However, gender differences in the gastric metabolism of ethanol may also be relevant.

Effects of Food on BEC In a two-part crossover study, 10 healthy men drank ethanol (0.80 g/kg; 56 g or 7 units for a 70 kg man) either after an overnight fast or immediately after standardized breakfast (Jones and Jönsson, 1994). The BEC was determined from venous samples taken at various times after drinking. The peak BEC was 67 mg/dl (standard deviation, SD 9.5; 14.4 mmol/l SD 2) after ethanol and breakfast compared with 104 mg/dl (SD 14.5; 23.7 mmol/l SD 3.1) when drinking occurred after an overnight fast ($p < 0.001$). The mean area under the BEC vs. time curve (AUC; 0–6 h) was 398 mg/dl × h (SD 56) in fasting subjects compared with 241 mg/dl × h (SD 34) when ethanol was ingested after breakfast ($p < 0.001$). The time required to metabolize the ethanol was approximately 2 h less if breakfast was eaten before drinking (Jones and Jönsson, 1994).

This study demonstrates that when ethanol is consumed with or after food the peak BEC is reduced. Food delays gastric emptying into the duodenum and reduces the sharp early rise in BEC seen when ethanol is taken on an empty stomach. However, food also increases elimination of ethanol from the blood. The area under the BEC vs. time curve (AUC) is reduced (Figure 41.4). This was confirmed in a separate experiment when a meal was eaten 5 h after drinking, that is, in the post-absorptive phase of ethanol metabolism. The mean rate of clearance of ethanol from blood was increased by up to 50% after eating (Jones, 1993).

The contributions of various nutrients to these effects have been studied, but small often conflicting differences have been found. It appears that the caloric value of the meal is more important than the precise balance of nutrients (Carbonnel *et al.*, 1994). However, food increases splanchnic blood flow which maintains the ethanol diffusion gradient in the small intestine (Kalant, 2004). Food-induced impairment of gastric emptying may be partially offset by faster absorption of ethanol in the duodenum (Kalant, 2004).

In animal studies ethanol is often administered with other nutrients in liquid diets. The AUC is less when ethanol is given in a liquid diet, than with the same dose of ethanol in water (de Fiebre *et al.*, 1994). The different blood ethanol profile in these models could affect the expression of pathology in these models (Kalant, 2004).

First-Pass Metabolism of Ethanol The AUC after oral dosing of ethanol (i.e. AUC_{oral}) is significantly lower than after intravenous administration (i.e. AUC_{iv}) or intraperitoneal administration (i.e. AUC_{ip}). The total dose of intravenously administered ethanol is available to the systemic circulation. The difference between AUC_{oral} and AUC_{iv} represents the fraction of the oral dose that was either not absorbed or metabolized before entering the systemic circulation, that is first-pass metabolism (FPM). The ratio of AUC_{oral} to AUC_{iv} reflects the oral bioavailability of ethanol.

The investigation of ethanol metabolism has primarily focused on the liver and its relationship to liver pathology. The role of the stomach in ethanol metabolism has been controversial. However, the presence of multiple ADH isoenzymes in human gastric mucosa suggests that the stomach metabolizes ethanol and contributes to FPM (Yin *et al.*, 1990; Moreno and Pares, 1991; Yasunami *et al.*, 1991; Lieber, 2005).

Approximately 90% of the rate of all ethanol elimination is performed by the liver (Utne and Winkler, 1980). However, several factors including ethnicity (Dohmen *et al.*, 1996), gender (Frezza *et al.*, 1990) and alcoholism (Di Padova *et al.*, 1987) alter FPM, despite an opposite effect on the total hepatic metabolism of ethanol. The observations that their effects on FPM correlate with those on gastric ADH activity (Di Padova *et al.*, 1987; Frezza *et al.*, 1990; Dohmen *et al.*, 1996) is further evidence for the contribution of the stomach to ethanol metabolism.

When gastric ADH activity is measured with BEC below 100 mM, it is negligible compared to liver ADH activity. The gastric cells, however, are close to the lumen of the stomach and thus exposed not only to the BEC, but also to gastric juices, in which the ethanol concentration is much higher (Lieber, 2005). Increasing the ethanol concentration used to test for ADH activity results in reduction of hepatic ADH activity as a result of saturation and substrate inhibition of Classes 1 and 2 ADH (Lieber, 2005). However in the stomach, activity progressively increases (Lieber, 2005).

Vmax is the maximum enzyme velocity in units of concentration of product per unit of time. σ-ADH has a high activity, with a Vmax considerably higher than that of the other enzymes, and a *K*m around 40 mM (Kwo and Crabb, 2002). Thus, although, hepatic oxidation of ethanol cannot increase once ADH is saturated, gastric ADH can significantly metabolize ethanol at the high concentrations in the stomach after initial ingestion. Thus, the function of gastric ADH could be to protect the body from excessive consumption of ethanol. If gastric emptying of ethanol is delayed, prolonged contact with gastric ADH increases FPM. Conversely, increasing the speed of gastric emptying by fasting virtually eliminates gastric FPM (Di Padova *et al.*, 1987).

Contribution of FPM to Overall Ethanol Metabolism FPM increases with decreasing amounts of alcohol, for example, a dose of 0.15 g ethanol/kg b.w. results in greater FPM than 0.3 or 0.8 g ethanol/kg b.w. When ethanol is given at a high dose, the presystemic contribution to its metabolism is relatively small, as hepatic metabolism dominates. In contrast, when small doses of alcohol are administered, the relative contribution of FPM to overall ethanol metabolism is greater (Gentry *et al.*, 1994; Crabb, 1997).

Beverage Ethanol Content and BEC The ethanol concentration of the beverage consumed (Table 41.7) affects ethanol absorption and can affect BEC. Absorption is fastest when the concentration is 10–30%. However, the ethanol concentration of most beers is below 6%. After drinking beer, diffusion of ethanol is slow because ethanol concentration in the GI tract is low and the large volume of liquid slows gastric emptying.

The concentration of ethanol in the GI tract also affects FPM. Gastric ADH requires a high ethanol concentration for optimal activity. The ethanol concentration in the beverage consumed affects oxidation of ethanol to acetaldehyde (Roine *et al.*, 1991). After ingestion of equivalent amounts of ethanol less FPM and higher blood levels occur after consumption of beer than whiskey (Roine *et al.*, 1993).

Quantification of Ethanol Absorption and FPM Many groups have attempted to develop models of ethanol pharmacokinetics to define and quantify the absorption and

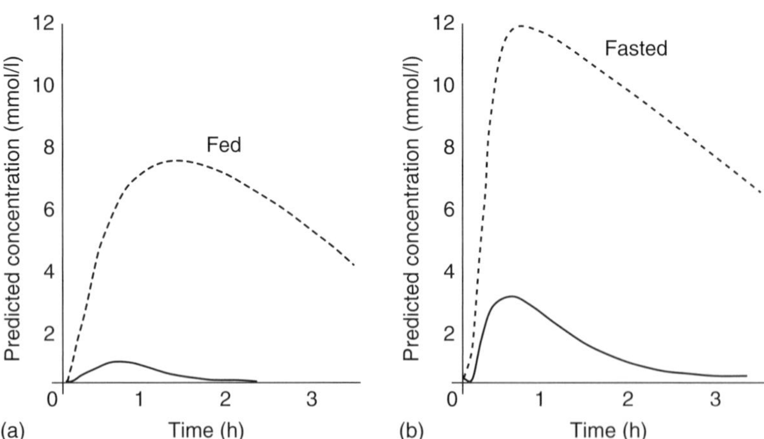

Figure 41.5 Predicted BEC profiles after ingestion of beer. The effect of food on BEC after oral dosing of ethanol as beer. Predicted venous ethanol concentration for an oral intake of one can of beer (260 mmol ethanol; solid black line) or three cans of beer (780 mmol ethanol; broken black line) over a 20 min period. (a) Coincident with a standard meal. (b) Without food. The peak BEC and the area under the curve are reduced if ethanol is consumed with food. *Source*: Adapted from Levitt (2002) with permission.

FPM of ethanol (e.g. see Levitt, 2002). However it has been difficult to produce accurate models, perhaps because there are several pathways of ethanol metabolism. Levitt (2002) applied a physiologically based pharmacokinetic computer program to human ethanol data and suggested that the predominant factors which affect ethanol absorption and FPM are the rate of gastric emptying and the dose of ethanol. When ethanol is ingested with food absorption is slow and for a dose of 0.15 g/kg (12 g for an 80 kg man) the predicted fractional FPM was 36%, but only 7% for a dose of 0.3 g/kg (24 g for an 80 kg man; Levitt, 2002). For comparison, in fasting subjects the absorption of oral ethanol is rapid and the predicted FPM was small. Levitt (2002) used this computer program to predict BEC profiles after consumption of one and three cans of beer over 20 min either with or without food. These BEC profiles are illustrated in Figure 41.5.

Summary

Ethanol in the form of beer is one of the most commonly used recreational drugs worldwide. When beer is consumed, ethanol is absorbed from the GI tract by diffusion and is rapidly distributed around the body in the blood before entering tissues by diffusion. Ethanol is metabolized to acetaldehyde mainly in the stomach and liver. Acetaldehyde is highly toxic and binds cellular constituents generating harmful acetaldehyde adducts. Acetaldehyde is further oxidized to acetate. The fate of acetate and its role in the effects of ethanol are much less well understood. Ethanol and the products of its metabolism affect nearly every cellular structure or function and is a significant cause of morbidity and mortality.

Summary Points

- The ethanol in beer is derived from the fermentation of malted grain by yeasts.
- The ethanol content of beer as ABV typically ranges from 3% to 8%.
- After ingestion of beer, ethanol travels along the GI tract until absorbed by diffusion.
- Absorbed ethanol is initially oxidized to acetaldehyde (FPM) by one of the three pathways: ADH, MEOS or catalase. Acetaldehyde is oxidized further to acetate.
- After consumption of beer, factors which affect the absorption, distribution and FPM of ethanol determine BEC. These factors include gender, beverage ethanol content, time over which ethanol is consumed and food.

References

Bode, C. and Bode, J.C. (2003). *Best Pract. Res. Clin. Gastroenterol.* 17, 575–592.

Bosron, W.F., Ehrig, T. and Li, T.K. (1993). *Semin. Liver Dis.* 13, 126–135.

Carbonnel, F., Lemann, M., Rambaud, J.C., Mundler, O. and Jian, R. (1994). *Am. J. Clin. Nutr.* 60, 307–311.

Cornier, M.-A. (2004). Disposal of ethanol carbon atoms. In Preedy, V.R. and Watson, R.R. (eds), *Comprehensive Handbook of Alcohol Related Pathology*, Vol. 1, pp. 103–110. Elsevier, London.

Crabb, D.W. (1997). *Hepatology* 25, 1292–1294.

de Fiebre, N.C., de Fiebre, C.M., Booker, T.K., Nelson, S. and Collins, A.C. (1994). *Alcohol* 11, 329–335.

Department of Health (1995). *Sensible Drinking: The Report of an Inter-departmental Working Group*. Department of Health, London.

Di Padova, C., Worner, T.M., Julkunen, R.J.K. and Lieber, C.S. (1987). *Gastroenterology* 92, 1169–1173.

Dohmen, K., Baraona, E., Ishibashi, K., Pozzato, G., Moretti, M., Matsunaga, C., Fujimoto, K. and Lieber, C.S. (1996). *Alcohol Clin. Exp. Res.* 20, 1569–1576.

Fisher, H.R., Simpson, R.I. and Kapur, B. (1987). *Can. J. Public Health* 78, 300–304.

Frezza, M., Di Padova, C., Pozzato, G., Terpin, M., Baraona, E. and Lieber, C.S. (1990). *New Engl. J. Med.* 322, 95–99.

Gentry, R.T., Baraona, E. and Lieber, C.S. (1994). *J. Lab. Clin. Med.* 123, 32–33.

Goist Jr., K.C. and Sutker, P.B. (1985). *Pharmacol. Biochem. Behav.* 22, 811–814.

Goldammer, T. (2000). *The Brewers' Handbook*. Apex Publishers, USA.

Halsted, C.H., Robles, E.A. and Mezey, E. (1973). *Am. J. Clin. Nutr.* 26, 831–834.

Hendriks, H.F.J., Veenstra, J., Velthuis-te Wierik, E.J.M., Schaafsma, G. and Kluft, C. (1994). *BMJ* 308, 1003–1006.

Jones, A.W. (1993). *J. Forensic Sci.* 38, 104–118.

Jones, A.W. and Jönsson, K.-Å. (1994). *J. Forensic Sci.* 39, 1084–1093.

Kalant, H. (2004). Effects of food and body composition on blood alcohol levels. In Preedy, V.R. and Watson, R.R. (eds), *Comprehensive Handbook of Alcohol Related Pathology*, Vol. 1, pp. 87–102. Academic Press, Elsevier, London.

Kroke, A. and Dierkes, J. (2005). Methods for measuring genetic variations in ADH and SLDH loci: A practical approach. In Preedy, V.R. and Watson, R.R. (eds), *Comprehensive Handbook of Alcohol Related Pathology*, Vol. 3, pp. 281–304. Elsevier, London.

Kwo, P.Y. and Crabb, D.W. (2002). Genetics of ethanol Metabolism and Alcoholic Liver Disease. In Sherman, D.I.N., Preedy, V.R. and Watson, R.R. (eds), *Ethanol and the Liver. Mechanisms and Management*, pp. 95–129. Taylor and Francis, London.

Levitt, D.G. (2002). *BMC Clin. Pharmacol.* 2, 4.

Lieber, C.S. (2005). Alcohol metabolism: General aspects. In Preedy, V.R. and Watson, R.R. (eds), *Comprehensive Handbook of Alcohol Related Pathology*, Vol. 1, pp. 15–26. Elsevier, Amsterdam.

Lieber, C.S. and DeCarli, L.M. (1968). *Science* 162, 917–918.

Lieber, C.S. and DeCarli, L.M. (1970). *J. Biol. Chem.* 245, 2505–2512.

Marshall, A.W., Kingstone, D., Boss, M. and Morgan, M.Y. (1983). *Hepatology* 3, 701–706.

Moreno, A. and Pares, X. (1991). *J. Biochem.* 266, 1128–1133.

Oxford Bottled Beer Database (2006). http://www.bottledbeer.co.uk/index.html (accessed December 1, 2006).

Pretorius, I.S. (2000). *Yeast* 16, 675–729.

Rajendram, R., Hunter, R., Peters, T.J. and Preedy, V.R. (2005). Alcohol: Absorption, metabolism and physiological effects. In Caballero, B., Allen, L. and Prentice, A. (eds), *Encyclopedia of Human Nutrition (2e)*, pp. 48–57. Elsevier, London.

Realbeer.com (2006). http://www.realbeer.com/edu/health/calories.php (accessed December 6, 2006).

Roine, R.P., Gentry, R.T., Lim Jr., R.T., Baraona, E. and Lieber, C.S. (1991). *Alcohol Clin. Exp. Res.* 15, 734–738.

Roine, R.P., Gentry, R.T., Lim Jr., R.T., Heikkonen, E., Salaspuro, M. and Lieber, C.S. (1993). *Alcohol Clin. Exp. Res.* 17, 709–711.

Royal College of Physicians, Royal College of Psychiatrists, Royal College of General Practitioners (1995). Alcohol and the Heart: Sensible Limits Reaffirmed. Royal Colleges of Physicians, London.

Savoie, T.M., Emory, E.K. and Moody-Thomas, S. (1988). *J. Stud. Alcohol* 49, 430–435.

Smith, G.D., Shaw, L.J., Maini, P.K., Ward, R.J., Peters, T.J. and Murray, J.D. (1993). *Alcohol Alcohol.* 28, 25–32.

Stone, C.L., Thomasson, H.R., Bosron, W.F. and Li, T.K. (1993). *Alcohol Clin. Exp. Res.* 17, 911–918.

Tsukamoto, S., Muto, T., Nagoya, T., Shimamura, M., Saito, M. and Tainaka, H. (1989). *Alcohol Alcohol.* 24, 101–106.

Utne, H.E., Winkler, K. (1980). *Scand. J. Gastroenterol.* 15, 297–304.

Wyeast Laboratories (2006). http://www.wyeastlab.com/beprlist.htm#1338 (accessed December 6, 2006).

Yasunami, M., Chen, C.S. and Yoshida, A. (1991). *Proc. Natl. Acad. Sci. USA* 88, 7610–7614.

Yin, S.J., Wang, M.F., Liao, C.S., Chen, C.M. and Wu, C.W. (1990). *Biochem. Int.* 22, 829–835.

42

What Contribution Is Beer to the Intake of Antioxidants in the Diet?

Fulgencio Saura-Calixto, José Serrano and Jara Pérez-Jiménez Department of Metabolism and Nutrition, CSIC, Ciudad Universitaria, Madrid, Spain

Abstract

Beer is a low-alcohol beverage brewed from natural ingredients and may contain appreciable amounts of bioactive compounds, mainly antioxidants, which are associated with health effects. Polyphenols and melanoidins are the major natural antioxidants in beer. Polyphenol and melanoidin contents are largely influenced by genetic and agricultural factors in the raw material and by technological factors in the brewing. Common beer polyphenols include flavonols, phenolic acids, catechins, procyanidins, tannins and chalcones. Beer also contains Maillard reaction products, largely formed during the malting and brewing process. Various assays have shown that beer has greater antioxidant capacity than white wine, but less than red wine. Nevertheless, in several countries the consumption of beer contributes significantly to the total intake of polyphenols and to the antioxidant capacity of the diet. Beer in Spain (150 ml/person/day) provides 7.2% of the daily dietary intake of polyphenols and accounts for around 3% of the total antioxidant capacity of the diet. Further research is needed to elucidate the potential role of beer in the prevention of chronic diseases associated with the intake of antioxidants.

List of Abbreviations

ABTS	2,2′-Azino-bis(3-ethylbenz-thiazoline-6-sulfonic acid)
DPPH	2,2-Diphenyl-1-picrylhydrazyl
FRAP	Ferric reducing/antioxidant power
HDLs	High density lipoproteins
ORAC	Oxygen radical absorbance capacity
ROS	Reactive oxygen species
TEAC	Trolox equivalent antioxidant capacity
TRAP	Total radical-trapping antioxidant parameter

Introduction

Epidemiological evidence from many studies overwhelmingly supports the hypothesis that moderate alcohol consumption is significantly associated with a reduction in cardiovascular disease incidence (Rimm *et al.*, 1991). In this context, alcoholic beverages that were identified as especially beneficial were red wine and beer. At the outset it was suggested that alcohol could be the main component responsible for the observed beneficial effects, since ethanol is able to increase the level of high density lipoproteins (HDL), decrease platelet aggregation and enhance blood fibrinolysis (Rotondo *et al.*, 2001). However, it was later suggested that the protective effects of red wine and beer may be the result of non-alcoholic components such as phenolics and antioxidants (Ghiselli *et al.*, 2000; Vinson *et al.*, 2001).

Nowadays, there is ample reason to believe that antioxidants provide protection from chronic diseases. In the last two decades, numerous biochemical and clinical studies have provided consistent evidence of the healthy properties of foods and beverages rich in antioxidants, such as olive oil, red wine, fish, citrus fruits and legumes (Halliwell, 1997). Dietary antioxidants are able to neutralize free radicals created during the aging process, thus preventing the onset of chronic diseases.

Free radicals may originate endogenously, basically from the respiratory chain, where the reduction of oxygen molecule gives rise to different radical species. They may also be of exogenous origin, from exposure to certain radiations (sunlight, ozone, electromagnetic radiations), some food additives, certain tobacco components, etc. Oxidative stress is involved in the pathology of many diseases, such as atherosclerosis, diabetes, neurodegenerative diseases, aging and cancer. The prevalent situation of an organism will be of health or of disease depending on the equilibrium between oxidants and antioxidants. Antioxidants are a group of compounds of varying chemical nature that can prevent oxidation. They can be natural or synthetic. Plant foods and beverages possess a large number of antioxidant compounds, and in recent years there has been considerable research into natural antioxidants prompted by consumer interest in natural rather than synthetic products.

Recent renewed interest has focused on beer, a common beverage rich in antioxidant compounds with moderate antioxidant activity coupled with low ethanol content. The compounds chiefly responsible for this antioxidant capacity are

Beer in Health and Disease Prevention
ISBN: 978-0-12-373891-2

polyphenols and Maillard compounds. It is therefore important to determine the antioxidant contents of natural products such as beer, their activity *in vitro* and *in vivo*, and the contribution of a given food item to the total antioxidant capacity of a diet. This chapter deals with the antioxidant capacity of beer, focusing mainly on the contribution of beer to the total antioxidant intake of a whole diet.

Beer Antioxidants: Contents and Antioxidant Power

Beer antioxidants mainly come from the two natural ingredients used in brewing: barley and hops. The antioxidant power of beer therefore presumably depends on the antioxidant contents in these two ingredients and on a number of parameters involved in brewing, namely the variety of barley and the malting process, temperature and pH during mashing, sparing, boiling, the variety of hops added during wort boiling and yeast fermentation.

The main antioxidant compounds in beer are phenolic compounds and Maillard compounds. In addition, some antioxidant additives used in beer (i.e. vitamin C) may also contribute to its antioxidant capacity.

Polyphenols

Polyphenols are a broad group of substances present in plant foods, with more than 8,000 compounds currently known. They are products of secondary metabolism of plants which may be classified, depending on their chemical structure into different groups, such as flavonoids, stilbenes, hydroxybenzoic acids, hydroxycinnamic acids, proanthocyanidins and hydrolysable tannins.

Most of the polyphenols present in beer come from barley. However, it should be noted that hops, although added in a proportion 100 times lower than malt, provide about 30% of the total polyphenols present in beer (Callemien *et al.*, 2005). The polyphenol content may range from 3% to 6% depending on the variety, geographic origin and freshness of the hops, the harvesting procedure and the manner in which hop cone is packaged.

Barley phenolics include phenolic acids derived from tyrosine and tyramine, their esters and glycosides, anthocyanins, proanthocyanidins, lignans and lignin-related substances (Salomonsson *et al.*, 1980; Yu *et al.*, 2001). Phenolics are mainly located in the outer layers (husk, pericarp, aleurone) of the grain (Nordkvist *et al.*, 1984; Hernanz *et al.*, 2001). Ferulic acid is the predominant free phenolic acid in barley seeds (Nordkvist *et al.*, 1984) and barley grains (Madhujith *et al.*, 2006). The proanthocyanidins from barley are implicated in the formation of haze in beer (Siebert *et al.*, 1996). These compounds are located in the testa of the grain and are a mixture of oligomeric prodelphinidins and procyanidins (McMurrough *et al.*, 1996).

Besides the polyphenols present in the different raw materials, it is important to note that the final phenolic compound content of beer may also be influenced by the processing. For example, mashing increases the concentrations of hydroxycinnamic acid derivatives as they are released from previously non-extractable combinations. Also, the extraction of phenolics from malt into the wort is highly dependent on malt to water ratios. And again, polymerization of phenolics and formation of polyphenols can occur during wort boiling, and possibly also during fermentation and storage of beer (Shahidi and Naczk, 2004).

There are many references in the literature to determine the total polyphenols content of beer. The results of some of these are summarized in Table 42.1. Dark beer contains more polyphenols, whereas the polyphenols content of lager beer – the most widely consumed type – is intermediate. And finally, low-alcohol beers contain much less polyphenols than the others.

Some authors have characterized beer polyphenols, identifying 78 different phenolics compounds in beer (Table 42.2), including simple phenolics, aromatic carboxylic and phenol carboxylic acids, hydroxycoumarins, catechins, leucoanthocyanidins, anthocyanidins, flavonols, flavonones, flavones, prenylated flavonoids and phenolic glycosides (Shahidi and Naczk, 2004; Gerhäuser, 2005).

Figure 42.1 shows the percentage of the different groups of polyphenols in lager beer. Proanthocyandins are the group with the highest presence (81%), followed by phenolics acids and flavonoids.

Proanthocyanidins are a particular kind of polyphenols which despite low bioavailability in the gastrointestinal tract can be fermented by the colonic microflora, producing an antioxidant status in the colon.

The most abundant phenolic acids in beer are gallic acid, ferulic acid and syringic acid. Some of these are present in beer mainly in free form, while others are mainly present in conjugated forms (Nardini *et al.*, 2004).

Beer also contains phenolic compounds of the flavonoid group such as catechin, epicatechin and quercetin, which come from the outer layers of malt and from hops. Total flavonoid content has been estimated at between 13.4 and 52.6 for lager beer (Gasowski *et al.*, 2004).

A number of *in vitro* studies have shown that polyphenols possess considerable antioxidant capacity, even more than other well-known natural antioxidants such as vitamin C or vitamin E (Sánchez-Moreno *et al.*, 1998). For example, when antioxidant capacity was measured by the 2,2-diphenyl-1-picrylhydrazyl (DPPH) assay, the EC_{50} (grams of compound needed to neutralize 1 g of the stable free radical DPPH) of these two vitamins was 76 ± 7 and 201 ± 11, respectively, while the EC_{50} of gallic acid, one of the main phenolic acids present in beer, was 26 ± 1; in other words, it was a more potent antioxidant compound. The antioxidant capacity of ferulic acid, another phenolic acid present in beer, was less than that of gallic acid

Table 42.1 Total polyphenols content of beer

Kind of beer	*Polyphenols content (mg/100 ml)*
Lager beer	31.2–37
Dark beer	47.3–57.2
Alcohol-free beer	18.9–21.8

Source: Gorinstein *et al.* (2000), Saura-Calixto *et al.* (2002), Lugasi and Hóvári (2003), Pulido *et al.* (2003) and Gasowski *et al.* (2004).

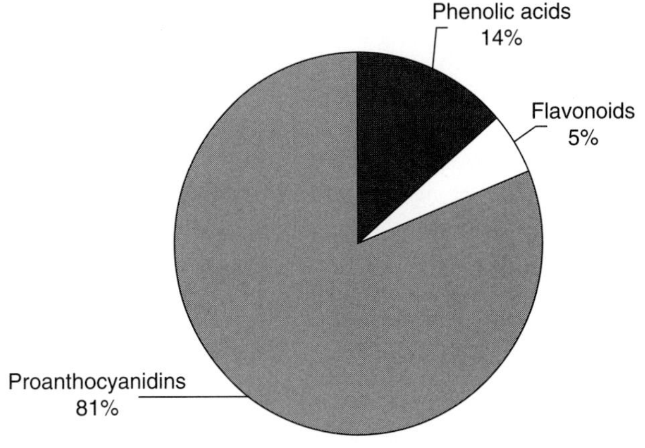

Figure 42.1 Distribution of phenolic acids, flavonoids and proanthocyanidins in lager beer.

Table 42.2 Summary of beer polyphenols

Simple phenols
- 4-Vinyl phenol
- 4-Vinyl guaiacol
- 4-Ethyl phenol
- Isoeugenol
- Tyrosol
- 4-Propyl syringol
- 2,3-Dihydroxy-guiacylpropane-1-one

Benzoic acid derivatives
- 4-Hydroxybenzoic acid
- Protocatechuic acid
- Vanillic acid
- Gallic acid
- Syringic acid
- Salicylaldehyde
- *o*-Vanillin
- Syringic aldehyde

Cinnamic acids
- Cinnamic acid
- *p*-Coumaric acid
- Caffeic acid
- Ferulic acid
- Sinapic acid

Coumarins
- Umbelliferon
- Scopoletin
- Daphnetin

Flavan-3-ols
- (+)-Catechin
- (−)-Epicatechin
- Gallocatechin
- Catechin gallate
- Epicatechin gallate
- 3′-*O*-methylcatechin
- Catechin-7-*O*-β-(6″-*O*-nicotinoyl)-β-D-glucopyranosid

Proanthocyanidins
- Procyanidin B1
- Procyanidin B2
- Procyanidin B3
- Procyanidin B4
- Procyanidin C2
- Prodelphinidin B3
- Prodelphinidin B9
- Prodelphinidin C
- *ent*-Epigallo-catechin-(4α→8, 2α→*O*→7)catechin
- *ent*-Epigallo-catechin-(4α→6, 2α→*O*→7)catechin
- 2,3-*cis*-3,4-*trans*-2-[2,3-*trans*-3,3′,4′,5,7-Pentahydroxyflavan-8-yl]-4-(3,4-dihydroxyphenyl)-3,5,7-trihydroxybenzopyran

Chalcones
- Xanthohumol
- Desmethylxanthohumol

Flavanones
- Isoxanthohumol
- Naringerin
- 8-Prenylnaringenin
- 6-Prenylnaringenin
- 6-Geranylnaringenin
- 5-Methyl-6″-dimethyl-4″,5″-dihydropyrano[2″,3″,7,8]naringenin
- Taxifolin

Flavones
- Apigenin
- Chrysoeriol
- Tricin
- Saponaretin
- Saponarin
- Vitexin

Flavanoles
- Kaempferol
- Kaempferol-3-rhamnosid
- Quercetin
- Quercitrin
- Isoquercitrin
- Rutin
- Myricetin
- Myricitrin

Alpha-acids
- Cohumulone
- *n*-Humulone
- Adhumulone
- *iso*-Cohumulone
- *iso*-*n*-Humulone
- *iso*-Adhumulone

Others
- Indole-3-carboxylic acid
- Indole-3-ethanol
- 1-Methyl-1,3,4,9-tetrahydropyrano[3,4]indol
- 4-Ketopinoresinol
- Syringaresinol
- 3-Acetoxy-propan-1,2-diol

as measured by the 2,2′-azino-bis(3-ethylbenz-thiazoline-6-sulfonic acid) (ABTS) and DPPH methods, but higher as measured by oxygen radical absorbance capacity (ORAC) assay (Villaño *et al.*, 2005). This shows that the same polyphenol may react in a different way with different radicals, and hence the antioxidant capacity of beer will be determined by the activity of all these compounds.

Different assays have shown that flavonoids present in beer, such as catechin, epicatechin and quercetin, also possess significant antioxidant capacity (Villaño *et al.*, 2005). And again, a DPPH assay of the antioxidant capacity of quercetin showed that it was more antioxidant than α-tocopherol and comparable to ascorbic acid (Sánchez-Moreno *et al.*, 1998).

Beer polyphenols seem to be bioavailable, since the ingestion of 500 ml of beer in a human study produced a significant temporary increase in plasma antioxidant activity (Ghiselli *et al.*, 2000). In general, phenolic acids from beer have been found to present maximum absorption peaks at 30 min. The rapidity of phenolic acid absorption indicates that it probably takes places in the proximal part of the intestine. Given the presence of both free and bound forms of phenolic acids in beer, plasma phenolic acids may be the result of direct absorption of the free forms or of enzymatic digestion of the bound forms.

The general consensus has been that many of these bound forms may not be available in the gastrointestinal tract but may be susceptible to fermentation by the colonic microflora, producing an antioxidant status in the colon. Nevertheless, some authors have suggested that some of these bound forms might be absorbed in the colon; for instance, Andreason *et al.* (2001) found that some diferulate esters could be detected in the plasma of rats after oral ingestion. Similarly, Nardini *et al.* (2002) suggested that chlorogenic acid, a bound form of caffeic acid, is absorbed in the colon, having found that after ingestion of coffee there was an increase in the plasmatic caffeic acid concentration despite the fact that coffee lacks free caffeic acid.

Finally, beer ethanol could play an important indirect role in the absorption of phenolic compounds. Phenolics are aromatic compounds which are not readily soluble in water but are readily soluble in ethanol. The increased solubility of these compounds in hydroalcoholic solution may affect the rate and the amount of their absorption (Ghiselli *et al.*, 2000).

Maillard compounds

The Maillard reaction is one of the most common processes in food products. It takes place between the amino groups of peptides and proteins and the aldehyde group of sugars, particularly in the presence of heat, and it is responsible for the characteristic color of many foodstuffs like bread or coffee.

In the case of beer, Maillard compounds are originated initially during the malting process, and later on in the extraction and boiling processes. These compounds, and especially melanoidins, influence the color, aroma and flavor characterizing some special styles of beers, and of course they also influence beer antioxidant capacity.

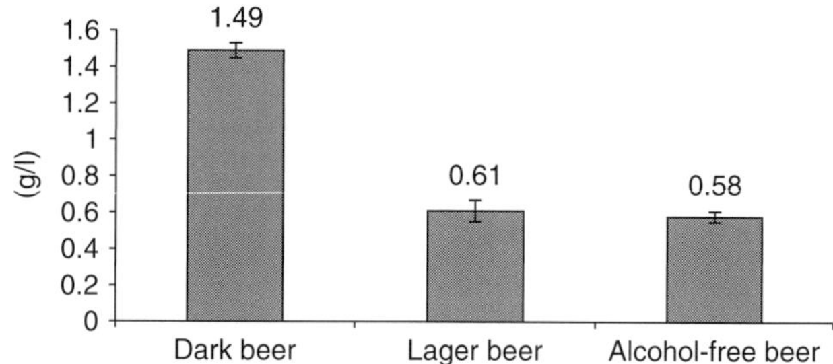

Figure 42.2 Melanoidins content of beer.

Rivero *et al.* (2005) quantified the melanoidin content of beer (see Figure 42.2). Dark beer obviously contains more of these compounds than lager or alcohol-free beer, since it is precisely that they are responsible for its characteristic color. There are no significant differences between the melanoidin contents of lager beer and alcohol-free beer.

From a nutritional point of view, various studies have also demonstrated the high antioxidant capacity of melanoidins, which act through a chain breaking, oxygen scavenging, free radical direct scavenging, metal chelating mechanism (Nicoli *et al.*, 1997; Borrelli *et al.*, 2003) without showing cytotoxic effects (Borrelli *et al.*, 2003). Also, Delgado-Andrade *et al.* (2005) recently measured the antioxidant capacity of certain pure melanoidins. The results showed that although melanoidins exhibit antioxidant capacity, this is much lower than the antioxidant capacity exhibited by certain phenolic compounds present in beer, such as catechin or epicatechin (Tsao *et al.*, 2005). Also, no relationship has been found between the antioxidant capacity of different melanoidins and the degree of browning (Morales and Babbel, 2002).

Melanoidins show a very low bioavailability in the upper gastrointestinal tract. However, it has recently been shown that they may be fermented by colonic microflora (Borrelli *et al.*, 2005). This is an aspect that should be widely studied, for a better understanding of the metabolism of these compounds and their relative contribution to the *in vitro* and *in vivo* antioxidant capacity of beer.

Antioxidant additives

The use of antioxidant additives in beers was first proposed by Gray and Stone in the United States, with the incorporation of ascorbic acid. Following its introduction into American breweries, ascorbic acid came to be used in various European countries (Moll and Joly, 1987). Ascorbic acid is a powerful antioxidant in beer, preventing color changes and alterations of aroma and flavor and prolonging the storage life of bottled beverages. Normally, between 30 and 50 mg of ascorbic acid is added to most beers (Leubolt and Klein, 1993). Nevertheless, several authors have analyzed the residual ascorbic acid content in commercial beers, finding a total amount between 18–33 mg/l (Moll and Joly, 1987; Wagner and McGarrity, 1991; Matos *et al.*, 1998; Luque-Pérez *et al.*, 2000). Ascorbic acid is a hydrophilic compound; it is able to scavenge peroxyl radicals and to inhibit the cytotoxicity induced by oxidants. Also, it can prevent or reduce H_2O_2-induced lipidic peroxidation and OH-deoxyguanosine formation, which occur as a consequence of DNA oxidation (Yen *et al.*, 2002).

Sulfite is another common preservative used in a wide variety of foods to prevent enzyme activity causing browning and to inhibit the growth of microorganisms during storage. Sulfur compounds such as cysteine, and glutathione and disulfide bridges in peptides and proteins occurring naturally in the raw materials used during the brewing process, may be oxidized to sulfite. Reactive oxygen species (ROS) are known to be deactivated by reaction with cellular thiols to form disulfides. The ready oxidation of thiols by ROS serves as an enzyme-based cellular antioxidant defence system. The amount of sulfite in commercial beers may range between 2.35 and 6.6 mg/l (Wagner and McGarrity, 1991; Leubolt and Klein, 1993). However, in recent years, it has been increasingly realized that sulfite can potentially cause an adverse reaction in sulfite-sensitive asthmatic individuals.

Antioxidant Capacity of Beer

The antioxidant capacity of a food is not the same as the sum of the antioxidant capacities of individual bioactive compounds. Antioxidant capacity is derived from synergistic effects between bioactive compounds, trace elements, metals and other food constituents (Liu, 2004). Antioxidants may act through very different mechanisms such as metal chelation, suppression of the first free radicals which initiate oxidative damage, capture of free radicals and formation of complexes or induction of the activity of antioxidant biological systems. They are also present in heterogeneous matrixes, as in the case of food products, and the existence of both factors means that their antioxidant capacity cannot be evaluated by a single method (Frankel and Meyer, 2000; Sánchez-Moreno, 2002; Aruoma, 2003; Prior *et al.*, 2005). Therefore, a number of procedures that take all these aspects into account have been developed to determine antioxidant capacity, and many of them have been applied to beer.

The antioxidant capacity of beer (Table 42.3) measured by two different assays: ferric reducing/antioxidant power (FRAP), which measures the reducing power of the sample, and ABTS or TEAC (Trolox equivalent antioxidant capacity), which is based on the ability of a sample to scavenge organic free radicals. Results are expressed as μmol Trolox/100 ml, Trolox being a hydrophilic analog of vitamin E that behaves as a potent antioxidant. As explained earlier in connection with polyphenols content, dark beers or higher-alcohol beers present greater antioxidant capacity, whereas low-alcohol or alcohol-free beers present the least antioxidant capacity, as measured by either ABTS or FRAP.

Table 42.3 Antioxidant capacity of beer

Kind of beer	*ABTS (μmol Trolox/100 ml)*	*FRAP (μmol Trolox/100 ml)*
Lager beer	220.0–305.6	139.6–149.5
Dark beer	259.0–536.5	278.8
Alcohol-free beer	155.8–175.3	75.6–91.2

Source: Saura-Calixto *et al.* (2002) and Lugasi and Hóvári (2003).

The effect of beer intake on plasma antioxidant capacity has also been studied. Ghiselli *et al.* (2000) found that 1 h after the consumption of 500 ml of beer there was a significant increase in plasma antioxidant capacity (measured by total radical-trapping antioxidant parameter (TRAP), which determines the ability of a sample to scavenge peroxyl radicals), which reverted to its basal value 2 h after ingestion. There was no such effect after intake of an aqueous solution with similar alcohol content, and the effect was not so pronounced after intake of dealcoholized beer. This is consistent with *in vitro* antioxidant capacity assays, in which ethanol presents no antioxidant capacity. The observed increase in plasma antioxidant capacity must therefore be caused by the antioxidant compounds present in beer.

Given that free radicals may also cause oxidative damage to DNA, one way to determine the antioxidant capacity that a sample may possess *in vivo* is to measure the inhibition of DNA damage, and specifically the inhibition of formation of the nucleotide 8-OH-dG, a product of DNA oxidation. Beer has been shown to have a positive effect on the inhibition of DNA oxidative damage, and the inhibiting effect was strongest in the case of dark beer. In this study, an inverse correlation was also observed between the levels of 8-OH-dG and the melanoidin content in beer, indicating how melanoidins may contribute to the overall antioxidant capacity of beer (Rivero *et al.*, 2005).

A possible explanation for these results is that the positive effects of beer intake may be associated not only with the presence of phenolic and other antioxidant compounds, but also with a combined effect of these compounds and ethanol, given that some large population studies have shown that the mortality rate is lower in people reporting moderate alcohol intake than in either non-drinkers or heavier drinkers.

Table 42.4 shows the antioxidant capacity of different beverages as measured by FRAP and ABTS assays (Pulido *et al.*, 2003). Coffee, red wine and tea exhibit the highest values. The antioxidant capacity of beer (Table 42.3) is similar to that of rose wine, higher than white wine, but lower than red

Table 42.4 Antioxidant capacity of beverages (FRAP and ABTS assays)

Beverage	*FRAP (μmol Trolox/100 ml)*	*ABTS (μmol Trolox/100 ml)*
Coffee	2,267 ± 18.9	1,328 ± 5.1
Tea	601 ± 5.5	631 ± 8.0
Red wine	1,214 ± 24.5	1,093 ± 54.2
White wine	154 ± 36.8	181 ± 22.2
Rose wine	286 ± 39.2	261 ± 23.7
Orange juice	515 ± 41.5	249 ± 3.4
Cola	20.7 ± 0.7	≤10

Source: Pulido *et al.* (2003) and Saura-Calixto and Goñi (2006).

wine, which is the most commonly consumed. These results agree with the findings of Lugasi and Hóvári (2003), who also found that the antioxidant capacity of beer and white wines is similar in terms of hydrogen-donating potency as determined by the DPPH assay. Table 42.4 also shows that the antioxidant capacity of beer (Table 42.3) is higher than that of orange juice when measured by ABTS assay.

Contribution of Beer to the Antioxidant Capacity of Diet

Many epidemiological studies have reported an association between diets with a high intake of plant food (which are rich in antioxidants in addition to other bioactive compounds) and a lower risk of certain chronic processes, such as cardiovascular disease (Serafini, 2006). However, intervention studies based on the intake of specific antioxidants have produced conflicting results. For example, in the Alpha-Tocopherol, Beta Carotene Cancer Prevention Trial conducted in Finland, smokers who received β-carotene presented a marked increase in lung cancer incidence compared with subjects who received a placebo (Woodside *et al.*, 2005). This led to an interest in the way that antioxidants are present in foods and diets, that is in complex matrixes where they are released by the action of enzymes and intestinal microbiota and may interact with other compounds; the global effect may then be due to the combined effect of all the bioactive compounds present in the foodstuff. It could also be that several of these compounds work together but have no effect individually, or that other dietary components, such as trace elements, act as effectors of micronutrient action (Woodside *et al.*, 2005).

Moreover, food products should not be considered individually, but globally as part of a diet. In this respect, it is important to know all the bioactive compounds that a whole diet contains and not only the ones supplied by a single food. Indeed, although the Mediterranean diet is considered a good pattern for the prevention of cardiovascular disease, no strong association has been found between any one of its individual dietary components and survival, suggesting that it is the overall pattern that is protective

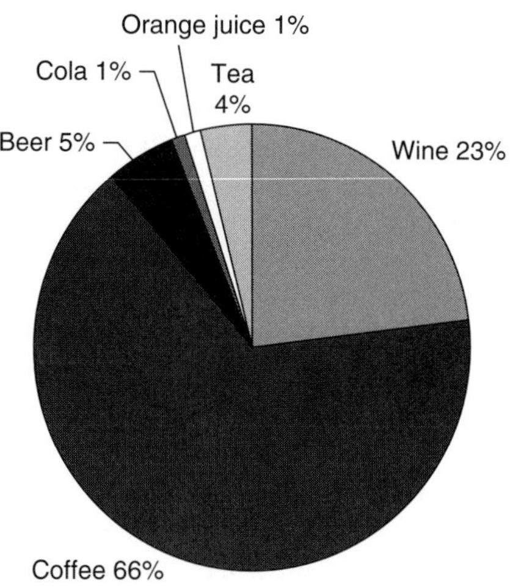

Figure 42.3 Contribution of beer to the antioxidant capacity intake in the beverage group of the Spanish Mediterranean diet.

(Trichopolou *et al.*, 2003). In the light of this, research was recently conducted to determine the total antioxidant capacity of the Spanish Diet as a type of Mediterranean diet (Saura-Calixto and Goñi, 2006). The antioxidant capacity of the whole diet was estimated at 6,014 and 3,549 μmol Trolox/day by FRAP and ABTS procedures, respectively. About 68% of the total dietary antioxidant capacity came from beverages and 20% from fruits and vegetables, with very little from cereals.

The per capita daily beer intake in Spain in 2001 was 150.4 ml, accounting for nearly one-third of the total intake of beverages. Beer contributes 84.2 mg of polyphenols, which is about 7.2% of the total polyphenol intake in the Spanish diet.

The contribution of beer to the total antioxidant capacity of beverages in the Spanish diet has also been evaluated by Pulido *et al.* (2003) (Figure 42.3). Coffee and wine were the principal contributors to antioxidant capacity of the beverage group, while beer accounted for 5% of the total antioxidant capacity intake from beverages, which is more than reported for tea and orange juice.

As regards the antioxidant capacity of the whole diet, following the same procedure it was found that beer provides 3% of the total antioxidant capacity of the Spanish diet as measured by ABTS assay (Figure 42.4). However, this means that as a single food item beer is a major contributor to the antioxidant capacity of the Spanish diet, considering that the entire nuts group supplies only 5% and fruits and vegetables 22% of the total antioxidant capacity of the Spanish diet. Note that this value represents the daily intake of antioxidants; but the biological effects would depend on their bioavailability, which is usually a fraction of the total intake. Comparative studies on bioavailability of antioxidants from different types of food groups are needed to elucidate their actual contribution to antioxidant status in humans.

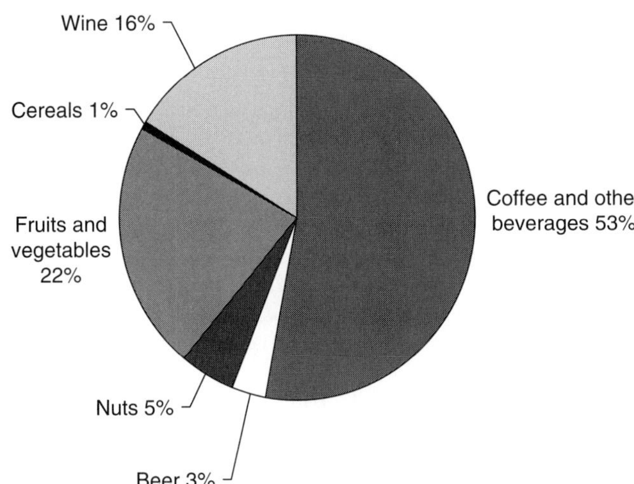

Figure 42.4 Contribution of beer to the total antioxidant capacity intake of the Spanish Mediterranean diet.

In the United States, daily per capita beer consumption in 1999 was 226.8 ml according to the Beverage Market Index (Beverage World Publications Group (2000), accounting for 19% of the total intake of beverages. This would mean a daily intake of 127.12 mg of polyphenols supplied by beer and an antioxidant capacity of 244 μmol Trolox/day by FRAP assay or 174 μmol Trolox/day by ABTS assay. Some researchers have studied the antioxidant capacity supplied by a large number of food products consumed in the United States (Wu *et al.*, 2004), as well as the daily intake of certain antioxidants such as anthocyanins (Wu *et al.*, 2006), but no exhaustive work has yet been done on the total antioxidant content and antioxidant capacity of the diet in the United States, including the contribution of beverages.

More studies dealing with the total antioxidant capacity of diets are needed, but the findings published so far show that beer is a significant contributor to the total antioxidant capacity of the diet. Whether moderate consumption could play a role in the prevention of several chronic diseases remains to be seen.

Summary Points

- Beer is a natural beverage with low alcohol content and appreciable antioxidant capacity.
- The antioxidant capacity of beer is mainly derived from polyphenols, Maillard compounds and vitamin C.
- Beer polyphenols come from the natural ingredients (barley and hops) employed in brewing. Maillard compounds are formed during malting, extraction and boiling processes. Vitamin C is incorporated exogenously to beer during the brewing process.
- Polyphenols, the main antioxidants in beer, are present in both free and bound forms. Several *in vivo* studies have shown that polyphenols in beer are bioavailable. Maillard compounds, particularly melanoidins, have been shown to have antioxidant effects *in vitro*.
- Beer antioxidants have been shown to have metal reducing power, the ability to scavenge free radicals and a protective effect against DNA oxidative damage.
- Beer antioxidant capacity, estimated at about 210 μmol Trolox/100 ml by FRAP assay (mean value between lager and dark beer), is lower than that of red wine and higher than that of white wine.
- Dark beer exhibits greater antioxidant capacity than lager and alcohol-free beers. The antioxidant capacity of alcohol-free beer is considerably lower than that of lager.
- Beer is a contributor to the total antioxidant capacity of diet. The consumption (150 ml/person/day) in Spain means around 3% of the total antioxidant capacity of the Spanish diet. A higher contribution can be expected in other countries where beer consumption is higher. For instance, the consumption in the United States (226.8 ml/person/day) is equivalent to 244 μmol Trolox/day by FRAP assay or 174 μmol Trolox/day by ABTS assay.
- Further research is needed to elucidate the contribution of beer to other diets, as well as its potential role in the prevention of chronic diseases, which is associated with the intake of antioxidants.

References

Andreason, M.F., Kroon, P.A., Williamson, G. and García-Conesa, M.T. (2001). *Free Radic. Biol. Med.* 31, 304–314.

Aruoma, O.I. (2003). *Mutation Res.*, 534–524, 9–20.

Beverage World Publications Group (2000). *Beverages World* 119, 51–60.

Borrelli, R.C., Mennella, C., Barba, F., Russo, M., Russo, G.L., Krome, K., Erbersdobler, H.F., Faist, V. and Fogliano, V. (2003). *Food Chem. Toxicol.* 41, 1367–1374.

Borrelli, R.C. and Fogliano, V. (2005). *Molec. Nutr. Food. Res.* 49, 673–78.

Callemien, D., Jerkovic, V., Rozenberg, R. and Collin, S. (2005). *J. Agric. Food Chem.* 53, 424–429.

Delgado-Andrade, C., Rufián-Henares, J.A. and Morales, F.J. (2005). *J. Agric. Food Chem.* 53, 7832–7836.

Frankel, E.N. and Meyer, A.S. (2000). *J. Sci. Food. Agric.* 80, 1925–1941.

Gasowski, B., Leontowicz, M., Leontowicz, H., Katrich, E., Lojek, A., Ciz, M., Trakhtenberg, S. and Gorinstein, S. (2004). *J. Nutr. Biochem.* 15, 527–533.

Gerhäuser, C. (2005). *Eur. J. Cancer* 41, 1941–1954.

Ghiselli, A., Natella, F., Guidi, A., Montanari, L., Fantozzi, P. and Scaccini, C. (2000). *J. Nutr. Biochem.* 11, 76–80.

Gorinstein, S., Caspi, A., Zemser, M. and Trakhtenberg, S. (2000). *Nutr. Res.* 20, 131–139.

Halliwell, B. (1997). *Nutr. Rev.* 5, 544–552.

Hernanz, D., Nuñez, V., Sancho, A.I., Faulds, C.B., Williamson, G., Bartolomé, B. and Gómez-Cordovés, C. (2001). *J. Agric. Food Chem.* 49, 4884–4888.

Leubolt, R. and Klein, H. (1993). *J. Chromatogr.* 640, 271–277.

Liu, R.H. (2004). *J. Nutr.* 134, 3458S–3479S.

Lugasi, A. and Hóvári, J. (2003). *Nahrung/Food* 47, 79–86.

Luque-Pérez, E., Ríos, A. and Valcárcel, M. (2000). *Fresenius J. Anal. Chem.* 366, 857–862.

Madhujith, T., Izydorczyk, M. and Shahidi, F. (2006). *J. Agric. Food Chem.* 54, 3283–3289.

Matos, R.C., Augelli, M.A., Pedrotti, J.J., Lago, C.L. and Angnes, L. (1998). *Electroanalysis* 10, 887–890.

McMurrough, I., Madigan, D. and Smyth, M.R. (1996). *J. Agric. Food Chem.* 44, 1731–1735.

Moll, N. and Joly, J.P. (1987). *J. Chromatogr.* 405, 347–356.

Morales, F.J. and Babbel, M.B. (2002). *J. Agric. Food. Chem.* 50, 2788–2792.

Nardini, M. and Ghiselli, A. (2004). *Food Chem.* 84, 137–143.

Nardini, M., Cirillo, E., Natella, F. and Scaccini, C. (2002). *J. Agric. Food Chem.* 50, 5735–5741.

Nicoli, M.C., Anese, M., Manzocco, L. and Lerici, C.R. (1997). *Lebensm. – Wiss. Technol.* 30, 292–297.

Nordkvist, E., Salomonsson, A.C. and Aman, P. (1984). *J. Sci. Food Agric.* 35, 657–661.

Prior, R.L., Wu, X. and Schaich, K. (2005). *J. Agric. Food Chem.* 53, 4290–4302.

Pulido, R., Hernández-García, M. and Saura-Calixto, F. (2003). *Eur. J. Clin. Nutr.* 57, 1275–1282.

Rimm, E.B., Giovannucci, E.L., Willet, W.C., Coldtiz, G.A., Ascherio, A., Rosner, B. and Stampfer, M.J. (1991). *Lancet* 35, 464–468.

Rivero, D., Pérez-Magariño, S., González-San José, M.L., Valls-Bellés, V., Codoñer, P. and Muñiz, P. (2005). *J. Agric. Food Chem.* 53, 3637–3642.

Rotondo, S., Di Castelnuovo, A. and de Gaetano, G. (2001). *Ital. Heart J.* 2, 1–8.

Salomonsson, A.C., Theander, O. and Aman, P. (1980). *Swed. J. Agric. Res.* 10, 11–16.

Sánchez-Moreno, C. (2002). *Food Sci. Technol. Int.* 8, 121–137.

Sánchez-Moreno, C., Larrauri, J.A. and Saura-Calixto, F. (1998). *J. Sci. Food Agric.* 76, 270–276.

Saura-Calixto, F. and Goñi, I. (2006). *Food Chem.* 94, 442–447.

Saura-Calixto, F., Goñi, I., Martín Albarrán, C. and Pulido Ferrer, R. (2002). *Fibra dietética en la cerveza: contenido, composición y evaluación nutricional.* Centro de Información Cerveza y Salud, Madrid.

Serafini, M. (2006). *Medicine* 34, 533–535.

Shahidi, F. and Naczk, M. (2004). *Phenolics in Foods and Nutraceuticals.* CRC Press LLC, Boca Raton, FL.

Siebert, K.J., Troukhanova, N.V. and Lynn, P.Y. (1996). *J. Agric. Food Chem.* 44, 80–85.

Trichopolou, A., Costacou, T., Bamia, C. and Trichopoulos, D. (2003). *NEJM* 348, 2599–2608.

Tsao, R., Yang, R., Xie, S., Sockovie, E. and Khanizhade, S. (2005). *J. Agric. Food Chem.* 53, 4989–4995.

Villaño, D., Fernández-Pachón, S., Troncoso, A.M. and García-Parrilla, M.C. (2005). *Anal. Chim. Acta* 538, 591–598.

Vinson, J.A., Teufel, K. and Wu, N. (2001). *Atherosclerosis* 156, 67–72.

Wagner, H.P. and McGarrity, M.J. (1991). *J. Chromatogr.* 546, 119–124.

Woodside, J.V., McCall, D., McGartland, C. and Young, I.S. (2005). *Proc. Nutr. Soc.* 64, 543–553.

Wu, X., Beecher, G.R., Holden, J.M., Haytowitz, D.B., Gebhardt, S.E. and Prior, R.L. (2004). *J. Agric. Food Chem.* 52, 4026–4037.

Wu, X., Beecher, G.R., Holden, J.M., Haytowitz, D.B., Gebhardt, S.E. and Prior, R.L. (2006). *J. Agric. Food Chem.* 54, 4069–4075.

Yen, G.C., Duh, P.D. and Tsai, H.L. (2002). *Food Chem.* 79, 307–313.

Yu, J., Vasanthan, T. and Temelli, F. (2001). *J. Agric. Food Chem.* 49, 4352–4358.

43

Antioxidant Activity of Beer's Maillard Reaction Products: Features and Health Aspects

Franco Tubaro Department of Chemical Sciences and Technology, University of Udine, Udine, Italy

Abstract

The capability of a mixture of compounds to quench peroxyl radicals is measured by comparing the kinetics of a reaction between these and the carotenoid crocin and the competition that other antioxidants have for the same peroxyl radicals. This kinetic approach uses a source of peroxyl radicals to evaluate the capacity of other compounds or a mixture of compounds to quench their intrinsic reactivity. Single compounds as well as complex mixtures may be analyzed by kinetic data processing. Overall antioxidant capacity, relative to that of Trolox C (the hydrophylic substitute of vitamin E) may be calculated. As examples of the use of this test, the antioxidant capacity of Maillard reaction products (MRPs are the condensation products of amino acids reacting with sugars when heated) from a standard mixture of glicine and glucose a model system cookie as close as possible to a real solid food the direct comparison of 12 craft beers with 10 commercial industrial beers were performed. Blood samples of 18 healthy volunteers were also withdrawn and analyzed before, during and after a 15-day period of daily intake of a beer particularly strong in antioxidants.

The solid model system was composed of wheat starch, glucose, lysine, water and butter. The antioxidative effect was compared with that of the reference antioxidant Trolox C; the maximum action of MRPs as peroxyl radical scavengers was found to be around 5% that of Trolox C. The contribution of sugar and an amino acid to antioxidant MRPs formation was evaluated by considering models without glucose or lysine. MRPs antioxidant action was found to increase with the browning of models up to a high browning level. The compounds formed when further browning occurred did not contribute to an increase in antioxidant activity. The model without added glucose showed slight browning due to starch hydrolysis or the reaction of lipids with lysine, but antioxidant action was negligible.

Liquids as beer and human plasma were easily compared to a 1 mM solution of Trolox C. Lagers had up to 2.8 mM equivalents of Trolox C, while in some dark craft beers the antioxidant activity reached 12 mM equivalents of Trolox C. Wide differences were noticed between industrial and craft beers, due to the much higher amounts of flavonoids in the latter. Human plasma rarely exceed 2 mM equivalents of Trolox C, but a 15% increase in the status of antioxidants has been observed after 2 weeks of treatment with a daily ingestion of 375 ml of a strong dark beer.

List of Abbreviations

ABAP	Azobis-amidinopropane
EDTA	Ethylen diamine tetra acetic acid
GC	Gas chromatography
HPLC	High performance liquid chromatography
KCl	Potassium chloride
MRP	Maillard reaction products
PUFA	Poly unsaturated fatty acids
TBA	Tiobarbituric acid
TRAP	Total radical trapping antioxidant potential

Introduction

Lipid oxidation of polyunsaturated fatty acids (PUFA) has been extensively analyzed in the last decades (Terao, 1990), in relation to their oxidative stability and the development of off-flavors in foods (Frankel, 1993), but also as a major important mechanism of cellular function derangement in many diseases (Halliwell and Gutteridge, 1990). Moreover, the toxicity of lipid oxidation products (Addis and Warner, 1991) highlights the relevance of technology of food processing in lowering the formation of toxic compounds.

Beer in Health and Disease Prevention
ISBN: 978-0-12-373891-2

The natural antioxidant content of foods is considered a major health-protecting factor, by supplying the human body with an exogenous antioxidant protection (Gey *et al.*, 1991; Block, 1992; Ames *et al.*, 1993). Furthermore, it is reasonable to assume that the reduction of the content of oxidized toxic components in foods, brought by the ingestion of antioxidants, must be significant for human health.

The capability of measuring overall antioxidant capacity of a food, therefore, may be very useful in food chemistry, to possibly expand information obtained from tests with single antioxidants.

Accelerated stability tests are the usual procedure for evaluating food antioxidants. A lipid matrix is exposed to various oxidizing conditions, and the effect of the antioxidant is calculated from the induction period prior to the rapid oxidation phase (Frankel, 1993). Oxidation is usually mea-sured by the production of specific compounds or oxygen consumption. Although useful for practical purposes, these procedures have been questioned for either the variability of conditions to produce oxidation products or the precision of the analytical procedure applied (Läubli and Bruttel, 1986).

There is a simple procedure for analyzing the antioxidant capacity of complex matrices (beers and Maillard reaction products – MRPs) which is expressed relative to the soluble analog of α-tocopherol, Trolox C on a concentration basis.

The description of the method needs a brief definition of the peroxidative process and of the antioxidant mechanism to which the analysis has been addressed, highlighting the kinetics of the reactions involved in the antioxidant effect. PUFA, after extraction of an allylic hydrogen atom by an initiator, react extremely fast with molecular oxygen, forming a peroxyl radical (Hasegawa and Patterson, 1978). Several different mechanisms are responsible for the initiation of peroxidation: the production of free radicals may happen by unimolecular homolysis of weak bonds, radiolysis, photolysis or electron transfer from transition metal ions (Pryor, 1976). The bond which most frequently undergoes a homolytic or heterolytic decomposition through the above mechanisms is the O—O bond of a hydroperoxide (Terao, 1990), thus this mechanism of initiation of lipid peroxidation is usually referred to as "hydroperoxide dependent" (Ursini *et al.*, 1991).

Peroxyl radicals react with other PUFA to yield hydroperoxides and a new carbon-centered radical, thus driving the peroxidation chain reaction (Ursini *et al.*, 1991). The reported rate constant for this propagation reaction is 36/M/s for linoleic acid (Barclay *et al.*, 1989) and increases exponentially by increasing up to six the number of double bonds (Micossi *et al.*, 1996). The length of the chain reaction is determined by the availability of substrates (PUFA and oxygen) and by the ratio between propagation and termination reactions by radical–radical interaction (Porter, 1990).

Inhibition of initiation, a primary antioxidant effect, is brought about by physical or chemical procedures preventing the formation of free radicals from pre-existing lipid hydroperoxides (reduction of hydroperoxides, protection from light, sequestration of metals, inhibition of lipoxygenases, etc.). On the other hand, free radical scavengers or chain breaking antioxidants are molecules which specifically quench peroxidation driving radicals, so shortening the chain reaction length. The theoretical targets of this antioxidant effect are carbon-centered radicals, peroxyl radicals and alkoxyl radicals.

As a matter of fact, it is almost impossible for an antioxidant to compete with oxygen for the interaction with a pentadienyl radical since the reaction is extremely fast (Hasegawa and Patterson, 1978), although reversible. The same kinetic limitation applies to alkoxyl radicals, which react with PUFA with a rate constant increasing with the insaturation of the fatty acid chain from 8.8×10^6 to 2.05×10^7/M/s (Small Jr. *et al.*, 1979). It is extremely difficult for the antioxidant reaction to kinetically overhelm the pro-oxidant reaction as the reactivity of the radical involved is very high. Moreover, the actual involvement of the reaction between alkoxyl radicals of fatty acids and a PUFA is questioned owing to their rearrangement. In fact, alkoxyl radicals may cyclize into the adjacent site of insaturation to form, upon oxygen addition, an epoxide-peroxyl radical (Labeque and Marnett, 1988), or undergo β-scission to form, in subsequent reactions, aldehydes and peroxyl radicals (Esterbauer *et al.*, 1990).

The propagation driving reaction between a peroxyl radical and a PUFA, on the other hand, has a limited rate constant (Barclay *et al.*, 1989; Micossi *et al.*, 1996), thus a competitive reaction may take place in which an antioxidant, reacting with a much higher rate constant, can actually spare PUFA.

The first requirement for a free radical scavenger to be an antioxidant is, therefore, the kinetic advantage of having the rate constant of the reaction with a peroxyl radical much higher than that of the propagation reaction between a peroxyl radical and a PUFA. The second requirement is that the radical of the antioxidant has to react with PUFA with a rate constant much lower than the one of peroxyl radical. This highlights the concept that the measurement of just the rate constant of the reaction between a compound and peroxyl radicals (often taken as an index of antioxidant capacity) could be misleading in terms of a real antioxidant effect, when the radical produced is still reactive enough to substitute for peroxyl radicals in the propagation reaction. In the case of an efficient antioxidant such as Trolox C, the rate constant of the antioxidant reaction is several orders of magnitude higher than the rate constants of the chain transfer pro-oxidant reactions (Mukai *et al.*, 1993).

The procedure for measuring antioxidant activity is based on kinetic constraints of the antioxidant effect: (i) the high rate constant of the reaction with peroxidation driving peroxyl radicals and (ii) the low rate constant of the propagation reaction (if any) of the radical of the antioxidant. By this procedure the capability of a compound (or the mixture of compounds) to quench peroxyl radicals, is measured in terms of Trolox C equivalents (on a concentration basis), by analyzing the kinetics of competition of a parallel reaction where peroxyl radicals bleach the carotenoid, crocin.

As an example, glucose and glycine undergo a Maillard reaction, and the products exhibit antioxidant properties. A high number of beers were also analyzed by this procedure, underlining the differences between simple lagers, amber beers and dark beers.

It is also well known that in a food product which undergoes a heat treatment, compounds with amine groups and free reducing functions of sugars may cause browning reactions, generally called the Maillard reaction. On the other hand, in a lot of foods containing only small amounts of lipids (about 1%), oxidation reactions may cause rancidity phenomena, almost always during storage, in such a way as to limit the shelf-life of foods themselves. Most often, in foods which undergo processing and/or storage, both reactions can occur. Intensive international research to study the antioxidative action of Maillard reaction intermediates and final products has been carried out (Eiserich *et al.*, 1992; Mastrocola and Munari, 2000).

It has been shown that the products obtained from heating model solutions of sugars and amino acids, are able to reduce the degree of oxidation in lipid substrates (Lingnert and Hall, 1986; Kitts and Hu, 2005). Among all of the mechanisms put forward to explain the antioxidative activity of the MRP, the following have been considered: the inactivation of free lipidic radicals, the inhibition of peroxide formation (Eichner, 1981), the ability of MRPs to sequestrate metallic ions, the catalysts of the first oxidation steps (Yamagushi *et al.*, 1981; Yen *et al.*, 2005) and their action as oxygen traps (Lingnert and Waller, 1983).

During heat treatment of a complex system such as in food, the development of interaction products is affected by the change of chemical and physical characteristics, so that the results obtained on models do not necessarily describe phenomena occurring in food. Several studies have been carried out to apply the results obtained on simple models to complex food systems. Furthermore, some conventional methods used to assess lipid oxidation are influenced by the presence of MRPs (tiobarbituric acid (TBA) formation of hexanal by gas chromatography (GC), etc.) and it is difficult to evaluate the action of MRPs on lipid oxidation.

The antioxidative activity of water-soluble compounds obtained by extraction from food model systems of various compositions heated for different times were studied. The methodology used in this work, which involved comparison with a reference antioxidant, demonstrates the antioxidative action of compounds which are able to interact with peroxyl radicals and thus act as radical scavengers.

The multiform nature of the primary antioxidant effect renders extremely vague its quantitative analysis, thus the measurement of "total radical trapping antioxidant potential" (TRAP) has been introduced for evaluating plasma antioxidant capacity (Ghiselli *et al.*, 1994; Rice-Evans and Miller, 1994). These tests adopt different free radical generating systems – thermo-labile diazocompounds or ferryl myoglobin – and the oxidation of either plasma lipids or of a reporter molecule as the event to be analyzed. Thus, as far as the formation of peroxyl radicals is concerned, these tests account for a "chain breaking antioxidant" effect, since the used radicals mimic the reactivity of peroxidation driving lipid-peroxyl radicals.

The basic requirement of lag-time based tests is that the rate constant of the reaction of an antioxidant with peroxyl radicals has to be much higher than that of the molecule to be protected, thus very limited oxidation of the latter takes place until the antioxidant is almost completely consumed. However, when different antioxidants are compared, this approach overlooks the difference among their rate constant for the reaction with peroxyl radicals. Different antioxidants, therefore, within a wide range of rate constants for the above reaction, produce the same lag.

Competition kinetics has been widely used in free radical research, for example in pulse radiolysis experiments (von Sonntag and Schuchmann, 1994) and the produced result is a relative rate constant for the reaction with a given radical. Since the chain breaking antioxidant capacity of a complex mixture, such as plasma, is the sum of the concentration of different antioxidants multiplied by their specific rate constant for the reduction of peroxyl radicals, the antioxidant effect can be reported with respect to the concentration of a reference antioxidant (Trolox C), the rate constant of which is known.

The Kinetic Competition Test

2,2′-Azobis (2-amidinopropane) dihydrochloride (ABAP) was purchased from Waco Chem. USA, Inc. Richmond VA; Trolox C, glucose and glycine from Janssen Chimica, Geel Belgium; potassium hydrogen phosphate from Carlo Erba, Milano Italy; Saffron and Trolox C from Sigma Chemical Co. St. Louis MI. All solvents for high performance liquid chromatography (HPLC grade) were from J.T. Baker Milano Italy. Crocin (8,8′-diapo-ψ,ψ-carotenedioic acid bis [6-*O*-β-D-glucopyranosyl-β-D-glucopyranosyl] ester) was prepared from saffron (Crocus sativus, Sigma, Italy) by methanolic extraction after being washed with ethylic ether to eliminate possible interferring substances (Bors *et al.*, 1984). The concentration of crocin in methanol was calculated from the absorbtion coefficient ($\varepsilon = 1.33 \times 10$/M/cm at 443 nm).

The original kinetic test (Bors *et al.*, 1984) was modified by introducing diazo-compounds to produce peroxyl radicals and by using solvents of different polarity to allow the analysis of either hydrophilic or lipophilic compounds.

Reactions were carried out at 40°C and the bleaching rate of crocin, linear 1–1.5 min after the addition of the diazocompound, was recorded for 10 min. Blanks without crocin were run to rule out spectral interferences between the molecule under analysis and crocin.

For hydrophilic compounds ABAP was the radical generator. The hydrophilic reaction mixture contained: 1 ml of 10% ethanol in water, 1 ml of 10 mM phosphate buffer pH 7, 12 μM crocin (from a 1.2 mM methanolic stock solution) and variable amounts of the sample containing the antioxidant to be analyzed. Samples were added either in water or ethanol, maintaining the final concentration of the latter constant. The reaction was started by the addition of 5 mM ABAP (from a fresh 0.5 M solution in water) to the complete reaction mixture pre-equilibrated at 40°C. This procedure was used for Trolox C (as reference compound), for Maillard reaction products in hydrophylic extracts and for beers and plasma samples.

Carbon-centered radicals, generated by thermal decomposition of the diazo-compound (reaction 1), add molecular oxygen yielding peroxyl radicals ($ROO^\bullet$), in a diffusion controlled reaction (reaction 2) (Bors *et al.*, 1987; Pryor *et al.*, 1993). These radicals bleach the carotenoid crocin, thus allowing the measurement of the reaction rate by following the specific absorbance decrease at 443 nm (Bors *et al.*, 1984). In the presence of an antioxidant, competing with crocin for the reaction with radicals, the bleaching rate (reaction 3) slows down, providing that: (i) the antioxidant is able to react with peroxyl radicals (reaction 4) and (ii) the rate of the interaction between the radical of the antioxidant and crocin (reaction 5) is slower than the rate of reaction 3.

$$R-N=N-R \xrightarrow{\text{(heat)}} 2R^\bullet + N_2 \quad (1)$$

$$R^\bullet + O_2 \longrightarrow ROO^\bullet \quad (2)$$

$$ROO^\bullet + \text{Crocin} \longrightarrow ROOH + \text{Crocin}^\bullet\text{ (bleached)} \quad (3)$$

$$ROO^\bullet + \text{AntiOx} \longrightarrow ROOH + \text{AntiOx}^\bullet \quad (4)$$

$$\text{AntiOx}^\bullet + \text{Crocin} \longrightarrow \text{AntiOx} + \text{Crocin}^\bullet\text{(bleached)} \quad (5)$$

The crocin bleaching by a peroxyl radical ($-\Delta A_o$), corresponding to $V_o = K_c[C]$, decreases in the presence of an antioxidant competing for the peroxyl radical and, according to the competition kinetics (Bors *et al.*, 1984, Tubaro *et al.*, 1996), the new bleaching rate (V) corresponds to:

$$V = V_o \times \frac{K_c[C]}{K_c[C] + K_a[A]}$$

where:

$$V_o = K_1 \times [ROO^\bullet] \times [C] \qquad K_c = K_1 \times [ROO^\bullet]$$

$$V_a = K_2 \times [ROO^\bullet] \times [A] \qquad K_a = K_2 \times [ROO^\bullet]$$

and:

V_o = rate of the reaction of crocin with $ROO^\bullet$
V_a = rate of the reaction of the antioxidant under study with $ROO^\bullet$
K_1 = rate constant for the reaction between $ROO^\bullet$ and crocin
K_2 = rate constant for the reaction between $ROO^\bullet$ and antioxidant
[C] = concentration of crocin
[A] = concentration of antioxidant

By transforming, the bleaching rate of crocin ($-\Delta A_o$) decreases in the presence of an antioxidant to a new value ($-\Delta A_a$) fitting the straight line equation:

$$\frac{-\Delta A_o}{-\Delta A_a} = \frac{V_o}{V} = \frac{K_c[C] + K_a[A]}{K_c[C]} = 1 + \frac{K_a}{K_c} \times \frac{[A]}{[C]}$$

The slope K_a/K_c, calculated from the linear regression of the plot of [A]/[C] vs. V_o/V, indicates the relative capacity of different molecules to interact with $ROO^\bullet$. When molecules which, although reacting with peroxyl radicals, are transformed into radicals able to react with crocin and thus, by analogy, to propagate peroxidation, this kinetic approach produces ratios K_a/K_c lower than the actual ratio between the absolute rate constants. Thus, this test averages the antioxidant capacity with a possible pro-oxidant effect of the sample.

Experimental Maillard reaction products

A procedure for preparing a mixture of Maillard reaction products was adopted by dissolving 13.3 g of glucose and 6.7 g of glycine in 80 ml of water and heating the mixture at 90°C in closed vials. The antioxidant capacity was analyzed on samples taken at 0, 3, 6 and 15 h and diluted 1:10 with 0.1 M phosphate buffer pH 7.

A more complex model system (model A) was made to simulate a butter biscuit formulation by mixing together 70.25 g of pure wheat starch with 3.4 g of anhydrous glucose (Carlo Erba, Milan, Italy), 1.35 g of l-lysine (Sigma, Italy), 21 g of concentrated butter (Prealpi, Varese, Italy) and 4 g of distilled water. In the same way, two reference systems were prepared, respectively, without glucose or lysine (models B and C), keeping the proportion of the other components unchanged.

Small amounts of each dough (10 g ± 0.5) were placed in small paper containers and then cooked at 140°C for 0, 10, 20, 30 or 40 min.

After cooking, water soluble compounds formed in the biscuits during the heat treatment, were extracted with a solution of 0.4 M KCl (Carlo Erba, Milan, Italy). The salt is used to increase the polarity of the medium and so promote the extraction of the hydrosoluble compounds. For each kind of dough, 5 g of pounded biscuit were dissolved in 20 ml of KCl solution. The system was homogenized using a Polytron apparatus (Kinematica AG, PT 3,000) for 1 min to facilitate suspension of the particles and the successive phase of extraction. Samples were centrifuged for 5 min at 5,000 rpm at 0°C (refrigerated centrifuge ALC, R.C.F. Meter, 4,233R) and the aqueous phase was filtered through filter paper (Whatman No. 4), mixed again with 10 ml of the KCl solution and centrifuged again as described above. The aqueous phase was then frozen and stored (−18°C) for about 15 h in hermetically sealed containers. Each extraction was carried out twice.

Before each determination of the antioxidative capacity of the extract, potential interference by the compounds of the extracts, on both rate and evolution of the crocin bleaching was evaluated. It has been shown that the variation of absorption of the extracts after reaction with the free radicals, under the experimental conditions described above, was negligible (Abs = 0.043–0.048).

To express the molar concentration of the antioxidative substances present in the extracts, it was necessary to acknowledge that all the dry matter of the extracts was able to exert an antioxidative action. As the nature and the concentration of these substances in the extracts were unknown, the results have been expressed as equivalents of antioxidative efficiency in comparison with the reference antioxidant: Trolox (6-hydroxy-2,5,7,8-tetramethylchroman-2-carbonsalt, Aldrich, Germany), even though it is not present in the extracts. Consequently, extracts were compared with a 1 mM solution of Trolox C.

Since the antioxidant capacity of a complex mixture is the sum of the products of each antioxidant multiplied by its rate constant, it can be functionally expressed as $K_a \times [A]$, where [A] is the concentration of a given antioxidant and K_a its rate constant for the reaction with peroxyl radicals. Thus, the antioxidant capacity of a complex mixture such as plasma is analyzed as follows.

According to the competition kinetics, by plotting the bleaching rates obtained using the solution under analysis (e.g. plasma) as it would be 1 mM of antioxidant, a ratio ka/kc is obtained. By dividing this value by the K_a/K_c of Trolox C, a millimolar concentration of Trolox C accounting for plasma antioxidant capacity is calculated.

Plasma samples

Blood samples were obtained from 18 healthy subjects (12 men and 6 women equally distributed between who would have beer to drink all 15 days of the trial and who would swap to a hydroalcoholic beverage after the first week). Plasma was immediately prepared using 5 mM EDTA (ethylen diamino tetra acetic acid) or 200 mg/l heparin. Plasma samples were analyzed immediately or frozen at −20°C and analyzed within 3 days.

Beer samples

The antioxidant capacity of different beers was measured by the same procedure. Craft beers and industrial beers were centrifuged at 3,000 rpm for 5 min, and immediately analyzed.

The kinetic competition test was applied to all samples. Chain breaking antioxidants are molecules which interact with free radicals produced during lipid peroxidation, thus inhibiting the free radical chain propagation. Their efficiency depends on several factors, among which the kinetic constraints of the reaction involved are particularly relevant. The described kinetic procedure was addressed to the capacity of a compound or a complex mixture of compounds to react with peroxidation driving peroxyl radicals, producing a hydroperoxide and the radical of the antioxidant, the reactivity of which affects the final result. Thus, this kinetic analysis provides information on the average between antioxidant and pro-oxidant effects. This extends information obtained just from the measurement of the rate constant of the interaction between antioxidant and peroxyl radical, and could be particularly relevant in analyzing complex mixtures.

Competition kinetics has been used for the analysis of radical reactions induced by pulse radiolysis (von Sontag and Schuchmann, 1994) and for the measurement of relative rate constant of antioxidants reacting with hydroxyl and alkoxyl radicals (Bors *et al.*, 1984). The latter test has been modified by introducing diazo-compounds as a source of peroxyl radicals at a constant rate, a procedure widely adopted for analyzing antioxidants (van Amsterdam *et al.*, 1992).

The results of the analyses of the antioxidant capacity of the water soluble analog of α-tocopherol, Trolox C in the hydrophilic system is reported in Figure 43.1. In these plots, V_0/V indicates the ratio of bleaching rates in the presence of different molar ratios between the antioxidant and crocin. These data indicate that experimental results fit the kinetic model (R values > 0.98 and intercept close to 1). Thus, according to the kinetic equation, the slope of the regression fitting of experimental data indicates the antioxidant capacity of the analyzed compound (Tubaro *et al.*, 1996). It is worth noting that, in different solvents the relative efficiency of the chromanol ring with respect to crocin slightly changes. This highlights the concept that different antioxidants must be compared under the same experimental conditions. Nevertheless, these observed differences of chromanol (or crocin) reactivity as a function of the solvent are minimal in comparison with the differences among different antioxidants (van Amsterdam *et al.*, 1992; Ursini *et al.*, 1994).

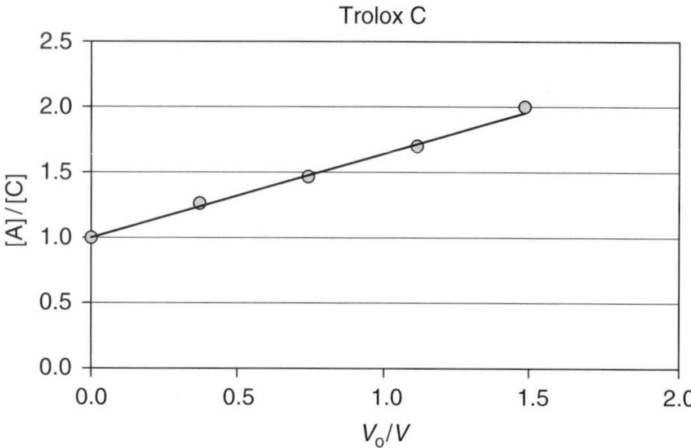

Figure 43.1 Kinetic plot for the competition between crocin and Trolox C for peroxyl radicals. The slope of the regression fitting indicates, according to the kinetic equation, the antioxidant capacity of the antioxidant. In three repeated measurements the interassay variability was <10%. The equation for Trolocx C was $y = 0.667x + 0.994$; $R^2 = 0.997$.

Antioxidant activity of Maillard reaction products

The described kinetic procedure, set up for the analysis of the antioxidant capacity of single molecules, was extended to complex mixtures (extracts from biscuits, craft and industrial beers, human plasma) where neither the concentration of antioxidants present nor their actual number were known. In fact, the overall antioxidant capacity of a complex mixture corresponds to the sum of each antioxidant concentration times its rate constant for the interaction with a peroxyl radical. Moreover, compounds possibly present in the mixture, which, upon interaction with the peroxyl radical, produce new radicals, reactive with crocin, by affecting crocin bleaching rate, decrease the antioxidant capacity of the mixture, as measured by the kinetic test (as an example, Figures 43.2 and 43.3 shows how craft beers are more antioxidant than industrial beers).

Trolox C as reference compound and the hydrophilic solvent have been used to analyse MRP which are known to play an antioxidant effect (Eichner, 1981).

The antioxidant capacity was measured on a mixture of glucose and glycine, heated to produce a mixture of MRP and analyzed at 3, 6 and 15 h. In this test the hydrophilic reaction mixture was used and, for the competition kinetics analysis, the molar concentration of the antioxidant was calculated by dividing the slope of the kinetic test of the mixture of glucose and glycine content by the slope of the kinetic test of Trolox C. Table 43.1 shows that the antioxidant capacity of the mixture progressively increases: after 3 h of heating, almost 600 g of glucose–glycine contained the antioxidant effect of one gram of Trolox, while just 31 g had the same effect after 15 h (0.667/0.0215 = 31). This result was supported by controls showing that at room temperature, or when glucose or glycine were heated independently, no antioxidant effect was produced (not shown).

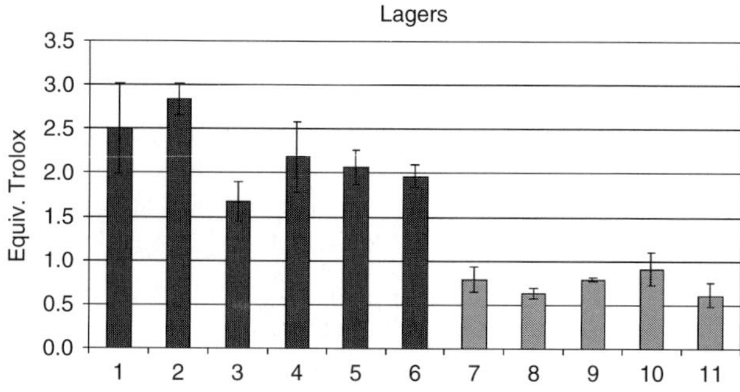

Figure 43.2 Antioxidant activity of lagers. Six craft beers (lagers; dark histograms) were compared to five industrial beers light found on the local markets. Antioxidant activity is expressed in mM equivalents of Trolox C. Bars indicate mean and the standard deviation of three measurements.

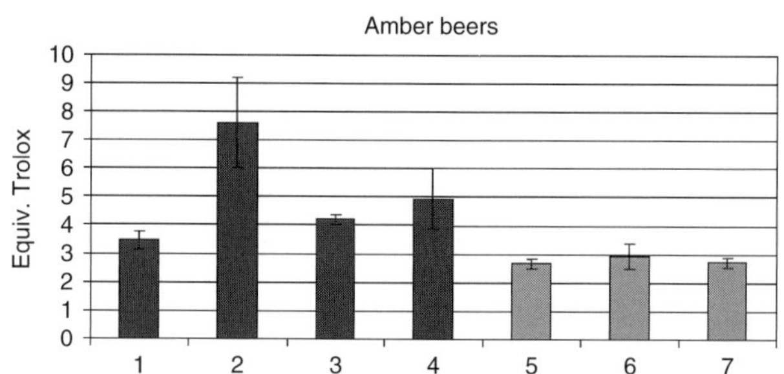

Figure 43.3 Antioxidant activity of amber beers. Four craft beers (amber beers idark histograms) were compared to three industrial beers light found on the local markets. Antioxidant activity is expressed in mM equivalents of Trolox C. Bars indicate the mean and standard deviation of three measurements.

It is possible to assert that hydrosoluble substances produced by heat treatment of the complex model system (defined as non-enzymatic browning products) are able to exert a radical scavenger effect. This antioxidative activity is proportional to the browning of the model and the variations of both parameters are statistically correlated ($r = 0.8872$; $p \leq 0.05$).

Table 43.2 shows the values of the antioxidative activity of the extracts deriving from the more complex MRP system. While model A had both ingredients necessary for the production of MRPs, the other reference model systems had the Maillard reaction limited or prevented by absence of the sugar (model B) or of the amino acid (model C) in the formulation. In both cases, it can be seen that products extracted from systems submitted to heat treatment for 40 min did not display significant antioxidative activity.

This test is, therefore, particularly appropriate for analyzing the antioxidant capacity of complex mixtures, such as plasma, where several molecules could react with peroxyl radicals producing radicals with different oxidation potential. The final fate of the radical of the antioxidant will discriminate between good antioxidants and propagators of chain reaction, and the analysis of the antioxidant capacity of a complex mixture must take in account all these effects.

Table 43.1 Kinetics of crocin bleaching inhibition by MRP[a]

Sample time	*Competition kinetics equation*	*R*	*MRP/Trolox C*
MRP 3h	$y = 1.12 \times 10^{-3}x + 1.007$	0.99	0.0017
MRP 6h	$y = 5.39 \times 10^{-3}x + 0.808$	0.99	0.0081
MRP 15h	$y = 21.50 \times 10^{-3}x + 1.007$	0.99	0.0322

Notes: The slope of the regression fitting indicates, according to the kinetic equation, the antioxidant capacity of the antioxidant. In three repeated measurements the interassay variability was <10%. MRP antioxidant activity is related to that of Trolox C measured in the same conditions.

[a]The simple hydrophilic reaction mixture was used. The ratio MRP/Trolox C indicates the relative slope differences between MRPs at different times and Trolox C measured in the same conditions.

Table 43.2 Kinetics of crocin bleaching inhibition by MRP[a] for models B and C total sample time is 40 minutes as for model A

Sample time	*Competition kinetics equation*	*R*	*MRP/Trolox C*
Model A			
MRP 0min	$y = 1.02 \times 10^{-4}x + 1.02$	0.98	Undetectable ($<10^{-3}$)
MRP 10min	$y = 2.29 \times 10^{-3}x + 1.01$	0.99	0.0034
MRP 20min	$y = 1.03 \times 10^{-2}x + 1.01$	0.99	0.0154
MRP 30min	$y = 1.67 \times 10^{-2}x + 1.01$	0.99	0.0250
MRP 40min	$y = 1.30 \times 10^{-2}x + 0.99$	0.99	0.0195
Model B			
MRP (?)	$y = 2.34 \times 10^{-4}x + 1.007$	0.98	Undetectable ($<10^{-3}$)
Model C			
MRP (?)	$y = 6.30 \times 10^{-5}x + 1.007$	0.66	Undetectable ($<10^{-3}$)

Notes: The slope of the regression fitting indicates, according to the kinetic equation, the antioxidant capacity of the antioxidant. In three repeated measurements the interassay variability was <10%. MRP antioxidant activity is related to that of Trolox C.

[a]The complex hydrophilic reaction mixture was used. The ratio MRP/Trolox C indicates the relative slope differences between MRPs at different times and Trolox C measured in the same conditions. See text for details.

Although the pro-oxidant effects so far observed are actually rather limited it is worth noting that they could be relevant when analyzing plasma under different nutritional and pathological conditions.

The antioxidant capacity of plasma is obtained by measuring its bleaching ratio after measuring that of a 1 mM solution of Trolox C. This has been calculated by dividing the slope of the plot obtained with plasma (considered as a 1 mM solution of antioxidant) by the slope obtained with Trolox C.

The procedure is extremely simple and rapid, one sample being fully processed in 10 min if a multiple cell spectrophotometer is used. The intra-assay variation of plasma samples in repeated measurements was less than 8%.

Plasma, when quickly and carefully prepared, taking care to avoid hemolysis, can be stored at −20°C for 3–5 days without any appreciable loss of antioxidant capacity.

No major differences have been noticed by using 5.0 mM EDTA or 200 mg/l heparin as anti-coagulant. However, since EDTA has some antioxidant capacity, although appreciable at concentrations much higher than those used in the test, heparin has been preferred for the standardized procedure.

One of the most attractive applications of this procedure is the analysis of the post prandial plasma, when several components introduced with diet could play relevant antioxidant or pro-oxidant effects. We report here the effect of beer, taken daily for 15 days, as an example of application of the procedure.

Plasma antioxidant capacity has been measured before, during and after the ingestion by nine healthy subjects of a dark beer (12 mM equivalents of Trolox C) for 15 days, and differences were measured comparing their antioxidant plasma levels to those of other nine subjects who interrupted the beer ingestion after 1 week and passed onto an hydroalcoholic mixture of 8% ethanol in water. In all subjects, the dark beer produced a pronounced increase of plasma antioxidant capacity (15% respect to the original value) after the first week of the trial, which was mantained constant at this level for the rest of the testing period. Those who consumed ethanol after the first week had slightly lower capacity at the end of the trial (Figures 43.4 and 43.5). A typical pattern, where an increase was followed by a steady constant level, was observed in all subjects, although the time course presented an individual variability suggesting different rates of uptake and clearance of antioxidant compounds (not shown).

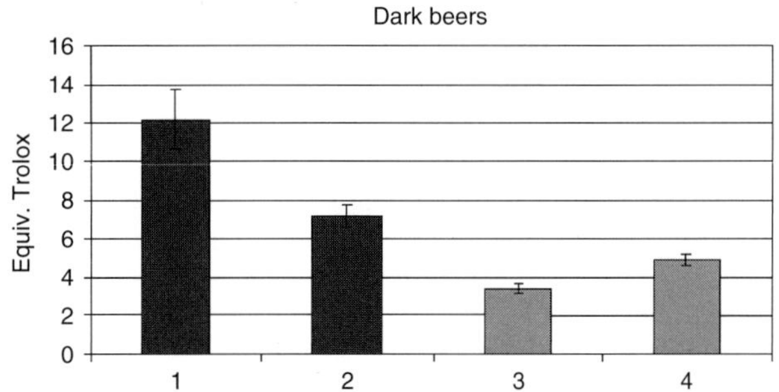

Figure 43.4 Antioxidant activity of dark beers. Two craft beers (dark bars) were compared to two industrial beers found on the local markets. Antioxidant activity is expressed in mM equivalents of Trolox C. Bars indicate the mean and standard deviation of three measurements.

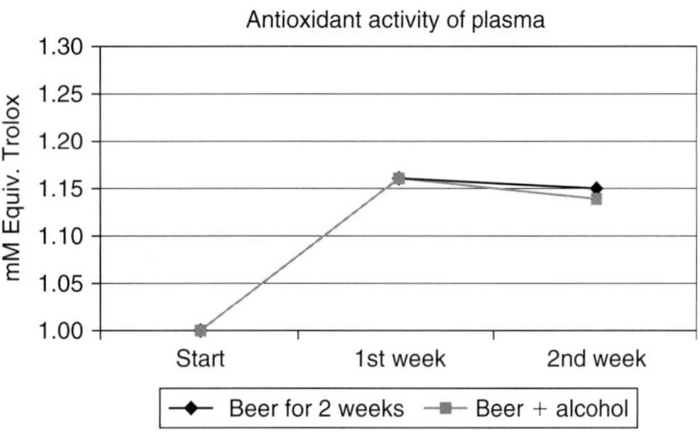

Figure 43.5 Human plasma antioxidant variations due to the ingestion of dark beer. A panel of nine volunteers consumed dark craft beer no. 1 (see Figure 43.4) for 2 weeks, while another nine volunteers consumed an alcohol solution (8%) after 1 week. Antioxidant activity are expressed by the ratio between mM equivalents of Trolox C at the beginning of the test and after 1 and 2 weeks.

The assessment of plasma antioxidant status is a fundamental parameter to define an oxidative stress produced by either a reduced intake or an increased consumption of antioxidants.

From a thermodynamic point of view, every couple of species with a reduction potential lower than that of the couple peroxyl radical/hydroperoxide could play an antioxidant role since the radical nature is transferred to a species with a decreased tendency to propagate the reaction. This is the thermodynamic support to the well-known sequence of redox reactions from a hydroperoxyl radical, to tocopherol to ascorbate (Scarpa *et al.*, 1984). Nonetheless, during this progressive "discharge of the oxidation capacity" from strong oxidants to progressively weaker oxidants (Cadenas, 1997), some intermediates could still promote the oxidation of targets which are supposed to be protected, and consequently it has been shown that tocopheroxyl radical can oxidize lipids (Bowry and Stocker, 1993).

From a kinetic point of view, the antioxidant must react faster than the target to be protected with the oxidant, and the radical of the antioxidant must be minimally reactive or, more frequently, undergo one of the reactions leading to annihilation of its radical nature (reaction with another radical, disproportion, reaction with another antioxidant), at a rate faster than that of its reaction with the target to be protected.

In conclusion, a very complex array of reactions could take place when a biological matrix as plasma is challenged with a free radical generating system. Our analytical approach is addressed to the kinetic evaluation of the antioxidant effect, taking also in account the effect of molecules, possibly present, which, following fast free radical oxidation, are transformed into radicals which are still oxidant.

In agreement with the most popular TRAP tests, the kinetic approach shows that the large majority of antioxidant capacity of plasma from fasting subjects, as analyzed by this test, is accounted for by ascorbate, urate and proteins, while the effect of vitamin E is minimal, due to its low concentration (Tubaro *et al.*, 1998).

Nevertheless, this test is more precise than lag-time based tests, taking in to the correct account also the weak antioxidant which is overestimated when the antioxidant capacity is measured at the time before massive oxidation of the target.

This analytical approach seems ideal for assessing the effect of nutrition on plasma antioxidant status as far as it concerns the reduction of peroxidation driving peroxyl radicals. In this respect, the evidence of a substantial increase of antioxidant capacity brought about by drinking beer confirms that this very popular beverage could be an important source of physiologically relevant antioxidants.

Conclusion

The principal aim of this experimental work was the evaluation of the antioxidative activity regarding the peroxyl radical scavenging capacity of compounds developed during the heat treatment of a complex food system. Simple and more complex MRPs have been considered (Bressa *et al.*, 1996; Tubaro *et al.*, 1996), and the real application on a popular drink such as dark beer, with many flavonoids and MRPs has been studied. Differences between industrial and craft beers have been underlined, and the influence of a powerfull beer on the antioxidant activity of plasma in human subjects has been quantified (Tubaro *et al.*, 2005).

Summary Points

- Antioxidants are able to quench peroxyl radicals, which are responsible for many degenerative processes in human beings.
- A kinetic competition test is used to measure the antioxidant capacity of many different types of foods, beverages and biological samples.

- MRPs are formed when amino acids (from proteins) and sugars (from polysaccarides) interact in the presence of heat.
- The total amount and exact chemical nature of MRPs in any food is unknown, as any cooking process forms them.
- A relevant antioxidant activity in these products is easily measured, and the potential benefits on humans can be evaluated in controlled conditions. The measurement of a total antioxidant status of volunteers before and after the ingestion of antioxidants may underline how a beer can increase the body's protection from free radicals.

References

Addis, P.B. and Warner, G.J. (1991). The potential health aspects of lipid oxidation products in food. In Aruoma, O.I. and Halliwell, B. (eds), *Free Radicals and Food Additives*, pp. 77–119. Taylor & Francis, London.

Ames, B.N., Shigenaga, M.K. and Hagen, T.M. (1993). *Proc. Natl. Acad. Sci. USA* 90, 7915–7922.

Barclay, L.R.C., Baskin, K.A., Locke, S.J. and Vinquist, M.R. (1989). *Can. J. Chem.* 67, 1366–1369.

Block, G. (1992). *Nutr. Rev.* 50, 207–213.

Bors, W., Michel, C. and Saran, M. (1984). *Biochim. Biophys. Acta* 796, 312–319.

Bors, W., Erben-Russ, M. and Saran, M. (1987). *Biolectrochem. Bioenerg.* 18, 37–49.

Bowry, V.W. and Stocker, R. (1993). *J. Am. Chem. Soc.* 115, 6029–6044.

Bressa, F., Tesson, N., Della Rosa, M., Sensidoni, A. and Tubaro, F. (1996). *J. Agric. Food Chem.* 44, 692–695.

Cadenas, E. (1997). *Biofactors* 6, 391–397.

Eichner, K. (1981). *Prog. Food Nutr. Sci.* 5, 441–451.

Eiserich, J.P., Machu, C. and Shibamoto, T. (1992). *J. Agric. Food Chem.* 40, 1982–1988.

Esterbauer, H., Zollner, H. and Jörg Schaur, R. (1990). Aldehydes formed by lipid peroxidation: Mechanisms of formation, occurrence, and determination. In Vigo-Pelfrey, C. (ed.), *Membrane Lipid Oxidation*, 1, pp. 239–268. CRC Press, Boca Raton, FL.

Frankel, E.N. (1993). *Trends Food Sci. Technol.* 4, 220–225.

Gey, K.F., Puska, P., Jordan, P. and Moser, U.K. (1991). *Am. J. Clin. Nutr.* 53, 326S–334S.

Ghiselli, A., Serafini, M., Maiani, G., Azzini, E. and Ferro-Luzzi, A. (1994). *Free Radic. Biol. Med.* 18, 29–39.

Halliwell, B. and Gutteridge, M.C. (1990). *Meth. Enzymol.* 186, 1–85.

Hasegawa, K. and Patterson, L.K. (1978). *Photochem. Photobiol.* 28, 817–823.

Kitts, D.D. and Hu, C. (2005). *Ann. N.Y. Acad. Sci.* 1043, 501–512.

Labeque, R. and Marnett, L.J. (1988). *Biochemistry* 27, 7060–7070.

Läubli, M.W. and Bruttel, P.A. (1986). *J. Am. Oil Chem. Soc.* 63, 792–795.

Lingnert, H. and Hall, G. (1986). Formation of antioxidative maillard reaction products during food processing. In Fujimaki, M., Namiki, M. and Kato, H. (eds), *Amino-Carbonyl Reactions in Food and Biological Systems*, pp. 273–279. Elsevier Science Publishers B. V., Amsterdam.

Lingnert, H. and Waller, G.R. (1983). *J. Agric. Food Chem.* 31, 27–30.

Mastrocola, D. and Munari, M. (2000). *J. Agric. Food Chem.* 48, 3555–3559.

Micossi, E., Tubaro, F., Magnabosco, P., Ciani, F. and Ursini, F. (1996). *Rivista di Suinicoltura* 3, 97–101.

Mukai, K., Sawada, K., Kohno, Y. and Terao, J. (1993). *Lipids* 28, 747–752.

Porter, N.A. (1990). Autoxidation of polyunsaturated fatty acids: initiation, propagation, and product distribution (Basic Chemistry). In Pryor, W.A. (ed.), *Free Radicals in Biology*, Vol. 1, pp. 1–49. Academic Press, New York.

Pryor, W.A., Cornicelli, J.A., Devall, L.J., Tait, B., Trivedi, B.K., Witiak, D.T. and Wu, M. (1993). *J. Org. Chem.* 58, 3521–3532.

Rice-Evans, C. and Miller, N.J. (1994). *Meth. Enzymol.* 234, 279–293.

Scarpa, M., Rigo, A., Maiorino, M., Ursini, F. and Gregolin, C. (1984). *Biochim. Biophys. Acta* 801, 215–219.

Small Jr., R.D., Scaino, J.C. and Patterson, L.K. (1979). *Photochem. Photobiol.* 29, 49–51.

Terao, J. (1990). Reactions of lipid hydroperoxides. In Vigo-Pelfrey, C. (ed.), *Membrane Lipid Oxidation*, I, pp. 219–238. CRC Press, Boca Raton, FL.

Tubaro, F., Micossi, E. and Ursini, F. (1996). *J. Am. Oil Chem. Soc.* 73, 173–179.

Tubaro, F., Ghiselli, A., Rapuzzi, P., Miorino, M. and Ursini, F. (1998). *Free Radic. Biol. Med.* 24, 1228–1234.

Tubaro, F., Buiatti, S. and Fiotti, N. (2005). *First European Conference on Chemistry for Life Sciences*, Rimini, October 4–8.

Ursini, F., Maiorino, M. and Sevanian, A. (1991). Membrane hydroperoxides. In Sies, H. (ed.), *Oxidative Stress: Oxidants and Antioxidants*, pp. 319–336. Academic Press, London.

Ursini, F., Maiorino, M., Morazzoni, P., Roveri, A. and Pifferi, G. (1994). *Free Rad. Biol. Med.* 16, 547–553.

van Amsterdam, F.T.M., Roveri, A., Maiorino, M., Ratti, E. and Ursini, F. (1992). *Free Radic. Biol. Med.* 12, 183–187.

von Sonntag, C. and Schuchmann, H.P. (1994). *Meth. Enzymol.* 233, 3–20.

Yamagushi, N., Koyama, Y. and Fujimaki, M. (1981). *Prog. Food Nutr. Sci.* 5, 429–439.

Yen, W.J., Wang, B.S., Chang, L.W. and Duh, P.D. (2005). *J. Agric. Food Chem.* 53, 2658 2663.

44

Beer Affects Oxidative Stress Due to Ethanol: A Preclinical and Clinical Study

Giovanni Addolorato, Lorenzo Leggio, Anna Ferrulli, Giovanni Gasbarrini, #Antonio Gasbarrini and Alcohol Related Diseases Study Group*
Institutes of Internal Medicine, and #Pathology, Catholic University of Rome, Rome, Italy
Antonio Gasbarrini Institutes of Pathology, Catholic University of Rome, Rome, Italy

Abstract

The oxidation of ethanol (ETOH) and its metabolites increase the production of superoxide anion and hydrogen peroxide, leading to initiation of peroxidation. The sensitivity to peroxidation is due to the overall balance between prooxidants and antioxidants. On the other hand, an increase of the antioxidant activity in blood of subjects with a moderate alcohol intake has been recently indicated as a possible protective mechanism. Beer has many non-alcoholic components with antioxidant properties such as vitamins, minerals, organic and inorganic salts, and phenolic compounds. The present chapter summarizes the results obtained by our laboratory on the effects of different alcoholic beverages, including beer, in both animals and humans. In particular, both preclinical and clinical studies showed that ETOH *per se* seems to decrease antioxidant parameters and increase lipoperoxidation. However, some of these changes appear to be attenuated when ETOH is consumed in beer. This aspect could be related to the counteracting effects of other antioxidant components.

List of Abbreviations

ADP	Adenosine diphosphate
ATP	Adenosine triphosphate
CD	Conjugated diene
ETOH	Ethanol
FFM	Free fat mass
FM	Fat mass
GSH	Reduced glutathione
HDL-C	High-density lipoprotein cholesterol
LPO	Lipid hydroperoxide production
MDA	Malondialdehyde
MEOS	Microsomal ethanol oxidation system
NADPH	Nicotinamide adenine dinucleotide phosphate
OFR	Oxygen-free radicals
TBA-RS	Acid-reactive substance
TRAP	Total plasma antioxidant potential

Introduction

Consumption of high doses of alcohol is able to damage several organ systems in the body (Lieber, 1992). A relationship exists between patterns of alcohol intake and the development of clinical manifestations (Lieber, 1995). Among the possible mechanisms involved in the pathogenesis of tissue injury, mortality and morbidity related to alcohol abuse, great attention has been recently devoted both to alcohol induced nutritional disorders (Preedy *et al.*, 1997; Addolorato *et al.*, 1997a, 1998, 2006) and alcohol related oxidative stress (Addolorato *et al.*, 2001; Lieber, 2005). The oxidation of ethanol (ETOH) and its metabolites increase the production of superoxide anion and hydrogen peroxide, leading to initiation of peroxidation (Krikun *et al.*, 1984; Gasbarrini *et al.*, 1996). The sensitivity to peroxidation is due to the overall balance between prooxidants and antioxidants (Gasbarrini *et al.*, 1996). Antioxidant protection includes both enzymatic and non-enzymatic defense systems (Gasbarrini *et al.*, 1996). In alcoholics a depletion of ascorbic acid, glutathione, selenium and vitamin E that the body stores has also been reported (Addolorato *et al.*, 1997b).

A synergistic hepatotoxic effect between alcohol and ischemia–reperfusion injury has been reported (Addolorato *et al.*, 2001). Alcohol metabolism and long-term anoxia

*Abenavoli, L., Vonghia, L., Cardone, S., D'Angelo, C., Mirijello, A., Leso, V. and Ojetti, V. Institute of Internal Medicine, Catholic University of Rome, Rome, Italy.
Capristo, E. and Malandrino, N. Metabolic Unit, Institute of Internal Medicine, Catholic University of Rome, Rome, Italy.
Caputo, F., Francini, S., Stoppo, M., Vignoli, T. and Bernardi, M. "G. Fontana" Centre for the Study and Multidisciplinary Treatment of Alcohol Addiction, University of Bologna, Italy.
Nardini, M., Scaccini, C. and Ghiselli, A. Free Radical Research Group, National Institute for Food and Nutrition Research, Rome, Italy.

Beer in Health and Disease Prevention
ISBN: 978-0-12-373891-2

are both able to induce a final perturbation of different cellular functions mediated by the production of oxygen-free radicals (OFR) (Caraceni *et al.*, 1997; Rouach *et al.*, 1997; Mantle and Preedy, 1999). In particular, the chronic administration of high doses of ETOH is associated with an increase in the production of superoxide, hydroxyl radical, hydrogen peroxide and alcohol-derived free radicals and a decrease in both enzymatic and non-enzymatic antioxidant systems (Shaw *et al.*, 1983; Tanner *et al.*, 1986; Addolorato *et al.*, 1997b). Moreover, the reoxygenation phase that follows a period of prolonged anoxia is characterized by a massive formation of OFR which is considered a major cause of liver injury occurring in post-ischemic reperfusion (McCord, 1985; Koo *et al.*, 1992; Gasbarrini *et al.*, 1997; Addolorato *et al.*, 2001).

On the other hand, an increase in the antioxidant activity in blood of subjects with a moderate alcohol intake has been recently indicated as a possible protective mechanism against coronary heart disease mortality (Gorinstein *et al.*, 1997), in addition to the alcohol related action on the high-density lipoprotein (HDL), cholesterol (Rapaport, 1989) and on platelet aggregation (Renaud and De Lorgeril, 1992). Wine and beer – the most common ETOH-containing beverages in developed countries – have many non-alcoholic components with antioxidant properties (Maxwell *et al.*, 1994; Rimm *et al.*, 1996). Wine has been found to contain antioxidants, vasorelaxants and stimulants to antiaggregatory mechanisms (Maxwell *et al.*, 1994; Rimm *et al.*, 1996). Beer also contains many different substances with nutritional value, such as vitamins, minerals, organic and inorganic salts, and phenolic compounds. Among these compounds, phenols, essential in determining the taste and in maintaining the foam, are well-documented antioxidants (Bors *et al.*, 1984; De Whalley *et al.*, 1990; Chimi *et al.*, 1991; Nardini *et al.*, 1995) contributing to physical and chemical stability of the packaged beer. Phenolic acids from beer seems to be absorbed from the gastrointestinal tract and extensively metabolized in humans (Nardini *et al.*, 2006).

The present chapter summarizes the recent results obtained by our laboratory on the effects of different alcoholic beverages, including beer, in both animals and humans.

Beer Affects Oxidative Stress Due to ETOH: A Preclinical Study

Animal studies suggested that the daily consumption of beer may have beneficial effects, including the prevention of carcinogenesis and osteoporosis (Kondo, 2004).

As regard to oxidative stress, a preclinical study was conducted by our laboratory to evaluate some parameters of redox status in liver and antioxidant status in plasma of rats chronically fed a beer-containing diet (Gasbarrini *et al.*, 1998). Plasma antioxidant capacity, resistance of lipoproteins to oxidative modifications and sensitivity of the livers to an oxidative stress such as the ischemia–reperfusion injury were investigated. The clamping of the hepatic hilus for a prolonged period of time, in leading to a consumption of reduced substrates coupled with a loss of adenosine triphosphate (ATP), is a prelude to the formation of free radicals when the liver is newly exposed to reoxygenation.

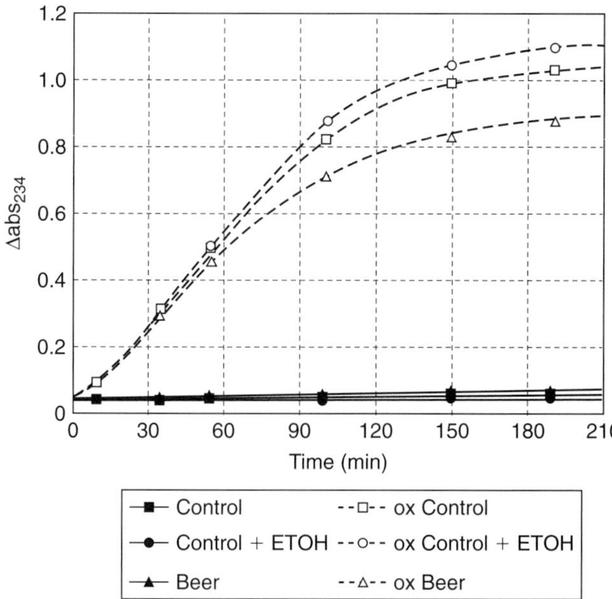

Figure 44.1 Resistance of lipoproteins in control conditions (continuous line) and to oxidative modification (dashed line). *Source*: Reprinted from Gasbarrini *et al.* (1998), with kind permission of Springer Science and Business Media.

In this study, sixty Wistar male rats were divided in three groups fed with three different isocaloric diets for 6 weeks: group A with an alcohol-free diet; group B with a beer-containing diet (30% w/w) and group C with an ETOH-supplemented diet (1.1/100 g, the same as in the beer diet). At the end of the feeding period, rats were analyzed for plasma and liver oxidative status. Some livers were isolated and exposed to ischemia–reperfusion to assess the additional oxidative stress determined by reperfusion.

The results of the study evidenced that there were no statistically significant differences among the three dietary groups for thiobarbituric acid-reactive substance (TBA-RS) and total phenols. Uric acid was markedly higher in group C than in groups A and B. Total plasma antioxidant potential (TRAP) was significantly higher in groups B and C than in group A. Conversely, α-tocopherol appeared to be significantly higher in the control group than in the two alcohol groups. The resistance of lipoproteins to oxidative modification was measured both by recording the kinetics of conjugated diene (CD) formation (Figure 44.1) and by measuring lipid hydroperoxides and TBA-RS concentration after a 1-h incubation (Figure 44.2). Lipoproteins from

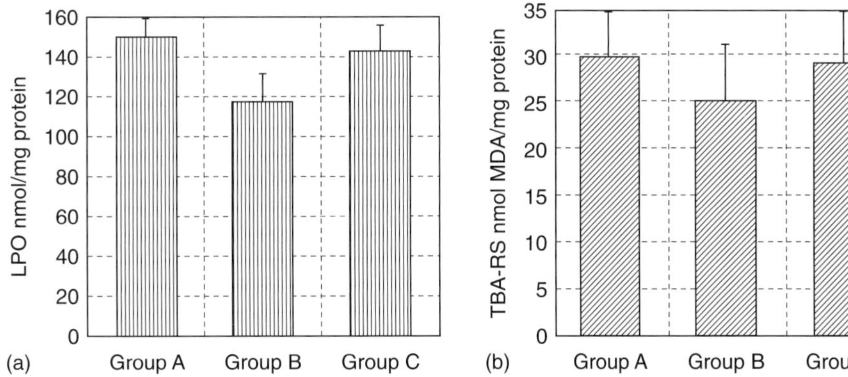

Figure 44.2 Resistance of lipoproteins to oxidative modification assessed by measuring (a) lipid hydroperoxides (LPO) and (b) acid-reactive substance (TBA-RS) concentrations after a 1-h incubation. *Source*: Reprinted from Gasbarrini *et al.* (1998), with kind permission of Springer Science and Business Media.

Table 44.1 Reduced glutathione (GSH), ATP and TBA-RS concentrations in the livers of rats exposed to the beer and ETOH diets and in controls

	N	*GSH (nmol/mg protein)*	*ATP (pmol/mg protein)*	*TBA-RS (nmol MDA/mg protein)*
Group A (control)	6	1.07 ± 0.04	1.14 ± 0.06	0.99 ± 0.05
Group B (beer)	18	1.10 ± 0.10	1.17 ± 0.10	1.01 ± 0.04
Group C (ETOH)	6	0.99 ± 0.02	1.00 ± 0.02	1.18 ± 0.02
P		NS	NS	NS

Source: Modified from Gasbarrini *et al.* (1998), with kind permission of Springer Science and Business Media.

group B showed a slight (although not statistically significant) propensity to resist lipid peroxidation with respect to groups A and C. In fact, as regards the kinetics of CD formation (Figure 44.1), lipoproteins from group B were the most resistant. Moreover, lipid hydroperoxide production (LPO) and TBA-RS concentration after a 1-h incubation (Figure 44.2) tended to be lowest in lipoproteins from group B.

As regard to the sensitivity of liver to ischemia–reperfusion injury, liver concentrations of reduced glutathione (GSH) and TBA-RS did not differ in the three groups after 6 weeks of experimental diet. Conversely, ATP appeared to be slightly lower in the livers of rats exposed to the ETOH diet (Table 44.1). After 60 min of ischemia, liver concentration of GSH and ATP decreased significantly in all groups ($p < 0.01$). GSH values at the end of ischemia did not differ between groups. In livers of rats exposed to ETOH diet (group C), ATP was significantly lower ($p < 0.05$) when compared to the control (group A) and to the beer group (group B) (Figure 44.3). During reperfusion, ATP and GSH recovered progressively in all groups. TBA-RS remained almost stable after ischemia, while it increased significantly during reperfusion (Figure 44.3) in all groups ($p < 0.01$). The livers obtained from rats of group C appear to be more sensitive to ischemia–reperfusion injury, showing a higher formation of TBA-RS during reperfusion (even if not statistically significant when compared to the other groups) (Figure 44.3).

The results of our preclinical study are in line with previous studies that reported no changes in lipid peroxidation values in rats chronically supplemented with ETOH when they were fed a well-balanced diet (Shaw *et al.*, 1984). However, we observed a certain amount of oxidant damage represented by the significantly lower plasma values of vitamin E in groups B and C than in group A. In liver, the basal TBA-RS values did not show any significant difference in any group; nevertheless its significant increase after the ischemia–reperfusion injury supported the toxic effect of ETOH. A toxic effect of ETOH in our study was also represented by the low values of ATP found in the livers of ETOH-fed rats which, probably, resulted from a direct effect of ETOH on ATP degradation (Puig and Fox, 1984; Addolorato *et al.*, 1997b) with consequent increase of plasma uric acid, responsible for a paradoxical action on plasma antioxidant capacity (Lieber, 1988). Since ETOH *per se* does not have any antiperoxidative capacity, vitamin E decreased and total phenolics did not show any modification, uric acid was responsible – at least in part – for the increase in plasma antioxidant capacity found in ETOH-fed rats.

LPO and TBA-RS concentration in lipoproteins tended to be lowest in the beer group with a 20% inhibition of the production of intermediate and end products of lipid

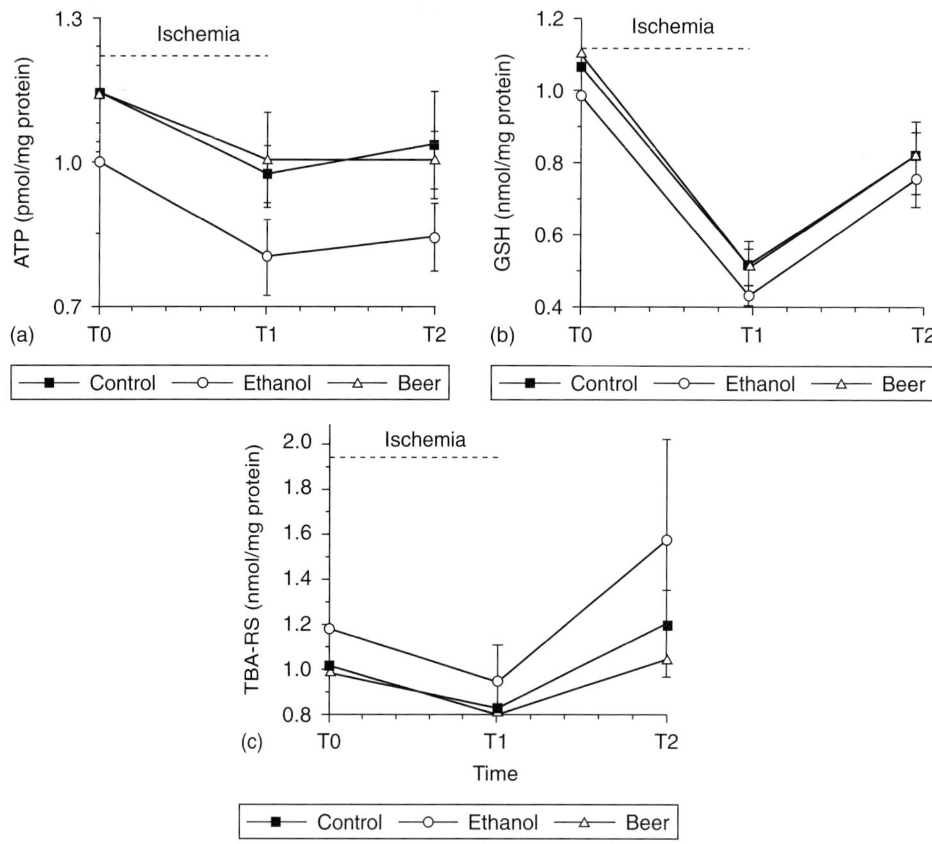

Figure 44.3 (a) ATP, (b) GSH and (c) TBA-RS of rat livers measured at baseline (T0), during ischemia (T1) and reperfusion (T2). *Source*: Reprinted from Gasbarrini *et al*. (1998), with kind permission from Springer Science and Business Media.

peroxidation, indicating a possible propensity to resist lipid peroxidation in the group of rats exposed to the beer-containing diet. When the livers were exposed to ischemia–reperfusion, the beer diet appeared to influence the event. In particular, after ischemia, liver concentrations of GSH and ATP decreased significantly in all groups, in livers of ETOH-fed rats. However, energy status appeared to be significantly lower when compared to the control and to the beer group.

Reoxygenation represents an event characterized by hyperproduction of free radicals, probably triggered by a high concentration of oxidizable substrates and the restored availability of oxygen (Caraceni *et al.*, 1994a, b). In our study, after reperfusion, ATP and GSH progressively recovered in all groups studied; lipid peroxidation was observed in all groups. However, in livers of ETOH-fed rats a greater increase of lipid peroxidation was observed when compared to the control and to the beer group. In conclusion, the minor compounds present in beer appeared to be able to counteract some of the toxic action exerted by ETOH itself. In this connection, a subsequent study has been performed by Rodriguez *et al.* (2001) to verify the real antioxidant role of some beer compounds. These authors have used rat liver microsomes to compare the effectiveness of prenylated chalcones and flavones from hops and beer to inhibit lipid peroxidation induced by Fe^{2+}/ascorbate, Fe^{3+}-adenosine diphosphate/nicotinamide adenine dinucleotide phosphate (Fe^{3+}-ADP/NADPH) and tert-butyl hydroperoxide. All the chalcones, with or without prenyl groups, were found to exhibit antioxidant activity in the iron/ascorbate system. Moreover, the results showed that some of flavonoids inhibited the system of lipid peroxidation in almost the same degree as the Fe^{2+}/ascorbate system, but did not interfere with the activity of NADPH cytochrome P450 reductase activity of rat liver microsomes.

Beer Affects Oxidative Stress due to ETOH: A Clinical Study

In humans, the possible protective effect of alcoholic beverages has been reported in several studies. In particular, alcohol appears to be a protective factor if consumed in moderate amount (25–30 g/die) and regularly during meals (Vogel, 2002). Several studies suggested that this protective effect seems to be independent from the type

Table 44.2 Plasma concentrations of malondialdeide (MDA), GSH, alpha-tocopherol (vitamin E) and ATP of the four groups examined at the start of the study (T0) and after 30 days (T1)

Group	*Redox parameters*	*T0 (±SD)*	*T1 (±SD)*	%
A	MDA	0.94 ± 0.04	1.03 ± 0.05*	9.5
	GSH	1.19 ± 0.04	1.14 ± 0.03*	−4.2
	E vitamin	10.33 ± 1.08	8.83 ± 1.34*	−14.5
	ATP	0.83 ± 0.11	0.81 ± 0.02	−2.4
B	MDA	0.89 ± 0.07	1.06 ± 0.05*	19.0
	GSH	1.17 ± 0.05	1.11 ± 0.03*	−5.1
	E vitamin	9.82 ± 0.64	6.63 ± 0.84*	−32.4
	ATP	0.82 ± 0.03	0.80 ± 0.02	−2.3
C	MDA	0.95 ± 0.04	1.02 ± 0.03*	7.3
	GSH	1.20 ± 0.04	1.10 ± 0.05*	−9.0
	E vitamin	10.47 ± 0.83	8.62 ± 1.07*	−17.6
	ATP	0.91 ± 0.04	0.80 ± 0.03*	−12.0
D	MDA	0.98 ± 0.05	1.02 ± 0.04	4
	GSH	1.17 ± 0.04	1.16 ± 0.04	−0.8
	E vitamin	9.74 ± 1.15	9.72 ± 1.53	−0.2
	ATP	0.91 ± 0.04	0.92 ± 0.05	1

Notes: No significant difference in ATP, GSH, MDA and vitamin E was found in controls before and after the 30-day study period. MDA significantly increased in all subjects exposed to ETOH ($p < 0.05$); a significant decrease in plasma levels of GSH and of vitamin E was found in all subjects which assumed ETOH ($p < 0.05$). ATP significantly decreased in group C ($p < 0.05$). %: variation between T1 and T0 expressed in percentage.

*p < 0.05 (respect to T0).

of beverage consumed (Gaziano *et al.*, 1999) although microcompounds contained in the alcohol beverages result involved in this mechanism (Renaud *et al.*, 1999). Other than the antioxidant action of the microcompounds (Miyagi *et al.*, 1997), several factors have been suggested to maintain the protective effects of the moderate intake of alcohol beverages, including the increase of high-density lipoprotein cholesterol (HDL-C) (Gaziano *et al.*, 1993), of the fibrinolysis processes (Aikens *et al.*, 1997; Dimmitt *et al.*, 1998; Grenett *et al.*, 1998), of vasodilation (Venkow *et al.*, 1999), decrease in blood pressure levels (Hatton *et al.*, 1992), protection against ischemia–reperfusion injury (Chen *et al.*, 1999; Addolorato *et al.*, 2001), inhibition of proliferation and migration of vascular smooth cells (Hendrickson *et al.*, 1998, 1999).

Taking into account our preclinical results, a clinical study has been more recently conducted by our laboratory (Addolorato *et al.*, 2008). In particular, the influence of 30 days of a moderate amount of beer, wine and spirit administration in healthy subjects on oxidant/antioxidant status and body composition has been evaluated. Forty non-smoking male healthy social drinker subjects were randomly divided into four groups. Group A: received 40 g of ETOH per day in lager type beer; group B: 40 g of ETOH per day in red wine; group C: 40 g of ETOH per day in spirit and group D (control group): maintained abstinence from alcohol during the study period. Plasma malondialdehyde (MDA, a lipoperoxidation marker), GSH, α-tocopherol (E vitamin) and ATP were evaluated at the start and at the end of the study. Moreover, the main biochemical blood parameters including total cholesterol, triglycerides, HDL-C and liver parameters were assessed. All subjects underwent to nutritional status evaluation. The results of the study (Table 44.2) evidenced a significant increase of MDA and a significant decrease in GSH in all subjects exposed to ETOH ($p < 0.05$) (Figure 44.4). Moreover, plasmatic levels of ATP significantly decreased in group C ($p < 0.05$) while this parameter was stable in groups A and B (Figure 44.4). In the control group (D), all the investigated blood parameters remained unmodified while in the three alcohol exposed groups some modifications were observed, in particular in HDL-C ($p < 0.05$). As regard to nutritional status evaluation, fat mass (FM) resulted increased in subjects who drank beer (group A) and wine (group B) and decreased in subjects exposed to spirit (group C) (Table 44.3). Free fat mass (FFM) was stable in subjects exposed to beer and wine and increased in subjects exposed to spirit (Table 44.3).

The clinical data obtained in our laboratory showed that a short-term (30 days) ETOH consumption – although in low doses – was able to determine a decrease of antioxidant status in plasma. However, while a significant ATP reduction was observed in subjects exposed to spirit, ATP levels were unmodified when ETOH consumed by beer or wine, at the same way of subjects not exposed to alcohol (group D). Since ATP represents a parameter of the energy level and antioxidant status (Gasbarrini *et al.*, 1996), these results could indicate that the decrease in plasma parameters of antioxidant status appear to be attenuated when

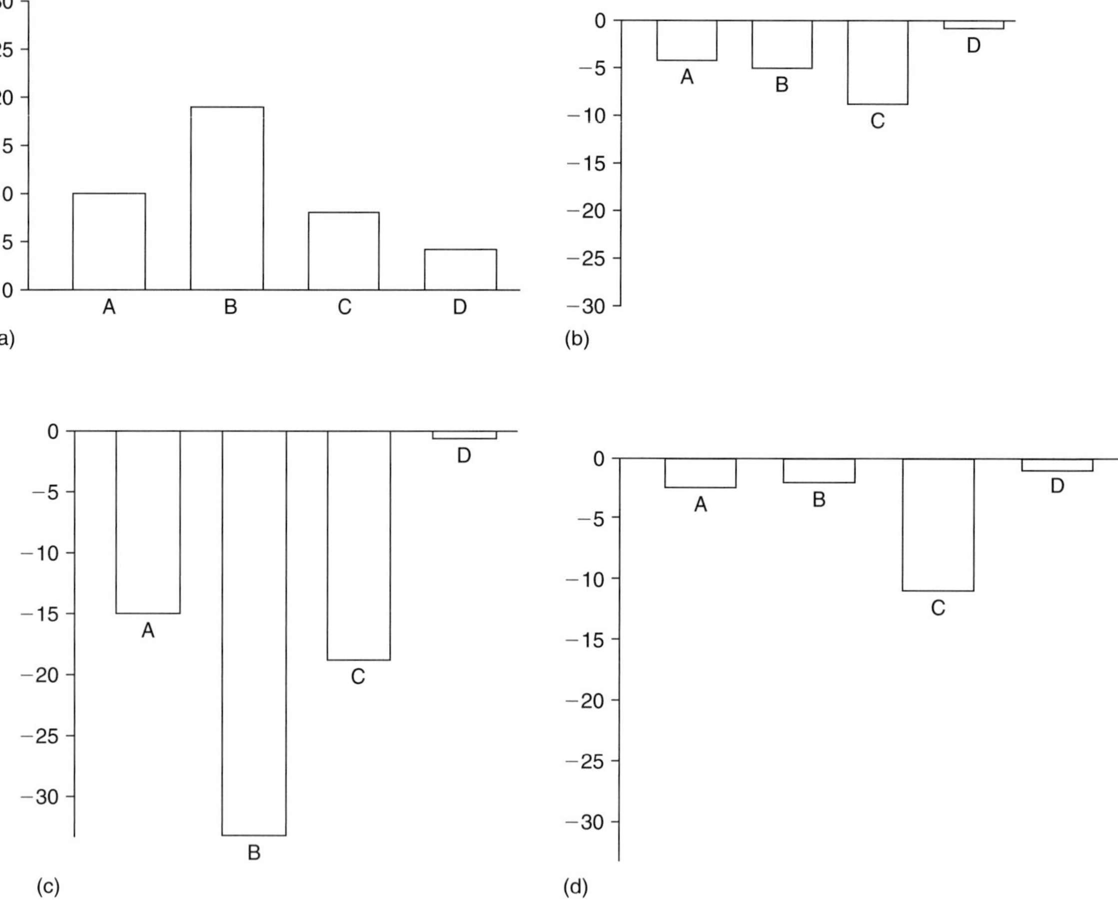

Figure 44.4 Plasma concentrations of (a) malondialdehyde (MDA), (b) GSH, (c) α-tocopherol (vitamin E) and (d) ATP of the groups examined at the start (T0) and the end (T1) of the study. A significant increase of MDA was found in all subjects exposed to ETOH (group A: +9.5%; group B: +19.0%; group C: +7.3%) ($p < 0.05$). On the other hand, GSH (group A: −4.2%; group B: −5.1%; group C: −9.0%) and vitamin E (group A: −14.5%; group B: −32.4%; group C: −17.6%) significantly decreased in all subjects exposed to ETOH ($p < 0.05$). A significant decrease of plasma levels of ATP was found only in group C (−12.0%; $p < 0.05$).

ETOH is consumed in beer or wine. Moreover, these clinical data are also in line with the alcohol related oxidative stress reported both in animals (Addolorato *et al.*, 2001) and humans (Lieber, 2005).

A previous clinical study was performed in healthy non-smoking men, consuming red wine, beer or spirit, investigating the effects of low alcohol doses on antioxidant compounds (Van der Gaad *et al.*, 2000) showed different results from our data with respect to glutathione and E vitamin. The differences between the two studies could be partially related to the possible different genetic and/or environmental factors between the two population evaluated (The Netherlands and Italy). Another possible difference could be related to the different antioxidant capacity of alcoholic beverages originating from different countries, as recently suggested (Meynell *et al.*, 2006).

Another interesting feature observed in our study is represented by the increase of HDL-C, observed in all subjects exposed to ETOH but not in the control group. This result is in line with previous similar data by Gaziano *et al.* (1993, 1999) and could be related to the possible protective effects of moderate amount alcohol intake on cardiovascular diseases (Lucas *et al.*, 2005).

Finally, as regard to the possible effects of moderate alcohol intake on nutritional status, FM decreased in subjects drinking spirit and increased in subjects drinking wine and beer, although these modifications were not significant. ETOH represents a high energy substrate providings 7.2 kcal (29.7 kJ) per gram; however, these calories are defined "empty," since they are not fully utilizable (Lieber, 1993). Accordingly, a previous study from our laboratory showed malnutrition and decrease in FM in chronic alcoholic patients (Addolorato *et al.*, 1997a). These effects were mainly due both to an increase of energetic expenditure related to the microsomal ethanol oxidation system (MEOS) induction, and to an increase of fat oxidation related to the mitochondria system induction due to free radicals action (Addolorato *et al.*, 1998). These data seem

Table 44.3 Weight, body mass index (BMI), fat mass (FM), free fat mass (FFM) and total body water examined in the four groups at the start (T0) and at the end of the study (T1)

Group	*Nutritional parameters*	*T0 (±SD)*	*T1 (±SD)*
A	Weight (kg)	80 ± 9	80 ± 9
	BMI (kg/m^2)	25.76 ± 2.46	25.88 ± 2.4
	FM (kg)	17.01 ± 6.62	17.48 ± 6.29
	FFM (kg)	62.84 ± 4.44	62.77 ± 4.31
	TBW (l)	44.03 ± 3.97	44.14 ± 3.84
B	Weight (kg)	73.05 ± 7.87	73.93 ± 7.46
	BMI (kg/m^2)	23.36 ± 1.96	23.65 ± 1.82
	FM (kg)	12.9 ± 5.3	14.3 ± 5.9
	FFM (kg)	60.1 ± 4.7	59.6 ± 4.3
	TBW (l)	42.08 ± 3.33	41.72 ± 3.29
C	Weight (kg)	77.1 ± 8.03	77.72 ± 8.36
	BMI (kg/m^2)	24.02 ± 2.14	22.22 ± 2.3
	FM (kg)	16.2 ± 4.35	14.62 ± 4.91
	FFM (kg)	60.9 ± 6.15	63.1 ± 6.33
	TBW (l)	42.5 ± 5	44.2 ± 5.5
D	Weight (kg)	76 ± 6	76 ± 6
	BMI (kg/m^2)	24.19 ± 2.02	24.26 ± 2.09
	FM (kg)	14.23 ± 5.49	14.4 ± 5.78
	FFM (kg)	62.01 ± 3.79	62.08 ± 3.89
	TBW (l)	43.71 ± 2.96	43.77 ± 3.03

Note: No significant changes in BMI, FM, FFM and TBW were found in all subjects before and after the study period. FM resulted increased in subjects of groups A and B and decreased in group C.

to be similar to the ones of the present study (Addolorato *et al.*, 2008). Consequently, it could be supposed that these mechanisms may occur also with moderate doses of ETOH consumed by itself. Conversely, when the same quantities of ETOH are contained in alcohol beverages as beer or wine, it is conceivable that the free radical action on the MEOS and mitochondria systems could be counterbalanced by the non-alcoholic compounds with antioxidant action. In this case FM could be increased since drinking during meals determines a prompt alcohol oxidation in competition with the metabolism of other nutrients (Sonko *et al.*, 1994; Addolorato *et al.*, 1997a).

Conclusion

In conclusion, ETOH *per se* seem to be able to increase oxidative damage both in animals and humans, even if it is consumed in moderate amounts. However, both animal and human data suggest that these damages appear to be attenuated when ETOH is assumed in beer. This aspect could be related to the counteracting effects of other antioxidant components.

Summary Points

- The oxidation of ETOH and its metabolites produce superoxide anion and hydrogen peroxide, leading to initiation of peroxidation.
- On the other hand, a moderate alcohol intake increases the antioxidant activity in blood and it has been recently indicated as a possible protective mechanism.
- Beer has many non-alcoholic components with antioxidant properties such as vitamins, minerals, organic and inorganic salts and phenolic compounds.
- Both animal and human studies showed that ETOH *per se* seems to decrease antioxidant parameters and increase lipoperoxidation.
- When ETOH is assumed in beer, some of these alterations appear to be attenuated.
- This aspect seems to be related to the counteracting effects of other antioxidant components present in the beer.

References

Addolorato, G., Capristo, E., Greco, A.V., Stefanini, G.F. and Gasbarrini, G. (1997a). *Alcohol. Clin. Exp. Res.* 21, 962–967.

Addolorato, G., Gasbarrini, A., Marcoccia, S., Simoncini, M., Baccarini, P., Vagni, G., Greco, A., Sbricioli, A., Granato, A., Stefanini, G.F. and Gasbarrini, G. (1997b). *Alcohol* 14, 569–573.

Addolorato, G., Capristo, E., Greco, A.V., Stefanini, G.F. and Gasbarrini, G. (1998). *J. Int. Med.* 244, 387–395.

Addolorato, G., DiCampli, C., Simoncini, M., Pasini, P., Nardo, B., Cavallai, A., Pola, P., Roda, A., Gasbarrini, G. and Gasbarrini, A. (2001). *Dig. Dis. Sci.* 46, 1057–1066.

Addolorato, G., Capristo, E., Leggio, L., Ferrulli, A., Abenavoli, L., Malandrino, N., Farnetti, S., Domenicali, M., D'Angelo, C., Vonghia, L., Mirijello, A., Cardone, S. and Gasbarrini, G. (2006). *Alcohol. Clin. Exp. Res.* 30, 1933–1937.

Addolorato, G., Leggio, L., Ojetti, V., Capristo, E., Gasbarrini, and Gasbarrini, A. (2008). *Appetite* 50, 50–56.

Aikens, M.L., Benza, R.L., Grenett, H.E., Tabengwa, E.M., Davis, G.C. and Booyse, F.M. (1997). *Alcohol. Clin. Exp. Res.* 21, 1471–1478.

Bors, W., Michel, C. and Saran, M. (1984). *Biochem. Biophys. Acta* 796, 312–319.

Caraceni, P., Gasbarrini, A., Van Thiel, D.H. and Borle, A.B. (1994a). *Am. J. Physiol.* 266, G451–G458.

Caraceni, P., Gasbarrini, A., Nussler, A., Di Silvio, M., Batoli, F., Borle, A.B. and Van Thiel, D.H. (1994b). *Hepatology* 20, 1247–1250.

Caraceni, P., Ryu, H.S., Subbotin, V., De Maria, N., Colantoni, A., Roberts, L., Trevisani, F., Bernardi, M. and Van Thiel, D.H. (1997). *Hepatology* 25, 943–949.

Chen, C.H., Gray, M.O. and Mochly-Rosen, D. (1999). *Proc. Natl. Acad. Sci. USA* 96, 12784–12789.

Chimi, H., Cillard, J. and Cillard, P. (1991). *J. Am. Oil Chem. Soc.* 68, 307–312.

De Whalley, C.V., Rankin, S., Hoult, J.R.A., Jessup, W. and Leake, D.S. (1990). *Biochem. Pharmacol.* 39, 1743–1750.

Dimmitt, S.B., Rakic, V., Puddey, I.B., Baker, R., Oostryck, R., Adams, M.J., Chesterman, C.N., Burke, V. and Beilin, L.J. (1998). *Blood Coagul. Fibrinolysis* 9, 39–45.

Gasbarrini, A., Borle, A.B., Caraceni, P., Colantoni, A., Farghali, H., Trevisani, F., Bernardi, M. and Van Thiel, D.H. (1996). *Dig. Dis. Sci.* 41, 2204–2212.

Gasbarrini, A., Colantoni, A., Di Campli, C., De Notariis, S., Masetti, M., Iovine, E., Mazziotti, A., Massari, I., Gasbarrini, G., Pola, P. and Bernardi, M. (1997). *Free Rad. Biol. Med.* 23, 1067–1072.

Gasbarrini, A., Addolorato, G., Simoncini, M., Gasbarrini, G., Fantozzi, P., Mancini, F., Montanari, L., Cardini, M., Ghiselli, A. and Scaccini, C. (1998). *Dig. Dis. Sci.* 43, 1332–1338.

Gaziano, J.M., Buring, J.E., Breslow, J.L., Goldhaber, S.Z., Rosner, B., VanDenburgh, M., Willett, W. and Hennekens, C.H. (1993). *New Engl. J. Med.* 329, 1829–1834.

Gaziano, J.M., Hennekens, C.H., Godfried, S.L., Sesso, H.D., Glynn, R.J., Breslow, J.L. and Buring, J.E. (1999). *Am. J. Cardiol.* 83, 52–57.

Gorinstein, S., Zemser, M., Lichman, I., Berebi, A., Kleipfish, A., Libman, I., Trakhtenberg, S. and Caspi, A. (1997). *J. Int. Med.* 241, 47–51.

Grenett, H.E., Aikens, M.L., Torres, J.A., Demissie, S., Tabengwa, E.M., Davis, G.C. and Booyse, F.M. (1998). *Alcohol. Clin. Exp. Res.* 22, 849–853.

Hatton, D.C., Bukoski, R.D., Edgar, S. and McCarron, D.A. (1992). *J. Hypertens.* 10, 529–537.

Hendrickson, R.J., Cahill, P.A., McKillop, I.H., Sitzmann, J.V. and Redmond, E.M. (1998). *Eur. J. Pharmacol.* 362, 251–259.

Hendrickson, R.J., Okada, S.S., Cahill, P.A., Yankah, E., Sitzmann, J.V. and Redmond, E.M. (1999). *J. Surg. Res.* 84, 64–70.

Kondo, K. (2004). *Biofactors* 22, 303–310.

Koo, A., Komatsu, H., Tao, G., Inoue, M., Guth, P.H. and Kaplowitz, N. (1992). *Hepatology* 15, 507–514.

Krikun, G., Lieber, C.S. and Cederbaum, A.I. (1984). *Biochem. Pharmacol.* 33, 3306–3309.

Lieber, C.S. (1988). *New Engl. J. Med.* 319, 1639–1650.

Lieber, C.S. (1992). *Medical and Nutritional Complications of Alcoholism: Mechanism and Management.* Plenum Publishing, New York.

Lieber, C.S. (1993). *Baillieres Clin. Gastroenterol.* 7, 581–608.

Lieber, C.S. (1995). *New Engl. J. Med.* 333, 1058–1065.

Lieber, C.S. (2005). *Clin. Liver Dis.* 9, 1–35.

Lucas, D.L., Brown, R.A., Wassef, M. and Giles, T.D. (2005). *J. Am. Coll. Cardiol.* 45, 1916–1924.

Mantle, D. and Preedy, V.R. (1999). *Adverse Drug React. Toxicol. Rev.* 18, 235–252.

Maxwell, S., Cruickshank, A. and Thorpe, G. (1994). *Lancet* 344, 193–194.

McCord, J.M. (1985). *New Engl. J. Med.* 312, 159–163.

Meynell, R., Wong, M.C.Y., Mahalingam, S., Fegredo, J.A., Arno, M.J., Wiseman, H. and Preedy, V.R. (2006). *Alcohol. Clin. Exp. Res.* 30, 139A.

Miyagi, Y., Miwa, K. and Inoue, H. (1997). *Am. J. Cardiol.* 80, 1627–1631.

Nardini, M., D'Aquino, M., Tomassi, G., Gentili, V., Di Felice, M. and Scaccini, C. (1995). *Free Rad. Biol. Med.* 19, 541–552.

Nardini, M., Natella, F., Scaccini, C. and Ghiselli, A. (2006). *J. Nutr. Biochem.* 17, 14–22.

Preedy, V.R., Peters, T.J. and Why, H. (1997). *Adverse Drug React. Toxicol. Rev.* 16, 235–256.

Puig, J.G. and Fox, I.H. (1984). *J. Clin. Invest.* 74, 936–941.

Rapaport, E. (1989). *New Engl. J. Med.* 320, 861–864.

Renaud, S. and De Lorgeril, M. (1992). *Lancet* 339, 1523–1526.

Renaud, S.C., Guéguen, R., Siest, G. and Salomon, R. (1999). *Arch. Int. Med.* 159, 1865–1870.

Rimm, E.B., Klatsky, A., Grobbee, D. and Stampfer, M.J. (1996). *BMJ* 312, 731–736.

Rodriguez, R.J., Miranda, C.L., Stevens, J.F., Deinzer, M.L. and Buhler, D.R. (2001). *Food Chem. Toxicol.* 39, 437–445.

Rouach, H., Fataccioli, V., Gentil, M., French, S.W., Morimoto, M. and Nordmann, R. (1997). *Hepatology* 25, 351–355.

Shaw, S., Rubin, K.P. and Lieber, C.S. (1983). *Dig. Dis. Sci.* 28, 585–589.

Shaw, S., Jayatilleke, E. and Lieber, C.S. (1984). *Biochem. Biophys. Res. Commun.* 118, 233–238.

Sonko, B.J., Prentice, A.M., Murgatroyd, P.R., Goldberg, G.R., van de Ven, M.L. and Coward, W.A. (1994). *Am. J. Clin. Nutr.* 59, 619–625.

Tanner, A.R., Bantock, I., Hinks, L., Lloyd, B., Turner, N.R. and Wright, R. (1986). *Dig. Dis. Sci.* 31, 1307–1312.

van der Gaad, M.S., van den Berg, R., van der Berg, H., Schaafsma, G. and Hendriks, H.F.J. (2000). *Eur. J. Clin. Nutr.* 54, 586–591.

Venkow, C.D., Myers, P.R., Tanner, M.A., Su, M. and Vaughan, D.E. (1999). *Thromb. Haemost.* 81, 638–642.

Vogel, R.A. (2002). *Rev. Cardiovasc. Med.* 3, 7–13.

45

Antioxidant Capacity of Hops

C. Proestos and M. Komaitis Laboratory of Food Chemistry, Agricultural University of Athens, Iera Odos, Athens, Greece

Abstract

Beer is a polyphenol-rich beverage that has recently been reported to reduce the incidence of coronary heart disease and cancer. Some of the mechanisms by which this effect occurs have already been elucidated and include antioxidant, antiinflammatory, antimutagenic, antiangiogenic, estrogen-interfering, and cell cycle regulating actions of its phenolic compounds. The antioxidant capacity of hop polyphenols is probably one of the main reasons for the health-promoting properties attributed to beer. In the present paper, the phenolic substances of hops were identified and quantified by RP-HPLC-UV-vis (reversed-phase–high-performance liquid chromatography–ultraviolet–visible), after comparison with reference standards. The antioxidant capacity tests can be categorized into two groups: assays for radical scavenging ability and assays that test the ability to inhibit lipid oxidation under accelerated conditions. The inhibition of lipid oxidation of the extracts was determined with the Rancimat test using sunflower oil as a substrate. Protection factors (PF) were greater than 1 (1.3 and 1.1 for ground material and methanol extracts) which indicates inhibition of lipid oxidation. Free radical scavenging activity was measured using the stable free radical 1, 1-diphenyl-2-picrylhydrazyl (DPPH). Results were compared with standard compounds (butylated hydroxytoluene (BHT) and ascorbic acid). IC_{50} value (concentration of substrate that causes 50% loss of the DPPH activity) of hop methanol extract (49.8) was found to be similar to BHT (18.5) and to other standard phenolic compounds for example ferulic acid (32.4). On the contrary, ascorbic acid IC_{50} value was lower than of hop extracts. The higher the antioxidant capacity, the lower is the value of EC_{50}. The FRAP (ferric-reducing antioxidant power) assay was also employed to measure the reducing power of antioxidants in hops. The change of absorbance ($\Delta A = A_{4\,\text{min}} - A_{0\,\text{min}}$ and $\Delta A = A_{30\,\text{min}} - A_{0\,\text{min}}$) was calculated. It can be seen from the results that the change in absorbance between 0 and 30 min for the 60% ethanol hop extract is significantly higher ($p < 0.05$) than the other extracts. Between 0 and 4 min the ethanol extract has significantly lower ($p < 0.05$) change in absorbance than the other extracts. There is also a significant difference ($p < 0.05$) in ΔA for the methanol extracts after 4 and 30 min. Total phenol concentration of the extracts was estimated with Folin–Ciocalteu reagent using gallic acid as a standard.

Introduction

Beer is a complex alcoholic beverage made from barley (malt), hop, water, and yeast. It is rich in nutrient as well as non-nutrient components including carbohydrates, amino acids, minerals, vitamins, and phenolic compounds. Phenolic constituents of beer are derived from malt (70–80%) and hops (20–30%) (Knorr, 1978; De Keukeleire, 2000). Structural classes include simple phenols, benzoic- and cinnamic-acid derivatives, coumarins, catechins, di-, tri- and oligomeric proanthocyanidins, (prenylated) chalcones, and flavonoids as well as alpha- and *iso*-alpha-acids derived from hops. Compounds belonging to different structural classes have distinct profiles of biological activity in *in vitro* test systems, and in combination might lead to enhanced effects. Scientific evidence has accumulated over the past 10 years pointing to the cancer and coronary heart disease preventive potential of selected hop-derived beer constituents, i.e. prenylflavonoids including xanthohumol and isoxanthohumol, and hop bitter acids.

The hop plant (*Humulus lupulus* L., Cannabinaceae) is used as a tranquilizer or is used to add bitterness to the beer. The hop cones (female inflorescences), are widely used in the brewing industry to add bitterness and aroma to beer. Several flavonoids such as chalcones and flavanones with prenyl or geranyl side chains have been identified in hops and beer (Stevens *et al.*, 1997, 1998, 1999b). As phenolic compounds, these flavonoids may be responsible for the antioxidant activity of beer, which is higher than that of green tea, red wine or grape juice (Vinson *et al.*, 1999). The dried hop cones contain 4–14% polyphenols, mainly phenolic acids, chalcones, flavonoids, catechins, and

Beer in Health and Disease Prevention
ISBN: 978-0-12-373891-2

proanthocyanidins (Stevens *et al.*, 1998; De Keukeleire *et al.*, 1999; Taylor *et al.*, 2003). In addition, hops provides a resin containing monoacyl phloroglucides, which are converted to hop bitter acids during the brewing process (De Keukeleire, 2000; De Keukeleire *et al.*, 2003). Barley polyphenols undergo changes during the malting and brewing process and are less well characterized than phenolic compounds from hops. However, specific proanthocyanidins from barley and malt have been separated and quantified (Madigan *et al.*, 1994; McMurrough and Baert, 1994; Friedrich *et al.*, 2000).

Interest in employing antioxidants from natural sources to increase the shelf life of foods is considerably enhanced by consumer preference for natural ingredients and concerns about the toxic effects of synthetic antioxidants. Selection of a suitable extraction procedure can increase the antioxidant concentration relative to the plant material. In view of the differences between the extraction techniques, it is obvious that extracts from the same plant material may widely vary with respect to their antioxidant concentration and pattern. The concentration of individual antioxidants in plant extracts determined by HPLC is the preferred way to provide standardized information. However, the antioxidant pattern is usually rather complex, thus making the prediction of a mixture's potency based on compositional data difficult. Therefore, the employment of specific assays to test the antioxidant capacity of the extracts – including synergistic effects is required. A variety of tests expressing antioxidant capacity has been suggested. The tests can be categorized into two groups: assays for radical scavenging ability and assays that test the ability to inhibit lipid oxidation under accelerated conditions. The antioxidant reactions involve multiple steps including the initiation, propagation, branching, and termination of free radicals. The antioxidants which inhibit or retard the formation of free radicals from their unstable precursors (initiation) are called the "preventive" antioxidants, and those which interrupt the radical chain reaction (propagation and branching) are the "chain-breaking" antioxidants (Ou *et al.*, 2001). Test systems that evaluate the radical scavenging ability of antioxidants aim to simulate basic mechanisms involved in lipid oxidation by measuring either the reduction of stable radicals or radicals generated by radiolysis, photolysis, or the Fenton reaction (Blois, 1958; Madsen *et al.*, 1996). Accelerated test systems mainly include lipids, which rapidly oxidize to simulate a long induction period in a short time. To accelerate oxidation, an increase in temperature is often used. This study compares assays used in the laboratories of the authors for the assessment of the antioxidant capacity of hops.

The method of reversed-phase HPLC coupled with a UV-vis multiwavelength detector was used for the determination of hop polyphenols. This method enables the collection of on-line spectra and simultaneous quantification in several wavelengths of the phenolic compounds examined.

Experimental techniques used in the analysis of hops

Standards Gallic acid, gentisic acid, *p*-coumaric acid, vanillic acid, ferulic acid, syringic acid, (+)-catechin, quercetin, apigenin, naringenin, eriodictyol were purchased from Sigma-Aldrich (Steinheim, Germany). Luteolin was from Roth (Karlsruhe, Germany). Caffeic acid was from Merck (Darmstadt, Germany). (−)-Epicatechin and ascorbic acid were from Fluka AG (Buchs, Switzerland). Rutin was from Alexis Biochemicals (Lausen, Switzerland). Hydroxytyrosol, *p*-hydroxybenzoic acid, and BHT (butylated hydroxytoluene) were a kind donation from the National Agricultural Research Foundation (N.AG.RE.F., Greece). Quantification was done via a calibration with standards (external standard method). All standards were prepared as stock solutions in methanol. Working standards were made by diluting stock solutions in 62.5% aqueous methanol containing BHT 1 g/l, and 6 mol/l HCl to yield concentrations ranging between 0.5 and 25 mg/l. Stock/working solutions of the standards were stored in darkness at −18°C.

Solvents and Reagents Methanol, acetone, acetic acid, dichloromethane were pro analysis (p.a.), acetonitrile and glacial acetic acid were HPLC grade, and sodium acetate and iron chloride all purchased from Sigma-Aldrich (Steinheim, Germany). Water was supplied by a Milli-Q water purifier system from Milipore (Bedford, MA, USA). The Folin–Ciocalteu reagent was from Merck (Darmstadt, Germany), 1, 1-diphenyl-2-picrylhydrazyl (DPPH) was obtained from Sigma-Aldrich (Steinheim, Germany), and TPTZ, 2,4,6-Tri(2-pirydil)-*s*-triazine was from Fluka (Buchs, Switzerland).

Plant Material Hop (*Humulus lupulus* L.) was obtained commercially and dried in the air (at 25°C in the dark). It was analyzed within 3 months of collection.

Sample Preparation The extraction method used for dried samples had as follows: 40 ml of 62.5% aqueous methanol containing BHT (1 g/l) was added to 0.5 g of dried sample. Then 10 ml of 6 mol/l HCl were added. The mixture was stirred carefully. In each sample nitrogen was bubbled for ca. 40–60 s. The extraction mixture was then sonicated for 15 min and refluxed in a water bath at 90°C for 2 h. The mixture was then filtered and made up to 100 ml with methanol (Justesen *et al.*, 1998), furthermore filtered quickly through a 0.45 μm membrane filter (Millex-HV) and injected to HPLC. To prevent enzymic oxidation, extraction of the polyphenols from plants with boiling alcohol is essential and should be adopted routinely (Harborne, 1998). For this reason all steps were carried out in dark (flasks were covered with aluminum foil) and under nitrogen atmosphere (the headspace above the plant extract was under an inert atmosphere created by a stream of nitrogen).

HPLC Analysis The analytical HPLC system employed consisted of a JASCO high-performance liquid chromatograph coupled with a UV-vis multiwavelength detector (MD-910 JASCO). The analytical data were evaluated using a JASCO data processing system (DP-L910/V). The separation was achieved on a Waters Spherisorb® 5 μm ODS2 4.6 × 250 mm column at ambient temperature. The mobile phase consisted of water with 1% glacial acetic acid (solvent A), water with 6% glacial acetic acid (solvent B), and water-acetonitrile (65:30 v/v) with 5% glacial acetic acid (solvent C). The gradient used was similar to that used for the determination of phenolics in wine (Parrilla *et al.*, 1999) with some modifications: 100% A 0–10 min, 100% B 10–30 min, 90% B/10% C 30–50 min, 80% B/20% C 50–60 min, 70% B/30% C 60–70 min, 100% C 70–105 min, 100% A 105–110; post time 10 min before next injection. The flow rate was 0.5 ml/min and the injection volume was 20 μl. The monitoring wavelength was 280 nm for the phenolic acids and 320 and 370 nm (flavones, flavonoles). The identification of each compound was based on a combination of retention time and spectral matching.

Antioxidant Capacity Tests

Rancimat Test This assay tests the ability to inhibit lipid oxidation under accelerated conditions.

Samples of sunflower oil (3.5 g) containing 0.02% w/w methanol or acetone extract or 2% w/w ground material were subjected to oxidation at 110°C (air flow 20 l/h). The standard compounds (0.02% addition) were also examined. Induction periods, *IP* (h), were recorded automatically. The protection factors (PF) were calculated according to the following formula: ($PF = IP_{extract}/IP_{extract}$) (Exarchou *et al.*, 2002).

Determination of the Total Phenolic Content Total phenolic content was measured by the Folin–Ciocalteu assay (Kähkönen *et al.*, 1999). Quantification was performed with the hydrolyzed samples. Results were expressed as mg of gallic acid/g dry sample.

DPPH Assay The DPPH$^•$ (Figure 45.1) radical is one of the few stable organic nitrogen radicals, commercially available, which bears a deep purple color. This assay is based on the measurement of the reducing ability of antioxidants toward DPPH$^•$. The ability can be evaluated by measuring the decrease of its absorbance. The widely used decoloration assay was first reported by Brand-Williams *et al.* (1995). This antioxidant assay is based on measurement of the loss of DPPH color at 517 nm after reaction with test compounds (Bondet *et al.*, 1997) and the reaction is monitored by a spectrometer. Experiments were carried out according to the method of Blois (1958) with a slight modification. Briefly, a 1 mmol/l solution of DPPH radical solution in methanol was prepared and then, 1 ml of this solution was mixed with 3 ml of sample solution in different concentrations after extraction with different solvents (methanol, water, dichloromethane). Dichloromethane was removed in a rotary evaporator at 40°C and the residue was dissolved in methanol. After 30 min, the absorbance was measured at 517 nm. The %DPPH radical scavenging is calculated from the equation: %DPPH radical − scavenging = $[(Abs_{control} - Abs_{sample})/Abs_{control}] \times 100$.

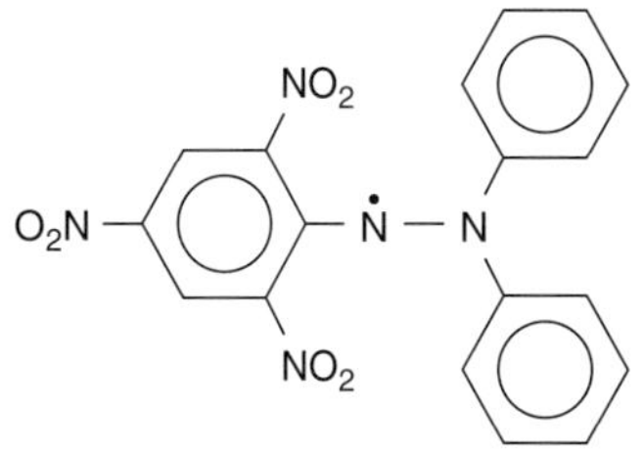

Figure 45.1 The structure of DPPH$^•$ radical.

The DPPH solution without sample solution was used as a control. The inhibitory concentration 50 (IC_{50} or EC_{50}) value of extracts (the concentration that causes a decrease in the initial DPPH concentration by 50%) was calculated by using the calibration %DPPH radical − scavenging =f (concentration (μg/ml) and expressed in μg/ml). Results were compared with ascorbic acid, BHT and some phenolic compounds which were used as standards.

Ferric-Reducing Antioxidant Power The FRAP assay was originally developed by Benzie and Strain (1996) to measure reducing power in plasma, but the assay subsequently has also been adapted and used for the assay of antioxidants in botanicals (Benzie and Szeto, 1999; Gil, 2000; Ou *et al.*, 2002; Proteggente *et al.*, 2002; Pellegrini *et al.*, 2003). The reaction measures reduction of ferric 2,4,6-tripyridyl-*s*-triazine (TPTZ) to a colored product (Figure 45.2) (Benzie, 1996).

Herein a ferric salt, TPTZ is used as an oxidant. FRAP is carried out under acidic (pH 3.6) conditions. The assay involves the following procedures: The oxidant is prepared by mixing TPTZ (2.5 ml, 10 mmol/l in 40 mmol/l HCl), 25 ml of acetate buffer, and 2.5 ml of $FeCl_3.H_2O$ (20 mmol/l). The conglomerate is referred to as "FRAP reagent." To measure FRAP value, 300 μl of freshly prepared FRAP reagent is warmed to 37°C and a reagent blank reading is taken at 593 nm; then 10 μl of sample (extracted with water, ethanol, 60% ethanol and methanol) and 30 μl of water are added. Absorbance readings are taken at 0, 4, and 30 min. The change of absorbance ($\Delta A = A_{4\,min} - A_{0\,min}$ and $\Delta A = A_{30\,min} - A_{0\,min}$) is calculated.

Fe^{3+} – TPTZ + reducing antioxidant ⟹ Fe^{2+} – TPTZ (intense blue at 595 nm)

Figure 45.2 Reaction for FRAP assay.

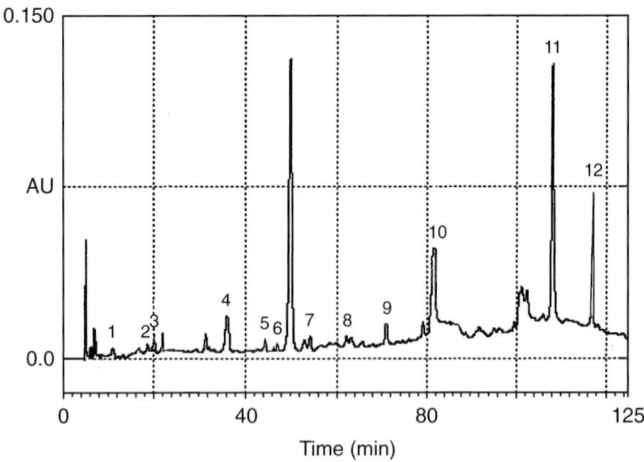

Figure 45.3 A typical HPLC chromatogram of hop extract.

Results derived form HPLC Analysis Using the aforementioned procedure, the phenolic substances present in hop extract were separated and quantified. HPLC with a UV-vis multiwavelength detector was used since all phenolic compounds show intense absorption in the UV region of the spectrum. The present method is simple, easy to use, and effective enough for the identification and quantification of major phenolic compounds. A similar technique has been reported by other authors, for the analysis of major flavonoid aglycones (Mattila *et al.*, 2000; Justesen and Knuthsen, 2001). Spherisorb® ODS2 stationary phase, which was used in this study to separate phenolic acids and flavonoids in the aforementioned wavelengths, produced satisfactory results. After extraction and acid hydrolysis the content of phenolic substances was determined. Quantification was done via a calibration with standards (external standard method). A typical HPLC chromatogram of hop extract is presented in Figure 45.3.

The amount of phenolic compounds (phenolic acids and flavonoids) detected in the analyzed sample is shown in Table 45.1. Results are expressed in mg/100 g dry sample. The most abundant phenolic acids were ferulic (6.4 mg/100 g dry sample) and vanillic acid (2.9 mg/100 g dry sample). Flavan-3-ols (Catechins), (+)-Catechin, and (−)-epicatechin were also detected (4.9 and 1.1 mg/100 g dry sample, respectively). Kaempferol, quercetin and rutin (quercetin 3-o-rhamnose glycoside) were the most abundant flavonoids detected (14.2, 8.1, and 2.0 mg/100 g dry sample, respectively). The levels of phenolic compounds were similar to those reported in previous investigations of these compounds in hop plant (Stevens *et al.*, 1998; De Keukeleire *et al.*, 1999; Stevens *et al.*, 2002).

Table 45.1 Summary of the amount of detected phenolic constituents (mg/100 g dry sample) of hops

Structural classes		*mg/100 g dry sample*
Benzoic acidderivatives		
	p-Hydroxy benzoic acid	0.8
	Vanillic acid	2.9
	Gallic acid	0.3
	Syringic acid	0.5
Cinnamic acids		
	p-Coumaric acid	0.7
	Caffeic acid	0.6
	Ferulic acid	6.4
Flavan-3-ols (Catechins)		
	(+)-Catechin	4.9
	(−)-Epicatechin	1.1
Flavonoles		
	Kaempferol	14.2
	Quercetin	8.1
	Rutin	2.0

Phenolic compounds are found usually in nature as esters and rarely as glycosides or in free form (Rice-Evans *et al.*, 1996). Thus hydrolysis was needed for their identification and quantitative determination. Flavonoids are also present in plants in the form of glycosides. Any flavonoid may

Table 45.2 Total phenolics in hops (*Humulus lupulus* L.) extracts and their antioxidant capacity (expressed as PF values)

Family species	*Part examined*	*Drying method*	*Total phenolics[b] (mg gallic acid/g dry sample)*	*PF[c] (ground material)*	*PF (methanol extracts)*	*PF (acetone extracts)*
Cannabinaceae *Humulus lupulus*	Leaves + flowers	Air[a]	6.9 ± 0.1	1.3	1.1	1.0

[a] Air: air drying.
[b] Mean of triplicate assays.
[c] PF: protection factor.

occur in a plant in several glycosidic combinations. For this reason, hydrolysis was used to release the aglycones which can be further investigated by HPLC. The data presented in Tables 45.1 are considered as indicative of phenolic content of these aromatic plants. Among others, time of harvest, and storing conditions, are considered responsible for the observed variations in the phenolic contents.

Antioxidant Capacity Tests

Total Phenolic Content (Folin–Ciocalteu (F-C) Assay) and Rancimat Test The antioxidant capacity (expressed as PF values) and the total phenolic content of hop extract are shown in Table 45.2. There is always the controversy over what is being detected in total antioxidant capacity assays only phenols, or phenols plus reducing agents plus possibly metal chelators. The F-C assay has for many years been used as a measure of total phenolics in natural products, but the basic mechanism is an oxidation/reduction reaction and, as such, can be considered another antioxidant method. The original F-C method developed by Folin (1927) originated from chemical reagents used for tyrosine analysis in which oxidation of phenols by a molybdotungstate reagent yields a colored product with λ_{max} at 745–750 nm. The method is simple, sensitive, and precise. However, the reaction is slow at acid pH, and it lacks specificity. Singleton and Rossi (1965) improved the method with a molybdotungstophosphoric heteropolyanion reagent that reduced phenols more specifically; the λ_{max} for the product is 765 nm. They also imposed mandatory steps and conditions to obtain reliable and predictable data: (1) proper volume ratio of alkali and F-C reagent; (2) optimal reaction time and temperature for color development; (3) monitoring of optical density at 765 nm; and (4) use of gallic acid as the reference-standard phenol. Lack of standardization of methods can lead to several orders of magnitude difference in detected phenols. Hence, continued efforts to standardize the assay are clearly warranted.

The outcome of the Rancimat test supports the hypothesis that hop extracts are good sources of natural antioxidants such as phenolic compounds. This method offers an efficient, simple and automated assay. Chain-breaking antioxidants react with peroxyl radicals, introducing a lag period into the peroxidation process that corresponds with the time taken for the antioxidant to be consumed. Hop methanol and acetone extracts, at the low concentration tested, produced good protection against autoxidation for sunflower oil. When ground material was added to sunflower oil, PF were slightly higher compared to the addition of methanol and acetone extracts (Table 45.2). In the same table the PF values for the standard compounds (0.02% addition) examined ranged from 1.2 to 1.5 for all phenolic acids, except for gallic acid which had $PF = 4.5$. (+)-Catechin hydrated and (−)-epicatechin had PF values 1.8 and 2.5, respectively, whereas the flavonoids (rutin, quercetin, apigenin, luteolin, eriodictyol, and naringenin) had PF values ranging from 1 to 1.2. The PF value for hydroxytyrosol was 1.4 and 1.8 for BHT. PF were greater than 1 (1.3 and 1.1 for ground material and methanol extracts) which indicates inhibition of lipid oxidation. The higher the PF, the better the antioxidant capacity. The effect of hop methanolic extract on the stability of sunflower oil during accelerated oxidation conditions was comparable with the effect of BHT. Bearing in mind that BHT is a pure compound while the extracts are complex mixtures containing ineffective substances in terms of their antioxidant activity or even some amount of pro-oxidant compounds, it could be supposed that hops contains very strong constituents retarding lipid peroxidation.

DPPH Assay The DPPH method is widely used to test the ability of compounds to act as free radical scavengers or hydrogen donors, and to evaluate antioxidant capacity. The parameter EC_{50} ("efficient concentration" value) otherwise called the IC_{50} value, is used for the interpretation of the results from the DPPH method and is defined as the concentration of substrate that causes 50% loss of the DPPH activity (color). The higher the antioxidant capacity, the lower is the value of EC_{50}. This can be a disadvantage in interpretation of results. That is why results are presented graphically as a bar chart and in numerical form. IC_{50} values of hop extracts were found to be similar to BHT and ascorbic acid values (Table 45.3). In the same table the IC_{50} values of some standard phenolic compounds are also presented.

All the IC_{50} values of the hop extracts (extracted with methanol, water, and dichloromethane) were determined

Table 45.3 Representative IC_{50} values of hop extracts and standard compound tested

Hops and standard compounds	$IC_{50}{}^{a}$ (μg/ml)		
	Methanol	*Water*	*Dichloromethane*
Humulus lupulus L.	49.8	98.6	505.5
Quercetin	16.6	–	–
(−)-epicatechin	15.1	–	–
(+)-catechin	19.5	–	–
Kaempferol	21.2	–	–
Ferulic acid	32.4	–	–
Ascorbic acid	3.9	–	–
BHT	18.5	–	–

[a] IC_{50}: (inhibitory concentration 50, expressed in μg/ml).

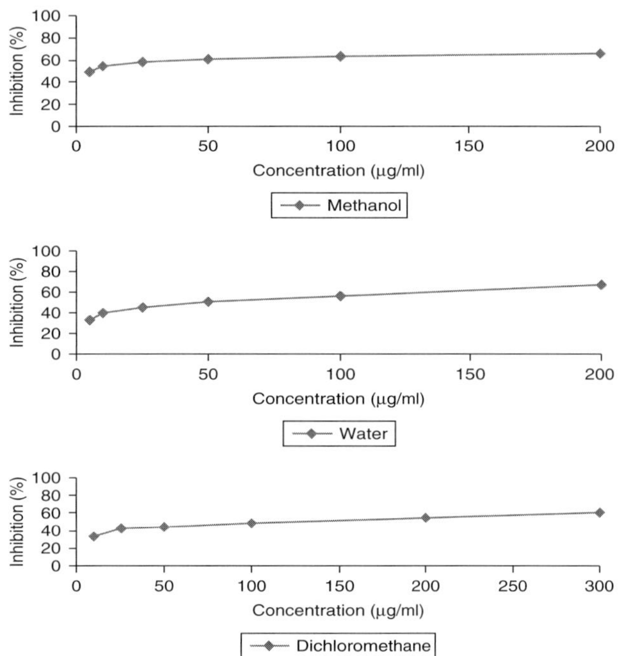

Figure 45.4 %DPPH radical scavenging against concentration (μg/ml) curves used to determine the IC_{50} values of hop extracts.

from the curves plotted in Figure 45.4. These curves show the %DPPH radical scavenging against concentration (μg/ml). The IC_{50} values of hop extracts for all solvents were much higher than the values of all the standard compounds tested. Hence, the antioxidant capacity of hops was not as high as the standard compounds. Methanol extract has given better antioxidant capacity compared to other solvent extracts.

The test is simple and rapid and needs only a UV-vis spectrophotometer to perform, which probably explains its widespread use in antioxidant screening. The assay is not a competitive reaction because DPPH is both a radical probe and oxidant. DPPH color can be lost via either radical reaction (HAT) or reduction (SET) as well as unrelated reactions, and steric accessibility is a major determinant of the reaction. Thus, small molecules that have better access to the radical site have higher apparent antioxidant capacity with this test. DPPH is a stable nitrogen radical that bears no similarity to the highly reactive and transient peroxyl radicals involved in lipid peroxidation. Many antioxidants that react quickly with peroxyl radicals may react slowly or may even be inert to DPPH due to steric inaccessibility. DPPH is also decolorized by reducing agents as well as H transfer, which also contributes to inaccurate interpretations of antioxidant capacity.

Ferric-Reducing Antioxidant Power It has been argued that the ability to reduce iron has little relationship to the radical quenching processes (H transfer) mediated by most antioxidants. However, oxidation or reduction of radicals to ions still stops radical chains, and reducing power reflects the ability of compounds to modulate redox tone in plasma and tissues. The FRAP mechanism is totally electron transfer rather than mixed SET and HAT, so in combination with other methods can be very useful in distinguishing dominant mechanisms with different antioxidants. In addition, because reduced metals are active propagators of radical chains via hydroperoxide reduction to $RO^{\bullet}$, it would be interesting to evaluate whether high FRAP values correlate with the tendency of polyphenols to become pro-oxidants under some conditions. This has been shown for some flavones and flavanones (Cao *et al.*, 1997) which also have high FRAP values.

The experiments were based in the measurement of the absorbance of the hop extracts after extraction with four different solvents at time 0 (beginning of the measurement) and after 4 and 30 min. The change of absorbance ($\Delta A = A_{4\,min} - A_{0\,min}$ and $\Delta A = A_{30\,min} - A_{0\,min}$) was calculated. In Figure 45.5 the change in absorbance from 0 to 30 minutes for all solvent extracts is presented, as well as with the effect of the solvent to the change of absorbance (ΔA) for the two time measurements (4 and 30 min). It can be seen from the results that the change in absorbance between 0 and 30 min for the 60% ethanol hop extract is significantly higher ($p < 0.05$) than the other extracts. Between 0 and 4 min the ethanol extract has significantly lower ($p < 0.05$) change in absorbance than the other extracts. There is also a significant difference ($p < 0.05$) in ΔA for the methanol extracts after 4 and 30 min. No other significant difference was observed. 60% ethanol and methanol extracts changed significantly the reducing capacity of antioxidants present in hops based on the ferric ion.

The FRAP assay evolves from assays that rely on the hypothesis that the redox reactions proceed so rapidly that all reactions are complete within 4 and 6 min, respectively, but in fact this is not always true. FRAP results can vary tremendously depending on the time scale of analysis. Fast-reacting phenols that bind the iron or break down to compounds with lower or different reactivity are best

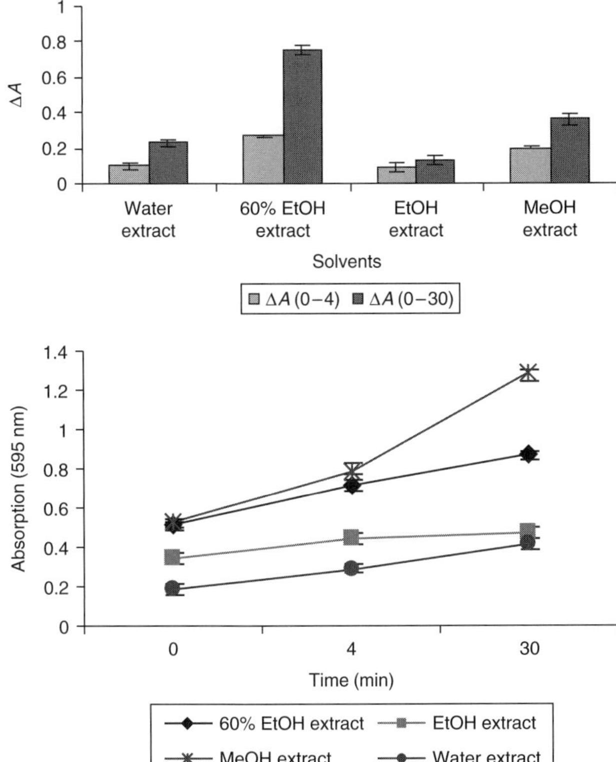

Figure 45.5 Change of absorbance ($\Delta A = A_{4\,\text{min}} - A_{0\,\text{min}}$ and $\Delta A = A_{30\,\text{min}} - A_{0\,\text{min}}$) and absorption readings taken at 0, 4, and 30 min.

analyzed with short reaction times (e.g. 4 min). However, some polyphenols react more slowly and require longer reaction times for detection (e.g. 30 min). That is why in our experiment absorbance was measured at 4 min as well as at 30 min. The order of reactivity of a series of antioxidants can vary tremendously and even invert, depending on the analysis time (Pulido *et al.*, 2000). These authors recently examined the FRAP assay of dietary polyphenols in water and methanol. The absorption (A_{593}) slowly increased for polyphenols such as caffeic acid, tannic acid, ferulic acid, ascorbic acid, and quercetin, even after several hours of reaction time. Thus, a single-point absorption endpoint may not represent a completed reaction. In contrast to other tests of total antioxidant capacity, the FRAP assay is simple, speedy, inexpensive, and robust and does not require specialized equipment.

Acknowledgments

We thank European Social Fund (ESF), Operational Program for Educational and Vocational Training II (EPEAEK II) and particularly the Program PYTHAGORAS, for funding the above work, and the National Agricultural Research Foundation (N.AG.RE.F., Greece), for providing some of the standards used in the research.

Summary Points

- Hops (*Humulus lupulus* L.) contains polyphenols (natural antioxidants), which are believed to be effective nutrients in the prevention of oxidative stress-related diseases such as cancer and heart diseases.
- Hops and its extracts retard oxidative degradation of lipids as it is shown by the Rancimat test.
- Hops antioxidant constituents, mainly phenolic compounds, are free radical scavengers as shown by the DPPH assay. Hence, they can protect foods against spoilage caused by radical chain reactions.
- Antioxidant capacity of hops was also determined by the FRAP assay, which was used to measure reducing power of hop antioxidants.
- Antioxidant capacity tests can be categorized into two groups: assays for radical scavenging ability and assays that test the ability to inhibit lipid oxidation under accelerated conditions.
- Antioxidants can deactivate radicals by two major mechanisms, HAT and SET. The end result is the same, regardless of mechanism, but kinetics and potential for side reactions differ.
- The F-C assay, which was used to determine the total phenolic compounds, has for many years been used as a measure of total phenolics in natural products, but the basic mechanism is an oxidation/reduction reaction and, as such, can be considered as another method to determine antioxidant capacity.
- The influence of the hop variety, storage, and production procedures still has to be investigated in detail to be able to draw the utmost benefit for the brewing technology.

References

Benzie, I.F.F. (1996). *Clin. Biochem.* 19, 111–116.

Benzie, I.F.F. and Strain, J.J. (1996). *Anal. Biochem.* 239, 70–76.

Benzie, I.F.F. and Szeto, Y.T. (1999). *J. Agric. Food Chem.* 47, 633–636.

Blois, M.S. (1958). *Nature* 181, 1199–1200.

Bondet, V., Brand-Williams, W. and Berset, C. (1997). *Lebensm. Wiss. Technol.* 30, 609–615.

Brand-Williams, W., Cuvelier, M.E. and Berset, C. (1995). *Lebensm. Wiss. Technol.* 28, 25–30.

Cao, G., Sofic, E. and Prior, R.L. (1997). *Free Radical Biol. Med.* 22, 749–760.

De Keukeleire, D. (2000). *Quím Nova* 23, 108–112.

De Keukeleire, D., De Cooman, L., Rong, H. *et al.* (1999). In Gross, *Plant Polyphenols 2: Chemistry, Biology, Pharmacology, Ecology*, pp. 739–760. Kluwer Academics/Plenum Publishers, New York.

De Keukeleire, J., Ooms, G. and Heyerick, A. (2003). *J. Agric. Food Chem.* 51, 4436–4441.

Exarchou, V., Nenadis, N., Tsimidou, M., Gerothanasis, I.P., Troganis, A. and Boskou, D. (2002). *J. Agric. Food Chem.* 50, 5294–5299.

Folin, O. (1927). *J. Biol. Chem.* 73, 649–672.

Friedrich, W., Eberhardt, A. and Galensa, J. (2000). *Eur. Food Res. Technol.* 211, 56–64.

Gil, M.I. (2000). *J. Agric. Food Chem.* 48, 4581–4589.

Harborne, J.B. (1998). In Harborne, J.B. (ed.), *Phytochemical Methods: A Guide to Modern Techniques of Plant Analysis*, pp. 40–106. Chapman and Hall, London, United Kingdom.

Justesen, U. and Knuthsen, P. (2001). *Food Chem.* 73, 245–250.

Justesen, U., Knuthsen, P. and Leth, T. (1998). *J. Chromatogr. A* 913, 101–110.

Kähkönen, M.P., Hopia, A.I., Heikki, J.V., Rauha, J.P., Pihlaja, K., Kujala, T.S. and Heinonen, M. (1999). *Agric. Food Chem.* 47, 3954–3962.

Knorr, F. (1978). *Z. Lebensm. Unters. For.* 166, 228–233.

Madigan, D., McMurrough, I. and Smyth, M.R. (1994). *Analyst* 119, 863–868.

Madsen, H.L., Nielsen, B.R., Bertelsen, G. and Skibsted, L.H. (1996). *Food Chem.* 57, 331–337.

Mattila, P., Astola, J. and Kumpulainen, J. (2000). *J. Agric. Food Chem.* 48, 5834–5841.

McMurrough, I. and Baert, T. (1994). *J. Inst. Brew.* 100, 409–416.

Ou, B., Hampsch-Woodill, M. and Prior, R.L. (2001). *J. Agric. Food Chem.* 49, 4619–4626.

Ou, B., Huang, D., Hampsch-Woodill, M., Flanagan, J. and Deemer, E. (2002). *J. Agric. Food Chem.* 50, 3122–3128.

Parrilla, M.C.G., Heredia, J.F. and Troncoso, M.A. (1999). *Food Res. Inter.* 32, 433–440.

Pellegrini, P., Serafini, M., Colombi, B., Del Rio, D., Salvatore, S., Bianchi, M. and Brighenti, F. (2003). *J. Nutr.* 133, 2812–2819.

Proteggente, A.R., Pannala, A.S., Paganga, G., Van Buren, L., Wagner, E., Wiseman, S., Van De Put, F., Pulido, R., Bravo, L. and Saura-Calixto, F. (2000). *J. Agric. Food Chem.* 48, 3396–3402.

Pulido, R., Bravo, L. and Saura-Calixto, F. (2000). *J. Agric. Food Chem.* 48, 3396–3402.

Rice-Evans, C.A., Miller, N.J. and Paganga, G. (1996). *Free Radical Biol. Med.* 20, 933–956.

Singleton, V.L. and Rossi, J.A. (1965). *Am. J. Enol. Viticult.* 16, 144–158.

Stevens, J.F., Ivancic, M., Hsu, V.L. and Deinzer, M.L. (1997). *Phytochemistry* 44, 1575–1585.

Stevens, J.F., Miranda, C.L., Buhler, D.R. and Deinzer, M.L. (1998). *J. Am. Soc. Brew. Chem.* 56, 136–145.

Stevens, J.F., Taylor, A.W. and Deinzer, M.L. (1999). *J. Chromatogr. A* 832, 97–107.

Stevens, J.F., Miranda, C.L., Wolthers, K.R., Schimerlik, M., Deinzer, M.L. and Buhler, D.R. (2002). *J. Agric. Food Chem.* 50, 3435–3443.

Taylor, A.W., Barofsky, E. and Kennedy, J.A. (2003). *J. Agric. Food Chem.* 51, 4101–4110.

Vinson, J.A., Jang, J., Yang, J., Dabbagh, Y.A., Liang, X., Serry, M., Proch, J. and Cai, S. (1999). *J. Agric. Food Chem.* 47, 2502–2504.

46

The Antioxidant Capacity of Beer: Relationships Between Assays of Antioxidant Capacity, Color and Other Alcoholic and Non-alcoholic Beverages

Justin A. Fegredo, Rachel Meynell, Alan K.H. Lai, Max C.Y. Wong, Colin R. Martin, Helen Wiseman and Victor R. Preedy Department of Nutrition and Dietetics, King's College London, London, UK

Abstract

The antioxidant capacity of foods and beverages has attracted considerable interest, since antioxidants are believed to possess protective properties against numerous pathologies. However, research into the antioxidant capacity of beers worldwide is limited. In Britain, beers represent approximately half of the alcoholic beverage market and are therefore a significant contributor to dietary antioxidant intake. The major antioxidants, phenolic compounds, are derived from the "hop" and malt components, and their concentration has been shown to correlate with total antioxidant capacity (TAC). As a result, assays to determine TAC are useful tools to derive the antioxidant potential of foods and beverages.

In this chapter, we present our findings on the TAC of several types of alcoholic beverage including ales and lagers (both bottled and draft), fruit beers and red wines. In addition, we investigate the relationship between beer color and TAC, and comment on the validity of systems such as that devised by the European Brewery Convention. For example, we show correlations between TAC when assessed by the ferric reducing ability of plasma assay with the darkness ($p < 0.01$), chroma ($p < 0.05$) and chromaticity x or relative redness ($p < 0.01$).

We intend that this chapter provides sufficient insight and motivation to investigate the specific role of beer in health and disease prevention.

List of Abbreviations

CIE	Commission Internationale de l'Eclairage
EBC	European Brewery Convention
FRAP	Ferric reducing ability of plasma
ORAC	Oxygen radical absorbance capacity
TAC	Total antioxidant capacity
TP-FCR	Total phenols by Folin–Ciocalteu reagent

Introduction

In recent years the role played by antioxidants and free radicals in health and aging has been increasingly acknowledged. One area of particular advancement is the degree of interest into dietary sources of antioxidants. Whilst red wine has been the target of much scientific interest (Frankel *et al.*, 1995), beer is increasingly recognized as a rich source of bioavailable dietary antioxidants (Montanari *et al.*, 1999; Nardini *et al.*, 2006), which are able to exert several positive effects on health (Halliwell and Gutteridge, 1999).

Antioxidants in Beer

Beer is composed of numerous constituents including a variety of phenolic and non-phenolic compounds (Gerhauser, 2005). The former, which are naturally occurring substances in fruit, vegetables, nuts, seeds and beverages (Katalinic *et al.*, 2004), are the most widely studied constituents of beer's antioxidant fraction, and are derived from both the "hop" (20–30%) and malt (70–80%) components (Gerhauser, 2005). "Hops," the dried ripe flowers of a twining vine (*Humulus lupulus* Linnaeus), are added to beer to prevent bacterial activity and provide the characteristic bitter taste (De Keukeleire, 2000), and contain 4–14% phenolic compounds by weight. These include phenolic acids, prenylated chalcones, flavanoids, catechins and proanthocyanidins (Gerhauser, 2005). The malt component, derived from the germination of grains, such as barley, contains an overall phenolic mass of 1.0–1.9 mg/g of dry matter (Maillard *et al.*, 1996). Aside from ingredients used in the brewing process, some authors have suggested that phenolic compounds such as gallic acid (Barroso *et al.*, 1996) may be leached from the oak casks or kegs used in the storage of alcoholic beverages (Escalona *et al.*, 2002). However, at present such research is confined to studies involving red wines and spirits.

Beer in Health and Disease Prevention
ISBN: 978-0-12-373891-2

Phenolic Compounds and Antioxidant Protection

The concentration of phenolic compounds is correlated well with total antioxidant capacity (TAC) (Minussi *et al.*, 2003; Pellegrini *et al.*, 2003; Pulido *et al.*, 2003; Katalinic *et al.*, 2004), and is therefore of substantial importance when considering the antioxidant potential of beverages such as beer. The ability of phenolic compounds to act as reducing agents (and hence antioxidants) is mediated by the hydrogen donating properties of their hydroxyl groups, in addition to their metal chelating ability (Brown *et al.*, 1998). The correlation between phenolic content and TAC can be extended across both alcoholic and non-alcoholic beverages ($r^2 = 0.849-0.981$) (Pulido *et al.*, 2003).

Several studies have demonstrated the high *in vitro* TAC of beers (Montanari *et al.*, 1999; Pellegrini *et al.*, 2003) and subsequent investigation has shown that this antioxidant component is indeed bioavailable (Ghiselli *et al.*, 2000). Preliminary studies have revealed a rapid rise in plasma phenolic compounds which peaks at 30 min following ingestion of beer, suggesting an absorption mechanism located in the proximal gastrointestinal tract (Nardini *et al.*, 2006). However, much further clarification is required regarding the kinetic handling of antioxidant compounds, including the time and site of absorption and the influence of ethanol on their metabolic fate (Vinson *et al.*, 2003).

Assessment of Antioxidant Protection

The quantification of TAC is perhaps of greater meaning than measurement of individual antioxidant constituents (such as phenolic compounds) because TAC acknowledges both synergistic interactions between antioxidant compounds and the contribution of antioxidant components which are at present unidentified. We have measured the TAC of numerous beers from around the world using the ferric reducing ability of plasma (FRAP), oxygen radical absorbance capacity (ORAC) and total phenols by Folin and Ciocalteu's reagent (TP-FCR) assays (Benzie and Strain, 1996; Re *et al.*, 1999; Singleton *et al.*, 1999; Naguib, 2000). Details of the procedures used can be found in Chapter 97.

Validity of Assays for Total Antioxidant Capacity

No well-established consensus exists regarding the choice of assay for measurement of TAC, and as a result studies employ a variety of different techniques thereby rendering their results incomparable. For example, the FRAP and TP-FCR assays measure solely the reducing capacity of a test substrate in the absence of free radicals (Huang *et al.*, 2005), whilst the ORAC assay offers superior measurement of the "radical scavenging ability" of an antioxidant substrate (Huang *et al.*, 2005). Furthermore, assay conditions are non-physiological (e.g. the TP-FCR assay is conducted at room temperature; the FRAP assay is conducted at pH 3.6; all assays are conducted in the absence of biological matrix (Pulido *et al.*, 2003); etc.) making the results interpretable with only limited biological relevance. Finally, only the ORAC assay is allowed to reach completion and thus incorporate both length and degree of inhibition of oxidation into a final value; the FRAP and TP-FCR assays employ an endpoint technique in which time of completion is arbitrarily set (Huang *et al.*, 2005). Due to the differential meaning of each assay, it is recommended that at least two discrete methods should be employed in the quantification of TAC (Schlesier *et al.*, 2002; Huang *et al.*, 2005) for example one to measure "radical quenching ability" and another to measure "reducing ability." Further details on both the mechanism and limitations of each assay may be found in Chapter 97.

Total Antioxidant Capacity of Beverages

We have measured the TAC of ale ($n = 31$), lager ($n = 37$), fruit beer ($n = 1$), orange juice ($n = 8$) and red wine ($n = 43$), using the FRAP, ORAC and TP-FCR assays. Significant correlations exist between the FRAP and ORAC ($p < 0.01$) and FRAP and TP-FCR ($p < 0.01$) assays, as can been seen in Figures 46.1 and 46.2. We will thus use the FRAP assay as the basis for further discussion.

Analysis revealed that the FRAP value (in mmol per liter) of red wine was over four times than that of any other beverage ($p < 0.01$), and that the mean FRAP of ale was approximately 16% (although non-significantly) higher than that of lager (Figure 46.3). The fruit beer (FRAP, 6.4 mM) was noted

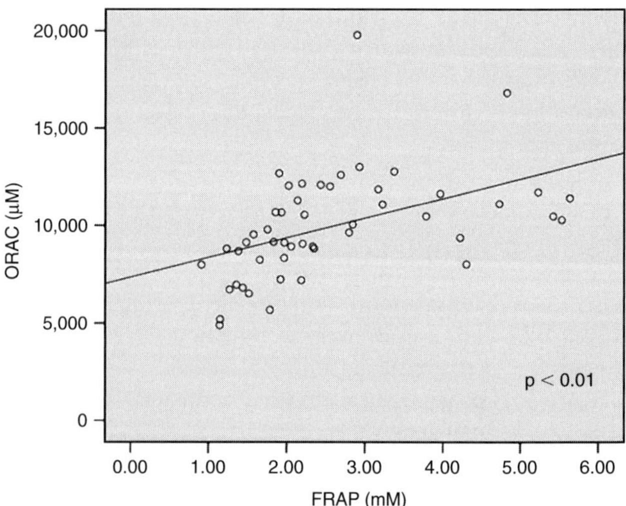

Figure 46.1 Correlation between the FRAP and ORAC assays. FRAP and ORAC were used to assess the TAC of ales and lagers from around the world.

to have a higher TAC than orange juice, ale or lager. The particular fruit beer tested was a blend of 70% white beer with 30% pure fruit juice (Specialist Brand Development, 2007), with the latter probably serving to explain the higher observed TAC. Orange juice was noted to have a higher TAC than either ale or lager, perhaps due to its greater concentration of carotenoids, terpenes and free radical scavenging vitamins (such as ascorbic acid – naturally occurring but sometimes added artificially) (Pulido *et al.*, 2003). After controlling for the portion size in which each beverage is commonly consumed (bottled ale, 500 ml; bottled lager, 330 ml; draft beer, 1 UK pint or 568 ml; glass of orange juice, 250 ml; large glass of red wine, 175 ml), the FRAP (in mmol per serving) provided by red wine was still substantially larger than that of any other beverage, however the quantity of antioxidants was less than three times that provided by a typical portion of draft ale. In addition, one portion of draft ale provided a greater (though non-significant) antioxidant mass than a portion of orange juice (Figure 46.4). Notwithstanding, one must exercise caution in such calculations, because serving size is highly variable. As an example, bottles of both ale and lager may be 330 or 500 ml capacity whilst servings of wine in UK pubs may range from 125 to 175 ml.

The "hop" component, which provides the characteristic bitter taste of beer, may be more abundant in bitter ales (Gorinstein *et al.*, 2000). Hop extracts release several phenolic compounds during brewing (e.g. procyanidins, epicatechin and ferulic acid) and may thus account for the increased antioxidant capacity of beers with "bitter" properties (Gorinstein *et al.*, 2000). In mild ales, the opposite

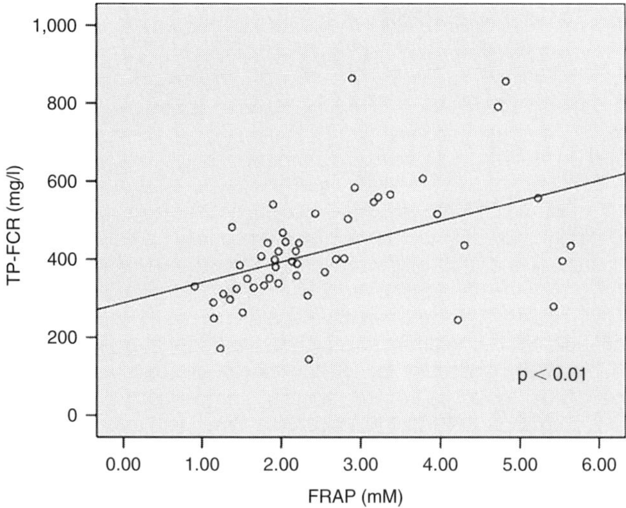

Figure 46.2 Correlation between the FRAP and TP-FCR assays. FRAP and TP-FCR were used to assess the TAC of ales and lagers from around the world.

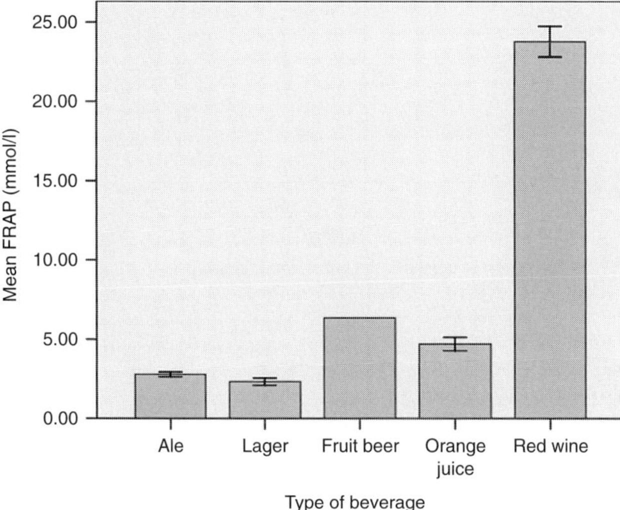

Figure 46.3 FRAP of beer, orange juice and red wine. Data are expressed as mean ± SEM (ale, $n = 31$; lager, $n = 37$; fruit beer, $n = 1$; orange juice, $n = 8$; red wine, $n = 43$). The FRAP assay was used to assess the TAC of several beverages. One-way analysis of variance (ANOVA; fruit beer excluded) found a significant difference in FRAP between beverage groups ($p < 0.001$). *Post hoc* analysis using Bonferroni adjustment revealed that FRAP of red wine was significantly higher than that of any other beverage ($p < 0.05$).

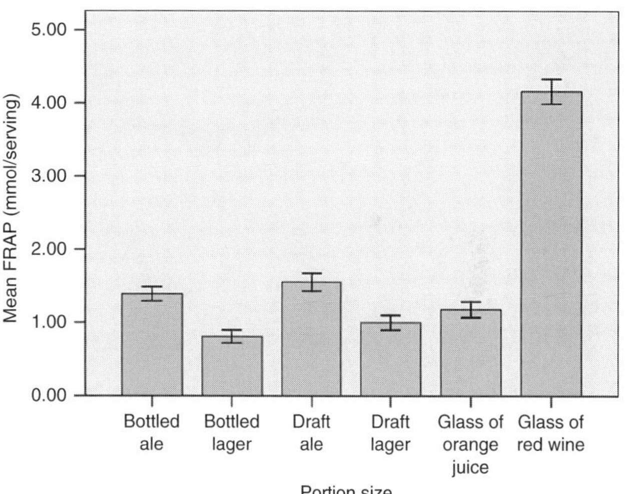

Figure 46.4 FRAP of beer, orange juice and red wine by serving size. Data are expressed as mean ± SEM (bottled ale, $n = 20$; bottled lager, $n = 30$; draft ale, $n = 11$; draft lager, $n = 7$; orange juice, $n = 8$; red wine, $n = 43$). The FRAP assay was used to assess the TAC of several beverages. TAC measured was subsequently controlled for by the portion size in which these beverages are commonly served (bottled ales, 500 ml; bottled lagers, 330 ml; draft ales and lagers, 1 UK pint = 568 ml; orange juice, 250 ml; red wine, 175 ml). One-way analysis of variance (ANOVA) found a significant difference in FRAP per portion size between beverage groups ($p < 0.001$). *Post hoc* analysis using Bonferroni adjustment revealed that FRAP of red wine was significantly higher than that of any other beverages ($p < 0.05$). There were no significant differences between FRAP obtained from ales, lagers or orange juices. In interpreting this, one needs to consider that there is a great deal of variability in "serving" size. For example, in the UK, bottled beer may be in servings of 300 or 500 ml, whilst red wine may be served in portions of 125–175 ml.

is true, and the phenolic profile is occupied by a greater proportion of malt than hop polyphenols (Gorinstein *et al.*, 2000). Malt phenols comprise 70–80% of the phenolic compounds sourced from beer and their antioxidant potential is, as a general rule, less than hop derived polyphenols (Mikyska *et al.*, 2002). This may explain why Asian beers, which are generally less bitter (and thus contain lower quantities of hop), have lower FRAP values (Figure 46.5).

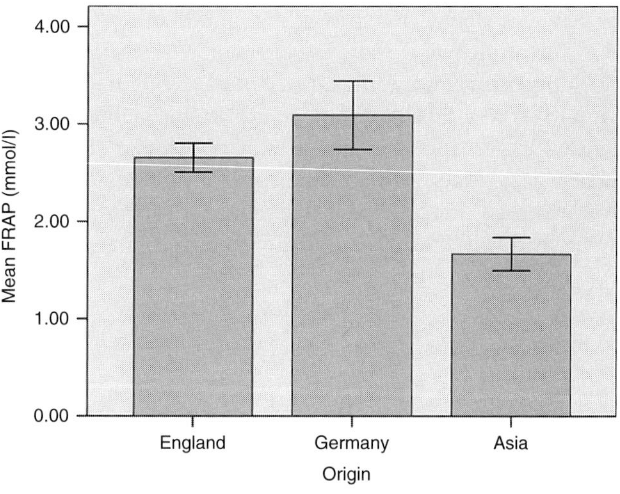

Figure 46.5 FRAP of bottled beer according to area of origin. Data are expressed as mean ± SEM. The FRAP assay was used to assess the TAC of bottled beers from Britain, Germany and Asia. One-way analysis of variance (ANOVA) found a significant difference in FRAP between beverage groups ($p < 0.01$). *Post hoc* analysis using Bonferroni adjustment revealed that FRAP of Asian beers was significantly lower than that of UK or German beers ($p < 0.05$). Asian beers were sourced from a variety of countries including Japan, Korea, Thailand, India, Singapore and Vietnam.

The Color of Beer

Beer color is the result of several compounds such as Maillard reaction products (especially melanoidins), polyphenols and artificial coloring agents. Color is influenced by brewing conditions such as temperature and pH. The intensity of beer color has been suggested to reflect phenolic content (Mann and Folts, 2004) and offer some indication of *in vivo* antioxidant protectiveness (Begolli *et al.*, 1996). Indeed, several systems, for example the European Brewery Convention (EBC) color scheme (Committee of the EBC, 1975), have used optical density to grade beers according to their color. In our studies we have noted correlations between the TAC and absorbance (four wavelengths: 420, 430, 520, 620 nm; Figure 46.6)

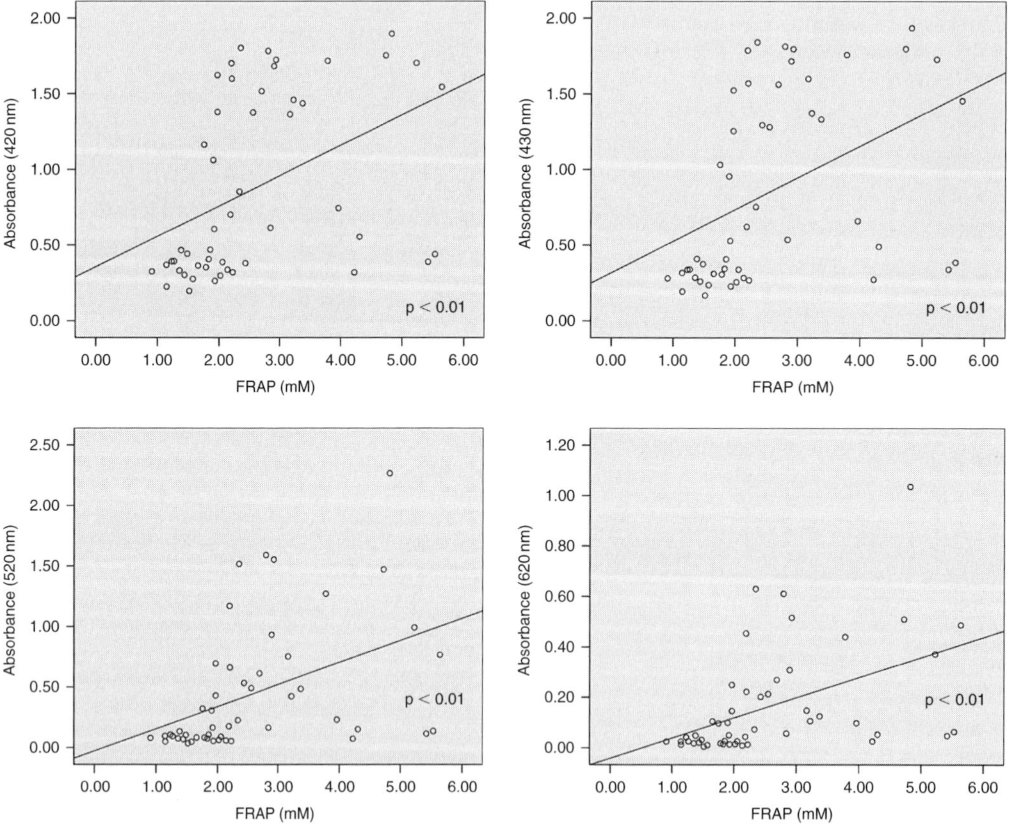

Figure 46.6 Correlation between the FRAP assay and absorbance at 420, 430, 520 and 620 nm. Data demonstrate the significant correlation between the FRAP assay (a widely used assay for TAC and spectrophotometric absorbance of beers at 420, 430, 520 and 620 nm using a cell with a 10 mm light path).

and between TAC and EBC grading (Figure 46.7). Optical density alone, however, cannot be used to quantify the color of a beer, since color perception involves a complex interplay between the spectral reflectance curve, nature of illumination and biological variation in retinal physiology (International Commission on Illumination, 2004). Several models have been proposed to describe color, for example the widely used Commission Internationale de l'Eclairage (CIE) $L^*a^*b^*$ (*L*, lightness; *a*, location on red–green continuum; *b*, location on yellow–blue continuum) and CIE $L^*C^*h^*$ (*L*, lightness; *C*, chroma; *h*, hue) systems (International Commission on Illumination, 2004) which involve the use of Cartesian coordinates to define color by pointing to a unique point in a three-dimensional color space (Figure 46.8). Other systems, for example chromaticity (International Commission on Illumination, 2004), seek to qualify color according to its dominant wavelength (corresponds to hue) and purity (corresponds to saturation or chroma); details given in Figure 46.9. Whilst some authors have used the CIE $L^*a^*b^*$ system to characterize beer color (Coghe *et al.*, 2003), we felt that lightness, *L*, was the only reliable variable in this system because use of *a* (red–green) or *b* (yellow–blue) introduced the confounding factors of whether increased antioxidant capacity was due to, for example, increased redness or decreased greenness (Figure 46.8). We did not correlate *h* (hue) from the CIE $L^*C^*h^*$ system for a similar reason. Using the CIE chromaticity values (*x*, *y* and *z*; collectively correspond to hue) we found that TAC was significantly and positively correlated with relative redness (x, $p < 0.01$) and greenness (y, $p < 0.05$) but inversely correlated with blueness (z, $p < 0.01$) (Figure 46.10). Furthermore, we found that FRAP was negatively correlated with lightness *L* of the beer (hence positively correlated with darkness, $p < 0.01$; Figure 46.11) and positively correlated with color saturation or chroma *C* ($p < 0.05$; Figure 46.12).

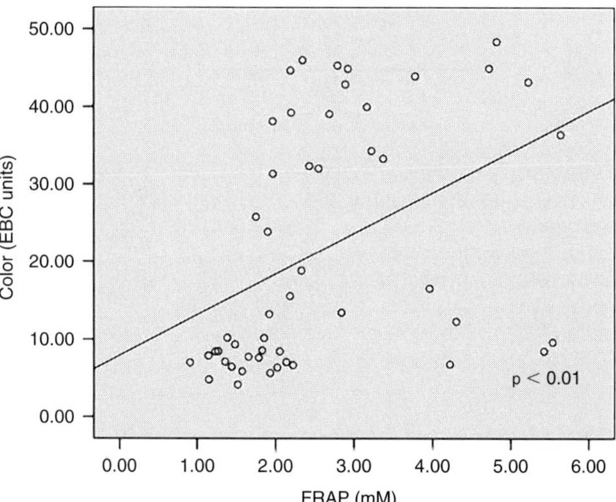

Figure 46.7 Correlation between the FRAP assay and EBC color. Data demonstrate the significant correlation between the FRAP assay and the EBC color rating (Committee of the EBC, 1975). EBC color is calculated by measuring absorbance at 430 nm with a light path of 10 mm and multiplying the result by 25.

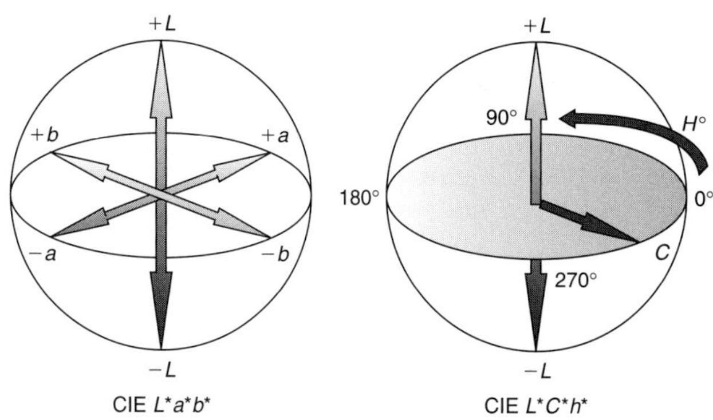

Figure 46.8 Three-dimensional color spaces: CIE $L^*a^*b^*$ and CIE $L^*C^*h^*$. Figure adapted from an online source (The Tintometer Ltd, 2006), where color images are available.

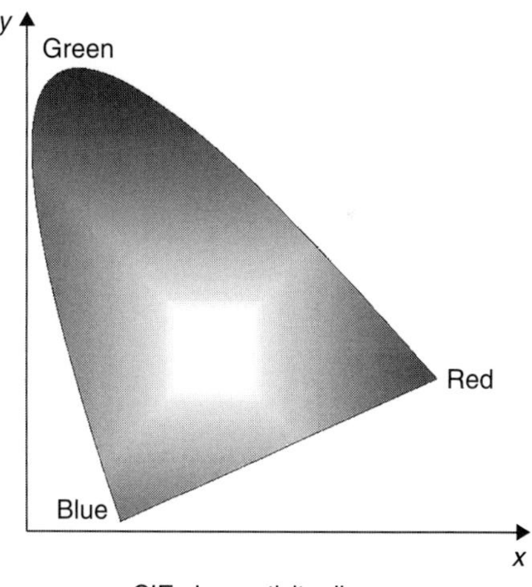

Figure 46.9 Two-dimensional color: CIE chromaticity (International Commission on Illumination, 2004). Any color may be said to be comprised of three primary colors; the tristimulus values of a color are the quantities of each primary color component (*X*, corresponds to red; *Y*, corresponds to green; *Z*, corresponds to blue). The use of tristimulus values to define color is inherently fragile, because color is affected by luminance. Chromaticity, on the other hand, expresses each primary color as a ratio to the total (e.g. $x = X/X + Y + Z$) and is thus irrespective of luminance. Given measurements of *x* and *y*, it is therefore mathematically possible to calculate *z*, ($x + y + z = 1$) which is therefore somewhat redundant. Consequently, the hue of a color can now be expressed in a two-dimensional color space. The value for tristimulus *Y* is approximately proportional to luminosity, thus chromaticity expressed as *Yxy* accounts for both hue and luminosity. Figure adapted from an online source (The Tintometer Ltd, 2006), where a color version is available.

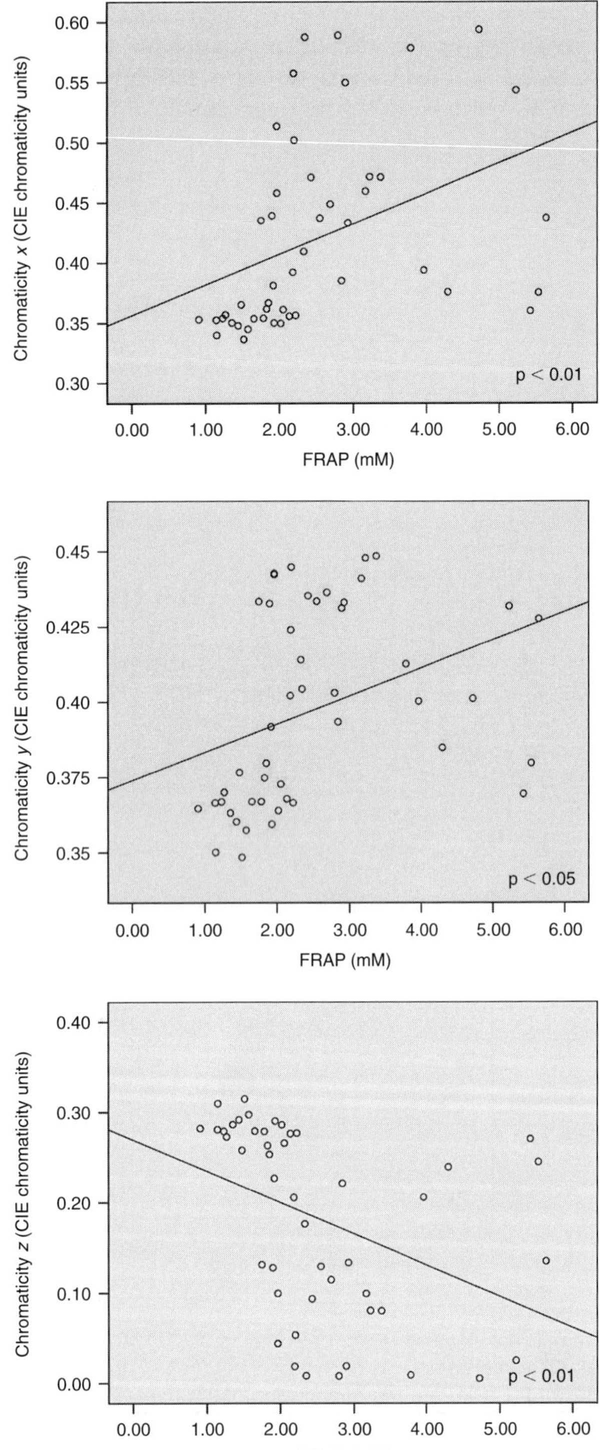

Figure 46.10 Correlation between the FRAP value and chromaticity *x*, *y* and *z* of beer. Data demonstrate the correlation between the FRAP assay and the chromaticity coordinates *x*, *y* and *z* of several beers ($n = 50$). Chromaticity is a system used to quantify color by way of dominant wavelength (hue) and luminosity (International Commission on Illumination, 2004). Positive correlations between FRAP and chromaticity *x* and *y* demonstrate that TAC is greater in redder and greener beers, respectively. The negative correlation between FRAP and chromaticity *z* demonstrates that TAC is lower in beers with a more bluish hue.

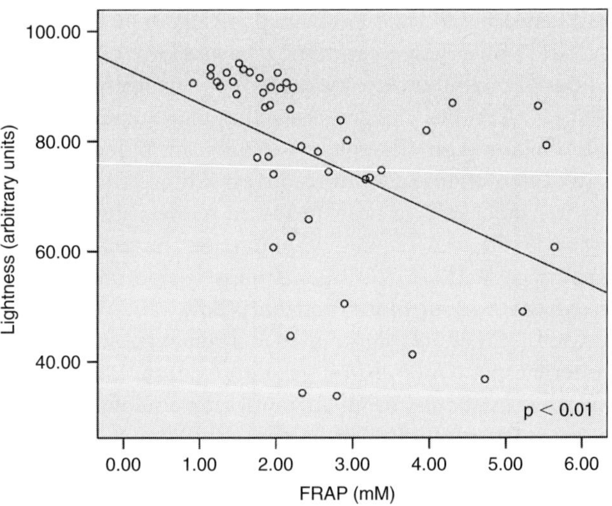

Figure 46.11 Correlation between the FRAP assay and lightness of beer. Data demonstrate the correlation between the FRAP assay and the lightness "*L*" of several beers ($n = 50$). The negative correlation between FRAP and lightness demonstrates that TAC is greater in darker beers.

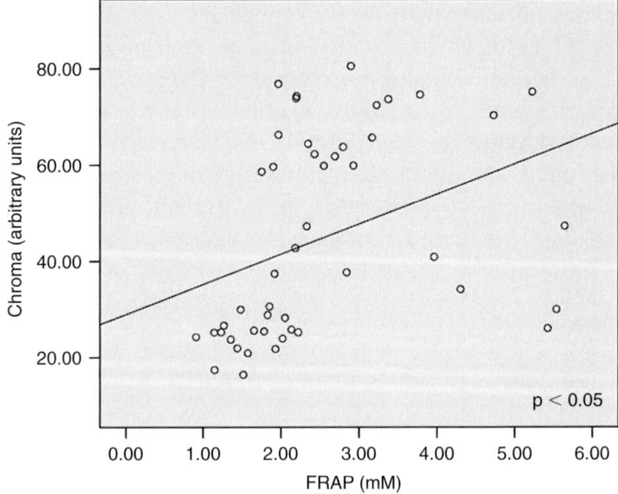

Figure 46.12 Correlation between the FRAP assay and chroma of beer. Data demonstrate the correlation between the FRAP assay and the chroma "*C*" of several beers ($n = 50$). Chroma can be defined as the saturation or vividness of color (International Commission on Illumination, 2004). The positive correlation between FRAP and chroma demonstrates that TAC is greater in more vivid and color-saturated beers.

Conclusion and Future Directions

A number of interesting and contemporary topic areas in the fields of biochemistry, public health and nutrition are involved in the assessment of the antioxidant capacity of beer. On a public health basis, it is important to realize the paradox that exists between any health recommendations made on consumption of certain types of beers over other beverages, and knowledge of the highly detrimental binge-drinking culture that has evolved in Britain. Nonetheless, the importance of dietary antioxidants in the prevention of disease is well recognized, and it is our intention that this chapter provides sufficient insight and motivation to investigate further the specific role of beer in health and disease prevention.

Summary Points

- Beer is a complex beverage with a high TAC which is comparable to fruit juice.
- Different types of beer exhibit different TAC: ales are higher than lagers.
- The TAC of high-antioxidant beverages cannot be considered in isolation, but must be evaluated with respect to the portion size in which the beverage is consumed.
- When portion size is taken into account, a draft portion of the fruit beer we tested provided 98% of the antioxidant content found in a large (175 ml) glass of red wine. Draft portions of ale and lager provided 42% and 27%, respectively.
- The color of beers serves as an indicator of TAC: darker, more saturated, vivid and redder beers contain the highest quantity of antioxidants.

Acknowledgments

The authors would like to thank the staff of the Department of Nutrition and Dietetics, and Dr. Matt Arno of the Genomics Centre, King's College London. We also extend our gratitude to The Wellington (351 The Strand, London, WC2R 0HS, UK) for providing the draft beers, Ian Dixon of Shepherd Neame Limited (17 Court Street, Faversham, Kent, ME13 7AX, UK) for supplying many of the bottled beers free of charge, and The Tintometer Ltd (The Color Laboratory, Waterloo Road, Salisbury, Wiltshire, SP1 2JY, UK) for performing the color measurements.

References

Barroso, C.G., Rodríguez, D.A., Guillén, D.A. and Pérez-Bustamante, J.A. (1996). *J. Chromatogr. A* 724, 125–129.

Begolli, B.P., Folts, J.D., Trella, B.C. and Waterhouse, A.L. (1996). *FASEB J.* 10, A43–A249.

Benzie, I.F. and Strain, J.J. (1996). *Anal. Biochem.* 239, 70–76.

Brown, J.E., Khodr, H., Hider, R.C. and Rice-Evans, C.A. (1998). *Biochem. J.* 330, 1173–1178.

Coghe, S., Vanderhaegen, B., Pelgrims, B., Basteyns, Av. and Delvaux, Fr. (2003). *J. Am. Soc. Brew. Chem.* 61, 125–132.

Committee of the EBC (1975). *Analytica EBC.* Schweizer Brauerei-Rundschau, Zurich, Switzerland.

De Keukeleire, D. (2000). *Química Nova.* 23, 108–12.

Escalona, H., Birkmyre, L., Piggott, J.R. and Paterson, A. (2002). *Anal. Chim. Acta.* 458, 45–54.

Frankel, E.N., Waterhouse, A.L. and Teissedre, P.L. (1995). *J. Agric. Food Chem.* 43, 890–894.

Gerhauser, C. (2005). *Eur. J. Cancer* 41, 1941–1954.

Ghiselli, A., Natella, F., Guidi, A., Montanari, L., Fantozzi, P. and Scaccini, C. (2000). *J. Nutr. Biochem.* 11, 76–80.

Gorinstein, S., Caspi, A., Zemser, M. and Trakhtenberg, S. (2000). *Nutr. Res.* 20, 131–139.

Halliwell, B. and Gutteridge, J.M.C. (1999). *Free Radicals in Biology and Medicine.* Clarendon Press, Oxford, UK.

Huang, D., Ou, B. and Prior, R.L. (2005). *J. Agric. Food Chem.* 53, 1841–1856.

International Commission on Illumination (2004). *Colorimetry.* CIE, Vienna, Austria.

Katalinic, V., Milos, M., Modun, D., Music, I. and Boban, M. (2004). *Food Chem.* 86, 593–600.

Maillard, M.N., Soum, M.H., Boivin, P. and Berset, C. (1996). *Lebensm. Wiss. Technol.* 29, 283–344.

Mann, L.B. and Folts, J.D. (2004). *Pathophysiology* 10, 105–112.

Mikyska, A., Hrabak, M., Haskova, D. and Srogl, J. (2002). *J. Inst. Brew.* 108, 78–85.

Minussi, R.C., Rossi, M., Bologna, L., Cordi, L., Rotilio, D., Pastore, G.M. and Duran, N. (2003). *Food Chem.* 82, 409–416.

Montanari, L., Perretti, G., Natella, F., Guidi, A. and Fantozzi, P. (1999). *Lebensm.-Wiss. Technol.* 32, 535–539.

Naguib, Y.M. (2000). *Anal. Biochem.* 284, 93–98.

Nardini, M., Natella, F., Scaccini, C. and Ghiselli, A. (2006). *J. Nutr. Biochem.* 17, 14–22.

Pellegrini, N., Del Rio, D., Colombi, B., Bianchi, M. and Brighenti, F. (2003). *J. Agric. Food Chem.* 51, 260–264.

Pulido, R., Hernandez-Garcia, M. and Saura-Calixto, F. (2003). *Eur. J. Clin. Nutr.* 57, 1275–1282.

Re, R., Pellegrini, N., Proteggente, A., Pannala, A., Yang, M. and Rice-Evans, C. (1999). *Free Radic. Biol. Med.* 26, 1231–1237.

Schlesier, K., Harwat, M., Bohm, V. and Bitsch, R. (2002). *Free Radic. Res.* 36, 177–187.

Singleton, V.L., Orthofer, R. and Lamuela-Raventós, R.M. (1999). *Methods Enzymol.* 299, 152–178.

Specialist Brand Development (2007). Früli. Viewed 25 April 2007, <http://www.specialist-brand-development.com/products/Fruli.html>.

The Tintometer Ltd (2006). A guide to understanding colour communication. The Tintometer Ltd. Viewed 10 May 2007, <http://www.lovibond.com/PDFS/COLOUR%20COMMUNICATION.pdfg>.

Vinson, J.A., Mandarano, M., Hirst, M., Trevithick, J.R. and Bose, P. (2003). *J. Agric. Food Chem.* 51, 5528–5533.

47

Biological Properties of Beer and Its Components Compared to Wine

Giuseppe Iacomino, Idolo Tedesco and Gian Luigi Russo Institute of Food Sciences, National Research Council, Avellino, Italy

Abstract

Increasing evidence supports the health benefits of moderate consumption of alcohol as part of a healthy lifestyle. Numerous studies suggest that moderate drinking of beer is associated with lower rates of cardiovascular disease, cancer and osteoporosis. Recent researches in bioactive principles revealed many notable properties of hop compounds. Scientific evidence has accumulated over the last years pointing to the potential anticancer activities of selected hop-derived beer constituents. A generalized radical scavenging activity was described for most beer polyphenolic components, and a protection against DNA oxidative damage was reported. In this chapter, we will discuss the potential chemopreventive role and helpful effects on health of beer and its constituents compared to wine.

List of Abbreviations

ROS	Reactive oxygen species
NF-κB	Nuclear factor-kappa B
Akt	Serine/threonine protein kinase
CYP1A1	Cytochrome P450, family 1, subfamily A, polypeptide 1
CYP1B1	Cytochrome P450, family 1, subfamily B, polypeptide 1
CYP1A2	Cytochrome P450, family 1, subfamily A, polypeptide 2
PhIP	2-amino-1-methyl-6-phenylimidazo [4,5-*b*]pyridine
FRAP	Ferric reducing antioxidant power
EGCG	Epigallocatechin gallate
DMBA	Dimethylbenz[a]antracene
PMA	Phorbol myristate acetate
ERK1/2	Extracellular signal-regulated kinase 1/2
PKC	Protein kinase C
Cdk1/4	Cyclin-dependent kinase 1/4
pRb	Retinoblastoma protein
Bax	Bcl-2-associated X protein
Bcl	B-cell leukemia

Introduction

Growing evidence supports the health benefits of moderate consumption of alcohol as part of a healthy lifestyle, whereas it is widely recognized that alcohol abuse exerts negative effects on health (Rehm *et al.*, 2003). Numerous studies evaluating the relative benefits of wine, beer and spirits, suggest that moderate drinking of any alcoholic beverage is associated with lower rates of cardiovascular disease (Corrao *et al.*, 1999). Apparently, beer drunk in moderation can help protect again heart disease, cancer and osteoporosis (Kondo, 2004). The positive association between moderate intake of alcoholic beverages and low risk for cardiovascular diseases has been linked to their polyphenol content. A recent study showed that the acute consumption of dealcoholized beer may reduce thrombogenic activity in young adults with beneficial effects on coronary artery disease development (Bassus *et al.*, 2004). Urologists suggest beer as an antidote agent against kidney stones formation (Curhan *et al.*, 1996).

Alcoholic beverages are produced from raw materials by fermentative processes (Rainbow and Float, 1990). The most consumed types of commercially alcoholic products are wine, beer and spirits. Beer and wine contain vitamins and other nutrients usually absent from distilled spirits: in addition, beer also contains large quantities of carbohydrates (Moll, 1991). Beer is obtained from malted cereal grains (typically barley and corn or rice) by yeast fermentation. Hops (*Humulus lupulus*) and water are added. Temperature and pH during mashing can affect color, flavor, alcohol content and other fine changes in the beer.

In Table 47.1, the national beer consumptions *per capita* is reported and compared to those of wine.

Except for Luxemburg, where both beer and wine consumption is relatively high, it is worthwhile to note that countries traditionally drinking wine (e.g. France and Italy) consume only modest amounts of beer, and vice versa (e.g. Czech Republic and Germany), whereas moderate consumption of red wine generates the "French Paradox"

Beer in Health and Disease Prevention
ISBN: 978-0-12-373891-2

Table 47.1 Worldwide beer consumption

Countries	*Per capita annual consumption (l)*	
	Beer[a]	*Wine*[b]
Czech Republic	156.5	6.3
Germany	115.8	24.2
Australia	109.9	20.5
Austria	109.0	30.4
Ireland	106.0	12.4
Luxemburg	106.0	59.2
United Kingdom	95.6	16.9
Belgium	91.5	24.1
Slovakia	88.4	11.8
Lithuania	87.5	5.6
Denmark	86.7	28.9
Finland	84.0	7.4
United States	81.6	8.7
Spain	80.6	34.5
The Netherlands	78.1	20.9
New Zealand	77.0	15.8
Poland	75.0	1.3
Estonia	75.0	6.1
Hungary	72.2	31.5
Canada	68.3	8.9
Cyprus	62.2	15.2
Portugal	61.7	46.7
South Africa	59.2	9.1
Russia	58.9	3.4
Sweden	50.5	15.8
Greece	40.0	27.7
Latvia	36.6	4.9
France	33.5	57.2
Italy	29.7	52.9
China	22.1	0.8

Source: [a]Adapted from Assobirra (2006) and referred to 2004–2005 data. [b]Adapted from the Wine Institute, California (www.wineinstitute.org). Data are referred to 2001 consumption and include both white and red wines.

(Constant, 1997), referring to its beneficial effect on health – quite little is known about the effects of moderate consumption of beer on human health (Kondo, 2004). The positive activity of red wine has usually been associated to its high content in polyphenols (Tedesco *et al.*, 2000; Scalbert *et al.*, 2005). Recent papers indicate that beer components might also exert similar beneficial effects on health (Gerhauser, 2005; Rivero *et al.*, 2005) and moderate beer consumption is supposed to be part of a healthy diet (Romeo *et al.*, 2006). A recent search on PubMed (http://www.pubmed.com) revealed that more than 3,700 studies have been published on this topic.

In this chapter, we will focus on the antithetical relation between beer drinking and the increase risk of diseases, as far as the potential chemopreventive role and helpful effects on health of beer or its constituents, compared to wine.

Beer Components Compared to Wine

Beer has a low alcohol content, but an extremely complex chemical composition; in fact, several hundred beer constituents have been so far characterized, as reviewed (Gerhauser, 2005). From a nutritional point of view, beer is more abundant in proteins (ranging 2.0–4.8 g/l) and vitamins compared to wines. Beer contains B type vitamins, including B12, B6 and folate derived from the barley used during production of beer (Flanzy, 1970; Romeo *et al.*, 2006). Beer does not contain fat or cholesterol and is low in free sugars. Furthermore, it is lower in calories than other drinks; calories, ranging from 15 (non-alcoholic beer) to 41 kcal/100 ml (lager beer), come largely from its alcohol content. Beer is a good source of soluble fiber derived from the cell walls of malted barley (Biles and Emerson, 1968). A liter of beer contains an average of 20–60% of the recommended daily intake of fiber, depending on the specific type. In fact, significant amounts of soluble dietary fiber are found in beer (0.4 and 6.2 g/l) (Gromes *et al.*, 2000) compared to red wine (0.94–1.37 g/l) and white wine (0.19–0.39 g/l) (Díaz-Rubio and Saura-Calixto, 2006).

In addition, beer contains a well-balanced array of minerals, such as phosphoric acid (90–400 mg/l), potassium (330–1,100 mg/l), magnesium (60–200 mg/l) and a very low amount of sodium (40–230 mg/l) (Bamforth, 2002). Finally, beer is a good source of bioavailable silicon extracted during the mashing process (Bellia *et al.*, 1994; Powell *et al.*, 2005). The median silicon level of beer is 18.0 mg/l, with no significant difference in the levels of the different beers by geographical origin or type of beer. Recent studies confirmed that serum and urinary silicon levels increased considerably following beer consumption indicating that the mineral in beer is present chiefly in a monomeric form and is readily bioavailable (Sripanyakorn *et al.*, 2004).

Natural antioxidants are found in fruits, vegetables and beverages such as wine and tea. They are also present in high levels in beer, deriving from both the malt (barley) and hops used as ingredients (Shahidi and Naczk, 1995; Paganga *et al.*, 1999). The total amount of antioxidants in the beverage depends on the beer types and therefore the raw materials and the brewing process used. Beer contains more than twice as many antioxidants as white wine per drink, although only half the amount in red wine (Suter, 2001). Relatively recent studies showed that the antioxidant content of blood is raised following beer consumption suggesting that the antioxidants in beer are readily absorbed (Ghiselli *et al.*, 2000). Moreover, phenolic components of wine and beer are quantitatively and qualitatively different because grape contains polyphenols different from those present in barley and hops used in beer production. Furthermore, polyphenols derived from hop are likely to be different from those of malt, about 20–30% of beer polyphenols derive from hop, whereas 70–80% originate from malt (Benitez *et al.*, 1997).

Table 47.2 Comparison between phenolic constituents of beer and wines

Structural classes	*Beer (mg/l)*	*Red wine (mg/l)*	*White wine (mg/l)*
Benzoic acid derivatives			
Gallic acid	Up to 0.2[a]	Up to 19.77[b]	Up to 0.57[b]
Protocatechuic acid	Up to 0.3[a]	Up to 2.36[b]	Up to 0.45[b]
Flavan-3-ols			
(+)-Catechin	Up to 5.4[a]	Up to 18.76[b]	Up to 11.23[b]
(−)-Epicatechin	Up to 1.1[a]	Up to 23.19[b]	Up to 16.95[b]
Cinnamic acids			
Caffeic acid	Up to 0.3[a]	Up to 5.60[b]	Up to 3.66[b]
Ferulic acid	Up to 6.5[a]	Up to 0.27[b]	Up to 0.52[b]
Flavonoles			
Quercetin	Up to 10[a]	Up to 21.06[c]	8.35[c]
Kaempferol	16.4[a]	Up to 2.37[c]	2.69[c]
Flavanones			
Isoxanthohumol	0.04–3.44[a]	–	–
8-Prenylnaringenin	0.001–0.24[a]	–	–
6-Prenylnaringenin	0.001–0.56[a]	–	–
Chalcones			
Xanthohumol	0.002–1.2[a]	–	–
Alpha-acids	~1.7[a]	–	–
iso-Alpha-acids (cis and trans)	0.6–100[a]	–	–
Proanthocyanidins	21–25[d]	105.45–366.08[e]	2.76–13.30[e]
Stilbenes			
trans-Resveratrol	–	0.114.3[f]	0.026–0.142[g]

Source: [a]Gerhauser (2005); [b]del Alamo *et al.* (2004); [c]Rodriguez-Delgado *et al.* (2001); [d]Gu *et al.* (2004); [e]Sanchez-Moreno *et al.* (2003); [f]Mark *et al.* (2005); [g]Dourtoglou *et al.* (1999).

Major, structural constituents of beer include simple phenols, benzoic and cinnamic acid derivatives, coumarins, catechins, oligomeric proanthocyanidins, prenylated chalcones, flavonoids (flavanones, flavones, flavonoles), alpha- and iso-alpha-acids derived from hop (Gerhäuser *et al.*, 2002) (Chapter X). Dark beer contains the highest total phenolic (489 ± 52 mg/l) and melanoidin (1.49 ± 0.02 g/l) contents with a 2-fold difference observed when compared to the alcohol-free beer. Beer antioxidant activity is strongly correlated with the total polyphenol content and with the melanoidin content (Rivero *et al.*, 2005; Tedesco *et al.*, 2005).

The main flavanols found in beer are (+)catechin, (−)epicatechin, gallocatechin and epigallocatechin, found either as monomers, or commonly connected to form flavanoids (dimers, trimers or larger polymers). Flavanoids (oligomers of flavanols), found at level of approximately 15 mg/l, have a basic structure of two aromatic rings linked by a three carbon unit and are variously hydroxylated and sometimes glycosylated or methylated. Alpha-acids or humulones are converted during wort boiling to iso-alpha-acids or isohumulones, which impart the typical bitter taste to beer (De Keukeleire, 2000). Table 47.2 summarizes the different phenolic composition between beer and wines.

It is clear that few classes of compounds, such as flavan-3-ols and flavonoles (Table 47.2), are present in comparable amounts in both beverages. Others are preferentially contained in red wine (benzoic acid derivatives), while ferulic acid is higher in beer compared to wines (Table 47.2). On the opposite, there are classes of molecules mainly present in red wines (stilbenes and proanthocyanidins), or exclusively in beer (flavanones and chalcones; Table 47.2).

Risks Associated to Beer Consumption Compared to Wine

Potential chemopreventive benefits deriving from beer consumption cannot leave out the analysis of the negative health effects deriving from alcohol consumption (Rehm *et al.*, 2003; Hingson *et al.*, 2005). The amount of alcohol in "a drink" can vary considerably depending on the size of the glass and the alcoholic strength. It will differ slightly across world according to historic traditions and customs. "A drink" of beer is usually defined as a 350 ml glass. Its resulting alcohol content is of about 18 g, very similar to a wine serving.

Beer drinking is obviously associated to alcohol consumption, since alcohol-free beer represents only the 2–3% of the beer market. Alcohol abuse contributes to a variety of acute and chronic illness, from injuries resulting from traffic accident to cardiovascular disease and cancer (Rehm *et al.*, 2001, 2003). An exhaustive analysis on alcohol consumption and cardiovascular disease found that this association can be described as a J-shaped curve, to indicate that, low-moderate consumption, compared with abstinence from alcohol, is associated with lower risk for cardiovascular disease and mortality, with the lowest risk set at 20 g/day (about one drink of beer) (Corrao *et al.*, 2000). The relationship reverses in the case of an averaged intake of more than 72–89 g/day, where the risk significantly increases over the abstainers (Corrao *et al.*, 2000). Chronic alcoholism leads to the obverse effect, although beer drinkers had significantly lower serum concentrations of homocysteine than did those consuming wine or spirits (Blasco *et al.*, 2005), it is worthwhile to note that hyperhomocysteinemia is considered a significant risk factor for vascular diseases.

There is also convincing evidence that high alcohol consumption is related to increased incidence in different types of cancer (Smith-Warner *et al.*, 1998; Dennis, 2000; Bagnardi *et al.*, 2001; Ellison *et al.*, 2001).

Moderate alcohol consumption increases the risk of breast cancer (Linos *et al.*, 2007), most probably by elevating estrogen and androgen levels, suggesting that alcohol drinking might also influence other hormone-related malignancies, such as ovarian cancer (Genkinger *et al.*, 2006). The latter has been reported to be associated with increased cancer risk in wine, but not in beer consumption (Chang *et al.*, 2007).

Alcohol abuse is also related to chronic health costs other than cardiovascular disease and cancer, such as cirrhosis or pancreatitis (Kozarevic *et al.*, 1983; Rodés *et al.*, 1999). However, it has been described a link between cirrhosis and excessive consumption of liquor, but not beer or wine (Gruenewald and Ponicki, 1995).

Differently than wine, beer may contain undesired components, such as nitrosamine that has been shown to increase the risk of cancer in animals and humans (Riboli *et al.*, 1991). Food constituents and the physical make-up of the beverage can provoke nitrosamine formation. Volatile *N*-nitrosamines were known to be generated during the traditional malting process in beer. Fortunately, modern techniques in malt drying process drastically reduces molecule content to ~0.074 μg/kg (about 2–3% respect to the original concentration) (Izquierdo-Pulido *et al.*, 1996). For moderate beer drinkers, these levels of nitrosamines are unlikely to constitute a hazard (Tricker and Preussmann, 1991). In fact, nitrates and nitrites originating from beer are quite lower than those in vegetables and meat products (Dich *et al.*, 1996).

Beer may also contain biogenic amines, notably tyramine; thus, the consumption of beer must be restricted in patients receiving monoamine oxidase inhibitor drugs (Izquierdo-Pulido *et al.*, 2000). Other risks that may derive from beer consumption are gout (Eastmond *et al.*, 1995) and sensitivity to cereal proteins (Ellis *et al.*, 1990).

Since beer originates from cereals, it is at risk of ochratoxin contamination, a class of compounds with teratogenic, genotoxic, mutagenic and carcinogenic capacities (Creppy, 1999). However, the vast majority of industrial beers are produced from uncontaminated grain and do not contain significant levels of ochratoxins (Long, 1999).

Chemopreventive Effects of Hops and Beer Compounds Compared to Bioactive Molecules Present in Wine

A modern and complete definition of chemoprevention includes the use of natural or pharmacological agents to suppress, arrest or reverse carcinogenesis at its early stages (Sporn and Suh, 2002). Many dietary compounds have been identified as potential chemopreventive agents (Russo *et al.*, 1999; Iacomino *et al.*, 2001; Russo *et al.*, 2005). These include vitamins, minerals, carotenoids, antioxidants, anti-inflammatory agents, *n*-3 polyunsaturated fatty acids and the large class of phytochemicals (polyphenols, isothiocyanates, organosulfur compounds) (Liu, 2004; Gerhauser *et al.*, 2006). The majority of chemopreventive agents are available in, and consumed from, vegetables and also from beverages, such as green tea, beer and wine (Meydani, 2001; Liu, 2003; Polidori, 2003; Lee *et al.*, 2004; Liu, 2004; Daviglus *et al.*, 2005). However, the mode of action of many of these agents is not completely understood (Russo, 2007). Chemopreventers exert a variety of biological activities and can be divided into two major groups: cancer-blocking and cancer-suppressing agents. The former prevents carcinogens to hit their cellular targets by several mechanisms including enhancing carcinogen detoxification, modifying carcinogen uptake and metabolism, scavenging reactive oxygen species (ROS) and other oxidative species, enhancing DNA repair mechanisms (Furst, 2002). Cancer-suppressing agents inhibit cancer promotion and progression after that the formation of pre-neoplastic cells occurred.

In the next paragraphs, we are going to review selected biological effects of specific beer components and beer extract which can result beneficial in preventing chronic and degenerative pathologies, underlying the differences existing with respect to bioactive molecules present in wine. We will not discuss antioxidant and cardio-protective activities of beer since extensively reported in different sections of the present book (Chapters X and Y).

Chemopreventive activity of compounds specifically present in beer

Recent studies revealed many notable properties of bioactive compounds present in hops, that justify the increasing interest of pharmaceutical firms in hops (or derivatives), as a potential source of novel drugs. Almost all hop secondary metabolites exhibit measurable bioactive effects (Kondo, 2004). Scientific evidence accumulated over the last years are in agreement with the potential anticancer activities of selected hop-derived beer constituents, such as prenylflavonoids (including xanthohumol, isoxanthohumol and hop bitter acids), exclusively present in beer compared to wine (Table 47.2) (Chapter X).

Based on the previous definition, potential chemopreventive effects have been suggested for the following beer components: vitamins, soluble fiber, silicon and polyphenolic antioxidant compounds (Bamforth, 2002).

Recently, attention has been devoted to hop prenylflavonoids, a group of plant secondary metabolites that are significantly and, among alcoholic beverages, exclusively present in beer with respect to wine (Table 47.2).

Xanthohumol (3′-[3,3-dimethylallyl]-2′,4′,4-trihydroxy-6′-methoxychalcone) is the principal prenylated flavonoid of the female inflorescences of the hop plant. The molecule is formed in lupulin glands by a specialized branch of flavonoid biosynthetic pathway that involves prenylation and *O*-methylation of the polyketide intermediate chalconaringenin (Stevens and Page, 2004). The fate of xanthohumol as hops is processed into beer has been investigated, about 20–30% is transformed in isoxanthohumol (Stevens *et al.*, 1999) (Chapter X).

Xanthohumol exhibits protective effects against a variety of disease including osteoporosis, cardiovascular pathologies and cancer (Vanhoecke *et al.*, 2005; Albini *et al.*, 2006). It has been characterized as a broad-range anticancer agent in *in vitro* and *ex vivo* in B-chronic lymphocytic leukemia cells (Miranda *et al.*, 1999; Lust *et al.*, 2005). There are several ways by which xanthohumol may exert its activities. As an example, the molecule may cause apoptosis of cancer cells, and it may also prevent angiogenesis or blood vessel growth by repressing both the NF-κB and Akt pathways (Albini *et al.*, 2006). Furthermore, xanthohumol inhibits the family of cytochromes P450 enzymes (Henderson *et al.*, 2000a, b). It also induces activity of the phase II enzymes quinone reductase (Miranda *et al.*, 2000), which contributes to cellular detoxification from carcinogens. Recent studies demonstrated that xanthohumol inducing downregulation of NF-κB activation in benign prostate hyperplasia can prevent prostate cancer cell proliferation (Colgate *et al.*, 2007). Substitutions on the chalcone structure have been found to profound influence the anticarcinogenic effects of derivatives. Xanthohumol metabolism in rat and human liver microsomes has also been investigated (Yilmazer *et al.*, 2001). Preliminary studies have shown that xanthohumol is absorbed from the digestive tract in rats (Hanske *et al.*, 2005; Hussong *et al.*, 2005; Hijova, 2006); more investigations are necessary to evaluate the bioavailability of the molecule in humans.

In addition, the chemopreventive effects of beer flavanones (i.e. isoxanthohumol and 8-prenylnaringenin) and chalcones (i.e. xanthohumol) (Table 47.2) have been associated to the inhibition, at nanomolar concentration, of phase I cytochrome P450 (phase I monooxygenase enzymes), responsible for the activation of procarcinogens. Cytochrome P450 enzymes are known for their role in the metabolism of drugs and other foreign compounds. Therefore, modulation of this enzymatic system can interfere with the metabolism of xenobiotics, producing effects of pharmacological and toxicological importance (Nebert and Dalton, 2006). Some prenylflavonoids such as xanthohumol, isoxanthohumol and 8-prenylnaringenin have been shown to inhibit the ethoxyresorufin-*O*-deethylase activity of recombinant human CYP1A1 and CYP1B1, and acetanilide 4-hydroxylase activity of CYP1A2 (Henderson *et al.*, 2000b). These enzymatic activities are involved in heterocyclic amines activation, such as 2-amino-3-methylimidazo[4,5-*f*]quinoline) and PhIP (2-amino-1-methyl-6-phenylimidazo[4,5-*b*]pyridine), among the most potent mutagens found in cooked food and potentially carcinogenic in humans (Felton and Knize, 1991; Hatch *et al.*, 1992; Sugimura, 1997). The metabolic activation of aflatoxin B1 as measured by aflatoxin B1-protein binding mediated by human CYP1A2 was also markedly inhibited by 8-prenylnaringenin and isoxanthohumol (Henderson *et al.*, 2000b).

As an example of the synergistic activity of beer components in inhibiting cell proliferation and inducing programmed cell death, we recently investigated the cytotoxic effects of several lyophilized beer extract on HL-60 cell line, derived from a human leukemia (Tedesco *et al.*, 2005). Firstly, we screened 48 commercially available beers for total polyphenol content. We found a strong correlation between the beer antioxidant activity, evaluated by the ferric reducing antioxidant power assay (FRAP assay), and the total phenolic content (Folin–Ciocalteau's assay). In addition, it was worthwhile to note that: (i) the antiproliferative and apoptogenic activity of lyophilized extracts was only associated to beers with high polyphenol content; (ii) these effects were synergic, since single molecules present in the lyophilized extract, when tested on HL-60 cells at exactly the same concentrations present in the original beer (usually in the micromolar range), did not show the same effect on cell growth and/or apoptosis, as the whole extract and (iii) among three different sources of polyphenolic antioxidants tested (beer, wine and green tea), only beer extracts did not increase peroxide concentration in the cell medium. On the opposite, preparation of crude polyphenols from other sources, such as green tea and red wine, increased enormously H_2O_2 concentration (Tedesco *et al.*, 2005).

Chemopreventive activity of compounds exclusively present in wine, not in beer

According to Table 47.2, three classes of compounds are abundantly present in red wine compared to beer: benzoic acids derivatives, catechins and epicatechins, proanthocyanidins and stilbenes. For all of them chemopreventive activities have been described.

Gallic acid and its structurally related compounds are found widely distributed in fruits and plants. Many published studies report the *in vitro* effects of gallic acid, its esters and gallic acid catechin derivatives on phase I and phase II enzymes. An antimutagenic effect (Ames test) may be observed through inhibition of CYP activation of indirectly acting mutagens and/or by scavenging of metabolically generated mutagenic electrophiles (Ow and Stupans, 2003). Similarly, grape seed proanthocyanidins are active in chemoprevention with particular emphasis on the involvement of matrix metalloproteinases in prostate cancer (Katiyar, 2006) and intestinal neoplasia (Hoensch and Kirch, 2005). The class of flavan-3-ols, including catechins, epicatechins and EGCG (catechin (–)-epigallocatechin-3-gallate, abundantly present in green tea polyphenols) represent main targets in anticancer research (Moyers and Kumar, 2004). Several studies suggest that EGCG and other catechins are poorly absorbed and undergo substantial biotransformation to species that include glucuronides, sulfates and methylated compounds. However, preclinical research is promising, and EGCG appears to be ready for further study in phase II and III trials (Moyers and Kumar, 2004). Finally, resveratrol is the main stilbene present in red wine. Several *in vivo* studies, recently reviewed, sustain resveratrol efficacy in inhibiting or retarding tumor growth and/or progression in animal models inoculated with malignant cell lines, or treated with tumorigenesis-induced drugs (benzo-[α]pyrene, DMBA, azoxymethane) (Ulrich *et al.*, 2005). *In vitro*, resveratrol and its analogs trigger numerous intracellular pathways leading to cell growth arrest. These include inhibition of ERK1/2-mediated signal transduction pathways, inhibition of PMA-dependent PKC activation, downregulation of β-catenin expression, block of cell cycle progression by inhibition of Cdk1 and Cdk4 kinase activities, activation of pRb, induction of apoptotic events, such as activation of caspases, p53 and Bax and inhibition of Bcl2 (Aziz *et al.*, 2003; Ulrich *et al.*, 2005).

Conclusion

Beer contains molecules positively associated with health. Recently, attention has been devoted to prenylflavonoids, a group of plant secondary metabolites that are significantly present in hop plant. Xanthohumol is the principal prenylated flavonoid of the female inflorescences of the hops and it is of general interest to humans since it is present in diet, possesses significant biological activities and an exceptional broad spectrum of inhibitory mechanisms of carcinogenesis. Consistently, xanthohumol modulates the activity of enzymes involved in carcinogen metabolism and detoxification. Furthermore, the molecule is able to scavenge ROS, including hydroxyl- and peroxyl radicals, and to inhibit superoxide anion radical and nitric oxide production.

Much has been written about the favorable impact on health of moderate consumption of wine. Critical assessment of the literature, however, indicates that among alcoholic beverages, beer also possesses such beneficial effects in countering cardiovascular heart disease (Chapters XXX). Additionally, beer can positively contribute to a healthy diet providing B vitamins, minerals, antioxidants and fiber. Urologists recommend beer as an ideal beverage to control kidney stones formation. Finally, numerous studies showed the anticancer effects of beer and beer components. Besides these encouraging data, more case-control studies are necessary to fully evaluate the favorable aspects of beer drinking.

Summary Points

- Moderate beer consumption is supposed to be part of a healthy diet.
- From a nutritional point of view, beer is more abundant in proteins (ranging 2.0–4.8 g/l) and vitamins derived from the barley used during its production, compared to wines.
- Beer is a good source of soluble fiber derived from the cell walls of malted barley. A liter of beer contains an average of 20–60% of the recommended daily intake of fiber.
- Phenolic components of wine and beer are quantitatively and qualitatively different because grape contains polyphenols different from those present in barley and hops used in beer production. A generalized radical scavenging activity was observed in most of beer polyphenolic component.
- Beer antioxidant activity is strongly correlated with the total polyphenol content.
- Recent studies revealed many notable properties of bioactive compounds present in hops, that justify the increasing interest of pharmaceutical firms in hops (or derivatives), as a potential source of novel drugs.
- Scientific evidence accumulated over the last years is in agreement with the potential anticancer activities of selected hop-derived beer constituents, such as xanthohumol and isoxanthohumol, and hop bitter acids.

Acknowledgment

This work was partially supported by a grant from Regione Campania, Italy, entitled "Effetto protettivo della componente polifenolica del vino rosso verso patologie croniche e degenerative" (L.R. n. 5/2002 – Year 2003).

References

Albini, A., Dell'Eva, R., Vene, R., Ferrari, N., Buhler, D.R., Noonan, D.M. and Fassina, G. (2006). *FASEB J.* 20, 527–529.

Assobirra (2006). *Annual Report 2006*, Roma.

Aziz, M.H., Kumar, R. and Ahmad, N. (2003). *Int. J. Oncol.* 23, 17–28.

Bagnardi, V., Blangiardo, M., La Vecchia, C. and Corrao, G. (2001). *Br. J. Cancer* 85, 1700–1705.

Bamforth, C.W. (2002). *Nutr. Res.* 22, 227–237.

Bassus, S., Mahnel, R., Scholz, T., Wegert, W., Westrup, D. and Kirchmaier, C.M. (2004). *Alcohol. Clin. Exp. Res.* 28, 786–791.

Bellia, J.P., Birchall, J.D. and Roberts, N.B. (1994). *Lancet* 343, 235.

Benitez, J.R., Forster, A., De Keukeleire, D., Moir, M., Sharpe, R., Verhagen, L.C. and Westwood, K.T. (1997). *Hops and Hop Products*. Verlag Hans Carl, Nürnberg, Germany.

Biles, B. and Emerson, T.R. (1968). *Nature* 219, 93–94.

Blasco, C., Caballeria, J., Deulofeu, R., Lligona, A., Pares, A., Lluis, J.M., Gual, A. and Rodes, J. (2005). *Alcohol. Clin. Exp. Res.* 29, 1044–1048.

Chang, E.T., Canchola, A.J., Lee, V.S., Clarke, C.A., Purdie, D.M., Reynolds, P., Bernstein, L., Stram, D.O., Anton-Culver, H., Deapen, D., Mohrenweiser, H., Peel, D., Pinder, R., Ross, R.K., West, D.W., Wright, W., Ziogas, A. and Horn-Ross, P.L. (2007). *Cancer Causes Control* 18, 91–103.

Colgate, E.C., Miranda, C.L., Stevens, J.F., Bray, T.M. and Ho, E. (2007). *Cancer Lett.* 246, 201–209.

Constant, J. (1997). *Clin. Cardiol.* 20, 420–424.

Corrao, G., Bagnardi, V., Zambon, A. and Arico, S. (1999). *Addiction* 94, 1551–1573.

Corrao, G., Rubbiati, L., Bagnardi, V., Zambon, A. and Poikolainen, K. (2000). *Addiction* 95, 1505–1523.

Creppy, E. (1999). *J. Toxic. Toxin Rev.* 18, 277–293.

Curhan, G.C., Willett, W.C., Rimm, E.B., Spiegelman, D. and Stampfer, M.J. (1996). *Am. J. Epidemiol.* 143, 240–247.

Daviglus, M.L., Liu, K., Pirzada, A., Yan, L.L., Garside, D.B., Wang, R., Van Horn, L., Manning, W.G., Manheim, L.M., Dyer, A.R., Greenland, P. and Stamler, J. (2005). *J. Am. Diet. Assoc.* 105, 1735–1744.

De Keukeleire, D. (2000). *Quím. Nova* 23, 108–112.

del Alamo, M., Casado, L., Hernandez, V. and Jimenez, J.J. (2004). *J. Chromatogr. A* 1049, 97–105.

Dennis, L.K. (2000). *Prostate* 42, 56–66.

Díaz-Rubio, M.E. and Saura-Calixto, F. (2006). *Am. J. Enol. Vitic.* 57, 69–72.

Dich, J., Jarvinen, R., Knekt, P. and Penttila, P.L. (1996). *Food Addit. Contam.* 13, 541–552.

Dourtoglou, V.G., Makris, D.P., Bois-Dounas, F. and Zonas, C. (1999). *J. Food Compos. Anal.* 12, 227–233.

Eastmond, C.J., Garton, M., Robins, S. and Riddoch, S. (1995). *Br. J. Rheumatol.* 34, 756–759.

Ellis, H.J., Freedman, A.R. and Ciclitira, P.J. (1990). *Clin. Chim. Acta* 189, 123–130.

Ellison, R.C., Zhang, Y., McLennan, C.E. and Rothman, K.J. (2001). *Am. J. Epidemiol.* 154, 740–747.

Felton, J.S. and Knize, M.G. (1991). *Mutat. Res.* 259, 205–217.

Flanzy, M. (1970). *Ann. Nutr. Aliment.* 24, B327–B331.

Furst, A. (2002). *Int. J. Toxicol.* 21, 419–424.

Genkinger, J.M., Hunter, D.J., Spiegelman, D., Anderson, K.E., Buring, J.E., Freudenheim, J.L., Goldbohm, R.A., Harnack, L., Hankinson, S.E., Larsson, S.C., Leitzmann, M., McCullough, M.L., Marshall, J., Miller, A.B., Rodriguez, C., Rohan, T.E., Schatzkin, A., Schouten, L.J., Wolk, A., Zhang, S.M. and Smith-Warner, S.A. (2006). *Br. J. Cancer* 94, 757–762.

Gerhauser, C. (2005). *Eur. J. Cancer* 41, 1941–1954.

Gerhäuser, C., Alt, A.P., Klimo, K., Knauft, J., Frank, N. and Becker, H. (2002). *Phytochemistry Rev.* 1, 369–377.

Gerhauser, C., Bartsch, H., Crowell, J., De Flora, S., D'Incalci, M., Dittrich, C., Frank, N., Mihich, E., Steffen, C., Tortora, G. and Gescher, A. (2006). *Eur. J. Cancer* 42, 1338–1343.

Ghiselli, A., Natella, F., Guidi, A., Montanari, L., Fantozzi, P. and Scaccini, C. (2000). *J. Nutr. Biochem.* 11, 76–80.

Gromes, R., Zeuch, M. and Piendl, A. (2000). *Brau Int.* 18, 24–28.

Gruenewald, P.J. and Ponicki, W.R. (1995). *J. Stud. Alcohol* 56, 635–641.

Gu, L., Kelm, M.A., Hammerstone, J.F., Beecher, G., Holden, J., Haytowitz, D., Gebhardt, S. and Prior, R.L. (2004). *J. Nutr.* 134, 613–617.

Hanske, L., Hussong, R., Frank, N., Gerhauser, C., Blaut, M. and Braune, A. (2005). *Mol. Nutr. Food Res.* 49, 868–873.

Hatch, F.T., Knize, M.G., Moore II, D.H. and Felton, J.S. (1992). *Mutat. Res.* 271, 269–287.

Henderson, C.J., Sahraouei, A. and Wolf, C.R. (2000a). *Biochem. Soc. Trans.* 28, 42–46.

Henderson, M.C., Miranda, C.L., Stevens, J.F., Deinzer, M.L. and Buhler, D.R. (2000b). *Xenobiotica* 30, 235–251.

Hijova, E. (2006). *Bratisl. Lek. Listy* 107, 80–84.

Hingson, R., Heeren, T., Winter, M. and Wechsler, H. (2005). *Annu. Rev. Public Health* 26, 259–279.

Hoensch, H.P. and Kirch, W. (2005). *Int. J. Gastrointest. Cancer* 35, 187–195.

Hussong, R., Frank, N., Knauft, J., Ittrich, C., Owen, R., Becker, H. and Gerhauser, C. (2005). *Mol. Nutr. Food Res.* 49, 861–867.

Iacomino, G., Tecce, M.F., Grimaldi, C., Tosto, M. and Russo, G.L. (2001). *Biochem. Biophys. Res. Commun.* 285, 1280–1289.

Izquierdo-Pulido, M., Barbour, J.F. and Scanlan, R.A. (1996). *Food Chem. Toxicol.* 34, 297–299.

Izquierdo-Pulido, M., Marine-Font, A. and Vidal-Carou, M. (2000). *Food Chem.* 70, 329–332.

Katiyar, S.K. (2006). *Endocr. Metab. Immune Disord. Drug Targets* 6, 17–24.

Kondo, K. (2004). *Biofactors* 22, 303–310.

Kozarevic, D., Vojvodic, N., Gordon, T., Kaelber, C.T., McGee, D. and Zukel, W.J. (1983). *Int. J. Epidemiol.* 12, 145–150.

Lee, K.W., Lee, H.J. and Lee, C.Y. (2004). *Crit. Rev. Food Sci. Nutr.* 44, 437–452.

Linos, E., Holmes, M.D. and Willett, W.C. (2007). *Curr. Oncol. Rep.* 9, 31–41.

Liu, R.H. (2003). *Am. J. Clin. Nutr.* 78, 517S–520S.

Liu, R.H. (2004). *J. Nutr.* 134, 3479S–3485S.

Long, D. (1999). *J. Inst. Brew.* 105, 79–84.

Lust, S., Vanhoecke, B., Janssens, A., Philippe, J., Bracke, M. and Offner, F. (2005). *Mol. Nutr. Food Res.* 49, 844–850.

Mark, L., Nikfardjam, M.S., Avar, P. and Ohmacht, R. (2005). *J. Chromatogr. Sci.* 43, 445–449.

Meydani, M. (2001). *Ann. NY Acad. Sci.* 928, 226–235.

Miranda, C.L., Stevens, J.F., Helmrich, A., Henderson, M.C., Rodriguez, R.J., Yang, Y.H., Deinzer, M.L., Barnes, D.W. and Buhler, D.R. (1999). *Food Chem. Toxicol.* 37, 271–285.

Miranda, C.L., Aponso, G.L., Stevens, J.F., Deinzer, M.L. and Buhler, D.R. (2000). *Cancer Lett.* 149, 21–29.

Moll, M. (1991). *Bieres and Coolers*. Tec & Doc-Lavoisier, Paris.

Moyers, S.B. and Kumar, N.B. (2004). *Nutr. Rev.* 62, 204–211.

Nebert, D.W. and Dalton, T.P. (2006). *Nat. Rev. Cancer* 6, 947–960.

Ow, Y.Y. and Stupans, I. (2003). *Curr. Drug Metab.* 4, 241–248.

Paganga, G., Miller, N. and Rice-Evans, C.A. (1999). *Free Radic. Res.* 30, 153–162.

Polidori, M.C. (2003). *J. Postgrad. Med.* 49, 229–235.

Powell, J.J., McNaughton, S.A., Jugdaohsingh, R., Anderson, S.H., Dear, J., Khot, F., Mowatt, L., Gleason, K.L., Sykes, M., Thompson, R.P., Bolton-Smith, C. and Hodson, M.J. (2005). *Br. J. Nutr.* 94, 804–812.

Rainbow, C. and Float, G.E.S. (1990). *An Introduction to Brewing Science and Technology*. The Institute of Brewing, London.

Rehm, J., Monteiro, M., Room, R., Gmel, G., Jernigan, D., Frick, U. and Graham, K. (2001). *Eur. Addict. Res.* 7, 138–147.

Rehm, J., Gmel, G., Sempos, C.T. and Trevisan, M. (2003). *Alcohol Res. Health* 27, 39–51.

Riboli, E., Cornee, J., Macquart-Moulin, G., Kaaks, R., Casagrande, C. and Guyader, M. (1991). *Am. J. Epidemiol.* 134, 157–166.

Rivero, D., Perez-Magarino, S., Gonzalez-Sanjose, M.L., Valls-Belles, V., Codoner, P. and Muniz, P. (2005). *J. Agric. Food Chem.* 53, 3637–3642.

Rodés, J., Salaspuro, M. and Sorensen, T.I.A. (1999). *Alcohol and Liver Disease*. Blackwell Science, Oxford.

Rodriguez-Delgado, M.A., Malovana, S., Perez, J.P., Borges, T. and Garcia Montelongo, F.J. (2001). *J. Chromatogr. A* 912, 249–257.

Romeo, J., Diaz, L., Gonzalez-Gross, M., Warnberg, J. and Marcos, A. (2006). *Nutr. Hosp.* 21, 84–91.

Russo, G.L. (2007). *Biochem. Pharmacol.* 74, 533–544.

Russo, G.L., Della Pietra, V., Mercurio, C., Palumbo, R., Iacomino, G., Russo, M., Tosto, M. and Zappia, V. (1999). *Adv. Exp. Med. Biol.* 472, 131–147.

Russo, M., Tedesco, I., Iacomino, G., Palumbo, R., Galano, G. and Russo, G.L. (2005). *Curr. Med. Chem. Immun. Endoc. Metab. Agents* 5, 61–72.

Sanchez-Moreno, C., Cao, G., Ou, B. and Prior, R.L. (2003). *J. Agric. Food Chem.* 51, 4889–4896.

Scalbert, A., Manach, C., Morand, C., Remesy, C. and Jimenez, L. (2005). *Crit. Rev. Food Sci. Nutr.* 45, 287–306.

Shahidi, F. and Naczk, M. (1995). Food phenolics. Technomic Publishing Co, Lancaster, Basel.

Smith-Warner, S.A., Spiegelman, D., Yaun, S.S., van den Brandt, P.A., Folsom, A.R., Goldbohm, R.A., Graham, S., Holmberg, L., Howe, G.R., Marshall, J.R., Miller, A.B., Potter, J.D., Speizer, F.E., Willett, W.C., Wolk, A. and Hunter, D.J. (1998). *JAMA* 279, 535–540.

Sporn, M.B. and Suh, N. (2002). *Nat. Rev. Cancer* 2, 537–543.

Sripanyakorn, S., Jugdaohsingh, R., Elliott, H., Walker, C., Mehta, P., Shoukru, S., Thompson, R.P. and Powell, J.J. (2004). *Br. J. Nutr.* 91, 403–409.

Stevens, J.F. and Page, J.E. (2004). *Phytochemistry* 65, 1317–1330.

Stevens, J.F., Taylor, A.W., Clawson, J.E. and Deinzer, M.L. (1999). *J. Agric. Food. Chem.* 47, 2421–2428.

Sugimura, T. (1997). *Mutat. Res.* 376, 211–219.

Suter, P.M. (2001). *Nutr. Rev.* 59, 293–297.

Tedesco, I., Russo, M., Russo, P., Iacomino, G., Russo, G.L., Carraturo, A., Faruolo, C., Moio, L. and Palumbo, R. (2000). *J. Nutr. Biochem.* 11, 114–119.

Tedesco, I., Nappo, A., Petitto, F., Iacomino, G., Nazzaro, F., Palumbo, R. and Russo, G.L. (2005). *Nutr. Cancer* 52, 74–83.

Tricker, A.R. and Preussmann, R. (1991). *J. Cancer Res. Clin. Oncol.* 117, 130–132.

Ulrich, S., Wolter, F. and Stein, J.M. (2005). *Mol. Nutr. Food Res.* 49, 452–461.

Vanhoecke, B., Derycke, L., Van Marck, V., Depypere, H., De Keukeleire, D. and Bracke, M. (2005). *Int. J. Cancer* 117, 889–895.

Yilmazer, M., Stevens, J.F. and Buhler, D.R. (2001). *FEBS Lett.* 491, 252–256.

48

The Absorption and Metabolism of Phenolic Acids from Beer in Man

Mirella Nardini, Fausta Natella, Andrea Ghiselli and Cristina Scaccini National Research Institute for Food and Nutrition Research, Via Ardeatina, Rome, Italy

Abstract

In spite of the wide literature describing the biological effects of phenolic compounds, scarce data are available on their absorption from diet and metabolism in humans. Recently, a renewal interest has been focused on beer, a common beverage with low ethanol content and rich in phenolic compounds, particularly caffeic, vanillic, *p*-coumaric, sinapic, syringic and ferulic acids. In this study, the absorption in humans of phenolic acids from beer was studied. Firstly, a recently developed hydrolytic procedure was applied to quantitatively measure total (free plus bound) phenolic acids in beer. Secondly, we measured plasma concentration of phenolic acids in samples collected before and 30 and 60 min after beer administration in healthy humans. The results obtained show that the most of phenolic acids are present in beer as bound forms and only a small portion can be detected as free forms. Moreover, phenolic acids from beer are absorbed from the gastrointestinal tract and are present in blood after being largely metabolized to the form of glucuronide and sulfate conjugates. The extent of conjugation is related to the chemical structure of phenolic acids, the monohydroxy derivatives showing the lowest conjugation degree and the dihydroxy derivatives showing the highest one.

List of Abbreviations

CAF	Caffeic acid
p-COU	*p*-Coumaric acid
EDTA	Ethylendiaminetetracetic acid
FER	Ferulic acid
HPLC-ECD	High pressure liquid chromatography with electrochemical detection
4-OH-PA	4-Hydroxyphenylacetic acid
SIN	Sinapic acid
SPE	Solid-phase extraction
VAN	Vanillic acid

Introduction

Oxidative stress has been recognized to be involved in several pathological conditions, such as atherosclerosis, diabetes, neurodegenerative diseases, cancer and in the aging. Antioxidants present in our daily diet may afford protection against oxidative-related diseases. In particular, beverages account for a very high proportion of dietary antioxidant intake in the Mediterranean diet (Pulido *et al.*, 2003). Among dietary antioxidants, phenolics are by far the most abundant in human diet. Plant phenolics received particular attention in the past 10 years due to their putative role in the prevention of several human diseases associated with oxidative stress, including atherosclerosis and cancer (Block *et al.*, 1992; Renaud and deLorgeril, 1992; Scalbert and Williamson, 2000). The total polyphenols intake has been reported to be in the order of 1 g/day (Scalbert and Williamson, 2000). For individuals regularly consuming wine, coffee, beer and tea, these beverages are likely to be the major sources of phenolic compounds. Coffee is the main contributor, followed by red wine, fruit juice, beer, tea. A major class of polyphenols is represented by phenolic acids, which are widely distributed in diet, mostly in fruits, vegetables, coffee, wine, beer and olive oil (Herrmann, 1989; Clifford, 1999). The average phenolic acids intake has been reported to be in the order of 200 mg/day within a large range, depending on the nutritional habits (Herrmann, 1989; Clifford, 1999; Scalbert and Williamson, 2000). Phenolic acids occur in food mainly as esterified forms with organic acids, sugar, lipids (Herrmann, 1989). Recently, a renewal interest has been focused on beer, a common beverage rich in phenolic compounds, with low ethanol content. In a previous study we demonstrated that beer is able to increase human plasma antioxidant capacity, probably through its phenolic components (Ghiselli *et al.*, 2000). In this study, the absorption in humans of phenolic acids from beer was studied, focusing on the measurements of plasma concentrations of both free (non-conjugated)

Beer in Health and Disease Prevention
ISBN: 978-0-12-373891-2

and conjugated forms of phenolic acids. Moreover, a new hydrolytic procedure to measure the total phenolic acids content of beer was successfully applied (Nardini *et al.*, 2002a). Most of the procedures described in the literature to detect bound phenolic acids in food take advantage of alkaline hydrolysis to release bound forms of phenolic acids (Fenton *et al.*, 1980; Krygier *et al.*, 1982; Kozlowska *et al.*, 1983; Maillard and Berset, 1995). However these procedures lead to a considerable loss of several phenolic acids, particularly caffeic acid (Krygier *et al.*, 1982; Maillard and Berset, 1995), which is one of the most abundant phenolic acids in plant-derived food and beverages. The new hydrolytic procedure used allowed the qualitative and quantitative measurement of total (free plus bound) phenolic acids in beer (Nardini and Ghiselli, 2004).

Study Design and Samples Treatments

The study was approved by the Ethical Committee of the National Institute for Food and Nutrition Research. Ten healthy subjects (25–45 years) were recruited. Participants were non-smokers, either non-drinkers or social drinkers (<28 and <14 g ethanol/day, for males and females, respectively). They were asked to avoid coffee, wine, beer, tea and fruit juices the day preceding the experiment. Fasting subjects received 500 ml of beer in combination with 27 g of crackers in the morning. The beer used in this study was an Italian brand containing 4.5% ethanol. The phenolic acids content of crackers, given to avoid undesirable effects of ethanol in fasting conditions, was not relevant with respect to the amount of phenolic acids present in beer. In a subsample of three subjects, 500 ml beer without crackers, or 27 g crackers without beer, were administered in fasting conditions as control. Blood was collected into ethylendiaminetetracetic acid (EDTA)-containing vacutainers before (time 0) and 30 and 60 min after ingestion of beer, crackers or beer plus crackers. Plasma prepared by centrifugation (1,000 × *g* for 20 min at 4°C) was acidified at pH 3.0 and stored at –80°C.

Plasma samples were treated for phenolic acids extraction essentially as previously described (Nardini *et al.*, 2002b), with minor modifications concerning the source and purity of the enzymes used to hydrolyze conjugated phenolic acids. Aliquots of plasma (1 ml), added with 200 ng *o*-coumaric acid as internal standard, were deproteinized as previously described (Nardini *et al.*, 2002b), then the dried residues treated according to one of the following four procedures: no hydrolytic treatment, to detect free (non-conjugated) phenolic acids; β-glucuronidase treatment, to hydrolyze glucuronide conjugates; sulfatase treatment, to hydrolyze sulfate conjugates; sequential β-glucuronidase–sulfatase treatment, to hydrolyze glucuronide, sulfate and sulfoglucuronide conjugates.

Plasma non-conjugated phenolic acids

The dried residue from deproteinization was extracted with ethyl acetate as already reported (Nardini *et al.*, 2002b). The residue obtained after extraction was dissolved in 0.5 ml water, vortexed for 5 min, the pH brought to 7–8 with NaOH and loaded on a LC-SAX tube (Supelco, Bellefonte, PA, USA) for solid-phase extraction (SPE). After washing with 1 ml water, phenolic acids elution was eluted with 1 ml of buffer containing 1N acetic acid/methanol (90:10). The eluant was brought to pH 3.0, filtered and aliquots analyzed by high pressure liquid chromatography with electrochemical detection (HPLC-ECD). This procedure allows the detection of free, non-conjugated phenolic acids in plasma sample.

Plasma glucuronides

The dried residue obtained by deproteinization was dissolved in 0.5 ml 0.2M K-phosphate buffer pH 6.8, vortexed for 5 min then incubated at 37°C for 2 h with 776U β-glucuronidase (EC 3.2.1.31, type IX A from *E. coli*). At the end of incubation, the pH was brought to 3.0, 300 mg NaCl added and the sample was extracted as already described (Nardini *et al.*, 2002b). The final residue was suspended in 0.5 ml water and processed for SPE as above described. This procedure allows the measure of free plus glucuronide conjugates of phenolic acids present in plasma sample. The amount of glucuronides was calculated by subtracting the value of free, non-conjugated phenolic acids obtained with the above reported procedure.

Plasma sulfates

The dried residue obtained by deproteinization was dissolved in 0.5 ml of 0.1M Na-acetate buffer pH 5.0, vortexed 5 min then incubated at 37°C for 2 h with 70U sulfatase (type H-1 from Helix pomatia, containing β-glucuronidase) and 26 mM D-saccharic acid 1,4-lactone monohydrate, an inhibitor of β-glucuronidase. At the end of incubation, the pH was brought to 3.0, 300 mg NaCl added and the sample was extracted as already described (Nardini *et al.*, 2002b). The final residue was resuspended in 0.5 ml water and processed for SPE as above described. This procedure allows the measure of free plus sulfates conjugates of phenolic acids present in plasma sample. The amount of sulfates was calculated by subtracting the value of free, non-conjugated phenolic acids obtained with the above reported procedure.

Plasma total phenolic acids

The dried residue obtained by deproteinization was dissolved in 0.5 ml 0.2M K-phosphate buffer pH 6.8, vortexed for 5 min then incubated at 37°C for 2 h with 776U β-glucuronidase (EC 3.2.1.31, type IX A from *E. coli*). At the end of incubation, the pH was brought to 5.0 with HCl and sample incubated at 37°C for 2 h with 70U sulfatase (type H-1 from Helix pomatia, containing β-glucuronidase). After incubation, the pH was brought to pH 3.0 with HCl, 300 mg NaCl added and sample extracted as already described (Nardini *et al.*, 2002b). The final residue was resuspended in 0.5 ml water and processed for SPE as above described. This procedure allows the measure of total phenolic acids (non-conjugated, glucuronides, sulfates and possible mixed sulfate/glucuronide conjugates) present in plasma sample. For each single phenolic acid, the amount obtained with this incubation, subtracted the amount of the respective non-conjugated form, glucuronides and sulfates derivatives obtained with the above reported procedures, should represent the amount of mixed sulfate/glucuronide conjugates in the sample.

Beer treatment for phenolic acid extraction

Beer samples were degassed by sonication and treated for free (non-hydrolyzed samples) and total (free plus bound, hydrolyzed samples) phenolic acids determination.

For free phenolic acids measurements, beer (0.5 ml) was added with 1 μg isoferulic acid as internal standard, acidified at pH 3.0 and added with 300 mg NaCl. Samples were extracted three times with ethyl acetate (4 × vols) by 5 min vortexing. After each extraction samples were centrifuged and supernatant collected. The pooled organic phases were dried under nitrogen flow. The residue was dissolved in methanol and diluted with sample buffer (1.25% glacial acetic acid, 7% methanol in water) prior to HPLC-ECD analysis. For total phenolic acids measurements, beer (0.5 ml) was subjected to alkaline hydrolysis with 4.5 ml 2N NaOH containing 10 mM EDTA and 1% ascorbic acid, in the presence of 1 μg isoferulic acid as internal standard. After incubation at 30°C for 30 min, 0.5 ml aliquot was acidified to pH 3 with HCl, added with 300 mg NaCl and extracted as above reported. Phenolic acids recovery, performed by adding known amounts of pure phenolic acids to beer samples (protocatechuic, vanillic, caffeic, syringic, *p*-coumaric, ferulic, sinapic, *o*-coumaric, 4-hydroxyphenylacetic acids, as representative of beer phenolics), was found to be in the range of 95.4–104.0% and 94.0–102.9% in non-hydrolyzed and hydrolyzed beer samples, respectively. Further, the addition of known amounts of chlorogenic acid to beer samples resulted in the almost complete recovery of caffeic acid released upon hydrolysis (98.7 ± 4.3% of expected value).

HPLC instrumentation

The HPLC consists of a Perkin-Elmer Series 4 Liquid Chromatograph (Perkin-Elmer, Norwalk, CT, USA) with a gradient pump, column thermoregulator and autosampling injector (Gilson, Beltline, Middleton, WI, USA) equipped with an electrochemical coulometric detector (Coulochem II, ESA, Bedford, MA, USA). Turbochrom chromatography workstation software was used for data processing. Operating conditions were as follows: column temperature, 30°C; flow rate, 1 ml/min; ECD at +600 mV; sensitivity range 100–200 nA. Chromatographic separation was performed on a Supelcosil LC-18 C_{18} column (5 μm particle size, 250 × 4.6 mm i.d.) including a C_{18} guard column (Supelco, Bellefonte, PA, USA). For gradient elution mobile phases A and B were employed. Solution A contained 1.25% glacial acetic acid in water; solution B was absolute methanol. For beer samples analyses the following gradient was used: 0–25 min, from 98%A, 2%B to 76%A, 24%B, linear gradient; 26–45 min, 76%A, 24%B; 46–53 min, from 76%A, 24%B to 55%A, 45%B, linear gradient; 54–55 min, 55%A, 45%B; 56–86 min, 98%A, 2%B. For plasma samples analyses the following gradient was used: 0–25 min, from 93%A, 7%B to 76%A, 24%B, linear gradient; 26–45 min, 76%A, 24%B; 46–53 min, from 76%A, 24%B to 55%A, 45%B, linear gradient; 54–55 min, 55%A, 45%B; 56–86 min, 93%A, 7%B. Prior to HPLC analysis, all samples were filtered using Millex-HV filters (Millipore) with 0.45 μm pore size. Stock solutions of standard phenolic acids prepared in methanol (1 mg/ml) were stored at −80°C and used within 1 week. Working standard solutions were prepared daily by dilution in sample buffer (1.25% glacial acetic acid, 7% methanol in water).

Data evaluation, quantitation and statistical analysis

For calibration curve, appropriate volumes of the stock standard solutions were diluted with sample buffer. Three replicates of standards at four concentration levels (20, 100, 200 and 500 ng/ml) were analyzed. For quantitative determination, peak areas in the sample chromatogram were correlated with the concentrations according to the calibration curve. Data presented are means ± SD or SE as specified. Statistical analysis was performed by a one-factor analysis of variance (ANOVA, Scheffe's method) for multiple comparison or paired *t*-test as specified. Probability of $p < 0.05$ was considered statistically significant.

Results

Phenolic acids in beer

Beer contains appreciable amounts of several phenolic acids whose chemical structures are shown in Figure 48.1. Figure 48.2 shows the beer content of both free and total (free plus bound) phenolic acids and their derivatives. 4-Hydroxyphenylacetic acid and *p*-coumaric acid were present in beer mainly as free, unbound forms (76.2% and 69.8% of the total, respectively). A moderate increase of

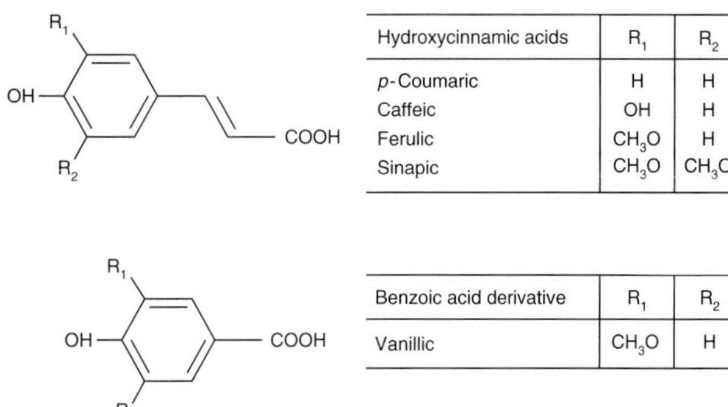

Hydroxycinnamic acids	R_1	R_2
p-Coumaric	H	H
Caffeic	OH	H
Ferulic	CH_3O	H
Sinapic	CH_3O	CH_3O

Benzoic acid derivative	R_1	R_2
Vanillic	CH_3O	H

Figure 48.1 Chemical structures of the main phenolic acids present in beer. Caffeic acid: 3,4-dihydroxycinnamic acid; ferulic acid: 4-hydroxy-3-methoxycinnamic acid; vanillic acid: 4-hydroxy-3-methoxybenzoic acid; *p*-coumaric acid: 4-hydroxycinnamic acid; sinapic acid: 3,5-dimethoxy-4-hydroxycinnamic acid.

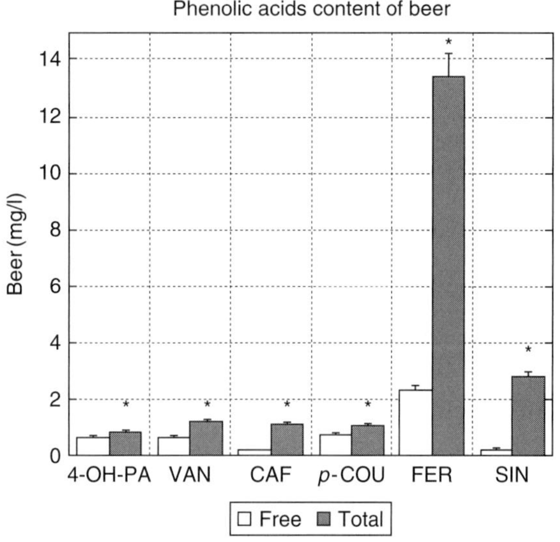

Figure 48.2 Phenolic acids content of beer before and after hydrolysis. Phenolic acids content was measured in non-hydrolyzed samples and in samples submitted to alkaline hydrolysis as reported in Methods section. Values are expressed as mg/l of beer and represent means ± SD (n = 3). 4-OH-PA, 4-hydroxyphenylacetic acid; VAN, vanillic acid; CAF, caffeic acid; *p*-COU, *p*-coumaric acid; FER, ferulic acid; SIN, sinapic acid. *Values are significantly different from those measured in non-hydrolyzed samples ($p \leq 0.05$ by ANOVA).

these compounds after hydrolysis was observed. Differently, the amount of vanillic, caffeic, ferulic and sinapic acids dramatically increased (≥100% of the value measured in non-hydrolyzed samples) in hydrolyzed beer in the respect of non-hydrolyzed samples. Caffeic, ferulic and sinapic acids were present in beer mainly as conjugated forms, the free and non-conjugated forms amounting to 18.6%, 17.3% and 7.8% of total, respectively. Vanillic was present in beer equally as bound and free forms, the latter amounting to 52.5% of total. The content of free phenolic acids measured in our beer is in agreement with data reported in the literature (Hayes *et al.*, 1987; Achilli *et al.*, 1993; Shahidi and Naczk, 1995; Gorinstein *et al.*, 2000). Ferulic acid was by far the most abundant phenolic acid in beer.

Absorption of phenolic acids from beer in humans

To study the absorption of phenolic acids from beer, plasma samples were collected before and after beer plus crackers administration and analyzed for phenolic acids content, both as free (non-conjugated) and conjugated forms. The different procedures applied allowed the detection of non-conjugated phenolic acids, glucuronide conjugates, sulfate conjugates and total phenolic acids (non-conjugated + glucuronide conjugates + sulfate conjugates + sulfoglucuronide conjugates). Beer plus crackers administration resulted in a fast, significant increase of phenolic acids concentrations in plasma. The concentration of total 4-hydroxyphenylacetic acid increased three- to fourfold at both 30 and 60 min with respect to time 0, the free, non-conjugated forms amounting to 70.8%, 82.2% and 77.4% of total at time 0, 30 and 60 min, respectively (Figure 48.3a). A slight, not significant increase in the concentration of sulfate conjugates was measured at 30 and 60 min, with respect to time 0. Non-conjugated and total *p*-coumaric acid significantly increased 30 min after beer and crackers administration with respect to time 0, the non-conjugated form amounting to 54.4%, 54.7% and 59.5% of total at time 0, 30 and 60 min, respectively (Figure 48.3b). Glucuronate derivatives of *p*-coumaric acid significantly increased at 60 min after ingestion with respect to time 0, while no significant change was observed for sulfate conjugates at any time after ingestion. A significant increase in non-conjugated form, sulfate conjugates and total vanillic acid was observed at 30 min after beer plus crackers administration with respect to time 0, while a slight, not significant increase in the glucuronate conjugates was observed at 30 and 60 min with respect to time 0. Differently from 4-hydroxyphenylacetic and *p*-coumaric acids, vanillic acid was present in plasma mainly as conjugated forms, the non-conjugated forms amounting to 17.2%, 31.6% and 39.3% of total at time 0, 30 and 60 min, respectively (Figure 48.3c). The most of caffeic acid was present in plasma as sulfate and glucuronate derivatives, the non-conjugated forms amounting to 0%, 4.4% and 12.7% of total at time 0, 30 and 60 min, respectively (Figure 48.3d). In particular, a significant increase in sulfate and glucuronate conjugates and total caffeic acid was observed at 30 min after beer plus crackers administration with respect to time 0, while at 60 min a significant increase in sulfate conjugates and total caffeic acid was measured with respect to time 0. A significant increase in non-conjugated form, sulfate conjugates, glucuronate

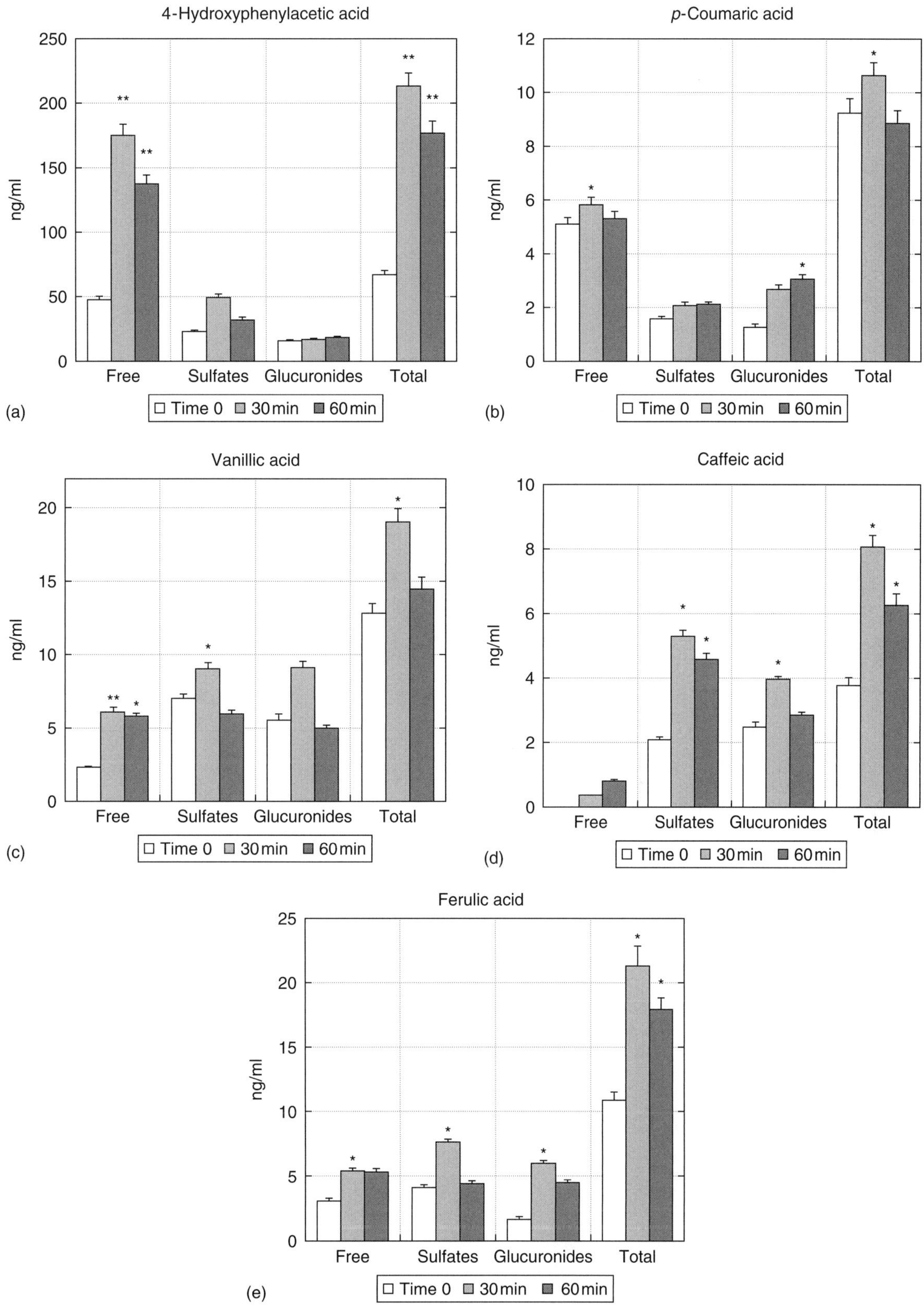

Figure 48.3 Plasma phenolic acids levels in 10 different subjects before and after beer plus crackers administration. Plasma samples separated from blood collected just before (time 0) or after (30 and 60 min) beer plus crackers administration were analyzed for non-conjugated and conjugated phenolic acids as reported in Methods section. (a): 4-hydroxyphenylacetic acid; (b): *p*-coumaric acid; (c): vanillic acid; (d): caffeic acid; (e): ferulic acid. Values are means ± SE. $^{*}p \leqslant 0.05$; $^{**}p \leqslant 0.01$ with respect to time 0 by paired *t*-test.

conjugates and total ferulic acid was measured at 30 min after beer plus crackers administration with respect to time 0, the non-conjugated form amounting to 27.8%, 25.2% and 29.0% of total at time 0, 30 and 60 min, respectively (Figure 48.3e). Total ferulic acid was also significantly higher at 60 min after ingestion with respect to time 0.

We failed to quantitatively measure sinapic acid in plasma due to both the low amount present in the samples and the interference from other unidentified components in the chromatograms.

Administration of crackers alone did not result in any significant increase of plasma phenolic acids concentrations at 30 and 60 min after ingestion with respect to time 0. Further, administration of beer alone resulted in plasma phenolic acids levels similar to those obtained after beer plus crackers ingestion in three different subjects (data not shown).

Discussion

The results obtained show that phenolic acids from beer are rapidly absorbed and circulate in human plasma as both free and conjugated forms, mainly glucuronates and sulfates. The fast absorption of phenolic acids, with a maximum peak at 30 min, suggests that it could take place in the proximal part of the intestine. Due to the presence of both free and bound forms of phenolic acids in beer, plasma circulating phenolics might be derived from the direct absorption of the free forms present in beer, by *in vivo* hydrolysis of the bound forms present in beer as well, or both. In the past, conjugated forms of phenolic compounds, although widely present in our diet, were considered not bioavailable in humans. However, more recently phenolic acids have been described to be absorbed from their bound forms present in food, both in humans and in rats (Azuma *et al.*, 2000; Andreason *et al.*, 2001a, b; Rechner *et al.*, 2001; Nardini *et al.*, 2002b; Lafay *et al.*, 2006). Esterases with the ability to hydrolyze hydroxycinnamate esters at appreciable rates have been described in humans and rats (Andreason *et al.*, 2001a). The cinnamoyl esterase activity is distributed all along the small and large intestine and it is present both in the mucosa and in the lumen. Moreover, bacteria in the gastrointestinal tract of mammals are also capable of releasing free phenolic acids from their bound complexes (Buchanan *et al.*, 1996; Kroon *et al.*, 1997; Wende *et al.*, 1997; Plumb *et al.*, 1999; Andreason *et al.*, 2001b; Couteau *et al.*, 2001). Both glucuronidation and sulfation occur at various extents during absorption of phenolic acids from beer. Glucuronidation and sulfation are two well-known ways of detoxification leading to increased solubility of compounds to promote their excretion. The most of 4-hydroxyphenylacetic acid was present in plasma as non-conjugated form (>70%) and this is in agreement with the hydrophilic feature of this compound, due to the presence of a polar acetyl group and one hydroxyl group on the aromatic ring. *p*-Coumaric acid, which possesses a propenoic side chain and an hydroxyl group on the aromatic ring, was present as free, non-conjugated form at levels lower than that observed for 4-hydroxyphenylacetic acid (54–59% of the total), but considerably higher than those observed for ferulic, vanillic and caffeic acids, which instead circulate mainly as conjugated forms, with a slight prevalence of sulfates with respect to glucuronate forms. The presence of a methoxyl group in addition to the hydroxyl group on the aromatic ring of both vanillic acid and ferulic acid decreases their hydrophilicity, with respect to both 4-hydroxyphenylacetic acid and *p*-coumaric, and may account for the extensive conjugation observed (61–83% of the total for vanillic acid; 71–75% of the total for ferulic acid). Similar results have been obtained after ferulic acid administration in rats, with plasma levels of conjugated ferulic acid amounting to 76% of the total ferulic acid (Rondini *et al.*, 2002). Caffeic acid, in spite of the two hydroxyl groups in the ortho position on the aromatic ring, was present in plasma almost exclusively as conjugated forms (87–100% of the total) with a prevalence of sulfates with respect to glucuronates. A similar result has been obtained for plasma caffeic acid after coffee drinking in humans (Nardini *et al.*, 2002b). Our results demonstrated that once absorbed from beer, phenolic acids are extensively conjugated to sulfates and glucuronates. Likely, the differences in the extent of conjugation are related to the different chemical features of phenolic acids and may reflect differences in the activity and specificity of both glucuronosyltransferases and sulfotransferases enzymes toward different phenolic acids. From our results, the monohydroxy derivatives showed the lowest degree of conjugation and the dihydroxy derivative showed the highest one, while the 3-methoxy-4-hydroxy derivatives (vanillic and ferulic acids) fell in the middle. On this regard, the evidence that caffeic acid circulates in human plasma almost exclusively as conjugated forms, particularly sulfate, may be explained by the high activity of intestine sulfotransferase SULT1A3 on catechol group (3,4-dihydroxy moiety) (Scalbert and Williamson, 2000). Moreover, human intestine glucuronosyltransferases appeared to be especially effective in conjugating the catechol unit. Since the antioxidant action as well as the prooxidant toxicity of caffeic acid is mainly related to its catechol unit (Shahidi and Wanasundara, 1992; Nardini *et al.*, 1995), it is of interest to note that the conjugating enzymes in human intestine seem to be especially active in conjugating this structure. This would imply that during the transport across the intestinal border, the catechol-type phenolic compounds might loose a significant part of their biological activity, due to glucuronidation and sulfation. Regarding the effect of the carbon side chain on the degree of conjugation, only minor differences were observed between ferulic acid, with a propenoic side chain, and vanillic acid, endowed with a carboxylic side chain. *p*-Coumaric acid, with a propenoic side chain, was conjugated to a higher degree with respect to

4-hydroxyphenylacetic acid, endowed with an acetyl group instead of the propenoic chain. From our data, mixed sulfate/glucuronide conjugates are present, if any, at very low levels, being the amount of total phenolic acids measured not significantly different from the theoretical amount calculated by addition of non-conjugated, glucuronide and sulfate conjugates.

The most relevant conclusion of our study is that the plasma concentration of conjugated forms of vanillic, ferulic and caffeic acids largely exceeds that of free, non-conjugated forms. While the biological activity of phenolic acids has been widely studied and described in the literature in the last decade, scarce or no data are available on the potential biological activity of their metabolites. Indeed, glucuronidation and sulfation might affect the biological activity of the parent free, non-conjugated compounds. As mentioned above, the conjugation of the catechol unit might result in a partial lost of biological activity for those phenolics endowed with a 3,4-dihydroxy unit. It has been described that quercetin glucuronides and quercetin 3-*O*-sulfate still retain antioxidant activity, although to a less degree with respect to non-conjugated quercetin (Manach *et al.*, 1998). Ferulic acid glucuronide, endowed with a sugar moiety beside the hydrophobic ferulic acid unit, showed an antioxidant activity stronger than that of ferulic acid (Ohta *et al.*, 1997).

From our results, plasma concentration of phenolic acids ranged between 0.05 and 0.07 μM for caffeic acid and *p*-coumaric acid and reached 0.11 μM for vanillic and ferulic acid at 30 min after beer plus crackers administration. 4-Hydroxyphenylacetic acid reached higher concentration in plasma in respect to the other phenolic acids, amounting to 1.40 and 1.17 μM at 30 and 60 min, respectively. 4-Hydroxyphenylacetic acid is a metabolite of tyrosine other than of various phenolic compounds (Mani *et al.*, 2003) and a discrete amount of tyrosine is present in beer (Pulido *et al.*, 2003). Hence, plasma 4-hydroxyphenylacetic acid might be derived either from the absorption of 4-hydroxyphenylacetic acid present in beer as such, or from the post-absorption metabolism of phenolic acids and tyrosine contained in beer as well. Noteworthy, no appreciable increase in plasma concentration of 4-hydroxyphenylacetic acid and other phenolic acids was observed at 30 and 60 min after ingestion of crackers alone with respect to time 0. Although the plasma concentrations of phenolic acids measured seem quite low, it must be kept in mind that they were obtained after a single administration of 500 ml beer, containing about 10 mg of the phenolic acids under study. This value is quite far from the average daily intake of phenolic acids, which has been calculated in the order of 200 mg/day (Herrmann, 1989; Scalbert and Williamson, 2000).

Synergistic effects might also occur *in vivo*. Further, an accumulation of phenolic acids and their metabolites might occur in many tissues (lung, heart, liver) as reported for 3-palmitoyl-catechin, epigallocatechin gallate and resveratrol (Das and Griffiths, 1969; Bertelli *et al.*, 1996; Suganuma *et al.*, 1998).

The antioxidant and biological activity of the metabolites of phenolic acids with respect to the parent compounds and possible synergistic interactions *in vivo* need to be investigated.

Summary Points

- Dietary antioxidants afford protection against oxidative-related human diseases, such as atherosclerosis, aging and cancer.
- Plant phenolics are by far the most abundant dietary antioxidants.
- Beer is a common beverage rich in phenolic compounds, mainly phenolic acids (caffeic, ferulic, vanillic, *p*-coumaric, 4-hydroxyphenylacetic acids).
- The content of phenolic acids has been quantitatively measured in beer, taking advantage of a specific hydrolytic procedure.
- Phenolic acids from a single beer administration are absorbed and extensively metabolized in man. Phenolic acids and their metabolites are found in human plasma at concentrations ranging from 0.05 to 1.4 μM within 1 h from beer drinking.

References

Achilli, G., Cellerino, G.P. and Gamache, P.H. (1993). *J. Chromatogr.* 632, 111–117.

Andreason, M.F., Kroon, P., Williamson, G. and Garcia-Conesa, M.T. (2001a). *J. Agric. Food Chem.* 49, 5679–5684.

Andreason, M.F., Kroon, P., Williamson, G. and Garcia-Conesa, M.T. (2001b). *Free Radic. Biol. Med.* 31, 304–314.

Azuma, K., Ippoushi, K., Nakayama, M., Ito, H., Higashio, H. and Terao, J. (2000). *J. Agric. Food Chem.* 48, 5496–5500.

Bertelli, A.A.E., Giovannini, L., Stradi, R., Bertelli, A. and Tillement, J.P. (1996). *Int. J. Tissue React.* 18, 67–71.

Block, G., Patterson, B. and Subar, A. (1992). *Nutr. Cancer* 18, 1–30.

Buchanan, C.J., Wallace, G. and Fry, S.C. (1996). *J. Sci. Food Agric.* 71, 459–469.

Clifford, M.N. (1999). *J. Sci. Food Agric.* 79, 362–372.

Couteau, D., Mc Cartney, A.L., Gibson, G.R., Williamson, G. and Faulds, C.B. (2001). *J. Appl. Microbiol.* 90, 873–881.

Das, N.P. and Griffiths, L.A. (1969). *Biochem. J.* 115, 831–836.

Fenton, T.W., Leung, J. and Clandinin, D.R. (1980). *J. Food Sci.* 45, 1702–1705.

Ghiselli, A., Natella, F., Guidi, A., Montanari, L., Fantozzi, P. and Scaccini, C. (2000). *J. Nutr. Biochem.* 11, 76–80.

Gorinstein, S., Caspi, A., Zemser, M. and Trakhtenberg, S. (2000). *Nutr. Res.* 20, 131–139.

Hayes, P.J., Smyth, M.R. and McMurrough, I. (1987). *Analyst* 112, 1205–1207.

Herrmann, K. (1989). *Crit. Rev. Food Sci. Nutr.* 28, 315–347.

Kozlowska, H., Rotkiewicz, D.A. and Zadernowski, R. (1983). *J. Am. Oil Chem. Soc.* 60, 1119–1123.

Kroon, P.A., Faulds, C.B., Ryden, P., Robertson, J.A. and Williamson, G. (1997). *J. Agric. Food Chem.* 5, 661–667.

Krygier, K., Sosulski, F. and Hogge, L. (1982). *J. Agric. Food Chem.* 30, 330–334.

Lafay, S., Gil-Izquierdo, A., Manach, C., Morand, C., Besson, C. and Scalbert, A. (2006). *J. Nutr.* 136, 1192–1197.

Maillard, M.N. and Berset, C. (1995). *J. Agric. Food Chem.* 43, 1789–1793.

Manach, C., Morand, C., Crespy, V., Demigné, C., Texier, O., Regerat, F. *et al.* (1998). *FEBS Lett.* 426, 331–336.

Mani, A.R., Pannala, A.S., Orie, N.N., Ollosson, R., Harry, D., Rice-Evans, C.A. *et al.* (2003). *Biochem. J.* 374, 521–527.

Nardini, M. and Ghiselli, A. (2004). *Food Chem.* 84, 137–143.

Nardini, M., D'Aquino, M., Tomassi, G., Gentili, V., Di Felice, M. and Scaccini, C. (1995). *Free Radic. Biol. Med.* 19, 541–552.

Nardini, M., Cirillo, E., Patella, F., Mencarelli, D., Comisso, A. and Scaccini, C. (2002a). *Food Chem.* 79, 119–124.

Nardini, M., Cirillo, E., Natella, F. and Scaccini, C. (2002b). *J. Agric. Food Chem.* 50, 5735–5741.

Ohta, T., Nakano, T., Egashira, Y. and Sanada, H. (1997). *Biosci. Biotechnol. Biochem.* 61, 1942–1943.

Plumb, G., Garcia-Conesa, M.T., Kroon, P., Rhodes, M., Saxon, R. and Williamson, G. (1999). *J. Sci. Food Agric.* 79, 390–392.

Pulido, R., Hernandez-Garcia, M. and Saura-Calixto, F. (2003). *Eur. J. Clin. Nutr.* 57, 1275–1282.

Rechner, A.R., Spencer, J.P.E., Kuhnle, G., Hahn, U. and Rice-Evans, C. (2001). *Free Radic. Biol. Med.* 30, 1213–1222.

Renaud, S. and deLorgeril, M. (1992). *Lancet* 339, 1523–1526.

Rondini, L., Peyrat-Maillard, M.N., Marsset-Baglieri, A. and Berset, C. (2002). *J. Agric. Food Chem.* 50, 3037–3041.

Scalbert, A. and Williamson, G. (2000). *J. Nutr.* 130, 2073S–2085S.

Shahidi, F. and Naczk, M. (1995). *Food Phenolics, Sources, Chemistry, Effects, Applications*, pp. 128–136. Technoming Publishing Co., Lancaster, PA.

Shahidi, F. and Wanasundara, P.K.J. (1992). *Crit. Rev. Food Sci. Nutr.* 32, 67–103.

Suganuma, M., Okabe, S., Oniyama, M., Tada, Y., Ito, H. and Fujiki, H. (1998). Carcinogenesis. 19, 1771–1776.

Wende, G., Buchanan, C.J. and Fry, S.C. (1997). *J. Sci. Food Agric.* 73, 296–300.

49

Caloric Compensation in Response to Beer Consumption

Neil E. Rowland Department of Psychology, University of Florida, Gainesville, FL, USA

Abstract

Excessive caloric intake, leading to obesity and associated metabolic diseases, is one of the most urgent health care problems facing many nations with post-industrial economies. In this chapter, we discuss critically the premise that caloric intake is in fact regulated, and the ways in which calories in liquid beverages including beer may or may not be offset by compensatory reductions in food intake.

List of Abbreviations

kcal Kilocalorie
NA Non-alcoholic
ml Milliliter

Introduction

It is generally acknowledged that ingestion of food and water is under the joint control of factors internal and external to the organism.

So reads the opening sentence of an insightful theoretical review written by Toates (1981). And now we find ourselves a quarter century downstream, awash in an obesity epidemic. Environmental factors are often ignored *viz*: "Although environmental factors contribute to changes in the incidence of obesity over time, individual differences in weight are largely attributable to genetic factors" (Friedman, 2004). Others believe that the environment has a much more influential role, but as Astrup *et al.* (2004) note, exactly which environmental factors can or do have an effect on body weight in free-living average humans are not clear.

The incidence of obesity in the human population, defined by the body mass index, is a threat to the health and health prospects of individuals in many nations ranging from post-industrial like the United States to the Pacific Islands in which the traditional lifestyle has been transformed almost overnight (Shell, 2002). While ethnic and presumptive genetic factors are of some importance, the increased incidence of obesity in countries of long-standing adequacy in the public food supply is of great concern and is almost certainly due to environmental pressures. So how has our food world changed in the past 25 years? I see three major types of change:

1. Easier or more continuous food availability, for example vending machines, "TV dinners."
2. Increased caloric yield, as fat content or portion size, of popular fast or junk foods.
3. Increased consumption of beverages containing calories, especially soft drinks.

Beer is, of course, also a caloric beverage and in this chapter I will consider the effects of beer within the context of overall caloric consumption and possible weight gain.

Homeostasis

The word homeostasis was introduced by Canon in the 1920s to describe the ensemble of physiological mechanisms that underlie the observed state of relative constancy found in many physiological measurements in healthy people and animals. In modern medicine, blood tests are common and substantial deviations from these norms are used to diagnose illness. Canon recognized that the concentrations of some of these substances seem tightly regulated – for example, deviations in blood sodium concentration of only a few percent are lethal – and others such as blood glucose have a much wider allowed range. However, the idea that these systems have ideal or average values (also known as set points) that are actively defended was intuitively appealing and was widely applied.

Beer in Health and Disease Prevention
ISBN: 978-0-12-373891-2

In the case of food intake, two major theories were advanced about 50 years ago. These are the glucostatic (Mayer, 1953) and the lipostatic (Kennedy, 1953) hypotheses. Both recognized two essential points. First, since food intake in most species occurs as meals or episodically then the rate at which digested food is entering the body will fluctuate from very high just after a meal to zero during a prolonged fast. Second, the needs of our tissues for metabolic fuels are continuous; even when we are at rest or asleep, our brain, heart, kidneys, and many other tissues consume energy at a rate only slightly slower than when we are awake and active. To manage this physiological problem, the body has internal stores of energy which serve as buffers. Soon after a meal, nutrients are entering the body faster than the tissues need energy, so the excess is stored as fat or glycogen. Hours after a meal or during fasting, nutrients are no longer entering, so fat or glycogen stores are mobilized to meet the fuel needs. This is in many ways similar to the way most of us try to manage our money: we are paid episodically but have continuous expenses so we use a bank or credit account as a buffer. Mayer and Kennedy realized that for this to work in the realm of energy balance, the body must have mechanisms to sense either circulating and/or stored energy status. Mayer (1953) focused on blood glucose level as a correlate that these sensors could use to assess energy status (i.e. body weight), while Kennedy (1953) focused on overall regulation of body fat. Fat is by far the largest energy stored in the body and changes in the body weight of adults reflect mostly changes in body fat mass.

These theories are fundamentally homeostatic insofar as deviations of correlate(s) of body weight from a biologically programmed range initiate proportional corrective changes in feeding behavior and energy expenditure to bring the weight back to that range. Numerous blood-borne correlates of weight and feeding, as well as many direct neural pathways, have since been discovered and studied as candidate mechanisms by which the brain can be appraised of peripheral nutrient status and adjust behavior (for reviews, see Schwartz *et al.*, 2000; Berthoud, 2002).

The problem is this: if homeostasis were a powerful mechanism, then none of us would be obese and we would maintain the same weight throughout our adult lives. Unfortunately, this does not seem to be the case. What is true is that if energy (measured in joules or kilocalories where 1 kcal = 4.2 J) consumed over a representative period of time exceeds energy expenditure (metabolism, muscular effort, etc.) over the same time then most or all of the excess calories will end up stored as fat. And even a very small error in balancing this equation over time will add up to a lot of fat! There have been many studies performed to examine constancy of caloric intake over time, and in particular what factors produce poor regulation of overall intake. Note that in the homeostatic model level of exercise is irrelevant because increases or decreases in energy expended should automatically produce parallel changes in food consumption. This also does not seem to be the real state of affairs, but discussion of this is beyond the scope of the present chapter. In the present chapter, I will consider specifically the compensation for liquid calories, including alcohol and beer.

Laboratory Animal Experiments

Behavioral experiments in animals can tell us a lot about the physiological capabilities of the systems that produce feeding but without the high level social and cognitive factors that are additionally prominent in human consumption. The studies I will report below all use rats; their advantages include availability of domesticated strains with genetic homogeneity, and that their omnivorous style of feeding behavior and digestive systems are similar to humans.

Sugar solutions

Many investigators have shown that providing rats with a concentrated solution of a sweet sugar in addition to their standard maintenance chow diet produces obesity. A typical result from Ackroff and Sclafani (1988) is shown in Figure 49.1. In this experiment, two groups of adult female rats were fed chow (11% fat, 26% protein, 63% carbohydrate, in powdered form) or chow plus a bottle of concentrated sucrose solution (32%) for 30 days. These were both freely available at all times, along with water. Figure 49.1 shows that the group with sucrose consistently consumed approximately 25% more calories than the chow group, and as a result gained about four times as much weight. These rats were initially ~240 g, so the weight gain in the sucrose group represents almost a 1% increase in body weight per day, with no signs of slowing. These investigators also reported the separate intakes from chow and sucrose. The sucrose group decreased their intake of chow by about 75% relative to chow only controls, a decrease of some 60 kcal per day, but their 80 kcal per day intake of sucrose led to a net increase in calories consumed. Another way of stating this is that their compensatory reduction in chow intake was about 0.75 kcal per kcal of sucrose consumed.

It could be argued that the rats were forced into this situation because they have to eat at least some chow to get essential protein and minerals, but an important counterargument is that the animals were under no obligation to consume any sucrose. Similar results are seen with other maintenance diets and using solutions or gels of other carbohydrates (reviewed by Sclafani, 1987). More important is the observation that giving rats a similar choice but with the sucrose (or other pure sugars) in a solid or powdered form does not produce overeating and subsequent weight gain (Sclafani, 1987; Sclafani *et al.*, 1988). Thus, sugars that are in concentrated solution or hydrated gels seem to selectively override normal mechanisms that regulate caloric

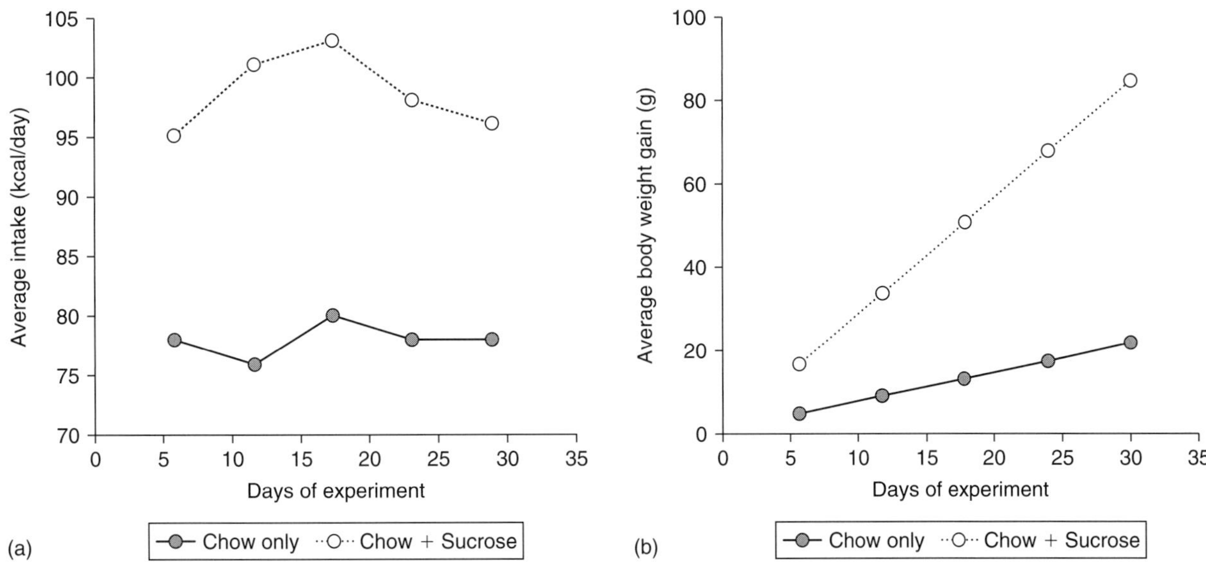

Figure 49.1 (a) Left panel shows average daily energy intake (kcal) of rats fed chow only (filled symbols) or with access to chow and a 32% solution of sucrose (open symbols). (b) Right panel shows the mean weight gain from initial during the course of the study by the rats in these two dietary conditions. The intakes and weight gains were significantly higher in the sucrose + chow condition. *Source*: These graphs are redrawn from data in Figures 1 and 2 in Ackroff and Sclafani (1988).

intake. This effect is often ascribed to the sweet taste and high palatability of these commodities.

Beer

Beer is a complex solution containing several carbohydrates, a small amount of protein, and numerous trace compounds including polyphenols, flavonoids, and isohumulones (e.g. Yajima *et al.*, 2005; Jastrzebski *et al.*, 2007), and alcohol typically around 5% by volume. The carbohydrates alone impart a partly sweet flavor, but the isohumulones in particular impart the characteristic bitter component. Alcohol alone also has a slightly unpleasant taste. Thus, experiments using beer in rats cannot be interpreted easily in terms of overall sweet or bitter taste. The component of alcohol can largely be removed by using non-alcoholic (NA) beer which has also been termed near-beer, although I will use the term NA beer.

Richter (1953) was the first to report the intake of beer in rats. The beer in his study was reported to be 4.4% by volume ethanol and 4.0% sugars and dextrins. Male rats had free access to dry McCollum diet (a forerunner of today's chows) and either water or beer. When water was available, during the initial phase, their daily intake was ~30 ml, but when beer only was available their intake rose over weeks from ~40 to ~70 ml/day. They also showed a concurrent reduction in food intake of ~1 kcal per kcal beer consumed, and as a result their weight gain was normal.

Richter (1940) earlier had found similar results for caloric compensation using plain ethanol solutions, results repeated more comprehensively by Cornier *et al.* (2002). The overall conclusion is that rats will consume large amounts of alcohol, and notably beer, when it is the only fluid available and at least over several weeks show no increase in weight gain. Rats often consume in excess of 25% of their body weight per day in beer and as a result exhibit signs of intoxication (Lancaster *et al.*, 1987; see McGregor and Gallate, 2004, for review). McGregor and Gallate have also shown that rats will show beer-motivated behavior, for example, by licking a spout many times to obtain a small drop of beer.

Table 49.1 Approximate energy content of NA and alcoholic beer

Beverage	*kcal/ml*	*Fraction of calories contained as alcohol*
NA beer[a]	0.21	<10
NA beer + 5% by volume ethanol[b]	0.45	57
NA beer + 10% by volume ethanol	0.71	73

[a]NA beer data from Coors website. Energy yield of ethanol = 5.24 kcal/ml.
[b]A 5% by volume ethanol solution is ~4% by weight ethanol.

We have used a protocol in which beer consumption was voluntary rather than forced (Rowland *et al.*, 2005). In our study, adult male and female rats were given continuous access to powdered rat chow from a jar in their home cage. In the first phase of the study, only water was available to drink, and intakes were measured over several days. In the second phase, the rats received chow and a choice of water and NA beer (Table 49.1). And in the last two phases of the experiment, 5% and 10% by volume ethanol was added to

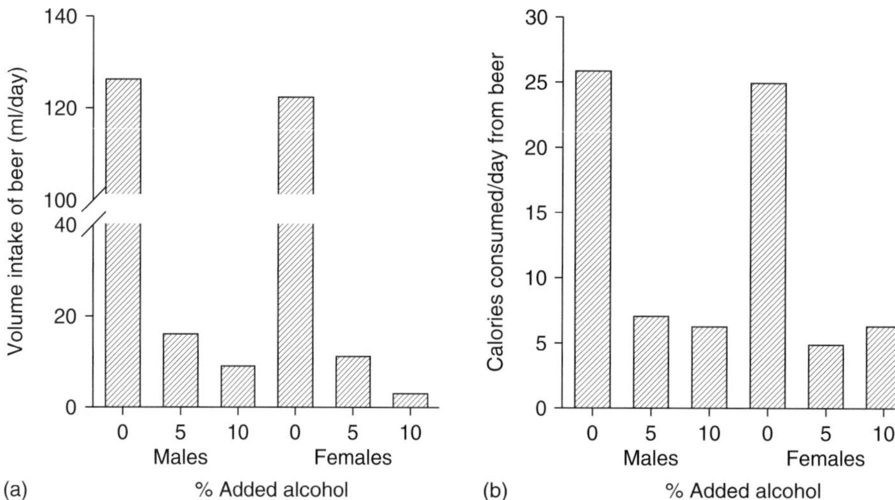

Figure 49.2 (a) Left panel shows the mean daily volume of NA beer with either 0%, 5%, or 10% added alcohol in adult male and female Sprague–Dawley rats. Each bar is the average of 4 days of data collection and five to six animals. (b) The right panel shows the number of kilocalories estimated to be contained in that beer. The rats also had free access to chow and water, but those intakes are not shown. *Source*: These graphs are redrawn from data in Table 1 and Figure 1 of Rowland *et al.* (2005).

the beer. Food intake was measured daily, but there were few changes across days, so the intakes for each phase were averaged and are shown in Figure 49.2. During the water only phase, rats consumed 40–50 ml water. When NA beer was also available, they consumed almost three times this volume per day. Even though the caloric density of NA beer is low, the high volume consumed ensured that almost 30% of their normal caloric intake came from the fluid. Concurrently, they reduced food intake, slightly more accurately in males than in females. When alcohol was added to the beer (5% is close to an average beer), volume intakes dropped dramatically, and the calories became only a small fraction of the total intake. Nonetheless, caloric compensation was accurate. These findings are consistent with the result of Lancaster *et al.* (1987) in which rats voluntarily drinking beer initially ate more but later ate less than control rats with no beer, but there were no group differences in body weight.

Although water intake was not measured in our published study (Rowland *et al.*, 2005), in a pilot study we did measure concurrent intakes of water and NA beer, and NA beer with 5% or 10% alcohol added. The preferences for beer over water are shown in Figure 49.3, along with results that were obtained in a similar protocol by Samson *et al.* (1998). In both cases, the preference for NA beer was attenuated as alcohol was added, although the slope was steeper in our study. There were some procedural differences that might account for this including the fact that Samson *et al.* used young male rats while we used older and heavier males as well as females. Also, the brand of NA used was different (O'Doul's by Samson *et al.* and Coors in our work) and in very preliminary tests we found that rats drank more NA Coors than O'Doul's – which is why we used Coors in our published studies.

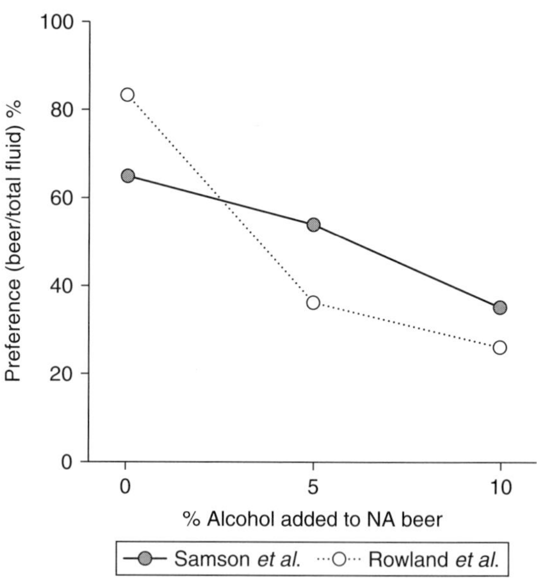

Figure 49.3 Intakes of beer relative to concurrently available water, expressed as % of total intake from beer; as a function of the amount of alcohol added to NA beer. *Source*: Shown are data redrawn from Samson *et al.* (1998) and unpublished data (2003) from a similar study from our laboratory.

In additional studies, to try to increase the amount of ethanol consumed, we mixed alcohol with a sweet vehicle (Polycose® comprised of oligosaccharides) in either a liquid or a gel form (Rowland *et al.*, 2005). This did increase caloric intake, but the calories so consumed were accurately compensated by reductions in chow intake. Body weights were not recorded routinely in these studies, but since intake was conserved there is no reason to expect major weight changes.

To summarize the main findings with beer in rats:

- Rats drink large amounts of NA beer, presumably because they like the taste, and compensate accurately for the calories in it by reducing chow intake.
- Rats do not like the taste of alcohol, and so addition of alcohol to NA beer decreases its intake substantially, but again there is accurate caloric compensation.
- When rats have no choice of fluid other than beer (Richter's work), they consume larger volumes than if water was available, and again compensate for calories.
- These results contrast with findings using solutions or gels of pure concentrated carbohydrates, when caloric intakes are very high and are not compensated, and so cause increased daily caloric intake and resultant weight gain.

Human Experiments

To what extent do these findings extrapolate to the much more varied and socially complex alimentary world of humans? It is much more difficult to assess accurately over a long period the compensation in food intake for alcohol consumed in humans. Buemann *et al.* (2002) performed a short-term study in which young men ate a dinner served with beer, wine, or a soft drink, and the total calories consumed were monitored. They found that under some conditions, energy intake was slightly higher with alcoholic drinks than in the soft drink condition, but there was no control when a non-caloric beverage was available.

In another study, Orozco and de Castro (1994) studied adults who habitually consumed low to moderate amounts of alcohol during a 6-day normal (alcohol) period and for a 6-day period when they abstained from alcohol. Subjects maintained food and beverage diaries to report energy consumption as well as estimates of energy expenditure. Energy intake was higher by about 10% (241 kcal/day) during the alcohol phase than during the abstinence phase. However, energy expenditure was also higher during the alcohol phase; for example, heart rate was higher, subjects had increased waking time and increased overall exercise level. Thus, little or no net change in energy balance was observed between the two conditions. Other evidence suggests that, in addition to any effects on movement-related expenditure, alcohol directly influences one or several metabolic processes to decrease overall efficiency (Camargo *et al.*, 1987; Lieber, 1991; Suter *et al.*, 1994) and therefore minimize weight gain.

Complementary conclusions have been drawn from studies in which body mass index or other estimates of obesity have been examined along with estimates of alcohol consumption in cross-sections of specific populations. The common result, in both males and females of several ethnicities, is that low to moderate alcohol consumption is not associated with an increased level of obesity (Wannamethee *et al.*, 2004, 2005; Pucarin-Cvetkovic *et al.*, 2006). However, high levels of consumption, often defined as three or more drinks per day, are associated with higher levels of obesity. These studies are unable to assess concurrent food intake with any degree of accuracy, so the similarity of body mass index in low or moderate drinkers and non-drinkers suggests that over years there is no net change in energy balance. It is not clear whether this is because the alcohol calories reduce food intake or because the drinkers increase energy expenditure. Lastly, in these studies, there did not seem to be a significant difference between drinkers for whom beer was the main beverage or those who consumed different alcoholic beverages.

In humans:

- Low to moderate alcohol consumption may be associated with increased energy intake, thus an incomplete compensation for the calories in the beverage.
- This seems to be offset by increased energy expenditure in the form of exercise or other activity, and decreased metabolic efficiency.
- Cross-sectional studies also indicate that low to moderate alcohol consumption is not associated with weight gain relative to age matched non-drinkers.
- Beer is no more or less likely to influence weight than other alcoholic beverages.

Conclusions

Animals seem to be able to monitor their energy intake relatively accurately and that at low levels of energy in beverages, with or without alcohol, they reduce their food intake by a commensurate amount. However, when the beverage is of high density and palatability (e.g. sucrose) then compensation breaks down and animals gain weight. It should be noted that the rat studies differ from the human environment insofar as they have not been performed when highly palatable alternative foods to the sucrose are available. The evidence in humans suggests that low to moderate habitual alcohol consumption does not lead to increased weight gain, but this may be a result of increased energy expenditure rather than compensation in food intake. Human studies have not been performed under conditions in which people are asked to restrain their food intake (i.e. diet), but it would be interesting to know whether the energy expenditure or other metabolic effects of alcohol carry over into mild caloric restraint or restriction and thus could actually improve weight loss on a diet.

References

Ackroff, K. and Sclafani, A. (1988). *Physiol. Behav.* 44, 181–187.

Astrup, A., O'Hill, J. and Rossner, S. (2004). *Obes. Rev.* 5, 125–127.

Berthoud, H.R. (2002). *Neurosci. Biobehav. Rev.* 26, 393–428.

Bobak, M., Skodova, Z. and Marmot, M. (2003). *Eur. J. Clin. Nutr.* 57, 1250–1253.

Buemann, B., Toubro, S. and Astrup, A. (2002). *Int. J. Obes. Metab. Disord.* 26, 1367–1372.

Camargo, C.A., Vranizan, K.M., Dreon, D.M., Frey-Hewitt, B. and Wood, P.D. (1987). *J. Am. Coll. Nutr.* 6, 271–278.

Cornier, M.A., Gayles, E.C. and Bessesen, D.H. (2002). *Metabolism* 51, 787–791.

Friedman, J.M. (2004). *Nature Med.* 10, 563–569.

Jastrzebski, Z., Gorinstein, S., Czyzewska-Szafran, H., Leontowicz, H., Leontowicz, M., Trakhtenberg, S. and Remiszewska, M. (2007). *Food Chem. Toxicol* 45, 296–302.

Kennedy, G.C. (1953). *Proc. Roy. Soc. B* 140, 578–592.

Lancaster, F., Spiegel, K. and Zaman, M. (1987). *Alcohol Drug Res.* 7, 393–403.

Lieber, C.S. (1991). *Am. J. Clin. Nutr.* 54, 976–982.

Mayer, J. (1953). *New Engl. J. Med.* 249, 13–16.

McGregor, I.S. and Gallate, J.E. (2004). *Addictive Behav.* 29, 1341–1357.

Orozco, S. and de Castro, J.M. (1994). *Pharmac. Biochem. Behav.* 49, 629–638.

Pucarin-Cvetkovic, J., Mustajbegovic, J., Doko Jelinic, J., Senta, A., Nola, I.A., Ivankovic, D., Kaic-Rak, A. and Milosevic, M. (2006). *Croat. Med. J.* 47, 619–626.

Richter, C.P. (1940). *Q. J. Stud. Alcohol* 1, 650–662.

Richter, C.P. (1953). *Q. J. Stud. Alcohol* 14, 525–539.

Rowland, N.E., Nasrallah, N. and Robertson, K.L. (2005). *Pharmac. Biochem. Behav.* 80, 109–114.

Samson, H.H., Denning, C. and Chappelle, A.M. (1998). *Alcohol* 13, 365–368.

Schwartz, M.W., Woods, S.C., Porte Jr., D., Seeley, R.J. and Baskin, D.G. (2000). *Nature* 404, 661–670.

Sclafani, A. (1987). *Neurosci. Biobehav. Rev.* 11, 131–153.

Sclafani, A., Vigorito, M. and Pfeiffer, C.L. (1988). *Physiol. Behav.* 42, 409–415.

Shell, E.R. (2002). *The Hungry Gene: The Science of Fat and the Future of Thin.* Atlantic Monthly Press.

Suter, P.M., Jequier, E. and Schutz, Y. (1994). *Am. J. Physiol. Regulat. Integ. Comp. Physiol.* 266, R1204–R1212.

Toates, F.M. (1981). *Appetite* 2, 35–50.

Wannamethee, S.G., Field, A.E., Colditz, G.A. and Rimm, E.B. (2004). *Obes. Res.* 12, 1386–1396.

Wannamethee, S.G., Shaper, A.G. and Whincup, P.H. (2005). *Int. J. Obes. Metab. Disord.* 29, 1436–1444.

Yajima, H., Noguchi, T., Ikeshima, E., Shiraki, M., Kanaya, T., Tsuboyama-Kasoka, N., Ezaki, O., Oikawa, A. and Kondo, K. (2005). *Int. J. Obes. Metab. Disord.* 29, 991–997.

50
Beer and Adiposity

S. Goya Wannamethee Department of Primary Care and Population Sciences, Royal Free and University College Medical School, London, UK

Abstract

The relationship between alcohol and adiposity has been conflicting. There is a widespread belief that drinking beer promotes abdominal fat ("beer belly") and that wine has little or no such effect. This chapter reviews the epidemiological evidence in population studies on the influence of the type of alcohol on adiposity measures including body weight and central adiposity. The association between alcohol and adiposity appears to be greater for abdominal adiposity (waist circumference and waist-to-hip-ratio) than for general adiposity (body mass index). Overall, evidence from cross-sectional and prospective studies supports the concept that alcohol, in particular beer and spirits, is a risk factor for obesity, as one might expect if the energy derived from alcohol consumption was added to the usual dietary calorie intake. There is no convincing evidence that wine is protective against abdominal fat deposition.

List of Abbreviations

BMI	Body mass index
BRHS	British Regional Heart Study
WC	Waist circumference
WHR	Waist-to-hip ratio

Introduction

Increased body weight and, in particular, abdominal obesity are associated with increased cardiovascular disease risk (Rimm *et al.*, 1995; Lakka *et al.*, 2002). In many developed countries the average alcohol intake in those who drink is about 10–30 g/day or 3–9% of the total energy intake (Westerterp *et al.*, 1999) and the efficiency of alcohol for the maintenance of metabolizable energy is the same as for carbohydrate (Rumpler *et al.*, 1996). Alcohol suppresses the oxidation of fat, favoring fat storage and can serve as a precursor for fat synthesis (Prentice, 1995; Suter *et al.*, 1997a). Moderate alcohol consumers usually add alcohol to their daily energy intake rather than substituting it for food, thus increasing energy balance (Suter *et al.*, 1997a). On the basis of this it would seem surprising if alcohol did not contribute directly to body weight. However, the relationship between "alcohol consumption and body weight remains an enigma to nutritionists and in many instances paradoxical" (Jequier, 1999). While laboratory studies on energy and nutrient balances show that alcohol is a nutrient that is efficiently utilized by the body and that alcohol calories do count, the epidemiological evidence is conflicting (Prentice, 1995; Suter *et al.*, 1997a; Westerterp *et al.*, 1999). In several reviews of studies of the alcohol and obesity relation, most of which are cross-sectional in nature, the association between alcohol intake and body weight has been inconsistent and has varied between men and women (Hellerstedt *et al.*, 1990; McDonald *et al.*, 1993; Suter *et al.*, 1997a; Westerterp *et al.*, 1999). In men the association between alcohol and body weight has been found to be almost equally positive or non-existent but in women the majority of cross-sectional studies report an inverse relationship (Hellerstedt *et al.*, 1990; Colditz *et al.*, 1991; Wannamethee and Shaper, 1992; McDonald *et al.*, 1993; Gutierrez-Fisac *et al.*, 1995; Suter *et al.*, 1997a; Rosmond *et al.*, 1999; Westerterp *et al.*, 1999; Bobak *et al.*, 2003; Lukasiewicz *et al.*, 2003; Wannamethee *et al.*, 2003, 2005; Nicolosi *et al.*, 2006). Evidence from a number of studies suggests that in drinkers, fat is preferentially deposited in the abdominal area (Suter *et al.*, 1997a) and that alcohol may be more associated with abdominal obesity than with general obesity (Dallongeville *et al.*, 1998; Wannamethee *et al.*, 2005). Several factors have been proposed which may explain the inconsistencies between studies, including the suggestion that the effect of alcohol on adiposity is influenced by the type of drink (Suter *et al.*, 1997a). There is a widespread belief that drinking beer promotes abdominal fat ("beer belly") (McDonald *et al.*, 1993) and that wine has little or no such effect (Duncan *et al.*, 1995; Vadstrup *et al.*, 2003). Beer's fattening reputation may have more to do with the lifestyle of those who drink it (Barefoot *et al.*, 2002; Ruidavets *et al.*, 2004; Johansen *et al.*, 2006). It has also been postulated that the effects of alcohol on body weight and fat distribution may also differ according to whether the alcohol is consumed with meals or not

Beer in Health and Disease Prevention
ISBN: 978-0-12-373891-2

(Suter *et al.*, 1997a) and by the pattern of drinking (Dorn *et al.*, 2003). The aim of this chapter is to review the epidemiological evidence in population studies for beer as a risk factor for overweight and obesity, and compare the effects of beer drinking with other types of beverage including wine and spirits.

Total alcohol and body weight

In the majority of cross-sectional studies, inverse associations between alcohol and body mass index (BMI) have been shown in women (Hellerstedt *et al.*, 1990; Colditz *et al.*, 1991; McDonald *et al.*, 1993; Gutierrez-Fisac *et al.*, 1995; Suter *et al.*, 1997a; Dallongeville *et al.*, 1998; Rosmond *et al.*, 1999; Westerterp *et al.*, 1999) whereas in men positive or no associations have been reported (Hellerstedt *et al.*, 1990; Wannamethee and Shaper, 1992; McDonald *et al.*, 1993; Gutierrez-Fisac *et al.*, 1995; Suter *et al.*, 1997a; Dallongeville *et al.*, 1998; Westerterp *et al.*, 1999; Bobak *et al.*, 2003; Wannamethee *et al.*, 2003, 2005). It is not clear why alcohol may promote leanness in women although it has been suggested that the calories from alcohol are added to energy intake from other sources in men, and that the energy from alcohol intake displaces sucrose in women (Howarth *et al.*, 2001). Cross-sectional analyses are limited in assessing cause and effect. The patterns of higher obesity rates in non-drinkers compared to drinkers commonly seen in women may reflect history of dieting or current dieting to lose weight. The higher BMI levels in non-drinkers may in part be due to self-selection bias. Women who are more prone to weight gain for reasons other than alcohol may abstain from drinking because of their belief that alcohol causes weight gain.

There have been relatively few prospective studies of the relation between type of alcohol and weight gain in men and women, and the findings have been inconsistent. Early data from the Framingham study showed that both men and women who took up drinking have increased their alcohol intake during follow-up experienced weight gain (Gordon *et al.*, 1983). In a study of over 12,000 Finns, heavier drinking (>75 g/week) in men and (>10 g/week) in women were associated with increased risk of weight gain (>5 kg), although the prevalence of obesity was inversely associated with alcohol intake in women (Rissanen *et al.*, 1991). This suggests that the higher BMI levels in female non-drinkers in cross-sectional studies may in part be due to self-selection bias. In a study of over 2,000 Chinese adults, alcohol was associated with a significant weight gain in men; in women only a small but positive association was seen (Bell *et al.*, 2001). Strong evidence supporting the effects of alcohol on obesity and weight gain comes from the British Regional Heart Study (BRHS) (Wannamethee *et al.*, 2003). The prevalence of men with high BMI (≥28 kg/m^2) tended to increase with increasing alcohol intake. An examination of the association between changes in alcohol intake and body weight over 5 years showed stable heavy drinkers (≥30 g/day; 1 UK unit is approximately 10 g/alcohol) and new heavy drinkers to have the greatest weight gain and the highest prevalence of obesity (Wannamethee *et al.*, 2003). Light and moderate drinkers showed no increased risk in weight gain compared to non-drinkers. These positive findings in heavier drinkers have been confirmed in recent prospective analyses carried out in a US cohort of over 40,000 female nurses aged 29–42 years at baseline in 1989 (Nurses II Health Study) (Wannamethee *et al.*, 2004). An inverse relationship was seen between alcohol and BMI in cross-sectional analyses but in prospective analyses light-to-moderate drinkers (up to 30 g/day) had significantly lower risk of weight gain (>5 kg) over 8 years than non-drinkers, but heavy drinkers (≥30 g/day/3 UK units/day) had the highest risk of weight gain (>5 kg). These prospective data support the concept of alcohol as a risk factor for obesity. However, weak positive or no association has been reported between alcohol and weight change and weight gain in five prospective studies from the United States (French *et al.*, 1993; Gerace *et al.*, 1996; Kahn *et al.*, 1997; Fogelholm *et al.*, 2000; Sherwood *et al.*, 2000). In these studies, data by levels of alcohol consumption were not presented and the average intake in these populations is not known. In two US studies an inverse association was seen between alcohol and weight gain (Colditz *et al.*, 1990; Liu *et al.*, 1994). This may be due to the small number of subjects who drank >2 drinks/day and the characteristics of the non-drinkers. It appears likely that higher levels on a regular basis are required to have an effect on body weight. Intervention studies are inconclusive. Cordain *et al.* (1997) reported that the addition of 35 g/day of wine to the daily energy requirements during a period of 6 weeks does not affect body weight or energy metabolism. This is consistent with the findings in the BRHS and Nurses II Health Study in which up to 30 g (3 UK units) was not associated with weight gain.

Alcohol and body fat distribution

Evidence from a number of studies suggests that in drinkers, fat is preferentially deposited in the abdominal area (Suter *et al.*, 1997a). In contrast to the cross-sectional relationship between alcohol and body weight, which has been found to be almost equally positive or non-existent in men and negative in women, more recent studies tend to report positive associations between alcohol and body fat distribution in men and women. In the French MONICA study, no association was seen between alcohol and BMI in men and an inverse association was seen in women (Dallongeville *et al.*, 1998). However, alcohol consumption was positively associated with waist-to-hip ratio (WHR) independent of BMI in both men and women (Dallongeville *et al.*, 1998). Positive associations between alcohol and fat distribution have also been reported in studies from Switzerland (Suter *et al.*, 1995, 1997b), US men and women (Laws *et al.*, 1990; Slattery *et al.*, 1992; Duncan *et al.*, 1995), Italian women (Armellini *et al.*, 1993) and in Japanese men (Sakurai *et al.*, 1998). In the Italian Bollate Eye Study, alcohol was inversely associated with BMI in women with non-drinkers showing the highest BMI and light drinkers the lowest. But moderate-to-heavy drinking was associated with higher waist circumference (WC) than both non-drinkers and light drinkers (Leite *et al.*, 2006). In men, moderate-to-heavy drinkers showed the highest mean levels of BMI and WC. The findings of a stronger and more positive association between alcohol and central adiposity as measured by the WHR or WC than with BMI in several of these studies suggest that alcohol is more associated with abdominal obesity than with general obesity. In the BRHS a positive relationship was seen with both central and general adiposity but the effects as measured by the standardized regression coefficients were greater for WC and WHR than for BMI and % body fat (measures of total adiposity) and the increase in percentage of men with large WC was more marked than the increase in rates of obesity as measured by BMI (Wannamethee *et al.*, 2005).

Beer and calories

It has been suggested that the type of alcohol consumed might explain the discrepant results in studies of alcohol and body weight. Alcohol contains almost twice the calories of protein and carbohydrate foods (7 cal/g of alcohol). According to the British Beer and Pub Association (BBPA), a glass of beer with a typical 4.6% alcoholic volume has not only fewer calories than a similar measure of wine, but also milk or fruit juice. Spirits, meanwhile, contain more than six times the calories of beer, and when mixed with a soft drink, the calorie-count soars even higher. Although beer has fewer calories than wine, it comes in pints while wine is served in smaller measures (Table 50.1).

Beer and lifestyle characteristics

Alcohol is metabolized primarily by the liver and used immediately as energy or stored in the liver or in the rest of the body as fat. Since beer contains more carbohydrate and thus more usable energy per unit of ethanol than most wines or spirits, the common belief is that beer drinkers are on average more obese than either wine or spirit drinkers (Suter *et al.*, 1997a). For example in the BRHS of men aged 60–79 years, beer drinkers overall showed the highest mean WC and BMI supporting the beer belly concept. Wine drinkers were the lightest (Figure 50.1). Research into drinking suggests that this may have more to do with the lifestyle of those who drink beer. Alcoholic beverage preference has found to be associated with dietary habits, social class and lifestyle factors including smoking, exercise

Table 50.1 Alcohol and calories

Beer	4.6% alc	41 calories
Wine	12.0% alc	77 calories
Spirits	40% alc	250 calories
Milk	0	64 calories
Orange juice	0	42 calories
Standard measure alcohol		
Beer	12 oz.	150 calories
Lite beer	12 oz.	110 calories
Wine	5 oz.	90 calories
Spirits	$1\frac{1}{2}$ oz.	90 calories
Spirits + carbonated drink	$1\frac{1}{2}$ oz.	(Add 75 calories)

Note: Calories per 100 ml.
Source: BBPA.

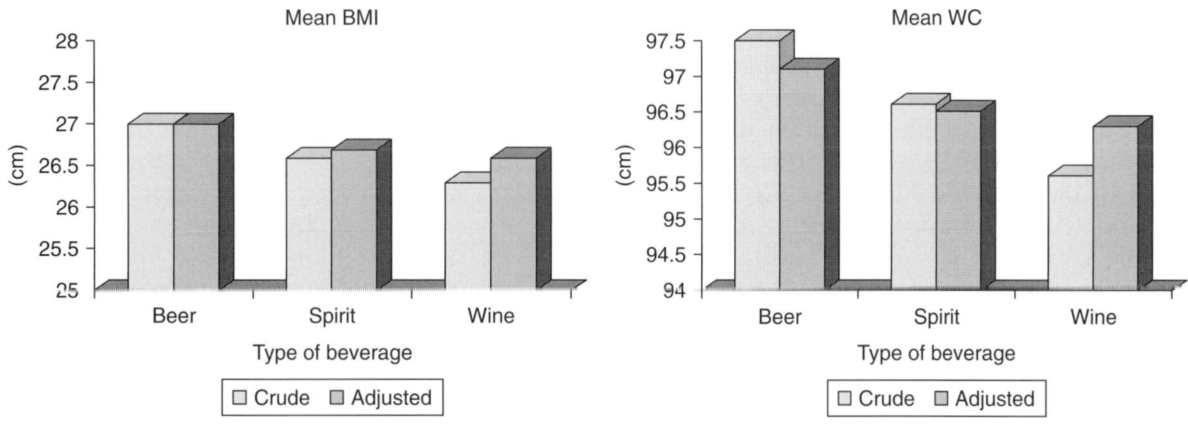

Figure 50.1 Preference of beverage type and unadjusted and adjusted mean BMI and WC in men aged 60–79 years with no diagnosed myocardial infarction, stroke or diabetes. Adjusted for age, social class, smoking, physical activity, other pre-existing cardiovascular disease, total fat intake, average weekly intake and time relation with meal. *Source*: Data extracted from Wannamethee *et al.* (2005).

Table 50.2 Alcoholic beverage preference (Q20) in men drinking at least 1 unit/week and diet and lifestyle characteristics

	Predominant type of drink		
N	*Beer* *1,037*	*Wine* *303*	*Spirit* *198*
Average number (drinks/week)	12.4	9.6	12.0
Total non-alcohol calories (kcal)	2,126	1,928	1,990
Percent with meal dietary nutrients (g/day)	28.5	83.7	22.5
Total fat	75.5	66.4	70.1
Protein	25.1	26.5	24.5
Carbohydrate	284.3	264.4	268.6
Vitamin C	78.3	87.5	76.2
Non-manual workers (%)	34.7	72.0	45.1
Inactive (%)	32.0	27.8	32.8
Smokers (%)	17.4	5.0	14.4

Source: Data from the BRHS (1998–2000).

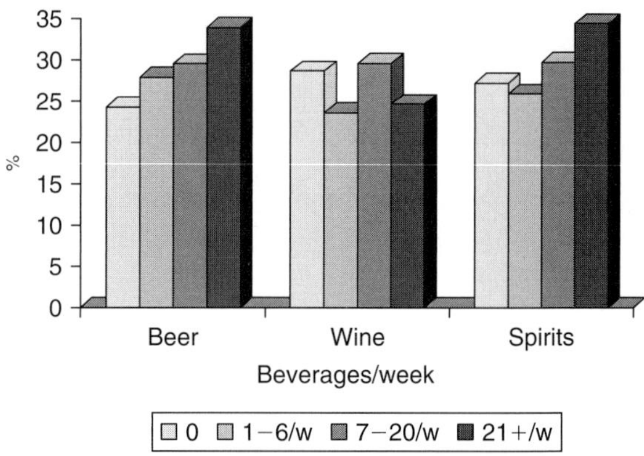

Figure 50.2 Prevalence (%) of central obesity (WC > 102 cm) in relation to weekly beer, wine and spirits consumption in men aged 60–79 years. 1 drink = 10 g/alcohol. *Source*: Data from the BRHS (1998–2000).

and BMI. Table 50.2 shows the characteristics of beer, wine and spirit drinkers using data from the rescreening phase of the BRHS in men aged 60–79 years. There is evidence that wine drinkers have healthier diets and are less likely to smoke and tend to be of higher socioeconomic status. Wine drinkers had lower total fat intake and higher intakes of vitamin C reflecting higher intake of fruits. Beer drinkers had the highest fat and carbohydrate intake. These findings are consistent with previous observations reported in the United States (Barefoot *et al.*, 2002), France (Ruidavets *et al.*, 2004) and Denmark (Johansen *et al.*, 2006) indicating that wine drinkers have healthier diets than other drinkers. Adjustment for total calories and lifestyle characteristics attenuated the differences and the findings were not significant although beer drinkers still showed the highest mean WC and BMI (Figure 50.1).

Beer, spirits, wine and adiposity

The common belief is that drinking beer promotes abdominal fat distribution and that wine in contrast has no such effect and may even have beneficial effects on metabolism.

Some studies have reported differing effects of type of beverage on body weight and fat distribution and observed no effect or even an adverse effect with wine (Duncan *et al.*, 1995; Vadstrup *et al.*, 2003). Others have not and shown a positive effect of wine on abdominal fat (Slattery *et al.*, 1992; Dallongeville *et al.*, 1998; Wannamethee *et al.*, 2005).

Cross-sectional Studies In a US study of 12,000 men and women aged 45–64 years, the WHR of those consuming >6 beer drinks/week was significantly greater than non-drinkers, while those drinking >6 wine drinks/week the WHR was significantly lower than non-drinkers. The findings were regarded as supporting the popular concept of the "beer belly" (Duncan *et al.*, 1995). By contrast, in another US study (CARDIA), beer, wine and liquor were all positively associated with WHR in white men (Slattery *et al.*, 1992). In a study of some 3,500 French men and women aged 35–64 years drawn from three distinct geographic areas of France (MONICA centers), wine was the main source of alcohol (67% of intake). Wine and beer consumption was positively and strongly associated with WHR in women, but only poorly associated with WHR in men (Dallongeville *et al.*, 1998). In the Czech MONICA survey, where beer was the predominant drink, beer was positively associated with WHR in non-smokers but not with the BMI (Bobak *et al.*, 2003). No association was seen between beer and WHR in women but an inverse association was seen for BMI. Findings from the BRHS show a strong positive relationship between alcohol intake and central obesity (WC > 102 cm) in beer and spirit drinkers; no association was seen with wine drinking (Figure 50.2). In the adjusted analyses, after adjustment for lifestyle characteristic, dietary fat, time taken with meal and each of the other type of alcohol, a positive association was seen between weekly alcohol intake and mean WC for all types of drink although the effect was strongest in beer drinkers (Figure 50.3) which suggests that alcohol *per se* rather than any alcoholic beverage consumption is associated with increased abdominal fat deposition.

Several studies have however failed to find any association between beer and adiposity. In the SU.VI.MAX intervention study on the effects of antioxidant supplement on chronic diseases in men and women, spirit was positively associated with BMI and WHR in both men and women, a J-shaped relationship was seen for wine but no association was seen for beer drinking (Lukasiewicz *et al.*, 2003). In the Nurses I Health Study and the Health Professionals Follow-up study, the lack of relationship between alcohol

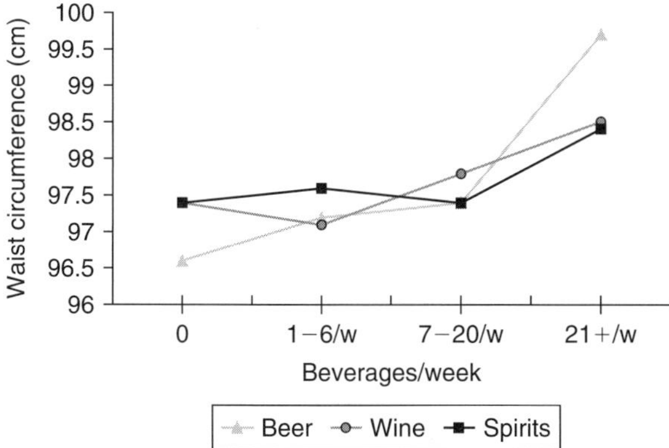

Figure 50.3 Adjusted mean WC in relation to weekly beer, wine and spirits consumption in men with no diagnosed myocardial infarction, stroke or diabetes. Adjusted for age, social class, smoking, physical activity, other pre-existing cardiovascular disease, total fat intake, time taken with meal and other types of alcohol. 1 drink = 10g/alcohol. *Source*: Adapted from Wannamethee et al. (2005).

intake and BMI was similar for men who drank only wine and those who drank only beer (Colditz *et al.*, 1991). In the Spanish national survey (Gutierrez-Fisac *et al.*, 1995) there appeared to be a positive association between wine intake and the prevalence of obesity in women and between spirit intake and obesity in men. No significant trends of association were observed for beer or wine in men, or for beer or spirits in women. In a cohort of Swedish women (Rosmond *et al.*, 1999), wine was inversely associated with BMI while beer and spirits showed no association. In another Swedish study in women, spirits were associated with WHR but no association was seen between beer and wine consumption (Lapidus *et al.*, 1989). In a study of Caucasian-American and African-American men, liquor drinking was associated with a greater tendency for greater central adiposity but beer drinking was unrelated (Dorn *et al.*, 2003). In the Japanese study of male self-defense, officials' abdominal obesity was associated with Japanese spirits but not with other types of alcohol (Sakurai *et al.*, 1998). The differences in findings between studies may be associated with unrecorded differences in lifestyle or differences in nutritional characteristics between wine, spirit and beer drinkers. It may also be due to the type of beverage which is most common. It is also suggested that the lack of association between beer and fat distribution in some studies may be due to mean consumption per day being too low to show any association (Lukasiewicz *et al.*, 2003), as a minimum level of alcohol may be required (>3 drinks/day) to increase fat distribution.

Prospective Studies Only a few studies have examined the association between type of alcohol intake and obesity on a prospective basis. Strong evidence to support beer as a risk factor for overweight and obesity comes from the Copenhagen City Heart Study (Vadstrup *et al.*, 2003). In this population-based study of 6,886 men and women, the authors explored the relations between both total alcohol intake and different types of alcoholic drinks and WC after 10 years. The subjects were asked about the average weekly number of drinks of beers, wines and spirits, and assigned according to their total alcohol consumption to one of seven groups ranging from <1 drink/week to >69 drinks/week. Moderate-to-high consumption of alcohol was associated with later high WC in both men and women and this was seen for beer and spirit consumption. The odds ratios of having a high WC (<102 cm in men, >88 cm in women—levels associated with increased CVD risk) showed a linear increase in both men and women. The adjusted relative odds (95% CI) were 1.65 (1.07–2.55) in men and 2.16 (0.86–5.14) in women who drank >28 beverages/week of total alcohol compared to those who drank 1–6 beverages/week. Men who drank >21 beers/week had odds ratio of having a large WC after 10 years of 1.63 (0.99–2.67) and women drinking >14 beers/week had odds ratio of 2.53 (0.92–6.34), compared to men and women who drank no beer. Additionally, for spirits, there was an increase in both men and women. The relative odds for having a large WC for men who drank 14–21 glasses of spirits/week compared to those who drank <1/week was 1.89 (95% CI 0.81–4.36) and 3.12 (95% CI 1.12–8.52) for women who drank >14 glasses of spirits/week. By contrast, moderate-to-high wine consumption showed no positive effect and may have the opposite effect. The relative odds for having a large WC for men who drank 14–20 glasses wine/week compared to those who drank <1/week was 0.88 (95% CI 0.39–1.94) and 0.88 (95% CI 0.44–1.69) for women who drank >14 glasses of wine/week. In the recent Danish MONICA study of men and women, beer and spirits were associated with increases in WC in women but not in men (Halkjaer *et al.*, 2004).

Influence of drinking with meals

It has also been postulated that the effects of alcohol on body weight and fat distribution may differ according to whether the alcohol is consumed with meals or not (Suter *et al.*, 1997a) although data are limited. There has been suggestion that wine drinkers may take their alcohol more frequently with meals than other drinkers and consume it more slowly which in consequence may have lesser effect on adiposity (Suter *et al.*, 1997a). Regular alcohol use at meals may increase total energy expenditure by potentiating normal-dietary-induced thermogenesis (Suter *et al.*, 1997a). In the BRHS, wine drinkers were more likely to drink with meals than other drinkers (see Table 50.2) but total alcohol intake (≥21 drinks/week) is positively associated with adiposity irrespective of whether the alcohol is usually drunk with meals or separately, and is thus unlikely to explain the

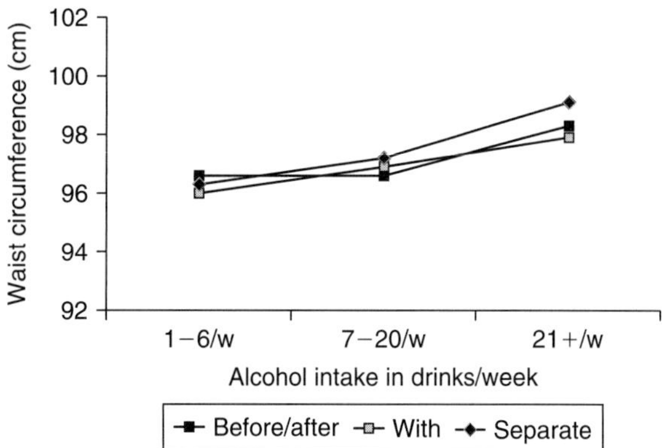

Figure 50.4 Total alcohol intake and adjusted mean WC in relation to timing of alcohol intake in relation to meals. Adjusted for age, social class, smoking, physical activity, pre-existing cardiovascular disease, dietary intake and type of drink. *Source*: Adapted from Wannamethee *et al.* (2005).

differences in finding between studies (Figure 50.4). The lack of heavy wine drinkers and the multiple healthy lifestyle characteristics associated with light-to-moderate wine drinking (Barefoot *et al.*, 2002; Ruidavets *et al.*, 2004) are more likely to explain why many studies have shown no association or even inverse associations with adiposity for wine.

Mechanisms

The mechanisms involving alcohol and abdominal fat deposition are not clearly established but endocrine changes reflected by various hormonal changes including increased cortisol secretion appear to be involved (Zakhari, 1993; Kissebah *et al.*, 1994). These hormones are involved to a certain extent in the regulation of energy balance and affect fat-tissue enzymatic activities which may promote abdominal fat deposition (Suter *et al.*, 1997a).

Conclusion

Higher total alcohol intake (≤21 UK units/week) is associated with increased adiposity and the effects appear to be greater for abdominal adiposity (WC and WHR) than for general adiposity (BMI). Findings from more recent prospective population studies suggest that light-to-moderate drinking is not associated with weight gain but that heavier levels (>3 drinks/day; >30 g alcohol/day) contribute to weight gain and obesity in men and women. *There is no clear evidence that the effects of alcohol differ according to the type of drink.* It appears that central and general adiposity are increased at ≥3 drinks/day. In many studies, the number of heavier wine drinkers (≥21 UK units/week) is very small and this may explain the lack of positive effect in wine drinkers. There is no convincing evidence that wine is protective against abdominal fat deposition. Overall evidence from cross-sectional and prospective studies support the concept that alcohol, in particular beer and spirits, is a risk factor for obesity, as one might expect if the energy derived from alcohol consumption was added to the usual dietary calorie intake.

Summary Points

- Higher total alcohol intake (≥21 UK units or 30 g alcohol/week) is associated with increased adiposity.
- The association between alcohol and adiposity appears to be greater for abdominal adiposity (WC and WHR) than for general adiposity (BMI).
- There is no clear evidence that the effects of alcohol on adiposity differ according to the type of drink.
- Evidence from cross-sectional and prospective studies suggests that alcohol in particular beer and spirits are a risk factor for obesity.
- There is no clear evidence that wine protects against abdominal fat deposition.

References

Armellini, F., Zamboni, M., Frigo, L., Mandragona, R., Robbi, R., Micciolo, R. *et al.* (1993). *Eur. J. Clin. Nutr.* 47, 52–60.

Barefoot, J.C., Gronbaek, M., Feagenes, J.R., Mcpherson, R.S., Williams, R.B. and Siegler, I.C. (2002). *Am. J. Clin. Nutr.* 76, 466–472.

Bell, A.C., Ge, K. and Popkin, B.M. (2001). *Int. J. Obes.* 25, 1079–1086.

Bobak, M., Skodova, Z. and Marmot, M. (2003). *Eur. J. Clin. Nutr.* 57, 1250–1253.

Colditz, G.A., Willett, W.C., Stampfer, M.J., London, S.J., Segal, M.R. and Speizer, F. (1990). *Am. J. Clin. Nutr.* 51, 1100–1105.

Colditz, G.A., Giovannucci, E., Rimm, E.B., Stampfer, M.J., Rosner, B., Speizer, F.E., Gordis, E. and Willett, W.C. (1991). *Am. J. Clin. Nutr.* 54, 49–55.

Cordain, L., Bryan, E.D., Melby, C.L. and Smith, M.J. (1997). *J. Am. Coll. Nutr.* 16, 134–139.

Dallongeville, J., Marecaux, N., Ducimetiere, P., Ferrieres, J., Arveiler, D., Bingham, A., Ruidavets, J.B., Simon, C. and Amouyel, P. (1998). *Int. J. Obes. Relat. Met. Disorders* 22, 1178–1183.

Dorn, J.M., Hovey, K., Muti, P., Freudenheim, J.L., Russell, M., Nochajski, T.H. and Trevisan, M. (2003). *J. Nutr.* 133, 2655–2662.

Duncan, B.B., Chambless, L.E., Schmidt, M.I., Folsom, A.R., Szklo, M., Crouse III, J.R. and Carpenter, M.A. (1995). *Am. J. Epidemiol.* 142, 1034–1038.

Fogelholm, M., Kujala, U., Kaprio, J. and Sarna, S. (2000). *Obes. Res.* 8, 367–373.

French, S.A., Jeffery, R.W., Forster, J.L., McGovern, P.G., Kelder, S.H. and Baxter, J.E. (1993). *Int. J. Obes.* 18, 145–154.

Gerace, T.A. and George, V.A. (1996). *Prev. Med.* 25, 593–600.

Gordon, T., Kannell W.B. (1983). Drinking and its relation to smoking, blood pressure, blood lipids and uric acid: the Framingham study. *Arch. Int. Med.* 143, 1366–1374.

Gutierrez-Fisac, J.L., Rodriguez-Artalejo, F., Rodriguez-Blas, C. and del Rey-Calero, J. (1995). *J. Epidemiol. Commun. Health* 49, 108–109.

Halkjaer, J., Sorensen, T.I.A., Tjonneland, A., Togo, P., Holst, C. and Heitmann, B.L. (2004). *Br. J. Nutr.* 92, 735–748.

Hellerstedt, W.L., Jeffery, R.W. and Murray, D.M. (1990). *Am. J. Epidemiol.* 132, 594–611.

Howarth, N.C., Saltzman, E. and Roberts, S.B. (2001). *Nutr. Rev.* 59, 129–139.

Jequier, E. (1999). *Am. J. Clin. Nutr.* 69, 173–174.

Johansen, D., Friis, K., Skovenborg, E. and Gronbaek, M. (2006). *BMJ.*

Kahn, H., Tatham, L.M., Rodriguez, C., Eugenia, E., Thun, M.J. and Clark, C.W. (1997). *Am. J. Publ. Health* 87, 747–754.

Kissebah, A. and Krakower, G.R. (1994). *Physiol. Rev.* 74, 761–811.

Lapidus, L., Bengtsson, C., Hallstrom, T., Bjorntop, P. (1989). Obesity, adipose tissue distribution and health in women – results form a population study in Gothenburg, Sweden. *Appetite* 13: 25–35.

Lakka, H.M., Lakka, T.A., Tuomilehto, J. and Salonen, J.T. (2002). *Eur. Heart J.* 23, 706–713.

Laws, A., Terry, R.B. and Barrett-Connor, E. (1990). *Am. J. Publ. Health* 80, 1358–1362.

Leite, M.K.C. and Nicolosi, A. (2006). *Int. J. Obes.*, 1–9. Advanced online publication.

Liu, S., Serdula, M.K., Williamson, D.F., Mokdad, A.H. and Byers, T. (1994). *Am. J. Epidemiol.* 140, 912.

Lukasiewicz, E., Mennen, L.I., Bertrais, S., Arnault, N., Preziosi, P., Galan, P. and Hercberg, S. (2003). *Publ. Health Nutr.* 8, 315–320.

McDonald, I., Debry, G. and Westerterp, K. (1993). Alcohol and overweight. In Verschuren, P.M. (ed.), *Health Issues Related to Alcohol Consumption*, pp. 263–279. Brussels, ILSI Europe.

National Institutes of Health (1998). *Obes. Res.* 6(Suppl 2), S51–S210.

Nicolosi, A. and Leite, M.L.C. (2006). *Int. J. Obes.*, 1–9.

Prentice, A.M. (1995). *Int. J. Obes.* 19(Suppl 5), S44–S50.

Rimm, E.B., Stampfer, M.J., Giovannucci, E. *et al.* (1995). *Am. J. Epidemiol.* 141, 1117–1127.

Rissanen, A.M., Heliovaara, M., Knekt, P., Reunanen, A. and Aromaa, A. (1991). *Eur. J. Clin. Nutr.* 45, 419–430.

Rosmond, R. and Bjorntorp, P. (1999). *Int. J. Obes. Relat. Met. Dis.* 23, 138–145.

Ruidavets, J.B., Bataille, V., Dallongeville, J., Simon, C., Bingham, A., Amouyel, P., Arveiler, D., Ducimetiere, P. and Ferrieres, J. (2004). *Eur. Heart J.* 25, 1153–1162.

Rumpler, W.V., Rhodes, D.G., Baer, D.J., Conway, J.M. and Seale, J.L. (1996). *Am. J. Clin. Nutr.* 64, 108–114.

Sakurai, Y., Umeda, T., Shinchi, K., Honjo, S., Wakabayashi, K., Todoroki, I., *et al.* (1997). Relations of total and beverage-specific alcohol intake to body mass index and waist-to-hip ratio: a study of self-defense officials in Japan. *European J. Epidemiol.* 13, 893–898.

Sherwood, N.E., Jeffery, R.W., French, S.A., Hannan, P.J. and Murray, D.M. (2000). *Int. J. Obes.* 24, 395–403.

Slattery, M.L., McDonald, A., Bild, D.E., Caan, B.J., Hilner, J.E., Jacobs, D.J., *et al.* (1992). *Am. J. Clin. Nutr.* 55, 943–949.

Suter, P.M., Maire, R. and Vetter, W. (1995). *J. Hypertens* 13, 1857–1862.

Suter, P.M., Hasler, E. and Vetter, W. (1997a). *Nutr. Rev.* 55, 157–171.

Suter, P.M., Maire, R. and Vetter, W. (1997b). *Addiction Biol.* 2, 101–103.

Vadstrup, E.S., Petersen, L., Sorensen, T.I.A. and Gronbaek, M. (2003). *Int. J. Obes.* 27, 238–246.

Wannamethee, G. and Shaper, A.G. (1992). *J. Epidemiol. Comm. Health* 46, 197–202.

Wannamethee, S.G. and Shaper, A.G. (2003). *Am. J. Clin. Nutr.* 77, 1312–1317.

Wannamethee, S.G., Field, AE., Colditz, G.A. and Rimm, E.B. (2004). *Obes. Res.* 12, 1386–1396.

Wannamethee, S.G., Shaper, A.G. and Whincup, P.H. (2005). *Int. J. Obes.*

Westerterp, K.R., Prentice, A.M. and Jequier, E. (1999). In McDonald, I. (ed.), *Health Issues Related to Alcohol Consumption*, 2nd edn., pp. 103–123. Brussels, ILSI Europe.

Zakhari, S. (1993). Alcohol and the endocrine system. Research Monograph No. 23. Bethesda, MD. National Institutes of Health, National Institute on Alcohol Abuse and Alcoholism (NIH–NIAAA), p. 411.

51

Relationship Between Exercise and Beer Ingestion in Regard to Metabolism

Tetsuya Yamamoto Division of Endocrinology and Metabolism, Department of Internal Medicine, Hyogo College of Medicine, Nishinomiya, Japan

Abstract

Beer contains various substances, such as water, ethanol, purines, and carbohydrates, which, especially ethanol, may affect the metabolism of carbohydrates, lipids, and purines in the body, while physical activity including exercise is also an important factor. Therefore, the effect of the relationship between exercise and beer ingestion on body metabolism is important. Exercise increases the serum concentration of urate by enhanced adenine nucleotide degradation and elevated lactate concentration in blood, while beer ingestion increases the serum concentration of urate by enhancing adenine nucleotide degradation and elevating lactate concentration in blood because of the ethanol and purines contained in beer. Accordingly, exercise combined with beer ingestion increases the serum concentration of urate synergistically. In addition, exercise increases the plasma concentration and urinary excretion of oxypurines (hypoxanthine and xanthine) by enhanced adenine nucleotide degradation, while the ingestion of beer also increases those by enhanced adenine nucleotide degradation and a slight inhibition of xanthine dehydrogenase. However, in our previous study, the increases in plasma concentration and urinary excretion of xanthine were lower with the combination of exercise and beer ingestion as compared to beer ingestion alone, which indicated that exercise reduces the beer-induced inhibition of xanthine dehydrogenase activity and abrogates the increase of xanthine induced by beer. Exercise also increases the plasma concentration of uridine (a pyrimidine nucleoside), presumably by adenosine triphosphate (ATP) consumption-induced pyrimidine degradation, while beer ingestion also increases it presumably by that same process as well as because of the uridine contained in beer. Therefore, a combination of exercise and beer ingestion may increase the plasma concentration of uridine synergistically. Further, exercise increases insulin sensitivity and improves hyperglycemia, while long-term beer ingestion has been shown to decrease fasting insulin levels, though the carbohydrate contents in beer transiently raise insulin and plasma glucose levels. Accordingly, a combination of beer ingestion and exercise may improve the metabolism of carbohydrates including insulin and glucose, if moderate beer ingestion and aerobic exercise are performed separately. Exercise decreases the levels of low density lipoprotein (LDL), triglyceride, and total cholesterol, while both exercise and beer increase high density lipoprotein (HDL). Therefore, a combination of exercise and beer ingestion may reduce the risk of cardiovascular diseases through their synergistic effects on serum lipoprotein levels. In addition, in regard to the effects of exercise on beer ingestion and vice versa, it is suggested that moderate amounts of beer consumed during an evening will not significantly compromise physiological functioning the next morning, while individuals who exercise may consume larger quantities of beer as compared to them who do not.

List of Abbreviations

ATP	Adenosine triphosphate
LDL	Low density lipoprotein
HDL	High density lipoprotein
MSU	Monosodium urate monohydrate
URT1	Urate transporter 1
ADP	Adenosine diphosphate
AMP	Adenosine monophosphate
IMP	Inosine monophosphate
XMP	Xanthosine monophosphate
S-AMP	Adenylosuccinic acid
NAD	Nicotinamide adenine dinucleotide
NADH	Nicotinamide adenine dinucleotide reduced form
NH_3	Ammonia
UDP	Uridine diphosphate
UTP	Uridine triphosphate
VLDL	Very low density lipoprotein
LDLr	LDL receptor
VO_2max	Maximal oxygen consumption or maximal oxygen uptake

Beer in Health and Disease Prevention
ISBN: 978-0-12-373891-2

Introduction

Throughout the world, people consume beer as an alcoholic beverage. Beer contains various substances, such as water, ethanol, electrolytes, protein, and carbohydrates (Table 51.1) (Mangum *et al.*, 1986), as well as considerable amounts of purines, which contribute to hyperuricemia, as compared to other alcoholic beverages. (Table 51.2) (Kaneko, 2006). Each of these substances, especially ethanol, may have effects on the metabolism of carbohydrates, lipids, and purines in the body (Hartung *et al.*, 1990; Rimm *et al.*, 1999; Carlsson *et al.*, 2000; Koppes *et al.*, 2005; Yamamoto *et al.*, 2005). On the other hand, physical activity including exercise is an important factor, which has an effect on metabolism (Yamamoto *et al.*, 1997b; Jennings *et al.*, 1986; Thompson *et al.*, 2001; Herzberg, 2004; Kelley *et al.*, 2006). Therefore, it was considered important to investigate the effects of a combination of exercise and beer on metabolism, and determine whether beer affects exercise capacity and if exercise is related to beer ingestion volume. In this chapter, findings regarding these points will be reviewed.

Effects of Exercise and Beer on Uric Acid

Gout is a disease, manifested by recurrent attacks of acute arthritis, deposits of monosodium urate monohydrate (MSU) in and around the joints of the extremities, renal disease involving interstitial tissues and blood vessels, and uric acid nephrolithiasis with a background of hyperuricemia (Figures 51.1 and 51.2), while it is also associated with conditions related to metabolic syndrome (Choi *et al.*, 2005). Thus, it is important for patients with gout to control the plasma concentration of urate. Rigorous muscle exercise increases urate concentration in plasma by two major mechanisms, one of which is abrupt adenosine

Table 51.1 Contents analysis of Budweiser beer

Iron	0.03 ppm
Copper	0.05 ppm
Silica	35 ppm
Calcium	40 ppm
Magnesium	100 ppm
Potassium	500 ppm
Sodium	40 ppm
Alcohol	4.7%
Protein	0.38% (by weight)
Carbohydrate	3.2% (by weight)
Fat	0

Note: Data provided by Anheuser-Busch, Inc. ppm = parts per million. Main contents of beer are alcohol and carbohydrate.

Table 51.2 Purine contents and calories in various alcoholic beverages

	Total purines (mg/l)	*Purine nitrogen (mg/l)*	*Calories (kcal/100 g)*
Brewage beverage			
Japanese beer	54.4 (43.5–68.6)	23.9 (20.0–31.5)	40–46
Sake	12.1	4.6	103–109
Wine	3.9	1.6	73–77
Happo-shu	38.3	17.6	45
Distilled liquor beverage			
Japanese whisky	1.2	0.5	237
Japanese brandy	3.8	1.6	237
Shouchu	0.3	0.1	146–206

Note: Happo-shu: a low malt liquor, which has a taste that is similar to beer. Shouchu: a traditional Japanese distilled spirits, which has a high alcohol concentration at about 20–45%. Beer contains considerable amounts of purines, as compared to other alcoholic beverages.

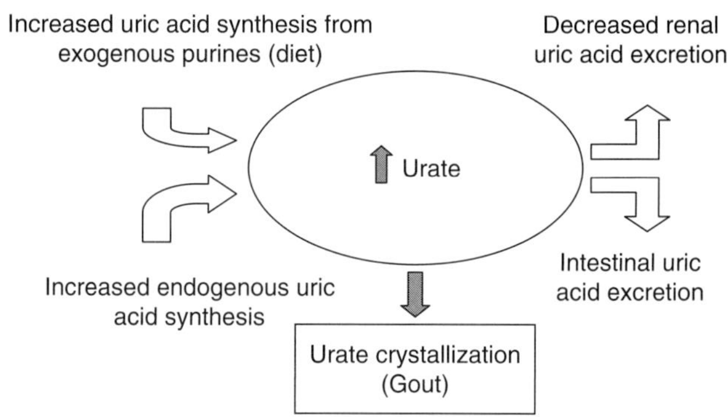

Figure 51.1 Mechanisms of hyperuricemia causing gouty arthritis. Hyperuricemia is ascribable to increased uric acid synthesis and/or decreased renal uric acid excretion.

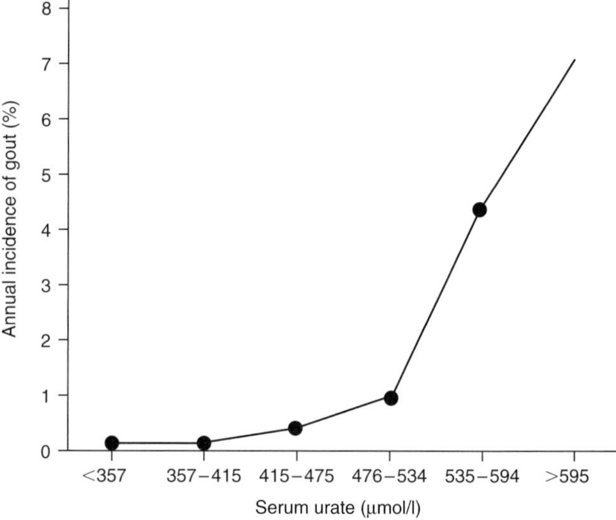

Figure 51.2 Relationship between serum urate and incidence of gout. Direct positive association between serum urate levels and a future risk of gout is shown.

triphosphate (ATP) degradation (Figure 51.3). In human muscle tissue in which xanthine dehydrogenase activity is negligible, the end-product of ATP degradation is hypoxanthine, which leaks into the blood stream and is transported to the liver, where it is converted to xanthine and uric acid by xanthine dehydrogenase. Muscular exercise increases ATP degradation in muscles. As a result, excessively produced hypoxanthine is converted to uric acid and increases the plasma concentration of urate. The other mechanism that increases the plasma concentration of urate is lactic acid production. During urate anion exchanger (URAT1) in the proximal tubules, lactate is secreted. Since the secretion of lactate is coupled with the reabsorption of uric acid during URAT1 (Figure 51.4) (Enomoto *et al.*, 2002), an increased blood concentration of lactate causes a decreased urinary excretion of uric acid. Further, exercise increases lactic acid production via increased glycolysis and leads to hyperuricemia. Therefore, both accelerated ATP degradation and lactic acid produced in exercising muscles increase the plasma concentration of urate following rigorous exercise.

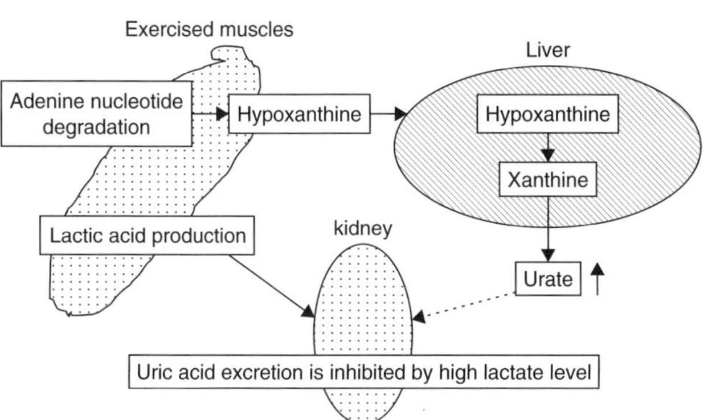

Figure 51.3 Mechanism of exercise-induced hyperuricemia. Rigorous exercise accelerates ATP degradation (ATP -> ADP -> AMP -> IMP -> inosine -> hypoxanthine -> xanthine -> uric acid) and lactic acid production, both leading to hyperuricemia.

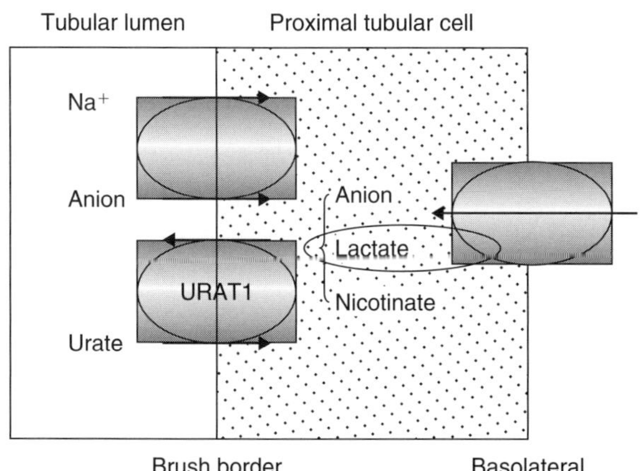

Figure 51.4 Urate anion exchanger.

Alcoholic beverages, especially beer, increase the concentration of urate in serum (Lieber, 1965; Faller and Fox, 1982; Yamamoto *et al.*, 1993; Yamamoto *et al.*, 1995; Yamamoto *et al.*, 1997a; Yamamoto *et al.*, 2002) and the ethanol in alcoholic beverages increases ATP degradation in the liver (ATP -> ADP -> AMP -> IMP -> inosine -> hypoxanthine -> xanthine -> uric acid) (Figure 51.5). Further, large amounts of ethanol increase the blood concentration of lactate (Figure 51.6) (Lieber, 1965). Beer contains considerable amounts of various purines, especially guanosine, as compared to other alcoholic beverages (Table 26.1) (Yamamoto *et al.*, 2002), and those purines are metabolized to uric acid in the body after beer ingestion. In our previous study (Yamamoto *et al.*, 2002), regular beer (10 ml/kg body weight) increased the plasma concentration of urate by 30 μmol/l, while freeze-dried beer (0.34 g/kg body weight) also increased that by 20 μmol/l. Since 10 ml of regular beer contains 0.34 g of content when freeze-dried, the amount of purines in freeze-dried beer are the

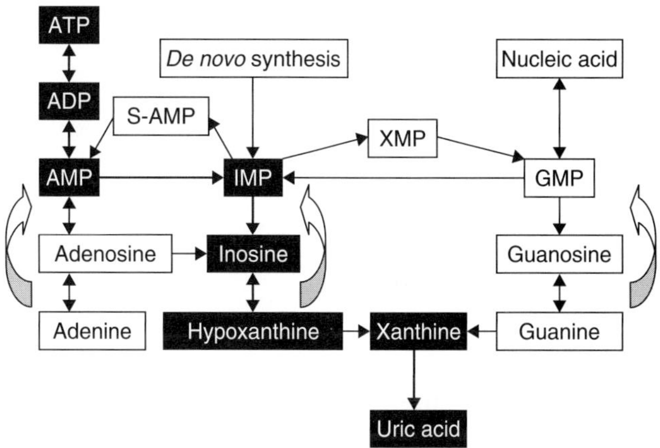

Figure 51.5 Adenine nucleotide degradation due to ethanol. Words in white indicate pathway of adenine nucleotide degradation.

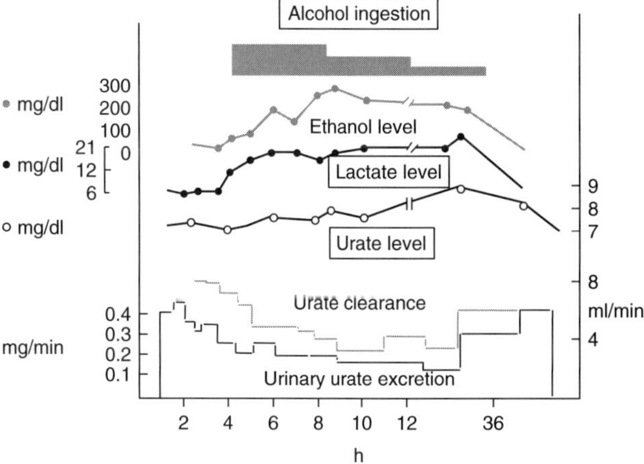

Figure 51.6 Effects of alcohol ingestion on lactate and urate levels. Large amounts of ethanol increase the concentration of lactate in blood, leading to decreased urinary urate excretion.

same as those in regular beer. These results indicate that the contents of beer contribute to an increase in urate in blood (Figure 51.7). Accordingly, beer may cause a greater increase in the plasma concentration of urate than other alcoholic beverages.

Since exercise is similar to beer ingestion in terms of the mechanism of increase in plasma concentration of urate, it was considered important to determine to what degree a combination of the two increased the plasma concentration of urate and a study was recently conducted (Ka *et al.*, 2003), with the protocol which is shown in Figure 51.8. Six healthy males participated in the experiments, which included a combination of exercise for 30 min (VO_2max 70%) and beer ingestion (10 ml/kg body weight), as well as each of those alone.

In the exercise alone experiment, the plasma concentration of urate was increased by 12% at 1 h after exercise, as compared with the reference value before the exercise (Figure 51.9). On the other hand, in the experiment of beer ingestion alone, the plasma concentration of urate was increased by 8% 1 h after the beginning of the beer ingestion, as compared with the reference value obtained before ingestion. In contrast, in the combination experiment (beer ingestion following exercise), the plasma concentration of urate was increased by 29% at 1 h after exercise, as compared with the reference value obtained before exercise. The increase in plasma concentration of urate ($87 \pm 16\,\mu$mol/l) in the combination experiment was greater than the sum of increases measured during the same period in the beer ingestion and exercise alone experiments ($58 \pm 25\,\mu$mol/l) ($p < 0.05$). Beer ingestion (10 ml/kg body weight) increased the plasma

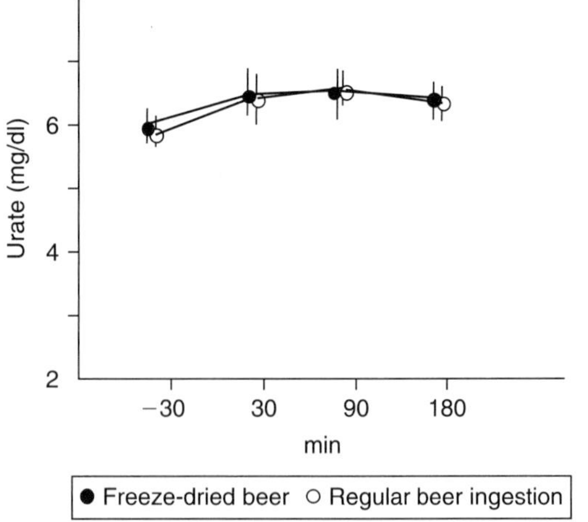

Figure 51.7 Effect of freeze-dried beer ingestion on the plasma concentration of urate.

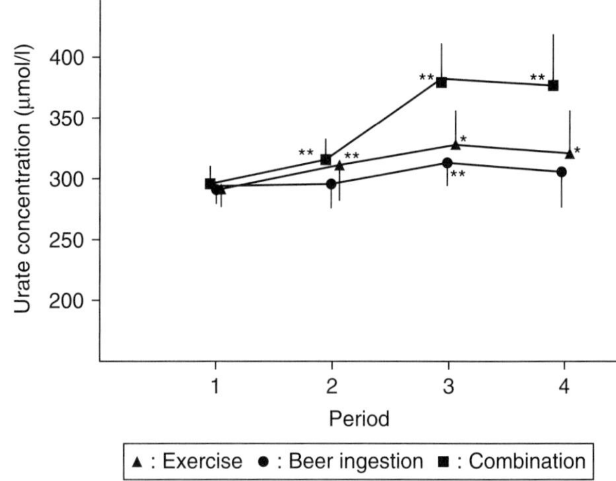

Figure 51.9 Effect of combination of exercise and beer ingestion on the plasma concentration of urate. * and ** denotes $p < 0.05$ and $p < 0.01$, respectively, as compared with the reference value in the first period. First period, second period, third period, and fourth period are the same as shown in Figure 51.8.

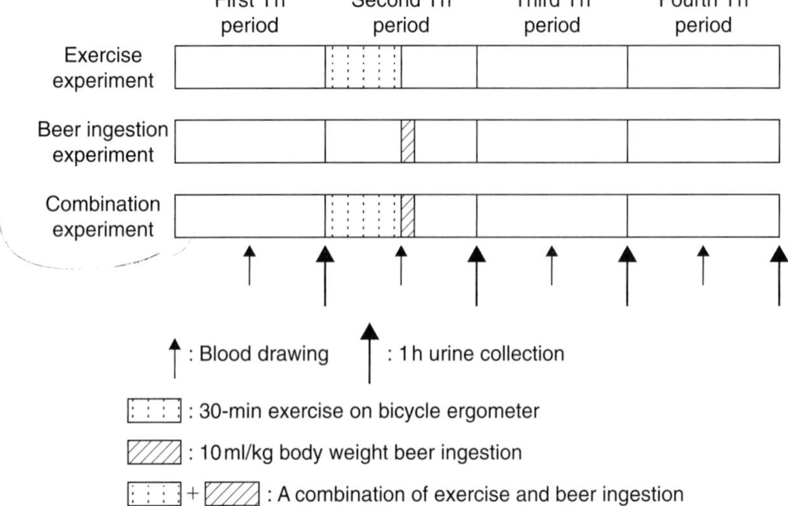

Figure 51.8 Experimental protocol for beer ingestion alone, exercise alone, and those in combination experiments.

concentration of urate by both ethanol-induced purine degradation and purine ingestion, and also increased the urinary excretion of uric acid (Table 51.3). Further, the increase in urinary excretion of uric acid in the combination experiment was less than the sum of increases over the same period in the beer ingestion and exercise alone experiments (11 ± 17 vs. 53 ± 38 μmol/h).

Those findings indicated that the plasma concentration of urate increased synergistically with the combination of beer ingestion and exercise, as the amount was greater than the sum of increases by each separately.

Uric acid is the end-product of purine degradation in humans and its plasma concentration is regulated by both the production and excretion of uric acid. Although an increased lactate concentration in blood inhibits urinary uric acid, a moderate amount of beer ingestion does not increase the blood concentration of lactate enough to significantly inhibit the urinary excretion of uric acid. Therefore, the production of uric acid by beer ingestion mainly caused an increase in the plasma concentration of urate. In contrast, the high blood concentration of lactate caused by exercise seems to enhance the increase in plasma concentration of urate caused by the beer-induced production of uric acid, as well as that induced by exercise, via a hyperlactatemia-induced inhibition of urinary uric acid excretion. In addition, though the blood concentration of lactate in the subjects immediately after exercising for 30 min in exercise alone experiment was not different from that in the combination experiment (Table 51.4), it was higher at 1 h after finishing exercise in the combination experiment than at the same period in the exercise and beer ingestion alone experiments (Table 51.4). This finding suggests that the decrease in blood concentration of lactate after exercise is disturbed by the metabolism of ethanol in the liver. Further, the production of uric acid induced by a combination of exercise and beer ingestion as well as the prolonged high blood lactate concentration may have a synergistic effect on the increase of plasma urate concentration.

In fact, the urinary excretion of uric acid did not increase in the third period of the combination experiment, though it was increased in the third period of the beer ingestion experiment (Table 51.3). In addition, the increase in urinary excretion of uric acid from the first to the third period of the combination experiment was less than the sum of increases over the same periods in the beer ingestion and exercise experiments (11 ± 17 vs. 53 ± 38 μmol/h).

From these results, we concluded that the production of uric acid induced by a combination of exercise and beer ingestion, as well as a prolonged high blood lactate concentration, provide a synergistic effect toward an increase of plasma urate concentration. Beer ingestion following exercise is a common habit of Japanese men and those in combination seems to

Table 51.3 Urinary excretion of uric acid in beer ingestion alone, exercise alone, and those in combination experiments

	First period	*Second period*	*Third period*	*Fourth period*
Exercise	168 ± 45	84 ± 45*	185 ± 32	184 ± 17
Beer ingestion	193 ± 23	210 ± 24	230 ± 27**	201 ± 20
Combination	180 ± 51	80 ± 26*	191 ± 54	201 ± 38

Notes: Values are expressed as the mean ± SD (μmol/h).

*Denotes $p < 0.01$ as compared with the reference value in the first period.
**Denotes $p < 0.05$ as compared with the reference value in the first period.

First period, second period, third period, and fourth period are the same as shown in Figure 51.8.

The urinary excretion of uric acid was decreased at the second period in the exercise alone and combination experiments.

Table 51.4 Concentrations of lactate in blood in beer ingestion alone, exercise alone, and those in combination experiments

	First period	*Second period*	*Third period*	*Fourth period*
Beer ingestion	0.96 ± 0.27	1.04 ± 0.24	1.26 ± 0.36	1.12 ± 0.35
Exercise	1.00 ± 0.41	7.11 ± 0.98*	1.32 ± 0.25	0.93 ± 0.18
Combination	0.75 ± 0.36	7.21 ± 0.73*	2.19 ± 0.31*a	1.70 ± 0.23*

Notes: Values are expressed as the mean ± SD (mmol/l).

*Denotes $p < 0.01$ as compared with the reference value in the first period.
[a] Denotes that the blood concentration of lactate was higher at 1 h after finishing exercise in the combination experiment than at the same period in the exercise and beer ingestion alone experiments.

First period, second period, third period, and fourth period are the same as shown in Figure 51.8.

increase the plasma concentration of urate to a greater degree than either one alone, which may induce a gouty attack in patients with gout. Therefore, it is better for such patients to refrain from beer ingestion following exercise.

Effects of Exercise and Beer Ingestion on Oxypurines (Hypoxanthine and Xanthine)

Oxypurines (hypoxanthine and xanthine) are precursors of uric acid, which is produced via purine degradation (Figure 51.5). The plasma concentration and urinary excretion of uric acid are markedly increased in patients with xanthine dehydrogenase deficiency, as well as gout patients treated with xanthine dehydrogenase inhibitor (allopurinol). On the other hand, the plasma concentration and urinary excretion of hypoxanthine are also markedly increased by enhanced purine degradation in the organ, in which xanthine dehydrogenase activity is negligible. A typical scenario is muscular exercise (Yamamoto *et al.*, 1994; Ka *et al.*, 2003). Hypoxanthine as a purine degradation end-product is excessively produced in muscles during exercise and leaks into blood stream, when the intensity is beyond the anaerobic threshold, where it is transported to the liver, and then converted to xanthine and uric acid by xanthine dehydrogenase (Figure 51.3). As a result, the plasma concentrations of xanthine and uric acid, as well as hypoxanthine, are increased by muscle exercise. On the other hand, beer containing ethanol and purines increases the plasma concentration and urinary excretion of oxypurines, especially xanthine, as well as the ratio of lactate/pyruvate, which suggests an increase in the level of the cytosolic nicotinamide

Table 51.5 Plasma concentrations of hypoxanthine and xanthine in beer ingestion alone, exercise alone, and those in combination experiments

	First period	*Second period*	*Third period*	*Fourth period*
Hypoxanthine				
Exercise	0.65 ± 0.08	16.16 ± 7.78*	6.59 ± 3.70**	2.78 ± 1.76**
Beer ingestion	0.67 ± 0.21	0.65 ± 0.24	1.69 ± 0.79**	0.98 ± 32**
Combination	0.74 ± 0.10	15.03 ± 6.82*	6.78 ± 4.16**	2.89 ± 1.98**
Xanthine				
Exercise	0.68 ± 0.12	1.37 ± 0.52**	1.31 ± 0.0.43*	1.05 ± 0.27*
Beer ingestion	0.53 ± 0.08	0.54 ± 0.10	3.10 ± 1.10*	2.64 ± 1.47**
Combination	0.64 ± 0.17	1.51 ± 0.62*	1.84 ± 0.67*	1.60 ± 0.77**

Notes: Values are expressed as the mean ± SD (μmol/l).

* Denotes $p < 0.01$ as compared with the reference value in the first period.

** Denotes $p < 0.05$ as compared with the reference value in the first period.

First period, second period, third period, and fourth period are the same as shown in Figure 51.8.

The increase in plasma concentration of xanthine from the first to the third period in the beer ingestion experiment was greater than that in the combination experiment.

Table 51.6 Urinary excretion of hypoxanthine and xanthine in beer ingestion alone, exercise alone, and those in combination experiments

	First period	*Second period*	*Third period*	*Fourth period*
Hypoxanthine				
Exercise	3.74 ± 1.16	43.35 ± 19.88*	36.76 ± 13.28*	13.47 ± 7.59**
Beer ingestion	4.26 ± 1.77	9.56 ± 0.92*	15.77 ± 6.74*	5.84 ± 1.25**
Combination	4.27 ± 1.57	46.21 ± 21.08*	43.60 ± 14.32*	15.29 ± 7.67**
Xanthine				
Exercise	2.73 ± 0.58	2.99 ± 1.37	5.95 ± 1.41*	4.56 ± 1.45**
Beer ingestion	2.97 ± 1.61	7.72 ± 2.76*	17.04 ± 5.81*	11.93 ± 4.53**
Combination	3.02 ± 0.64	4.30 ± 2.36	8.65 ± 2.00*	7.65 ± 4.08**

Notes: Values are expressed as the mean ± SD (μmol/h).

* Denotes $p < 0.01$ as compared with the reference value in the first period.

** Denotes $p < 0.05$ as compared with the reference value in the first period.

First period, second period, third period, and fourth period are the same as shown in Figure 51.8.

The increase in the urinary excretion of xanthine from the first to the third period in the beer ingestion experiment was greater than that in the combination experiment.

adenine dinucleotide reduced form (NADH) (Yamamoto *et al.*, 1995; Yamamoto *et al.*, 1997a; Yamamoto *et al.*, 2002).

Both the degradation of purines in beer and the ethanol-induced degradation of adenine nucleotide increase the plasma concentration of purine bases. However, an increase in NADH slightly inhibits xanthine dehydrogenase activity during beer ingestion (Yamamoto *et al.*, 1995), and the plasma concentration and urinary excretion of xanthine are increased to a greater degree than those of hypoxanthine by ethanol ingestion, as demonstrated in our recent beer ingestion study (Yamamoto *et al.*, 2002).

Nevertheless, our recent study of a combination of exercise and beer ingestion disclosed that the increase in plasma concentration and urinary excretion of xanthine was lower in the combination experiment than in the beer ingestion alone experiment, indicating that exercise relieves the increase of xanthine induced by beer (Tables 51.5 and 51.6) (Ka *et al.*, 2003).

Further, beer ingestion decreased the blood concentration of pyruvate, though the combination of exercise and beer did not do so (Table 51.7). Exercise produces pyruvic acid together with lactic acid via glycolysis in exercised muscles, after which the pyruvic acid is partly transported to the liver and metabolized to lactic acid with the conversion of NADH to nicotinamide adenine dinucleotide (NAD). Further, exercise increases adenine nucleotide degradation and produces NH_3 by the deamination of adenosine monophosphate (AMP) in exercised muscles. In the combination experiment, the blood concentration of NH_3 markedly increased (Table 51.8). Such produced NH_3 is transported to the liver and removed through the mediation of glutamate dehydrogenase to form glutamate and NAD from 2-ox-oglutarate, NH_3, and NADH. As a result, NAD may increase and NADH may decrease in the cytosol of liver cells (Tischler *et al.*, 1977). Therefore, it is suggested that a decrease in the concentration of NADH in cytosol reduces the beer-induced inhibition of xanthine dehydrogenase activity, leading to decreases in the plasma concentration and urinary excretion of xanthine.

Effects of Exercise and Beer on Uridine

Uridine is a pyrimidine nucleoside, that consists of uracil and ribose, and forms a part of RNA that is not necessary for endogenous synthesis of nucleic acids, though it plays

Table 51.7 Concentrations of pyruvate in blood in beer ingestion, exercise alone, and those in combination experiments

	First period	*Second period*	*Third period*	*Fourth period*
Exercise	0.077 ± 0.020	0.225 ± 0.024*	0.082 ± 0.018	0.066 ± 0.023
Beer ingestion	0.072 ± 0.036	0.075 ± 0.036	0.033 ± 0.012**	0.029 ± 0.011**
Combination	0.069 ± 0.026	0.238 ± 0.023*	0.053 ± 0.007	0.042 ± 0.007**

Notes: Values are expressed as the mean ± SD (mmol/l).

* Denotes $p < 0.01$ as compared with the reference value in the first period.

** Denotes $p < 0.05$ as compared with the reference value in the first period.

First period, second period, third period, and fourth period are the same as shown in Figure 51.8.

The blood concentration of pyruvate decreased at the third period in the beer ingestion experiment, whereas that of pyruvate at the same period did not change in the combination experiment.

Table 51.8 Concentrations of NH_3 in blood in beer ingestion, exercise alone, and those in combination experiments

	First period	*Second period*	*Third period*	*Fourth period*
Exercise	0.047 ± 0.004	0.087 ± 0.015*	0.047 ± 0.006	0.044 ± 0.008
Beer ingestion	0.044 ± 0.013	0.042 ± 0.012	0.035 ± 0.001	0.037 ± 0.007
Combination	0.047 ± 0.008	0.089 ± 0.011*	0.046 ± 0.012	0.043 ± 0.005

Notes: Values are expressed as the mean ± SD (mmol/l).

*Denotes $p < 0.01$ as compared with the reference value in the first period.

First period, second period, third period, and fourth period are the same as shown in Figure 51.8.

The blood concentration of NH_3 did not change in the beer ingestion experiment, whereas that of NH_3 at the second period increased in the combination experiment.

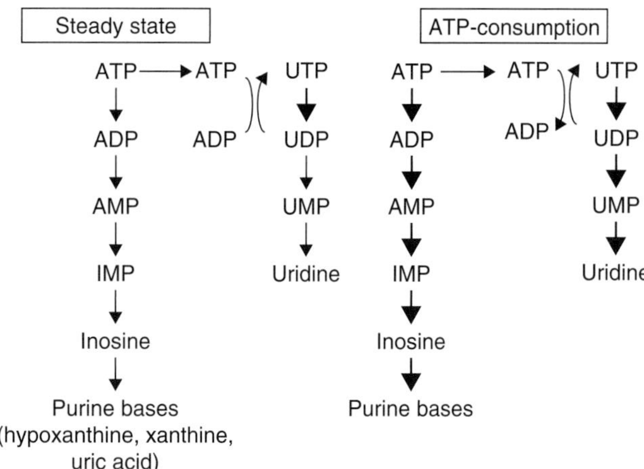

Figure 51.10 Purine and pyrimidine degradation due to ATP consumption. Thick arrows indicate increased purine and pyrimidine degradation.

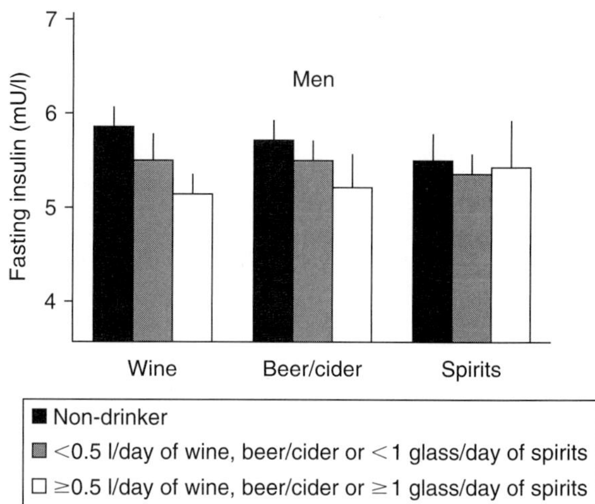

Figure 51.11 Insulin concentrations in men according to alcohol intake and type of alcoholic beverage consumed. Wine and beer decreased insulin concentrations in men.

an important role in the synthesis of glycogen. Further, it has been suggested that uridine has an action that causes vascular muscle constriction (Macdonald *et al.*, 1987).

Plasma uridine is increased by muscular exercise, ethanol ingestion, fructose infusion, and xylitol infusion, which are well known to enhance adenine nucleotide degradation and lead to an increase in the plasma concentration of purine bases (Yamamoto *et al.*, 1997a, b, 1998). Since uridine diphosphate (UDP) is phosphorylated to uridine triphosphate (UTP) using ATP as a phosphate donor, an abrupt decrease in ATP reduces the production of UTP and enhances pyrimidine degradation (UDP -> UMP -> uridine), resulting in an increase in the plasma concentration of uridine (Figure 51.10). Exercise increases uridine in exercised muscles, while ethanol ingestion also increases uridine in the liver. The uridine produced in these organs leaks into the blood stream, causing an increase in plasma concentration. In addition, beer, which contains considerable amounts of uridine, increases the plasma concentration of uridine. Therefore, a combination of exercise and beer ingestion seems to increase the plasma concentration of uridine to a greater degree than exercise or beer ingestion alone, though there are no data known to have been reported to support that speculation.

Effects of Exercise and Beer on Insulin and Glucose

A number of studies have demonstrated that exercise increases insulin sensitivity and improves hyperglycemia (Jennings *et al.*, 1986; Thompson *et al.*, 2001), while others have shown that insulin-mediated glucose is increased in the whole body and skeletal muscles in humans by physical training (Rodnick *et al.*, 1987; Mikines *et al.*, 1989; Dela *et al.*, 1992; Dela *et al.*, 1995). In addition, it was reported that adipose tissues as well as muscles play a role in the increase in insulin-mediated glucose uptake caused by exercise (Stallknecht *et al.*, 2000). These favorable effects seem to provide cardiovascular benefits.

Ethanol ingestion causes hyperglycemia or hypoglycemia depending on whether glycogen stores are adequate. However, since beer contains carbohydrates, its ingestion increases the plasma concentration of glucose. In a previous study (Nishioka *et al.*, 2002), beer (0.8 ml of ethanol equivalent/kg body weight) increased the levels of blood glucose by 26.7% and insulin by 5.1-fold. On the other hand, in another study of the relationship between alcohol intake and fasting insulin (Konrat *et al.*, 2002), an inverse relationship between beer or cider consumption and fasting insulin level, as well as that between wine consumption and fasting insulin level, were shown in non-diabetic French men (Figure 51.11). Further, in a report on the relationship between alcohol consumption and Type 2 diabetes mellitus (Carlsson *et al.*, 2000), it was speculated that consumption of large quantities of beer may increase the occurrence of Type 2 diabetes. Together, these results (acute effects of beer ingestion, effects of long-term beer ingestion, and effects of consumption of large quantities of beer) suggest that though the carbohydrate content in beer transiently raises insulin and plasma glucose levels, the decrease in fasting insulin level caused by long-term beer ingestion is associated with a cardio-protective effect in non-diabetic moderate drinkers, but not heavy drinkers, as reported by Keil *et al.* (1997).

Although the effects of a combination of exercise and beer ingestion have not been reported by others, the effects of a combination of alcohol consumption and exercise have been shown (Heikkonen *et al.*, 1998). According to that study, acute alcohol intake (1.5 g/kg of body weight) immediately before exercise inhibited an increase in the level of glucose in plasma after a single bout of rigorous exercise and slightly decreased plasma glucose levels during recovery from exercise, indicating that alcohol interferes with the metabolism of carbohydrates during and after anaerobic exercise. However, since consumption of moderate amounts of alcoholic beverages including beer may improve the metabolism of carbohydrates (Carlsson *et al.*, 2000) and aerobic exercise also improves that metabolism (Jennings *et al.*, 1986; Thompson *et al.*, 2001), a combination of moderate beer ingestion and exercise may improve the metabolism of carbohydrates including insulin and glucose, if performed separately.

Effects of Exercise and Beer Ingestion on Serum Lipids

Aerobic exercise has been shown to reduce the risk of cardiovascular disease (CVD) (Berlin and Colditz, 1990; Kohl II, 2001), which is at least partially mediated by changes in circulating lipoproteins. Aerobic exercise decreases low density lipoprotein (LDL), triglyceride, and total cholesterol levels, while it increases high density lipoprotein (HDL) (Tran *et al.*, 1983; Halbert *et al.*, 1999; Hata and Nakajima, 2000; Leon and Sanchez, 2001), though prolonged exercise is needed to reduce LDL-cholesterol. In addition, chronic exercise was shown to decrease oxidized LDL (Herzberg, 2004). It is considered that these changes may reduce the risk of CVD. The acute effects of exercise on triglycerides and HDL-cholesterol seem to be ascribable to energy expenditure, leading to reductions in levels of intramuscular triglycerides (Thompson *et al.*, 2001), which in turn may decrease serum triglyceride and increase serum HDL-cholesterol levels.

On the other hand, moderate alcohol consumption has also been shown to reduce the risk of CVD (Moore and Pearson, 1986; Marmot and Brunner, 1991; Maclure, 1993), which might be partially mediated by an increase in the level of HDL. A previous study found that beer, wine, and spirits consumption each increased HDL-cholesterol levels (Koppes *et al.*, 2005). Further, a recent animal study (Degrace *et al.*, 2006) demonstrated that moderate levels of beer consumption reduced liver triglycerides and aortic cholesterol deposits in LDL receptor-deficient and apo B-expressing [LDLr(-/-) apoB(100/100)] mice. Moderate beer (0.57 g of ethanol/kg of body weight/day) or ethanol-free beer consumption over a period of 12 weeks each increased HDL-cholesterol and VLDL-cholesterol levels, with no changes in LDL-cholesterol. In addition, liver triglyceride contents were decreased in both experiments. In contrast, cholesterol accumulation was attenuated in the whole aortas of mice with moderate beer consumption, but not in those that received ethanol-free beer. These results suggest the beneficial effects from unidentified components in beer toward atherosclerosis development, which are ascribable to changes in lipoprotein levels that are slightly enhanced by the ethanol in beer. From these findings, we concluded that a combination of exercise and beer ingestion may reduce the risk of CVD through their synergistic effects on serum lipoproteins.

Beer Ingestion-Induced Change in Exercise Capacity

In a previous study (Mangum *et al.*, 1986), acute effects of beer on physical responses following submaximal exercise were reported. Beer (1.25 ml/kg of body weight) was administered 15 min prior to exercise, which was performed for 45 min at 50% VO_2max at 5 min intervals. Heart rate, Na, K, and Cl values determined following exercise were not different between subjects who ingested beer and those who did not, suggesting that beer has no obvious benefit as a replacement fluid during exercise. In another study, ingestion of moderate amounts of beer over an evening did not significantly compromise physiological functioning in adult females the next morning. However, the number and severity of hangover symptoms (headache, dizziness, nausea, upset stomach, tremors, fatigue, dry mouth, and irritability) were increased, as was the rate of decision-making errors. Those results suggested that a mild hangover has little effect of maximal muscle strength like grip strength. On the other hand, O'Brien (1993) showed that alcohol consumption at night decreased VO_2max the next afternoon, though it was unclear from the results whether residual fatigue or hangover caused aerobic performance to decrease, or if there was an interaction between fatigue and hangover that produced the observed effects since the subjects were subjected to two different VO_2max tests in less than 24 h.

Exercise-Induced Changes in Beer Ingestion Volume

Several studies (Segovia *et al.*, 1989; Thorlindsson *et al.*, 1990) have reported that physical exercise was negatively related to the frequency of drinking. Those results suggested that favorable outcomes of exercise, such as increased academic performance, emotional stability, memory, and job satisfaction, along with decreases in work-related stress and negative emotions such as depression, might be associated with a lowered consumption of alcohol (Watten, 1995). On the other hand, results of a nationwide survey comprising more than 13,000 Norwegian inhabitants aged 15–60 years old (Saglie, 1994) suggested that sports participation was positively correlated with beer consumption. In addition, in another general population study conducted in Norway comprising 994 women and 1,000 men (Watten, 1995), it was found that the frequency of exercise, irrespective of type of sport, was related to increased consumption of wine, but not of beer, liquor, or total yearly consumption of alcohol among men and women. These two studies suggest that men and women who exercise regularly might consume more beer or wine, as compared to those who do not.

Summary points

- Exercise combined with beer ingestion increases the serum concentration of urate synergistically.
- Exercise reduces the beer-induced inhibition of xanthine dehydrogenase activity and abrogates the increase of xanthine induced by beer.
- Exercise combined with beer ingestion increases the plasma concentration of uridine.
- A combination of exercise and beer ingestion may improve the metabolism of carbohydrates including insulin and glucose, if moderate beer ingestion and aerobic exercise are performed separately. In addition, it may reduce the risk of cardiovascular diseases through their synergistic effects on serum lipoprotein levels.

References

Berlin, J.A. and Colditz, G.A. (1990). *Am. J. Epidemiol.* 132, 612–628.

Carlsson, S., Hammar, N., Efendic, S., Persson, P.G., Ostenson, C.G. and Grill, V. (2000). *Diabet. Med.* 17, 776–781.

Choi, H.K., Mount, D.B. and Reginato, A.M. (2005). *Ann. Intern. Med.* 143, 499–516.

Degrace, P., Moindrot, B., Mohamed, I., Gresti, J. and Clouet, P. (2006). *Atherosclerosis* 189, 328–335.

Dela, F., Mikines, K.J., von Linstow, M., Secher, N.H. and Galbo, H. (1992). *Am. J. Physiol.* 263, E1134–E1143.

Dela, F., Larsen, J.J., Mikines, K.J., Ploug, T., Petersen, L.N. and Galbo, H. (1995). *Diabetes* 44, 1010–1020.

Enomoto, A., Kimura, H., Chairoungdua, A., Shigeta, Y., Jutabha, P., Cha, S.H., Hosoyamada, M., Takeda, M., Sekine, T., Igarashi, T., Matsuo, H., Kikuchi, Y., Oda, T., Ichida, K., Hosoya, T., Shimokata, K., Niwa, T., Kanai, Y. and Endou, H. (2002). *Nature* 417, 447–452.

Faller, J. and Fox, I.H. (1982). *New Engl. J. Med.* 307, 1598–1602.

Halbert, J.A., Silagy, C.A., Finucane, P., Withers, R.T. and Hamdorf, P.A. (1999). *Eur. J. Clin. Nutr.* 53, 514–522.

Hartung, G.H., Foreyt, J.P., Reeves, R.S., Krock, L.P., Patsch, W., Patsch, J.R. and Gotto Jr., A.M. (1980). *Metabolism.* 39, 81–86.

Hata, Y. and Nakajima, K. (2000). *J. Atheroscler. Thromb.* 7, 177–197.

Heikkonen, E., Ylikahri, R., Roine, R., Valimaki, M., Harkonen, M. and Salaspuro, M. (1998). *Alcohol Clin. Exp. Res.* 22, 437–443.

Herzberg, G.R. (2004). *Can. J. Appl. Physiol.* 29, 800–807.

Jennings, G., Nelson, L., Nestel, P., Esler, M., Korner, P., Burton, D. and Bazelmans, J. (1986). *Circulation* 73, 30–40.

Ka, T., Yamamoto, T., Moriwaki, Y., Kaya, M., Tsujita, J., Takahashi, S., Tsutsumi, Z., Fukuchi, M. and Hada, T. (2003). *J. Rheumatol.* 30, 1036–1042.

Kaneko, K. (2006). *Hyperuricemia and Gout* 14, 38–43. (Japanese)

Keil, U., Chambless, L.E., Doring, A. and Filipiak, B. (1997). *Stieber J. Epidemiol.* 8, 150–156.

Kelley, G.A., Kelley, K.S. and Franklin, B. (2006). *J. Cardiopulm. Rehabil.* 26, 131–139. quiz 140–141, discussion 142–144

Kohl III, H.W. (2001). *Med. Sci. Sports Exerc.* 33, S472–S483. discussion S493–494.

Konrat, C., Mennen, L.I., Caces, E., Lepinay, P., Rakotozafy, F., Forhan, A. and Balkau, B. (2002). *D.E.S.I.R. Diabetes Metab.* 28, 116–123.

Koppes, L.L., Twisk, J.W., Van Mechelen, W., Snel, J. and Kemper, H.C. (2005). *J. Stud. Alcohol* 66, 713–721.

Leon, A.S. and Sanchez, O.A. (2001). *Med. Sci. Sports Exerc.* 33, S502–S515. discussion S528–529.

Lieber, C.S. (1965). *Arthritis Rheumatol.* 8, 786–798.

Macdonald, G., Assef, R., Watkins, S. and Burrell, J. (1987). *Clin. Exp. Pharmacol. Physiol.* 14, 253–257.

Maclure, M. (1993). *Epidemiol. Rev.* 15, 328–351.

Marmot, M. and Brunner, E. (1991). *BMJ* 303, 565–568.

Mangum, M., Gatch, W., Cocke, T.B. and Brooks, E. (1986). *J. Sports Med. Phys. Fitness* 26, 301–305.

Mikines, K.J., Sonne, B., Farrell, P.A., Tronier, B. and Galbo, H. (1989). *J. Appl. Physiol.* 66, 695–703.

Moore, R.D. and Pearson, T.A. (1986). *Medicine (Baltimore)* 65, 242–267.

Nishioka, K., Sumida, T., Iwatani, M., Kusumoto, A., Ishikura, Y., Hatanaka, H. and Yomo, H. (2002). *Alcohol Clin. Exp. Res.* 26, 20S–25S.

O'Brien, C.P. (1993). *Sports Med.* 15, 71–77.

Rimm, E.B., Williams, P., Fosher, K., Criqui, M. and Stampfer, M.J. (1999). *BMJ* 319, 1523–1528.

Rodnick, K.J., Haskell, W.L., Swislocki, A.L., Foley, J.E. and Reaven, G.M. (1987). *Am. J. Physiol.* 253, E489–E495.

Saglie, J. (1994). *SIFA rapport nr. 1/94/ ISBN 2-7171-179-2.* National Institute for Alcohol and Drug Research, Oslo.

Segovia, J., Bartlett, R.F. and Edwards, A.C. (1989). *Can. J. Public Health* 80, 32–37.

Stallknecht, B., Larsen, J.J., Mikines, K.J., Simonsen, L., Bulow, J. and Galbo, H. (2000). *Am. J. Physiol. Endocrinol. Metab.* 279, E376–E385.

Thompson, P.D., Crouse, S.F., Goodpaster, B., Kelley, D., Moyna, N. and Pescatello, L. (2001). *Med. Sci. Sports. Exerc.* 33, S438–S445. discussion S452–S453.

Thorlindsson, T., Vilhjalmsson, R. and Valgeirsson, G. (1990). *Soc. Sci. Med.* 31, 551–556.

Tischler, M.E., Hecht, P. and Williamson, J.R. (1977). *FEBS Lett.* 76, 99–104.

Tran, Z.V., Weltman, A., Glass, G.V. and Mood, D.P. (1983). *Med. Sci. Sports Exerc.* 15, 393–402.

Watten, R.G. (1995). *Scand. J. Med. Sci. Sports* 5, 364–368.

Yamamoto, T., Moriwaki, Y., Takahashi, S., Suda, M. and Higashino, K. (1993). *Metabolism.* 42, 1212–1216.

Yamamoto, T., Moriwaki, Y., Takahashi, S., Ishizashi, H. and Higashino, K. (1994). *Horm. Metab. Res.* 26, 504–508.

Yamamoto, T., Moriwaki, Y., Takahashi, S., Suda, M. and Higashino, K. (1995). *Metabolism* 44, 779–785.

Yamamoto, T., Moriwaki, Y., Takahashi, S., Yamakita, J., Tsutsumi, Z., Ohata, H., Hiroishi, K., Nakano, T. and Higashino, K. (1997a). *Metabolism* 46, 544–547.

Yamamoto, T., Moriwaki, Y., Takahashi, S., Tsutsumi, Z., Yamakita, J. and Higashino, K. (1997b). *Metabolism* 46, 1339–1342.

Yamamoto, T., Moriwaki, Y., Takahashi, S., Tsutsumi, Z., Yamakita, J., Nakano, T., Hiroishi, K. and Higashino, K. (1998). *Metabolism* 47, 739–743.

Yamamoto, T., Moriwaki, Y., Takahashi, S., Tsutsumi, Z., Tuneyoshi, Ka. and Hada, T. (2002). *Metabolism* 51, 1317–1323.

Yamamoto, T., Moriwaki, Y. and Takahashi, S. (2005). *Clin. Chim. Acta* 356, 35–57.

52

Estrogenicity of Beer: The Role of Intestinal Bacteria in the Activation of the Beer Flavonoid Isoxanthohumol

Sam Possemiers, Willy Verstraete and Tom Van de Wiele Laboratory of Microbial Ecology and Technology (LabMET), Ghent University, Gent, Belgium

Abstract

For many centuries, hops (*Humulus lupulus* L.) have been used as essential ingredient in beers, providing the typical bitterness and hoppy flavor. However, for the last few years the plant has gained increasing attention as a source of prenylflavonoids and in 1999, 8-prenylnaringenin was identified as the most potent phytoestrogen known so far. However, despite this high activity, health effects related to the presence of 8-prenylnaringenin in beers were always considered negligible because of the concentrations ($<100\,\mu g/l$). In this chapter we show that introducing the aspect of bioavailability into the discussion of estrogen exposure after beer consumption can drastically change this vision. Upon ingestion, prenylflavonoids reach the liver and large intestine, where they can be transformed into metabolites with different biological activity. Special attention is given to isoxanthohumol, the main prenylflavonoid in beers present in 10–30 higher concentrations than 8-prenylnaringenin, in the role of a potential pro-estrogen by virtue. After all, isoxanthohumol has the potential for a substantial degree of metabolic activation: *O*-demethylation into 8-prenylnaringenin would increase its relative estrogenic potency from 0.001 to 0.4. Recent work shows that some isoxanthohumol indeed might be activated into 8-prenylnaringenin in the liver. However, the most important activation would occur in the colon. Here, intestinal bacteria can produce 8-prenylnaringenin from isoxanthohumol with high efficiency. As it was shown that a large fraction of ingested isoxanthohumol reaches the colon, this process could easily 10-fold increase the 8-prenylnaringenin exposure after beer consumption. One drawback is that this process only occurs in one-third of humans due to interindividual differences in intestinal microbiota. Therefore, new strategies are now being developed to increase the 8-prenylnaringenin production in all individuals. In conclusion, these recent findings about increased 8-prenylnaringenin exposure can give new insights in the scientific question whether moderate beer consumption can lead to specific health outcomes.

List of Abbreviations

DMX	Desmethylxanthohumol
E_2	17β-Estradiol
ERα/β	Estrogen receptor α/β
ADME	Absorption, distribution, metabolism and excretion
CYP	Cytochrome P450 enzyme
T_{max}	Time needed to reach maximum plasma concentrations of an ingested compound
O-DMA	*O*-Desmethylangolensin
SECO	Secoisolariciresinol
SHIME	Simulator of the human intestinal microbial ecosystem
UGT	UDP-glucuronosyltransferases

Historical Perspective

History of hop use

Hops (*Humulus lupulus* L.) are known since ancient times and nowadays mainly used in the beer industry because of the presence of favorable secondary metabolites, produced in yellow glandular trichomes, termed lupulin glands, that cover the bracteoles of the female inflorescences (hop cones) (Figure 52.1). Although several hundreds of metabolites are being produced in these unique glands, the most important compounds for the brewing industry are the bitter acids, which give beer its typical bitter flavor and ensure foam and bacterial stability, and the hop essential oils, which give beer its typical "hoppy" aroma.

However, despite its long history of cultivation, the use of hop in beers is not as old as the history of beer itself, dating back to at least 1750 BC when the Sumerians discovered how to use yeast for the fermentation of barley into beer (Ross *et al.*, 2002). Prior to the use in beer, hops were cultivated as early as 736 BC by German monks for medicinal

Beer in Health and Disease Prevention
ISBN: 978-0-12-373891-2

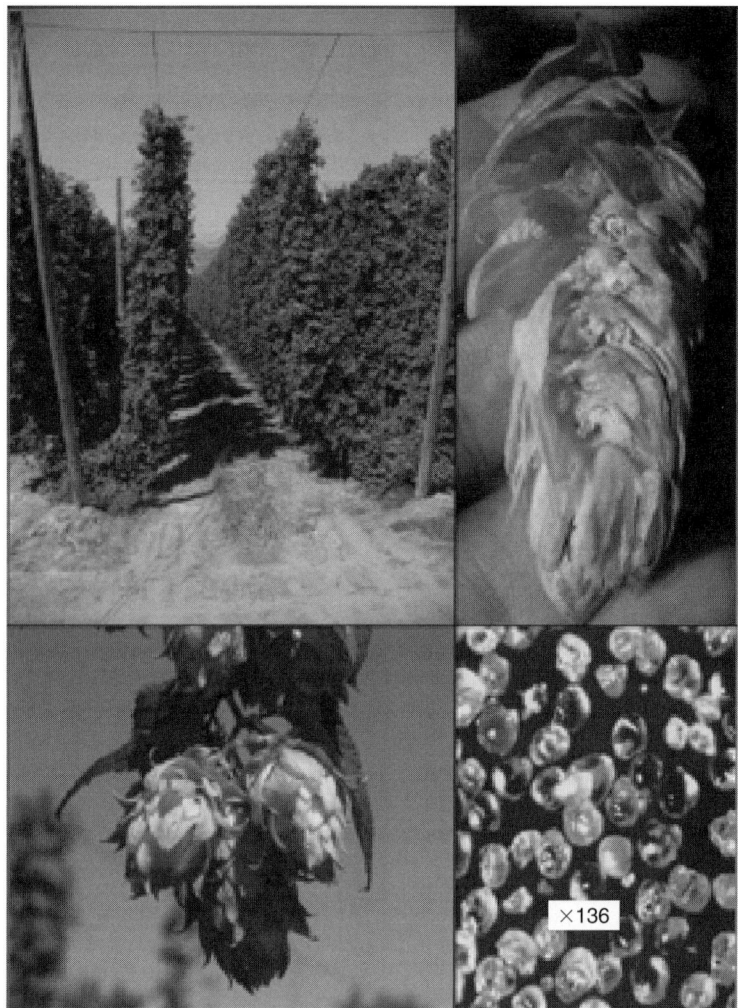

Figure 52.1 Lupulin glands from hops, present in the female hop cone. In commercial hop production, female hop vines are trained to climb strings up to 5–10 m high. On lateral arms, the plants produce the typical female inflorescences, called hop cones. Covering the bracteoles of these cones, the plant produces numerous yellow glandular trichomes. In these trichomes, called lupulin glands, hops can efficiently secrete large amounts of specific secondary metabolites. At harvest, the vines are cut down and the cones are stripped off.

purposes. Probably one of the first historical applications of hops was the treatment of insomnia, stress and anxiety because of its mild sedative effects. Some other reported applications include stimulation of the digestive tract, the use as diureticum or to clean the blood and as bacteriostatic and anti-inflammatory agent (Neve, 1991). Burgess (1964) writes that hop sprouts were already used as a salad in the first century AD. And hop sprouts were also eaten by the poor in medieval times as a substitute for asparagus. Next to this, hop stems were used in some cases to make cloth and paper and in a number of other traditional applications.

Hops were probably first added to beer in the twelfth century by German monks (Burgess, 1964; Neve, 1991). In those days, it was popular to use a variety of fruits, herbs and spices to flavor beer (so-called gruit beer). In northern central Europe and north-west Europe, *Myrica gale* L. (sweet gale or bog myrtle) was used since ancient times as principal beer additive (Behre, 1999). However, when the production of beer increased in the fourteenth century and the brewers started to export their beer, the importance of hops in beer was more and more appreciated. Because of the bacteriostatic properties of hops, hopped beers could be preserved much longer than gruit beer and the use of hops allowed the brewers to market their beers further from its production site (Burgess, 1964). When finally rumors were spread that drinking beer from sweet gale was harmful and could lead to blindness and even death, the use of *Mirica* completely declined (Behre, 1999). The enacting of the "Reinheitsgebot" (Purity law) by Wilhelm IV, the Lord of Bayern, eventually made from hops a standard ingredient in beer. Many aspects of this law, ordering that beer must be made from barley, water and hops, were adapted by other countries and since the nineteenth century, the main application of hops is to make beer.

Renewed interest in hops as a source of prenylflavonoids

Renewed interest in the alternative use of hops arose at the end of the last century when hops were acknowledged to be a source of prenylflavonoids with possible health beneficial effects, mainly related to its estrogenic properties (Milligan *et al.*, 1999). However, even before this discovery a recurring suggestion has been for many years that hops have a powerful estrogenic activity. Already in 1953, Koch and Heim reported that hops contain "the equivalent of 20–300 μg estradiol/g" (Koch and Heim, 1953). In those days, hops were picked by hand and the need for massed labor at harvest time led to the migration of many whole families from the entire region surrounding the hop region to the hop fields. According to folk legends, women who started picking hops regularly began to menstruate 2 days after arriving to pick hops, indicating the presence of an estrogenic substance. Other reports stated that brewery sludge baths, containing about 30% hop extracts were taken in Germany for the treatment of gynecological disorders (Fenselau and Talalay, 1973). However, the lack of identification of the responsible compound resulted in contradictory reports whether or not hops would really show estrogenic activity.

A first attempt for structure identification was made by Verzele *et al.* (1957) and Verzele (1986), who isolated the chalcone xanthohumol (X) from hops and, without any proof, attributed the estrogenic properties of hops to this compound. However, the real identification of the structure was only established in 1988 by Hänsel and Schulz (1988). Earlier, in 1972, Nastainczyk reported in his Ph.D. thesis the isolation of a "pro-estrogen" from hops which could be isomerized to a mixture he called the "hop estrogen" (Chadwick *et al.*, 2006). Hänsel and Schulz showed that a new chalcone, desmethylxanthohumol (DMX), was Nastainczyk's pro-estrogen, which can be isomerized into a mixture of 8-prenylnaringenin and 6-prenylnaringenin. Finally, the definitive unambiguous identification was made in 1999 when Milligan *et al.* (1999) identified 8-prenylnaringenin as a potent phytoestrogen present in hops.

The final discovery of 8-prenylnaringenin as a phytoestrogen immediately led to numerous studies in which the estrogenic activity of 8-prenylnaringenin was elucidated *in vitro* and *in vivo*. This showed that 8-prenylnaringenin was the first ERα selective phytoestrogen with only 25-fold lower affinity for the latter receptor than 17β-estradiol (E_2), the endogenous female reproductive hormone (Overk *et al.*, 2005). Its *in vitro* biological activity on the ERα receptor would be in the range of 5–600 times weaker than E_2 (Milligan *et al.*, 1999; Schaefer *et al.*, 2003; Matsumura *et al.*, 2005; Zierau *et al.*, 2005), making it far more active compared to the other known phytoestrogens. Interestingly, the concentrations needed to cause (negative) *in vivo* biological effects, such as uterine growth and vaginal mitosis, were 20,000 times higher compared to E_2.

Estrogenicity of Beer: Fact or Fiction?

Prenylflavonoids in hops

As hops are mainly used for beer production, beer is the most important dietary source of hop compounds. Prenylated flavonoids are found in a limited number of plant families, of which the Moraceae–Cannabaceae (with *Humulus lupulus* L.), Leguminosae and Asteraceae host about 80% of the ca. 1,100 known prenylflavonoids (Barron and Ibrahim, 1996). However, as none of the other plants can be identified as rich nutritional sources of prenylated flavonoids in the Western diet, beer may very well represent the most important dietary source of prenylflavonoids.

Within the female hop cone, xanthohumol would be the principal flavonoid (Figure 52.2), present at high concentrations in the lupulin glands (0.1–1% of cone dry weight) (Stevens *et al.*, 1999b) with large differences depending on the variety and flowering stage (De Keukeleire *et al.*, 2003). This prenylated chalcone is accompanied by at least 13 related chalcones, present in 10–100-fold lower concentrations, from which desmethylxanthohumol is the most important (Stevens and Page, 2004). The hop chalcones are accompanied by a number of prenylated flavanones, from which isoxanthohumol (IX), 8-prenylnaringenin and 6-prenylnaringenin are the most important. Although concentrations of these flavanones have been determined in different hop varieties (Stevens *et al.*, 1997; Rong *et al.*, 2000), some authors question whether the array of prenylflavonoids are in part the result of decomposition during drying and storage (Hänsel and Schulz, 1988; Stevens *et al.*, 1997). The presence of chalcone isomerases, enzymes which convert chalcones in the corresponding flavanones by ring closure, has been shown in hops, yet not in the lupulin glands (Stevens *et al.*, 1997). However, even without the presence of a chalcone isomerase, chalcones would isomerize chemically. Xanthohumol has one free hydroxyl available for ring closure, yielding the prenylflavanone IX, whereas desmethylxanthohumol has two free hydroxyls that can participate in cyclization, yielding two flavanones 8-prenylnaringenin and 6-prenylnaringenin. This could explain the small amounts of the flavanones in comparison to xanthohumol and desmethylxanthohumol (Stevens *et al.*, 1997). Furthermore, it has been shown that the exposure to alkali during the extraction and purification process further favor the isomerization, yielding higher prenylflavanone amounts (Verzele *et al.*, 1957). Therefore, some authors now consider 8-prenylnaringenin as an artifact, rather than a real compound present in hops (Chadwick *et al.*, 2004).

Exposure to 8-prenylnaringenin after beer consumption

The final content of prenylflavonoids in beer strongly depends on the production process and more specifically

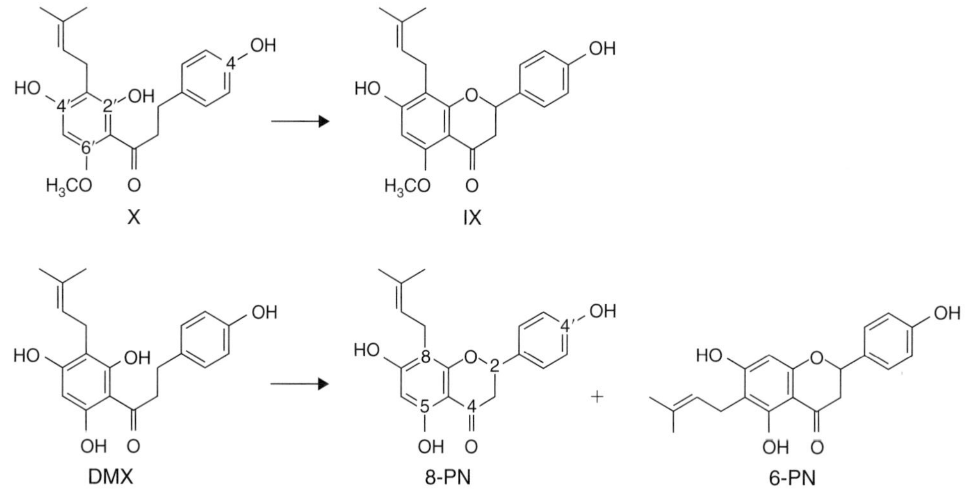

Figure 52.2 Prenylflavonoids in hops. The main prenylflavonoid in the female hop cone is the prenylchalcone xanthohumol (X) next to low concentrations of desmethylxanthohumol (DMX). During extraction of the hop cones and further processing, the chalcones can isomerize into the prenylflavanones isoxanthohumol (IX), 8-prenylnaringenin and 6-prenylnaringenin (6-PN).

Table 52.1 Prenylflavonoid contents (g/100g; average ± standard deviation) in different hop products

	Hop products		
	Pellets (type 45)	*Ethanolic extract*	*CO_2 extract*
Xanthohumol	0.62 ± 0.01	3.75 ± 0.05	0.089 ± 0.001
Isoxanthohumol	<LOD	0.17 ± 0.01	<LOD

LOD: limits of detection.
Source: After Magalhaes *et al.* (2007).

on the way hops are introduced in the brewing kettle. Hops are either introduced as pellets or as extracts. Pellets are basically hop cones which are ground and pressed into a small form, facilitating storage, handling and dosage (Magalhaes *et al.*, 2007). Hop extraction involves milling, pelleting and remilling, passing a solvent through a column to collect the resin components and finally remove the solvent. Ethanol was one of the first solvents used to extract flavor and bitter compounds from hops but has the disadvantage of low selectivity resulting in high impurity and solvents are difficultly removed. Therefore, the selected and easily removable supercritical CO_2 is currently the most accepted solvent (Gardner, 1993). However, as hop pellets and extracts differ in the concentration of prenylflavonoids, the choice for one form has a crucial impact on the final prenylflavonoid content (Table 52.1). Pellets of course still contain all flavonoids and so do ethanolic extracts because of the low selectivity of the solvent. On the contrary, polar compounds such as flavonoids cannot be excreted with supercritical CO_2 leading to very low prenylflavonoid concentrations in the extract (Magalhaes *et al.*, 2007) and in the final beers brewed with these extracts (Stevens *et al.*, 1999b; Rong *et al.*, 2000).

Although xanthohumol and (lower amounts of) desmethylxanthohumol are the main prenylflavonoids in the hop cone, their abundance in beer is much lower in favor of the corresponding prenylflavanones. This is also related to the production process. Stevens *et al.* (1999a) showed that upon introducing hops, 95% of the prenylflavonoid fraction consists of X, desmethylxanthohumol and 3′-geranylchalconaringenin. However, during the wort boiling much of the xanthohumol and all of the desmethylxanthohumol is converted by thermal isomerization into isoxanthohumol and a mixture of 6-prenylnaringenin and 8-prenylnaringenin. Later in the production process the isomerization of xanthohumol continues leading in their example to a 98% conversion into IX. Therefore, isoxanthohumol and lower quantities of 6-prenylnaringenin and 8-prenylnaringenin are the main prenylflavonoids in beers (Table 52.2).

Although isoxanthohumol concentrations often are in the range of 1 mg/l depending on the origin of the hops and brewing process, the 8-prenylnaringenin concentrations generally are much lower and normally below 100 μg/l. This is in agreement with other groups who quantified 8-prenylnaringenin concentrations in Belgian, German and other European beers and found concentrations in the range of undetected up to 20 μg/l (Tekel *et al.*, 1999), 21 μg/l (Rong *et al.*, 2000) and 138 μg/l (Schaefer *et al.*, 2005).

Biological relevance of 8-prenylnaringenin exposure?

There is currently a considerable interest whether moderate beer consumption can influence human health (De Keukeleire, 2003). Because of the risks associated with high alcohol intake (Fund, 1997), clinical guidelines

Table 52.2 Prenylflavonoid contents in beer and dietary supplements

Beer (μg/l)[a]	*X*	*IX*	*8-prenylnaringenin*	*Total*[b]
US major brand				
Lager/pilsner	34	500	13	590
Lager/pilsner	9	680	14	750
Lager/pilsner	14	400	17	460
Lager/pilsner	–	–	–	–
Northwest/US microbrews				
American porter	690	1,330	240	2,900
American hefeweizen	5	300	8	330
Strong ale	240	3,440	110	4,000
India Pale Ale	160	800	39	1,160
Imported beers				
European stout	340	2,100	69	2,680
European lager	2	40	1	43
European pilsner	28	570	21	680
European pilsner	12	1,060	8	1,100
Czech lager	28	1,350	150	1,834
Czech lager	28	1,180	175	1,688
Czech lager	26	1,910	116	2,342
Czech draught	<0.2	<20	<2.0	<24
Other				
Non-alcohol beer	3	110	3	120
Dietary supplements[c] *(daily dose)*				
Breast enhancement	3,220–4,830	792–1,188	103–155	4,388–6,582
Menopausal complaints	2,500–3,000	1,000–1,500	100	3,700–4,700

[a] Most beers contain no desmethylxanthohumol due to thermal isomerization in the brew kettle.
[b] Minor prenylflavonoids contributing to the total include 6-geranylnaringenin and 6-/8-geranylnaringenin.
[c] Selection of two commercially available dietary supplements claiming specific beneficial effects.
Source: After Stevens *et al.* (1999b).

generally do not recommend the consumption of alcohol-containing beverages. Red wine is about the only beverage escaping this judgment, often referred to as the "French Paradox" (Kopp, 1998; Avellone *et al.*, 2006). However, more and more studies now conclude that moderate beer consumption would equally protect against these lifestyle-related diseases (Klatsky *et al.*, 1997; Cleophas, 1999; Di Castelnuovo *et al.*, 2002) indicating that moderate beer consumption should not unconditionally be contemplated as negative. This may be related to direct protective effects of moderate alcohol consumption (Giles and Sander, 2005), but additional benefits might also be associated with specific non-alcohol components in beer, such as isohumulones (Kondo, 2004; Nozawa *et al.*, 2006).

In view of the recent findings on the potent biological activity of 8-prenylnaringenin, an extra question was recently added to this discussion: Are any (positive or negative) endocrine effects to be expected related to moderate beer consumption? Much attention has recently been given to the presence of endocrine-active substances in the human diet and possible associated health risks (Jefferson and Newbold, 2000; Rasier *et al.*, 2006). As previously mentioned, 8-prenylnaringenin would be the most potent phytoestrogen currently known with much higher activity than other dietary compounds with estrogenic activity, and therefore this question should indeed be carefully considered when assessing the health effects of moderate beer consumption. Yet, the final 8-prenylnaringenin concentrations in beers are generally below 100 μg/l, resulting in a total estrogenicity of beers which is still 500–1,000-fold lower than the concentration needed for harmful *in vivo* activity (~100 mg/l) in rat experiments (Milligan *et al.*, 2002). Therefore, it is generally agreed that with the current knowledge, no detrimental health effects are to be expected through moderate beer consumption (Milligan *et al.*, 1999; Stevens and Page, 2004).

But what about the positive effects of long term exposure to very low concentrations of dietary estrogens? Many reports now conclude positive effects on for instance bone density of long term exposure to ultra-low doses (0.25 mg/day) of E_2 (Prestwood *et al.*, 2003; Kenny *et al.*, 2005; Peeyananjarassri and Baber, 2005; Appt *et al.*, 2006). Based on the absolute 8-prenylnaringenin concentrations in beer, even these kinds of effects probably should not be expected. However, one important factor often is not taken into consideration: the aspect of bioavailability and possible biotransformation reactions inside the human body. Biotransformation of food components has evolved to facilitate the elimination of potentially toxic substances through the production of polar, and usually less active, metabolites (Coldham *et al.*, 2002). However, in certain cases, biotransformation may confer a substantial increase in the biological activity. Therefore, the rest of this chapter will handle with all possible aspects of the bioavailability and biotransformation of prenylflavonoids from hops with respect to question whether uptake of hops can lead to significant exposure to the potent phytoestrogen 8-prenylnaringenin. Special attention will be given to IX, the main prenylflavonoid in beers and hop products, in the role of a potential pro-estrogen by virtue. After all, isoxanthohumol has the potential for a very substantial degree of metabolic activation: *O*-demethylation into 8-prenylnaringenin would increase its relative estrogenic potency from 0.001 to 0.4 (Coldham *et al.*, 2002).

Isoxanthohumol as Pro-estrogen: Activation into 8-Prenylnaringenin

Bioavailability

The term bioavailability has been the subject of much debate. Originally, the term mainly related to the extent and rate of absorption from the gut. Subsequently, the importance of distribution, metabolism and excretion were recognized, leading to a "biodelivery" concept of bioavailability. Current definitions have been extended to encompass the concept of "bioefficacy." Therefore, for flavonoids bioavailability now refers to the effectiveness of a compound to elicit a biological response in a target tissue (Rowland *et al.*, 2003). Ideally, this response should be monitored with a sensitive functional marker (e.g. plasma homocysteine for folate). In reality, however, no such marker is available for flavonoids and bioavailability can only be assessed based on data from absorption, distribution, metabolism and excretion (ADME).

Absorption and distribution of flavonoids

Flavonoids mainly occur in food as glycosides, bound to sugar moieties, but sometimes also as aglycones. For instance, naringenin is present in citrus fruits bound to glucose or rutinose molecules, but in tomatoes it is present as free naringenin. Many aglycones can readily be absorbed in the small intestine and depending on the sugar moiety and position on the flavonoid, deglycosilation of flavonoid glycosides can occur by mammalian β-glucosidases in the small intestine, followed by absorption of the aglycon (Bugianesi *et al.*, 2002; Walle, 2004; Wang *et al.*, 2006). Others, however, reach the colon intact where deglycosilation occurs by bacterial enzymes (Erlund *et al.*, 2001; Cermak *et al.*, 2006; Wang *et al.*, 2006). Due to extensive phase I and II metabolism in the intestinal wall during absorption and in the liver (see below), a major fraction of the absorbed flavonoids is excreted back into the intestine through the bile as glucuronides and/or sulfates and reaches the colon where bacterial β-glucuronidases and sulfatases can release the flavonoid aglycon (Hu *et al.*, 2003a; Liu *et al.*, 2003; Walle *et al.*, 2004). In most cases flavonoids mainly occur in plasma as phase II conjugates which can be excreted in urine or reach specific target organs to exert biological activity.

Few studies have been performed on the pharmacokinetics of hop prenylflavonoids. Whereas the absorption of xanthohumol would be low (Avula *et al.*, 2004; Nookandeh *et al.*, 2004) 8-prenylnaringenin is easily taken up from the gut, probably by passive diffusion (Nikolic *et al.*, 2006). After 8-prenylnaringenin administration to rats, dogs and postmenopausal women, rapid almost complete absorption ($T_{max} = 1.5$ h) was noted, followed however by extensive presystemic elimination (>50%) via the bile. Enterohepatic circulation resulted in a secondary plasma peak ($T_{max} = 7–10$ h) (Rad *et al.*, 2006). This rapid elimination would be due to extensive phase II metabolism. This was confirmed *in vivo* as conjugates dominated over free 8-prenylnaringenin in both plasma and urine (Schaefer *et al.*, 2005; Rad *et al.*, 2006). Plasma concentrations showed a good dose response relation but conjugation was less efficient at high dose. Within 48 h, respectively 5–10% and 20–30% of the ingested dose were excreted in urine and feces, in the latter predominantly as free 8-prenylnaringenin (Rad *et al.*, 2006). Although no data are published on isoxanthohumol absorption and distribution, one of our recent studies with germ-free rats indicates that isoxanthohumol would also be well absorbed, but that presystemic elimination also excretes a major fraction of the absorbed isoxanthohumol back into the intestine. Therefore, about 35% of the ingested dose was excreted in the feces of germ-free rats. This would mean that, in the presence of intestinal bacteria, a large fraction of the ingested isoxanthohumol becomes substrate for the bacterial enzymes in the colon.

Liver metabolism of flavonoids: production of 8-prenylnaringenin from IX?

Liver metabolism of dietary compounds can include a variety of reactions including condensation, cyclization, hydroxylation, dehydroxylation, alkylation, *O*-dealkylation, halogenation, dehydrogenation, double-bond reduction, carbonyl reduction and ring degradation (Das and Rosazza, 2006). For flavonoids, cytochrome P450 (CYP) hydroxylation of the B ring, leading to catechol formation, and/or A ring would be the major site of hepatic metabolism (Nielsen *et al.*, 1998). For instance, naringenin, the non-prenylated analog of 8-prenylnaringenin, mainly is hydroxylated on the 3′ position, yielding eriodictyol (Breinholt *et al.*, 2002) and also for the isoflavone phytoestrogens daidzein and genistein A and B ring hydroxylation is the main route of hepatic metabolism (Hu *et al.*, 2003b). Methylated flavonoids often are demethylated in the liver. The methylated isoflavones formononetin and biochanin A are *O*-demethylated into respectively daidzein and genistein (Hu *et al.*, 2003b; Lania-Pietrzak *et al.*, 2005) and demethylation on both the A and B rings has been shown for a number of flavonoids (Nielsen *et al.*, 1998; Breinholt *et al.*, 2002; Kagawa *et al.*, 2004; Wen and Walle, 2006).

However, due to the presence of the prenyl side chain, hepatic metabolism seems to be different for prenylflavonoids. Using rat liver microsomes as a model, Yilmazer *et al.* (2001) showed that phase I metabolism of xanthohumol yielded four metabolites. The formation of three of them involved epoxidation of the prenyl group in the A ring. The fourth metabolite was formed by hydroxylation of the B ring of X, yielding a catechol structure. This shows that the prenyl group in the A ring of prenylflavonoids would be the major site of hepatic phase I metabolism by CYP enzymes and not hydroxylation of the B ring. In a recent study on xanthohumol transformation by human liver microsomes, the prenyl group also was the primary site of metabolism (Nikolic *et al.*, 2005). However, the most abundant metabolite was not a cyclization product of xanthohumol but a *trans*-X alcohol after oxidation of the terminal methyl group of the prenyl chain.

Phase I metabolism of the flavanones isoxanthohumol and 8-prenylnaringenin also mainly took place on the prenyl chain. 8-Prenylnaringenin metabolism yielded four major metabolites (Nikolic *et al.*, 2004). Two were identified as *cis*- and *trans*-8-prenylnaringenin alcohol, from which the latter was more abundant and could further be oxidized to *trans*-8-prenylnaringenin aldehyde. The fourth was oxidized on the 3′ position yielding 8-prenyleriodictyol. Incubation of human hepatocytes with 8-prenylnaringenin revealed that phase II metabolism mainly involved 7-*O*-glucuronidation on the A ring of 8-prenylnaringenin and its alcohol metabolites (Nikolic *et al.*, 2006). Isoxanthohumol metabolism showed to be very similar as for 8-prenylnaringenin (Nikolic *et al.*, 2005), yielding the *cis*- and *trans*-IX alcohol as main metabolites (Figure 52.3).

The most interesting finding however was that, although not the most abundant, one metabolite of isoxanthohumol was identified as 8-prenylnaringenin, indicating demethylation of isoxanthohumol in the liver. Although *O*-demethylation of chalcones (Sanchez-Gonzalez and Rosazza, 2004) and

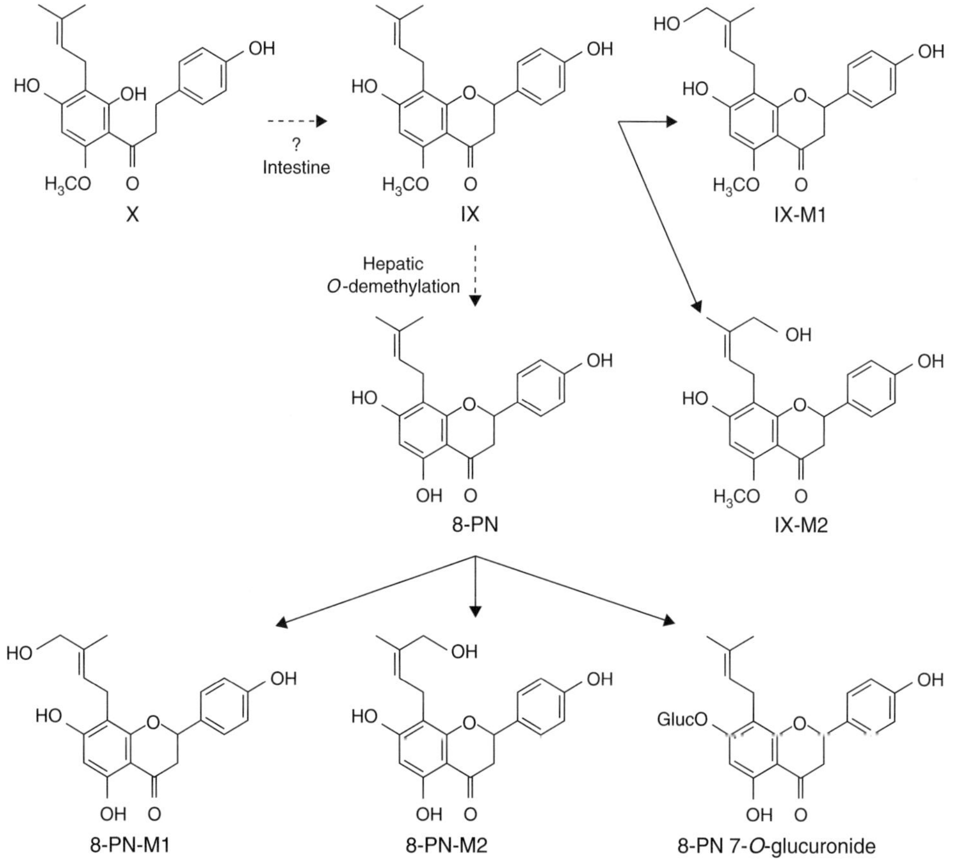

Figure 52.3 Liver metabolism of 8-prenylnaringenin. Main phase I and II metabolites of 8-prenylnaringenin. Xanthohumol (X) may chemically be converted into isoxanthohumol (IX) in the intestine, increasing the isoxanthohumol concentration. Phase I metabolism of isoxanthohumol mainly yields *cis*- and *trans*-alcohols of the prenyl group but may also be an extra source of 8-prenylnaringenin by hepatic *O*-demethylation of IX.

non-prenylated analogs of 8-prenylnaringenin on the A ring (Nielsen *et al.*, 1998; Ibrahim *et al.*, 2003) has been shown, no demethylation of xanthohumol into desmethylxanthohumol was found (Yilmazer *et al.*, 2001) and previous attempts to activate isoxanthohumol into 8-prenylnaringenin with liver enzymes were unsuc-cessful (Coldham *et al.*, 2002). Therefore, although 8-prenylnaringenin was only a minor metabolite in this study, this was the first report of the role of isoxanthohumol as a pro-estrogen, being activated into the potent phytoestrogen 8-prenylnaringenin by human liver enzymes such as CYP1A2 (Guo *et al.*, 2006).

Metabolism of flavonoids by intestinal bacteria

While many recent studies focus on the absorption of flavonoids and the importance of liver phase I and II metabolism toward their final biological activity, it is often forgotten that a major fraction of ingested flavonoids reaches the colon directly or through enterohepatic circulation (see above). Here, the aglycones can be absorbed from the colon or act as substrate for the indigenous bacterial community with their extensive metabolic potential. In many cases bacterial metabolism of polyphenols leads to a decrease in biological activity. However, in some cases specific bacterial transformations give products with increased biological properties compared to the parent compounds. Therefore, bacterial degradation and specific transformation will be discussed separately.

Microbial Biotransformation Activity When considering the metabolism of hop components by intestinal bacteria, it is important to first give an overview of their metabolic potency toward compounds that reach the large intestine. The human large intestine harbors an incredibly diverse microbial ecosystem comprising 400–500 species at concentrations of 10^{12} microorganisms per gram gut content, the highest recorded for any microbial habitat (Whitman *et al.*, 1998). For many years it was believed that the main purpose of the large intestine was the resorption of water and salt by the body and the facilitated disposal of waste materials. However, it has now become clear that this diverse group of colon bacteria play a key role in many processes that are in direct relationship with our body. Numerous studies show the role of intestinal microorganisms in the synthesis of short chain fatty acids that provide energy to the colon epithelium (Cummings and Englyst, 1987), the stimulation of the gut immune system (Salminen *et al.*, 1998), the synthesis of vitamins K and B (Conly and Stein, 1992) and the colonization resistance against exogenous pathogens (Hopkins and Macfarlane, 2003).

Most resident colon microbiota typically perform fermentation processes taking care of carbohydrate and protein breakdown, but it has become clear that many bacterial groups are also capable of transforming xenobiotic compounds (Macdonald *et al.*, 1983; Ilett *et al.*, 1990; Aura *et al.*, 2002). The metabolic potency of the intestinal microbiota is considered to be enormous, rivaling that of the liver in the number of biochemical reactions and transformations in which it participates (Macfarlane and Macfarlane, 1997). In contrast to the oxidative and conjugative reactions from the phase I and II enzymes in the enterocytes and hepatocytes, the bacterial metabolism is more reductive, hydrolytic and even of degradative nature with a great potential for both bioactivation as detoxification of xenobiotics (Table 52.3) (Ilett *et al.*, 1990). Additionally, intestinal microbiota also interferes with the human biotransformation process through the enterohepatic circulation of xenobiotic compounds. Once released in the intestinal lumen, liver conjugates may be hydrolyzed again by bacterial enzymes such as β-glucuronidase, sulfatase and glucosidases. This would negate the detoxification cycle and delay the excretion of many exogenous compounds since the original compounds or phase I metabolites are more prone to intestinal absorption than their phase II conjugates.

Degradation of Flavonoids in the Colon Colonic metabolism of dietary flavonoids has been extensively studied and associations between the urinary excretion of simple phenolic structures, such as hippuric acid derivatives, and bacterial degradation of flavonoids have been shown in many studies (Gonthier *et al.*, 2003; Gao *et al.*, 2006). It is clear that the metabolites are formed by microbial action, as lower recovery was found in human and animal studies where antibiotics were dosed prior to the flavonoid uptake (Gott and Griffiths, 1987; Kohri *et al.*, 2001) and as phenolic metabolites were not detected in germ-free rats (Griffiths and Barrow, 1972).

Bacterial flavonoid degradation follows a very general pattern in which many non-specific metabolites are formed, such as hydroxylated phenylpropionic acids. The consequence is that a relatively small number of phenolic degradation products are formed in the colon from the extremely diverse group of natural flavonoids (Rechner *et al.*, 2004). Already in 1956 it was shown that flavonoid degradation involves ring fission of the heterocyclic C ring (Booth *et al.*, 1956). More studies have elucidated the complete degradation pathway (Braune *et al.*, 2001; Cermak *et al.*, 2006). With naringenin as example, the degradation starts with isomerization of the flavanone's C ring at the hetero atom into the corresponding chalcone phloretin (Figure 52.4). After reduction into a dihydrochalcone, further splicing takes place at the carbonyl moiety, yielding phloroglucinol and 3-(4-hydroxyphenyl)propionic acid. The metabolite 3-(4-hydroxyphenyl)propionic acid may be dehydroxylated into 3-phenylpropionic acid and the mixture can be absorbed from the colon. Both components often are recovered as such or conjugated in urine (Felgines *et al.*, 2000), but may also be subjected to β-oxidation and glycination in

Table 52.3 Metabolic potency of human gastrointestinal microbiota

Reactions	*Enzyme*	*Bacterial species/origin of sample*
Hydrolysis		
Glucuronides	β-Glucuronidase	*E. coli*
Glycosides	β-Glucosidase	*Enterococcus faecalis*, *Eubacterium rectale*, *Clostridium sphenoides*
Amides	Amide hydrolase	*E. coli*, *B. subtilis*
Esters	Deacetylase	*Enterococcus faecalis*
Sulfamates	Arylsulfotransferase	Clostridia, enterobacteria, enterococci
Reduction		
Azo-compounds	Azoreductase	Clostridia, lactobacilli
Unsaturated lactone	Unsaturated glycoside hydrogenase	*Eubacterium lentum*
Aliphatic double bounds	Unsaturated fatty acid hydrogenase	*Enterococcus faecalis*
Nitro-compounds	Nitroreductase	*E. coli*, bacteroides
N-oxides	*N*-oxide reductase	Human colon
S-oxides	Sulfoxide reductase	*E. coli*
Ketones	Hydrogenase	Rat caecum
Hydroxylamines	Nitroreductase	Rat GIT
Dehydroxylation		
Demethylation	Demethylase	Enterococci, lactobacilli, clostridia
Deamination	Deaminase	Bacteroides, clostridia
Decarboxylation	Decarboxylase	*Enterococcus faecalis*
Dehydrogenation	Dehydrogenase	*Clostridium welchii*
Dehalogenation	Dehalogenase	*E. coli*, *Aerobacter aerogenes*
Synthetic reactions		
Esterification	Acetyltransferase	*E. coli*
N-nitrosation		*Enterococcus faecalis*, *E. coli*
Other reactions		
Oxidation	Oxidase	*E. coli*, *Enterococcus faecalis*
Isomerization	Isomerase	*Eubacterium rectale*, *clostridium sphenoides*
Fission aliphatic	Tryptophanase	*E. coli*, *Bacillus alvei*
Fission ring	C–S lyase	Pig GIT, *Eubacterium aerofaciens*

GIT: gastrointestinal tract.

Source: After Ilett *et al*. (1990).

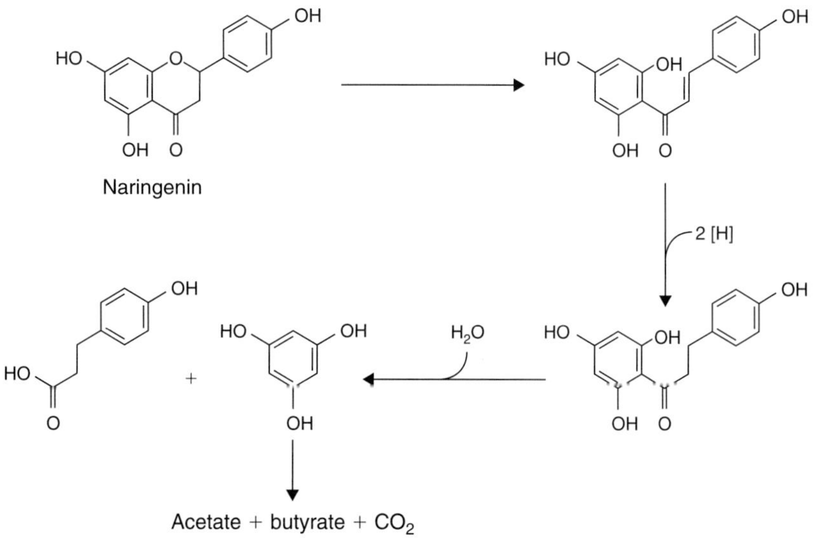

Figure 52.4 Colonic degradation of naringenin by intestinal bacteria. Degradation of naringenin by intestinal bacteria yields 3-(4-hydroxyphenyl)propionic acid and phloroglucinol. Whereas the former may further be transformed to 3-phenylpropionic acid, the latter is completely degraded by intestinal bacteria.

the liver, yielding hippuric acid and 4-hydroxyhippuric acid (Rechner *et al.*, 2004). In contrast, phloroglucinol hardly ever is recovered as final metabolite, as it can be degraded into acetate, butyrate and CO_2 (Krumholz and Bryant, 1986; Brune and Schink, 1992).

Important to notice is that colonic degradation of flavonoids is highly variable because of two main reasons. Firstly, small differences in substitution pattern of flavonoids lead to major changes in colonic degradation (Griffiths and Smith, 1972; Lin *et al.*, 2003; Simons *et al.*, 2005). The major factor determining rapid degradation is the presence of a 5- and 7-OH on the A ring plus a 4′-OH on the B ring. Methoxy groups however, both on A or B ring significantly slow bacterial degradation. A good example of these differences is the degradation of the isoflavone phytoestrogens. Genistein, having all necessary OH groups, is rapidly degraded into 2-(4-hydroxyphenyl)propionic acid and phloroglucinol (Schoefer *et al.*, 2002), whereas daidzein, lacking the 5-OH, may be transformed into *O*-desmethylangolensin (*O*-DMA) but is not fully degraded into phenolic acids (Schoefer *et al.*, 2002). Secondly, large interindividual differences were noted in the degradation of specific flavonoids. This has led to the separation of individuals into high, moderate and low flavonoid degraders (Erlund, 2004; Simons *et al.*, 2005).

As degradation of flavonoids leads to a decrease in biological activity, especially when the structure of the parent compound is necessary to interact with specific targets in the human body such as estrogen receptors, knowledge about the intestinal degradation of prenylflavonoids from hops is crucial toward the understanding of possible health-related effects of these beer compounds. In our first report about intestinal metabolism of prenylflavonoids from hops (Possemiers *et al.*, 2005), we showed that isoxanthohumol and xanthohumol would have a high metabolic stability, whereas 8-prenylnaringenin was sensitive toward bacterial degradation. However, these preliminary conclusions were based on long term (8 days) batch incubations. Short term experiments under more relevant intestinal conditions (Possemiers *et al.*, 2006) showed that 8-prenylnaringenin also has a remarkably high intestinal metabolic stability compared to the non-prenylated naringenin. These results would have the important implication that, in contrast with easily degradable flavonoids (Rechner *et al.*, 2004; Cermak *et al.*, 2006), the fraction of 8-prenylnaringenin reaching the colon would have an increased bioavailability, as high metabolic stability favors the possibility of being absorbed from the colon to exert systemic biological effects.

Colonic Activation of Phytoestrogens: Activation of Isoxanthohumol into 8-Prenylnaringenin Next to degrading active dietary compounds into less active metabolites, a number of bacterial transformations are also known leading to the production of metabolites with increased biological activity. The best example of a transformation leading to more active metabolites is the activation of phytoestrogens inside the human intestine (Figure 52.5). Until recently, the two most dominant well-known dietary phytoestrogens were the isoflavones from soy and the lignans present in flaxseed, grains, nuts, fruit . . .. For these two groups, it is now commonly accepted that the biological activity of these compounds largely depends on the metabolic potential of the intestinal bacteria (Rowland *et al.*, 1999; Raffaelli *et al.*, 2002; Turner *et al.*, 2003).

The isoflavones daidzein and genistein are present predominantly as glucosides in most commercially available soy products. Glucosides originating from food which escaped deconjugation in the small intestine, as well as phase II glucuronides and sulfates excreted in the gut through enterohepatic circulation, can be deconjugated (De Boever, 2001; Choi *et al.*, 2002; Tsangalis *et al.*, 2002). It was previously mentioned that genistein is much more susceptible to bacterial degradation than daidzein. Many reports have shown however, that the latter isoflavone not only can partially be degraded into *O*-DMA, but may also be transformed into equol. The production of equol, named after *equus* (Pike *et al.*, 1999) as it was first found in horse urine (Marrian and Haslewood, 1932), was shown to be performed exclusively by bacteria as antibiotic treatment decreased equol production (Blair *et al.*, 2003) and as equol was not produced in germ-free rats (Bowey *et al.*, 2003). As many *in vitro* (Lund *et al.*, 2004; Muthyala *et al.*, 2004; Turner *et al.*, 2004; Messina *et al.*, 2006) and *in vivo* studies (reviewed in Atkinson *et al.*, 2005) indicate that equol would exert increased health beneficial effects, the intestinal bacteria have a crucial role in the activation of soy phytoestrogens.

A similar story is true for lignans. These plant compounds are present in foods as inactive glycoside precursors (Liggins *et al.*, 2000) but can be activated inside the human intestine into the active mammalian lignans (enterolignans) enterodiol and enterolactone (Setchell *et al.*, 1981a, b;

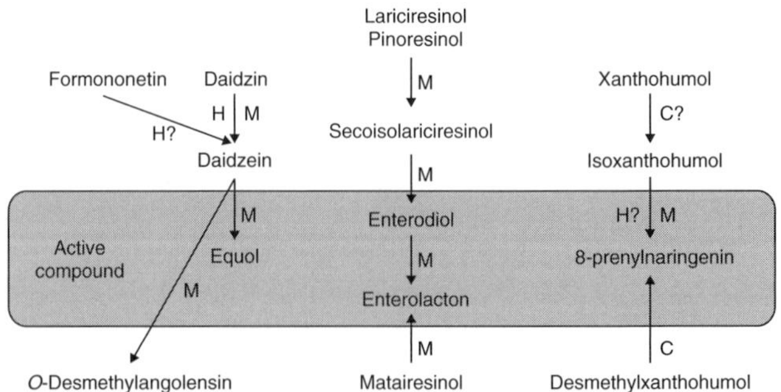

Figure 52.5 Metabolism of phytoestrogens in the human body. The most relevant groups of phytoestrogens, the isoflavones, lignans and prenylflavonoids, are present in food as less active precursors. Inside the human body, they can be activated into the respective active metabolites equol, enterodiol + enterolactone and 8-prenylnaringenin. Although some transformations are of chemical origin (C) or catalyzed by human enzymes (H), microbial enzymes (M) have a crucial role in the generation of the final metabolites for each group of phytoestrogens.

Clavel *et al.*, 2006). The main dietary precursors are identified as secoisolariciresinol (SECO), matairesinol and recently lariciresinol and pinoresinol (Milder *et al.*, 2005). As this transformation again was shown to be performed uniquely by bacteria (Bowey *et al.*, 2003) and as the enterolignans would have increased biological activity (McCann *et al.*, 2005; Kuijsten *et al.*, 2006; Saarinen *et al.*, 2006; Zeleniuch-Jacquotte *et al.*, 2006), it can be concluded that intestinal bacteria also determine health effects related to lignan intake.

But might this also be happen with this new group of phytoestrogens from hops? In 2002, it was suggested that isoxanthohumol might act as a pro-estrogen *in vivo* supposing it could be demethylated into 8-prenylnaringenin after uptake in the human body (Coldham *et al.*, 2002) and in 2005, urinary 8-prenylnaringenin excretion was indeed detected after isoxanthohumol consumption by healthy men (Schaefer *et al.*, 2005). Although this was attributed to liver metabolism (see above), the intestinal microbial community might very well be responsible for this transformation, as a number of bacteria have been identified as capable to demethylate methoxylated aromates (Table 52.4).

And indeed, incubation of fecal samples with isoxanthohumol learned that intestinal bacteria are capable of *O*-demethylation of isoxanthohumol into 8-prenylnaringenin (Possemiers *et al.*, 2005). Using a dynamic *in vitro* model of the intestinal tract, designated the simulator of the human intestinal microbial ecosystem (SHIME) (Figure 52.6), we further unravelled this process and showed activation of isoxanthohumol mainly occurs in the distal part of the colon, leading up to 80% 8-prenylnaringenin production (Possemiers *et al.*, 2006). And whereas 8-prenylnaringenin was only a minor liver metabolite of IX, the only intestinal metabolism of the latter compound was the activation into 8-prenylnaringenin. Moreover, the definitive role of bacterial enzymes in this process was recently shown by the fact that no 8-prenylnaringenin production was noted in germ-free rats (manuscript submitted). Therefore, we were the first to show that intestinal processes not only determines the activity of isoflavones and lignans, but that this is also valid for this new group of phytoestrogens, the prenylflavonoids.

But we discovered also another interesting parallel with the other groups of phytoestrogens. For isoflavones and lignans it is well known that the extent of bacterial metabolism is highly variable between individuals. It has been observed that only about 30–50% of humans have the intestinal metabolic potential to produce equol (Lampe *et al.*, 1994; Atkinson *et al.*, 2004; Atkinson *et al.*, 2006).

Table 52.4 Overview of bacteria having *O*-demethylation capacity

Strain	*References*
Desulfitobacterium hafniense	Neumann *et al.* (2004)
Sphingomonas paucimobilis	Masai *et al.* (2004)
Pseudomonas putida	Furukawa *et al.* (2003)
Clostridium coccoides	Kamlage *et al.* (1997)
Clostridium formoaceticum	Frank *et al.* (1998)
Acetobacterium dehalogenans	Kaufmann *et al.* (1998)
Thermoanaerobacter kivui	Kevbrina and Pusheva (1996)
Sporomusa ovata	Stupperich *et al.* (1996)
Sporomusa sphaeroides	Muller and Bowien (1995)
Acetobacterium woodii	Muller and Bowien (1995)
Sporomusa paucivorans	Hermann *et al.* (1987)
Butyribacterium methylotrophicum	Kerby and Zeikus (1987)
Clostridium aceticum	Lux and Drake (1992)
Clostridium formicoaceticum	Lux and Drake (1992)
Eubacterium limosum	Hur and Rafii (2000)
Peptostreptococcus productus	Clavel *et al.* (2005)
Eubacterium aggregans	Mechichi *et al.* (1998)
Clostridium methoxybenzovorans	Mechichi *et al.* (2005)
Holophaga foetida	Kreft and Schink (1997)

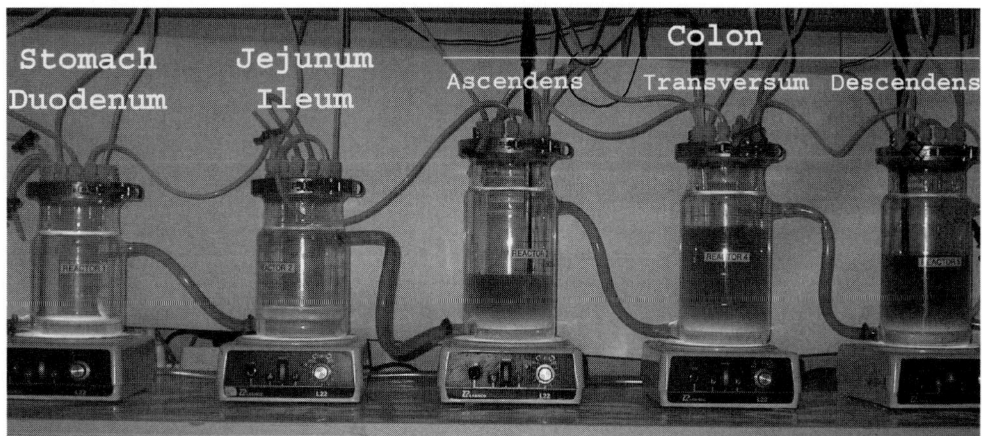

Figure 52.6 Simulator of the human intestinal microbial ecosystem. The SHIME consisting of five reactors which simulate the different parts of the human intestinal tract. The model was developed at the Laboratory of Microbial Ecology and Technology (LabMET), UGent, Belgium.

O-DMA production would occur in 80–90% of the individuals (Kelly *et al.*, 1993). As wide ranges in the production of the mammalian lignans also have been observed (Lampe *et al.*, 1994; Hutchins *et al.*, 2000; Atkinson *et al.*, 2006), interindividual differences in the intestinal bacterial community result in interindividual differences in the exposure to certain phytoestrogen metabolites.

Very similar observations were made for hop phytoestrogens. Only about 35% of *in vitro* tested intestinal microbial communities produced medium or high amounts of 8-prenylnaringenin from isoxanthohumol (Possemiers *et al.*, 2005; Possemiers *et al.*, 2006), separating individuals in high, moderate and low 8-prenylnaringenin producers (Figure 52.7). As clear cut correlations were found between the intestinal potential to activate isoxanthohumol and urinary 8-prenylnaringenin excretion after isoxanthohumol administration *in vivo* (Possemiers *et al.*, 2006), it was shown that differences in the intestinal bacterial community also for hop phytoestrogens result in interindividual differences in the exposure to the active phytoestrogen.

Probiotics to Increase 8-Prenylnaringenin Exposure After Beer Consumption? Because of these marked interindividual differences in the metabolism of and exposure to phytoestrogens, differences in the health outcome of phytoestrogen consumption can also be expected. As this indicates that increased exposure to the active metabolite is favorable, the next question therefore would be: What can we do about it? How can one change the phytoestrogen metabolism status in individuals, making them exposed to increased amounts of the active metabolites? The answer could be simple: by introducing bacteria capable of metabolizing the precursors from food inside the intestine of non-producers, or in other words the use of specific probiotics to increase the intestinal production of bioactive metabolites.

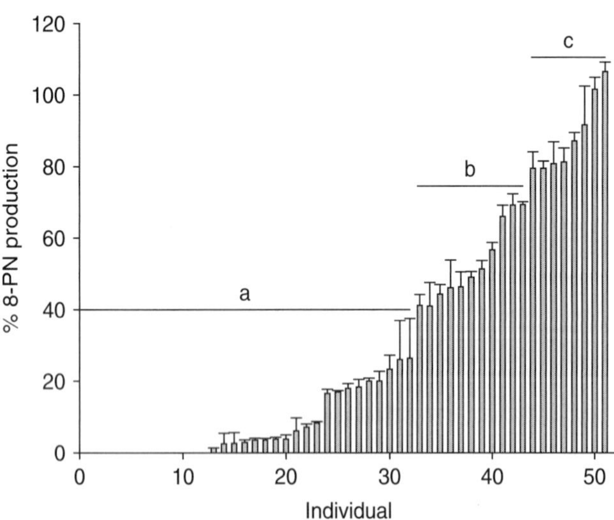

Figure 52.7 Interindividual differences in intestinal production of 8-prenylnaringenin. Interindividual differences in the conversion of isoxanthohumol into 8-prenylnaringenin by intestinal bacteria derived from 51 individuals. Statistical two-step cluster analysis revealed three groups with significantly different means ($p < 0.01$). Individuals were separated in low (a), moderate (b) and high (c) 8-prenylnaringenin producers. *Source*: After Possemiers *et al.* (2006).

A first attempt to apply this strategy to phytoestrogen metabolism has been made in our group by Decroos *et al.* who isolated a consortium capable of equol production (Decroos *et al.*, 2005, 2006). These positive results encouraged us to apply the same strategy for hop phytoestrogens. After screening a number of candidate demethylating bacteria strains (Table 52.4), only one bacterium, *Eubacterium limosum*, was found which could efficiently convert isoxanthohumol into 8-prenylnaringenin after a selection procedure. Administration of the strain to fecal samples increased the 8-prenylnaringenin production in these samples (Possemiers *et al.*, 2005). Last years, this bacterium has gained increasing attention because of its beneficial effects on the colonic environment in inflammatory bowel disease, possibly attributed to its butyrate-producing capacity (Kanauchi *et al.*, 2002, 2005). Therefore, the bacterium would be a suitable candidate probiotic to increase intestinal 8-prenylnaringenin production. Administration of the bacterium to the SHIME and rats increased both butyrate and 8-prenylnaringenin production, confirming this potential application (manuscript submitted).

Estrogenicity of Beers: A New Perspective

Consequences of bioavailability on biological activity

Because of the extremely diverse metabolic potential of the liver, many studies now focus on the influence of liver phase I metabolism toward final biological activity, mainly by using liver microsomes. However, although CYP-mediated metabolism of flavonoids has been shown *in vitro* in liver microsomes, it has never been shown to be important *in vivo* or in intact hepatocytes where conjugative metabolism may be expected to compete with oxidation (Otake *et al.*, 2002; Walle, 2004). This was also observed for 8-prenylnaringenin. Whereas, liver microsome incubations yielded a number of phase I metabolites (Nikolic *et al.*, 2004), 80% of the 8-prenylnaringenin metabolites produced by hepatocytes consisted of the phase II 7-*O*-glucuronide of 8-prenylnaringenin. In view of the exposure to 8-prenylnaringenin after beer consumption, one consequence of this would be that phase I activation only plays a minor role and that mainly isoxanthohumol conjugates can be expected after passage through the liver. This is confirmed by the fact that no 8-prenylnaringenin could be detected after administering isoxanthohumol to germ-free rats.

A second consequence of extensive phase II metabolism is the observation that the oral bioavailability of flavonoid aglycones generally is very low (Liu *et al.*, 2003; Walle *et al.*, 2004). This means that mainly the conjugates circulate through the body and can exert systemic effects. Although glucuronides/sulfates sometimes remain biologically active or even have increased activity (Manach *et al.*, 1998; Fang *et al.*, 2003), conjugation can also decrease the biological activity. However, two remarks should be made. A number of flavonoids might already have effects in the intestine itself, for example protective effects of xanthohumol against colon cancer (Gerhauser *et al.*, 2002), leading to a high biological activity independent of (low) oral bioavailability (Scalbert *et al.*, 2002; Walle *et al.*, 2004). Moreover, many reports now describe that both conjugation and deconjugation can occur in the tissues at cellular level, which may influence the amount of active aglycon in the tissues (Santner *et al.*, 1984; Zhu *et al.*, 1996; Spencer *et al.*, 2004).

A last, and for hops most important, consequence of enterohepatic circulation is that a major fraction of the ingested flavonoids reach the colon where they become substrates for bacterial enzymes. Hop prenylflavonoids were shown to be metabolically stable against colonic degradation, making them good substrates for absorption from the colon or specific metabolic processes, in this case the demethylation of the pro-estrogen isoxanthohumol into the highly potent 8-prenylnaringenin. As our studies showed that the intestinal bacteria are responsible for *in vivo* demethylation of IX, the combination of an extensive liver first-pass effect, a high metabolic stability of prenylflavonoids and a good absorption of 8-prenylnaringenin from the gut create ideal circumstances for efficient intestinal activation of isoxanthohumol and increased exposure to 8-prenylnaringenin after beer consumption.

Beers and estrogens

Estrogen Exposure After Beer Consumption When reviewing the prenylflavonoid composition of beers (Table 52.2) and taking the recent knowledge about isoxanthohumol transformation into account, it is clear that the picture now looks completely different. These recent findings show that the final exposure to the potent phytoestrogen is not only dependent on the original 8-prenylnaringenin concentrations in beers, but also on the amount of isoxanthohumol which is being transformed into 8-prenylnaringenin inside the human colon. As the isoxanthohumol concentrations in beers often are in the range of one to a few mg/l, the amount of isoxanthohumol in beers is generally 10–30 times higher than the 8-prenylnaringenin amounts. If isoxanthohumol is efficiently transformed in the intestine and if 8-prenylnaringenin is well absorbed from the colon, this process could easily 10-fold increase the circulating 8-prenylnaringenin concentrations.

As further studies are needed to investigate the final biological relevance of these findings, one can now only hypothesise about whether or not regular moderate beer consumption could lead to exposure to biologically active 8-prenylnaringenin concentrations. Even when all isoxanthohumol would be converted into 8-prenylnaringenin, the final 8-prenylnaringenin concentrations will still be much below the reported concentrations leading to negative effects in rats, 100 mg/l drinking water (Milligan *et al.*, 1999) or 68 mg/kg body weight (Christoffel *et al.*, 2006; Rimoldi *et al.*, 2006). Conclusions about positive effects of long term exposure to low 8-prenylnaringenin concentrations are even more difficult to make as extrapolation of *in vitro* results is very difficult and no long term studies have been published in which low 8-prenylnaringenin concentrations were dosed. However, some indications of biological activity can be given based on data from hop-based dietary supplements. These supplements generally contain a daily dose of about 100 μg 8-prenylnaringenin (Table 52.2) and claim specific biological effects such as alleviating menopausal discomforts. Although many of these claims lack thorough scientific background (Coldham and Sauer, 2001), a first prospective placebo controlled study was recently published which indicated that a hop supplement, standardized on 100 μg 8-prenylnaringenin/day, exerted favorable effects on vasomotor symptoms and other menopausal discomforts after 6 weeks (Heyerick *et al.*, 2006). However, these supplements also contain 10–20-fold higher isoxanthohumol concentrations. In view of the recent findings, the active 8-prenylnaringenin dose inducing the effect may be higher due to intestinal activation of IX. But nevertheless, if further studies show that these hop supplements really have beneficial health outcome, similar effects might also be expected from moderate beer consumption as the prenylflavonoid composition in beers are similar as in these medicinal products (Table 52.2).

Interindividual Variability One major drawback for positive biological effect of both beers and hop-based supplements, based on *in vivo* activation of the pro-estrogen IX, is the reported interindividual variation in the intestinal potential to produce 8-prenylnaringenin. If this process only efficiently occurs in one-third of humans, this would imply that, after consumption of identical amounts of hop-containing products, some people could be exposed to at least 10-fold higher 8-prenylnaringenin doses because of their intestinal capacity to transform IX. This would then also lead to interindividual differences in biological health effects. The fact that in the previously mentioned study on the effect of hops on menopausal complaints (Heyerick *et al.*, 2006), high variability was found in the response to the product, separating individuals in responders and non-responders, is a further indication of the importance of the (variable) intestinal activation of isoxanthohumol and absorption of 8-prenylnaringenin.

Future Perspectives From the brewers point of view, the valuable constituents of hops are mainly the bitter (alpha) acids and hop oils. Normally, hops are added to the boiling wort as the alpha acids isomerize under these conditions into the bitter isoalpha acids. As the hop oils, providing the hoppy flavor to beer, are evaporated or degraded during wort boiling, "late hopping" (hop dosage at the end of the wort boiling) can be used to increase the hoppy flavor. However, in view of the recent findings on the biological activity of hop prenylflavonoids, it might also be interesting to increase the polyphenol content in beers to create "bioactive beers." Because of the beneficial properties attributed to X, strategies are now being developed to increase the xanthohumol concentrations in beer up to several mg X/l (Wunderlich *et al.*, 2005). But in the same line of thinking it would also be interesting to increase the amounts of isoxanthohumol in beers, which can be activated in the intestine. Diverse extraction methods by ethanol and CO_2 at different pressures lead to residues that contain more than 30% X. Using these X-enriched hop products, several brewing studies led to the production of beers with isoxanthohumol concentrations greater than 8 mg/l (Wunderlich *et al.*, 2005).

However, this would imply the efficient intestinal conversion of isoxanthohumol into 8-prenylnaringenin and this is exactly hampered by interindividual differences in the intestinal transformation potential. Therefore, two extra strategies could be developed to ensure that everybody would be exposed to similar 8-prenylnaringenin concentrations. One could try to increase the 8-prenylnaringenin concentrations in beer by implementing a prefermentation step in the process to convert isoxanthohumol with our selected bacterium into 8-prenylnaringenin in the hop extract or beer intermediate. An alternative would be to create a "probiotic beer" by combining an IX-rich beer with the appropriate bacterium which can activate the isoxanthohumol in the intestine. There is currently already interest toward possible probiotic effects of beer consumption. Some beers still contain living yeast to which probiotic properties are now attributed (Kuhle *et al.*, 2005). Moreover, some beers are produced by lactic acid fermentation, so there might be interest in the exploration of "probiotic healthy beers."

In conclusion, even though these recent findings may have important biological consequences, the final question remains whether beer will ever have a "healthy image" or in other words: Does the average beer consumer like to associate drinking a beer with health effects? A recent survey among menopausal women to investigate a possible market for a beer which would relieve menopausal complaints, learnt that women cannot imagine to buy or order a special "menopause beer" but rather buy pharmaceuticals (personal communication). Therefore, the recent findings about intestinal activation of isoxanthohumol might mainly find its applications among the producers of hop-based dietary supplements and pharmaceuticals.

Summary Points

- Hop is an essential ingredient in beer providing bitterness and taste.
- It contains the most potent phytoestrogen, 8-prenylnaringenin. This compound mimics the activity of the female sex hormone estradiol and may be applied in the relief of menopausal complaints.
- The concentration in beer is too low for eliciting a positive health effect.
- Recent research has shown that another hop compound, isoxanthohumol (IX), can be converted by gut bacteria to the more potent 8-prenylnaringenin.
- This isoxanthohumol is present at much higher concentrations in beer. As it was shown that a large fraction of ingested isoxanthohumol reaches the colon, this process could easily 10-fold increase the 8-prenylnaringenin exposure.
- New strategies are being developed to increase the conversion of isoxanthohumol into 8-prenylnaringenin by means of health-promoting bacteria.
- These recent findings about increased 8-prenylnaringenin exposure can give new insights in the scientific question whether moderate beer consumption can lead to specific health outcomes.

Acknowledgments

The authors would like to thank the Fund for Scientific Research – Flanders (FWO Vlaanderen) for supporting Sam Possemiers during his Ph.D. and Tom Van de Wiele during his postdoctoral work.

References

Appt, S.E., Clarkson, T.B., Lees, C.J. and Anthony, M.S. (2006). *Maturitas* 55, 187–194.

Atkinson, C., Berman, S., Humbert, O. and Lampe, J.W. (2004). *J. Nutr.* 134, 596–599.

Atkinson, C., Frankenfeld, C.L. and Lampe, J.W. (2005). *Exp. Biol. Med.* 230, 155–170.

Atkinson, C., Lampe, J.W., Scholes, D., Chen, C., Wahala, K. and Schwartz, S.M. (2006). *Am. J. Clin. Nutr.* 84, 587–593.

Aura, A.M., O'leary, K.A., Williamson, G., Ojala, M., Bailey, M., Puupponen-Pimia, R., Nuutila, A.M., Oksman-Caldentey, K.M. and Poutanen, K. (2002). *J. Agric. Food Chem.* 50, 1725–1730.

Avellone, G., Di Garbo, V., Campisi, D., De Simone, R., Raneli, G., Scaglione, R. and Licata, G. (2006). *Eur. J. Clin. Nutr.* 60, 41–47.

Avula, B., Ganzera, M., Warnick, J.E., Feltenstein, M.W., Sufka, K.J. and Khan, I.A. (2004). *J. Chromatogr. Sci.* 42, 378–382.

Barron, D. and Ibrahim, R.K. (1996). *Phytochemistry* 43, 921–982.

Behre, K.E. (1999). *Veg. Hist. Archaeobot.* 8, 35–48.

Blair, R.M., Appt, S.E., Franke, A.A. and Clarkson, T.B. (2003). *J. Nutr.* 133, 2262–2267.

Booth, A.N., Murray, C.W., Jones, F.F. and De Eds, F. (1956). *J. Biol. Chem.* 223, 251–260.

Bowey, E., Adlercreutz, H. and Rowland, I. (2003). *Food Chem. Toxicol.* 41, 631–636.

Braune, A., Gutschow, M., Engst, W. and Blaut, M. (2001). *Appl. Environ. Microbiol.* 67, 5558–5567.

Breinholt, V.M., Offord, E.A., Brouwer, C., Nielsen, S.E., Brosen, K. and Friedberg, T. (2002). *Food Chem. Toxicol.* 40, 609–616.

Brune, A. and Schink, B. (1992). *Arch. Microbiol.* 157, 417–424.

Bugianesi, R., Catasta, G., Spigno, P., D'uva, A. and Maiani, G. (2002). *J. Nutr.* 132, 3349–3352.

Burgess, A.H. (1964). Hops: Botany, cultivation, and utilization. Interscience Publishers Inc., New York.

Cermak, R., Breves, G., Lupke, M. and Wolffram, S. (2006). *Arch. Anim. Nutr.* 60, 180–189.

Chadwick, L.R., Nikolic, D., Burdette, J.E., Overk, C.R., Bolton, J.L., Van Breemen, R.B., Frohlich, R., Fong, H.H.S., Farnsworth, N.R. and Pauli, G.F. (2004). *J. Nat. Prod.* 67, 2024–2032.

Chadwick, L.R., Pauli, G.F. and Farnsworth, N.R. (2006). *Phytomedicine* 13, 119–131.

Choi, Y.B., Kim, K.S. and Rhee, J.S. (2002). *Biotechnol. Lett.* 24, 2113–2116.

Christoffel, J., Rimoldi, G. and Wuttke, W. (2006). *J. Endocrinol.* 188, 397–405.

Clavel, T., Henderson, G., Alpert, C.A., Philippe, C., Rigottier-Gois, L., Dore, J. and Blaut, M. (2005). *Appl. Environ. Microbiol.* 71, 6077–6085.

Clavel, T., Henderson, G., Engst, W., Dore, J. and Blaut, M. (2006). *FEMS Microbiol. Ecol.* 55, 471–478.

Cleophas, T.J. (1999). *Biomed. Pharmacother.* 53, 417–423.

Coldham, N.G. and Sauer, M.J. (2001). *Food Chem. Toxicol.* 39, 1211–1224.

Coldham, N.G., Horton, R., Byford, M.F. and Sauer, M.J. (2002). *Food Addit. Contam.* 19, 1138–1147.

Conly, J.M. and Stein, K. (1992). *Am. J. Gastroenterol.* 87, 311–316.

Cummings, J.H. and Englyst, H.N. (1987). *Am. J. Clin. Nutr.* 45, 1243–1255.

Das, S. and Rosazza, J.P.N. (2006). *J. Nat. Prod.* 69, 499–508.

De Boever, P. (2001). *Interaction Between Soy, Bile Salt Hydrolytic Lactobacilli and in vitro Cultured Gut Microbiota. Faculty of Agricultural and Applied Biological Sciences,* RUG, Gent.

De Keukeleire, D. (2003). *Scand. Brewers' Rev.* 60, 10–17.

De Keukeleire, J., Ooms, G., Heyerick, A., Roldan-Ruiz, I., Van Bockstaele, E. and De Keukeleire, D. (2003). *J. Agric. Food Chem.* 51, 4436–4441.

Decroos, K., Vanhemmens, S., Cattoir, S., Boon, N. and Verstraete, W. (2005). *Arch. Microbiol.* 183, 45–55.

Decroos, K., Eeckhaut, E., Possemiers, S. and Verstraete, W. (2006). *J. Nutr.* 136, 946–952.

Di castelnuovo, A., Rotondo, S., Iacoviello, L., Donati, M.B. and De Gaetano, G. (2002). *Circulation* 105, 2836–2844.

Erlund, I. (2004). *Nutr. Res.* 24, 851–874.

Erlund, I., Meririnne, E., Alfthan, G. and Aro, A. (2001). *J. Nutr.* 131, 235–241.

Fang, S.H., Hou, Y.C., Chang, W.C., Hsiu, S.L., Chao, P.D.L. and Chiang, B.L. (2003). *Life Sci.* 74, 743–756.

Felgines, C., Texier, O., Morand, C., Manach, C., Scalbert, A., Regerat, F. and Remesy, C. (2000). *Am. J. Physiol. Gastrointest. Liver Physiol.* 279, G1148–G1154.

Fenselau, C. and Talalay, P. (1973). *Food Cosmetics Toxicol.* 11, 597–603.

Frank, C., Schwarz, U., Matthies, C. and Drake, H.L. (1998). *Arch. Microbiol.* 170, 427–434.

Fund, W.C.R. (1997). Food, nutrition and the prevention of cancer: A global perspective. American Institute of Cancer Research, Washington, DC.

Furukawa, H., Morita, H., Yoshida, T. and Nagasawa, T. (2003). *J. Biosci. Bioeng.* 96, 401–403.

Gao, K., Xu, A.L., Krul, C., Venema, K., Liu, Y., Niu, Y.T., Lu, J.X., Bensoussan, L., Seeram, N.P., Heber, D. and Henning, S.M. (2006). *J. Nutr.* 136, 52–57.

Gardner, D.S. (1993). Commercial scale extraction of alpha-acids and hop oils with compressed CO_2. In King, M.B. and Bott, T.R. (eds), *Extraction of Natural Products Using Near-Critical Solvents.* Blackie Academic and Professional, London.

Gerhauser, C., Alt, A., Heiss, E., Gamal-eldeen, A., Klimo, K., Knauft, J., Neumann, I., Scherf, H.R., Frank, N., Bartsch, H. and Becker, H. (2002). *Mol. Canc. Therapeut.* 1, 959–969.

Giles, T.D. and Sander, G.E. (2005). *Am. J. Geriatr. Cardiol.* 14, 154–158.

Gonthier, M.P., Verny, M.A., Besson, C., Remesy, C. and Scalbert, A. (2003). *J. Nutr.* 133, 1853–1859.

Gott, D.M. and Griffiths, L.A. (1987). *Xenobiotica* 17, 423–434.

Griffiths, L.A. and Barrow, G. (1972). *Biochem. J.* 130, 1161–1162.

Griffiths, L.A. and Smith, G.E. (1972). *Biochem. J.* 128, 901–911.

Guo, J., Nikolic, D., Chadwick, L.R., Pauli, G.F. and Van Breemen, R.B. (2006). *Drug Metabol. Dispos.* 34, 1152–1159.

Hänsel, R. and Schulz, J. (1988). *Arch. Pharmazie* 321, 37–40.

Hermann, M., Popoff, M.R. and Sebald, M. (1987). *Int. J. Syst. Bacteriol.* 37, 93–101.

Heyerick, A., Vervarcke, S., Depypere, H., Bracke, M. and De Keukeleire, D. (2006). *Maturitas* 54, 164–175.

Hopkins, M.J. and Macfarlane, G.T. (2003). *Appl. Environ. Microbiol.* 69, 1920–1927.

Hu, M., Chen, J. and Lin, H.M. (2003a). *J. Pharmacol. Exp. Therapeut.* 307, 314–321.

Hu, M., Krausz, K., Chen, J., Ge, X., Li, J.Q., Gelboin, H.L. and Gonzalez, F.J. (2003b). *Drug Metabol. Dispos.* 31, 924–931.

Hur, H.G. and Rafii, F. (2000). *FEMS Microbiol. Lett.* 192, 21–25.

Hutchins, A.M., Martini, M.C., Olson, B.A., Thomas, W. and Slavin, J.L. (2000). *Canc. Epidemiol. Biomarkers Prev.* 9, 1113–1118.

Ibrahim, A.R.S., Galal, A.M., Ahmed, M.S. and Mossa, G.S. (2003). *Chem. Pharmaceut. Bull.* 51, 203–206.

Ilett, K.F., Tee, L.B.G., Reeves, P.T. and Minchin, R.F. (1990). *Pharmacol. Therapeut.* 46, 67–93.

Jefferson, W.N. and Newbold, R.R. (2000). *Nutrition* 16, 658–662.

Kagawa, H., Takahashi, T., Ohta, S. and Harigaya, Y. (2004). *Xenobiotica* 34, 797–810.

Kamlage, B., Gruhl, B. and Blaut, M. (1997). *Appl. Environ. Microbiol.* 63, 1732–1738.

Kanauchi, O., Suga, T., Tochihara, M., Hibi, T., Naganuma, M., Homma, T., Asakura, H., Nakano, H., Takahama, K., Fujiyama, Y., Andoh, A., Shimoyama, T., Hida, N., Haruma, K., Koga, H., Mitsuyama, K., Sata, M., Fukuda, M., Kojima, A. and Bamba, T. (2002). *J. Gastroenterol.* 37, 67–72.

Kanauchi, O., Matsumoto, Y., Matsumura, M., Fukuoka, M. and Bamba, T. (2005). *Curr. Pharmaceut. Des.* 11, 1047–1053.

Kaufmann, F., Wohlfarth, G. and Diekert, G. (1998). *Eur. J. Biochem.* 257, 515–521.

Kelly, G.E., Nelson, C., Waring, M.A., Joannou, G.E. and Reeder, A.Y. (1993). *Clin. Chim. Acta* 223, 9–22.

Kenny, A.M., Kleppinger, A., Wang, Y. and Prestwood, K.M. (2005). *J. Am. Geriatr. Soc.* 53, 1973–1977.

Kerby, R. and Zeikus, J.G. (1987). *J. Bacteriol.* 169, 5605–5609.

Kevbrina, M.V. and Pusheva, M.A. (1996). *Microbiology* 65, 10–14.

Klatsky, A.L., Armstrong, M.A. and Friedman, G.D. (1997). *Am. J. Cardiol.* 80, 416–420.

Koch, W. and Heim, G. (1953). *Munch. Med. Wochenschr.* 95, 845.

Kohri, T., Matsumoto, N., Yamakawa, M., Suzuki, M., Nanjo, F., Hara, Y. and Oku, N. (2001). *J. Agric. Food Chem.* 49, 4102–4112.

Kondo, K. (2004). *Biofactors* 22, 303–310.

Kopp, P. (1998). *Eur. J. Endocrinol.* 138, 619–620.

Kreft, J.U. and Schink, B. (1997). *Arch. Microbiol.* 167, 363–368.

Krumholz, L.R. and Bryant, M.P. (1986). *Arch. Microbiol.* 144, 8–14.

Kuhle, A., Skovgaard, K. and Jespersen, L. (2005). *Int. J. Food Microbiol.* 101, 29–39.

Kuijsten, A., Arts, I.C.W., Hollman, P.C.H., Van't Veer, P. and Kampman, E. (2006). *Canc. Epidemiol. Biomarkers Prev.* 15, 1132–1136.

Lampe, J.W., Martini, M.C., Kurzer, M.S., Adlercreutz, H. and Slavin, J.L. (1994). *Am. J. Clin. Nutr.* 60, 122–128.

Lania-Pietrzak, B., Hendrich, A.B., Zugaj, J. and Michalak, K. (2005). *Arch. Biochem. Biophys.* 433, 428–434.

Liggins, J., Grimwood, R. and Bingham, S.A. (2000). *Anal. Biochem.* 287, 102–109.

Lin, Y.T., Hsiu, S.L., Hou, Y.C., Chen, H.Y. and Chao, P.D.L. (2003). *Biol. Pharmaceut. Bull.* 26, 747–751.

Liu, Y., Liu, Y., Dai, Y., Xun, L.Y. and Hu, M. (2003). *J. Alternative Compl. Med.* 9, 631–640.

Lund, T.D., Munson, D.J., Haldy, M.E., Setchell, K.D.R., Lephart, E.D. and Handa, R.J. (2004). *Biol. Reprod.* 70, 1188–1195.

Lux, M.F. and Drake, H.L. (1992). *FEMS Microbiol. Lett.* 95, 49–56.

Macdonald, I.A., Mader, J.A. and Bussard, R.G. (1983). *Mutat. Res.* 122, 95–102.

Macfarlane, G.T. and Macfarlane, S. (1997). *Scand. J. Gastroenterol.* 32, 3–9.

Magalhaes, P.J., Guido, L.F., Cruz, J.M. and Barros, A.A. (2007). *J. Chromatogr. A* 1150, 295–301.

Manach, C., Morand, C., Crespy, V., Demigne, C., Texier, O., Regerat, F. and Remesy, C. (1998). *FEBS Lett.* 426, 331–336.

Marrian, G.F. and Haslewood, G.A.D. (1932). *Biochem. J.* 26, 1227–1232.

Masai, E., Sasaki, M., Minakawa, Y., Abe, T., Sonoki, T., Miyauchi, K., Katayama, Y. and Fukuda, M. (2004). *J. Bacteriol.* 186, 2757–2765.

Matsumura, A., Ghosh, A., Pope, G.S. and Darbre, P.D. (2005). *J. Steroid Biochem. Mol. Biol.* 94, 431–443.

Mccann, M.J., Gill, C.I.R., Mcglynn, H. and Rowland, I.R. (2005). *Nutr. Canc. Int. J.* 52, 1–14.

Mechichi, T., Labat, M., Woo, T.H.S., Thomas, P., Garcia, J.L. and Patel, B.K.C. (1998). *Anaerobe* 4, 283–291.

Mechichi, T., Patel, B.K.C. and Sayadi, S. (2005). *Int. Biodet. Biodeg.* 56, 224–230.

Messina, M., Kucuk, O. and Lampe, J.W. (2006). *J. AOAC Int.* 89, 1121–1134.

Milder, I.E.J., Feskens, E.J.M., Arts, I.C.W., De Mesquita, H.B.B., Hollman, P.C.H. and Kromhout, D. (2005). *J. Nutr.* 135, 1202–1207.

Milligan, S., Kalita, J., Pocock, V., Heyerick, A., De Cooman, L., Rong, H. and De Keukeleire, D. (2002). *Reproduction* 123, 235–242.

Milligan, S.R., Kalita, J.C., Heyerick, A., Rong, H., De Cooman, L. and De Keukeleire, D. (1999). *J. Clin. Endocrinol. Metabol.* 84, 2249–2252.

Muller, V. and Bowien, S. (1995). *Arch. Microbiol.* 164, 363–369.

Muthyala, R.S., Ju, Y.H., Sheng, S.B., Williams, L.D., Doerge, D.R., Katzenellenbogen, B.S., Helferich, W.G. and Katzenellenbogen, J.A. (2004). *Bioorg. Med. Chem.* 12, 1559–1567.

Neumann, A., Engelmann, T., Schmitz, R., Greiser, Y., Orthaus, A. and Diekert, G. (2004). *Arch. Microbiol.* 181, 245–249.

Neve, R.A. (1991). Hops. Chapman and Hall, New York.

Nielsen, S.E., Breinholt, V., Justesen, U., Cornett, C. and Dragsted, L.O. (1998). *Xenobiotica* 28, 389–401.

Nikolic, D., Li, Y.M., Chadwick, L.R., Grubjesic, S., Schwab, P., Metz, P. and Van Breemen, R.B. (2004). *Drug Metabol. Dispos.* 32, 272–279.

Nikolic, D., Li, Y., Chadwick, L.R., Pauli, G.F. and Van Breemen, R.B. (2005). *J. Mass Spectrom.* 40, 289–299.

Nikolic, D., Li, Y.M., Chadwick, L.R. and Van Breemen, R.B. (2006). *Pharmaceut. Res.* 23, 864–872.

Nookandeh, A., Frank, N., Steiner, F., Ellinger, R., Schneider, B., Gerhauser, C. and Becker, H. (2004). *Phytochemistry* 65, 561–570.

Nozawa, H., Nakao, W., Takata, J., Arimoto-Kobayashi, S. and Kondo, K. (2006). *Cancer Lett.* 235, 121–129.

Otake, Y., Hsieh, F. and Walle, T. (2002). *Drug Metabol. Dispos.* 30, 576–581.

Overk, C.R., Yao, P., Chadwick, L.R., Nikolic, D., Sun, Y.K., Cuendet, M.A., Deng, Y.F., Hedayat, A.S., Pauli, G.F., Farnsworth, N.R., Van Breemen, R.B. and Bolton, J.L. (2005). *J. Agric. Food Chem.* 53, 6246–6253.

Peeyananjarassri, K. and Baber, R. (2005). *Climacteric* 8, 13–23.

Pike, A.C.W., Brzozowski, A.M., Hubbard, R.E., Bonn, T., Thorsell, A.G., Engstrom, O., Ljunggren, J., Gustafsson, J.K. and Carlquist, M. (1999). *EMBO J.* 18, 4608–4618.

Possemiers, S., Heyerick, A., Robbens, V., De Keukeleire, D. and Verstraete, W. (2005). *J. Agric. Food Chem.* 53, 6281–6288.

Possemiers, S., Bolca, S., Grootaert, C., Heyerick, A., Decroos, K., Dhooge, W., De Keukeleire, D., Rabot, S., Verstraete, W. and Van De Wiele, T. (2006). *J. Nutr.* 136, 1862–1867.

Prestwood, K.M., Kenny, A.M., Kleppinger, A. and Kulldorff, M. (2003). *JAMA* 290, 1042–1048.

Rad, M., Humpel, M., Schaefer, O., Schoemaker, R.C., Schleuning, W.D., Cohen, A.F. and Burggraaf, J. (2006). *Br. J. Clin. Pharmacol.* 62, 288–296.

Raffaelli, B., Hoikkala, A., Leppala, E. and Wahala, K. (2002). *J. Chromatogr. B Anal. Technol. Biomed. Life Sci.* 777, 29–43.

Rasier, G., Toppari, J., Parent, A.S. and Bourguignon, J.P. (2006). *Mol. Cell. Endocrinol.* 254, 187–201.

Rechner, A.R., Smith, M.A., Kuhnle, G., Gibson, G.R., Debnam, E.S., Srai, S.K.S., Moore, K.P. and Rice-Evans, C.A. (2004). *Free Radic. Biol. Med.* 36, 212–225.

Rimoldi, G., Christoffel, J. and Wuttke, W. (2006). *Menopause J. North Am. Menopause Soc.* 13, 669–677.

Rong, H., Zhao, Y., Lazou, K., De Keukeleire, D., Milligan, S.R. and Sandra, P. (2000). *Chromatographia* 51, 545–552.

Ross, R.P., Morgan, S. and Hill, C. (2002). *Int. J. Food Microbiol.* 79, 3–16.

Rowland, I., Wiseman, H., Sanders, T., Adlercreutz, H. and Bowey, E. (1999). *Biochem. Soc. Trans.* 27, 304–308.

Rowland, I., Faughnan, M., Hoey, L., Wahala, K., Williamson, G. and Cassidy, A. (2003). *Br. J. Nutr.* 89, S45–S58.

Saarinen, N.M., Power, K., Chen, J.M. and Thompson, L.U. (2006). *Int. J. Canc.* 119, 925–931.

Salminen, S., Bouley, C., Boutron-Ruault, M.C., Cummings, J.H., Franck, A., Gibson, G.R., Isolauri, E., Moreau, M.C., Roberfroid, M. and Rowland, I. (1998). *Br. J. Nutr.* 80, S147–S171.

Sanchez-Gonzalez, M. and Rosazza, J.P.N. (2004). *J. Nat. Prod.* 67, 553–558.

Santner, S.J., Feil, P.D. and Santen, R.J. (1984). *J. Clin. Endocrinol. Metabol.* 59, 29–33.

Scalbert, A., Morand, C., Manach, C. and Remesy, C. (2002). *Biomed. Pharmacother.* 56, 276–282.

Schaefer, O., Humpel, M., Fritzemeier, K.H., Bohlmann, R. and Schleuning, W.D. (2003). *J. Steroid Biochem. Mol. Biol.* 84, 359–360.

Schaefer, O., Bohlmann, R., Schleuning, W.-D., Schulze-Forster, K. and Humpel, M. (2005). *J. Agric. Food Chem.* 53, 2881–2889.

Schoefer, L., Mohan, R., Braune, A., Birringer, M. and Blaut, M. (2002). *FEMS Microbiol. Lett.* 208, 197–202.

Setchell, K.D.R., Lawson, A.M., Borriello, S.P., Harkness, R., Gordon, H., Morgan, D.M.L., Kirk, D.N., Adlercreutz, H., Anderson, L.C. and Axelson, M. (1981a). *Lancet* 2, 4–7.

Setchell, K.D.R., Lawson, A.M., Conway, E., Taylor, N.F., Kirk, D.N., Cooley, G., Farrant, R.D., Wynn, S. and Axelson, M. (1981b). *Biochem. J.* 197, 447–458.

Simons, A.L., Renouf, M., Hendrich, S. and Murphy, P.A. (2005). *J. Agric. Food Chem.* 53, 4258–4263.

Spencer, J.P.E., El Mohsen, M.M.A. and Rice-Evans, C. (2004). *Arch. Biochem. Biophys.* 423, 148–161.

Stevens, J.F. and Page, J.E. (2004). *Phytochemistry* 65, 1317–1330.

Stevens, J.F., Ivancic, M., Hsu, V.L. and Deinzer, M.L. (1997). *Phytochemistry* 44, 1575–1585.

Stevens, J.F., Taylor, A.W., Clawson, J.E. and Deinzer, M.L. (1999a). *J. Agric. Food Chem.* 47, 2421–2428.

Stevens, J.F., Taylor, A.W. and Deinzer, M.L. (1999b). *J. Chromatogr. A* 832, 97–107.

Stupperich, E., Konle, R. and Eckerskorn, C. (1996). *Biochem. Biophys. Res. Commun.* 223, 770–777.

Tekel, J., De Keukeleire, D., Rong, H.J., Daeseleire, E. and Van Peteghem, C. (1999). *J. Agric. Food Chem.* 47, 5059–5063.

Tsangalis, D., Ashton, J.F., Mcgill, A.E.J. and Shah, N.P. (2002). *J. Food Sci.* 67, 3104–3113.

Turner, N.J., Thomson, B.M. and Shaw, I.C. (2003). *Nutr. Rev.* 61, 204–213.

Turner, R., Baron, T., Wolffram, S., Minihane, A.M., Cassidy, A., Rimbach, G. and Weinberg, P.D. (2004). *Free Radic. Res.* 38, 209–216.

Verzele, M. (1986). *J. Inst. Brew.* 92, 32–48.

Verzele, M., Stockx, J., Fontijn, F. and Antheunis, M. (1957). *Bulletin des Sociétés des Chimiques Belges* 66, 452–475.

Walle, T. (2004). *Free Radic. Biol. Med.* 36, 829–837.

Walle, T., Hsieh, F., Delegge, M.H., Oatis, J.E. and Walle, U.K. (2004). *Drug Metabol. Dispos.* 32, 1377–1382.

Wang, M.J., Chao, P.D.L., Hou, Y.C., Hsiu, S.L., Wen, K.C. and Tsai, S.Y. (2006). *J. Food Drug Anal.* 14, 247–253.

Wen, X. and Walle, T. (2006). *Drug Metabol. Dispos.* 34, 1786–1792.

Whitman, W.B., Coleman, D.C. and Wiebe, W.J. (1998). *Proc. Nat. Acad. Sci., USA* 95, 6578–6583.

Wunderlich, S., Zurcher, A. and Back, W. (2005). *Mol. Nutr. Food Res.* 49, 874–881.

Yilmazer, M., Stevens, J.F., Deinzer, M.L. and Buhler, D.R. (2001). *Drug Metabol. Dispos.* 29, 223–231.

Zeleniuch-Jacquotte, A., Lundin, E., Micheli, A., Koenig, K.L., Lenner, P., Muti, P., Shore, R.E., Johansson, I., Krogh, V., Lukanova, A., Stattin, P., Afanasyeva, Y., Rinaldi, S., Arslan, A.A., Kaaks, R., Berrino, F., Hallmans, G., Toniolo, P. and Adlercreutz, H. (2006). *Int. J. Canc.* 119, 2376–2381.

Zhu, B.T., Evaristus, E.N., Antoniak, S.K., Sarabia, S.F., Ricci, M.J. and Liehr, J.G. (1996). *Toxicol. Appl. Pharmacol.* 136, 186–193.

Zierau, O., Hamann, J., Tischer, S., Schwab, P., Metz, P., Vollmer, G., Gutzeit, H.O. and Scholz, S. (2005). *Biochem. Biophys. Res. Commun.* 326, 909–916.

53

Effects of Beer Ingestion on Body Purine Bases

Yuji Moriwaki and Tetsuya Yamamoto Division of Endocrinology and Metabolism, Department of Internal Medicine, Hyogo College of Medicine, Nishinomiya, Japan

Abstract

Increased adenosine triphosphate (ATP) degradation and diminished uric acid elimination are considered to be the major causes of alcohol-induced hyperuricemia. In addition, the ingestion of beer, which contains considerable amounts of various purines that might augment the hyperuricemic effect of alcohol, may lead to a greater increase in the plasma concentration of uric acid than other alcoholic beverages. A clinical study of the effects of beer drinking on plasma concentration and urinary excretion of oxypurine (hypoxanthine and xanthine, precursors of uric acid) clearly showed that increased ATP degradation followed beer ingestion. However, freeze-dried beer, which contains no alcohol, and low-malt beer also increased the plasma concentration of uric acid, while purine-free low-malt beer did not, which clearly indicated that the purines present in beer cause an increase in the plasma concentration of uric acid. Further, epidemiological studies and experiments regarding the effects of long-term beer drinking have shown that beer has a deleterious effect on serum uric acid concentration. Therefore, patients with gout should be encouraged to refrain from drinking large amounts of beer regularly.

Introduction

Alcohol consumption increases adenosine triphosphate (ATP) degradation in the liver, leading to an increased production of uric acid (Faller and Fox, 1982; Yamamoto *et al.*, 1995; Nishioka *et al.*, 2002; Yamamoto *et al.*, 2002), while large amounts of alcohol increases the blood concentration of lactic acid, which inhibits uric acid excretion by the kidneys (Lieber, 1965). These two mechanisms, uric acid overproduction and uric acid under excretion, are considered to be the major contributors to alcohol-induced hyper uricemia. In addition, fermented drinks are considered to augment the hyperuricemic effect of alcohol and increase the risk of gout, since they contain greater concentrations of purines than distilled drinks (Gibson *et al.*, 1984). Among alcoholic beverages, beer contains considerably greater amounts of various purines, including guanosine, adenosine, xanthine, and guanine (Yamamoto *et al.*, 2002). Although findings of a case-control study suggested that the high purine content in beer might play an important role in the risk of gout by augmenting the hyperuricemic effect of alcohol (Gibson *et al.*, 1983), definitive data have become available only recently. According to recent studies, beer seems to affect the concentrations of body purine bases to a greater degree than other alcoholic beverages.

Little is known regarding the effects of beer drinking on the plasma concentration and urinary excretion of purine bases other than uric acid, though there are several studies on the effect of beer on plasma uric acid (Eastmond *et al.*, 1995; Nishioka *et al.*, 2002; Yamamoto *et al.*, 2002). In the present review, the effects of beer drinking on the plasma concentration and urinary excretion of oxypurine (hypoxanthine and xanthine), as well as those of uric acid, are described. However, before discussing the effects of beer drinking on body purine bases, it is important to separately examine the effects of alcohol and purines present in beer.

Effects of Alcohol on Body Purine Bases

Lieber administered alcohol to non-gouty heavy drinkers and found an increase in blood lactic acid and uric acid levels, along with a concomitant decrease in urinary uric acid excretion. From those results, he proposed that lactic acid formed during the metabolism of alcohol interfered with the urinary excretion of uric acid, leading to increased plasma levels of uric acid (Lieber, 1965).

Thereafter, Puig and Fox proposed that alcohol-enhanced abrupt ATP consumption was also involved in increased levels of plasma purine bases as a mechanism of alcohol-induced hyperuricemia (Puig and Fox, 1984), as they had earlier found increases in both plasma oxypurine levels and urinary oxypurine excretion after the administration of acetate (Faller and Fox, 1982). During the conversion of acetate to acetyl-CoA, ATP is dephosphorylated to adenosine monophosphate (AMP) and, since ATP is converted

Beer in Health and Disease Prevention
ISBN: 978-0-12-373891-2

to AMP in this pathway, 2 mol of high-energy phosphate is consumed for each mole of alcohol metabolized. Although most of the AMP formed is re-synthesized to ATP, a small part of AMP may enter the pathway of adenine nucleotide degradation, leading to uric acid production.

Later, it was shown that acetaldehyde decreased ATP, while it increased AMP, adenosine diphosphate (ADP), glyceraldehyde 3-phosphate + dihydroxyacetone phosphate, and hypoxanthine levels in erythrocytes (Yamamoto *et al.*, 1995). Further, the addition of pyruvate to erythrocyte incubation medium prevented the acetaldehyde-induced changes described above, indicating that pyruvate was converted to lactic acid by lactic dehydrogenase together with the conversion of nicotinamide adenine dinucleotide reduced form (NADH) to nicotinamide adenine dinucleotide (NAD) in erythrocytes (Yamamoto *et al.*, 1993). These results suggest that the conversion of NAD to NADH plays an important role in glycolysis and glycolytic ATP production. Since acetaldehyde is metabolized to acetate, coupled with the conversion of NAD to NADH in erythrocytes, it is strongly suggested that inhibition of the reduction in redox potentials of nicotinamide adenine nucleotides by pyruvate prevents acetaldehyde-induced inhibition of glycolysis, glycolytic ATP production, and adenine nucleotide degradation. In fact, after consuming alcohol, the concentrations of AMP, ADP, and glyceraldehyde 3-phosphate + dihydroxyacetone phosphate in erythrocytes increase and that of pyruvic acid in blood decreases significantly, with a concomitant increase in the plasma concentration and urinary excretion of oxypurine in healthy subjects (Yamamoto *et al.*, 1993), suggesting that acetaldehyde-induced adenine nucleotide degradation in erythrocytes may contribute to the increase in plasma concentration of oxypurine caused by alcohol. Therefore, it is also considered that glycolysis inhibition reduces glycolytic ATP synthesis, while a decrease in the concentration of inorganic phosphate in the cytosol enhances adenine nucleotide degradation.

In addition, purines present in beer contribute to increases in plasma concentration and urinary excretion of purine bases. Therefore, in the following section, the effects of beer on body purine bases are discussed from the viewpoint of purines present in beer, since the effects of alcohol on body purine bases are commonly observed with the consumption of all alcoholic beverages.

Effects of Purines in Beer on Body Purine Bases

Effects of short-term beer drinking on body purine bases

In a previous study (Gibson *et al.*, 1983), patients with gout were found to drink greater amounts of alcoholic beverages than control subjects. Although the daily intake of most nutrients, including total purine nitrogen, was similar, 41% of the subjects with gout consumed more than 60 g of alcohol daily. Further, it was demonstrated that the intake of purine nitrogen, half of which was derived from beer, was higher in those with gout who consumed more than 60 g of alcohol daily. From those results, it was suggested that the effects of ingested purines, half of which were derived from beer, had a clinical effect on serum uric acid, augmenting the hyperuricemic effect of alcohol. They also demonstrated that consumption of beer containing 53 g of ethanol and 70.6 mg of purine nitrogen over 4 h increased the plasma concentration of uric acid, though an equal volume of artificial fruit juice sweetened with glucose did not, suggesting that both the purines and alcohol in beer contributed to the increases in plasma concentration and urinary excretion of uric acid (Gibson *et al.*, 1984). In addition, the same study group suggested that the relatively large amounts of guanosine present in beer may be more quickly reabsorbed and rapidly converted to uric acid in humans, since guanosine is more readily absorbed than other nucleosides, nucleotides, or bases in animals (Gibson *et al.*, 1983). In another study, it was demonstrated that beer (0.8 ml ethanol equivalent/kg body weight) increased the serum concentration of uric acid by 13.6%, while whisky or Japanese distilled liquor (0.8 ml ethanol equivalent/kg body weight), which contains very low levels of purines, did not affect the serum concentration of uric acid (Nishioka *et al.*, 2002). Together, these results strongly suggest that the effects of purines present in beer on plasma uric acid levels are not negligible. Consequently, regular beer is considered to have a deleterious effect on uric acid metabolism and patients with gout are recommended to severely regulate their consumption.

Studies on the effects of beer on plasma concentration and urinary excretion of purine bases (hypoxanthine, xanthine, and uric acid) are scarce. However, one study demonstrated that regular beer (10 ml/kg body weight) significantly increased the plasma concentrations of hypoxanthine and xanthine by 3.5- and 4.7-fold, respectively, 30 min after ingestion, and increased the urinary excretion of hypoxanthine and xanthine by 4.0- and 4.5-fold, respectively, when measured 1 h after ingestion (Figures 53.1 and 53.2).

Further, in those subjects the plasma concentration of uric acid increased by 6.5% at 30 min, 9.6% at 60 min, and 4.2% at 90 min after ingestion. On the other hand, the urinary excretion of uric acid was not changed throughout the experimental period (Yamamoto *et al.*, 2002) (Figures 53.3 and 53.4).

Low-alcohol and alcohol-free beer are becoming popular, and various kinds of non-alcoholic beer from various countries are available to consumers, however, there has been no detailed study regarding the effects of non-alcoholic beer on the plasma concentration and urinary excretion of purine bases. It was previously demonstrated that ingestion of regular beer (10 ml/kg body weight) by healthy male subjects increased the plasma concentration of uric acid

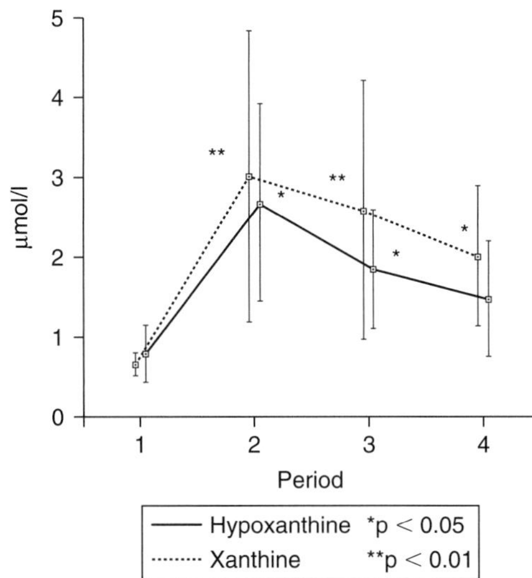

Figure 53.1 Changes in plasma concentrations of hypoxanthine and xanthine after ingestion of regular beer.

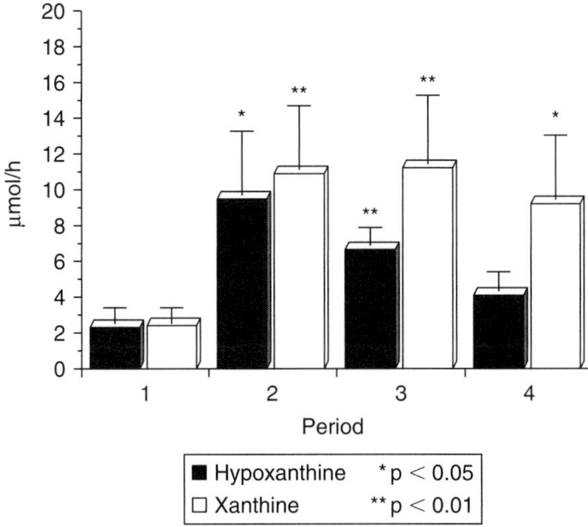

Figure 53.2 Changes in urinary excretion of hypoxanthine and xanthine after ingestion of regular beer.

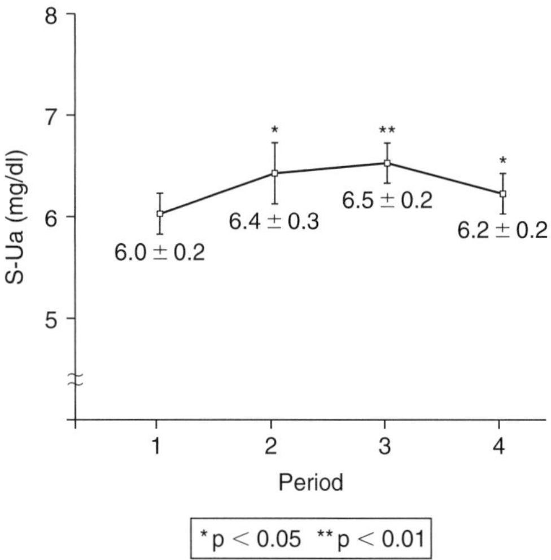

Figure 53.3 Changes in plasma concentrations of uric acid after ingestion of regular beer.

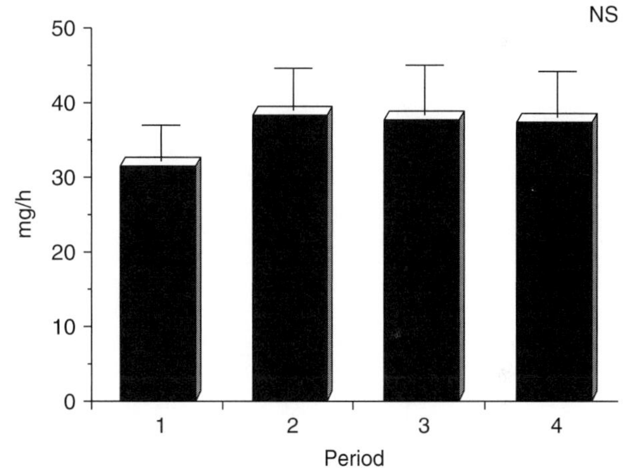

Figure 53.4 Changes in urinary excretion of uric acid after ingestion of regular beer. Regular beer did not have an effect.

by approximately 0.50 mg/dl, while freeze-dried beer (0.34 g/kg body weight), which contained no alcohol, also increased that by approximately 0.34 mg/dl (Yamamoto *et al.*, 2002) (Figure 53.5).

Since 10 ml of regular beer contains 0.34 g of content when freeze-dried, the amount of purines in freeze-dried beer is the same as in regular beer. However, freeze-dried beer did not have an effect on the plasma concentrations and urinary excretion of hypoxanthine and xanthine, suggesting that the purines were converted to uric acid via hypoxanthine and xanthine in the liver and small intestine with the absence of alcohol in the freeze-dried beer (Yamamoto *et al.*, 2002) (Figures 53.6 and 53.7).

In another study, the effect of alcohol-free beer (1.5 l) on uric acid metabolism was studied in four gout patients, and

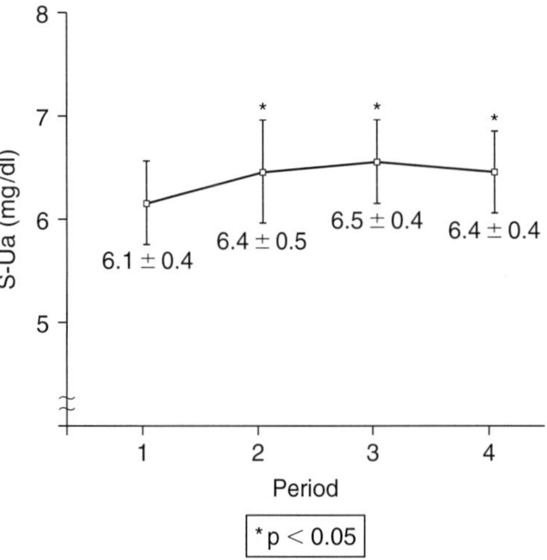

Figure 53.5 Effects of non-alcoholic (freeze-dried) beer on the plasma concentration of uric acid.

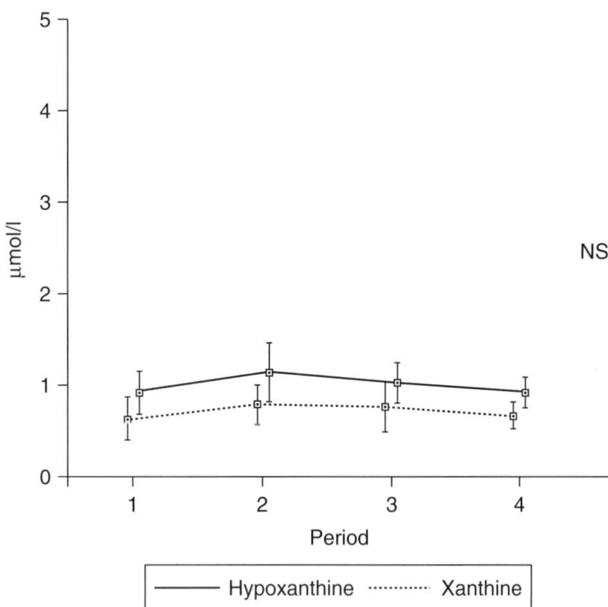

Figure 53.6 Effects of non-alcoholic (freeze-dried) beer on the plasma concentrations of hypoxanthine and xanthine.

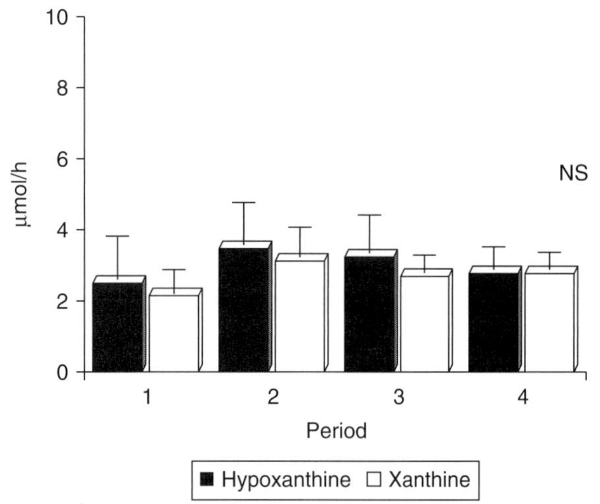

Figure 53.7 Effects of non-alcoholic (freeze-dried) beer on the urinary excretion of hypoxanthine and xanthine.

the results showed that there was no increase in the plasma concentration of uric acid (Eastmond *et al.*, 1995). However, the discrepancies between those findings remain unclear.

Beer contains isohumulones, bittering agents derived from hops, which may also have some unknown effects on body purine bases. Since favorable effects of isohumulones on lipid metabolism have been reported, further studies of their effects on purine metabolism are required.

In light of the hyperuricemic effect of purines in beer, low-malt beer (*happo-shu*) and purine-free *happo-shu* have been recently developed in Japan. The former contains a lower amount of malt and a considerable amount of purines, while the latter contains the same lower amount of malt and a very low level of purines (Yamamoto *et al.*, 2004).

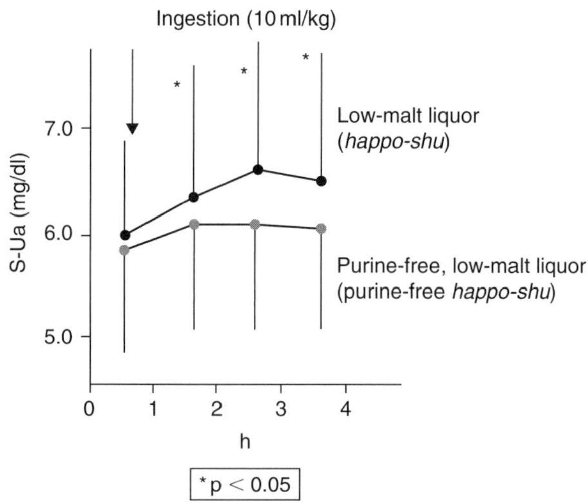

Figure 53.8 Effects of regular and purine-free *happo-shu* (low-malt beer) on the plasma concentration of uric acid.

Ingestion of regular *happo-shu* (10 ml/kg body weight) increased the plasma concentration of uric acid, while that of purine-free *happo-shu* did not, which clearly indicates that the purines present in the former caused an increase in the plasma concentration of uric acid (Figure 53.8).

That study also demonstrated the effects of purines in regular *happo-shu* on the plasma concentration and urinary excretion of oxypurine. The urinary excretion of hypoxanthine and xanthine increased after drinking regular *happo-shu*, as did the plasma concentration of xanthine, as compared with purine-free *happo-shu*, whereas the plasma concentration of hypoxanthine with regular *happo-shu* was not significantly different from that following drinking of purine-free *happo-shu*. These results indicate that purines in regular *happo-shu* increase the production of oxypurine (Figures 53.9 and 53.10).

The plasma concentrations of uric acid and oxypurine may increase as blood alcohol level increases (6.5–10 mmol/l). Therefore, purine-free *happo-shu* seems to be better than beer in regards to its effect on plasma uric acid only within a range of 6.5–10 mmol/l of blood alcohol, since an increase in the ingested volume of purine-free *happo-shu* raises the plasma concentration of uric acid.

Both alcohol-free beer and purine-free *happo-shu* have deleterious effects on uric acid metabolism, though to a lesser degree than regular beer. Therefore, even when ingesting non-alcohol beer or purine-free *happo-shu*, consumption of a large amount of these beverages as an alternative to regular beer should be avoided by gout patients.

Effects of long-term beer drinking on body purine bases

Present knowledge of beer-induced hyperuricemia is mainly based on data obtained from a variety of short-term experiments, and it remains unclear whether long-term beer

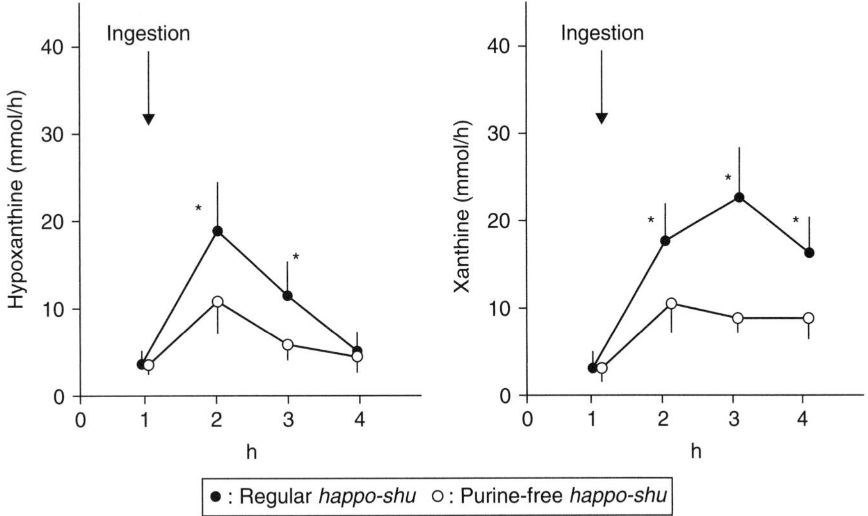

Figure 53.9 Effects of regular and purine-free *happo-shu* (low-malt beer) on the urinary excretion of hypoxanthine and xanthine.

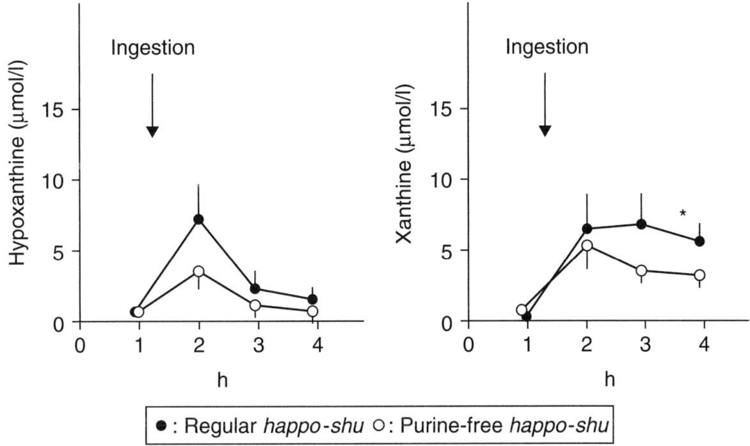

Figure 53.10 Effects of regular and purine-free *happo-shu* (low-malt beer) on the plasma concentrations of hypoxanthine and xanthine.

drinking has the same effect on uric acid that has been found in short-term studies. It is considered important to investigate the effect of long-term moderate beer drinking on the increase of uric acid concentration in plasma, since such an increase may induce a gouty attack in patients with pre-existing hyperuricemia. According to Ka *et al.*, who studied the effects of long-term moderate beer drinking on the plasma concentrations and urinary excretion of purine bases, daily consumption of 15 ml/kg body weight of beer for 3 months significantly increased the plasma concentration and urinary excretion of uric acid, as compared with the values before starting the experiment (Ka *et al.*, 2005).

In contrast, uric acid and creatinine clearance remained unchanged throughout the study. Accordingly, it was suggested that the enhanced adenine nucleotide degradation induced by beer plays a role in the increases in plasma concentration and urinary excretion of uric acid. In addition, when the subjects were divided into two groups, those who did not regularly drink more than 15 ml/kg body weight of beer and those who regularly drank more than 15 ml/kg body weight daily, the plasma concentration and urinary excretion of uric acid were significantly increased only in the latter group (Figures 53.11 and 53.12).

However, values for the 24-h urinary excretion of oxypurines and plasma concentration of oxypurines were not increased during the 3-month-experimental period, suggesting that the effects of long-term moderate beer drinking on the plasma concentrations and urinary excretion of oxypurines are limited, and have a short duration. These results indicate that the production of uric acid caused by beer drinking is a significant contributor to the increase in plasma uric acid concentration in subjects who regularly drink more than 15 ml/kg body weight of beer daily. Therefore, patients with gout should be encouraged to refrain from drinking large amounts of beer on a daily basis.

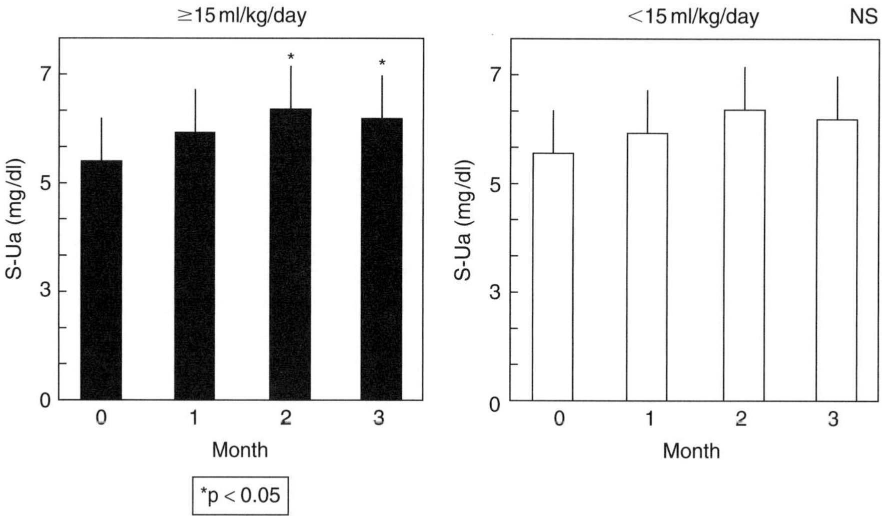

Figure 53.11 Effects of long-term beer drinking (3 months) on the plasma concentration of uric acid according to drinking habits.

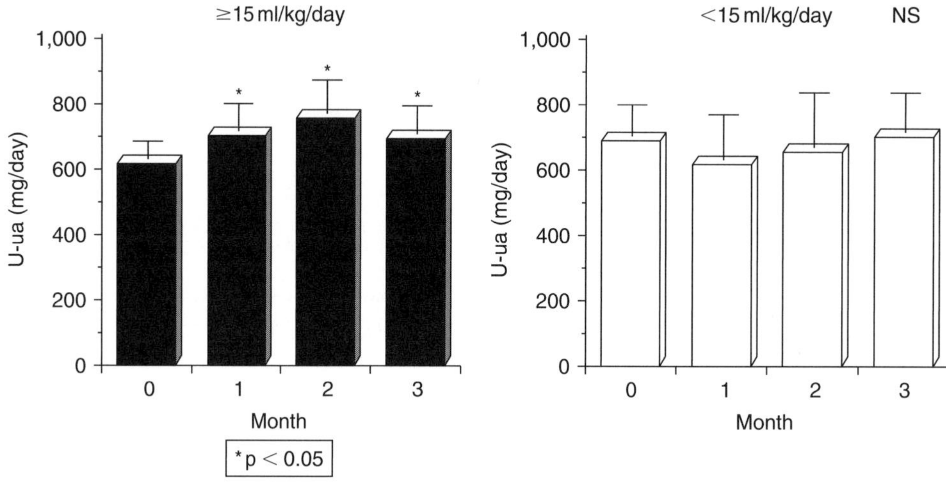

Figure 53.12 Effects of long-term beer drinking (3 months) on the urinary excretion of uric acid according to drinking habits.

Epidemiological studies of the effect of beer drinking on serum uric acid

Using data from a retirement health examination of 2,487 male Japan Self Defence Force officials, it was demonstrated that among four different types of alcoholic beverages (beer, shochu, sake, and whisky) only beer consumption was significantly associated with an elevated level of serum uric acid (Kono *et al.*, 1994). On the contrary, results of a cross-sectional study of Japanese male office workers suggested that the increased risk of alcohol-induced hyperuricemia did not vary according to the type of alcoholic beverage consumed (Sugie *et al.*, 2005).

Recently, a retrospective study using data from 14,809 participants over the age of 20 in The Third National Health and Nutrition Examination Survey (NHANES III) in the United States demonstrated that alcohol consumption, especially beer, was significantly associated with serum uric acid level (Choi and Curhan, 2004). Moreover, their prospective study of 47,150 male health professionals aged 40–75 years old conducted over 12 years showed that the risk of gout varied depending on the type of alcoholic beverage, as beer increased the risk of gout more than twice as much as did spirits, even though the alcohol content per serving was less for beer than spirits (12.8 g vs. 14.0 g), while two 4-oz glasses or more of wine per day was not associated with an increased risk of gout (Choi *et al.*, 2004). These findings suggest that the large purine content present in beer may play an important role in increased serum uric acid concentration and the incidence of gout, though whether other non-alcoholic offending factors are present in beer or some defending factors in wine remains unknown.

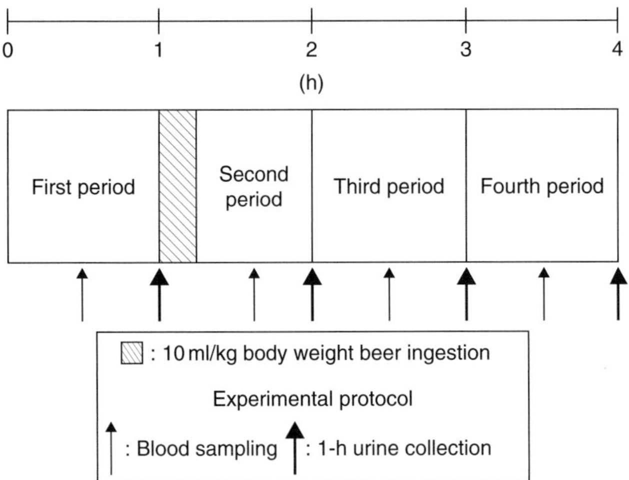

Figure 53.13 Experimental protocol used to investigate the short-term effects of various kinds of beer drinking on the plasma concentration and urinary excretion of purine bases. After an overnight fast except for water consumption, the subjects completely void their urine, after which the first 1-h urine samples are collected (first period). After the first urine samples are collected, beer (10 ml/kg body weight) containing 5.5% alcohol is ingested within 10 min. The second urine samples are collected after 1 h (second period), the third between 1 and 2 h (third period), and the fourth between 2 and 3 h (fourth period) after beer ingestion. The first, second, third, and fourth blood samples are drawn with heparinized syringes at the mid-point of the respective 1-h urine collections.

Prevention of Beer-Induced Increases in Plasma and Urinary Excretion of Purine Bases: Effects of Allopurinol

It has been suggested that ingestion of alcohol together with allopurinol (xanthine dehydrogenase inhibitor that inhibits the conversion of hypoxanthine to xanthine and xanthine to uric acid) decreases the conversion of allopurinol into oxypurinol, an active metabolite of allopurinol, while it increases the urinary excretion of allopurinol, which may reduce the hypouricemic effect of oxypurinol (Kaneko *et al.*, 1990). In a recent study, the effects of allopurinol (300 mg) administered 13 h prior to ingesting beer (10 ml/kg body weight) on plasma and urinary excretion of purine bases were compared with beer drinking (10 ml/kg body weight) alone and allopurinol (300 mg) intake alone (Ka *et al.*, 2006). With the pre-administration of allopurinol, the beer-induced increases in plasma concentration and urinary excretion of hypoxanthine were markedly increased as compared with beer alone. On the other hand, the sum of increases in plasma concentrations of purine bases by beer alone was greater than that by the pre-administration of allopurinol. In addition, allopurinol administration inhibited the beer-induced increase in plasma concentration of uric acid. These results suggest that abrupt adenine nucleotide degradation may increase the plasma concentration and urinary excretion of hypoxanthine under a condition of low xanthine dehydrogenase activity, which is mostly ascribable to allopurinol. Further, the differences in the sum of increases in plasma concentrations of purine bases with and without the pre-administration of allopurinol were largely ascribable to a greater increase in urinary excretion of hypoxanthine. Also, allopurinol intake is suggested to be effective to control the rapid increase in plasma uric acid caused by drinking alcoholic beverages.

A common experimental protocol used to study the short-term effects of various kinds of beer on the plasma concentration and urinary excretion of purine bases is indicated in Figure 51.13.

Summary Points

- Beer contains considerable amounts of various purines as compared to other alcoholic beverages.
- The high purine content augments the hyperuricemic effect of alcohol contained in beer.
- Beer consumption increases the plasma concentrations and urinary excretion of hypoxanthine and xanthine.
- Both alcohol-free beer and *happo-shu* (low-malt beer) have deleterious effects on uric acid metabolism.
- Long-term alcohol consumption, especially beer, is significantly associated with increased serum uric acid levels.
- An epidemiological study showed that serum uric acid levels increased with increasing amounts of beer or liquor intake, though beer caused a larger increase.
- Pre-administration of allopurinol was found to be effective to control the rapid rise in plasma uric acid concentration caused by beer drinking.

References

Choi, H.K. and Curhan, G. (2004). *Arthritis Rheum.* 51, 1023–1029.
Choi, H.K. *et al.* (2004). *Lancet* 363, 1277–1281.
Eastmond, C.J. *et al.* (1995). *Br. J. Rheumatol.* 34, 756–759.
Faller, J. and Fox, I.H. (1982). *New Engl. J. Med.* 307, 1598–1602.
Gibson, T. *et al.* (1983). *Ann. Rheum. Dis.* 42, 123–127.
Gibson, T. *et al.* (1984). *Br. J. Rheumatol.* 23, 203–209.
Ka, T. *et al.* (2005). *Horm. Metab. Res.* 37, 641–645.
Ka, T. *et al.* (2006). *Horm. Metab. Res.* 38, 188–192.
Kaneko, K. *et al.* (1990). *Clin. Chim. Acta* 193, 181–186.
Kono, S. *et al.* (1994). *Int. J. Epidemiol.* 23, 517–522.
Lieber, C.S. (1965). *Arthritis Rheum.* 8, 786–798.
Nishioka, K. *et al.* (2002). *Alcohol Clin. Exp. Res.* 26, 20S–25S.
Puig, J.G. and Fox, I.H. (1984). *J. Clin. Invest.* 74, 936–941.
Sugie, T. *et al.* (2005). *J. Epidemiol.* 15, 41–47.
Yamamoto, T. *et al.* (1993). *Metabolism* 42, 1212–1216.
Yamamoto, T. *et al.* (1995). *Jpn. J. Rheumatol.* 5, 355–361.
Yamamoto, T. *et al.* (1995). *Metabolism* 44, 779–785.
Yamamoto, T. *et al.* (2002). *Metabolism* 51, 1317–1323.
Yamamoto, T. *et al.* (2004). *Horm. Metab. Res.* 36, 231–237.

54

Neuropharmacological Activity of *Humulus Lupulus* L.

Paola Zanoli and Manuela Zavatti Department of Biomedical Sciences, Section of Pharmacology and National InterUniversity Consortium for the Study of Natural Active Principles (CINSPAN), University of Modena and Reggio Emilia, Modena, Italy

Abstract

The traditional use of hops in the treatment of sleep disturbances has been supported by experimental studies performed in rodents, as described in the present chapter. An inhibitory influence on the central nervous system was suggested by the finding of a reduction in locomotor behavior together with an enhancement of pentobarbital hypnotic activity, following the oral administration of hop extracts. A lipophilic hop extract showed an antidepressant-like activity in an animal model of behavioral despair, without a significant anxiolytic activity. Among hop components, the bitter acids have been carefully investigated for their role in the neuropharmacological activities of hops. In particular, the fraction containing α-acids has been recognized to be mainly responsible for the sedative effects of hops. On the other hand the fraction containing β-acids appears to exert a central stimulatory activity, probably due to a reduction in the GABAergic activity. This hypothesis is supported by its effects in animal models of sedation and convulsions as well as in electrophysiological studies on cerebellar granule cells in culture.

Clinical trials specifically related to the sedative properties of hops are still inadequate since human studies were mainly performed using valerian–hop combination extracts.

List of Abbreviations

H. lupulus	*Humulus lupulus*
i.p.	Intraperitoneally
b.w.	Body weight
GABA	γ-Aminobutyric acid
CNS	Central nervous system
EPM	Elevated plus maze
FST	Forced swimming test
5-HT_6	5-Hydroxy-triptamine (serotonin) receptor type 6
ML_1	Melatoninergic receptor type 1
A_1	Adenosine receptor type 1

Introduction

Humulus lupulus L. (Cannabinaceae) is a dioecious twining perennial plant, widely cultivated throughout the temperate regions of the world. The female inflorescences (hop cones or "hops") (Figure 54.1) made up of membranaceous bracts contain a resinous yellow substance named lupulin. Hops are collected in the late summer and used in the brewing industry to add bitterness, flavor and aroma to beer.

In the traditional medicine the dried flowers were recommended for the treatment of sleep disturbances, restlessness, mania, toothache and earache.

The use of hops as a mild sedative came from the observation of fatigue, tiredness and sleepiness symptoms in the hop pickers, apparently due to resin absorption during harvesting or processing hops (Tyler, 1987). The tranquilizing and sleep-enhancing properties of *H. lupulus* were cited in old manuals of *Pharmacology and Pharmacognosy* (Fluckiger and Hanbury, 1879; Maisch, 1892; Schleif and Galludet, 1907; Greenish, 1909; Culbreth, 1927; Gathercoal and Wirth, 1936) as well as in modern textbooks of *Phytotherapy* (Newall *et al.*, 1996; Schulz *et al.*, 2001; Capasso *et al.*, 2003). The German Commission E Monographs advised to use the plant in the treatment of "discomforts during restlessness or anxiety and sleep disturbances" (Blumenthal, 1998).

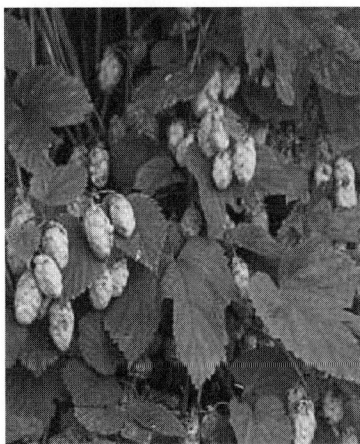

Figure 54.1 The female inflorescences (hops) of *Humulus Lupulus* L.

Beer in Health and Disease Prevention
ISBN: 978-0-12-373891-2

A sedative-like activity of hops was observed in different animal species: frog (Staven-Groenberg, 1928), pigeon (Sikorski and Rusiecki, 1938), goldfish (Bouchardy, 1953) and golden carp (Grumbach and Mirimanoff, 1955). The administration of single components of hops allowed to suggest humulone and lupulone as responsible for the marked sedative effects observed in pigeons and small birds (Sikorski and Rusiecki, 1938). The prenylated acylphloroglucinols (humulone, lupulone and their analogs) are still under investigation for their neuropharmacological properties, as further described in the present chapter. On the other hand, prenylated flavonoids of hops are receiving an increasing attention primarily for the antioxidant and chemopreventive properties (xanthohumol) (Stevens and Page, 2004) and for the estrogenic activity (8-prenylnaringenin) (Chadwick *et al.*, 2006).

Experimental Studies

The first investigation on the neuropharmacological effects of *H. lupulus* was performed by Hänsel and Wagener (1967). The oral administration of lupulone or ethanol hop extract (500 mg/kg body weight) in mice failed to influence motor activity and pentobarbital sleeping time. The lack of a clear sedative effect was also reported in human subjects treated with 250 mg of a lipophilic hop extract for 5 days (Stocker, 1967).

Subsequently, Bravo *et al.* (1974) intraperitoneally (i.p.) injected different types of the plant extract in mice for evaluating locomotor behavior. A different reduction in the spontaneous motor activity without a myorelaxant effect was observed in dependence of the solvent used in the extraction procedure. The ether extract was the most active in comparison with the aqueous and alcoholic ones. However, this effect was seen only at high doses (1 ml of hop extract 10%/20 g. b.w.).

In the study of Lee *et al.* (1993) a not well-identified hop extract was i.p. injected in mice at doses from 100 to 500 mg/kg b.w. Hypothermic, analgesic and anticonvulsant effects were found 30 min after the injection. Moreover, a reduction in the spontaneous motor activity together with a prolonged pentobarbital-induced sleeping time suggested a mild hypnotic activity.

The results of these studies, summarized in Table 54.1, might suggest a neurodepressant property of *H. lupulus*; but the different extraction procedures as well as the undefined composition of the administered preparations make still questionable the identity of the active sedative principle/s.

A degradation product deriving from hop constituents during storage, 2-methyl-3-butene-2-ol, was examined by Wohlfart *et al.* (1983). A high dose of the compound (206.5 mg/kg i.p. in rats) was needed to obtain a decline of motility by 50%. A higher dose (800 mg/kg i.p.) produced a narcotic effect in mice for about 8 h (Hänsel *et al.*, 1980). Considering the small amount of 2-methyl-3-butene-2-ol detected in the commercially available hop extracts (maximum content 0.15%), a significant contribution of this compound to the sedative activity of hops can be reasonably excluded (Hänsel *et al.*, 1982).

Few studies investigated the effects of hop flavonoids. Myrcene displayed analgesic activity in mice (Rao *et al.*, 1990; Lorenzetti *et al.*, 1991) but it was excluded to be responsible for the sedative effects of hops (Hänsel *et al.*, 1980). During boiling wort with hops, myrcene gives rise to myrcenol which has been shown to prolong pentobarbital-induced sleeping time, when injected in mice, and to potentiate GABA receptor response *in vitro* (Aoshima *et al.*, 2006).

Table 54.1 Behavioral effects of hop extracts or single components in laboratory animals

Effect	*Hop extract/component*	*Laboratory animal*	*References*
Reduced spontaneous motor activity	Ether > alcoholic > aqueous extract	Mice	Bravo *et al.* (1974)
Hypothermic, analgesic, anticonvulsant, reduced motor activity, prolonged pentobarbital-induced sleeping time	Non-identified hop extract	Mice	Lee *et al.* (1993)
Narcotic	2-Methyl-3-butene-2-ol	Mice	Hänsel *et al.* (1980)
Reduced motility	2-Methyl-3-butene-2-ol	Rat	Wohlfart *et al.* (1983)
Analgesic	Myrcene	Mice	Rao *et al.* (1990), Lorenzetti *et al.* (1991)
Prolonged pentobarbital-induced sleeping time	Myrcenol (produced from myrcene during boiling)	Mice	Aoshima *et al.* (2006)
Prolonged pentobarbital sleeping time, antidepressant	CO_2 extract, α-acid fraction	Rat	Zanoli *et al.* (2005)
Increased animal ambulation, increased rearings, reduced percentage of sleeping rats, antidepressant, worsened picrotoxin-induced seizures	β-Acid fraction	Rat	Zanoli *et al.* (2007)
Reduced spontaneous locomotor activity, increased ketamine-induced sleeping time, hypothermic	Ethanolic, CO_2 extract, α-acids, β-acids, hop pure oil	Mice	Schiller *et al.* (2006)

Our recent studies examined the neuropharmacological effects of a CO_2 hop extract and two single fractions containing α-acids (humulone and its analogs) and β-acids (lupulone and its analogs). The CO_2 extract was dissolved in Tween 80 (10%) and water, β-acid fraction in Tween 80 (5%) and water, while the α-acid fraction was solubilized in peanut oil. The activity of each substance was compared with one of the respective vehicles. The solutions were administered at different dosages (from 2.5 to 20 mg/kg b.w.) by oral gavage 60 min before the behavioral tests. We utilized a series of experimental models widely validated for the analysis of substances affecting central nervous system (CNS) functions. The evaluation of locomotor behavior was performed placing the single rats in the center of a square black-painted arena (100 × 100 cm) with 50 cm high walls. The animals were continuously filmed for 10 min by a camera and a detailed analysis was carried out by a computerized system. The results reported in Figure 54.2 show that only β-acid fraction was able to alter the locomotor activity of rats. This fraction increased ($p < 0.05$ vs. vehicle group) animal ambulation, particularly in the central area of the open field, while the CO_2 extract and the α-acid fraction did not significantly affect the length of rat pathways (Zanoli *et al.*, 2005, 2007). Examples of rat pathways in the open field arena following the different pharmacological treatments are reported in Figure 54.3. The rats placed in the unfamiliar environment of the open field are used to rear upon their hind feet. Comparing the rearings displayed by the different experimental groups of rats, it is clearly evident that only β-fraction significantly increased the number of rearings during the test (Figure 54.4). The results of these experiments suggested a different pharmacological profile of the two fractions of bitter acids: β-fraction appears to exert a stimulatory effect, while α-acids had no significant influence on animal locomotor behavior. With the aim of clarifying this crucial point, the influence on pentobarbital-induced sleeping time was investigated. The three substances were orally administered 60 min before the i.p. injection of pentobarbital sodium (35 mg/kg). As reported in Table 54.2, the CO_2 extract and the α-fraction significantly prolonged sleeping time in comparison with pentobarbital plus vehicle treated rats. On the other hand β-fraction did not affect sleeping time but strongly reduced the percentage of sleeping rats. Therefore, the fraction containing β-acids appears to exert

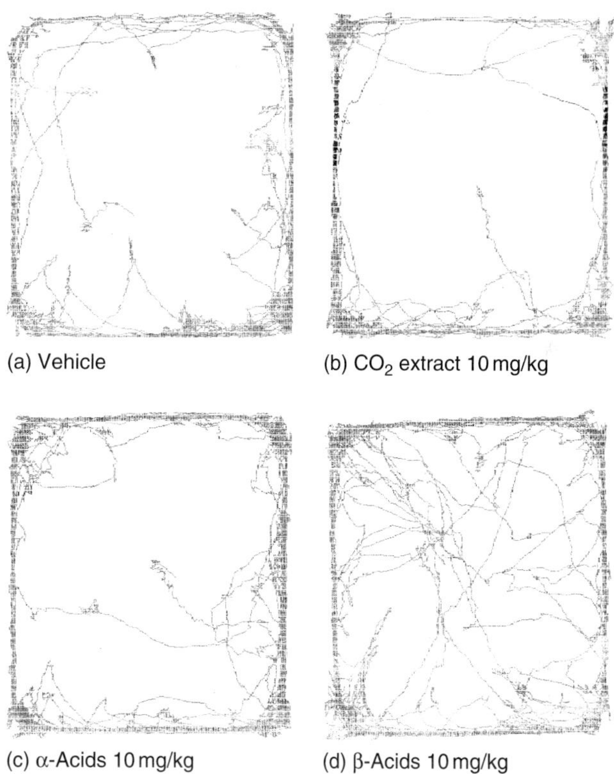

Figure 54.3 Examples of rat pathways in the open field. Pathways traveled by rats during 10-min test in the square arena of the open field.

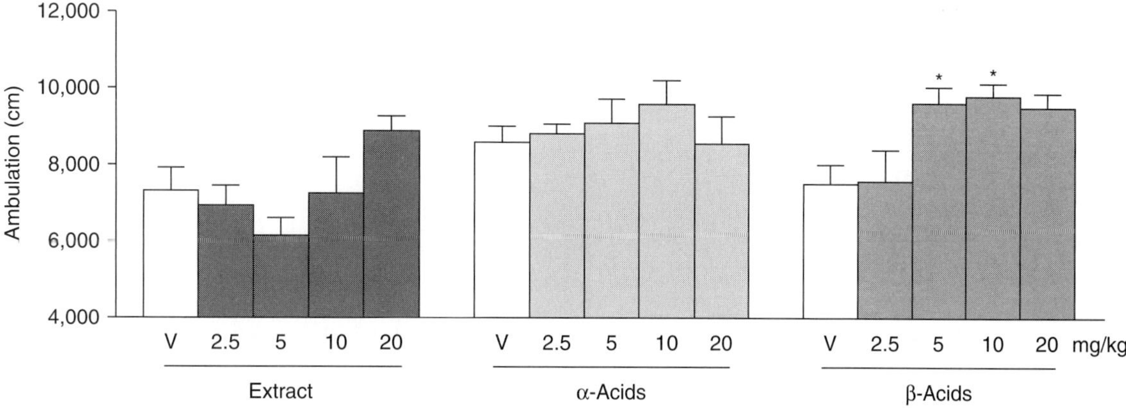

Figure 54.2 Ambulatory activity of rats in the open field. The substances (CO_2 hop extract, α-acids, β-acids) were orally administered 60 min before the test. Each column represents the mean ± SEM ($n = 8$); $^*p < 0.05$ in comparison with the respective vehicle group (V) (Anova followed by Dunnett's test). *Source*: The data were adapted from our previous papers (Zanoli *et al.*, 2005, 2007).

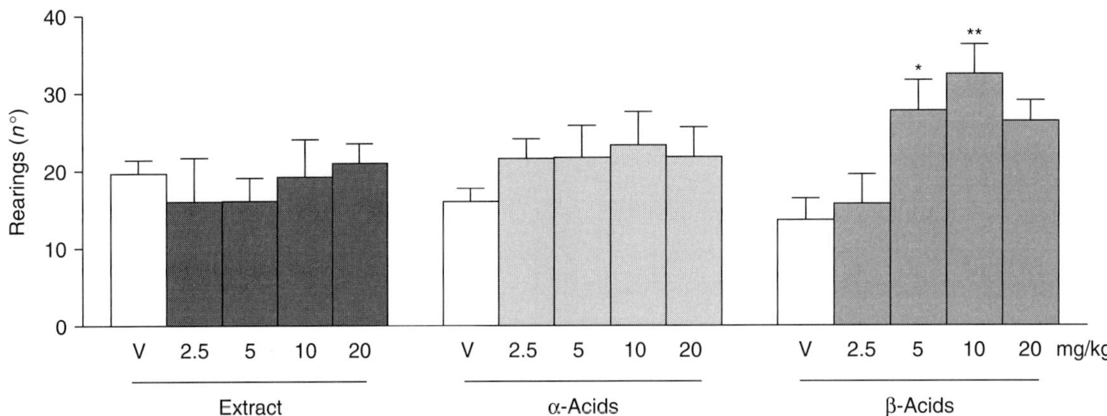

Figure 54.4 Vertical activity of rats during the open field test. Each column represents the number of rearings (mean ± SEM, $n = 8$) of rats treated with CO_2 extract, α- and β-acids; $^*p < 0.05$, $^{**}p < 0.01$ in comparison with the respective vehicle group (V) (Anova followed by Dunnett's test). *Source*: The data were adapted from our previous papers (Zanoli *et al.*, 2005, 2007).

Table 54.2 Influence of CO_2 hop extract, α- and β-acids on pentobarbital induced sleep

Pretreatment (mg/kg)	*Sleeping time (min)*	*Sleeping rats (%)*
Vehicle	38.9 ± 1.9	90.0
Extract 5	38.7 ± 3.3	80.0
Extract 10	49.7 ± 3.5*	87.5
Extract 20	56.8 ± 4.0**	100.0
Vehicle	38.1 ± 2.1	100.0
α-acids 5	43.4 ± 2.1	87.5
α-acids 10	55.1 ± 2.2**	100.0
α-acids 20	67.6 ± 4.4**	100.0
Vehicle	38.0 ± 1.7	100.0
β-acids 2.5	46.9 ± 2.0	80.0
β-acids 5.0	39.0 ± 4.2	66.7
β-acids 10	46.7 ± 2.7	46.7†

Notes: All rats were i.p. treated with pentobarbital sodium (35 mg/kg) 60 min after the oral administration of CO_2 extract, α- and β-acids. The data represent the mean ± SEM ($n = 8$–15) of sleeping time (the interval between the loss of the righting reflex and its recovery) and the percentage of sleeping animals.
$^*p < 0.05$.
$^{**}p < 0.01$ (Anova followed by Dunnett's test).
$^{\dagger}p < 0.05$ (Fisher test) vs. respective vehicle group.
Source: The data were adapted from our previous papers (Zanoli *et al.*, 2005, 2007).

Table 54.3 Effect of CO_2 hop extract, α- and β-acids on open arm exploration in the elevated plus maze

Treatment (mg/kg)	*Open arm entries (%)*	*Time spent in open arms (%)*
Vehicle	21.7 ± 4.2	15.2 ± 3.2
Extract 2.5	24.0 ± 5.0	14.7 ± 3.5
Extract 5	29.4 ± 5.6	17.0 ± 4.5
Extract 10	25.0 ± 6.6	12.8 ± 3.6
Vehicle	15.4 ± 4.5	10.6 ± 3.3
α-Acids 2.5	20.9 ± 7.0	24.0 ± 7.7
α-Acids 5	20.9 ± 8.2	20.1 ± 7.7
α-Acids 10	19.6 ± 7.4	15.1 ± 4.5
Vehicle	13.9 ± 3.7	6.4 ± 1.7
β-Acids 2.5	11.7 ± 5.5	8.8 ± 4.6
β-Acids 5	20.6 ± 4.4	9.5 ± 2.0
β-Acids 10	34.2 ± 7.0*	14.6 ± 4.6
Diazepam 1	40.4 ± 2.8*	40.0 ± 4.8**

Notes: The substances (CO_2 extract, α-acids, β-acids) were orally administered 60 min before the test. Diazepam, used as reference drug, was i.p. injected at the dose of 1 mg/kg, 20 min before the test. The data are mean ± SEM of the entries and the time spent in the open arms ($n = 6$–10).
$^*p < 0.05$.
$^{**}p < 0.01$ vs. respective vehicle group (Anova followed by Dunnett's test).
Source: The data were adapted from our previous papers (Zanoli *et al.*, 2005, 2007).

an opposite effect (stimulatory) in comparison with α-fraction and CO_2 extract, both displaying a sedative effect.

For evaluating the anxiolytic activity of hop extract and its fractions, rats were submitted to the elevated plus maze (EPM) test, which is extensively validated as a tool to screen anxioselective effects of drugs. Animals were tested in a plus-shaped maze elevated above the floor level, with two wall-closed arms and two opposite open arms. Rats exposed to EPM tend to avoid the open arms and prefer to stay in the enclosed arms: there is an inverse correlation between anxiety levels and the exploration of the open arms. Thus, the substances that elicit an increase in the number of entries and in the time spent in open arms are considered anxiolytic drugs.

During the 5-min test, the number of entries and the time spent in open and closed arms were recorded. The hop extract and α-fraction were unable to affect these parameters, while β-fraction significantly increased the open arm entries only at the highest dose (10 mg/kg), suggesting hence a modest anxiolytic-like activity (Table 54.3). The effect of a classic anxiolytic drug (diazepam) is reported for comparison.

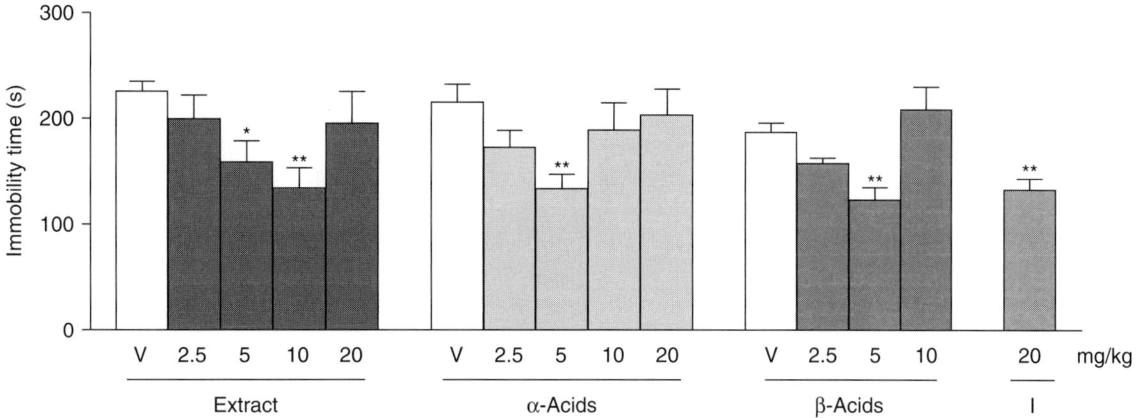

Figure 54.5 Immobility time of rats during forced swimming test. The substances (CO_2 extract, α- and β-acids) were orally administered three times (24 h, 5 h and 1 h) before the test. Imipramine (I), used as standard antidepressant drug, was orally administered (24 h, 5 h and 1 h before the test) at the dose of 20 mg/kg. The histograms represent the mean ± SEM ($n = 8$) of the immobility time of rats during 5-min test. $^{*}p < 0.05$, $^{**}p < 0.01$ vs. vehicle treated animals (V) (Anova followed by Dunnett's test). *Source*: The data were adapted from our previous papers (Zanoli *et al.*, 2005, 2007).

For a better knowledge about the neuropharmacological activity of hop extract and its fractions, we submitted rats to the forced swimming test (FST), a standard method for screening potential antidepressant agents. In the FST, animals are placed in a cylinder of water, from which they cannot escape during a 15-min pretest. This condition is thought to induce a state of behavioral despair, since the animals become immobile, remaining in a floating position without swimming or climbing. The duration of immobility is evaluated in a 5-min test session performed 24 h after the pretest. Antidepressant drugs, administered between the pretest and test periods, decrease the duration of immobility. The histograms reported in Figure 54.5 show that all the three substances at the dose of 5 mg/kg (and also at 10 mg/kg for the extract) significantly reduced the immobility time of rats. It must be underlined that a repeated schedule of administration (24 h, 5 h and 1 h before the test) was adopted for all compounds, including imipramine used as reference drug.

The results obtained in FST clearly demonstrate an antidepressant activity of hop extract as well as the two fractions. At our knowledge, it is the first demonstration of this type of activity for *H. lupulus*. Moreover these findings demonstrate a similar effect of the three substances, differently from the results related to the locomotor behavior and to pentobarbital-induced sleep.

The issue related to the sedative activity of hops and its constituents has been resumed very recently by Schiller *et al.* (2006). Ethanolic and CO_2 extracts were orally administered in mice with the aim of checking their influence on body temperature, locomotor activity and ketamine-induced sleeping time. A hypothermic effect together with a reduction in motility and an increase in sleeping time brought the Authors to confirm the traditional use of hops in sleep disorders. In the same experimental conditions the authors tested the effects of different fractions of hop extract. Both fractions containing α- and β-acids were able to prolong ketamine-induced sleeping time, but it must be stressed that the fraction containing β-acids needed an approximately six times higher dosage to significantly potentiate the narcotic event. This last result seems to suggest a contribution of β-acids to the sedative activity of the plant. The discrepancy between these results and our findings should be elucidated taking into consideration several factors (raw material, condition of storage, extraction procedure, type of solvent), besides the different applied dosages.

Molecular Mechanisms

Till now we have investigated a possible interaction of β-acid fraction with the GABA-benzodiazepine neurotransmitter system. The reduction in the hypnotic effect of pentobarbital in β-acids treated rats, suggested a decreased GABAergic activity. To validate our hypothesis we investigated the influence of β-acids on picrotoxin-induced seizures. The significant increase in the seizure severity and in the lethal effect observed in β-acids pretreated rats, in comparison with control ones, demonstrated that a reduction in the GABAergic activity could play an important role in the behavioral effect of β-acids (Figure 54.6). Electrophysiological studies performed on cerebellar granule cells in culture showed a reduction in GABA currents when β-acid fraction was applied together with GABA (Figure 54.7). On the other hand the capacity of hop extract to interact with benzodiazepine recognition sites was excluded by radioreceptor binding assays performed in our laboratories (Zanoli *et al.*, 2007).

Studies previously performed by Abourashed *et al.* (2004) demonstrated the capacity of a hop dried extract to bind serotoninergic 5-HT_6 receptors as well melatoninergic ML_1 receptors. The involvement of these receptors in sleep disturbances or in the regulation of circadian rhythm, respectively, has been demonstrated (Pickering and Niles, 1990; Shen *et al.*,

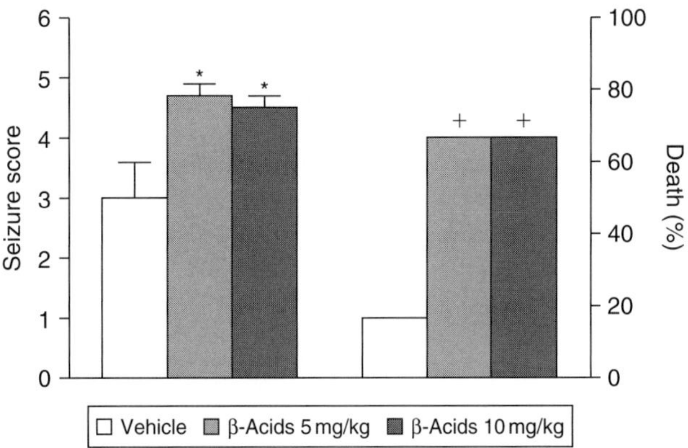

Figure 54.6 Influence of β-acids on picrotoxin-induced seizures. The animals pretreated with vehicle or β-acids were subcutaneously injected, after 60 min, with picrotoxin (5 mg/kg). The severity of picrotoxin-induced seizures was evaluated according to a modified behavioral scale (for details see Zanoli *et al.*, 2007). Each column represents the mean ± SEM ($n = 6$). *$p < 0.05$ (Anova followed by Dunnett's test), **$p < 0.05$ (Fisher test). *Source*: The data were adapted from our previous papers (Zanoli *et al.*, 2007).

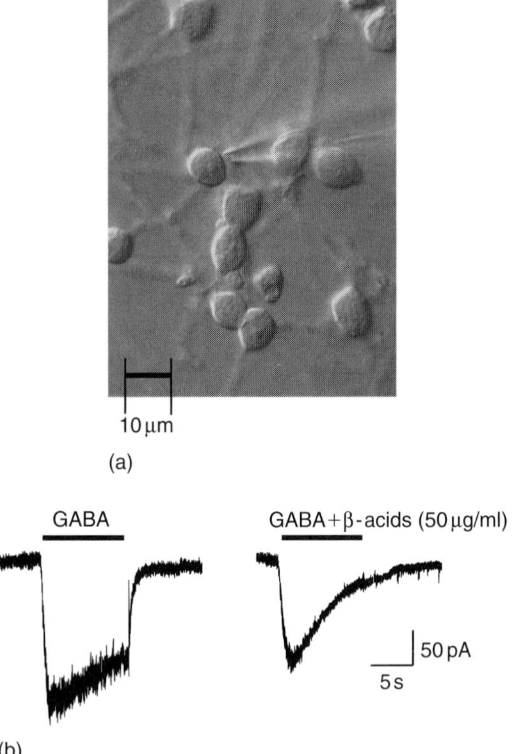

Figure 54.7 Influence of β-acids on GABA currents in cultured cerebellar granule neurons. (a) Cerebellar granule cells in culture at 8 days *in vitro*. Calibration bar: 10 µm. (b) Whole-cell recordings of currents evoked by GABA 1 µM alone or in presence of hop β-acids 50 µg/ml (holding potential –60 mV). pA = picoAmpère; s = seconds. *Source*: The data were adapted from our previous papers (Zanoli *et al.*, 2007).

1993). It must be underlined that the tested extract did not contain bitter acids, because a hydrophilic solvent was used in the extraction procedure (Abourashed *et al.*, 2004).

The role of adenosine receptors in the sleep-inducing activity of a valerian–hop combination (Ze 91019) has been investigated by Müller *et al.* (2002). Ze 91019 as well as the valerian extract therein exhibited a partial agonist activity at A_1 adenosine receptors, while hop extract alone failed to exert a similar effect. Therefore an adenosine-mediated mechanism can be excluded to play a role in the sedative property of hops.

Clinical Studies

The clinical investigations on the efficacy of hop preparation in sleep disturbances generally refer to hops given in combination with other sedative herbs. A randomized, double-blind, controlled trial in patients suffering from sleep disorders showed equivalent efficacy and tolerability between a hop–valerian preparation and a benzodiazepine drug (Schmitz and Jackel, 1998). Sleep quality was determined by psychometric tests, psychopathologic scales and sleep questionnaires. This study pointed out the lack of withdrawal symptoms following hop–valerian treatment for 2 weeks, differently from benzodiazepine therapy.

The pharmacodynamic effects of a commercially available mixture of valerian and hops (Ze 91019) were studied in young adult patients using quantitative topographical electroencephalography (Vonderheid-Guth *et al.*, 2000). A clear effect at the CNS level was observed 4 h after the intake of high dosage of the mixture (1,500 mg valerian plus 360 mg hops).

A multicenter, randomized and placebo-controlled study was conducted in 184 patients with mild insomnia, nightly administered with a combination of standardized extracts of hops (83.8 mg) and valerian (374 mg) for 28 days (Morin *et al.*, 2005). Sleep parameters were measured by daily diaries and polysomnographic assays. The combination hops–valerian showed to have a modest hypnotic effect, improving sleep without producing significant residual effects and rebound insomnia. The lack of residual sedative effects had been previously stressed by Gerhard *et al.* (1996) in healthy volunteers, receiving a hop–valerian combination or flunitrazepam, used as reference drug. The objective measurement of cognitive psychomotor performance and the subjective questionnaires on well-being led to emphasize impairment of vigilance in the morning after ingestion of the benzodiazepine drug, while more alertness and activity were observed in patients treated with the herbal remedy. Therefore, the valerian–hop combination can be considered, a useful and safe alternative to the classic sedative drugs (Gerhard *et al.*, 1996; Schmitz and Jackel, 1998; Kubish *et al.*, 2004; Morin *et al.*, 2005). However, no meaningful information regarding the potential clinical efficacy of hops alone can be extrapolated from these studies due to the presence of valerian in the clinical formulations.

Conclusions

Since a long time *H. lupulus* has been traditionally a reputed sedative herbal remedy and is used in the treatment of sleep disturbances. Previous (Bravo *et al.*, 1974; Lee *et al.*, 1993) and recent (Zanoli *et al.*, 2005, 2007; Schiller *et al.*, 2006) experimental studies performed in rodents confirmed the sedative properties of hops, even if there are some discrepancies in the results. As a whole, a reduced motility together with a prolonged pentobarbital-induced sleeping time was found. In our experimental conditions, hop extract failed to affect locomotor behavior, but it must be stressed that our dosages were much lower than the ones used in the other studies. However, the sleep-promoting activity of hops was confirmed by our findings of an enhanced pentobarbital hypnotic activity in hop extract treated rats.

Among hop components, the bitter acids have been studied to check their role in the sedative effect of the plant. The authors (Zanoli *et al.*, 2005; Schiller *et al.*, 2006) agree on the sedative property of α-acids, but they found opposite effects following the administration of β-acids. In fact, our experiments showed a stimulatory influence of β-fraction on CNS, probably due to an antagonistic effect on GABA neurotransmission (Zanoli, 2007).

The other hop components have been poorly investigated. Only one study reported an increase in ketamine- and ether-induced sleeping time by administering hop oil in mice, suggesting its contribution to the sedative effect of *H. lupulus* (Schiller *et al.*, 2006). In addition hop oil was demonstrated to cause a small potentiation of GABA response *in vitro* (Aoshima *et al.*, 2006).

In conclusion, the sedative effect of hops is confirmed by several experimental studies, but the antidepressant activity has been recognized only recently (Zanoli *et al.*, 2005, 2007). The common antidepressant effect of the bitter acids and the extract opens up new therapeutic perspectives for this medicinal plant. It might be an alternative herbal medication with a beneficial profile of efficacy and safety. In fact, St. John's Wort is commonly used in the treatment of moderate depressive disorders, but in recent years its pharmacological interactions with several drugs have been reported. More experimental studies are needed to further elucidate the neuropharmacological properties of *H. lupulus*, with particular attention for the antidepressant activity.

Summary Points

- Hop cones have been used in traditional medicine to treat sleep disturbances since a long time.
- Experimental evidence of the sedative property of hop extract has been supported by the finding of a reduced motor behavior and an enhanced pentobarbital hypnotic activity in hop extract treated animals.
- A CO_2 hop extract, as well as its α- and β-acid fractions, showed an antidepressant effect in an animal model of behavioral despair.
- Among hop components the fraction containing α-bitter acids has been recognized to play a main role in the sedative effect of hops.
- On the other hand, the fraction containing β-bitter acids seems to exert a stimulatory influence on CNS.
- No clinical trials utilizing hop extract alone have been performed till now.

References

Abourashed, E.A., Koetter, U. and Brattström, A. (2004). *Phytomedicine* 11, 633–638.

Aoshima, H., Takeda, K., Okita, Y., Hossain, S.J., Koda, H. and Kiso, Y. (2006). *J. Agric. Food Chem.* 54, 2514–2519.

Blumenthal, M. (1998). *The Complete German Commission E Monograph: Therapeutic Guide to Herbal Medicines.* American Botanical Council, Austin, TX. p. 147.

Bouchardy, M. (1953). *Pharm. Acta Helv.* 28, 183–206. (*Chem. Abstr.* 48, 12144).

Bravo, L., Cabo, J., Fraile, A., Jimenez, J. and Villar, A. (1974). *Boll. Chim. Farm.* 113, 310–315.

Capasso, F., Gaginella, T.S., Grandolini, G. and Izzo, A.A. (2003). *Phytotherapy.* Springer-Verlag, Berlin, Heidelberg, New York.

Chadwick, L.R., Pauli, G.F. and Farnsworth, N.R. (2006). *Phytomedicine* 13, 119–131.

Culbreth, D.M.R. (1927). In Hop, N.F. (ed.), *Manual of Materia Medica and Pharmacology.* Lea and Febiger, Philadelphia.

Fluckiger, F.A. and Hanbury, D. (1879). Strobili humuli. *Pharmacographia.* Macmillan and Co., London.

Gathercoal, E.N. and Wirth, E.H. (1936). In Humulus, N.F., *Pharmacognosy.* Lea and Febiger, Philadelphia.

Gerhard, U., Linnenbrink, N., Georghiadou, C. and Hobi, V. (1996). *Schweiz. Rundsch. Med. Prax.* 85, 473–481.

Greenish, H.C. (1909). Hops. *A Textbook of Materia Medica.* J. and A. Churchill, London.

Grumbach, P. and Mirimanoff, A. (1955). *Bull. Soc. Pharm. (Bordeaux)* 94, 196–202. (*Chem. Abstr.* 51, 7268).

Hänsel, R. and Wagener, H.H. (1967). *Arzeneimittelforshung* 17, 79–81.

Hänsel, R., Wohlfart, R. and Coper, H. (1980). *Z. Naturforsch.* 35, 1096–1097.

Hänsel, R., Wohlfart, R. and Schmidt, H. (1982). *Planta Med.* 45, 224–228.

Kubish, U., Ullrich, N. and Müller, A. (2004). *Schweiz. Zeitsch. Ganz. Med.* 16, 348–354.

Lee, K.M., Jung, J.S., Song, D.K., Kräuter, M. and Kim, Y.H. (1993). *Planta Med.* 59, A691.

Lorenzetti, B.B., Souza, G.E.P., Sarti, S.J., Santos Filho, D. and Ferreira, S.H. (1991). *J. Ethnopharmacol.* 34, 43–48.

Maisch, J.M. (1892). Humulus. *Organic Materia Medica.* Lea Brothers and Co., Philadelphia.

Morin, C.M., Koetter, U., Bastien, C., Ware, J.C. and Wooten, V. (2005). *Sleep* 28, 1465–1471.

Müller, C.E., Schumacher, B., Brattström, A., Abourashed, E.A. and Koetter, U. (2002). *Life Sci.* 71, 1939–1949.

Newall, C.A., Anderson, L.A. and Phillipson, J.D. (1996). *Herbal Medicines: A Guide for Health-Care Professionals.* The Pharmaceutical Press, London. pp. 162–163.

Pickering, D.S. and Niles, L.P. (1990). *Eur. J. Pharmacol.* 175, 71–77.

Rao, V.S., Mezenes, A.M. and Viana, G.S. (1990). *J. Pharm. Pharmacol.* 42, 877–878.

Schiller, H., Forster, A., Vonhoff, C., Hegger, M., Biller, A. and Winterhoff, H. (2006). *Phytomedicine* 13, 535–541.

Schleif, W. and Galludet, B.B. (1907). Humulus, US. In: *Materia Medica, Therapeutics, Pharmacology and Pharmacognosy*. Lea Brothers and Co., Philadelphia.

Schmitz, M. and Jackel, M. (1998). *Wien. Med. Wochenschr.* 148, 291–298.

Schulz, V., Hänsel, R. and Tyler, V.E. (2001). Hop strobiles and hop glands. In: *Rational Phytotherapy*. Springer, Berlin, Germany.

Shen, Y., Monsma, F.J., Metcalf, M.A., Jose, P.A., Hamblin, M.W. and Sibley, D.R. (1993). *J. Biol. Chem.* 268, 18200–18204.

Sikorski, H. and Rusiecki, W. (1938). *Bull. Int. Acad. Polon Sci. Classe Med.* 1936, 73–83. (*Chem. Abstr.* 32, 66011).

Staven-Groenberg, A. (1928). *Arch. Exp. Path. Pharm.* 1927, 272–281. (*Chem. Abstr.* 22, 2362).

Stevens, J.F. and Page, J.E. (2004). *Phytochemistry* 65, 1317–1330.

Stocker, H.R. (1967). *Schweizer Brauerei Rundschau* 78, 80–89.

Tyler, V.E. (1987). The new honest herbal. *A Sensible Guide to Herbs and Related Remedies*, 2nd edn., pp. 125–126. Stickley Co., Philadelphia.

Vonderheid-Guth, B., Todorova, A., Brattström, A. and Dimpfel, W. (2000). *Eur. J. Med. Res.* 5, 139–144.

Wohlfart, R., Hänsel, R. and Schmidt, H. (1983). *Planta Med.* 48, 120–123.

Zanoli, P., Rivasi, M., Zavatti, M., Brusiani, F. and Baraldi, M. (2005). *J. Ethnopharmacol.* 102, 102–106.

Zanoli, P., Zavatti, M., Rivasi, M., Brusiani, F., Losi, G., Puia, G., Avallone, R. and Baraldi, M. (2007). *J. Ethnopharmacol.* 109, 87–92.

55

Beer: Effects on Saliva Secretion and Composition

H.S. Brand, M.L. Bruins, E.C.I. Veerman and A.V. Nieuw Amerongen Section of Oral Biochemistry, Department of Basic Dental Sciences, Academic Centre for Dentistry (ACTA), Amsterdam, The Netherlands

Abstract

We investigated the effects of beer consumption on salivary secretion rate, pH, uric acid and amylase concentration. Ten healthy volunteers consumed either 300 ml top-fermented beer or the same volume of non-alcoholic beer at 1 week intervals. The consumption of beer induced a transient reduction in the volume of chewing-stimulated whole saliva after 15 min. No significant changes were observed in the salivary pH and concentrations of uric acid and amylase.

Introduction

Uric acid (Figure 55.1), the final oxidation product of purine metabolism, is normally excreted in urine. Excessive accumulation of uric acid in tissues leads to a type of arthritis known as gout. This disease is characterized by deposition of large crystalline aggregates in joints leading to an agonizingly painful attack (Kumar *et al.*, 1997).

Alcohol intake is associated with an increased risk of gout. This risk varies substantially according to the type of alcoholic beverage: beer confers a higher risk than spirits or wine (Choi *et al.*, 2004). This is probably related to a beer-induced increase in plasma concentration of uric acid. The ingestion of regular beer by healthy volunteers resulted in a statistical significant increase in the plasma concentration of uric acid after 30 min (Yamamoto *et al.*, 2002; Ka *et al.*, 2003). An elevation of plasma uric acid concentration was also reported for patients with gout drinking beer (Gibson *et al.*, 1984).

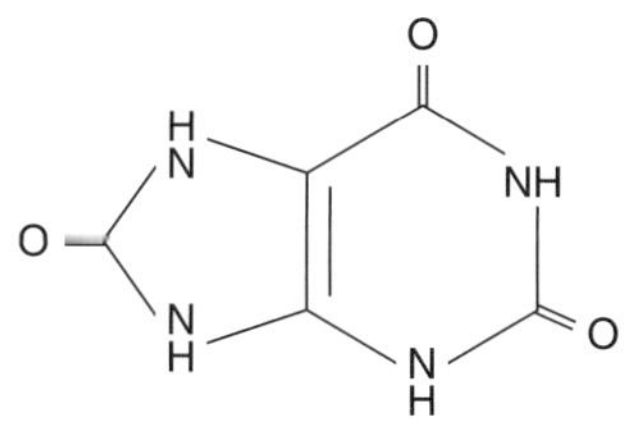

Figure 55.1 Uric acid. Structural formula of uric acid.

Recently, it has been shown that uric acid can be quantified in saliva (Meucci *et al.*, 1998; Inoue *et al.*, 2003). The concentration of uric acid in saliva correlates significantly with the serum concentration (Veerman *et al.*, manuscript in preparation). Therefore, the aim of this study was to investigate whether consumption of beer affects the salivary uric acid concentration.

Materials and Methods

Ten healthy volunteers participated in this study: seven men and three women with a mean age of 32 years (ranging from 23 to 50 years). They were instructed to abstain from alcohol at least 16 h prior to the experiment and to abstain from smoking, eating and drinking caffeine containing beverages and tooth brushing at least 1 h prior to the experiment (Hoek *et al.*, 2002). All experiments took place between 9.30 and 12.30 a.m. to avoid potential effects of diurnal variation on the composition of saliva (Hardt *et al.*, 2005). This study was approved by the Medical Ethic Committee of the Vrije Universiteit Medical Centre, Amsterdam, The Netherlands.

In a crossover design, the volunteers consumed either 300 ml top-fermented beer (Palm, Steenhuffel Breweries, Belgium, 5.2% alcohol) or 300 ml non-alcoholic beer (Amstel Malt, Zoeterwoude, The Netherlands, <0.1% alcohol) within 5 min. Both beers were served at 8°C. The time interval between both experimental conditions was 1 week.

Immediately before the consumption of beer and 15, 30, 45, 60, 90 and 120 min later, chewing-stimulated whole saliva was collected in pre-weighed tubes for 5 min (Bots *et al.*, 2004; Brand *et al.*, 2004). During the collection of saliva, the volunteers chewed one flat piece of 5×5 tasteless wax (Parafilm "M," Pechiney Plastic Packaging, Chicago, USA).

The salivary flow rates were determined gravimetrically, assuming 1 g = 1 ml, using an analytical balance (Sartorius MP8, Göttingen, Germany). Within 5 min of collection,

Beer in Health and Disease Prevention
ISBN: 978-0-12-373891-2

the salivary pH was measured using a PHM 240 Sentron 1001 (Radiometer, Copenhagen, Denmark). Subsequently, the salivary samples were transferred to Eppendorf vials and centrifuged at 10,000 g for 10 min. The clarified supernatant was stored at −20°C.

The salivary concentrations of uric acid and amylase were quantified by capillary electrophoresis, using benzoic acid as an internal standard (BioFocus C2000, Biorad, Hercules, USA).

All data are expressed as mean ± SD. The overall differences of the salivary parameters were statistically analyzed with analysis of variance (ANOVA) for repeated measures, followed by paired Student's *t*-tests where appropriate. The statistical analysis was performed using the statistical software package SPSS version 10.0. All levels of significance were set at $p < 0.05$.

Results

Consumption of 300 ml top-fermented beer induced changes in the flow rate of parafilm-chewing-stimulated whole saliva (Figure 55.2). A transient decrease in flow rate was observed 15 min after beer consumption (−15% vs. baseline values), which was not observed after consumption of non-alcoholic beer. The salivary pH did not differ between both experimental conditions (Figure 55.3).

Neither top-fermented beer nor non-alcoholic beer did induce significant changes in the salivary uric acid concentration (Figure 55.4) or uric acid output (Figure 55.5). The salivary amylase concentration (Figure 55.6) and amylase output (Figure 55.7) were not significantly affected too.

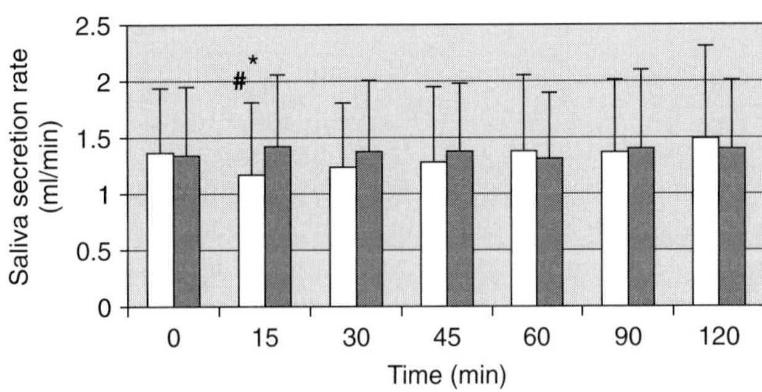

Figure 55.2 Saliva secretion rate after beer consumption. Flow rate of chewing-stimulated whole saliva before and after consumption of 300 ml beer (white bars) or non-alcoholic beer (gray bars). Data are expressed as mean ± SD ($n = 10$). *$p < 0.05$ vs. top-fermented beer at $T = 0$, #$p < 0.05$ vs. non-alcoholic beer at $T = 15$.

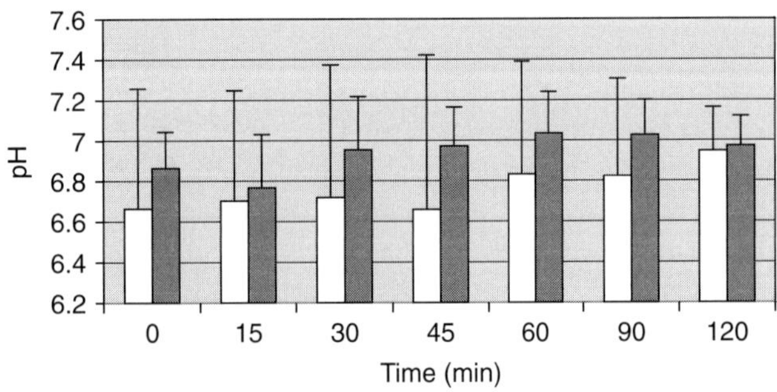

Figure 55.3 Salivary pH after beer consumption. The pH of chewing-stimulated whole saliva before and after consumption of 300 ml beer (white bars) or non-alcoholic beer (gray bars). Data are expressed as mean ± SD ($n = 10$). No statistical significant differences were observed between beer and non-alcoholic beer.

Discussion

This study demonstrated that consumption of a relatively small amount of top-fermented beer induced a transient decrease in saliva secretion after 15 min (Figure 55.2). This result is in agreement with a previous study by Enberg

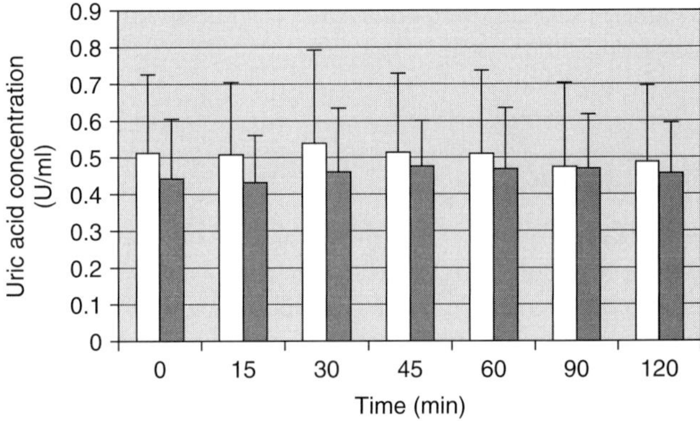

Figure 55.4 Salivary uric acid concentration after beer consumption. Uric acid concentration of chewing-stimulated whole saliva before and after consumption of 300 ml beer (white bars) or non-alcoholic beer (gray bars). Data are expressed as mean ± SD ($n = 10$). No statistical significant differences were observed between beer and non-alcoholic beer.

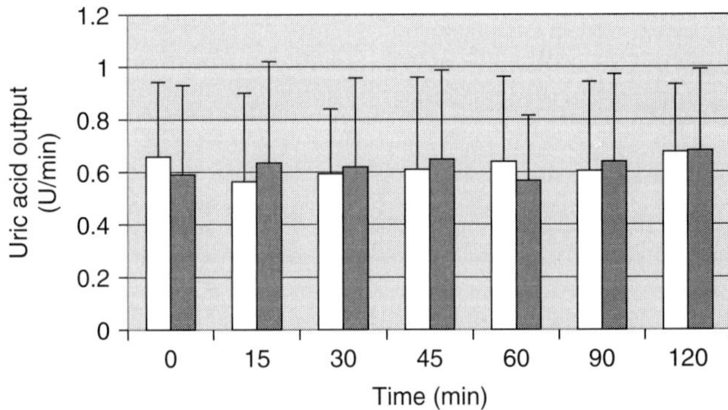

Figure 55.5 Salivary uric acid output after beer consumption. Uric acid output of whole saliva before and after consumption of 300 ml beer (white bars) or non-alcoholic beer (gray bars). Data are expressed as mean ± SD ($n = 10$). No statistical significant differences were observed between beer and non-alcoholic beer.

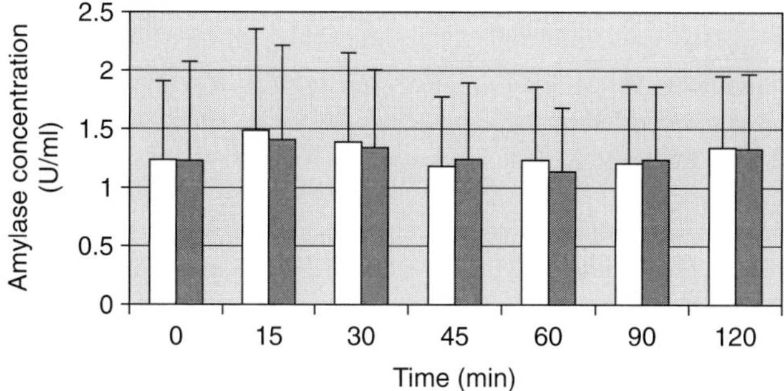

Figure 55.6 Salivary amylase concentration after beer consumption. Amylase concentration of whole saliva before and after consumption of 300 ml beer (white bars) or non-alcoholic beer (gray bars). Data are expressed as mean ± SD (*n* = 10). No statistical significant differences were observed between beer and non-alcoholic beer.

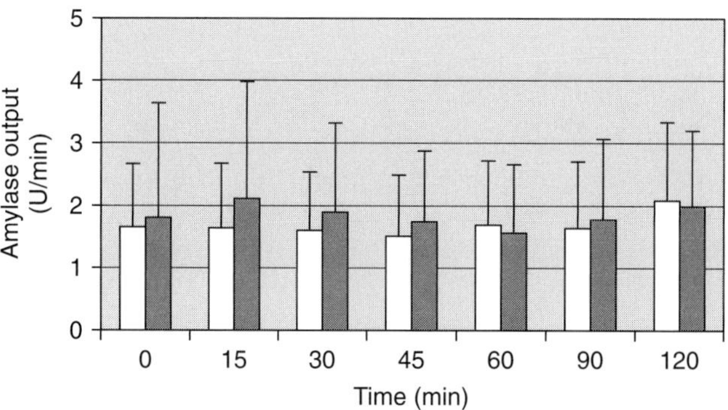

Figure 55.7 Salivary amylase output after beer consumption. Amylase output of whole saliva before and after consumption of 300 ml beer (white bars) or non-alcoholic beer (gray bars). Data are expressed as mean ± SD (*n* = 10). No statistical significant differences were observed between beer and non-alcoholic beer.

et al. (2001), who observed a decrease in parafilm-chewing-stimulated saliva secretion after acute consumption of 0.6–0.7 g alcohol/kg body weight in a soft drink. After consumption of that much higher amount of alcohol than in our study (0.2–0.3 g alcohol/kg body weight), a maximum decrease in parafilm-chewing-stimulated saliva secretion (−40%) was observed after 45 min. A reduction of 50% in parotid salivary flow rate after ingestion of a large dose of alcohol has also been reported (Dutta *et al.*, 1984). On the other hand, rinsing of the mouth with 15 ml beer (Coors, 4% alcohol) induced a 93% increase in unstimulated parotid saliva secretion during 5 min (Guinard *et al.*, 1998). However, one has to realize that under non-stimulated conditions, the secretion rate of parotid saliva is very low and will react rapidly to any type of stimulus.

Consumption of 300 ml beer did not induce significant changes in salivary uric acid concentrations (Figure 55.4). Probably, the increase in the plasma concentration of uric acid after consumption of beer (Yamamoto *et al.*, 2002; Ka *et al.*, 2003) is too limited to affect the saliva concentration.

We also did not observe a statistical significant change in salivary amylase concentration (Figure 55.6) or output after the consumption of beer (Figure 55.7). This may be related to the relatively small volume amount of alcohol consumed in our study. In rats, acute administration of a high dose of alcohol caused a significant reduction in stimulated parotid secretion (Scott *et al.*, 1989) and reduced the protein synthesis in all major salivary glands (Proctor *et al.*, 1993). Ingestion of a high dose of alcohol by humans also caused a decrease in parotid salivary flow rate (Dutta *et al.*, 1984) and stimulated whole saliva flow rate (Enberg *et al.*, 2001), with a concomitant reduction in salivary amylase activity and output (Enberg *et al.*, 2001).

Saliva is of paramount importance for the maintenance of oral health (Nieuw Amerongen and Veerman, 2002). Although our study showed that acute consumption of 300 ml of beer has only a limited effect on salivary secretion, frequent intake of beer may reduce salivary flow rate more extensively and for a longer time. This may impair the beneficial effects of saliva on oral health, especially in adolescents with a high frequency of (binge) drinking (Andersson *et al.*, 2002).

Summary Points

- Consumption of 300 ml top-fermented beer induces a transient decrease in salivary flow rate after 15 min.
- Consumption of 300 ml beer has no effect on salivary uric acid concentration and output.
- Consumption of 300 ml beer has no effect on salivary amylase concentration and output.

References

Andersson, B., Hansagi, H., Damstrom-Thakker, K. and Hibell, B. (2002). *Drug Alcohol Rev.* 21, 253–260.

Bots, C.P., Brand, H.S., Veerman, E.C.I., van Amerongen, B.M. and Nieuw Amerongen, A.V. (2004). *Int. Dent. J.* 54, 143–148.

Brand, H.S., Ligtenberg, A.J.M., Bots, C.P. and Nieuw Amerongen, A.V. (2004). *Int. J. Dent. Hyg.* 2, 137–138.

Choi, H.K., Atkinson, K., Karlson, E.W., Willett, W. and Curhan, G. (2004). *Lancet* 363, 1277–1281.

Dutta, S.K., Parasher, V. and Smalls, U. (1984). *Gastroenterology* 86, 1065.

Enberg, N., Alho, H., Loimaranta, V. and Lenander-Lumikari, M. (2001). *Oral Surg. Oral Med. Oral Pathol. Oral Radiol. Endod.* 92, 292–298.

Gibson, T., Rodgers, A.V., Simmonds, H.A. and Toseland, P. (1984). *Br. J. Rheumatol.* 23, 203–209.

Guinard, J.X., Zoumas-Morse, C. and Walchak, C. (1998). *Physiol. Behav.* 63, 109–118.

Hardt, M., Witkowska, H.E., Webb, S., Thomas, L.R., Dixon, S.E., Hall, S.C. and Fisher, S.J. (2005). *Anal. Chem.* 77, 4947–4954.

Hoek, G.H., Brand, H.S., Veerman, E.C.I. and Nieuw Amerongen, A.V. (2002). *Eur. J. Oral Sci.* 110, 480–481.

Inoue, K., Namiki, T., Iwasaki, Y., Yoshimura, Y. and Nakazawa, H. (2003). *J. Chromatogr. B Analyt. Technol. Biomed. Life Sci.* 785, 57–63.

Meucci, E.R., Littarru, C., Deli, G., Luciani, G., Tazza, L. and Littarru, G.P. (1998). *Free Radic. Res.* 29, 367–376.

Ka, T., Yamamoto, T., Moriwaki, Y., Kaya, M., Tsujita, J., Takahashi, S., Tsutsumi, Z., Fukuchi, M. and Hada, T. (2003). *J. Rheumatol.* 30, 1036–1042.

Kumar, V., Cotran, R.S. and Robbins, S.L. (1997). *Basic Pathology*, 6th edn. Saunders, Philadelphia, PA.

Nieuw Amerongen, A.V. and Veerman, E.C.I. (2002). *Oral Dis.* 8, 12–22.

Proctor, G.B., Shori, D.K. and Preedy, V.R. (1993). *Arch. Oral Biol.* 38, 971–978.

Scott, J., Berry, M.R. and Woods, K. (1989). *Alcohol Clin. Exp. Res.* 13, 560–563.

Yamamoto, T., Moriwaki, K., Takahashi, S., Tsutsumi, Z., Ka, T., Fukuchi, M. and Hada, T. (2002). *Metabolism* 51, 1317–1323.

56

Beer and Celiac Disease

Glen P. Fox Department of Primary Industries & Fisheries, Queensland Grains Research Laboratory, Plant Science – Wheat, Barley and Oats, Toowoomba Qld., Australia

Abstract

Celiac disease is a serious disease which can cause a number of symptoms including headache, nausea, cramps and diarrhea. The disease affects thousands of individuals in our communities. Like a number of diseases, celiac disease appears to be on the rise in the Western world. Celiacs react to particular peptides sequences found in a protein group found in barley, wheat and related species. As barley and wheat are the dominant cereals used in the production of beer, and the toxic peptides survive the brewing process, then celiacs can suffer reactions to beer. Grains such as sorghum or buckwheat are suitable alternatives and have the necessary grain components to provide full bodied beer that celiacs can enjoy without the risk of reaction. While, there may be limited choices for suitable beers, improvements in plant genetics as well as understanding of brewing with alternative grains should allow celiacs to enjoy their favorite drop in the future.

What Is Celiac (Coeliac) Disease?

A roman physician, Galen, first described the condition in about 250 AD and Samuel Gee again noted a similar condition in 1888. However, Dickie (1950), a doctor from The Netherlands, was the first to identify the link between wheat and his celiac patients. The food shortages during World War II had a positive impact on his patients during which they presented themselves less frequently with symptoms. After the war, when bread was more available, the incidence of their symptoms increased.

Celiacs react to a particular protein group found in some cereal grains, namely wheat, barley, rye and triticale. This protein group, gluten, is a mixture of gliadin and glutenin protein subgroups. These proteins stimulate T cells in the intestinal lamina proporia of celiac patients, although a minimum length and specific sequences of the protein are required for the T cells to recognize the toxic protein (Solid, 2002). The result for the patients is a range of symptoms including malabsorption of food and chronic diarrhea associated with anemia, rickets, inhibited growth, bloating, bulky stools, a blistering rash on the buttocks and mouth ulcers. Recently, Wiesner (2004) presented an excellent review of the disease symptoms as well as links between celiac disease and other serious diseases such as diabetes and possibly some cancers. Wiesner (2004) also highlighted the causative protein sequences from problematic plant species that were responsible for inducing reactions.

Celiac disease affects the small intestine. In a healthy body, the small intestine has "villi," tiny finger-like projections, visible under the microscope (Figure 56.1a). They provide a large surface area over which we absorb nutrients such as vitamins, folic acid, iron and calcium. In sufferers of celiac disease, the villi are attacked by the immune system (Figure 56.1b) and are eventually destroyed (Figure 56.1c). This results in nutrients in food passing through the digestive system without being absorbed (malabsorption), leading to vitamin and mineral deficiencies. In addition, a particular component of wheat (and related species) protein (gluten) causes the more serious symptoms of the disease.

Individuals can be born with celiac disease but the results of this type of immune system attack on the intestine can also appear in fully grown adults. Small children usually become symptomatic when they are weaned off liquids onto solids. They present with weight loss, refusal to feed, irritability, abdominal swelling and diarrhea. Certain groups of people are at greater risk for developing celiac disease and it is more common in individuals from families that already have the condition (being linked to the HLA DQ3 gene).

Celiac Disease Linked to Other Diseases

Celiac disease is more likely to occur in insulin dependent diabetics, people with Down's syndrome, sarcoidosis, infertility, IgA antibody deficiency and certain autoimmune diseases such as thyroid disease, rheumatoid arthritis, Addison's disease and Sjorgens syndrome of dry eyes and mouth. Celiac sufferers absorb fewer nutrients from their diet and so may develop nutritional deficiencies. Fifty percent are at risk of developing osteoporosis or fractures from calcium deficiency. There is a twofold increased risk

Beer in Health and Disease Prevention
ISBN: 978-0-12-373891-2

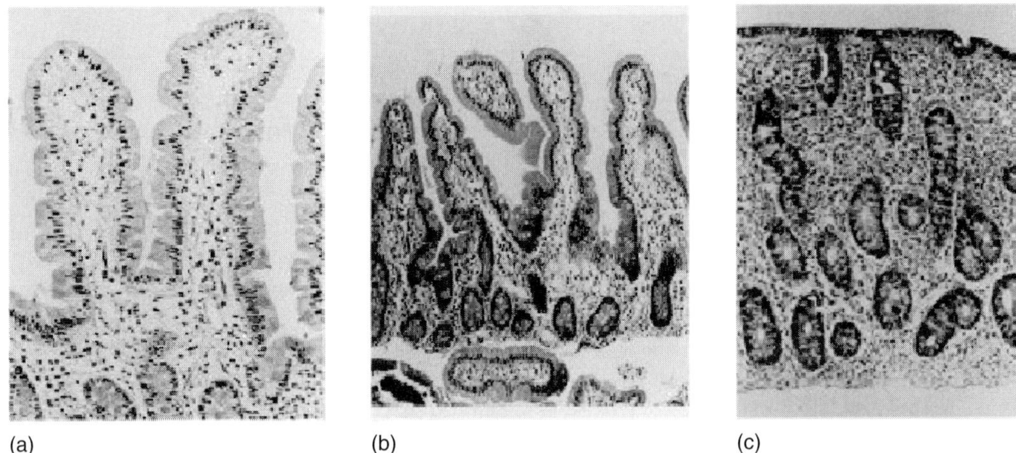

Figure 56.1 Healthy (a), damaged (b) and destroyed (c) villi of the small intestine (as seen under the microscope) (Fraser, 2005: www.netdoctor.co.uk).

of cancers of the mouth, throat and gullet as well as intestinal lymphomas and carcinomas. There is a strong link with insulin dependant diabetes through the HLA DQ3 gene. People with Down's syndrome are 43 times more likely to develop celiac disease but will often develop a milder spectrum of symptoms.

A certain amount of cross-reactivity occurs between grains, fruits and vegetables of similar classes and this should be borne in mind when trying to understand the various effects of different food groups. For example if a person is allergic to peanuts, then there is a high risk of being allergic to other members of the legume family including beans, peas, lentils, carob, senna and liquorice. However, foods from divergent food families may also cross-react, for example "celery-spice-carrot-mugwort syndrome." This may be due to the presence of other allergens such as lipid transfer protein (LTP), common to fruit, grasses and vegetables. LTP is heat and digestion resistant and can cause more severe systemic allergic reactions. As stated above, LTP is present in grasses (including barley) and, with its thermolabile properties, it survives the malting and brewing process to be present in beer. LTP has been shown to inhibit protease enzymes (Jones, 2005) and may have a positive contribution to beer foam (Evans and Sheehan, 2002).

Testing Your Foods

For celiacs to adhere to a strict gluten diet, they must be confident that the food labeled "gluten-free" is not contaminated with even trace amounts of gluten. A number of tests have been developed to screen "gluten-free" foods.

Enzyme-linked immunosorbant assays

Denery-Papini *et al.* (1999) reviewed a number of immunochemical assays for their efficacy at testing food products containing gluten. Enzyme-linked immunosorbant assays (ELISA) have been used for a number of years with success based on the development of antibodies to the suspected peptide. These assays have been applied to raw materials as well as the processed food products. However, there have been problems with ELISA. Kanerva *et al.* (2006) demonstrated the use of ELISA where by using different substrates the level of gluten protein groups could be under- or over-estimated. This work was shown when screening for barley contamination in oats samples adulterated with barley flour.

In specific relation to barley, malt or beer, ELISA has successfully been used to detect storage proteins in barley and malt (Skerritt, 1988; Skerritt and Henry, 1988) as well as to detect residual barley and malt protein in beers (Sheehan and Skerritt, 1997; Kanerva *et al.*, 2005), particularly in beer foam (Evans and Sheehan, 2002). Sorell *et al.* (1998) developed an ELISA specifically for detecting the "celiac" peptide in barley hordeins (the homologous protein group to the wheat gliadin protein). This ELISA also detected the common peptide between wheat, rye and oats. Kanerva *et al.* (2005) used an ELISA system, designed to detect gluten, to determine the presence of peptides in beer. There was considerable variation between beer types as the beer was produced from a range of cereals including barley, corn, rice, wheat and buckwheat. A number of beers had levels of gluten below the threshold recommended by the World Health Organization (WHO). These results suggest that beers can be produced from barley, with the appropriate adjunct source, may be suitable for celiacs.

Polymerase chain reaction

An alternative to the protein detection systems described above is the use of DNA. A number of the genes that are translated into the proteins that cause the celiac response have been sequenced. The use of DNA markers rather than protein markers may offer a more accurate measure of the "celiac" peptides. Dahinden *et al.* (2001) reported a new DNA-based method using the polymerase chain reaction (PCR) to identify contamination of wheat, barley or rye gluten components in "gluten-free" food products. Sandberg *et al.* (2003) used real time (RT) PCR to detect gluten contamination in "gluten-free" foods. While Olexová *et al.* (2006) also described a PCR method to detect gluten proteins in the so-called "gluten-free" flours and bakery products.

Statistics

Celiac disease has been reported in countries around the world, with varying levels of occurrence between 1:80 in Australia, 1:130 in the United States and Canada and 1:300 in the United Kingdom. However, actual diagnosis of suspected patients varies between countries including 1:2 in Finland, 1:8 in Australia and 1:20 in the United States. Of particular note is that most of these countries also have a strong affinity with beer consumption. However, the increasing level of celiac disease or gluten intolerance within these populations means that many people cannot enjoy beer that has been produced using conventional techniques and grain sources.

Celiacs and Beer

Beer has been consumed as either a social beverage or for medicinal purposes for over 10,000 years. Traditionally, beer has been produced from barley although it can be brewed from a number of different grains, including wheat, sorghum, rice or maize. The process of making beer has been described in detail in previous chapters. However, the composition of the raw materials and the brewing style has a significant impact on final flavor and quality. Barley is the most common solid raw material used in brewing. Through a series of complex biochemical reactions (carried out in temperature controlled vessels), it is structurally modified to produce a food source for yeast to ferment as well as provide compounds that impact on color, flavor and taste.

Protein is one of the important components in barley that impacts on quality. There are four groups of proteins:

1. albumins,
2. globulins,
3. glutenins and
4. prolamins.

Each of these groups have differing solubilities but more importantly, differing functionalities. In cereals, the major protein component is the prolamin group. However, there are many protein groups or individual proteins that contribute to the final product of beer, such as enzymes responsible for the degradation of storage proteins and starch to produce amino acids or glucose which will be a food source for yeast or individual barley proteins (foam-positive proteins, LTPs or protein Z) that can survive the rigors of the malting and brewing processes more or less intact – impacting on product quality (Evans and Sheehan, 2002). In addition, a number of protein inhibitors as well as storage protein groups have been identified in foam using the latest mass spectrometry techniques (Hao *et al.*, 2006).

The most abundant protein group in barley consists of the prolamin storage proteins (called hordeins in barley) located in the endosperm around starch granules. During malting and brewing these proteins provide a food source, either to the growing embryo or to the growing yeast cells throughout fermentation, as well as providing amino acids for enzyme synthesis. The prolamins are large water-insoluble molecules that are made up of all amino acids but especially rich in *prol*ine and glut*amin*e (prolamins). These are the antagonistic proteins in barley, wheat, rye and triticale that are responsible for the celiac reaction when suffers eat food or drink beverages produced from these grains. While other grains such as sorghum or maize may have high ratios of glutamine and proline, it is the amino acid sequence that lends itself to being problematic. It has been reported that a few small peptides are responsible for the reaction by celiacs. These small peptide sequences are PSQQ, PQQP and QQQP. These peptides occur in varying quantities within each of the storage protein families (which are usually characterized by molecular weight and/or presence of sulfur amino acids). Brewing grains such as wheat and barley have a high proportion of these repeat motifs. Tatham and Shewry (1995) highlight that the S-poor barley hordeins had no PQQP peptide. However, this and the other peptides exist in the S-rich hordein fractions. This also applies to the various wheat gliadin and glutenin protein groups, while other grains such as rice, maize and sorghum have no PQQP sequences.

Evolution and Homology of Proteins

Modern grass species are thought to have evolved from a single ancient family of grains (Figure 56.2) and as such there is considerable similarity in their structure and composition. The more closely related species, wheat, rye, triticale, barley and oats, evolved from the Pooideae subfamily and as such have similar properties in starch and protein. Importantly those species in the Pooideae family appear to be the grains solely responsible for the celiac reaction. The more distantly related tropical species such as sorghum, maize and rice have starch and protein properties that are different to the related wheat species. This evolutionary divergence has resulted in a variation in the protein and as a consequence these tropical crop species do not affect celiacs.

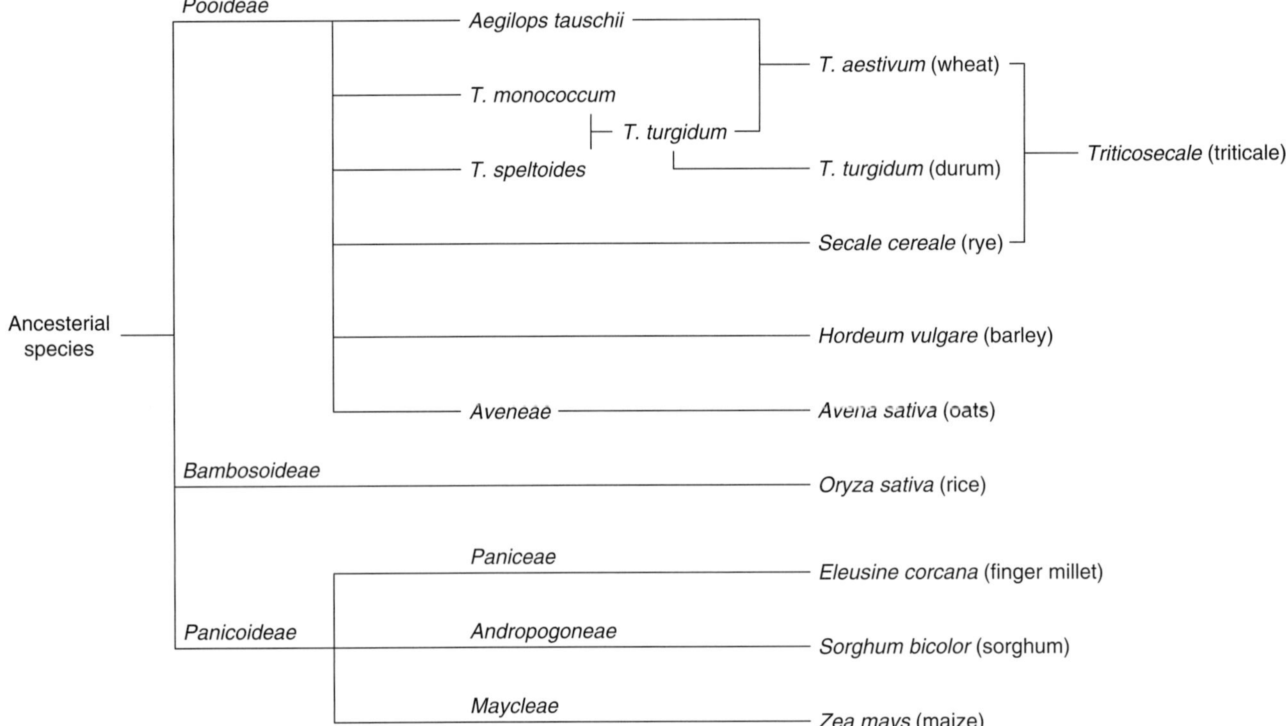

Figure 56.2 Evolutionary relationship between economically important species that impact on celiac disease.

Surviving the Brewing Process

This group of proteins, whether in a barley or wheat malt beer, are degraded during the production of malt as well as during the initial brewing stages. However, small residual peptides survive in the beer and play a role in foaming properties. These peptides are soluble in initial stages otherwise they would precipitate out during mashing or boiling. However, under certain conditions they can become hydrophobic and be involved in foam formation (bubble size and stability, retention time) and foam lacing/cling, after a period they again become soluble.

In addition, there are varying quantities of hordein peptides in different beer styles (ales and lagers) as well as within beer styles (stouts, bitters or brown ales). This is a result of the malting process, modifying the grain that is optimal for the beer style being produced, as well as the brewing process to produce that beer style. Ellis *et al.* (1990) used specifically designed ELISAs to detect residual hordein proteins and peptides in beer. The results showed that regardless of beer style (ales or lagers) or within a group of ale styles (brown, bitter or stout), there were still toxic levels of peptides. Kanerva *et al.* (2005) also demonstrated the presence of prolamin fractions in a range of beers using barley, wheat, corn, rice and buckwheat as raw materials. There was considerable variation between the lager and wheat beers but of note is that the wheat beers using barley and wheat had over 6,000 units of prolamin while the lager beers from barley, corn, rice or buckwheat ranged from not detected to 12 units. Again this shows that the brewing style as well as raw material will impact on final prolamin content in the beer. The selection of the appropriate raw materials and brewing style could produce beer with little or no prolamin content.

In addition, toxic levels were also detected in wort and hence concentrated wort (malt extract). As malt extract is used as a color or flavoring agent in foods or confectionery products, the presence of prolamins makes any product containing malt extract a problem to any celiac or gluten sensitive person.

Suitable Grains for Brewing

Over the last decade or so, as celiac disease has been more precisely diagnosed and food manufacturers have customized their products, brewers have also investigated the options of "gluten-free" beers. Recently, a number of studies have shown how to optimize malt production and brewhouse performance using non-traditional brewing grains such as sorghum, millet and buckwheat to produce beer that is acceptable not only in aroma, color and flavors but more importantly it is "gluten-free."

Sorghum

Sorghum (*Sorghum bicolor*) is a common summer crop used as a food source in African countries but only as animal feed in Western countries such as the United States and Australia. Beer has been produced from sorghum in many African countries for decades, either because there was no other grain source available or through preference. However, compared to barley or wheat beers, sorghum beers have been historically lower in quality. Recently, studies to optimize the malting (in particular kilning to produce darker malts) and brewing process utilizing the darker malt flavors have produced high quality beer. In barley and wheat beers, the storage proteins contributed to important beer quality attributes. However, for sorghum the structure of the storage proteins differs somewhat to barley and wheat in that sorghum has lower levels of proline and there are no reported toxic protein sequences.

Buckwheat

Buckwheat is a traditional feed crop in Central and Eastern Europe and Asia, with China currently the largest producer followed by the Russia and the Ukraine (Death, 2004). There are three species of buckwheat, with common buckwheat (*Fagopyrum esculentum* Moench) being the dominant species while *F. tataricum* and *F. emargimatum* are the minor species (Marshall and Pomeranz, 1981; Mazza and Oomah, 2005). Buckwheat is a pseudo-cereal and does not actually belong to the cereal family. It is a dicotyledon rather than a monocotyledon but does exhibit similar characteristics to cereals in that it seed with a starchy endosperm and non-starch aleurone layer (Aufhammer, 2000; Bonafaccia *et al.*, 2003).

The protein composition and structure of buckwheat is quite different to that of cereals. Globulins are the most abundant protein found with less than 3% prolamins (Ikeda *et al.*, 1991). Within the globulin family there are two major groups, namely 13S and 8S globulins. Compositionally these proteins show high levels of lysine, arginine and aspartic acid. There is a low level of glutamic acid and a particularly low level of proline, compared to barley or wheat (Pomeranz and Robbins, 1972), resulting in the protein being non-reactive.

Options for the Future

The incidence of celiac disease and gluten intolerance appears to be on the rise. This suggests that a larger proportion of beer consumers will be unable to consume beer produced from barley or wheat. Hence, an increase in the production of beer manufactured from celiac friendly grains will be required. However, as stated previously, these species are often either inefficient for processing or exhibit flavor problems.

A number of options exist to remedy this situation. Firstly, through genetic engineering it may be possible to change the structure of barley and wheat so as the protein structure and composition does not cause the celiac reaction. Also using the same approach it may also be viable to improve the structure of sorghum or other grains that currently produce beer with less desirable flavors or are less efficient in producing high-quality malt and beer.

A second approach that utilizes mutation breeding may produce celiac friendly grains from barley or wheat and not therefore fall under the legal minefield of genetic modification technology. Mutation breeding is not subject to the same legal constraints as genetic modification. While the process of nuclear or chemical treatment may be considered by some undesirable, these grains are not considered to be genetically modified. This approach is also possible for those celiac friendly grains such as sorghum, where mutation breeding increases the malting enzyme levels or reduces tannins that produce off-flavors.

A third option is to carry out detailed studies on wild (ancestral) germplasm. Some of these wild types may be structurally or compositionally distinct from their domesticated descendants. However, one such study has shown that for a wheat related species (*Triticum monococcum*) this may not be possible (Pogna, 2002).

A fourth option may be the use of medication. Hartmann *et al.* (2006) showed that endogenous enzymes (proteases) produced from germinating grains break down the toxic peptides. These enzymes are active at temperatures and pH conditions that could allow them to be used as an oral medication for celiacs.

Conclusion

The incidence of celiac disease appears to be increasing and is linked to a number of other disorders. As a consequence for the brewing industry, celiac suffers cannot enjoy flavorsome and healthy beer produced from wheat or barley. While beer can be produced from other grain species, there are differences in the malt and beer quality. In addition, some of these other species, such as buckwheat or millet, are not produced in broadacre farming systems, like wheat or barley.

Genetic improvement in the protein composition of the traditional grains, barley and wheat, would assist in acceptance for raw materials in beers that celiacs could consume as these grains are well known and processing for beer is understood. However, improvements in the non-traditional grains will also ensure adoption into traditional malting and brewing production systems.

Summary Points

- Celiac disease is a serious disorder that affects around 1:100 people.
- Serious health effects include headaches, malabsorption of food, diarrhea and bloating.
- A group of small peptides found in barley, wheat and related species cause the reactions.

- These peptides survive the brewing process and have been identified in beer.
- Beer can be produced from grains such as sorghum or buckwheat as they do not have these "toxic" peptides.

References

Aufhammer, W. (2000). *Pseudogetreidearten – Buchweizen, Reismelde and Amarant.* Verlag Eugen Ulmer, Stuttgart, Germany.

Bonafaccia, G., Marocchin, M. and Kreft, I. (2003). *Food Chem.* 80, 9–15.

Dahinden, I., Buren, M. and Luthy, J. (2001). *Eur. Food Res. Tech.* 212, 228–233.

Denery-Papini, S., Nicholas, Y. and Popineau, Y. (1999). *J. Cer. Sci.* 30, 121–131.

Dickie, W. (1950). Ph.D. Thesis, University of Utrecht, The Netherlands.

Death, R. (2004). RIRDC Publication No 04/019, http://www.rirdc.gov.au/reports/NPP/04-019sum.html.

Ellis, H.J., Freedman, A.R. and Ciclitira, P.J. (1990). *Clin. Chim. Acta* 189, 123–130.

Evans, D.E. and Sheehan, M.C. (2002). *J. Am. Soc. Brew. Chem.* 60, 47–57.

Fraser, J.S. (2005). http://www.netdoctor.co.uk.

Hao, J., Li, Q., Dong, J., Yu, J., Gu, G., Fan, W. and Chen, J. (2006). *J. Am. Soc. Brew. Chem.* 64, 166–174.

Hartmann, G., Koehler, P. and Wieser, H. (2006). *J. Cer. Sci.* 44, 368–371.

Ikeda, K. and Kishida, M. (1993). *Fagopyrum* 13, 21–24.

Jones, B.L. (2005). *J. Cereal Sci.* 42, 271–280.

Kanerva, P., Sontag-Strohm, T. and Lehtonen, P. (2005). *J. Inst. Brew.* 111, 61–64.

Kanerva, P.M., Sontag-Strohm, T.S., Ryöppy, P.H., Alho-Lehto, P. and Salovaara, H.O. (2006). *J. Cer. Sci.* 44, 347–353.

Marshall, H.G. and Pomeranz, Y. (1981). *Adv. Cereal Sci. Tech.* 5, 157–210.

Mazza, G. and Oomah, B.D. (2005). In Abdel-Aal, E. and Wood, P. (eds), *Speciality grains for food and feed*, pp. 375–393. AACC Press, USA.

Olexová, L., Dovi ovi ová, L., Švec, M., Siekel, P. and Kuchta, T. (2006). *Food Cont.* 17, 234–237.

Pogna, N.E. (2002). *Dig. Liver Dis.* 34, S154–S158.

Pomeranz, Y. and Robbins, G.S. (1972). *J. Ag. Food. Chem.* 20, 270–274.

Sandberg, M., Lundberg, L., Ferm, M. and Yman, I.M. (2003). *Eur. Food Res. Tech.* 217, 344–349.

Sheehan, M. and Skerritt, J.H. (1997). *J. Inst. Brew.* 103, 297–306.

Skerritt, J.H. (1988). *J. Cer. Sci.* 7, 251–263.

Skerritt, J.H. and Henry, R.J. (1988). *J. Cer. Sci.* 7, 265–281.

Solid, L.M. (2002). *Nat. Rev. Imm.* 2, 647–655.

Sorell, L., Antonio, J.A., Valdes, I., Alfonso, P., Camafeita, E., Acevedo, B., Fernando, C., Gavilondo, J. and Mendez, E. (1998). *FEBS Lett.* 439, 46–50.

Tatham, A.S. and Shewry, P.R. (1995). *J. Cer. Sci.* 22, 1–16.

Wiesner, H. (2004). In Wrigley, C., Walker, C. and Corke, H. (eds), *Encyclopaedia of Grains Sciences*, pp. 179–187. Academic Press, London, UK.

57

The Effect of Beer and Other Alcoholic Beverages on the Esophagus with Special Reference to Gastroesophageal Reflux

H. Seidl and C. Pehl Department of Gastroenterology, Hospital Bogenhausen, Academic Teaching Hospital, Munich, Germany

Abstract

Patients with gastroesophageal reflux disease (GERD) complain often about heartburn after ingestion of beer and other alcoholic beverages. In several studies, an induction of gastroesophageal reflux (GER) was observed after intake of beer and other alcoholic beverages like white wine, red wine, whiskey, and vodka in healthy volunteers and/or in patients with GERD. The magnitude of reflux after consumption of beer is significantly less than white wine and comparable to red wine in healthy volunteers. In contrast, the amount of reflux induced by beer seems to be similar to that of white wine in patients with GERD.

The ingredients responsible for the reflux induction by beer and the other alcoholic beverages are unknown. It could be demonstrated that the ethanol content *per se*, the acidic pH of the beverages and their high osmolality are not responsible for its effect on the esophagus. GER seems to be induced locally by alcoholic beverages and not systemically via the blood stream.

Thera are no data in the literature about the effects of beer on esophageal motory function, while there are several data about the effects of white wine. White wine depresses the lower esophageal sphincter pressure and disturbs esophageal primary and secondary peristalsis.

Chronic intake of alcoholic beverages like beer increases the risk of squamous cell cancer of the esophagus, while it is unclear whether alcoholic beverages increase also the risk for esophageal adenocarcinoma.

List of Abbreviations

GER Gastroesophageal reflux
GERD Gastroesophageal reflux disease
LES Lower esophageal sphincter

Introduction

Gastroesophageal reflux (GER) is the reflux of gastric contents – mainly gastric acid secretions – into the esophagus. GER can occur postprandially in healthy people without symptoms. In contrast, gastroesophageal reflux disease (GERD) is characterized by an increased magnitude of reflux which provokes symptoms (heartburn, acid regurgitation) and/or damages the esophageal mucosa (reflux esophagitis).

Feldman and Barnett reported that intake of beer, white wine, and red wine provoke heartburn in 60%, 63%, and 68%, respectively, of patients with GERD (Feldman and Barnett, 1995). The induction of heartburn by alcoholic beverages might be the result of a local irritating effect on the damaged mucosa as seen after ingestion of orange juice (Lloyd and Borda, 1981). On the other hand, alcoholic beverages might favor the occurrence of GER by stimulating gastric acid secretion which has been demonstrated for beer and wine (McArthur *et al.*, 1982; Lenz *et al.*, 1983; Peterson *et al.*, 1986; Singer *et al.*, 1987; Teyssen *et al.*, 1997). In chronic alcoholics with upper GI-complaints, reflux esophagitis is one of the most common findings in upper GI endoscopy pointing to a relationship between the intake of alcoholic beverages and GER (Tonnesen *et al.*, 1987).

The following article will report on the effects of alcoholic beverages on the esophagus with special focus on the effects of beer.

Alcoholic Beverages and GER

The induction of GER was reported for the first time after intake of high-proof alcoholic beverages like whiskey and vodka in healthy volunteers (Kaufman and Kaye, 1978; Vitale *et al.*, 1987). After this initial reports, further studies in healthy volunteers observed also an induction of GER after ingestion of commonly consumed alcoholic beverages like white wine, red wine, and beer (Pehl *et al.*, 1993; Grande *et al.*, 1997; Pehl *et al.*, 1998). Pehl *et al.* (1993) directly compared the effects of white wine and beer on GER in healthy volunteers. The volunteers received 300 ml of white wine (Kluesserather St. Michael, Winzergenossenschaft Moselland eG, Bernkastel-Rues, FRG; 7.5 v/v, pH 3.2), beer

Beer in Health and Disease Prevention
ISBN: 978-0-12-373891-2

(Heller Bock, Augustiner-Braeu Wagner KG, Munich, FRG; 7.0 v/v, pH 4.5) and tap water (pH 6.4), each, together with a standardized meal. Both alcoholic beverages induced GER compared to tap water in the first hour after intake, but the amount of GER was significantly higher after intake of white wine than after intake of beer (Figure 57.1). Despite being a short lasting effect (Figure 57.2), more than half of the healthy volunteers would be classified as pathologic refluxers when drinking wine during the investigation period (300 ml white wine with lunch and 400 ml white wine at night). Keeping in mind that red wine and beer were not administered to the same healthy volunteers, it seems that the magnitude of GER induction by these two alcoholic beverages is comparable (Figures 57.1 and 57.3). Both alcoholic beverages induce significantly more GER than water and significantly less GER than white wine (Pehl *et al.*, 1993, 1998). The assumption of a comparable effect of beer and red wine on GER induction is strengthened by an abstract of Pehl *et al.* (2004) presented at the German Congress for Internal Medicine. They compared the effect of white wine, red (rose-colored) wine, beer, and water on GER and on the duodeno-GER in healthy volunteers. All alcoholic beverages induced significantly more GER than water. The magnitude of GER was highest after ingestion of white wine (significant compared to both other alcoholic beverages) and nearly identical after ingestion of red wine and beer. None of the alcoholic beverages induced duodeno-GER.

GERD patients demonstrate higher reflux parameters, measured by esophageal 24 pH-metry, than healthy volunteers (Stein *et al.*, 1992; Vaezi *et al.*, 1995). Therefore, it could be speculated whether the already increased reflux in these patients will be further increased by ingestion of an alcoholic beverage. Pehl *et al.* (2006) tested this hypothesis in 25 GERD patients, 7 females and 18 males (median age 54 years, range 24–84 years). A reflux esophagitis was seen in 15 of these patients during endoscopy (nine grade I, four grade II, one grade III, and one grade IVb (Barrett's esophagus) according to Savary Miller classification (Savary and Miller, 1978). The other 10 patients had a pathological result of 24-h pH-metry according to the authors normal values. All patients consumed alcoholic beverages weekly to daily (<40 g/day in males, <30 g/day in females), but nobody was addicted to alcohol. Each patient was studied twice with a minimum of 2 days apart for 3 h by pH-measurement after ingestion of 300 ml white wine (Kluesserather St. Michael, Moselland Winzergenossenschaft, Bernkastel-Kues, Germany; $n = 17$), 500 ml beer (Augustiner Hell, Augustiner Braeu, Munich, Germany; $n = 8$), or tap water (all patients) within 30 min in a randomized order together with a standardized meal. Five hundred milliliter beer (1 bottle) was administrated, since this is the usual ingested volume of the kind of offered beer. Furthermore, different volumes of wine and beer were applied to compensate for the different alcohol concentration (wine 8.6 v/v, 300 ml = 20.64 g ethanol; beer 5.2 v/v, 500 ml = 20.8 g ethanol).

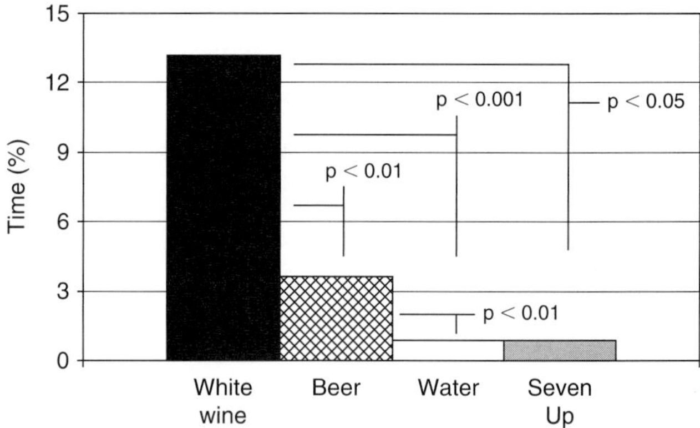

Figure 57.1 Effect of beer, white wine, an acid beverage, and water on GER in healthy volunteers. Percentage of time (%) with esophageal pH < 4 (data represent median) in the first hour after ingestion of 300 ml white wine, beer, water, and Seven Up together with a standardized meal in healthy volunteers (adapted from Pehl *et al.* (1993), reprinted with kind permission of Springer Science and Business Media).

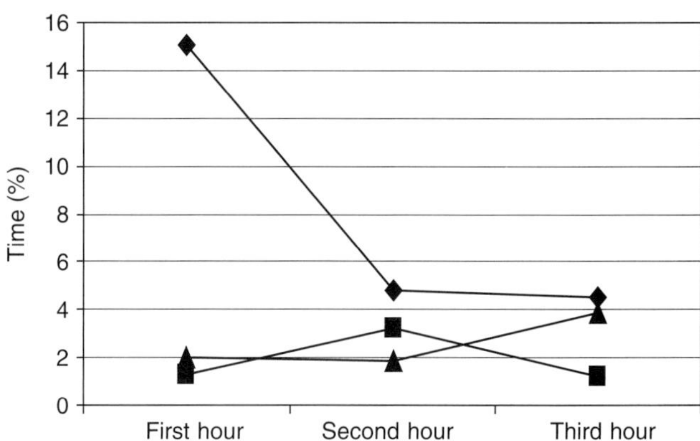

Figure 57.2 Time course of reflux induction in healthy volunteers. Percentage of time (%) with esophageal pH < 4 (data represent median) in the first, second, and third hour after ingestion of 300 ml white wine, an adapted ethanol solution, and water together with a standardized meal in healthy volunteers (adapted from Pehl *et al.* (1993), reprinted with kind permission of Springer Science and Business Media).

The percentage of time esophageal pH < 4, that is, GER, during the postprandial hours was significantly increased after both alcoholic beverages compared to tap water (Figure 57.4). An increase of the percentage of time pH < 4 was observed in 14 out of 17 patients after ingestion of wine and in all but one patient after ingestion of beer (Figure 57.5). Statistical analysis revealed no difference in the magnitude of reflux induction between wine and beer. However, it has to be realized that no direct comparison of beer and white wine was done in the GERD patients, while beer and white wine were applied to every healthy volunteer in the above mentioned study of Pehl *et al.* (1993). A decrease in

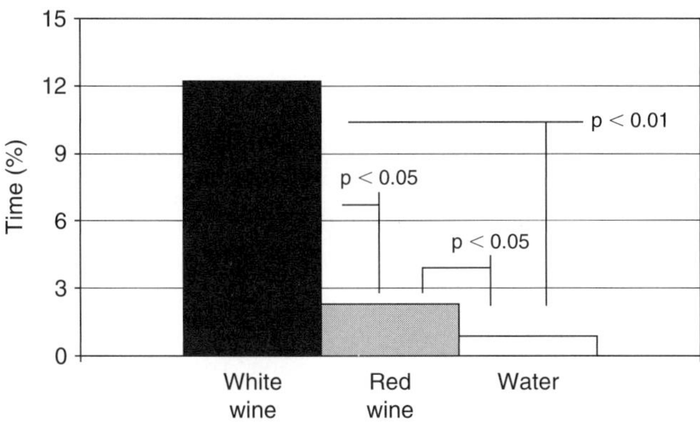

Figure 57.3 Differences in reflux induction between white wine and red wine. Percentage of time (%) with esophageal pH < 4 (data represent median) in the first hour after ingestion of 300 ml white wine, red wine, and water together with a standardized meal in healthy volunteers (adapted from Pehl *et al.* (1998), reprinted with permission).

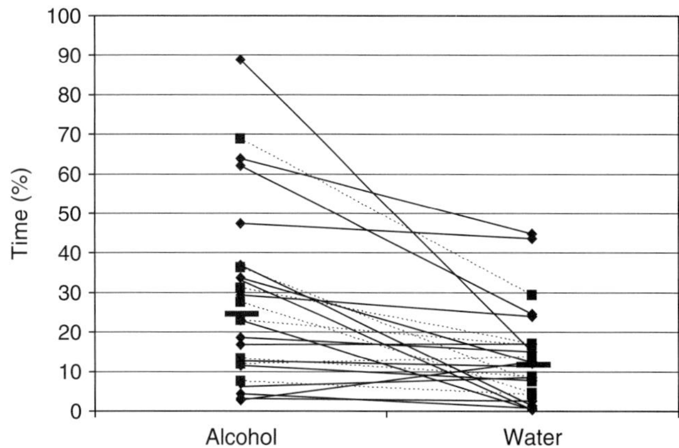

Figure 57.5 Individual reflux data with and without ingestion of an alcoholic beverage. Scatter graph of the percentage of time (%) esophageal pH < 4 during 3 h after ingestion of an alcoholic beverage (rhombic points = white wine, square points = beer) and tap water together with a standardized meal in 25 patients with GERD (Pehl *et al.*, 2006), reprinted with permission.

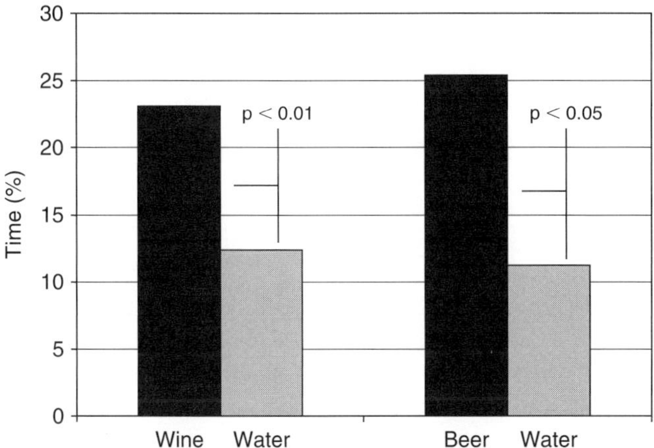

Figure 57.4 Induction of GER in patients with reflux disease. Percentage of time (%) esophageal pH < 4 (data represent median) during 3 h after ingestion of 300 ml white wine, beer, and water together with a standardized meal in patients with GERD (adapted from Pehl *et al.* (2006)), reprinted with permission.

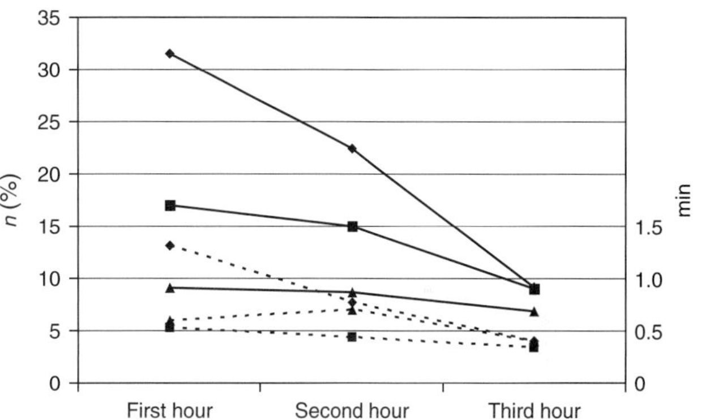

Figure 57.6 Time course of reflux induction in patients with GERD. Percentage of time (%) esophageal pH < 4 (rhombic points), number of reflux episodes (square points), and mean reflux duration (triangle) during the first, second, and third hour after ingestion of an alcoholic beverage (white wine or beer; dark line) and tap water (dotted line) together with a standardized meal in patients with GERD (data represent median; Pehl *et al.* (2006)), reprinted with permission.

the percentage of time pH < 4, in reflux frequency, and in mean reflux duration was seen postprandially over time after ingestion of all three beverages (Figure 57.6). Nevertheless, all three reflux parameters remained increased during each of the three postprandial hours after both alcoholic beverages compared to tap water. Thus, it seems that the GER enhancing effect of alcoholic beverages acts for a longer time period in GERD patients (Figure 57.6) than in healthy volunteers (Figure 57.2). Separating the GERD patients in those with and without reflux esophagitis, a significant induction of GER was observed in both groups by ingestion of an alcoholic beverage. Postprandial percentages of time pH < 4 were slightly higher in patients with compared to those without reflux esophagitis after ingestion of water as well as after intake of an alcoholic beverage in this study. However, the magnitude of reflux induction was not significantly different in patients with and without reflux esophagitis. Considering gender, ingestion of alcoholic beverages induced GER in women as well as in men.

It might be assumed that the ethanol content is responsible for the effects of alcoholic beverages on GER. In line with this assumption are data about a decrease in lower esophageal sphincter (LES) pressure and an increase in simultaneous contractions and in failed peristalsis provoked by intravenous administration of ethanol in healthy volunteers (Hogan *et al.*, 1972; Keshavarzian *et al.*, 1990).

However, the administered volume of ethanol in these studies resulted in signs of intoxication in nearly all volunteers. No effect on sphincter pressure and the frequency of abnormal esophageal contractions was seen by intravenous administration of a lower dose of ethanol (Mayer *et al.*, 1978). Pehl *et al.* (1993, 1994) directly compared the effects of white wine and an ethanol solution, adapted in alcohol content to white wine, on GER in healthy volunteers. Significant differences in the magnitude of reflux induction were observed between white wine and the ethanol solution despite similar blood levels of alcohol, while no significant difference was detectable between the ethanol solution and tap water (Figure 57.2). These data demonstrate that the ethanol content of an alcoholic beverage is, at least alone, not responsible for the effects of an alcoholic beverage on GER. However, esophageal exposure to ethanol might potentiate the deleterious effects of refluxed acid to the esophageal mucosa (Salo, 1983; Bor *et al.*, 1999). Yet, the ethanol concentration which is necessary for this co-toxic effect remains unclear. Bor *et al.* reported noxious effects of 10% ethanol on rabbit esophagus, while Salo did not observe noxious effects on rabbit esophagus for 20% ethanol, but for 40% ethanol.

Another mechanism which is assumed to be responsible for the induction of heartburn after intake of a beverage is its pH, since Feldman and Barnett (1995) observed a relationship between heartburn and low pH of non-alcoholic beverages. Therefore, the reported difference in the magnitude of reflux induction between white wine and beer might be the result of its different pH. However, several data argue against an effect of the pH of a beverage on the genesis of GER and heartburn. First, white wine induced a much higher amount of GER in healthy volunteers than red wine despite only small differences in pH (3.2 and 3.4, respectively) (Pehl *et al.*, 1998). Second, intake of Seven Up® with a similar pH of 3.2 like white wine did not induce GER in healthy volunteers (Pehl *et al.*, 1993). Third, orange juice and tomato juice provoke GER in GERD patients even after neutralization to a pH of 7 (Lloyd and Borda, 1981). Thus, beverages can provoke heartburn by a direct irritating effect independent of its pH. The local irritating effect may be amplified in GERD patients by the break-down of intercellular tight junctions by GER facilitating the entrance of acid and beverages into the epithelial layer where these substances come into contact with sensory nerve endings (Tobey *et al.*, 1996).

One of these substances, respectively, mechanisms which are responsible for the stimulation of the sensory nerve endings might be the osmolality of beverages, since Lloyd and Borda (1981) demonstrated a relationship between high osmolality of beverages and the occurrence of heartburn. While osmolality seems to be related to the induction of heartburn in sensitized patients by local irritation, it seems not to be related to the induction of GER. The amount of GER induced by white wine, red wine, and beer in healthy volunteers is significantly different (Pehl *et al.*, 1993, 1998), while all these alcoholic beverages are characterized by high osmolalities. In the studies of Pehl *et al.* (1993, 1998), the osmolalities of the applied white wine was 1,710 mosmol/l, of red wine 1,805 mosmol/l, and of beer 1,650 mosmol/l. Similarly, Becker *et al.* (1989) did not report an effect of meals with different osmolalities on GER in healthy volunteers and GERD patients. In addition, neither an ethanol solution with low osmolality nor an isovolumetric ethanol solution with high osmolality induces significantly more GER than tap water (Pehl *et al.*, 1993, 1994).

Alcoholic Beverages and Lower Esophageal Sphincter

The LES is a high-pressure zone at the junction between esophagus and stomach created by tonically active muscle fibers of the esophageal wall. The LES acts as a barrier against GER. A progressive decrease of LES pressure is seen in relation to an increasing severity of GERD (Stein *et al.*, 1992). In healthy volunteers, a decrease of LES pressure was reported after whiskey, but not after vodka (Hogan *et al.*, 1972; Keshavarzian *et al.*, 1990). Different effects on LES pressure were also observed after intake of white wine and red wine in healthy volunteers (Pehl *et al.*, 1998). While red wine did not decrease LES pressure, an impairment of LES pressure was seen after ingestion of white wine. These different effects of white wine and red wine might be the reason for the enhanced GER after white wine compared to red wine in healthy volunteers. No data exist in the literature to the effect of beer on LES pressure in healthy volunteers, GERD patients or chronic alcoholics. Moreover, the effect of alcoholic beverages on LES pressure might be habituation dependent. Keshavarzian *et al.* (1990) demonstrated that the inhibitory effect of intravenous ethanol on LES pressure was less in chronic alcoholics compared to healthy volunteers, indicating the development of tolerance. In addition, the infusion of ethanol returned the increased contraction amplitude seen in withdrawing alcoholics to normal values.

Reflux across the LES can be the result of three mechanisms (Dent *et al.*, 1988). Most of the reflux episodes occur during a LES relaxation, either swallow induced or transient. Transient LES relaxations are a vagal reflex triggered by gastric distension, for example, to permit belching after meal. In GERD, transient LES relaxations are increased in number and/or more often accompanied by a reflux event (Sifrim and Holloway, 2001). GERD patients with a lowered LES pressure can further reflux during an increase in abdominal pressure, for example during bending down, so-called "stress reflux." "Free reflux" can occur during prolonged periods of absent LES pressure which can be observed in some GERD patients postprandially. Pehl *et al.* (1998) could demonstrate that the decrease in LES pressure provoked by the intake of white wine changed the reflux pattern of the healthy volunteers with occurrence of stress and free reflux. In contrast, reflux after intake of red wine, which did not decrease LES pressure, was nearly exclusively during LES relaxations as seen normally in healthy volunteers. This data demonstrate together with the reported unchanged number of LES relaxations after white wine and red wine compared to tap water that the main mechanism of GER induction after alcoholic beverages must be a higher percentage of LES relaxations accompanied by a reflux event. Since beer increases GER comparable to red wine and less than white wine in healthy volunteers, it can be assumed that beer does not decrease LES pressure and induce GER by a higher number of reflux events during LES relaxations.

As already stated, beer and white wine induce GER in GERD patients to the same magnitude (16), while white wine is a more potent stimulator of GER in healthy volunteers (Pehl *et al.*, 1993, 1998). It can be speculated that the different effects of these beverages on LES pressure and the reflux pattern seen in healthy volunteers will not be relevant in GERD patients with an already preexisting decreased LES pressure. In these patients, beer and white wine might stimulate each type of reflux equally or the pressure reducing effect of white wine is equalized by the stronger stimulatory effect of beer on gastric acid secretion (Singer *et al.*, 1987).

Alcoholic Beverages and Esophageal Motility

Alcoholic beverages do not only increase the frequency of reflux episodes, their intake seems also to impair reflux clearance resulting in a prolonged reflux duration. A prolongation of the mean reflux duration, in part significantly, was seen after ingestion of beer, white wine, and red wine in healthy volunteers and GERD patients (Pehl *et al.*, 1998, 2006). In a reflux model with installation of 15 ml 0.1N HCl into the esophagus, a significantly enhanced number of swallows were needed to rise esophageal pH above five after oral ingestion of whiskey or white wine (Dent *et al.*, 1988; Pehl *et al.*, 2000). In line with these data, Pehl *et al.* (2002) registered a significantly increased number of peristaltic contractions necessary to rise esophageal pH > 4 after white wine induced reflux episodes. Esophageal acid clearance is a two step process (Helm *et al.*, 1983, 1984). Initially, volume clearance takes place which needs one to two peristaltic sequences, either swallow induced ("primary") or induced by esophageal distension due to reflux ("secondary"). This volume clearance is the prerequisite before saliva, swallowed with every primary peristaltic sequence, can neutralize the residual acidic layer occupying the esophageal mucosa.

Data regarding the effect of alcohol on salivary output are controversial. A diminished, an unchanged, and an increased basal and/or stimulated salivary flow is reported in chronic alcoholics with and without liver cirrhosis (Bonnin *et al.*, 1950; Kissin and Kaley, 1974; Duerr *et al.*, 1975; Abelson *et al.*, 1976; Silver *et al.*, 1986; Dutta, 1989, 1992). A stimulation of salivary flow was observed after oral intake but not after intragastric instillation of high-proof alcoholic beverages such as whiskey, brandy, sherry, and gin (Winsor and Strongin, 1933; Chittenden *et al.*, 1898). Thus, these beverages seem to stimulate salivation by local irritation. No data exist in the literature on the effect of beer on salivary flow. For wine, only data after ingestion of red wine are reported. Martin and Pangborn (1971) observed a stimulation of salivary flow with a greater stimulatory effect of red wine with an ethanol content of 12 v/v than with either 6 or 20 v/v. To our knowledge, no data exist about the effect of beer on salivary output.

Defects in esophageal peristalsis are reported in chronic alcoholics (Winship *et al.*, 1968; Keshavarzian *et al.*, 1987; Keshavarzian *et al.*, 1992). In short-time stationary esophageal manometry in healthy volunteers, an impaired wet swallow induced primary peristalsis with increased frequencies of simultaneous contractions and failed peristalsis were reported after ingestion of high-proof alcoholic beverages (Hogan *et al.*, 1972; Mayer *et al.*, 1978). In contrast, Pehl *et al.* (2000, 2002) did not observe an influence of ingestion of white wine on wet swallow induced primary peristalsis. Similarly, no disturbance of peristalsis but even an increase in contraction amplitude was seen after intake of red wine during 24-h manometry (Grande *et al.*, 1997). Likewise, by continuous measurement of pH and motility during 90 min, Pehl *et al.* (2002) also did not observe any effect of white wine on swallowing rate, contraction rate, contraction amplitude, and the rate of primary, secondary, simultaneous, and non-propagated contractions. However, when they separately analyzed the periods with esophageal pH < 4, an increased incidence of simultaneous contractions and of failed peristalsis, which insufficiently cleared reflux (Kahrilas *et al.*, 1988; Massey *et al.*, 1991), was seen after ingestion of white wine compared to tap water. Thus, at least ingestion of white wine results in a disturbed motility response after onset of GER which prolongs acid clearance. While primary peristalsis is thought to be the predominant motility pattern which clears the esophagus from refluxed material during daytime (Bremner *et al.*, 1993; Anggiansah *et al.*, 1997), secondary peristalsis seems to become more important for esophageal acid clearance during sleep (Orr *et al.*, 1981; Schoeman *et al.*, 1995) when saliva production and swallow induced primary peristalsis are strongly decreased (Schneyer *et al.*, 1956; Castiglione *et al.*, 1993). The reported disturbance in triggering secondary peristalsis by intra-esophageal air injection after ingestion of white wine (Pehl *et al.*, 2000) could therefore become important for acid clearance when wine is ingested in the evening shortly before going to bed. Unfortunately, no data on the effect of beer on esophageal motility are reported in the literature.

Beside a disturbed acid clearance, prolonged reflux episodes can also be the result of repeated reflux events ("re-reflux") into the esophagus when luminal pH is still acidic from the previous reflux event (Shay and Richter, 1998; Shay *et al.*, 2003). Shay and Richter (1998) demonstrated that re-reflux is even the main mechanism for long-lasting GER episodes. In a study in healthy volunteers (Pehl *et al.*, 2002), signs of re-reflux were observed during half of the reflux episodes after ingestion of white wine but only during 20% of the reflux episodes after ingestion of tap water. Thus, induction of reflux episodes seems to be more important than a disturbance of acid clearance for the increased percentage of time with esophageal pH < 4 after intake of alcoholic beverages.

Local or Systemic Action of Alcoholic Beverages on Esophageal Function

Hogan *et al.* (1972) and Mayer *et al.* (1978) demonstrated that ethanol can influence esophageal function systemically via the blood stream. In healthy volunteers, they observed an increase in failed esophageal peristalsis and in simultaneous contractions as well as a decrease in pentagastrin stimulated LES pressure after intravenous application of an ethanol solution resulting in blood ethanol concentrations of 0.7% to 2.0%. However, several data argue against a systemic action of alcoholic beverages on esophageal function. No correlation between the blood ethanol concentration and the observed esophageal effects was determined in the Hogan's study (1972). Additionally, white wine exerted deleterious effects on esophageal function, while an ethanol solution did not effect esophageal function despite similar blood ethanol concentrations (Pehl *et al.*, 1994). Furthermore, the reported time effects are strong arguments for a local mechanism. An increase in GER is already observed in the first 10 min after intake of beer (Shoenut *et al.*, 1998). Similarly, the decrease in LES pressure is already seen in the first 10 min after ingestion of white wine and does not further decrease in the next 10-min periods (Pehl *et al.*, 1994). Acid clearance is also prolonged immediately after ingestion of white wine and the disturbance of acid clearance diminishes within 1 h after ingestion, while blood ethanol concentration increases within the first hour after drinking (Pehl *et al.*, 2000). Last, no disturbance in triggering of secondary peristalsis was seen in healthy volunteers and chronic alcoholics by intravenous administration of ethanol (0.8 g/kg) (Keshavarzian *et al.*, 1992), while a disturbed triggering was observed after ingestion of 300 ml white wine in healthy volunteers (Pehl *et al.*, 2000).

Locally, alcoholic beverages can act by a direct toxic effect or via nerves or GI hormones. Direct depressive effects on smooth muscle cells and on nerve function are reported for ethanol (Inove and Frank, 1967; Sunano and Miyazaki, 1968; Littleton, 1978; Keshavarzian *et al.*, 1994). However, as stated above, the ethanol content is not the main ingredient responsible for the effects of alcoholic beverages on esophageal function. There are no data in the literature on the effect of alcoholic beverages on smooth muscle function. Effects of alcoholic beverages on nerve function are only reported in abstract form (Pehl *et al.*, 1996). In the reported study, white wine did not influence the EEG potentials evoked by intra-esophageal electrical stimulation. These evoked esophageal potentials are transferred to the CNS by vagal afferents.

Another mechanism by which alcoholic beverages might exert its effects is the release of GI hormones. Several data exist about the release of gastrin by alcoholic beverages. A release of gastrin is seen after ingestion of beer, white wine, and red wine, but not after intake of high-proof alcoholic beverages like whiskey, gin, and cognac (Lenz *et al.*, 1983; Singer *et al.*, 1983, 1987, 1991; Peterson *et al.*, 1986; Hajnal *et al.*, 1989, 1990, 1993; Chari *et al.*, 1996). The release of gastrin was, at least in some studies, higher after intake of beer than after intake of wine. Straathof *et al.* (1997) observed a decrease in LES pressure and an increased percentage of GER during transient LES relaxations by administration of gastrin in a dose resembling the postprandial state. However, three other studies did not find a decrease of LES pressure by gastrin (Freeland *et al.*, 1976; Jensen *et al.*, 1980; Allescher *et al.*, 1995). Another GI hormone acting on esophageal function is cholecystokinin (CCK). The CCK release postprandially seems to be related to the meal-induced decrease of LES pressure. Beer is a potent stimulator of CCK release (Masclee *et al.*, 1993; Katschinski *et al.*, 1994; Zerbib *et al.*, 1998), while only a small stimulation is seen by intake of white wine and no release after ingestion of Gin (Hajnal *et al.*, 1989, 1990, 1993; Chari *et al.*, 1996). Since white wine induces GER even stronger than beer, CCK cannot be the sole substance responsible for the effects of alcoholic beverages on GER induction.

Alcoholic Beverages and Esophageal Cancer

Chronic consumption of alcoholic beverages is a risk factor for esophageal cancer (Bagnardi *et al.*, 2001). This risk increases with an increasing daily dose of ingested alcoholic beverages (Tuyns *et al.*, 1977; Bagnardi *et al.*, 2001). Bagnardi *et al.* performed a meta-analysis of published data about the relation between alcohol consumption and the risk of cancer. From 28 studies with 7,239 cases, they calculated a pooled relative risk (and 95% confidence interval) of 1.51 (1.48–1.55), 2.21 (2.11–2.31), and 4.23 (3.91–4.59) for esophageal cancer in patients consuming 25, 50, or 100 g of alcohol per day. They calculated an especially increased risk of esophageal cancer in women with regular intake of alcoholic beverages. Smoking strongly enhances the esophageal cancer risk of drinkers by acting synergistically in carcinogenesis (Tuyns *et al.*, 1977; Bagnardi *et al.*, 2001). According to type of esophageal cancer, alcoholic beverages are surely a risk factor for esophageal squamous cell cancer (Brown *et al.*, 1994; Vaughan *et al.*, 1995; Wu *et al.*, 2001; Bollschweiler *et al.*, 2002; Lindblad *et al.*, 2005), while there are conflicting data whether consumption of alcoholic beverages are a risk factor for esophageal adenocarcinoma.

Several researchers attempted to determine whether different types of alcoholic beverages have different effects on cancer risk. Compared to wine, the cancer risk of beer was reported to be similar (Williams and Horn, 1977; Doll *et al.*, 1999), increased (Graham *et al.*, 1990; Gammon *et al.*, 1997) or decreased (Barra *et al.*, 1990; Bosetti *et al.*, 2000). Other alcoholic beverages possibly linked to the esophageal cancer risk are the intake of liquor (Williams and Horn, 1977; Brown *et al.*, 1994; Bahmanyar and Ye, 2006), spirits (Doll *et al.*, 1999), apple brandy, and hard cider (Tuyns *et al.*, 1979; Yamada *et al.*, 1992).

There is no evidence that alcohol by itself can cause cancer by acting as a complete carcinogen. However, animal studies have indicated that alcohol can have a co-carcinogenic or cancer-promoting effect. For example, Yamada *et al.* (1992) observed an exaggerated nitrosamine bioactivation by intake of beer and other alcoholic beverages in rats. Nitrosamines and other carcinogens like polycyclic hydrocarbon or acetaldehyde can be found in alcoholic beverages (Blot, 1992; Poschl *et al.*, 2004). In addition, metabolism of ethanol by alcohol dehydrogenase results in the formation of acetaldehyde, which is a potent carcinogen (Salaspuro, 2003). The enzyme alcohol dehydrogenase is, beside the liver, already localized in the upper GI tract (Vaglenova *et al.*, 2003). Bacterial flora of the oropharynx and in the upper GI tract can contribute to the local accumulation of acetaldehyde due to bacterial metabolism of ethanol (Homann *et al.*, 1997a, b, 2000). Smoking can further increase the formation of acetaldehyde by inducing changes in the oral bacterial flora (Homann *et al.*, 2000; Poschl *et al.*, 2004). It becomes obvious from these data why drinking and smoking potentiate its cancer risks. In addition, genetic polymorphisms of the alcohol dehydrogenase gene and the acetaldehyde dehydrogenase gene seem to be linked to an increased risk of esophageal (squamous cell) cancer risk due to higher blood and salivary acetaldehyde levels (Yokoyama *et al.*, 1996; Visapaa *et al.*, 2004).

Summary

Beer, like other alcoholic beverages, has deleterious effects on esophageal function. Its intake can induce heartburn and GER in healthy volunteers and GERD patients. The effects of beer seem to be locally transmitted by acting on acid secretion, reflux induction, and esophageal motility. In addition, chronic consumption of beer increases the risk for esophageal cancer, especially for squamous cell cancer.

Summary Points

- Intake of beer induces GER in healthy volunteers.
- Intake of beer induces GER in patients with GERD.
- The magnitude of reflux induction is less after beer than after white wine in healthy volunteers, but seems to be similar in reflux patients.
- There are no data on the effect of beer on esophageal peristalsis, while depressive effects were reported for whiskey, vodka, and white wine, but not for red wine.
- Other ingredients than ethanol are responsible for the effects of alcoholic beverages on esophageal function.
- The effects of alcoholic beverages on esophageal function seem to be induced locally.
- Chronic consumption of beer and other alcoholic beverages increase the risk for esophageal cancer (i.e. of squamous cell cancer).
- The cancer risk of alcoholic beverages is potentiated by smoking.

References

Abelson, D.C., Mandel, I.D. and Karmiol, M. (1976). *Oral Surg. Oral Med. Oral Pathol.* 41, 188–192.

Allescher, H.D., Stoschus, B., Wunsch, E., Schusdziarra, V. and Classen, M. (1995). *Z. Gastroenterol.* 33, 385–391.

Anggiansah, A., Taylor, G., Marshall, R.E., Bright, N.F., Owen, W.A. and Owen, W.J. (1997). *Gut* 41, 600–605.

Bagnardi, V., Blangiardo, M., La Vecchia, C. and Corrao, G. (2001). *Alcohol Res. Health* 25, 263–270.

Bahmanyar, S. and Ye, W. (2006). *Nutr. Cancer* 54, 171–178.

Barra, S., Franceschi, S., Negri, E., Talamini, R. and La Vecchia, C. (1990). *Int. J. Cancer* 46, 1017–1020.

Becker, D.J., Sinclair, J., Castell, D.O. and Wu, W.C. (1989). *Am. J. Gastroenterol.* 84, 782–786.

Blot, W.J. (1992). *Cancer Res.* 52, 2119s–2123s.

Bollschweiler, E., Wolfgarten, E., Nowroth, T., Rosendahl, U., Monig, S.P. and Holscher, A.H. (2002). *J. Cancer Res. Clin. Oncol.* 128, 575–580.

Bonnin, H., Morretti, G. and Geyer, A. (1950). *Presse Med* 62, 1449–1451.

Bor, S., Bor-Caymaz, C., Tobey, N.A., Abdulnour-Nakhoul, S. and Orlando, R.C. (1999). *Dig. Dis. Sci.* 44, 290–300.

Bosetti, C., La Vecchia, C., Negri, E. and Franceschi, S. (2000). *Eur. J. Clin. Nutr.* 54, 918–920.

Bremner, R.M., Hoeft, S.F., Costantini, M., Crookes, P.F., Bremner, C.G. and DeMeester, T.R. (1993). *Ann. Surg.* 218, 364–369. discussion 369–370.

Brown, L.M., Silverman, D.T., Pottern, L.M., Schoenberg, J.B., Greenberg, R.S., Swanson, G.M., Liff, J.M., Schwartz, A.G., Hayes, R.B., Blot, W.J. *et al.* (1994). *Cancer Causes Control* 5, 333–340.

Castiglione, F., Emde, C., Armstrong, D., Schneider, C., Bauerfeind, P., Stacher, G. and Blum, A.L. (1993). *Gut* 34, 1653–1659.

Chari, S.T., Harder, H., Teyssen, S., Knodel, C., Riepl, R.L. and Singer, M.V. (1996). *Dig. Dis. Sci.* 41, 1216–1224.

Chittenden, R., Mendel, L. and Jackson, H. (1898). *Am. J. Physiol.* 1, 164–209.

Dent, J., Holloway, R.H., Toouli, J. and Dodds, W.J. (1988). *Gut* 29, 1020–1028.

Doll, R., Forman, D., La Vecchia, C. and Woutersen, R. (1999). In Macdonal, I. (ed.), *Health Issues Related to Alcohol Consumption*, pp. 351–393. Blackwell Science Ltd, Oxford.

Duerr, H., Bode, J. and Gieseking, R. (1975). *Verh. Dtsch. Ges. Inn. Med.* 81, 1322–1324.

Dutta, S.K., Dukehart, M., Narang, A. and Latham, P.S. (1989). *Gastroenterology* 96, 510–518.

Dutta, S.K., Orestes, M., Vengulekur, S. and Kwo, P. (1992). *Am. J. Gastroenterol.* 87, 350–354.

Feldman, M. and Barnett, C. (1995). *Gastroenterology* 108, 125–131.

Freeland, G.R., Higgs, R.H., Castell, D.O. and McGuigan, J.E. (1976). *Gastroenterology* 71, 570–574.

Gammon, M.D., Schoenberg, J.B., Ahsan, H., Risch, H.A., Vaughan, T.L., Chow, W.H., Rotterdam, H., West, A.B., Dubrow, R., Stanford, J.L., Mayne, S.T., Farrow, D.C., Niwa, S., Blot, W.J. and Fraumeni Jr, J.F. (1997). *J. Natl. Cancer Inst.* 89, 1277–1284.

Graham, S., Marshall, J., Haughey, B., Brasure, J., Freudenheim, J., Zielezny, M., Wilkinson, G. and Nolan, J. (1990). *Am. J. Epidemiol.* 131, 454–467.

Grande, L., Manterola, C., Ros, E., Lacima, G. and Pera, C. (1997). *Dig. Dis. Sci.* 42, 1189–1193.

Hajnal, F., Flores, M.C. and Valenzuela, J.E. (1989). *Pancreas* 4, 486–491.

Hajnal, F., Flores, M.C., Radley, S. and Valenzuela, J.E. (1990). *Gastroenterology* 98, 191–196.

Hajnal, F., Flores, M.C. and Valenzuela, J.E. (1993). *Dig. Dis. Sci.* 38, 12–17.

Helm, J.F., Dodds, W.J., Riedel, D.R., Teeter, B.C., Hogan, W.J. and Arndorfer, R.C. (1983). *Gastroenterology* 85, 607–612.

Helm, J.F., Dodds, W.J., Pelc, L.R., Palmer, D.W., Hogan, W.J. and Teeter, B.C. (1984). *New Engl. J. Med.* 310, 284–288.

Hogan, W.J., Viegas de Andrade, S.R. and Winship, D.H. (1972). *J. Appl. Physiol.* 32, 755–760.

Homann, N., Jousimies-Somer, H., Jokelainen, K., Heine, R. and Salaspuro, M. (1997a). *Carcinogenesis* 18, 1739–1743.

Homann, N., Karkkainen, P., Koivisto, T., Nosova, T., Jokelainen, K. and Salaspuro, M. (1997b). *J. Natl. Cancer. Inst.* 89, 1692–1697.

Homann, N., Tillonen, J., Meurman, J.H., Rintamaki, H., Lindqvist, C., Rautio, M., Jousimies-Somer, H. and Salaspuro, M. (2000). *Carcinogenesis* 21, 663–668.

Inove, F. and Frank, G. (1967). *Br. J. Pharmacol.* 30, 186–193.

Jensen, D.M., McCallum, R.W., Corazziari, E., Elashoff, J. and Walsh, J.H. (1980). *Gastroenterology* 79, 431–438.

Kahrilas, P.J., Dodds, W.J. and Hogan, W.J. (1988). *Gastroenterology* 94, 73–80.

Katschinski, M., Schirra, J., Koppelberg, T., Arnold, R., Rovati, L.C., Beglinger, C. and Adler, G. (1994). *Dig. Dis. Sci.* 38, 983–989.

Kaufman, S.E. and Kaye, M.D. (1978). *Gut* 19, 336–338.

Keshavarzian, A., Iber, F.L. and Ferguson, Y. (1987). *Gastroenterology* 92, 651–657.

Keshavarzian, A., Polepalle, C., Iber, F.L. and Durkin, M. (1990). *Alcohol. Clin. Exp. Res.* 14, 561–567.

Keshavarzian, A., Polepalle, C., Iber, F.L. and Durkin, M. (1992). *Dig. Dis. Sci.* 37, 517–522.

Keshavarzian, A., Zorub, O., Sayeed, M., Urban, G., Sweeney, C., Winship, D. and Fields, J. (1994). *J. Pharmacol. Exp. Ther.* 270, 1057–1062.

Kissin, B. and Kaley, M. (1974). In Kissin, B. and Begleiter, H. (eds), *The Biology of Alcoholism*, pp. 481–511. Plenum Publishing, New York.

Lenz, H.J., Ferrari-Taylor, J. and Isenberg, J.I. (1983). *Gastroenterology* 85, 1082–1087.

Lindblad, M., Rodriguez, L.A. and Lagergren, J. (2005). *Cancer Causes Control* 16, 285–294.

Littleton, J. (1978). *Clin. Endocrinol. Metab.* 7, 369–384.

Lloyd, D.A. and Borda, I.T. (1981). *Gastroenterology* 80, 740–741.

Martin, S. and Pangborn, R.M. (1971). *J. Dent. Res.* 50, 485–490.

Masclee, A.A., Jansen, J.B., Rovati, L.C. and Lamers, C.B. (1993). *Dig. Dis. Sci.* 38, 1889–1892.

Massey, B.T., Dodds, W.J., Hogan, W.J., Brasseur, J.G. and Helm, J.F. (1991). *Gastroenterology* 101, 344–354.

Mayer, E.M., Grabowski, C.J. and Fisher, R.S. (1978). *Gastroenterology* 75, 1133–1136.

McArthur, K., Hogan, D. and Isenberg, J.I. (1982). *Gastroenterology* 83, 199–203.

Orr, W.C., Robinson, M.G. and Johnson, L.F. (1981). *Dig. Dis. Sci.* 26, 423–427.

Pehl, C., Wendl, B., Pfeiffer, A., Schmidt, T. and Kaess, H. (1993). *Dig. Dis. Sci.* 38, 93–96.

Pehl, C., Pfeiffer, A., Wendl, B., Schmidt, T. and Kaess, H. (1994). *Neurogastroenterol. Mot.* 6, 43–47.

Pehl, C., Pfeiffer, A., Schmidt, T. and Kaess, H. (1996). *Neurogastroenterol. Mot.* 8, 186.

Pehl, C., Pfeiffer, A., Wendl, B. and Kaess, H. (1998). *Scand. J. Gastroenterol.* 33, 118–122.

Pehl, C., Frommherz, M., Wendl, B., Schmidt, T. and Pfeiffer, A. (2000). *Scand. J. Gastroenterol.* 35, 1255–1259.

Pehl, C., Frommherz, M., Wendl, B. and Pfeiffer, A. (2002). *Am. J. Gastroenterol.* 97, 561–567.

Pehl, C., Czekalla, R. and Schepp, W. (2004). *Med. Klinik.* 99, 86.

Pehl, C., Wendl, B. and Pfeiffer, A. (2006). *Aliment. Pharmacol. Ther.* 23, 1581–1586.

Peterson, W.L., Barnett, C. and Walsh, J.H. (1986). *Gastroenterology* 91, 1390–1395.

Poschl, G., Stickel, F., Wang, X.D. and Seitz, H.K. (2004). *Proc. Nutr. Soc.* 63, 65–71.

Salaspuro, M.P. (2003). *Best Pract. Res. Clin. Gastroenterol.* 17, 679–694.

Salo, J.A. (1983). *Scand. J. Gastroenterol.* 18, 713–721.

Savary, M. and Miller, G. (ed.) (1978). *Handbook and Atlas of Endoscopy*. Gassmann Ltd, Solothurn, Switzerland.

Schneyer, L.H., Pigman, W., Hanahan, L. and Gilmore, R.W. (1956). *J. Dent. Res.* 35, 109–114.

Schoeman, M.N., Tippett, M.D., Akkermans, L.M., Dent, J. and Holloway, R.H. (1995). *Gastroenterology* 108, 83–91.

Shay, S.S. and Richter, J.E. (1998). *Dig. Dis. Sci.* 43, 95–102.

Shay, S.S., Johnson, L.F. and Richter, J.E. (2003). *Dig. Dis. Sci.* 48, 1–9.

Shoenut, J.P., Duerksen, D. and Yaffe, C.S. (1998). *Dig. Dis. Sci.* 43, 834–839.

Sifrim, D. and Holloway, R. (2001). *Am. J. Gastroenterol.* 96, 2529–2532.

Silver, L.S., Worner, T.M. and Korsten, M.A. (1986). *Am. J. Gastroenterol.* 81, 423–427.

Singer, M.V., Eysselein, V. and Goebell, H. (1983). *Digestion* 26, 73–79.

Singer, M.V., Leffmann, C., Eysselein, V.E., Calden, H. and Goebell, H. (1987). *Gastroenterology* 93, 1247–1254.

Singer, M.V., Teyssen, S. and Eysselein, V.E. (1991). *Gastroenterology* 101, 935–942.

Stein, H.J., Barlow, A.P., DeMeester, T.R. and Hinder, R.A. (1992). *Ann. Surg.* 216, 35–43.

Straathof, J.W., Lamers, C.B. and Masclee, A.A. (1997). *Dig. Dis. Sci.* 42, 2547–2551.

Sunano, S. and Miyazaki, E. (1968). *Sapporo. Igaku. Zasshi.* 34, 292–301.

Teyssen, S., Lenzing, T., Gonzalez-Calero, G., Korn, A., Riepl, R.L. and Singer, M.V. (1997). *Gut* 40, 49–56.

Tobey, N.A., Carson, J.L., Alkiek, R.A. and Orlando, R.C. (1996). *Gastroenterology* 11, 1200–1205.

Tonnesen, H., Andersen, J.R., Christoffersen, P. and Kaas-Claesson, N. (1987). *Digestion* 38, 69–73.

Tuyns, A.J., Pequignot, G. and Jensen, O.M. (1977). *Bull. Cancer* 64, 45–60.

Tuyns, A.J., Pequignot, G. and Abbatucci, J.S. (1979). *Int. J. Cancer* 23, 443–447.

Vaezi, M.F., Singh, S. and Richter, J.E. (1995). *Gastroenterology* 108, 1897–1907.

Vaglenova, J., Martinez, S.E., Porte, S., Duester, G., Farres, J. and Pares, X. (2003). *Eur. J. Biochem.* 270, 2652–2662.

Vaughan, T.L., Davis, S., Kristal, A. and Thomas, D.B. (1995). *Cancer Epidemiol. Biomarkers Prev.* 4, 85–92.

Visapaa, J.P., Gotte, K., Benesova, M., Li, J., Homann, N., Conradt, C., Inoue, H., Tisch, M., Horrmann, K., Vakevainen, S., Salaspuro, M. and Seitz, H.K. (2004). *Gut* 53, 871–876.

Vitale, G.C., Cheadle, W.G., Patel, B., Sadek, S.A., Michel, M.E. and Cuschieri, A. (1987). *JAMA* 258, 2077–2079.

Williams, R. and Horn, J. (1977). *J. Natl. Cancer Inst.* 58.

Winship, D.H., Caflisch, C.R., Zboralske, F.F. and Hogan, W.J. (1968). *Gastroenterology* 55, 173–178.

Winsor, A. and Strongin, E. (1933). *J. Exp. Psych.* 16, 589–597.

Wu, A.H., Wan, P. and Bernstein, L. (2001). *Cancer Causes Control* 12, 721–732.

Yamada, Y., Weller, R.O., Kleihues, P. and Ludeke, B.I. (1992). *Carcinogenesis* 13, 1171–1175.

Yokoyama, A., Muramatsu, T., Ohmori, T., Makuuchi, H., Higuchi, S., Matsushita, S., Yoshino, K., Maruyama, K., Nakano, M. and Ishii, H. (1996). *Cancer* 77, 1986–1990.

Zerbib, F., Bruley Des Varannes, S., Scarpignato, C., Leray, V., D'Amato, M., Roze, C. and Galmiche, J.P. (1998). *Am. J. Physiol.* 275, G1266–G1273.

58

Effects of Beer on the Gastric Mucosa as Determined by Endoscopy

Andreas Franke and Manfred V. Singer Department of Medicine II (Gastroenterology, Hepatology and Infectious Diseases), University Hospital of Heidelberg at Mannheim, Mannheim, Germany

Abstract

It is clinically well known that alcohol consumption, especially in excess, may cause acute gastrointestinal bleeding and hemorrhagic gastritis. Induction of hemorrhagic lesions was endoscopically proven for pure ethanol solutions in concentrations between 40% and 80% by several studies. However, the data on the effect of alcoholic beverages and their corresponding ethanol concentrations is rare. Only in one study the effect of beer, some other alcoholic beverages and their appropriate control solutions (4% and 10% v/v ethanol and isotonic saline) was endoscopically examined in humans. Additionally, the time-dependent course of potential lesions was determined. According to these results, beer induces gastric mucosal injury in healthy non-alcoholic volunteers that are endoscopically detectable 30, 60 and 240 min after the application. After 24 h those lesions are completely healed. However, the injury by 4% ethanol is significantly stronger than that of beer. Beer may contain ingredients that protect the gastric mucosa against the damaging action of ethanol.

Introduction

In some, mostly uncontrolled, endoscopic studies in humans ethanol in high concentrations (40–80% v/v) was shown to damage gastric mucosa (Agrawal *et al.*, 1986; Tarnawski *et al.*, 1987; Cohen *et al.*, 1989, 1990; Kobayashi *et al.*, 1991; Konturek *et al.*, 1992; Loguercio *et al.*, 1993). However, the physiological relevance has been challenged since in everyday life it is not pure ethanol that is consumed, but palatable alcoholic beverages. Moreover, beer and wine contain ethanol in much lower concentrations.

As early as 1833, William Beaumont (1833) observed in a patient suffering from a gastric stoma due to a gunshot injury that consumption of different alcoholic beverages caused gastric mucosal erythema and erosions, which appeared after 4–5 days of abstinence. Over 100 years later, Palmer (1954) investigated 34 subjects within 6 h after ingestion of alcoholic beverages, the type of beverage is not specified in the publication. Thirty (of 34) had acute gastritis findings, based on patchy hyperemia, erosions, petechiae and purulent exsudate. In 22 subjects, gastroscopy was repeated after 7–20 days of abstinence from alcohol, at which point gastric mucosa appeared normal. Laine and Weinstein (1988) characterized the endoscopic features of hemorrhagic and erosive gastric lesions in 148 alcoholic patients (50–330 g mean pure ethanol consumption), who underwent upper gastrointestinal endoscopy for gastrointestinal bleeding. In 20 patients, subepithelial hemorrhages were predominantly found in the proximal stomach.

The effect of moderate amounts of beer in non-alcoholic individuals was uninvestigated until Knoll *et al.* (1998) studied the effect of some commonly consumed alcoholic beverages and their corresponding ethanol concentrations and amounts on gastric mucosa in healthy humans.

Study Design

Knoll *et al.* (1998) carried out the first endoscopy between 9.00 a.m. and 10.00 a.m. on day 1 (Figure 58.1), after the healthy volunteers have fasted overnight. All remaining gastric juice was carefully aspirated through the suction channel of the endoscope. One of the following test solutions (100 ml each) was sprayed onto the mucosa of the anterior wall of the antrum: beer (4.5% v/v), 4% (v/v) ethanol and isotonic saline solutions. Moreover, white wine, whiskey and their corresponding ethanol solutions (10% and 40% (v/v), respectively) were tested. Endoscopists and subject were blinded to the kind of instilled solution; 30 min later a second endoscopy was done to aspirate the remaining test solution out of the stomach. The endoscopic appearance of fundic, antral and duodenal mucosa was assessed before, immediately after, and 30, 60, 240 min and 24 h after instillation. The endoscopically visible mucosal lesions were scored by three independent endocopists using the Tarnawski grading system (Table 58.1). The integrated endoscopic scores over the examination time were calculated and compared between the test solutions.

Beer in Health and Disease Prevention
ISBN: 978-0-12-373891-2

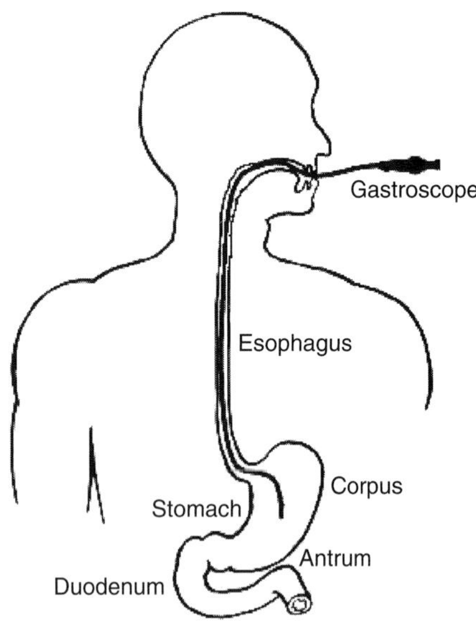

Figure 58.1 Gastroscopy. Anatomy and endoscopy of the upper gastrointestinal tract.

Table 58.1 Classification of gastric mucosal inflammation

0	Normal mucosa
1	Marked diffuse hyperemia
2	Single hemorrhagic lesion (1 mm or larger)
3	2–5 hemorrhagic lesions
4	6–9 hemorrhagic lesions
5	10 or more hemorrhagic lesions or larger area of confluent hemorrhage

Source: Tarnawski endoscopic grading system (Tarnawski *et al.*, 1987).

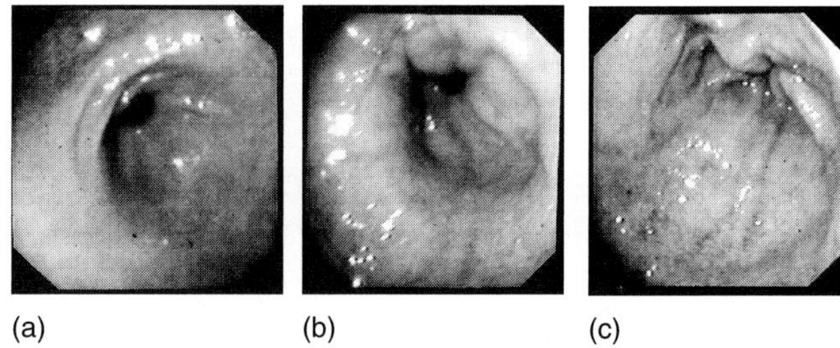

Figure 58.2 Changes of gastric mucosa after alcoholic beverages: (a) gastric mucosa of the antrum as seen before, (b) after instillation of beer and (c) after instillation of whiskey.

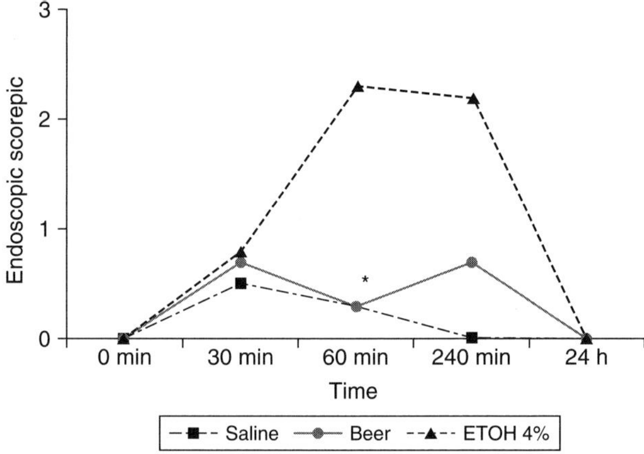

Figure 58.3 Effect of beer and its control solutions on gastric mucosa. Mean endoscopic scores in response to beer, 4% (v/v) ethanol and isotonic saline on the mucosa of the fundus. *$p < 0.05$ vs. corresponding ethanol solution (4% v/v).

Effect of Beer and Its Control Solutions

Intragastric beer instillation induced 30 and 60 min after instillation of single erosions in the antrum and fundus (Figure 58.2a and b). After 240 min, these findings were nearly unchanged, and after 24 h normal mucosa was detected in all subjects (Figure 58.3). Duodenal mucosa was normal at all time points.

After intragastric instillation of isotonic saline either no or up to five lesions in the antrum and fundus were observed at 30 min (Figure 58.3). After 60 min these lesions were still present and after 240 min they were disappeared in the fundus. At 24 h normal mucosa was observed in all subjects. Duodenal mucosa was normal at all time points.

Intragastric instillation of 4% ethanol produced either no lesions, hyperemia or single lesions in the antrum and hyperemia in the fundus in all subjects at 30 min (Figure 58.3). These findings were unchanged after 60 and 240 min and they were no longer demonstrable after 24 h. Again, duodenal mucosa was normal at all time points.

Comparison between the mean endoscopic score for beer and its corresponding ethanol content (4% (v/v)) resulted in a significant higher score for 4% ethanol than for beer at 60 min in the fundus (Figure 58.3). At all other time points the mean scores in the antrum and fundus in response to beer and 4% ethanol were not significantly different. However, 4% ethanol significantly increases the 24-h integrated endoscopic score in the fundus, but not in the antrum, as compared to beer (Figure 58.4).

Effect of Other Alcoholic Beverages and Higher Ethanol Concentrations

White wine, whiskey, 10% and 40% (v/v) ethanol induced also significant hyperemia and hemorrhagic lesions after intragastric application.

Intragastric instillation of white wine induced hyperemia and/or up to five erosions in the antrum and fundus at 30 min, with a maximum at 60 min. At 240 min, these lesions were still present, but to a lesser degree. Normal mucosa was found after 24 h.

The corresponding ethanol solution (10% v/v) produced two to more than ten erosions in the antrum and fundus at 30 min. After 60 and 240 min, these findings were unchanged. Lesions were still present, but to a lesser degree after 24 h.

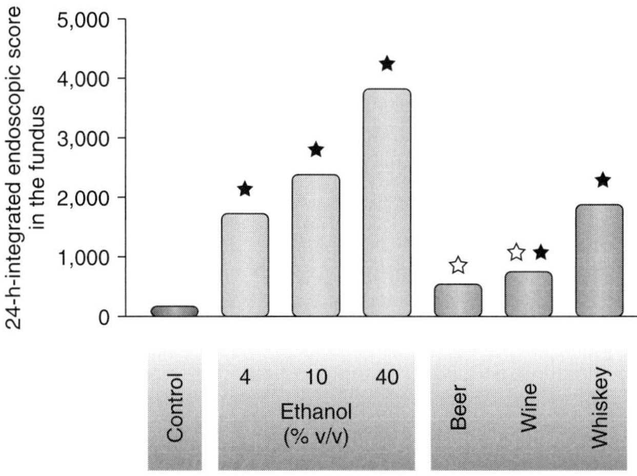

Figure 58.4 Effect of some alcoholic beverages and corresponding ethanol concentrations on gastric mucosa. Integrated endoscopic scores over 24h in the fundus in response to beer, wine and whiskey and the corresponding ethanol content (4%, 10% and 40% v/v) in comparison with the control. The results are expressed as means of 6 subjects and 11 subjects (whiskey). #$p < 0.05$ compared with control (★) or with corresponding ethanol content (☆).

The comparison between white wine and 10% ethanol resulted in a significantly higher score in the antrum at 24h and in a significantly higher 24-h integrated endoscopic score in the antrum and fundus (Figure 58.4).

Whiskey caused hyperemia and up to more than 10 erosions in the fundus and antrum within 30min (Figure 58.2c). This was still present after 60min and to a lesser degree after 240min and 24h. The corresponding ethanol solution (40% v/v) resulted in a significantly higher score in the fundus at 240min and in a significantly increased 24-h integrated endoscopic score in the antrum and fundus (Figure 58.4).

Conclusions

This study demonstrates that beer induces gastric mucosa injury. Other alcoholic beverages like wine and whiskey also damage the gastric mucosa. Hemorrhagic lesions can last for more than 24h after consumption of whiskey. Ingestion of ethanol also in lower concentrations (4% and 10% v/v) causes hemorrhagic erosions in the antral and fundic gastric mucosa. In case of 10% (v/v) ethanol and higher concentration (40% v/v), but not after 4% (v/v) ethanol, erosions were still present after 24h. This suggests that ethanol in concentrations of over 10% breaks the gastric mucosal barrier. Davenport found in dogs that ethanol in concentrations higher than 8–14% damages the mucosal barrier and allow thereby diffusion of hydrogen ions from the lumen into the mucosa, which induced a potential difference (Davenport, 1967; Singer *et al.*, 1983).

Alcoholic beverages and pure ethanol may induce gastric lesions by direct toxic effects as well as by an increased gastric acid response (Singer *et al.*, 1983, 1987, 1991). Pure ethanol in low concentrations (1.4% and 4%) is a mild stimulant of gastric acid secretion, whereas in higher concentrations (5–40%), it has either no inhibitory effect, or a mild one (Singer *et al.*, 1983). On the other hand, alcoholic beverages with low ethanol content (beer and wine) are strong stimulants of gastric acid output and gastrin release (Singer *et al.*, 1987, 1991). It is possible that alcoholic beverages may contain some unknown non-alcoholic ingredients that protect the mucosa against the damaging effect of ethanol and hydrochloric acid. It is also possible that the high buffer capacity of the proteins, and other ingredients of alcoholic beverages, reduces the damaging effect of the ethanol.

Summary Points

- Beer and other alcoholic beverages (e.g. wine and whiskey) may induce gastric mucosal injury.
- Intragastric administration of ethanol in concentrations of 4%, 10%, 40% and higher also causes mucosal lesions in the gastric fundus and antrum, but not in the duodenum.
- Mucosal lesions after beer or corresponding ethanol concentration occur within 30min, reach maximum after 60–240min and are disappeared after 24h, whereas lesions after 10% and 40% or after whiskey last more than 24h.
- Mucosal injury caused by alcoholic beverages is less pronounced than by the corresponding ethanol concentrations.
- Non-alcoholic ingredients in beer (and other alcoholic beverages) may have protective effects on ethanol-induced mucosal injury.

References

Agrawal, N.M., Godiwala, T., Arimura, A. and Dajani, E.Z. (1986). *Gastrointest. Endosc.* 32, 67–70.

Beaumont, W. (1833/1959). *Experiments and Observations on the Gastric Juice and the Physiology of Digestion* [facsimile of the original edition of 1833], pp. 108–237. Dover, New York.

Cohen, M.M., Bowdler, R., Gervais, P., Morris, G.P. and Wang, H.R. (1989). *Gastroenterology* 96, 292–298.

Cohen, M.M., Yeung, R., Wang, H.R. and Clark, L. (1990). *Gastroenterology* 99, 45–50.

Davenport, H.W. (1967). *Proc. Soc. Exp. Biol. Med.* 126, 657–662.

Davenport, H.W. (1969). *Gastroenterology* 56, 439–449.

Knoll, M.R., Kölbel, C.B., Teyssen, S. and Singer, M.V. (1998). *Endoscopy* 30, 293–301.

Kobayashi, K., Arakawa, T., Higuchi, K. and Nakaruma, H. (1991). *J. Clin. Gastroenterol.* 13, 32–36.

Konturek, S.J., Maczka, J., Kaminski, K., Sito, E., Torres, J. and Oleksy, J. (1992). *Scand. J. Gastroenterol.* 27, 438–442.

Laine, L. and Weinstein, W.M. (1988). *Gastroenterology* 94, 1254–1262.

Loguercio, C., Taranto, D., Beneduce, F., del Vecchio Blanco, C., de Vincentiis, A., Nardi, G. and Romano, M. (1993). *Gut* 34, 161–165.

Palmer, E.D. (1954). *Medicine* 33, 199–290.

Singer, M.V., Eysselein, V.E. and Goebel, H. (1983). *Digestion* 26, 73–79.

Singer, M.V., Leffmann, C., Eysselein, V.E., Calden, H. and Goebell, H. (1987). *Gastroenterology* 93, 1247–1254.

Singer, M.V., Teyssen, S. and Eysselein, V.E. (1991). *Gastroenterology* 101, 935–942.

Tarnawski, A., Hollander, D., Stachura, J., Klimszyk, B., Mach, T. and Bogdal, J. (1987). *Clin. Invest. Med.* 3, 259–263.

59

The Effect of Beer and Its Non-alcoholic Ingredients on Secretory and Motoric Function of the Stomach

Andreas Franke and Manfred V. Singer Department of Medicine II (Gastroenterology, Hepatology and Infectious Diseases), University Hospital of Heidelberg, Mannheim, Germany

Abstract

Alcoholic beverages produced by fermentation like beer and wine strongly stimulate gastric acid secretion, whereas those produced by distillation (e.g. whisky, gin) have no stimulatory effect. Pure ethanol affects gastric acid secretion dose dependently: lower ethanol concentrations (1.4% and 4% v/v) have a mild, but significant stimulatory effect, whereas higher ethanol concentrations have no effect (5–10% v/v) or even a mild inhibitory effect (20% and 40% v/v). Non-alcoholic ingredients in alcoholic beverages produced by fermentation have to be responsible for the strong stimulation of gastric acid secretion. After separation by chromatography maleic acid and succinic acid could be identified to be responsible for the strong stimulatory effect of beer on gastric acid secretion.

Alcoholic beverages and corresponding pure ethanol concentrations (4%, 10% and 40% v/v) are significantly slower emptied from the stomach than water: Gastric emptying of beer and wine, alcoholic beverages produced by fermentation, but not that of alcoholic beverages produced by distillation (e.g. whisky), is significantly slower than that of their corresponding ethanol solutions. Beer, other alcoholic beverages such as wine and whisky, and corresponding ethanol solutions (4% and 10% v/v) also inhibit gastric emptying of solid meals. The inhibitory effect results from a decelaration of the emptying phase, whereas in the initial lag-phase, the period of time between the end of consumption and the start of gastric emptying is unaffected by the alcoholic beverages.

List of Abbreviations

w/v Weight per volume
v/v Volume per volume
MAO Maximal acid output

Introduction

It is a popular belief that alcoholic beverages (e.g. beer and wine) improve digestive functions when consumed alone or together with meals. However, information about the effects of alcoholic beverages on gastric secretion and motility were scanty for a long time. Controlled studies on the effect of alcoholic beverages as well as their alcoholic and non-alcoholic content on gastric secretory and motor function were only published during the last two decades.

It is about 100 years ago that after uncontrolled experiments with alcohol a stimulatory effect on gastric acid secretion was suggested (Chittenden *et al.*, 1898; Beazell and Ivy, 1940). In the early 1980s the first systematic and controlled studies on the effect of pure ethanol and commonly ingested alcoholic beverages on gastric acid secretion have been published (McArthur *et al.*, 1982; Lenz *et al.*, 1983; Singer *et al.*, 1983; Peterson *et al.*, 1986). Singer *et al.* (1987) compared the effect of different ethanol concentrations with the maximal acid output (MAO) induced by pentagastrin stimulation. They found that the effect of ethanol on gastric acid secretion in healthy humans is differentiated and concentration dependent: low concentrations (1.4% and 4.0% v/v) have a mild stimulatory effect on gastric acid output. Higher concentrations of pure ethanol (up to 40% v/v) have either no or if at all a mild inhibitory effect (Figure 59.1).

In contrast, alcoholic beverages with low ethanol concentration such as beer and wine are powerful stimulants of gastric acid output (Figure 59.2) (Singer *et al.*, 1991). Oral ingestion or gastric instillation of beer causes a stimulation of acid output to 95% of the MAO produced by pentagastrin stimulation (MAO). Red and white wines increase gastric acid output to 61% of MAO (Singer *et al.*, 1991).

On the other hand, beverages with a higher alcohol content, such as whisky, gin or cognac (ethanol concentration of approximately 40% v/v), do not stimulate gastric acid output (Singer *et al.*, 1987) (Figure 59.2).

The ethanol content in beer (4% v/v) and wine (10% v/v) is only partially or not at all responsible for the marked gastric acid secretory response to beer and wine. Thus, non-alcoholic ingredients in beer and wine are most likely responsible for the stimulatory effect of these alcoholic beverages.

Beer in Health and Disease Prevention
ISBN: 978-0-12-373891-2

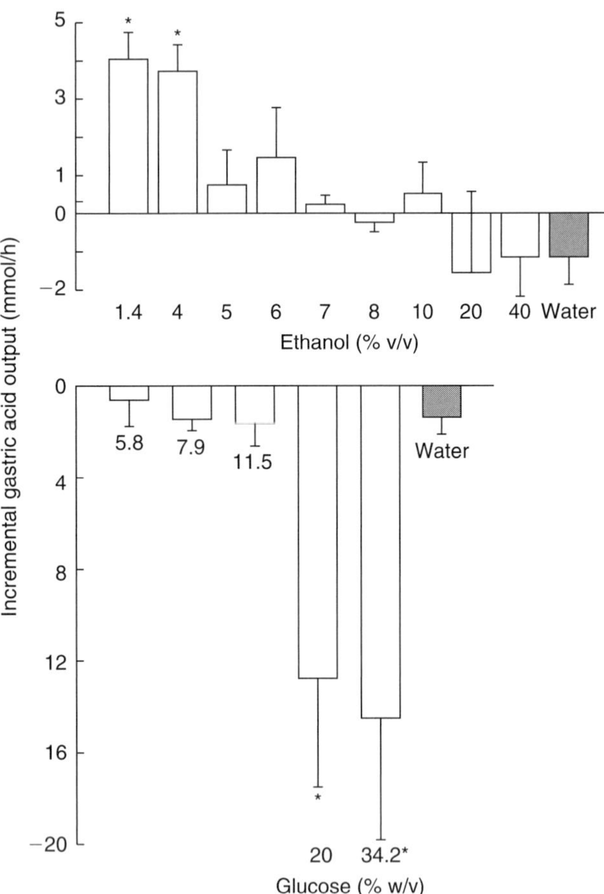

Figure 59.1 Effect of ethanol and glucose on gastric acid secretion. Effect of intragastric instillation of ethanol, distilled water and glucose on incremental 1-h gastric acid output. The 7.9%, 11.5%, 20% and 34.2% (w/v) glucose solutions are equivalent to 1.4%, 4%, 10% and 20% ethanol (v/v), respectively. Results are mean ± SEM of six subjects. *$p < 0.05$ compared with both distilled water and the isotonic glucose control solution. *Source*: Reprinted from Singer *et al.* (1987). Copyright 1987, with permission from the American Gastroenterological Association.

Singer *et al.* (1991) studied the effect of beer and its known ingredients before and after fermentation on gastric acid secretion (Figure 59.3). The effect of magnesium, calcium, amines, vitamins, organic acids, purines, amino acids and phenols in concentrations and amounts comparable to beer was examined. They found that none of the 11 tested ingredients of fermented beer (alone or in combination) nor hop extract had any significant effect (Table 59.1). However, finished beer (6 weeks old) and new beer were potent stimuli of acid output. Before the addition of yeast, preproducts of beer were considerably less potent. Thus, first and finished wort caused only a minor acid response (48% and 46% of MAO, respectively). Foreign fermentation in first and finished wort is presumably the reason for the stimulatory effect because glucose solution in concentrations seen in wort (11.5% w/v) does not stimulate acid secretion (Figure 59.1). However, after addition of yeast which results in fermentation of the glucose solution, it is a potent stimulator of acid secretion. Lyophilization of beer at pH 11.0 and dialysis (cutoff molecular weight 1,000) removed the stimulatory substances. The addition of yeast to finished wort and the following alcoholic fermentation are the essential steps for the stimulatory effect of beer (Singer *et al.*, 1991).

Teyssen *et al.* (1999) further separated and specified the gastric acid stimulatory ingredients of beer. They used yeast-fermented glucose which has the same stimulatory effect on gastric acid secretion than beer (Table 59.1) as a simple model of fermented alcoholic beverages. Yeast-fermented glucose was stepwise separated by liquid chromatography and the separated solutions were tested in volunteers for their effect on gastric acid secretion (Table 59.1). Lyophilized-fermented glucose, substances with a molecular weight lower than 1,000, anions with a molecular weight lower than 1,000, anions with a molecular weight lower than 700 and the non-bound fractions of anions at pH 1.0 with a molecular weight lower than 700 had significant stimulatory effect on gastric acid secretion (Table 59.1). The fraction of non-bound anions at pH 1.0 with a molecular weight lower than 700 was further separated until five carboxylic and dicarboxylic acids were left: acetic acid, L(+)-lactic acid, oxalic acid, maleic acid and succinic acid. Their mixture at the same concentrations as in beer significantly stimulated gastric acid output. All acids together increased gastric acid output up to 94% of incremental MAO and 99% of the response to fermented glucose. When tested separately, oxalic acid, acetic acid and L(+)-lactic acid had no stimulatory effect. However, maleic acid and succinic acid significantly increased gastric acid output by 76% and 70%, respectively (Table 59.1). Given together in concentrations present in beer, maleic acid and succinic acid significantly increased gastric acid output by 100% of fermented glucose. Thus, the dicarboxylic acids, maleic acid and succinic acid were identified to be responsible for the strong stimulatory effect of alcoholic beverages produced by fermentation like beer or wine. The mechanisms of actions remain to be elucidated.

Motility

Only few studies have examined the effect of alcoholic beverages like beer on gastric motility, although consumption of alcoholic beverages before, after or with a meal is commonly thought to improve digestive functions. There exist some studies on the effect of pure ethanol on gastric motility. All studies on the effect of alcoholic beverages or ethanol on gastric motility relate on the gastric emptying rate of the gastric content, since it is the clinical decisive parameter of gastric motility and represents the sum of gastric motor activity. The mechanism and the regulation is different between the gastric emptying of liquids and that of solid meal. Gastric emptying of liquids is mainly under the

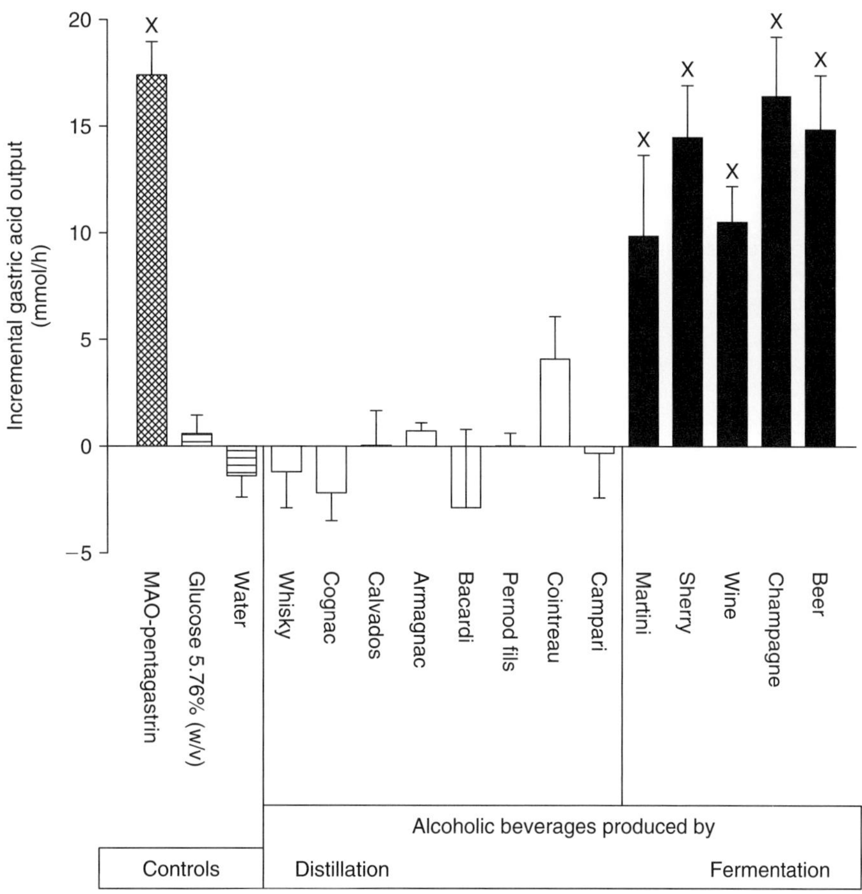

Figure 59.2 Effect of alcoholic beverages on gastric acid secretion. Gastric acid secretion (mmol/h) after instillation of different types of alcoholic beverages (hard liquors, aperitifs, wine, champagne and beer) compared to the MAO of pentagastrin. Results represent means ± SEM from six subjects. $^{x}p < 0.05$ for the difference compared to glucose control (5.76% w/v). *Source*: Reprinted from Singer *et al.* (1987). Copyright 1987, with permission from the American Gastroenterological Association.

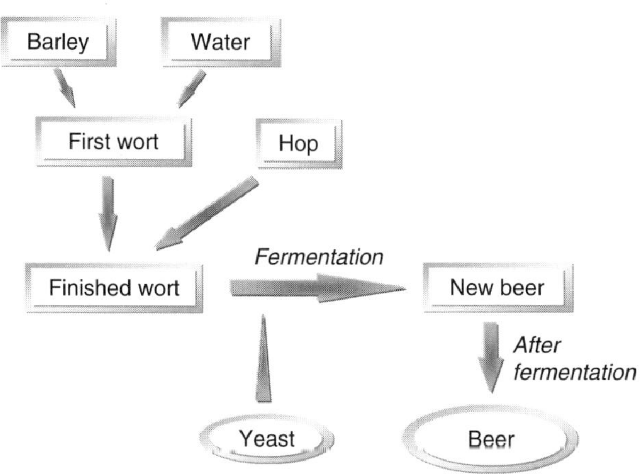

Figure 59.3 Brewing. Primary and intermediate products.

influence of the tone of the fundus, whereas gastric emptying of solids is regulated by the activity of the antrum and the pylorus. This has to be considered when the effect of alcoholic beverages and ethanol on gastric emptying is studied.

In 1970, the first study on the gastric emptying rate of ethanol was conducted by Cooke (1970). He examined different ethanol solutions (6, 8, 12 and 16 g/100 ml) and found that ethanol concentrations of 8 g/100 ml and more (12 and 16 g/100 ml) were delayed emptied from the stomach when compared to water or the lowest ethanol concentration tested (6 g/100 ml). However, there was no dose-dependent effect of the higher ethanol concentrations.

Kaufmann and Kaye (1979) studied the gastric emptying of ethanol and isocaloric glucose solutions to identify the impact of the caloric content of ethanol for its inhibitory effect. They compared gastric emptying of three isocaloric solutions (each with a volume of 750 ml): pure ethanol (80 ml), a mixture of ethanol (40 ml) and dextrose (63.3 g) and pure dextrose (126.6 g). They found that dextrose had a more pronounced inhibitory effect than its isocaloric ethanol amount.

Moore *et al.* (1981) examined the role of the ethanol content of red wine for its gastric emptying rate. They compared gastric emptying of red wine (9.5 g ethanol/dl) with that of a low-alcoholic red wine solution (1.3 g ethanol/dl), in

Table 59.1 Effect of beer and its constituents on gastric acid secretion

Test solution	*Effect*	*Reference*
Beer	>93% of MAO	Singer *et al.* (1987)
First wort	48% of MAO	Singer *et al.* (1991)
Hop extract	No effect	
Finished wort	46% of MAO	
New beer	76% of MAO	
Ingredients of beer: 4% ethanol, amines, phenoles, magnesium, calcium, amino acids, phenols, vitamins, organic acids, purines, pyrimidines (alone or in combination)	No effect	Singer *et al.* (1991)
Beer, lyophilized	pH dependent	Singer *et al.* (1991)
pH 2.5	67% of beer	
pH 7.0	53% of beer	
pH 11.0	20% of beer	
Beer, dialyzed (mol wt > 1,000)	No effect	Singer *et al.* (1991)
Unfermented glucose (11.5% w/v)	No effect	Singer *et al.* (1991), Teyssen *et al.* (1997)
Fermented glucose (11.5% w/v)	97% of MAO	Singer *et al.* (1991), Teyssen *et al.* (1997)
Ingredients of fermented glucose		Teyssen *et al.* (1999)
Lyophilized fermented glucose	100% of FG	
Substances with mol wt > 1,000	No effect	
Substances with mol wt < 1,000	102% of FG	
Cations and neutral substances (mol wt < 1000)	No effect	
Anions (mol wt < 1,000)	104% of FG	
Anions (mol wt < 700)	72% of FG	
Anions (mol wt < 700) at pH 1.0	78% of FG	
Fractions of anions with mol wt < 700 at pH 1.0		Teyssen *et al.* (1999)
Acetic acid	No effect	
Oxalic acid	No effect	
L(+)-lactic acid	No effect	
Succinic acid	70% of FG	
Maleic acid	76% of FG	
Maleic acid and succinic acid	100% of FG	

Note: Effect of beer, modified beer and selected ingredients of beer or fermented glucose (11.5% w/v) on gastric acid secretion in relation to maximal acid output, or to that of beer or fermented glucose. mol wt = molecular weight, FG = fermented glucose.

which major parts of the ethanol were exchanged by isocaloric amounts of medium-chain triglycerides. Gastric emptying rates were not significantly different if normal or dealcoholized, isocaloric red wine were applicated.

The first controlled study on the effect of alcoholic beverages was conducted by Franke *et al.* (2004). They studied the gastric emptying of beer, red wine, whisky, corresponding ethanol solutions (4%, 10%, 40% v/v) and isocaloric and isovolumetric controls. Ethanol solutions even in low concentrations (4% v/v) were slower emptied from the stomach than water (Figure 59.4). There was no dose-dependent effect between 4% and 10% (v/v). Beer, red wine and whisky were also slower emptied. Alcoholic beverages produced by fermentation (beer and red wine) were significantly slower emptied than their corresponding ethanol concentrations (4% and 10% v/v). However, whisky, an alcoholic beverage produced by distillation, inhibited gastric emptying to the same degree than the corresponding ethanol solution (40% v/v). Presumably, non-alcoholic ingredients in those alcoholic beverages produced by fermentation alone are important additional inhibitory factors.

Jian *et al.* studied in 1986 the effect of an ethanol solution (approximately 25% v/v) on gastric emptying of a solid meal and found an inhibitory effect by ethanol (Jian *et al.*, 1986). Barboriak and Meade (1970) showed that whisky also inhibited gastric emptying of a solid meal.

The effect of beer, red wine, corresponding ethanol solutions (4% and 10% v/v) and isocaloric and isovolumetric control solutions on gastric emptying of solid meals were studied by Franke *et al.* (2005): beer and red wine induced a significant prolongation of gastric emptying of the meal (Figure 59.5). Corresponding ethanol solutions (4% and 10% v/v) also inhibited gastric emptying. However, red wine, but not beer, induced a significantly slower emptying than their corresponding ethanol solutions (10% and 4%, respectively). No differences between the ethanol solutions and isocaloric glucose solutions concerning the gastric half emptying time of the meal were detected, but the slope of gastric emptying was different: whereas the initial lag-phase (the period of time between end of consumption of the meal and begin of gastric emptying) was prolonged by glucose solutions, the lag-phase was nearly unchanged by

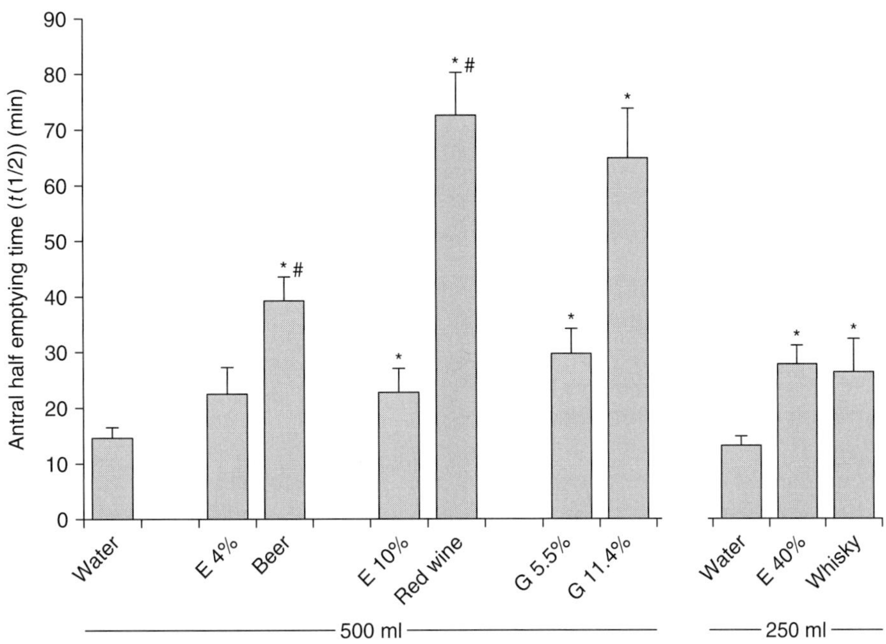

Figure 59.4 Gastric emptying of alcoholic beverages. Antral half emptying time (t(1/2)) of the test and control solutions as determined by ultrasonography. Results are means ± SEM of 10 subjects. G = glucose (w/v), E = ethanol (v/v). Whisky (125 ml) and E 40% (125 ml) were diluted with 125 ml water. $^{*}p < 0.05$ compared with water, $^{\#}p < 0.05$ compared with respective pure ethanol solution.

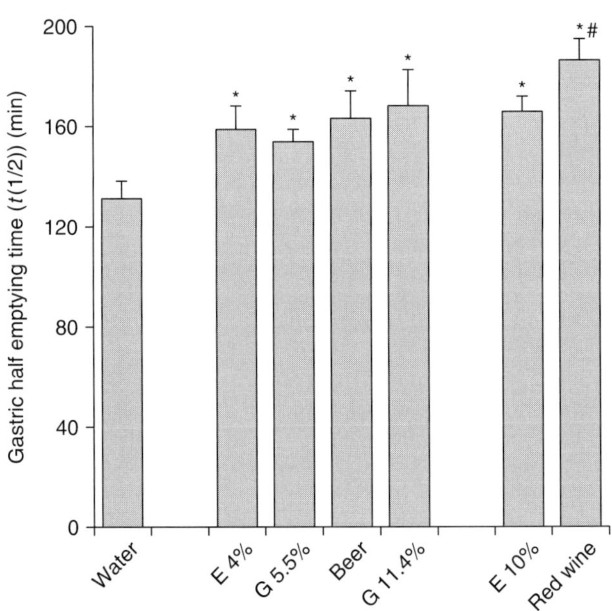

Figure 59.5 Effect of alcoholic beverages on gastric emptying of a meal. Gastric half emptying time (t(1/2)) of a solid meal with the test solutions. Results are means ± SEM of eight subjects with each meal. G = glucose (w/v), E = ethanol (v/v). $^{*}p < 0.05$ compared with water, $^{\#}p < 0.05$ compared with the corresponding ethanol solution.

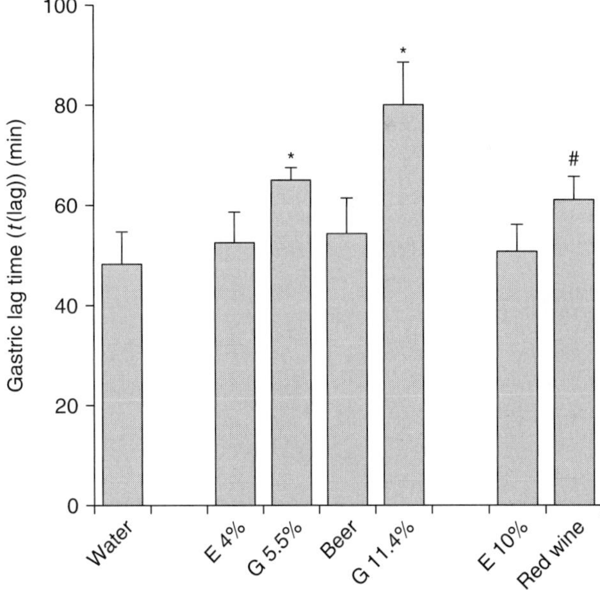

Figure 59.6 Effect of alcoholic beverages on the lag-phase of gastric emptying. Gastric lag time (t(lag)) of a solid meal with the test solutions. Results are means ± SEM of eight subjects with each meal. G = glucose (w/v), E = ethanol (v/v). $^{*}p < 0.05$ compared with water, $^{\#}p < 0.05$ compared with the corresponding pure ethanol solution.

ethanol or alcoholic beverages (Figure 59.6). Thus, compared to isocaloric glucose solutions alcohol induces an earlier begin of a slower gastric emptying. The mechanism by which this is mediated remains elucidated.

Concerning chronic effects of alcohol on gastric motility the data is scanty and inconsistent. While Keshvarzian *et al.* (1986) did not detect any effect on gastric emptying of solid test meals 3–10 days after alcohol abstinence,

Wegener *et al.* (1991) found a dose-related inhibitory effect on gastric emptying rate of solid test meals in actively drinking and symptomatic alcoholics. However, gastric retention may play a role in the development of malnutrition in alcoholics (Sankaran *et al.*, 1994).

Summary Points

- Beer and other alcoholic beverages produced by fermentation (e.g. wine) are powerful stimulators of gastric acid secretion.
- Corresponding ethanol concentrations (4% and 10% v/v) have only a mild stimulatory effect on gastric acid secretion.
- Alcoholic beverages produced by distillation (e.g. whisky, gin) have no stimulatory effect on gastric acid secretion.
- Maleic acid and succinic acid, non-alcoholic contents of alcoholic beverages produced by fermentation (especially beer), are responsible for the strong stimulatory effect.
- Beer and other alcoholic beverages produced by fermentation (e.g. wine), but not alcoholic beverages produced by distillation (e.g. whisky), are significantly slower emptied from the stomach than their corresponding ethanol solutions (4%, 10% and 40% v/v).
- Non-alcoholic ingredients in beer and red, which still have to be identified, are responsible for this additional effect compared to pure ethanol solutions.
- Beer and other alcoholic beverage, as well as corresponding ethanol solutions (4% and 10% v/v) prolong gastric emptying of solid meals.
- The inhibitory effect of beer is induced by a slower emptying phase, whereas the initial lag-phase is unchanged.

References

Barboriak, J.J. and Meade, R.C. (1979). *Am. J. Clin. Nutr.* 23, 1151–1153.

Beazell, J.M. and Ivy, A.C. (1940). *J. Stud. Alcohol.* 1, 45–60.

Chittenden, R.H., Mendel, L.B. and Jackson, H.C. (1898). *Am. J. Physiol.* 1, 164–209.

Cooke, A.R. (1970). *Am. J. Dig. Dis.* 15, 449–454.

Franke, A., Teyssen, S., Harder, H. and Singer, M.V. (2004). *Scan. J. Gastroenterol.* 39, 638–644.

Franke, A., Nakchbandi, I.A., Schneider, A., Harder, H. and Singer, M.V. (2005). *Alcohol Alcohol.* 40, 187–193.

Jian, R., Cortot, A., Ducrot, F., Jobin, G., Chayvialle, J.A. and Mosigliani, (1986). *Dig. Dis. Sci.* 31, 604–614.

Kaufmann, S.E. and Kaye, M.D. (1979). *Gut* 20, 688–692.

Keshvarzian, A., Iber, F.L., Greer, P. and Wobbleton, J. (1986). *Alcohol. Clin. Exp. Res.* 10, 432–435.

Lenz, H.J., Ferrari-Taylor, J. and Isenberg, J.I. (1983). *Gastroenterology* 85, 1082–1087.

McArthur, K., Hogan, D. and Isenberg, J.I. (1982). *Gastroenterology* 83, 199–203.

Moore, J.G., Christian, F.L., Datz, F.L. and Coleman, R.E. (1981). *Gastroenterology* 81, 1072–1075.

Peterson, W.L., Barnett, C. and Walsh, J.H. (1986). *Gastroenterology* 91, 1390–1395.

Pfeiffer, A., Högl, B. and Kaess, H. (1992). *J. Clin. Investig.* 70, 487–491.

Sankaran, H., Larkin, E.C. and Rao, G.A. (1994). *Med. Hypotheses* 42, 124–128.

Singer, M.V., Eysselein, V.E. and Goebell, H. (1983). *Digestion* 26, 73–79.

Singer, M.V., Leffmann, C., Eysselein, V.E., Calden, H. and Goebell, H. (1987). *Gastroenterology* 93, 1247–1254.

Singer, M.V., Teyssen, S. and Eysselein, V.E. (1991). *Gastroenterology* 101, 935–942.

Teyssen, S., Lenzing, T., González-Calero, G., Korn, A., Riepl, R.L. and Singer, M.V. (1997). *Gut* 40, 49–56.

Teyssen, S., González-Calero, G., Schimiczek, M. and Singer, M.V. (1999). *J. Clin. Invest.* 103, 707–713.

Wegener, M., Schaffstein, J., Dilger, U., Coenen, C., Wedmann, B. and Schmidt, G. (1991). *Dig. Dis. Sci.* 36, 917–923.

60

The Effect of Beer and Its Non-alcoholic Constituents on the Exocrine and Endocrine Pancreas as Well as on Gastrointestinal Hormones

Peter Feick, Andreas Gerloff and Manfred V. Singer Department of Medicine II (Gastroenterology, Hepatology and Infectious Diseases), University Hospital of Heidelberg at Mannheim, Mannheim, Germany

Abstract

The possible adverse effect of excessive alcohol consumption on the pancreas has been known since many years. Alcohol (ethanol) is generally consumed in the form of alcoholic beverages which contain numerous non-alcoholic compounds. On gastric acid secretion it has been convincingly demonstrated that alcohol and alcoholic beverages have markedly different effects. In this chapter we provide an overview about the effect of beer and different non-alcoholic constituents of beer on the pancreas and their possible interaction with molecular mechanisms leading to "alcoholic" pancreatitis, diabetes and pancreatic carcinoma. The present data indicate that pancreatic enzyme secretion in humans is stimulated by non-alcoholic constituents of beer which are generated by alcoholic fermentation of glucose. Natural phenolic compounds (e.g. quercetin, resveratrol) of beer have been shown to exert different effects on the pancreas in *in vitro* experiments, such as inhibition of pancreatic enzyme output, of pancreatic stellate cell activation and of pancreatic cancer growth. However, some compounds, for example resveratrol and catechins, showed also protective effects against oxidative stress and on experimentally induced acute pancreatitis or experimentally induced diabetes in rats. Bioavailability and efficacy of these compounds are summarized at the end of this chapter.

List of Abbreviations

α-SMA	α-Smooth muscle actin
AP-1	Activator protein 1
BB/E rat	Biobreeding/Edinburgh rat
BSDL	Bile salt-dependent lipase
b.w.	Body weight
cAMP	Adenosine-3′,5′-cyclic monophosphate
CCK-OP	Cholecystokinin octapeptide
COX	Cyclooxygenase
ERK	Extracellular signal-regulated kinase
GST	Glutathione *S*-transferase
GTC	Green tea catechin
IL	Interleukin
iNOS	Inducable nitric oxide synthase
MAO	Maximal acid output
MAP kinase	Mitogen activated protein kinase
MCP-1	Monocyte chemoattractant protein 1
NF-κB	Nuclear factor-kappa B
PDGF	Platelet derived growth factor
PKC	Protein kinase C
PSC	Pancreatic stellate cell
RWE	Red wine polyphenolic extract
SAP	Severe acute pancreatitis
SD-rats	Sprague–Dawley rats
SEM	Standard error of the mean
SOD	Superoxide dismutase
STZ	Streptozotocin
TNF	Tumor necrosis factor
TPA	12-*O*-tetradecanoylphorbol-13-acetate

Introduction

Chronic excessive consumption of alcoholic beverages is clearly associated with chronic pancreatitis. While the role of alcohol (ethanol) in the development of pancreatitis has been intensively investigated over the past 30 years, the role of non-alcoholic constituents was hardly considered. However, alcoholic beverages contain numerous non-alcoholic compounds. For example, up to now in beer more than 2,000 and in wine more than 1,000 organic and inorganic constituents were identified. As outlined briefly below and described by Franke *et al.* in detail in another chapter of this encyclopedia, evidence has been conclusively provided that alcoholic beverages and ethanol have markedly different effects on gastric acid secretion.

Some of the non-alcoholic constituents have been shown to be biologically active, although these compounds were

Beer in Health and Disease Prevention
ISBN: 978-0-12-373891-2

often not studied in respect of the effects of alcoholic beverages. Evidences accumulate that these compounds could have a critical role in inducing metabolic, pathological and functional changes *in vivo* and *in vitro*.

This chapter summarizes the published data about the effect of beer on the pancreas in comparison to ethanol. Furthermore, it will focus on the impact of different non-alcoholic constituents of beer on the pancreas and it will discuss their possible beneficial or adverse effects on molecular mechanisms leading to "alcoholic" pancreatic diseases.

Alcohol Consumption and Pancreatitis

Chronic calcifying pancreatitis is the alcohol-related disease of the pancreas (for review see Sarles, 1991; Singer and Müller, 1995). It is characterized by progressive and irreversible destruction of pancreatic structure and function: loss of acinar tissue, dilated and distorted ducts and significant fibrosis (DiMagno *et al.*, 1993). The disease usually begins as an acute process of a sudden and severe inflammation. Recurrent attacks of acute pancreatitis, which may last for several years, lead to the chronic phase of disease characterized by the development of chronic pain, pancreatic calcifications and exocrine as well as endocrine insufficiency (Apte and Wilson, 2003).

Epidemiological data indicate that heavy alcohol consumption causes pancreatitis in humans. Patients develop clinical manifestations of chronic pancreatitis after the consumption of more than 80 g alcohol per day (equivalent to approximately 2 l of beer) for average 18 ± 11 years for men and 11 ± 8 years for women (Durbec and Sarles, 1978). An increased risk to develop the disease has already been reported in patients with moderate alcohol consumption as low as 20 g ethanol/day. This risk increases logarithmically with higher amounts of alcohol consumption (Durbec and Sarles, 1978). However, only about 5–10% of clinically documented alcoholics develop symptoms of pancreatitis (Gumaste, 1995). Thus, a simple dose-related injury model for the development of the disease must be rejected (Durbec and Sarles, 1978; Worning, 1998).

Another issue which has been proposed to lead to chronic pancreatitis is the consumption of a specific type of alcoholic beverage. However, alcoholic chronic pancreatitis is observed in patients with a dominant consumption of beer, wine, hard liquor as well as other alcoholic beverages (Wilson *et al.*, 1985; Haber *et al.*, 1995). Therefore, the development of pancreatitis does not seem to be related to a specific type of alcoholic beverage. While alcohol exposure is obviously necessary, several lines of evidence suggest that alcohol alone cannot explain pancreatic inflammation, and that one or more additional factors must be also involved in the development of chronic pancreatitis. The other cofactors are yet to be determined, but could be environmental, genetic, race or concomitant risk factors such as smoking and nutrition (for reviews see Schneider and Singer, 2005; Schneider *et al.*, 2005; Chowdhury and Gupta, 2006).

Effects of ethanol and alcoholic beverages on the exocrine pancreas

The normal function of the exocrine pancreas is synthesis and release of digestive enzymes such as trypsin, chymotrypsin, amylase and lipase after stimulation by a meal. Altered secretion of these enzymes can lead to pancreatitis. Because hypersecretion of pancreatic enzymes has been observed in chronic alcoholics, a general impression is that ethanol stimulates basal (interdigestive) pancreatic exocrine secretion (Niebergall-Roth *et al.*, 1998). However, in the literature alcohol consumption demonstrates various effects on pancreatic exocrine secretion (Table 60.1) which may be due to different experimental conditions (Schneider *et al.*, 2005). The action of ethanol is affected by several variables such as: duration of alcohol consumption, administration route, the secretory state of the gland, species and accompanying dietary regimen. In addition, alcohol is commonly consumed as a tasteful beverage that is a complex mixture of non-alcoholic compounds with possible influence on pancreatic secretion.

Table 60.1 Major findings in studies with humans and ethanol-fed animals on pancreatic exocrine secretion

Acute ethanol administration
- Oral and intragastric ethanol administration increases pancreatic bicarbonate and protein secretion
- Intravenous ethanol administration reduces basal and hormonally stimulated pancreatic bicarbonate and protein secretion
- Non-alcoholic constituents of beer may increase pancreatic secretion

Chronic ethanol administration
- In human alcoholics, the basal pancreatic enzyme secretion is increased
- In human alcoholics, the viscosity of the pancreatic juice is enhanced
- In human alcoholics, the pancreatic juice contains a higher concentration of proteins
- In human alcoholics, the pancreatic bicarbonate secretion is decreased
- In human alcoholics, an enhanced ratio of trypsinogen levels to pancreatic secretory trypsin inhibitor levels is present in the pancreatic juice
- In ethanol-fed animals, a diet rich in fat and protein increases the concentrations of enzymes in the pancreatic juice

Note: Acute and chronic ethanol administration results in changes in pancreatic exocrine secretion in humans and animals which may contribute to the development of pancreatic damage.

Source: Reviewed in Niebergall-Roth *et al.* (1998); originally published by Schneider *et al.* (2005).

Effects of Ethanol, Alcoholic Beverages and Their Non-alcoholic Constituents on Gastric Acid Secretion Before describing their effects on the pancreatic enzyme output, the different effects of ethanol and beer on gastric acid output will be described first.

Low concentrations (<4% v/v) of pure ethanol are only a mild stimulant of gastric acid output with a response equal to about 23% of the pentagastrin-stimulated gastric acid output (maximal acid output, MAO) (Figure 60.1). Higher concentrations of ethanol (5–40% v/v) have either no effect or a mildly inhibitory one (Singer *et al.*, 1987). None of the ethanol concentrations tested increase plasma gastrin concentrations.

In contrast, beer is a powerful stimulant of gastric acid output with a response equal to about 85% of MAO (Figure 60.1) as well as of gastrin release. Other alcoholic beverages with low ethanol content produced by fermentation (e.g. wine and champagne) are also powerful stimulants whereas distilled alcoholic beverages with a higher ethanol content (e.g. whisky and cognac) do not stimulate gastric acid output (Figure 60.1) or release of gastrin (Singer *et al.*, 1987; Teyssen *et al.*, 1997).

The ethanol content in beer (4% v/v) can be only partially responsible for the marked gastric acid secretory response to beer. Therefore, non-alcoholic ingredients are most likely responsible for the stimulatory gastric action of beer and the other alcoholic beverages.

The gastric-stimulatory substances have been identified as the dicarboxylic acids, maleic acid and succinic acid, which are produced during the process of alcoholic fermentation (Teyssen *et al.*, 1999). The surprising outcome of this investigation was that these dicarboxylic acids do not stimulate gastrin release. Therefore, it is hypothesized that maleic acid and succinic acid induce gastric acid output by a direct yet unknown mechanism.

Effects of Ethanol, Alcoholic Beverages and Their Non-alcoholic Constituents on Pancreatic Exocrine Function Ethanol can be metabolized by the pancreas by different pathways. Oxidative metabolism generates acetaldehyde and non-oxidative metabolism generates fatty acid ethyl esters with both having damaging effects on the pancreas (reviewed in Schneider *et al.*, 2002). The role of ethanol and its metabolites in pancreatitis has been studied since many years and is summarized in several reviews (Go *et al.*, 2005; Schneider and Singer, 2005; Schneider *et al.*, 2005; Chowdhury and Gupta, 2006). It is also not in the focus of this chapter and, thus, the effects of pure ethanol on the exocrine pancreas will be outlined only briefly (Table 60.2).

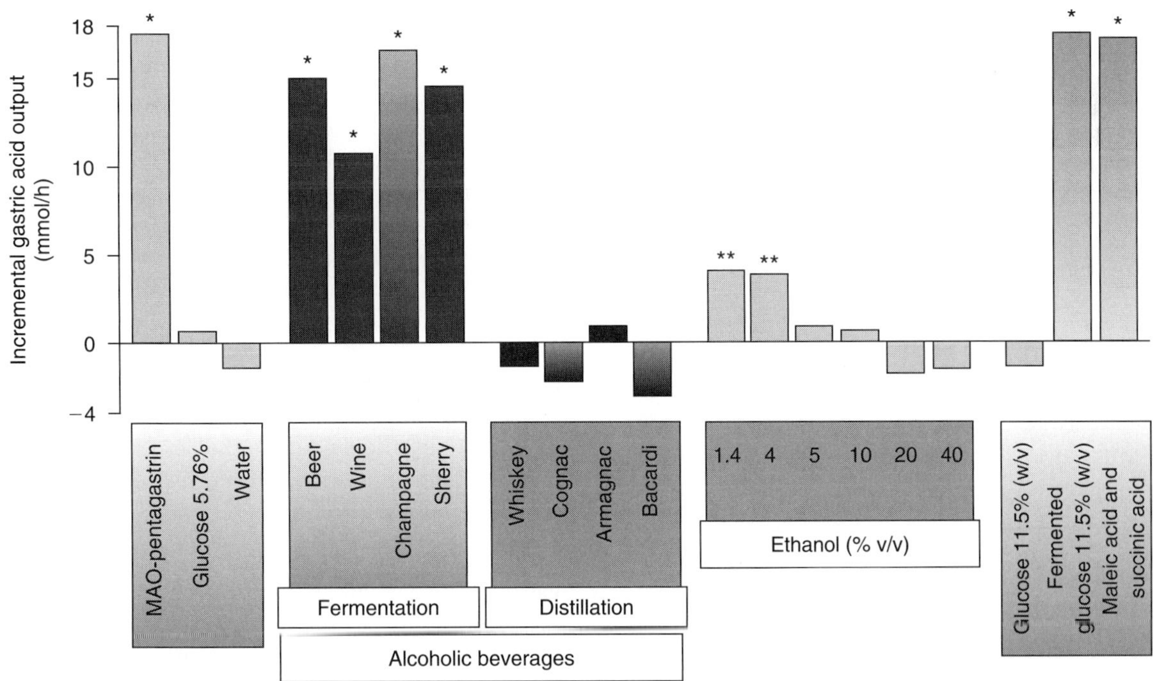

Figure 60.1 Effect of beer, different types of alcoholic beverages and ethanol on gastric acid secretion of healthy human subjects. One hour incremental gastric acid output in response to beer and various alcoholic beverages produced by fermentation or distillation, and to different concentrations of ethanol as well as to fermented glucose and to the combination of maleic acid and succinic acid in concentrations found in finished beer. For comparison the maximal acid output in response to pentagastrin and gastric acid output to control solutions (isotonic glucose, 5.76 w/v, and distilled water) are also shown. Results are means ± SEM from at least six subjects. *$p < 0.05$ for the difference with isotonic glucose control solution, **$p < 0.05$ in comparison to isotonic glucose control solution and distilled water. *Source*: Adapted from Singer *et al.* (1987) and Teyssen *et al.* (1997, 1999).

Acute Effects of Ethanol In Vivo Intravenous administration of ethanol appears to be the most adequate method to investigate direct effects of alcohol on pancreatic cells *in vivo* (Singer, 1985; Singer and Goebell, 1985; Singh and Simsek, 1990). With this route of administration, ethanol leads to a dose-dependent inhibition of the basal and hormonally stimulated pancreatic bicarbonate and enzyme output in humans and different animal species (Niebergall-Roth *et al.*, 1998). Although the inhibitory action of ethanol on pancreatic secretion has been suggested to be a consequence of a cholinergic mediation, this mechanism was never proven in humans. Thus, the exact mechanisms remain unclear. Ethanol has no further inhibitory effects on pancreatic amylase output after premedication with atropine (Kolbel *et al.*, 1986).

Acute Effects of Ethanol In Vitro The application of ethanol to isolated pancreatic acini led to an increase of basal amylase secretion, but decreased the cholinergic or secretagogue-mediated amylase release (Uhlemann *et al.*, 1979; Ponnappa *et al.*, 1987; Nakamura *et al.*, 1991). These investigations have shown that acute ethanol administration influences pancreatic secretion through the production of cAMP, an increase of cytosolic free calcium concentrations, an inhibition of calcium efflux, the inhibition of cholecystokinin-receptor binding and impairment of microtubule function (Niebergall-Roth *et al.*, 1998).

Table 60.2 Major findings with animal models of acute and chronic ethanol administration on pancreatic morphology

Major findings with animal models of acute ethanol administration
- Ethanol administration (intragastrically, intraperitoneally, intravenously) with physiological stimulation (CCK, secretin) and obstruction of the pancreatic duct results in acute pancreatitis
- Ethanol administration enhances the vulnerability of the pancreas to develop acute pancreatitis and limits pancreatic regeneration from acute pancreatitis
- Ethanol administration selectively reduces pancreatic blood flow and microcirculation
- Cigarette smoke enhances ethanol-induced pancreatic ischemia
- Ethanol administration increases free oxygen radical generation in the pancreas
- Ethanol metabolites directly damage the pancreas

Major findings with animal models of chronic ethanol administration
- Dietary fat potentiates ethanol-induced pancreatic injury
- Ethanol administration increases free oxygen radical generation in the pancreas
- Ethanol administration increases pancreatic acinar cell mRNA expression and glandular content of digestive and lysosomal enzymes
- Ethanol administration decreases the number of muscarinic receptor sites
- Ethanol administration limits pancreatic regeneration after temporary obstruction of the pancreatic duct and further aggravates already induced pancreatic damage
- Ethanol administration sensitizes pancreatic acinar cells to endotoxin-induced injury
- Ethanol administration enhances the vulnerability of the pancreas to pancreatitis caused by CCK-OP

Note: Experimental studies have provided various insights into the mechanisms, whereby alcohol damages the pancreas. It is likely that several mechanisms act together and increase the risk to develop alcoholic chronic pancreatitis.

Source: Reviewed in Schneider *et al.* (2002); originally published by Schneider *et al.* (2005).

Chronic Effects of Ethanol In Vivo In human alcoholics, basal pancreatic enzyme output was increased compared with non-alcoholics (Sahel and Sarles, 1979; Renner *et al.*, 1980; Planche *et al.*, 1982; Brugge *et al.*, 1985). Viscosity of the pancreatic juice was enhanced in alcoholic subjects and this rise was correlated with increased protein concentrations (Harada *et al.*, 1980). The volume of pancreatic juice was similar in controls and alcoholics, thereby indicating a true hypersecretion of pancreatic proteins in chronic alcoholics (Sahel and Sarles, 1979). The pancreatic bicarbonate secretion was significantly lower in human alcoholics than in non-alcoholics (Sahel and Sarles, 1979; Renner *et al.*, 1980), whereas basal plasma concentrations of secretin, cholecystokinin (CCK) and gastrin remained unchanged (Singer *et al.*, 1985; Singh and Simsek, 1990; Niebergall-Roth *et al.*, 1998). Administration of a diet rich in fat and protein resulted in an increase of the concentrations of enzymes in the pancreatic juice in animals (Devaux *et al.*, 1990; Niebergall-Roth *et al.*, 1998). In some dogs, a decreased flow rate of the pancreatic juice together with protein plug formation was found (Devaux *et al.*, 1990).

Studies of the effects of chronic alcohol intake on hormonally stimulated pancreatic secretion revealed that pancreatic bicarbonate output remains unaffected. However, alcoholics have an increased enzyme response on exogenous administration of CCK (Sahel and Sarles, 1979; Rinderknecht *et al.*, 1985). In addition, an enhanced ratio of trypsinogen levels to pancreatic secretory trypsin inhibitor levels was found in the pancreatic juice from chronic alcoholics (Rinderknecht *et al.*, 1985). This alteration of the normal ratio in favor of trypsinogen may facilitate premature activation of pancreatic proenzymes within the pancreas with an increased risk of subsequent pancreatic autodigestion (Rinderknecht *et al.*, 1985).

In summary, the ethanol-induced altered pancreatic secretion might contribute to the development of alcoholic chronic pancreatitis. However, the exact mechanisms still remain to be identified.

Effects of Beer on Pancreatic Exocrine Function In Vivo Intragastric administration of beer in a volume (250 ml) that does not alter plasma ethanol concentrations causes a significant stimulation of basal pancreatic enzyme output (Figure 60.2) (Chari *et al.*, 1996). The stimulatory effect might be mediated by the hormones CCK and gastrin which are released after oral or intragastric administration of beer (Table 60.3) (Chari *et al.*, 1996). Intragastric administration of ethanol in concentrations similar to beer (4% v/v) has no effect on pancreatic enzyme output (Figure 60.2). Therefore, non-alcoholic constituents might be responsible for the stimulatory effect of beer on pancreatic enzyme secretion in humans. Intragastric administration of fermented glucose in a concentration (11.5% w/v) found in finished wort, a preproduct of beer, but not non-fermented glucose induced an increase in pancreatic enzyme secretion similar to that of beer (Figure 60.2). This finding indicates that alcoholic fermentation of glucose might be the essential event generating as yet unknown pancreatic secretagogues in beer (Chari *et al.*, 1996).

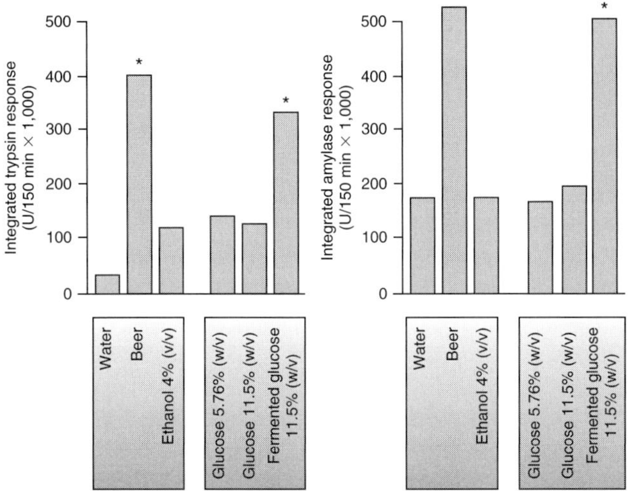

Figure 60.2 Effect of beer, ethanol and fermented glucose on pancreatic enzyme output of healthy human subjects. The 150 min integrated trypsin response (left) and amylase response (right) to intragastric beer, ethanol (4% v/v) and fermented glucose (11.5% w/v) as well as to the corresponding caloric (glucose, 5.76% w/v), osmotic (glucose, 11.5% w/v) and volumetric (water) control solutions were determined. Results are means ± SEM of six subjects. *$p < 0.05$ in comparison to ethanol and all control solutions. *Source*: Adapted from Chari *et al.* (1996).

The intragastric administration of an higher amount of beer (850 ml) elevated plasma ethanol concentrations but did not affect the basal pancreatic enzyme output (Hajnal *et al.*, 1989). It was suggested that the direct inhibitory effect of circulating ethanol neutralized the stimulatory effect of non-alcoholic components of beer. The basal enzyme output also remained unchanged after intragastric application of white wine and gin.

In addition, the meal-stimulated pancreatic enzyme output was inhibited by intragastric beer, but also by white wine and gin, although postprandial plasma CCK and gastrin concentrations were increased by beer and wine (Table 60.4) (Hajnal *et al.*, 1990; Niebergall-Roth *et al.*, 1998). Since ethanol plasma levels were concurrently elevated in these studies, the inhibitory effect of circulating ethanol on pancreatic secretion might have neutralized the stimulatory effect of a meal as well as that of beer and white wine.

Effects of Beer on Pancreatic Exocrine Function In Vitro

In vitro experiments with the rat pancreatic acinar tumor cell line AR4-2J which in its differentiated state retains much of the characteristics of pancreatic acinar cells and is a common model to study stimulus-secretion coupling have shown that beer dose dependently increased amylase release (Figure 60.3). Incubation of AR4-2J cells with ethanol (10–400 mM) had no effect on basal protein secretion whereas hormone-stimulated amylase secretion was dose dependently inhibited at ethanol concentrations of more than 100 mM (Feick *et al.*, 2003). Maleic acid and succinic acid, the non-alcoholic compounds of beer and other fermented alcoholic beverages that maximally increase gastric acid output, had alone or in combination with ethanol in concentrations found in beer no effect on basal protein

Table 60.3 Effect of alcoholic beverages on the basal plasma concentration of several gastrointestinal hormones in humans, compared with equicaloric–equiosmotic control solutions

Hormone	*Beverage*	*Volume (ml)*	*Route of administration*	*Effect*	*Reference*
Gastrin	Beer	250–850	Oral/intragastric	Strong stimulation	Chari *et al.* (1996); Hajnal *et al.* (1989); Singer *et al.* (1983a); Singer *et al.* (1987); Kölbel *et al.* (1988)
		250	Intraduodenal	No effect	Kölbel *et al.* (1988)
	White wine	240–500	Intragastric	Strong stimulation	Hajnal *et al.* (1989); Singer *et al.* (1983a); Peterson *et al.* (1986); Singer *et al.* (1987)
	Gin	120	Intragastric	No effect	Hajnal *et al.* (1989)
CCK	Beer	250–850	Oral/intragastric	Stimulation	Hajnal *et al.* (1989); Hajnal *et al.* (1990)
	White wine	400	Intragastric	Stimulation	Hajnal *et al.* (1989)
	Gin	120	Intragastric	No effect	Hajnal *et al.* (1989)
Pancreatic polypeptide	Beer	250	Oral	No effect	Singer *et al.* (1983b)
	Wine	250	Oral	No effect	Singer *et al.* (1983b)

Source: Adapted from Niebergall-Roth *et al.* (1998).

Table 60.4 Effect of intragastric alcoholic beverages on the postprandial release of several gastrointestinal hormones in humans

Hormone	*Beverage*	*Volume (ml)*	*Effect*	*Reference*
Gastrin	Beer	850	Increase	Hajnal *et al.* (1990)
	White wine	400	Increase	Hajnal *et al.* (1990)
	Gin	120	No effect	Hajnal *et al.* (1990)
CCK	Beer	850	Increase	Hajnal *et al.* (1990)
	White wine	400	No effect	Hajnal *et al.* (1990)
	Gin	120	No effect	Hajnal *et al.* (1990)

Source: Adapted from Niebergall-Roth *et al.* (1998).

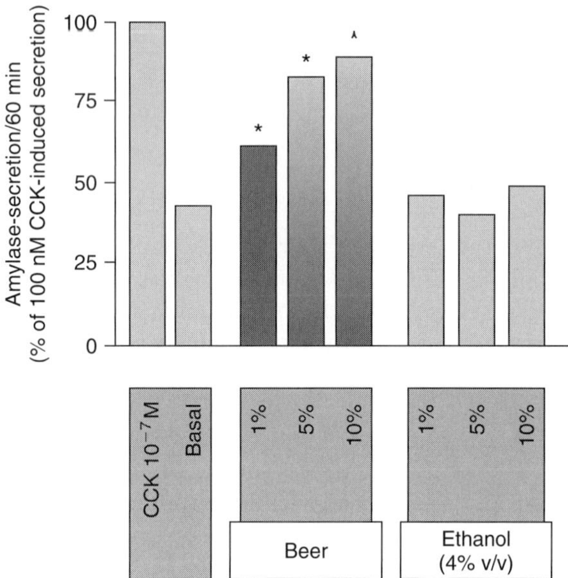

Figure 60.3 Effect of beer and ethanol on enzyme output of differentiated pancreatic acinar AR4-2J cells. The 60-min amylase release induced by 1%, 5% and 10% (v/v) of beer in incubation medium as well as by equivalent ethanol concentrations was determined. The results are expressed as percentage of maximal amylase secretion induced by 100 nM cholecystokinin (CCK). $^*p < 0.01$ in comparison to basal secretion from unstimulated cells.

secretion (Gerloff *et al.*, unpublished). Therefore, non-alcoholic substances of beer other than these dicarboxylic acids might be responsible for the stimulatory effect of beer on pancreatic enzyme output.

Polyphenolic compounds of beer

One of the differentiating characteristics among alcoholic beverages is their polyphenol composition. In this context wine contains more abundant polyphenols – more than beer and liquors (Bujanda, 2000). In beer more than 50 polyphenolic compounds were identified (Piendl, 2005). About 75–85% of these polyphenols derive from malt and 15–25% from hop. The polyphenol content of each beer is largely affected by the type and the sort of corn (barley, wheat), the type of hop as well as by the different processes to get malt, wort and hop extract. Table 60.5 shows the concentrations

Table 60.5 Concentrations of various non-alcoholic compounds found in beer

Compound	*Concentration (mg/l)*	*Reference*
Quercetin	0.7–20	Piendl (2005)
Resveratrol	0.34–3.4	Tedesco *et al.* (2005)
Maleic acid	110	Piendl (1980)
Succinic acid	16	Piendl (1980)
Rutin	Under 0.1	Piendl (2005)
Catechin	0.5 to over 20	Piendl (2005)
Epicatechin	0.8 to over 20	Piendl (2005)
Ellagic acid	1.0–10	Piendl (2005)
Folic acid	0.086	Piendl (2005)
Ascorbic acid	20	Moll and Joly (1987)
Salicylic acid	0.02–5	Piendl (2005)

mg/l: milligram per liter.

of some phenolic substances and other non-alcoholic constituents found in beer. The first such polyphenols studied were *quercetin* and *rutin* followed more recently by *resveratrol* (*Deschner et al.*, 1991; Bujanda, 2000).

Quercetin is a naturally occurring flavonoid present in a variety of plants and in beer and wine and has important anti-degenerative properties (Maxwell *et al.*, 1994). *Rutin* is the glycosidic form of quercetin and is one of the flavonoids most abundantly consumed in foods. It has anti-inflammatory and anti-mutagenic properties (Janbaz *et al.*, 2002). *Resveratrol* is a phenolic phytoalexin present in grape skins and wines (especially red wines) and was also found in beer. Among a variety of biological effects it has a potent anti-inflammatory function *in vitro* (Bujanda, 2000). *Ellagic acid* is a polyphenol mainly found in fruits (raspberries, strawberries), nuts (walnuts) and wood, but also in beer and wine (Masamune *et al.*, 2005; Piendl, 2005). It has a variety of biological activities including anti-oxidant, anti-inflammatory and anti-fibrotic effects (Masamune *et al.*, 2005). *Catechins* are phytoalexins which are found in green tea, various vegetables and fruits and particularly in paring of grapes of red wines as well as beer. In several studies the anti-oxidative and radical-scavenging properties of *catechins* have been reported (Yang and Wang, 1993; Noroozi *et al.*, 1998). In the following sections the effects of different polyphenols on the pancreas are described (Table 60.6).

Table 60.6 Studies on the effects of non-alcoholic constituents of beer on the pancreas

Compound	*Experimental design*	*Effect on pancreas*	*Species*	*Reference*
Quercetin	*In vitro* 10–100 μM Isolated pancreatic acini	Inhibition of agonist-induced amylase release and of PKC activity	Rat (SD)	Lee *et al.* (1988)
Resveratrol	*In vitro* 10–100 μM	Inhibition of bile salt-dependent lipase (BSDL) activity Reduction of secreted and intracellular BSDL	Human (purified BSDL), rat (purified BSDL, AR4-2J cell line)	Sbarra *et al.* (2005)
	In vivo 20 mg/kg b.w. Experimentally induced pancreatitis	Decrease of elevated amylase, malondialdehyde and myeloperoxidase levels Increase of pancreatic superoxide dismutase Reduction of turbidity ascitic fluid, pancreatic edema, necrosis and inflammatory cell infiltration	Rat (SD)	Li *et al.* (2006)
	In vivo 10 mg/kg b.w. Experimentally induced pancreatitis	Reduction of elevated serum amylase and lipase activities and reduction of changes of serum glucose, calcium and creatinine and aspartate aminotransferase Increase of serum concentration of triglyceride and urea nitrogen to normal level Reduction of extent of tissue edema, acinar vacuolization and total histological damage	Rat (Wistar)	Szabolcs *et al.* (2006)
	In vivo 2 mg/day Experimentally induced pancreatitis	Decrease of elevated serum activity of amylase Less pronounced necrotic changes of pancreata	Rat (Wistar)	Lawinski *et al.* (2005)
	In vivo 10 mg/kg b.w. Experimentally induced pancreatitis	Decrease of NF-κB activation in peritoneal macrophages Reduction of iNOS expression and of TNF-α, IL-1 and NO serum levels	Rat (SD)	Ma *et al.* (2005)
	In vivo 30 mg/kg b.w. Experimentally induced pancreatitis	Reduction of NF-κB expression and of TNF-α and IL-8 level in pancreatic tissue	Rat (SD)	Meng *et al.* (2005)
Ellagic acid	*In vivo* 1% w/w	Increase of glutathione *S*-transferase expression	Rat (Wistar)	Nijhoff and Peters (1994)
	In vitro ≤25 μg/ml PSCs	Inhibition of PDGF-induced proliferation and migration of PSCs and of phosphorylation of PDGF β-receptor, ERK and Akt Decrease of expression of α-SMA, procollagen I and III and MCP-1 Inhibition of transformation of freshly isolated PSCs	Rat (Wistar)	Masamune *et al.* (2005)
Catechin (green tea extract)	*In vivo* 0.1% solution (80% catechins)	Protective effect against *N*-nitrosobis(2-oxopropyl)amine-induced oxidative damage	Syrian golden hamster	Takabayashi *et al.* (1997, 2004)
	In vivo 0.2% solution (91.2% catechins) Experimentally-induced pancreatitis	Decrease of elevated serum amylase activity and lipid peroxides concentration Protection of pancreatic tissue	Rat (Wistar)	Takabayashi *et al.* (1995)

α-SMA: α-smooth muscle actin; BSDL: bile salt-dependent lipase; b.w.: body weight; ERK: extracellular signal-regulated kinase; IL: interleukin; iNOS: inducible nitric oxide synthase; MCP-1: monocyte chemoattractant protein 1; NF-κB: nuclear factor-kappa B; PDGF: platelet derived growth factor; PKC: protein kinase C; PSC: pancreatic stellate cell; SD: Sprague–Dawley; TNF: tumor necrosis factor.

Effects of different non-alcoholic constituents of beer on the exocrine pancreas

As described above chronic ethanol consumption significantly increases basal pancreatic enzyme output, protein concentration in the pancreatic juice and the viscosity of pancreatic juice. Investigation of the effects of non-alcoholic compounds of alcoholic beverages have been undertaken to facilitate our understanding of their direct effects.

In a former study the effect of quercetin on stimulated amylase release in isolated rat pancreatic acini was investigated (Lee *et al.*, 1988). Quercetin inhibited amylase release stimulated by carbachol in a time- and dose-dependent manner. In addition, quercetin partially inhibited amylase release induced by various agonists such as cholecystokinin C-terminal octapeptide (CCK-OP), calcium ionophore A23187 and protein kinase C (PKC) activator 12-*O*-tetradecanoylphorbol-13-acetate (TPA) whereas vasoactive intestinal polypeptide-induced amylase release was potentiated. Since quercetin also inhibited PKC activity in a dose-dependent manner, the ability of quercetin to decrease agonist-stimulated amylase release may be ascribed – at least in part – to quercetin-induced inhibition of PKC activity.

A recent study compared the effects of resveratrol and a whole red wine polyphenolic extract (RWE) on the pancreatic bile salt-dependent lipase (BSDL) *in vitro* (Sbarra *et al.*, 2005). Resveratrol and RWE inhibited human and rat BSDL activity in a dose-dependent manner. Furthermore, resveratrol (but not RWE) decreased the expression and secretion of BSDL in AR4-2J cells. Our own data suggest that resveratrol induces activation of an actin cytoskeleton-controlled protein tyrosine phosphatase leading to a decrease of protein tyrosine phosphorylation in AR4-2J cells which is involved in bombesin-stimulated amylase secretion (Feick *et al.*, 2006).

Effects of Non-alcoholic Constituents of Beer upon Oxidative Stress Oxidative stress is another important event that may play a role in pancreatic injury. Evidence of oxidative stress has also been reported in the pancreas of patients with alcoholic chronic pancreatitis (Schneider *et al.*, 2005). In general, oxidative stress results from an imbalance between the production of free radicals or reactive oxygen species (highly reactive molecules with the potential to damage lipid membranes, intracellular proteins and DNA) and the anti-oxidant defense mechanisms within the cell (including glutathione, the enzymes glutathione peroxidase, superoxide dismutase (SOD, an internal anti-oxidase) and catalase) (Apte *et al.*, 2005).

The effect of resveratrol on pancreatic oxygen free radicals was investigated in rats with severe acute pancreatitis (SAP) (Li *et al.*, 2006). Histological examinations showed that the resveratrol treatment after SAP induction led to a significant reduction of turbidity ascitic fluid, pancreatic edema, necrosis and inflammatory cell infiltration as compared to the SAP group. In addition, serum amylase was significantly diminished by resveratrol. Furthermore, resveratrol treatment inhibited the formation of the lipid peroxidation product malondialdehyde and increased the pancreatic SOD. Measurement of myeloperoxidase (MPO) as degree for neutrophil sequestration which is another source of oxygen free radicals during acute pancreatitis showed a reduction of this enzyme in the resveratrol-treated group. In conclusion, resveratrol had a protective effect on pancreatic damage by lowering oxidative free radicals and reducing tissue infiltration of neutrophils.

A chemoprotective effect of ellagic acid and flavone has been shown by enhancing the glutathione *S*-transferase (GST) detoxification system in the pancreas of male Wistar rats (Nijhoff and Peters, 1994). Studies on GST isozyme expression levels showed an ellagic acid-increased expression of GST-μ by 160% and a flavone-induced increase of GST-π expression by 200%. Ellagic acid and flavone had no significant effect on pancreatic GST enzyme activity and glutathione content.

Certain catechins have anti-oxidative properties by eliminating superoxide and hydroxyl radicals. Thus, it could be shown that a 0.1% solution of green tea catechins (GTC) as drinking water had a protective effect against the oxidative stress in pancreas and liver induced by the carcinogen *N*-nitrosobis(2-oxopropyl)amine in Syrian golden hamsters (Takabayashi *et al.*, 1997). GTC inhibited the increase of 8-hydroxydeoxyguanosine content in nuclear DNA which is a biomarker of DNA oxidative damage, as well as lipid peroxidation confirming the protective effect of catechins on oxidative stress. In contrast, GTC in combination with a high fat diet may increase oxidative stress in pancreas but may slightly suppress oxidative stress in liver (Takabayashi *et al.*, 2004).

Effects of Ethanol and Non-alcoholic Constituents of Beer upon Pancreatic Stellate Cells Pancreatic stellate cells (PSCs) are the main source of extracellular matrix synthesis leading to pancreatic fibrosis and are activated by growth factors, inflammatory cytokines, alcohol, its metabolites and oxidative stress (Apte *et al.*, 2006).

Recently, it has been shown, that ellagic acid has crucial effects on a number of cell functions of PSCs *in vitro* (Masamune *et al.*, 2005). Ellagic acid inhibited the platelet derived growth factor (PDGF)-induced proliferation and migration in a dose-dependent manner without affecting cell viability. At a concentration of 10 μg/ml ellagic acid inhibited PDGF-induced tyrosine phosphorylation of PDGF β-receptor and the activation of the downstream signaling pathways (ERK and Akt). Furthermore, ellagic acid significantly inhibited several key functions of PSCs including AP-1 and MAP kinases activation, α-SMA gene expression, MCP-1 production and collagen expression in a dose-dependent manner. In addition, ellagic acid blocked the transformation of freshly isolated PSCs from quiescent to myofibroblast-like phenotype in culture. Taken altogether ellagic acid seems to be a potential candidate for the treatment of pancreatic fibrosis and inflammation.

Effects of Non-alcoholic Constituents of Beer upon Pancreatitis Induced in Animals Several animal models have been developed to induce acute pancreatitis (Siegmund *et al.*, 2005). In some recent studies a protective effect of resveratrol on experimentally induced acute pancreatitis could be demonstrated.

Szabolcs *et al.* (2006) examined the effect of resveratrol on CCK-OP-induced acute pancreatitis in male Wistar rats. Pretreatment with resveratrol ameliorated CCK-induced changes of laboratory parameters such as amylase, lipase, glucose, calcium, creatinine and aspartate aminotransferase activities as well as the serum concentration of triglyceride and urea nitrogen. However, resveratrol showed no effect on the reduced pancreatic Cu/Zn-SOD and glutathione peroxidase activity and on the elevated MPO activity and tumor necrosis factor alpha (TNF-α) concentration in the pancreatitis rats. Histopathologically, the pancreas showed a reduced extent of tissue edema, acinar cell vacuolization and focal tissue necrosis after resveratrol treatment. Since no inhibition of nuclear factor-kappa B (NF-κB) activation by resveratrol has been found, it was concluded that the beneficial effects of resveratrol seem to be mediated by the anti-oxidant effect of resveratrol or by an anti-inflammatory mechanism independent of NF-κB.

In contrast to this, activation of NF-κB in macrophages is involved in the inflammatory response of rats with sodium taurocholate-induced SAP. Resveratrol decreased the NF-κB activation as well as iNOS expression in peritoneal macrophages (Ma *et al.*, 2005). In addition, in resveratrol-treated SAP rats serum levels of TNF-α, IL-1 and NO were also reduced. Histological examinations of the pancreas showed an attenuation of various pathological manifestations by resveratrol as compared to SAP group. These results were confirmed by a second study showing an inhibitory effect of resveratrol on expression of NF-κB and the levels of TNF-α and IL-8 in pancreatic tissues of SAP-rats (Meng *et al.*, 2005).

Less pronounced necrotic changes of rat pancreata as well as a decrease of serum amylase activity were also found by treatment with resveratrol for 8 days before induction of acute pancreatitis with free radicals (tert-butyl hydroperoxide) in male Wistar rats (Lawinski *et al.*, 2005). In summary, resveratrol may be considered as an agent for reducing the inflammatory response in acute pancreatitis.

Similar results were found for the effect of catechins on DL-ethionine-induced acute pancreatitis (Takabayashi *et al.*, 1995) and on cerulein-induced pancreatitis (Takabayashi and Harada, 1997) in male Wistar rats showing a protective effect of catechins on experimental-induced pancreatitis in rats, too.

Alcohol Consumption and Diabetes

Diabetes mellitus is a metabolic disorder that is rapidly reaching epidemic proportions, and the World Health Organization has predicted that by 2025, 300 million people will be affected worldwide (Su *et al.*, 2006). Alcohol consumption is associated with type 2 diabetes in a U-shaped manner, indicating a decreased risk of moderate consumers (5–30 g of alcohol per day in the order of 30%) compared with heavier consumers (30 g or more of alcohol per day) or abstainers (Carlsson *et al.*, 2005; Koppes *et al.*, 2005). The beneficial effect of moderate alcohol consumption seems to be equal in women and men as well as consistent across different ethnic groups. High consumers have an increased risk of type 2 diabetes compared to moderate consumers, but whether they have an increased risk compared to low consumers or abstainers is less clear (Carlsson *et al.*, 2005). In patients with type 1 diabetes alcohol is a recognized risk factor for hypoglycemia 12–16 h after the consumption of an alcoholic beverage (Lange *et al.*, 1991). While it seems that the kind of beverage does not influence the association between alcohol consumption and the risk of diabetes for older women with type 2 diabetes (Beulens *et al.*, 2005), Wannamethee *et al.* (2003) showed different effects of various alcoholic beverages on serum insulin concentration in men. Depending on the number of drinks per day, beer and wine showed an inverse effect on blood insulin concentration, whereas spirit had no significant influence.

Recently there has been renewed interest in the use of plant compounds (flavonoids) as antidiabetic compounds since they possess strong anti-oxidant effects resulting in the regeneration of β-cells and protection of pancreatic islets against cytotoxic effects such as oxidative stress (Ihara *et al.*, 1999). Streptozotocin (STZ) and alloxan are the most common substances to induce experimental diabetes in rat to mimic the human situation and to simplify studies on the effects of therapeutic substances on diabetes (Table 60.7).

Effects of non-alcoholic compounds of beer on experimentally induced diabetes in rats

Effects of Epicatechin Chakravarthy and co-workers examined the regeneration of β-cells in alloxan-induced diabetic rats by (–)-epicatechin (Chakravarthy *et al.*, 1981, 1982). Treatment of albino rats with epicatechin for 5 days after alloxan administration resulted in blood sugar levels, β-cell counts and serum insulin levels within normal range. In contrast, untreated diabetic rats showed necrosis and reduction of β-cells, increased blood sugar level and decreased serum insulin level. Epicatechin *per se* had no effect on these parameters and did not cause any toxic effect, too. Another study of Kim *et al.* (2003) investigated the effect of epicatechin on the toxic effect, too STZ in Sprague–Dawley (SD)-rats. The intraperitoneal administration with epicatechin twice a day over a 6-day period resulted in significantly reduced blood glucose level as compared to the diabetic rats. Immunohistochemical analysis showed a significant decline of β-cells to 8.5 ± 2.1% in STZ-rats whereas the pretreatment with epicatechin caused a recovery to 60% as compared to normal control rats. The increase of insulin release

Table 60.7 Effects of non-alcoholic compounds of beer upon diabetes

Compound	*Experimental design*	*Results*	*Species*	*Reference*
Epicatechin (30 mg/kg b.w., twice a day, 24 h after alloxan treatment for 5 days)	*In vivo* Alloxan-induced diabetes Intraperitoneal administration	Reduction of increased blood glucose levels Increase of glucose-induced insulin secretion Increase β-cell counts	Rat (albino)	Chakravarthy *et al.* (1981, 1982)
Epicatechin (30 mg/kg b.w., twice a day, 6 h after STZ treatment for 6 days)	*In vivo/in vitro* STZ-induced diabetes Intraperitoneal administration Isolated islets of Langerhans	Reduction of increased blood glucose levels Protection of β-cells Increased reduced insulin release Inhibited nitrite production	Rat (SD)	Kim *et al.* (2003)
Epicatechin (30 mg/kg b.w., twice a day, for 9 days after STZ-treatment)	*In vivo* STZ-induced diabetes Spontaneous diabetes Intraperitoneal/oral administration	No significant effect on increased blood glucose levels Failed to maintain body weight	Rat (Wistar, BB/E)	Bone *et al.* (1985)
Quercetin (10 and 15 mg/kg b.w./day, for 10 days after STZ-treatment)	*In vivo* STZ-induced diabetes Intraperitoneal administration	Reduction of increased levels of blood glucose, plasma cholesterol and triglyceride Increase of hexokinase activity	Rat (SD)	Vessal *et al.* (2003)
Quercetin (15 mg/kg b.w./day, 3 days pretreatment and for 4 weeks after STZ-treatment)	*In vivo* STZ-induced diabetes Intraperitoneal administration	Reduction of increased blood glucose levels Protection of β-cells Increase of reduced serum insulin levels and anti-oxidant enzyme activities Decrease of elevated blood malondialdehyde levels	Rat (SD)	Coskun *et al.* (2005)
Resveratrol (0.1–0.75 mg/kg b.w., up to three applications/day, 7 days after STZ-treatment for 2 weeks)	*In vivo* STZ-induced and STZ + nicotineamide-induced diabetes Gastric intubation	Reduction of increased levels of blood glucose and of plasma triglyceride Prevention of decreased body weight Increase of glucose uptake by insulin-sensitive tissues	Rat (SD)	Su *et al.* (2006)

b.w.: body weight; BB/E rat: biobreeding/Edinburgh rat; SD: Sprague–Dawley; STZ: Streptozotocin.

as well as the decrease of nitrite concentration indicated a protective effect of epicatechin against the diabetogenic activity of STZ. However, in the study of Bone *et al.* (1985) epicatechin failed to reverse and to halt the progression of diabetes in STZ-induced diabetic Wistar rats and spontaneously diabetic BB/E rats *in vivo*.

Effects of Quercetin Intraperitoneal administration of quercetin showed no effect on plasma glucose concentration in control animals, but significantly reduced elevated blood glucose level of STZ-induced diabetic rats within 8–10 days (Vessal *et al.*, 2003). Lowering of plasma cholesterol and triglyceride levels as well as the significant increase of hexokinase activity by quercetin supplied further evidences for the regenerative action of quercetin on pancreatic islet cells. Coskun *et al.* (2005) showed an increase of the lowered serum insulin levels in STZ-diabetic Wistar rats by quercetin. Quercetin also significantly decreased the elevated blood malondialdehyde level and increased the reduced anti-oxidant enzyme activities. Immunohistological staining of pancreatic islet cells showed a decrease in hydropic degeneration, degranulation, necrosis and an increase of the area of insulin immunoreactive β-cells (Coskun *et al.*, 2005).

Effects of Resveratrol Studies in STZ-induced and STZ plus nicotinamide-induced (strong vs. moderate inducer of diabetes) diabetic SD-rats showed that oral administration of resveratrol resulted in a dose-dependent decrease of the plasma glucose concentrations with a maximal glucose-lowering activity at a dose of 0.5 mg/kg b.w. (Su *et al.*, 2006). Moreover, hypoglycemic activity of resveratrol was confirmed in normal rats. Chronic administration of resveratrol over a period of 14 days significantly reduced plasma glucose and plasma triglyceride concentrations in both types of diabetic rats compared with resveratrol-untreated control animals. In addition, resveratrol generally ameliorated diabetic symptoms in STZ-rats: it prevented decrease of b.w., increased glucose uptake by insulin-sensitive tissues (soleus muscle, hepatocytes and adipocytes) and promoted glycogen synthesis by hepatocytes (Su *et al.*, 2006).

Effects on non-alcoholic compounds of beer on insulin release *in vitro*

Effects of Epicatechin Since insulin deficiency is the main reason for the development of diabetes mellitus various studies on the effect of flavonoids on insulin release were performed (Table 60.8). Hii and Howell (1984) showed that (–)epicatechin increased glucose-induced insulin secretion from isolated islet cells in a dose-dependent manner whereby 1 mM epicatechin produced the greatest response to both 2 and 20 mM glucose. The addition of 0.05 mM epicatechin to culture medium of adult rat islets containing 5.5 or 20 mM glucose caused an increase in DNA synthesis suggesting that the regenerative effect of epicatechin in experimental diabetic rats may be a direct effect on β-cell replication (Hii and Howell, 1984). The stimulatory effect of epicatechin on insulin secretion in pancreatic islet cells seems to be mediated, at least in part, via alterations in Ca^{2+} fluxes (Hii and Howell, 1985) and in cyclic nucleotide metabolism (Ahmad *et al.*, 1991) and depends on the age of the experimental rats (Ahmad *et al.*, 1991).

Other flavonoids have different effects on insulin secretion of islet cells (Hii and Howell, 1985). They were able to stimulate (quercetin), or to reduce (chrysin, naringenin) insulin secretion or they had no significant effect (catechin, flavone). The stimulation occurred only in the presence of 20 mM glucose, suggesting that cell functions are affected by flavonoids only when the cells are fully activated. Quercetin may, at least in part, exert its effect on insulin release via changes in Ca^{2+} uptake (Hii and Howell, 1985).

Effects of Resveratrol Resveratrol showed no effect on insulin secretion from INS-1 cells (Zhang *et al.*, 2004), whereas incubation of freshly isolated islets from Wistar rats with resveratrol resulted in a significant and concentration-dependent inhibition of glucose-induced insulin secretion (Szkudelski, 2006). Insulin secretion induced by insulin secretagogues other than glucose (leucine and glutamine) was also inhibited by resveratrol, suggesting that glucose transport or metabolism is not crucial for the inhibition of insulin secretion by resveratrol. However, the PKC activator TPA completely suppressed the inhibitory effect of resveratrol on glucose-induced insulin secretion suggesting that the effect of resveratrol on insulin secretion involves the inhibition of PKC activity.

Effects of Anthocyanins and Anthocyanidins Proanthocyanidins are polyphenols which are present mainly in cacao liquor but also in beer and wine (Madigan *et al.*, 1994; Stevens *et al.*, 2002). Proanthocyanidins are effective scavengers of radicals which are cleaved to anthocyanidins by oxidative hydrolysis (Cheynier, 1992). Jayaprakasam *et al.* (2005) studied the effect of 50 μg/ml of various anthocyanins (cyanidin-3-glucoside, delphinidin-3-glucoside, cyanidin-3-galactoside and pelargonidin-3-galactoside) and anthocyanidins (cyanidin, delphinidin, pelargonidin, malvidin and petunidin) on glucose-induced insulin release from INS-1 cells. Both, anthocyanins and anthocyanidins increased glucose-induced insulin secretion whereby the most potent anthocyanin was delphinidin-3-glucoside. The comparison of different anthocyanins indicated that the number of hydroxyl groups at the second ring played an important role in their ability to stimulate insulin secretion. Among the anthocyanidins tested, pelargonidin was the most active one whereas the others did not significantly increase insulin secretion.

Effects of Salicylic Acid Salicylic acid is the primary immune hormone in plants and is among other things a non-alcoholic constituent of beer. Sodium salicylate is known to be a cyclooxygenase inhibitor. In this regard Walsh and Pek (1984) investigated the effect of sodium salicylate on glucose (16.7 mM)-stimulated insulin secretion from isolated perfused pancreas of SD-rats. Glucose-induced insulin release was slightly but not significantly increased by sodium salicylate. Since sodium salicylate decreased the total prostaglandin 2 release to less than 1% of control, the authors concluded that inhibition of cyclooxygenase did not play any role in glucose-induced insulin release (Walsh and Pek, 1984).

Tran *et al.* (2002) showed that pretreatment of isolated pancreatic islets with 20 mg/dl sodium salicylate for 45 min prevented the IL-1β-induced decrease in insulin secretion in such a rate that glucose-stimulated insulin secretion was not significantly different from control. Furthermore, treatment of islets with sodium salicylate prevented IL-1β-induced NF-κB activation. Sodium salicylate also inhibits IL-1β-induced increase of COX-2 and EP3 gene expression indicating that its positive effect on pancreatic β-cell function includes inhibition of prostaglandin signaling pathways (Tran *et al.*, 2002). Sodium salicylate (250 μM) prevented also the increased apoptosis rate of human islets cultured on extracellular matrix induced by either IL-1β or high glucose concentration (Zeender *et al.*, 2004). Furthermore, sodium salicylate decreased cAMP release (Metz *et al.*, 1982), and showed effects on ionic fluxes (decrease in Ca^{2+} influx, activation of K^+ channels) and β cell membrane potential that can partly account for the sodium salicylate-induced changes in pancreatic β-cell function (Fujimoto and Metz, 1984; Chapman and Pattinson, 1987; Drews *et al.*, 1992).

In conclusion, flavonoids showed insulin-like and insulin-stimulatory effects when tested on insulin target tissues *in vitro* and *in vivo* and had protective effects on experimental diabetes possibly by reduction of oxidative stress and/or by conservation of pancreatic β-cell viability.

Table 60.8 Effects of non-alcoholic constituents of beer upon insulin secretion

Compound	*Experimental design*	*Results*	*Species*	*Reference*
Epicatechin (30 mg/kg b.w. twice a day for 4 days *in vivo*, <1,000 μM *in vitro*)	*In vivo/in vitro* Isolated islets of Langerhans	Increase of glucose-induced insulin secretion via changes in Ca^{2+}-uptake Increase of DNA replication of β-cells	Rat (Wistar)	Hii and Howell (1984, 1985)
Epicatechin (200 μM–1 mM)	*In vitro* Isolated islets of Langerhans	Increase of cAMP content Biological activity depends on age of rats	Rat (Charles Foster)	Ahmad *et al.* (1991)
Quercetin (10 and 100 μM)	*In vitro* Isolated islets of Langerhans	Increase of glucose-induced insulin secretion via changes in Ca^{2+}-uptake	Rat (Wistar)	Hii and Howell (1985)
Resveratrol (1–100 μM)	*In vivo* Isolated islets of Langerhans	Decrease of glucose-, leucine- and glutamine-induced insulin secretion	Rat (Wistar)	Szkudelski (2006)
Catechin (0.1 and 1.0 mM)	*In vitro* Isolated islets of Langerhans	No effect on glucose-induced insulin secretion	Rat (Wistar)	Hii and Howell (1985)
Flavone (100 μM)	*In vitro* Isolated islets of Langerhans	No effect on glucose-induced insulin secretion	Rat (Wistar)	Hii and Howell (1985)
Anthocyanins/anthocyanidins (50 μg/ml)	*In vitro* INS-1 cell line	Increase of glucose-induced insulin secretion	Rat	Jayaprakasam *et al.* (2005)
Sodium salicylate (1.2 mM)	*In vitro* Isolated perfused pancreas	Increase of glucose-induced insulin secretion Decrease of prostaglandin 2 release	Rat (SD)	Walsh and Pek (1984)
Sodium salicylate (1.25 mM)	*In vitro* Isolated islets of Langerhans	Prevention of IL-1β-induced decrease in insulin secretion and NF-κB activation Inhibition of IL-1β-induced COX-2 and EP3 gene expression	Rat (Wistar)	Tran *et al.* (2002)
Sodium salicylate (250 μM)	*In vitro* Isolated islets of Langerhans	Protection of human β-cells against IL-1β- or high glucose-induced apoptosis and loss of function	Human	Zeender *et al.* (2004)
Sodium salicylate (1.25 mM)	*In vitro* Isolated islets of Langerhans	Increase of glucose-induced insulin secretion Inhibition of basal and theophylline-induced cAMP accumulation	Rat (SD)	Metz *et al.* (1982)
Sodium salicylate (0.5–10 mM)	*In vitro* Isolated islets of Langerhans	Increase of glucose-induced insulin release Decrease of Ca^{2+}-efflux Inhibition of glucose-induced electrical activity in β-cells	Mouse (Naval Medical Research Institute)	Drews *et al.* (1992)
Sodium salicylate (1.25 mM)	*In vitro* Isolated neonatal islets of Langerhans	Increase of glucose-induced insulin secretion	Rat (SD)	Fujimoto and Metz (1984)

b.w.: body weight; cAMP: adenosine-3′,5′-cyclic monophosphate; COX: Cyclooxygenase; EP3: prostaglandin E3 receptor; SD: Sprague–Dawley.

Bioavailability of Polyphenols

An important aspect of critical consideration of *in vitro* results and their transferability to *in vivo* models is the fact that non-alcoholic constituents are extensively altered during metabolism so that, in general, the molecular forms reaching the peripheral circulation and tissues are different from those in foods. In the case of polyphenols the resulting metabolites are conjugates which are chemically distinct from their parent compounds, differing in size, polarity and ionic form displaying a different physiologic behavior as compared to the native compounds (for review see Kroon *et al.*, 2004). For example, Day *et al.* (2001) showed that the plasma of volunteers fed fried onions (containing quercetin-4-glucoside and quercetin-3,4-di-glucoside) contained a mixture of 12 discrete quercetin conjugates. The same authors demonstrated *in vitro* that the anti-oxidant activity of quercetin conjugates is, on average, about half of aglycone, and that there are significant variations according to the position of conjugation (Day *et al.*, 2000).

In addition, a recent study showed that, at least for quercetin and quercetin-3-glucoside, the alcohol content of red wine is a major factor responsible for the uptake of polyphenols in mucosal tissue of Wistar rats (Dragoni *et al.*, 2006). Vice versa, Hey and Haslund-Vinding (2006) showed that the type of alcoholic beverage consumed determines the amount of absorbed alcohol. Therefore, it is crucial to use only physiologically relevant compounds and their metabolites at appropriate concentrations in the study of biological responses to non-alcoholic constituents of alcoholic beverages.

Summary Points

- Beer has a stimulatory effect on exocrine pancreas secretion whereas ethanol in concentration found in beer (4% v/v) has no effect.
- Non-alcoholic constituents of beer seem to be responsible for the stimulatory effect of beer. These substances are generated during fermentation.
- Maleic acid and succinic acid, the non-alcoholic compounds of beer and other fermented alcoholic beverages that maximally increase gastric acid output, have alone or in combination with ethanol in concentrations found in beer no effect on basal protein secretion.
- Non-alcoholic constituents of beer other than these dicarboxylic acids must be responsible for the stimulatory action of beer on exocrine pancreas.
- There is accumulating evidence that natural phenolic compounds of plants found in alcoholic beverages exert different effects on the pancreas.
- Particularly *resveratrol* protects the pancreas against pro-oxidative activity of hydroperoxide and inhibits inflammation. It is anticipated that *resveratrol* could serve as a therapeutic compound in managing acute pancreatitis through different pathways.
- Other non-alcoholic constituents of alcoholic beverages such as quercetin, epicatechin exert also protective effects *in vitro*.
- In *in vitro* studies bioavailability and efficacy of non-alcoholic constituents has to be considered because the compounds are extensively altered *in vivo* after ingestion.
- Alcoholic beverages contain much more non-alcoholic ingredients. The effects of these ingredients are still unknown.
- The effect of the combination of the different substances acting alone on the pancreas has been scarcely or not at all examined.
- Therefore, caution is required in attempting to draw firm conclusions on the effect of alcoholic beverages on defining alcoholic etiology of pancreatic diseases.

References

Ahmad, F., Khan, M.M., Rastogi, A.K., Chaubey, M. and Kidwai, J.R. (1991). *Indian J. Exp. Biol.* 29, 516–520.

Apte, M.V. and Wilson, J.S. (2003). *Best Pract. Res. Clin. Gastroenterol.* 17, 593–612.

Apte, M.V., Pirola, R.C. and Wilson, J.S. (2005). *Dig. Dis.* 23, 232–240.

Apte, M.V., Pirola, R.C. and Wilson, J.S. (2006). *J. Gastroenterol. Hepatol.* 21, S97–S101.

Beulens, J.W., Stolk, R.P., van der Schouw, Y.T., Grobbee, D.E., Hendriks, H.F. and Bots, M.L. (2005). *Diabetes Care* 28, 2933–2938.

Bone, A.J., Hii, C.S., Brown, D., Smith, W. and Howell, S.L. (1985). *Biosci. Rep.* 5, 215–221.

Brugge, W.R., Burke, C.A., Brand, D.L. and Chey, W.Y. (1985). *Dig. Dis. Sci.* 30, 431–439.

Bujanda, L. (2000). *Am. J. Gastroenterol.* 95, 3374–3382.

Carlsson, S., Hammar, N. and Grill, V. (2005). *Diabetologia* 48, 1051–1054.

Chakravarthy, B.K., Gupta, S., Gambhir, S.S. and Gode, K.D. (1981). *Lancet* 2, 759–760.

Chakravarthy, B.K., Gupta, S. and Gode, K.D. (1982). *Life Sci.* 31, 2693–2697.

Chapman, B.A. and Pattinson, N.R. (1987). *Biochem. Pharmacol.* 36, 3353–3360.

Chari, S.T., Harder, H., Teyssen, S., Knodel, C., Riepl, R.L. and Singer, M.V. (1996). *Dig. Dis. Sci.* 41, 1216–1224.

Cheynier, V. (1992). Structure of procyanidin oligomers isolated from grape seeds in relation of some of their chemical properties. In Hemingway, R.W. and Laks, P.E. (eds), *Plant Polyphenols*, pp. 281–294. Plenum Press, New York.

Chowdhury, P. and Gupta, P. (2006). *World J. Gastroenterol.* 12, 7421–7427.

Coskun, O., Kanter, M., Korkmaz, A. and Oter, S. (2005). *Pharmacol. Res.* 51, 117–123.

Day, A.J. Mellon, F., Barron, D., Sarrazin, G., Morgan, M.R. and Williamson, G. (2001). *Free Radic. Res.* 35, 941–952.

Day, A.J., Bao, Y., Morgan, M.R. and Williamson, G. (2000). *Free Radic. Biol. Med.* 29, 1234–1243.

Deschner, E.E., Ruperto, J., Wong, G. and Newmark, H.L. (1991). *Carcinogenesis* 12, 1193–1196.

Devaux, M.A., Lechene de la Porte, P., Johnson, C. and Sarles, H. (1990). *Pancreas* 5, 200–209.

DiMagno, E.P., Layer, P. and Clain, J.E. (1993). Chronic Pancreatitis. In Go, V.L.W., DiMagno, E.P., Gardner, J.D., Lebenthal, L., Reber, H.A. and Scheele, G.A. (eds), *The Pancreas: Biology, Pathobiology and Disease*, pp. 665–706. Plenum Press, New York.

Dragoni, S., Gee, J., Bennett, R., Valoti, M. and Sgaragli, G. (2006). *Br. J. Pharmacol.* 147, 765–771.

Drews, G., Garrino, M.G. and Henquin, J.C. (1992). *Diabetes* 41, 620–626.

Durbec, J.P. and Sarles, H. (1978). *Digestion* 18, 337–350.

Feick, P., Henn, E. and Singer, M.V. (2003). *Gastroenterology* 124, M2211.

Feick, P., Haas, S., Böcker, U. and Singer, M.V. (2006). *Alcohol. Clin. Exp. Res.* 30, A141.

Fujimoto, W.Y. and Metz, S.A. (1984). *Diabetes* 33, 872–878.

Go, V.L., Gukovskaya, A. and Pandol, S.J. (2005). *Alcohol* 35, 205–211.

Gumaste, V.V. (1995). *Gastroenterology* 108, 297–299.

Gerloff et al. (unpublished)

Haber, P., Wilson, J., Apte, M., Korsten, M. and Pirola, R. (1995). *J. Lab. Clin. Med.* 125, 305–312.

Hajnal, F., Flores, M.C. and Valenzuela, J.E. (1989). *Pancreas* 4, 486–491.

Hajnal, F., Flores, M.C., Radley, S. and Valenzuela, J.E. (1990). *Gastroenterology* 98, 191–196.

Harada, H., Takeda, M., Yabe, H., Hanafusa, E., Hayashi, T., Kunichika, K., Kochi, F., Mishima, K., Kimura, I. and Ubuga, T. (1980). *Gastroenterol. Jpn.* 15, 520–526.

Hey, H. and Haslund-Vinding, P. (2006). *Ugeskr. Laeger* 168, 470–475.

Hii, C.S. and Howell, S.L. (1984). *Diabetes* 33, 291–296.

Hii, C.S.T. and Howell, S.L. (1985). *J. Endocrinol.* 107, 1–8.

Ihara, Y., Toyokuni, S., Uchida, K., Odaka, H., Tanaka, T., Ikeda, H., Hiai, H., Seino, Y. and Yamada, Y. (1999). *Diabetes* 48, 927–932.

Janbaz, K.H., Saeed, S.A. and Gilani, A.H. (2002). *Fitoterapia* 73, 557–563.

Jayaprakasam, B., Vareed, S.K., Olson, L.K. and Nair, M.G. (2005). *J. Agric. Food Chem.* 53, 28–31.

Kim, M.J., Ryu, G.R., Chung, J.S., Sim, S.S., Min do, S., Rhie, D.J., Yoon, S.H., Hahn, S.J., Kim, M.S. and Jo, Y.H. (2003). *Pancreas* 26, 292–299.

Kolbel, C.B., Singer, M.V., Mohle, T., Heinzel, C., Eysselein, V. and Goebell, H. (1986). *Pancreas* 1, 211–218.

Kolbel, C.B., Singer, M.V., Dorsch, W., Krege, P., Eysselein, V.E., Layer, P. and Goebell, H. (1988). *Pancreas* 3, 89–94.

Koppes, L.L., Dekker, J.M., Hendriks, H.F., Bouter, L.M. and Heine, R.J. (2005). *Diabetes Care* 28, 719–725.

Kroon, P.A., Clifford, M.N., Crozier, A., Day, A.J., Donovan, J.L., Manach, C. and Williamson, G. (2004). *Am. J. Clin. Nutr.* 80, 15–21.

Lange, J., Arends, J. and Willms, B. (1991). *Med. Klin. (Munich)* 86, 551–554.

Lawinski, M., Sledzinski, Z., Kubasik-Juraniec, J., Spodnik, J.H., Wozniak, M. and Boguslawski, W. (2005). *Pancreas* 31, 43–47.

Lee, P.C., Shimizu, K., Rossi, T.M. and Cumella, J.C. (1988). *Pancreas* 3, 317–323.

Li, Z.D., Ma, Q.Y. and Wang, C.A. (2006). *World J. Gastroenterol.* 12, 137–140.

Ma, Z.H., Ma, Q.Y., Wang, L.C., Sha, H.C., Wu, S.L. and Zhang, M. (2005). *Inflamm. Res.* 54, 522–527.

Madigan, D., McMurrough, I. and Smyth, M.R. (1994). *Analyst* 119, 863–868.

Masamune, A., Satoh, M., Kikuta, K., Suzuki, N., Satoh, K. and Shimosegawa, T. (2005). *Biochem. Pharmacol.* 70, 869–878.

Maxwell, S., Cruickshank, A. and Thorpe, G. (1994). *Lancet* 344, 193–194.

Meng, Y., Ma, Q.Y., Kou, X.P. and Xu, J. (2005). *World J. Gastroenterol.* 11, 525–528.

Metz, S., Fujimoto, W. and Robertson, R.P. (1982). *Metabolism* 31, 1014–1022.

Moll, N. and Joly, J.P. (1987). *J. Chromatogr.* 405, 347–356.

Nakamura, T., Okabayashi, Y., Fujii, M., Tani, S., Fujisawa, T. and Otsuki, M. (1991). *Pancreas* 6, 571–577.

Niebergall-Roth, E., Harder, H. and Singer, M.V. (1998). *Alcohol. Clin. Exp. Res.* 22, 1570–1583.

Nijhoff, W.A. and Peters, W.H. (1994). *Carcinogenesis* 15, 1769–1772.

Noroozi, M., Angerson, W.J. and Lean, M.E. (1998). *Am. J. Clin. Nutr.* 67, 1210–1218.

Peterson, W.L., Barnett, C. and Walsh, J.H. (1986). *Gastroenterology* 91, 1390–1395.

Piendl, A. (1980). *Brauwelt* 120, 518–532.

Piendl, A. (2005). Inhaltsstoffe des bieres, dargestellt am beispiel des pilsener lagerbieres. In Singer, M.V. and Teyssen, S. (eds), *Alkohol und Alkoholfolgekrankheiten*, pp. 65–69. Springer Verlag Berlin, Heidelberg.

Planche, N.E., Palasciano, G., Meullenet, J., Laugier, R. and Sarles, H. (1982). *Dig. Dis. Sci.* 27, 449–453.

Ponnappa, B.C., Hoek, J.B., Waring, A.J. and Rubin, E. (1987). *Biochem. Pharmacol.* 36, 69–79.

Renner, I.G., Rinderknecht, H., Valenzuela, J.E. and Douglas, A. P. (1980). *Scand. J. Gastroenterol.* 15, 241–244.

Rinderknecht, H., Stace, N.H. and Renner, I.G. (1985). *Dig. Dis. Sci.* 30, 65–71.

Sahel, J. and Sarles, H. (1979). *Dig. Dis. Sci.* 24, 897–905.

Sarles, H. (1991). *Pancreas* 6, 470–474.

Sbarra, V., Ristorcelli, E., Petit-Thevenin, J.L., Teissedre, P.L., Lombardo, D. and Verine, A. (2005). *Biochim. Biophys. Acta* 1736, 67–76.

Schneider, A. and Singer, M.V. (2005). *Dig. Dis.* 23, 222–231.

Schneider, A., Haas, S.L. and Singer, M.V. (2005). Alcohol and Pancreatitis. In Preedy, V.R. (ed.), *Comprehensive Handbook of Alcohol Related Pathology*, Vol. 2, pp. 577–597. Elsevier Ltd, Amsterdam.

Schneider, A., Whitcomb, D.C. and Singer, M.V. (2002). *Pancreatology* 2, 189–203.

Siegmund, S.V., Haas, S. and Singer, M.V. (2005). *Dig. Dis.* 23, 181–194.

Singer, M.V. (1985). *Schweiz. Med. Wochenschr.* 115, 973–987.

Singer, M.V. and Goebell, H. (1985). Acute and chronic effects of alcohol on pancreatic exocrine secretion in humans and animals. In Seitz, H.K. and Kommerell, B. (eds), *Alcohol Related Diseases in Gastroenterology*, pp. 376–414. Springer, Berlin.

Singer, M.V. and Müller, M.K. (1995). Epidemiologie, Ätiologie und Pathogenese der chronischen Pankreatitis. In Mössner, J.,

Adler, G., Fölsch, U.R. and Singer, M.V. (eds), *Erkrankungen des exkretorischen Pankreas*, pp. 313–324. Gustav Fischer Verlag, Jena.

Singer, M.V., Eysselein, V. and Goebell, H. (1983a). *Digestion* 26, 73–79.

Singer, M.V., Eysselein, V. and Goebell, H. (1983b). *Regul. Pept.* 6, 13–23.

Singer, M.V., Gyr, K. and Sarles, H. (1985). *Gastroenterology* 89, 683–685.

Singer, M.V., Leffmann, C., Eysselein, V.E., Calden, H. and Goebell, H. (1987). *Gastroenterology* 93, 1247–1254.

Singh, M. and Simsek, H. (1990). *Gastroenterology* 98, 1051–1062.

Stevens, J.F., Miranda, C.L., Wolthers, K.R., Schimerlik, M., Deinzer, M.L. and Buhler, D.R. (2002). *J. Agric. Food Chem.* 50, 3435–3443.

Su, H.C., Hung, L.M. and Chen, J.K. (2006). *Am. J. Physiol. Endocrinol. Metab.* 290, E1339–E1346.

Szabolcs, A., Varga, I.S., Varga, C., Berko, A., Kaszaki, J., Letoha, T., Tiszlavicz, L., Sari, R., Lonovics, J. and Takacs, T. (2006). *Eur. J. Pharmacol.* 532, 187–193.

Szkudelski, T. (2006). *Eur. J. Pharmacol.* 552, 176–181.

Takabayashi, F. and Harada, N. (1997). *Pancreas* 14, 276–279.

Takabayashi, F., Harada, N. and Hara, Y. (1995). *Pancreas* 11, 127–131.

Takabayashi, F., Harada, N., Tahara, S., Kaneko, T. and Hara, Y. (1997). *Pancreas* 15, 109–112.

Takabayashi, F., Tahara, S., Kaneko, T. and Harada, N. (2004). *Biofactors* 21, 335–337.

Tedesco, I., Nappo, A., Petitto, F., Iacomino, G., Nazzaro, F., Palumbo, R. and Russo, G.L. (2005). *Nutr. Cancer* 52, 74–83.

Teyssen, S., Lenzing, T., Gonzalez-Calero, G., Korn, A., Riepl, R.L. and Singer, M.V. (1997). *Gut* 40, 49–56.

Teyssen, S., Gonzalez-Calero, G., Schimiczek, M. and Singer, M.V. (1999). *J. Clin. Invest.* 103, 707–713.

Tran, P.O., Gleason, C.E. and Robertson, R.P. (2002). *Diabetes* 51, 1772–1778.

Uhlemann, E.R., Robberecht, P. and Gardner, J.D. (1979). *Gastroenterology* 76, 917–925.

Vessal, M., Hemmati, M. and Vasei, M. (2003). *Comp. Biochem. Physiol. C Toxicol. Pharmacol.* 135C, 357–364.

Walsh, M.F. and Pek, S.B. (1984). *Life Sci.* 34, 1699–1706.

Wannamethee, S.G., Lowe, G.D., Shaper, G., Whincup, P.H., Rumley, A., Walker, M. and Lennon, L. (2003). *Thromb. Haemost.* 90, 1080–1087.

Wilson, J.S., Bernstein, L., McDonald, C., Tait, A., McNeil, D. and Pirola, R.C. (1985). *Gut* 26, 882–887.

Worning, H. (1998). Alcoholic chronic pancreatitis. In Beger, H.G., Warshaw, A.L. and Büchler, M.W. (eds), *The Pancreas*, pp. 672–682. Blackwell Science, Malden, MA.

Yang, C.S. and Wang, Z.Y. (1993). *J. Natl. Cancer Inst.* 85, 1038–1049.

Zeender, E., Maedler, K., Bosco, D., Berney, T., Donath, M.Y. and Halban, P.A. (2004). *J. Clin. Endocrinol. Metab.* 89, 5059–5066.

Zhang, Y., Jayaprakasam, B., Seeram, N.P., Olson, L.K., DeWitt, D. and Nair, M.G. (2004). *J. Agric. Food Chem.* 52, 228–233.

61

Beer and the Liver

Rajaventhan Srirajaskanthan Centre of Gastroenterology, Royal Free Hospital, London, UK
Victor R. Preedy Nutritional Sciences Research Division, School of Biomedical and Health Sciences, Department of Nutrition and Dietetics, King's College London, London, UK

Abstract

This chapter examines the evidence supporting the link between alcohol and liver disease. There is clear evidence that excessive alcohol consumption is associated with liver disease; this is true for all different types of alcoholic beverages. However, it is apparent that some beverages are more harmful, particularly spirits compared to wine or beer, although this is contentious. For example, the threshold value for the increases in serum gamma glutamyl transferase is higher with beer than alcohol in general. The interpretation of this is complicated by the evidence showing that alcoholics change their preference for a particular beverage type as liver disease progresses. Thus, in one study on cirrhotic patients, pre-alcoholics preferred beer as opposed to more ardent spirits in chronic alcoholics. There are other confounding issues. For example, there is a substantial body of evidence to support the notion that wine and beer drinkers have different diets. The importance of this relates to the observation that diet modulates the effect of alcohol. Thus, in patients with cirrhosis there is a positive correlation with beer consumption and ingestion of pork-related products. In contrast, there is a negative correlation between wine consumption and ingestion of pig products in patients with cirrhosis. There is also evidence that beer alters the biochemistry of the liver directly, for example modulating the response to ischemic stress and increasing enzymes involved in detoxification. However, light beers and dark beers have different effects on the liver. Unfortunately, this distinction between beer types has not been investigated in depth in clinical studies and this merits further investigation.

List of Abbreviations

ATP	Adenosine triphosphate
GGT	Gamma glutamyl transferase
RR	Relative risk
SDR	Standard death rate
WHO	World Health Organization

Introduction

The first section of this chapter will focus on the rise in cirrhosis related to alcohol consumption. Thereafter the putative role of beer in liver disease is examined. Confounding factors including the contribution of the diet are also discussed, particularly the differences between beer and wine drinkers. Finally we review the effects of beer on liver biochemistry. This data show that beer has specific effects on the liver, compared to ethanol alone and there are also differences in the responses to consumption of light and dark beers.

Liver Disease Associated with Alcohol Consumption

There is a general consensus regarding the causal role of alcohol and risk of alcoholic liver disease, especially cirrhosis (Preedy and Watson, 2005). Alcohol is thought to be the underlying cause of cirrhosis in 39% of men and 18% of women worldwide (Rehm *et al.*, 2003a). It is accepted that long-term heavy alcohol intake is required to cause cirrhosis; however, there are still questions regarding the minimal threshold above which alcoholic liver disease can occur. It has been shown that a consumption of 20 g of alcohol a day led to a twofold increase in cirrhosis when compared to individuals with no intake (Anderson, 1995). This issue is further complicated by underlying influences of body weight and gender. Studies have shown that ethanol intakes of 3.2 g/kg for males and 2.0 g/kg for females are required to cause cirrhosis (Mezey *et al.*, 1988). Other studies have shown that between 0.5 and 1.0 g/kg of alcohol per day can lead to cirrhosis in females (Norton *et al.*, 1997).

Within the United Kingdom, there has been a steady state of alcohol consumption from the 1980s to 2004, with a total rise of 2.5%. However, interestingly there has been a much higher increase in liver cirrhosis (Figure 61.1).

Beer in Health and Disease Prevention
ISBN: 978-0-12-373891-2

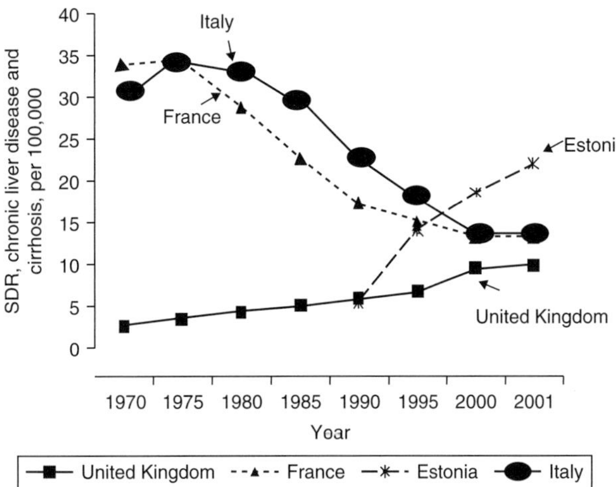

Figure 61.1 The changing rates of cirrhosis. The falling rates of cirrhosis in France and Italy are associated with a fall in alcohol consumption over the corresponding time period. There is a worrying rise in cirrhosis rates in some countries like Estonia. In the United Kingdom there has been a rise in cirrhosis rates over the last 10 years, this rise is marked and has not correlated with a dramatic rise in alcohol consumption. Note that the data report 5-year intervals except for the last two entry points which depict a 1-year interval. SDR, standard death rate.

A recent paper showed that cirrhosis rates have increased greatly, by 64% in England and Wales over the period from 1987–1991 to 1997–2001 (Leon and McCambridge, 2006). Of particular concern is the observation that cirrhosis rates in Scotland have doubled (increased 104%) over the period from 1987–1991 to 1997–2001. Why this has occurred remains unclear. Some cases of cirrhosis will be related to increased prevalence of hepatitis C which has been on the rise; however, this will only account for a small percentage of the total increase.

Other non-alcohol-related causes of cirrhosis have remained at a stable level over the past decade (Leon and McCambridge, 2006); however, there are increasing numbers of patients being diagnosed with non-alcoholic steatohepatitis and consequent cirrhosis, for example in the United States (Clark, 2006; Farrell and Larter, 2006). It is possible that the number of individuals drinking may have reduced and yet the total consumption has increased. However, studies have shown no significant change in the number of people abstaining from alcohol within the United Kingdom. The pattern of drinking in the United Kingdom has changed over the last few years and this is thought to be partly responsible for the increased rate of cirrhosis. The number of individuals involved in binge drinking and heavy drinking has increased markedly.

There has been a 924% increase in cirrhosis rates in women between ages 25 and 44 years, between 1970 and 1990 (WHO, 2004). This increase is mainly due to an increase in alcohol consumption *per se* women and a change in drinking practices. The effects of alcohol on women occur at different levels of consumption than in males. Beneficial mortality rates have been noted to occur in women with an intake of 1.5–4.9 g of alcohol a day (i.e. 1–3 drinks per week). However, increased mortality was noted with an intake of 30 g a day (i.e. 18 drinks per week) (Sijbrands *et al.*, 1995).

Beer and Other Beverage Consumption Within Europe

Within Europe there have been clear trends and changes in consumption of alcohol, and more importantly there is a clear difference in drinking patterns within countries in Europe (Figures 61.2 and 61.3). There is evidence supporting that the "binge" drinking culture which is particularly problematic in the United Kingdom is related to the higher incidence of alcohol-related morbidity and mortality (Mukamal *et al.*, 2005). It has been shown that mortality rates are higher in binge beer drinkers when compared to non-binge drinkers, independent of the total alcohol consumption of alcoholic drinks (Kauhanen *et al.*, 1997). Deaths due to injuries and external causes were increased in binge drinkers; however, in addition there were an increased number of deaths secondary to myocardial infarction.

In Sweden there had also been a small rise in alcohol consumption over the last few years, however, there has been a decrease in cirrhosis rates. So the cause of this difference is unclear but it may be related to the type of beverage being consumed or the nature of alcohol consumption (Stokkeland *et al.*, 2006) or other hitherto unexplained factors.

In Central Europe there are a group of previous communist countries including Maldova Romania and Hungary in which rates of cirrhosis have increased even though legal alcohol sales have not increased. In these countries studies looking into the use of privately/homemade alcohol have found that these confer a greater risk of developing cirrhosis (Szucs *et al.*, 2005). Since there is no formal method of assessing total consumption of illegal or homemade ethanol, then only estimates can be made (Leon *et al.*, 1997; Rehm *et al.*, 2003b). Figure 61.4 clearly shows that unrecorded beverage consumption can be very high, and values range from 11% to 53% per region.

Beer in Relation to Wine and Spirits and Their Beneficial Effects

There is clear evidence that moderate intake of alcohol on a regular basis has a protective effect on overall mortality (Thun *et al.*, 1997). Alcohol consumption and mortality show a J-shaped curve, so moderate drinkers have a lower overall mortality than non-drinkers and then as alcohol consumption increases there is a sharp rise in mortality (Thakker, 1998; Gutjahr *et al.*, 2001). There has been a clear trend in many European countries over the last 20 years that although alcohol consumption has increased slightly, there has been an overall decrease in cirrhosis rates (Stokkeland *et al.*, 2006).

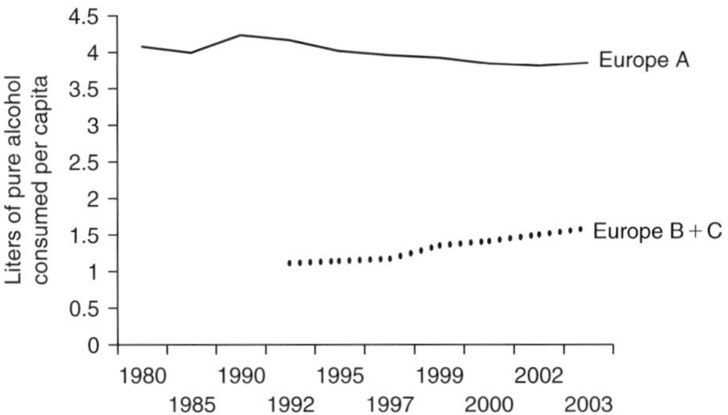

Figure 61.2 Consumption of beer within Europe between 1980 and 2003. It can be seen that there is a general trend to harmonization between Europe A countries (e.g. United Kingdom, France and Spain) and Europe B + C countries (e.g. Albania, Estonia and Poland). Note that year-related data sets are episodic, that is, dates are not sequentially patterned. Europe A covers Andorra, Austria, Belgium, Croatia, Czech Republic, Denmark, Finland, France, Germany, Greece, Iceland, Ireland, Israel, Italy, Luxembourg, Malta, Monaco, The Netherlands, Norway, Portugal, San Marino, Slovenia, Spain, Sweden, Switzerland and the United Kingdom. Europe B covers Albania, Armenia, Azerbaijan, Bosnia and Herzegovina, Bulgaria, Georgia, Kyrgyzstan, Poland, Romania, Slovakia, the Former Yugoslav Republic of Macedonia, Tajikistan, Turkmenistan, Turkey, Uzbekistan and Yugoslavia. Europe C covers Belarus, Estonia, Hungary, Kazakhstan, Latvia, Lithuania, Republic of Moldova, Russian Federation and Ukraine. Data from WHO Health Trends in Europe database.

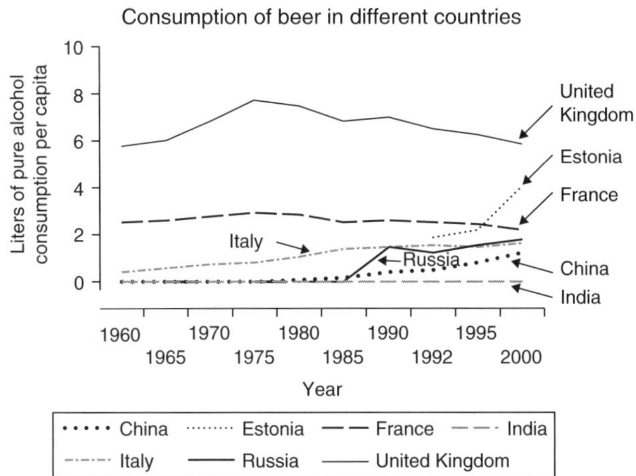

Figure 61.3 Trends in consumption of beer in specific countries around the world. The fall in beer consumption seen in the United Kingdom has been offset by an increased wine consumption. The reverse has occurred in Italy, where increased beer consumption has been associated with a decrease in wine consumption. Note that year-related data sets are episodic, that is, dates are not sequentially patterned in that a 1992 entry is included. Data sets for India, China and Russia in the period leading up to the 1980s are difficult to distinguish on these graphical scales since they are very low (though increasing in recent years).

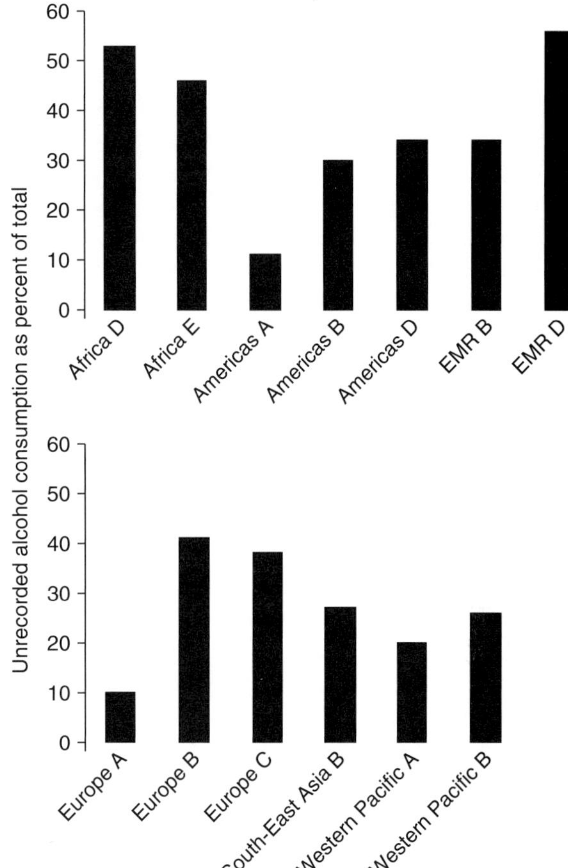

Figure 61.4 The percentage of the total unrecorded alcohol consumption. There is a large proportion of unrecorded alcohol intake from countries in Africa and South-East Asia. The high levels of consumption per drinker relative to the total consumption in some regions are due to the percentage of the population that abstain from alcohol and the number of children under the age of 15 years which contributes to the population. *Source*: Figure adapted from data in Rehm *et al.* (2003a, b).

There is some evidence to suggest that different alcoholic beverages have different overall protective effects; most research has looked into wine and its apparent cardio-protective effect. Furthermore work has illustrated that wine drinkers have a lower risk of death from all causes (Gronbaek *et al.*, 2000; Klatsky *et al.*, 2003). The cause for this difference in mortality between wine, beer and spirits has been postulated to be related to the possible carcinogenic nitrosamines present in beer (Castegnaro, 1988; Kubacki *et al.*, 1989; Tricker and Preussmann, 1991) and whether wine has additional cardio-protective or anticarcinogenic properties beyond that of ethanol (Gronbaek *et al.*, 2004). There have been some studies looking into mortality and cirrhosis in patients with a predominant intake of beer, wine and spirits. A longitudinal study has been carried out on 30,000 plus individuals looking at their drinking habits and beverage preference (Gronbaek *et al.*, 2004). Of this cohort of individuals, 282 developed cirrhosis and the study concluded that wine drinkers appeared to be at a lower risk of becoming heavy and excessive drinkers. It also suggested that a person who prefers beer is more likely to become a heavy or excessive drinker (Gronbaek *et al.*, 2004).

In a cohort study of 128,934 patients over a 20-year follow-up, they found that the mortality was lowest in the wine drinking group in comparison to the beer and spirits groups (Klatsky *et al.*, 2003). There was no difference between types of wine consumed. Interestingly from this study they looked at frequency of beer, wine and liquor consumption, it was found that liver cirrhosis was not increased in individuals drinking beer or wine more than once a month; however, it was increased in individuals consuming spirits. However, this result is of questionable significance since there is no clarification of exact frequency of drinking or the quantity of alcohol being consumed (Klatsky *et al.*, 2003).

A Swedish study looking at mortality in relation to liver disease secondary to alcohol concluded that the increase in cirrhosis that occurred in the early 1970s coincided with an increase in sales of spirits; however, though spirit sales declined, the cirrhosis rates remained stable. The sale of beer is currently the same as it was in 1970; however, the sale of wine has increased over this time period, though this increase in wine consumption has not led to the increase in cirrhosis that was seen in the 1970s with the increased sale of beer (Stokkeland *et al.*, 2006).

An examination of different types of alcoholic beverages and their associated mortality has been conducted where the relative risk was set at 1.00 for subjects that never drank wine (Becker *et al.*, 2002). The data showed that individuals who drank between three and five glasses of wine a day have a reduced risk of all cause mortality (0.51 relative risk, RR) (Becker *et al.*, 2002). Though this beneficial effect was not illustrated with beer at the same level of consumption, spirits showed an increased mortality at this consumption. There was a slight significant decrease in relative risk in individuals who drank beer weekly (0.95 RR). However, wine consumption is not associated with a decreased risk of alcoholic cirrhosis in heavy drinkers (Pelletier *et al.*, 2002).

Further analysis of the large Copenhagen study, the results of which were discussed earlier, has been done by the same group. They looked specifically at the risk of alcohol-induced cirrhosis in patients who consume different beverages. The results from their study concluded that increased alcohol consumption was associated with increased alcohol-induced cirrhosis. They found individuals who drank more than 5 drinks a day had a much higher risk (14–20 RR) of developing cirrhosis than those who did not drink or were light drinkers. Within the cohort that drank they found that individuals who had no intake of wine, that is, were predominately drinking spirits or beer, had a higher risk of developing cirrhosis than those who had 30% or 50% of their intake as wine (Gronbaek *et al.*, 2004).

Specific Beverage Intake and Association with Cirrhosis

Prior to the early 1970s there was a clear association between alcohol consumption and the cirrhosis mortality rates; however, as stated earlier with the Swedish study there has been an increase in alcohol consumption and yet a decrease in cirrhosis mortality rates. The cause of this is unclear, some have postulated that it is related to increased alcoholism treatment and the medical management of cirrhosis (Noble *et al.*, 1993; Smart and Mann, 1993). The other cause is thought to be related to a change in the distribution of alcohol consumption and the type of alcohol consumed. The analysis of beverage specific associations with cirrhosis is important because certain beverages may indicate certain drinking patterns associated with cirrhosis. Studies showed wine and spirits to be associated with cirrhosis (Whitlock, 1974; Smith and Burvill, 1985). A time series analysis looking at the United States from 1949 to 1994 also showed spirits to be associated with cirrhosis rates (Roizen *et al.*, 1999).

There is evidence that spirit drinkers are more likely to have a poorer nutritional state which would in turn makes them at increased risk to develop cirrhosis. Using a combined cross-sectional time series method for a group of predominantly beer consuming countries, Kerr *et al.* (2000) concluded that alcohol consumption is the best marker of predicting cirrhosis mortality rates. Spirit consumption was found to have a significant association with cirrhosis mortality. However, there was no association between beer and cirrhosis mortality in this group of countries where beer is the predominant beverage. The cause of this link between spirits and cirrhosis rates is yet to be elucidated; it may be related to the beverage or could be related to habits and associated social state of the individuals who consume spirits. Since heavy drinkers may not have a large income they may drink the cheapest available alcohol, which would be spirits, considering their high alcohol content per bottle, although this would be subjected to geographical variations in availability, drinking culture and taxation (the latter effectively dictating affordability in some countries with high taxes on alcohol). In some countries (say in wine producing regions), individuals who drink exclusively spirits are rare (see below; Hoffmeister *et al.*, 1999).

Threshold Values for Inducing Changes in the Liver

One population-based study from Germany has addressed the issue of whether beers confer a protective effect on the liver by examining drinking histories and serum gamma glutamyl transferase (GGT) activities of 15,000 individuals (Hoffmeister *et al.*, 1999). Of the male and female subjects 50% and 12% were mainly beer drinkers, respectively, whereas wine drinkers comprised 30% and 42% of the male and female population, respectively. Only 2.3% and 1.9% of the male and female subjects, respectively, were classified as mainly spirit drinkers. As expected, the study showed increasing GGT activities in response to increasing levels in alcohol intake. Effectively, increases in serum GGT provide a surrogate measured of liver damage. However, the threshold value (defined as "the point within a model at which GGT concentrations start to rise after a linear performance before") (Hoffmeister *et al.*, 1999) for beer in men was 42 g/day compared to 26 g/day for unspecified alcohol intake, in general. This suggests that compared to unspecified alcohol ingestion, beer is less damaging. For wine the threshold value for men was 51 g/day but this was not significant (Figure 61.5). For women threshold values for the three beverage categories were much lower and a similar pattern was observed: that is, in the order of unspecified alcohol, beer and wine intakes. However, none of these data for threshold values for women attained statistical significance (Figure 61.5; Hoffmeister *et al.*, 1999).

Changes in Beverage Preference in Disease: From Beer to Spirits

Part of the problem in ascribing a particular beverage type to the development of a specific disease entity relates to the changing pattern of beverage preference. In one study drinking histories were examined prospectively in 70 patients with alcohol-derived cirrhosis (those with cirrhosis of viral origin were excluded) (Campollo *et al.*, 2001). Patients were classified as either (i) pre-alcoholics, (ii) critical alcoholics or (iii) chronic alcoholics in their periods of alcoholism (Figure 61.6). Weekly mean alcohol ingestion rates were 3, 48 and 252 g/day for the three categories, respectively. Subjects in the early pre-alcoholic stage clearly showed a preference for beer whereas those classified as chronic alcoholics had a preference for beverages with higher alcohol contents such as tequila and pure ethanol (Figure 61.6; Campollo *et al.*, 2001).

However, the aforementioned study does not prove that beer is less harmful than more potent alcoholic drinks, and more controlled and detailed studies are required. For example, there are periods of overlapping drinking preference and also diet has a role in the development of liver disease. It is very unusual for individuals to consume a single beverage type. In a study of over 50,000 men and women in Northern California, only 15% of drinkers had a preference for a beverage type. Furthermore just over 20% of those with a particular preference used exclusively their preferred beverage (Klatsky *et al.*, 1990).

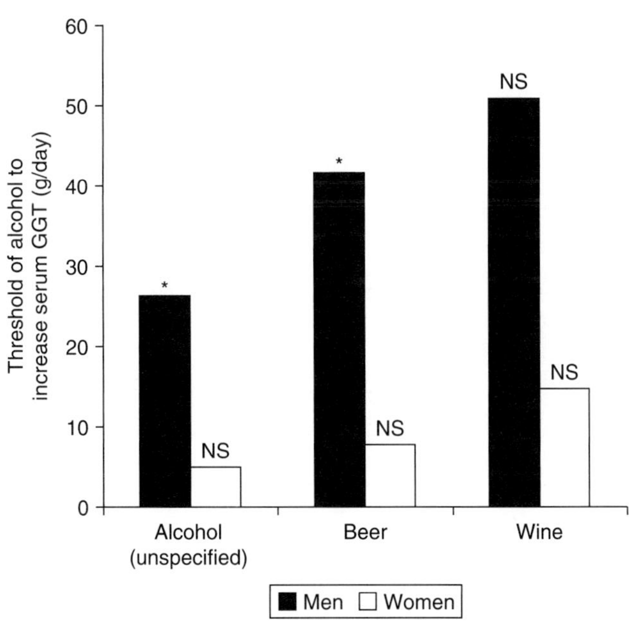

Figure 61.5 The relationship between beverage types and threshold levels for increasing serum GGT. Drinking histories and GGT activities were obtained for 15,000 individuals. Threshold values were defined as "the point within a model at which GGT concentrations start to rise after a linear performance before" (Hoffmeister *et al.*, 1999). For beer in men threshold value was 41.6 g/day compared to 26.3 g/day for overall alcohol intake in general. Other threshold values did not attain statistical significance. *, significant; NS, not significant. *Source*: Data adapted from Hoffmeister *et al.* (1999).

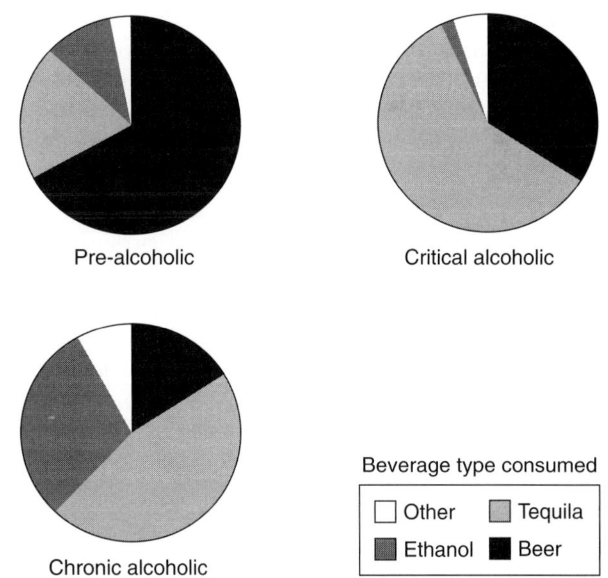

Figure 61.6 Changes in beverage preference in liver disease. Changes in beverage preference in a set of 70 alcoholics with cirrhosis were examined prospectively (those with cirrhosis of viral origin were excluded). Those classified as "pre-alcoholic" showed periods of drunkenness of 1–6 times a year and those classified as "critical" were drunk 1–3 times a month. "Chronic alcoholics" were drunk 1 or more times a week. Weekly mean alcohol ingestion rates were 3, 48 and 252 g/day for the three categories, respectively. The early pre-alcoholic stage clearly shows a preference for beer, whereas those classified as chronic alcoholics had a preference for beverages with higher alcohol contents (tequila and pure ethanol). *Source*: Data adapted from Campollo *et al.* (2001).

Changes in drinking preference during the stages of alcohol could reflect the socio-geographical circumstances of the individual: for example, beverage cost is a modulating factor in drinking preference (Cook and Moore, 2002). Supply by family members also increases alcohol consumption in the form of beer, wine and spirits whereas those receiving education about alcohol misuse is an important modulator in reducing the consumption of beer, but not wine and spirits (Lundborg, 2002).

The Compounding Influence of Diet

There is a substantial body of evidence to suggest that diet is an important modulatory of disease and alcohol is no exception. There is a positive correlation between pork consumption and cirrhosis mortality (Nanji and French, 1985; Bode *et al.*, 1998). In an analysis of beer and wine drinking in relation to alcoholic liver disease, it was shown that in patients with alcoholic hepatitis there was a significant correlation between beer consumption and pork intake ($r = 0.43$; $p = 0.004$), offal ($r = 0.36$; $p = 0.016$) and total pig products ($r = 0.47$; $p = 0.001$) (Bode *et al.*, 1998). In subjects with alcoholic cirrhosis, positive correlations were significant for beer consumption vs. offal intake ($r = 0.36$; $p = 0.032$) and beer consumption vs. intake of total pig products ($r = 0.45$; $p = 0.007$) (see also Figure 61.7 where simple regression analysis data are displayed) (Bode *et al.*, 1998). In contrast, only one statistically significant relationship for wine drinkers was observed, namely for total pig products and wine consumption but the data were negatively correlated ($r = -0.37$; $p = 0.027$) (Bode *et al.*, 1998). Overall the data show that there is a correlation between pig product consumption and cirrhosis, and this relationship is modulated by beverage type, particularly with respect to beer (Bode *et al.*, 1998).

More recent studies have investigated the difference between the diet of beer and wine drinkers (Johansen *et al.*, 2006). These studies show that beer drinkers consumed foods that were less healthy than the wine drinkers: that is, beer drinkers ate more butter, carbonated drinks, chips, lamb, margarine or butter, pork, sausages and sugar but less cooking oil, fruit and vegetables, low fat cheese, meat, milk, olives and poultry (Johansen *et al.*, 2006).

The importance of this putative diet–beer interaction merits concern only if there is sufficient direct evidence to support the contention that the severity of alcoholic liver disease can indeed be modulated by diet. Well-controlled systematic laboratory animal studies have compared the effects of alcohol feeding with different dietary fats in the form of either corn oil, pork lard or beef tallow (Nanji *et al.*, 1989). Surprisingly, features of alcoholic liver disease were not apparent in rats fed beef fat and ethanol. On the other hand, rats fed alcohol with pork fat had minimal to moderate features. Rats fed corn oil diet developed the most severe lesions in response to alcohol (Nanji *et al.*, 1989). These results show that the type of fat is instrumental in contributing to the severity of the lesions in alcohol-fed rats possibly via Ito cell activation (Nanji *et al.*, 1989).

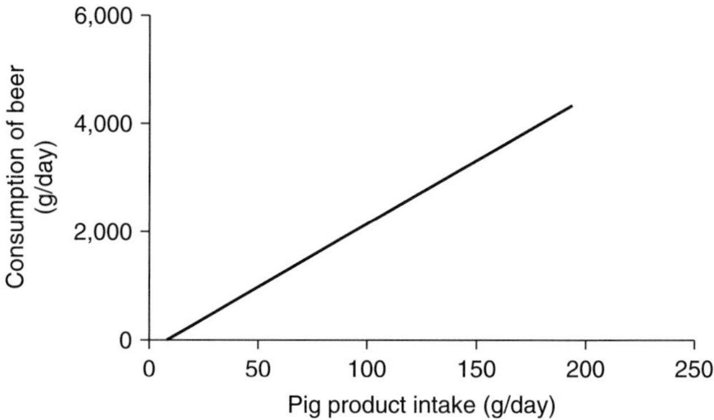

Figure 61.7 The relationship between beer intake and ingestion of pig products. The data show the relationship between ingestion of beer and pig products in cirrhotic subjects. The line is best-fit obtained using regression analysis from a data set encompassing 35 cirrhotic subjects where p = 0.001. *Source*: Data adapted from Bode *et al.* (1998).

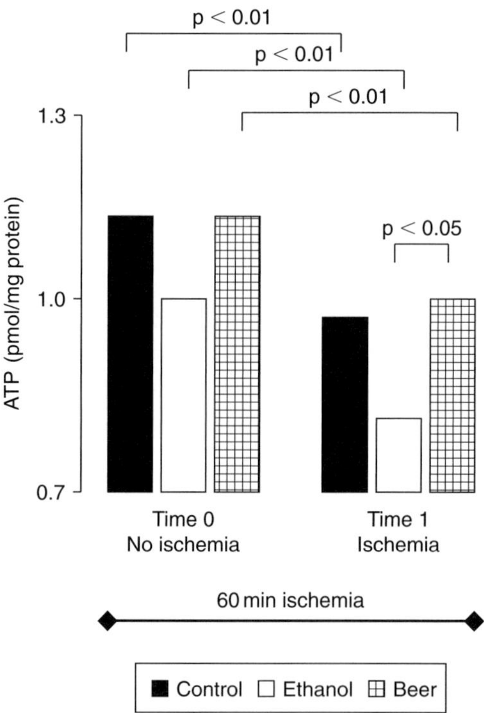

Figure 61.8 The effect of ischemia on liver ATP in control, ethanol- and beer-fed animals. The data show mean ATP levels in livers of rats fed a control diet or a diet containing beer. Ethanol provided 2.5% of total energy intake. In response to ischemia (clamping of the hepatic pedicle for 60 min) liver ATP in liver of control, ethanol- and beer-fed rats decreased. However, ATP levels in beer-fed animals were higher than levels fed the ethanol-containing diet. *Source*: Data adapted from Gasbarrini *et al.* (1998).

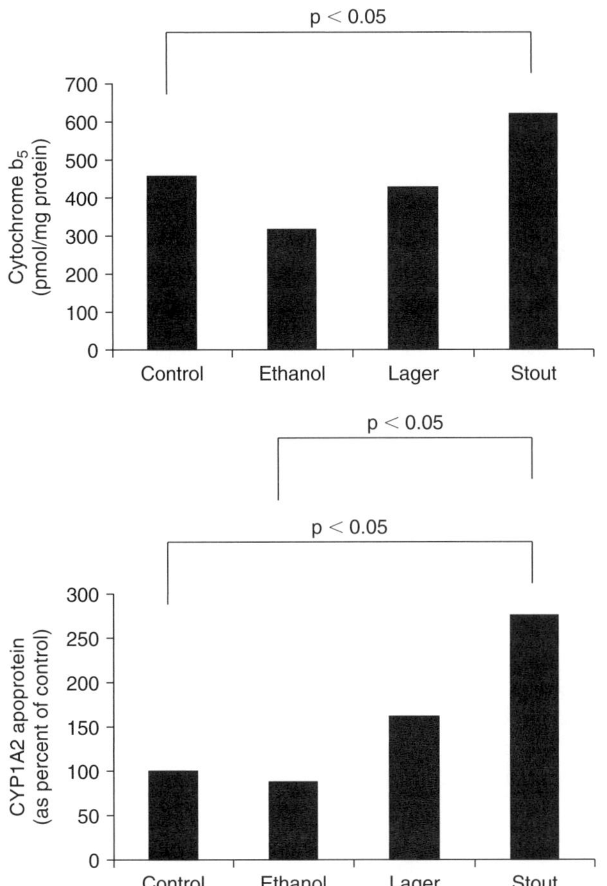

Figure 61.9 The effect of different beer types on liver cytochrome b_5 and CYP1A2 apoprotein. Animals were infused for 21 days with a total enteral preparation fed either 3.5% ethanol or an equivalent amount of ethanol in the form of either light (lager) or dark (stout) beer. The data show mean cytochrome b_5 and CYP1A2 apoprotein in livers of control and treated rats which was increased in liver of rats fed the dark beer. *Source*: Data adapted from Hidestrand *et al.* (2005).

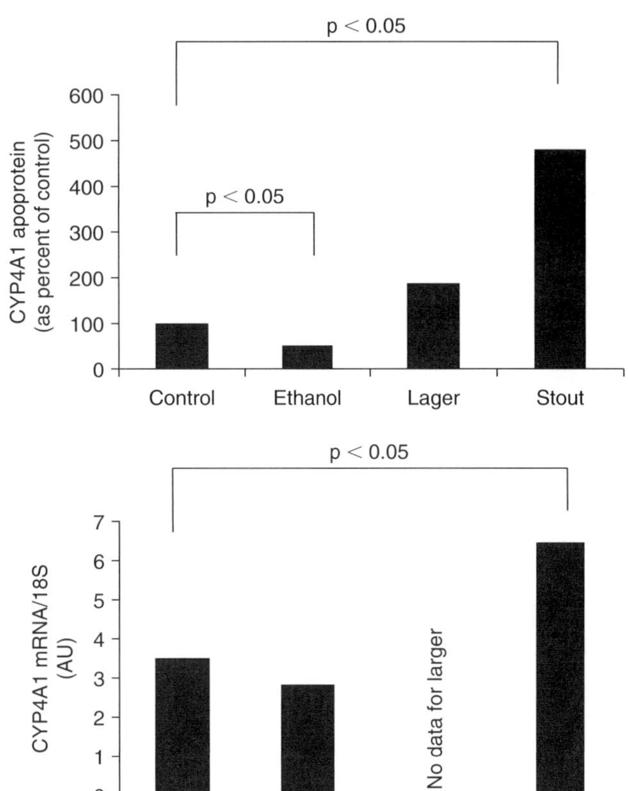

Figure 61.10 The effect of different beer types on the liver CYP4A1 apoprotein and mRNA. Animals were infused for 21 days with a total enteral preparation containing either 3.5% ethanol or an equivalent amount of ethanol in the form of either light (lager) or dark (stout) beer. The data show mean CYP4A1 apoprotein and mRNA levels in livers of control and treated rats which was increased in rats fed the dark beer. Note that no data for the CYP4A1 mRNA in the lager group were presented by the authors. *Source*: Data adapted from Hidestrand *et al.* (2005).

Protective Components in Beer: Are They Beneficial to the Liver?

A number of studies have shown that beer contains protective elements on the form of anti-oxidants (Bourne *et al.*, 2000; Denke 2000; Pulido *et al.*, 2003). Thus, it would not be surprising to find that, compared to say pure alcohol, consumption of moderate amounts of beer is protective to the liver. This was addressed in a study where animals were fed a diet containing pure ethanol or the same amount of ethanol in the form of beer (Gasbarrini *et al.*, 1998). In these aforementioned studies the contribution of ethanol to the overall energy ingested was low, that is, at 2.5% of total energy; or 1.1 g ethanol per 100 ml of diet. At the end of 6 weeks there were no significant changes in adenosine triphosphate (ATP), glutathione, or thiobarbituric acid reacting substances in liver of rats fed ethanol or beer compared to controls (Figure 61.8; Gasbarrini *et al.*, 1998).

In response to ischemia (clamping of the hepatic pedicle for 60 min) liver ATP in liver of control, ethanol- and beer-fed rats decreased ($p < 0.01$). However, ATP concentrations in beer-fed animals were higher than levels fed the ethanol-containing diet (Figure 61.8; Gasbarrini *et al.*, 1998). This suggests that protective element within beer may be hepato-protective.

Interestingly there has been some work on the biochemical effects of different beers (i.e. light and dark beers) on enzyme induction (Hidestrand *et al.*, 2005). Dark beer increased cytochrome b_5, CYP1A2 apoprotein, CYP4A1 apoprotein and CYP4A1 mRNA in liver of rats fed (Figures 61.9 and 61.10). In contrast, the activity of and CYP4A was reduced in *in vitro* activity assays which were subsequently ascribe to a blocking mechanism where a component of stout or stout metabolism blocked CYP4A activity (Hidestrand *et al.*, 2005). Thus light and dark beers have different effects on the liver: dark beers appear to have components that interact with hepatic metabolism.

The relevance of this relates to the suggestion that consumption of darker beers is associated with an increased risk of rectal cancer. Roasting grain, used in darker beers and stouts, produces pro-carcinogen compounds such as aromatic amines and polycyclic aromatic hydrocarbons (Hidestrand *et al.*, 2005). These induce P450 CYP1A1 enzymes, which convert the aforementioned pro-carcinogenic compounds to analytes (i.e. carcinogens) that induce cancer. However, contrary evidence also suggests that induction of CYP1A1 imparts a biological advantage as CYP1A1 facilitates a faster clearance rate of toxic compounds (Hidestrand *et al.*, 2005). Unfortunately, there are few or no clinical studies which have investigated the effects of beer types on liver disease.

Conclusion

There is a beneficial effect in morbidity and mortality with low to moderate alcohol consumption in both men and women, this applies to beer, wine and spirits; however, the evidence supporting wine is the strongest and most studied. High consumption of alcohol leads to alcoholic liver disease, and no specific beverage has been shown to be less harmful than any other. However, there is some evidence that the nutritional value of beer and its possible anti-oxidant properties are of additional benefit beyond that of alcohol alone.

Summary Points

- Liver disease is clearly correlated with high levels of alcohol intake; however, the exact threshold required to cause disease is not known. The threshold is different for men and women.
- One population study shows the threshold value (defined as "the point within a model at which GGT concentrations start to rise after a linear performance before") for beer in men is higher than for overall alcohol.
- Subjects in the early pre-alcoholic stage show preference for beer whereas those classified as chronic alcoholics had a preference for beverages with higher alcohol contents.
- It is very unusual for individuals to consume a single beverage type.
- Beer drinkers consumed foods that are less healthy than the wine drinkers.
- Overall the data show that there is a correlation between pig product consumption and cirrhosis, and this relationship is modulated by beverage type, particularly with respect to beer.
- In response to ischemia, liver ATP in liver of control, ethanol- and beer-fed rats decreased. However, ATP concentrations in the liver of beer-fed animals were higher than levels found in the livers of animals fed the ethanol-containing diet, suggestive of hepato-protection by beer.
- Light and dark beers have different effects on the liver: dark beers appear to have components that interact with hepatic metabolism.
- There are few or no clinical studies that have investigated the effects of beer types on liver disease.

References

Anderson, P. (1995). Alcohol and risk of physical harm. In Holder, H.D. and Edwards, G. (eds), *Alcohol and Public Policy: Evidence and Issues*, pp. 82–113. Oxford University Press, Oxford, UK.

Becker, U., Gronbaek, M., Johansen, D. and Sorensen, T.I.A. (2002). *Hepatology* 35, 868–875.

Bode, C., Bode, J.C., Erhardt, J.G., French, B.A. and French, S.W. (1998). *Alcohol Clin. Exp. Res.* 22, 1803–1805.

Bourne, L., Paganga, G., Baxter, D., Hughes, P. and Rice-Evans, C. (2000). *Free Radic. Res.* 32, 273–280.

Campollo, O., Martinez, M.D., Valencia, J.J. and Segura-Ortega, J. (2001). *Subst. Use Misuse* 36, 387–398.

Castegnaro, M. (1988). *Food Addict. Contam.* 5, 283–288.

Clark, J.M. (2006). *J Clin. Gastroenterol.* 40, S5–S10.

Cook, P.J. and Moore, M.J. (2002). *Health Aff. (Millwood)* 21, 120–133.

Denke, M.A. (2000). *Am. J. Med. Sci.* 320, 320–326.

Farrell, G.C. and Larter, C.Z. (2006). *Hepatology* 43, S99–S112.

Gasbarrini, A., Addolorato, G., Simoncini, M., Gasbarrini, G., Fantozzi, P., Mancini, F., Montanari, L., Nardini, M., Ghiselli, A. and Scaccini, C. (1998). *Dig. Dis. Sci.* 43, 1332–1338.

Gronbaek, M., Becker, U., Johansen, D., Gottschau, A., Schnohr, P., Hein, H.O., Jensen, G. and Sorensen, T.I. (2000). *Ann. Intern. Med.* 133, 411–419.

Gronbaek, M., Jensen, M.K., Johansen, D., Sorensen, T.I.A. and Becker, U. (2004). *Biol. Res.* 37, 195–200.

Gutjahr, E., Gmel, G. and Rehm, J. (2001). *Eur. Addict. Res.* 7, 117–127.

Hidestrand, M., Shankar, K., Ronis, M.J.J. and Badger, T.M. (2005). *Alcohol Clin. Exp. Res.* 29, 888–895.

Hoffmeister, H., Schelp, F.-P., Mensink, G.B.M., Dietz, E. and Bohning, D. (1999). *Int. J. Epidemiol.* 28, 1066–1072.

Johansen, D., Friis, K., Skovenborg, E. and Gronbaek, M. (2006). *BMJ* 332, 519–521.

Kauhanen, J., Kaplan, G.A., Goldberg, D.E. and Salonen, J.T. (1997). *BMJ* 315, 846–851.

Kerr, W.C., Fillmore, K.M. and Marvy, P. (2000). *Addiction* 95, 339–346.

Klatsky, A.L., Armstrong, M.A. and Kipp, H. (1990). *Br. J. Addict.* 85, 1279–1289.

Klatsky, A.L., Friedman, G.D., Armstrong, M.A. and Kipp, H. (2003). *Am. J. Epidemiol.* 158, 585–595.

Kubacki, S.J., Havery, D.C. and Fazio, T. (1989). *Food Addict. Contam.* 6, 29–53.

Leon, D.A., Chenet, L., Shkolnikov, V.M., Zakharov, S., Shapiro, J., Rakhmanova, G., Vassin, S. and McKee, M. (1997). *Lancet* 1, 383–388.

Leon, D.A. and McCambridge, J. (2006). *Lancet* 367, 52–56.

Lundborg, P. (2002). *Addiction* 97, 1573–1582.

Mezey, E., Kolman, C.J., Diehl, A.M., Mitchell, M.C. and Herlong, H.F. (1988). *Am. J. Clin. Nutr.* 48, 148–151.

Mukamal, K.J., Maclure, M., Muller, J.E. and Mittleman, M.A. (2005). *Circulation* 112, 3839–3845.

Nanji, A.A. and French, S.W. (1985). *Lancet* 1, 681–683.

Nanji, A.A., Mendenhall, C.L. and French, S.W. (1989). *Alcohol Clin. Exp. Res.* 13, 15–19.

Noble, J.A., Caces, M.F., Steffens, R.A. and Stinson, F.S. (1993). *Publ. Health Rep.* 108, 192–197.

Norton, G.R., Rockman, G.E., Ediger, J., Pepe, C., Goldberg, S., Cox, B.J. and Asmundson, G.J.G. (1997). *Behav. Res. Ther.* 35, 859–862.

Pelletier, S., Vaucher, E., Aider, R., Martin, S., Perney, P., Balmes, J.L. and Nalpas, B. (2002). *Alcohol Alcohol.* 37, 618–621.

Preedy, V.R. and Watson, R.R. (2005). *Comprehensive Handbook of Alcohol-Related Pathology*. Academic Press, London, UK. Vols. 1–3.

Pulido, R., Hernandez-Garcia, M. and Saura-Calixto, F. (2003). *Eur. J. Clin. Nutr.* 57, 1275–1282.

Rehm, J., Gmel, G., Sempos, C.T. and Trevisan, M. (2003a). *Alcohol Res. Health* 27, 39–51.

Rehm, J., Rehn, N., Room, R., Monteiro, M., Gmel, G., Jernigan, D. and Frick, U. (2003b). *Eur. Addict. Res.* 9, 147–156.

Roizen, R., Kerr, W.C. and Fillmore, K.M. (1999). *BMJ* 319, 666–670.

Sijbrands, E.J.G., Smelt, A.H.M., Westendorp, R.G.J., Lowenfels, A.B., Fuchs, C.S., Stampfer, M.J. and Willett, W. C. (1995). *New Engl. J. Med.* 333, 1081–1082.

Smart, R.G. and Mann, R.E. (1993). *Addiction* 88, 193–198.

Smith, D.I. and Burvill, P.W. (1985). *Drug Alcohol Depend.* 15, 35–45.

Stokkeland, K., Brandt, L., Ekbom, A., Osby, U. and Hultcrantz, R. (2006). *Scand. J. Gastroenterol.* 41, 463–468.

Szucs, S., Sarvary, A., McKee, M. and Adany, R. (2005). *Addiction* 100, 536–542.

Thakker, K.D. (1998). *Alcohol Clin. Exp. Res.* 22, 285S–298S.

Thun, M.J., Peto, R., Lopez, A.D., Monaco, J.H., Henley, S.J., Heath Jr., C.W. and Doll, R. (1997). *New Engl. J. Med.* 337, 1705–1714.

Tricker, A.R. and Preussmann, R. (1991). *J. Cancer Res. Clin. Oncol.* 117, 130–132.

Whitlock, F.A. (1974). *Q. J. Stud. Alcohol* 35, 586–605.

WHO (2004). *Global Status Report on Alcohol.* World Health Organization, Geneva.

(ii) Cardiovascular and Cancer

62

Beer Consumption and Homocysteine

D.A. de Luis and R. Aller Institute of Endocrinology and Nutrition, Medicine School and Unit of Investigation, Hospital Rio Hortega, University of Valladolid, Valladolid, Spain

Abstract

Hyperhomocysteinemia has received increasing attention during the past decade and has joined hypertension, obesity, dyslipemia, smoking, and diabetes mellitus as an independent risk factor for cardiovascular disease. Chronic alcohol ingestion has also been associated with increased homocysteine levels. However, drinking beer may have a special health benefit not attributable to other alcohol-containing beverages. Contrary to wine, little is known about potential cardio protective effect of beer whose high content of vitamins B may have beneficial effects on homocysteine metabolism. One of the first studies, which showed an inverse relation between beer consumption and homocysteine levels, were designed by our group in patients with diabetes mellitus type 2. Our study's hypothesis is based on previous studies. Folate, vitamins B12 and B6 were assessed in chronic alcoholics and healthy volunteers. Mean serum homocysteine was twice as high in chronic alcoholics than in non-drinkers. However, beer consumers had significantly lower concentrations of homocysteine compared with drinkers of wine or spirits. Other cross-sectional population study with a high amount of patients has been performed with residents of Pilsen (Czech Republic). By categories of beer intake, subjects with intake of 1 l daily or more had significantly lower tHcy and higher folate concentrations than those that reporting lower daily beer intake. However, some studies have not demonstrated this inverse association. The conflicting results may derive in part from confounding by the interaction of alcoholic beverage consumed. Other confounding factors may play a role in all studies, changing direction of the results secondary to bias such as race-ethnicity, genetic background, age, cigarette smoking, and amount of ethanol. As we can see interaction in different factors present in some type of patient could modify the results of previous and further studies in this topic area to relate beer consumption and homocysteine.

List of Abbreviations

BHMT	Betaine–homocysteine methyltranspherase
B12	Vitamin B12
CBS	Cistathionine-β-sintetase
CI	Confidence interval
MAT	Methionine adenosiltranspherase
MTHFR	Methylentetrahydrofolato reductase
OR	Odds ratio
P5P	Pyridoxal 5′-phosphate
SAM	*S*-adenosyl-methionine
tHcy	Total homocysteine

Introduction

Homocysteine is a non-essential sulfur-containing amino acid formed from the demethylation of an essential amino acid, methionine (Figure 62.1). Epidemiologic studies have

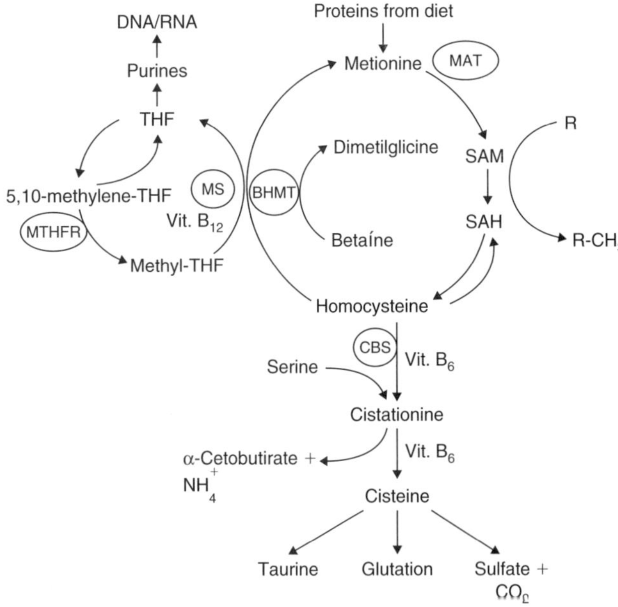

Figure 62.1 Metabolism of homocysteine. MAT, methionine adenosiltranspherase; SAM, S-adenosyl-methionine; CBS, cistathionine-β-sintetase; BHMT, Betaine–homocysteine methyltranspherase.

Beer in Health and Disease Prevention
ISBN: 978-0-12-373891-2

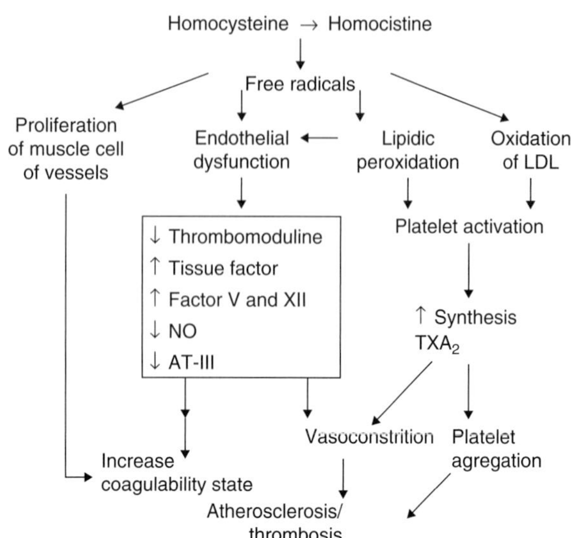

Figure 62.2 Association between homocysteine concentration and risk for heart disease.

Table 62.1 Clinical conditions associated with hyperhomocysteinemia

Neural tube defects
Placental abruption
Low birth weight
Spontaneous abortion
Renal failure
Diabetes mellitus
Reumatoid arthritis
Alcoholism
Osteoporosis
Neuropsychiatric disorders

shown that elevated total homocysteine (tHcy) concentration in the blood is an independent risk factor for occlusive vascular diseases. Several possible mechanisms that may underlie the positive association between homocysteine concentration and risk for heart disease include oxidation of cholesterol, toxic effects on endothelial cells, impaired platelet activity, and increased smooth cell proliferation (Figure 62.2).

Coenzymes of folate, vitamin B12, riboflavin, and pyridoxine vitamins are essential in homocysteine metabolism. Homocysteine is either remethylated to methionine or transsulfurated to cysteine. Folate, riboflavin, and vitamin B12 coenzymes are needed for the remethylation pathway, whereas pyridoxine coenzyme is required for the transsulfuration pathway (Figure 62.1). Decreased circulating concentrations of folate, riboflavin, vitamin B12, and pyridoxine are associated with increased serum tHcy concentration. Hyperhomocysteinemia has received increasing attention during the past decade and has joined hypertension, obesity, dyslipemia, smoking, and diabetes mellitus as an independent risk factor for cardiovascular disease. In addition to its main role in cardiovascular disease, hyperhomocysteinemia has been implicated in a variety of other clinical conditions (de Luis *et al.*, 2004) (Table 62.1).

Studies of healthy men and women indicate that certain genetic and acquired determinants can modify total plasma homocysteine. For example, women tend to have lower basal levels than men (Tucker *et al.*, 1996), and neither contraceptives nor hormone replacement therapy seem to significantly alter the levels. The above-mentioned sex differences in homocysteine concentrations persist even in elderly populations. Nevertheless, epidemiological evidence has shown homocysteine levels to be 45% lower in westernized adult black South Africans than in age-matched white adults, revealing racial genetic differences in homocysteine metabolism too (Vermaak *et al.*, 1991).

Nutrition impacts homocysteine concentrations in both men and women. Those individuals in the lowest quartiles for serum folate and vitamin B12 (nutrients which impact homocysteine metabolism) have significantly higher concentrations of homocysteine, and men in the lowest quartile of serum pyridoxal 5′-phosphate (P5P, the bioactive form of vitamin B6) also have increased homocysteine concentrations (Lusier Cacan *et al.*, 1996).

The objective of this chapter is to review the evidence in the literature in this interesting association between beer consumption and homocysteine levels and the theorical heart protective effect of regular beer consumption.

Drinking Habits and Homocysteine

Coffee consumption and homocysteine

Drinking habits have been associated with homocysteine levels. An association between coffee consumption and the concentration of tHcy in plasma has been reported. A positive dose–response relation between coffee consumption and plasma homocysteine levels was observed. This association was most marked in males and females consuming greater than eight cup of coffee per day (Nygard *et al.*, 1997). Chronic alcohol ingestion has also been associated with increased homocysteine levels (Cravo *et al.*, 1996).

Beer consumption and homocysteine

However, drinking beer may have a special health benefit not attributable to other alcohol-containing beverages, according to results of a Dutch trial published (Van der Gaag *et al.*, 2000). In that report, consumption of red wine and gin raised blood levels of homocysteine, an above-mentioned product linked to increased risks of several diseases but most definitively to heart disease. The increase in homocysteine resulting from wine or gin consumption, almost 10%, was statistically significant. Beer drinking, in contrast, had no detrimental effect on homocysteine levels. Contrary to wine, little is known about potential cardio protective effect of beer whose high content of vitamins B may have beneficial effects on homocysteine metabolism. It was proved that group B vitamins originate in beer from the malted barley. Germination promotes a three to sixfold increase in the level of riboflavin, a doubling of the level of niacin and almost a doubling of the level of folate (Walker and Baxter, 2000). The cyanocobalamin, that is vitamin B12, as a corrinoid compound is known to be produced only in animals and micro-organisms. It originates in beer from yeasts. Therefore, its content in different beers may vary largely according to the brewing process. The largest amount of vitamin B12 is contained in some type of beers, where yeasts are added at the end of the brewery yeasts.

Table 62.2 Clinical characteristics of diabetic pa-tients studied (mean ± SD)

n	*155*
Age (years)	57.4 ± 15.7
Sex (male/female)	65/90
BMI (Kg/m^2)	28.6 ± 5.9
Diabetes course (years)	8.4 ± 6.7
Glucose (mmol/l)	9.72 ± 3.1
Retinopathy (%)	41.9
Nefropathy (%)	18.7
Neuropathy (%)	3.8
Stroke (%)	3.3
Peripheral arteriopathy (%)	5.2
Coronary heart disease (%)	5.8

Note: Basal parameters of the studied sample of patients with diabetes mellitus type 2.

Source: de Luis *et al.* (2003).

Epidemiological Studies

Results of our group

One of the first studies, which showed an inverse relation between beer consumption and homocysteine levels, realized in this topic area were designed by our group in patients with diabetes mellitus type 2, a model of disease with high cardiovascular risk (de Luis *et al.*, 2003) (Tables 62.2 and 62.3). In previous studies, high homocysteine levels (tHcy) have been associated with an increased risk of cardiovascular events and microangiopathy in diabetic patients (Smulders *et al.*, 1999; Stabler, 1999). This association between homocysteine and chronic complications of diabetes mellitus could be explained with different mechanisms; direct toxic effect on vascular endothelium and an indirect effect on the normal methylation in endothelial cells (Weir and Molloy, 2000). Direct toxic effects of homocysteine could be mediated by damage to vascular endothelial cells, resulting in vascular events, such as microvascular disease and cardiovascular events (Figure 62.2).

Studies in diabetic populations

The relationship between tHcy levels and dietary intake remained controversial. Above-mentioned relation with coffee consumption may be clear. The postprandial as well as long-term effect of methionine intake from proteins has been investigated, and probably only causes a marginal change in the tHcy levels (Stolzenberg *et al.*, 1999). In contrast it is clear that dietary intakes (Allen *et al.*, 1993) or plasma levels of folate and vitamin B12 are inversely related to tHcy concentration. Deficiencies of these vitamins may cause a moderate or even severe hyperhomocysteinemia, and an increased tHcy level is a sensitive marker of disturbed function or both folate and vitamin B12. Few studies have been realized in diabetic populations; it has been reported that ethanol consumption, especially heavy alcohol drinking, increases the risk of atherosclerosis assessed

Table 62.3 Percentage of recommended dietary allowances (RDA) in our population of patients with diabetes mellitus type 2

	Mean (SD)	*% RDA*
Macronutrients		
Carbohydrates (g/day)	145.1 ± 40.9	–
Lipids (g/day)	49.5 ± 19	–
Total proteins (g/day)	80.7 ± 17	–
Total calories (cal/day)	1327 ± 295	–
Gram of proteins/kg	1.08 ± 0.4	–
Calories/kg	20 ± 8.1	–
Vitamins		
Vitamin A (μg)	732 ± 78	74
Vitamin D (μg)	1.9 ± 4.6	18
Vitamin E (mg)	7.1 ± 2.3	71
Vitamin K (μg)	134.1 ± 73.8	167
Vitamin C (mg)	144.6 ± 79.1	240
Tiamine (mg)	1.15 ± 1.2	76.7
Riboflavine (mg)	1.7 ± 0.6	100
Niacine (mg)	29.5 ± 11.2	155
Vitamin B6 (mg)	1.8 ± 0.6	90
Vitamin B12 (μg)	5.6 ± 4.2	280
Folic acid (μg)	197.4 ± 2.3	108.9
Minerals		
Calcium (mg)	907 ± 298	90.6
Fosforum (mg)	1,250.8 ± 404	156.3
Magnesium (mg)	227.5 ± 60.8	64.9
Fe (mg)	9.98 ± 3.3	98
Zn (mg)	10.2 ± 4.5	68.1
Y (μg)	423 ± 191	282
Se (μg)	41.9 ± 20.6	59.9
Other nutrients		
Fiber (g)	15.5 ± 7.7	
Beer (ml)	105 ± 205	
Other alcoholic drinks (ml)	49.7 ± 85	
Cholesterol (mg)	310.8 ± 198	

Note: Comparation of dietary intakes in our sample of patients with diabetes mellitus and RDA, showing a high intake of folic acid and vitamin B12.

Source: de Luis *et al.* (2003).

Table 62.4 Vitamin composition in different drinks (per 100 ml) in our area

	Folic acid (μg)	*B12 (μg)*
Beer	4.1	0.14
Wine	0.1	0
Spirits	0	0
Vermut	0	0
Natural juices	3	0

Note: Vitamin B12 and folic acid of different drinks in Spain.

Table 62.5 Beer composition of vitamin as per 50 ml

	MG	*% RDA*
Tiamine (B1)	0.0145	1.21
Riboflavine (B2)	0.1675	11.96
Niacine (B3)	3.86	24.16
Pantotenic acid	0.745	12.5
Piridoxin (B6)	0.3095	20.63
Biotin	0.006	10–20
Folic acid (B9)	0.043	10.75
B12	0.0004	13.2
Vitamin A	0.002	0.2
Vitamin D	0.0005	8
Vitamin E	0.035	0.25

Note: Percentage of recommended dietary allowance (RDA) with 50 ml of beer consumption.

by intimal medial thickness in type 2 diabetic patients (Cooper *et al.*, 2002). However, the mechanism by which heavy alcohol drinking accelerates the development of atherosclerosis in diabetic patients is not known. Type of alcoholic beverages has been related with different decrease in cardiovascular risk (Wannamethee and Shaper, 1999), perhaps beer with a high concentration of folic acid and vitamin B12 could modify tHcy levels (Jayasinghe, 2000).

In a population of young adults with type 1 diabetes, chronic cigarette smoking seems to adversely affect plasma tHcy levels (Targher *et al.*, 2000). In our population (patients with diabetes mellitus type 2), no correlation was detected with smoking habit and tHcy levels (de Luis *et al.*, 2003). Alcohol consumption has been related with tHcy, a moderate consumption may be associated with reduced tHcy levels, whereas a chronic high alcohol consumption is associated with elevated tHcy (Huktberg *et al.*, 1993; Cravo *et al.*, 1996), possibly via impaired folate or vitamin B12 function (Gloria *et al.*, 1997). An elevation of tHcy was detected in a diabetic population (Sakuta *et al.*, 2005). In this study, the mechanisms by which ethanol consumption leads to tHcy elevation is not clear, a 42% of ethanol consumed from beer, whereas 41% was from spirits (whiskey and shochu). Beer, as above-mentioned, is a rich source of folate (Table 62.4). However, the elevation of tHcy in heavy drinking diabetic subjects may not be ascribed to folate in beer as it is known that tHcy is inversely associated with folate. Thus, these authors postulate that ethanol consumption itself, rather than nutrients in alcoholic beverage, are associated with the observed interaction effect between ethanol consumption and diabetes prevalence for tHcy. This effect between ethanol consumption and diabetes prevalence for tHcy cannot be explained by decrease levels of vitamin B12 (plasma levels of vitamin B12 in this group of diabetic patients was increased). The association is not explained by renal dysfunction or glycaemic control, this interaction may be explained by a direct effect of ethanol consumption of diabetic patients.

In our area (Spain), the composition of locally consumed beers is high in folic acid 4.1 μg/100 ml and 0.14 μg/100 ml of vitamin B12. This inverse relation between beer consumption and tHcy concentrations in our diabetic patients (de Luis *et al.*, 2003) has been described by Mayer *et al.* (2001), too. Beer is a beverage with a high ratio of vitamin B12 and folic acid (Table 62.5) and an interaction between nutrients composition of beer and tHcy may explain this association.

Studies in other populations

Our study's hypothesis is based on previous studies. In this previous study (Cravo *et al.*, 1996), folate, vitamins B12, and B6 were assessed in 32 chronic alcoholics and 31 healthy volunteers by measuring blood vitamin concentrations as well as serum homocysteine concentrations. In chronic alcoholics, serum P5P and red blood cell folate concentrations were significantly lower than in the control subjects. Mean serum homocysteine was twice as high in chronic alcoholics than in non-drinkers. However, beer consumers had significantly lower concentrations of homocysteine compared with drinkers of wine or spirits. These results suggest that by interfering with folate or vitamin B6 metabolism, chronic alcohol intake may impair the disposal of homocysteine through the transmethylation or transsulfuration pathways, but beer consumers could improve this fact secondary to a better vitamin dietary intakes from beer (Table 62.6).

Other studies with a high amount of patients have been performed. For example, Mayer *et al.* (2001) designed a cross-sectional population-based survey, residents of Pilsen (Czech Republic). Population series included 292 males and 251 females aged 35–65 years, with a mean age of 53.4 years. Beer intake was associated with blood folate and vitamin B12 concentrations positively and with tHcy concentration negatively. By categories of beer intake, subjects with intake of 1 l daily or more had significantly lower tHcy and higher folate concentrations than those that reporting lower daily beer intake. These authors concluded that moderate beer consumption may help to maintain the tHcy levels in the normal range due to high folate content. These data are in agreement with a previous large epidemiological

Table 62.6 % RDA of folic acid with 500 ml of beer consumption

	Mg of folic acid as RDA	*Per 500 ml of beer*
Male	200	1.21
Female	200	11.96
Female with lactancy	400	24.16
Female with pregnancy	300	12.5

Note: Percentage of recommended dietary allowance (RDA) with 500 ml of beer consumption in different situations and gender.

study (the Caerphilly cohort), this cohort has suggested a link between beer consumption and lower tHcy concentration in men aged 50–64 years (Ubbink *et al.*, 1998).

Physiology of Beer Consumption and Homocysteine Levels

This association between beer intake and homocysteine levels could have other implications on the endothelial function. In a cross-over study (Zilkens *et al.*, 2003), 16 healthy men either substituted their usual alcohol intake with a 0.9% alcohol beer or maintained their usual alcohol intake during sequential 4-week periods. At the end of each period homocysteine and endothelial function (E-selectin, von Willebrand factor, endothelin-1) were assessed. The subjects reduced their alcohol intake from 72 to 8 g per day. The decrease in alcohol intake resulted in reductions in total cholesterol, high-density lipoprotein cholesterol and homocysteine. There was no effect of alcohol on endothelial function. These authors summarized that reduction in alcohol intake in healthy moderate-to-heavy drinkers did not improve endothelial function but improved cholesterol and homocysteine levels. The improvement of homocysteine levels could be secondary to the decrease of alcohol consumption or to the increase of folate intake with beer (two hypotheses with the same result).

The kinetics of homocysteine metabolism after beer consumption has been studied, too (Beulens *et al.*, 2005). Ten healthy men and nine healthy postmenopausal women were studied in a controlled randomized trial. They consumed beer or alcohol-free beer (men: 4 units/day; women: 3 units/day) during 3 weeks, separated by a 1-week washout. On days 5, 10, 15, and 20 of each period, homocysteine (tHcy) levels were measured. Plasma tHcy and *S*-adenosyl methionine/*S*-adenosyl homocysteine ratio were not affected by consumption of beer or alcohol-free beer. Plasma P5P (microgram/liter) increased during consumption of beer, whereas it decreased during consumption of alcohol-free beer. Changes over time of plasma vitamin B6 (microgram/liter) were similar to changes in plasma pyridoxal-5-phosphate. Serum vitamin B12 was higher after 3 weeks consumption of alcohol-free beer as compared with beer consumption. Changes in serum methionine, cysteine, cystathionine, and plasma folate were not different between beer-drinking and alcohol-free beer-drinking periods. As we can see the alcohol–homocysteine interaction is complex, perhaps with different effects depending on type of beverage and course of drinking habit (acute or chronic). Although chronic alcohol consumption clearly increases Hcy concentration, the effects of moderate and regular consumption of alcohol are debated in epidemiological studies. This is paradoxical since the coronary protective effect of alcoholic beverages has been established. However, a negative correlation between Hcy and alcoholic beverages has been described in some above-mentioned studies, more especially in beer-drinkers (Schlienger, 2003).

Some authors have explored different drinking patterns with tHcy levels. In a cross-sectional study of 2,126 men have been tested the relationship between preference of alcoholic beverages and atherosclerotic risk factors (tHcy) (Rouillier *et al.*, 2006), using a complicated statistical method (hierarchical clustering method), determined six drinking patterns, "low drinkers," "high quality wines," "beer and cider," "digestives," "local wines," and "table wines," according to the intake of alcoholic beverages. Logistic models estimated the relative risk of abnormal markers in the drinking patterns compared with low drinkers. The results showed that abstainers had high total plasma homocysteine (tHcy), even after full adjustment (odds ratio (OR) = 1.6, 95% confidence interval (CI): 1.0–2.8). Drinkers of high quality wine had low lipoprotein (a) (a new cardiovascular risk factor), high tHcy and high body mass index; beer drinkers had high tHcy and waist circumference. Drinkers of digestives had high triacylglycerol; after adjustment they were at risk of low apolipoprotein A-I. Local wine drinkers were similar to low drinkers. Table wine drinkers had high apolipoprotein B, high triacylglycerol, and high waist-to-hip ratio. These authors suggest that preference of alcoholic beverage could indicate groups at specific risks of atherosclerotic disease with complex relationships between drinking patterns and homocysteine levels and other cardiovascular risk factors.

Other study in this unclear area (Sakuta *et al.*, 2005) analyzed the relation between tHcy and daily ethanol consumption (beer and others) in middle-aged Japanese men (974 subjects). These authors detected that plasma tHcy was positively associated with consumption of whiskey but not with consumption of shochu (Japanese spirits), sake, beer, or wine. ORs of an increase in daily intake of 30 ml ethanol for hyperhomocysteinemia (>14.0 μmol/l) were 2.58 (95% CI, 1.29–5.14) for whiskey, 1.08 (0.78–1.50) for shochu, 0.99 (0.59–1.66) for sake, 0.98 (0.58–1.63) for beer, and 1.70 (0.31–9.50) for wine in a multivariate logistic regression analysis adjusted by other cardiovascular risk factors such as the daily number of cigarettes smoked, physical activity, and vegetable consumption. These data show that local drinking pattern and perhaps genetic background of each ethnicity could modify the relation between beverage type and tHcy levels (Sakuta *et al.*, 2005).

Analysis of Confounding Factors

Drinking habits as a confounding factor

The conflicting results may derive in part from confounding by the interaction of alcoholic beverage consumed or type of beer (Table 62.7). In 1996, a cross-sectional study measuring tHcy and red blood cell folate concentrations was conducted in 1,196 middle-aged women and men from the French Supplementation with Antioxidant Vitamins and Minerals Study. Intakes of alcohol, energy, coffee, and B vitamins were assessed by six separate 24-h dietary records from the previous year. In this study, tHcy concentrations were positively associated with wine intake in the women and with beer intake in the men, without association with the consumption of spirits was observed. The association between beer consumption and tHcy concentrations in the men was modified by the consumption of wine; the association was positive in wine drinkers, whereas an inverse trend was seen in those who drank no wine (Mennen *et al.*, 2003). This data confirm the hypothesis that beer drinking is inversely related to tHcy in persons who drink no wine. It is possible that B-vitamin content of beer (vitamins B6 and B12 and folate) is enough to counteract the tHcy-increasing effect of the alcohol in the beer, but not enough to compensate the effects of the alcohol in wine consumed in the same period. Apparently, the betaine content in wine is too low to counteract the negative effects of alcohol on tHcy. Nevertheless, in the same area the beer and wine consumptions can change with the time as in Spain (Figure 62.3), with a high increase in beer consumption.

Other confounding factors

Other confounding factors may play a role in all studies, changing direction of the results secondary to bias. Some of above-mentioned studies have demonstrated different results due to no control in these factors. For example, an age-dependent increase in tHcy can be related to a decline in renal function, all studies without creatinin as a control factor could misclassify the results of association of beer consumption and tHcy (Norlund, 1998). Furthermore, elevated serum tHcy in older populations can also be attributed to low blood folate concentrations and an increased incidence of vitamin B12 deficiency resulting from malabsorption of vitamin B12 by the aging gut (Van Asselt *et al.*, 1998).

Race-ethnicity was associated with serum tHcy, too. Among all the race-ethnicity groups examined, non-Hispanic whites had the highest serum tHcy concentrations. Mean serum tHcy concentrations in non-Hispanic whites were 0.8 and 1.1 μmol/l higher than those of non-Hispanic blacks and Mexican-Americans, respectively (Ganji and Kafai, 2006).

Other confounding factor is genetic background. Elevated tHcy can be attributed to point mutation (cytosine to thymidine substitution at nucleotide 677) in the gene that encodes N^5,N^{10}-methylenetetrahydrofolate reductase (MTHFR; EC 1.7.99.5). The 677C→T mutation results in reduced activity of MTHFR; activity is reduced to 34% in *TT* and 71% in *CT* relative to *CC* (Ma *et al.*, 1996). MTHFR is required for the conversion of N^5,N^{10}-methylenetetrahydrofolate to 5-methyltetrahydrofolate, which is a methyl donor for remethylation of homocysteine to methionine. Individuals who are homozygous for the 677C→T mutation have increased circulating tHcy when dietary folate intake is low (Jacques *et al.*, 1996). As far as we have known, all the studies mentioned in our chapter did not have a genetic background analysis to explain relation between beer consumption and tHcy levels.

Several studies have reported a positive association between cigarette smoking and tHcy concentration. A positive association between serum cotinine concentration and serum tHcy has been described. Cotinine is a metabolite of nicotine with a half-life of 20 h. Absorbed nicotine is directly related to the serum cotinine concentration. Serum cotinine is a better indicator of smoking than is self-reported information because individuals tend to underreport cigarette smoking and different persons inhale cigarette smoke differently. Also, serum cotinine reflects passive smoking. Serum cotinine concentration was correlated with number of cigarettes smoked in the NHANES III. By using serum cotinine rather than number of cigarettes smoked as a

Table 62.7 Vitamin composition in different type of beers (per 100 ml) in our area

	Folic acid (μg)	*B12 (μg)*	*B6 (mg)*
Normal beer	10	0.14	0.10
Dark beer	4	0.11	0.01
Blond beer	10	0.12	0.03

Note: Vitamin B12, vitamin B6, and folic acid of different beers in Spain.

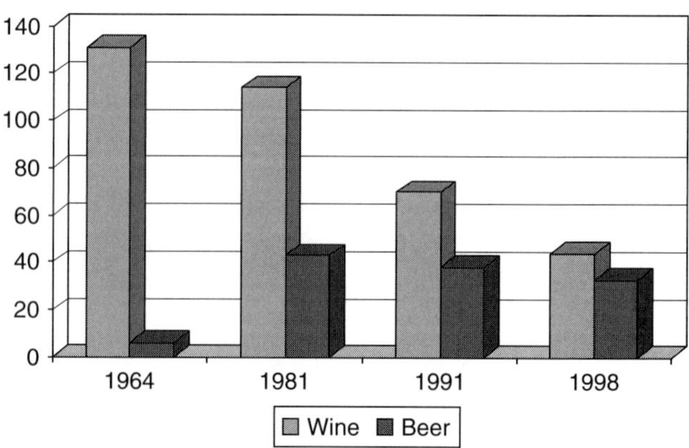

Figure 62.3 Changes in beer consumption in our country. A decrease of wine consumption and an increase of beer consumption in ml/person/day in Spain is observed above. (National Institute of Statistical Sciences).

measure of smoking, association between biochemical smoke and serum tHcy has been demonstrated (Ganji and Kafai, 2006). The exact mechanism by which cigarette smoking increases tHcy is not known. However, the association between smoking and tHcy can be explained by low concentrations of blood folate, vitamin B12, and vitamin B6 in smokers. Consumption of beverage and smoking habit goes joint in almost all subjects; the lack of analysis of this association can bias the results. As we can see, interaction in different factors present in some type of patient could modify the results of previous and further studies in this topic area.

The last confounding factor could be the amount of ethanol. Status of vitamin B12, B6, and folate is related with tHcy levels, but amount of ethanol disturbs vitamin metabolism. For example, the etiology of folate deficiency in alcoholism can be ascribed to several causes, such as poor absorption, decreased hepatic uptake and retention, and increase urinary excretion. The effects could be due to a direct toxic effect or a poor nutrition status. For example, a low jejunal uptake of labeled folic acid has been detected in malnourished alcoholic patients (Halsted *et al.*, 1971). An inhibition of jejunal folate hydroxilase in miniature pigs fed ethanol for 11 months has been later demonstrated, suggesting that toxic effect of ethanol could also play an important role in the pathogenesis of folate malabsorption. Liver concentrations of vitamin B12 were significantly lower in alcoholics compared with non-drinkers, perhaps alcoholism is associated with impaired retention of cobalamins in tissues, followed by an accumulation of this vitamin in the plasma. Intracellular depletion of vitamin B12 could lead to an intracellular accumulation of N^5-methyltetrahydrofolate because of the irreversible reaction that forms it and because its removal is prevented by impairment of the vitamin B12-dependent methylation of homocysteine. Intracellular accumulation of N^5-methyltetrahydrofolate would ultimately lead to intracellular depletion of folate because N^5-methyltetrahydrofolate is a poor substrate for polyglutamation, which is a vitamin B12-dependent process required for cellular retention of folates.

Chronic alcoholics have low concentrations of vitamin B6, too. This deficiency is due in part to acetaldehyde, a product of ethanol oxidation, which displaces protein-bound vitamin B6, thereby exposing this coenzyme to the action of phosphatases. Vitamin B6 serves as a coenzyme for cystathionine beta synthase and serine transhydroxymethylase; therefore, the hyperhomocysteinemia in alcoholics could be due in part to the impairment of one or both of these enzymes. Serine transhydroxymethylase catalyzes the conversion of tetrahydrofolate into methylenetetrahydrofolate. After reduction, the resulting methylenetetrahydrofolate will then donate its methyl group to homocysteine in a vitamin B12-dependent reaction. Therefore, inhibition of serine transhydroxymethylase could ultimately affect the remethylation of homocysteine.

Summary Points

- Homocysteine is a non-essential sulfur-containing amino acid formed from the demethylation of an essential amino acid, methionine.
- Hyperhomocysteinemia has received increasing attention during the past decade and has joined hypertension, obesity, dyslipemia, smoking, and diabetes mellitus as an independent risk factor for cardiovascular disease.
- Chronic alcohol ingestion has also been associated with increased homocysteine levels. However, drinking beer may have a special health benefit not attributable to other alcohol-containing beverages, with an inverse relation with homocysteine levels.
- The hypothesis of a reduction in Hcy induced by the beer contents has been described in an interventional study. The vitamins contained in beer may well be at the origin of this beneficial effect.
- Subjects with intake of 1 l daily or more had significantly lower tHcy and higher folate concentrations than those that reporting lower daily beer intake.

However, some studies have not demonstrated this inverse association. The conflicting results may derive in part from confounding by the interaction of alcoholic beverage consumed. Other confounding factors may play a role in all studies, changing direction of the results secondary to bias such as race-ethnicity, genetic background, age, cigarette smoking, and amount of ethanol.

References

Allen, R.H., Stabler, S.P., Savage, D.G. and Lindenbaum, J. (1993). *FASEB J.* 7, 1344–1353.

Beulens, J.W., Sierksma, A., Schaafsma, G., Kok, F.J. and Struys, E.A. (2005). *Alcohol Clin. Exp. Res.* 29, 739–745.

Cravo, M.L., Gloria, L.M. and Selhud, J. (1996). *Am. J. Clin. Nutr.* 63, 220–224.

Cooper, D.E., Goff, D.C. and Bell, R.A. (2002). *Diabetes Care* 25, 1425–1431.

de Luis, D.A., Fernandez, N. and Aller, R. (2003). *Ann. Nutr. Metabol.* 47, 119–123.

de Luis, D.A., Fernandez, N. and Aller, R. (2004). *Med. Clin. (Barc.)* 122, 27–32.

Ganji,, V. and Kafai, M.R. (2006). *J. Nutr.* 136, 153–158.

Gloria, L., Cravo, M. and Camilo, M.E. (1997). *Am. J. Gastroenterol.* 92, 485–489.

Halsted, C.H., Robles, E.A. and Mezey, E. (1971). *New Engl. J. Med.* 285, 701–706.

Huktberg, B., Berglund, M., Andersson, A. and Frank, A. (1993). *Alcohol Clin. Exp. Res.* 17, 687–689.

Jacques, P.F., Bostom, A.G. and Williams, R.R. (1996). *Circulation* 93, 7–9.

Jayasinghe, S. (2000). *Lancet* 356, 1522.

Lusier Cacan, S., Xhignesse, M. and Piolot, A. (1996). *Am. J. Clin. Nutr.* 64, 587–593.

Ma, J., Stampfer, M.J. and Hennekens, C.H. (1996). *Circulation* 94, 2410–2416.

Mayer Jr., O., Simon, J. and Rosolova, H. (2001). *Eur. J. Clin. Nutr.* 55, 605–609.
Mennen, L.I., de Courcy, G.P., Ducros, V., Zarebska, M. and Bertrais, S. (2003). *Am. J. Clin. Nutr.* 78, 334–338.
Norlund, L., Grubbb, A. and Flex, G. (1998). *Clin. Chem. Lab. Med.* 36, 175–178.
Nygard, O., Refsum, H. and Ueland, P.M. (1997). *Am. J. Clin. Nutr.* 65, 136–143.
Rouillier, P., Bertrais, S., Daudin, J.J., Bacro, J.N. and Hercberg, S. (2006). *Eur. J. Nutr.* 45, 79–87.
Sakuta, H. and Suzuki, T. (2005). *Alcohol* 37, 73–77.
Sakuta, H., Suzuki, T., Katayama, Y. and Yasuda, H. (2005). *Diabet. Med.* 22, 1359–1363.
Smulders, Y.M., Rakic, M., Slaats, E.H., Treskes, M., Sijbrands, E.J., Odekerken, D.A., Stehouwer, C.D. and Silberbush, J. (1999). *Diabetes Care* 22, 125–132.
Schlienger, J.L. (2003). *Presse Med.* 32, 262–267.
Stabler, S.P., Estacio, R., Jeffers, B.W., Cohen, J.A., Allen, R.H. and Schrier, R.W. (1999). *Metabolism* 48, 1096–1101.
Stolzenberg-Solomon, R.Z., Miller, E.R., Maguire, M.G., Selhub, J. and Appel, L.J. (1999). *Am. J. Clin. Nutr.* 69, 467–475.
Targher, G., Bertolini, L., Zenarini, L., Cacciatori, V., Muggeo, M., Faccini, G. and Zoppini, G. (2000). *Diabetes Care* 23, 524–528.
Tucker, K.L., Selhub, J. and Wilson, P.W. (1996). *J. Nutr.* 126, 3025–3031.
Ubbink, J.B., Fehily, A.M. and Pickering, J. (1998). *Atherosclerosis* 140, 349–356.
Van Asselt, D.Z., de Groot, L.C. and van Staveren, W.A. (1998). *Am. J. Clin. Nutr.* 68, 328–334.
Van der Gaag, M.S., Ubbink, J.B. and Sillanaukee, P. (2000). *Lancet* 355, 1522.
Vermaak, W.J., Ubbink, J.B. and Delport, R. (2001). *Atheroscleoris* 89, 155–162.
Walker, C. and Baxter, E.E. (2000). *Tech. Q. Master Brew. Assoc. Am.* 37, 301–305.
Wannamethee, S.G. and Shaper, A.G. (1999). *Am. J. Public Health* 89, 685–690.
Weir, D. and Molloy, A. (2000). *Am. J. Clin. Nutr.* 71, 859–860.
Zilkens, R.R., Rich, L., Burke, V. and Beilin, L.J. (2003). *J. Hypertens.* 21, 97–103.

63

Alcohol, Beer, and Ischemic Stroke

Kenneth J. Mukamal Division of General Medicine & Primary Care Beth Israel Deaconess Medical Center, Boston, MA, USA

Abstract

In contrast to the consistent associations of beer and alcohol intake with lower risk of coronary heart disease, their corresponding associations with risk of stroke are more complex and nuanced. In recent cohort studies of alcohol use and ischemic stroke, the association is of modest magnitude, with risk ratios approximating 0.8, and the lowest risk among less-than-daily drinkers. Consumers of 3 or more drinks per day clearly have a higher risk of ischemic stroke, and heavy intake may also acutely trigger strokes. In addition, alcohol use is generally associated with a roughly dose-dependent higher risk of hemorrhagic stroke throughout the full range of intake. These same relationships have generally been seen with both beer and other alcoholic beverages, with only limited evidence that beer intake may not confer as low a risk as wine. The mechanisms that underlie the lower risk of ischemic stroke among moderate drinkers have not yet been definitively explored. The higher risks of hypertension and atrial fibrillation that accompany heavy drinking may explain its association with ischemic stroke, and the antithrombotic effects of alcohol may mediate its link with hemorrhagic stroke.

List of Abbreviations

ADH	Alcohol dehydrogenase
CI	Confidence interval
HDL-C	High-density lipoprotein cholesterol
INR	International normalized ratio

Introduction

Although the relationship of alcohol consumption and coronary heart disease has been extensively addressed in literally dozens of studies (Maclure, 1993; Corrao *et al.*, 2000; Di Castelnuovo *et al.*, 2002), alcohol consumption has also been associated with other cardiovascular diseases, including congestive heart failure and peripheral arterial disease (Djousse *et al.*, 2000; Walsh *et al.*, 2002; Bryson *et al.*, 2006). Among the most challenging of the cardiovascular diseases to be associated with beer and alcohol intake is stroke (or cerebrovascular accident). In fact, Arthur Klatsky, a pioneer in the study of population-wide health effects of alcohol intake including stroke (Klatsky *et al.*, 2001, 2002) has termed this association an "epidemiological labyrinth" (Klatsky, 2005).

In this chapter, we review the difficulties inherent in the study of risk of stroke, current epidemiological evidence regarding the relationships of beer and alcohol intake with risk of ischemic and hemorrhagic stroke, and review both experimental and observational evidence regarding potential mechanisms that may play important roles in the etiology of observed associations.

A primary consideration in understanding the association of alcohol and beer intake with stroke is the extraordinary heterogeneity inherent in the clinical syndrome of stroke (Table 63.1). In general, stroke comprises two main types – ischemic and hemorrhagic – and several subtypes of each (e.g. atherothrombotic, lacunar, embolic, subarachnoid hemorrhage, intracerebral hemorrhage). The pathogeneses of these main and subtypes differ substantially, and hence alcohol appears to have decidedly different associations with each.

Main Text

Alcohol use and ischemic stroke

Ischemic stroke, the most common type in the United States and Europe, is the result of vascular occlusion of an intracerebral artery, whether by local thrombosis or distal embolism. It is noteworthy that two of the strongest chronic risk factors for ischemic stroke are hypertension and atrial fibrillation (AF)(Manolio *et al.*, 1996), both of which have been attributed to heavy drinking (see below). Thus, even though ischemic stroke shares an atherosclerotic and thrombotic etiology with coronary heart disease, the particular factors that most strongly predict ischemic stroke risk appear to be the subset of cardiovascular risk factors exacerbated by heavy alcohol use. As a consequence, it may not be surprising that the apparent inverse association of moderate alcohol intake with ischemic stroke risk occurs at a lower

Beer in Health and Disease Prevention
ISBN: 978-0-12-373891-2

Table 63.1 Major types and subtypes of stroke

Type	*Lay definition*	*Subtype*	*Characteristics*
Ischemic stroke or cerebral	Blockage in an artery feeding the brain	Atherothrombotic	Narrowing in large outer arteries, often by cholesterol plaques
Infarction		Embolic	Blockage by clots or other material becoming free and lodging downstream in arteries
		Lacunar	Blockage in small, deep arteries of the brain
Hemorrhagic	Bleeding from an artery into or around the brain	Subarachnoid	Leakage from blood vessels coursing outside the brain
		Intracerebral	Disruption of blood vessels inside the brain itself

Note: Stroke, or cerebrovascular accident, occurs when brain tissue dies related to loss of blood providing it with nutrients and oxygen. Two major types, and five major subtypes of these, are commonly recognized, based on their causes and characteristics.

dose of alcohol, and with a lower magnitude of risk reduction, than does the corresponding association with coronary heart disease risk. It is also unsurprising that heavy drinking is consistently associated with higher stroke risk.

For many years, observational studies of the relationship of alcohol consumption and risk of ischemic stroke, in substantial part case-control studies, suggested a relatively strong inverse relationship (Camargo, 1989; Reynolds *et al.*, 2003). For example, in the Nurses' Health Study cohort, Stampfer and colleagues documented 66 incident ischemic strokes and found relative risks of 0.3 (95% confidence interval (CI), 0.1–0.7) for intake of 5–14 g of alcohol per day, and 0.5 (95% CI, 0.2–1.1) for intake of 15 g/day or more (Stampfer *et al.*, 1988). Another excellent early example is a large case-control study from Gill and colleagues in Birmingham, UK, who documented 621 cases of stroke and a similar number of employed controls from the general population (Figure 63.1) (Gill *et al.*, 1991). In this study, the relative risks for ischemic stroke were 0.6 among consumers of 1–90 g/week and 0.7 among consumers of 100–390 g/week; the relative risks for total stroke (of which ischemic strokes comprised over half) were similar.

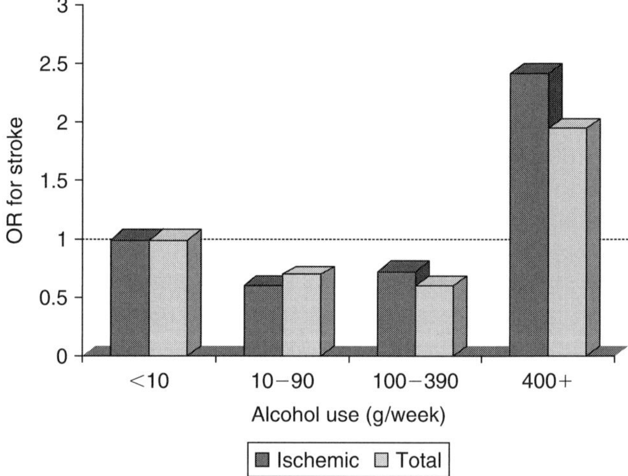

Figure 63.1 The relationship of alcohol use and risk of total and ischemic stroke in a case-control study conducted in Birmingham, UK. Consumers of <10 g/week (~1 drink per week) were the reference category (dotted line). The *y*-axis indicates odds ratios (OR) for ischemic (■ bars) and all-cause stroke (□ bars). In this older but very large case-control study, light drinking categories were associated with lower risk of total or ischemic stroke, but heavy drinking (32 drinks per week or more) was associated with a twofold higher risk.

However, more recent studies have called this magnitude of lower risk into question. In particular, the reliance on case-control methodology in earlier studies may have introduced bias in at least three ways. First, case subjects with stroke may not recall their usual alcohol consumption with the same accuracy that control subjects do, especially if the stroke has influenced their cognitive or expressive functions in even subtle ways. Second, some patients with stroke may cut back on their alcohol intake in the days or weeks prior because of transient ischemic symptoms that herald the onset of the index stroke. Because of biases in reporting, such patients are apt to recall recent intake more adeptly and to report their usual intake as lower than it may have been prior to such symptoms. Finally, case-control studies are limited to interviewing relatively healthy stroke survivors. If alcohol consumption influences stroke severity in addition to stroke incidence, then the observed effects of alcohol in such studies will be combinations of effects of alcohol on the likelihood of having and of surviving a stroke.

Data from recent cohort studies have indeed suggested that the apparent benefit of moderate intake of alcohol or specific alcoholic beverages may have been overestimated. For example, in a meta-analysis restricted to 19 cohort studies, Reynolds and colleagues found that light drinking

(<12 g/day) was associated with a relative risk of 0.82 (95% CI, 0.73–0.92), but consumption of 12–50 g/day was not associated with lower or higher risk (Reynolds *et al.*, 2003). In contrast, among case-control studies, the relative risk associated with light drinking was 0.80 (95% CI, 0.67–0.97), but intake of 12–24 g/day was associated with a relative risk of 0.65 (95% CI, 0.44–0.96). Thus, light drinking was associated with ~20% lower risk of stroke in all studies, but only case-control studies suggested a lower risk with more moderate drinking.

Ischemic stroke vs. coronary heart disease

As described above, there are some similarities in the pathogenesis of ischemic stroke and coronary heart disease, and they are often grouped together as forms of "cardiovascular disease." Indeed, both coronary heart disease and ischemic stroke are vascular diseases characterized by the acute onset of tissue injury related to blood vessel occlusion superimposed on the chronic process of atherosclerosis within the vessel wall. Standard risk factors for coronary heart disease, such as tobacco smoking, diabetes, and hypertension, are risk factors for ischemic stroke as well.

However, they differ in important ways, and it is worthwhile to contrast the relationships of alcohol use and ischemic stroke with the corresponding relationship of alcohol use and coronary heart disease. Luckily, several large cohort studies have studied both outcomes with relationship to alcohol use, so the effects of alcohol on the two outcomes can be directly contrasted. A recent example is shown in Figure 63.2 that illustrates the differences in these relationships well.

In a cohort study among members of a single Californian insurance plan (Figure 63.2), Klatsky and colleagues reported that alcohol intake has a U-shaped association with hospitalization for ischemic stroke, with relative risks of 0.8 (95% CI, 0.7–1.0) among those who consumed 1 drink monthly-to-daily and 1.0 (95% CI, 0.8–1.2) among those who consumed 3 or more drinks per day (Klatsky *et al.*, 2001). In contrast, these authors found a direct inverse association between alcohol use and risk of coronary heart disease hospitalization, with relative risks of 0.6 among women and 0.7 among men who consumed 3 or more drinks per day (Klatsky *et al.*, 1997).

In results that are strikingly similar, we performed analyses of the Cardiovascular Health Study, a cohort study of 5,888 older adults funded by the National Heart, Lung, and Blood Institute. There was a lower risk of ischemic stroke confined to consumers of 1–6 drinks per week (hazard ratio 0.75; 95% CI, 0.53–1.06) (Mukamal *et al.*, 2005b). Again, there was direct, dose-dependent relationship between alcohol intake and risk of myocardial infarction, with the lowest risk among consumers of 14 or more drinks per week. Interestingly, we also found a U-shaped relationship of alcohol intake with prevalence of white matter lesions (a radiographic finding on MRI images of the brain thought to reflect tiny ischemic lesions) in this population, with the lowest risk among consumers of 1–6 drinks per week (Mukamal *et al.*, 2001).

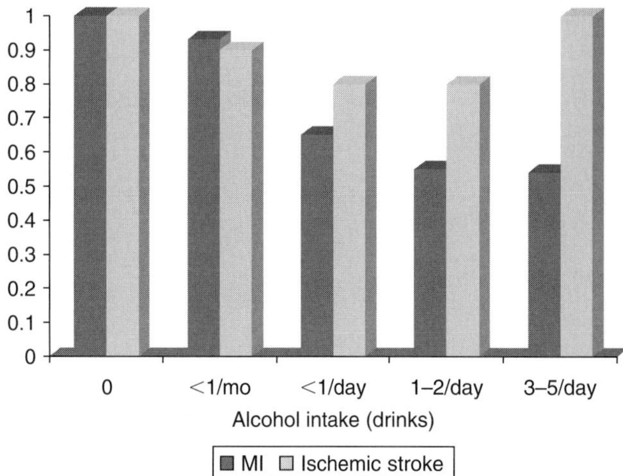

Figure 63.2 The dual relationships of alcohol intake with risks of hospitalization for myocardial infarction (MI) or ischemic stroke among members of the Kaiser Permanente cohort in northern California, US. Abstainers were the reference category. The *y*-axis indicates hazard ratios for myocardial infarction (■ bars) and ischemic stroke (■ bars). The relationship between alcohol intake and risk of myocardial infarction (or heart attack) was linear, with lower risk with higher intake. In contrast, the relationship with ischemic stroke was U-shaped, with a much smaller benefit and at a smaller level of intake.

Ischemic stroke subtypes

Even within the category of ischemic stroke, several subtypes exist. These are sometimes classified as atherothrombotic, lacunar, and embolic. Atherothrombotic strokes reflect large-vessel *in situ* occlusion, most closely related to coronary heart disease. Lacunar infarcts are generally small, deep areas of infarction following small-vessel occlusion of penetrating arteries, while embolic strokes occur when clots or friable atherosclerotic deposits break free from the heart, aorta, or venous system (through right-to-left shunts). Dulli has emphasized how the heterogeneity of ischemic stroke may influence its association with alcohol intake (Dulli, 2002), but relatively few data exist to confirm this hypothesis.

To address this, we examined ischemic stroke risk in the Health Professionals Follow-up Study (Mukamal *et al.*, 2005a). Concordant with previous work, lower risk was restricted to consumers of an average of 0.1–9.9 g/day, and particularly those whose consumption was spread out over 3–4 days per week (hazard ratio 0.56; 95% CI, 0.31–1.02). This finding matches well with the other recent cohort studies described above, all of which point to consumption at least weekly but less than daily as conferring lowest risk. However, stroke subtype appeared to modify risk substantially. Compared with abstention, the hazard ratios associated with intake of 0.1–9.9 g/day were 0.76 (0.50–1.15) for confirmed thrombotic stroke, but 2.20 (95% CI, 0.84–5.76) for confirmed embolic stroke, much as predicted from their respective pathogeneses. Unfortunately, large numbers of strokes cannot be conclusively categorized using standard classification schemes, and larger studies that attempt to classify ischemic stroke subtypes are needed to confirm these findings.

Adverse effects of heavy drinking on ischemic stroke

Little controversy exists regarding the relationship of heavier drinking with a higher risk of ischemic stroke (Reynolds *et al.*, 2003; Mukamal *et al.*, 2005a). This has long been a feared consequence of heavy drinking and again differs from the relationship of heavy drinking with coronary heart disease, where the existence of a true J-shape is far less clear (Maclure, 1993).

However, there has been some clarification in the magnitude of higher risk associated with heavy drinking over time. As seen in Figure 63.1, Gill and colleagues found that the risks of ischemic and total stroke were increased two- to threefold among the heaviest drinkers relative to abstainers in their case-control study (Gill *et al.*, 1991). In contrast, in our cohort study of health professionals, we found that consumers of 30.0 g or more per day of alcohol had approximately 45% higher risk than did abstainers (Mukamal *et al.*, 2005a). Some of this difference may reflect the greater extremes of drinking behavior found in case-control studies than among participants in long-term cohort studies, but it also likely reflects better control of confounding factors that tend to track with heavy drinking, including poor diet and smoking, and the advantages of a prospective design. In their meta-analysis of older cohort studies, Reynolds and colleagues found a relative risk associated with intake of >60 g/day of 1.98 among case-control studies but 1.63 among cohort studies (Reynolds *et al.*, 2003). Thus, while there is unequivocally higher ischemic stroke associated with heavy drinking, its magnitude is apt to be in the range of 50–60% above abstainers. Nonetheless, because heavy drinkers also tend to have other risk factors, their absolute risk can be sizable indeed.

Another development in this field has been a better understanding of the risk associated with individual episodes of heavy drinking, or binge drinking. Because binge drinking is extremely common even among otherwise moderate drinkers (Naimi *et al.*, 2003), any potential effects of such episodes can have widespread public health import. Hillbom and colleagues have evaluated the risk of recent drinking in a series of studies (Hillbom and Kaste, 1978, 1981, 1983; Hillbom *et al.*, 1995, 1999). In general, even single episodes of intake of 3 or more drinks or drinking to intoxication may acutely and transiently increase risk of ischemic stroke for the ensuing 24 h. For example, in a study of Finnish younger adults (who are particularly apt to consume alcohol in binges), ischemic stroke patients were five- to sevenfold more likely to report heavy alcohol use in the preceding 24 h than were other hospitalized young adults (Figure 63.3).

Specific relationships of beer and other alcohol beverages with ischemic stroke

There has long been interest in whether specific non-alcoholic constituents of alcoholic beverages influence cardiovascular risk, with the greatest attention paid to polyphenolic constituents of red wine (Waddington *et al.*, 2004). A substantial amount of basic research has investigated the potentially protective properties of the diverse constituents of such beverages, reviewed elsewhere in this volume. In observational studies, this has generally taken the form of analyses examining the relative associations of beer, wine, and spirits with cardiovascular risk. Interestingly, for coronary heart disease, this approach has not necessarily shown a particular benefit for any given beverage (Rimm *et al.*, 1996; Cleophas, 1999), perhaps because the effects of ethanol itself make it difficult to detect the smaller effects of other components that are present in smaller concentrations. For stroke, this issue remains under active investigation.

We have investigated the relative effects of different beverage types with risk of ischemic stroke in two cohort studies.

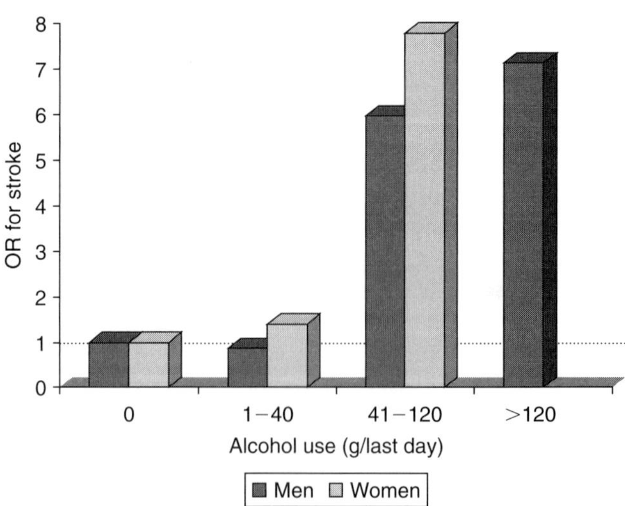

N = 75 stroke cases, 133 controls

Figure 63.3 The relationships of alcohol intake in the preceding 24 h with risk of hospitalization for ischemic stroke among adults aged 16–40 in Helsinki, Finland. Controls were hospitalized for other acute illnesses. Abstainers were the reference category (dotted line). The *y*-axis indicates odds ratios for men (■ bars) and women (□ bars). Patients hospitalized with ischemic stroke with severalfold more likely to report alcohol intake of more than 3 drinks in the last day than were other patients, suggesting that heavy alcohol intake can acute precipitate (or trigger) ischemic stroke.

In the Health Professionals Follow-up Study (Figure 63.4) (Mukamal *et al.*, 2005a), in which the beverages consumed in greatest quantity are beer and spirits (as is typical for American men), we found a significant difference between red wine and other beverages in their relationships with ischemic stroke risk. For beer, there was a relatively direct relationship, with a slight increase in risk with greater exposure. This contrasted with the dose-dependent lower risk associated with red wine intake.

We employed a similar approach in the Cardiovascular Health Study (Figure 63.5), where the relative levels of alcohol intake were considerably lower (as expected from the older age of participants) (Mukamal *et al.*, 2005b). In this case, wine intake (including both red and white) was again associated with a dose-dependent lower ischemic stroke risk. However, beer intake too was associated with significantly lower risk, particularly at intake of 1–6 drinks per week (hazard ratio 0.57).

Other cohort studies have tended to support the notion that beer intake is unlikely to confer lower risk of ischemic stroke than do other alcoholic beverages. In the Kaiser Permanente cohort, there was a slightly higher risk associated only with liquor intake after adjustment for total alcohol consumption, with no independent effects of wine or beer intake (Klatsky *et al.*, 2001). In the Copenhagen City Heart Study, another large prospective cohort study comprising over 13,000 adults, beer intake was not associated with risk of stroke, including the category of ischemic/other strokes, while wine intake between weekly and daily was associated with lowest risk (hazard ratio 0.59); liquor intake was also unassociated with risk (Truelsen *et al.*, 1998). However, wine intake in Denmark is strongly associated with favorable dietary and other lifestyle characteristics (Tjonneland *et al.*, 1999; Johansen *et al.*, 2006), making it likely that the lower risk observed for wine intake is at least partly the product of other factors.

In sum, at the present time, there is suggestive but clearly not definitive evidence that wine intake might be more strongly associated with lower ischemic stroke risk than other beverages, while beer intake tends to mirror the overall effects of alcohol intake.

Hemorrhagic stroke

Although not as common in Western countries, hemorrhagic stroke is a common stroke type in Asia, where most studies have been performed, and comprises subarachnoid and intracerebral subtypes. Hemorrhagic and ischemic stroke share some common risk factors – most notably hypertension – but also some important differences. Most important of these is thrombotic tendency, for antithrombotic medications tend to decrease risk of ischemic stroke but increase risk for hemorrhagic stroke. It has generally been assumed to be a dose-dependent increase in risk of

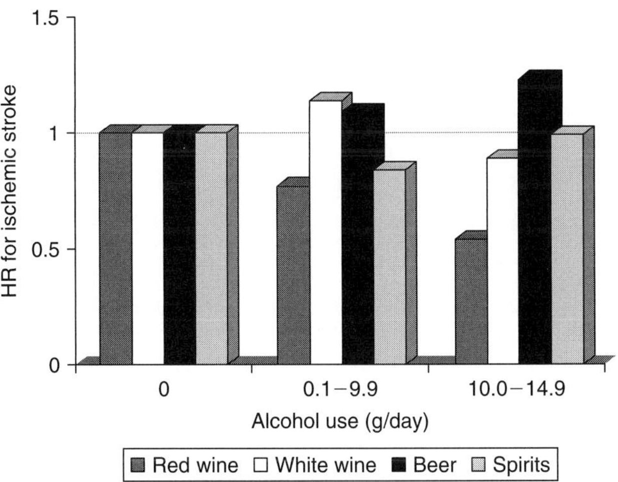

Figure 63.4 The relationships of alcoholic beverage intake with risk of incident ischemic stroke among men who were free of cardiovascular disease in the Health Professionals Follow-up Study. Abstainers from each beverage were the reference category. The *y*-axis indicates hazard ratios for red wine (■ bars), white wine (□ bars), beer (■ bars), and spirits (□ bars). Pairwise tests of the linear trends were significant for the comparisons of red wine with beer and liquor, suggesting that red wine (which appears to be associated with a lower risk of ischemic stroke in a dose-dependent manner) differs significantly from beer and spirits (where little relationship at all is seen).

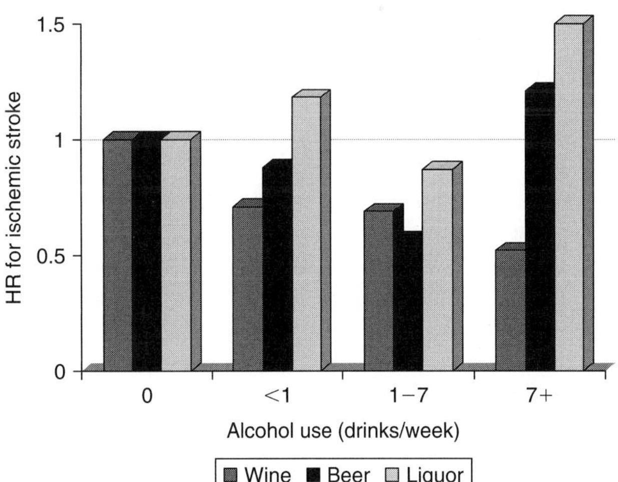

Figure 63.5 The relationships of alcoholic beverage intake with risk of incident ischemic stroke among older adults who were free of cardiovascular disease in the Cardiovascular Health Study. Abstainers from each beverage were the reference category. The *y*-axis indicates hazard ratios for wine (■ bars), beer (■ bars), and liquor (□ bars). In this population of older adults, both beer and wine were associated with lower risk of ischemic stroke, particularly with intake of 1–7 drinks per week. The differences among beverages in the highest category appear to reflect residual differences in how much of each beverage was actually consumed.

hemorrhagic stroke associated with alcohol use (Camargo, 1996). In a meta-analysis of case-control studies of intracerebral hemorrhage, Ariesen found summary odds ratios of 2.05 (95% CI, 1.35–3.11) for intake ≤56 g/day, and 4.11 (95% CI, 2.54–6.65) for intake >56 g/day (Ariesen *et al.*, 2003). However, in a comparable meta-analysis of cohort studies of subarachnoid hemorrhage, Feigin found an increased risk restricted to heavier intake (>150 g/week), with a summary relative risk of 2.1 (95% CI, 1.5–2.8) (Feigin *et al.*, 2005). In one of the largest studies to date, Klatsky and his colleagues at Kaiser Permanente found higher risk associated only with intake of 6 or more drinks per day (Klatsky *et al.*, 2002).

The contrasting associations of light-to-moderate drinking with ischemic and hemorrhagic stroke are largely consistent with Renaud's hypothesis that moderate drinking mediates its effects, at least in part, through activity on platelets and prothrombotic factors (Renaud and De Lorgeril, 1992). If this hypothesis is correct, light drinking would be expected to decrease risk of thrombotic events, such as myocardial infarction and ischemic stroke, but increase risk of bleeding in the brain and potentially other sites (Kaufman *et al.*, 1999), much as has been observed. An outstanding example of these contrasting associations was reported by Iso and colleagues in the Japan Public Health Center-based Prospective Study on Cancer and Cardiovascular Disease (Iso *et al.*, 2004), a sample of nearly 20,000 men with approximately equal numbers of hemorrhagic and ischemic strokes. Compared with occasional drinking, there was a clear dose-dependent increase in risk of hemorrhagic stroke with heavier alcohol use, with a 56–83% increase in risk even among consumers of 1–149 g/week. For ischemic stroke, the relationship was U-shaped, with lower risk among the lightest drinkers but 12% higher risk among the heaviest drinkers.

To date, there has not been extensive information available on whether beer differs from other alcoholic beverages in its association with hemorrhagic stroke. Klatsky and colleagues did not find evidence that beverage type was independently related to risk in their prospective cohort study, but this remains an important area of investigation, especially because of early evidence that homocysteine levels (which are beneficially lowered by beer) may be a risk factor for hemorrhagic stroke (Li *et al.*, 2003; Van Guelpen *et al.*, 2005).

Risk factors for stroke

Understanding the relationships of beer and alcohol intake with various risk factors for stroke may provide insight into the relatively complex set of associations observed in epidemiological studies. Four of the most prominent of these, based on their links to either stroke risk or beverage intake, are high-density lipoprotein cholesterol (for atherothrombotic stroke), atrial fibrillation (for embolic stroke), hypertension (for all types of ischemic stroke), and subclinical carotid atherosclerosis (for atherothrombotic stroke) (Table 63.2). We briefly review the effects of alcohol and beer on these risk factors – and how they are apt to influence ischemic stroke risk – below.

Atrial fibrillation

Atrial fibrillation is the most common chronic arrhythmia. It leads to ischemic stroke by disrupting the co-ordinated atrial contraction that characterizes atrial systole, leading to stasis and thrombus formation within the atrium. Risk of ischemic stroke is elevated as much as four- to fivefold among individuals with AF (Kannel *et al.*, 1998). Physicians have long recognized that binge drinking can trigger the onset of AF, sometimes termed the "holiday heart" syndrome (Greenspon and Schaal, 1983; Rich *et al.*, 1985). In a variety of observational studies, most analyses have suggested that only heavy drinking is clearly associated with higher risk (i.e. a threshold exists) (Rich *et al.*, 1985; Koskinen *et al.*, 1987; Ruigomez *et al.*, 2002; Djousse *et al.*, 2004; Mukamal *et al.*, 2005c). The largest such study to date suggested that AF risk does not increase until a chronic level of intake of at least 28 and probably 35 drinks per week (Mukamal *et al.*, 2005c). In this study, beer intake tended to be associated with higher risk only at the highest levels of intake, with a pattern similar to intake of spirits and to overall alcohol intake. Although other studies have suggested that risk may also be higher even among more moderate alcohol drinkers (Frost and Vestergaard, 2004), whether this reflects an effect of moderate drinking or occasional binge drinking among moderate drinkers is uncertain.

A related issue is whether alcohol can be consumed safely among adults with chronic AF, most of whom should be taking warfarin or similar anticoagulants. Although guidelines have often explicitly recommended that individuals taking

Table 63.2 Qualitative associations of alcohol and beer intake with ischemic stroke and four of its major risk factors

	Light–moderate alcohol intake	*Heavier alcohol intake*	*Evidence that beer and alcohol differ?*
Ischemic stroke	↑	↑↑	±
HDL-cholesterol	↑↑	↑↑	No
Atrial fibrillation	↔	↑↑	No
Blood pressure	↔	↑↑	No
Carotid atherosclerosis	↓	↑↑	No

Notes: Different amounts of beer and alcohol intake have varying effects on stroke and its major risk factors. Beer generally appears to be similar to other alcoholic beverages. Light–moderate drinking (less than 2 drinks daily for younger men, 1 drink daily for women and men over 65) often is linked to benefits in risk for ischemic stroke, good cholesterol (HDL), and atherosclerosis in the carotid arteries. Heavy drinking (3 drinks or more per day) is linked to detrimental effects on ischemic stroke risk and most of its risk factors.

warfarin abstain entirely (Weathermon and Crabb, 1999), the limited available data suggest that moderate drinkers do not have a higher risk of excessive anticoagulation than do abstainers, although binge drinkers may (Fihn *et al.*, 1993; Hylek *et al.*, 1998). In fact, in the Post CABG Trial, where participants were randomly assigned to low-dose warfarin or placebo following coronary artery bypass graft surgery, we found no evidence that alcohol intake adversely influenced average levels of the International Normalized Ratio (INR), a measure of anticoagulation, and the heaviest drinkers actually had the lowest risk of excessive INR values (Mukamal *et al.*, 2006).

Hypertension

Hypertension is, on a population basis, the most important risk factor for stroke. Almost 80% of individuals with a first stroke have hypertension (American Heart Association, 2007), and it increases the risk of both ischemic and hemorrhagic strokes. Approximately one in three US adults has hypertension, and it increases stroke risk as much as fourfold.

Somewhat similar to atrial fibrillation, alcohol intake has chiefly been associated with elevated blood pressure in a threshold manner, with higher risk predominately at levels of intake of 3 or more drinks per day or more (Klatsky, 1996). Lower levels of intake have even been associated with lower risk of hypertension in some cohort studies (Witteman *et al.*, 1990; Thadhani *et al.*, 2002), although this has not been universal (Trevisan *et al.*, 1987). The mechanism for the increase in blood pressure is uncertain, but a biphasic effect on blood pressure has been noted in experimental studies of alcohol administration (Abe *et al.*, 1994; Rosito *et al.*, 1999), with both higher and lower blood pressure noted depending on when measurement occurs. Randomized trials to lower blood pressure by encouraging reduction in alcohol intake have been encouraging (Puddey *et al.*, 1987, 1992), but the large PATHS trial found little effect of cognitive-behavioral alcohol reduction intervention program on blood pressure (Cushman *et al.*, 1998). Beer is not thought to differ from other alcoholic beverages in its effect on blood pressure (Stranges *et al.*, 2004).

A few cohort studies have addressed the effects of alcohol consumption among individuals with established hypertension. These have generally supported an inverse association with at least cardiovascular disease mortality (Palmer *et al.*, 1995; Malinski *et al.*, 2004), similar to that seen in the general population. How alcohol intake influences stroke risk among hypertensive individuals has not yet been conclusively studied.

High-density lipoprotein cholesterol

High-density lipoprotein cholesterol (HDL-C), commonly thought of as the "good cholesterol," is a key component of reverse cholesterol transport, the process of returning cholesterol to the liver for excretion in bile. HDL-C levels are strongly inversely associated with risks of both coronary heart disease and stroke (Boden, 2000; Sacco *et al.*, 2001).

Alcohol intake unequivocally increases levels of HDL-C. In a large meta-analysis of randomized trials of alcohol administration, there was a dose-dependent increase in HDL-C with greater alcohol intake, with a roughly 4 g/dl increase with consumption of 30 g/day (Rimm *et al.*, 1999). In observational studies, alcohol consumption is the lifestyle factor most closely correlated with HDL-C levels, with correlation coefficients of 0.2–0.4 in most studies (Giovannucci *et al.*, 1991; Ellison *et al.*, 2004). The effect may be non-linear at high doses of alcohol, where direct toxic effects of alcohol upon the liver may influence HDL production (Johansen *et al.*, 2003). Beer appears to have similar effects to other alcoholic beverages, based both on the similarity in its effect in the meta-analysis and based on a rigorous randomized trial that compared multiple alcoholic beverages using a Latin square design (Rimm *et al.*, 1999; van der Gaag *et al.*, 2001).

Carotid atherosclerosis

Unsurprisingly, atherosclerosis of the carotid arteries (typically measured by ultrasound) is a strong risk factor for stroke (O'Leary *et al.*, 1999; Lorenz *et al.*, 2006), presumably on the basis of its eventual role in vascular stenosis and occlusion and because it reflects atherosclerosis developing in other cerebral beds as well. In fact, it appears to predict stroke well even after accounting for traditional atherosclerotic risk factors (O'Leary *et al.*, 1999) and hence is particularly a key factor to evaluate in understanding the role of alcohol consumption in the occurrence of ischemic stroke.

A large number of studies have evaluated the cross-sectional or longitudinal association of alcohol intake with carotid intima-media thickness, a widely used measure of atherosclerosis in the common and internal carotid arteries (Demirovic *et al.*, 1993; Kiechl *et al.*, 1998; Kauhanen *et al.*, 1999; Bo *et al.*, 2001; Djousse *et al.*, 2002; Jerrard-Dunne *et al.*, 2003; Mukamal *et al.*, 2003; Zureik *et al.*, 2004; Schminke *et al.*, 2005). These have generally (Kiechl *et al.*, 1998; Bo *et al.*, 2001; Mukamal *et al.*, 2003), but clearly not universally (Demirovic *et al.*, 1993; Djousse *et al.*, 2002; Zureik *et al.*, 2004), yielded J-shaped associations, with the least atherosclerosis among light drinkers and the most among the heaviest drinkers, although it is often difficult to determine how well the associations with heavy drinking are controlled for the adverse lifestyle features of heavy drinkers. In those studies that have identified less carotid atherosclerosis among light drinkers, beer intake has generally been at least as strongly associated with lower intima-media thickness as other beverages (Figure 63.6) (Kiechl *et al.*, 1998; Mukamal *et al.*, 2003).

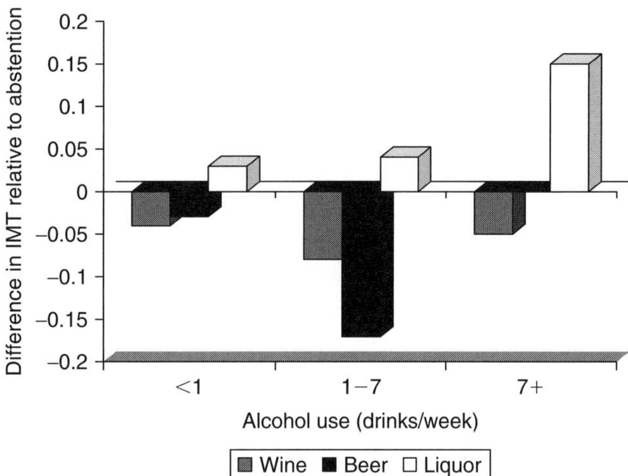

N = 4,247 older adults free of cardiovascular disease

Figure 63.6 The relationships of alcoholic beverage intake with carotid intima-media thickness among older adults who were free of cardiovascular disease in the Cardiovascular Health Study. Abstainers from each beverage were the reference category. The *y*-axis indicates differences in atherosclerosis of the carotid artery (based on intima-media thickness) associated with intake of wine (▩ bars), beer (■ bars), and liquor (□ bars), compared with abstention from each beverage. Beer intake at 1–7 drinks per week was associated with the greatest decrease in atherosclerosis.

Genetic vulnerability to alcohol-related stroke

There is currently limited information on the degree to which specific variation in specific genes influences the relationship of alcohol intake with risk of stroke. The few studies that have evaluated specific variants provide some intriguing insights into pathways by which alcohol use may influence risk of stroke, both positively and negatively.

An important influence on the metabolism of ethanol from beer and other alcoholic beverages is genetic variation in the alcohol dehydrogenase (ADH) set of genes, located on chromosome 4q. One of these genes, ADH1C, encodes a Class I ADH enzyme product that has a common functional variant in Caucasian populations. Although this variant appears to influence risk of coronary heart disease among consumers of ethanol (Hines *et al.*, 2001; Djousse *et al.*, 2005), a nested case-control study of the Physicians' Health Study cohort found no such interaction with risk of total or ischemic stroke (Zee *et al.*, 2004), even though moderate alcohol intake was associated with a lower risk of stroke in this cohort (Berger *et al.*, 1999).

A gene of increasing interest for studies of alcohol use and chronic disease is apoE. The apoE lipoprotein is a key component of HDL particles and has a strong link to Alzheimer's disease. The carriers of the apoE4 allele of this gene appear to have an attenuated response to alcohol intake in their levels of HDL-C (Djousse *et al.*, 2002) and inflammatory markers (Mukamal *et al.*, 2004). Most importantly, we found that this gene appears to modify the association of alcohol use with risk of ischemic stroke in the Cardiovascular Health Study (Mukamal *et al.*, 2005b). Among apoE4-negative participants, there was a typical U-shaped relationship, with lower risk among consumers of 1–6 drinks per week and similar risk among abstainers and the heaviest drinkers. In contrast, among apoE4 carriers, no level of intake was associated with lower risk, and consumers of 7 or more drinks per week had a significant twofold increase in risk relative to abstainers.

Finally, a gene–alcohol interaction has been noted in the Carotid Atherosclerosis Progression Study, where a variant in the interleukin-6 gene appears to modify the association of alcohol use with carotid atherosclerosis and interleukin-6 levels (Jerrard-Dunne *et al.*, 2003). This variant, located in the promoter, has been associated with interleukin-6 levels itself (Jenny *et al.*, 2002). In this study, alcohol intake had J-shaped relationships with both interleukin-6 levels and with carotid intima-media thickness, and the relationship with atherosclerosis was quite consistent across genotypes through intake of 30 g/day. Above this level, however, CC homozygotes had increased intima-media thickness relative to abstainers, while GG homozygotes had decreased thickness. Given the key role of interleukin-6 in systemic inflammation, this finding implicates inflammation as yet another potential mechanism by which alcohol may influence ischemic stroke risk.

The caffeinol hypothesis

A particularly novel application of alcohol to ischemic stroke in an entirely different context has been proposed by Aronowski and colleagues (Strong *et al.*, 2000; Aronowski *et al.*, 2003; Piriyawat *et al.*, 2003). Drawing on the concept of ischemic neuroprotection, in which neuronal death can be averted even after a transient ischemic insult by administration of neuroprotective agents, this group developed and tested a novel combination of caffeine and ethanol dubbed "caffeinol." Neither ethanol nor caffeine alone induced neuroprotection (Strong *et al.*, 2000). However, caffeinol at a dose of only 0.2 mg/kg of ethanol consistently reduced the volume of infarcted cerebral cortex when administered after occlusion of the common carotid and middle cerebral arteries. Daily ethanol administration prior to the ischemic insult produced tolerance to this neuroprotective effect (Aronowski *et al.*, 2003). A second group has confirmed this finding of neuroprotection (Belayev *et al.*, 2004), but a third group using a rabbit model found that it increased the incidence of intracerebral hemorrhage associated with administration of thrombolytic therapy (Lapchak *et al.*, 2004). Pilot studies to evaluate this combination in the treatment of acute stroke patients are underway, although early experience suggests that considerable vigilance may be necessary to maintain blood levels of ethanol in a relatively narrow therapeutic window (Piriyawat *et al.*, 2003).

Conclusions

In summary, there are complex relationships of alcohol use with different types of stroke, in part reflecting their heterogeneity. To date, evidence generally suggests a J-shaped relationship of alcohol use with ischemic stroke, with lower risk limited to consumers of approximately 1 drink every other day and clearly higher risk among consumers of 3 or more drinks per day, an association quite different from that seen for coronary heart disease. The risk of hemorrhagic stroke appears to rise in a graded fashion with greater alcohol intake. Beer intake seems to mirror the overall associations of alcohol use with these outcomes. The risks of hypertension and atrial fibrillation, two key risk factors for ischemic stroke, seem to be related primarily to alcohol use of 3 drinks per day or higher, while beer and other alcoholic beverages raise levels of HDL-C even at moderate doses. Ongoing work is needed to identify how particular genetic variants may modify these associations, and whether alcohol can also be harnessed as a neuroprotective agent to modify the potentially devastating outcomes of ischemic stroke.

Summary Points

- Alcohol intake of approximately 1 drink every other day is associated with a roughly 20% lower risk of ischemic stroke than abstention.
- Regular intake of 3 drinks per day or more increases risk of ischemic stroke by at least 45–50%, and binge drinking also acutely increases stroke risk.
- Beer appears to be similar to other alcoholic beverages in these associations.
- Alcohol intake increases risk of hemorrhagic stroke in a dose-dependent manner.
- Beer and alcohol intake increase risk of atrial fibrillation, a key stroke risk factor, but only at high levels of chronic consumption.
- Beer and alcohol intake increase risk of high blood pressure at levels of 3 drinks per day or more.
- Beer and alcohol intake increase levels of HDL-C, which may lower risk of ischemic stroke.
- The apoE4 allele, which increases risk of Alzheimer's disease, may also blunt the benefits and increase the risks of alcohol consumption.
- Alcohol combined with caffeine is currently being tested as a protective agent among patients who sustain acute ischemic strokes; in animals, this combination reduces stroke severity considerably.

Acknowledgments

I have no competing interests to disclose. My research to date has been funded entirely by the National Institutes of Health and the American Heart Association.

References

Abe, H., Kawano, Y., Kojima, S., Ashida, T., Kuramochi, M., Matsuoka, H. and Omae, T. (1994). Biphasic effects of repeated alcohol intake on 24-hour blood pressure in hypertensive patients. *Circulation* 89, 2626–2633.

American Heart Association (2007). *Heart Disease and Stroke Statistics – 2007 Update*, American Heart Association, Dallas, TX.

Ariesen, M.J., Claus, S.P., Rinkel, G.J. and Algra, A. (2003). Risk factors for intracerebral hemorrhage in the general population: a systematic review. *Stroke* 34, 2060–2065.

Aronowski, J., Strong, R., Shirzadi, A. and Grotta, J.C. (2003). Ethanol plus caffeine (caffeinol) for treatment of ischemic stroke: preclinical experience. *Stroke* 34, 1246–1251.

Belayev, L., Khoutorova, L., Zhang, Y., Belayev, A., Zhao, W., Busto, R. and Ginsberg, M.D. (2004). Caffeinol confers cortical but not subcortical neuroprotection after transient focal cerebral ischemia in rats. *Brain Res.* 1008, 278–283.

Berger, K., Ajani, U.A., Kase, C.S., Gaziano, J.M., Buring, J.E., Glynn, R.J. and Hennekens, C.H. (1999). Light-to-moderate alcohol consumption and risk of stroke among U.S. male physicians. *New Engl. J. Med.* 341, 1557–1564.

Bo, P., Marchioni, E., Bosone, D., Soragna, D., Albergati, A., Micieli, G., Trotti, R. and Savoldi, F. (2001). Effects of moderate and high doses of alcohol on carotid atherogenesis. *Eur. Neurol.* 45, 97–103.

Boden, W.E. (2000). High-density lipoprotein cholesterol as an independent risk factor in cardiovascular disease: assessing the data from Framingham to the Veterans Affairs High-Density Lipoprotein Intervention Trial. *Am. J. Cardiol.* 86, 19L–22L.

Bryson, C.L., Mukamal, K.J., Mittleman, M.A., Fried, L.P., Hirsch, C.H., Kitzman, D.W. and Siscovick, D.S. (2006). The association of alcohol consumption and incident heart failure: the Cardiovascular Health Study. *J. Am. Coll. Cardiol.* 48, 305–311.

Camargo Jr., C.A. (1989). Moderate alcohol consumption and stroke. The epidemiologic evidence. *Stroke* 20, 1611–1626.

Camargo Jr., C.A. (1996). Case-control and cohort studies of moderate alcohol consumption and stroke. *Clin. Chim. Acta.* 246, 107–119.

Cleophas, T.J. (1999). Wine, beer and spirits and the risk of myocardial infarction: a systematic review. *Biomed. Pharmacother.* 53, 417–423.

Corrao, G., Rubbiati, L., Bagnardi, V., Zambon, A. and Poikolainen, K. (2000). Alcohol and coronary heart disease: a meta-analysis. *Addiction* 95, 1505–1523.

Cushman, W.C., Cutler, J.A., Hanna, E., Bingham, S.E., Follmann, D., Harford, T., Dubbert, P., Allender, P.S., Dufour, M., Collins, J.F., Walsh, S.M., Kirk, G.F., Burg, M., Felicetta, J.V., Hamilton, B.P., Katz, L.A., Perry, H.M., Willenberg, M.L., Lakshman, R. and Hamburger, R.J. (1998). Prevention and Treatment of Hypertension Study (PATHS) – Effects of an alcohol treatment program on blood pressure. *Arch. Intern. Med.* 158, 1197–1207.

Demirovic, J., Nabulsi, A., Folsom, A.R., Carpenter, M.A., Szklo, M., Sorlie, P.D. and Barnes, R.W. (1993). Alcohol consumption and ultrasonographically assessed carotid artery wall thickness and distensibility. The Atherosclerosis Risk in Communities (ARIC) Study Investigators. *Circulation* 88, 2787–2793.

Di Castelnuovo, A., Rotondo, S., Iacoviello, L., Donati, M.B. and De Gaetano, G. (2002). Meta-analysis of wine and beer consumption in relation to vascular risk. *Circulation* 105, 2836–2844.

Djousse, L., Levy, D., Murabito, J.M., Cupples, L.A. and Ellison, R.C. (2000). Alcohol consumption and risk of intermittent claudication in the Framingham Heart Study. *Circulation* 102, 3092–3097.

Djousse, L., Myers, R.H., Province, M.A., Hunt, S.C., Eckfeldt, J.H., Evans, G., Peacock, J.M. and Ellison, R.C. (2002). Influence of apolipoprotein E, smoking, and alcohol intake on carotid atherosclerosis: National Heart, Lung, and Blood Institute Family Heart Study. *Stroke* 33, 1357–1361.

Djousse, L., Levy, D., Benjamin, E.J., Blease, S.J., Russ, A., Larson, M.G., Massaro, J.M., D'Agostino, R.B., Wolf, P.A. and Ellison, R.C. (2004). Long-term alcohol consumption and the risk of atrial fibrillation in the Framingham Study. *Am. J. Cardiol.* 93, 710–713.

Djousse, L., Levy, D., Herbert, A.G., Wilson, P.W., D'Agostino, R.B., Cupples, L.A., Karamohamed, S. and Ellison, R.C. (2005). Influence of alcohol dehydrogenase 1C polymorphism on the alcohol–cardiovascular disease association (from the Framingham Offspring Study). *Am. J. Cardiol.* 96, 227–232.

Dulli, D.A. (2002). Alcohol, ischemic stroke, and lessons from a negative study. *Stroke* 33, 890–891.

Ellison, R.C., Zhang, Y., Qureshi, M.M., Knox, S., Arnett, D.K. and Province, M.A. (2004). Lifestyle determinants of high-density lipoprotein cholesterol: the National Heart, Lung, and Blood Institute Family Heart Study. *Am. Heart J.* 147, 529–535.

Feigin, V.L., Rinkel, G.J., Lawes, C.M., Algra, A., Bennett, D.A., Van Gijn, J. and Anderson, C.S. (2005). Risk factors for subarachnoid hemorrhage: an updated systematic review of epidemiological studies. *Stroke* 36, 2773–2780.

Fihn, S.D., McDonell, M., Martin, D., Henikoff, J., Vermes, D., Kent, D. and White, R.H. (1993). Risk factors for complications of chronic anticoagulation. A multicenter study. Warfarin Optimized Outpatient Follow-up Study Group. *Ann. Intern. Med.* 118, 511–520.

Frost, L. and Vestergaard, P. (2004). Alcohol and risk of atrial fibrillation or flutter: a cohort study. *Arch. Intern. Med.* 164, 1993–1998.

Gill, J.S., Shipley, M.J., Tsementzis, S.A., Hornby, R.S., Gill, S.K., Hitchcock, E.R. and Beevers, D.G. (1991). Alcohol consumption – a risk factor for hemorrhagic and non-hemorrhagic stroke. *Am. J. Med.* 90, 489–497.

Giovannucci, E., Colditz, G., Stampfer, M.J., Rimm, E.B., Litin, L., Sampson, L. and Willett, W.C. (1991). The assessment of alcohol consumption by a simple self-administered questionnaire. *Am. J. Epidemiol.* 133, 810–817.

Greenspon, A.J. and Schaal, S.F. (1983). The "holiday heart": electrophysiologic studies of alcohol effects in alcoholics. *Ann. Intern. Med.* 98, 135–139.

Hillbom, M. and Kaste, M. (1978). Does ethanol intoxication promote brain infarction in young adults? *Lancet* 2, 1181–1183.

Hillbom, M. and Kaste, M. (1981). Ethanol intoxication: a risk factor for ischemic brain infarction in adolescents and young adults. *Stroke* 12, 422–425.

Hillbom, M. and Kaste, M. (1983). Ethanol intoxication: a risk factor for ischemic brain infarction. *Stroke* 14, 694–699.

Hillbom, M., Haapaniemi, H., Juvela, S., Palomaki, H., Numminen, H. and Kaste, M. (1995). Recent alcohol consumption, cigarette smoking, and cerebral infarction in young adults. *Stroke* 26, 40–45.

Hillbom, M., Numminen, H. and Juvela, S. (1999). Recent heavy drinking of alcohol and embolic stroke. *Stroke* 30, 2307–2312.

Hines, L.M., Stampfer, M.J., Ma, J., Gaziano, J.M., Ridker, P.M., Hankinson, S.E., Sacks, F., Rimm, E.B. and Hunter, D.J. (2001). Genetic variation in alcohol dehydrogenase and the beneficial effect of moderate alcohol consumption on myocardial infarction. *New Engl. J. Med.* 344, 549–555.

Hylek, E.M., Heiman, H., Skates, S.J., Sheehan, M.A. and Singer, D.E. (1998). Acetaminophen and other risk factors for excessive warfarin anticoagulation. *JAMA* 279, 657–662.

Iso, H., Baba, S., Mannami, T., Sasaki, S., Okada, K., Konishi, M. and Tsugane, S. (2004). Alcohol consumption and risk of stroke among middle-aged men: the JPHC Study Cohort I. *Stroke* 35, 1124–1129.

Jenny, N.S., Tracy, R.P., Ogg, M.S., Luong Le, A., Kuller, L.H., Arnold, A.M., Sharrett, A.R. and Humphries, S.E. (2002). In the elderly, interleukin-6 plasma levels and the -174G>C polymorphism are associated with the development of cardiovascular disease. *Arterioscler. Thromb. Vasc. Biol.* 22, 2066–2071.

Jerrard-Dunne, P., Sitzer, M., Risley, P., Steckel, D.A., Buehler, A., Von Kegler, S. and Markus, H.S. (2003). Interleukin-6 promoter polymorphism modulates the effects of heavy alcohol consumption on early carotid artery atherosclerosis: the Carotid Atherosclerosis Progression Study (CAPS). *Stroke* 34, 402–407.

Johansen, D., Andersen, P.K., Jensen, M.K., Schnohr, P. and Gronbaek, M. (2003). Nonlinear relation between alcohol intake and high-density lipoprotein cholesterol level: results from the Copenhagen City Heart Study. *Alcohol Clin. Exp. Res.* 27, 1305–1309.

Johansen, D., Friis, K., Skovenborg, E. and Gronbaek, M. (2006). Food buying habits of people who buy wine or beer: cross sectional study. *BMJ* 332, 519–522.

Kannel, W.B., Wolf, P.A., Benjamin, E.J. and Levy, D. (1998). Prevalence, incidence, prognosis, and predisposing conditions for atrial fibrillation: population-based estimates. *Am. J. Cardiol.* 82, 2N–9N.

Kaufman, D.W., Kelly, J.P., Wiholm, B.E., Laszlo, A., Sheehan, J. E., Koff, R.S. and Shapiro, S. (1999). The risk of acute major upper gastrointestinal bleeding among users of aspirin and ibuprofen at various levels of alcohol consumption. *Am. J. Gastroenterol.* 94, 3189–3196.

Kauhanen, J., Kaplan, G.A., Goldberg, D.E., Salonen, R. and Salonen, J.T. (1999). Pattern of alcohol drinking and progression of atherosclerosis. *Arterioscler. Thromb. Vasc. Biol.* 19, 3001–3006.

Kiechl, S., Willeit, J., Rungger, G., Egger, G., Oberhollenzer, F. and Bonora, E. (1998). Alcohol consumption and atherosclerosis: what is the relation? Prospective results from the Bruneck Study. *Stroke* 29, 900–907.

Klatsky, A.L. (1996). Alcohol and hypertension. *Clin. Chim. Acta.* 246, 91–105.

Klatsky, A.L. (2005). Alcohol and stroke: an epidemiological labyrinth. *Stroke* 36, 1835–1836.

Klatsky, A.L., Armstrong, M.A. and Friedman, G.D. (1997). Red wine, white wine, liquor, beer, and risk for coronary artery disease hospitalization. *Am. J. Cardiol.* 80, 416–420.

Klatsky, A.L., Armstrong, M.A., Friedman, G.D. and Sidney, S. (2001). Alcohol drinking and risk of hospitalization for ischemic stroke. *Am. J. Cardiol.* 88, 703–706.

Klatsky, A.L., Armstrong, M.A., Friedman, G.D. and Sidney, S. (2002). Alcohol drinking and risk of hemorrhagic stroke. *Neuroepidemiology* 21, 115–122.

Koskinen, P., Kupari, M., Leinonen, H. and Luomanmaki, K. (1987). Alcohol and new onset atrial fibrillation: a case-control study of a current series. *Br. Heart J.* 57, 468–473.

Lapchak, P.A., Song, D., Wei, J. and Zivin, J.A. (2004). Pharmacology of caffeinol in embolized rabbits: clinical rating scores and intracerebral hemorrhage incidence. *Exp. Neurol.* 188, 286–291.

Li, Z., Sun, L., Zhang, H., Liao, Y., Wang, D., Zhao, B., Zhu, Z., Zhao, J., Ma, A., Han, Y., Wang, Y., Shi, Y., Ye, J. and Hui, R. (2003). Elevated plasma homocysteine was associated with hemorrhagic and ischemic stroke, but methylenetetrahydrofolate reductase gene C677T polymorphism was a risk factor for thrombotic stroke: a Multicenter Case-Control Study in China. *Stroke* 34, 2085–2090.

Lorenz, M.W., Von Kegler, S., Steinmetz, H., Markus, H.S. and Sitzer, M. (2006). Carotid intima-media thickening indicates a higher vascular risk across a wide age range: prospective data from the Carotid Atherosclerosis Progression Study (CAPS). *Stroke* 37, 87–92.

Maclure, M. (1993). Demonstration of deductive meta-analysis: ethanol intake and risk of myocardial infarction. *Epidemiol. Rev.* 15, 328–351.

Malinski, M.K., Sesso, H.D., Lopez-Jimenez, F., Buring, J.E. and Gaziano, J.M. (2004). Alcohol consumption and cardiovascular disease mortality in hypertensive men. *Arch. Intern. Med.* 164, 623–628.

Manolio, T.A., Kronmal, R.A., Burke, G.L., O'Leary, D.H. and Price, T.R. (1996). Short-term predictors of incident stroke in older adults. The Cardiovascular Health Study. *Stroke* 27, 1479–1486.

Mukamal, K.J., Longstreth Jr., W.T., Mittleman, M.A., Crum, R.M. and Siscovick, D.S. (2001). Alcohol consumption and subclinical findings on magnetic resonance imaging of the brain in older adults: the cardiovascular health study. *Stroke* 32, 1939–1946.

Mukamal, K.J., Kronmal, R.A., Mittleman, M.A., O'Leary, D.H., Polak, J.F., Cushman, M. and Siscovick, D.S. (2003). Alcohol consumption and carotid atherosclerosis in older adults: the Cardiovascular Health Study. *Arterioscler. Thromb. Vasc. Biol.* 23, 2252–2259.

Mukamal, K.J., Cushman, M., Mittleman, M.A., Tracy, R.P. and Siscovick, D.S. (2004). Alcohol consumption and inflammatory markers in older adults: the Cardiovascular Health Study. *Atherosclerosis* 173, 79–87.

Mukamal, K.J., Ascherio, A., Mittleman, M.A., Conigrave, K.M., Camargo Jr., C.A., Kawachi, I., Stampfer, M.J., Willett, W.C. and Rimm, E.B. (2005a). Alcohol and risk for ischemic stroke in men: the role of drinking patterns and usual beverage. *Ann. Intern. Med.* 142, 11–19.

Mukamal, K.J., Chung, H., Jenny, N.S., Kuller, L.H., Longstreth Jr., W.T., Mittleman, M.A., Burke, G.L., Cushman, M., Beauchamp Jr., N.J. and Siscovick, D.S. (2005b). Alcohol use and risk of ischemic stroke among older adults: the cardiovascular health study. *Stroke* 36, 1830–1834.

Mukamal, K.J., Tolstrup, J.S., Friberg, J., Jensen, G. and Gronbaek, M. (2005c). Alcohol consumption and risk of atrial fibrillation in men and women: the Copenhagen City Heart Study. *Circulation* 112, 1736–1742.

Mukamal, K.J., Smith, C.C., Karlamangla, A.S. and Moore, A.A. (2006). Moderate alcohol consumption and safety of lovastatin and warfarin among men: the post-coronary artery bypass graft trial. *Am. J. Med.* 119, 434–440.

Naimi, T.S., Brewer, R.D., Mokdad, A., Denny, C., Serdula, M.K. and Marks, J.S. (2003). Binge drinking among US adults. *JAMA* 289, 70–75.

O'Leary, D.H., Polak, J.F., Kronmal, R.A., Manolio, T.A., Burke, G.L. and Wolfson Jr., J.S. (1999). Carotid-artery intima and media thickness as a risk factor for myocardial infarction and stroke in older adults. Cardiovascular Health Study Collaborative Research Group. *New Engl. J. Med.* 340, 14–22.

Palmer, A.J., Fletcher, A.E., Bulpitt, C.J., Beevers, D.G., Coles, E.C., Ledingham, J.G., Petrie, J.C., Webster, J. and Dollery, C.T. (1995). Alcohol intake and cardiovascular mortality in hypertensive patients: report from the Department of Health Hypertension Care Computing Project. *J. Hypertens.* 13, 957–964.

Piriyawat, P., Labiche, L.A., Burgin, W.S., Aronowski, J.A. and Grotta, J.C. (2003). Pilot dose-escalation study of caffeine plus ethanol (caffeinol) in acute ischemic stroke. *Stroke* 34, 1242–1245.

Puddey, I.B., Beilin, L.J. and Vandongen, R. (1987). Regular alcohol use raises blood pressure in treated hypertensive subjects. A randomised controlled trial. *Lancet* 1, 647–651.

Puddey, I.B., Parker, M., Beilin, L.J., Vandongen, R. and Masarei, J.R. (1992). Effects of alcohol and caloric restrictions on blood pressure and serum lipids in overweight men. *Hypertension* 20, 533–541.

Renaud, S. and De Lorgeril, M. (1992). Wine, alcohol, platelets, and the French paradox for coronary heart disease. *Lancet* 339, 1523–1526.

Reynolds, K., Lewis, B., Nolen, J.D., Kinney, G.L., Sathya, B. and He, J. (2003). Alcohol consumption and risk of stroke: a meta-analysis. *JAMA* 289, 579–588.

Rich, E.C., Siebold, C. and Campion, B. (1985). Alcohol-related acute atrial fibrillation. A case-control study and review of 40 patients. *Arch. Intern. Med.* 145, 830–833.

Rimm, E.B., Klatsky, A., Grobbee, D. and Stampfer, M.J. (1996). Review of moderate alcohol consumption and reduced risk of coronary heart disease: is the effect due to beer, wine, or spirits. *BMJ* 312, 731–736.

Rimm, E.B., Williams, P., Fosher, K., Criqui, M. and Stampfer, M.J. (1999). Moderate alcohol intake and lower risk of coronary heart disease: meta-analysis of effects on lipids and haemostatic factors. *BMJ* 319, 1523–1528.

Rosito, G.A., Fuchs, F.D. and Duncan, B.B. (1999). Dose-dependent biphasic effect of ethanol on 24-h blood pressure in normotensive subjects. *Am. J. Hypertens.* 12, 236–240.

Ruigomez, A., Johansson, S., Wallander, M.A. and Rodriguez, L.A. (2002). Incidence of chronic atrial fibrillation in general practice and its treatment pattern. *J. Clin. Epidemiol.* 55, 358–363.

Sacco, R.L., Benson, R.T., Kargman, D.E., Boden-Albala, B., Tuck, C., Lin, I.F., Cheng, J.F., Paik, M.C., Shea, S. and Berglund, L. (2001). High-density lipoprotein cholesterol and ischemic stroke in the elderly: the Northern Manhattan Stroke Study. *JAMA* 285, 2729–2735.

Schminke, U., Luedemann, J., Berger, K., Alte, D., Mitusch, R., Wood, W.G., Jaschinski, A., Barnow, S., John, U. and Kessler, C. (2005). Association between alcohol consumption and subclinical carotid atherosclerosis: the Study of Health in Pomerania. *Stroke* 36, 1746–1752.

Stampfer, M.J., Colditz, G.A., Willett, W.C., Speizer, F.E. and Hennekens, C.H. (1988). A prospective study of moderate alcohol consumption and the risk of coronary disease and stroke in women. *New Engl. J. Med.* 319, 267–273.

Stranges, S., Wu, T., Dorn, J.M., Freudenheim, J.L., Muti, P., Farinaro, E., Russell, M., Nochajski, T.H. and Trevisan, M. (2004). Relationship of alcohol drinking pattern to risk of hypertension: a population-based study. *Hypertension* 44, 813–819.

Strong, R., Grotta, J.C. and Aronowski, J. (2000). Combination of low dose ethanol and caffeine protects brain from damage produced by focal ischemia in rats. *Neuropharmacology* 39, 515–522.

Thadhani, R., Camargo Jr., C.A., Stampfer, M.J., Curhan, G.C., Willett, W.C. and Rimm, E.B. (2002). Prospective study of moderate alcohol consumption and risk of hypertension in young women. *Arch. Intern. Med.* 162, 569–574.

Tjonneland, A., Gronbaek, M., Stripp, C. and Overvad, K. (1999). Wine intake and diet in a random sample of 48763 Danish men and women. *Am. J. Clin. Nutr.* 69, 49–54.

Trevisan, M., Krogh, V., Farinaro, E., Panico, S. and Mancini, M. (1987). Alcohol consumption, drinking pattern and blood pressure: analysis of data from the Italian National Research Council Study. *Int. J. Epidemiol.* 16, 520–527.

Truelsen, T., Gronbaek, M., Schnohr, P. and Boysen, G. (1998). Intake of beer, wine, and spirits and risk of stroke: the Copenhagen City Heart Study. *Stroke* 29, 2467–2472.

Van Der Gaag, M.S., Van Tol, A., Vermunt, S.H., Scheek, L.M., Schaafsma, G. and Hendriks, H.F. (2001). Alcohol consumption stimulates early steps in reverse cholesterol transport. *J. Lipid Res.* 42, 2077–2083.

Van Guelpen, B., Hultdin, J., Johansson, I., Stegmayr, B., Hallmans, G., Nilsson, T.K., Weinehall, L., Witthoft, C., Palmqvist, R. and Winkvist, A. (2005). Folate, vitamin B12, and risk of ischemic and hemorrhagic stroke: a prospective, nested case-referent study of plasma concentrations and dietary intake. *Stroke* 36, 1426–1431.

Waddington, E., Puddey, I.B. and Croft, K.D. (2004). Red wine polyphenolic compounds inhibit atherosclerosis in apolipoprotein E-deficient mice independently of effects on lipid peroxidation. *Am. J. Clin. Nutr.* 79, 54–61.

Walsh, C.R., Larson, M.G., Evans, J.C., Djousse, L., Ellison, R. C., Vasan, R.S. and Levy, D. (2002). Alcohol consumption and risk for congestive heart failure in the Framingham Heart Study. *Ann. Intern. Med.* 136, 181–191.

Weathermon, R. and Crabb, D.W. (1999). Alcohol and medication interactions. *Alcohol Res. Health* 23, 40–54.

Witteman, J.C., Willett, W.C., Stampfer, M.J., Colditz, G.A., Kok, F.J., Sacks, F.M., Speizer, F.E., Rosner, B. and Hennekens, C.H. (1990). Relation of moderate alcohol consumption and risk of systemic hypertension in women. *Am. J. Cardiol.* 65, 633–637.

Zee, R.Y., Ridker, P.M. and Cook, N.R. (2004). Prospective evaluation of the alcohol dehydrogenase gamma1/gamma2 gene polymorphism and risk of stroke. *Stroke* 35, e39–e42.

Zureik, M., Gariepy, J., Courbon, D., Dartigues, J.F., Ritchie, K., Tzourio, C., Alperovitch, A., Simon, A. and Ducimetiere, P. (2004). Alcohol consumption and carotid artery structure in older French adults: the Three-City Study. *Stroke* 35, 2770–2775.

64

Beer: Is It Alcohol, Antioxidants, or Both? Animal Models of Atherosclerosis

Joe A. Vinson Department of Chemistry, Loyola Hall, University of Scranton, Scranton, PA, USA

Abstract

Beer is the most consumed alcoholic beverage in the world and also historically the oldest. There are several possible active ingredients, especially alcohol which has been amply demonstrated by epidemiological studies. In addition the polyphenol antioxidants may be bioactive. Beer contains moderate amounts of these antioxidants but the large per capita consumption of beer makes it a substantial contributor to beverage antioxidants. In the United States it ranks third and ahead of wine which is in fourth place. Ethanol may be an antioxidant depending on the model. The polyphenols are always antioxidants and are active at sub-micromolar levels in an *in vitro* model of atherosclerosis, the oxidation of lower-density lipoproteins. Beer polyphenols also bind to these proteins potentially protecting them from *in vivo* oxidation and slowing down the atherosclerosis process. Short-term animal studies have shown that beer without alcohol is indeed an *in vivo* antioxidant and that beer is equally as protective as red wine. Beer countered the oxidative stress of alcohol and was an antioxidant in several rat models. Animal atherosclerosis studies with beer gave mixed results. In a hamster model at equal dilution of red wine and beer, beer proved to be an equivalent inhibitor of atherosclerosis by hypocholesterolemic and/or antioxidant mechanisms. Lager beer at a human-equivalent dose in this model was a significant anti-atherosclerotic agent. In a genetic mouse model with a lipid profile similar to humans, beer without alcohol was an effective anti-atherosclerotic agent but beer combined with alcohol was more effective. Both types of beer influenced protein expression that could beneficially impact atherosclerosis. Alcohol enhances the protective effect of beer in this model. Long-term human studies are needed to compare beer with and without alcohol and thus determine the bioactive ingredient(s).

List of Abbreviations

HDL	High-density lipoprotein
LDL	Low-density lipoprotein
VLDL	Very low-density lipoprotein
HPLC	High-performance liquid chromatography
CVD	Cardiovascular disease
AAPH	2,2′-Azobis(2-amidinopropane)
SR-B1	Scavenger receptor-B1
LRP	LDL receptor-related protein
LCAT	Lecithin–cholesterol acyltransferase
ABCA1	ATP-binding cassette transporter A1
SREBP2	Sterol-regulatory element binding protein 2

Introduction

Beer is man's oldest fermented beverage made from malt and hops and produced in the Mesopotamia region around 4000 BC (Kondo, 2004) and is the most popular alcoholic beverage in the world today. In the United States beer is the most consumed alcoholic beverage (224 ml/day) and is far ahead of wine (24 ml/day) and distilled spirits (15 ml/day). This is 2004 availability data, not strictly consumption, from the US government (Economic Research Service, 2005). In most laymen's opinion, wine, especially red wine, would be considered the healthiest alcoholic beverage to consume because of the French paradox. This same view would be taken by many medical doctors and scientists. There have been several systematic reviews in the last 10 years comparing beer, wine, and spirits with respect to cardiovascular disease (CVD) with differing results. For instance Di Castelnuovo *et al.* (2002) found a stronger inverse association with wine (32% reduction) compared to beer (22%). An older review gave the same high marks for both beer and wine whose benefits were equal (Rimm *et al.*, 1996). The most recent meta-analysis of men with follow-up since 1986 found moderate alcohol consumption of either beer, wine, or spirits equally reduced risk of CVD (Mukamal *et al.*, 2006). However, all of these epidemiological studies are subject to confounding variables such as lifestyle which is typically healthier for wine drinkers as opposed to those who drink beer. The human trials

Beer in Health and Disease Prevention
ISBN: 978-0-12-373891-2

are flawed as they are short-term studies (usually last only 4 weeks) and typically use young subjects (20–40 years) and have not provided conclusive evidence to the question of which alcoholic beverage, wine or beer, is better for the heart (Rimm *et al.*, 2002) and whether alcohol is a necessary ingredient for CVD protection.

This review will include some information about the ethanol and the antioxidants in wine and beer and their relative antioxidant effectiveness. The oxidative theory of atherosclerosis will be explored and the *in vitro* and *ex vivo* experimental data relating beer and wine will be discussed. We have attempted to separate the antioxidants of beer from the alcohol in beer in this chapter. It will also cover animal studies which have involved beer and especially those which have compared wine and beer.

In Vitro Antioxidants

Polyphenol antioxidants in fruits, vegetables, and whole grains may well be the active ingredients responsible for the CV benefits of these foods and the beverages made from them including beer and wine. These compounds may act as antioxidants *in vivo* but also have the possibility of being cardio-protective by other mechanisms (Manach *et al.*, 2005a, b) such as endothelial function and hemostasis. The oxidative theory of atherosclerosis, first promulgated by Steinberg (1989), indicates the possible effectiveness of antioxidants for protection of the heart. Low density lipoprotein (LDL) oxidation in the sub-endothelial space is the initiating event of atherosclerosis. This theory has come under attack with the failure of tocopherol (vitamin E) in human supplementation trials to affect atherosclerosis and thus heart disease risk as reviewed by Bleys *et al.* (2006). It is our contention that antioxidants work best, not as isolated compounds consumed alone, but in the complete milieu of the food or beverage matrix containing a potpourri of nutrients and antioxidants.

Beer, like any plant-derived material, contains hundreds of compounds. Phenolic constituents of beer are derived from malt (70–80%) and hops (20–30%). Structural classes include simple phenols, benzoic and cinnamic acid derivatives, coumarins, catechins, di-, tri- and oligomeric proanthocyanidins (prenylated) chalcones, and flavonoids. One indication of this complexity is a recent high performance liquid chromatography (HPLC) examination of a freeze dried Israeli beer as shown in Table 64.1 (Jastrzebski *et al.*, 2007) indicated a total of over 9 mg/g of phenols yet only about 5 mg/g were identified. A more complete HPLC examination with electrochemical detection identified 27 phenolic compounds in beer (Jandera *et al.*, 2005). Phenolic acids make up the bulk of the individual compounds and these are the ones found as the metabolites (glucuronides and sulfates) after human consumption (Nardini *et al.*, 2006).

It is our hypothesis that alcoholic beverages that contain significant antioxidants should be more beneficial than those that have substantially less. For instance distilled spirits are very low in polyphenols. Red wine is substantially higher in these compounds than beer. We have compared wine and beer for free phenolic antioxidants. Next we examined consumption data. Using our Folin colorimetric assay, we averaged the results for red and white wines 3397 μM (Vinson, 1998) since market research indicates about equal preference (Tordsen *et al.*, 2004). We used the government data for consumption (Economic Research Service, 2005) and assumed consumption of lager beer which averaged 677 μM polyphenols. Porter beers have almost three times more polyphenols than lager beers and the difference is significant, $p < 0.001$. Beer provides 42 mg of catechin equivalents/day while wine has 24 mg per capita. Thus in spite of beer having considerably less antioxidant content than wine, it still was the number one source of antioxidants from alcoholic beverages in the US diet.

Table 64.1 Free polyphenols in an Israeli beer

Components	*Concentration (mg/g)*
Epicatechin	1.77
Quercetin	0.03
p-Coumaric acid	0.06
Gallic acid	0.08
Ferulic acid	0.18
Procyanidins	1.68
Flavonoids	1.40
Total polyphenols	9.33

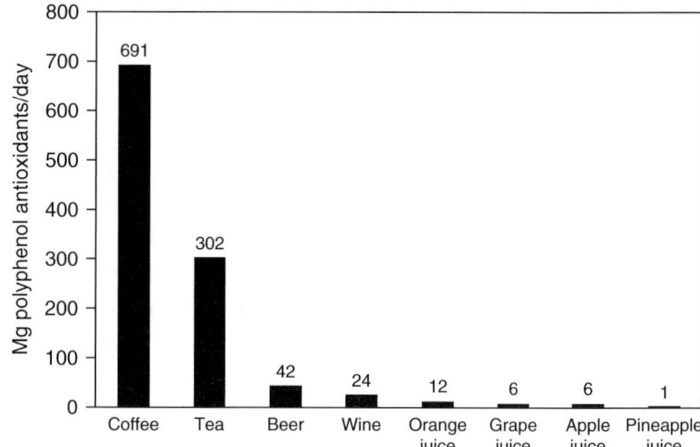

Figure 64.1 Per capita contribution of polyphenol antioxidants from commonly consumed beverages in the United States in 2004.

However, to put beer's contribution in perspective, we have measured polyphenols in a number of fruit juices (Vinson, 1998) and most recently tea and coffee. The per capita beverage consumption from beverages in the US diet is shown in Figure 64.1.

Beer is a distant third compared to coffee and tea. Thus comparing per capita consumption data would not find beer to be an important source of antioxidants in spite of its reputed cardiovascular benefits. However, it is the *in vivo*

Table 64.2 Comparison of antioxidant quality (IC_{50}) and lipoprotein-bound antioxidant effectiveness (CLT_{50}) of vitamins, beer and wine polyphenols, and beer and red wine. The lower number indicates the higher quality and greater effectiveness

Components	IC_{50} (μM)	CLT_{50} (μM)
Ascorbic acid	1.45	Not active
Tocopherol	2.40	54
Ferulic acid (beer)	0.54	N/A
Epicatechin (beer)	0.19	85
Gallic acid (wine)	1.25	N/A
Cyanidin (wine)	0.21	120
Catechin (wine)	0.67	N/A
Lager beer	0.30	390
Red wine	0.45	27

N/A = not analyzed.

effectiveness of beer that clearly deems it superior to tea and coffee with respect to heart disease. The mechanism of beer's polyphenols may not be as antioxidants in the body but by other mechanisms.

Alcohol, the other ingredient in both beer and wine, is in fact an *in vitro* antioxidant in some models. For instance, ethanol protected LDL from oxidation initiated by superoxide and hydroxyl radicals by conversion of these to the less oxidizing ethanoxy radical (Bonnefont-Rousselot *et al.*, 2001). We also saw an *in vitro* effect from ethanol and other alcohols in a chemiluminescence assay of albumin oxidation (Trevithick *et al.*, 1999). However, when LDL + VLDL is oxidized by cupric ions in a mechanism which produces peroxy radicals, then ethanol has no effect since it cannot produce a less oxidizing radical (Vinson and Hontz, 1995). The larger molecules in beer, the proanthocyanidins, were found to have antioxidant activity more than 10 times that of ascorbic acid or tocopherol for the inhibition of neuronal nitric oxidase synthase activity (Stevens *et al.*, 2002).

We compared wine and beer as to their effectiveness in preventing LDL + VLDL oxidation by cupric ion using our standard model for heart disease in a test tube (Vinson *et al.*, 2001a, b). The measure of antioxidant quality is the IC_{50} value which is the concentration to inhibit the lipoprotein oxidation 50%. Values for beer and wine polyphenols, a representative lager beer and red wine, and vitamin antioxidants are shown in Table 64.2 (Vinson *et al.*, 1999). The beer and wine polyphenols are better antioxidants than the vitamins. Ferulic acid has been found in human plasma after beer ingestion (Nardini *et al.*, 2006) and gallic acid and catechin have been found after red wine ingestion (Cartron *et al.*, 2003). Beer is a better antioxidant than red wine and the concentrations that would be active are possible physiologically since polyphenols (mostly metabolites) seldom reach a concentration in plasma $>1\,\mu M$ (Manach *et al.*, 2005a, b).

A second and more relevant measure of antioxidants is lipoprotein-bound antioxidant effectiveness (Table 64.2). This is the plasma concentration to increase the lag time of oxidation of LDL + VLDL isolated after equilibration for 2 h of plasma with the antioxidant(s) (Vinson *et al.*, 2001a). The lag time in minutes is the time for all the bound antioxidants incorporated in the lipoprotein to become oxidized at which time the oxidation rate becomes much faster. These would include the vitamin E, retinol, and beta carotene from the diet as well as polyphenols from the diet and those polyphenols incorporated during plasma equilibration. Vitamin C is inactive as it does not bind to lipoproteins, being too water-soluble. The order of antioxidants is red wine > tocopherol > epicatechin > cyanidin (anthocyanins) ≫ lager beer ≫ ascorbic acid. In this assay red wine is much more potent than beer.

Animal Studies

Short term

Animal models represent a means to do the equivalent of large-scale long-term studies with humans and alcoholic beverages, a task only feasible with government funding.

One Japanese study focused on the comparison of alcohol-free red wine and beer given to rats (Kondo, 2004). They were given the same equivalent dose of alcohol, although alcohol was removed to determine the effect of the antioxidants in the two beverages. An equivalent of 150 ml of beer or 58 ml of red wine was given per kg of body weight to the animals and there was a control group given water. Plasma taken at 0 and 1 h was examined by oxidation with a peroxy initiator, 2,2′-azobis(2-amidinopropane) (AAPH). Tocopherol is oxidized in the plasma and its disappearance kinetics were followed. Beer and red wine equally and significantly protected the plasma tocopherol from oxidation. In addition the intake of beer or red wine for 6 weeks equally suppressed the elevation of plasma lipid peroxides in animals given a vitamin E-deficient diet. These results indicate that the polyphenolic antioxidants in beer and red wine were absorbed into the plasma as seen in human studies and are equal in plasma antioxidant protection at the same dose of alcohol.

In this rat experiment the animals were given either a normal diet, ethanol-supplemented diet (1.1 g/100 g of food), or a beer-containing diet (30% w/w) containing the same concentration of ethanol for 6 weeks (Gasbarrini *et al.*, 1998). This is equivalent to a moderate consumption of beer for humans. Plasmas of the ethanol group were significantly elevated in uric acid. Urate is an antioxidant but also a risk factor for heart disease and stroke in humans (Bos *et al.*, 2006). LDL oxidation was exacerbated in the ethanol group and decreased in the beer group compared to the control group. Thus beer (presumable the polyphenol component) was an *in vivo* antioxidant and ethanol was a pro-oxidant in this animal model. Beer thus overcame and surpassed the oxidant effects of alcohol.

A comprehensive study with rats examined the effect of alcohol-containing red wine and beer and lyophilized and thus dealcoholized red wine and beer (Gorinstein *et al.*, 1998). This was a 4-week supplementation with 2 ml of wine and 6 ml of beer or their lyophilized equivalents. The human dose equivalent was 350 ml of red wine or 1050 ml of beer/day. Compared to the control group given no alcohol, all treatments significantly decreased low density lipoprotein (LDL), high density lipoprotein (HDL), and triglycerides, and there was no difference among the experimental groups. The cholesterol/HDL ratio was increased by the wine and beer but the change was not significant. This animal study points out the differences between human and animal metabolism and biochemistry. Another positive benefit from this study was the significant 60% decrease in plasma lipid peroxides indicating that the beer and wine components were *in vivo* antioxidants. The fact that the results were equivalent for the alcohol and the non-alcohol groups indicates the lipid and antioxidant effects were probably due to the polyphenols in the wine and beer and not the alcohol.

Alcohol is proposed to be the cause of an HDL increase from alcoholic beverages in human studies. However, in the rat study just described, HDL was decreased by the alcohol-containing beer and wine. Interestingly, a recent mouse study investigated isohumulones, some of the bitter components of beer (Miura *et al.*, 2005). These are hop-derived compounds formed from humulones during the wort boiling step of the brewing process. The mice were given an atherogenic diet for 1 week with or without the isohumulones. Although the dose was supra-physiological (1–3 g/kg diet), these compounds were found to raise plasma HDL in a dose–response manner by activating peroxisome proliferator-activated receptors and beneficially affected the expression of genes involved in lipid metabolism. The control group given the atherogenic diet suffered a 27% decrease in HDL and the group given the high dose of isohumulones had a 39% increase in HDL. Isohumulones in beer may provide some of the HDL-raising effect in humans and perhaps work in cooperation with the alcohol-raising mechanism.

Long term

Rabbit Model The first comparative examination of alcoholic beverage and animal atherosclerosis was conducted in 1981 (Klurfeld and Kritchevsky, 1981). This elegant study examined alcohol, red wine, white wine, whisky, and beer given to cholesterol-fed rabbits. All alcohol groups experienced an increase in plasma HDL except for beer. The beer group had significantly lower liver cholesterol than the control and was superior to the other beverages in this respect. The red wine group had significantly less atherosclerosis than the controls, white wine, or whiskey. White wine, whiskey, and beer had no significant effect on atherosclerosis in this model although beer had less atherosclerosis than the control (30% reduction). The rabbit model has been criticized for having lipid metabolism dissimilar for humans, and for being a lipid storage disease rather than an atherosclerosis model since cholesterol levels are very high, in excess of 20 mM, an impossible level in humans. In addition pathogen-free rabbits do not develop atherosclerosis even with a high cholesterol diet, thus it is not a very relevant atherosclerosis model (Russell and Proctor, 2006).

Mouse Models A mouse study compared the effect of lager beer and dark beer in two models: C57BL/6 mice given a high fat Western diet for 24 weeks for early atherosclerosis and the apoE-deficient given a normal diet for 12 weeks for mature atherosclerosis (Escola-Gil *et al.*, 2004). The dosing of the ethanol control was 1.62% in the drinking water and the 5.4% beers were diluted appropriately to give the same ethanol dose. Water was also used for another control group. Red wine in the apoE model was previously shown to inhibit early but not mature (late) atherosclerosis (Hayek *et al.*, 1997; Bentzon *et al.*, 2001). Neither ethanol nor any type of beer had any significant effect on early or late atherosclerosis. Unfortunately, beer was not tested for early atherosclerosis by means of a short-term supplementation to apoE animals as was done by Hayek. In the apoE model of early atherosclerosis red wine was beneficial. The apoE model can be viewed as analogous to untreated, severely dyslipidemic humans (Russell and Proctor, 2006).

Illustrative of the different animal models of atherosclerosis is the study which used the human atherogenic lipoprotein profile LDLr$^{-/-}$ apoB$^{100/100}$ mouse (Degrace *et al.*, 2006). They used a moderate dose of lager beer (0.57 g of ethanol/kg of body weight) or the equivalent volume of ethanol-free beer. Animals were supplemented for 12 weeks with a single dose given during 5 min. There was no effect on serum glucose, cholesterol, LDL, or triglyceride or on liver toxicity (alanine aminotransferase). Liver triglycerides were significantly decreased by both beers. As a measure of atherosclerosis the authors used total cholesterol in the aorta which had been previously validated by correlational analysis with histology of the aorta. Cholesterol accumulation was slightly reduced in the ethanol-free beer and significantly reduced in the beer group. Ethanol had a very slight protective effect in addition to the beer components. Both beer groups equally and significantly raised HDL and VLDL levels in the serum but beer was significantly more effective than ethanol-free beer in raising VLDL, the major carrier of triglycerides.

The mechanism of beer's beneficial effect on this model of atherosclerosis was investigated by gene expression analysis and the pertinent data are shown in Table 64.3.

Among all the genes studies, only SR-B1 was significantly down-regulated by both beers compared to the control. Ethanol-containing beer significantly down-regulated LDL receptor-related protein (LRP), lecithin–cholesterol acyltransferase (LCAT), and sterol-regulatory element binding protein 2 (SREBP2). This study used one-fifth of the

Table 64.3 Effect of beer (0.57 g ethanol/kg body weight) and an equivalent amount of ethanol-free beer on gene expression in a human atherogenic lipoprotein mouse model of atherosclerosis compared to the water control given for 12 weeks

Gene RNA levels	*Beer*	*Ethanol-free beer*
Liver lipoprotein uptake		
Scavenger receptor-B1 (SR-B1)	Down-regulates*	Down-regulates*
LDL receptor related protein (LRP)	Up-regulates	Down-regulates*
Hepatic lipase (HL)	No effect	No effect
VLDL receptor (VLDLr)	No effect	Down-regulates
Lipoprotein cholesterol transfer		
Lecithin–cholesterol acyltransferase (LCAT)	Down-regulates*	Down-regulates
ATP-binding cassette transporter AI (ABCA1)	No effect	No effect
Sterol-regulatory element binding protein 2 (SREBP2)	Down-regulates*	No effect

*Significantly different from control, $p < 0.05$.

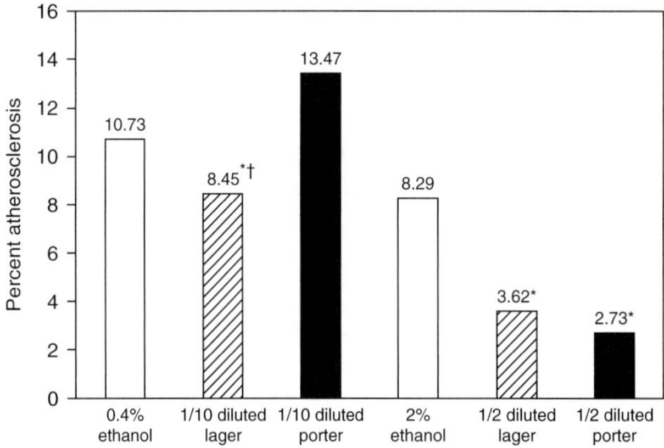

Figure 64.2 Percent of aortal coverage by foam cells in hamster given an atherogenic diet for 10 weeks. The control groups were given different doses of ethanol and the experimental groups were given diluted lager and porter beer at two different dilutions. *Significantly different from the corresponding control group, †significantly different from the corresponding lager group. Note the dose-related reduction in atherosclerosis with ethanol and the beers.

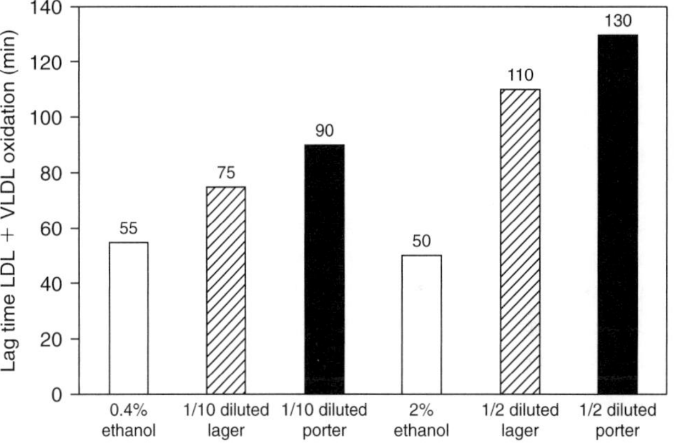

Figure 64.3 Lag time of LDL + VLDL isolated from pooled plasmas from each of the hamster groups and oxidized under standard conditions at physiological pH and temperature. This time represents the amount of antioxidants bound to the lipoproteins with the longer time indicating more antioxidant activity. Note the dose–response effect of the two varieties of beer.

dose of ethanol as is the previous genetic mouse model, but the lipid profile and lack of effect of ethanol on the lipids in this study are more representative of the effect of moderate alcohol on humans. The benefits of the beer components, probably the polyphenols, are amplified by the presence of ethanol in the beverage.

Hamster Model The hamster is often used as a model of atherosclerosis as its lipid profile, when given a cholesterol and saturated fat diet, resembles humans with a preponderance of LDL compared to HDL. This is an early atherosclerosis model as aortic lesions are confined to fatty streaks and there are no advanced intimal lesions of myocardial infarcts (Russell and Proctor, 2006). Our hamster atherosclerosis study was the first to compare lager with a dark beer at two different doses. There were two control groups given 0.4% and 2% alcohol and four experimental groups given a Czech Urquell lager and porter at 1/10 and 1/2 dilutions. All liquids were sweetened with an artificial sweetener. The diets were supplemented with 0.2% cholesterol/10% coconut oil. The beer groups drank significantly more liquid with the ethanol groups. Yes, beer is better tasting than plain alcohol even to hamsters. There was no significant effect of the beers on HDL compared to the ethanol controls. Both beers at the high dose significantly decreased triglycerides and cholesterol. There was no effect of either beer at the low dose on lipids.

Figure 64.2 illustrates the effect of the beers on atherosclerosis (% of aorta covered with foam cells) and the lag time of LDL + VLDL oxidation of pooled plasmas in Figure 64.3. Ethanol seemed to have beneficial effect as the high ethanol control had less atherosclerosis than the low ethanol control. This was also seen in our hamster atherosclerosis study with red wine (Vinson *et al.*, 2001b). In the red wine study ethanol increased triglycerides compared to the water control. Although we did not have a water control group in the beer study, there was one in the red wine hamster study. Ethanol was an *in vivo* antioxidant and significantly decreased lipid peroxides in the plasma relative to water and also increased the lag time of LDL + VLDL oxidation. Both beers significantly decreased atherosclerosis at the high dose, 56–67%. At the low dose only lager beer significantly decreased atherosclerosis, 21% vs. the control, $p < 0.05$. At this dose the lager beer was significantly more effective than the dark beer, $p < 0.001$. The human-equivalent dose is 1.25 l. The inability of dark beer to inhibit atherosclerosis may be due to the fact that some of its antioxidants, such as the melandoins and Maillard products, are non-phenolic and may not be absorbed or be bioactive. Both beers increased the lag time, indicating an *in vivo* antioxidant effect of the polyphenols from the beer. There was a negative correlation of lag times with atherosclerosis at the high dose, Pearson correlation coefficient 0.9577, $p = 0.07$. This indicates a significant proportion of the atherosclerosis inhibition can be attributed to the antioxidants in the two beers at this dose. Although we did not compare beer to red wine during the same study, beer with 2% alcohol (half diluted) decreased atherosclerosis by 56% while red wine with 6.75% alcohol (half diluted) decreased it by 53%. Thus beer is certainly equal if not greater in effectiveness to red wine in the hamster model of atherosclerosis.

Summary Points

- Beer contains substantial levels of polyphenols antioxidants and beer is the number three source of beverage antioxidants in the US diet on a daily per capita basis.
- Compared to red wine, beer provides almost twice as many antioxidants in the US daily diet.
- In a rat study red wine and beer given at the same dose of alcohol were equally protective as *in vivo* plasma antioxidants.
- At the same dose of alcohol given to rats in a short-term study, beer was an *in vivo* antioxidant and ethanol was a pro-oxidant *in vivo*.
- In a 4-week study rats were given alcohol-containing red wine and beer at the same alcohol dose, or without alcohol. The beneficial lipid and antioxidant effects were equal for wine and beer and were not due to the alcohol.
- A mouse study given an atherogenic diet for a short period investigated the effect of isohumulones, the bitter principles in beer. These compounds at a high dose raised HDL and may work with ethanol in humans to improve that risk factor for CVD.
- A rabbit model was the first comparison of different alcoholic beverages on atherosclerosis. Red wine had the only significant benefit compared to ethanol control. Beer had no effect on atherosclerosis.
- Two genetic mouse models were examined at a fairly high dose of ethanol and beer. Neither ethanol nor any type of beer had any significant effect on early or late atherosclerosis.
- The most human relevant mouse model had a lipoprotein profile similar to humans. Beer significantly inhibited atherosclerosis and ethanol-free beer was almost as effective. Both beer groups significantly increased HDL. Beer and ethanol-free beer affected several genes involved in lipid receptor uptake and lipid metabolism. Beneficial effects of the beer polyphenols (hypothesized by this author) were amplified by the presence of ethanol.
- Beer polyphenols appear to contribute a large degree of CVD protection in the short- and long-term supplementation of animal models of atherosclerosis although ethanol is also beneficial.
- Long-term human supplementation studies must be performed to compare beer with and without alcohol and thus determine the bioactive ingredient(s).

References

Bentzon, J.F., Skovenborg, E., Hansen, C., Moller, J., de Gaulejac, N.S., Proch, J. and Falk, E. (2001). *Circulation* 103, 1681–1687.

Bleys, J., Miller III, E.R., Pastor-Barriuso, R., Appel, L.J. and Guallar, E. (2006). *Am. J. Clin. Nutr.* 84, 880–887.

Bonnefont-Rousselot, D., Rouscilles, A., Bizard, C., Delattre, J., Jore, D. and Gardes-Albert, M. (2001). *Radiat. Res.* 155, 279–287.

Bos, M.J., Koudstaal, P.J., Hofman, A., Witteman, J.C. and Breteler, M.M. (2006). *Stroke* 37, 1503–1507.

Cartron, E., Fouret, G., Carbonneau, M.A., Lauret, C., Michel, F., Monnier, L., Descomps, B. and Leger, C.L. (2003). *Free Radic. Res.* 37, 1021–1035.

Degrace, P., Moindrot, B., Mohamed, I., Gresti, J. and Clouet, P. (2006). *Atherosclerosis* 189, 328–335.

Di Castelnuovo, A., Rotondo, S. and Iacoviello, L. (2002). *Circulation* 105, 2836–2844.

Economic Research Service (2005). USDA/ERS, Washington, DC, last updated December 21, 2005.

Escola-Gil, J.C., Calpe-Berdiel, L., Ribas, V. and Blanco-Vaca, F. (2004). *Nutr. J.* 3, 1.

Gasbarrini, A., Addolorato, G., Simoncini, M., Gasbarrini, G., Fantozzi, P., Mancini, F., Montanari, L., Nardini, M., Ghiselli, A. and Scaccini, C. (1998). *Dig. Dis. Sci.* 43, 1332–1338.

Gorinstein, S., Zemser, M., Weisz, M., Halevy, S., Martin-Belloso, O. and Trakhtenberg, S. (1998). *J. Nutr. Biochem.* 9, 682–686.

Hayek, T., Fuhrman, B., Vaya, J., Rosenblat, M., Belinky, P., Coleman, R., Elis, A. and Aviram, M. (1997). *Arterioscler. Thromb. Vasc. Biol.* 17, 2744–2752.

Jandera, P., Skeifikova, V., Rehova, L., Hajek, T., Baldrianova, L., Skopova, G., Kellner, V. and Horna, A. (2005). *J. Sep. Sci.* 28, 1005–1022.

Jastrzebski, Z., Gorinstein, S., Czyzewska-Szafran, H., Leontowicz, H., Leontowicz, M., Trakhtenberg, S. and Remiszewska, M. (2007). *Food Chem. Toxicol.* 45, 296–302.

Klurfeld, D.M. and Kritchevsky, D. (1981). *Exp. Mol. Pathol.* 34, 62–71.

Kondo, K. (2004). *Biofactors* 22, 303–310.

Manach, C., Mazur, A. and Scalbert, A. (2005a). *Curr. Opin. Lipidol.* 16, 77–84.

Manach, C., Williamson, G., Morand, C., Scalbert, A. and Remesy, C. (2005b). *Am. J. Clin. Nutr.* 81, 230S–242S.

Miura, Y., Hosono, M., Oyamada, C., Odai, H., Oikawa, S. and Kondo, K. (2005). *Br. J. Nutr.* 93, 559–567.

Mukamal, K.J., Chiuve, S.E. and Rimm, E.B. (2006). *Arch. Intern. Med.* 166, 2145–2150.

Nardini, M., Natella, F., Scaccini, C. and Ghiselli, A. (2006). *J. Nutr. Biochem.* 17, 14–22.

Rimm, E.B., Klatsky, A. and Grobbee, D. (1996). *BMJ* 312, 731–736.
Rimm, E.B. and Stampfer, M.J. (2002). *Circulation* 105, 2806–2807.
Russell, J.C. and Proctor, S.D. (2006). *Cardiovasc. Pathol.* 15, 318–330.
Steinberg, D., Parthasarathy, S., Carew, T.E., Khoo, J.C. and Witztum, J.L. (1989). *New Engl. J. Med.* 320, 915–924.
Stevens, J.F., Miranda, C.L., Wolthers, K.R., Schimerlik, M., Deinzer, M.L. and Buhler, D.R. (2002). *J. Agric. Food Chem.* 50, 3435–3443.
Tordsen, C., Clause, R. and Holz-Clause, M. (2004). Value-Added Agriculture Extension, Agricultural Marketing Resource Center, Iowa State University Extension, Ames, IA, USA.
Trevithick, C.C., Vinson, J.A., Caulfield, J., Rahman, F., Derksen, T., Bocksch, L., Hong, S., Stefan, A., Teufel, K., Wu, N., Hirst, M. and Trevithick, J.R. (1999). *Redox Rep.* 4, 89–93.
Vinson, J.A. and Hontz, B.A. (1995). *J. Agric. Food Chem.* 43, 401–403.
Vinson, J.A. (1998). *Adv. Exp. Med. Biol.* 439, 151–164.
Vinson, J.A., Jang, J., Yang, J., Dabbagh, Y., Liang, X., Serry, M., Proch, J. and Cai, S. (1999). *J. Agric. Food Chem.* 47, 2502–2504.
Vinson, J.A., Proch, J. and Bose, P. (2001a). *Meth. Enzymol.* 335, 103–114.
Vinson, J.A., Teufel, K. and Wu, N. (2001b). *Atherosclerosis* 156, 67–72.
Vinson, J.A., Mandarano, M., Hirst, M., Trevithick, J.R. and Bose, P. (2003). *J. Agric. Food Chem.* 51, 5528–5533.

65

Beer Inhibition of Heterocyclic Amines-Induced Carcinogenesis

Hajime Nozawa and Keiji Kondo Central Laboratories for Frontier Technology, Research Section for Applied Food Science, Kirin Holdings Co., Ltd., Takasaki, Gunma, Japan

Abstract

Antimutagenic and anticarcinogenic effects of beer on heterocyclic amines (HCAs)-induced carcinogenesis were studied *in vitro* and *in vivo*. Four commercial beers (two pilsner-type, black and stout) showed inhibitory effects against five HCAs, MeIQx, PhIP, Trp-P-2, Glu-P-1 and IQ, in the Ames assay using *Salmonella typhimurium* TA98 in the presence of rat S9 mix. The inhibitory effects of dark-colored beers (stout and black beers) were greater than those of pilsner-type beers. Dark-colored beers suppressed CYP1A2 activity in a dose-dependent manner, suggesting that inhibition of HCA activation is partly responsible for their strong antimutagenic effects. Single cell gel electrophoresis assay (comet assay) revealed that oral ingestion of pilsner-type and stout beers for 1 week significantly inhibited DNA damage in the liver cells of male ICR mice exposed to MeIQx (13 mg/kg, i.p.). Male Fischer 344 rats were orally received PhIP (75 mg/kg, 5 times a week for 2 weeks) and aberrant crypt foci (ACF) formation in the colon was analyzed after 5 weeks. The number of ACF was significantly reduced in rats fed a diet containing freeze-dried (FD) beer. Female Sprague-Dawley rats were orally received PhIP (85 mg/kg, 4 times a week for 2 weeks) and the tumors were pathologically examined at the end of the 22 weeks experiment. Tumor development was inhibited by FD beer intake in a dose-dependent manner. Tumor incidence (38.5%) and tumor multiplicity (0.8 ± 0.4) for the group fed a diet containing 4% FD beer were significantly reduced as compared with the control group (73.3% and 1.8 ± 0.7). In conclusion, our results suggest that intake of beer ingredients may reduce the risk of carcinogenesis caused by HCAs.

List of Abbreviations

ACF	Aberrant crypt foci
ACs	Aberrant crypts
FD beer	Freeze-dried beer
(I/PI)	Initiation and post-initiation
AIN	AIN-76A
AD	Adenomas
ADC	Adenocarcinomas
HCAs	Heterocyclic amines
IQ	2-Amino-3-methylimidazo[4,5-*f*]-quinoline
MeIQx	2-Amino-3,8-dimethylimidazo[4,5-*f*] quinoxaline
Trp-P-2	3-Amino-1-methyl-5*H*-pyrido[4,3-*b*]indole
PhIP	2-Amino-1-methyl-6-phenylimidazo[4,5-*b*] pyridine
Glu-P-1	2-Amino-6-methyldipyrido[1,2-*a*:3′,2′-*d*] imidazole
MROD	Methoxy resorufin-*O*-demethylase
Comet assay	Single cell gel electrophoresis assay

Introduction

Heterocyclic amines (HCAs) exist in cooked meat and fried fish (Felton *et al.*, 1997) and this family of compounds exert a strong mutagenic effect in the Ames *Salmonella* mutagenicity assay (Sugimura, 1997). Carcinogenic studies in rodents demonstrated that they are carcinogens in colon, mammary, liver and prostate, and they may cause cancer in human (Ito *et al.*, 1991; Shirai *et al.*, 1997). Approximately 20 HCAs have been purified from the pyrolysates of amino acids and proteins; they are categorized as IQ type and non-IQ type. IQ type includes aminoimidazoles, such as IQ (2-amino-3-methylimidazo[4,5-*f*]-quinoline), MeIQx (2-amino-3,8-dimethylimidazo[4,5-*f*]quinoxaline) and PhIP (2-amino-1-methyl-6-phenylimidazo[4,5-*b*]pyridine), and non-IQ type includes pyridoindoles and dipyridoimidazoles, such as Trp-P-1 (3-amino-1,4-dimethyl-5*H*-pyrido

Beer in Health and Disease Prevention
ISBN: 978-0-12-373891-2

[4,3-*b*]indole) and Glu-P-1 (2-amino-6-methyldipyrido[1,2-*a*:3′,2′-*d*]imidazole) (Nagao *et al.*, 1996; Sugimura *et al.*, 1996). HCAs are activated to mutagenic intermediates by *N*-oxidation reactions, which are catalyzed by hepatic cytochrome P-450 enzymes (especially CYP1A2). Further activation of these metabolites involves enzymatic esterification with acetyltransferases or sulfotransferases to produce reactive nitrenium ions, which form covalent bonds with DNA mainly at the N2 and C8 positions of guanine, and thereby cause mutation in cells (Minchin *et al.*, 1992; Turesky *et al.*, 1992; Chou *et al.*, 1995; Turesky *et al.*, 1998). Among them, PhIP is one of the most abundant HCAs (Felton *et al.*, 1986) and has been shown in rodents to cause colon, mammary and prostate cancers (Ito *et al.*, 1991; Shirai *et al.*, 1997). A high incidence of PhIP-DNA adducts in exfoliated ductal epithelial cells from human breast milk has indicated that humans are exposed to this mutagen daily (Gorlewska-Roberts *et al.*, 2002). PhIP is reasonably anticipated to be a human carcinogen based on sufficient evidence of carcinogenicity in experimental animals and supporting genotoxicity data by the US National Toxicology Program. Therefore, there is a growing interest in finding dietary factors with anticarcinogenic effects to reduce the mutagenic and carcinogenic risks caused by PhIP and other HCAs (Ohta *et al.*, 2000; Hagiwara *et al.*, 2002; Tavan *et al.*, 2002; Yamagishi *et al.*, 2002; Yang *et al.*, 2003; Hikosaka *et al.*, 2004).

It has been reported that many components from plant sources reduce the mutagenic activities of HCAs (Apostolides *et al.*, 1997; Edenharder *et al.*, 1997). Several molecular processes are involved in the defense against HCAs, such as direct interaction with non-activated or activated HCAs (Dashwood *et al.*, 1996), inhibition of enzymes involved in the activation of HCAs (Edenharder *et al.*, 1997), induction of detoxifying enzymes (Kensler, 1997) and amelioration of DNA repair or replication (Sanyal *et al.*, 1997). The Ames test using the bacteria *Salmonella* can be used to find chemopreventive agents with antimutagenic effects on HCAs. Although *in vitro* methods are convenient and used widely, it is important to assess antimutagenic activity with *in vivo* experiments since metabolism of a mutagen may be changed by chemopreventive agent or the chemopreventive agent itself may be metabolized after absorption. Single cell gel electrophoresis assay (comet assay) has been used to characterize chemopreventive agents against DNA damage in organs of rodents exposed to mutagens (Singh *et al.*, 1988; Sasaki *et al.*, 1997; Tice *et al.*, 2000; Kassie *et al.*, 2003). Detection of DNA adducts, which are considered to be an initiating event in chemical carcinogenesis induced by HCAs, is useful for evaluation of chemopreventive efficacy *in vivo* (Lin *et al.*, 2003). Aberrant crypt foci (ACF) are early morphological changes or hyperproliferative lesions found in the colon of carcinogen-treated rodents and considered to be putative preneoplastic lesions for colon cancer (Bird, 1987; Wargovich *et al.*, 2000). Oral administration of PhIP induces ACF in male F344 rats; thus, chemopreventive effects were assessed in this model (Takahashi *et al.*, 1997; Chewonarin *et al.*, 1999). It has been shown that PhIP induces mammary tumors in female rats, and this carcinogenesis model has been used to study anticarcinogenic effects of many dietary factors (Ohta *et al.*, 2000; Schut and Yao, 2000; Futakuchi *et al.*, 2002; Hirose *et al.*, 2002; Yamagishi *et al.*, 2002). Therefore, in this chapter, we evaluated the modulating effects of freeze-dried (FD) beer on PhIP-induced mammary carcinogenesis.

Beer is a low alcohol beverage brewed from natural ingredients, rich in vitamins, amino acids and minerals, and contains a number of micronutrients such as phenolic acids and polyphenols (Madigan *et al.*, 1994; Lapcik *et al.*, 1998). Beer or extracts of raw materials are cancer preventive against azoxymethane-induced carcinogenesis (Nozawa *et al.*, 2004b, 2005). Furthermore, previous studies demonstrated that the antimutagenic effects of beer against activated HCAs (Trp-P-2(NHOH), Trp-P-1(NHOH) and Glu-P-1(NHOH)) were exerted in the Ames assay. In addition, beer intake reduced the number of DNA adducts generated in the liver of mice by Trp-P-2 treatment (Arimoto-Kobayashi *et al.*, 1999; Kimura *et al.*, 1999; Yoshikawa *et al.*, 2002). Glycine-betaine and pseudouridine, both present in beer, have been identified as antimutagens against 2-chloro-4-methylthiobutanoic acid and *N*-methyl-*N*′-nitro-*N*-nitrosoguanidine, respectively (Kimura *et al.*, 1999; Yoshikawa *et al.*, 2002). It has also been reported that several phenolic compounds derived from hops exert antimutagenic effect against HCAs through inhibition of CYP1A2 (Miranda *et al.*, 2000). In addition, hot water extract of hops showed antimutagenic effects against Trp-P-2(NHOH) (Arimoto-Kobayashi *et al.*, 1999). Therefore, the antimutagenic and anticarcinogenic activities of beer against HCAs were extensively studied using *in vitro* cell-based mutagenicity assays, *in vivo* mutagenicity assays (comet assay) and *in vivo* carcinogenesis experiment (Nozawa *et al.*, 2004a, 2006).

Beer Inhibition of HCAs-Induced Mutagenesis in the Ames Test

Two pilsner-type beers, P1 (beer B) and P2 (beer A, same beer as used in AOM-induced carcinogenesis experiments), a black beer (D) and a stout beer (S) were used for the antimutagenicity experiments. Ames test was conducted according to the method established by Ames *et al.* (1975). As shown in Figure 65.1, all samples of beer showed antimutagenic effects against all HCAs tested (MeIQx, PhIP, Glu-P-1, Trp-P-2 and IQ). For example, addition of 100 μl black, stout and two pilsner-type beers into the reaction mixture with MeIQx decreased the number of revertants by 75%, 95%, 53% and 60%, respectively (Figure 65.1a). Growth inhibitions and mutagenic effects of beer samples on bacterial cells were not observed. Dark-colored beers (stout and black beers)

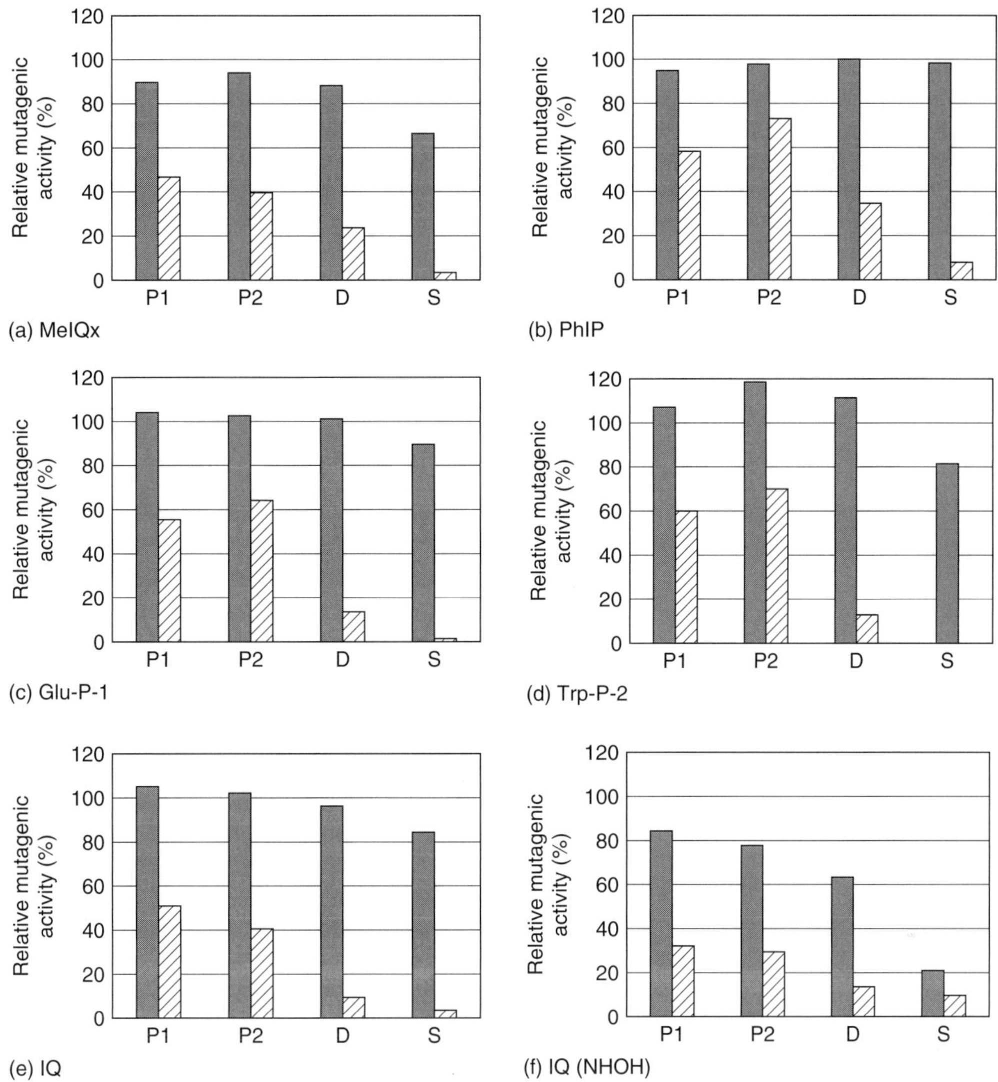

Figure 65.1 Antimutagenic effects of beer against HCAs in *Salmonella typhimurium* TA98. Assays were performed in the presence (a–e) or absence (f) of rat S9, using duplicate plates per sample. Two pilsner-type beers (P1 and P2), black beer (D) and stout beer (S) were used. Beer samples were mixed at 10 μl (closed bar) or 100 μl (slashed bar) in reactions. Results are given as relative mutagenic activities in comparison with ethanol controls. MeIQx, PhIP, Glu-P-1, Trp-P-2, IQ and activated IQ were used at 30 pmol, 10 nmol, 300 pmol, 50 pmol, 80 pmol and 20 pmol per plate, respectively (a–e). One hundred percent mutagenicity of ethanol control corresponds to 466(a), 286(b), 1,661(c), 1,417(d), 967(e) and 735(f) revertants.

had a greater antimutagenic effect than the pilsner-type beers (Figure 65.1a–e). Moreover, antimutagenicity of the beer samples was also observed against activated IQ (IQ-NHOH); black and stout beers exhibited stronger antimutagenic effects than pilsner type beers (Figure 65.1f).

Beer Inhibition of CYP1A2 Activity

The inhibitory effect of beer on the activity of CYP1A2, an enzyme involved in the activation of HCAs, was examined by measuring methoxy resorufin-*O*-demethylase activity (Xu *et al.*, 1996). Dose-dependent inhibition of CYP1A2 by dark-colored beers (black and stout beers) was observed, but the pilsner-type beers had no inhibitory effects (Figure 65.2). This suggests that the strong antimutagenic effects observed with dark-colored beers in the Ames tests could be partly attributed to the inhibition of CYP1A2.

Beer Inhibition of MeIQx-Induced DNA Damage in Liver Cells by Single Cell Gel Electrophoresis Assay

Male ICR mice at 8 weeks of age were fed a basal diet of AIN-76A and experimental drinks (stout beer (2 times diluted by water) and pilsner-type beer) or control drinks (5% ethanol and water) *ad libitum* for 1 week. Each

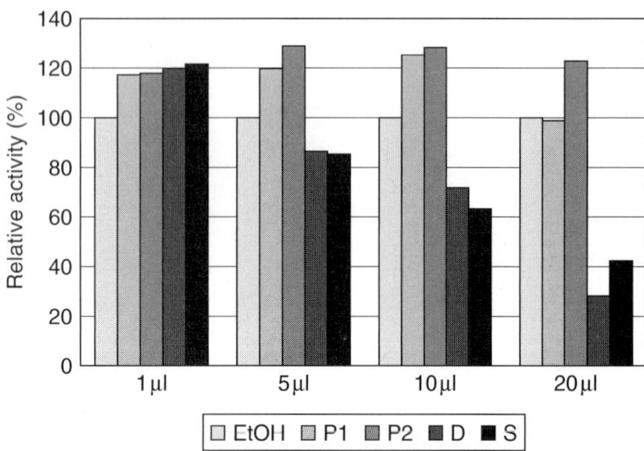

Figure 65.2 Inhibition of CYP1A2 activity with beer. Methoxy resorufin was used as a substrate for CYP1A2 in rat S9. Two pilsner-type beers, one black and one stout beer were added to the 100 µl of reaction mix at indicated amounts. Results are given as relative inhibitory activities in comparison with ethanol controls.

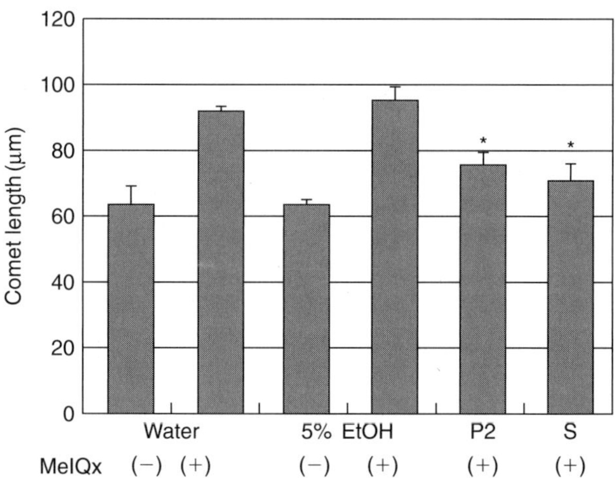

Figure 65.3 Induction of DNA damage in liver cells by MeIQx and its prevention by beer. Male ICR mice (n = 3) were given beer samples for 1 week and received intraperitoneal injections with MeIQx (13 mg/kg b.w.) or saline 3 h before sacrifice. One hundred nuclei were analyzed for each animal in the comet assay. Results are given as mean comet length ± SD. Statistical significance comparison results between experimental groups and controls are shown by * for $p < 0.05$.

treatment group consisted of three animals. They received intraperitoneal injections of MeIQx at a dose of 13 mg/kg body weight at 3 h before sacrifice (Sasaki *et al.*, 1997). Liver cells were prepared and analyzed by comet assay (Singh *et al.*, 1988; Pool-Zobel *et al.*, 1993; Tice *et al.*, 2000). MeIQx treatment induced significant DNA damage in liver cells: comet lengths in groups fed 5% ethanol or water as a drink were approximately 1.5-fold longer than those in the saline-treated control (Figure 65.3). Comet lengths in the groups fed either pilsner-type beer or stout beer were significantly shorter than those in the group fed 5% ethanol (20% and 26% reduction, respectively), indicating DNA damage induced by MeIQx was reduced by the intake of beer as a drink before administration of this mutagen.

Beer Inhibition of PhIP-Induced ACF Formation in Rat Colon

Analysis of ACF formation was performed according to previous reports (Takahashi *et al.*, 1997; Chewonarin *et al.*, 1999). Male Fischer 344 rats at 5 weeks of age (n = 8) were fed the AIN-76A basal diet or experimental diets containing FD samples of pilsner-type beer A for the experimental period of 5 weeks. The powder of FD beer A was mixed in the basal diet at a concentration of 0.5%, 1%, 2% and 4%. One week after the start of feeding experimental diets, PhIP in saline was given to the rats at a dose of 75 mg/kg body weight by daily oral gavage; the dose was given 10 times (days 8–12 and 15–19). All rats were weighed weekly and the animals were sacrificed at the end of the 5-week experimental period. ACF were distinguished from normal crypts by their increased size, prominent epithelial cells and increased pericryptal area according to established criteria (Bird, 1987). The numbers of ACF and aberrant crypts (ACs) per rat were quantified (Nozawa *et al.*, 2004a, b). There were no significant differences in the daily consumption of diets and final body weights among the experimental and control groups (Table 65.1). The incidence of ACF was 100% in the control and experimental groups. Ingestion of FD beer at 1% and 2% in the basal diet during the whole experimental period (I/PI) reduced the number of ACF/colon by 54% and 45%, respectively (Table 65.1). Diets containing 0.5% and 4% FD beer were less effective in reducing the number of ACF/colon (33% and 19% reduction, respectively), suggesting the optimal effective dose to be between 1% and 2% (Table 65.1). The number of ACs/colon was significantly reduced in the groups fed FD beer at 0.5%, 1% and 2% (55%, 70% and 55% reduction, respectively). In addition, a significant reduction in the number of ACs/focus was observed in the group fed sample containing 1% FD beer (Table 65.1). The dosing level at 1% of FD beer in this animal experiment was estimated as 220 ml beer intake for humans (Nozawa *et al.*, 2004a).

Beer Inhibition of PhIP-Induced Mammary Carcinogenesis in Rats

Carcinogenesis experiments were conducted according to the established method reported previously (Ohta *et al.*, 2000; Kawamori *et al.*, 2001, 2002). Six-week-old female Sprague-Dawley rats were divided into four groups. They were fed either a basal high fat diet (control group, n = 30) or basal high fat diets containing FD beer A at 1% (n = 30), 2% (n = 30) or 4% (n = 26) (Table 65.2). One week after the start of feeding, rats received PhIP suspension in corn

Table 65.1 Effects of beer P2 (beer A) on PhIP-induced ACF formation in rat colon

Group	*Incidence*	*Body weight (g)*	*Daily diet intake (g/rat)*	*Number of ACF/colon*	*Number of ACs/colon*	*Number of ACs/focus*
AIN (control)	8/8	177.6 ± 12.0[a]	10.2	8.4 ± 3.3	18.5 ± 15.0	2.1 ± 0.8
0.5% FD Beer	8/8	182.8 ± 13.5	10.3	5.6 ± 3.0	8.4 ± 4.5[b]	1.5 ± 0.3
1% FD Beer	8/8	179.9 ± 3.2	10.1	3.9 ± 2.1[c]	5.6 ± 3.5[c]	1.4 ± 0.3[b]
2% FD Beer	8/8	182.3 ± 7.9	10.5	4.6 ± 2.2[b]	8.3 ± 4.5[b]	1.8 ± 0.6
4% FD Beer	8/8	176.1 ± 10.1	10.1	6.8 ± 2.7	12.0 ± 5.3	1.8 ± 0.3

[a] Results are shown in the table indicating mean ± SD.
[b,c] Statistical significance comparison results between experimental groups and controls are shown by $p < 0.05$ and $p < 0.01$, respectively.

Table 65.2 The composition of experimental diet

	g/kg Diet			
Ingredient	*Group 1 (control)*	*Group 2 (1% FD beer)*	*Group 3 (2% FD beer)*	*Group 4 (4% FD beer)*
Casein	235	235	235	235
DL-methionine	3.5	3.5	3.5	3.5
Corn starch	95	95	95	95
Sucrose	317	307	297	277
Cellulose	59	59	59	59
Corn oil	235.2	235.2	235.2	235.2
Salt mixture	41.1	41.1	41.1	41.1
Vitamin mixture	11.8	11.8	11.8	11.8
Choline bitartrate	2.4	2.4	2.4	2.4
ED beer	0	10	20	40

Note: Calorific content in each experimental group was same as control group by adjusting the sucrose content in each diet.

oil at a dose of 85 mg/kg by gavage 4 times weekly for 2 weeks. Palpable tumors were recorded weekly until 21 weeks. At 22 weeks all rats were sacrificed, and neoplastic lesions were examined macroscopically and scored. Then the lesions were measured with calipers, and the tumor volume was calculated using the formula (length)*(width)*(depth)*π/6 (Tayek *et al.*, 1986). After measuring the tumor size, they were immediately fixed with 10% neutral buffered formalin. The lesions were embedded in paraffin blocks, sectioned and stained with hematoxylin and eosin (H&E) for histopathological examination according to established criteria (Russo *et al.*, 1990).

Palpable breast tumors were observed in all groups of rats 8 weeks after the administration of PhIP (experimental week 11). The time courses of tumor incidence (the percentage of rats with tumors) and multiplicity (the number of tumors per rat) are shown for each experimental group in Figure 65.4. Tumor incidence in the groups fed diets containing 2% and 4% FD beer was lower than in the control group throughout the carcinogenesis experiment (Figure 65.4a). While tumor incidence in the group treated with 1% FD beer was higher than in the control group from 10 to 14 weeks, by 20 weeks it reached a similar value. The changes in tumor multiplicity mirrored those of tumor incidence. Feeding the rats diets with 2% or 4% FD beer greatly reduced the tumor multiplicity compared to the control group, while only a slight decrease was noticed in the group fed the diet with 1% FD beer after 16 weeks (Figure 65.4b). Furthermore, there was a noticeable delay in the appearance of tumors in the group fed the diet with 4% FD beer until 13 weeks, when only one palpable tumor was found in one rat. The results of mammary tumor development in each group examined at week 22 are summarized in Table 65.3. Dose-dependent inhibition of tumor incidence and tumor multiplicity was observed following intake of FD beer. Tumor incidence in the control group and the groups fed FD beer at 1%, 2% and 4% was 73.3%, 63.3%, 53.3% and 38.5%, respectively. As compared to the control group, the tumor incidence of the 4% FD beer-fed group was significantly reduced to 53% of the control value ($p < 0.05$). Tumor multiplicity in the control group and the groups fed FD beer at 1%, 2% and 4% was 2.0 ± 0.4, 2.0 ± 0.5, 1.4 ± 0.3 and 0.8 ± 0.4, respectively. The decrease in the 4% FD beer group was also significant as it was reduced to 40% of the control value ($p < 0.01$). Dose-dependent suppression was also observed in tumor volumes. The values were 1.8 ± 0.7 cm^3, 1.5 ± 0.5 cm^3, 0.9 ± 0.3 cm^3 and 0.8 ± 0.4 cm^3 for the control, 1% FD beer, 2% FD beer and 4% FD beer groups, respectively.

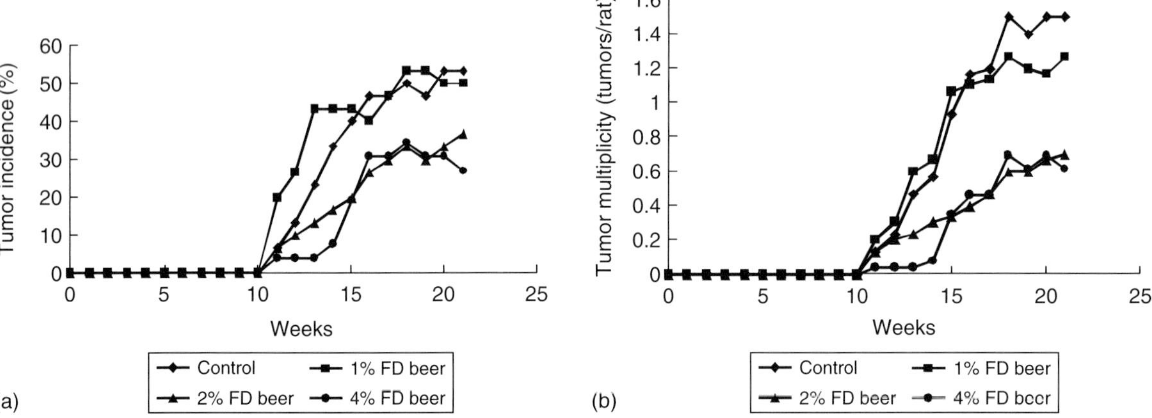

Figure 65.4 Intake of FD beer dose-dependently inhibited mammary carcinogenesis in rats. Tumor incidence (a) and tumor multiplicity (b) were measured in female rats treated with PhIP and fed experimental diets, control (rhombus), 1% (square), 2% (triangle) or 4% (circle) FD beer.

Table 65.3 Tumor volume, tumor incidence and tumor multiplicity in carcinogenesis experiment

	Animals (n)	*Average tumor volume (cm³)*	*Tumor incidence (%)*	*Tumor multiplicity*
Control	30	1.8 ± 0.7^a	22/30 (73.3)	2.0 ± 0.4
1% FD beer	30	1.5 ± 0.5	19/30 (63.3)	2.0 ± 0.5
2% FD beer	30	0.9 ± 0.3	16/30 (53.3)	1.4 ± 0.3
4% FD beer	26	0.8 ± 0.4	10/26 $(38.5)^c$	0.8 ± 0.4^b

[a] Values are given as the mean ± SEM.
Significantly different from Group 1: $^b p < 0.05$; $^c p < 0.01$.

Summary Points

- Antimutagenic activities of beer (two pilsner, black and stout) were observed against five HCAs, including MeIQx, PhIP, Glu-P-1, Trp-P-2 and IQ in the presence of rat S9 activation system in the Ames mutagenicity assay. Dark-colored beers (black and stout beers) exerted stronger antimutagenic effects than that of pilsner beer.
- These inhibitory effects were also observed when activated HCAs (IQ) were used in the Ames experiment, suggesting that some components with desmutagenic activity are present in all beers.
- Dark-colored beers inhibited CYP1A2 activity *in vitro*, however, pilsner-type beers did not show any inhibitory effects. It is indicated that the strong antimutagenic effects of dark-colored beers against HCAs observed in the Ames assays with S9 mix are partly due to inhibition of the activation of HCAs by CYP1A2.
- DNA damage in liver cells induced by MeIQx was protected by intake of both pilsner and stout beers in the single cell gel electrophoresis assay (comet assay). These antimutagenic effects of pilsner and stout beers *in vivo* were approximately the same degree.
- Intake of beer A inhibited the PhIP-induced ACF formation in rat colon. It is suggested that beer components with antimutagenic activity may contribute to the inhibition of ACF formation. Moreover, beer components exerted anticancer promotion activity by the decreased average ACF size.
- In the PhIP-induced mammary carcinogenesis experiment, intake of beer A reduced the tumor incidence and tumor multiplicity. Overall, from these results, it is indicated that beer may reduce the risk of carcinogenesis caused by HCAs, the food-borne carcinogens.

References

Ames, B.N., McCann, J. and Yamasaki, E. (1975). *Mutat. Res.* 31, 347–364.

Apostolides, Z., Balentine, D.A., Harbowy, M.E., Hara, Y. and Weisburger, J.H. (1997). *Mutat. Res.* 389, 167–172.

Arimoto-Kobayashi, S., Sugiyama, C., Harada, N., Takeuchi, M., Takemura, M. and Hayatsu, H. (1999). *J. Agric. Food Chem.* 47, 221–230.

Bird, R.P. (1987). *Cancer Lett.* 37, 147–151.

Chewonarin, T., Kinouchi, T., Kataoka, K., Arimochi, H., Kuwahara, T., Vinitketkumnuen, U. and Ohnishi, Y. (1999). *Food Chem. Toxicol.* 37, 591–601.

Chou, H.C., Lang, N.P. and Kadlubar, F.F. (1995). *Cancer Res.* 55, 525–529.

Dashwood, R., Yamane, S. and Larsen, R. (1996). *Environ. Mol. Mutagen.* 27, 211–218.

Edenharder, R., Rauscher, R. and Platt, K.L. (1997). *Mutat. Res.* 379, 21–32.

Felton, J.S., Knize, M.G., Shen, N.H., Lewis, P.R., Andresen, B.D., Happe, J. and Hatch, F.T. (1986). *Carcinogenesis* 7, 1081–1086.

Felton, J.S., Malfatti, M.A., Knize, M.G., Salmon, C.P., Hopmans, E.C. and Wu, R.W. (1997). *Mutat. Res.* 376, 37–41.

Futakuchi, M., Cheng, J.L., Hirose, M., Kimoto, N., Cho, Y.M., Iwata, T., Kasai, M., Tokudome, S. and Shirai, T. (2002). *Cancer Lett.* 178, 131–139.

Gorlewska-Roberts, K., Green, B., Fares, M., Ambrosone, C.B. and Kadlubar, F.F. (2002). *Environ. Mol. Mutagen.* 39, 184–192.

Hagiwara, A., Yoshino, H., Ichihara, T., Kawabe, M., Tamano, S., Aoki, H., Koda, T., Nakamura, M., Imaida, K., Ito, N. and Shirai, T. (2002). *J. Toxicol. Sci.* 27, 57–68.

Hikosaka, A., Asamoto, M., Hokaiwado, N., Kato, K., Kuzutani, K., Kohri, K. and Shirai, T. (2004). *Carcinogenesis* 25, 381–387.

Hirose, M., Nishikawa, A., Shibutani, M., Imai, T. and Shirai, T. (2002). *Environ. Mol. Mutagen.* 39, 271–278.

Ito, N., Hasegawa, R., Sano, M., Tamano, S., Esumi, H., Takayama, S. and Sugimura, T. (1991). *Carcinogenesis* 12, 1503–1506.

Kassie, F., Uhl, M., Rabot, S., Grasl-Kraupp, B., Verkerk, R., Kundi, M., Chabicovsky, M., Schulte-Hermann, R. and Knasmuller, S. (2003). *Carcinogenesis* 24, 255–261.

Kawamori, T., Uchiya, N., Nakatsugi, S., Watanabe, K., Ohuchida, S., Yamamoto, H., Maruyama, T., Kondo, K., Sugimura, T. and Wakabayashi, K. (2001). *Carcinogenesis* 22, 2001–2004.

Kawamori, T., Nakatsugi, S., Ohta, T., Sugimura, T. and Wakabayashi, K. (2002). *Adv. Exp. Med. Biol.* 507, 371–376.

Kensler, T.W. (1997). *Environ. Health Perspect.* 105, 965–970.

Kimura, S., Hayatsu, H. and Arimoto-Kobayashi, S. (1999). *Mutat. Res.* 439, 267–276.

Lapcik, O., Hill, M., Hampl, R., Wahala, K. and Adlercreutz, H. (1998). *Steroids* 63, 14–20.

Lin, D.X., Thompson, P.A., Teitel, C., Chen, J.S. and Kadlubar, F.F. (2003). *Mutat. Res.* 523–524, 193–200.

Madigan, D., McMurrough, I. and Smyth, M.R. (1994). *Analyst* 119, 863–868.

Minchin, R.F., Reeves, P.T., Teitel, C.H., McManus, M.E., Mojarrabi, B., Ilett, K.F. and Kadlubar, F.F. (1992). *Biochem. Biophys. Res. Commun.* 185, 839–844.

Miranda, C.L., Aponso, G.L., Stevens, J.F., Deinzer, M.L. and Buhler, D.R. (2000). *Cancer Lett.* 149, 21–29.

Nagao, M., Wakabayashi, K., Ushijima, T., Toyota, M., Totsuka, Y. and Sugimura, T. (1996). *Environ. Health Perspect.* 104, 497–501.

Nozawa, H., Tazumi, K., Sato, K., Yoshida, A., Takata, J., Arimoto-Kobayashi, S. and Kondo, K. (2004a). *Mutat. Res.* 559, 177–187.

Nozawa, H., Yoshida, A., Tajima, O., Katayama, M., Sonobe, H., Wakabayashi, K. and Kondo, K. (2004b). *Int. J. Cancer* 108, 404–411.

Nozawa, H., Nakao, W., Zhao, F. and Kondo, K. (2005). *Mol. Nutr. Food Res.* 49, 772–778.

Nozawa, H., Nakao, W., Takata, J., Arimoto-Kobayashi, S. and Kondo, K. (2006). *Cancer Lett.* 235, 121–129.

Ohta, T., Nakatsugi, S., Watanabe, K., Kawamori, T., Ishikawa, F., Morotomi, M., Sugie, S., Toda, T., Sugimura, T. and Wakabayashi, K. (2000). *Carcinogenesis* 21, 937–941.

Pool-Zobel, B.L., Bertram, B., Knoll, M., Lambertz, R., Neudecker, C., Schillinger, U., Schmezer, P. and Holzapfel, W.H. (1993). *Nutr. Cancer* 20, 271–281.

Russo, J., Russo, I.H., Rogers, A.E., van Zwieten, M.J. and Gusterson, B. (1990). *IARC Sci. Publ.*, 47–78.

Sanyal, R., Darroudi, F., Parzefall, W., Nagao, M. and Knasmuller, S. (1997). *Mutagenesis* 12, 297–303.

Sasaki, Y.F., Tsuda, S., Izumiyama, F. and Nishidate, E. (1997). *Mutat. Res.* 388, 33–44.

Schut, H.A. and Yao, R. (2000). *Nutr. Cancer* 36, 52–58.

Shirai, T., Sano, M., Tamano, S., Takahashi, S., Hirose, M., Futakuchi, M., Hasegawa, R., Imaida, K., Matsumoto, K., Wakabayashi, K., Sugimura, T. and Ito, N. (1997). *Cancer Res.* 57, 195–198.

Singh, N.P., McCoy, M.T., Tice, R.R. and Schneider, E.L. (1988). *Exp. Cell Res.* 175, 184–191.

Sugimura, T. (1997). *Mutat. Res.* 376, 211–219.

Sugimura, T., Nagao, M. and Wakabayashi, K. (1996). *Environ. Health Perspect.* 104, 429–433.

Takahashi, M., Totsuka, Y., Masuda, M., Fukuda, K., Oguri, A., Yazawa, K., Sugimura, T. and Wakabayashi, K. (1997). *Carcinogenesis* 18, 1937–1941.

Tavan, E., Cayuela, C., Antoine, J.M., Trugnan, G., Chaugier, C. and Cassand, P. (2002). *Carcinogenesis* 23, 477–483.

Tayek, J.A., Istfan, N.W., Jones, C.T., Hamawy, K.J., Bistrian, B.R. and Blackburn, G.L. (1986). *Cancer Res.* 46, 5649–5654.

Tice, R.R., Agurell, E., Anderson, D., Burlinson, B., Hartmann, A., Kobayashi, H., Miyamae, Y., Rojas, E., Ryu, J.C. and Sasaki, Y.F. (2000). *Environ. Mol. Mutagen.* 35, 206–221.

Turesky, R.J., Rossi, S.C., Welti, D.H., Lay Jr., J.O. and Kadlubar, F.F. (1992). *Chem. Res. Toxicol.* 5, 479–490.

Turesky, R.J., Constable, A., Richoz, J., Varga, N., Markovic, J., Martin, M.V. and Guengerich, F.P. (1998). *Chem. Res. Toxicol.* 11, 925–936.

Wargovich, M.J., Jimenez, A., McKee, K., Steele, V.E., Velasco, M., Woods, J., Price, R., Gray, K. and Kelloff, G.J. (2000). *Carcinogenesis* 21, 1149–1155.

Xu, M., Bailey, A.C., Hernaez, J.F., Taoka, C.R., Schut, H.A. and Dashwood, R.H. (1996). *Carcinogenesis* 17, 1429–1434.

Yamagishi, M., Natsume, M., Osakabe, N., Nakamura, H., Furukawa, F., Imazawa, T., Nishikawa, A. and Hirose, M. (2002). *Cancer Lett.* 185, 123–130.

Yang, H., Holcroft, J., Glickman, B.W. and De Boer, J.G. (2003). *Mutagenesis* 18, 195–200.

Yoshikawa, T., Kimura, S., Hatano, T., Okamoto, K., Hayatsu, H. and Arimoto-Kobayashi, S. (2002). *Food Chem. Toxicol.* 40, 1165–1170.

66

Maize Beer Carcinogenesis: Molecular Implications of Fumonisins, Aflatoxins and Prostaglandins

Zodwa Dlamini, Zukile Mbita and Lindiwe Skhosana University of the Witwatersrand, Wits Medical School, Johannesburg, South Africa

Abstract

The most thirst-quenching beverage at the end of a hard-working day is beer, yet it is associated with detrimental effects to human health in many instances. Consumption of maize in the form of beer or food has risks associated with it. This is because of contaminations that are found in maize and the most prevalent contaminant found in maize is the fungus, *Fusarium*. Unfortunately this fungus is associated with cancer predisposition in both Africa and the rest of the world. These fungi are the sources of mycotoxins that have been shown to be cancer causing toxins as exemplified by fumonisin B_1 produced by another species of the genus *Fusarium*, that is *F. verticilloides*. These mycotoxins inhibit the apoptotic machinery by inhibiting the ceramide synthase thus leading to cell proliferation and tumorigenesis. Genetic alterations contribute hugely in the development of cancer in humans, such as the cancer of the esophagus, Kaposi's sarcoma and liver cancer. These alterations are abnormally found in tumor suppressors and oncogenes. Tumor suppressors like p53 are very important in the cell cycle control of which deregulation results in cancer development. Mutations in codon 249 of p53 have been linked to contamination of maize by aflatoxins.

Other mycotoxins, fumonisins, are involved in the production of reactive nitrogen species, which induce nitrative stress and are main contributors to carcinogenesis by inducing DNA damage leading to mutations of tumor suppressor gene like p53.

High intake of linoleic acid in a diet deficient in other polyunsaturated fatty acids and in riboflavin results in high tissue production of prostaglandin E2 (PGE2), which in turn causes inhibition of the proliferation and cytokine production. It has been postulated that this association is due to the conversion, in the stomach mucosa, of the linoleic acid contained in maize meal to PGE2. The proportion of non-esterified linoleic acid available in the stomach is therefore being an important factor in cancer predisposition. High levels of non-esterified linoleic acid in the diet cause increased production of PGE2 and profoundly affect the normal pH and fluid content that creates a predisposition to carcinogenesis. High linoleic acid diet contributes to oxidative stress leading to a marginal increase in oxidative DNA damage.

Intervention strategies that aim to reduce dietary exposure in the population need to focus on maize consumption in particular and educating communities that are main consumers of maize beer/products.

Introduction

Maize is a staple food in many African countries. In these countries, it is also used in the making of traditional maize beer. In the process of traditional beer making, the maize is fermented, cooked and fermented again. After the second fermentation, the product is sieved to produce a thick opaque liquid containing solid suspensions. In South Africa, mainly those with low socio-economic standards consume this type of beer because it is readily available and cost effective. Beer is the most thirst-quenching beverage at the end of a hard-working day or during festive seasons, yet it is associated with detrimental effects in most cases. Evolution of beer brewing dates back some thousand years during which there was poor sanitation in contrast to modern times. But during those days, there were few illnesses as compared to modern life, may be this can be attributed to other factors rather than beer drinking.

Fumonisins are a group of mycotoxins produced primarily by *Fusarium moniliforme*. *Fusarium* is a family of fungi that grow freely in maize (Isaacson, 2005). The occurrence of these organisms in maize is dependent on environmental factors and the storage of maize, for example, *Fusarium* grows maximally when the moisture content of the harvested corn is between 18% and 23% (Musser and Plattner, 1997). This shows that the way traditional maize beer is prepared, which involves double fermentation process, favors the growth of the *Fusarium* species. *Fusarium* produces a wide range of mycotoxins (about 28 types) called fumonisins,

Beer in Health and Disease Prevention
ISBN: 978-0-12-373891-2

fumonisin B_1 (FB_1) being the most prevalent in contaminated corn and the most toxic one (Musser and Plattner, 1997). This is a world problem; it does not only affect third world countries but also first world counties like Italy (Francheschi *et al.*, 1990). Unfortunately this fungus is associated with cancer predisposition in both Africa, where maize is used on a daily basis, and the rest of the world. These mycotoxins have been linked to carcinogenesis as exemplified by FB_1 produced by another species of the genus *Fusarium*, that is *F. verticilloides*. This toxin increases the risk of developing esophageal cancer. Beer drinking may not be a problem but contaminated maize that the beer is made from is being the bearer of the problem. Other crops like a hop plant have been documented to have a protective ability against different cancers (Miranda *et al.*, 1999; Chen and Lin, 2004). This does not mean that drinking beer from hops is completely safe because it also contains carcinogenic metabolites like acetaldehyde that has been documented to be responsible for promoting tumor growth (Salaspuro, 2003) (Figure 66.1).

FB_1, FB_2 and FB_3 are the ones present in naturally contaminated foods, with B_1 being the most toxic of the three. The toxicity of FB_1 is through inhibition of ceramide synthase that catalyzes the formation of dihydroceramide from sphingosine. This mechanism of action leads to antiapoptotic effects resulting to a variety of pathologies observed when this mycotoxin is consumed and backed by a high rate of human esophageal cancer and promotion of primary liver cancer (Figure 66.2) (Soriano *et al.*, 2005).

Fumonisins are also known to produce reactive nitrogen species (RNS). It has been reported that free radicals such as reactive oxygen species (ROS) and reactive nitrogen species (RNS), which induce oxidative and nitrative stress, are main contributors to oral carcinogenesis. The RNS (nitrosamines: nitrates and nitrites) are also produced by the reaction of ROS and other free radicals with nitric oxide (NO). The increase in ROS and RNS leads to the oxidative damage of the DNA and proteins, and possibly the promotion of esophageal squamous cell carcinoma. The oxidized proteins and DNA is a direct link between free radicals, antioxidants and esophageal squamous cell carcinoma (Bahar *et al.*, 2006) (Figure 66.3).

Aflatoxins are another family of fungal toxins that are carcinogenic to man and cause immunosuppression and growth reduction in animals. The consumption of maize is an important source of aflatoxin exposure. Higher AF-alb adducts have been correlated with higher *A. flavus* (CFU) infestation of maize ($p = 0.006$), higher aflatoxin contamination (ppb) of maize ($p < 0.0001$) and higher consumption frequencies of maize ($p = 0.053$) (Egal *et al.*, 2005).

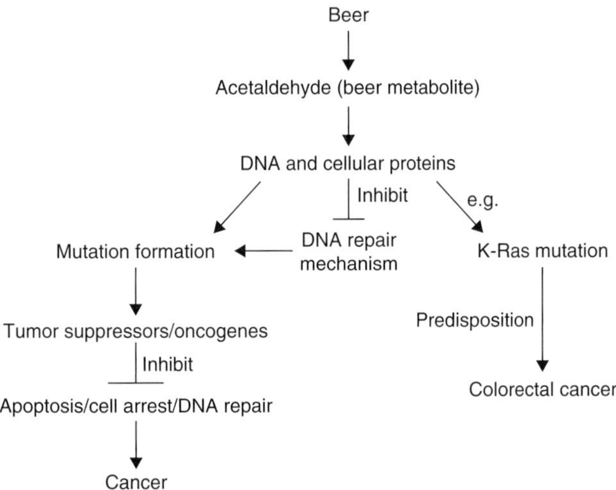

Figure 66.1 General effects of beer consumption. Alcohol metabolite, acetaldehyde, causes mutations in tumor suppressors and oncogenes by inducing replication errors and mutations and also aggravates the situation by interfering with the DNA repair mechanism to damage caused by alkylating agents. An example of predisposition to cancer development due to resultant mutation is the formation of K-Ras mutation where there may be either G to A transition or G to T transversion.

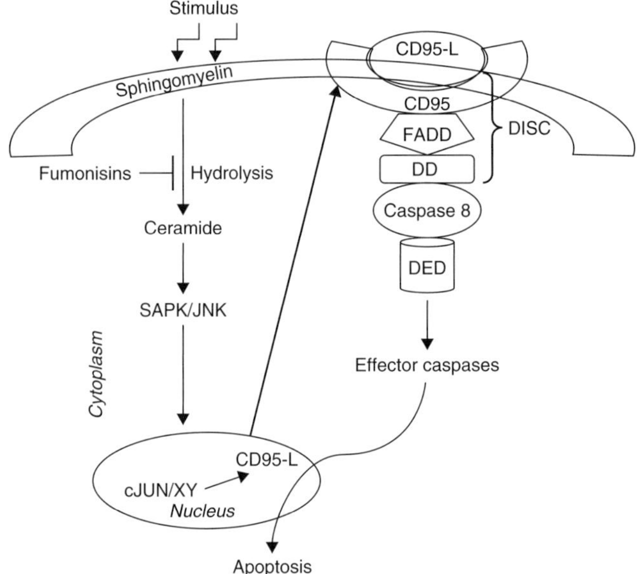

Figure 66.2 The effects of fumonisins on the apoptotic machinery. FB_1 inhibits the activity of sphingosine *N*-acyltransferase (ceramide synthase) and this reduces the conversion of [3H]sphingosine to [3H]ceramide. This inhibits the ceramide apoptotic pathway and this inhibition promotes cell growth and carcinogenesis.

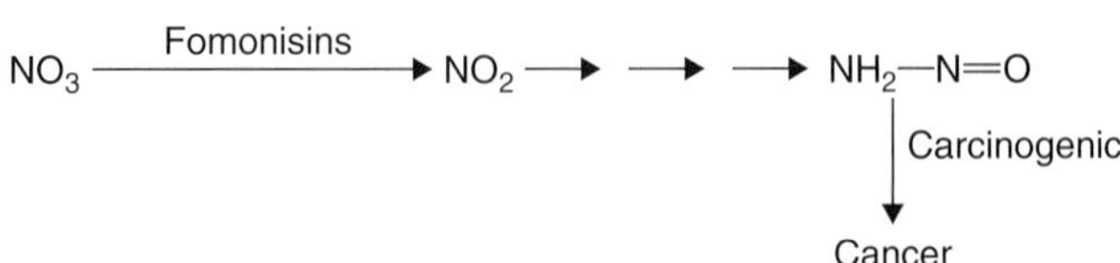

Figure 66.3 The effects of RNS resulting from fumonisins contaminated maize. Fumonisins reduce nitrates that are prevalent in the maize like in the vegetables, to nitrite that in turn form nitrosating agents in the stomach and form nitrosamines. High levels of nitrosamines induce tumor formation.

Interactions between hepatitis B virus (HBV) infection and exposure to aflatoxins have been linked to the development of hepatocellular carcinoma (HCC). Aflatoxins and HBV are major risk factors for HCC in high incidence areas for this cancer, namely South East Asia and parts of Africa. There is evidence from both epidemiological studies and animal models that the two factors can act synergistically to increase the risk of HCC (Sylla *et al.*, 1999). Aflatoxin contamination has been linked to mutation in a p53, a tumor suppressor gene responsible for cell cycle regulation. In several cancers, the distribution of mutation types and sites follow a specific pattern reflecting the effects of environmental mutagens. An example for such a "mutagen fingerprint" is p53 mutation at codon 249 in HCC in regions of the world characterized by high levels of the mutagen aflatoxin B_1 and endemic HBV infection (Le Roux *et al.*, 2005). Chronic infection with the HBV and exposure to aflatoxins in foodstuff are the main risk factors. A G to T transversion at codon 249 of the p53 gene {249(ser)} is commonly found in HCCs from patients in regions with dietary aflatoxins exposure (Stern *et al.*, 2001) (Figure 66.4).

Maize meal has also been reported to predispose to prevalent squamous cancer of the esophagus in Africa: The breakdown of esterified linoleic acid to the free form in stored meal leads to increased intragastric prostaglandin E2 (PGE2) production and a low-acid reflux. It has been reported that prevalent esophageal cancer in Africa is associated with the use of maize meal as a staple food and it is also used in making beer. This cancer has been shown to have a strong statistical association with the intake of foods based on maize in the meal form. The prevalence of esophageal cancer and association with the consumption of maize meal have also been shown in a region of Italy. An important factor is the breakdown of esterified linoleic acid to the free form in stored maize meal. And this leads to excess production of PGE2 in the stomach. The excess of PGE2 is a basis for a low-acid duodenogastroesophageal reflux and that predisposes to tumorigenesis (Sammon and Iputo, 2006) (Figure 66.5).

The carcinogenic effects of fumonisins, aflatoxins and PGE2 are summarized in Table 66.1.

Health measures including poverty alleviation, health education, monitoring and control of maize meal storage and content may be required to reduce the incidence of this disease in Africa and worldwide. Intervention strategies that aim to reduce dietary exposure in the population need to focus on maize consumption in particular. Specific hepatitis virus B (HBV), hepatitis virus C (HCV) and aflatoxins biomarkers reveal the complexity of risks contributing to HCC and suggest further application of these biomarkers as intermediate end points in prevention, intervention trials and etiologic investigations. It should be remembered that alcohol works synergistically with smoking in cancer predisposition as is supported by many previous studies (Dlamini and Bhoola, 2005).

Maize Beer and Esophageal Cancer

Esophageal cancer is the sixth most common cancer in the world and the second most common in Black South African men (Dlamini and Bhoola, 2005). Esophageal cancer is caused by several factors: genetic (Wu *et al.*, 1979), lifestyle (like smoking) and socio-economic status (Craddock, 1992; Shepard *et al.*, 2005).

The content of fumonisins in the maize beer ranges between 43 and 1,329 ng/ml (Shepard *et al.*, 2005), and the FB_1 being the major analog. Regular drinkers take between 1,050 and 4,130 ml/day of the traditional beer. When these

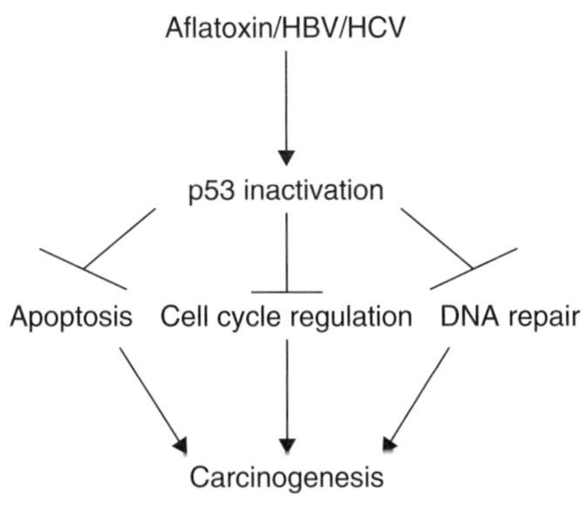

Aflatoxin/HBV/HCV

p53 inactivation

Apoptosis Cell cycle regulation DNA repair

Carcinogenesis

Figure 66.4 The effects of aflatoxin contamination and HBV co-infection. The tumor suppressor protein p53 mediates cell cycle arrest, DNA repair and apoptosis when stimulated by different forms of cellular stresses. When activated, this "master protein" modulates its response depending on the type and intensity of the stress. When this master regulator is inactivated by possible effects of aflatoxins or hepatitis virus infection, the consequences are increased cell proliferation and tumor formation.

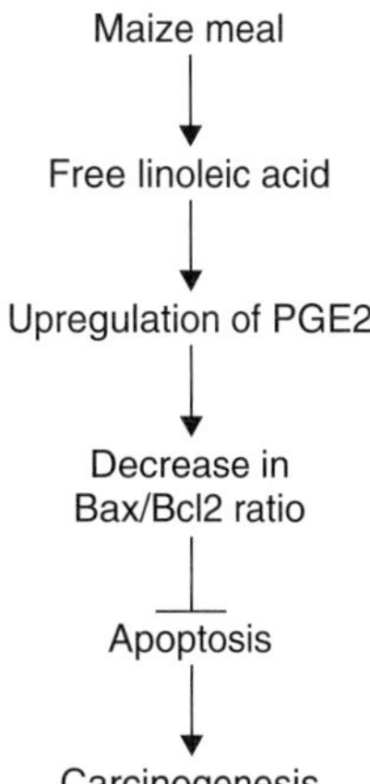

Figure 66.5 Effects of free linoleic acid from maize meal used for brewing maize beer. Free linoleic acids found in maize meal result in excess production of PGE2, lead to the decrease of the Bax/Bcl2 ratio resulting in the inhibition of the intrinsic apoptotic pathway, and this result in cancer.

Table 66.1 Predisposition to cancer due to maize contamination

Maize contaminant	*Mode of action*	*Effect/s*
Fumonisins	1. Reduce nitrates to reactive nitrogen species (nitrosamines) 2. Inhibit ceramide synthase	DNA damage and cancer predisposition Inhibition of ceramide apoptotic pathway leading to cell proliferation and carcinogenesis
Aflatoxins	p53 inactivation by mutations mostly at codon 249	p53 mutations lead to deregulation in the apoptotic machinery, cell cycle leading to tumorigenesis
Increased free linoleic acid in maize meal (used for making maize beer)	Leads to decrease in the Bax/Bcl2 ratio	Increased Bcl2 anti-apoptotic gene products lead to decrease in apoptosis and increased cell proliferation resulting in cancer formation

Note: Summary of effects of maize contaminants (aflatoxins, fumonisins) and increased levels of prostaglandins in maize meal used in maize beer brewing.

are translated into FB_1 consumption, the per capita exposure is between 6.5 and 25.4 μg/kg b.w./day, which is way above the recommended exposure limit of 2 μg/kg b.w./day set by the Food and Agriculture Organization (Shepard *et al.*, 2005).

Fumonisins present a threat in both human and animal health. In humans, these mycotoxins have been implicated in esophageal cancer (Nikander *et al.*, 1991; Rheeder *et al.*, 1992; Shepard *et al.*, 2005). The prevalence of esophageal cancer coincides with maize beer consumption in South Africa (Shepard *et al.*, 2005) and Tanzania (Nikander *et al.*, 1991). These mycotoxins reduce nitrate to nitrite, which leads to the synthesis of the carcinogenic nitrosamines (Isaacson, 2005). Nitrosamines are present in cigarette and alcoholic beverages including maize beer, hence cigarette smoking is always implicated in cancer development. *N*-nitrosamines have been reported to induce tumors of the esophagus (Myburg *et al.*, 2002) (Figure 66.3).

Fumonisins are also the causative agents of leukophalomacia in horses and pulmonary edema in pigs (Harrison *et al.*, 1990). In rats, fumonisins have been reported to cause lesions on the liver and esophageal cancer (Gelderblom *et al.*, 2001). Comparative toxicity studies of the *Fusarium* in different animal species showed that the major target organs differ in each species (Kriek *et al.*, 1981).

Predisposition to esophageal carcinoma is also linked to the form in which maize is consumed, for example, maize meal. Maize is milled before it can be used in a beer making process. In this form the esterified linoleic acid is broken down into free form. In the stomach freed linoleic acid promotes the excess production of PGE2, a proinflammatory bioactive lipid (Sammon and Iputo, 2006). Too much PGE2 predisposes the esophagus and the stomach to carcinogenesis. Downregulation of PGE2 is associated to an increased inhibition of cell growth and increased apoptosis in cancer cells (Lev-Ari *et al.*, 2006). Apoptosis inhibition in the body is a major cause of cancer development. Any substance that alters the apoptotic gene expression will cause carcinogenesis.

Free linoleic acid is responsible for cancer predisposition of the esophagus and the stomach. This contrasts the effect of conjugated linoleic acids have. These have been reported to possess an anticarcinogenic effect (Park *et al.*, 2004). These linoleic acids exert this by decreasing the levels of PGE2 produced. Free linoleic acid has been implicated in the progression of breast cancer cell solid tumors in athymic nude mice through excess PGE2 production (Connolly *et al.*, 1999). PGE2 plays a key role in carcinogenesis by modulating different pathways like apoptosis induced by tumor necrosis-alpha (Nishimura *et al.*, 2006), mitochondrial apoptotic pathway through alteration of Bax/Bcl2 ratio to favor apoptosis (Park *et al.*, 2004) and interaction with prostaglandin dehydrogenase, PGDH (Mann *et al.*, 2006) (Figure 66.5).

Maize Beer and Kaposi's Sarcoma

Kaposi's sarcoma is a mesenchymal tumor associated with human herpes virus-8 (HHV-8) infection. Given the association between consumption of traditional maize beer and high serum ferritin, iron concentration, the association between Kaposi's sarcoma and maize beer consumption has been reported. The association between maize traditional beer and the development of Kaposi's sarcoma has been reported in East and Central Africa (Ziegler *et al.*, 2001). In South Africans, the association was also found, but it was marginal (Wojcicki *et al.*, 2003). The association can be explained by high concentration of ionized, bioavailable iron as a result of being brewed and fermented in iron-clad pots. The concentration of iron in traditional beer prepared in iron-clad pots is about 82 mg/l (Goedert *et al.*, 2002).

The pathogenic role of iron in cancer development and/or progression has been documented. Several pathways leading to cancer development that involve iron have been described (Reichard and Ehrenberg, 1983; Cazzola *et al.*, 1990; Weinberg, 1996).

Iron and cell division

Iron is an essential element for dividing cells. It is involved in the incorporation of the enzymes that play a role in cellular metabolism. Iron also directly promotes the growth of some cancer cells by facilitating the reduction of ribonucleotides to deoxyribonucleotides (Cazzola *et al.*, 1990).

Iron and mutagenic hydroxyl radicals

Iron may promote the formation of mutagenic hydroxyl radicals (Weinberg, 1996). In humans excess iron has harmful consequences. Excess iron also accelerates oxidative catabolism of ascorbic acid (vitamin C), leading to deficiency of this vitamin (Kasvosve *et al.*, 2000). Vitamin C provides antioxidant protection because it is a free radical scavenger. In the presence of excess iron, vitamin C has a pro-oxidant activity. Iron gets trapped within ferritin as Fe^{3+} and enters the pores of the ferritin where it is converted to Fe^{2+}; vitamin C becomes oxidized in the process. Fe^{2+} then leaks out of the ferritin protein and generates free radicals (Delanghe *et al.*, 1998).

Iron and CD4 activity inhibition

Iron excess diminishes host defenses through inhibition of the activity of CD4 lymphocytes and through the suppression of the tumoricidal action of macrophages (Weinberg, 1996). During iron overload, excess iron is stored in parenchymal cells and macrophages, which interferes with $CD4^{+}$ proper functioning (Weinberg, 1996).

Iron and viral nucleic acid production by host cell

Iron can enhance the production of viral nucleic acids by the host (Boelaert *et al.*, 1996). The process involves free radicals and the activation of NF-κB (Gaynor, 1992). This may lead to development of Kaposi sarcoma, which is caused by HHV-8 (Wojcicki *et al.*, 2003).

Maize and Liver Carcinoma

Maize seems to be the target of fungal contaminations that consequently results in accumulation of aflatoxins, for example, aflatoxin B_1 (AB_1). Many staple food crops (maize, rice and wheat) are contaminated by *Aspergillus* molds that produce aflatoxin B_1. This toxin has been linked to prevalence of primary liver cancer in the Eastern Cape region of South Africa (van Rensburg *et al.*, 1990). Apparently this region uses maize as its staple food crop. Aflatoxins have been characterized as one of the major risk factors of HCC (Hsia *et al.*, 1992; Wild *et al.*, 1993; Sylla *et al.*, 1999; Turner *et al.*, 2002). These studies suggest that maize beer drinking predisposes to liver cancer due to the maize contamination by aflatoxins.

Consumption of food contaminated with aflatoxins B_1 is enough to promote carcinogenic phenotypes. Different reports from different regions have highlighted the effects these aflatoxins have on carcinogenesis. It is probably not only due to aflatoxins consumption because these cases also have HBV and HCV infections. It is apparent that aflatoxins, HBV and HCV affect p53 cell death regulation, apoptotic modulation through mutation formation. Association of these mutations with aflatoxins and hepatitis virus accumulation suggests their involvement in hepatic carcinogenesis through p53 inactivation. Tumor suppressor, p53, mediates cell cycle arrest, DNA repair and apoptosis in response to different cellular stresses (Le Roux *et al.*, 2005). A common mutation that is found in p53 worldwide in HCC is at codon 249. This mutation may be the bases of pathogenesis caused by aflatoxins and hepatitis viruses. In China (Stern *et al.*, 2001) and India (Katiyar *et al.*, 2000), this type of mutation has been reported in HCC and also other parts of the world. This strongly points to p53 mutation involvement in HCC pathogenesis (Figure 66.5).

Summary Points

- Consumption of maize in the form of home brewed beer has major health risks associated with it.
- The health risks are associated with mainly the effects of mycotoxins associated with maize used in making home brewed maize beer in most low socio-economic populations.
- Mycotoxins that are culprits include both fumonisins and aflatoxins and these are linked to the pathogenesis of cancers that are prevalent in countries where maize is a staple diet and its storage leaves much to be desired.
- According to our knowledge in low socio-economic communities stored rotting maize is not discarded but is mainly used in making home brewed beer. This rotting maize is highly contaminated with mycotoxins that have a predisposition to cancer especially esophageal squamous cell carcinoma and liver cancer.
- Fumonisins are involved in generating RNS that are involved in DNA damage and mutations involving the tumor suppressors.
- The aflatoxins contaminated beer consumption and co-infection with HBV lead to liver cancer. HBV and aflatoxins are said to work synergistically in predisposition to liver cancer. The contamination with aflatoxins is associated with mutation in codon 249 of p53 tumor suppressor protein that is involved in cell cycle regulation.
- Grinding of maize corn to maize meal powder form (milling) that is used in home brewed beer making is also detrimental to human health. The process converts

esterified linoleic acid to a free form which leads to the accumulation of PGE2 that is implicated in carcinogenesis especially esophageal squamous cell carcinoma. This is attributed to the increased Bcl2 to Bax ratio leading to antiapoptotic effects.

- Storage of maize meal should be done in a way that inhibits its contamination with mycotoxins. The public should be encouraged to avoid making maize as staple food and also avoid, or at least limit, the consumption of maize beer. It can be a challenge to do this in poverty stricken third world countries that mainly depend on maize related foods for their survival.

References

Bahar, G., Feinmesser, R., Shpitzer, T., Popovtzer, A. and Nagler, R.M. (2006). *Med. Hypotheses* 67, 1431–1436.

Boelaert, J.R., Weinberg, G.A. and Weinberg, E.D. (1996). *Infect. Agents Dis.* 5, 36–46.

Cazzola, M., Bergamaschi, G., Dezza, L. and Arosio, P. (1990). *Blood* 75, 1903–1919.

Chen, W.J. and Lin, J.K. (2004). *J. Agric. Food Chem.* 52, 55–64.

Connolly, J.M., Gilhooly, E.M. and Rose, D.P. (1999). *Nutr. Cancer* 35, 44–49.

Craddock, V.M. (1992). *Eur. J. Cancer Prev.* 2, 89–103.

Delanghe, J.R., Langlois, M.R., Boelaert, J.R. *et al.* (1998). *AIDS* 12, 1027–1032.

Dlamini, Z. and Bhoola, K. (2005). *Ethn. Dis.* 15, 786–789.

Egal, S., Hounsa, A., Gong, Y.Y., Turner, P.C., Wild, C.P., Hall, A.J., Hell, K. and Cardwell, F. (2005). *Int. J. Food Microbiol.* 104, 215–224.

Francheschi, S., Bidoli, E., Baron, A.E. and Vecchia, C. (1990). *J. Natl. Cancer Inst.* 82, 1407–1411.

Gaynor, R. (1992). *AIDS* 6, 347–363.

Gelderblom, W.C., Abel, S., Smuts, C.M., Marnewick, J., Marasas, W.F., Lemmer, E.R. and Ramljak, D. (2001). *Environ. Health Perspect.* 109, 291–300.

Goedert, J.J., Vitale, F., Lauria, C., Serriano, D., Tamburini, M., Montella, M., Messina, A., Brown, E.E., Rezza, G., Gafa, L. and Roamano, N. (2002). *J. Natl. Cancer Inst.* 20, 1712–1718.

Harrison, L.M., Colvin, B.M., Greene, J.T., Newman, L.E. and Cole Jr., J.R. (1990). *J. Vet. Diagn. Invest.* 2, 217–221.

Hsia, C.C., Kleiner Jr., D.E., Axiotis, C.A., Di Bisceglie, A., Nomura, A.M., Stemmermann, G.N. and Tabor, E. (1992). *J. Natl. Cancer Inst.* 84, 1619–1620.

Isaacson, C. (2005). *Med. Hypotheses* 64, 658–660.

Kasvosve, I., Gomo, Z.A., Mvundura, E., Moyo, V.M., Saungweme, T., Khumalo, H., Gordeuk, V.R., Boelaert, J.R., Delanghe, J.R., De Bacquer, D. and Gangaidzo, I.T. (2000). *Int. J. Tuberc. Lung Dis.* 4, 771–775.

Katiyar, S., Dash, B.C., Thakur, V., Guptan, R.C., Sarin, S.K. and Das, B.C. (2000). *Cancer* 89, 2322–2323.

Kriek, N.P.J., Kelleman, T.S. and Marasas, W.F.O. (1981). *Onderstepoort. J. Vet. Res.* 48, 129–131.

Le Roux, E., Gormally, E. and Hainaut, P. (2005). *Rev. Epidemiol. Sante Publique* 53, 257–266.

Lev-Ari, S., Maimon, Y., Strier, L., Kazanov, D. and Arber, N. (2006). *J. Soc. Integr. Oncol.* 4, 21–26.

Mann, J.R., Backlund, M.G., Buchanan, F.G., Daikoku, T., Holla, V.R., Rosenberg, D.W., Dey, S.K. and DuBois, R.N. (2006). *Cancer Res.* 66, 6649–6656.

Miranda, C.L., Stevens, J.F., Helmrich, A., Henderson, M.C., Rodriquez, R.J., Yang, Y.H., Deinzer, M.L., Barnes, D.W. and Buhler, D.R. (1999). *Food Chem. Toxicol.* 37, 271–285.

Musser, S.M. and Plattner, R.D. (1997). *J. Agric. Food Chem.* 45, 1169–1173.

Myburg, R.B., Dutton, M.F. and Chutergoon, A.A. (2002). *Environ. Health Perspect.* 10, 813–815.

Nikander, P., Seppälä, T., Kilonzo, G.P., Huttunen, P., Saarinen, L., Kilima, E. and Pitkanen, T. (1991). *Trans. R. Soc. Trop. Med. Hyg.* 85, 133–135.

Nishimura, K., Setoyama, T., Tsumagari, H., Miyata, N., Hatano, Y., Xu, L., Jisaka, M., Nagaya, T. and Yokota, K. (2006). *Biosci. Biotechnol. Biochem.* 70, 2145–2153.

Park, H.S., Cho, H.Y., Ha, Y.L. and Park, J.H. (2004). *J. Nutr. Biochem.* 15, 229–235.

Reichard, P. and Ehrenberg, A. (1983). *Science* 221, 514–519.

Rheeder, J.P., Mararas, W.F.O., Thiel, P.G., Sydenham, E.W., Shephard, G.S. and van Schalkwyk, D.J. (1992). *Phytopathology* 82, 353–357.

Salaspuro, M.P. (2003). *Best Pract. Res. Clin. Gastroenterol.* 17, 679–694.

Sammon, A.M. and Iputo, J.E. (2006). *Med. Hypotheses* 67, 1431–1436.

Shepard, G.S., van der Westhuizen, L., Gatyeni, P.M., Somdyala, N.I.M., Burger, H. and Marasas, W.F.O. (2005). *J. Agric. Food Chem.* 53, 9634–9637.

Soriano, J.M., Gonzalez, L. and Catala, A.I. (2005). *Prog. Lipid Res.* 44, 345–356.

Stern, M.C., Umbach, D.M., Yu, M.C., London, S.J., Zhang, Z.Q. and Taylor, J.A. (2001). *Cancer Epidemiol. Biomarkers Prev.* 10, 617–625.

Sylla, A., Diallo, M.S., Castegnaro, J. and Wild, C.P. (1999). *Mutat. Res.* 428, 187–196.

Turner, P.C., Sylla, A., Diallo, M.S., Castegnaro, J. and Wild, C.P. (2002). *J. Gastroenterol. Hepatol.* 17, S441–S448.

van Rensburg, S.J., van Schalkwyk, G.C. and van Schalkwyk, D.J. (1990). *Cancer Epidemol. Biomarker Prev.* 1, 229–234.

Weinberg, E.D. (1996). *Eur. J. Cancer Prev.* 5, 19–36.

Wild, C.P., Jansen, L.A., Cova, L. and Montesano, R. (1993). *Environ. Health Perspect.* 99, 115–122.

Ziegler, J.L., Simonart, T. and Snoeck, R. (2001). *J. Clin. Virol.* 20, 127–130.

67
The Relationship Between Beer Consumption and Lung Cancer

Douglas E. Paull and Alex G. Little Department of Surgery, Boonshoft School of Medicine, Wright State University, Dayton, OH, USA

Abstract

The study of beer consumption and the risk of lung cancer is complicated by the fact that beer drinkers have increased rates of cigarette smoking. Nonetheless, roughly one-half of all the retrospective case control and prospective cohort studies performed, in which the confounding effects of cigarette smoking have been carefully adjusted for, demonstrate a significant increase in the risk of the development of lung cancer among beer drinkers compared to non-drinkers. The increased risk is relatively moderate, odds ratio/relative risks between 1.3 and 2. The increased risk of lung cancer is most often limited to the heaviest beer consumers. Similar increases in lung cancer risk are demonstrated for consumers of hard liquor (whiskey, vodka, "spirits"). Moderate consumption of red wine clearly decreases the risk of lung cancer. Alcohol consumption is associated with worse outcomes among patients with established lung cancer. Data regarding lung cancer treatment outcomes and specific beer consumption are not available. Heavy alcohol consumption leads to more postoperative complications, primarily respiratory and infectious, among patients undergoing resection for early stage lung cancer. Further, heavy alcohol consumption correlates with less response to chemotherapy and worse survival in patients treated for advanced lung cancer. There are a number of molecular mechanisms that account for the increased risk of lung cancer among alcohol and beer consumers and the poor outcomes among alcohol consumers with lung cancer.

Abbreviations/Definitions

AWS – Alcohol withdrawal syndrome. Syndrome consisting of tremor; elevated pulse, respiratory rate, and temperature; insomnia; anxiety; and seizures associated with a sudden decrease in alcohol intake in an alcoholic patient.

Case control study. Unlike prospective cohort studies, case control studies are done after the fact. Patients who experienced an outcome (the *cases*) (e.g. lung cancer) are identified and then the number exposed to some risk factor (e.g. alcohol abuse) are counted. The *controls* are patients similar in relevant ways to the cases, but who did not experience the outcome (e.g. do not have lung cancer). The number of *controls* exposed to the risk factor can be counted and compared to the *case* group.

CI – Confidence interval. The probability that the *true* average, as opposed to the *observed* average, of a population is within the given limits. For example, if the *observed* mean age of a population is reported as 62 years (95% CI 58–64) then there is a 95% probability that the *true* mean age for the population lies between 58 and 64 years. The larger the population studied, the more powerful the study, and the more "narrow" the CI becomes for any given observation.

Cohort, prospective study. Two groups of patients, similar in most aspects except for some risk factor (e.g. alcohol usage) are followed over time for the development of a disease (e.g. lung cancer). The number of patients developing the disease are counted and compared among the two groups who differ only in exposure to the risk factor. Note the difference between this type of study and a case control study.

ECOG – Eastern Cooperative Oncology Group.

HR – Hazard ratio. Suppose we are comparing survival rates of lung cancer among alcohol abusers and non-abusers. Let us say that alcohol abusers are dying at twice the rate than non-abusers. The HR for alcohol abuse would be 2.0. The *HR* can be calculated for any given variable (e.g. alcohol abuse (yes/no), age, etc.). For every unit increase in the value of the variable studied, the risk of the event (in this case, death) changes by a factor equal to the *HR*.

Multivariate analysis. A more advanced statistical analysis that permits looking at variables all together rather than just one at a time. Let us consider the example of the dependent variable/outcome of respiratory failure following resection of lung cancer. Independent variables which might be associated with such an outcome include preoperative pulmonary function tests such as the forced expiratory volume in 1 s (FEV1) measured in liters, pack year smoking history (pack years), and/or alcohol abuse (drinks/day). This could be described in an equation as follows during a multivariate analysis:

Respiratory failure = (−2.0) FEV1 + (1.2) pack years + (2.3) drinks/day.

Beer in Health and Disease Prevention
ISBN: 978-0-12-373891-2

The coefficients in the equation state that any unit increase in the independent variable (e.g. increase of 1 pack year of smoking) results in an increase in the mean value of the respiratory failure by a factor equal to the coefficient (e.g. 1.2 units for each increase in 1 pack year). In the example given, a larger preoperative FEV1 is associated with less respiratory failure following resection (negative coefficient), whereas an increase in preoperative smoking or drinking is associated with an increase in postoperative respiratory failure (positive coefficients).

NSCLC – Non-small cell lung cancer. Histologic type of lung cancer. Vast majority of lung cancer consists of NSCLC. Small cell lung cancer makes up the smaller remainder of cases. Treatment strategies are different for non-small cell and small cell lung cancer. There are a number of histologic sub-types making up NSCLC including: adenocarcinoma, squamous cell carcinoma, and large cell carcinoma.

NK cells – Natural killer cells. Lymphocytes, white blood cells, which attack and kill malignant cells in the body.

OR – Odds ratio. Used in comparing data from case control studies. The OR is the odds of exposure in cases/odds of exposure in controls. For example, in a case control study involving alcohol abuse and lung cancer, the following data were obtained:

Group	*Lung cancer*	*No lung cancer*
Alcohol abusers	10	90
Non-abusers	5	95
Total	15	185

Odds of alcohol abuse among *cases* (patients with lung cancer) = (10/15)/(5/15) = 2.0.

Odds of alcohol abuse among controls (patients without lung cancer) = (90/185)/(95/185) = 1.0.

The *OR* would be 2.0/1.0 = 2.0.

In this study, patients with lung cancer were twice as likely to be alcohol abusers compared to patients without lung cancer, suggesting a relationship between alcohol abuse and the development of lung cancer.

p-value. The probability of obtaining a value of the test statistic as large or larger than the one computed from the data when in reality there is no difference between the two groups. For example, a study shows that the 5-year-survival rate was 30% for alcohol abusing patients with lung cancer and 60% for non-abusing patients, with a p-value of <0.05. The question is whether the observed survival differences between the two groups of patients are *real*, or simply due to the *random* variation associated with placing patients in one of the two groups. The smaller the p-value the more likely the differences are real. By convention, a p-value < 0.05 is considered statistically significant. In the study example above, there is less than a 5% chance that the observed differences in survival rates were simply random events, and one would conclude that alcohol abuse was associated with worse survival among patients with lung cancer.

RR – Relative risk. The *RR* is similar to the OR. Whereas the OR is used for case control studies, the *RR* is utilized in cohort, prospective studies. The probability of an event (e.g. lung cancer) among people exposed to a risk factor (e.g. alcohol abuse) is compared to people who are not exposed to the risk factor (e.g. non-abusers). The data from such a hypothetical study are shown below:

Group	*Lung cancer*	*No lung cancer*	*Total*
Alcohol abuse	20	180	200
No alcohol abuse	5	195	200
Total	25	375	

The *RR* would be (20/200)/(5/200) = 4.0.

In this hypothetical study, alcohol abuse was associated with a 4 times greater chance of developing lung cancer.

Introduction

The purpose of this chapter is to examine the effects of alcohol-containing beverages, including beer, upon the epidemiology and treatment of lung cancer. Specifically, we hope to demonstrate that beer consumption: (1) increases the incidence of lung cancer and (2) leads to worse outcomes in the treatment of lung cancer.

For the purposes of this chapter, "alcohol," "total alcohol," and "overall alcohol" consumption refer to ingestion of any alcohol-containing beverage including beer, hard liquor, wine, or combination thereof. Consumption is converted into a universal unit since an individual may drink more than one type of alcohol-containing beverage. For example, in a given study, a patient drinking one glass of hard liquor and four cans of beer per day has a total alcohol consumption of five "drinks per day." Other studies have reported total alcohol consumption in grams/day, ounces/day, "whiskey equivalents"/day, and a variety of other units. "Hard liquor" consumption refers to ingestion of whiskey, vodka, or "spirits." Studies may variably report data for only total alcohol consumption, only specific beverage consumption (e.g. beer, wine, hard liquor), or both total alcohol and specific beverage consumption.

In reporting the risk associated with alcohol consumption and lung cancer, retrospective case control studies will report an odds ratio (OR), odds of exposure to alcohol in lung cancer patients (cases)/odds of exposure in patients without lung cancer (controls), while prospective cohort studies report a relative risk (RR), probability of lung cancer in patients drinking alcohol/probability of lung cancer in non-drinking patients (Glantz, 2005). These ratios are derived by comparing the incidence of lung cancer at a given drinking level with the incidence of lung cancer among non-drinkers or to the lowest drinking level.

Lung cancer represents the most common cause of cancer death in most Western countries (Ahrendt *et al.*, 2000). The most important risk factor is cigarette smoking which accounts for over 90% of all lung cancer (Woodson *et al.*, 1999). Nonetheless, there is accumulating evidence suggesting a relationship between alcohol consumption, particularly beer or liquor, and the development of lung cancer, even when the confounding variable of cigarette smoking is carefully adjusted for. The relationship between alcohol use and the development of lung cancer is complicated by the fact that alcohol drinkers have different lifestyles than non-drinkers. Alcohol drinkers are more likely to be cigarette smokers, eat less fruits and vegetables, consume less vitamin A and folate, and have lower socioeconomic status than non-drinkers (Bandera *et al.*, 1992, 2001; Hu *et al.*, 2002; Benedetti *et al.*, 2006). Each of these co-variables is associated with a higher incidence of lung cancer. Even if alcohol consumption were not independently associated with the development of lung cancer, its modulation of other risk factors such as smoking and lifestyle would have important implications in the prevention of lung cancer.

Alcohol is not considered a carcinogen, but rather a promoter or co-carcinogen. Alcohol has been postulated to induce lung cancer by a number of molecular mechanisms. Acetaldehyde, the primary metabolite of alcohol, impairs DNA repair. Alcohol induces free radicals which cause cell membrane damage. Alcohol, via the cytochrome P450 system, alters the liver's metabolism of carcinogens, such as benzopyrenes, in cigarette smoke. The consumption of alcohol is associated with dietary deficiencies which lead to immunosuppression, impaired immunosurveillance, and the development of cancer. Finally, other substances contained within the alcohol beverages are carcinogenic, including asbestos, aromatic hydrocarbons, and pesticide residues (Bandera *et al.*, 2001). The relevant exposure period of alcohol in the development of lung cancer is different than for cigarette smoking. Lung cancer risk is closely associated with cigarette smoking levels 15 years prior to lung cancer mortality whereas recent alcohol consumption is more closely associated with lung cancer risk, again emphasizing smoking as a carcinogen, and alcohol as a promoter (Potter and McMichael, 1984). Alcohol use has been associated with p53 mutations in human lung cancer (Ahrendt *et al.*, 2000). The tumor suppressor protein p53 is the most commonly mutated gene in human cancers, including lung cancer. Gene expression profile analysis of lung cancer specimens has shown that alcohol drinkers have higher p53 mutation rates than non-drinkers. The results are not explained by cigarette smoking. Alcohol drinkers, who are non-smokers, have more frequent p53 mutations than non-drinkers.

The most conservative epidemiologic view is that any relationship between alcohol use and lung cancer is either explained by the confounding effects of cigarette smoking in non-adjusted studies, or by residual confounding even in those studies carefully adjusting for cigarette smoking (Carpenter *et al.*, 1998; Woodson *et al.*, 1999; Bandera *et al.*, 2001; Djousse *et al.*, 2002). However, on balance, there seems to be a relationship between alcohol consumption and the incidence of lung cancer after careful adjustment for cigarette smoking and other covariates. In those studies supporting a relationship, heavy alcohol consumption is most closely associated with an increased risk of lung cancer (Prescott *et al.*, 1999).

Total Alcohol Consumption and the Risk of Lung Cancer

Overview

Several collective reviews and meta-analyses regarding alcohol consumption and lung cancer have been published. Potter and McMichael were the first to emphasize the relationship between alcohol use and lung cancer risk (Potter and McMichael, 1984). Eight out of ten prospective studies they reviewed demonstrated that high alcohol consumers and alcoholics were at greater risk for lung cancer, even after adjustment for levels of cigarette smoking. Bandera reviewed eight case control and nine prospective cohort studies (Bandera *et al.*, 2001). Four of eight case control studies demonstrated a positive relationship between alcohol consumption and lung cancer risk. The results from cohort studies were inconsistent, and in those studies where a positive correlation was demonstrated, it was generally limited to higher levels of alcohol consumption. In the two studies of never smokers, one study demonstrated a positive relationship between alcohol consumption and lung cancer risk. Overall, it was concluded that the cumulative evidence suggested a relation between alcohol use and lung cancer. Similarly, another meta-analysis of 7 prospective studies and 3,137 lung cancer patients using pooled, adjusted RR demonstrated an association between lung cancer and alcohol use in never-smoking men (Freudenheim *et al.*, 2005).

Studies favoring a relationship between *total alcohol consumption* and lung cancer risk

A number of studies suggest a relationship between alcohol use and lung cancer (Table 67.1). Pollack investigated a cohort of 7,837 males of whom 89 developed lung cancer as part of the Honolulu Heart Study (Pollack *et al.*, 1984). A dose response was demonstrated between increasing alcohol consumption and increasing risk of lung cancer, even when adjusted for age and smoking. The adjusted incidence of lung cancer for those drinking ≥40 oz./month of alcohol was 130/100,000 person years as compared to 70/100,000 for non-drinkers. Interestingly, patients in this

Table 67.1 Results of studies of *total alcohol consumption* and the risk of lung cancer[a]

Study (year)[b]	*Location*	*Number of lung cancer cases*	*Adjusted RR or OR of lung cancer*	*95% CI*
Woodson (1999)	Finland	1,059	1.0	0.8–1.1
Bandera (1992)	New York	280	1.60	1.0–2.5
Benedetti (2006)	Canada	699	1.5	1.0–2.10
Hu (2002)	Canada	161	0.8	0.5–1.2
Potter (1984)	Hawaii	89	1.86	n/a
Carpenter (1998)	Los Angeles	261	0.68	0.33–1.41
Djousse (2002)	Massachusetts	269	1.3	0.7–2.4
Prescott (1999)	Denmark	480	1.57	1.06–2.33
Freudenheim (2005)	United States, Canada, Europe	3,137	1.21	0.91–1.61
Nishino (2006)	Japan	377	0.97	0.66–1.43
Zang (2001)	United States	4,575	1.2	1.0–1.4
Freudenheim (2003)	New York	273	1.35	0.54–3.41
DeStefani (2002)	Uruguay	160	1.2	0.6–2.1

Notes: All results reported are adjusted for smoking. In addition, studies variably adjusted for age, sex, race, education, body mass index, income, dietary intake of fruits and vegetables, dietary fat, exposure to environmental smoke, and/or family history of lung cancer. Adjusted RR (prospective cohort studies) or OR (retrospective case control studies) reported compares highest risk drinking level to either lowest risk drinking level or to non-drinkers. Table reflects highest value of adjusted RR or OR reported from study whether among men and women combined, men only, or women only.

n/a: not available/reported.

[a] *Total alcohol consumption* refers to the ingestion of any combination of alcohol-containing beverages including beer, wine, and hard liquor.

[b] Studies listed in order in which they appear in text of chapter. Every study cited in the text in which an OR or RR is reported for total alcohol consumption and lung cancer risk is listed in table.

study were light drinkers, suggesting that heavy consumption was not a prerequisite for increased lung cancer risk. Nonetheless, even in this carefully performed study, the authors warn of residual confounding from cigarette smoking. In a series of three prospective studies from Denmark involving 28,160 men and women, heavy alcohol consumption (≥41 drinks/week) was correlated with increased lung cancer risk, RR = 1.57 (95% confidence interval (CI) 1.06–2.33, p = 0.002, adjusted for age, smoking, and education) (Prescott *et al.*, 1999).

In a case control study of 280 white male lung cancer patients and 564 controls, as part of the Western New York Diet Study, Bandera reported an OR of 1.6 (CI 1.0–2.5, p = 0.03, adjusted for age, education, and dietary intake of carotenoids and fat) among consumers of >22 drinks/month vs. those taking in 0–1 drinks/month (Bandera *et al.*, 1992). This relationship was limited to patients smoking ≥41 pack years.

Studies that do not favor a relationship between *total alcohol consumption* and lung cancer risk

Several prospective studies have failed to demonstrate a correlation between alcohol consumption and lung cancer risk. As part of the Alpha-Tocopherol Beta-Carotene Cancer Prevention Study in Finland, 1,059 lung cancer patients among 27,111 male smokers were studied (Woodson *et al.*, 1999). They found no association between total alcohol consumption and lung cancer in a regression model adjusted for age, smoking, and intervention. In the Japan Collaborative Study for the Evaluation of Cancer Risk, a cohort study of 28,536 Japanese males including 377 lung cancer deaths, there was no association of increased mortality from lung cancer for light (<25 g/day), moderate (25–49.9 g/day), or heavy drinking (≥50 g/day) (Nishino *et al.*, 2006). Data from the Framingham Study and the Framingham Offspring Study including 9,238 participants and 269 cases of observed lung cancer, demonstrated similar overall findings (Djousse *et al.*, 2002). Although in crude analysis increasing alcohol consumption correlated strongly with an increasing incidence of lung cancer; these differences disappeared once adjusted for smoking. However, 89% of patients in that study drank <3 drinks per day, and therefore the influence of heavy alcohol use and lung cancer risk could not be fully evaluated. Interestingly, in the Offspring cohort, drinking >24 g/day was associated with an increased risk of lung cancer (RR = 2.0, CI 0.7–5.7, adjusted for age, sex, and smoking status).

A number of case control studies have demonstrated no relationship between alcohol use and lung cancer risk (Zang *et al.*, 2001; Freudenheim *et al.*, 2003). A study of 261 lung cancer patients and 615 population-based controls in Los Angeles County, found no association between total alcohol intake and lung cancer risk (Carpenter *et al.*, 1998). Pack years smoking was closely associated with the level of alcohol consumption. The number of pack years smoking was highest for those with highest alcohol consumption, again emphasizing the importance of residual confounding by cigarette use. In a study of males in

Uruguay involving 160 patients with adenocarcinoma of the lung and 520 hospitalized controls, there was an OR of 2.4 (CI 1.4–4.2, $p < 0.001$) for the risk of lung cancer in the crude analysis comparing the highest quartile of alcohol use to the lowest quartile of alcohol use (DeStefani *et al.*, 2002). However, after adjustment for smoking, the effect was lost. The authors demonstrated that the greater care used to adjust for levels of smoking (pack years, current smoker, years since quitting, age started smoking) the less the effect of alcohol use upon the risk of lung cancer. The National Enhanced Cancer Surveillance System studied Canadian women who never smoked (Hu *et al.*, 2002). There were 161 patients with lung cancer compared to 483 population-based controls matched for age and residence. Lung cancer patients had lower education level, income, and social class compared to controls. After adjustment for covariates, there was no association of total alcohol consumption and lung cancer risk.

Other aspects of *total alcohol consumption* and lung cancer risk

A case control study from the MD Anderson Cancer Center of 470 lung cancer patients and 472 population-based controls demonstrated a significant reduction of lung cancer risk among alcohol drinkers with increasing dietary folate consumption (OR = 0.48, CI 0.28–0.82, $p = 0.002$, highest vs. lowest quartile folate consumption, adjusted for age, sex, ethnicity, total energy intake, body mass index, family history of lung cancer, and pack years smoking) (Shen *et al.*, 2003). These results support the hypothesis that the increased risk of lung cancer seen among alcohol consumers may be at least partly due to folate deficiency, and that the increased risk may be ameliorated by folate supplementation.

Among patients undergoing liver transplantation, Jimenez reported a higher incidence of lung cancer among alcoholic patients than among non-alcoholic patients (4.3% vs. 0.7%, $p < 0.001$) (Jimenez *et al.*, 2005). The association, however, was largely attributed to heavy cigarette smoking among the alcoholic group. Alcoholic transplant recipients who developed lung cancer had uniformly advanced disease on presentation, and all died despite treatment with a mean survival of only 5.3 months. Such studies, as well as our own to be discussed later, suggest that not only does total alcohol consumption lead to an increased incidence of lung cancer, but that such consumption also leads to worse survival in patients with lung cancer.

Summary: *total alcohol consumption* and lung cancer risk

There are data from carefully performed prospective and case control studies, adjusting for cigarette smoking, to suggest that alcohol use is associated with an increased incidence of lung cancer. Taking into account the studies that fail to show this causative relationship, a reasonable conclusion is that the association between alcohol use and lung cancer risk is not great, and the effect is most evident among heavy alcohol users and abusers rather than mild to moderate users. Any association between alcohol use and lung cancer is weaker than that confirmed between alcohol use and, for example, oral cancers. The RR for oral cancer among alcohol users even after adjustment for smoking is much higher (RR = 8.8, CI 5.4–14.3, among males drinking ≥30 drinks/week vs. ≤1 drink/week, adjusted for smoking, age, race, study location, and respondent status) (Blot *et al.*, 1988).

Although the independent effect of alcohol consumption upon the risk of lung cancer is relatively small, alcohol consumption is associated with lifestyles that are associated with lung cancer development. Efforts to curb alcohol consumption would be expected to favorably affect such additional behaviors and indirectly decrease lung cancer incidence. In the Working Well Trial in Washington State, a cohort study of 6,867 participants, a dose response between smoking and drinking alcohol was demonstrated (McClure *et al.*, 2002). Baseline drinking level was the best predictor of the ability of an individual to quit smoking at a 4-year follow-up. These results demonstrate that efforts to curb alcohol drinking will lead to less cigarette smoking, and ultimately reduce lung cancer risk.

Beer Consumption and the Risk of Lung Cancer

Overview

Geography is important in investigation of specific alcohol-containing beverages and the incidence of lung cancer. Individuals of different cultures and regions in the world vary in which beverage is most popular. For example, beer, the most common alcoholic drink in the United States, has frequently been associated with an increased risk of lung cancer in US studies (Bandera *et al.*, 2001). In these studies, the number of individuals drinking other beverages, such as wine, is often so limited as to exclude them from statistical analysis. In studies from Poland, where vodka drinking is more prevalent, that beverage has been associated with an increased risk of lung cancer (Rachtan, 2002). There are also different lifestyles, behaviors, and diets associated with the consumption of specific alcohol-containing beverages. Beer drinkers consume more total alcohol, smoke more cigarettes, have less education, and eat less vegetables and fruits than individuals who drink wine (McCann *et al.*, 2003). Moreover, even among individuals within the same location, there can be widely different behaviors associated with consumption of sub-types of the same beverage. For example, malt liquor

Table 67.2 Results of studies of *beer consumption* and the risk of lung cancer[a]

Study (year)[b]	*Location*	*Number of lung cancer cases*	*Adjusted RR or OR of lung cancer*	*95% CI*
Woodson (1999)	Finland	1,059	0.9	0.7–1.1
Bandera (1992)	New York	280	1.6	1.0–2.4
Benedetti (2006)	Canada	699	1.9	1.3–2.9
Hu (2002)	Canada	161	1.2	0.6–2.4
Carpenter (1998)	Los Angeles	261	0.95	0.48–1.86
Prescott (1999)	Denmark	480	1.36	1.02–1.82
Freudenheim (2005)	United States, Canada, Europe	3,137	1.88	1.45–2.42
Freudenheim (2003)	New York	273	1.36	0.82–2.27
DeStefani (2002)	Uruguay	160	0.9	0.1–5.6
Potter (1992)	Iowa	109	2.0	1.02–3.80
Zatloukal (2003)	Czechloslavkia	366	1.32	0.83–2.09
Ruano-Ravina (2004)	Spain	132	1.10	0.59–2.08
Chow (1992)	United States	219	1.8	1.1–3.0

Notes: All results reported are adjusted for smoking. In addition, studies variably adjusted for age, sex, race, education, body mass index, income, dietary intake of fruits and vegetables, dietary fat, exposure to environmental smoke, and/or family history of lung cancer. Adjusted RR or OR reported compares highest risk beer drinking level to either lowest risk beer drinking level or to non-drinkers. Table reflects highest value of adjusted RR or OR reported from study whether among men and women combined, men only, or women only.

[a] Only studies where *beer consumption* specifically studied included.

[b] Studies listed in order in which they appear in text of chapter. Every study cited in the text in which an OR or RR is reported specifically for beer consumption and lung cancer risk is listed in table.

beer drinkers in Los Angeles County consume more total alcohol, combine smoking and drinking more often, and exhibit adverse social behaviors compared to "regular" beer drinkers (Bluthenthal *et al.*, 2005). Depending on the population studied, the beverage of choice, and the confounding variables involved and adjusted for; the results linking a specific beverage to lung cancer may appear inconsistent, especially if any true association is weak. Nonetheless, there are multiple studies implicating beer consumption with an increased risk of lung cancer, Table 67.2.

Studies favoring a relationship between *beer consumption* and lung cancer risk

In a collective review, 7 of 11 epidemiologic studies reviewed demonstrated a relationship between beer consumption and an increased risk of lung cancer and in two of those studies a dose response relationship was established (Bandera *et al.*, 2001). In a carefully performed study, adjusting for smoking/age/education/dietary intake of carotenoids, drinkers of >12 beers/month had a RR of 1.6 (CI 1–2.4, p = 0.003) compared to non-drinkers of beer (Bandera *et al.*, 1992). In a Canadian case control study involving 1,793 cases and 1,975 age/sex matched controls, there was an increasing OR of lung cancer with increasing beer intake (Benedetti *et al.*, 2006). The lung cancer OR was 1.2 (CI 0.9–1.7) and 1.5 (1.1–2.1) for men drinking 1–6 beers/week and ≥7 beers/week, respectively. These data were adjusted for age, smoking, ethnicity, income, and education. In a cohort study of 41,837 Iowa women, the RR of lung cancer after adjustment for smoking was 2.0 (1.02–3.80) among those drinking ≥1 beer/week compared to those drinking <1 beer/week (Potter *et al.*, 1992).

Studies that do not favor a relationship between *beer consumption* and lung cancer risk

Several studies have failed to demonstrate a relationship between beer consumption and an increased risk of lung cancer (Pollack *et al.*, 1984; Woodson *et al.*, 1999; DeStefani *et al.*, 2002; Zatloukal *et al.*, 2003; Ruano-Ravina *et al.*, 2004), and in at least one study an inverse relationship was found (Carpenter *et al.*, 1998). In a study demonstrating no increased risk of lung cancer among "current" beer drinkers, an increased risk of lung cancer was demonstrated among "former" drinkers of beer (RR = 1.8, CI 1.1–3.0, adjusted for age, smoking, and occupation). The authors believed former beer drinkers had heavy consumption in the past, and that drinking cessation may have been due to health related problems (Chow *et al.*, 1992).

Summary: *beer consumption* and lung cancer risk

Mechanisms postulated to explain observed increases in lung cancer risk among beer drinkers include: higher levels of nitrosamines in beer (Bandera *et al.*, 2001); residual confounding due to smoking (Carpenter *et al.*, 1998; Zang

Table 67.3 Results of studies of *hard liquor consumption* and the risk of lung cancer[a]

Study (year)[b]	*Location*	*Number of lung cancer cases*	*Adjusted RR or OR of Lung Cancer*[a]	*95% CI*
Woodson (1999)	Finland	1,059	1.1	0.9–1.3
Bandera (1992)	New York	280	1.1	0.7–1.6
Benedetti (2006)	Canada	699	1.5	0.9–2.6
Hu (2002)	Canada	161	1.1	0.6–2.1
Carpenter (1998)	Los Angeles	261	1.87	1.02–3.42
Prescott (1999)	Denmark	480	1.46	0.99–2.14
Freudenheim (2005)	United States, Canada, Europe	3,137	1.34	1.09–1.66
Freudenheim (2003)	New York	273	1.21	0.77–1.91
DeStefani (2002)	Uruguay	160	2.1	0.9–4.9
Potter (1992)	Iowa	109	1.1	0.6–2.3
Zatloukal (2003)	Czechloslavkia	366	0.85	0.53–1.37
Ruano-Ravina (2004)	Spain	132	1.64	0.79–3.40
Chow (1992)	United States	219	1.9	1.1–3.1
Rachtan (2002)	Poland	242	4.64	1.19–18.06

Notes: All results reported are adjusted for smoking. In addition, studies variably adjusted for age, sex, race, education, body mass index, income, dietary intake of fruits and vegetables, dietary fat, exposure to environmental smoke, and/or family history of lung cancer. Adjusted RR or OR reported compares highest risk hard liquor drinking level to either lowest risk drinking level or to non-drinkers. Table reflects highest value of adjusted RR or OR reported from study whether among men and women combined, men only, or women only.

[a] Only studies where *hard liquor consumption* specifically studied included. Hard liquor includes whiskey, vodka, and spirits. It does not include beer or wine consumption.

[b] Studies listed in order in which they appear in text of chapter. Every study cited in the text in which an OR or RR is reported specifically for hard liquor consumption and lung cancer risk is listed in table.

and Wynder, 2001; DeStefani *et al.*, 2002; McCann *et al.*, 2003); low fruit/vegetable consumption among beer drinkers (Benedetti *et al.*, 2006); and specific lifestyles among beer drinkers (McCann *et al.*, 2003). In summary, beer consumption, especially heavy beer consumption, even when adjusted for smoking, is associated with a moderately increased risk of lung cancer.

Hard Liquor Consumption and Lung Cancer Risk

The relationship between hard liquor consumption and the risk of lung cancer is similar to, if not greater in magnitude than, that described for beer. In studies demonstrating an association, there is usually an increased risk of lung cancer associated with heavy consumption of hard liquor. Confounding variables, especially cigarette smoking, are just as problematic.

In the Honolulu Heart Study where beer consumption was not associated with lung cancer risk, there was an increased risk of lung cancer for heavy whiskey consumption (≥50 oz. whiskey/month, RR = 2.62, p = 0.01, adjusted for age and smoking) compared to non-drinkers (Pollack *et al.*, 1984). Likewise, in the Los Angeles County Study in which beer consumption demonstrated a weak inverse correlation with lung cancer risk, consumption of hard liquor (≥1 drink/day) was strongly associated with lung cancer risk compared to consumers of 0–3 drinks/month (OR = 1.87, CI 1.02–3.42, p = 0.06, adjusted for smoking, diet, age, race, and sex) (Carpenter *et al.*, 1998).

In a case control study of Polish women involving 242 cases of lung cancer and 352 healthy controls, drinking of vodka was strongly associated with an increased risk of lung cancer even among lifetime non-smokers (RR = 15.0, CI 2.34–96.0, p = 0.000, adjusted for age, passive smoking, diet, residence, and occupational exposure) (Rachtan, 2002). This study also yielded a comparison of the individual and collective effects of hard liquor consumption and cigarette smoking upon the increased risk of lung cancer. Lifelong non-drinkers who smoked had a RR of 10.5 (CI 5.75–19.2, p = 0.000), and those who both drank vodka and smoked had a RR of 20.2 (CI 11.7–35.0, p = 0.000). These trends are similar to those demonstrated for hard liquor consumption, cigarette smoking, and oral cancer (Kabat and Wynder, 1989; Castellsague *et al.*, 2004). Additional studies have supported a positive correlation between hard liquor consumption and lung cancer risk (Prescott *et al.*, 1999) (Table 67.3).

Several studies have demonstrated no association between hard liquor consumption and an increased risk of lung cancer (Hu *et al.*, 2002; Ruano-Ravina *et al.*, 2004). In one such study demonstrating no association between current hard liquor use and lung cancer risk, past use of hard liquor correlated with increased lung cancer risk (Chow *et al.*, 1992).

Table 67.4 Results of studies of wine consumption and the risk of lung cancer[a]

Study (year)[b]	*Location*	*Number of lung cancer cases*	*Adjusted RR or OR of lung cancer*[a]	*95% CI*
Woodson (1999)	Finland	1,059	0.8	0.6–1.1
Bandera (1992)	New York	280	0.7	0.5–1.1
Benedetti (2006)	Canada	699	0.3	0.2–0.4
Hu (2002)	Canada	161	0.7	0.4–1.2
Carpenter (1998)	Los Angeles	261	0.60	0.29–1.25
Prescott (1999)	Denmark	480	0.44	0.22–0.86
Freudenheim (2005)	United States, Canada, Europe	3,137	0.66	0.51–0.87
Freudenheim (2003)	New York	273	0.80	0.51–1.25
DeStefani (2002)	Uruguay	160	0.4	0.2–1.1
Zatloukal (2003)	Czechloslavkia	366	0.46	0.23–0.92
Ruano-Ravina (2004)	Spain	132	0.43	0.19–0.96

Notes: All results reported are adjusted for smoking. In addition, studies variably adjusted for age, sex, race, education, body mass index, income, dietary intake of fruits and vegetables, dietary fat, exposure to environmental smoke, and/or family history of lung cancer. Adjusted RR or OR reported compares lowest risk wine drinking level to non-drinkers of wine. Table reflects lowest value of adjusted RR or OR reported from study whether among men and women combined, men only, or women only.

[a] Only studies where *wine consumption* specifically studied included.
[b] Studies listed in order in which they appear in text of chapter. Every study cited in the text in which an OR or RR is reported specifically for wine consumption and lung cancer risk is listed in table.

Wine Consumption **and Lung Cancer Risk**

Whereas beer and hard liquor consumption are associated with an increased risk of lung cancer, mild to moderate wine consumption is associated with a decreased risk of lung cancer (Prescott *et al.*, 1999; DeStefani *et al.*, 2002; Freudenheim *et al.*, 2005; Benedetti *et al.*, 2006) (Table 67.4). More specifically, red wine is associated with a decreased lung cancer risk, and white wine is not (Ruano-Ravina *et al.*, 2004). Additionally, the dose response curve for wine and lung cancer risk is U-shaped (Bandera *et al.*, 2001). Mild to moderate consumption decreases the risk whereas heavy wine consumption increases the risk. Authors have speculated that red wine contains antioxidants including flavonoids and resveratrol which inhibit carcinogenesis (DeStefani *et al.*, 2002). Alternative explanations include the fact that mild to moderate wine drinkers have higher education, greater incomes, lower smoking, higher dietary fruits/vegetables, and less dietary fat than those who do not drink wine (McCann *et al.*, 2003).

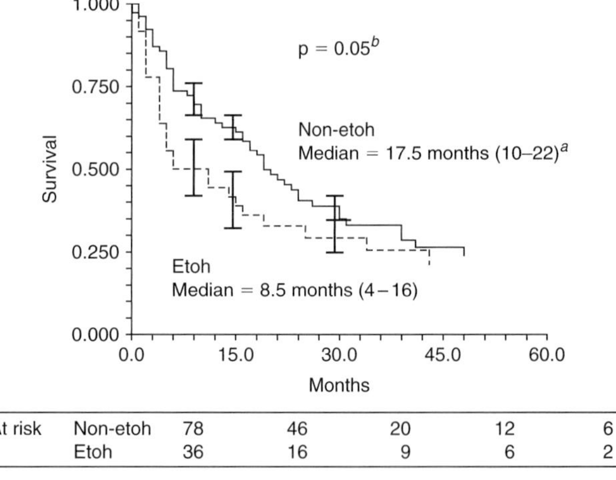

At risk						
	Non-etoh	78	46	20	12	6
	Etoh	36	16	9	6	2

Figure 67.1 Overall survival of 36 alcoholic patients and 78 non-alcoholic patients with non-small cell lung cancer. *Source*: Reprinted from Paull *et al.* (2005), Copyright (2005), with permission from the Society of Thoracic Surgeons. Etoh = alcoholic (broken line) patients defined as having any of the following: (1) CAGE screening questionnaire ≥2; (2) consuming ≥5 drinks/day; or (3) having a current DSM IV diagnosis of alcohol abuse/dependence. Non-etoh = non-alcoholic (solid line). [a] Median survival in months (95% CI). [b] Gehans-Wilcoxon log rank test.

Alcohol Consumption and Treatment Outcomes for Lung Cancer

Introduction

In addition to the risk of lung cancer development, there is evidence that alcohol use is an independent risk factor for poor outcomes in patients being treated for lung cancer (Paull *et al.*, 2005) (Figure 67.1). Heavy alcohol use specifically increases the morbidity and mortality of pulmonary resection among patients with early stage, resectable lung cancer (Neuenschwander *et al.*, 2002; Paull *et al.*, 2004a). Alcohol abusers have more respiratory and infectious complications than non-abusing controls undergoing similar operations. Among patients with more advanced, unresectable lung cancer, alcohol abuse may decrease response rates to chemotherapy (Paull *et al.*, 2004b). These adverse outcomes are not due to clinical cirrhosis, as these studies specifically excluded such patients. Furthermore, the worse outcomes associated with alcohol abuse do not appear to be solely due to differences in smoking, comorbidity, performance status, or nutritional status as these covariates have been adjusted for in multivariate analyses.

Alcohol abuse and the risk of pulmonary resection for lung cancer

Our group at University Affiliated VA Medical Center has studied alcohol abusing patients undergoing treatment for non-small cell lung cancer (NSCLC). Patients were classified as alcohol abusers if they exhibited any one of the following: CAGE screening questionnaire ≥ 2, consumption of ≥ 5 alcohol-containing drinks/day, or a current DSM IV diagnosis of alcohol dependence/abuse (303.90, 305.00). Using this classification, 32% of patients undergoing pulmonary resection for NSCLC were alcohol abusers. The alcohol-containing beverages consumed in this population included beer alone (47%), beer and hard liquor (33%), and hard liquor alone (20%).

Nineteen alcohol abusers were compared to 37 non-abusers undergoing resection for NSCLC. Despite similar pack years smoking, performance status, Charlson comorbidity, pulmonary function, stage of disease, operation, and operative blood loss, the two groups of patients had different postoperative outcomes (Paull *et al.*, 2004a). Alcohol abusers had an increase in infectious complications (37% vs. 5%, $p = 0.001$) and respiratory failure (42% vs. 5%, $p = 0.001$). These data closely resembled that reported several years earlier (Neuenschwander *et al.*, 2002) where patients consuming ≥ 5 drinks/day had a higher rate of infectious and respiratory complications (OR = 3.38, CI 1.02–11.2, $p = 0.047$). Whereas transfusion was believed to explain the findings in the latter study, in our study alcohol abuse was an independent and even stronger predictor of infectious and respiratory complications than transfusion in multivariate analysis. Alcohol abusers undergoing resection for NSCLC, as compared to non-abusers, had worse secondary outcomes including greater increase in postoperative Apache II scores (98% vs. 27%, $p = 0.008$), ventilator days (11.7 ± 7.4 vs. 0.7 ± 0.4, $p = 0.04$), fever days (3.9 ± 1.4 vs. 0.9 ± 0.3, $p = 0.007$), hospital days (26.1 ± 8.4 vs. 10.6 ± 1.8, $p = 0.02$), and costs (\$49,526 ± 17,525 vs. \$18,385 ± 3,260). Perioperative mortality was 16% (3/19) among abusers and 0% (0/37) for non-abusers.

Other studies support an increase of complications in alcohol abusing patients undergoing resection for NSCLC. One such study investigated the development of acute lung injury (ALI) following resection in 879 patients with NSCLC. ALI occurred in 4.2% patients (37/879), but was responsible for 43% of all perioperative deaths. In addition, ALI was associated with an increase in ICU and hospital stays. In a multivariate analysis, there were four independent risk factors identified for the development of ALI: high intraoperative airway pressures, excess perioperative fluid administration, pneumonectomy, and alcohol abuse (OR = 1.9, CI 1.1–4.6, $p = 0.01$) (Licker *et al.*, 2003).

Even in the absence of cirrhosis, alcohol abuse has a profound effect on postoperative physiology. Alcohol abuse is associated with immunosuppression, hematologic abnormalities, an exaggerated stress response, hypertension, cardiomyopathy, smoking, and comorbidities, all of which contribute to the 2–5 times increase in morbidity and mortality following surgeries (Tonnesen, 1992). In addition, the development of the alcohol withdrawal syndrome (AWS), which can occur despite prophylaxis, is associated with complications and death, as it was in one of three of the deaths in our study.

Despite the increase in postoperative morbidity and mortality experienced by alcohol abusers, long term survival following resection among operative survivors in our cohort of patients was similar for alcohol abusers and non-abusers (Paull *et al.*, 2004a). Three-year survival was 58% and 61% for abusers and non-abusers, respectively. In a Cox Proportional Hazards Model, stage of disease (hazard ratio (HR) = 3.29, $p = 0.03$), not alcohol abuse (HR = 1.36, $p = 0.61$), was the best predictor of long term survival.

A patient with early stage NSCLC who is reasonably fit and has resectable disease should not be denied operation because of alcohol abuse. Efforts should focus upon the early identification of the alcohol abusing patient preoperatively, followed by detoxification and counseling, AWS prophylaxis, and an awareness of the increase in infectious and respiratory complications. The immunosuppression associated with alcohol abuse abates within 4 weeks, during which time smoking cessation efforts can be instituted.

Alcohol abuse and treatment outcomes in patients with advanced lung cancer

Few studies have examined the effect of alcohol abuse upon outcomes in patients with advanced, unresectable NSCLC. In a study of 74 such patients with stage III and IV NSCLC, 24 alcohol abusers have worse outcomes than 50 non-abusers (Paull *et al.*, 2004b). Overall survival (9.5 vs. 13.8 months, $p < 0.05$) and progression-free survival (7.0 vs. 12.5 months, $p = 0.02$) were worse for abusers compared to non-abusers. In a Cox Proportionate Hazards Model, independent predictors of survival included alcohol abuse (HR = 1.82, $p = 0.03$) and ECOG performance status. Despite similar doses and toxicity of platin-based chemo-therapy, alcohol abuse was associated with lack of response to chemotherapy (response rates of 23% (3/13) for abusers vs. 59% (17/29) for non-abusers, $p = 0.05$). Alcohol abusers, compared to non-abusers were more likely to refuse at least one recommended component of their care (44%

Table 67.5 Multivariate analysis. Lung cancer outcome among 114 patients with NSCLC

	Univariate analysis	*Multivariate analysis*		
Outcome predictor variable	*p-value*	*Coefficient*	*Hazard/OR (95% CI)*	*p-value*
Overall survival[a,b]				
Stage	0.000	0.63	1.88 (1.49–2.36)	0.000
ECOG	0.000	0.46	1.58 (1.18–2.12)	0.002
Etoh	0.15			
Comorbidity	0.64			
Pack years smoking	0.82			
Disease-specific survival[a,c]				
Stage	0.000	0.67	1.95 (1.52–2.51)	0.000
ECOG	0.000	0.42	1.53 (1.12–2.08)	0.008
Etoh[b]	0.03	0.52	1.65 (1.01 2.80)	0.05
Comorbidity	0.89			
Pack years smoking	0.59			
Progression-free survival[a,d]				
Stage	0.000	0.69	1.99 (1.58–2.51)	0.000
ECOG	0.000	0.37	1.44 (1.08–1.93)	0.01
Etoh	0.06	0.58	1.79 (1.12–2.86)	0.01
Comorbidity	0.59			
Pack years smoking	0.48			
Progression of disease or death within 12 months[e]				
Stage	0.000	0.98		0.000
ECOG	0.000	1.12		0.002
Etoh	0.03	1.23	3.44 (1.17–10.1)	0.02
Comorbidity	0.58			
Pack years smoking	0.84			

CI: confidence interval; comorbidity: Charlson comorbidity score; ECOG: Eastern Cooperative Oncology Group performance index; Etoh = [b]CAGE ≥ 2, ≥5 drinks/day, or a current DSM IV diagnosis of alcohol dependence/abuse (303.90, 305.00).

[a] Cox proportional hazard regression with hazard ratio reported.
[b] Overall survival calculated from date of lung cancer tissue diagnosis to date of death due to any cause.
[c] Disease-specific survival calculated from date of lung cancer tissue diagnosis to date of death by lung cancer.
[d] Progression defined as a 20% increase in size of measurable disease or any new lesions. Progression-free survival calculated from date of lung cancer tissue diagnosis to date of progression.
[e] Logistic regression with OR reported.

Source: Reprinted from Paull *et al.* (2005), Copyright (2005), with permission from the Society of Thoracic Surgeons.

vs. 3%, $p = 0.001$), less likely to receive multimodality treatment (50% vs. 80%, $p = 0.05$), and received a lower total dose of radiation (4,145 ± 611 vs. 5,468 ± 238 cGy, $p = 0.03$). These outcome disparities between alcohol abusers and non-abusers were not explained by differences in performance status, stage, comorbidity, smoking history, pulmonary function, liver enzymes, or nutrition.

Summary: alcohol consumption and treatment outcomes for lung cancer

In a study of 114 consecutive patients with NSCLC, of whom 36 were abusers, we examined the effect of alcohol abuse upon outcomes for patients while adjusting for covariates stage of disease, comorbidity, performance status, and smoking history (Paull *et al.*, 2005). Alcohol abuse was an independent predictor of disease-specific survival, progression-free survival, and progression of disease or death within 12 months (Table 67.5).

Although this study would suggest otherwise, others have argued that alcohol abusers with lung cancer have worse outcomes as a function of increased comorbidities. In a study from the Josephine Ford Cancer Center of 1,155 lung cancer patients, alcohol abuse was an independent risk factor for an increase in comorbidity count (Tammemagi *et al.*, 2004). Furthermore, patients with a >3 comorbidity count were 4 times less likely to receive surgery for localized lung cancer and 5 times less likely to receive chemotherapy for advanced lung cancer.

The worse survival noted among alcohol abusers with lung cancer does not appear to be simply due to residual confounding by smoking or comorbidity. Alternative explanations include worse biologic behavior of tumors and/or impaired natural killer (NK) cell activity in alcohol abusers compared to non-abusers with lung cancer.

In a study of 188 patients with operable NSCLC, specimens were analyzed for p53 mutations using GeneChip and direct sequencing (Ahrendt *et al.*, 2003). Alcohol intake of even 1 drink/day was associated independently, after covariate adjustment, with an increase in p53 mutations. Furthermore, stage I NSCLC patients with p53 mutations had worse 4-year survival than wild-type patients (52% vs. 78%, respectively, $p = 0.009$).

In a laboratory animal model of lung tumor metastases, alcohol ingestion is associated with NK cell inhibition, and an increase in the number of metastases (Wu and Pruett, 1999). Studies in humans have demonstrated depressed NK cell activity in patients with alcoholic cirrhosis (Laso *et al.*, 1997) as well as in healthy volunteers consuming alcohol (Ochshorn-Adelson *et al.*, 1994). A study of social drinking examined the effects of drinking two cans of beer upon killer cell activity. Although NK cell activity was unaffected, interleukin 2-induced lymphokine activated killer cell activity was reduced compared to pre-alcohol blood samples ($p < 0.01$) (Bounds *et al.*, 1994). These studies would suggest that alcohol consumption impedes the immune system's ability to clear neoplastic cells, leading to either the development or progression of cancer. These findings, however, cannot be taken as definitive as other studies have not confirmed NK cell inhibition in chronic alcoholic patients or in healthy volunteers ingesting alcohol (Kronfol *et al.*, 1993; Li *et al.*, 1997).

Summary Points

- Alcohol consumption, even when adjusted for cigarette smoking, is associated with an increased risk of lung cancer.
- The study of alcohol consumption and lung cancer risk is complicated by the confounding effect of greater cigarette smoking among drinkers.
- The adjusted RR for lung cancer due to alcohol consumption (1–2 × non-drinkers) is less in magnitude than the RR for oral cancer due to alcohol consumption (8 × non-drinkers).
- Beer consumption is associated with an increased risk of lung cancer.
- Residual confounding by smoking is a major problem in the study of lung cancer among beer drinkers, as beer drinkers tend to have the greatest exposure to cigarette smoking.
- Heavy beer consumption (≥5 drinks/day, 60 oz.) is most closely related to the increased risk of lung cancer.
- The RR of lung cancer due to beer consumption is 1.2–2 times that of non-drinkers.
- Though the RR for lung cancer among beer drinkers is not high, the impact on society may be great in those countries, such as the United States, where the prevalence of beer drinking is high.
- The relationship between hard liquor and lung cancer is similar to that for beer.
- Wine, specifically red wine, consumed in mild to moderate quantities, reduces the adjusted risk of lung cancer roughly in half compared to wine non-drinkers.
- Heavy alcohol consumption, including beer, is associated with worse outcomes in the treatment of patients with lung cancer.
- Worse outcomes have been demonstrated for alcohol abusing patients receiving surgery for early stage as well as for those receiving chemotherapy for advanced stage lung cancer.
- The poor outcomes associated with heavy alcohol use are not solely due to differences in smoking history, comorbidity, performance status, or stage of disease.
- Alcoholic beverages, including beer, either promote the development of or lead to progression of lung cancer by a number of biologic mechanisms.

References

Ahrendt, S.A., Chow, J.T., Yang, S.C., Wu, L., Zhang, M., Jen, J. and Sidransky, D. (2000). *Cancer Res.* 60, 3155–3159.

Ahrendt, S.A., Hu, Y., Buta, M., McDermott, M.P., Benoit, N., Yang, S.C., Wu, L. and Sidransky, D. (2003). *J. Natl. Cancer Inst.* 95, 926–927.

Bandera, E.V., Freudenheim, J.L., Graham, S., Marshall, J.R., Haughey, B.P., Swanson, M., Brasure, J. and Wilkinson, G. (1992). *Cancer Causes Control* 3, 361–369.

Bandera, E.V., Freudenheim, J.L. and Vena, J.E. (2001). *Cancer Epidemiol. Biomarkers Prev.* 10, 813–821.

Benedetti, A., Parent, M.E. and Siemiatycki, J. (2006). *Cancer Causes Control* 17, 469–480.

Blot, W.J., McLaughlin, J.K., Winn, D.M., Austin, D.F., Greenberg, R.S., Preston-Martin, S., Bernstein, L., Schoenberg, J.B., Stemhagen, A. and Fraumeni, J.F. (1988). *Cancer Res.* 48, 3282–3287.

Bluthenthal, R.N., Brown-Taylor, D., Guzman-Becerra, N. and Robinson, P.L. (2005). *Alcohol. Clin. Exp. Res.* 29, 402–409.

Bounds, W., Betzing, K.W., Stewart, R.M. and Holcombe, R.F. (1994). *Am. J. Med. Sci.* 307, 391–395.

Carpenter, C.L., Morgenstern, H. and London, S.J. (1998). *J. Nutr.* 128, 694–700.

Castellsague, X., Quintana, M.J., Martinez, M.C., Nieto, A., Sanchez, M.J., Juan, A., Monner, A., Carrera, M., Agudo, A., Quer, M., Munoz, N., Herrero, R., Franceschi, S. and Bosch, F.X. (2004). *Int. J. Cancer* 108, 741–749.

Chow, W.H., Schuman, L.M., McLaughlin, J.K., Bjelke, E., Gridley, G., Wacholder, S., Co Chien, H.T. and Blot, W.J. (1992). *Cancer Causes Control* 3, 247–254.

DeStefani, E., Correa, P., Deneo-Pellegrini, H., Boffetta, P., Gutierrez, L.P., Ronco, A., Brennan, P. and Mendilaharsu, M. (2002). *Lung Cancer* 38, 9–14.

Djousse, L., Dorgan, J.F., Zhang, Y., Schatzkin, A., Hood, M., D'Agostino, R.B., Copenhafer, D.L., Kreger, B.E. and Ellison, R.C. (2002). *J. Natl. Cancer Inst.* 94, 1877–1882.

Freudenheim, J.L., Ram, M., Nie, J., Muti, P., Trevisan, M., Shields, P.G., Bandera, E.V., Campbell, L.A., McCann, S.E., Schunemann, H.J., Carosella, A.M., Vito, D., Russell, M., Nochajski, T.H. and Goldman, R. (2003). *J. Nutr.* 133, 3619–3624.

Freudenheim, J.L., Ritz, J., Smith-Warner, S.A., Albanes, D., Bandera, E.V., van den Brandt, P.A., Colditz, G., Feskanich, D., Goldbohm, R.A., Harnack, L., Miller, A.B., Rimm, E., Rohan, T.E., Sellers, T.A., Virtamo, J., Willet, W.C. and Hunter, D.J. (2005). *Am. J. Clin. Nutr.* 82, 657–667.

Glantz, S.A. (2005). *Primer of Biostatistics*, 6th edn. McGraw-Hill, New York. pp. 163–168.

Hu, J., Mao, Y., Dryer, D. and White, K. (2002). *Cancer Detect. Prev.* 26, 129–138.

Jimenez, C., Marques, E., Manrique, A., Loinaz, C., Gomez, R., Meneu, J.C., Perez, B., Moreno, A., Garcia, I. and Moreno, E. (2005). *Transplant. Proc.* 37, 3970–3972.

Kabat, G.C. and Wynder, E.L. (1989). *Int. J. Cancer* 43, 190–194.

Kronfol, Z., Nair, M., Hill, E., Kroll, P., Brower, K. and Greden, J. (1993). *Alcohol. Clin. Exp. Res.* 17, 279–283.

Laso, F.J., Madruga, J.I., Giron, J.A., Lopez, A., Ciudad, J., San Miguel, J.F., Alvarez-Mon, M. and Orfao, A. (1997). *Hepatology* 25, 1096–1100.

Li, F., Cook, R.T., Alber, C., Rasmussen, W., Stapleton, J.T. and Ballas, Z.K. (1997). *Alcohol. Clin. Exp. Res.* 21, 981–987.

Licker, M., de Perrot, M., Spiliopoulos, A., Robert, J., Diaper, J., Chevalley, C. and Tschopp, J.M. (2003). *Anesth. Analg.* 97, 1558–1565.

McCann, S.E., Sempos, C., Freudenheim, J.L., Muti, P., Russell, M., Nochajski, T.H., Ram, M., Hovey, K. and Trevisan, M. (2003). *Nutr. Metab. Cardiovasc. Dis.* 13, 2–11.

McClure, J.B., Wetter, D.W., de Moor, C., Cinciripini, P.M. and Gritz, E.R. (2002). *Addict. Behav.* 27, 367–379.

Neuenschwander, A.U., Pedersen, J.H., Krasnik, M. and Tonnesen, H. (2002). *Eur. J. Cardiothorac. Surg.* 22, 287–291.

Nishino, Y., Wakai, K., Kondo, T., Seki, N., Ito, Y., Suzuki, K., Ozasa, K., Watanabe, Y., Ando, M., Tsubono, Y., Tsuji, I. and Tamkoshi, A. (2006). *J. Epidemiol.* 16, 49–56.

Ochshorn-Adelson, M., Bodner, G., Toraker, P., Albeck, H., Ho, A. and Kreek, M.J. (1994). *Alcohol. Clin. Exp. Res.* 18, 1361–1367.

Paull, D.E., Updyke, G.M., Davis, C.A. and Adebonojo, S.A. (2004a). *Am. J. Surg.* 188, 553–559.

Paull, D.E., Updyke, G.M., Pacheco, J., Chin, H.W., Baumann, M. and Adebonojo, S.A. (2004b). *Chest* 126, 769S–770S.

Paull, D.E., Updyke, G.M., Baumann, M.A., Chin, H.W., Little, A.G. and Adebonojo, S.A. (2005). *Ann. Thorac. Surg.* 80, 1033–1039.

Pollack, E.S., Nomura, A.M.Y., Heilbrun, L.K., Stemmermann, G.N. and Green, S.B. (1984). *New Engl. J. Med.* 310, 617–621.

Potter, J.D. and McMichael, A.J. (1984). *Int. J. Epidemiol.* 13, 240–242.

Potter, J.D., Sellers, T.A., Folsom, A.R. and McGovern, P.G. (1992). *Ann. Epidemiol.* 2, 587–595.

Prescott, E., Gronbaek, M., Becker, U. and Sorensen, T.I.A. (1999). *Am. J. Epidemiol.* 149, 463–470.

Rachtan, J. (2002). *Lung Cancer* 35, 119–127.

Ruano-Ravina, A., Figueiras, A. and Barros-Dios, J.M. (2004). *Thorax* 59, 981–985.

Shen, H., Wei, Q., Pillow, P.C., Amos, C.I., Hong, W.K. and Spitz, M.R. (2003). *Cancer Epidemiol. Biomarkers Prev.* 12, 980–986.

Tammemagi, C.M., Neslund-Dudas, C., Simoff, M. and Kvale, P. (2004). *J. Clin. Epidemiol.* 57, 597–609.

Tonnesen, H. (1992). *Acta Psychiatr. Scand.* 86, 67–71.

Woodson, K., Albanes, D., Tangrea, J.A., Rautalahti, M., Virtamo, J. and Taylor, P.R. (1999). *Cancer Causes Control* 10, 219–226.

Wu, W.J. and Pruett, S.B. (1999). *Int. J. Cancer* 82, 886–892.

Zang, E.A. and Wynder, E.L. (2001). *Prev. Med.* 32, 359–370.

Zatloukal, P., Kubik, A., Pauk, N., Tomasek, L. and Petruzelka, L. (2003). *Lung Cancer* 41, 283–293.

68

Phenolic Beer Compounds to Prevent Cancer

Clarissa Gerhäuser German Cancer Research Center, Division Toxicology and Cancer Risk Factors, Workgroup Chemoprevention, Heidelberg, Germany

Abstract

Beer is a rich source of dietary polyphenols that are derived from malt (70–80%) and hop (20–30%). Structural classes include simple phenols, benzoic- and cinnamic acid derivatives, coumarins, catechins, di-, tri- and oligomeric proanthocyanidins, (prenylated) chalcones and various flavonoids. We have tested 48 beer phenolics representing 10 different structural classes in a series of test systems indicative of cancer preventive potential. These test systems measured (i) antioxidant effects, for example scavenging of DPPH, superoxide anion, peroxyl and hydroxyl radicals, (ii) modulation of carcinogen metabolism by reducing phase 1 Cyp1A activity and induction of phase 2 NAD(P)H:quinone reductase (QR) activity, (iii) anti-inflammatory mechanisms through inhibition of inducible nitric oxide synthase induction and inhibition of cyclooxygenase 1 activity and (iv) estrogenic and anti-estrogenic effects in Ishikawa cell culture. Gallic acid, catechins, proanthocyanidins and flavonols such as quercetin demonstrated the broadest range of antioxidant activity with scavenging potential against all radicals tested. Quercetin and the hop-derived chalcone xanthohumol were most potent in modulating xenobiotics metabolism. Gallic acid and xanthohumol inhibited iNOS induction, whereas (+)-catechin and (−)-epicatechin were the most potent Cox-1 inhibitors. Overall it became clear that beer compounds belonging to different structural classes have distinct profiles of biological activity in these *in vitro* test systems. Since carcinogenesis is a complex process, combination of compounds with complimentary activities may lead to enhanced preventive effects.

List of Abbreviations

AAPH	2,2,-Azobis-(2-amidinopropane) dihydrochloride
ALP	Alkaline phosphatase
β-PE	β-Phycoerythrin
CD	Concentration required to double the specific enzyme activity
CEC	3-Cyano-7-ethoxycoumarin
CHC	3-Cyano-7-hydroxycoumarin
Cox-1	Cyclooxygenase 1
Cyp1A	Cytochrome P450 1A
DPPH	1,1-Diphenyl-2-picrylhydrazyl radicals
Em	Emission
Ex	Excitation
HHBSS	Hanks balanced salt solution containing 30 mM Hepes, pH 7.8
IC_{50}	Half-maximal inhibitory concentration
iNOS	Inducible nitric oxide synthase
NBT	Nitro blue tetrazolium
$O_2^{-\bullet}$	Superoxide anion radical
OD	Optical density
$OH^{\bullet}$	Hydroxyl radical
ORAC	Oxygen radical absorbance capacity
PMA	Phorbol myristate acetate
PMS	Phenazine methosulfate
QR	NAD(P)H:quinone reductase
$ROO^{\bullet}$	Peroxyl radical
SC_{50}	Half-maximal scavenging concentration
SOD	Superoxide dismutase
XO	Xanthine oxidase

Introduction

Advances in our understanding of the carcinogenic process at the cellular and molecular level made over the past few decades have led to the development of a promising new approach to cancer prevention, termed "chemoprevention" (Sporn and Newton, 1979). Chemoprevention aims to halt or reverse the development and progression of precancerous cells through use of non-cytotoxic nutrients and/or pharmacological agents during the time period between tumor initiation and malignancy (Kelloff *et al.*, 2006). There is a considerable time frame wherein the carcinogenic process could potentially be halted or reversed. Taking this into consideration, the validation and utilization of dietary components, natural products or their synthetic analogs as potential cancer chemopreventive agents in the form of

Beer in Health and Disease Prevention
ISBN: 978-0-12-373891-2

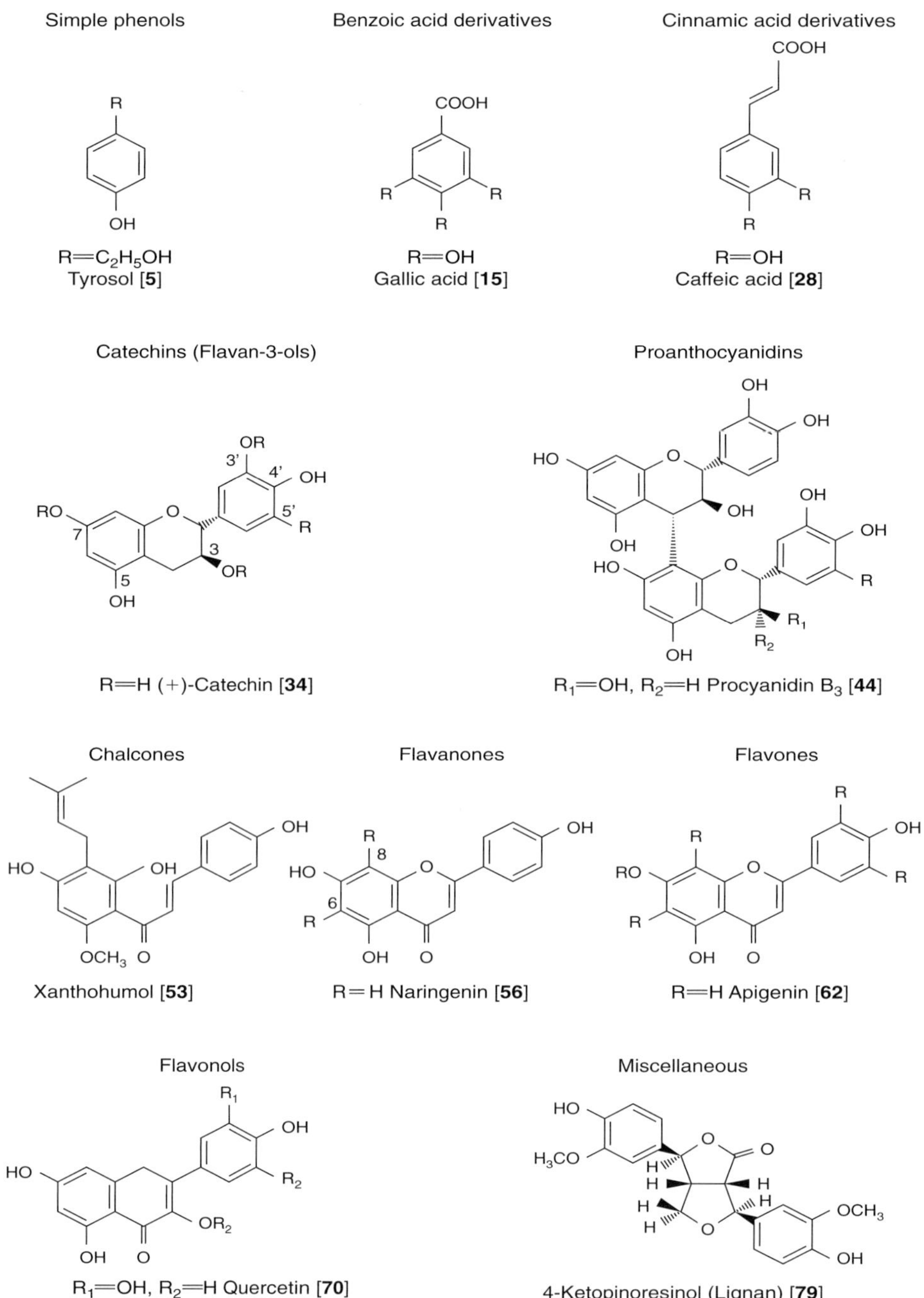

Figure 68.1 Chemical structures of typical phenolic compounds from beer, derived from 10 different structural classes. One typical representative of each class is given as an example.

functional foods or nutraceuticals has become an important issue in current health- and cancer-related research.

There are several lines of evidence suggesting beer as an interesting starting material for chemopreventive agent development. Beer is one of the most consumed beverages worldwide. It is a rich source of nutrient as well as non-nutrient components including vitamins. Beer contains a complex mixture of phenolic constituents, which are derived from malt (70–80%) and hop (20–30%). Structural classes include simple phenols, benzoic- and cinnamic acid derivatives, coumarins, catechins, di-, tri- and oligomeric proanthocyanidins, (prenylated) chalcones and several classes of flavonoids (Figure 68.1).

Polyphenols have been linked to health promoting aspects including the prevention of cancer based on their antioxidant activity and other mechanisms (Yang *et al.*, 2001; Surh, 2003). Recently, several reports have demonstrated that feeding beer or freeze dried beer inhibited chemically induced mammary and colonic carcinogenesis in rats (Nozawa *et al.*, 2004a, b; Nozawa *et al.*, 2006).

Scientific evidence accumulated over the past 10 years points to the cancer preventive potential of selected hop-derived beer constituents including prenylated flavonoids and hop bitter acids (reviewed in Gerhauser, 2005), but a general comparison of beer constituents based on multiple activities relevant for cancer prevention has not been performed so far. To this end, we have investigated the potential cancer chemopreventive activity of 48 beer constituents belonging to 10 different classes of phenolics. Here we summarize the antioxidant activities of these compounds in five different test systems, their influence on the metabolic activation and detoxification of carcinogens, as well as anti-inflammatory properties. Selected hop compounds were also tested for estrogenic and anti-estrogenic properties. Parts of these results have been described previously (Gerhauser *et al.*, 2002a, b; Gerhauser, 2005).

Materials and Methods

Chemicals

All cell culture media and supplements were obtained from Invitrogen (Eggenstein, Germany). Fetal calf serum was provided by PAA Laboratories (Pasching, Austria). β-Phycoerythrin (4 mg/ml), calcein AM, 4-methylumbelliferyl phosphate (MUP), 7-hydroxy-4-methylcoumarin, 3-cyano-7-ethoxycoumarin (CEC) and 3-cyano-7-hydroxycoumarin (CHC) were purchased from Molecular Probes (Mobitec, Göttingen, Germany). The human Ishikawa cell line was obtained from S. Mader, Department of Biochemistry, University of Montreal (Montreal, Canada). All other chemicals were purchased from Sigma Chemical Co. (Deisenhofen, Germany).

Source of phenolic beer compounds

The phytochemical analysis of unstabilized beer and a polyvinylpolypyrrolidone residue obtained during beer stabilization led to the isolation of a total of 51 compounds (Gerhauser *et al.*, 2002b). Tyrosol, salicylaldehyde, vanillin, 4-hydroxyphenylacetic acid, *o*-coumaric acid, *m*-coumaric acid, chlorogenic acid, epicatechin gallate, kaempferol, quercetin, quercitrin, isoquercitrin, rutin and myricetin were also purchased from Sigma Chemical Co. (Deisenhofen, Germany). Syringic aldehyde was obtained from Fluka (Deisenhofen, Germany).

Test Systems to Detect Potential Cancer Chemopreventive Activity

Scavenging of diphenyl-picrylhydrazyl radicals

Radical scavenging potential was determined spectrophotometrically by reaction with 1,1-diphenyl-2-picrylhydrazyl (DPPH) free radicals in a microplate format at 515 nm (van Amsterdam *et al.*, 1992, with modifications). Briefly, test compounds dissolved in DMSO were treated with a solution of 100 μM DPPH in ethanol for 30 min at 37°C. Scavenging potential was compared with a solvent control (0% radical scavenging) and ascorbic acid (250 μM final concentration, 100% radical scavenging, used as a blank), and the half-maximal scavenging concentration (SC_{50}) was generated from data obtained with 8 serial 2-fold dilutions in a final concentration range of 2–250 μM tested in duplicates. Correction for colored samples was achieved by preparing identical dilutions of the sample in ethanol instead of DPPH solution.

Scavenging of superoxide anion radicals generated non-enzymatically by NADH and phenazine methosulfate

Ewing and Janero (1995) have developed a microassay system suitable for the rapid detection of superoxide anion radical ($O_2^{\bullet-}$) scavengers. Aerobic mixtures of NADH and phenazine methosulfate (PMS) generate $O_2^{\bullet-}$ via the univalent oxidation of reduced PMS. Nitro blue tetrazolium (NBT) can serve as a detector molecule for $O_2^{\bullet-}$ through reduction to a stable formazan product. The reaction mixture (in 0.25 ml total volume) consists of 50 mM phosphate buffer, pH 7.4, containing 0.1 mM EDTA, 50 μM NBT, 78 μM NADH and 3.3 μM PMS (final concentrations). For the assay, 25 μl test sample (stock solution of test compound or superoxide dismutase (SOD) enzyme as a positive control) is pipetted into a microplate well containing 200 μl freshly prepared 0.1 mM EDTA, 62 μM NBT and 98 μM NADH in 50 mM phosphate buffer, pH 7.4. The reaction is initiated by the addition of 25 μl freshly prepared 33 μM PMS in 50 mM phosphate buffer, pH 7.4, containing 0.1 mM EDTA. NBT reduction is continuously monitored at 560 nm over 5 min using a SpectraMax 340PC microplate reader (Molecular Devices, Sunnyvale, CA) in the kinetic mode and with the "automix" function activated. Alternatively, the optical density (OD) at 560 nm can be measured as an endpoint after 5 min of incubation. The percent inhibition of $O_2^{\bullet-}$-dependent NBT reduction by the test sample is calculated, and SC_{50} values are generated from data obtained with 8 serial 2-fold dilutions in a final concentration range of 8–1,000 μM tested in duplicates. SOD (3 U/well) is used as a positive control.

Scavenging of superoxide anion radicals formed enzymatically by xanthine oxidase

Superoxide anion radicals were generated by oxidation of hypoxanthine to uric acid by xanthine oxidase (XO) and quantitated by the concomitant reduction of NBT (Ukeda *et al.*, 1997) adjusted to a 96-well microplate format. The reaction mixture (170 μl), consisting of 50 mM sodium carbonate buffer, pH 9.4, 100 μM EDTA, 25 μM NBT and 50 μM hypoxanthine, was mixed with test compounds (10 μl, in 100% DMSO, 5% final DMSO concentration) or DMSO (10 μl) as a solvent control. 1 U SOD (in 10 μl 50 mM sodium carbonate buffer, pH 9.4) was used as a positive control. The reaction was started by addition of 12 mU XO (in 10 μl buffer), and the rate of reduction of NBT was monitored for 6 min at 550 nm in a microplate reader (Spectramax 340, Molecular Devices). Alternatively, the yellow tetrazolium salt XTT [2,3-bis(2-methoxy-4-nitro-5-sulfophenyl)-2H-tetrazolium-5-carboxanilide], which forms a soluble orange formazan dye, was used. Under these conditions, the amount of XO was reduced to 3 mU and measurements were performed at 480 nm. V_{max} values were computed, and the SC_{50} was generated from the data obtained with 8 serial 2-fold dilutions of inhibitors in a final concentration range of 0.8–100 μM tested in duplicates. To exclude a direct inhibitory effect on XO, formation of uric acid was monitored directly at 290 nm under identical conditions as described above without addition of NBT or XTT. In the reaction mixture, 50 μM hypoxanthine was replaced by 100 μM xanthine.

Inhibition of phorbol myristate acetate-induced superoxide anion radical formation in HL-60 cells

Inhibition of phorbol myristate acetate (PMA)-induced superoxide radical formation in HL-60 human promyelocytic leukemia cells differentiated to granulocytes was detected by photometric determination of cytochrome c reduction (Pick and Mizel, 1981; Takeuchi *et al.*, 1994). Briefly, HL-60 cells at a density of 2×10^5 cells/ml were treated with 1.3% DMSO in RPMI 1640 medium containing 100 units/ml penicillin G sodium and 100 units/ml streptomycin sulfate supplemented with 10% fetal bovine serum at 37°C in a 5% CO_2 atmosphere for 4 days to induce terminal differentiation to granulocytes. Cells were harvested by centrifugation, washed twice with Hanks balanced salt solution containing 30 mM Hepes, pH 7.8 (HHBSS) and adjusted to a density of 2×10^6/ml. 2×10^5 cells/well (100 μl) were pre-incubated with test compounds (25 μl, in 10% DMSO) for 5 min prior to addition of 75 μl cytochrome c solution in HHBSS (5 mg/ml, 1.25 mg/ml final concentration); 25 μl SOD (600 U/ml in HHBSS, 12 U/well final concentration) was used as a positive control, all other wells obtained 25 μl HHBSS. Superoxide anion radical formation was started by addition of 25 μl PMA (0.55 mg/ml in HHBSS, 55 ng/ml final concentration). The plates were briefly shaken. After an incubation period of 30 min at 37°C, the reaction was stopped by chilling the plates on ice for 15 min. Finally, the plates were centrifuged, and cytochrome c reduction in the supernatant was determined at 550 nm using a microplate reader (Spectramax 340, Molecular Devices). The cell pellet was washed twice with PBS, and cell viability was measured fluorimetrically by enzymatic hydrolysis of the fluorogenic esterase substrate calcein AM (250 nM in PBS, 100 μl/well) at 37°C in a Cytofluor 4000 microplate fluorescence reader (PE Applied Biosystems; excitation 485 nm, emission 620 nm). Using this method, we could avoid unspecific effects of reducing test compounds which falsify commonly used viability assays based on MTT [3-(4,5-dimethylthiazo-2-yl)-2,5-diphenyltetrazolium bromide] or XTT [2,3-bis(2-methoxy-4-nitro-5-sulfophenyl)-2H-tetrazolium-5-carboxanilide] bioreduction. The reaction was linear for at least 30 min. SC_{50} values (half-maximal scavenging concentration of PMA-induced superoxide burst) were generated from the results of 8 serial dilutions of inhibitors tested in duplicate. Only non-toxic inhibitor concentrations resulting in greater than 50% cell viability were considered to calculate scavenging potential.

Measurement of oxygen radical absorbance capacity

For the determination of peroxyl or hydroxyl radical absorbance capacity of test compounds, the oxygen radical absorbance capacity (ORAC) assay (Cao and Prior, 1999) was modified and adapted to a 96-well plate format. β-Phycoerythrin (β-PE) was used as a redox-sensitive fluorescent indicator protein, 2,2,-azobis-(2-amidinopropane) dihydrochloride (AAPH) as a peroxyl radical generator and H_2O_2-$CuSO_4$ as a hydroxyl radical generator. Results were expressed as ORAC units, where 1 ORAC unit equals the net protection of β-PE produced by 1 μM Trolox, a water-soluble Vit. E analog used as a reference compound. Briefly, for the $ORAC_{ROO}$ assay, reaction mixtures contained 170 μl 75 mM sodium potassium phosphate buffer, pH 7.0, 10 μl 9.43 nM β-PE in phosphate buffer and 10 μl of the inhibitor solution (1–5 μM final concentration) or phosphate buffer as a negative control, respectively. The reaction was initiated by addition of 10 μl 320 mM AAPH in phosphate buffer. For the $ORAC_{OH}$ assay, the reaction mixture contained 175 μl 75 mM sodium potassium phosphate buffer, pH 7.0, 10 μl 9.43 nM β-PE in phosphate buffer and 10 μl of the inhibitor solution (1–5 μM final concentration) or phosphate buffer as a negative control. The reaction was initiated by addition of 10 μl of a 1:1 mixture of H_2O_2 (12%) and $CuSO_4$ (0.36 mM in phosphate buffer). The decline of β-PE fluorescence was measured at 37°C until completion for 100 min using a Cytofluor 4000 fluorescent microplate reader (excitation wavelength Ex 530/25 nm, emission wavelength Em 585/30 nm). Results were expressed as ORAC units, where 1 ORAC unit equals the net protection of β-PE produced by 1 μM Trolox. Scavenging capacities > 1 ORAC unit were considered as positive. Current ORAC experiments are performed following the improved protocols by Ou *et al.* (2001, 2002) with fluorescein replacing β-PE as the fluorescent sensor.

Inhibition of Cyp1A activity

β-Naphthoflavone-induced H4IIE rat hepatoma cell preparations were used as a source of cytochrome P450 1A (Cyp1A) enzyme activity. Cyp1A activity was determined *via* the time-dependent dealkylation of CEC to CHC based on the method of Crespi *et al.* (1997, with modifications). Briefly, H4IIE rat hepatoma cells were cultured in 100 mm tissue culture dishes at a density of 5×10^4 cells/ml in MEME medium containing 100 units/ml penicillin G sodium, 100 units/ml streptomycin sulfate and 250 ng/ml amphotericin B supplemented with 10% fetal bovine serum at 37°C in a 5% CO_2 atmosphere. After a preincubation period of 24 h, Cyp1A was induced by addition of 10 μM β-naphthoflavone (dissolved in DMSO, 0.1% final concentration). Cells were harvested after 38 h by scraping in 1 ml/plate buffer P (200 mM potassium phosphate buffer, pH 7.4 containing 10 mM $MgCl_2$) and snap frozen in liquid nitrogen. For determination of Cyp1A activity, test compounds dissolved in 10% DMSO (10 μl, final concentration 0.5%) were pipetted to a 96-well microplate. A freshly prepared reaction mixture (100 μl), consisting of 5.2 μl 50 mm $NADP^+$ in water, 4.4 μl 150 mM glucose-6-phosphate in water, 0.5 U glucose-6-phosphate dehydrogenase, 0.1 μl 10 mM CEC (in DMSO) and 90.25 μl buffer P, was then added to each well. The reaction was started by addition of 90 μl cell lysate, passed once through a 27-gauge needle and diluted with buffer P to a final protein concentration of 50–100 μg/ml depending on Cyp1A activity. The rate of dealkylation of CEC to fluorescent CHC was measured for 45 min at 37°C in a Cytofluor 4000 microplate fluorescence reader (PE Applied Biosystems, reading every 2.5 min with prior shaking, excitation 408/20 nm, emission 460/40 nm). V_{max} values were computed, and the half-maximal inhibitory concentration (IC_{50}) was generated from the data obtained with 8 serial 2-fold dilutions of inhibitors in a final concentration range of 0.004–0.5 μM or 0.04–5 μM, respectively, tested in duplicates. Enzyme activities were calculated in comparison with a CHC standard curve and normalized to protein content determined by the BCA method (Smith *et al.*, 1985). α-Naphthoflavone as a known Cpy1A inhibitory compound was used as a positive control.

Determination of NAD(P)H:quinone reductase activity in mouse hepatoma cell culture

For the detection of phase 2 enzyme inducers, quinone reductase (QR) activity was measured in Hepa 1c1c7 cells as described previously (Prochaska and Santamaria, 1988). QR activity was determined by measuring the NADPH-dependent menadiol-mediated reduction of MTT [3-(4,5-dimethylthiazo-2-yl)-2,5-diphenyltetrazolium bromide] to a blue formazan. Protein was determined by crystal violet staining of an identical set of test plates. Induction of QR activity was calculated from the ratio of specific enzyme activities of compound-treated cells in comparison with a solvent control, and CD values (concentration required to double the specific enzyme activity in μM) were generated. In addition, IC_{50} values for the inhibition of cell proliferation were calculated. Only non-toxic inhibitor concentrations resulting in greater than 50% cell viability were considered to calculate inducing potential.

Inhibition of LPS-mediated inducible nitric oxide synthase induction in murine macrophages

Inhibition of lipopolysaccharide (LPS)-mediated inducible nitric oxide synthase (iNOS) induction in murine Raw 246.7 macrophages was determined *via* the Griess reaction (Heiss *et al.*, 2001). Briefly, murine macrophages were cultured in DMEM medium containing 100 units/ml penicillin G sodium, 100 units/ml streptomycin sulfate and 250 ng/ml amphotericin B supplemented with 10% fetal bovine serum at 37°C in a 5% CO_2 atmosphere. Cells were plated at a density of $1-2 \times 10^5$ cells/well in DMEM in 96-well plates. After a preincubation period of 24 h, the medium was replaced by 170 μl serum-free DMEM. Inhibitors (10 μl in 10% DMSO, 8 serial 2-fold dilutions, final concentration range 0.8–50 μM) were added, and iNOS was induced by addition of 20 μl LPS solution (500 ng/ml in serum-free DMEM). After 24 h, iNOS activity was determined *via* the quantitation of nitrite levels according to the Griess reaction. Briefly, 100 μl aliquots of cell culture supernatants were incubated with an equal volume of Griess reagent (1% sulphanilamide/0.1% naphthylethylene diamine dihydrochloride/2.5% H_3PO_4) at room temperature for 10 min. The absorbance at 550 nm was determined in a microplate reader and compared to a nitrite standard curve. To determine cytotoxic effects of test compounds, residual cell culture medium was removed, cells were fixed at 4°C for 30 min with 50 μl ice-cold 10% trichloroacetic acid solution in water, washed five times with tap water and briefly dried. Cell numbers were estimated by sulforhodamin B staining (Skehan *et al.*, 1990). Generally, compounds were tested at non-toxic concentrations (cell staining > 50% of LPS-treated control cells).

Inhibition of cyclooxygenase activity

Cox activity was measured at 37°C by monitoring oxygen consumption during conversion of arachidonic acid to prostaglandins in a 1.0 ml incubation cell of an Oxygen Electrode Unit (Hansatech DW, based on a Clark-type O_2 electrode) according to Jang and Pezzuto (1997) with modifications. The reaction mixture, containing 0.1 M sodium potassium phosphate buffer, pH 7.4, 1 mM hydroquinone, 0.01 mM hemin and approximately 0.2 U Cox-1 in 100 μl microsome fraction derived from ram seminal vesicles as a crude source of Cox-1 (specific activity 0.2–1 U/mg protein), was incubated with 10 μl DMSO (negative control) or inhibitor solution (10 mM in DMSO), respectively, for 90 s. The reaction was started by addition of 2 μl 50 mM arachidonic acid in ethanol (100 μM final concentration), and oxygen consumption was monitored for 20 s. For calculation, the rate of O_2 consumption was compared to a DMSO control (100% activity).

Determination of estrogenic and anti-estrogenic capacity in cultured Ishikawa cells

Measurement of the enhancement of alkaline phosphatase (ALP) activity in the Ishikawa human endometrial adenocarcinoma line allows the assessment of intrinsic estrogenic activity of test compounds. Anti-estrogenic effects are determined by co-treatment with β-estradiol and inhibitors. Cell culture conditions were essentially as described earlier (Littlefield *et al.*, 1990; Markiewicz *et al.*, 1992). Ishikawa cells were routinely maintained in α-MEM medium containing 100 units/ml penicillin G sodium, 100 units/ml streptomycin sulfate and 250 ng/ml amphotericin B supplemented with 10% charcoal-stripped fetal bovine serum at 37°C in a 5% CO_2 atmosphere. One day before the start of an experiment, the medium was changed to an estrogen- and phenol-red-free D-MEM/F-12 mix (1:1) (estrogen-free mix) containing L-glutamate and pyridoxine HCl (Gibco BRL), supplemented with 100 units/ml penicillin G sodium, 100 units/ml streptomycin sulfate, 250 ng/ml amphotericin B and 5% charcoal-stripped fetal bovine serum. For the determination of estrogenic activity, cells were trypsinized with 0.25% phenol-red-free trypsin/EDTA, passed through a 27-gauge injection needle to obtain a single-cell suspension, and plated in 96-well microplates at a density of 2×10^4/well in 200 μl estrogen-free mix. After a preincubation period of 24 h, the medium was replaced by 190 μl fresh estrogen-free mix. Test compounds (10 μl in 10% DMSO, 8 serial 2- or 5-fold dilutions, final concentration range 10^{-12}–10^{-5} M in duplicate) were added to a final volume of 200 μl, and the plates were incubated at 37°C in a humidified 5% CO_2 atmosphere for 72 h. Plates were washed three times with PBS (pre-warmed to 37°C), 50 μl/well 0.5% Triton X in PBS were added, and plates were kept at −80°C overnight. To determine ALP activity, plates were thawed at 37°C for 2 min, 100 μl/well 15 μM MUP in 1 M diethanolamine buffer, pH 9.8, containing 0.24 mM $MgCl_2$ were added, and plates were shaken thoroughly for 5 min on a microplate shaker. Dephosphorylation of MUP to fluorescent 4-methyl-7-hydroxy-coumarin (4-methylumbelliferon) was monitored for 45 min at 37°C (excitation 360 nm, emission 460 nm). ALP activity was determined from the rate of product formation (in arbitrary fluorescent units/min). Protein was determined by SRB staining of an identical set of test plates. For calculation of estrogenic activity, results were expressed as a percentage in comparison with a control sample treated with 50 nM β-estradiol (set as 100%) to determine the half-maximal effective concentration.

For the determination of anti-estrogenic activity, the medium pre-incubated cells (as described above) were changed to 170 μl estrogen-free mix, and cells were treated simultaneously with test samples (10 μl in 10% DMSO) on 10 μl 10% DMSO as a solvent control, respectively, and 20 μl 50 nM β-estradiol in estrogen-free mix. Inhibition of ALP induction was calculated in comparison with the result obtained with the β-estradiol control set as 100%. Tamoxifen was used as a known anti-estrogenic reference compound and produced an inhibition of >50% at a test concentration of 0.5 μM.

Results

We have tested 48 beer constituents for cancer preventive potential in a battery of nine test systems suitable to detect antioxidant and radical scavenging activity (**5.1**), potential to inhibit the metabolic activation of xenobiotics by Cyp1A and to enhance phase 2 detoxification (**5.2**), anti-inflammatory and estrogenic/anti-estrogenic effects (**5.4**).

Antioxidant and radical scavenging capacity

It is well established that excessive production of reactive oxygen species (ROS) caused by immune diseases, chronic inflammation and infections leads to continuous oxidative stress and is causally linked with processes during tumor initiation, promotion and progression (Bartsch and Nair, 2006).

There are three major types of ROS: Hydroxyl radicals (•OH) are very reactive oxidants which attack all biomolecular targets (DNA, proteins, lipids ...). Superoxide anion radicals ($O_2^{\bullet-}$) do not directly react with biological molecules, but are linked to toxic effects by secondary radical reactions. Other free radicals of the peroxyl type (ROO•) contribute by enhancement to oxidative stress (Valko *et al.*, 2006). We have established multiple test systems, including the DPPH radical scavenging assay, three systems to generate superoxide anion radicals (non-enzymatically, enzymatically and cellularly), and the oxygen radical absorbance capacity (ORAC) assay with peroxyl and hydroxyl radicals, to investigate the radical scavenging and antioxidant capacity of phenolic beer compounds. An overview of all tested compounds and their activities in these test systems is given in Table 68.1. To allow a comparison with chemical structures, numbering of the compounds was kept consistent with the Chapter 48. Some examples of phenolic beer constituents are shown in Figure 68.1.

DPPH Radical Scavenging The DPPH assay was included as it is a very simple test system which gives a first indication of radical scavenging potential of a test compound. Due to the bulky structure of the stable DPPH

Table 68.1 Antioxidant and radical scavenging activities of beer constituents

		DPPH scavenging[b]	*Superoxide radical scavenging*			
	Compound[a]	SC_{50} *(μM*[c]*)*	*PMS/NADH* SC_{50} *(μM)*	*X/XO* SC_{50} *(μM)*	$ORAC_{ROO}$ *(units)*	$ORAC_{OH}$ *(units)*
	Simple phenols					
5	Tyrosol	>250	>100	>100	2.2	3.8
	Benzoic acid derivatives					
10	*p*-Hydroxy benzoic acid	>250	>1,000	>100	0.9	3.8
13	Protocatechuic acid	**44.8**	**664.6**	**51.9**	**2.8**	**5.6**
15	Gallic acid	**8.5**	**503.7**	>100	**3.1**	3.3
16	Vanillic acid	>250	>1,000	>100	0.5	1.2
17	Syringic acid	44.2	>1,000	>100	1.7	**5.8**
18	Salicylaldehyde	>250	>1,000	n.b.		
20	Vanillin	>250	>1,000	>100	0.3	2.5
21	Syringic acid	>250	>1,000	>100	0.6	3.5
	Phenylacetic acids					
22	4-Hydroxy-phenylacetic acid	>250	>1,000	>100	1.0	4.4
	Cinnamic acids					
24	Cinnamic acid	>250	>1,000	>100	0.1	**8.0**
25	*o*-Coumaric acid	>250	>1,000	>100	0.2	**5.5**
26	*m*-Coumaric acid	>250	>1,000	>100	0.3	3.8
27	*p*-Coumaric acid	>250	>1,000	>100	1.4	**7.9**
28	Caffeic acid	**20.5**	**310.4**	**21.1**	**2.7**	**8.3**
29	Ferulic acid	**47.5**	>1,000	>100	**3.5**	**4.9**
30	Sinapic acid	**31.2**	>1,000	>100	1.0	1.5
31	Chlorogenic acid	**25.6**	n.d.	**75.1**	**2.4**	n.d.
	Flavan-3-ols (catechins)					
34	(+)-Catechin	**16.9**	**116.7**	**23.3**	**4.0**	4.4
35	(−)-Epicatechin	**13.7**	**299.7**	>100	**4.7**	**4.7**
36	Gallocatechin	**15.4**	**52.1**	**11.7**	**2.6**	**7.0**
38	Epicatechin gallate	**12.7**	**116.7**	**23.3**	**7.8**	**4.5**
39	3′-*O*-methylcatechin	**170.6**	>1,000	>100	**4.0**	**5.2**
40	Catechin-7-*O*-β-D-glucopyranosid	**33.1**	**253**	18.2	**2.3**	**4.8**
	Proanthocyanidins					
44	Procyanidin B_3	**7.6**	**55.2**	>100	**5.3**	2.9
49	Procyanidin C	**9.7**	**18.5**	**6.6**	**5.2**	2.5
50	*ent*-Epigallocatechin-(4α→8, 2α→O→7)-catechin	**16**	**77.4**	n.b.	**5.2**	2.6
52	2,3-*Cis*-3,4-*trans*-2-[2,3*trans*-3,3′,4′,5,7-pentahydroxyflavan-8-yl]-4-(3,4-dihydroxyphenyl)3,5,7-trihydroxybenzopyran	**11**	>1,000	**14.7**	**3.0**	2.6
	Chalcones					
53	Xanthohumol	>250	>1,000	**31.1**	**2.9**	**8.9**
	Flavanones					
55	Isoxanthohumol	>250	**563.4**	>100	**2.8**	2.1
56	Naringenin	>250	**395.3**	>100	**3.7**	**6.1**
57	8-Prenylnaringenin	>250	**506.7**	>100	1.0	**5.6**
58	6-Prenylnaringenin	>250	**309.4**	**88.5**	1.3	**3.1**
60	5-Methyl-6′-dimethyl-4′,5′-dihydropyrano[2′,3′,7,8]naringenin	>250	>1,000	>100	1.8	**4.3**
	Flavones					
62	Apigenin	>250	>1,000	>100	0.7	**2.7**
64	Tricin	>250	>1,000	70.8	1.0	1.0
65	Apigenin-6-*C*-glucoside (saponaretin)	>250	**157.0**	>100	0.8	1.9
66	Apigenin-6-*C*-glucoside 7-*O*-glucoside (saponarin)	**114.8**	**183.1**	77.6	1.2	1.8
	Flavonols					
68	Kaempferol	**23.7**	**228.8**	**46**	0.9	2.6
70	Quercetin	**8.6**	**67.1**	**18.3**	**5.5**	**4.3**
71	Quercitrin (quercetin-3-*O*-rhamnoside)	**22.4**	n.b.	>100	**2.2**	n.b.
72	Isoquercitrin (quercetin-3-*O*-glucoside)	**15.7**	n.b.	>100	**2.1**	n.b.
73	Rutin (quercetin-3-*O*-rutinoside)	**15**	**65**	**29.7**	**2.6**	**6.1**

Table 68.1 (Continued)

	Compound [a]	DPPH scavenging [b]	Superoxide radical scavenging			
		SC_{50} (μM)[c]	PMS/NADH SC_{50} (μM)	X/XO SC_{50} (μM)	$ORAC_{ROO}$ (units)	$ORAC_{OH}$ (units)
74	Myricetin	**10.4**	**24**	**5.3**	**4.2**	**8.2**
	Miscellaneous compounds					
76	Indole-3-carboxylic acid	>250	>1000	>100	1.7	**4.3**
77	Indole-3-ethanol (tryptophol)	>250	n.d.	>100	n.d.	n.d.
78	1-Methyl-1,3,4,9-tetrahydropyrano [3,4b]indole	>250	>1,000	>100	1.9	3.2
79	4-Ketopinoresinol (lignan)	**191.3**	>1,000	>100	3.7	2.7

Notes: n.d.: not determined; bold print indicates most potent activities.

[a] For chemical structures and further information see Chapter 48. Compounds 1, 2, 3, 4, 6, 7, 8, 9, 11, 12, 14, 19, 23, 32, 33, 37, 41, 42, 43, 45, 46, 47, 48, 51, 54, 59, 61, 63, 67, 69, 75, 80 have not been tested.

[b] The following *in vitro* test systems have been utilized: DPPH: Scavenging of the stable free radical diphenylpicrylhydrazyl; PMS/NADH: Scavenging of superoxide anion radicals generated non-enzymatically by phenazine methosulfate and NADH; X/XO: Scavenging of superoxide anion radicals generated enzymatically during the oxidation of hypoxanthine to uric acid by xanthine oxidase; ORAC: Oxygen radical absorbance capacity assay with peroxyl (ROO) and hydroxyl radicals ($OH^•$).

[c] SC_{50}: Halfmaximal scavenging concentration; one ORAC unit equals the net protection of β-PE produced by 1 μM Trolox.

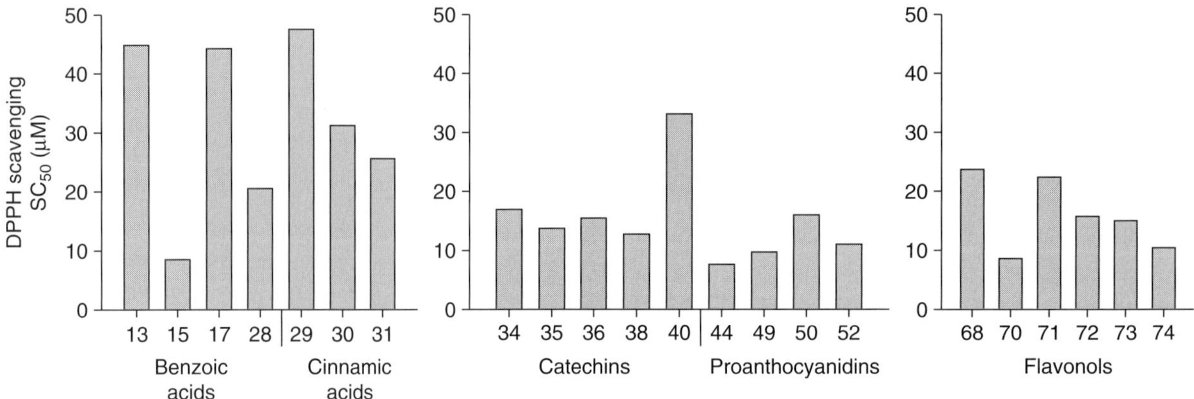

Figure 68.2 DPPH radical scavenging potential of phenolic beer compounds, expressed as the SC_{50}. Only classes with active representatives are shown.

radical, interaction with radical scavengers is sometimes hindered, leading to false negative results.

SC_{50} values of active DPPH scavengers are depicted in Figure 68.2. Overall, it became apparent that the structural classes of catechins (flavan-3-ols), proanthocyanidins and flavonols were most potent in scavenging DPPH radicals.

Gallic acid [**15**] as a benzoic acid derivative with three hydroxyl groups was identified as potent DPPH radical scavenger. The catechins (+)-catechin [**34**], (−)-epicatechin [**35**], gallocatechin [**36**], epicatechin gallate [**38**] and 3′-*O*-methyl-catechin [**39**] were almost equally active in DPPH scavenging with SC_{50} values of 12.7–16.9 μM. A glucosidic linkage at the OH group in position 7 as in [**40**] reduced the SC_{50} in comparison with (+)-catechin [**34**] by about 50%. Procyanidin B_3 [**44**] and prodelphinidin C [**49**] were even more potent than the respective subunits (+)-catechin [**34**] and gallocatechin [**36**], with SC_{50} values of 7.6 and 9.7 μM. Interestingly, neither flavanones such as naringenin [**56**] nor flavones such as apigenin [**62**] were able to scavenge DPPH radicals. In contrast, the flavonols quercetin [**70**] and myricetin [**74**], which have an additional hydroxyl group in position 3 in comparison with flavones, were identified as good scavengers. A glycosidic linkage at the OH group in position 3 as in quercitrin [**71**], isoquercitrin [**72**] and rutin [**73**] reduced the scavenging potential by a factor of 2–3.

Superoxide Anion Radical Scavenging Superoxide anion radicals can be generated chemically, enzymatically or in living cells. We established test systems for all three methods.

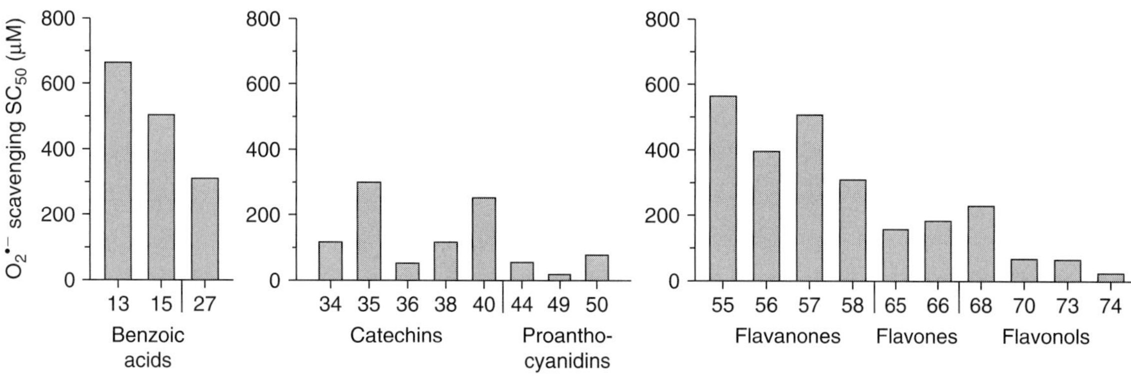

Figure 68.3 Scavenging of superoxide anion radicals generated non-enzymatically in the PMS/NADH system by phenolic beer compounds. The antioxidant potential was expressed as the SC_{50}. Only classes with active representatives are compared.

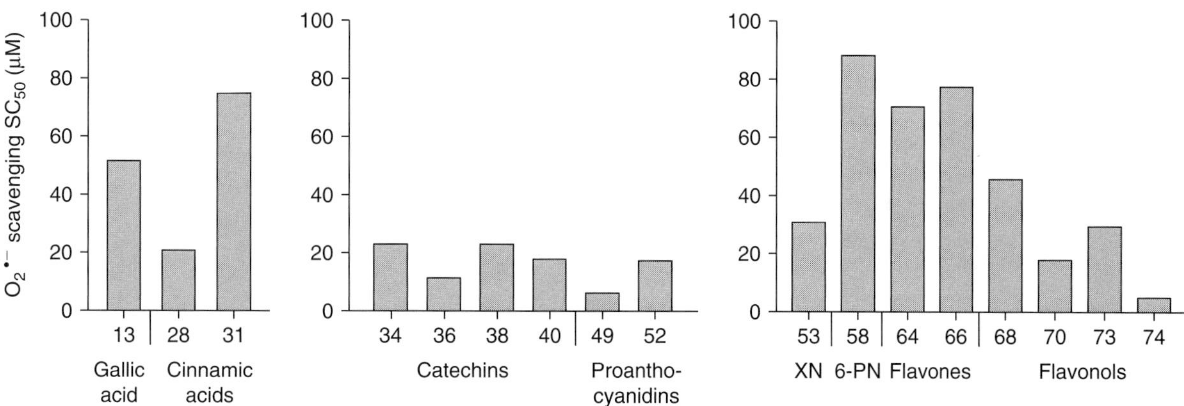

Figure 68.4 Scavenging of superoxide anion radicals generated enzymatically in the xanthine/xanthine oxidase (X/XO) system by phenolic beer compounds. The antioxidant potential was expressed as the SC_{50}. Only results of active compounds are depicted. XN: xanthohumol [**53**]; 6-PN: 6-prenylnaringenin [**58**].

Non-enzymatic PMS/NADH System Non-enzymatically, an aerobic solution of PMS and NADH generates $O_2^{\bullet-}$. The assay was established according to Ewing and Janero (1995). In comparison with the other two $O_2^{\bullet-}$ assays described below, this method apparently generated the highest amount of $O_2^{\bullet-}$, since compounds had to be tested in an about 10-fold higher concentration range up to 1 mM to reach 50% radical scavenging. Results are summarized in Figure 68.3.

In good agreement with DPPH radical scavenging potential, the catechins (+)-catechin [**34**], gallocatechin [**36**] and epicatechin gallate [**38**] potently scavenged superoxide anion radicals, whereas the glucoside [**40**] was less active than the aglycon [**34**]. Again, procyanidin B_3 [**44**] and especially the trimeric proanthocyanidin prodelphinidin C [**49**] were more potent than the respective subunits (+)-catechin [**34**] and gallocatechin [**36**]. The flavanones isoxanthohumol [**55**] as well as naringenin [**56**] and its prenylated derivatives [**57**] and [**58**] showed weak potential to scavenge superoxide anion radicals in this system. Apigenin derivatives saponaretin [**65**] and saponarin [**66**] were more potent scavengers. Overall, the flavonol myricetin [**74**] with three OH groups in positions 3′, 4′ and 5′of the flavonoid structure was identified as the most potent $O_2^{\bullet}-$ scavenger in this assay with a SC_{50} value of 24 μM.

Enzymatic X/XO System Oxidation of hypoxanthine to uric acid by XO leads to the enzymatic generation of superoxide anion radicals. Compounds were tested in a concentration range of up to 100 μM. Most consistently with the previous assays, catechins and proanthocyanidins were identified as the most potent superoxide radical scavengers as shown in Figure 68.4.

(+)-Catechin [**34**], gallocatechin [**36**], epicatechin gallate [**38**] and the glucoside [**40**] all resulted in about 50% scavenging at a concentration of 20 μM. The trimeric prodelphinidin C [**49**] as well as dimer [**52**] were even more potent scavengers, with SC_{50} values of 6.6 and 14.7 μM, respectively, whereas procyanidin B_3 [**44**] was not able to scavenge superoxide anion radicals efficiently at concentrations below 100 μM. The hop-derived chalcone xanthohumol [**53**] was identified as a superoxide radical scavenger in the X/XO system, but not in the PMS/NADH assay. Consistently with the results obtained in the latter test system, flavanones and flavones were less potent scavengers than flavonols, and myricetin [**74**] was identified as the most potent $O_2^{\bullet -}$ radical scavenger with 50% scavenging of the generated radicals at a concentration of 5.3 μM. Concomitant detection of uric acid proved that the result was not falsified by direct inhibition of XO activity (data not shown).

Cellular System: PMA-Induced Superoxide Burst in Granulocytes Alternatively, superoxide anion radical formation was detected in differentiated HL-60 human promyelocytic leukemia cells stimulated with PMA to generate superoxide anion radicals. Out of 48 compounds tested, only three were more than 50% inhibitory at a test concentration of 100 μM. Dose-dependent inhibition by xanthohumol [**53**], the flavone saponaretin [**65**] and the lignan 5-ketopinoresinol [**79**] is shown in Figure 68.5. These compounds inhibited the PMA-mediated superoxide production with SC_{50} values of 5.5 μM [**53**], 4.7 μM [**65**] and 7.1 μM [**79**]. Interestingly, the lignan 5-ketopinoresinol [**79**] did not show potential to scavenge superoxide anion radicals in the two other assays. This indicated that 5-ketopinoresinol [**79**] may inhibit the signal transduction cascade induced by PMA.

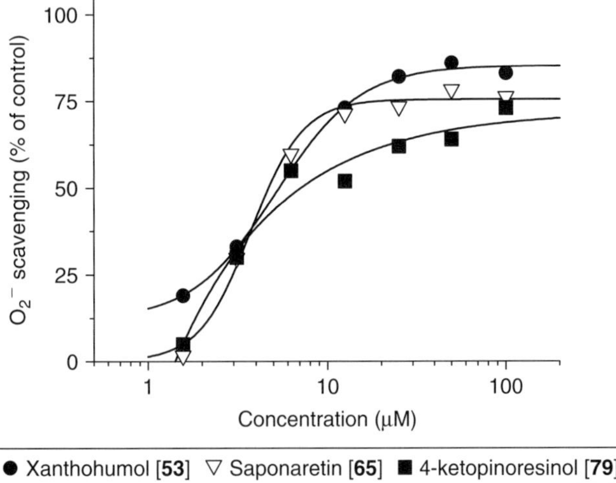

Figure 68.5 Dose-dependent inhibition of phorbol ester-induced superoxide burst in granulocytes by xanthohumol [**53**], saponaretin [**65**] and 4-ketopinoresinol [**79**]. Scavenging of superoxide anion radicals is shown as a percentage in comparison with a solvent control.

Oxygen Radical Absorbance Capacity The ORAC assay is a well-established test system to identify peroxyl and hydroxyl radical scavengers. In the present study, the protocol using β-phycoerythrin (β-PE) as a redox-sensitive fluorescent indicator was adapted to a 96-well plate format. In our current screening assay, we have replaced β-phycoerythrin by fluorescein, due to higher stability of the fluorescence signal and lower price.

$ORAC_{ROO}$ Peroxyl radicals are generated at 37°C by the peroxyl radical generator AAPH. Trolox, a water-soluble Vit. E derivative, is generally used as a reference compound, and one ORAC unit is defined as the net protection of β-PE produced by 1 μM Trolox. For comparison, beer phenolics were also tested at a concentration of 1 μM. 35 out of 48 compounds demonstrated a higher peroxyl radical scavenging potential than Trolox at this concentration. Figure 68.6 summarizes only those compounds which were twice as potent as Trolox (equivalent to at least 2 ORAC units at 1 μM).

The simple phenol tyrosol [**5**], the benzoic acid derivatives protocatechuic acid [**13**] and gallic acid [**15**] as well as caffeic [**28**], ferulic [**29**] and chlorogenic acid [**31**]

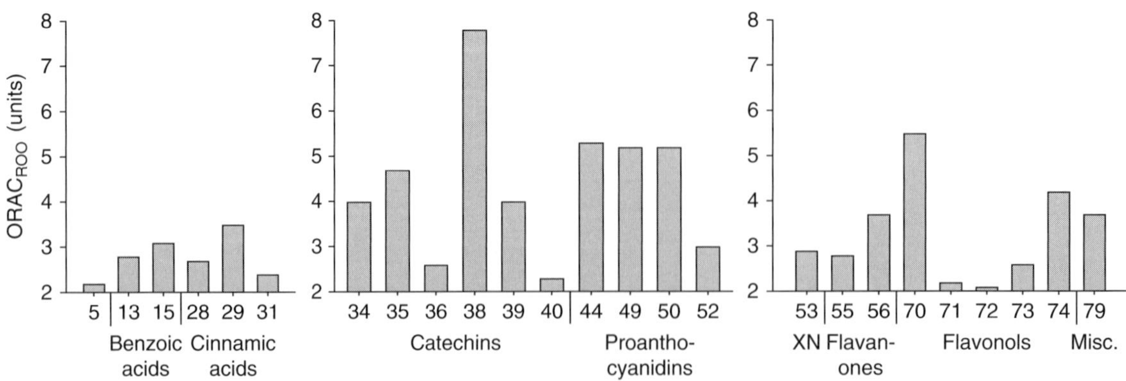

Figure 68.6 Peroxyl radical absorbance capacity ($ORAC_{ROO}$) of phenolic beer compounds. Peroxyl radicals were generated by AAPH and β-phycoerythrin was used as a fluorescent indicator. One ORAC unit is defined as the net protection provided by 1 μM Trolox, a water-soluble Vit. E analog. Compounds were tested at a concentration of 1 μM.

were more potent peroxyl radical scavengers than Trolox. Overall, catechins and proanthocyanidins were the most potent antioxidants in the $ORAC_{ROO}$ assay. Gallocatechin [**36**] was only about half as active as (+)-catechin [**34**] and (−)-epicatechin [**35**], which had a peroxyl scavenging capacity of 4.0 and 4.7 $ORAC_{ROO}$ units, respectively. Esterification of gallic acid [**15**] with (−)-epicatechin [**35**] significantly increased peroxyl scavenging potential, and epicatechin gallate [**38**] was identified as the most potent compound with 7.8 $ORAC_{ROO}$ units. In contrast, blocking of free hydroxyl groups as in [**40**] reduced the scavenging potential in comparison with (+)-catechin [**34**]. Di- and trimeric proanthocyanidins procyanidin B_3 [**44**], prodelphinidin C [**49**] and [**50**] were more potent than the respective subunits (+)-catechin [**34**] and especially gallocatechin [**36**]. Quercetin [**70**], which produced 5.5 ORAC units, was identified as the most potent flavonol.

$ORAC_{OH}$ A combination of H_2O_2 and $CuSO_4$ was used in a Fenton-type reaction to generate hydroxyl radicals. Of notice, the potential of Trolox to scavenge hydroxyl radicals is quite low. Therefore the factor generated from the area between the fluorescence decay curve of the control reaction and that of 1 μM Trolox, which represents 1 $ORAC_{OH}$ unit, was quite low. Consequently, normalization to this factor produced relatively high $ORAC_{OH}$ values for most phenolic beer compounds. In 2002, the authors of the original $ORAC_{OH}$ assay published an improved method termed HORAC, which utilizes fluorescein as a fluorescent sensor, Co(II) fluoride/picolinic acid-H_2O_2 to generate hydroxyl radicals and gallic acid as a reference standard (Ou *et al.*, 2002). In our hands, 1 μM gallic acid was 3.3-fold more potent than 1 μM Trolox. For comparison with gallic acid equivalents (GAE), $ORAC_{OH}$ units summarized in Table 68.1 should be divided by 3.3.

Due to the high number of active compounds, Figure 68.7 shows only those compounds with $ORAC_{OH}$ values above 4. Cinnamic [**24**], caffeic [**27**] and ferulic acid [**28**], gallocatechin [**36**], xanthohumol [**53**] and myricetin [**74**] were identified as the most potent hydroxyl radical scavengers of all beer phenolics investigated.

Modulation of carcinogen metabolism

In addition to the broad spectrum of antioxidant tests, we also investigated the influence of beer compounds to modulate activation and detoxification of xenobiotics. Cyp1A, which is, for example, involved in the activation of carcinogens from cigarette smoke or grilled meat, was used as a model phase 1 enzyme, and NAD(P)H:quinone reductase was tested as a phase 2 enzyme which is induced concomitantly with other phase 2 enzymes such as glutathione *S*-transferases. The results of all compounds which were able to modulate at least one of the activities of these enzymes are summarized in Table 68.2. Compounds which have not been tested in the assays described in Table 68.1 have also not been tested in these systems.

Cyp1A Inhibition Microsomes of β-naphthoflavone-induced rat hepatoma cells were used as a source for Cyp1A activity, and the dealkylation of CEC was monitored over 45 min. As indicated in Figure 68.8a, none of the benzoic and cinnamic acid derivatives [**10–31**], catechins [**34–40**] and proanthocyanidins [**44–52**] inhibited Cyp1A activity more than 50% at the concentration limit of 5 μM. In contrast, xanthohumol [**53**], apigenin [**62**] and quercetin [**70**] were identified as extremely potent Cyp1A inhibitors, with IC_{50} values of 0.02 μM. Glycosides such as saponaretin [**65**] and saponarin [**66**] as well as the quercetin derivatives quercitrin [**71**] and isoquercitrin [**72**] were considerable less active than the respective aglycons. The flavanones isoxanthohumol [**55**], naringenin [**56**] and 8- and 6-prenylnaringenin [**57, 58**] as well as the flavon tricin [**64**] potently blocked Cyp1A activity with IC_{50} values below 0.5 μM. In addition, 1-methyl-1,3,4,9-tetrahydropyrano[3,4-b]indole

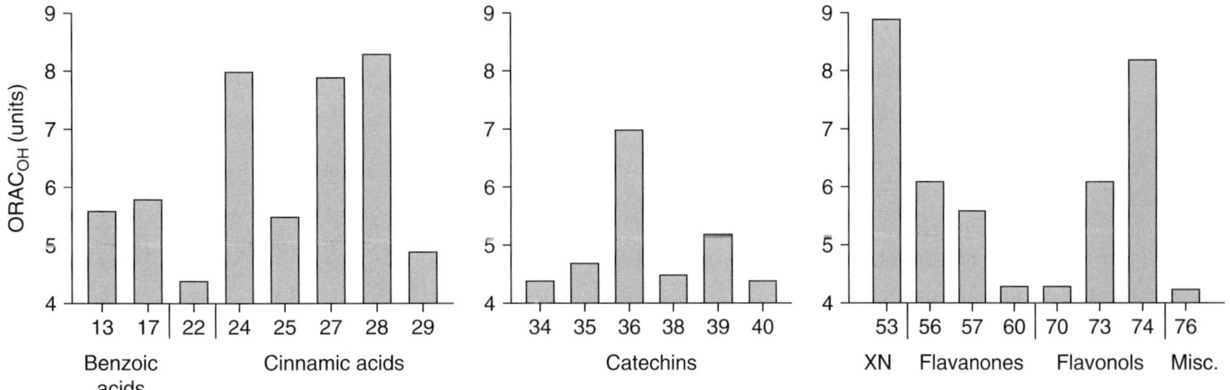

Figure 68.7 Hydroxyl radical absorbance capacity ($ORAC_{OH}$) of phenolic beer compounds. Hydroxyl radicals were generated by $CuSO_4$ and H_2O_2, and β-phycoerythrin was used as a fluorescent indicator. One ORAC unit is defined as the net protection provided by 1 μM Trolox, a water-soluble Vit. E analog. Compounds were tested at a concentration of 1 μM.

Table 68.2 Modulation of xenobiotics metabolism and anti-inflammatory potential of phenolic beer compounds

		Cyp1A inhibition[a]	*QR induction*		*Inhibition of iNOS induction*	*Cox-1 inhibition*
	Verbindung	*IC_{50} (μM)*[b]	*CD (μM)*[c]	*IC_{50}-T (μM)*[d]	*IC_{50} (μM)*	*IC_{50} (μM)*
	Benzoic acid derivatives					
15	Gallic acid	>5	>50	>50	**8.7**	>100 (6)[b]
	Flavan-3-ols (catechins)					
34	(+)-Catechin	>5	>50	>50	>50	**5.2**
35	(−)-Epicatechin	>5	>50	>50	>50	**7.5**
36	Gallocatechin	>5	>50	>50	>50	**45.3**
38	Epicatechin gallate	>5	>50	>50	>50	**26.5**
39	3′-*O*-methylcatechin	>5	>50	>50	>50	**24.8**
	Chalcones					
53	Xanthohumol	**0.02**	**1.7**	7.4	**12.9**	**16.6**
	Flavanones					
55	Isoxanthohumol	**0.3**	**6.5**	29.9	**21.9**	>100 (36)
56	Naringenin	**0.2**	>50	>50	>50	>100 (49)
57	8-Prenylnaringenin	**0.07**	**15.5**	>50	>50	**27.1**
58	6-Prenylnaringenin	**0.09**	**15.4**	>50	>50	>100 (52)
60	5-Methyl-6′-dimethyl-4′,5′-dihydropyrano[2′,3′,7,8]naringenin	**1.6**	**19.6**	>50	>50	>100 (0)
	Flavones					
62	Apigenin	**0.02**	>38.6	38.6	**17.5**	>100 (22)
64	Tricin	**0.13**	>50	>50	>50	>100 (38)
	Flavonols					
68	Kaempferol	>0.5	**5.5**	35.3	**40.6**	>100 (44)
70	Quercetin	**0.02**	2.6	14	**19.8**	>100 (47)
71	Quercitrin (quercetin-3-*O*-rhamnoside)	**3.6**	**5.1**	>50	**29.2**	>100 (15)
72	Isoquercitrin (quercetin-3-*O*-glucoside)	**4.3**	>50	>50	>50	>100 (8)
74	Myricetin	**0.05**	**11.7**	50	>50	>100 (36)
	Miscellaneous compounds					
78	1-Methyl-1,3,4,9-tetrahydropyrano[3,4b]indole	**1.5**	**33.9**	>50	>50	>100 (5)
79	4-Ketopinoresinol (lignan)	**2.2**	**6.0**	34.7	**33**	>100 (15)

Notes: Bold print indicates most potent activities.

[a]Cyp1A: Inhibition of the enzyme activity of cytochrome P450 1A; QR: Induction of the specific activity of NAD(P)H:quinone oxidoreductase (QR) in Hepa1c1c7 murine hepatoma cells; iNOS: Inhibition of lipopolysaccharide-mediated induction of inducible nitric oxide synthase (iNOS) in murine macrophages, measured *via* nitrite levels in cell culture supernatants; Cox-1: Inhibition of sheep-seminal vesicle-derived cyclooxygenase-1 enzymatic activity.
[b]IC_{50}: Halfmaximal inhibitory concentration. Values in parentheses indicate the percentage of inhibition at the indicated concentration.
[c]CD: Concentration required to double the specific activity of QR.
[d]IC_{50}: Concentration that results in 50% inhibition of cell viability.

[**78**] and 4-ketopinoresinol [**79**] displayed moderate Cyp1A inhibitory potential.

NAD(P)H:Quinone Reductase Induction The well-described model of QR induction in cultured Hepa 1c1c7 mouse hepatoma cells was used to characterize the potential of our series of test compound to induce phase 2 xenobiotics metabolism. Antioxidants may induce phase 2 enzymes *via* transcription factor binding to the so-called antioxidant response element. CD values of QR are summarized in Table 68.2 and Figure 68.8b.

The chalcone xanthohumol [**53**] and quercetin [**70**] were identified as most potent inducers of QR activity and we determined CD values of 1.7 and 2.6 μM, respectively. However, both compounds also displayed the highest cytotoxicity with IC_{50}-T values (concentration resulting in 50% inhibition of cell viability), of 7.4 and 14 μM (Table 68.2). Overall, the flavonols kaempferol [**68**], quercetin [**70**] and two quercetin glycosides quercitrin [**71**] and isoquercitrin [**72**] had a higher potential to induce QR activity than the flavanones isoxanthohumol [**55**], 8- and 6-prenylnaringenin [**57, 58**] and the naringenin derivative [**60**]. 1-Methyl-1,3,4,9-tetrahydropyrano[3,4b]indole [**78**] and the lignan 4-ketopinoresinol [**79**] induced QR activity with CD values of 33.9 and 6.0 μM, respectively.

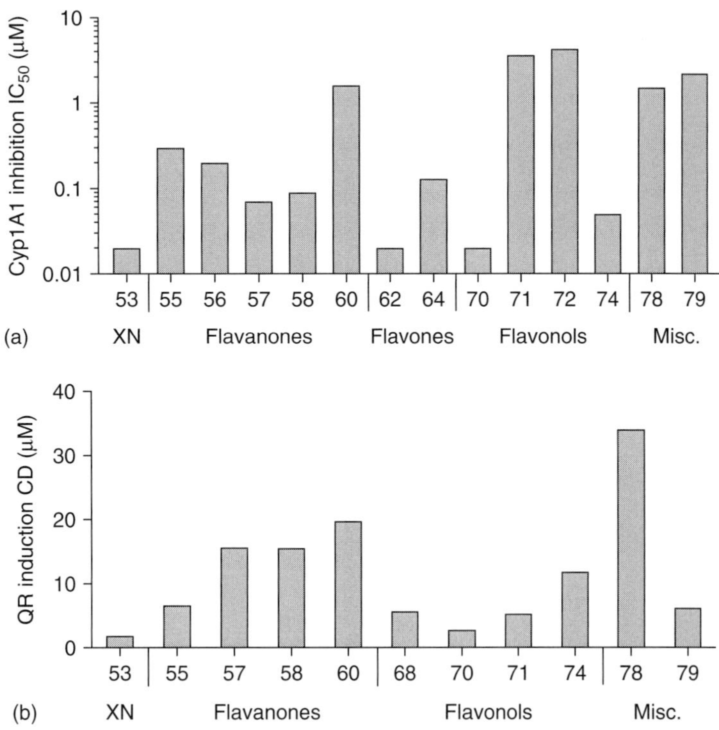

Figure 68.8 Modulation of xenobiotics metabolism. (a) Inhibition of phase 1 Cyp1A activity by beer compounds, measured in β-naphthoflavone-induced H4IIE rat hepatoma cell homogenates by dealkylation of CEC to fluorescent CHC. For comparison of inhibitory potential, IC_{50} are shown of all compounds which resulted in > 50% inhibition at a test concentration of 5 μM. (b) Induction of NAD(P)H: quinone reductase activity as a marker phase 2 enzyme in Hepa 1c1c7 cell culture by beer compounds. Given are CD values of QR in μM.

Anti-inflammatory mechanisms

It is estimated that 18% of all cancer cases are related to chronic inflammatory processes. We therefore tested for potential to inhibit the induction of iNOS and the activity of cyclooxygenase 1 (Cox-1). Both enzymes are involved in the generation of inflammatory mediators in the form of nitric oxide and prostaglandins.

Inhibition of iNOS Induction in Murine Macrophages Inhibition of iNOS induction was measured in LPS-stimulated Raw 264.7 murine macrophage cultures. As summarized in Table 68.2 and Figure 68.9a, only eight of all tested compounds were able to moderately inhibit iNOS induction, that is gallic acid [**15**], xanthohumol [**53**] and its cyclization product isoxanthohumol [**55**], apigenin [**62**], the flavonols kaempferol [**68**], quercetin [**70**] and quercitrin [**71**], as well as 4-ketopinoresinol [**79**], with IC_{50} values in the range of 18.7–40.6 μM. iNOS induction is mediated through activation of the NF-κB signaling pathway (Karin, 2006); therefore, it is likely that these compounds may inhibit iNOS induction by interfering with this pathway (Aggarwal and Shishodia, 2006).

Inhibition of Cox-1 Activity We utilized sheep seminal vesicle microsomes as a source of Cox-1 and measured oxygen consumption during the first step of prostaglandin production as an indication of Cox-1 activity. Notably, only the catechins [**34–39**], xanthohumol [**53**] and 8-prenylnaringenin [**57**] inhibited Cox-1 activity > 50% at concentrations below 100 μM. For (+)-catechin [**34**] and (−)-epicatechin [**35**] we determined IC_{50} values of 5.2 and 7.5 μM. Both compounds were clearly more potent than gallocatechin [**36**], epicatechin gallate [**38**] and 3′-*O*-methylcatechin [**39**]. A sugar linkage at the hydroxyl group in position 7 as in [**40**] completely abrogated Cox-1 inhibitory potential.

Estrogenic and anti-estrogenic activities

Hops have repeatedly been reported to possess estrogenic properties. Therefore, we investigated pro- and anti-estrogenic properties of xanthohumol [**53**] and the (prenylated) flavanones [**55–58**] derived from hops in Ishikawa cell culture. This human endometrial cancer cell line responds to estrogens with elevated ALP activity. Concomitant treatment with estrogens and test compounds allows the identification of anti-estrogens.

Dose-dependent induction of ALP activity is shown in Figure 68.10a. As reported previously (Gerhauser *et al.*, 2002a), xanthohumol [**53**] was identified as a pure anti-estrogen which did not induce ALP activity. In contrast,

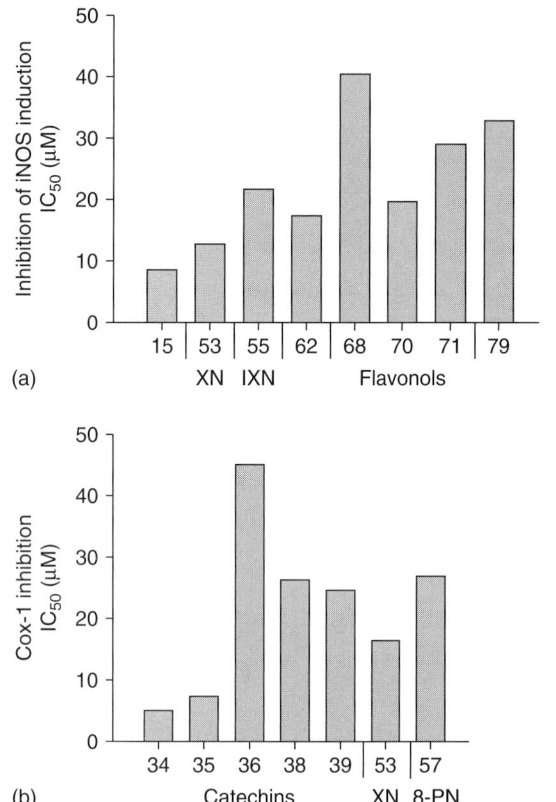

Figure 68.9 Anti-inflammatory mechanisms. (a) Inhibition of LPS-mediated nitric oxide production in Raw 264.7 murine macrophages. IC_{50} are given. XN: xanthohumol [**53**], IXN: isoxanthohumol [**55**]. (b) Inhibition of oxygen consumption during *in vitro* prostaglandin formation by Cox-1. IC_{50} are shown of all compounds which resulted in >50% inhibition at a test concentration of 100 μM. XN: xanthohumol [**53**]; 8-PN: 8-prenylnaringenin [**57**].

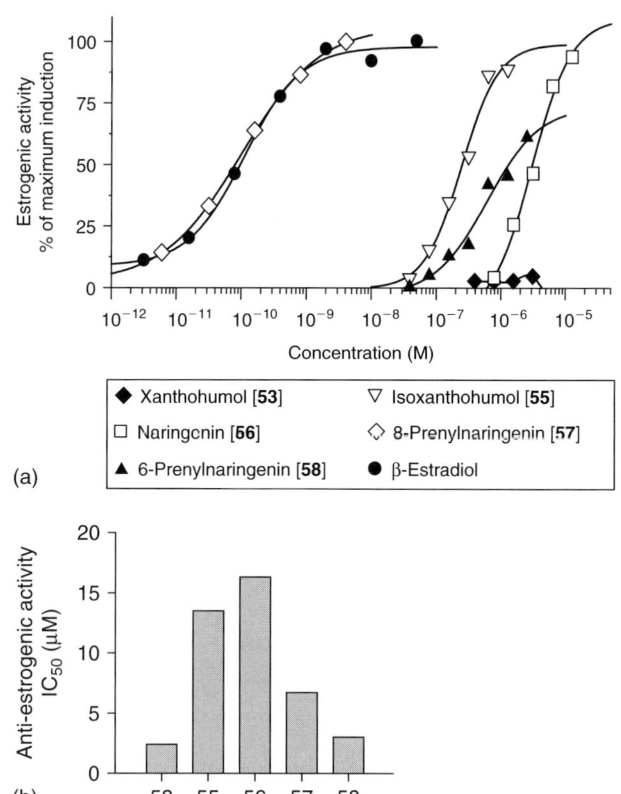

Figure 68.10 Demonstration of estrogenic and anti-estrogenic effects by xanthohumol and selected flavanones. (a) Induction of ALP activity in Ishikawa cell culture as a measure of estrogenic properties. Dose–response curves of xanthohumol [**53**], isoxanthohumol [**55**], naringenin [**56**], 8-prenylnaringenin [**57**], 6-prenylnaringenin [**57**] are shown in comparison with β-estradiol as a percentage of maximum induction. (b) Anti-estrogenic potential of xanthohumol [**53**], isoxanthohumol [**55**], naringenin [**56**], 8-prenylnaringenin [**57**] and 6-prenylnaringenin [**57**]. Ishikawa cells were treated concomitantly with test compounds and 5 nM β-estradiol. Anti-estrogenic activity was determined as inhibition of β-estradiol-induced ALP activity, and IC_{50} values are depicted.

isoxanthohumol [**55**] demonstrated estrogenic potential and induced ALP in a concentration range of 0.1–1 μM. Naringenin [**56**] was about one order of magnitude less active than isoxanthohumol. Prenylation in position C8 strongly increased the estrogenic activity of naringenin by a factor of 10.000, since 8-prenylnaringenin [**57**] was equally estrogenic as β-estradiol used for comparison as a reference compound. This was expected, as 8-prenyl-naringenin [**57**] has been described as one of the most potent phytoestrogens identified so far (Milligan *et al.*, 2002; and references cited in Gerhauser, 2005). On the contrary, prenylation in position C6 as in 6-prenylnaringenin [**58**] only weakly enhanced the estrogenic potential of naringenin [**56**].

All five compounds were also tested for potential anti-estrogenic activity by concomitant application of the compounds in combination with β-estradiol (Figure 68.10b). Xanthohumol [**53**] and 6-prenylnaringenin [**58**] were most effective in inhibiting β-estradiol-mediated induction of ALP activity with IC_{50} values of 2.5 and 3.1 μM. Isoxanthohumol [**55**], naringenin [**56**] and 8-prenylnaringenin [**57**] also inhibited ALP induction, although at higher concentrations. Under *in vivo* conditions the overall response will most likely be an estrogenic effect due to the lower concentrations required for induction of ALP activity in comparison with those required for inhibition of β-estradiol-mediated induction of ALP.

Further Investigations with Xanthohumol

Of all compounds tested, xanthohumol [**53**] was identified as the most promising lead compound for cancer chemoprevention. In addition to the described activities, xanthohumol was tested for anti-proliferative activity. It decreased human recombinant DNA polymerase α activity and inhibited DNA synthesis in MDA MB 435 human breast cancer cells. This led to an arrest of the cell cycle in S-phase (Gerhauser *et al.*, 2002a). Poly(ADP-ribose)polymerase

(PARP) cleavage, activation of caspases-3, -7, -8 and -9 and downregulation of Bcl-2 protein expression were found to contribute to apoptosis induction in cultured human colon cancer cells (Pan *et al.*, 2005). Xanthohumol was also shown to induce cell differentiation in HL-60 human leukemia cells (Gerhauser *et al.*, 2002a) and demonstrated anti-angiogenic potential in a human *in vitro* anti-angiogenesis assay (summarized in Gerhauser, 2005).

Importantly, xanthohumol at nanomolar concentrations prevented carcinogen-induced preneoplastic lesions in mouse mammary gland organ culture (MMOC), providing a first direct indication for its chemopreventive potential (Gerhauser *et al.*, 2002a). Ongoing investigations determine mammary cancer preventive potential of xanthohumol in a long-term carcinogenesis model.

Summary Points

- Beer contains a complex mixture of phenolic compounds belonging to at least 10 different structural classes. In the present study, 48 beer compounds were tested in a series of *in vitro* bioassays indicative of cancer preventive potential. Notably, various structural classes of compounds had quite distinct profiles of activities.
- Overall, catechins and proanthocyanidins were identified as the most potent radical scavengers against DPPH, superoxide anion and peroxyl radicals. Cinnamic acids, xanthohumol and myricetin were most potent in scavenging very reactive hydroxyl radicals.
  With respect to modulation of xenobiotics metabolism, especially xanthohumol and various classes of flavonoids demonstrated potent effects: Xanthohumol, (prenylated) flavanones and the aglycons apigenin, quercetin and myricetin were identified as very potent inhibitors of Cyp1A activity at nanomolar concentrations. On the other hand, xanthohumol, flavanones and flavonols enhanced NAD(P)H:quinone reductase activity as an indication for elevated detoxification.
- Anti-inflammatory activity by inhibition of LPS-induced iNOS activity was provided by gallic acid, xanthohumol, isoxanthohumol, apigenin, selected flavonols and 4-ketopinoresinol, whereas catechins, xanthohumol and 8-prenylnaringenin were identified as Cox-1 inhibitors.
- Based on these results, it is likely that the combination of compounds with different activity profiles might enhance a potential biological effect *in vivo*. This aspect should be paid more attention in future studies.

Acknowledgments

I would like to thank my current and former coworkers K. Klimo, J. Knauft, I. Neumann, A. Gamal-Eldeen, M. Späth and E. Heiss for their valuable results summarized in this report and our cooperation partners A. Alt and H. Becker for long-lasting fruitful cooperation.

References

Aggarwal, B.B. and Shishodia, S. (2006). *Biochem. Pharmacol.* 71, 1397–1421.
Bartsch, H. and Nair, J. (2006). *Langenbeck Arch. Surg.* 391, 499–510.
Cao, G. and Prior, R.L. (1999). *Method Enzymol.* 299, 50–62.
Crespi, C.L., Miller, V.P. and Penman, B.W. (1997). *Anal. Biochem.* 248, 188–190.
Ewing, J.F. and Janero, D.R. (1995). *Anal. Biochem.* 232, 243–248.
Gerhauser, C., Alt, A., Heiss, E., Gamal-Eldeen, A., Klimo, K., Knauft, J., Neumann, I., Scherf, H.R., Frank, N., Bartsch, H. and Becker, H. (2002a). *Mol. Cancer Ther.* 1, 959–969.
Gerhauser, C., Alt, A.P., Klimo, K., Knauft, J., Frank, N. and Becker, H. (2002b). *Phytochem. Rev.* 1, 369–377.
Gerhauser, C. (2005). *Eur. J. Cancer* 41, 1941–1954.
Heiss, E., Herhaus, C., Klimo, K., Bartsch, H. and Gerhauser, C. (2001). *J. Biol. Chem.* 276, 32008–32015.
Jang, M.S. and Pezzuto, J.M. (1997). *Method Cell Sci.* 19, 25–31.
Karin, M. (2006). *Nature* 441, 431–436.
Kelloff, G.J., Lippman, S.M., Dannenberg, A.J., Sigman, C.C., Pearce, H.L., Reid, B.J., Szabo, E., Jordan, V.C., Spitz, M.R., Mills, G.B., Papadimitrakopoulou, V.A., Lotan, R., Aggarwal, B.B., Bresalier, R.S., Kim, J., Arun, B., Lu, K.H., Thomas, M.E., Rhodes, H.E., Brewer, M.A., Follen, M., Shin, D.M., Parnes, H.L., Siegfried, J.M., Evans, A.A., Blot, W.J., Chow, W.H., Blount, P.L., Maley, C.C., Wang, K.K., Lam, S., Lee, J.J., Dubinett, S.M., Engstrom, P.F., Meyskens Jr., F.L., O'Shaughnessy, J., Hawk, E.T., Levin, B., Nelson, W.G. and Hong, W.K. (2006). *Clin. Cancer Res.* 12, 3661–3697.
Littlefield, B.A., Gurpide, E., Markiewicz, L., McKinley, B. and Hochberg, R.B. (1990). *Endocrinology* 127, 2757–2762.
Markiewicz, L., Hochberg, R.B. and Gurpide, E. (1992). *J. Steroid Biochem. Mol. Biol.* 41, 53–58.
Milligan, S., Kalita, J., Pocock, V., Heyerick, A., De Cooman, L., Rong, H. and De Keukeleire, D. (2002). *Reproduction* 123, 235–242.
Nozawa, H., Nakao, W., Takata, J., Arimoto-Kobayashi, S. and Kondo, K. (2006). *Cancer Lett.* 235, 121–129.
Nozawa, H., Tazumi, K., Sato, K., Yoshida, A., Takata, J., Arimoto-Kobayashi, S. and Kondo, K. (2004a). *Mutat. Res.* 559, 177–187.
Nozawa, H., Yoshida, A., Tajima, O., Katayama, M., Sonore, H., Wakabayashi, K. and Kondo, K. (2004b). *Int. J. Cancer* 108, 404–411.
Ou, B., Hampsch-Woodill, M., Flanagan, J., Deemer, E.K., Prior, R.L. and Huang, D. (2002). *J. Agric. Food Chem.* 50, 2772–2777.
Ou, B., Hampsch-Woodill, M. and Prior, R.L. (2001). *J. Agric. Food Chem.* 49, 4619–4626.
Pan, L., Becker, H. and Gerhauser, C. (2005). *Mol. Nutr. Food Res.* 49, 837–843.
Pick, E. and Mizel, D. (1981). *J. Immunol. Methods* 46, 211–226.
Prochaska, H.J. and Santamaria, A.B. (1988). *Anal. Biochem.* 169, 328–336.

Skehan, P., Storeng, R., Scudiero, D., Monks, A., McMahon, J., Vistica, D., Warren, J.T., Bokesch, H., Kenney, S. and Boyd, M.R. (1990). *J. Natl. Cancer Inst.* 82, 1107–1112.

Smith, P.K., Krohn, R.I., Hermanson, G.T., Mallia, A.K., Gartner, F.H., Provenzano, M.D., Fujimoto, E.K., Goeke, N.M., Olson, B.J. and Klenk, D.C. (1985). *Anal. Biochem.* 150, 76–85.

Sporn, M.B. and Newton, D.L. (1979). *Fed. Proc.* 38, 2528–2535.

Surh, Y.J. (2003). *Nat. Rev. Cancer* 3, 768–780.

Takeuchi, T., Nakajima, M. and Morimoto, K. (1994). *Cancer Res.* 54, 5837–5840.

Ukeda, H., Maeda, S., Ishii, T. and Sawamura, M. (1997). *Anal. Biochem.* 251, 206–209.

Valko, M., Rhodes, C.J., Moncol, J., Izakovic, M. and Mazur, M. (2006). *Chem. Biol. Interact.* 160, 1–40.

van Amsterdam, F.T., Roveri, A., Maiorino, M., Ratti, E. and Ursini, F. (1992). *Free Radical Biol. Med.* 12, 183–187.

Yang, C.S., Landau, J.M., Huang, M.T. and Newmark, H.L. (2001). *Annu. Rev. Nutr.* 21, 381–406.

69

Beer Inhibition of Azoxymethane-Induced Colonic Carcinogenesis

Hajime Nozawa and Keiji Kondo Central Laboratories for Frontier Technology, Research Section for Applied Food Science, Kirin Holdings Co., Ltd., Takasaki, Gunma, Japan

Abstract

Modulatory effects of beer intake on azoxymethane (AOM)-induced rat colonic carcinogenesis in male Fischer 344 rats were investigated. Single cell gel electrophoresis assay indicated that DNA damage of colonocytes, induced by a single AOM injection (15 mg/kg body weight), was significantly reduced in rats fed beer or malt extract for 2 weeks. Examination of aberrant crypt foci (ACF) formation in colonic mucosa, induced by AOM (15 mg/kg body weight, twice weekly), revealed that feeding of beer during the whole experimental period of 5 weeks significantly reduced the number of ACF by 35%. In the post-initiation protocol, a reduction in ACF formation by 26% was not significant. The efficacy in inhibition of ACF formation varied with the brand of beer. ACF formation was significantly reduced in rats treated with freeze-dried beer, but not with ethanol, suggesting that nonvolatile components of beer are responsible for the reduction. Significant suppression of ACF formation was observed in groups treated with hot water extract of malt, especially with extracts of colored malts, although no reduction was observed by feeding with hops extract. A long-term experiment of 42 weeks indicated that intake of beer decreased tumor incidence by 22% and decreased the number of neoplastic lesions, including adenocarcinomas and adenomas by 44%. These results suggest that components of beer have chemopreventive effects on colonic carcinogenesis induced by AOM and that intake of beer may contribute to a reduction in the risk of cancer susceptibility.

List of Abbreviations

ACF	Aberrant crypt foci
ACs	Aberrant crypts
AOM	Azoxymethane
FD beer	Freeze-dried beer
(I)	Initiation
(PI)	Post-initiation
(I/PI)	Initiation and post-initiation
AIN	AIN-76A
AD	Adenomas
ADC	Adenocarcinomas
Comet assay	Single cell gel electrophoresis assay

Introduction

The cancer process by which normal cells become progressively transformed to malignancy is now known to require the sequential acquisition of mutations that arise as a consequence of damage to the DNA. This damage may result from interactions of DNA with exogenous agents such as ionizing radiation, UV radiation, and chemical carcinogens. Around a century ago, it has already demonstrated that chemical carcinogens cause cancer in rodents, and it is now considered that cancer is caused by the process of sequenced steps summarized in Figure 69.1. The first step is called initiation process. This process includes multisteps of mutagenesis which leads normal cell to mutated (initiated) cell. The second process, promotion process, causes clonal expansion in initiated cell to form preneoplastic lesions or tumors. In the third process, progression process, tumors cause angiogenesis or metastasis to become more malignancy.

It is well recognized that in the fight against cancer, preventive strategies are in the long term better than therapy. The agents derived from dietary source or medicinal source are used for cancer chemoprevention to retard the progression of carcinogenesis or to inhibit carcinogenesis, leading to lowered risk of neoplastic diseases. Chemopreventive agents are generally categorized in five classes: antimutagens, antioxidants, antiinflammatory agents, signal transduction modulators, and hormone modulators by their molecular

Beer in Health and Disease Prevention
ISBN: 978-0-12-373891-2

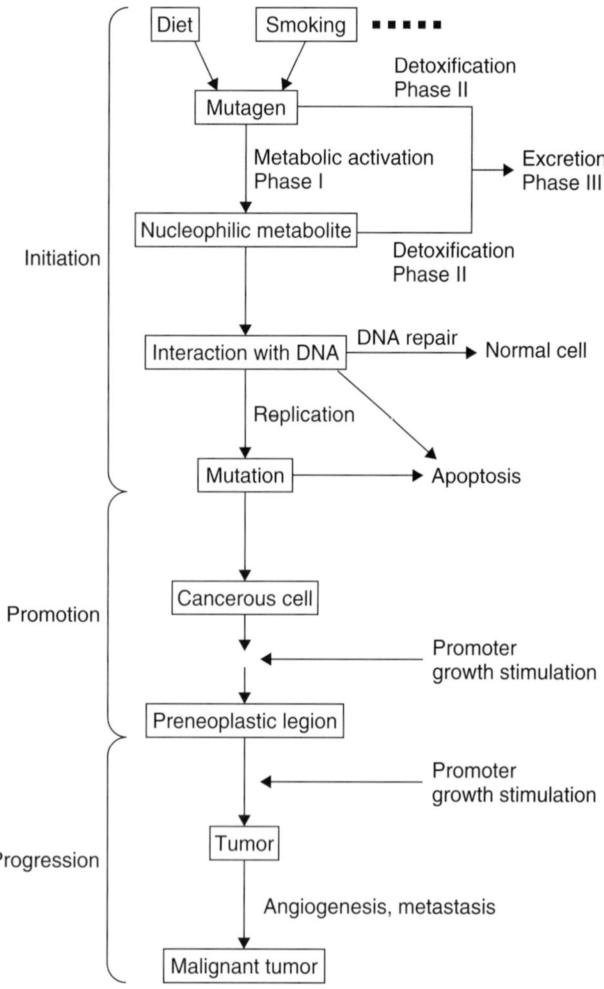

Figure 69.1 Schematic representation of carcinogenesis. There are several steps in carcinogenesis and many targets exist for the preventive strategies for cancer incidences.

action in cancer prevention (Lieberman *et al.*, 1998). Some plant constituents, including antioxidative vitamins and phenolics, possess many biological functions, such as anti-inflammatory (Middleton and Kandaswami, 1992), antioxidative (Ho *et al.*, 1992), antimutagenic (Shiraki *et al.*, 1994; Arimoto-Kobayashi *et al.*, 1999), and antiangiogenetic (Paper, 1998) actions, related to cancer chemopreventive activity. The famous bioactive plant constituents which exert cancer chemopreventive effects are catechins, isothiocyanates, and isoflavones. Tea catechins exert antimutagenic and antiangiogenic activities (Rodriguez *et al.*, 2005). Isothiocyanates, for example sulforaphane from broccoli sprout, activate nrf2 (nuclear factor-erythroid 2 p45-related factor) and then induce phase II detoxification enzymes to prevent cancer initiation (Morimitsu *et al.*, 2002). Soy isoflavones are excellent chemopreventive agents against breast cancer by which exhibit antiestrogenic action *in vivo* (Cotroneo *et al.*, 2002).

For evaluation of cancer preventive activity, the typical approach is to screen *in vitro* or cell-based mechanistic assays, and then, to confirm the efficacy in animal carcinogenesis models with cancers or precancerous lesions as end points. For the screen *in vitro* or cell-based mechanistic assays, the battery of assays is designed to address various specific activities associated with ability of cancer prevention, that is antimutagenicity, antiproliferation, and antioxidation. For the confirmation of the efficacy in animal carcinogenesis models, many chemically induced carcinogenesis models or transgenic and gene knockout models have been developed (Steele *et al.*, 1994). Among chemical carcinogenesis models, AOM-induced colonic carcinogene-sis model is well established and utilized for the evaluation of chemopreventive agents. In the chemically induced carcinogenesis, those carcinogens are introduced to the experimental animals at a dose level high enough to induce a significant incidence and number of cancers or preneoplastic lesions in a target tissue. The chemopreventive agents are administered to animals before, at the same time, or after the treatment of carcinogen. The relative timing of the treatment of carcinogen and chemopreventive agent is useful in interpreting mechanistic insights for chemoprevention. For example, if the chemopreventive agents inhibit carcinogenesis when they are administered to animals only before the carcinogen treatment, these agents most likely inhibit the initiation phase of carcinogenesis.

Beer, a low-alcohol beverage made primarily of malt and hops, is the most consumed type of alcohol in the world. Beer in moderation is recognized as a wholesome beverage because it is brewed by yeast from natural ingredients containing valuable substances in a harmonious composition nutritionally and some of which have been used in homeopathy for many hundreds of years. Beer is rich in amino acids, peptides, vitamins, and phenolic compounds derived from hops and malts, and thus may have some health benefits. In particular, it is rich in the B vitamins, for example niacin, riboflavin, pyridoxine (B6), and folate. The dried hop cones contain 4–14% polyphenols and these compounds are mainly phenolic acids, prenylated chalcones, flavonoids, catechins, and proanthocyanidins (Stevens *et al.*, 1998). In addition, hops provides a resin containing monoacyl phloroglucides, which are converted to hop bitter acids during the brewing process (De Keukeleire *et al.*, 2003). However, the majority (70–80%) of beer polyphenols are from malts. Barley polyphenols are not well characterized than hop polyphenols, although cathecins or proanthocyanidins are derived from barley or malts. Recent research suggests that vitamin B6 in beer gives beer drinkers additional protection against cardiovascular disease compared to drinkers of wine or spirits (Schlienger, 2003). Folate has been shown to be protective against cardiovascular disease and some cancers (Mayer *et al.*, 2001). In the epidemiological study, there is the evidence that high alcohol intake is related to carcinogenesis, especially to cancers of the mouth, pharynx, larynx, esophagus, and liver, and probable evidence for an association between heavy drinking and colorectal cancer in men, and breast cancer in women (Potter, 1997). On the other hand, beer consumption was reported to significantly decrease the risk of prostate and colon cancer (La Vecchia *et al.*, 1993; Jain *et al.*, 1998). In the carcinogenesis experiments in rodents, there are some evidences. Nelson reported that beer significantly reduced the incidence of DMH (1,2-dimethylhydrazine)-induced tumors by 33% and the number of gastrointestinal tumors per rat from 2.91 ± 0.52 in the control group to 1.33 ± 0.43 in the beer-fed group, significantly (Nelson and Samelson, 1985). Hamilton incorporated high or low amounts of beer (23% or 12% of calories as alcohol in beer) into a liquid diet and the high beer group showed a significantly reduced incidence of tumors in the right colon (Hamilton *et al.*, 1987). Moreover, beer intake reduced the chromosome damage of lymphocytes induced by X-ray radiation (Monobe and Ando, 2002). However, there are not enough evidences to clarify whether beer in moderation is cancer chemopreventive or not, and therefore, further detailed experiments are required. There are no experimental data for the relation between beer intake and whole steps of AOM-induced colonic carcinogenesis. In this chapter, modulating effects of beer on AOM-induced rat colonic carcinogenesis are stated (Nozawa *et al.*, 2004, 2005).

Beer Inhibition of AOM-Induced DNA Damage in Colon Cells by Single Cell Gel Electrophoresis Assay

The single cell gel electrophoresis assay (comet assay) can be used to monitor DNA damage in individual organs of rodents exposed to mutagens (Singh *et al.*, 1988; Sasaki *et al.*, 1997). This assay is based on the ability of denatured DNA fragments to migrate out of the nucleus to form comet tails during electrophoresis under alkaline conditions (pH > 12.6) and has been used to examine the efficacy of chemopreventive agents in the initiation stage of carcinogenesis (Kassie *et al.*, 2002; Guglielmi *et al.*, 2003; Lazze *et al.*, 2003). Male Fischer 344 rats at 5 weeks of age were fed a basal diet (CE2) and experimental drinks or a control drink (water) *ad libitum* for 2 weeks. In this experiment, experimental drinks were beer A (brewed from Munich malt, Pilsner malt, and hops), 1% (w/w) hot water extracts of hops and 5% (w/w) hot water extracts of malt. Each treatment group consisted of four animals and they received subcutaneous injections of AOM at a dose of 15 mg/kg body weight at 16 h before sacrifice. Three animals used as the vehicle controls were administered an equal volume of saline. Immediately after the sacrifice, colons were excised and colonocytes were prepared for comet assay (Singh *et al.*, 1988; Pool-Zobel *et al.*, 1993; Tice *et al.*, 2000).

As shown in Figure 69.2, comet lengths of the colonocytes from untreated control animals were, on average,

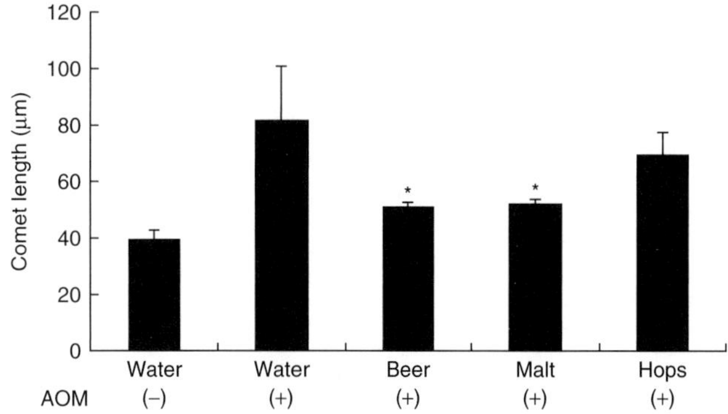

Figure 69.2 Effects of beer A, malt extract, and hops extract on DNA damage in the rat colonocyte induced by AOM. Experimental drinks were fed to the animals ($n = 4$ for AOM treated and $n = 3$ for saline treated) for 2 weeks and colons were excised 16 h after AOM injection; 100 nuclei were analyzed for each animal in the comet assay. Bars indicate means ± SD values. Significantly different from the AOM control at $^{*}p < 0.01$.

40 μm. AOM treatment induced significant DNA damage in colon cells: comet lengths in the group receiving water were 2-fold longer than those in the saline-treated control. Comet lengths in the groups fed either beer or malt extract were significantly shorter than those in the AOM-treated rats (37% and 36%, respectively), suggesting beer or malt extract inhibited AOM-induced DNA damage. A reduction in comet length of only 15% was observed in the hops extract group: this was not significant.

Beer Inhibition of AOM-Induced ACF Formation in Rat Colon

Aberrant crypt foci (ACF) are early morphological changes or hyperproliferative lesions found in the colon of humans and carcinogen-treated rodents: they are considered to be putative pre-neoplastic lesions for colon cancer (Bird, 1987; Roncucci *et al.*, 1991; Pretlow *et al.*, 1994). Azoxymethane (AOM)-induced colonic ACF in rats have been used to identify chemical agents that prevent colon cancer, including many dietary factors, especially those derived from plant sources (Olivo and Wargovich, 1998; Wargovich *et al.*, 2000). In this chapter, ACF formation was investigated by three protocols over 5 weeks. Test samples, beer in liquid form or freeze-dried one (FD beer), were given to the animals during the whole experimental period of 5 weeks (I/PI), during initiation phase (I) and during post-initiation phase (PI). For the initiation (I) protocol, experimental samples were given for 17 days from the beginning of the experiment. For the post-initiation (PI) protocol, experimental samples were given 3 days after the second AOM injection until the end of the experiment. In all protocols for 1 week after the start of experiments, rats were treated with subcutaneous injections of AOM (15 mg/kg body weight) once a week for 2 weeks. ACF were distinguished from normal crypts by their increased size, more prominent epithelial cells and their increased pericryptal area (Bird, 1987). The number of ACF and the number of aberrant crypts (ACs) per rat were quantified.

Typical ACF observed in rat colon by treatment with AOM are shown in Figure 69.3. Daily ingestion of beer A during the whole experimental period of 5 weeks (I/PI) significantly reduced the number of ACF/colon by 35%, the total number of ACs/colon by 40%, and the number of ACF with 4 or more crypts/focus by 67% (Table 69.1). The inhibitory effect was less pronounced when beer A was introduced after the second AOM injection (PI): 26% reduction in ACF/colon, 33% reduction in ACs/colon, and 62% reduction in ACF with 4 or more crypts/focus. In the post-initiation protocol, a reduction in the total number of ACF was not significant. Intake of 5% ethanol in both protocols slightly reduced the number of ACF/colon, ACs/colon, and ACF with 4 or more crypts, but these effects were not significant. It was observed that the extent of inhibition of beer on AOM-induced ACF formation varied among the brands of beer (Nozawa *et al.*, 2004).

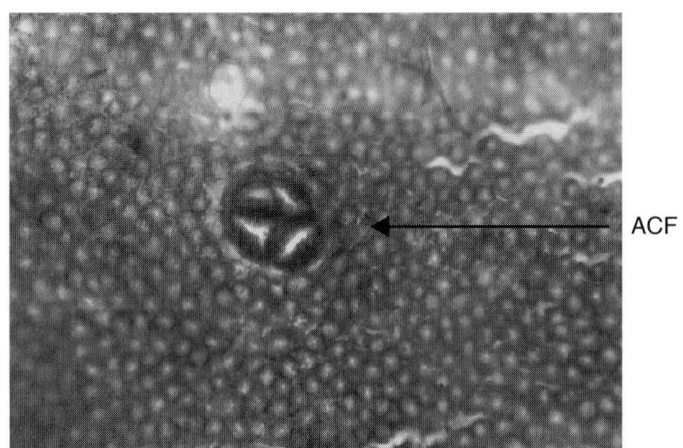

Figure 69.3 ACF with 4 ACs observed in the colonic mucosa of rat treated with AOM.

Inhibitory Effects of FD Beer A on AOM-Induced ACF Formation

Since ethanol had only a small effect on AOM-induced ACF formation, the inhibitory effects of beer were thought to be attributable to the solid components. We evaluated the effects of various concentrations of FD beer A on AOM-induced ACF formation (Table 69.2). Animals

Table 69.1 Effects of beer A on AOM-induced ACF formation in the (I/PI) and (PI) protocols

Group	*Incidence*	*Body weight (g)*	*No. of ACF/colon*	*No. of ACs/colon*	*No. of ACs/focus*	*No. of ACF > 3AC/colon*
AOM + water	8/8	221.4 ± 6.6^a	97.9 ± 25.7	213.3 ± 54.0	2.2 ± 0.1	8.8 ± 3.5
AOM + 5% ethanol (I/PI)	8/8	217.5 ± 8.2	92.6 ± 25.4	186.0 ± 46.4	2.0 ± 0.2	5.6 ± 2.4
AOM + beer A (I/PI)	8/8	212.5 ± 14.6	63.3 ± 12.7^b	126.6 ± 28.6^d	2.0 ± 0.2	2.9 ± 1.7^c
AOM + 5% ethanol (PI)	8/8	219.4 ± 7.4	95.3 ± 23.0	193.8 ± 47.2	2.0 ± 0.1	5.5 ± 3.3
AOM + beer A (PI)	8/8	217.6 ± 9.8	72.4 ± 18.7	142.8 ± 39.6^b	2.0 ± 0.2	3.3 ± 2.6^c

[a]Values are given as mean ± SD.
Significantly different from AOM + water group: $^b p < 0.05$; $^c p < 0.005$; $^d p < 0.001$.

Table 69.2 Effects of FD beer A on AOM-induced ACF formation in the (I/PI) protocol

Group	*Incidence*	*Body weight (g)*	*Daily diet intake (g/rat)*	*No. of ACF/colon*	*No. of ACs/colon*	*No. of ACs/focus*	*No. of ACF > 3AC/colon*
AOM + AIN	8/8	217.4 ± 14.5^a	12.2	97.5 ± 16.1	222.1 ± 40.7	2.3 ± 0.2	10.3 ± 4.2
AOM + 0.1%FD beer A (I/PI)	8/8	210.1 ± 12.7	11.8	100.9 ± 17.6	208.9 ± 31.9	2.1 ± 0.2	5.9 ± 4.3
AOM + 0.25%FD beer A (I/PI)	8/8	216.7 ± 14.3	12.1	86.3 ± 16.3	187.4 ± 34.9	2.2 ± 0.2	7.0 ± 3.7
AOM + 0.5%FD beer A (I/PI)	8/8	218.9 ± 13.5	11.7	83.9 ± 17.3	173.9 ± 42.0^b	2.1 ± 0.1	5.4 ± 3.2^b
AOM + 1%FD beer A (I/PI)	8/8	214.3 ± 12.7	12.1	69.8 ± 10.9^c	150.1 ± 23.5^c	2.2 ± 0.1	3.8 ± 2.4^c
AOM + 2%FD beer A (I/PI)	8/8	213.1 ± 11.4	11.3	67.0 ± 19.3^b	139.0 ± 39.1^c	2.1 ± 0.2	3.1 ± 1.1^c
AOM + 4%FD beer A (I/PI)	8/8	212.2 ± 6.0	11.5	77.8 ± 10.0^b	159.6 ± 18.2^c	2.1 ± 0.2	4.6 ± 2.5^c

[a]Values are given as mean ± SD.
Significantly different from the AOM + AIN group: $^b p < 0.05$; $^c p < 0.005$.

were fed the AIN76-A basal diet containing 0.1%, 0.25%, 0.5%, 1%, 2%, or 4% FD beer for 5 weeks (I/PI). There were no significant differences in the daily consumptions of diets and final body weights among the experimental and control groups. A significant decrease in the number of ACF was observed by feeding FD beer at 1%, 2%, and 4% in the basal diet (28%, 31%, and 20% reduction, respectively). Diets containing 0.1%, 0.25%, and 0.5% FD beer were less effective with the same protocol, suggesting the optimal effective dose to be between 1% and 2%. These dosing levels for animal experiments were estimated as 265 and 530 ml beer intake for humans (Nozawa *et al.*, 2004).

We then compared the inhibitory effect of FD beer on AOM-induced ACF formation with that of piroxicam, a nonsteroidal antiinflammatory drug, in the three different protocols (I/PI, I, and PI in Table 69.3). Results indicated that feeding of 1% FD beer in the basal diet during the whole experimental period (I/PI) and initiation phase (I) significantly suppressed ACF formation; the total number of ACF was decreased by 28% and 30%, respectively. A weak suppressive effect was observed when the experimental diet was fed in the post-initiation phase (PI) (14%). Piroxicam showed strong inhibition of ACF formation in the (I/PI) and (PI) protocols; the total number of ACF was decreased by 46% and 53%, respectively. No significant inhibition was observed in the (I) protocol.

Inhibitory Effects of Raw Materials on AOM-Induced ACF Formation

To investigate the nature of the inhibitory components in beer, AOM-injected animals were given malt or hops extracts during the experimental period of 5 weeks (I/PI). Treatment of animals with 5% malt extract significantly reduced the number of ACF, no decrease was observed in the group treated with 1% hops extract (Table 69.4). In addition, four different types of malt, Pilsner, Munich, Chocolate, and Caramel, were examined for their ability to inhibit ACF formation. While all types of malt extract significantly reduced the number of ACF, dark roasted malts were more effective than pilsner malt in reducing the number of ACF: Munich, Chocolate, and Caramel malts showed 28%, 28%, and 29% reduction, respectively (Table 69.5).

Table 69.3 Effects of FD beer A and piroxicam on AOM-induced ACF formation in the (I), (PI), and (I/PI) protocols

Group	*Incidence*	*Body weight (g)*	*No. of ACF/colon*	*No. of ACs/colon*	*No. of ACs/focus*	*No. of ACF > 3AC/colon*
AOM + AIN	8/8	217.4 ± 14.5^a	97.5 ± 16.1	222.1 ± 40.7	2.3 ± 0.2	10.3 ± 4.2
AOM + 1%FD beer A (I/PI)	8/8	214.3 ± 12.7	69.8 ± 10.9^c	150.1 ± 23.5^c	2.2 ± 0.1	3.8 ± 2.4^c
AOM + 200 ppm piroxicam (I/PI)	8/8	205.2 ± 6.3	44.8 ± 16.4^d	94.4 ± 38.7^d	2.1 ± 0.2	3.3 ± 2.4^c
AOM + 1%FD beer A (I)	8/8	217.3 ± 13.8	68.3 ± 17.4^c	136.1 ± 32.8^c	2.0 ± 0.3	4.8 ± 4.1^b
AOM + 200 ppm piroxicam (I)	8/8	209.2 ± 8.3	89.9 ± 17.1	189.1 ± 35.7	2.1 ± 0.1	6.6 ± 3.3
AOM + 1%FD beer A (PI)	8/8	214.7 ± 9.0	83.9 ± 16.9	172.1 ± 34.2^b	2.1 ± 0.1	3.9 ± 1.6^c
AOM + 200 ppm piroxicam (PI)	8/8	209.7 ± 6.5	46.9 ± 14.2^d	96.6 ± 31.3^d	2.1 ± 0.2	1.6 ± 2.6^d

[a] Values are given as mean ± SD.
Significantly different from the AOM + AIN group: $^b p < 0.05$; $^c p < 0.005$; $^d p < 0.001$.

Table 69.4 Effects of hot water extracts of hops and pilsner malt on AOM-induced ACF formation in the (I/PI) protocol

Group	*Incidence*	*Body weight (g)*	*No. of ACF/colon*	*No. of ACs/colon*	*No. of ACs/focus*	*No. of ACF > 3AC/colon*
AOM + water	6/6	236.9 ± 5.6^a	153.5 ± 19.5	350.5 ± 63.0	2.3 ± 0.2	15.7 ± 8.0
AOM + hops (I/PI)	6/6	229.0 ± 10.6	174.3 ± 60.8	380.2 ± 142.9	2.2 ± 0.1	12.7 ± 7.2
AOM + Pilsner Malt (I/PI)	6/6	240.6 ± 10.9	91.7 ± 23.5^b	221.7 ± 65.4	2.4 ± 0.2	11.8 ± 5.0

[a] Values are given as mean ± SD.
Significantly different from the AOM + water group: $^b p < 0.05$.

Table 69.5 Effects of hot water extracts of four types of malts on AOM-induced ACF formation in the (I/PI) protocol

Group	*Incidence*	*Body weight (g)*	*No. of ACF/colon*	*No. of ACs/colon*	*No. of ACs/focus*	*No. of ACF > 3AC/colon*
AOM + water	8/8	218.3 ± 4.9[a]	171.3 ± 27.0	390.1 ± 70.2	2.3 ± 0.2	20.1 ± 8.9
AOM + Pilsner malt (I/PI)	8/8	218.9 ± 14.9	139.3 ± 15.3[b]	309.8 ± 29.5[b]	2.2 ± 0.1	11.5 ± 4.4
AOM + Munich malt (I/PI)	8/8	213.6 ± 12.9	123.3 ± 30.3[c]	267.0 ± 70.4[c]	2.2 ± 0.1	11.9 ± 4.9
AOM + Chocolate malt (I/PI)	8/8	212.2 ± 8.6	124.0 ± 20.7[c]	287.9 ± 62.2[c]	2.3 ± 0.3	16.0 ± 7.2
AOM + Caramel malt (I/PI)	8/8	212.1 ± 9.6	121.5 ± 21.4[c]	256.3 ± 43.5[d]	2.1 ± 0.1	9.1 ± 5.5

Note: Effects of beer A on colonic carcinogenesis.
[a]Values are given as mean ± SD.
Significantly different from the AOM + water group: [b]$p < 0.05$; [c]$p < 0.01$; [d]$p < 0.005$.

Table 69.6 Effects of beer A on AOM-induced tumor incidence in the colon of F344 rats

			Tumor incidence (%)								
			Rectum		*Middle colon*		*Proximal colon*		*Entire colon*		
Group	*Animals (n)*	*Body weight (g)*	*AD*	*ADC*	*AD*	*ADC*	*AD*	*ADC*	*AD*	*ADC*	*Total*
Saline + water	13	416.2 ± 21.5[a]	0	0	0	0	0	0	0	0	0
AOM + water	22	393.7 ± 24.7[b]	14	9	32	64	9	32	46	82	86
AOM + beer A	22	385.2 ± 22.8[b]	0	9	5[c]	59	0	18	5[d]	64	64

[a]Values are given as mean ± SD.
Significantly different from the saline + water group: [b]$p < 0.05$.
Significantly different from the AOM + water group: [c]$p < 0.05$; [d]$p < 0.01$.

Table 69.7 Effects of beer A on AOM-induced tumor multiplicity in the colon of F344 rats

		Tumor multipulicity (tumors/animals)								
		Rectum		*Middle colon*		*Proximal colon*		*Entire colon*		
Group	*Animals (n)*	*AD*	*ADC*	*AD*	*ADC*	*AD*	*ADC*	*AD*	*ADC*	*Total*
Saline + water	13	0	0	0	0	0	0	0	0	0
AOM + water	22	0.14 ± 0.35[a]	0.14 ± 0.47	0.32 ± 0.48	0.86 ± 0.83	0.09 ± 0.29	0.41 ± 0.73	0.55 ± 0.67	1.41 ± 1.10	1.95 ± 1.50
AOM + beer A	22	0	0.13 ± 0.47	0.09 ± 0.43[b]	0.73 ± 0.70	0	0.14 ± 0.35[b]	0.09 ± 0.43[c]	1.00 ± 0.98[b]	1.09 ± 1.15[c]

[a]Values are given as mean ± SD.
Significantly different from the AOM + water group: [b]$p < 0.05$; [c]$p < 0.005$.

Beer Inhibition of AOM-Induced Colonic Carcinogenesis in Rats

Ninety-three rats were randomly divided into three groups, 40 rats for the AOM + water group, 40 rats for the AOM + beer A group, and 13 rats for the AOM untreated group (saline + water group). Rats received the basal diet (CE2) with water or beer *ad libitum* during the experimental period. Rats in the AOM + water and AOM + beer A groups received 2 subcutaneous injections of AOM (15 mg/kg body weight per week), rats in the saline + water group were injected with saline. Six rats each were taken from the AOM + beer A and AOM + water groups for the analysis of ACF at 5, 16, and 24 weeks. At 42 weeks, all rats were sacrificed and colons were excised and examined for the presence of neoplastic. Each colon was divided into three parts: rectum colon (3 cm from anus), middle colon (3–15 cm part), and proximal colon (rest of the colon including cecum). The locations of all lesions were scored and these lesions were embedded in paraffin blocks, sectioned, and stained with hematoxylin and eosin (H&E) for histopathological analysis. Tumors were classified into carcinomas and adenomas according to published criteria (Ward, 1974).

The results of colon tumor development examined at week 42 are summarized in Tables 69.6 and 69.7. Tumors in the colon were classified as adenomas or adenocarcinomas.

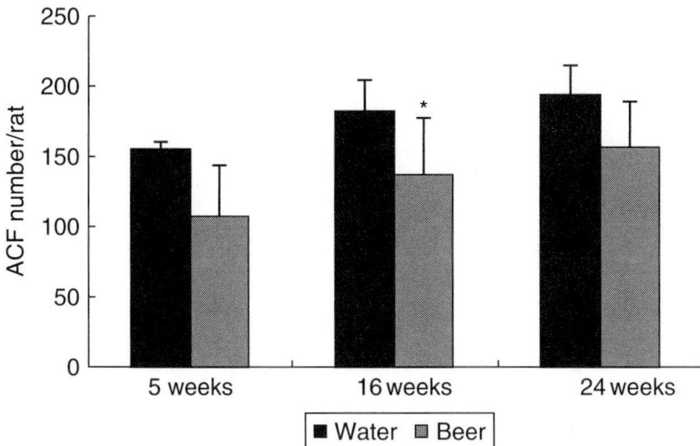

Figure 69.4 Effects of beer A on AOM-induced ACF formation in the long-term experiment. Six rats were taken from the water- and beer-fed groups at 5, 16, and 24 weeks after the start of the experiment. Bars indicate means ± SD values. Significantly different from the water-control at $^*p < 0.05$.

The incidence of adenomas and adenocarcinomas, and total tumor incidence in the entire colon were lower in the beer-fed rats than in the control group (41%, 18%, and 22% reduction, respectively). A decrease in the incidence of adenomas was detected in the proximal, middle, and rectum colons. The incidence of adenocarcinomas was not reduced in the middle and rectum colons, while there was a slight reduction in the proximal colon. Tumor multiplicity in the entire colon was significantly suppressed, by 44%, in the group given beer. The tumor multiplicity of adenocarcinomas in the proximal colon was significantly reduced by beer intake. A decrease in the number of ACF was observed at weeks 5, 16, and 24 in the beer-fed group (by 31%, 26%, and 20%, respectively) and the decrease was significant at week 16 (Figure 69.4). In conclusion, the cancer preventive effects of beer were observed using an AOM-induced colonic carcinogenesis model. Further studies are needed to clarify the components responsible and the underlying mechanisms. The results suggest that daily moderate consumption of beer may reduce the risk of cancer susceptibility in colon.

Summary Points

- Beer intake inhibited the AOM-induced colonic carcinogenesis in male Fischer 344 rats.
- Beer intake protected against DNA damage induced by AOM in the rat colonic mucosa by the single cell gel electrophoresis assay (comet assay).
- Beer intake inhibited the AOM-induced colonic ACF by the initiation treatment. Moreover, inhibitory trend in the ACF formation was observed by the post-initiation treatment. Taken together, beer ingredients exerted both antimutagenic and antipromotion activities.
- Beer intake inhibited the AOM-induced colonic tumor formation in the long-term experiments.
- Nonvolatile components of beer from raw materials are responsible for the inhibitory effects on AOM-induced colonic carcinogenesis. Alcohol in beer is not responsible for these inhibitory effects.

References

Arimoto-Kobayashi, S., Sugiyama, C., Harada, N., Takeuchi, M., Takemura, M. and Hayatsu, H. (1999). *J. Agric. Food Chem.* 47, 221–230.

Bird, R.P. (1987). *Cancer Lett.* 37, 147–151.

Cotroneo, M.S., Wang, J., Fritz, W.A., Eltoum, I.E. and Lamartiniere, C.A. (2002). *Carcinogenesis* 23, 1467–1474.

De Keukeleire, J., Ooms, G., Heyerick, A., Roldan-Ruiz, I., Van Bockstaele, E. and De Keukeleire, D. (2003). *J. Agric. Food Chem.* 51, 4436–4441.

Guglielmi, F., Luceri, C., Giovannelli, L., Dolara, P. and Lodovici, M. (2003). *Br. J. Nutr.* 89, 581–587.

Hamilton, S.R., Hyland, J., McAvinchey, D., Chaudhry, Y., Hartka, L., Kim, H.T., Cichon, P., Floyd, J., Turjman, N., Kessie, G. *et al.* (1987). *Cancer Res.* 47, 1551–1559.

Ho, C.T., Chen, Q., Shi, H., Zhang, K.Q. and Rosen, R.T. (1992). *Prev. Med.* 21, 520–525.

Jain, M.G., Hislop, G.T., Howe, G.R., Burch, J.D. and Ghadirian, P. (1998). *Int. J. Cancer* 78, 707–711.

Kassie, F., Rabot, S., Uhl, M., Huber, W., Qin, H.M., Helma, C., Schulte-Hermann, R. and Knasmuller, S. (2002). *Carcinogenesis* 23, 1155–1161.

La Vecchia, C., Negri, E., Franceschi, S. and D'Avanzo, B. (1993). *Nutr. Cancer* 19, 303–306.

Lazze, M.C., Pizzala, R., Savio, M., Stivala, L.A., Prosperi, E. and Bianchi, L. (2003). *Mutat. Res.* 535, 103–115.

Lieberman, R., Crowell, J.A., Hawk, E.T., Boone, C.W., Sigman, C.C. and Kelloff, G.J. (1998). *Clin. Chem.* 44, 420–427.

Mayer Jr., O., Simon, J. and Rosolova, H. (2001). *Eur. J. Clin. Nutr.* 55, 605–609.

Middleton Jr., E. and Kandaswami, C. (1992). *Biochem. Pharmacol.* 43, 1167–1179.

Monobe, M. and Ando, K. (2002). *J. Radiat. Res. (Tokyo)* 43, 237–245.

Morimitsu, Y., Nakagawa, Y., Hayashi, K., Fujii, H., Kumagai, T., Nakamura, Y., Osawa, T., Horio, F., Itoh, K., Iida, K., Yamamoto, M. and Uchida, K. (2002). *J. Biol. Chem.* 277, 3456–3463.

Nelson, R.L. and Samelson, S.L. (1985). *Dis. Colon Rectum* 28, 460–462.

Nozawa, H., Yoshida, A., Tajima, O., Katayama, M., Sonobe, H., Wakabayashi, K. and Kondo, K. (2004). *Int. J. Cancer* 108, 404–411.

Nozawa, H., Nakao, W., Zhao, F. and Kondo, K. (2005). *Mol. Nutr. Food Res.* 49, 772–778.

Olivo, S. and Wargovich, M.J. (1998). *In vivo* 12, 159–166.

Paper, D.H. (1998). *Planta Med.* 64, 686–695.

Pool-Zobel, B.L., Bertram, B., Knoll, M., Lambertz, R., Neudecker, C., Schillinger, U., Schmezer, P. and Holzapfel, W.H. (1993). *Nutr. Cancer* 20, 271–281.

Potter (1997). WCRF/AICR Report.

Pretlow, T.P., Cheyer, C. and O'Riordan, M.A. (1994). *Int. J. Cancer* 56, 599–602.

Rodriguez, S.K., Guo, W., Liu, L., Band, M.A., Paulson, E.K. and Meydani, M. (2005). *Int. J. Cancer.*

Roncucci, L., Stamp, D., Medline, A., Cullen, J.B. and Bruce, W.R. (1991). *Hum. Pathol.* 22, 287–294.

Sasaki, Y.F., Tsuda, S., Izumiyama, F. and Nishidate, E. (1997). *Mutat. Res.* 388, 33–44.

Schlienger, J.L. (2003). *Presse Med.* 32, 262–267.

Shiraki, M., Hara, Y., Osawa, T., Kumon, H., Nakayama, T. and Kawakishi, S. (1994). *Mutat. Res.* 323, 29–34.

Singh, N.P., McCoy, M.T., Tice, R.R. and Schneider, E.L. (1988). *Exp. Cell Res.* 175, 184–191.

Steele, V.E., Moon, R.C., Lubet, R.A., Grubbs, C.J., Reddy, B.S., Wargovich, M., McCormick, D.L., Pereira, M.A., Crowell, J.A., Bagheri, D. *et al.* (1994). *J. Cell Biochem. Suppl.* 20, 32–54.

Stevens, J.F., Miranda, C.L., Buhler, D.R. and Deinzer, M.L. (1998). *J. Am. Soc. Brew. Chem.* 56, 136–145.

Tice, R.R., Agurell, E., Anderson, D., Burlinson, B., Hartmann, A., Kobayashi, H., Miyamae, Y., Rojas, E., Ryu, J.C. and Sasaki, Y.F. (2000). *Environ. Mol. Mutagen.* 35, 206–221.

Ward, J.M. (1974). *Lab. Invest.* 30, 505–513.

Wargovich, M.J., Jimenez, A., McKee, K., Steele, V.E., Velasco, M., Woods, J., Price, R., Gray, K. and Kelloff, G.J. (2000). *Carcinogenesis* 21, 1149–1155.

Part III

Specific Effects of Selective Beer Related Components

(i) General Metabolism and Organ Systems

70

Biological Activities of Humulone

Hiroyasu Tobe Kochi National College of Technology, Department of Materials Science and Engineering, Nankoku City, Kochi, Japan

Abstract

In the screening test for the substance to inhibit bone resorption, we found that humulone (HU) from beer hop extracts showed a strong inhibitory activity to bone resorption. The value of IC_{50} (50% inhibition of bone resorption) was 5.9 nM in pit formation assay. To study the mechanism of the action of HU, we studied the biological activity of HU as a bone resorption inhibitor with reference to prostaglandin biosynthesis. We found that HU inhibited the transcription of cyclooxygenase-2 (COX-2) gene of osteoblast MC3T3-E1 with an IC_{50} of 30 nM. The recent reports demonstrated a close relationship between COX enzymes and angiogenesis. We showed also that HU as a COX-2 inhibitor inhibited angiogenesis in chick embryo chorioallantoic membrane (CAM). The value of ED_{50} was 1.5 μg/CAM.

HU enhanced effectively the differentiation-inducing action of vitamin D to myelogenous leukemia cells in the concentration of 0.5–2.5 μM. HU also induced apoptosis (DNA fragmentation and cell death) in HL-60 cells in the concentration of 1–100 μg/ml.

List of Abbreviation

HU	Humulone
XH	Xanthohumol
PG	Prostaglandin
COX	Cyclooxygenase
DEX	Dexamethasone
NFκB	Nuclear factor kappa B
GRE	Glucocorticoid response element
VEGF	Vascular endothelial growth factor
CAM	Chick embryo chorioallantoic membrane
bFGF	basic fibroblast growth factor
PDGF-B	Platelet-derived growth factor-B
VD3	Vitamin D3
NBT	Nitroblue tetrazolium
ATRA	All-*trans*-retinoic acid
TPA	12-*O*-tetradecanoylphorobol-13-acetate
TNFα	Tumor necrosis factor-α

Introduction

Hop is originally a herb (medicinal plant) and has been believed that it had a female hormone (Zenisek and Bedner, 1960; Fenselau and Talalay, 1973). On the other hand, there is a direct relationship between a female hormone (estrogen) and osteoporosis. We thought that there was a possibility to find out an effective compound from hop extract for the treatment of osteoporosis. To estimate the effectiveness of hop extract to osteoporosis, we employed a pit formation assay system (Kitamura *et al.*, 1993) which is a method to estimate the activities of osteoclast cell by counting the number of cavity (pit) on the surface of a dentine slice.

We speculated that the inhibitor, which interferes with the function of osteoclast, will express the inhibitory activity to the bone resorption of osteoclast.

Therefore, we started to screen the inhibitor against osteoclast function (bone resorption) by the pit formation assay.

Hop Extract and Osteoporosis

In the screening assay for the compound to inhibit bone resorption, we found two inhibitors from hop cake (Tobe *et al.*, 1997a). The hop cake (250 g) was extracted with acetone (2 l) to give a syrup (50 g) after the removal of the solvent. These two compounds in the syrup (17.5 g) were purified by Dowex-1 (x4, 200–400 mesh, CH_3COO^- type) column chromatography (stepwise elution with 0.5%, 5%, and 20% acetic acid in 80% methanol) and high performance liquid chromatography (reversed phase column; Chromatorex-ODS DM1020T) with 80% methanol. On the basis of ^{1}H-NMR, ^{13}C-NMR, and mass spectra, we concluded that one of the two inhibitors was to be xanthohumol (XH), and the other one was to be humulone (HU) (Tobe *et al.*, 1997a). The structure of HU is shown in Figure 70.1. The bone resorption inhibitory activities of the two compounds are shown in Table 70.1. The IC_{50} (the concentration of 50% inhibition to bone resorption) value

Beer in Health and Disease Prevention
ISBN: 978-0-12-373891-2

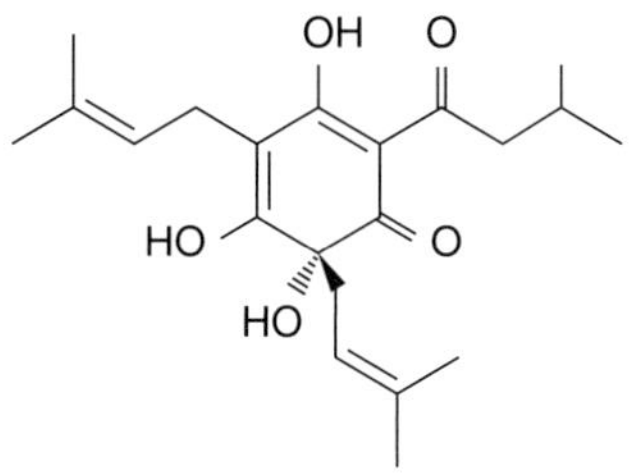

Figure 70.1 Structure of humulone.

Table 70.1 The bone resorption inhibitory activity of xanthohumol and humulone

Concentration of compound (M)		*Number of pits (average ± SD)*	*Inhibition (%)*
Xanthohumol	0	248.3 ± 35.7	–
	10^{-6}	162.7 ± 41.2*	34.5
	10^{-5}	15.8 ± 6.0*	93.6
	10^{-4}	0*	100
Humulone	0	328.0 ± 51.0	–
	10^{-11}	274.3 ± 91.6*	16.4
	10^{-10}	274.3 ± 54.9*	16.4
	10^{-9}	251.5 ± 135.4*	23.3
	10^{-8}	128.5 ± 23.1*	60.8
	10^{-7}	34.5 ± 7.4*	89.5
	10^{-6}	6.5 ± 3.8*	98.0
	10^{-5}	0.3 ± 0.5*	99.9

Notes: Dentin slices (6 mm diameter, 0.15 mm thickness) were placed in each well of a 96-well culture plate (Falcon, Becton Dickinson and Company, Lincoln Park, NJ). One hundred μl of α-MEM (minimum essential medium) containing 5% fetal bovine serum (Flow Laboratories, Scotland) and synthetic rat parathyroid hormone (residues 1–34, Backem, Inc., CA) were added to each well and each slice was overlaid with 100 μl of 1×10^6 mouse bone marrow cells suspension. The cells were then incubated for 3 days at 37°C in a humid atmosphere of 10% CO_2 and 90% air. After incubation, the cells on a slice were removed, and resorbed pits were stained with Coomassie brilliant blue. Bone resorption was assessed by counting the number of pits under a light microscope.

*$p < 0.01$ vs. 0 M ($n = 6$, Bonferroni/Dunn).

of XH and HU were 1.3 μM and 5.9 nM, respectively, in pit formation assay. HU was one of the strongest inhibitors to bone resorption.

HU and COX-2 Gene

The mechanism of the action of HU to bone resorption was unknown. The molecular model of HU was similar to that of prostaglandin (PG). Both HU and PG molecules have a cyclic (ring) structure and side chains in their molecules. We speculated, therefore, that HU might interfere with the cascade pathway of arachidonic acid-PG biosynthesis. On the other hand, it is reported that PGE2 is one of key factors for bone remodeling (Yokota *et al.*, 1986) and that PGE2 produced by osteoblastic cell line (MC3T3E1) is a chemical mediator to develop and differentiate osteoclast function (Yamamoto *et al.*, 1995, 1998).

Cyclooxygenase-1 (COX-1) and -2 are responsible enzymes for PG biosynthesis. COX-1 is a constitutive enzyme and COX-2 is an inducible enzyme for the biosynthesis of PG. It is reported that COX-2 enzyme is biologically and pathologically more important than COX-1 enzyme (Herschman, 1996; Smith *et al.*, 1996). Therefore, we studied the mechanism of the action of HU to bone resorption with reference of dexamethasone (DEX) in PG biosynthesis (Yamamoto *et al.*, 2000).

We estimated the effects of HU and DEX on tumor necrosis factor-α (TNFα)-mediated COX-2 induction. The results of PGE2 release assay (Figure 70.2a and b), the COX-2 activity assay (Figure 70.2c and d), the COX-2 mRNA assay (Figure 70.2e and f), and the luciferase assay (Figure 70.2g and h) showed that HU inhibited the production of PGE2 and the transcription of COX-2 gene of osteoblast MC3T3E1. As shown in Figure 70.2c and d, the value of IC_{50} of HU and DEX were 30 and 1 nM, respectively. We thought that HU inhibited the osteoclast function (bone resorption) through the inhibition of COX-2 gene expression (transcription) and then PGE2 production.

As shown in Figure 70.3, HU inhibited strongly COX-2 enzyme activity (IC_{50}: 1.6 μM) rather than COX-1 enzyme activity (IC_{50}: 70 μM). HU showed the specific affinity to COX-2 enzyme rather than COX-1 enzyme.

Figure 70.4 showed that both HU and DEX inhibited almost equally the NFκB and NF-IL6 response element activity induced by the addition of TNFα.

As shown in Figure 70.5a, HU inhibited more strongly the PGE2 release from MC3T3E1 cells induced by the addition of TNFα than DEX did. On the other hand, Figure 70.5b showed that DEX reacted strongly to glucocorticoid response element (GRE). But HU did not react strongly to GRE. Therefore, the mechanism of action of HU was different from that of DEX. These data suggested that the HU-dependent suppression of COX-2 induction was mediated by not glucocorticoid response but NFκB and NF-IL6 response element.

HU and Angiogenesis

According to the recent reports, there is a close relationship between COX-2 and angiogenesis (Masferrer *et al.*, 2000). We speculated that an inhibition of COX-2 gene expression might induce the inhibition of angiogenesis.

HU showed (Shimamura *et al.*, 2001) the strong *in vivo* antiangiogenic activity, clearly producing an avascular zone in chick embryo chorioallantoic membrane (CAM) (Figure 70.6b). In contrast, no avascular zones were observed in any of the control embryos treated with 0.9% NaCl alone (Figure 70.6a). The inhibitory activity of HU and NS-398 (positive control; an specific inhibitor to COX-2 enzyme) to

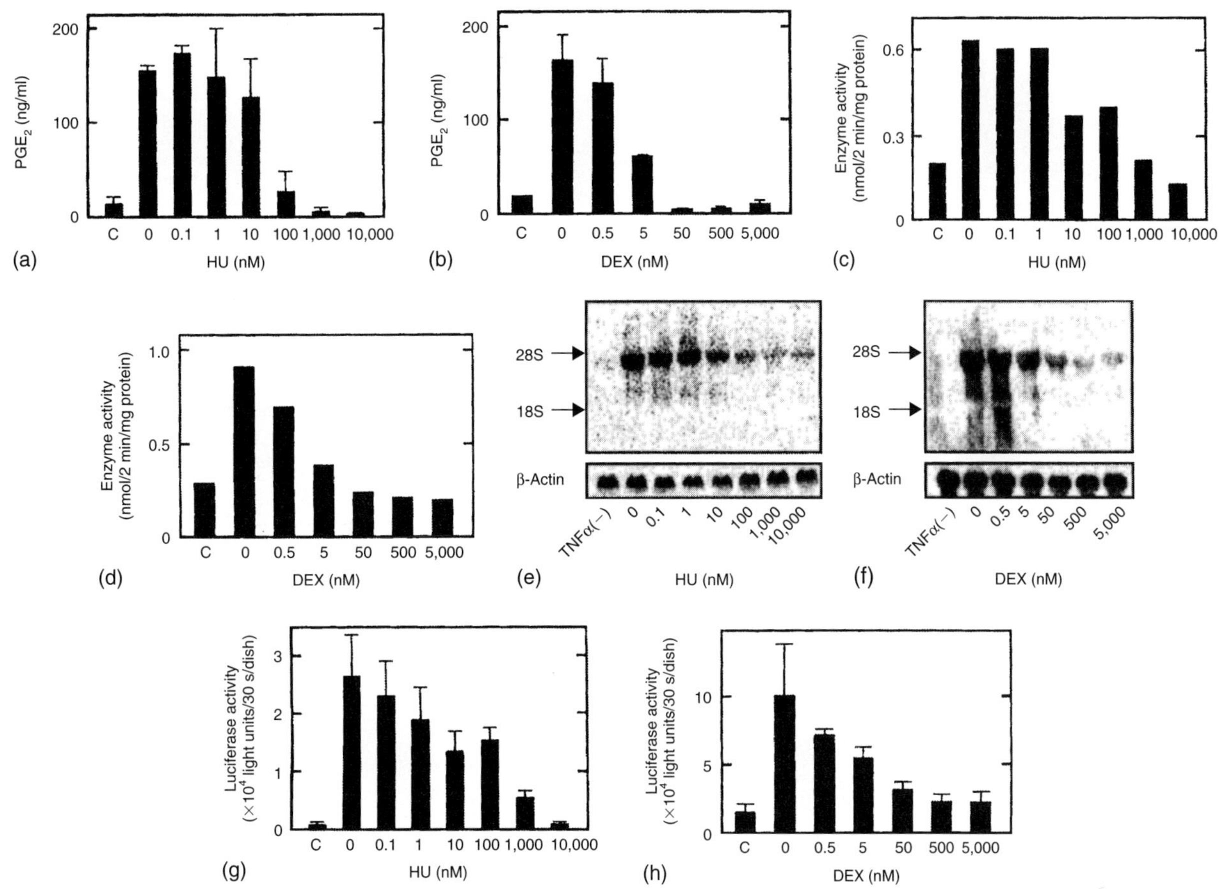

Figure 70.2 Effects of HU and DEX on TNFα-mediated COX-2 induction. TNFα was present at a concentration of 10 ng/ml for HU and 20 ng/ml for dexamethasone. HU (a, c, e, and g) or dexamethasone (b, d, f, and h) was added at various concentration. For the PGE2 release assay, 3×10^5 MC3T3-E1 cells were incubated with TNFα for 12 h (a and b). For the COX-2 activity assay, 2.2×10^6 cells were incubated with TNFα for 12 h (c and d). For the COX-2 mRNA assay, 2.2×10^6 cells were incubated with TNFα for 2 h (e and f). Total RNA (10 μg/ml) was applied to Northern blot analysis for COX-2 mRNA assay and β-actin mRNA. For the luciferase assay (g and h), 7.8×10^5 confluent cells were transfected with luciferase plasmid including promoter regions of mouse COX-2 gene. The cells were incubated with TNFα for 12 h. (a), (b), (g) and (h) are means ± SD of triplicate determination. (c), (d), (e) and (f) are typical results of the experiments each repeated three times giving similar results.

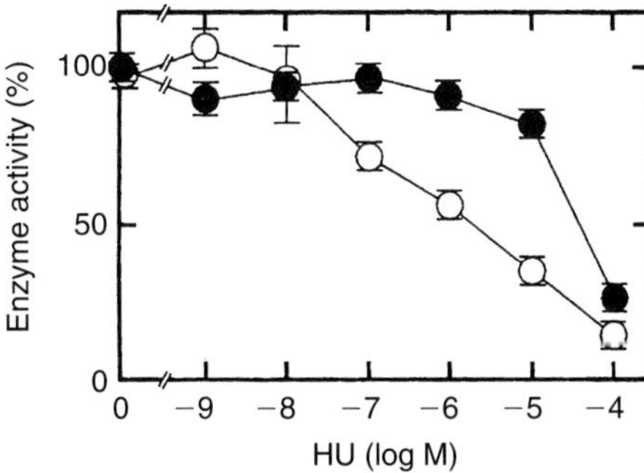

Figure 70.3 Effects of HU on COX-1 and -2 activities. The standard COX assays were performed with [1-14C]-arachidonic acid (10 μM) incubated with the COX-1 of sheep seminal vesicle microsome (4.3 μg protein) (closed circle) or the COX-2 of MC3T3-E1 cell lysate (50 μg protein) stimulated by phorbol 12-myristate and A23187 (open circle). HU was added at various concentrations. Data are means ± SD of duplicate determination.

angiogenesis by CAM assay is shown in Figure 70.6c. The dose-dependent inhibition of *in vivo* angiogenesis CAM assay by HU and NS-398 were observed and the value of ED_{50} of HU and NS-398 were 1.5 and 65 μg/CAM, respectively. The inhibitory activity of HU was stronger than that of NS-398 by 40 times.

We tested also an assay of rat lung endothelial cell growth inhibition (Shimamura *et al.*, 2001). Figure 70.7 showed the effect of HU and NS-398 on proliferation of endothelial cells using KOP2.16 (murine endothelial cell line) stimulated by 10 ng/ml basic fibroblast growth factor (bFGF). HU strongly inhibited the proliferation of endothelial cells. The value of ED_{50} of HU and NS-398 were 7 and 100 μM, respectively. The inhibitory activity of HU was stronger than that of NS-398 by 14 times.

Tumor cells are known to produce various factors, such as VEGF (vascular endothelial growth factor), bFGF, and

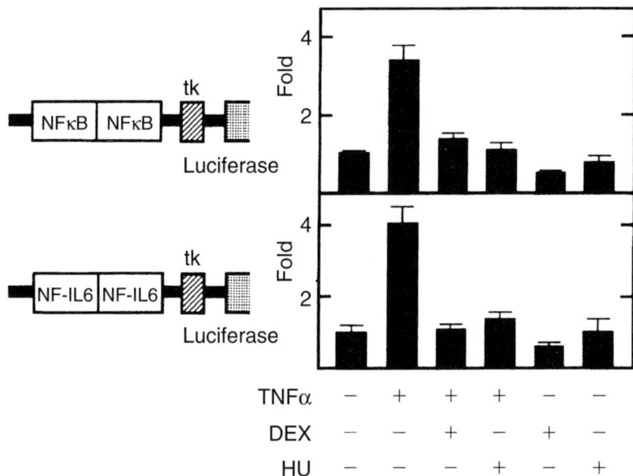

Figure 70.4 Effect of HU and DEX on NFκB and NF-IL6 response elements as examined by the luciferase analysis. Confluent MC3T3-E1 cells (7.8×10^5) were transfected with luciferase plasmid including NFκB or NF-IL6 response element. The cells were incubated for 12 h in the presence or absence of 10 ng/ml TNFα, 5 μM DEX, or 10 μM HU as indicated. Data are means ± SD of triplicate determination.

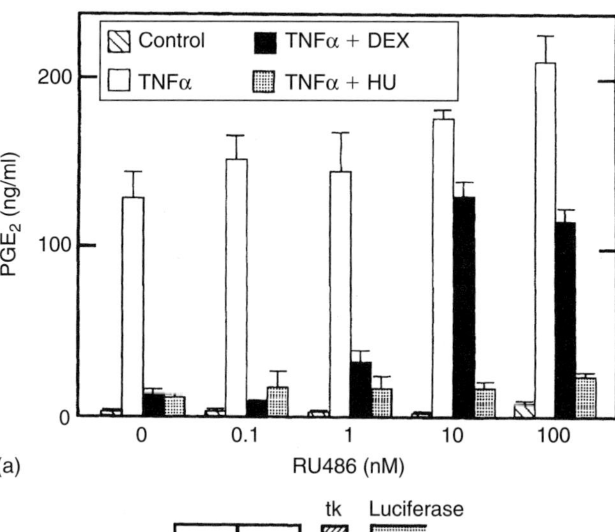

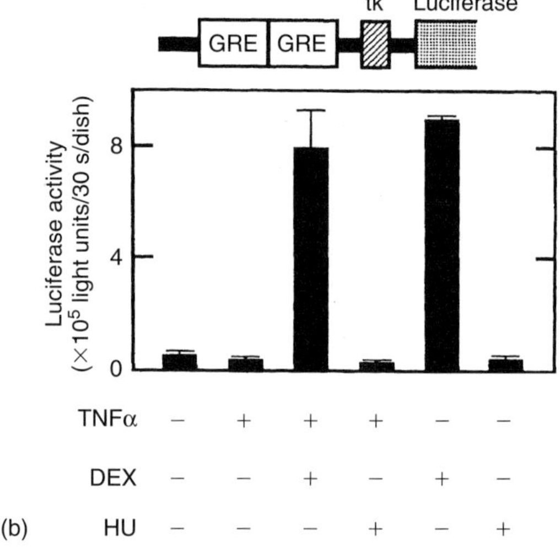

Figure 70.5 Possible binding of HU and DEX to glucocorticoid receptor. (a) MC3T3-E1 cells (3×10^5) were incubated with TNFα for 12 h in the presence or absence of 5 μM DEX or 10 μM HU. Various concentrations of RU486 were added. Produced PGE2 was measured using radioimmunoassay. Data are means ± SD of triplicate determination. (b) Confluent cells (7.8×10^5) were transfected with luciferase plasmid including two glucocorticoid response elements (GRE) and thymidine kinase gene (tk). The cells were incubated for 12 h in the presence or absence of TNFα, 5 μM DEX, or 10 μM HU. Data are means ± SD of triplicate determinations.

PDGF-B which contribute to angiogenesis. To evaluate if HU suppresses the production of VEGF by KOP2.16 endothelial cells or Co26 colon cancer cells which constitutively express COX-2 protein, we measured VEGF in the culture medium of these cells that were treated or not treated with HU. HU at 100 μM substantially inhibited the production of VEGF by KOP2.16 cells (Figure 70.8a) and Co26 cells (Figure 70.8b). The inhibition was more significant in tumor cells than in endothelial cells at 10–100 μM of HU.

HU and Myelogenous Leukemia

HU enhanced effectively the differentiation-inducing action of vitamin D to myelogenous leukemia (Honma *et al.*, 1998).

The active form of vitamin D (VD_3; 1α, 25-dihydroxyvitamin D_3) inhibits proliferation and induces differentiation of several leukemia and solid tumor cells (Hozumi, 1983; Koeffler, 1983; Niitsu *et al.*, 1997), but its hypercalcemic effects prevent it from the clinical use (Bikle, 1992). VD_3 mobilizes calcium store from bone by inducing the dissolution of bone mineral and matrix. VD_3 is a potent stimulator of bone resorption (Raisz *et al.*, 1972; The Southern California Leukemia Group *et al.*, 1985), whereas HU is a potent inhibitor of bone resorption (Tobe *et al.*, 1997a). Then we examined the effect of HU on the differentiation of human monoblastic leukemia U937 cells induced by VD_3. As shown in Figure 70.9a, in the presence of VD_3 (2 and 4 nM), HU at concentrations up to 2.5 μM induced the nitroblue tetrazolium (NBT)-reducing activity in the U937 cells, and HU effectively enhanced this activity induced by VD_3 and the enhancing effect was statistically significant (Figure 70.9b). VD_3 induced lysozyme and α-naphthyl acetate esterase activities, other markers of monocytic differentiation, and the combination of VD_3 with HU induced these activities more effectively than VD_3 alone (Figure 70.9c and d). Morphologically, HU enhanced the monocytic differentiation of U937 cells induced by suboptimal concentration of VD_3 (data not shown).

U937 cells are induced to differentiate by TPA (12-*O*-tetradecanoylphorobol-13-acetate), ATRA (all-*trans*-retinoic acid), and TNFα. We examined whether HU enhanced the differentiation of U937 cells induced by these compounds.

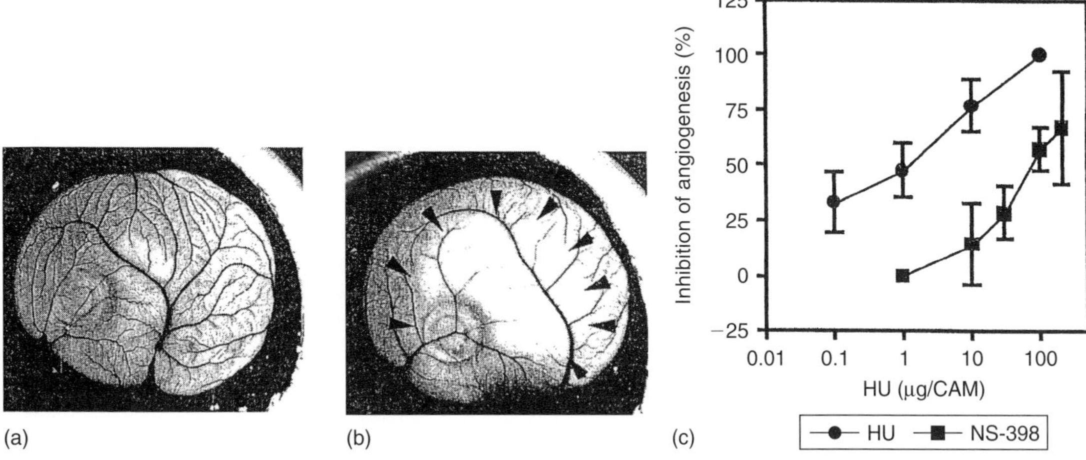

Figure 70.6 Inhibitory effect of HU on *in vivo* angiogenesis in CAM. No (a) or 10 μg/ml (b) HU was added to the CAM surfaces of 4-day-old fertilized eggs, and then the eggs were incubated for 46–48 h. HU produced an avascular zone (surrounded by arrows), indicating its antiangiogenic activity. (c) Dose-dependent inhibition of *in vivo* angiogenesis in CAM by HU and NS-398. The antiangiogenic activity was assessed. Values are the means of five experiments. HU potently inhibited angiogenesis in CAM in a dose-dependent manner.

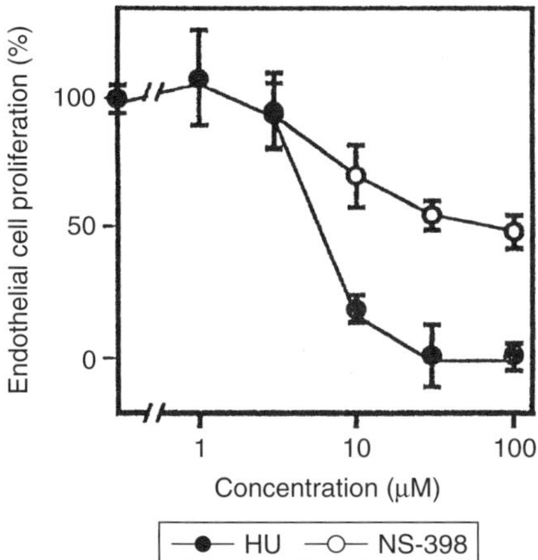

Figure 70.7 Effect of HU on proliferation of endothelial cells. KOP2.16 cells were treated for 48 h with HU or NS-398 at various concentrations indicated. Data are means ± SD from five separate wells. HU potently inhibited the proliferation of endothelial cells.

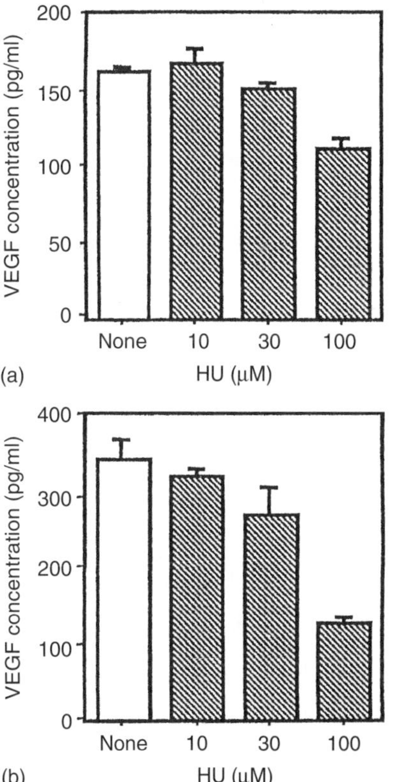

Figure 70.8 Effect of HU on production of VEGF by endothelial cells and tumor cells. KOP2.16 cells (a) and Co26 cells (b) were treated for 24 h with HU at various concentrations indicated. VEGF in conditioned medium was assayed by ELIZA. HU suppressed the production of VEGF by endothelial cells and tumor cells.

To access the effect on differentiation, we combined HU with suboptimal concentration of TPA, ATRA, and TNFα. HU also increased the NBT-reducing activity induced by these inducers (Table 70.2).

Other myelomonocytic leukemia cells (erythroid leukemia K562, HEL, and KU812) were induced to differentiation by the addition of VD_3 and this was also enhanced by the addition of HU as shown in Figure 70.10 (the case of K562).

These results indicated that the combination of VD3 derivatives with HU is a promising candidate for differentiation therapy of monocytic leukemia.

HU and Apoptosis

HU induced apoptosis in the promyelocytic leukemia cell line HL-60 in the concentration of 1–100 μg/ml (Tobe *et al.*, 1997b). The time-dependent cell death ratio and DNA fragmentation pattern are shown in Figures 70.11 and 70.12, respectively. In the hydrogen peroxide hemolysis test of antioxidants, IC_{50} value of HU and ascorbic acid

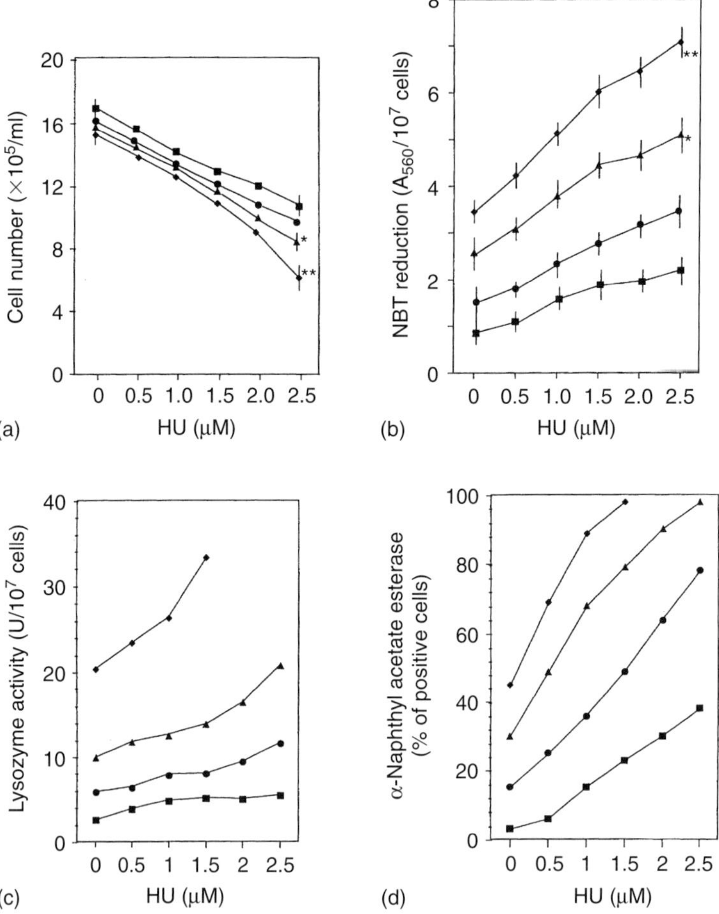

Figure 70.9 Growth inhibition and induction of NBT reduction in U937 cells by HU in combination with VD_3. Growth inhibition (a) and induction of NBT reduction (b) in U937 cells by HU in combination with VD_3. (c) Induction of lysozyme activity, and (d) α-naphthyl acetate esterase activity in U937 cells by HU in combination with VD_3. Values are means ± SD of three separate experiments. * $p < 0.05$ and ** $p < 0.005$ compared the data without VD_3. Cells were cultured with various concentrations of HU in the presence of 0 (■), 1 (●), 2 (▲), or 4 (◆) nM VD_3 for 6 days.

Table 70.2 Effect of humulone on NBT reduction of U937 cells treated with ATRA, TPA, or TNFα

Treatment	*NBT reduction*	*(A_{300} 10^7 cells)*
	−Humulone	+Humulone
None	1.2 ± 0.2	1.8 ± 0.2
ATRA	1.6 ± 0.2	3.1 ± 0.4
TPA	1.9 ± 0.3	3.6 ± 0.5
TNFα	1.8 ± 0.2	2.9 ± 0.3

Note: Cells were cultured with 8nM ATRA, 0.5ng/ml of TPA, or 1ng/ml of TNFα in the presence or absence of 2μM humulone for 5 days. Values are means ± SD from three separate experiments.

were 2.8×10^{-5} and 1.25×10^{-4}M, respectively. Other antioxidants, quercetin (Takahama, 1988; Whalley *et al.*, 1990) and genistein (Pratt and Watts, 1964; Letan, 1966), showed the apoptosis-inducing activity (Figure 70.13; DNA fragmentation and cell death). We speculated that the apoptosis-inducing activity of HU had a direct correlation with not its inhibitory activity to bone resorption but its antioxidant activity.

Summary Points

- The inhibition of COX-2 gene expression by HU caused the inhibitions of bone resorption and angiogenesis.
- The antioxidant activity of HU induced the apoptosis to the promyelocytic leukemia cell line HL-60.
- The biological activities of HU are useful for our health and the structure of HU presents the idea of the drug design for enzyme inhibitor.

Conclusion

HU had five different biological activities as described below:

1. HU showed the strong inhibitory activity to bone resorption (IC_{50}: 5.9nM) in pit formation assay. XH had the weaker inhibitory activity (IC_{50}: 1.3μM). HU might be a candidate for the treatment of osteoporosis.
2. HU inhibited both COX-2 gene transcription (IC_{50}: 5.9nM) and COX-2 enzyme activity (IC_{50}: 1.6μM).

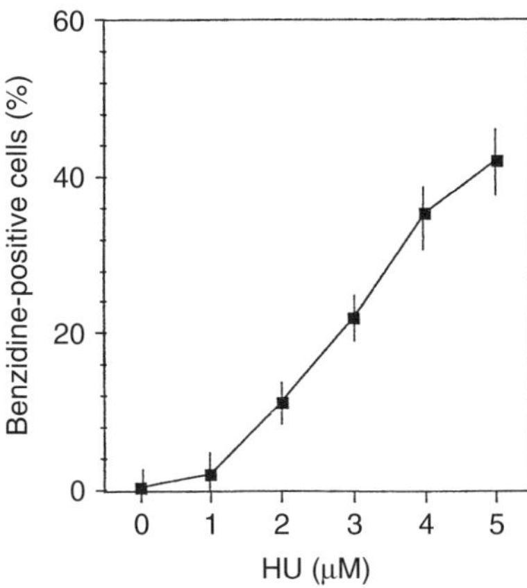

Figure 70.10 Effect of HU on induction of erythroid differentiation of K562 cells. Cells were cultured with various concentrations of HU for 4 days. Hemoglobin-producing cells were assayed by benzidine staining. Values are means ± SD from three separate experiments.

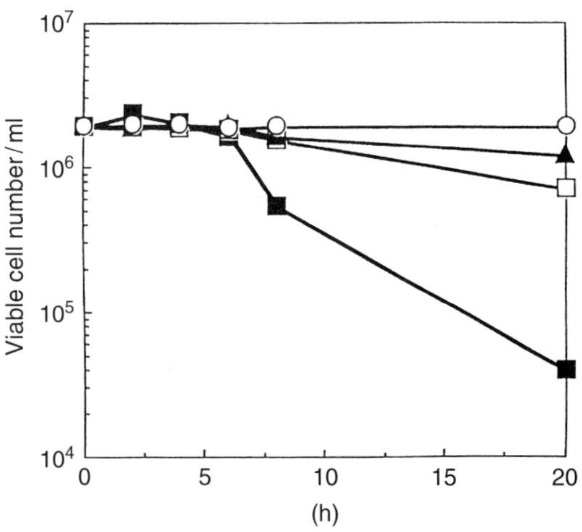

Figure 70.11 Growth inhibition of HL-60 by HU. HL-60 cells were incubated with or without HU in the concentration of 1, 10, and 100 g/ml, respectively. The final concentration of EtOH in the culture medium was below 1%. The samples (50 μl) of the culture medium were taken after 0, 2, 4, 6, 8, and 20 h of cultivation and used for counting the viable cell number of HL-60 by trypan blue staining. The four symbols present the viable cell number of HL-60 in the concentrations of 0 (○), 1 (▲), 10 (□), and 100 μg/ml (■).

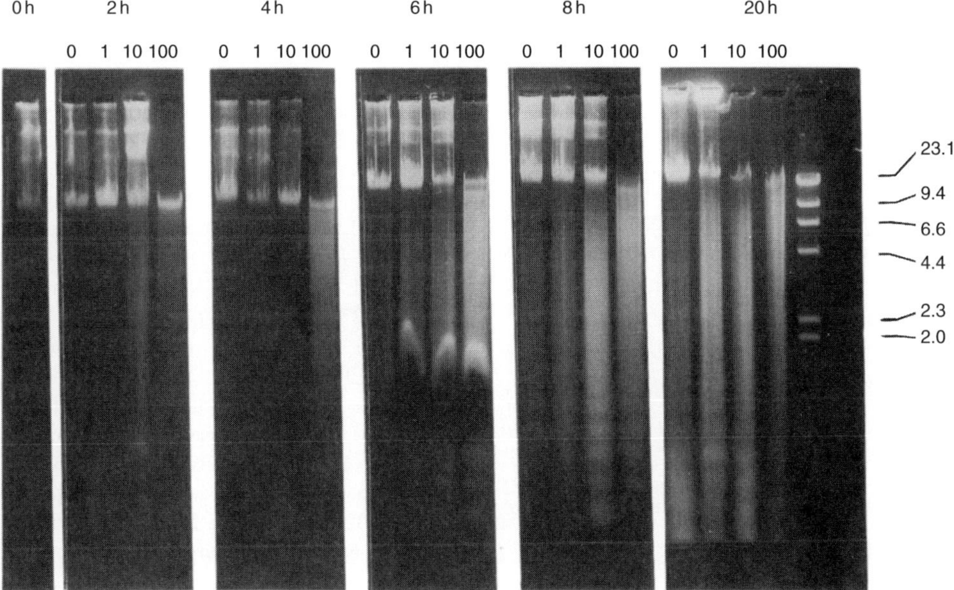

Figure 70.12 DNA fragmentation pattern of HL-60 by HU. HL-60 cells were treated as described in Figure 70.11. The samples (1 ml) of the culture medium were taken after 0, 2, 4, 6, 8, and 20 h of cultivation and used for the analysis of DNA fragmentation pattern of HL-60. After the samples were treated with RNase A and proteinase K, 10 μl from each sample was applied to 1.5% agarose gel and analyzed. We used λc1857 DNA digested with *Hind*III for DNA size standards.

The inhibition of signal transduction by HU may not involve in a glucocorticoid receptor but may be mediated by the NFκB and NFIL6 response element.

3. HU inhibited angiogenesis in CAM assay (ED_{50}: 1.5 μg/CAM). HU also inhibited *in vitro* tube formation of vascular endothelial cells. Moreover it suppressed the proliferation of endothelial cells and the production of VEGF, an angiogenic growth factor, in endothelial and tumor cells. Thus, HU was a potent angiogenic inhibitor both *in vitro* and *in vivo*. HU may be applied clinically as an antiangiogenic agent in the treatment of cancer, rheumatoid arthritis, and diabetic retinopathy.
4. HU enhanced effectively the differentiation-inducing action of vitamin D to myelogenous leukemia cells in

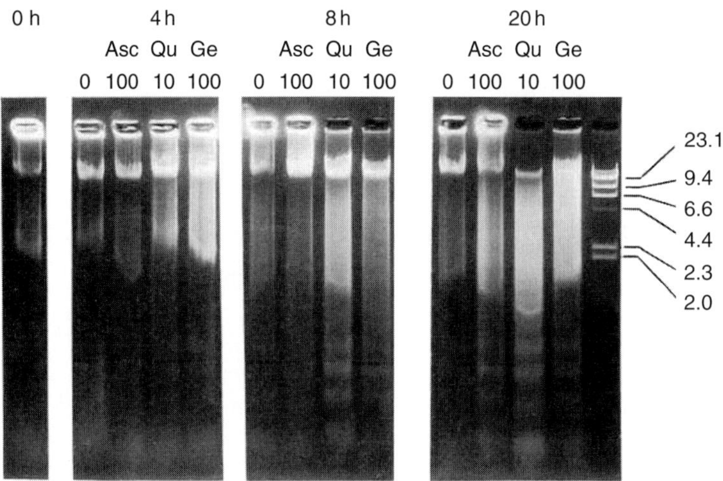

Figure 70.13 DNA fragmentation pattern of HL-60 by ascorbic acid, quercetin, and genistein. HL-60 cells were treated with or without ascorbic acid (100 μg/ml), quercetin (100 μg/ml) and genistein (100 μg/ml), as described in Figure 70.11. The samples (1 ml) of the culture medium were taken after 0, 4, 8, and 20 h of cultivation and used for the analysis of DNA fragmentation pattern of HL-60 as mentioned in Figure 70.12. Asc, ascorbic acid; Qu, Quercetin; Ge, genistein.

the concentration of 0.5–2.5 μM. The combination of VD_3 derivatives with HU is a promising candidate for differentiation therapy of monocytic leukemia.

5. HU had the activity to induce apoptosis (DNA fragmentation and cell death) in HL-60 cells in the concentration of 1–100 μg/ml.

We concluded that the primary target molecule of HU was COX-2 gene and that the inhibition of the gene transcription caused the inhibition of bone resorption and angiogenesis. The secondary biological activity of HU was its antioxidant activity, and this activity might induce the apoptosis in HL-60 cells.

Acknowledgments

This study was done in cooperation with Prof. Yamamoto, S., Dr. Yamamoto, K., Dr. Shimamura, M., Dr. Hazato, T., and Prof. Honma, Y. I appreciate their enthusiastic collaboration.

References

Bikle, D.D. (1992). *Endocr. Rev.* 13, 765.

Fenselau, C. and Talalay, P. (1973). *Food Cosmet. Toxicol.* 11, 597–603.

Herschman, H.R. (1996). *Biochem. Biophys. Acta* 1299, 125–140.

Honma, Y., Tobe, Y.H., Makishima, M., Yokoyama, A. and Okabekado, J. (1998). *Leukemia Res.* 22, 605–610.

Hozumi, M. (1983). *Adv. Cancer Res.* 38, 121.

Kitamura, K., Katoh, M., Komiyama, O., Kitagawa, H., Matubara, F. and Kumegawa, M. (1993). *Bone* 14, 829–834.

Koeffler, H.P. (1983). *Blood* 62, 709.

Letan, A. (1966). *J. Food Sci.* 31, 518–523.

Masferrer, J.L., Leahy, K.M., Koki, A.T., Zweifel, B.S., Settle, S.L., Woener, B.M., Edwers, D.A., Flickinger, A.G., Moore, R.J. and Seibert, K. (2000). *Cancer Res.* 60, 1306–1311.

Niitsu, N., Yamamoto-Yamaguchi, Y., Miyoshi, H., Shimizu, K., Ohki, M., Umeda, M. and Honma, Y. (1997). *Cell Growth Differ.* 8, 319.

Pratt, D.E. and Watts, B.M. (1964). *J. Food Sci.* 29, 27–33.

Raisz, L.G., Trummel, C.L., Horick, M.F. and DeLuca, H.F. (1972). *Science* 175, 768.

Shimamura, M., Hazato, T., Ashino, H., Yamamoto, Y., Iwasaki, E., Tobe, H., Yamamoto, K. and Yamamoto, S. (2001). *Biochem. Biophys. Res. Commun.* 289, 220–224.

Smith, W.L., Garavito, R.M. and DeWitt, D.L. (1996). *J. Biol. Chem.* 271, 33157–33160.

Takahama, U. (1988). *Protein Nucleic Acid Enzyme* 33, 2994–2999.

The Southern California Leukemia Group, Koeffler, H.P., Hiruji, K. and Itri, L. (1985). *Cancer Treat. Rep.* 69, 1399.

Tobe, H., Muraki, Y., Kitamura, K., Komiyama, O., Sato, Y., Sugioka, T., Maruyama, H.B., Matsuda, E. and Nagai, M. (1997a). *Biosci. Biotech. Biochem.* 61, 158–159.

Tobe, H., Kubota, M., Yamaguchi, M., Kocha, T. and Aoyagi, T. (1997b). *Biosci. Biotech. Biochem.* 61, 1027–1029.

Whalley, C.V., Rankin, S.M., Hoult, J.R.S., Jessup, W. and Leake, D.S. (1990). *Biochem. Pharmacol.* 39, 1743–1750.

Yamamoto, K., Arakawa, T., Ueda, N. and Yamamoto, S. (1995). *J. Biol. Chem.* 270, 31315–31320.

Yamamoto, K., Wang, J., Yamamoto, S. and Tobe, H. (2000). *FEBS Lett.* 465, 103–106.

Yamamoto, S., Yamamoto, K., Kurobe, H., Yamashita, R., Yamaguchi, H. and Ueda, N. (1998). *Int. J. Tissue React.* 20, 17–22.

Yokota, K., Kusaka, M., Ohshima, T., Yamamoto, S., Kurihara, N., Yoshino, T. and Kumegawa, M. (1986). *J. Biol. Chem.* 261, 15410–15415.

Zenisek, A. and Bedner, J. (1960). *Am. Perfumer Arom.* 75, 61–65.

71

Desmethylxanthohumol from Hops, Chemistry and Biological Effects

Reinhard A. Diller and Herbert M. Riepl Institute of Resource and Energy Technology, Technical University of Munich, Straubing, Germany
Oliver Rose, Corazon Frias, Günter Henze and Aram Prokop Department of Pediatric Oncology/Hematology, University Medical Center Charité, Campus Virchow, Berlin, Germany

Abstract

Desmethylxanthohumol is a chalcone-type compound isolated from hops. It is present in extracts in a concentration of about 1/5 of the xanthohumol content. It isomerizes easily in aequous media like beer to a mixture of 6- and 8-prenylnaringenin, a phytoestrogen with hormonal activity. Desmethylxanthohumol is a powerful apoptosis inducing agent in lymphoid leukemic cell assays and it acts as a chemoprotective compound activating oxidation and excretion of harmful xenobiotics.

List of Abbreviations

BJAB	Burkitt-type lymphoma cell line
CAD	Caspase-3-activated DNA fragmenting enzyme
EC_{50}	Half effective dosis
EIMS	Electron impact mass spectroscopy
LDH	Lactate dehydrogenase
MeOH	Methanol
MEM	2-Methoxyethoxymethyl-protecting group
MOM	Methoxymethyl-protecting group
6-PN	6-Prenylnaringenin
8-PN	8-Prenylnaringenin
TNF-α	Tumor necrosis factor
UV–VIS	Spectroscopy with ultraviolet and visible light
λ_{max}	Peak in the UV–VIS spectrum with top most intensity
log ε	Extinction of the λ_{max}-peak at logarithmic scale

Introduction

Hop is extracted at technical scale with supercritical carbondioxide since nearly 25 years. The knowledge of the cytoprotective effects of hop polyphenoles has triggered some interest how these compounds in beverages possibly can be enriched. It was seen easily that by using carbondioxide extracts of hops as wort, very little of the flavonoid content of the plant is available for the beverage since it is only sparingly soluble in this extractant. This can be overcome by addition of some dried hops. The best known polyphenole from hops is xanthohumol, besides that there are some minor compounds which differ slightly from xanthohumol with respect to their substitutions pattern and properties. Of particular importance due to its relation to hormonal activities of hop and hop containing preparations is desmethylxanthohumol, present in a concentration of 1/5 of the xanthohumol content of a plant.

Chemistry

Desmethylxanthohumol **1** or fully named 1-(2′,4′,6′-trihydroxy-3′(3″-methylbut-2″-enyl) phenyl-3-(4-hydroxyphenyl) prop-2-en-1-one, is one of the five to seven major polyphenoles existent in hop, which are distinguished by the length of their carbon side chains and methylation pattern.

Reactivity

Like xanthohumol, **1** belongs to the chalcone type of chemical compounds which means that there are two phenolic ring moieties (Figure 71.1, **3**, called ring A and B) connected by a three atom-membered carbon chain. This chain is a so-called vinylogous system composed of a ketone group and an adjacent carbon—carbon double bond, usually in the trans configuration. Vinylogous double bonds are very reactive at the β-carbon atom, this site in the molecule is deficient in electron density. Chalcone compounds, which have a suitable heteroatom like oxygen in position (2′) thus can close a ring with the activated carbon—carbon double bond to form a flavanone type of compound. The heterocyclic ring formed like this is saturated with respect to the vinylogous double bond and can decompose under suitable conditions to give back the original chalcone type of molecule. Desmethylxanthohumol differs in its chemical structure from xanthohumol in one particular point, at carbon 6′, where an oxygen is substituted with a methyl group. Xanthohumol **2** itself can thus form only isoxanthohumol **6** because the hydroxyl group at position 6′ is blocked (Figure 71.2).

Beer in Health and Disease Prevention
ISBN: 978-0-12-373891-2

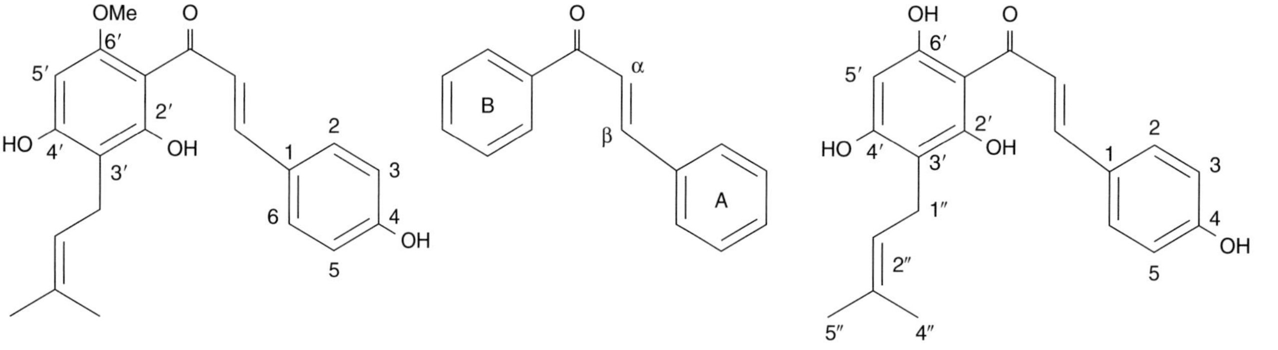

2, Xanthohumol 3, General chalcone formula 1, Desmethylxanthohumol

Figure 71.1 Chemical structure of the title compounds. Xanthohumol (**2**) and desmethylxanthohumol (**1**) are the main flavonoids in hop. Both compounds belong to the chalcone type of natural products characterized by a model structure (**3**).

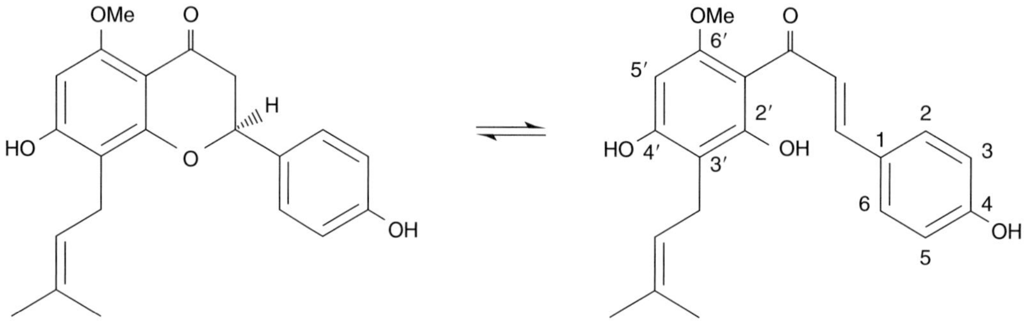

6, Isoxanthohumol 2, Xanthohumol

Figure 71.2 Ring-closure reaction xanthohumol. Solutions of chalcones in water are unstable. They have a tendency to close a ring by virtue of the carbon—carbon double bond, which is electron poor and thus reacts with a nearby 2′-hydroxylgroup. Xanthohumol (**2**) reacts in this manner to give isoxanthohumol (**6**).

In this manner, desmethylxanthohumol **1** can form two isomers due to the possibility of rotation around the carbon bond of the aromatic B ring to the keto-group. By this rotation, either oxygen at 6′or 2′can undergo the vinylogous reaction. These isomers are 6-prenylnaringenin and 8-prenylnaringenin. Principially, two enantiomeric molecules are formed by the ring closure, but the resulting prenylnaringenins are devoid of optical activity.

Physical and chemical data

Desmethylxanthohumol is a yellow powder. Its UV–VIS spectrum shows an absorption at $\lambda_{max} = 366\,nm$ ($\log\varepsilon = 4{,}591$, solv: MeOH). In the infrared spectrum, **1** shows a characteristic carbon–oxygen stretching vibration at $1{,}623\,cm^{-1}$. Its mass spectrum (electron impact mass spectroscopy, EIMS) has been reported to be *e*/*m* = 340 (M^+, 100%), 285 ($M\text{-}C4H7^+$), 26%, 220 (A^+-ring fragment), 13%, 165 (A ring fragment-$C4H7^+$), 51%, 120 (B^+-ring fragment), 16%. Nuclear magnetic resonance data (Hänsel and Schulz, 1988; Stevens *et al.*, 1997) can be found in Table 71.1. To determine the concentration of **1** in any solutions, high performance liquid chromatography (HPLC) analysis using reversed phase columns (C18) is applied, the mobile phases being composed of acetonitrile, another organic solvent and a trace of formic acid. Quantitative assessment by gaschromatography is not considered to be accurate, there is some discrimination and decomposition rendering this method unreliable.

Occurrence in beverages

Desmethylxanthohumol is more soluble in aqueous media than xanthohumol, thus during brewing it is extracted from hops preferably. At the same time, it is isomerized more quickly according to scheme **71.3**. Following addition of a sample of hop to hot brew, only after 15 min boiling its total content of **1** can be found in solution in form of 8-PN (**4**) and 6-PN (**5**) in a ratio of about 1:4, meaning 6-PN (**5**) is formed preferably (Stevens *et al.*, 1999a). From there on, substances **1**, **4**, **5** disappear from the solution due to absorption on precipitating proteins, carbohydrates or filtering media. Usually, only 10–15% of the original content remain in the beverage amounting to 35–15 μg/l in the form of **4** and **5** (Stevens *et al.*, 1999b) (Figure 71.3).

Table 71.1 Nuclear magnetic resonance data of desmethylxanthohumol

^{1}H-NMR assignment		*^{13}C-NMR assignment*	
Hydrogen atom no.	*NMR-shift (d^6-DMSO, ppm*)*	*Carbon atom no.*	*NMR-shift (d^6-DMSO, ppm*)*
		C—O	191.8
Hα	8.0	Cα	123.4
Hβ	7.66	Cβ	142.0
		C1	126.2
H2 and H6	7.53	C2 and C6	130.3
H3 and H5	6.84	C3 and C5	116.0
		C4	159.2
		C1′	104.1
		C2′	164.1
		C3′	106.0
		C4′	162.4
H5′	6.03	C5′	94.4
		C6′	159.8
H1″	3.11	C1″	21.0
H2″	5.14	C2″	124.1
		C3″	129.5
$(CH_3)4''$	1.61	C4″	17.0
$(CH_3)5''$	1.7	C5″	25.5
4 × OH	14.56; 10.66; 10.36; 10.08		

Note: ^{1}Hydrogen and ^{13}Carbon – Nuclear magnetic resonance-shift data of individual atoms in desmethylxanthohumol **1** in ppm* relative to tetramethylsilane, which is generally acknowlegded to be 0 ppm, calibration against a standard of deuterium containing solvent (d^6-DMSO = deuteriodimethylsulfoxide).

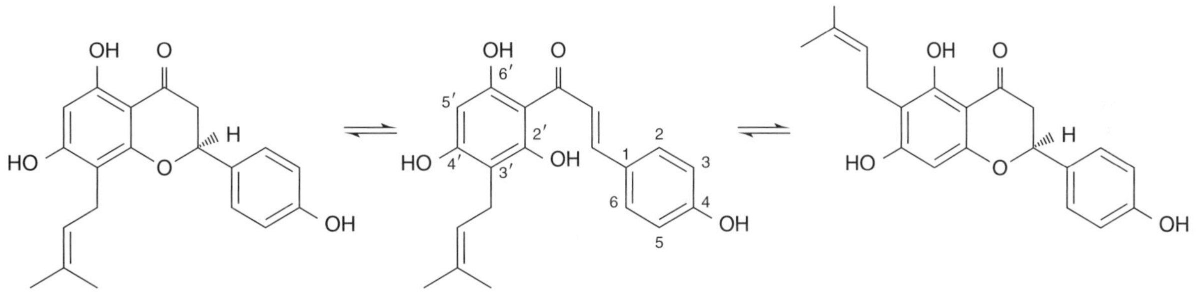

4,8-Prenylnaringenin   **1**, Desmethylxanthohumol   **5**,6-Prenylnaringenin

Figure 71.3 Ring-closure reaction of desmethylxanthohumol. Whereas xanthohumol in water only forms isoxanthohumol by a ring-closure reaction, desmethylxanthohumol (**1**) has the possibility to give two compounds because there are two hydroxylgroups. Either hydroxyl group at 2′ can react to give 6-prenylnaringenin (**5**) or hydroxyl group at 6′ reacts to give 8-prenylnaringenin (**4**).

Synthesis

In contrast to xanthohumol, there is a synthesis of **1** (Diller *et al.*, 2005). The key step of the synthesis of prenylated chalcones often relates to the appropriate acetophenone and benzaldehyde for aldol condensation. It is often complicated by interference of the protecting groups with the conditions of the aldol condensation. The lucky use of protecting groups is crucial for the outcome. After checking most of the usual methods without success, the hydroxy-functions of the educts were found to be protected by methoxymethyl-protecting groups (MOM) with advantage, the acid-catalysed deprotection turned out to occur at milder reaction conditions compared to the 2-methoxyethoxymethyl-protecting group (MEM) ethers. The resulting acetophenone was condensed with a *p*-hydroxybenzaldehyde derivative and deprotected (Figure 71.4).

Biological Activities

Hormonal effects

The chalcone–flavanone system of natural compounds from hops is active toward the estrogenic hormonal system in the human body (Milligan *et al.*, 2000; Zierau *et al.*, 2003). 8-PN is one of the most potent phytoestrogens, due to its activity at estradiol receptors, EC_{50} = 4.4 nmol/l compared to estradiol itself (0.82 nmol/l). Information about this issue with prenylated chalcones would become important

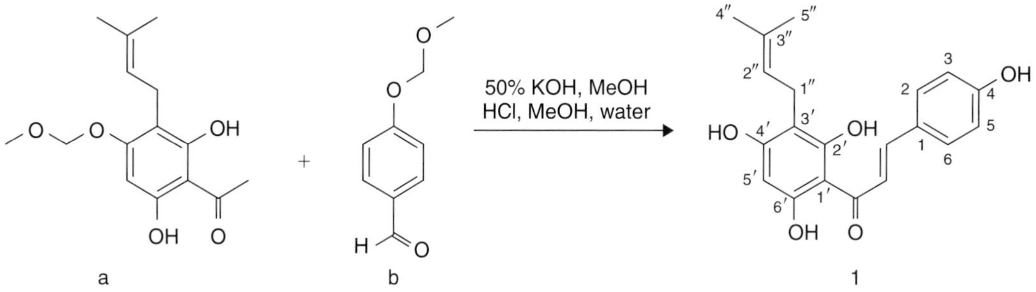

Figure 71.4 Synthesis of desmethylxanthohumol via aldol condensation. Many chalcone-type compounds were synthesized according to the scheme of an aldol condensation – reaction of a suitable aldehyde (b) with an acetophenone compound (a) bearing the right assembly of substituents. The problem is that the desired reaction conditions often lead to quite different product because of interference by the hydroxyl-substituents. In the case of desmethylxanthohumol, one hydroxyl group in position 4′ had to be protected as a methoxymethylether. In concentrated alkali in a water/methanol mixture, the desired reaction proceedes sufficiently. Desmethylxanthohumol was obtained finally by removing the protecting group with hydrochloric acid.

in connection with a prospective hormone replacement therapy to counteract osteoporosis. In contrast to 8-PN, desmethylxanthohumol – like xanthohumol – does not activate any estrogen receptors (De Keukeleire *et al.*, 1997; Milligan *et al.*, 2000). If there is any estrogenic activity from beverage preparations containing xanthohumol or desmethylxanthohumol, it may derive solely from an already observed isomerization or from unknown compounds. Concentration of circulating estradiol in the plasma (may amount up to 400 pM in women and 25 pM in men) is tightly regulated at the level of the synthesis of estradiol from androstenedione or testosterone by the enzyme aromatase. At least 8-PN itself, being able to activate estradiole receptors, can interfere substantially with aromatase activity. It is thus acting by a kind of pseudo product inhibition mechanism. Surprisingly, xanthohumol and isoxanthohumol, not being estrogen receptor agonists, inhibited aromatase as well, xanthohumol better than isoxanthohumol. Although for desmethylxanthohumol no data were available, one can assume some inhibition of aromatase which can account for the high aromatase inhibiting properties of some beers (Monteiro *et al.*, 2006).

Cancer protection and cytotoxic activities

Today, cancer is considered as an uncontrolled tissue growth which has two causes: Firstly, it may be induced by mutations or other genetic events resulting in impaired transcription from the DNA to yield ill functioning cell machinery not so severe to lead to cell death. Instead there can be continuous active growth inducing regulatory enzymes. Secondly, it may be caused by growth hormonal influences leading to deregulation at the level of signalization from the cellular environment to the intact cell nucleus. Breast cancer cells, for example, from post menopausal women most likely show hormonal-dependent growth activity. Not only is proliferation greatly induced by estradiol and every agent acting as an estradiol receptor agonist, but these cells also show very high aromatase activity enabling them to produce estradiol from its source. This type of early neoplastic tissue cells eventually can undergo cell death by so-called induced suicide mechanisms or apoptosis following lack of growth factors (among them – estradiole). Apoptosis is a mechanism for self-digestion of cells after some clearly defined stimuli from inside or outside the cell. It consists of condensation of chromatin, fragmentation of the DNA into small parts of about 180 base pairs, disintegration of the nucleus. Especially, the appearance of an array of small DNA fragments ("DNA ladder") is very characteristic of apoptosis and offers clear means of distinguishing from necrotic cell death by some toxic influence. Apoptosis is the most important mechanism in regulating tissue homeostasis (meaning the equal or nearly equal numbered replacement of cells during existence of an organism, when cells become aged and have to be replaced). Failure of apoptosis is among the most prominent reasons for uncontrolled cell proliferation.

Apoptotic stimuli can be: a lack of growth factors, missing contact to neighbor cells, ill replicated or severely damaged DNA and high or low molecular substances which contact sometimes very specific receptors. Apoptosis is only the last event in a series of signaling/regulating mechanisms. Tumor cells in the progression phase, for example, show uncontrolled cell proliferation, independent of growth factor stimulation, but susceptible to other means of apoptosis induction. This has given insight to the fact that there is more than one simple mechanism leading to apoptotic cell death. Following damage of a site of the DNA, repair/checking mechanisms are activated; especially a protein called P53 is involved, usually committing these cells to programmed cell death or apoptosis. This is called the "intrinsic" way of apoptosis induction. In the system of immune-competent cells (T-lymphocytes, B-cells, etc.), there is a cell surface receptor (Fas-receptor, "death"-receptor) which, upon contact with Fas-ligand protein from the surrounding medium, signalizes the "extrinsic" induction of apoptosis. Another important protein, able to induce apoptosis

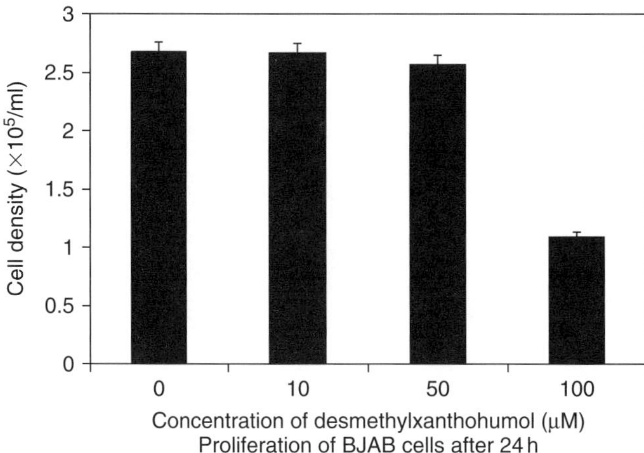

Figure 71.5 Decrease of proliferation of BJAB cells under influence of desmethylxanthohumol. Cell density (number of cells × 10^5/ml) at various concentrations of desmethylxanthohumol after 24 h. Beyond a concentration of 75 μM in the culture medium, **1** induces a significant inhibition of proliferation in BJAB cells after 24 h treatment. *Source*: From Diller *et al.* (2005).

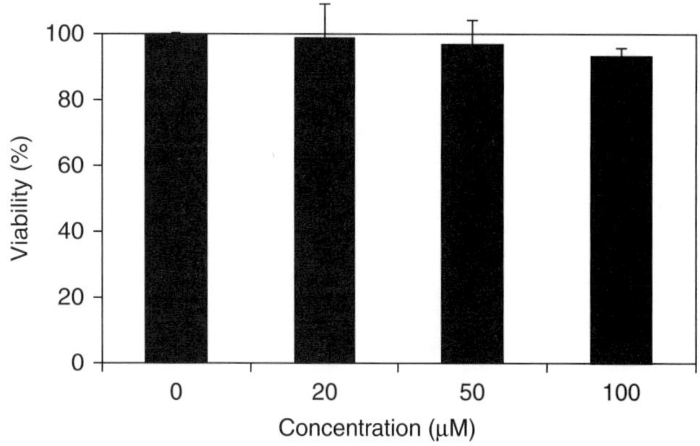

Figure 71.6 Viability assessment of BJAB cells after treatment with desmethylxanthohumol by measurement of LDH release. LDH is a cytosolic enzyme liberated only by rupture of the total cell wall. Cell death by apoptosis is not accompanied by disintergration of the cell. The graph indicates only a small effect of about 8% activity from this enzyme, so only very few cells are harmed by unspecific toxicity after treatment over 4 h. This shows that desmethylxanthohumol-induced cell death is a selectively induced process. *Source*: From Diller *et al.* (2005).

by docking to a death receptor is the tumor necrosis factor (TNF-α). Overconcentration of calcium ion or deterioration of cells by heat are additional means of apoptosis induction.

All these signals meet at the level of more central regulating proteins being pro-apoptotic or antiapoptotic. Whereas the cell surface death receptors are often tissue specific, these central regulating proteins are from tissue to tissue uniform. Some proteins of the Bcl-family are antiapoptotic, whereas proteins of the Bax type are pro-apoptotic. Both proteins are located at the surface of the mitochondria or nearby. Bax-proteins can open channels in the mitochondrial membrane; this mitochondrial permeability transition is crucial for apoptosis, since hereby reactive oxygen metabolites and cytochrome c-like proteins with oxidizing properties can be released into the cytosol to do the harmful work characteristic to apoptotic cell death. Bax and Bcl proteins usually form heterodimers, the permeating property of Bax is balanced by Bcl. Disturbing this equilibrium is a main switch of the signaling pathway during the induction of apoptosis.

Both signaling pathways merge at the level of cystein-rich proteolytic enzymes (caspase-3, 6 or 7) whose substrates are the different physiological structural proteins like chromatin that are digested in the process of apoptosis. DNA itself is fragmented by a special protein complex, the caspase-3-activated DNA fragmenting enzyme (CAD). (Hengartner, 2000).

To assess the antiproliferative acitivity of desmethylxanthohumol, the proliferation of BJAB cells, a Burkitt lymphoma cell line from the lineage of B-leucocytes, was measured. We observed a strong inhibition of BJAB cells after 24 h at a concentration of 100 μM (Figure 71.5).

Cell death in experimental systems can occur after two distinct events: cell death due to toxic necrosis or cell death by induction of apoptosis. We were able to show that there is not a significant cytotoxic effect of desmethylxanthohumol due to necrosis. Lactate dehydrogenase (LDH) is an enzyme in the cyclosol. Due to its high molecular weight (140 kDa) it cannot pass the cell membrane. LDH release can only be detected after cell membrane disruption caused by necrotic cell death. The release of LDH was measured 4 h after treatment with desmethylxanthohumol at a concentration of 20, 50 and 100 μM. There was no LDH release detectable after 4 h (Figure 71.6). Therefore, the antiproliferative properties as described above cannot be caused by a general cytotoxicity. Whether there is an apoptotic effect was examined by determination of DNA fragmentation.

The degree of cells undergoing apoptosis was estimated from the percentage of cells with DNA fragments. At a concentration of 100 μM desmethylxanthohumol, a remarkable fraction of cells (35%) in the subG1-phase of the cell division cycle is detected by flow cytometric determination of hypodiploid DNA (Figure 71.7).

At concentrations up to 50 μM desmethylxanthohumol, the amount of apoptotic cells is negligible after treatment for 72 h. In a concentration of 100 μM, desmethylxanthohumol induces apoptosis in BJAB cells. We further investigated the type of apoptotic pathway induced by desmethylxanthohumol. Therefore, we measured the extent of mitochondrial permeability transition. A decrease in the mitochondrial membrane potential indicates that desmethylxanthohumol is able to induce apoptosis via the intrinsic signaling pathway (Figure 71.8).

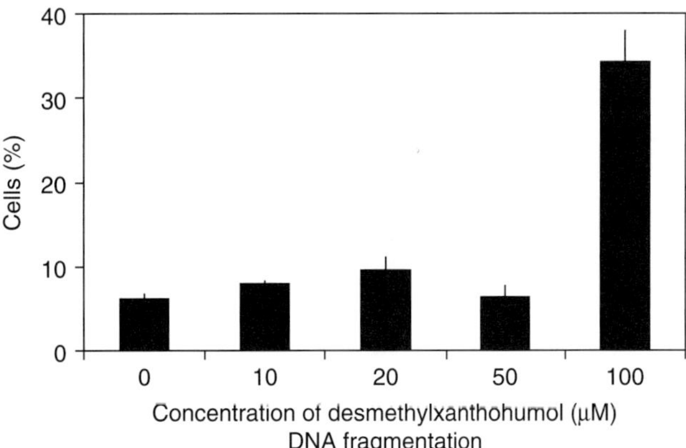

Figure 71.7 Assessment of cells undergoing apoptotic cell death. Apoptosis is characterized by extensive DNA fragmentation and occurrence of hypodiploid DNA (DNA in subG1-phase of the cell cycle). The latter can be assessed by flow cytometry via propidium iodide-staining. The graph reflects the number of apoptotic cells in relation to the concentration of desmethylxanthohumol. 100 μM is able to induce apoptosis in 36% of all BJAB cells. *Source*: From Diller *et al.* (2005).

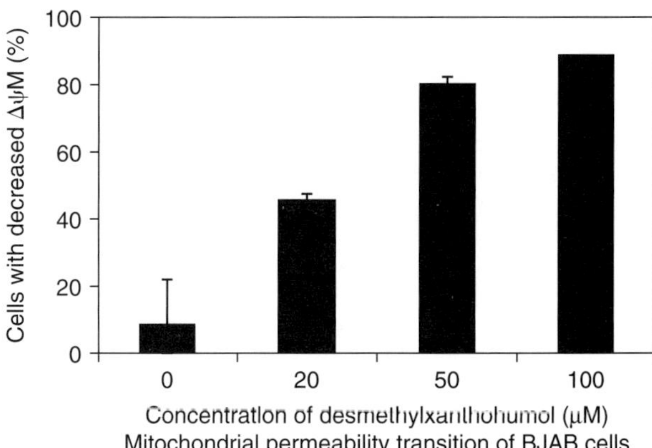

Figure 71.8 Assessment of the mitochondrial membrane potential. Mitochondrial membrane potential was determined by staining the cells with 5,5′,6,6′-tetrachloro-1,1′,3,3′-tetraethyl-benzimidazolylcarbocyanin iodide (JC-1) and flow cytometric cell count. The decrease of the mitochondrial membrane potential is induced even at 20 μM desmethylxanthohumol in BJAB Mock cells. Over 40% of all cells have a defect in mitochondrial membrane potential after this treatment. This shows that desmethylxanthohumol most probably is able to induce apoptosis via the mitochondrial-dependent pathway. *Source*: From Diller *et al.* (2005).

It could be demonstrated that there is a clearly shown concentration-dependent decrease in the mitochrondrial membrane potential, enabling oxygen radical species to penetrate into the cytosol and activating the apoptosome.

Anticarcinogenic activity is different from antiproliferative activity since in the latter case an already neoplastic transformed cell line is expected to undergo cell death. Anticarcinogenic activity means an inhibition of the event in a cell system to undergo neoplastic transformation to a fully developed, steadily dividing cancer cell line. An important milestone in this process of transformation is thought to be the presence in the cell of xenobiotics, substances exerting DNA damage. There are mechanisms in the cells to dispose these substances either by immediate expulsion using a transporter system or by the process of reduction, conjugation with glucuronic acid and the final excretion. With this respect, the enzyme quinone reductase has found to be of major importance. Nearly every plant-derived cancer-protective agent has found to be active in this system, either being a mono- or bifunctional inducer of the CYP-Genes encoding for quinone reductases. After Miranda (Miranda *et al.*, 2000) desmethylxanthohumol in a system of quinone reductase from mouse liver cells (Hepa 1c1c7) was able to greatly enhance the activity of quinone reduc-tase, but not so much than xanthohumol itself. Both substances being monofunctional inducers, do not require a functionally intact arylhydrocarbon receptor.

General assessment with respect to human nutrition

Up to the present day, studies of the physiological effects of hop constituents mostly have been done with tissue cultures or in animal studies with mouse models. To assess possible implications on human nutrition, one has to take into consideration the passage of the beverages through the intestinal system. For example, due to its ability easily to isomerize to 8-PN, only desmethylxanthohumol contributes to any hormonal effect of hop, but its concentration relative to xanthohumol is approximately 1/10. It has been shown by Possemiers (Possemiers *et al.*, 2005) that intestinal bacteria can demethylate cyclization products of xanthohumol, means isoxanthohumol to 8-PN. Considering this facts, it can be expected that the total hormonal effect of a hop ingestion will surely increase by such digestional activity.

Summary

Desmethylxanthohumol from hops is protective against mutagenesis by environmental harmful chemical and tumor-like tissue growth. It is unstable in beverages, whereby it contributes more than other compounds to a hormonal effect.

References

De Keukeleire, D., Milligan, S.R., De Cooman, L. and Heyerick, A. (1997). *Pharmaceut. Pharmacol. Lett.* 7, 83–86.

Diller, R.A., Riepl, H.M., Rose, O., Frias, C., Henze, G. and Prokop, A. (2005). *Chem. Biodiv.* 2, 1331.

Hengartner, M.O. (2000). *Nature* 407, 770.

Hänsel, R. and Schulz, J. (1988). *Archiv der Pharmazie* 321, 37.

Milligan, S.R., Kalita, J.C., Pocock, V., Van de Kauter, V., Stevens, J.F., Deinzer, M.L., Rong, H. and De Keukeleire, D. (2000). *J. Clin. Endocrin. Metab.* 85, 4912–4915.

Miranda, C.L., Alphonso, G.L., Stevens, J.F., Deinzer, M.L. and Buhler, D.R. (2000). *Cancer Lett.* 149, 21.

Monteiro, R., Becker, H., Azevedo, I. and Calhau, C. (2006). *J. Agric. Food Chem.* 54, 2938.

Possemiers, S., Heyerick, A., Robbens, V., De Keukelaire, D. and Verstraete, W. (2005). *J. Agric. Food Chem.* 53, 6281.

Stevens, J.F., Ivanic, M., Hsu, V.L. and Deinzer, M.L. (1997). *Phytochemistry* 44, 1575.

Stevens, J.F., Taylor, A.W., Clawson, J.E. and Deinzer, M.L. (1999a). *J. Agric. Food Chem.* 47, 2421.

Stevens, J.F., Taylor, A.W. and Deinzer, M.L. (1999b). *J. Chromatogr. A* 832, 97.

Zierau, O., Morrissey, C., Watson, R.W., Schwab, P., Kolba, S., Metz, P. and Vollmer, G. (2003). *Planta Med.* 69, 856–858.

72

Reproductive and Estrogenic Effects of 8-Prenylnaringenin in Hops

Stuart R. Milligan Division of Reproduction and Endocrinology, School of Biomedical Sciences, King's College London, Guy's Campus, London, UK

Abstract

Historical and anecdotal observations of the estrogenic activity of hops led to the identification of 8-prenylnaringenin (8PN) as one of the most potent phyto-oestrogens. As an estrogen, 8PN has the potential to interact with the estrogen-signaling systems within the body, including the reproductive system. In terms of normal exposure, only those situations in which there is large scale exposure to "raw" hops (e.g. hop workers) are likely to be of significance, with disturbances to menstrual cycles being most likely. There is no evidence, nor reason to suspect, that exposure to 8PN via the most common hop product, namely beer, is of any significance to the fertility of either sex. In terms of the potential exploitation of the estrogenic activity of 8PN, menopausal symptoms seems to offer some promise as a target. Treatment with a weak "natural" estrogen seems to be readily acceptable to many women and uncertainties about efficacy may be masked by strong placebo effects, at least for symptoms like hot flushes. Indeed, the relative weakness of the estrogenic activity of 8PN compared to pharmacological estrogen preparations may be of advantage as this would also reduce the risk of hormone-dependent cancer. However, as treatments for menopausal symptoms typically tend to involve continuous or long-term exposure regimens to otherwise healthy women, all treatments need careful monitoring in terms of both safety and efficacy, not least because other (non-estrogenic) bioactivities of 8PN and associated hop-derived compounds need to be considered.

List of Abbreviations

8PN	8 Prenylnaringenin
ERα	Estrogen receptor alpha
ERβ	Estrogen receptor beta
LH	Luteinizing hormone
SERM	Selective estrogen receptor modulator

Introduction

Over the last two decades there has been increasing scientific and public interest in the reproductive effects of the exposure of humans to compounds in the environment that may interfere with the hormonal control of development. The interest initially developed in relation to compounds with weak estrogenic activity (Routledge and Sumpter, 1996), but further studies soon widened the concept of "endocrine disruption" so that any compound interacting with hormonal signaling systems or interfering with hormonally controlled systems can be labeled as an "endocrine disruptor" (e.g. Zacharewski, 1998).

Reproductive disturbances in wildlife (e.g. feminization of fish downstream from sewage effluents; Sumpter, 1995) raised a general scientific interest. However, the main drive came from the suggestion that the increasing exposure to industrial chemicals with potential endocrine-disrupting activity (e.g. pesticides, phthalates, surfactants) was a cause of the increase in reproductive tract abnormalities in men (Toppari *et al.*, 1996; Sharpe, 2001). These abnormalities include a cluster of conditions under the banner of the "testicular dysgenesis syndrome": reduced sperm counts, increased testicular cancer, cryptorchidism and hypospadias (Skakkebaek *et al.*, 2001; Sharpe and Irvine, 2004). The various phenotypes of this syndrome are thought to derive from disturbances of fetal or early post-natal life, a time when the developing reproductive system is particularly sensitive to perturbations of the hormonal environment.

In seeming contrast to these concerns about the adverse effects of hormonally active, "industrial" chemicals, an alternative focus of interest has come from health beneficial effects attributed to "natural," plant-derived estrogenic compounds (phyto-oestrogens) in food (Adlercreutz, 1990). Phyto-oestrogens have been regularly implicated as protective factors against many of the so-called western diseases, including breast and prostate cancer, and cardiovascular disease in women (e.g. Setchell, 1998). Such potential

Beer in Health and Disease Prevention
ISBN: 978-0-12-373891-2

beneficial effects have been the rationale for the inclusion of plant extracts rich in phyto-oestrogens in a number of herbal supplements, "health foods" and complementary medicine products (Lee, 2006).

The apparent discrepancy between the potential adverse effects of industrial "endocrine disruptors" and the beneficial attributes of plant oestrogens is counter-intuitive and is due to a number of confounding factors. In part it reflects an unfortunate public perception that industrial chemicals are inherently unnatural and therefore "bad," while plants have "natural compounds." This confusion has been compounded by sometimes over-enthusiastic extrapolation by some scientists of the significance of their field of work and by commercial interests promoting "natural health products." Another complicating factor is that many of the putative hormonal activities of environmental chemicals have been demonstrated *in vitro*. The *in vitro* systems (e.g. effects on cell lines in culture) inevitably tend to focus on the specific effects of single chemicals in a single cell type. These studies are particularly useful in defining the precise cell signaling pathways through which the chemicals can act and in providing a guide to the concentrations that may require to produce any effect. However, trying to extrapolate from *in vitro* results to the whole body situation is notoriously difficult. A mono-culture of identical cells cannot imitate either the complexity of organs or the multifactorial, homeostatic control systems that operate throughout the body. Neither do *in vitro* systems mimic the kinetics of uptake, metabolism, breakdown and excretion. *In vivo* studies in experimental animals can help to bridge the gap in our understanding, but are limited in terms of their experimental design (e.g. the animal and the time of exposure in its life history; the mode, dose and duration of exposure; short or long-term effects evaluated). *In vivo* studies in humans are severely limited both by even more complex ethical and practical considerations. In view of such limitations, the influence of these chemicals on humans remains an area of speculation and sometimes over-hyped debate. The situation is additionally complicated by the fact that the body may be simultaneously exposed to many different endocrine-disrupting chemicals, each operating through different mechanisms in different cell types. For example, oestrogens may act genomically via the two estrogen receptors alpha and beta (ERα and ERβ), and/or non-genomically via cell surface receptors, and/or by modulation of other cell signaling systems, including epigenetic modifications (Crews and McLachlan, 2006).

There is no doubt that many plants provide a source of chemicals with estrogenic activity. The main groups of non-steroidal dietary "phyto-oestrogens" are: isoflavones (e.g. daidzein, genistein), lignans (e.g. secoisolariciresinol, enterodiol, enterolactone), coumestans (e.g. coumestrol) and resorcyclic acid lactones (Dixon, 2004). In addition, Miksicek (1993) originally reported that many of the common plant flavonoids (including some chalcones, flavanones and flavones) can bind to and activate the estrogen receptor (albeit very weakly). Resveratrol, a phytoalexin found in grapes and red wine was also shown to be a weak agonist for the estrogen receptor (Gehm *et al.*, 1997) and this provided further ammunition for those wishing to attribute health benefits to red wine drinking. Quantitatively, isoflavones (present in legumes, particularly soyabeans) and lignans are the most important dietary phyto-oestrogens (both in terms of magnitude and duration of exposure).

The ability of dietary phyto-oestrogens to affect mammalian reproduction was initially highlighted by the disruption of fertility in ewes grazing on pastures unusually rich in phyto-oestrogens. Similar observations have been made in a number of other farm and animal species exposed to high levels of phyto-oestrogens (Yang and Bittner, 2002), but disturbances to human fertility by normal levels of dietary phyto-oestrogens have not been reported. However, although dietary phyto-oestrogens may have no reproductive effects in humans, there is intense interest in the potential of estrogenic isoflavones to modulate other estrogen-dependent processes, particularly reducing the risk of breast cancer and cardiovascular disease and improving bone health and menopausal symptoms. It is not the place of the current chapter to detail these, but the reader is referred to other literature for current assessments on the role of dietary phyto-oestrogens in health and disease (e.g. cardiovascular disease: Cassidy and Hooper, 2006; breast cancer: Messina *et al.*, 2006; genistein and reproductive health: National Toxicology Program Center For The Evaluation Of Risks To Human Reproduction, 2006; menopausal symptoms: Nedrow *et al.*, 2006). Unfortunately, for those who want a definitive answer, the recurrent take-home message is that more work is needed to define the relative risks and benefits (if any) of dietary phyto-oestrogens to the health of either specific individuals or the general population!

How do hops feature in this context? Circumstantial evidence over many years has linked hops with potential hormonal activity in women, particularly in terms of affecting menstrual cyclicity. However, the scientific literature on the possible hormonal activity of hops ranged from suggestions that they may be one of the richest sources of oestrogens, to the failure to find any evidence of estrogenic activity. The studies eventually led to the identification of one specific chemical, 8-prenylnaringenin (8PN) as the major source of the estrogenic activity of hops. This chapter will review our current understanding of the biological activity of 8PN in terms of its ability to modulate reproductive processes in humans.

The Identification of the Estrogenic Activity of Hops

The use of hops for medicinal purposes dates back centuries and probably reflects the fact that hops are a very rich source of a variety of bioactive chemicals. Although hops have been used for the treatment of conditions ranging from indigestion to tuberculosis and nervous disorders, a recurring suggestion has been that hops could be used to treat gynecological problems. One early reference cites the following: "Half a dram of the seed in powder take in drink brings down women courses" (Culpepper, 1653; cited by Neve, 1991). Brewery sludge baths were used for many years in Germany, partly for their alleged healing and rejuvenating powers, and partly for the treatment of gynecological disorders (Zenisek and Bednar, 1960). Further observations consistent with some hormonal activity came from reports that changes occurred in the menstrual cycle of women engaged in picking hops. These claims included that menstrual cyclicity was synchronized soon after the start of hop harvesting, and that disturbances of menstrual cyclicity were common (Verzele, 1986). In reply to a query from the present author about the estrogenic activity of hops, Verzele wrote "In my country [Belgium] the notion of the 'hop devil' is well established. People used to gather in September in the hop growing fields for the harvest and the young men and women spent weeks together to do that. Much intercourse went on and these occasions (just like grape picking) were famous for this. The contact of the women with fresh hops … threw off their period and many got unintentionally, unexpectedly pregnant – therefore the term 'hop devil.' Also it seems because women in the hop gardens were unusually receptive to sexual advances" (Verzele, 1992, personal communication). Despite the delightful nature of this communication, it should be remembered that hop pickers were often very poor and suffered many health problems. Since menstrual cycles are notoriously sensitive to nutritional status, energy balance and stress, the causes of any menstrual disturbances in hop pickers must remain speculative. However, reports of modern day workers in hop processing plants suffering disruption of menstrual cyclicity (personal observations) are consistent with the original observations on hop pickers.

The historical reports of reproductive disturbances in female hop pickers were followed by a number of scientific studies on the hormonal activity of hops. Using the sensitive bioassay for oestrogens in rodents, Koch and Heim (1953) reported that a crude extract of hop cones contained estrogenic activity. These authors discovered that the extract of hop cones contained the equivalent of 20–300 μg 17β-oestradiol/g. This is an extraordinarily large amount in relation to other plants. The authors suggested that the high contents of phyto-oestrogens in hops could be of value for medicinal purposes. Zenisek and Bednar (1960) confirmed these findings and suggested that estrogenic activity of hops was much higher than in other plants. They found that the extract rich in the β-bitter acids contained the highest activity. Chury (1960) also reported estrogenic activity in hop extracts when saponified hops were extracted with 95% ethanol. However, in contrast to these positive reports of estrogenic activity, Fenselau and Talalay (1973) found no evidence of such activity in a wide range of hop extracts and hop derivatives (including essential oil fractions, the alpha and beta bitter acids, some commercial extracts and various organic extracts of different varieties of hops from both Europe and the United States). These negative findings were contradicted again by Hesse *et al.* (1981) who used an *in vitro* receptor binding bioassay based on calf uterine estrogen receptors and concluded that hops are one of the richest plant sources of oestrogens. In that study, the estrogenic activity was associated to the lipophilic fractions of hops.

What is the explanation of the apparent inconsistencies in some of the above studies? The *in vivo* assays used by Koch and Heim (1953), Zenisek and Bednar (1960) and Fenselau and Talalay (1973) were based on the stimulation of vaginal cornification or uterine growth in immature or ovariectomized rodents. The ability of these assays to detect weak estrogenic activity is very dependent on the route and frequency of administration of the material; negative results in these assays could easily be explained by an inappropriate treatment regimen. The *in vitro* receptor binding assay (as used by Hesse *et al.*, 1981) detects binding to estrogen receptor but binding activity does not necessarily reflect biological activity. The different investigators also used different hop extracts and the nature of the hop materials were not always adequately identified.

None of these studies had provided clear evidence of the chemical nature and biological activity of the putative estrogen(s). The progress toward its eventual identification has been well described by Chadwick *et al.* (2006). Xanthohumol, a chalcone present in hops at rather high concentrations, was suggested by some (without evidence) to be the active estrogenic compound (Verzele, 1986). Using an *in vitro* assay similar to that of Zenisek and Bednar (1960), Milligan (unpublished observations) was unable to confirm that xanthohumol was estrogenic and was also unable to detect any estrogenic activity in the the β-bitter acid fraction that had been reported as containing high activity by Zenisek and Bednar (1960). Nastainczyk (1972) isolated a hop constituent that could be isomerized into an active estrogen but did not identify it. Hansel and Schulz (1988) concluded that this hop constituent was desmethylxanthohumol and that this was converted into 8PN and 6-prenylnaringenin (6PN). Whilst 6PN was deemed not to have estrogenic activity, the activity of 8PN was not directly studied.

The work that led to the final identification of the chemical nature of the estrogenic activity of hops was initiated by present author following menstrual disturbances in the author's wife when working with hops. A collaboration between the author (with expertise of both *in vivo* and *in vitro* bioassays for oestrogens) and Professor Denis de Keukeleire (with expertise in hop chemistry) was initiated. A bioassay-guided fractionation of hop extracts was undertaken and led to the identification of 8PN as the principle

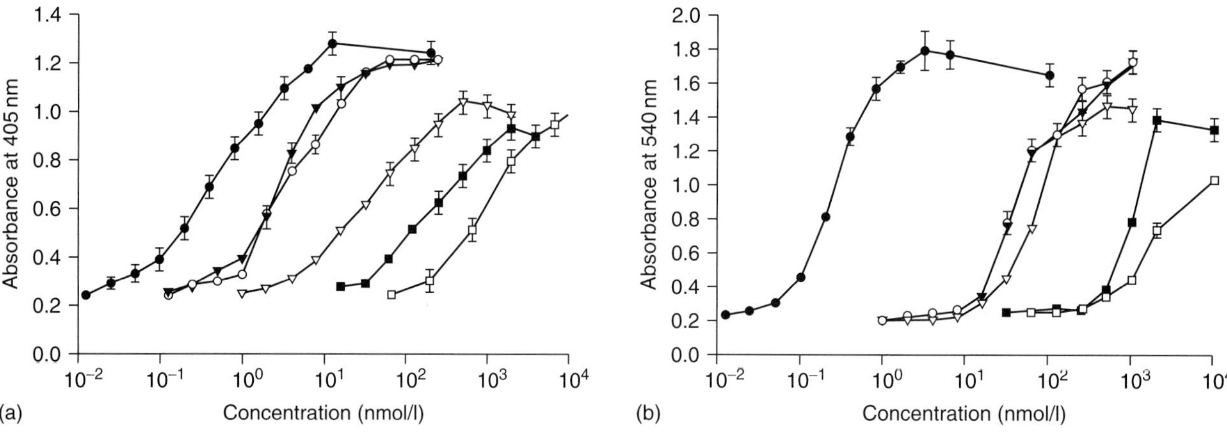

Figure 72.1 The estrogenic activity of 8PN *in vitro*. The relative estrogenic activity of oestradiol (•), 8PN (semi-synthetic; ○), 8PN (natural; ▾) and other phyto-oestrogens (coumestrol (▿), genistein (▪), daidzein (□)) in (a) human Ishikawa Var I cells (a uterine cell line) and (b) a yeast screen bearing the human estrogen receptor. Results are mean + SEM; $n = 6$ wells per point. Where no error bars are visible, the errors were smaller than the symbols. In both assays, 8PN exerts considerably greater bioactivity than the other established phyto-oestrogens. *Source*: From Milligan *et al.* (2002). © Society for Reproduction & Fertility. Reproduced by permission.

hop estrogen. The demonstration that synthetic 8PN also showed strong estrogenic activity confirmed that 8PN was one of the most potent phyto-oestrogens, with an activity far exceeding that of the established soy-derived phyto-oestrogens (Milligan *et al.*, 1999). In an *in vitro* bioassay based on human endometrial cells (Ishikawa Var 1), the EC_{50} for 17β-estradiol, 8PN, coumestrol, genistein and daidzein were 0.8, 4, 30, 200 and 1,500 nM, respectively, while in a yeast screen bearing human estrogen receptors, the results were 0.3, 40, 70, 1,200 and 2,200 nM, respectively (Figure 72.1). The bioactivity was completely blocked in the Ishikawa cells by the anti-estrogen ICI 182,780, confirming that the effects were mediated by estrogen receptors. Subsequently, it was shown that 8PN is able to bind to both ERα and ERβ (Milligan *et al.*, 2000), although Bovee *et al.* (2004) reported that 8PN was relatively more potent with ERα in yeast assays stably expressing the different human estrogen receptors.

Other hop constituents including 6-prenylnaringenin, 6,8-diprenylnaringenin and 8-geranylnaringenin exhibit some oestrogenicity, but their potency is less than 1% of that of 8PN (Milligan *et al.*, 2000). Isoxanthohumol was also weakly active in the Ishikawa cell assay (1% of 8PN) but showed no estrogenic activity in the yeast screen (Figure 72.1). Since it also showed no activity in the receptor binding assay, this was interpreted as suggesting its weak activity reflected metabolic conversion to 8PN in the human cells (Milligan *et al.*, 1999). The importance of this metabolic conversion of isoxanthohumol to 8PN was highlighted again some years later when Possemiers *et al.* (2005, 2006) showed that isoxanthohumol can be converted by intestinal microflora into 8PN, hence providing a much larger potential source of 8PN from beer or hop products than would be suspected by measuring the 8PN content alone (Figure 72.2).

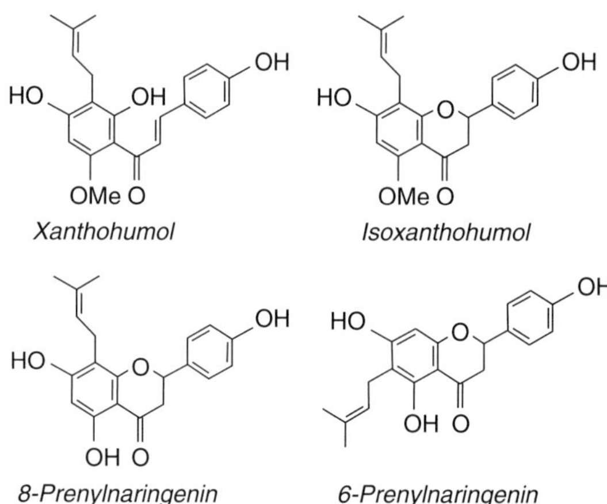

Figure 72.2 Structures of 8PN and related polyphenols. 8PN is the most potent hop estrogen. Isoxanthohumol shows no activity *per se*, but can be metabolized to 8PN. 6-Prenylnaringen shows <1% the estrogenic activity of 8PN. Xanthohumol shows no estrogenic activity.

Potential Sources of 8PN Exposure to Humans

The amount of 8-prenlnaringenin in hop flowers is relatively small but increases during cone development (Stevens *et al.*, 2000). An important route of formation is from the isomerization of desmethylxanthohumol (Stevens *et al.*, 1999; Chadwick *et al.*, 2004). The amount of 8PN in dry hops is in the order of 100 mg.kg^{-1} (Milligan *et al.*, 1999). In the brew kettle, desmethylxanthohumol has a half-life of less than 5 min, isomerizing to 8PN and 6PN (Stevens *et al.*, 1999). Although 8PN levels in beer are relatively low (normally <100 ug/l; Rong *et al.*, 2000; Stevens and Page, 2004; Schaeffer *et al.*, 2005), estimates by Schaeffer *et al.*

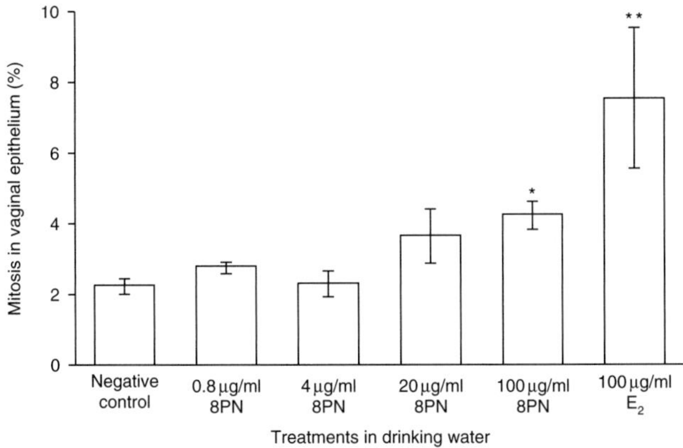

Figure 72.3 The stimulatory effects of 8PN in the drinking water on the vaginal epithelium of ovariectomized mice. The vaginal epithelium of mice is very sensitive to oestrogens and responds with cell proliferation. This figure shows the mitotic response of the vaginal luminal epithelium of ovariectomized mice to 8PN or oestradiol (E2) administered for 72 h in drinking water. Data are mean + SEM ($n = 6$ per treatment). Significant differences are denoted by *$p < 0.05$, **$p < 0.005$ (Kruskal–Wallis test on ranks and Dunn's multiple comparison test). *Source*: From Milligan *et al.* (2002). ©Society for Reproduction & Fertility. Reproduced by permission.

(2005) and Possemiers *et al.* (2006) suggested that conversion of isoxanthohumol by intestinal flora might increase 8PN exposure up to 10-fold in some subjects. In this case, exposure levels would be likely to reach 1–2 mg 8PN/day in association with moderate daily beer consumption.

Once formed, important factors influencing the bioavailability and activity of phyto-oestrogens include the route of exposure, the kinetics of absorption and excretion, and metabolic conversions (e.g. Zierau *et al.*, 2005). The pharmacokinetics of a single oral dose of 8PN in post-menopausal women showed that the compound was absorbed rapidly, after which plasma levels remained significantly elevated for many hours, probably reflecting enterohepatic circulation (Rad *et al.*, 2006). There is only a limited amount of data on the routes of metabolism of 8PN by human tissues, but these suggest that it is transformed into a wide variety of metabolites, some of which have very weak estrogenic activity (Nikolic *et al.*, 2004; Zierau *et al.*, 2004). In experimental animals, a variety of estrogenic effects of 8PN on the reproductive tract have been reported after dietary (in food or drinking water) exposure (Milligan *et al.*, 2002; Christoffel *et al.*, 2006). In mice, the minimal effective concentration to stimulate vaginal mitoses (a sensitive index of estrogenic activity) in the drinking water was about 100 μg/ml. This is about 1,000× greater than the levels of 8PN in beer (Figure 72.3).

For most humans, the dietary intake of beer represents the commonest source of 8PN exposure. For a few, the dietary intake of herbal supplements containing hops or hop extracts for the treatment of menopausal symptoms, "breast enlargement" or other "natural therapies" is another possible source. In both situations, the amount of 8PN exposure will reflect both the amount of 8PN *per se* in the raw product and possible conversion of isoxanthohumol into 8PN (Possemiers *et al.*, 2005, 2006). Individuals working with raw hops would be expected to have the most direct exposure to 8PN, both through transdermal absorption of 8PN and due to inhalation of hop dust.

The Need for Caution in Considering the Reproductive Effects of 8PN

Oestrogens are hormones controlling the development and function of the reproductive system of both sexes. There are many target sites for estrogenic activity, ranging from the reproductive tract and breast, through bone, fat and blood vessels, to the bladder and brain. The physiological significance of estrogenic effects at many of these sites is still unclear. Two estrogen receptors (ERα and ERβ) modulate the effects of the hormones: these receptors have differing affinities for different estrogen, differing tissue and cellular distributions, interact with a large array of different coactivators and corepressors (Kuiper *et al.*, 1997; Xiao *et al.*, 2006). Oestrogens can also act non-genomically. The recognition of such diverse modulators of estrogen action has opened a surprising new dimension in our ignorance of the effects of even the endogenous, potent hormone, 17β-oestradiol (Ciana *et al.*, 2006). In this atmosphere, understanding the molecular mechanisms and activity of the much weaker phyto-oestrogens still seems a long way off.

While much more potent than the traditional soy-based phyto-oestrogens (Milligan *et al.*, 1999, 2002), the bioactivity of 8PN is still relatively weak compared to endogenous oestrogens (e.g. ~ <1/10–1/100 that of oestradiol, depending on the assay technique; Milligan *et al.*, 2002). Crucially, the *in vivo* biological activity of weak oestrogens is very dependent on the route of administration and the duration of exposure. This is well illustrated by considering oestriol: a "weak" natural estrogen compared to oestradiol, but considerably more potent than any of the phyto-oestrogens, including 8PN. It was once assumed that oestriol would protect against breast cancer because it appeared to act only weakly in experiments on uterine growth. When its effects were measured 24 h after a single injection, oestriol appeared to have a low potency and a flat dose–response line. This was a misinterpretation: the low apparent potency was not due to a failure of oestriol to stimulate growth but from the failure of a single daily injection to sustain the resulting cells (Martin *et al.*, 1976). Using more a continuous treatment regimen of oestriol, premature cell death was avoided and oestriol produced as much uterine hypertrophy and hyperplasia as oestradiol. These discordant results arising simply from different treatment regimens of a "weak" estrogen should serve as a strong warning to others trying to extrapolate from the results of experiments involving any of the considerably weaker phyto-oestrogens. The issue of how treatment regimens may affect the responses of different tissues has also been highlighted by the studies of estrogen receptor activation *in vivo* (Ciana *et al.*, 2006). This discussion of the importance of treatment regimens is particularly relevant to the interpretation of the results of the study of Hümpel *et al.* (2005), showing apparent selective effects of 8PN on the bone rather than the uterus and implying a selective estrogen receptor modulator (SERM)-like action of 8PN. However, other studies have certainly shown strong and rapid effects of 8PN on the uterus (Milligan *et al.*, 2002) and the results of Hümpel *et al.* (2005) may simply reflect their particular experimental treatment regimen (single daily injections).

In view of the importance of continuous exposure to weak oestrogens to enhance their estrogenic effects, the potential slow-release reservoir effect provided by intra-intestinal conversion of isoxanthohumol to 8PN (Possemiers *et al.*, 2006) deserves particular emphasis. Such a reservoir effect would be consistent with the observations of Schaefer *et al.* (2005) that urinary 8PN excretion after beer consumption was slower than expected. An additional factor contributing to a more continuous *in vivo* exposure (and hence continuous estrogenic stimulation) would be the enterohepatic circulation (Rad *et al.*, 2006).

A final word of caution concerning 8PN is that, like most compounds, it exhibits a spectrum of different bioactivities (Stevens and Page, 2004; Effenberger *et al.*, 2005; Gerhauser, 2005; Monteiro *et al.*, 2006). It is beyond the scope of this chapter to detail these, but these other potential bioactivities should be considered in any experimental intervention.

8PN and Menstrual Cyclicity

Anecdotal observations about the effects of hop exposure on menstrual cyclicity are detailed above. While the identification of a potent phyto-estrogen in hops (8PN) provides an attractive potential explanation for the cause of such disturbances, there is no direct evidence for this. Dietary phyto-oestrogens (particularly soy-derived) have been implicated in only rather subtle effects on the menstrual cycle and its associated symptoms (Kurzer, 2002; Bryant *et al.*, 2005; Cassidy and Hooper, 2006) but these are not in the same league as the dramatic menstrual disturbances associated with hop exposure.

There are two obvious potential explanations for this difference. The first relates to the potency and method of exposure to phyto-oestrogens. Soy-derived phyto-oestrogens are relatively weak and exposure is via the diet. The impact of dietary phyto-oestrogens is severely modulated by both the kinetics of uptake from the gut and first-pass metabolism by the liver. In contrast, hop workers are likely to have been exposed to 8PN through absorption across the skin (which would be facilitated by the oily nature of hops) and/or through the lungs (with a very large, thin and well vascularized surface area) after the intake of hop dust. In both cases, the problems of first-pass metabolism would be avoided, resulting in direct exposure of tissues to relatively high levels of 8PN. The potential for 8PN to exert estrogenic effects on the body would be exacerbated by the relatively continuous exposure that hop pickers would have experienced. The importance of such continuous exposure for weak oestrogens to exert their effects is discussed above (see section "The Need for Caution in Considering the Reproductive Effects of 8PN"). Nowadays, premenopausal women are more likely to be exposed to 8PN through "natural" dietary products containing hops, particularly those targeting breast enhancement (see below) and some websites associated with these do warn of possible menstrual problems.

The most likely target sites for the action of 8PN for disrupting menstrual cycles would be either on the hypothalamic-pituitary control of the ovary or directly on the uterus itself. Both acute and chronic effects of weak phyto-oestrogens like 8PN can be envisaged. Milligan *et al.* (2002) reported rapid and dramatic increases in uterine vasculature within 6h of 8PN administration. Experimental studies in primates have shown that treatment with high doses of *Pueraria mirifica* (containing phyto-oestrogens) affected gonadotrophin levels and abolished or increased the length of cycles of monkeys (Trisomboon *et al.*, 2005). Rad *et al.* (2006) reported a small suppression of luteinizing hormone (LH) in post-menopausal women after a single oral dose of 750mg of 8PN, suggesting an effect on the hypothalamic-pituitary axis. In a long-term study over 3 months, Christoffel *et al.* (2006) showed that 8PN included in the diet of rats (providing them with 70mg/Kg bw) stimulated uterine growth, specific gene expression in the uterus, and affected serum levels of the pituitary hormones LH and prolactin in a similar manner to oestradiol (Figure 72.4).

The second possible reason why the effects on menstrual cyclicity in hop workers may have been more dramatic than those caused by soy phyto-oestrogens is that the effects in hop workers may not have been due to either 8PN or hops. The menstrual disturbances in hop workers may simply have reflected other lifestyle and nutritional factors associated with their poverty, poor health and lifestyle. In view of the almost complete disappearance of manual hop picking, it is unlikely that this question will ever be answered definitively.

Hops, 8PN and Menopausal Symptoms

The estrogenic activity of hops in general, and 8PN in particular, has provided a focus for their possible use as a "natural" treatment for post-menopausal symptoms. The menopause is caused by the functional failure of the ovaries in women and is associated with a loss of fertility and a host of symptoms resulting from the sharp decline in circulating estrogen levels. The loss of estrogenic stimulation causes

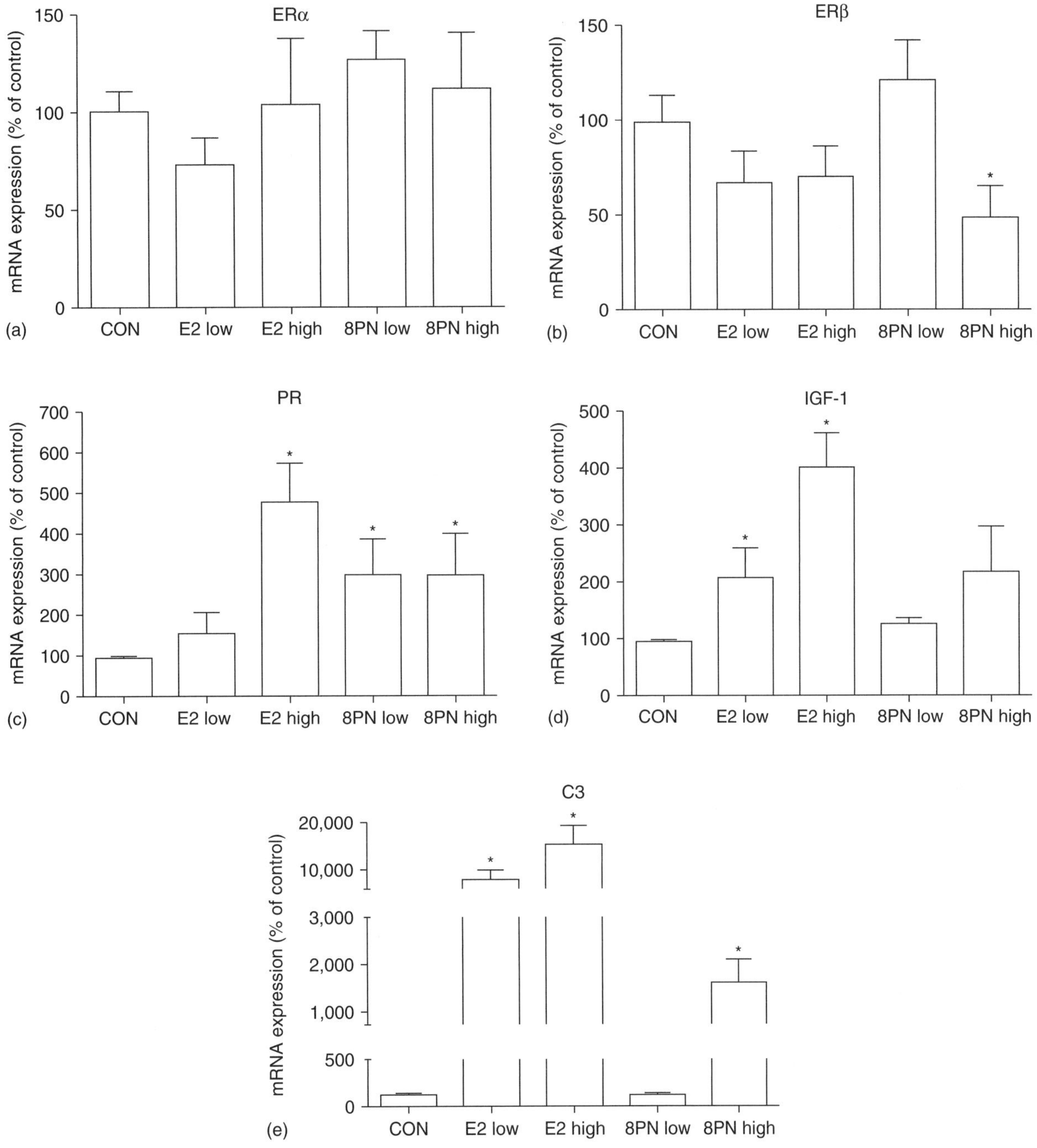

Figure 72.4 The effects of long-term 8PN exposure via the diet on gene expression in the uterus of ovariectomized rats. The effects of the two dietary doses (6.8 or 68 mg/kg body weight/day) of 17β-oestradiol (E2) and 8PN on uterine ERα (a), ERβ (b), PR (c), IGF-I (d) and complement protein C3 (e) gene expression. Significant effects of the high dose of 8PN were seen on ERβ, PR and C3, similar to those exerted by E2. *$p < 0.05$ vs. control. *Source*: From Christoffel *et al.* (2006). © Society for Endocrinology. Reproduced by permission.

the reproductive tract to atrophy; the vaginal wall thins and vaginal dryness, itching and painful intercourse are frequent complaints (Suckling *et al.*, 2006). The vaginal environment also becomes less acidic making it more susceptible to infection. The reduction in bone density leading to osteoporosis is a very serious effect of the withdrawal of estrogenic stimulation of bone. Other post-menopausal changes include an increase in cardiovascular disease, vasomotor changes (especially "hot flushes") and cognitive and psychological function (Morrison *et al.*, 2006). The seriousness and upsetting nature of these symptoms, coupled with the fact that more than a third of a woman's life in Western countries is post-menopausal, has led to the targeted treatment of the estrogen deficiency symptoms. Hormone replacement therapy with steroids is an extraordinarily effective treatment for osteoporosis and vasomotor problems, but may provide little protective effect against coronary heart disease and atherosclerosis (Lawlor and Smith, 2006). Recent large scale studies have also identified some risks of hormone replacement therapy to some women, highlighting adverse effects such as breast cancer, stroke and thromboembolism. These have raised concerns and anxiety amongst both patients and practitioners (Chen *et al.*, 2002; Rossouw, 2002; Rossouw *et al.*, 2002; ESHRE Capri Workshop Group, 2006). The recognition of these risks has reinforced the preference of many women to use so-called natural products as alternative therapies for menopausal symptoms, even though these natural products often have no proven effectiveness, contain uncontrolled constituents and may have had no critical safety evaluation. Indeed, there is little evidence from randomized controlled trials that soy protein and isolated isoflavones, or a number of other phyto-estrogen treatments (e.g. red clover, black cohosh), are effective at all (Shanafelt *et al.*, 2002; Krebs *et al.*, 2004).

The high estrogenic activity of hops (compared to many other plants) and 8PN (compared to other phyto-oestrogens) has led to the hope that these may offer better or alternative constituents for "natural" treatments for menopausal symptoms. This hope was reinforced by the report that 8PN may exert greater selectivity toward bone compared to the reproductive tract (Hümpel *et al.*, 2005), raising the possibility that 8PN could provide some of the advantages of estrogen-based hormone replacement therapy but with fewer of the disadvantages (Rad *et al.*, 2006). However, the reader is referred to the section above on "The Need for Caution in Considering the Reproductive Effects of 8PN" for a critical discussion of the interpretation of such results.

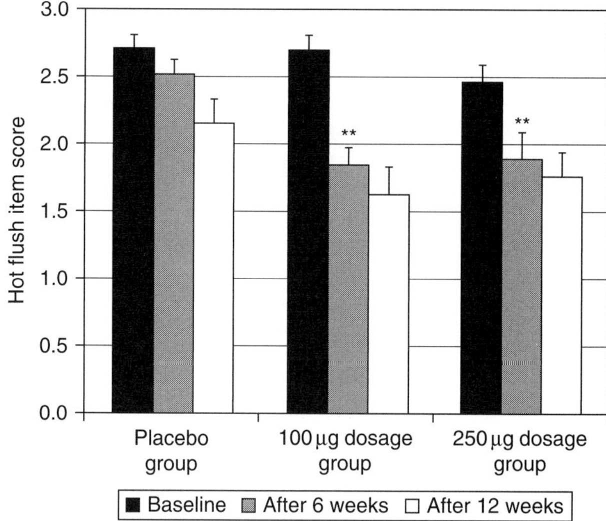

Figure 72.5 The effect of a hop extract containing standardized amounts of 8PN on hot flushes in menopausal women. The mean hot flush scores for the three groups of human subjects being given a hop extract containing either 100 or 200 µg 8PN. The scores are shown at the start of treatment (baseline), after 6 weeks, and after 12 weeks. The error bars represent SEM $^{**}p < 0.01$ as compared to placebo. *Source*: From Heyerick *et al.* (2006).

Hot flushes

The mechanisms underlying menopausal hot flushes are poorly understood, although it is generally assumed they result from disturbances in thermoregulatory control by the hypothalamus. Hot flushes are a distressing symptom of the menopausal syndrome, affecting over 75% of women, many of whom seek medical treatment (Shanafelt *et al.*, 2002). A number of treatments containing estrogenic isoflavones from soy or red clover have been marketed for treatment of hot flushes and a recent meta-analysis of the published studies found that such supplementation may produce a slight to modest benefit (Howes *et al.*, 2006), albeit with a strong placebo effect as well.

In an inadequately controlled study, a non-standardized hop extract was reported to reduce hot flashes in a small number (25) of menopausal women (Goetz, 1990). After 30 days of treatment with large doses of hops extract (1,600–2,600 mg/day), positive effects were reported. However, the study was not randomized, and the control group was apparently composed of five women who had been accidentally treated with a low dose of hops (300 mg), which (since it had no benefit) was considered a placebo. In 17 of the 20 treated subjects, the reduction of hot flush score was better than controls (but neither statistical test nor significance level was stated).

A more rigorous study (randomized, double blind, placebo-controlled) using a hop extract containing defined amounts of 8PN has been undertaken recently (Heyerick *et al.*, 2006). The results suggested that these hop extracts could produce positive benefits in alleviating the range of symptoms contributing to menopausal discomfort (as measured by the Kupperman index). The benefits were particularly evident for hot flushes (Figure 72.5), which were reduced by hop treatment. However, the ability to make firm conclusions is blurred by the known strong placebo effects of menopausal treatments. The potential for the use of 8PN for treating hot flushes is reinforced by the clear demonstration that 8PN reduces the raised skin temperatures in a well-defined experimental animal model of menopausal hot flushes (Bowe *et al.*, 2006) (Figure 72.6).

Vaginal treatment

The loss of estrogenic stimulation to the vagina post-menopausally results in a number of uncomfortable symptoms, as outlined above. These can be readily treated by local administration of oestrogens (e.g. via creams, pessaries, vaginal rings) usually without encountering the side effects and potential risks of systemic estrogen administration (Suckling *et al.*, 2006). There has been one report that good results

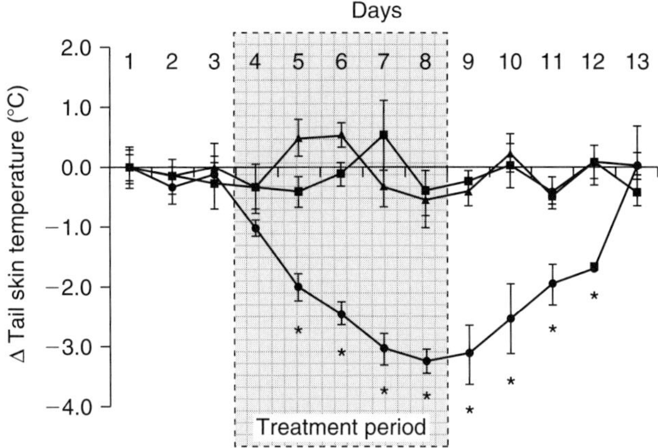

Figure 72.6 The effect of 8PN on tail temperature in an animal model of hot flushes. The effects of subcutaneous (sc) administration of 8PN; •400 μg/kg/day, 8PN and the anti-estrogen ICI 182,780 (▲; 400 μg/kg/day and 200 μg/kg/day, respectively) or peanut oil (■; 1 ml/kg) on tail skin temperature (TST) in the ovariectomized rat. The shaded area from day 4 to 8 indicates period during which treatment was given. The data show the mean changes in TST (±SEM) compared to the mean values on day 1 (ΔTST). Note that the elevation of temperature caused by ovariectomy (comparable to the hot flush phenomenon in postmenopausal women) is reversed by 8PN. Administration of ICI 182,780 completely blocked the effect of 8PN. *$p < 0.05$ vs. vehicle control on the same day; $n = 7$. *Source*: From Bowe *et al.* (2006). © Society for Endocrinology. Reproduced by permission.

can also be obtained using a vaginal gel containing hop extracts (Morali *et al.*, 2006). The gel contained hyaluronic acid, liposomes, hop extract and Vitamin E and the treatment was well accepted by one hundred post-menopausal women without any obvious adverse side effects. While this may raise hopes that 8PN *per se* may be similarly effective, the study of Morali *et al.* (2006) was not a double blind, placebo-controlled study, did not look at the efficacy of the individual constituents and there was no information provided about the amount of 8PN in the preparation.

Bone and osteoporosis

The control of bone deposition and resorption is complicated, and the reader is referred to other sources for more information on this (e.g. Raisz, 2005; Zallone, 2006). The important effects of oestrogens on bone are particularly clear in relation to the major biological transitions: the growth spurt at puberty and the reduction in bone density that occurs with ovarian failure in the perimenopausal period. These effects of estrogen stimulation and withdrawal are a consequence of reproductive events but are not strictly "reproductive effects" *per se* and are therefore beyond the scope of this chapter. However, in any context in which the risks or benefits of exposure to hop-derived oestrogens and 8PN are being considered, there is obviously a need to take bone effects into account.

As would be expected for an estrogenic compound, there is good evidence that 8PN can mimic oestradiol in terms of effects on bone (Miyamoto *et al.*, 1998). There is also evidence that other, less estrogenic, hop constituents (e.g. 6PN, xanthohumol, isoxanthohumol) can have similar effects on osteoblasts in culture (Effenberger *et al.*, 2005). The significance of understanding the role of oestrogens or phyto-estrogens in bone remodeling is complicated by the involvement of both estrogen receptors (ERα and ERβ) (Silvestri *et al.*, 2006). In view of the fact that one of the drives behind alternative therapies for menopausal symptoms is to find treatments that have selective beneficial effects on bone while reducing inappropriate risks in the reproductive tract and breast ("selective estrogen receptor modulators": SERMs), the findings of Hümpel *et al.* (2005) are of interest. These authors studied the effects of 8PN in the skeleton of female rats following ovariectomy, an animal model of osteoporosis. They found that injections of 8PN protected against the expected ovariectomy-induced bone loss, whilst exhibiting minimal trophic effects on the uterus. However, as already discussed, whether this apparent tissue selectivity is real, or whether it reflects their particular treatment regimen, needs reexamination.

8PN, Hops and Breast Tissue

The breast is an important target site for estrogen action, both in terms of stimulating normal growth and function, and in relation to breast cancer. The main drive to breast growth is the rising levels of circulating ovarian oestrogens at puberty. Local metabolism and synthesis of oestrogens are considered to be important in the pathogenesis and development of hormone-dependent breast cancer (Sasano *et al.*, 2006). The importance of oestrogens in breast cancer is the foundation of concerns about inappropriate exposure of the breast to oestrogens derived from estrogen replacement therapy for menopausal symptoms. The essential role of oestrogens in hormone-dependent breast cancer has led to the use of anti-oestrogens (blocking estrogen action), SERMs and aromatase inhibitors (blocking local synthesis of oestrogens from circulating androgens) in treatment regimens.

As an estrogen-responsive organ, the breast is a potential target site of 8PN. Human breast cancer cells (MCF-7) form the basis of a number of *in vitro* estrogen bioassays and are responsive to 8PN (e.g. Rong *et al.*, 2001; Effenberger *et al.*, 2005; Matsumura *et al.*, 2005; Overk *et al.*, 2005). *In vivo*, Rimoldi *et al.* (2006) showed that 8PN given via the diet (~70 mg/Kg bw/day) stimulated a range of reproductive tissues (uterus, vagina) and the mammary gland in ovariectomized rats.

Hops have been incorporated into a number of herbal preparations that claim the ability to enlarge breasts in women. These have included a variety of imaginatively named products (e.g. Natural Push-Up, 2Enhance, Breast Success and Newbust, amongst many)! The website of one of these (Natural Push Up, 1999) reported that it was originally developed following reports that cows eating large amounts of brewing waste from "got enormous udders" and observations that women in a small Italian village drinking a local beer that had never been boiled developed "larger and good looking breast" [sic]. Claims for the effectiveness of such herbal breast enlargement preparations have been based partly on their phyto-estrogen content (although these are not necessarily from hops alone). The concentration of 8PN in one type of these breast-enhancing preparations containing hops was found to be ~11 μg/g, producing a daily intake of approximately 130 μg/day (Coldham and Sauer, 2001). This value is less than that found in a liter of some beers. However, the content of 8PN itself is not the only factor to be considered: other phyto-oestrogens may be present and other hop prenylflavonoids may be converted to 8PN by gut microflora (Possemiers *et al.*, 2005, 2006). Nevertheless, it should be noted that the same hops-containing supplement studied by Coldham and Sauer (2001) showed no evidence of estrogenic activity in mice following administration either in the feed or by subcutaneous injection of the extract.

The essential question is that, if breast enhancement products do provide 8PN (or other phyto-oestrogens), are such products either effective or safe (Milligan, 2002)? In terms of efficacy, no peer-reviewed clinical trials appear to have been published. However, the concern would be that if any such effectiveness were to be shown, real fears over safety issues would then be raised. As noted above, the breast is an important site of hormone-dependent cancer and is very sensitive to oestrogens and inappropriate estrogenic stimulation would be of significant concern. In addition, estrogenic effects would be expected not to be limited to breast tissue alone; this is perhaps consistent with reports of menstrual disturbances associated with taking some of the supplements (see above). Any such disturbance of menstrual cyclicity would raise questions concerning effects on fertility as well as interactions with family planning/contraceptive methods. An additional concern would be that women may inadvertently take such breast enhancement products in the early stages of pregnancy, a time when fetal development is particularly susceptible to perturbations by xenobiotic chemicals (Milligan, 2002).

Are There Any Reproductive Effects of 8PN in Men?

For many years, oestrogens were considered to be primarily "female" hormones, contributing to female health and fertility. However, it is now clear that oestrogens play a variety of important roles in males, including modulating sexual development, the function of the testis, epididymis, brain and bone (Korach *et al.*, 1996; Hess *et al.*, 1997; Luconi *et al.*, 2002). In view of these roles of endogenous oestrogens, the question arises whether exposure to exogenous environmental or phyto-oestrogens can interfere or modulate estrogen-dependent processes within the body or contribute to the testicular dysgenesis syndrome described earlier (e.g. Skakkebaek *et al.*, 2001; Sharpe and Irvine, 2004). However, there have been no published reports of any effects of either 8PN or hop exposure either in this context or on the fertility and reproductive function of men. Neither are there any documented cases of gynecomastia directly attributable to hop exposure.

Injections of 8PN in mice induce estrogenic responses in the prostate (Hümpel *et al.*, 2005) indicating that this organ is a potential target site in males. While it has been suggested that phyto-oestrogens may offer a protective effect against prostate cancer (Hedelin *et al.*, 2006), there is no epidemiological information available about any association between this condition and exposure to hops. A variety of prenylflavonoids, including 8PN, showed anti-proliferative activity in prostate cancer cells lines, although the effective concentration required for 8PN was high (IC50 ~ 35–40 μM) (Delmulle *et al.*, 2006).

Based on anecdotal observations that many male hop workers seemed to have a preponderance of daughters, a question has been raised concerning whether the expected ~ 50:50 male:female sex ratio of offspring could be affected by exposure to the estrogenic activity of hops (Dr P. Darby, personal communication). There is certainly considerable general academic interest in the control of the sex ratios in a variety of mammalian species, and there is one report of an abnormal sex ratio in a human population possibly associated with pollutant exposure (Mackenzie *et al.*, 2005). However, even if a skewed sex ratio did exist in the offspring of male hop workers, any attribution as to its origin (hops, pesticides, solvents, etc.) would have to remain entirely speculative.

In vitro experimental studies have shown that 8PN can directly affect the function of sperm. A number of reports that spermatozoa may have binding sites or receptors for oestrogens (e.g. Misao *et al.*, 1997; Durkee *et al.*, 1998) and "non-genomic" effects of oestrogens have been reported (Luconi *et al.*, 1999, 2001). Whether such estrogen binding sites play any functional role in the fertilizing ability of sperm was recently investigated by Fraser *et al.* (2006). At the time of ejaculation, spermatozoa are unable to fertilize an egg (Yanagimachi, 1994) but after some time in an appropriate environment, spermatozoa acquire the capacity to fertilize and are said to be "capacitated" (Chang, 1951; Austin, 1952). Capacitated spermatozoa show hyperactivated motility, can undergo the acrosome reaction (involving the release of enzymes essential for egg penetration) and are able to fertilize an oocyte (Yanagimachi, 1994). Using mouse sperm, Fraser *et al.* (2006) found that oestradiol, two phyto-oestrogens (genistein and 8PN) and nonylphenol (a weakly active environmental estrogen) were all able to significantly stimulate mammalian sperm capacitation, acrosome reaction and fertilizing ability *in vitro*. Interestingly, the two phyto-oestrogens were effective at very low concentrations (1 nM) and were more potent than oestradiol itself. The mechanism(s) mediating such an effect remains unclear and, in the absence of any evidence that male fertility is directly affected *in vivo* by the acute exposure to such xenobiotic compounds, these observations may more reflect our ignorance of normal sperm physiology than imply any *in vivo* effect.

Conclusion

As an estrogenic chemical, 8PN has the potential to interact with the estrogen-signaling systems within the body. Therefore, demonstrations that experimentally administered 8PN can modulate responses in the reproductive tract, breast, bone or any other tissue is not surprising. However, there are two key questions. Firstly, is there any evidence that *normal* exposures to 8PN (either from hops, beer or other hop products) can have effects? Secondly, can the effects of 8PN be exploited for useful treatment of medical conditions in humans?

In terms of normal exposures, only those situations in which there is a large scale exposure to "raw" hops (e.g. hop workers) seem to be of significance, with disturbances to menstrual cycles being the most likely possible effect. There is no evidence, nor reason to suspect, that exposure to 8PN via the most common hop product, namely beer, is of any adverse significance. Any feminization effects of excessive drinking (e.g. in male alcoholics) is due to the effects of alcohol on the liver and steroid metabolism, rather than any hop-derived chemical.

In terms of the potential exploitation of the estrogenic activity of 8PN for use in human treatment, menopausal symptoms seem to offer some promise as a target. Treatment with a weak "natural" estrogen seems to be readily acceptable to many women and uncertainties about efficacy may be masked by strong placebo effects, at least for symptoms like hot flushes. Indeed, the relative weakness of the estrogenic activity of 8PN compared to pharmacological estrogen preparations may be of advantage in that this also minimizes the risks to hormone-dependent cancer. The administration of formulations locally (e.g. intravaginal: Morali *et al.*, 2006; Suckling *et al.*, 2006) may also be particularly useful in avoiding systemic risks. However, as treatments for menopausal symptoms typically tend to involve continuous or long-term exposure regimens to otherwise healthy women, all treatments need careful monitoring in terms of both safety and efficacy, not least because other (non-estrogenic) bioactivities of 8PN and associated hop-derived compounds need to be considered.

Summary Points

- 8PN is a phyto-estrogen with the potential to effect estrogenic responses in human reproductive tissues.
- As a weak estrogen (albeit relatively potent when compared to other, even weaker, phyto-oestrogens), the *in vivo* activity of 8PN is poorly understood.
- It is conceivable that the disturbances to menstrual cyclicity historically reported in hop workers was due to 8PN.
- There is no indication that exposure to 8PN in either hops or beer has any reproductive effect in men.
- The desire for exploitation of 8PN as a "natural" estrogen for the treatment on menopausal symptoms needs to be tempered with caution until clinical trials have justified its efficacy and confirmed its safety.

References

Adlercreutz, H. (1990). *Scand. J. Clin. Lab. Invest. Suppl.* 201, 3–23.

Austin, C.R. (1952). *Nature* 170, 326.

Bovee, T.F., Helsdingen, R.J., Rietjens, I.M., Keijer, J. and Hoogenboom, R.L. (2004). *J. Steroid. Biochem. Mol. Biol.* 91, 99–109.

Bowe, J., Li, X.F., Kinsey-Jones, J., Heyerick, A., Brain, S., Milligan, S. and O'Byrne, K. (2006). *J. Endocrinol.* 191, 399–405.

Bryant, M., Cassidy, A., Hill, C., Powell, J., Talbot, D. and Dye, L. (2005). *Br. J. Nutr.* 93, 731–739.

Cassidy, A. and Hooper, L. (2006). *J. Br. Menopause Soc.* 12, 49–56.

Chadwick, L.R., Nikolic, D., Burdette, J.E., Overk, C.R., Bolton, J.L., van Breemen, R.B., Frohlich, R., Fong, H.H., Farnsworth, N.R. and Pauli, G.F. (2004). *J. Nat. Prod.* 67, 2024–2032.

Chadwick, L.R., Pauli, G.F. and Farnsworth, N.R. (2006). *Phytomedicine* 13, 119–131.

Chen, C.L., Weiss, N.S., Newcomb, P., Barlow, W. and White, E. (2002). *JAMA* 287, 734–741.

Change, M.C. (1951). *Fertil. Steril.* 2, 205–222.

Christoffel, J., Rimoldi, G. and Wuttke, W. (2006). *J. Endocrinol.* 188, 397–405.

Chury, J. (1960). *Experientia* 16, 194–195.

Ciana, P., Scarlatti, F., Biserni, A., Ottobrini, L., Brena, A., Lana, A., Zagari, F., Lucignani, G. and Maggi, A. (2006). *Maturitas* 54, 315–320.

Coldham, N.G. and Sauer, M.J. (2001). *Food Chem. Toxicol.* 39, 1211–1224.

Crews, D. and McLachlan, J.A. (2006). *Endocrinology* 147, S4–S10.

Delmulle, L., Bellahcene, A., Dhooge, W., Comhaire, F., Roelens, F., Huvaere, K., Heyerick, A., Castronovo, V. and De Keukeleire, D. (2006). *Phytomedicine* 13, 732–734.

Dixon, R.A. (2004). *Annu. Rev. Plant Biol.* 55, 225–261.

Durkee, T.J., Mueller, M. and Zinaman, M. (1998). *Am. J. Obstet. Gynecol.* 178, 1288–1297.

Effenberger, K.E., Johnsen, S.A., Monroe, D.G., Spelsberg, T.C. and Westendorf, J.J. (2005). *J. Steroid. Biochem. Mol. Biol.* 96, 387–399.

ESHRE Capri Workshop Group (2006). *Hum. Reprod.* 12, 483–497.

Fenselau, C. and Talalay, P. (1973). *Food Cosmet. Toxicol.* 11, 597–603.

Fraser, L.R., Beyret, E., Milligan, S.R. and Adeoya-Osiguwa, S.A. (2006). *Hum. Reprod.* 21, 1184–1193.

Gehm, B.D., McAndrews, J.M., Chien, P.Y. and Jameson, J.L. (1997). *Proc. Natl. Acad. Sci. USA* 94, 14138–14143.

Gerhauser, C. (2005). *Eur. J. Cancer* 41, 1941–1954.

Goetz, P. (1990). *Revue de Phytothérapie Pratique* 4, 13–15.

Hansel, R.V. and Schulz, J. (1988). *Arch. Pharm. Weinheim.* 321, 37–40.

Hedelin, M., Balter, K.A., Chang, E.T., Bellocco, R., Klint, A., Johansson, J.E., Wiklund, F., Thellenberg-Karlsson, C., Adami, H.O. and Gronberg, H. (2006). *Prostate* 66, 1512–1520.

Hess, R.A., Bunick, D., Lee, K-H., Bahr, J., Taylor, J.A., Korach, K.S. and Lubahn, D.B. (1997). *Nature* 390, 509–511.

Hesse, R., Hoffman, B., Karg, H. and Vogt, K. (1981). *Zentralblatt fur Veterinärmedizin* 28, 422–454.

Heyerick, A., Vervarcke, S., Depypere, H., Bracke, M. and De Keukeleire, D. (2006). *Maturitas* 54, 164–175.

Howes, L.G., Howes, J.B. and Knight, D.C. (2006). *Maturitas* 55, 203–211.

Hümpel, M., Isaksson, P., Schaefer, O., Kaufmann, U., Ciana, P., Maggi, A. and Schleuning, W.D. (2005). *J. Steroid. Biochem. Mol. Biol.* 97, 299–305.

Koch, W. and Heim, G. (1953). *Brauwiss* 8, 132–133.

Korach, K.S., Couse, J.F., Curtis, S.W., Washburn, T.F., Lindzey, J., Kimbro, K.S., Eddy, E.M., Migliaccio, S., Snedeker, S.M. and Lubahn, D.B. (1996). *Recent Prog. Horm. Res.* 51, 59–186.

Krebs, E.E., Ensrud, K.E., MacDonald, R. and Wilt, T.J. (2004). *Obstet. Gynecol.* 104, 824–836.

Kuiper, G.G.J.M., Carlsson, B., Grandien, K., Enmark, E., Haggblad, J., Nilsson, S. and Gustafsson, J.A. (1997). *Endocrinology* 138, 863–870.

Kurzer, M.S. (2002). *J. Nutr.* 132, 570S–573S.

Lawlor, D.A. and Smith, G.D. (2006). *Curr. Opin. Obstet. Gynecol.* 18, 658–665.

Lee, N. (2006). *J. AOAC Int.* 89, 1135–1137.

Luconi, M., Bonaccorsi, M., Forti, G. and Baldi, E. (2001). *Mol. Cell. Endocrinol.* 178, 39–45.

Luconi, M., Forti, F. and Baldi, E. (2002). *J. Ster. Biochem. Mol. Biol.* 80, 369–381.

Luconi, M., Muratori, M., Forti, G. and Baldi, E. (1999). *J. Clin. Endocrinol. Metab.* 84, 1670–1678.

Mackenzie, C.A., Lockridge, A. and Keith, M. (2005). *Environ. Health Perspect.* 113, 1295–1298.

Martin, L., Pollard, J.W. and Fagg, B. (1976). *J. Endocrinol.* 69, 103–115.

Matsumura, A., Ghosh, A., Pope, G.S. and Darbre, P.D. (2005). *J. Steroid. Biochem. Mol. Biol.* 94, 431–443.

Messina, M., McCaskill-Stevens, W. and Lampe, J.W. (2006). *J. Natl. Cancer Inst.* 98, 1275–1284.

Meyer, O., Muller, J., Rajpert-De Meyts, E., Scheike, T., Sharpe, R., Sumpter, J. and Skakkebaek, N.E. (1996). *Environ. Health Perspect.* 104, 741–803.

Miksicek, R.J. (1993). *Mol. Pharmacol.* 44, 37–43.

Milligan, S.R., Kalita, J.C., Heyerick, A., Rong, H., De Cooman, L. and De Keukeleire, D. (1999). *J. Clin. Endocrinol. Metab.* 83, 2249–2252.

Milligan, S.R., Kalita, J.C., Pocock, V., Van de Kauter, V., Stevens, J.F., Deinzer, M.L., Rong, H. and De Keukeleire, D. (2000). *J. Clin. Endocrinol. Metab.* 85, 4912–4915.

Milligan, S.R., Kalita, J.C., Pocock, V., Heyerick, A., De Cooman, L., Rong, H. and De Keukeleire, D. (2002). *Reproduction* 123, 235–242.

Milligan, S.R. (2002). *Alternative Therapies in Womens' Health* 4, 44–47.

Misao, R., Niwa, K., Morishita, S., Fujimoto, J., Nakanishi, Y. and Tamaya, T. (1997). *Int. J. Fertil.* 42, 421–425.

Miyamoto, M., Matsushita, Y., Kiyokawa, A., Fukuda, C., Iijima, Y., Sugano, M. and Akiyama, T. (1998). *Planta Med.* 64, 516–519.

Monteiro, R., Becker, H., Azevedo, I. and Calhau, C. (2006). *J. Agric. Food Chem.* 54, 2938–2943.

Morali, G., Polatti, F., Metelitsa, E.N., Mascarucci, P., Magnani, P. and Marre, G.B. (2006). *Arzneimittelforschung.* 56, 230–238.

Morrison, J.H., Brinton, R.D., Schmidt, P.J. and Gore, A.C. (2006). *J. Neurosci.* 26, 10332–10348.

Nastainczyk, W. (1972). Ph.D. Thesis, University of Saarbrucken, Germany.

National Toxicology Program Center For The Evaluation Of Risks To Human Reproduction (2006). http://cerhr.niehs.nih.gov/chemicals/genistein-soy/SoyMeeting%20Summary.pdf (accessed November 16, 2006).

Natural Push Up (1999). http://pmcint.com/npu.htm (accessed June 07, 1999).

Nedrow, A., Miller, J., Walker, M., Nygren, P., Huffman, L.H. and Nelson, H.D. (2006). *Arch. Intern. Med.* 166, 1453–1465.

Neve, R.A. (1991). Hops. London, Chapman & Hall.

Nikolic, D., Li, Y., Chadwick, L.R., Grubjesic, S., Schwab, P., Metz, P. and van Breemen, R.B. (2004). *Drug Metab. Dispos.* 32, 272–279.

Overk, C.R., Yao, P., Chadwick, L.R., Nikolic, D., Sun, Y., Cuendet, M.A., Deng, Y., Hedayat, A.S., Pauli, G.F., Farnsworth, N.R., van Breemen, R.B. and Bolton, J.L. (2005). *J. Agric. Food Chem.* 53, 6246–6253.

Possemiers, S., Heyerick, A., Robbens, V., De Keukeleire, D. and Verstraete, W. (2005). *J. Agric. Food Chem.* 53, 6281–6288.

Possemiers, S., Bolca, S., Grootaert, C., Heyerick, A., Decroos, K., Dhooge, W., De Keukeleire, D., Rabot, S., Verstraete, W. and Van de Wiele, T. (2006). *J. Nutr.* 136, 1862–1867.

Rad, M., Hümpel, M., Schaefer, O., Schoemaker, R.C., Schleuning, W.-D., Cohen, A.F. and Burggraaf, J. (2006). *Br. J. Clin. Pharmacol.* 62, 288–296.

Raisz, L.G. (2005). *J. Clin. Invest.* 115, 3318–3325.

Rimoldi, G., Christoffel, J. and Wuttke, W. (2006). *Menopause* 13, 669–677.

Rong, H., Zhao, Y., Lazou, K., De Keukeleire, D., Milligan, S.R. and Sandra, P. (2000). *Chromatographia* 51, 545–552.

Rong, H., Boterberg, T., Maubach, J., Stove, C., Depypere, H., Van Slambrouck, S., Serreyn, R., De Keukeleire, D., Mareel, M. and Bracke, M. (2001). *Eur. J. Cell Biol.* 80, 580–585.

Rossouw, J.E. (2002). *J. Hyperten* 20, S62–S65.

Routledge, E.J. and Sumpter, J.P. (1996). *Environ. Toxicol. Chem.* 15, 241–258.

Rossouw, J.E., Anderson, G.L., Prentice, R.L., LaCroix, A.Z., Kooperberg, C., Stefanick, M.L., Jackson, R.D., Beresford, S.A., Howard, B.V., Johnson, K.C., Kotchen, J.M. and Ockene, J. (2002). *JAMA* 288, 321–333.

Sasano, H., Suzuki, T., Nakata, T. and Moriya, T. (2006). *Breast Cancer* 13, 129–136.

Schaefer, O., Bohlmann, R., Schleuning, W.D., Schulze-Forster, K. and Humpel, M. (2005). *J. Agric. Food Chem.* 53, 2881–2889.

Setchell, K.D. (1998). *Am. J. Clin. Nutr.* 68, 1333S–1346S.

Shanafelt, T.D., Barton, D.L., Adjei, A.A. and Loprinzi, C.L. (2002). *Mayo Clinic. Proc.* 77, 1207–1218.

Sharpe, R.M. (2001). *Toxicol. Lett.* 120, 221–232.

Sharpe, R.M. and Irvine, D.S. (2004). *BMJ* 328, 447–451.

Silvestri, S., Thomsen, A.B., Gozzini, A., Bagger, Y., Christiansen, C. and Brandi, M.L. (2006). *Menopause* 13, 451–461.

Skakkebaek, N.E., Rajpert-De Meyts, E. and Main, K.M. (2001). *Hum. Reprod.* 16, 972–978.

Stevens, J.F. and Page, J.E. (2004). *Phytochemistry* 65, 1317–1330.

Stevens, J.F., Taylor, A.W., Clawson, J.E. and Deinzer, M.L. (1999). *J. Agric. Food Chem.* 47, 2421–2428.

Stevens, J.F., Taylor, A.W., Nickerson, G.B., Ivancic, M., Henning, J., Haunold, A. and Deinzer, M.L. (2000). *Phytochemistry* 53, 759–775.

Suckling, J., Lethaby, A. and Kennedy, R. (2006). *Cochrane Database Syst Rev: CD001500.*

Sumpter, J.P. (1995). *Toxicol. Lett.* 82–83, 737–742.

Toppari, J., Larsen, J.C., Christiansen, P., Giwercman, A., Grandjean, P., Guillette Jr., L.J., Jegou, B., Jensen, T.K., Jouannet, P., Keiding, N., Leffers, H., McLachlan, J.A.,

Trisomboon, H., Malaivijitnond, S., Watanabe, G. and Taya, K. (2005). *Endocrine* 26, 33–39.

Verzele, M. (1986). *J. Inst. Brew.* 92, 32–48.

Xiao, C.W., Wood, C. and Gilani, S. (2006). *J. AOAC Int.* 89, 1207–1214.

Yanagimachi, R. (1994). In Knobil, E. and Neill, J.D. (eds), *The Physiology of Reproduction*, 2nd edn, pp. 189–317. Raven Press, New York.

Yang, C.Z. and Bittner, G.D. (2002). *Lab. Anim. (NY)* 31, 43–48.

Zacharewski, T. (1998). *Environ. Health Perspect.* 106, 577–582.

Zallone, A. (2006). *Ann. NY Acad. Sci.* 1068, 173–179.

Zenisek, A. and Bednar, I.J. (1960). *Am. Perfum. Arom.* 75, 61–62.

Zierau, O., Hauswald, S., Schwab, P., Metz, P. and Vollmer, G. (2004). *J. Steroid. Biochem. Mol. Biol.* 92, 107–110.

Zierau, O., Hamann, J., Tischer, S., Schwab, P., Metz, P., Vollmer, G., Gutzeit, H.O. and Scholz, S. (2005). *Biochem. Biophys. Res. Commun.* 326, 909–916.

73

Regulation of Gene Expression by Hop-Derived 8-Prenylnaringenin

Oliver Zierau and Günter Vollmer Molekulare Zellphysiologie und Endokrinologie, Institut für Zoologie, Technische Universität Dresden, Dresden, Germany

Abstract

Anecdotal stories, structural considerations and findings from *in vitro* assays suggested that 8-prenylnaringenin (8-PN) contained in the female hop (*Humulus lupulus* L.) flowers exhibits a strong estrogenic potency. Estrogens act through the two nuclear receptors estrogen receptor-α and -β (ER-α and -β). Hallmark of estrogen action in target cells or organs is regulation of gene expression. Here we first describe the experimental setup to test for estrogen dependent activation of gene expression *in vitro* and *in vivo*. With these assays we provide several pieces of evidence that 8-PN is a potent ligand for estrogen dependent gene regulation *in vitro* and *in vivo*, particularly on ER-α dependent processes. Based on findings *in vitro* by us and others human exposure to phytoestrogen levels contained in beer apparently does not pose a threat to human health. Whether or not 8-PN represents a natural compound which can be unrestrictedly recommended for pharmacological application particularly in menopausal applications remains to be further elucidated. However, based on the published *in vitro* and *in vivo* biological activities 8-PN has at least to be regarded as an interesting pharmacological lead compound.

List of Abbreviations

8-PN	8-prenylnaringenin
ER	Estrogen receptor
ER-α	Estrogen receptor-α
ER-β	Estrogen receptor-β
AP-1	Activator protein-1
NFκB	Nuclear factor kappa B
ERE	Estrogen responsive element
Nar	Naringenin
6-DMAN	6-Dimethylallylnaringenin
HT	Hormone therapy
PPAR	Peroxisome proliferators-activated receptor

Introduction

Identification of 8-prenylnaringenin

The main focus of this chapter is on putative hormonal activities of substances contained in hops. Since medieval times there are anecdotal stories which point to potential hormonal, particularly estrogenic activities of constituents of the female hop (*Humulus lupulus* L.) flowers. It was reported from Bohemia and Belgium that female hop pickers apparently did not become pregnant in the cropping season. When hops were hand picked, menstrual disturbances amongst women pickers were reportedly common (Verzele, 1986). Other stories followed up by Koch and Heim (1953), who were the first to describe hormonal activities for hops, tell the legend that women who normally live "a distance" from hop gardens regularly begin to menstruate 2 days after arrival to pick hops.

A series of applications published in the scientific literature comprise the use of brewery sludges as baths, cosmetic applications and applications in the folk medicine (for review see Chadwick *et al.*, 2006 and references therein).

The field went ahead when chemical structure of the estrogenic compounds in hops was solved by phytochemical means. Interestingly, almost at the same time the most potent chemical of hops was identified as 8-prenylnaringenin (8-PN) (Milligan *et al.*, 1999) and as isopentenylnaringenin from the Thai medicinal plant *Anaxagorea luzonensis* A. Gray (Annonaceae) (Kitaoka *et al.*, 1998). Soon after discovery it turned out that 8-PN represents the most potent phytoestrogen discovered so far with an IC_{50} value in the nanomolar range (Kitaoka *et al.*, 1998).

Exposure to 8-PN by consumption of beer

The anecdotal tales mentioned above suggest physiological, estrogen-like properties of 8-PN in humans. These

Beer in Health and Disease Prevention
ISBN: 978-0-12-373891-2

observations pose two important questions: (1) is 8-PN during the brewing process transferred into the beer? and (2) if so, what is the level of human exposure?

Analysis by different analytical protocols revealed that the quantities of 8-PN transferred to beer in the brewing process are low and sometimes undetectable. In selected Belgian beers and other beers of European origin levels between 5 and 20 μg/l were detected (Milligan *et al.*, 1999; Tekel *et al.*, 1999). The overall level apparently is dependent on the brand of beer and the respective brewing process. In this latter study 8-PN content of various North American brands and varieties was compared among each other with imported beers. Except for an American porter (240 μg/l) and a strong ale (110 μg/l) levels of 8-PN were far below 100 μg/l ranging between 1–69 μg/l (Stevens and Page, 2004) with the large majority of beer brands in the range of the Belgian study.

This means exposure by 8-PN through beer consumption is very low even in the beers with the highest content. However, depending on the type of beer isoxanthohumol levels are 5–30 times higher than those of 8-PN (Stevens and Page, 2004). Taking into consideration that isoxanthohumol is readily converted into 8-PN both *in vitro* and by the intestine (Possemiers *et al.*, 2005, 2006), exposure levels could be considerably higher. However, in a worst case consideration and according to the published literature a daily consumption of 1 l of beer by an 80 kg individual would amount to an exposure level of approximately 50 μg/mg/day.

Estrogen receptors

Estrogens and estrogen-like substances act through the two estrogen receptors (ER). Because of their hydrophobic character, estrogens like other steroid hormones are able to enter the cells by diffusion across the plasma membrane into the cell where they encounter their receptors.

Jensen first reported the existence of a protein that mediates the biological effects of estrogen in 1962 (Jensen, 1962). In 1986, two research groups reported the cloning of the first ER (Walter *et al.*, 1985; Greene *et al.*, 1986), which is now called estrogen receptor-α (ER-α). In 1996, a second ER, called estrogen receptor-β (ER-β), was cloned from rat (Kuipper *et al.*, 1996), mouse (Tremblay *et al.*, 1997) and human (Mosselman *et al.*, 1996).

The classical pathway for estrogen action involves the activation of the ERs as transcription factors (see Figure 73.1). After ligand binding, ERs undergo extensive conformational changes, which allow their dissociation from heat shock protein, and the homo- or heterodimerization of ERs (Pettersson and Gustafsson, 2001). Activated dimers diffuse into the nucleus and bind a specific DNA sequence named estrogen response element (ERE), which is located within the promoter region of estrogen target genes, and finally induce gene transcription (Klinge, 2000).

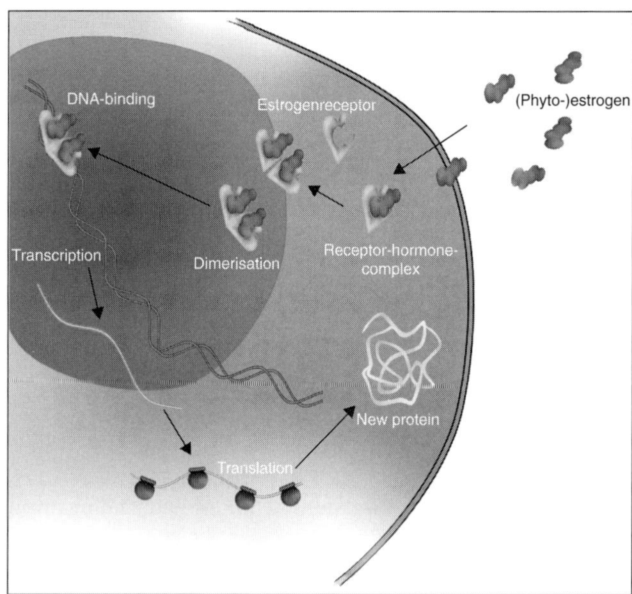

Figure 73.1 Estrogen action through nuclear ER. Estrogens function through genomic and non-genomic pathways. Shown is the "classical" genomic pathway of estrogen action.

Through its binding to ERE, the activated ER complex recruits co-regulators to the promoter through the concerted action of activation function domains. Activated ER complexes bind to the TATA box within the gene promoter, and trigger the expression of specific mRNAs and the subsequent production of proteins that are responsible for the effects of the ligand (Wolffe *et al.*, 1997).

Besides the direct binding of the ER-ligand complex to the ERE sequence, ER-α and -β can also modulate the expression of genes by a tethering mechanism thereby interacting indirectly with DNA. In this way, ER-α and -β act through binding to other DNA-bound transcription factors such as activator protein-1 (AP-1) transcription factors c-fos and c-jun (Paech *et al.*, 1997; Webb *et al.*, 1999), Sp1 (Porter *et al.*, 1997) or nuclear factor kappa B (Nilsson *et al.*, 2001). However, as a functional consequence ERs indirectly regulate the expression of a specific set of genes different from that regulated through ERE dependent mechanisms.

Finally, estrogens and estrogen-like substances act through membrane initiated signalling, also referred to as rapid action (Moriarty *et al.*, 2006). In a rough approximation two main pathways can be discriminated. The first involved recruitment of the nuclear ER to the membrane thereby activating various signal transduction cascades (Song and Santen, 2006), depending on the target cell. Second, the seven transmembrane G-protein coupled receptor GPCR30 for estrogens has been discovered (Rae and Johnson, 2005). Interaction between estrogens and their receptors depend on the number of receptors in the target tissue, the concentration of circulating estrogens and the affinity of estrogenic compounds to the ER. Generally speaking the affinity of hormone receptors does not change and thus the biological response depends on the number of receptors and the concentration of the estrogenic compounds.

Gene regulation as tool for the assessment of estrogenic activities

Estrogens like other steroid hormones and related molecules can directly regulate gene expression. This means that gene regulation has to be regarded as hallmark of estrogen action. Both *in vitro* and *in vivo* test systems use gene expression analysis as endpoint of estrogen action. This can be done on several levels of complexity.

For pure screening purposes and primary testing for estrogenicity very commonly so-called reporter gene assays are used. For this goal yeast (Routledge and Sumpter, 1996) or mammalian cells (Gagne *et al.*, 1994) are stably or transiently transfected with the respective ER and so-called reporter gene constructs. These reporter gene constructs represent artificial genes consisting either of an extended promoter region of estrogen responsive genes or of naked EREs in a tandem or triple arrangement. Either of these binding sites is capable to control the expression of an easily measurable reporter gene, for example β-galactosidase (Routledge and Sumpter, 1996) or luciferase (Demirpence *et al.*, 1993).

The next level of complexity comprises assays on regulation of endogenous gene expression in estrogen dependent cells in response to treatment with estrogenic compounds. In these assays total RNA, total protein or protein fractions are harvested and analyzed for altered expression levels of specific genes. The steady state mRNA-levels are measured by, for example, Realtime-rt-PCR and the alteration of protein levels by immunobiochemical means, for example Western blots (Strunck *et al.*, 2000).

The ultimate level of complexity is the uterotrophic assay in juvenile or adult ovariectomized rodents (Figure 73.2). The classical uterotrophic assay in ovariectomized rats involves castration, so-called ovariectomy, of animals, a period of hormonal decline of 7–10 days and a dose dependent treatment of animals for 3 days in comparison to a carrier treated negative control and a treatment with an appropriate positive control. Following ovariectomy and in response to the hormonal decline the uterus undergoes a reversible regression. If a test compound shows estrogenic activity, the weight loss by regression is counteracted depending on the potency of the estrogen and can be measured as uterine weight gain in comparison to untreated ovariectomized control animals (Owens and Ashby, 2002). The same holds true for the immature or juvenile rat uterotrophic assay, with the only difference, that there is no need of ovariectomy because the animals are not under the influence of endogenous estrogen production.

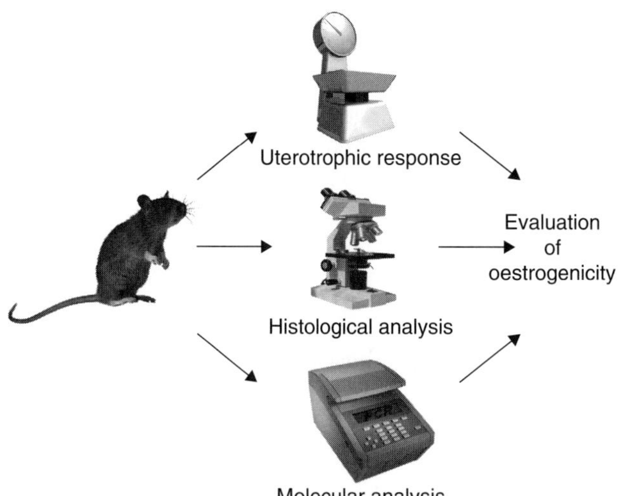

Figure 73.2 Work flow in the rodent uterotrophic assay. This assay is performed with castrated (ovariectomized) or juvenile female rats. In response to estradiol withdrawal by castration the uterus considerably regresses into an atrophic state. Starting from this situation estrogens reversibly stimulate uterine growth leading to a measurable uterine weight gain. To obtain a higher sensitivity and to assess organ specificity of estrogen action particularly by phytoestrogens, we and others have extended these assays to multiple organ systems and additionally assess histological and molecular endpoints of ER action.

This classical core uterotrophic assay can be modified in its duration (7 h to 3 month; Christoffel *et al.*, 2006) by the source of animals (e.g. transgenic knockout mice) (Hewitt *et al.*, 2003), by increasing the number of organs subjected to investigation (e.g. bone, capillary, pituitary gland and liver), and particularly by increasing the number of assessed morphologic and molecular endpoints (Diel *et al.*, 2002). Our group was one of the first research groups to use gene expression analysis for the assessment of estrogenicity (Diel *et al.*, 2000). This method is superior over others because it not only measures responsiveness but by the usage of pathway specific marker genes also provides clues toward the understanding mechanistic pathways in the hormonal response, for example discrimination between ERE dependent and ERE independent gene regulatory pathways.

Gene Regulation by 8-PN: A Comparative Assessment

Chemical access to test compounds

Although trivial to mention, prerequisite for the molecular characterization of a natural compound is availability of sufficient quantities of test substance. One way to overcome this hurdle is successful chemical synthesis of the compound. Starting from naringenin (Nar) Gester *et al.* were the first to describe a synthetic chemical approach yielding sufficient quantities of the racemic mixture of 8-PN for biological analysis (Gester *et al.*, 2001). The synthesis strategy consisted of a europium catalyzed Claisen rearrangement reaction yielding in addition to 8-PN significant quantities of 6-Dimethylallylnaringenin (6-DMAN). The latter also represents a natural compound found in the African tree *monotes engleri Gilg* (Seo *et al.*, 1997).

Reporter gene assays

With this tool in hand we could solve several questions: (1) to investigate the relative potency of 8-PN in comparison to estradiol and two structurally related compounds Nar and 6-DMAN (Figure 73.3). (2) To investigate potential preferences of 8-PN for one of the two ERs. Extensive investigations of other xenoestrogens showed that most of the phytoestrogens have a preference for the ER-β, whereas endocrine disruptors are more likely to act through the ER-α. (3) To investigate whether the compounds interact with other nuclear receptor systems and with the endogenous estrogen production.

Using two different reporter gene test system we could clearly confirm previous findings that 8-PN is the most potent ER-α agonist amongst the phytoestrogens known to date, although still some orders of magnitude less potent than estradiol (Table 73.1). In the comparative analysis, however, 8-PN was more potent in the yeast ER assay and in the MCF-7 cells stably transfected with a reporter gene consisting of the Vitellogenin-A2-promoter and the Luciferase reporter (MVLN) test than the parental compound Nar or the other substituted Nar 6-DMAN.

The ER-β activation by 8-PN points toward promoter and/or organ selectivity of the observed effects. Although the activation of ER-β systems requires higher doses of 8-PN, it is still capable to induce ER-β response. Interestingly, the ER-β effect appears to be dependent on the target cells and the promoter constructs used. In bone cells in combination with a reporter construct in consisting of a minimal promoter (ERE_2) and a reporter gene the overall activity picture for relative potencies of the three Nar

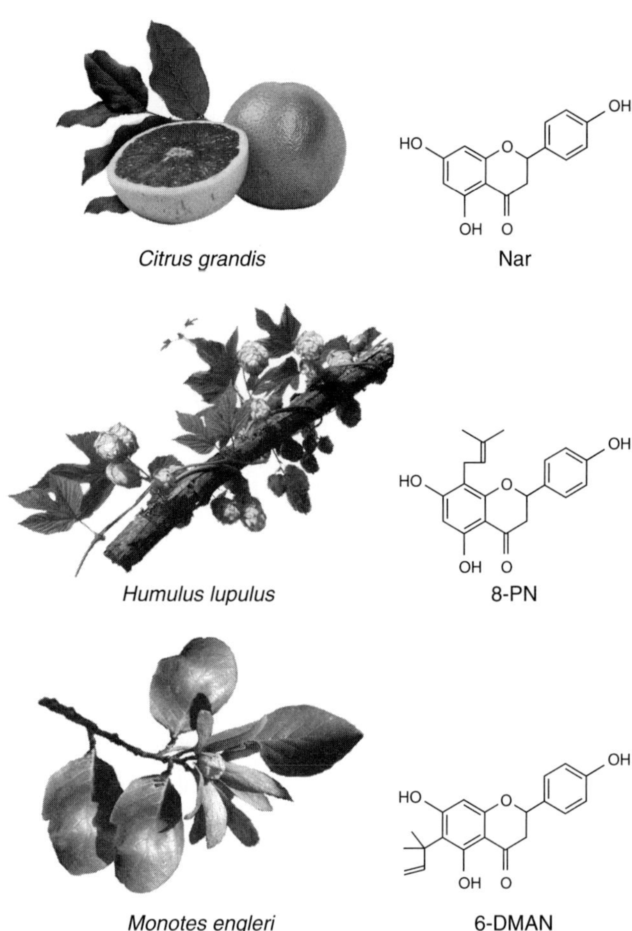

Figure 73.3 Natural occurring Nar. To date at least three Nar from natural sources are known. These comprise Nar from grapefruit (*Citrus grandis*), 8-PN from hops (*Humulus lupulus*) and 6-DMAN from the African tree *Monotes engleri*.

Table 73.1 Relative potency of 8-PN and other Nar in nuclear receptor assays

Test system	*Reference hormone*	*Biological effectiveness (sorted from weakest to strongest effect)*
Reporter gene assay ER-α		
Yeast estrogen receptor-α assay	Estradiol	Nar < 6-DMAN < 8-PN < E2
MVLN luciferase assay (ER-α)	Estradiol	Nar < 6-DMAN = 8-PN < E2
Reporter gene assay ER-β		
U2OS transfected by ER-β and (ERE)2-tk-Luc	Estradiol	Nar < 6-DMAN < 8-PN < E2
HEC-1B transfected by ER-β and mC3-tk-Luc	Estradiol	6-DMAN ≤ 8-PN < Nar < E2
Regulation of endogenous gene expression		
AP in endometrial Ishikawa cells (ER-α)	Estradiol	Nar < 6-DMAN < 8-PN < E2
pS2 and PR in MCF-7 cells	Estradiol	Nar < 6-DMAN = 8-PN < E2
Inhibition of yeast androgen receptor assay	Flutamide	Nar < 8-PN ≤ 6-DMAN < Flu

6-DMAN: 6-dimethylallylnaringenin; E2: estradiol; ER-α: estrogen receptor-α; ER-β: estrogen receptor-β; ERE: estrogen responsive element; Flu: Flutamide; Luc: Luciferase; mC3: murine complement C3 promoter; Nar: naringenin; 8-PN: 8-prenylnaringenin; tk: thymidine kinase.

compared is more or less the same as detectable for ER-α, however less potent (Table 73.1). The picture completely changes if the test is performed in HEC-1B human endometrial adenocarcinoma cells and a complex murine complement C3 promoter in front of the luciferase reporter. In this test system 8-PN is by far less effective than Nar or E2 (Table 73.1). These data are in line with a very recent data set on estrogenic activity following subtle side-chain modifications of the 8-position which resulted in very complex functional pattern of function ranging from a full ER-α agonist to pure antagonistic compounds (Roelens *et al.*, 2006).

Endogenous gene expression in target cells

To test for endogenous gene expression in a target cell requires that this particular target cell stably expresses at least one of the ERs and that genes, endogenously regulated by ER are known. For these kinds of assays we used two cell systems representing classical target organs for female sex steroids namely endometrial and breast tissue. We used the Ishikawa human endometrial adenocarcinoma cell line and human MCF-7 breast cancer cells which both endogenously express ER-α. Representing non-classical target organs we in addition investigated Fe33 rat hepatoma cells, which are stably transfected with the human ER-α and represent a liver model (Diel *et al.*, 1995).

A (semi)quantitative Realtime-rt-PCR of RNA from MCF-7 cells revealed that 8-PN potently stimulates increase of steady state mRNA-levels of the pS2 and the progesterone receptor gene (Figure 73.4; Table 73.2), although at 100-fold higher concentrations as estradiol. This effect was also observable for 6-DMAN (Table 73.1). Likewise both substituted Nar stimulated increase of alkaline phosphatase expression in Ishikawa cells, which was measured on the enzymatic activity level (Wober *et al.*, 2002). These findings clearly validate the findings from reporter gene assays in these more complex test systems (Table 73.2).

An important issue in all gene expression analyses is proof of the receptor mediation of the effect. For this purpose estrogenic effects are counteracted by co-incubation of cells

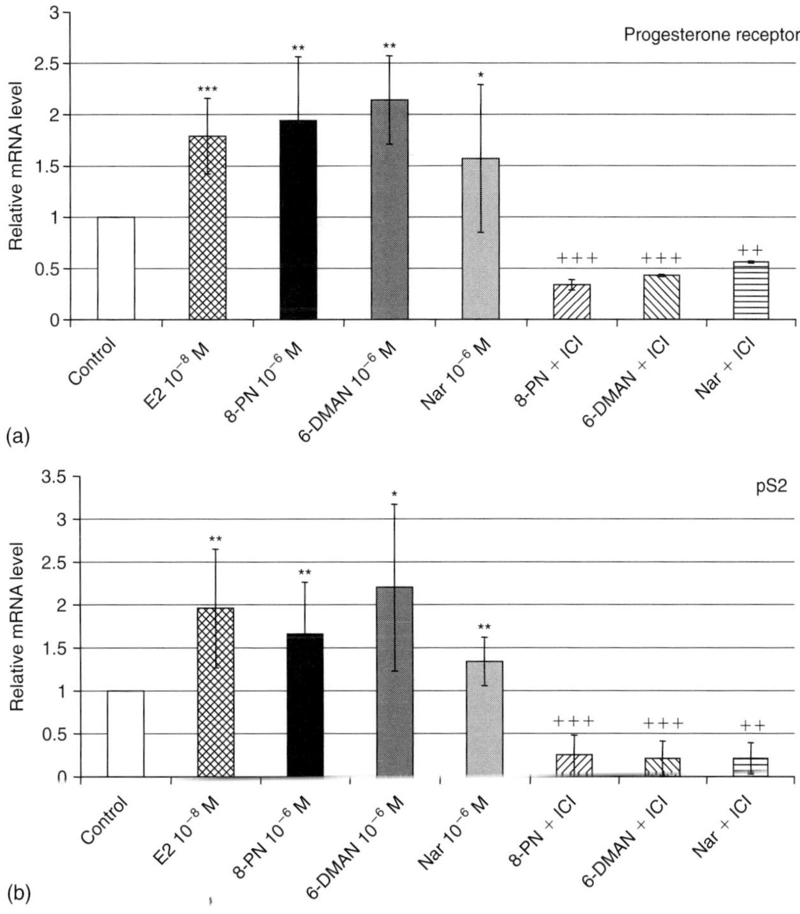

Figure 73.4 Comparative assessment of regulation of endogenous gene expression in MCF-7 breast cancer cells by 8-PN. This figure shows that 8-PN is capable to induce the estrogen dependent expression of the two marker genes progesterone receptor and pS2 in MCF-7 cells a well-known model cell line for breast tissue. The specificity of this effect is demonstrated by co-incubation of estrogens with the antiestrogen faslodex (ICI 182780) which inhibits estrogen induced gene regulation. E2: estradiol; 8-PN: 8-prenylnaringenin; 6-DMAN: 6-dimethylallylnaringenin; Nar: naringenin. Significance against untreated control $^{*}p < 0.05$, $^{**}p < 0.01$, $^{***}p < 0.001$; significance of ICI effects amongst treatment groups: $^{+}p < 0.05$, $^{++}p < 0.01$, $^{+++}p < 0.001$.

with an excess of a pure antiestrogen-like fulvestrant (ICI 182780) (Wakeling and Bowler, 1987, 1992). In all assays co-treatment of cells with an antiestrogen lead to inhibition of estrogen or 8-PN induced gene regulatory responses, as shown for pS2 and progesterone receptor up-regulation in MCF-7 cells (Figure 73.4).

Whereas the findings on regulation of endogenous gene expression in cells representing classical target organs are in line with those obtained in reporter gene assays, the results with hepatic cells deliver another picture. Whereas estradiol up-regulated all genes investigated, unlike in mammary gland derived and in endometrial cells 8-PN did not mimic this estrogenic response (Table 73.2). No effects of 8-PN following treatment of Fe33 cells were detectable for the expression of calcium binding protein 9 kD, apolipoprotein A1 and carbonic anhydrase II (Caldarelli *et al.*, 2005), whereas steady state mRNA-levels of insulin-like growth factor binding protein-1 were down-regulated by low doses of 8-PN and up-regulated by high doses of 8-PN. In summary, these findings provide another piece of evidence for an organ selective component of the bioactive function of the pure substance 8-PN.

While 8-PN clearly is estrogenic and activates preferentially ER-α it is questionable whether the estrogenic activity in beer, at least in part attributable to 8-PN, is sufficient to elicit estrogenic effects. One study directly addressed this question. One liter of various varieties of Austrian beers was extracted and the extract subjected to the yeast ER assay. The extracts were capable to induce the reporter gene activity, however, the highest activity corresponded to 43 ng of estradiol. From these low activities measured the authors concluded that there is no hazard for human health from drinking beer (Promberger *et al.*, 2001).

8-prenylnaringenins and other nuclear receptor systems

In other sets of experiments we addressed the question whether 8-PN is capable to induce other nuclear receptors. Some of the xenoestrogens described in the literature also interfere with the androgen receptor signalling pathway (Sohoni and Sumpter, 1998). However, none of the Nar was capable to induce an androgen receptor dependent reporter gene activity comparable to the positive control dihydrotestosterone. Conversely, both substituted Nar, unlike the parental compound Nar inhibited dihydrotestosterone induced reporter gene activity in a yeast androgen receptor assay (Table 73.1). Only for 6-DMAN but not for 8-PN this result could be confirmed in a second independent assay on androgen receptor dependent expression of prostate specific antigen (Zierau *et al.*, 2003).

Very important regarding regulation of general metabolism are "peroxisome proliferator-activated receptor" (PPAR), existing in the three subtypes α,γ,δ with activation of PPAR-γ leading to enhanced insulin sensitivity in type-II diabetes (Knouff and Auwerx, 2004). We tested whether Nar, particularly 8-PN activate PPAR-γ, but no activity was detectable.

In conclusion, these data show that 8-PN is a potent activator of ER-α with a preference for ER-α over ER-β, which is in line with data in the literature (Schaefer *et al.*, 2003). Further, there are first indications that the ER-β response may be tissue selective. Finally, prenylated Nar have also been regarded as week antiandrogens with 6-DMAN being superior over 8-PN regarding this activity.

Gene regulation by 8-PN *in vivo*

As mentioned above 8-PN is a potent *in vitro* activator of ER-α with a clear preference for ER-α over ER-β and therefore theoretically also qualifies for pharmacological application *in vivo*. The first important issue to be investigated *in vivo* is the proof of the principle of the biological activity determined *in vitro*. The *in vivo* effectiveness can be hampered for several reasons; most often this is caused by an insufficient bioavailability.

Phytochemicals, if ingested through an oral route first of all need to be taken up by the intestine and second are subject to massive bioconversion in the liver. Therefore, it is

Table 73.2 Regulation of endogenous gene expression by 8-PN

Cell line	*Target organ*	*Target gene*	*Estradiol*	*8-PN*
Ishikawa	Endometrium	Alkaline Phosphatase	↑↑	↑↑ (10^{-6}M)
MCF-7	Mammary gland	pS2	↑↑ (10^{-8}M)	↑↑ (10^{-6}M)
		Progesterone receptor	↑↑ (10^{-8}M)	↑↑ (10^{-6}M)
Fe33	Liver	Calcium binding protein 9 KD	↑↑↑ (10^{-8}M)	– (10^{-6}M)
		Insulin-like growth factor binding protein 1	↑↑(10^{-8}M)	↓ (10^{-8}M)/ – (10^{-7}M)/↑ (10^{-6}M)
		Apolipoprotein A1	↑↑ (10^{-8}M)	– (10^{-6}M)
		Carbonic anhydrase II	↑↑ (10^{-8}M)	– (10^{-6}M)

Note: In this table the relative potency of 8-PN in comparison to estradiol is shown for three independent cell culture systems representing three different target organs for estrogens. 8-PN: 8-prenylnaringenin.

important to test whether bioavailable levels of substance are sufficient to induce tissue specific responses. 8-PN for example has been shown to be readily taken up by intestinal mechanisms (Nikolic *et al.*, 2006) and to be subjected to phases I and II mechanisms in the liver (Nikolic *et al.*, 2006) which in other words means that its bioavailability should be reduced significantly by intestinal and hepatic metabolism (Nikolic *et al.*, 2004). On the other hand, two of the most abundant metabolites which are produced by liver microsomal preparations *in vitro*, namely (E)-8-(4″-hydroxyisopentenyl)naringenin and (E)-8-(4″-oxoiso pentenyl)naringenin are still quite potent estrogens on inducing reporter gene activation in transactivation assays (Zierau *et al.*, 2004).

As mentioned above, estrogenicity *in vivo* is primarily tested in the uterotrophic assay at pharmacological doses of the tested substance. In a first line of experiments a subcutaneous application route in ovariectomized rodents is taken to achieve significant exposure levels. Following proof of effectiveness usually a second animal study also in ovariectomized rats and mice is performed this time using an oral exposure route. The outcome of this assay shows whether bioavailability of the substance in question is sufficient to evoke responses even after passage of the substance through intestine and liver, including the enterohepatic circulation.

8-PN in a dosage of 10 mg/kg/day given subcutaneously for 3 days is clearly estrogenic *in vivo*. Like estradiol

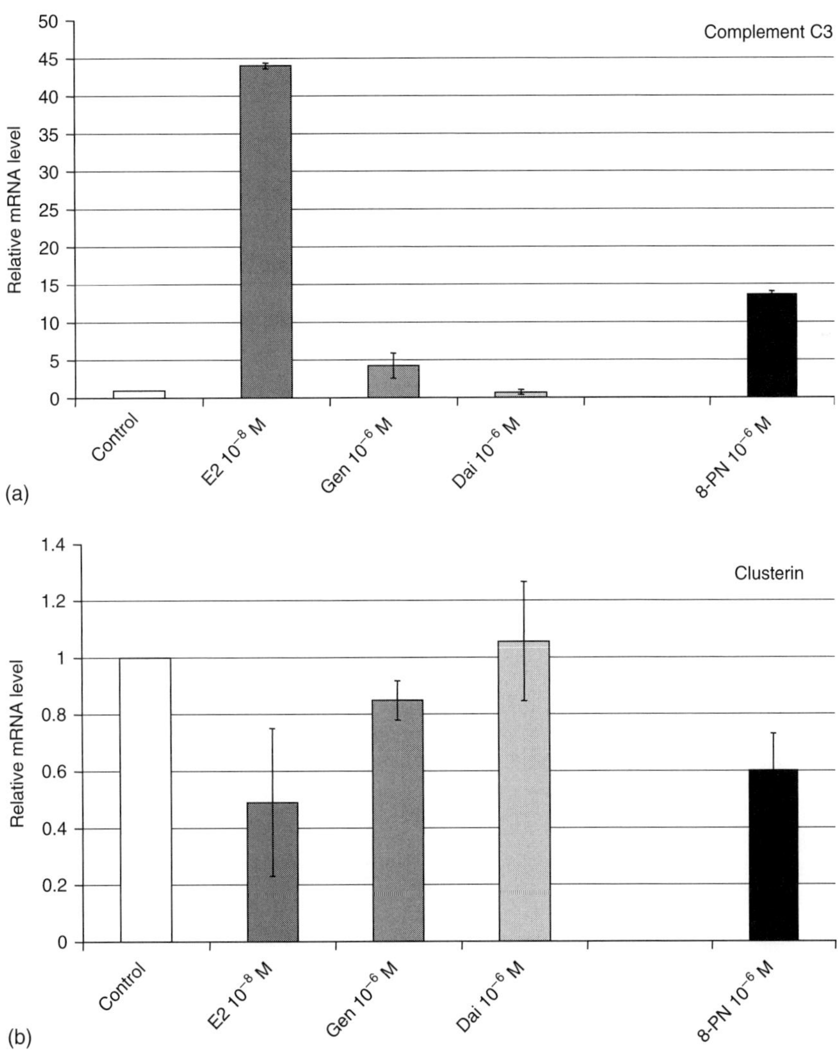

Figure 73.5 Regulation of uterine gene expression by 8-PN. Here the impact of 8-PN on the expression of rat uterine genes is shown. Complement C3 is up-regulated in response to estradiol (E2; 10 μg/kg/day), whereas clusterin is down-regulated. 8-PN mimics this pattern of regulation although at higher concentrations (10 mg/kg/day). However, its response is stronger than those observable for the isoflavones genistein (Gen) and daidzein (Dai), the latter being completely ineffective. Significance is not given because the results were obtained from two different experiments.

(10 μg/kg/day) 8-PN stimulates increase of uterine wet weight after 3 days of treatment (Diel *et al.*, 2004). In addition, it stimulates the modulation of estrogen responsive genes in the same way as estradiol, meaning, for example, stimulation of proliferation marker, up-regulation of complement C3 and down-regulation of clusterin (Figure 73.5). In a comparison to other phytoestrogens (e.g. genistein and daidzein), 8-PN could be shown to be a lot more potent (Diel *et al.*, 2004).

Menopausal applications of 8-PN

Due to its potent estrogenic profile it has been suggested to use hop extracts and/or 8-PN as an alternative for the classical hormone therapy (HT). HT is very effective in relieving climacteric complaints during postmenopause as well as preventing the long-term consequences of estrogen deficiency such as osteoporosis (Lindsay and Thome, 1990; Skafar *et al.*, 1997). HT replaces the female sex steroid estradiol alone or in combination with the other female sex steroid progestogen. Results from randomized controlled trials (Colditz *et al.*, 1995; Magnusson *et al.*, 1999; Schairer *et al.*, 2000; Beral *et al.*, 2002; Rossouw *et al.*, 2002; Beral, 2003; Chlebowski *et al.*, 2003) showed HT to be associated with an increased risk of endometrial cancer and venous thromboembolism (Ross *et al.*, 2000; Rosendaal *et al.*, 2002). In addition, if HT is started in perimenopause, the risk of developing breast cancer is increased (Aggarwal *et al.*, 2004). Thus, HT is not risk free, and since patients demand for alternative treatments that are free of the potential risks associated with HT, hops extracts and/or 8-PN have been proposed to represent such an alternative treatment regimen.

In perimenopause patients particularly suffer from hot flushes, insomnia and mood disorders. In a very recent animal study it was shown that 8-PN is capable to reverse estrogen deficiency – induce rise in skin temperature (Bowe *et al.*, 2006). Cessation of estrogen production in menopause in addition is accompanied by loss of bone mass and density. In a second study it was shown that 8-PN protects ovariectomized estrogen deficient rats from bone loss, with a minimal stimulation of the uterus (Humpel *et al.*, 2005). In a 3-month study with a threefold higher dose of 8-PN a clear estrogenic response in the uterus could be detected on the level of uterine weight gain and estrogen responsive uterine gene expression (Christoffel *et al.*, 2006). These physiological and molecular observations were further validated by histological means showing an unfavourable impact of 8-PN treatment on uterine and vaginal morphology (Rimoldi *et al.*, 2006).

In a pharmacokinetic study with postmenopausal women it was shown that single doses of up to 750 mg of 8-PN are well tolerated and exert systemic effects as measured by a decrease of luteinizing hormone serum concentrations (Rad *et al.*, 2006). While no further clinical studies have been conducted with pure 8-PN, there is a prospective randomized double blind placebo controlled study with an 8-PN enriched hop extract (MenoHop; 100 or 250 μg 8-PN). This trial showed favorable effects on vasomotor symptoms after 6 but not after 12 weeks of treatment and only for the low dose (Heyerick *et al.*, 2006). No dose response was detectable.

In summary, these data demonstrate that hop extracts and/or 8-PN are capable to alleviate menopausal complaint both in humans and animals. However, concerns come from studies on uterine effects, which clearly showed that 8-PN exerts the undesirable effect of uterine stimulation. One of the authors of the cited papers stated: *Human pharmacologic studies will show whether the stimulatory effect on the uterus that was found . . . . would require the concomitant administration of progestins to prevent endometrial overstimulation* (Christoffel *et al.*, 2006).

Summary Points

- 8-PN is the most potent phytoestrogen identified to date.
- 8-PN represents a highly efficient inductor of ER-α dependent reporter gene activity.
- Unlike other phytoestrogens 8-PN exhibits a clear preference for ER-α over ER-β, a rather unique feature for phytoestrogens.
- The prenylation of the 8-position appears to be particularly important for this feature since substitution of the 6-position also confers to a higher ER-β potency and to antiandrogenicity.
- 8-PN is a potent inducer of ER-α dependent gene regulation in cultured cells from classical target organs for female sex steroids (e.g. endometrium and mammary gland).
- The only cell system investigated so far in which 8-PN just induces a marginal response is a hepatic cell line. This is surprising since liver is believed to express ER-α only.
- 8-PN behaves as an ER-α agonist *in vivo* and induces ER-α dependent gene regulation in all target organs investigated.
- Overall, 8-PN and structural related derivatives represent highly interesting lead compounds for pharmacological applications, including the treatment of menopause associated problems.

References

Aggarwal, B.B., Bhardwaj, A., Aggarwal, R.S., Seeram, N.P., Shishodia, S. and Takada, Y. (2004). *Anticancer Res.* 24, 2783–2840.

Beral, V. (2003). *Lancet* 362, 419–427.

Beral, V., Banks, E. and Reeves, G. (2002). *Lancet* 360, 942–944.

Bowe, J., Li, X.F., Kinsey-Jones, J., Heyerick, A., Brain, S., Milligan, S. and O'Byrne, K. (2006). *J. Endocrinol.* 191, 399–405.

Caldarelli, A., Diel, P. and Vollmer, G. (2005). *J. Steroid Biochem. Mol. Biol.* 97, 251–256.

Chadwick, L.R., Pauli, G.F. and Farnsworth, N.R. (2006). *Phytomedicine* 13, 119–131.

Chlebowski, R.T., Hendrix, S.L., Langer, R.D., Stefanick, M.L., Gass, M., Lane, D., Rodabough, R.J., Gilligan, M.A., Cyr, M.G., Thomson, C.A., Khandekar, J., Petrovitch, H. and McTiernan, A. (2003). *JAMA* 289, 3243–3253.

Christoffel, J., Rimoldi, G. and Wuttke, W. (2006). *J. Endocrinol.* 188, 397–405.

Colditz, G.A., Hankinson, S.E., Hunter, D.J., Willett, W.C., Manson, J.E., Stampfer, M.J., Hennekens, C., Rosner, B. and Speizer, F.E. (1995). *New Engl. J. Med.* 332, 1589–1593.

Demirpence, E., Duchesne, M.J., Badia, E., Gagne, D. and Pons, M. (1993). *J. Steroid Biochem. Mol. Biol.* 46, 355–364.

Diel, P., Walter, A., Fritzemeier, K.H., Hegele-Hartung, C. and Knauthe, R. (1995). *J. Steroid Biochem. Mol. Biol.* 55, 363–373.

Diel, P., Schulz, T., Smolnikar, K., Strunck, E., Vollmer, G. and Michna, H. (2000). *J. Steroid Biochem. Mol. Biol.* 73, 1–10.

Diel, P., Schmidt, S. and Vollmer, G. (2002). *J. Chromatogr. B Analyt. Technol. Biomed. Life Sci.* 777, 191–202.

Diel, P., Thomae, R.B., Caldarelli, A., Zierau, O., Kolba, S., Schmidt, S., Schwab, P., Metz, P. and Vollmer, G. (2004). *Planta Med.* 70, 39–44.

Gagne, D., Balaguer, P., Demirpence, E., Chabret, C., Trousse, F., Nicolas, J.C. and Pons, M. (1994). *J. Biolumin. Chemilumin.* 9, 201–209.

Gester, S., Metz, P., Zierau, O. and Vollmer, G. (2001). *Tetrahedron* 57, 1015–1018.

Greene, G.L., Gilna, P., Waterfield, M., Baker, A., Hort, Y. and Shine, J. (1986). *Science* 231, 1150–1154.

Hewitt, S.C., Deroo, B.J., Hansen, K., Collins, J., Grissom, S., Afshari, C.A. and Korach, K.S. (2003). *Mol. Endocrinol.* 17, 2070–2083.

Heyerick, A., Vervarcke, S., Depypere, H., Bracke, M. and De Keukeleire, D. (2006). *Maturitas* 54, 164–175.

Humpel, M., Isaksson, P., Schaefer, O., Kaufmann, U., Ciana, P., Maggi, A. and Schleuning, W.D. (2005). *J. Steroid Biochem. Mol. Biol.* 97, 299–305.

Jensen, E.V. (1962). *Perspect. Biol. Med.* 6, 47–59.

Kitaoka, M., Kadokawa, H., Sugano, M., Ichikawa, K., Taki, M., Takaishi, S., Iijima, Y., Tsutsumi, S., Boriboon, M. and Akiyama, T. (1998). *Planta Med.* 64, 511–515.

Klinge, C.M. (2000). *Steroids* 65, 227–251.

Knouff, C. and Auwerx, J. (2004). *Endocr. Rev.* 25, 899–918.

Koch, W. and Heim, G. (1953). *Munch. Med. Wochenschr.* 95, 845.

Kuipper, G.G., Enmark, E., Pelto-Huikko, M., Nilsson, S. and Gustafsson, J.A. (1996). *Proc. Natl. Acad. Sci. USA* 93, 5925–5930.

Lindsay, R. and Thome, J.F. (1990). *Obstet. Gynecol.* 76, 290–295.

Magnusson, C., Baron, J.A., Correia, N., Bergstrom, R., Adami, H.O. and Persson, I. (1999). *Int. J. Cancer* 81, 339–344.

Milligan, S.R., Kalita, J.C., Heyerick, A., Rong, H., De Cooman, L. and De Keukeleire, D. (1999). *J. Clin. Endocrinol. Metab.* 84, 2249–2252.

Moriarty, K., Kim, K.H. and Bender, J.R. (2006). *Endocrinology* 147, 5557–5563.

Mosselman, S., Polman, J. and Dijkema, R. (1996). *FEBS Lett.* 392, 49–53.

Nikolic, D., Li, Y., Chadwick, L.R., Grubjesic, S., Schwab, P., Metz, P. and Van Breemen, R.B. (2004). *Drug Metab. Dispos.* 32, 272–279.

Nikolic, D., Li, Y., Chadwick, L.R. and Van Breemen, R.B. (2006). *Pharm. Res.* 23, 864–872.

Nilsson, S., Makela, S., Treuter, E., Tujague, M., Thomsen, J., Andersson, G., Enmark, E., Petterson, K., Warner, M. and Gustafsson, J.A. (2001). *Physiol. Rev.* 81, 1535–1565.

Owens, J.W. and Ashby, J. (2002). *Crit. Rev. Toxicol.* 32, 445–520.

Paech, K., Webb, P., Kuipper, G.G., Nilsson, S., Gustafsson, J., Kushner, P.J. and Scanlan, T.S. (1997). *Science* 277, 1508–1510.

Pettersson, K. and Gustafsson, J.A. (2001). *Annu. Rev. Physiol.* 63, 165–192.

Porter, W., Saville, B., Hoivik, D. and Safe, S. (1997). *Mol. Endocrinol.* 11, 1569–1580.

Possemiers, S., Heyerick, A., Robbens, V., De Keukeleire, D. and Verstraete, W. (2005). *J. Agric. Food Chem.* 53, 6281–6288.

Possemiers, S., Bolca, S., Grootaert, C., Heyerick, A., Decroos, K., Dhooge, W., De Keukeleire, D., Rabot, S., Verstraete, W. and Van De Wiele, T. (2006). *J. Nutr.* 136, 1862–1867.

Promberger, A., Dornstauder, E., Fruhwirth, C., Schmid, E.R. and Jungbauer, A. (2001). *J. Agric. Food Chem.* 49, 633–640.

Rad, M., Humpel, M., Schaefer, O., Schoemaker, R.C., Schleuning, W.D., Cohen, A.F. and Burggraaf, J. (2006). *Br. J. Clin. Pharmacol.* 62, 288–296.

Rae, J.M. and Johnson, M.D. (2005). *Breast Cancer Res.* 7, 243–244.

Rimoldi, G., Christoffel, J. and Wuttke, W. (2006). *Menopause* 13, 669–677.

Roelens, F., Heldering, N., Dhooge, W., Bengtsson, M., Comhaire, F., Gustafsson, J.A., Treuter, E. and De Keukeleire, D. (2006). *J. Med. Chem.* 49, 7357–7365.

Rosendaal, F.R., Helmerhorst, F.M. and Vandenbroucke, J.P. (2002). *Arterioscler. Thromb. Vasc. Biol.* 22, 201–210.

Ross, R.K., Paganini-Hill, A., Wan, P.C. and Pike, M.C. (2000). *J. Natl. Cancer Inst.* 92, 328–332.

Rossouw, J.E., Anderson, G.L., Prentice, R.L., Lacroix, A.Z., Koopenberg, C., Stefanick, M.L., Jackson, R.D., Beresford, S.A., Howard, B.V., Johnson, K.C., Kotchen, J.M. and Ockene, J. (2002). *JAMA* 288, 321–333.

Routledge, E. and Sumpter, J.P. (1996). *Environ. Toxicol. Chem.* 15, 241–248.

Schaefer, O., Humpel, M., Fritzemeier, K.H., Bohlmann, R. and Schleuning, W.D. (2003). *J. Steroid Biochem. Mol. Biol.* 84, 359–360.

Schairer, C., Lubin, J., Troisi, R., Sturgeon, S., Brinton, L. and Hoover, R. (2000). *JAMA* 283, 485–491.

Seo, E.K., Silva, G.L., Chai, H.B., Chagwedera, T.E., Farnsworth, N.R., Cordell, G.A., Pezzuto, J.M. and Kinghorn, A.D. (1997). *Phytochemistry* 45, 509–515.

Skafar, D.F., Xu, R., Morales, J., Ram, J. and Sowers, J.R. (1997). *J. Clin. Endocrinol. Metab.* 82, 3913–3918.

Sohoni, P. and Sumpter, J.P. (1998). *J. Endocrinol.* 158, 327–339.

Song, R.X. and Santen, R.J. (2006). *Biol. Reprod.* 75, 9–16.

Stevens, J.F. and Page, J.E. (2004). *Phytochemistry* 65, 1317–1330.

Strunck, E., Stemmann, N., Hopert, A., Wunsche, W., Frank, K. and Vollmer, G. (2000). *J. Steroid Biochem. Mol. Biol.* 74, 73–81.

Tekel, J., De Keukeleire, D., Rong, H., Daesleire, E. and Van Peteghem, C. (1999). *J. Agric. Food Chem.* 47, 5059–5063.

Tremblay, G.B., Tremblay, A., Copeland, N.G., Gilbert, D.J., Jenkins, N.A., Labrie, F. and Giguere, V. (1997). *Mol. Endocrinol.* 11, 353–365.

Verzele, M. (1986). *J. Inst. Brew.* 92, 32–48.

Wakeling, A.E. and Bowler, J. (1987). *J. Endocrinol.* 112, R7–R10.

Wakeling, A.E. and Bowler, J. (1992). *J. Steroid Biochem. Mol. Biol.* 43, 173–177.

Walter, P., Green, S., Greene, G., Krust, A., Bornert, J.M., Jeltsch, J.M., Staub, A., Jensen, E., Scrace, G., Waterfield, M., *et al.* (1985). *Proc. Natl. Acad. Sci. USA* 82, 7889–7893.

Webb, P., Nguyen, P., Valentine, C., Lopez, G.N., Kwok, G. R., McInerney, E., Katzenellenbogen, B.S., Enmark, E., Gustaffson, J.A., Nilsson, S. and Kushner, P.J. (1999). *Mol. Endocrinol.* 13, 1672–1685.

Wober, J., Weiswange, I. and Vollmer, G. (2002). *J. Steroid Biochem. Mol. Biol.* 83, 227–233.

Wolffe, A.P., Wong, J., Li, Q., Levi, B.Z. and Shi, Y.B. (1997). *Biochem. Soc. Trans.* 25, 612–615.

Zierau, O., Morrissey, C., Watson, R.W., Schwab, P., Kolba, S., Metz, P. and Vollmer, G. (2003). *Planta Med.* 69, 856–858.

Zierau, O., Hauswald, S., Schwab, P., Metz, P. and Vollmer, G. (2004). *J. Steroid Biochem. Mol. Biol.* 92, 107–110.

74

Hop-Derived Phytoestrogens Alter Osteoblastic Phenotype and Gene Expression

Katharina E. Effenberger Institute of Tumour Biology, Center of Experimental Medicine, University Medical Center-Hamburg Eppendorf, Hamburg, Germany
Johannes Westendorf Institute of Pharmacology and Toxicology, Center of Experimental Medicine, University Medical Center-Hamburg Eppendorf, Hamburg, Germany

Abstract

Certain plant-derived compounds show selective estrogen receptor modulator (SERM) activity and are therefore considered to have chemopreventive potential or to be an alternative to the conventional hormone replacement therapy. Most of the phytoestrogens identified so far have phenolic structures which are known to be able to bind estrogen receptors (ERs). In addition they have been shown to display desirable effects on hormone-related diseases like osteoporosis or cancer. We tested the effects of the hop-derived prenylflavonoids 8-prenylnaringenin, 6-prenylnaringenin, xanthohumol and isoxanthohumol to modulate markers of differentiation and gene expression in osteoblasts. Additionally, we analyzed the ER-binding affinities of these hop compounds as well as the ER-mediation of their effects. Bone-forming activity and ER-subtype specificity were investigated by measuring alkaline phosphatase (AP) activity in hFOB/ERα cells and regulation of gene transcription for AP, interleukin-6 (IL-6), presenelin-2 (pS2) and von Willebrand Factor (VWF) in U-2 OS/ERα and U-2 OS/ERβ cells.

Our results demonstrate that AP, pS2 and VWF mRNA levels are significantly increased by treatment with the compounds in an estrogen-like manner via both ERα and ERβ, while IL-6 is down-regulated in U-2 OS/ERα cells. Consistently, AP enzymatic activity is up-regulated by all compounds in hFOB/ERα9 cells. Except for 8-PN the hop constituents display an ERβ-preference. Reversal of estrogen-specific AP-induction in Ishikawa cells indicates an ER-regulated mechanism. Finally, the flavonoids display cytotoxic effects only at high concentrations ($\geqslant 10^{-4}$ M).

In summary, we have demonstrated for the first time that specific phytoestrogen compounds found in hop extracts exert estrogen-like activities on bone metabolism. Beer is the main dietary source of such prenylflavonoids. Regarding a potential for use of beer or isolated prenylflavonoids in osteoporosis-prevention therapy, the dosage and pharmacokinetics of these phytoestrogens will play an important role concerning a desired *in vivo* profile.

List of Abbreviations

AP	Alkaline phosphatase
CFE	Colony-forming efficiency
E_2	17β-Estradiol
EE	Ethinyl estradiol
ER	Estrogen receptor
HRT	Hormone replacement therapy
IXH	Isoxanthohumol
6-PN	6-Prenylnaringenin
8-PN	8-Prenylnaringenin
pS2	Presenelin-2
SERM	Selective estrogen receptor modulator
VWF	von Willebrand Factor
XH	Xanthohumol

Introduction

Bone remodeling is a dynamic process which is maintained by a balance between bone formation and bone resorption. It has long been recognized that the acute loss of estrogen at the onset of menopause is responsible for an accelerated bone loss in women, called Type I osteoporosis (Rizzoli and Bonjour, 1997). It is characterized by an imbalance in bone remodeling and leads to an increased fracture risk. Besides estrogen deficiency, there are other important factors which determine the extent of bone loss such as race, genetics and nutrition. The peak bone mass achieved during adolescence also influences the risk of developing osteoporosis during menopause (Bilezikian, 1998).

Hormone replacement therapy (HRT) is currently the most common therapy used for peri- and postmenopausal women to prevent bone loss. However, chronic estrogen therapy provides both benefits and hazards. While there are positive effects on bone, climacteric symptoms and possibly on the cardiovascular system, there are also increased risks of breast and endometrial cancers after a certain period of

Beer in Health and Disease Prevention
ISBN: 978-0-12-373891-2

application (Grodstein *et al.*, 1997; Rizzoli and Bonjour, 1997; Gustafsson and Warner, 2000). Thus, intensive investigation is currently underway to identify selective estrogen receptor modulators (SERMs) which display the desirable estrogenic effects but lack the undesirable side effects. Several plant-derived compounds, including isoflavones, lignans and coumestans, display SERM activity. Some plant extracts already commonly used against climacteric complaints include soy (*Glycine max* L.), black cohosh (*Cimicifuga racemosa* L.), red clover (*Trifolium pratense* L.) and derivatives of the hop plant (*Humulus lupulus* L.) (Khosla, 2002; Wuttke *et al.*, 2002; Zierau *et al.*, 2002a). The female flowers of the hop plant contain a variety of compounds whose structures have been shown to bind to the estrogen receptors (ERs) α and β such as the flavanones 8-prenylnaringenin (8-PN), 6-prenylnaringenin (6-PN) (Milligan *et al.*, 2000) and the isoflavone xanthohumol (XH), as well as its opened ring form isoxanthohumol (IXH) (Stevens *et al.*, 1999) (Figure 74.1). The hop plant *Humulus lupulus* L. (*Cannabaceae*) has traditionally been used as a sedative and flavoring agent for beer. Beer is the main dietary source of hop prenylflavonoids. Although its estrogenic effects have also been known and investigated (Kumai and Okamoto, 1984; Milligan, *et al.*, 1999; Liu *et al.*, 2001; Milligan *et al.*, 2002; Stevens and Page, 2004), very little is known about the molecular mechanism of action on bone and osteoblastic cell cultures. It is yet to be established if there is a causal link between the action of phytoestrogens and bone mass maintenance in humans. According to Tobe *et al.*, XH, at a concentration of 10^{-5} M, has a strong inhibitory effect on bone resorption, but the mechanism remains unclear. This is not surprising as XH is a precursor of 8-PN (Tobe *et al.*, 1997). 8-PN has been shown to act as an estrogen agonist in bone *in vivo* (Miyamoto *et al.*, 1998). Moreover, in different

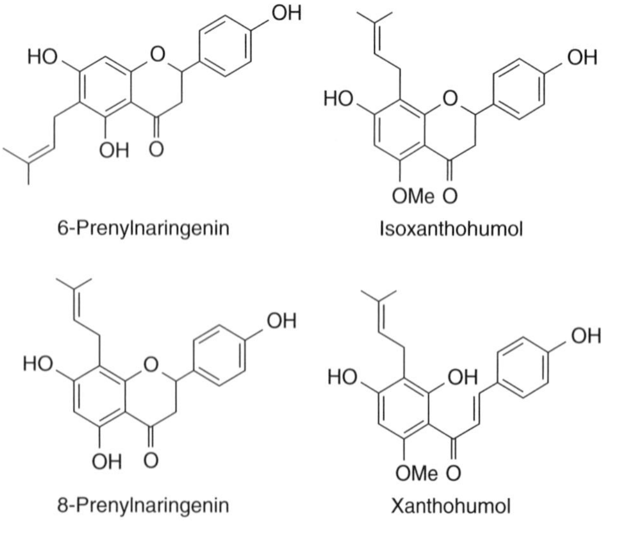

6-Prenylnaringenin

Isoxanthohumol

8-Prenylnaringenin

Xanthohumol

Figure 74.1 Chemical structures of the tested single constituents of the hop plant, *Humulus lupulus* L.

tissues 8-PN shows estrogenic effects with an activity about one order of magnitude greater than that of other established plant estrogens (e.g. genistein) (Kitaoka *et al.*, 1998; Milligan *et al.*, 1999, 2002). Genistein, a soybean isoflavone, behaves as a weak estrogen agonist in hFOB/ERα9 and hFOB/ERβ6 cells (Rickard *et al.*, 2003). Since 8-PN, like genistein, binds to both ER isoforms, it might be possible that 8-PN acts in a similar manner to genistein on bone *in vivo* (Morabito *et al.*, 2002; Li and Yu, 2003). Other *in vivo* experiments in ovariectomized rats have shown that certain isoflavones suppress ovariectomy-induced bone resorption in a manner similar to estrogen (Miyamoto *et al.*, 1998).

The action of 17β-estradiol (E_2) in bone occurs via its two receptor subtypes ERα and ERβ (Eriksen *et al.*, 1988; Komm *et al.*, 1988). Both are found in osteoblastic cells *in vivo*. ERα is mainly expressed in cortical bone and therefore responsible for longitudinal growth, whereas ERβ prevails in cancellous bone and may be important for the maintenance of bone substance (Bord *et al.*, 2001). *In vitro* ERα and ERβ are differentially expressed during osteoblast differentiation (Arts *et al.*, 1997). Both receptors exhibit differential ligand-dependent regulation of endogenous genes and markers characteristic for osteoblasts *in vitro* (Kuiper *et al.*, 1997; Waters *et al.*, 2001; Monroe *et al.*, 2003). The variety of target genes as well as the specific effect on gene expression depends on the particular receptor-ligand complex, the ratio of ERα and ERβ, and the steroid receptor coactivators in the specific cell type.

In this study we investigated the effects of several hop-derived compounds on cultured osteoblast-like cells in comparison to E_2. To examine the differential regulation via the two ER isoforms, we compared the responses of normal human fetal osteoblast cells (hFOB) and human osteosarcoma cells (U-2 OS) stably transfected with either ERα or ERβ following treatment with E_2 or the phytoestrogens. In addition, we tested the ER-binding affinity of the hop-derived compounds to the two ER-subtypes in a cell-free system using human recombinant receptor proteins of ERα and ERβ proteins, as well as the ER-mediation of their effects.

The purpose of this study was to investigate the effects of specific hop-derived phytoestrogen compounds on osteoblast-like cell phenotypes and determine if these effects are mediated by either ERα or ERβ (Effenberger *et al.*, 2005). We examined endogenous target gene regulation of four estrogen-regulated genes, alkaline phosphatase (AP), interleukin-6 (IL-6), presenelin-2 (pS2) and von Willebrand Factor (VWF). As AP is an excellent marker of osteoblast function (Waters *et al.*, 2001), we measured its enzymatic activity as well. Furthermore, co-treatment with an antiestrogen demonstrates that these compounds function in an ER-dependent manner. This is the case when induction of estrogen-specific marker AP can be reversed by the antiestrogen.

Regulation of Estrogen-Inducible Gene Expression by Estradiol and Phytoestrogens in U-2 OS/ER Cells

The ER isoforms ERα and ERβ are known to differ in their tissue specificity and response to various ER agonists and antagonists (Paech *et al.*, 1997). To determine the differential gene regulation, we used the human osteosarcoma cell lines U-2 OS/ERα and U-2 OS/ERβ (Monroe *et al.*, 2003). The advantages of these cell lines are that (1) they express comparable ER levels between the two cell lines, (2) the effects observed can directly be ascribed to one receptor subtype and (3) no interactions between the receptor subtypes such as ERα/β heterodimers have to be expected (Pace *et al.*, 1997).

The effects of treatment with the hop compounds (8-PN, 6-PN, XH and IXH) and E_2 on four estrogen-egulated genes AP, IL-6, pS2 and VWF were tested in the U-2 OS/ERα and U-2 OS/ERβ cell lines by semi-quantitative RT-PCR. Two of the genes, AP and IL-6, play an important role in bone metabolism. AP is a bone formation marker and is up-regulated by E_2 (Riggs and Khosla, 1995; Robinson *et al.*, 1997). In contrast, IL-6 is down-regulated by E_2 and is linked to a decreased bone resorption activity (Qu *et al.*, 1999).

The compound 6-PN increases AP gene expression to the same extent as 10^{-8}M E_2 in the U-2 OS/ERα cells in higher concentrations (Figure 74.2a and b). Interestingly, 8-PN up-regulates AP even stronger than E_2, with a peak induction at 1.0 μg/μl. In the U-2 OS/ERβ cells 8-PN has a similarly strong effect as compared to E_2, while 6-PN acts slightly weaker (Figure 74.2c and d). XH and IXH show a weaker effect than estrogen in both cell lines with 1.0 μg/ml displaying the strongest induction, respectively. Dose dependency is observed for 6-PN, XH and IXH in U-2 OS/ERα cells and for 6-PN in U-2 OS/ERβ cells.

IL-6, a marker of bone resorption, is down-regulated by all test samples in U-2 OS/ERα cells, in certain concentrations to the same extent as estrogen with the exception of IXH which acts slightly weaker. At 10.0 μg/ml, IXH seems to induce IL-6 (Figure 74.3a and b). Here 6-PN

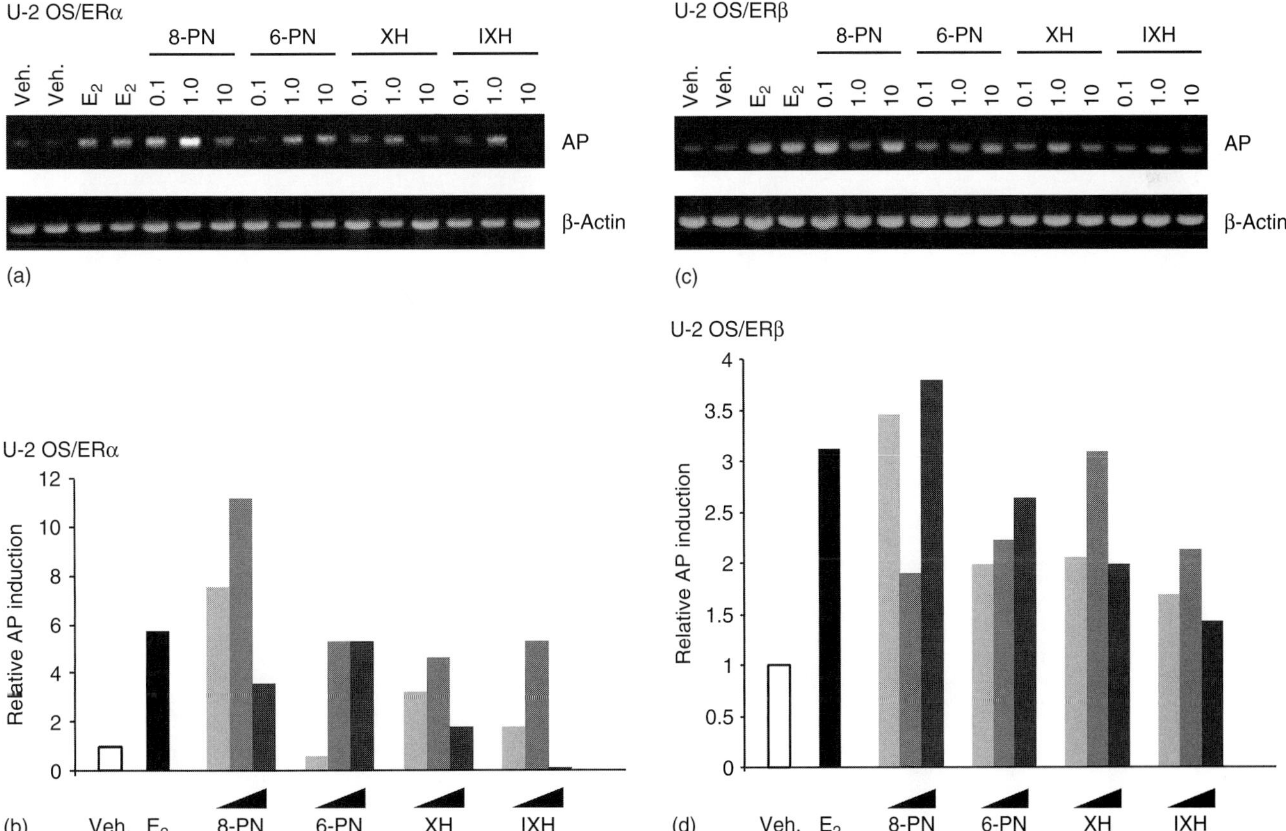

Figure 74.2 Regulation of AP mRNA expression by E_2 and plant-derived compounds. U-2 OS/ERα (a) and U-2 OS/ERβ (c) cells were grown in DMEM/F12 media containing 10% cs-FBS, treated overnight with 1 μg/μl doxycycline to induce ER expression and then treated for an additional 24 h with the indicated compounds in the concentrations 0.1, 1.0 or 10.0 μg/ml (i.e. 0.5×10^{-6}–0.5×10^{-4}M) and E_2 10^{-8}M. mRNA was harvested and RT-PCR was performed with cDNA templates using specific primers for human AP. β-actin gene expression serves as a control. Figure (b) (for U-2 OS/ERα) and (d) (for U-2 OS/ERβ) show the quantitated data, which results from densitometry of the bands as bar graphs.

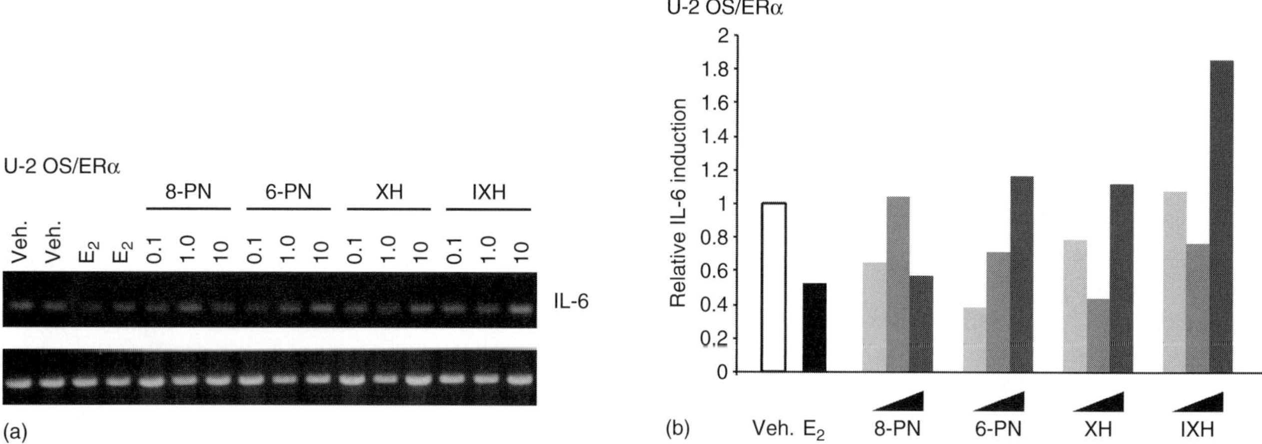

Figure 74.3 Regulation of IL-6 mRNA expression by E_2 and plant-derived compounds. RT-PCR was performed with cDNA from U-2 OS/ERα (a) and U-2 OS/ERβ (data not shown) cells as described in Figure 74.2 using specific primers for human VWF. β-actin gene expression serves as a control. Figure (b) shows the quantitated data for U-2 OS/ERα, which results from densitometry of the bands as bar graphs.

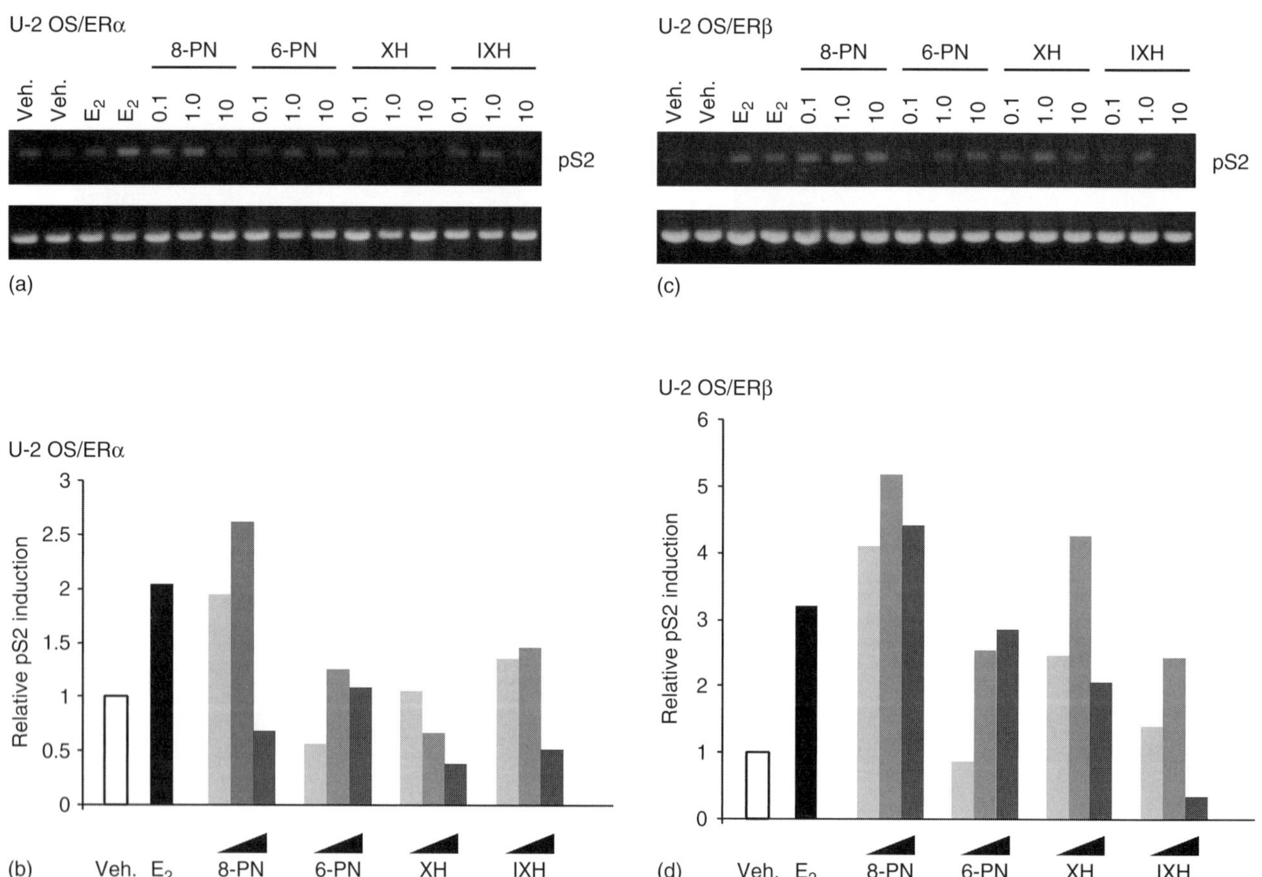

Figure 74.4 Regulation of pS2 mRNA expression by E_2 and plant-derived compounds. RT-PCR was performed with cDNA from U-2 OS/ERα (a) and U-2 OS/ERβ (c) cells as described in Figure 74.2 using specific primers for human pS2. β-actin gene expression serves as a control. Figure (b) (for U-2 OS/ERα) and (d) (for U-2 OS/ERβ) show the quantitated data, which results from densitometry of the bands as bar graphs.

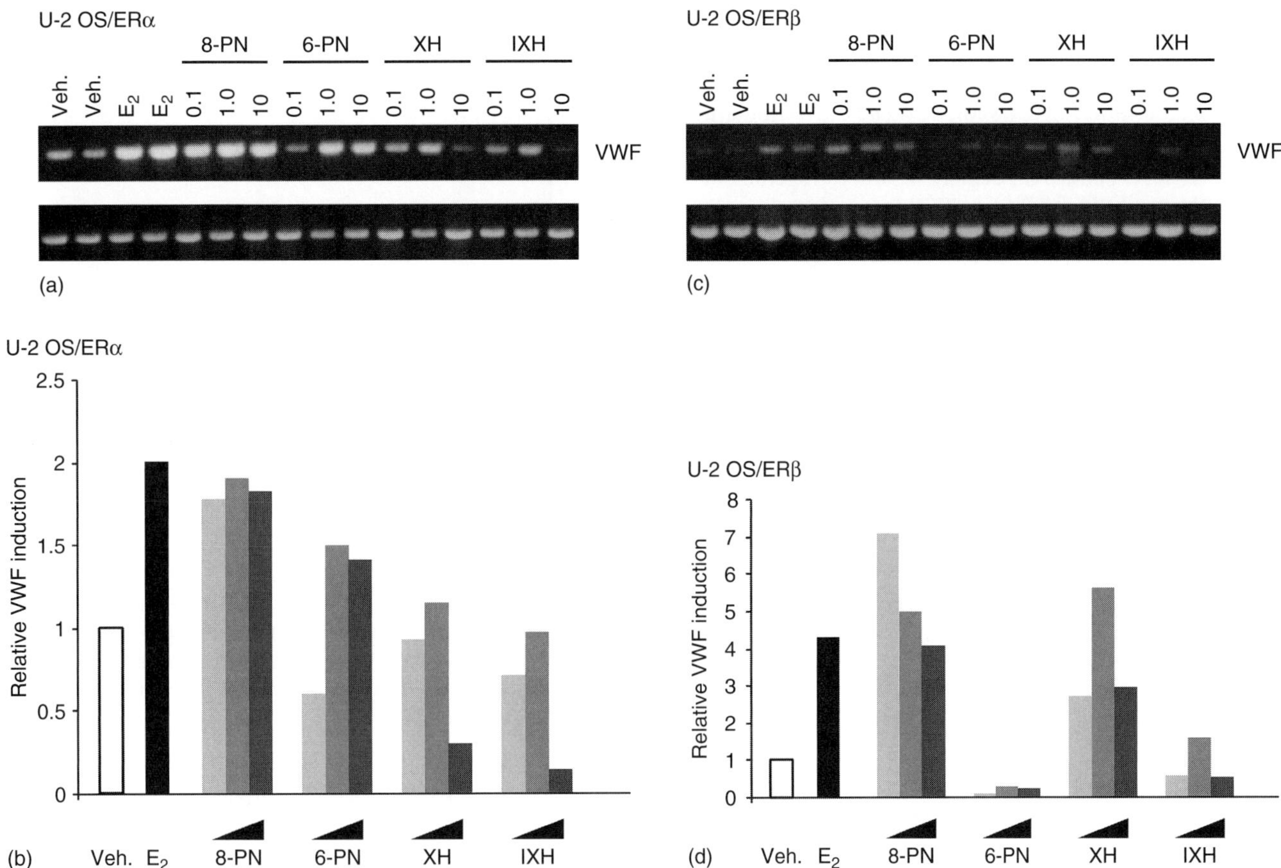

Figure 74.5 Regulation of VWF mRNA expression by E_2 and plant-derived compounds. RT-PCR was performed with cDNA from U-2 OS/ERα (a) and U-2 OS/ERβ (c) cells as described in Figure 74.2 using specific primers for human VWF. β-actin gene expression serves as a control. Figure (b) (for U-2 OS/ERα) and (d) (for U-2 OS/ERβ) show the quantitated data, which results from densitometry of the bands as bar graphs.

displays reverse dose dependency. Surprisingly, IL-6 expression remains unaltered by E^2 and all plant compounds in U-2 OS/ERβ (data not shown). This leads to the assumption that (1) the IL-6 gene in osteoblast-like cells might be ERα-regulated and (2) none of the tested hop constituents or estrogen enhances bone resorption via IL-6 regulation *in vitro*.

Another well-characterized estrogen-regulated gene is pS2. Only the lower doses of 8-PN (0.1 and 1.0 μg/ml) up-regulate pS2 to a similar degree as E_2 in U-2 OS/ERα (Figure 74.4a and b). IXH displays intermediate levels of induction while 6-PN and XH only weakly increase pS2 gene expression. 8-PN and E_2 markedly induce pS2 mRNA levels in U-2 OS/ERβ cells (Figure 74.4c). XH shows a slightly weaker up-regulation with a distinct peak at 1.0 μg/ml, but stronger than 6-PN and IXH. pS2 is a well-characterized estrogen-regulated marker in different cell systems (Brown *et al.*, 1984; Liu *et al.*, 2001; Barkhem *et al.*, 2002) and is over-expressed in certain breast cancers (Nunez *et al.*, 1987). Whether pS2 also plays a role in bone formation is not known. However, because of its robust inducibility by estrogen, we used it for determination of the estrogenicity of the phytoestrogens compared to E^2 in the U-2 OS/ER cell lines.

Finally, recent data demonstrated that the VWF gene is a very sensitive marker for estrogen regulation in the U-2 OS/ER cell lines (Monroe *et al.*, 2003). Therefore, VWF gene regulation was chosen in our study to further investigate the estrogenic effects of the phytoestrogens. In the U-2 OS/ERα cells, VWF is strongly up-regulated to a similar extent as E_2 by 8-PN followed by 6-PN (Figure 74.5a and b). XH and IXH show remarkably weaker effects. Dose dependency is observed for the three latter compounds for 0.1 and 1.0 μg/ml. In U-2 OS/ERβ cells, 8-PN induces VWF gene expression to a higher level than estrogen in a reverse dose-dependent manner (Figure 74.5c and d). XH has a similar effect as E_2 at 1.0 μg/ml, whereas 6-PN and IXH induce VWF gene expression, if at all, to a lesser degree. The VWF gene is a strongly regulated parameter for E_2 and the hop components. VWF is involved in blood clotting as a so-called antihemophilic factor (factor VIIIA) and interacts with factor VIIIC to enhance thrombocyte aggregation at the vascular endothelium. Monroe *et al.* (2003) suggested a possible function in the extracellular matrix of bone as VWF is known to associate with various collagen types during blood clotting (Budde and Schneppenheim, 2001). Collagen is an important constituent of bone extracellular matrix.

In summary, the results of this gene expression profile in the U-2 OS/ER cell lines reveal that the compound 8-PN has the strongest estrogen-like activity of the compounds tested. Furthermore, 8-PN shows potent estrogenic effects in a dose-dependent manner for the regulation of all tested genes. 6-PN, XH and IXH display weaker estrogenic effects than 8-PN. Regarding AP and VWF gene expression, 6-PN induces obviously stronger than XH and IXH.

In some cases a reverse dose dependency, for example 8-PN regulation of VWF in U-2 OS/ERβ, or a decreased effect of the 10.0 μg/ml concentration of the compound, for example XH or IXH in U-2 OS/ERα cells, can be observed while the lower concentrations 0.1 or 1.0 μg/ml show the strongest regulation. This might be due to a nonspecific cytotoxic effect of the higher phytoestrogen concentrations in cell culture as observed for IXH (Miranda *et al.*, 1999). For XH other mechanisms, like tyrosine kinase inhibition, might be crucial (Akiyama *et al.*, 1987; Yamagishi *et al.*, 2001).

We demonstrated for the first time that constituents of the hop plant display positive estrogen-like effects on osteoblast-like cell cultures. In some instances these effects are even stronger than those of E_2. Importantly, they also influence markers of bone metabolism (AP and IL-6) to a similar extent as E_2. The tested compounds can therefore be declared phytoestrogens because they display estrogenic activity in several independent assays.

Regulation of AP Activity by Ethinyl Estradiol and Phytoestrogens in hFOB/ER Cells

For the human fetal osteoblast cell line hFOB/ERα9 the previous statements (2) and (3) made for the U-2 OS/ER cells can be applied, respectively ((2) the effects observed can directly be ascribed to one receptor subtype and (3) no interactions between the receptor subtypes such as ERα/β heterodimers have to be expected). However, ER levels between the two cell lines are considerably different. Whereas hFOB/ERα9 cells express a fairly high level of receptor protein, the level of ERβ expressed in hFOB/ERβ6 is relatively low (Waters *et al.*, 2001). Consistent with this, AP activity was nearly undetectable.

Since AP is both a marker of bone formation and osteoblast differentiation in confluent osteoblast cell cultures (Waters *et al.*, 2001), we tested the effects of the hop compounds on AP activity. Ethinyl estradiol (EE) displays a nearly 5-fold increase in AP activity compared to media in the hFOB/ERα9 cells. All hop compounds or extracts induce the AP enzyme to a lesser extent than EE with AP activity being most strongly induced by 8-PN (Figure 74.6). In the concentrations 0.1 and 1.0 μg/ml 8-PN displays a nearly 3-fold increase compared to media. To a lesser extent XH dose dependently increases AP activity as well. In the concentration 10.0 μg/ml XH displays an approximately

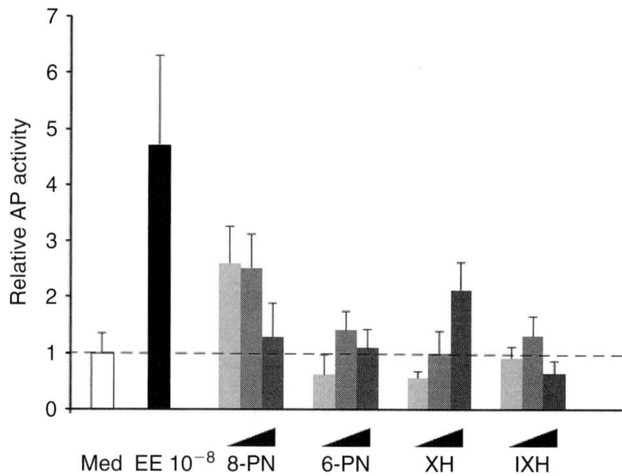

Figure 74.6 Regulation of AP activity by ethinyl estradiol (EE) and plant-derived compounds in hFOB/ERα9 cells. The cells were grown in media containing 10% cs-FBS and treated for 4 days with the indicated compounds (0.1, 1.0 and 10.0 μg/ml) or EE (10^{-8} M). AP activity was determined, normalized for protein content and expressed relative to control (media). The bars represent fold induction of AP ± standard deviation ($n = 8$). At $p < 0.005$ level these data are significantly different (*t*-test) from the EE control.

2.2-fold stimulation of AP activity compared to media. IXH and 6-PN display no significant effects compared to media.

Consistent with a previous report (Waters *et al.*, 2001), no stimulation of AP activity with EE-treatment is observed after 4 days in the hFOB/ERβ6 cells (data not shown).

Comparing AP gene expression and enzymatic activity we found that they were regulated in the same manner and to a similar extent in the U-2 OS/ER and hFOB/ERα9 cell lines, respectively. 8-PN most effectively up-regulates AP gene expression and activity.

This data demonstrates the consistency and reproducibility of the estrogenic effects of these compounds between different *in vitro* osteoblastic models.

Reversal of Phytoestrogen-Induced AP Up-regulation in Ishikawa Cells

Induction of AP in Ishikawa cells is used as an estrogen-specific marker to analyze the estrogenicity of (plant-derived) compounds (Holinka *et al.*, 1986; Kayisli *et al.*, 2002). To assess whether the observed phytoestrogen effects are tissue specific and ER-mediated, the potent estrogen derivative EE (10^{-9} M) and each compound at the concentration, which showed the strongest AP-induction in this system, were added to the cells together with the ERα-antagonist ICI 182780 (10^{-7} M). Figure 74.7 shows reversal of the inductions for EE as well as for all four hop ingredients. This implies a likely complete ER-mediated mechanism.

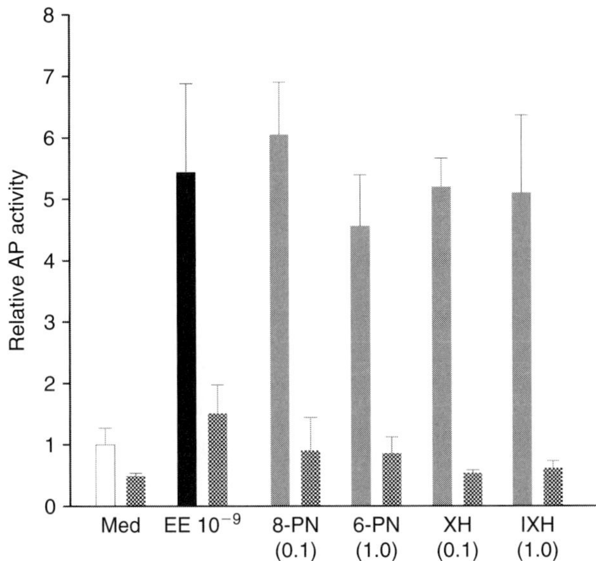

Figure 74.7 Reversal of phytoestrogen-induced AP up-regulation in Ishikawa cells. The cells were grown in media containing 10% cs-FBS and treated for 2 days with the indicated compound (μg/ml) or EE (10^{-9}M) with or without ICI182780 (10^{-7}M). AP activity was determined, normalized for protein content and expressed relative to control (media). The *y*-axis shows the fold activation of AP compared to control. Error bars indicate standard deviation ($n = 4$). Hatched bars display parallel treatment with ICI. The bars represent fold induction of AP ± standard deviation ($n = 4$). At $p < 0.005$ level the data point of each compound/EE for AP activity is significantly different (*t*-test) from its data resulting from co-treatment with ICI.

Relative Binding Affinities of Estradiol and Phytoestrogens to ERα and ERβ

In addition to these cell culture methods, we tested the ER-binding affinity of the hop compounds to the two ER-subtypes in a cell-free system. To characterize the affinity we calculated the IC_{50}-values for all compounds and E_2 (Figure 74.8; Table 74.1a). The relative binding potency of the phytoestrogens compared to the endogenous ligand is described by dividing the IC_{50} (compound, ERα) through the IC_{50} (E^2, ERα) (Table 74.1b). Further, ER-subtype specificity was determined and expressed by the ratio IC_{50} (compound, ERα) to IC_{50} (compound, ERβ) in Table 74.1c.

We could show that none of the isolated compounds from hops binds as efficiently as E_2. Apart from 8-PN, they display relative affinities of approximately 3 orders of magnitude lower than E_2. 8-PN shows the strongest ER-binding affinity which is only 0.5 orders of magnitude lower compared to E_2. An increased affinity for ERβ, as observed for the well-known phytoestrogen genistein, has been connected with a positive overall action, that is decreased risks of breast and endometrial cancers (Liu *et al.*, 2001; Morito *et al.*, 2001). In our study, 6-PN, XH and IXH, but not 8-PN, reveal a preference for ERβ (Table 74.1c).

Not only the affinity to the ER-subtype, but also the transactivation through the receptor compared to E^2, is important. For 8-PN a remarkable transactivation, even stronger than that of the well-known phytoestrogen genistein but less strong than for E_2, could be shown in reporter gene assays (data not shown; Milligan *et al.*, 2002; Zierau *et al.*, 2002b).

Taken together, 8-PN has to be regarded as a pure estrogen agonist. Shifting of the prenyl group from position 8 to 6 in the flavanone structure (Figure 74.1) goes along with the loss of estrogenic potency. Also ER-binding affinity of 6-PN is tremendously less compared to 8-PN (Milligan *et al.*, 2000).

Cytotoxic Effects of the Phytoestrogens in Cell Culture

To assess the potential toxic effects of the hop compounds and extracts in cell culture, V79 cells were treated with the test compounds and media as a control. The effects of increasing concentrations of the samples on the colony-forming ability were assessed over a 7-day incubation period. The results (Figure 74.9) show that no cells are viable after any treatment with the concentrations 30.0, 100.0 and 300.0 μg/ml. XH is the least cytotoxic treatment. But at a concentration of 10.0 μg/ml, only 65% of the media control colony-forming efficiency (CFE) is kept. XH displays a slight opposite effect at 3.0 μg/ml (120% CFE relative to control).

The highest number of colonies was counted for 1.0 μg/ml 8-PN (130% CFE compared to media control) with a rapid decrease of the colony number down to almost 0% at a concentration of 10.0 μg/ml. For 6-PN, this level is already reached at the concentration of 3.0 μg/ml, whereas 1.0 μg/ml still shows a 10% higher CFE than the control. Interestingly, IXH inhibits colony formation completely in all concentrations tested.

Summary Points

- Loss of estrogen at the onset of menopause results in an increased fracture risk and osteoporosis.
- HRT with E_2 or synthetic estrogens is able to reduce osteoporosis. However, side effects, such as an increased risk of breast and endometrial cancers render this therapy questionable. Alternative treatment schedules are therefore being investigated.
- In this study we investigated isolated components of hops (*Humulus lupulus* L.) concerning their phytoestrogen character: XH, IXH, 8-PN and 6-PN. For these components an estrogenic potency has already been known and partially analyzed.
- To assess the estrogenic effect of the plant-derived compounds vs. estrogen on bone we employed test systems

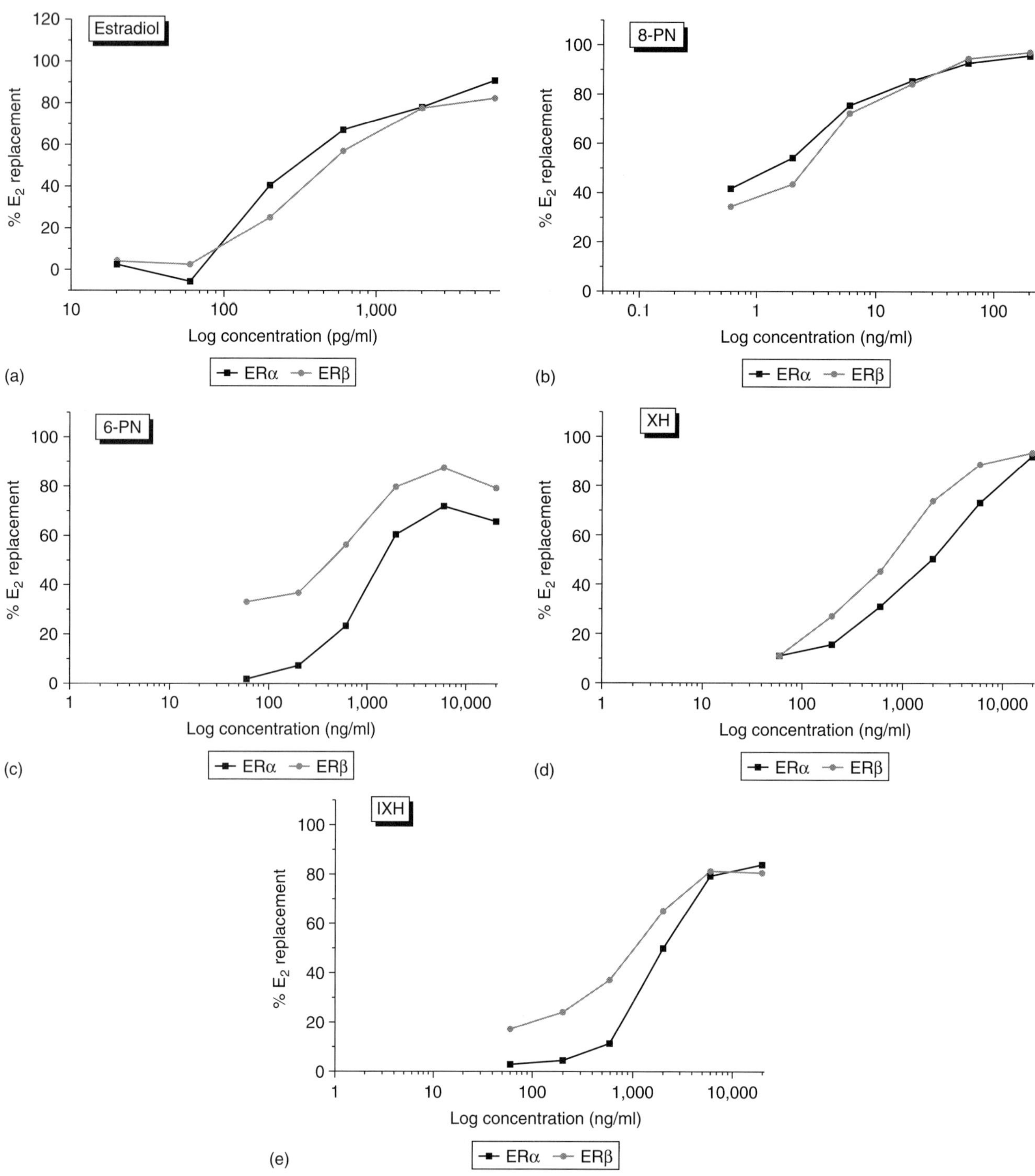

Figure 74.8 Relative binding affinities of E^2 and phytoestrogens to ERα and ERβ. ERα or ERβ was incubated with the indicated compound ((a)–(e); designated concentrations in μg/ml) or E_2 (Figure 74.9; designated concentrations in pg/ml), DES (1 μM) or solvent as well as ^3H-E_2 (1.2 pM) for 18 h. Any excessive ^3H-E_2 was then bound to HAP. The amount of ^3H-E_2 bound to an ER was determined using a scintillation counter ($n = 3$). Figure (a)–(e) show the replacement of ^3H-E_2 in percent through each compound for ERα (black line with squares) and ERβ (gray line with balls). From these graphs the IC_{50} of each compound was derived.

on the level of enzymatic activity (proteins) and on the level of gene regulation.

- The human osteosarcoma cell lines U2-OS/ERα and U2-OS/ERβ, stably expressing either ERα or ERβ, were assayed for regulation of the bone-specific genes, AP and IL-6, as well as two other estrogen-regulated genes, pS2 and VWF. These genes are also influenced by the hop components tested in this study.
- Most of the tested phytoestrogens displayed positive profiles in osteoblasts and osteoblast-like cell lines.

Table 74.1 Receptor binding behavior of E^2 and phytoestrogens to ERα and ERβ

(a) IC_{50}-values

Compound	*IC_{50} ERα (μg/ml)*	*IC_{50} ERβ (μg/ml)*
Estradiol	0.31×10^{-3}	0.48×10^{-3}
8-PN	1.53×10^{-3}	1.88×10^{-3}
6-PN	1.42	0.42
XH	1.94	0.73
IXH	2.0	1.04

Note: The smaller a compound's IC_{50}-value (μg/ml) the higher receptor's affinity.

(b) Relative potency of phytoestrogens compared to E^2

Compound	*IC_{50} (phytoestrogen, ERα)/IC_{50} (E_2, ERα)*	*IC_{50} (phytoestrogen, ERβ)/IC_{50} (E_2, ERβ)*
Estradiol	1	1
8-PN	4.9	3.9
6-PN	4.6×10^3	0.9×10^3
XH	6.3×10^3	1.5×10^3
IXH	6.5×10^3	2.2×10^3

Note: Dividing the IC_{50} (compound, ERα) through the IC_{50} (E_2, ERα) describes the phytoestrogen's relative potency regarding ER-replacement to the endogenous ligand E_2. Replacement through E_2 is characterized by the number "1". The higher this number the lower the sample's affinity for the ER.

(c) Receptor-specific affinity: ERα/ERβ

Compound	*IC_{50} (ERα)/IC_{50} (ERβ)*
Estradiol	0.65
8-PN	0.81
6-PN	3.38
XH	2.66
IXH	1.92

Note: A ratio <1 depicts a stronger affinity for ERα compared to ERβ. An ERβ-preference is described by a ratio >1.

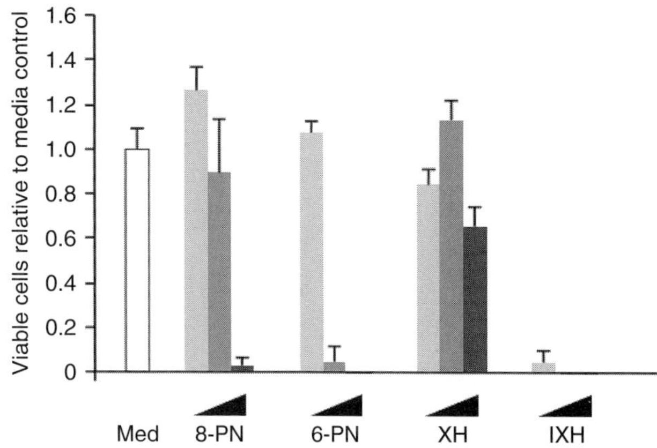

Figure 74.9 Cytotoxicity of hop compounds in V79 hamster fibroblasts. The cells were grown in DMEM/F12 media containing 10% FBS and treated for 7 days with the indicated compounds in the concentrations 1.0, 3.0, 10.0, 30.0, 100.0 and 300.0 μg/ml or media as control in serum-free media. The colony-forming efficiency was determined and expressed relative to control (media). The *y*-axis shows the factor of viable cells relative to media control. Error bars indicate standard deviation ($n = 3$). No columns are visible at high compound concentrations where no viable cells are left.

Therefore, a feasible potential of these compounds to effectively prevent osteoporosis *in vivo* might be concluded. This assumption is supported by previous investigations found in the literature (Fanti *et al.*, 1998; Ishimi *et al.*, 1999).

- Regarding the binding affinity to ERα and ERβ, none of the hop components binds as efficiently as E_2. 8-PN shows the strongest ER-binding affinity which is only 0.5 orders of magnitude lower compared to E_2. The other phytoestrogens are 2–3 orders of magnitude less potent.
- An increased relative affinity for ERβ has been connected with a positive overall action, that is bone conserving and decreasing risks of breast and endometrial cancers (Mori *et al.*, 2001; Milligan *et al.*, 2002). In our study, 6-PN, XH and IXH reveal a preference for ERβ.
- Beer is rich in certain flavonoles acting as phytoestrogens; however, the concentrations vary greatly between different brands.
- Serum concentrations of phytoestrogens depend on their dietary intake. Pharmacokinetic studies with these compounds will have to be carried out in the future to assess the serum concentrations after supply with beer or as part of a special, balanced diet. The concentrations applied in this study are commonly used to test the *in vitro* activity of phytoestrogens, as for example 8-PN (Kuiper *et al.*, 1998; Milligan *et al.*, 2002; Setchell and Lydeking-Olsen, 2003).
- Despite the observed positive effects on bone, the risk of breast cancer which might be implied in a phytoestrogen intake must be taken into account. So far a good deal of phytoestrogen supplementation of nutrition (in the diet) has been connected with a decreased risk of breast cancer (Ingram *et al.*, 1997) and positive effects on bone. Based on our results (data not shown), certain phytoestrogens consumed in low doses presumably have an enhancing effect on development and promotion of some hormone-dependent breast cancers. In contrast, at high concentrations they act antiestrogenic (e.g. 6-PN, XH, IXH). For other phytoestrogens (e.g. genistein) the opposite is true (Allred *et al.*, 2001; Morito *et al.*, 2001). This means that any recommendation of a phytoestrogen-rich diet or even medical substitution of phytoestrogens should be critically evaluated.

Amounts in Beer

XH	2 mg/l (European lager)–690 mg/l (American porter)
IXH	40 mg/l (European lager)–3,440 mg/l (strong ale)

8-PN	1 mg/l (European lager)–240 mg/l (American porter)
6-PN	–
Stevens and Page (2004)	

References

Akiyama, T., Ishida, J., Nakagawa, S., Ogawara, H., Watanabe, S., Itoh, N., Shibuya, M. and Fukami, Y. (1987). *J. Biol. Chem.* 262, 5592–5595.

Allred, C.D., Allred, K.F., Ju, Y.H., Virant, S.M. and Helferich, W.G. (2001). *Cancer Res.* 61, 5045–5050.

Arts, J., Kuiper, G.G., Janssen, J.M., Gustafsson, J.A., Lowik, C.W., Pols, H.A. and van Leeuwen, J.P. (1997). *Endocrinology* 138, 5067–5070.

Barkhem, T., Haldosen, L.A., Gustafsson, J.A. and Nilsson, S. (2002). *Mol. Pharmacol.* 61, 1273–1283.

Bilezikian, J.P. (1998). *J. Bone Miner. Res.* 13, 774–776.

Bord, S., Horner, A., Beavan, S. and Compston, J. (2001). *J. Clin. Endocrinol. Metab.* 86, 2309–2314.

Brown, A.M., Jeltsch, J.M., Roberts, M. and Chambon, P. (1984). *Proc. Natl. Acad. Sci. USA* 81, 6344–6348.

Budde, U. and Schneppenheim, R. (2001). *Rev. Clin. Exp. Hematol.* 5, 335–368.

Effenberger, K.E., Johnsen, S.A., Monroe, D.G., Spelsberg, T.C. and Westendorf, J. (2005). *J. Steroid Biochem. Mol. Biol.* 96, 387–399.

Eriksen, E.F., Colvard, D.S., Berg, N.J., Graham, M.L., Mann, K.G., Spelsberg, T.C. and Riggs, B.L. (1988). *Science* 241, 84–86.

Fanti, P., Monier-Faugere, M.C., Geng, Z., Schmidt, J., Morris, P.E., Cohen, D. and Malluche, H.H. (1998). *Osteoporos. Int.* 8, 274–281.

Grodstein, F., Stampfer, M.J., Colditz, G.A., Willett, W.C., Manson, J.E., Joffe, M., Rosner, B., Fuchs, C., Hankinson, S.E., Hunter, D.J., Hennekens, C.H. and Speizer, F.E. (1997). *New Engl. J. Med.* 336, 1769–1775.

Gustafsson, J.A. and Warner, M. (2000). *J. Steroid Biochem. Mol. Biol.* 74, 245–248.

Holinka, C.F., Hata, H., Kuramoto, H. and Gurpide, E. (1986). *Cancer Res.* 46, 2771–2774.

Ingram, D., Sanders, K., Kolybaba, M. and Lopez, D. (1997). *Lancet* 350, 990–994.

Ishimi, Y., Miyaura, C., Ohmura, M., Onoe, Y., Sato, T., Uchiyama, Y., Ito, M., Wang, X., Suda, T. and Ikegami, S. (1999). *Endocrinology* 140, 1893–1900.

Kayisli, U.A., Aksu, C.A., Berkkanoglu, M. and Arici, A. (2002). *J. Clin. Endocrinol. Metab.* 87, 5539–5544.

Khosla, S. (2002). Phytoestrogens and DHEA. In Cummings, SR., Cosman, F. and Jamal, SA. (eds), *Osteoporosis*, 5, pp. 169–180. American College of Physicians, Philadelphia.

Kitaoka, M., Kadokawa, H., Sugano, M., Ichikawa, K., Taki, M., Takaishi, S., Iijima, Y., Tsutsumi, S., Boriboon, M. and Akiyama, T. (1998). *Planta Med.* 64, 511–515.

Komm, B.S., Terpening, C.M., Benz, D.J., Graeme, K.A., Gallegos, A., Korc, M., Greene, G.L., O'Malley, B.W. and Haussler, M.R. (1988). *Science* 241, 81–84.

Kuiper, G.G., Carlsson, B., Grandien, K., Enmark, E., Haggblad, J., Nilsson, S. and Gustafsson, J.A. (1997). *Endocrinology* 138, 863–870.

Kuiper, G.G., Lemmen, J.G., Carlsson, B., Corton, J.C., Safe, S. H., van der Saag, P.T., van der Burg, B. and Gustafsson, J.A. (1998). *Endocrinology* 139, 4252–4263.

Kumai, A. and Okamoto, R. (1984). *Toxicol. Lett.* 21, 203–207.

Li, B. and Yu, S. (2003). *Biol. Pharm. Bull.* 26, 780–786.

Liu, J., Burdette, J.E., Xu, H., Gu, C., van Breemen, R.B., Bhat, K.P., Booth, N., Constantinou, A.I., Pezzuto, J.M., Fong, H.H., Farnsworth, N.R. and Bolton, J.L. (2001). *J. Agric. Food Chem.* 49, 2472–2479.

Milligan, S., Kalita, J., Pocock, V., Heyerick, A., De Cooman, L., Rong, H. and De Keukeleire, D. (2002). *Reproduction* 123, 235–242.

Milligan, S.R., Kalita, J.C., Heyerick, A., Rong, H., De Cooman, L. and De Keukeleire, D. (1999). *J. Clin. Endocrinol. Metab.* 84, 2249–2252.

Milligan, S.R., Kalita, J.C., Pocock, V., Van De Kauter, V., Stevens, J.F., Deinzer, M.L., Rong, H. and De Keukeleire, D. (2000). *J. Clin. Endocrinol. Metab.* 85, 4912–4915.

Miranda, C.L., Stevens, J.F., Helmrich, A., Henderson, M.C., Rodriguez, R.J., Yang, Y.H., Deinzer, M.L., Barnes, D.W. and Buhler, D.R. (1999). *Food Chem. Toxicol.* 37, 271–285.

Miyamoto, M., Matsushita, Y., Kiyokawa, A., Fukuda, C., Iijima, Y., Sugano, M. and Akiyama, T. (1998). *Planta Med.* 64, 516–519.

Monroe, D.G., Getz, B.J., Johnsen, S.A., Riggs, B.L., Khosla, S. and Spelsberg, T.C. (2003). *J. Cell. Biochem.* 90, 315–326.

Morabito, N., Crisafulli, A., Vergara, C., Gaudio, A., Lasco, A., Frisina, N., D'Anna, R., Corrado, F., Pizzoleo, M.A., Cincotta, M., Altavilla, D., Ientile, R. and Squadrito, F. (2002). *J. Bone Miner. Res.* 17, 1904–1912.

Mori, H., Niwa, K., Zheng, Q., Yamada, Y., Sakata, K. and Yoshimi, N. (2001). *Mutat. Res.* 480–481, 201–207.

Morito, K., Hirose, T., Kinjo, J., Hirakawa, T., Okawa, M., Nohara, T., Ogawa, S., Inoue, S., Muramatsu, M. and Masamune, Y. (2001). *Biol. Pharm. Bull.* 24, 351–356.

Nunez, A.M., Jakowlev, S., Briand, J.P., Gaire, M., Krust, A., Rio, M.C. and Chambon, P. (1987). *Endocrinology* 121, 1759–1765.

Pace, P., Taylor, J., Suntharalingam, S., Coombes, R.C. and Ali, S. (1997). *J. Biol. Chem.* 272, 25832–25838.

Paech, K., Webb, P., Kuiper, G.G., Nilsson, S., Gustafsson, J., Kushner, P.J. and Scanlan, T.S. (1997). *Science* 277, 1508–1510.

Qu, Q., Harkonen, P.L., Monkkonen, J. and Vaananen, H.K. (1999). *Bone* 25, 211–215.

Rickard, D.J., Monroe, D.G., Ruesink, T.J., Khosla, S., Riggs, B.L. and Spelsberg, T.C. (2003). *J. Cell. Biochem.* 89, 633–646.

Riggs, B.L. and Khosla, S. (1995). *Acta Orthop. Scand. Suppl.* 266, 14–18.

Rizzoli, R. and Bonjour, J.P. (1997). *Lancet* 349, sI20–sI23.

Robinson, J.A., Harris, S.A., Riggs, B.L. and Spelsberg, T.C. (1997). *Endocrinology* 138, 2919–2927.

Setchell, K.D. and Lydeking-Olsen, E. (2003). *Am. J. Clin. Nutr.* 78, 593S–609S.

Stevens, J.F. and Page, J.E. (2004). *Phytochemistry* 65, 1317–1330.

Stevens, J.F., Taylor, A.W., Clawson, J.E. and Deinzer, M.L. (1999). *J. Agric. Food Chem.* 47, 2421–2428.

Tobe, H., Muraki, Y., Kitamura, K., Komiyama, O., Sato, Y., Sugioka, T., Maruyama, H.B., Matsuda, E. and Nagai, M. (1997). *Biosci. Biotechnol. Biochem.* 61, 158–159.

Waters, K.M., Rickard, D.J., Riggs, B.L., Khosla, S., Katzenellenbogen, J.A., Katzenellenbogen, B.S., Moore, J. and Spelsberg, T.C. (2001). *J. Cell. Biochem.* 83, 448–462.

Wuttke, W., Jarry, H., Westphalen, S., Christoffel, V. and Seidlova-Wuttke, D. (2002). *J. Steroid Biochem. Mol. Biol.* 83, 133–147.

Yamagishi, T., Otsuka, E. and Hagiwara, H. (2001). *Endocrinology* 142, 3632–3637.

Zierau, O., Bodinet, C., Kolba, S., Wulf, M. and Vollmer, G. (2002a). *J. Steroid Biochem. Mol. Biol.* 80, 125–130.

Zierau, O., Gester, S., Schwab, P., Metz, P., Kolba, S., Wulf, M. and Vollmer, G. (2002b). *Planta Med.* 68, 449–451.

75

Antimalarials from Prenylated Chalcone Derivatives of Hops

Sonja Frölich, Carola Schubert and Kristina Jenett-Siems Institut für Pharmazie (Pharmazeutische Biologie), Freie Universität Berlin, Berlin, Germany

Abstract

There is an urgent need to discover new antimalarials, due to the spread of chloroquine resistance and the limited number of available drugs. Chalcones are one of the classes of natural products that are known to possess antiplasmodial properties. Therefore, the *in vitro* antiplasmodial activity of the main hop chalcone xanthohumol and seven derivatives was evaluated against two strains of *Plasmodium falciparum* (poW, Dd2). Four compounds possessed an activity with IC_{50} values below 25 μM against either strain. Xanthohumol was most active with IC_{50} values of 8.2 ± 0.3 (poW) and 24.0 ± 0.8 μM (Dd2). In addition, the influence of the compounds on the glutathione-dependent hemin degradation was analyzed to determine its contribution to the antimalarial effect of chalcones.

List of Abbreviations

CQ	Chloroquine
FP	Heme
GSH	Glutathione
GSSG	Glutathione disulfide
Hb	Hemoglobin
HZ	Hemozoin
IC	Inhibitory concentration

Introduction

Malaria still is the most dangerous parasitic disease, afflicting 40% of the world's population with an annual incidence of 300–500 million (Fidock *et al.*, 2005). It is caused by protozoan parasites of the genus *Plasmodium*, of which *P. falciparum* is the most important one, producing the highest mortality with 1–3 million people every year. Most of these victims are children in sub-Saharan Africa. Clinical manifestations include fever, prostration and anemia. Severe disease is characterized by delirium, metabolic acidosis, cerebral malaria and multi-organ system failure, leading to death if not treated. As standard antimalarials (e.g. chloroquine) are loosing efficacy due to spreading resistance of *P. falciparum*, the search for new drugs is increasingly important. New antimalarial drugs have to combine rapid efficacy, low toxicity and low cost. At the moment, artemisinin derivatives are high on the list for chloroquine replacement. However, these drugs have very short half-lives, which make it necessary to combine them with longer-acting drugs. Clearly, additional new drugs are needed.

Chalcones are phenolic secondary plant metabolites derived from the flavonoid pathway but lacking the central heterocyclic ring. Compared to flavonoids, which are nearly ubiquitous occurring plant constituents, chalcones and the closely related dihydrochalcones are much rarer. They are characteristic metabolites of plant families as, for example, Fabaceae, Piperaceae and Cannabaceae. Chalcones/dihydrochalcones are known to possess a variety of biological activities including antiplasmodial activity. Licochalcone A from Chinese licorice roots (*Glycyrrhiza* sp., Fabaceae) (Chen *et al.*, 1994) or the benzylated dihydrochalcone uvaretin from *Uvaria* species (Annonaceae) (Nkunya *et al.*, 1991) have shown *in vitro* IC_{50} values against *P. falciparum* between 4.5 and 0.6 μg/ml. The former also demonstrated activity against two *Leishmania* species, parasites that cause severe cutaneous and systemic diseases in tropical as well as sub-tropical countries. Li *et al.* (1995) analyzed the structure–activity relationships of a series of semi-synthetic antiplasmodial chalcone derivatives, suggesting them to act as parasitic cysteine protease inhibitors due to certain structural features. A similar study including also an antileishmanial assay has been conducted by Liu *et al.* (2001).

The hop plant, *Humulus lupulus* L., of the family Cannabinaceae is a large, dioecious climber often cultivated. Secretory glands on the surface of the female flowers contain a volatile oil and also a resin consisting of bitter compounds such as humulones and lupulones. In addition, polyphenols like flavonoids and chalcones are present,

Beer in Health and Disease Prevention
ISBN: 978-0-12-373891-2

especially the prenylated chalcone derivative xanthohumol (Figure 75.1) as a main constituent (Wohlfart, 1993).

In Vitro Antiplasmodial Activity of Hop Chalcones and Semi-synthetic Derivatives

To check the potential antimalarial efficacy of chalcones from hops, the *in vitro* antiplasmodial activity of the main hop chalcone xanthohumol and seven natural or semi-synthetic derivatives against two different strains of *Plasmodium falciparum* has been evaluated (Frölich *et al.*, 2005).

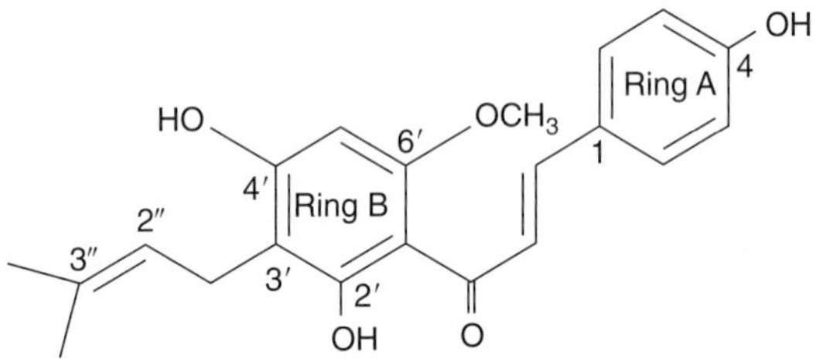

Figure 75.1 Structure of the main hop chalcone xanthohumol (**1**).

The employed bioassay is based on a continuous intra-erythrocytic culture of *P. falciparum*. Normally, two different strains of the parasite are used, one that is sensitive to the standard antimalarial drug chloroquine and another one that is chloroquine- or even multi-resistant. This procedure allows to judge already at this early stage whether an active compound is affected by the same resistance mechanisms as the known antimalarials or not. In this study a West African isolate of *P. falciparum* named poW, which is sensible to chloroquine with an IC_{50} value of 0.01 μM, and the chloroquine-resistant clone Dd2 with a 10-fold higher IC_{50} value were employed. Antiplasmodial activity tests were performed in 96-well culture plates and tritium-labeled hypoxanthin, a metabolite that is essential for the growth of the parasite was used to determine its viability.

Of the eight compounds tested (Figures 75.1 and 75.2), four possessed an activity with IC_{50} values (Figure 75.3) below 25 μM against either strain (Table 75.1; Figure 75.4). The main hop chalcone, xanthohumol (**1**), was most active, revealing IC_{50} values of 8.2 (poW) and 24.0 μM (Dd2), respectively. 2″,3″-Dihydroxanthohumol (**2**) gave an IC_{50} value of 12.9 μM against poW, and also two pyrano-derivatives (**3**, **4**) where the prenyl residue is forming an additional ring possessed antiplasmodial activity

6 $R^1=R^2=R^3=H$

7 $R^1=R^2=R^3=CH_3$

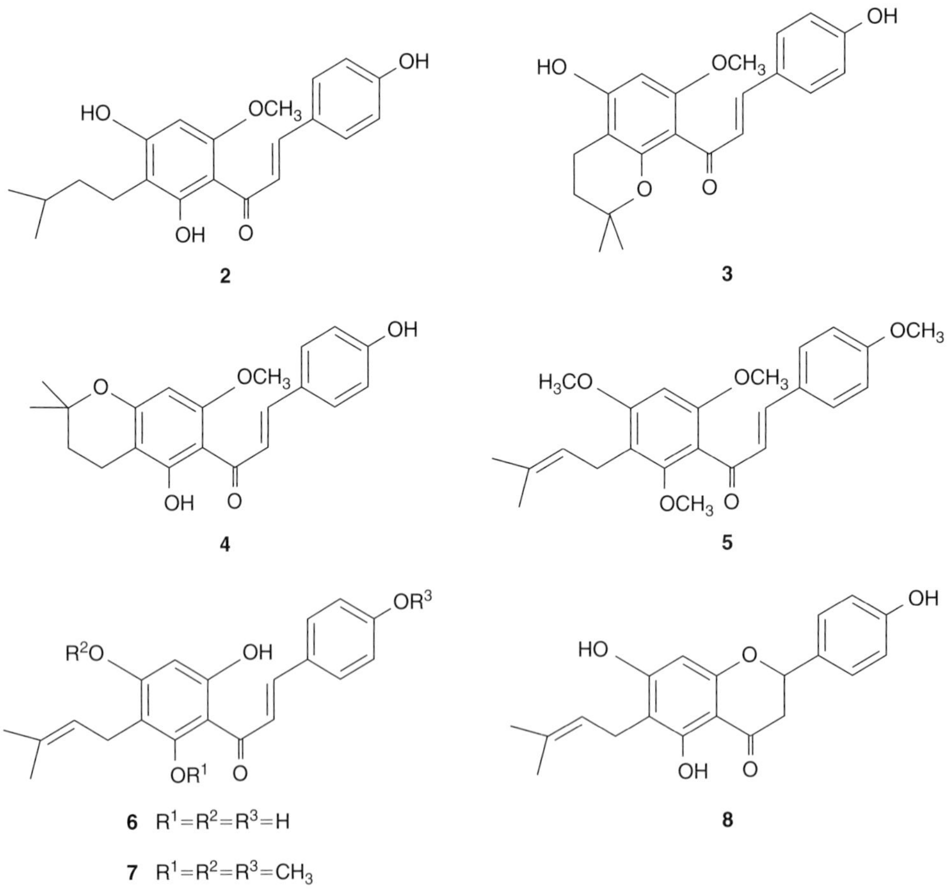

Figure 75.2 Chemical structures of chalcone and flavanone derivatives evaluated.

with IC_{50} values of 16.4 and 23.7 μM (poW), respectively. 6′-Desmethylxantohumol (**6**) on the other hand displayed only a moderate effect (IC_{50} values: 42.4 μM (poW); 92.1 μM (Dd2)). Compounds **5** (2′,4′,4-trimethylxanthohumol) and **7** (2′,4′,4-trimethyl-6′-desmethylxanthohumol) were inactive showing IC_{50} values >100 μM against both strains, whereas the flavanone derivative **8** revealed moderate activity against the multi-resistant clone Dd2 (IC_{50} value 55.3 μM), but no effect against poW (IC_{50} value >100 μM).

This is only the second time that prenylated natural chalcones were proven to possess antiplasmodial properties but in contrast to xanthohumol (**1**) with a prenyl side chain in ring B, the prenyl residue of licochalcone A, which was isolated from Chinese licorice roots, is attached to the ring A of the chalcone skeleton (Chen *et al.*, 1995). Nevertheless, the presence of the double bond in the prenyl side chain is irrelevant for the bioactivity, as indicated by the nearly identical potency of xanthohumol and its 2″,3″-dihydro derivative (**2**). Additionally, the two pyrano-derivatives **3** and **4** where the prenyl residue is cyclized to an additional ring also show antiplasmodial activity. Compared to **1**, desmethylxanthohumol (**6**), which only differs by the lack of the methyl residue at the C-6′-hydroxy group, is four to five times less active. This might be due to its higher hydrophilicity, which makes it more difficult to reach the site of action inside the parasite. Interestingly, the semisynthetic methylated derivatives **5** and **7** are totally inactive; thus, as synthetic 2′,4′-dimethoxychalcones revealed good antiplasmodial activity in an extensive structure–activity relationship study (Liu *et al.*, 2003), especially the methylation of the hydroxy group in position 4 seems to be less favorable.

When comparing these results with those obtained with human cells, *P. falciparum* is slightly more sensitive to xanthohumol (**1**) than are different cancer cell lines and also macrophages (Miranda *et al.*, 1999; Gerhäuser *et al.*, 2002). A real cytotoxic activity can only be observed at 100 μM, though antiproliferative effects become visible at lower concentrations in dependence on the cell line used. In the case of xanthohumol this cytotoxicity is not due to an estrogen-mimicking activity, since in contrast to the flavanone derivative 8-prenylnaringenin, which is also a major constituent of hop cones, xanthohumol does not display estrogenic effects (Milligan *et al.*, 2000). Instead, inhibition of DNA synthesis is discussed. Nevertheless, to develop xanthohumol as a new antiplasmodial lead compound, efforts to separate antiplasmodial and cytotoxic bioactivities have to be undertaken.

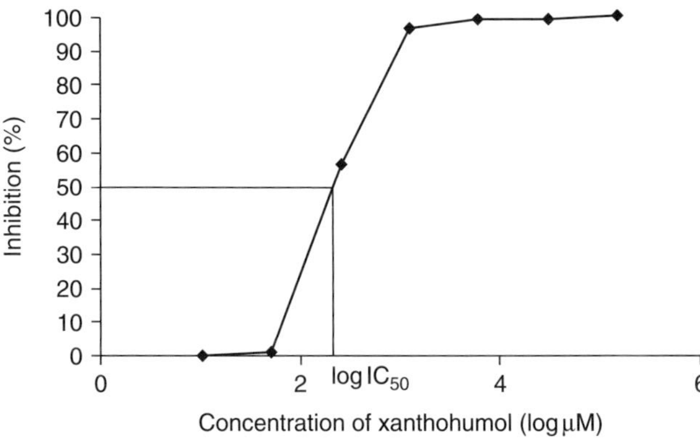

Figure 75.3 Growth inhibition of *Plasmodium falciparum* (strain poW) by different concentrations of xanthohumol. The IC_{50} value (concentration of a substance that causes 50% inhibition of a given system) can be calculated from the dose-response curve.

Table 75.1 Antiplasmodial activity

Compound	*PoW IC_{50} (μM)*	*Dd2 IC_{50} (μM)*
1 (xanthohumol)	8.2 ± 0.3	24.0 ± 0.8
2	12.9 ± 0.6	17.4 ± 0.6
3	16.4 ± 0.9	10.7 ± 0.3
4	23.7 ± 1.5	36.0 ± 2.9
5	>126	>126
6	42.4 ± 0.3	92.1 ± 2.4
7	>131	>131
8	>147	55.3 ± 2.1
Chloroquine	0.015 ± 0.002	0.14 ± 0.012
Artemisinin	0.003 ± 0.0002	0.015 ± 0.003

Note: IC_{50} values of xanthohumol and chalcone derivatives tested against *Plasmodium falciparum* (strains poW and Dd2, values are given as a mean of three experiments ± standard deviation). Artemisinin and chloroquine are given as references.

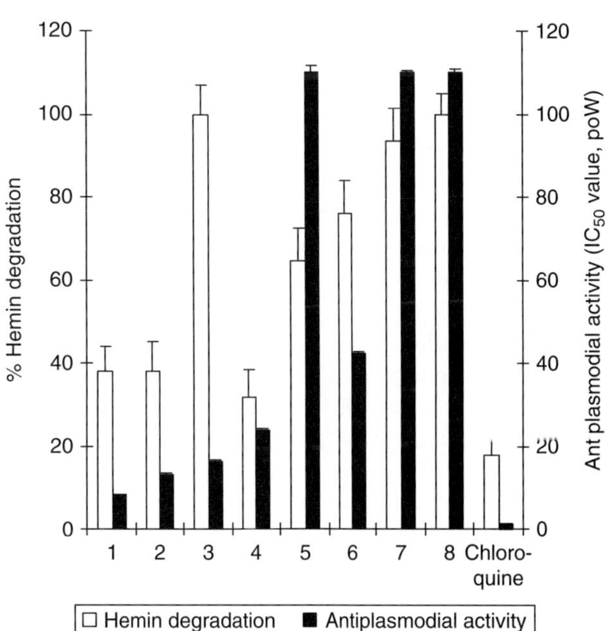

Figure 75.4 Comparison of antiplasmodial activity (IC_{50} value, μM, strain poW of *Plasmodium falciparum*) and influence on hemin degradation (%) of xanthohumol (**1**) and derivatives. Chloroquine is given as reference compound.

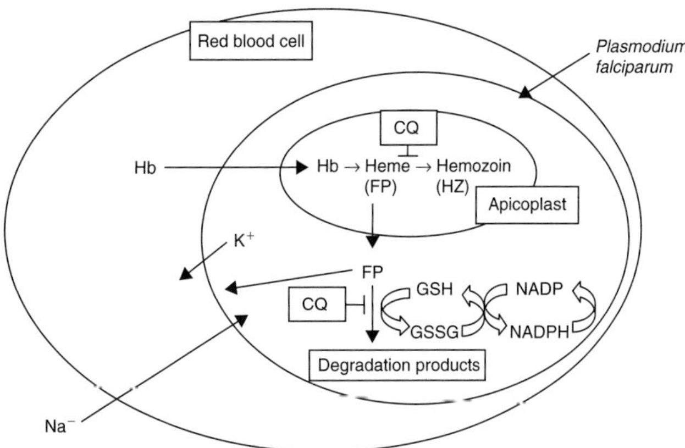

Figure 75.5 Heme detoxification and mechanism of action of chloroquine (CQ). When *Plasmodium falciparum* enters human erythrocytes (red blood cells), it feeds from enzymatic degradation of hemoglobin (Hb). Hb is ingested and digested inside the parasite's food vacuole. The by-product of this digestion, toxic heme (FP), is detoxified by forming an insoluble polymer, malaria pigment or hemozoin (HZ). Non-polymerized heme exits the food vacuole into the parasite's cytosol where it is degraded by glutathione (GSH). CQ has been shown to interfere with both detoxification pathways. It accumulates to high levels inside the acid food vacuole where it complexes with heme and prevents its polymerization. Free or complexed heme exits the food vacuole where its GSH-dependent degradation is also inhibited. Heme thus accumulates in membranes and permeabilizes them to cations, thus leading to parasite death. *Source*: Adapted from Ginsburg *et al.* (1998).

Influence of Hop Chalcones on the Glutathione-Dependent Hemin Degradation

When blood stages of the malaria parasite *Plasmodium falciparum* enter human erythrocytes, they feed from enzymatic degradation of hemoglobin. Hemoglobin is ingested from the host cell and is digested inside the parasites food vacuole (Goldberg *et al.*, 1992). The by-product of this digestion is toxic hemin or ferriprotoporphyrin IX, which is detoxified by forming an insoluble polymer, malaria pigment or hemozoin (Bohle *et al.*, 1997). Recently, an alternative heme detoxification mechanism has been described. Non-polymerized heme exits the food vacuole into the parasites cytosol where it is degraded by glutathione (Ginsburg *et al.*, 1998). Quinoline antimalarials like chloroquine have been shown to interfere with both detoxification pathways. Chloroquine accumulates to high levels inside the acid food vacuole where it complexes with heme and prevents its polymerization. Free or complexed heme exits the food vacuole where its glutathione-dependent degradation is also inhibited. Heme thus accumulates in membranes and permeabilizes them to cations, thus leading to parasites death (Ginsburg *et al.*, 1999; Zhang *et al.*, 1999) (Figure 75.5).

To test the ability of compounds to interfere with the parasites heme detoxification pathways, different *in vitro*

Table 75.2 GSH-hemin interaction assay

Compound	*% Inhibition of hemin degradation*
1 (xanthohumol)	62 ± 6
2	62 ± 7
3	1 ± 0.5
4	68 ± 7
5	7 ± 6
6	36 ± 8
7	1 ± 0.3
8	24 ± 8
Chloroquine	82 ± 3

Note: The effect of chalcone derivatives (11 μM) and chloroquine (11 μM) as reference compound on the interaction of 1 mM GSH with 5.7 μM hemin is given as % inhibition of hemin degradation compared to drug free control. Values are the mean of four assays ± standard deviation.

assays have been developed, thus allowing investigating possible modes of action of antiplasmodial compounds (Basilico *et al.*, 1998; Dorn *et al.*, 1998; Steele *et al.*, 2002). The reaction of hemin with glutathione and the interference of antimalarials can be monitored spectrophotometrically. The broad absorption of hemin is immediately changed to a peak at 364 nm upon addition of glutathione. During 30 min this peak decreases to approximately half without further decrease. Addition of quinoline antimalarials to hemin results first in the alteration of the hemin spectrum due to immediate formation of an alkaloid-hemin-complex and then leads to altered effects of glutathione. In the case of chloroquine the 364 nm peak is not formed and there is little change over 30 min. Based on these findings, Steele (2002) developed a microplate based assay to determine the influence of compounds on heme degradation. Compounds are tested at a concentration of 11 μM in 96-well flat-bottomed plates and are mixed with 5.7 μM hemin and glutathione. The absorbance at 360 nm is measured after 1 and 30 min to determine ΔA_{360} values. The effect of the hemin binding compounds is expressed as the percentage decrease compared with control absorbance.

The exact mechanism of action of antiplasmodial chalcones is not known, though they are often considered to be cysteine protease inhibitors (Li *et al.*, 1995). Nevertheless, natural congeners characterized by a carbonyl moiety in position 9 and a free hydroxy group in position 2 might also be able to form complexes with hemin, thus interfering with its detoxification pathways. Therefore, the influence of compounds **1–8** on the glutathione-dependent hemin degradation was evaluated. In the hemin-degradation assay, compounds **1**, **2** and **4** which also proved to be active in the antiplasmodial bioassay displayed an inhibition >60% at a concentration of 11 μM, compared to 82% for chloroquine (Table 75.2; Figure 75.4), whereas the inactive derivatives **5** and **7** did not inhibit hemin degradation. Compounds **6** and **8** were weakly active, inhibiting hemin degradation by 36% and 24%, respectively, which is also in agreement with the antiplasmodial findings. However, compound **3** is an exception insofar as it is active against *P. falciparum* but does not inhibit the hemin degradation.

Indeed, those compounds possessing a 2′-methoxy group (**5**, **7**) or a 2′,3′-pyrano ring system (**3**) instead of a free hydroxy group obviously were not able to interact with hemin, stressing the importance of this structural feature for this kind of bioactivity. Desmethylxanthohumol (**6**) and the flavanone derivative **8**, on the other hand, were only weakly active despite their free hydroxy group. In the case of cyclized chalcones such as flavanones and flavones a binding to hemin might not be possible via this structural feature due to less flexibility of the skeleton. Finally, desmethylxanthohumol (**6**) is more easily isomerized to the analogous flavanone derivative in aqueous solutions (Hänsel *et al.*, 1988), thus explaining its poor activity.

These results demonstrate for the first time the ability of chalcone derivatives to interfere with the hemin-degradation process of *P. falciparum*. This effect might contribute to their antiplasmodial activity. Nevertheless, as compound **3** showed inhibition of *P. falciparum* without being able to interact with the GSH-dependent hemin degradation, other modes of action must contribute to the observed antiparasitic activity of hop chalcones. Thus, further studies evaluating their possible inhibition of *P. falciparum* cysteine proteases seem to be worthwhile. Nevertheless, first results in this field indicate that xanthohumol is a poorer inhibitor of parasitic proteases than desmethylxanthohumol (**6**) leading to the assumption that a further up to now unknown mechanism has to be responsible for the antiplasmodial action of xanthohumol.

Is Beer an Antimalarial?

Beer is the most important dietary source of xanthohumol and related derivatives. However, despite the fact that xanthohumol is the major chalcone in hops, it is only a minor compound in beer due to thermal isomerization of chalcones into flavanones during the brewing process. Its content in beer varies between 0 and up to 700 μg/l (Stevens *et al.*, 2004) and may reach 1.2 or 3.4 μM/l in stout and porter beers (Gerhäuser *et al.*, 2005). Therefore, taking into account pharmacokinetic parameters as absorption, distribution and metabolism, it is unlikely that antiplasmodially active blood levels of xanthohumol could be reached by normal beer intake. Nevertheless, this chalcone derivative might be a promising candidate for the development of new antimalarials.

Summary Points

- Due to the spreading resistance of *Plasmodium falciparum* against standard antimalarials, there is an urgent need to discover new lead compounds.
- Xanthohumol, the main chalcone from hops, is active against *P. falciparum in vitro*.
- As a possible mode of action, influence on the glutathione-dependent heme-degradation pathway is discussed.
- Due to its low xanthohumol content, antiplasmodially active blood levels cannot be reached by beer intake.
- Nevertheless, this chalcone derivative might be a promising candidate for the development of new antimalarials.

Acknowledgments

The authors are indebted to Prof. R. Hänsel, Freie Universität Berlin, for providing the chalcone derivatives. Financial support by the DPhG to K. J.-S. is acknowledged.

References

Basilico, N., Pagani, E., Monti, D., Olliaro, P. and Taramelli, D. (1998). *JAC* 42, 55–60.

Bohle, D.S., Dinnebier, R.E., Madsen, S.K. and Stephens, P.W. (1997). *J. Biol. Chem.* 272, 713–716.

Chen, M., Theander, T.G., Christensen, S.B., Hviid, L., Zhai, L. and Kharazmi, A. (1994). *Antimicrob. Agents Chemother.* 38, 1470–1475.

Dorn, A., Vippagunta, S.R., Matile, H., Jaquet, C., Vennerstrom, J.L. and Ridley, R.G. (1998). *Biochem. Pharmacol.* 55, 727–736.

Fidock, D.A., Rosenthal, P.J., Croft, S.L., Brun, R. and Nwaka, S. (2004). *Nat. Rev. Drug Discov.* 3, 509–520.

Frölich, S., Schubert, C., Bienzle, U. and Jenett-Siems, K. (2005). *JAC* 55, 883–887.

Gerhäuser, C. (2005). *Eur. J. Cancer* 41, 1941–1954.

Gerhäuser, C., Alt, A., Heiss, E., Gamal-Eldeen, A., Klimo, K., Knauft, J., Neumann, I., Scherf, H.R., Frank, N., Bartsch, H. and Becker, H. (2002). *Mol. Cancer Ther.* 1, 959–969.

Ginsburg, H., Famin, O., Zhang, J. and Krugliak, M. (1998). *Biochem. Pharmacol.* 56, 1305–1313.

Ginsburg, H., Ward, S.A. and Bray, P.G. (1999). *Parasitol. Today* 15, 357–360.

Goldberg, D.E. and Slater, A.F.G. (1992). *Parasitol. Today* 8, 280–283.

Hänsel, R. and Schulz, J. (1988). *Arch. Pharm. (Weinheim)* 321, 37–40.

Li, R., Kenyon, G.L., Cohen, F., Chen, X., Gong, B., Dominguez, J.N., Davidson, E., Kurzban, G., Miller, R.E., Nuzumu, E.O., Rosenthal, P.J. and McKerrow, J.H. (1995). *J. Med. Chem.* 38, 5031–5037.

Liu, M., Wilairat, P. and Go, M.L. (2001). *J. Med. Chem* 44, 4443–4452.

Liu, M., Wilairat, P., Croft, S.L., Tan, A.L. and Go, M.L. (2003). *Bioorg. Med. Chem.* 11, 2729–2738.

Milligan, S.R., Kalita, J.C., Pocock, V., Van de Kauter, V., Stevens, J.F., Deinzer, M.L., Rong, H. and De Keukeleire, D. (2000). *J. Clin. Endocrinol. Metab.* 85, 4912–4915.

Miranda, C.L., Stevens, J.F., Helmrich, A., Henderson, M.C., Rodriguez, R.J., Yang, Y.H., Deinzer, M.L., Barnes, D.W. and Buhler, D.R. (1999). *Food Chem. Toxicol.* 37, 271–285.

Nkunya, M.H.H., Weenen, H., Bray, D.H., Mgani, Q.A. and Mwasumbi, L.B. (1991). *Planta Med.* 57, 341–343.

Steele, J.C.P., Phelps, R.J., Simmonds, M.S.J., Warhurst, D.C. and Meyer, D.J. (2002). *JAC* 50, 25–31.

Stevens, J.F. and Page, J.E. (2004). *Phytochemistry* 65, 1317–1330.

Wohlfart, R. (1993). In Hänsel, R., Keller, K., Rimpler, H. and Schneider, G. (eds), *Hagers Handbuch der Pharmazeutischen Praxis*, Vol. 5, pp. 447–458. Springer, Berlin, Heidelberg, Germany.

Zhang, J., Krugliak, M. and Ginsburg, H. (1999). *Mol. Biochem. Parasitol.* 99, 129–141.

76
Acylphloroglucinol Derivatives from Hops as Anti-inflammatory Agents

Hans Becker Pharmakognosie und Analytische Phytochemie, der Universität des Saarlandes, Saarbrücken, Germany
Clarissa Gerhäuser German Cancer Research Center, Chemoprevention, Im Neuenheimer Feld, Heidelberg, Germany
Gregor Bohr Pharmakognosie und Analytische Phytochemie, der Universität des Saarlandes, Saarbrücken, Germany

Abstract

Separation of a polyphenol-enriched fraction of an ethanolic hop extract (*Humulus lupulus* L.) provided four acylphloroglucinol-glucopyranosides (**1**)–(**4**), that is 1-(2-methylpropanoyl) phloroglucinol-glucopyranoside (**1**), 1-(2-methylbutyryl)phloroglucinol-glucopyranoside (**2**), previously known as multifidol-glucoside, 1-(3-methylbutyryl)phloroglucinol-glucopyranoside (**3**), and 5-(2-methylpropanoyl)phloroglucinol-glucopyranoside (**4**). The compounds show a substitution pattern similar to hop bitter acids; therefore we propose the following novel nomenclature: co-multifidol-glucoside for (**1**), ad-multifidol-glucoside for (**2**), and *n*-multifidol-glucoside for (**3**). For compound (**4**), we suggest co-iso-multifidol-glucoside as trivial name. The occurence of these acylphloroglucinol derivatives in beer has not yet been investigated. The compounds were tested for anti-inflammatory potential by inhibition of cyclooxygenase-1 activity. The aglycon (**5**), obtained by acid hydrolysis of (**1**), was equally effective as phloroglucinol with a half-maximal inhibitory concentration (IC_{50}) of 3.8 μM. The inhibitory potential of the glucosides decreased with increasing length of the acyl-side chain (IC_{50} values: (**1**) 23.7, (**2**) 131.3, (**3**) >100 μM). Compound (**4**) with an IC_{50} of 58.7 μM was about 2.5-fold less active than (**1**), indicating that the position of the sugar moiety also influences anti-inflammatory potential.

Introduction

Hops (*Humulus lupulus* L.) is added as a beer ingredient during beer brewing either as hops cones, as an alcoholic or supercritical fluid extract, or as a mixture of bitter acids. When hops cones or an alcoholic extract are added to wort, not only bitter acids, but also a variety of other hops constituents may occur in the end product. Recently, the hops-derived prenylated chalcone xanthohumol and its isomerization product isoxanthohumol were found to exert biological effects indicative of cancer chemopreventive potential in *in vitro* and *in vivo* studies (Gerhauser *et al.*, 2002a; Bertl *et al.*, 2004a, b; Pan *et al.*, 2005; Albini *et al.*, 2006). Other phenolic compounds from beer, such as benzoic and isoferulic acid derivatives, as well as indan and catechin derivatives also showed *in vitro* effects that correlate with cancer chemopreventive activities (Gerhauser *et al.*, 2002b). These results suggested that hops is a source very rich in bioactive phytochemicals.

One of the potential chemopreventive mechanisms of hops constituents is the inhibition of cyclooxygenase (Cox), a key enzyme in inflammatory processes. It is estimated that chronic inflammation and infections contributed to about 18% of all new cancer cases (Oshima *et al.*, 2005). Inflammation is mediated by prostaglandins, that is, hormone-like endogenous substances generated by Cox. The expression of Cox-2, the inducible form of Cox, is often elevated in tumor tissue in comparison to normal tissue. Excessive production of prostaglandins is thought to be a causative factor of cellular injury and may ultimately lead to carcinogenesis, since prostaglandins enhance cell proliferation and stimulate the formation of new blood vessels essential for tumor growth. Consequently, non-steroidal anti-inflammatory drugs like Aspirin® or selective Cox-2 inhibitions (e.g. celecoxib) are regarded as promising chemopreventive agents and inhibitors of tumor promotion (Furstenberger *et al.*, 2006).

The aim of the present study was to fractionate a polyphenol-enriched hop extract to isolate additional pure hops compounds and to test them for their anti-inflammatory activity using microsomes of ram seminal vesicles as a source of Cox-1 activity (Bohr *et al.*, 2005).

Starting Material

Hops is commercially extracted with ethanol. To obtain a fraction rich in bitter acids, the alcoholic extract is evaporated resulting in two phases, a lipophilic phase containing

Beer in Health and Disease Prevention
ISBN: 978-0-12-373891-2

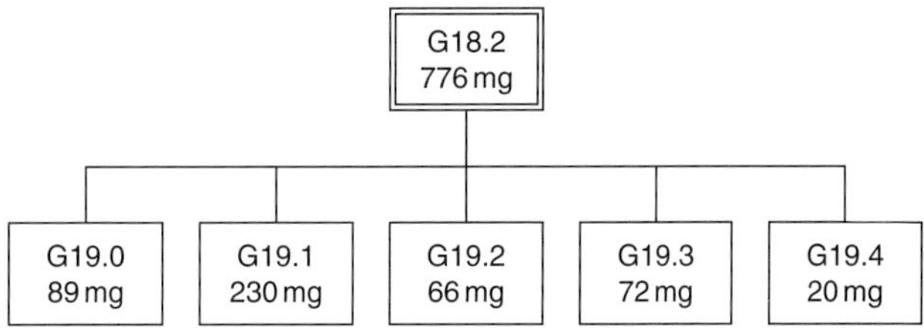

Figure 76.1 Fractionation scheme: the ethylacetate-extracted portion (G18.2) of an ethanolic hops extract was fractionated by column chromatography using Sephadex LH 20 and isocratic elution with methanol to provide four subfractions G19.1–G19.4.

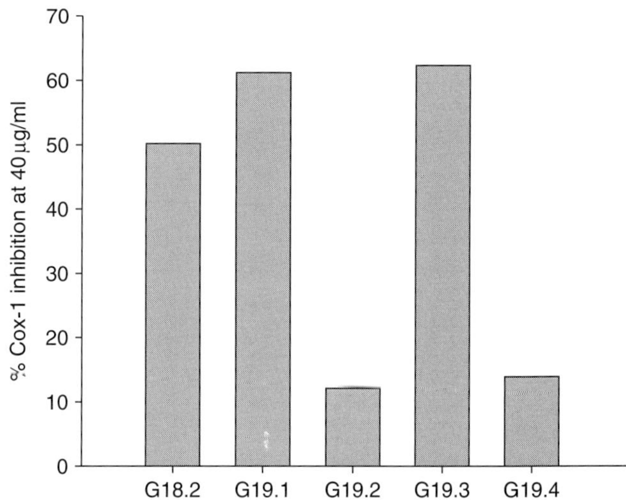

Figure 76.2 Cox-1 inhibitory effects of the fractions described in Figure 76.1.

bitter acids and a hydrophilic phase containing mostly water-soluble substances. Only about 20% of the latter fraction is used in brewery either to standardize hops extract (lipophilic fraction) for a certain bitter acid content or as addition to wort during the brewing process. The other 80% are used in agriculture as fertilizer because they contain a considerable amount of nitrate. The high nitrate content is the reason why this fraction has no broader use either in the brewing process or for other beverages. Nitrate may be transformed by sublingual or intestinal bacteria to nitrite, which can contribute to the formation of carcinogenic nitrosamines.

The ethanolic hops extract analyzed in this study was derived from the variety "Hallertauer Perle" and provided by Simon H. Steiner, Hopfen GmbH, Mainburg, Germany. The analytical data were as follows: dry weight 55%, nitrate content 56 g/kg, density 1.23 g/ml.

Determination of Cox-1 Activity

Inhibition of Cox-1 activity was measured by monitoring oxygen consumption during the conversion of arachidonic acid to prostaglandins using a Clark-type O_2-electrode (Hansatech Ltd., Kings Lynn, UK) (Jang *et al.*, 1997). The reaction mixture contained approximately 0.2 U Cox-1 in 100 μl microsome fraction derived from ram seminal vesicles as a crude source of Cox-1 (specific activity 0.2–1 U/mg protein). For calculation, the rate of O_2 consumption was compared to a solvent control (100% activity).

Activity-Guided Fractionation

The ethanolic hops extract was partitioned with *n*-hexane to remove lipophilic compounds such as remaining α- and β-bitter acids. The aqueous layer was partitioned with ethylacetate. After drying with Na_2SO_4, the organic layer was concentrated to dryness to provide a powder (G18.2) which yielded 1.3% of the dry weight of the starting aqueous extract. G18.2 was tested for its Cox-1 inhibitory activity. The fraction significantly inhibited Cox-1 activity by 50% at a final test concentration of 40 μg/ml. Further fractionation to identify compounds responsible for the inhibitory effect was done by column chromatography using Sephadex LH 20 and isocratic elution with methanol. The elution was monitored by thin layer chromatography and high-pressure liquid chromatography (HPLC) coupled with UV spectroscopy.

According to the chromatographic behavior, four subfractions (G19.1–G19.4) were obtained (Figure 76.1) and again tested for Cox-1 inhibitory potential. Good inhibition of Cox-1 activity was achieved with fractions G19.1 and G19.3 (Figure 76.2). Fraction G19.3 was not further investigated in the present study.

G19.1 showed one major and three minor peaks after analytical HPLC separation (Figure 76.3a) and was further subfractionated by semipreparative HPLC (VP 250/10 Nucleodur, 100-5, C 18 ec, Macherey and Nagel, Germany) under isocratic conditions (acetonitrile/water with 0.05% trifluoroacetic acid 25:75) to yield four subfractions G19.1.1–G19.1.4.

Fraction G19.1.2 contained one compound. The structure was elucidated with 1H and 13C NMR spectroscopy as 1-[(2-methylpropanoyl)phloroglucinyl]-β-D-glucopyranoside (**1**) which we named as "*co-multifidol-glucoside*" in comparison to the substitution pattern of hop bitter acids. Subfraction G19.1.3 also provided one pure compound. Structure elucidation identified a homolog of **1**, that is 1-[(2-methylbutyryl)phloroglucinyl]-β-D-glucopyranoside (**2**), which was named "*ad-multifidol-glucoside*." G19.1.1 and G19.1.4 consisted of a mixture of three respective two compounds with similar UV-spectroscopic properties as G19.1.2 and G19.1.3 (Figure 76.3b). As the amount of these two fractions was too low for isolation and consecutive structure elucidation of pure compounds, we started a second fractionation over Sephadex LH 20 material with 3 g of G18.2. Besides the two already identified compounds, we identified two additional minor phloroglucinol derivatives by further subfractionation using

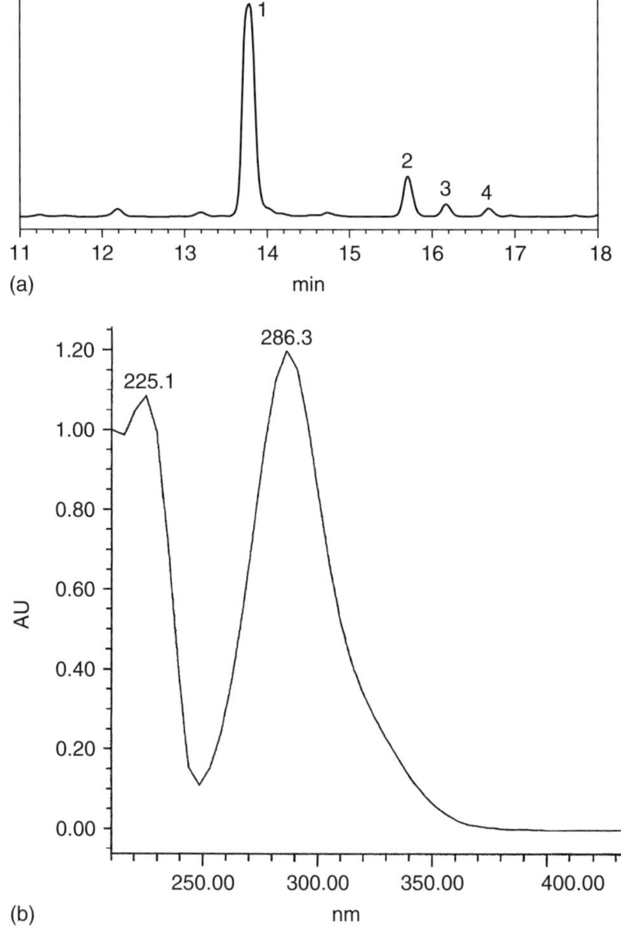

Figure 76.3 (a) HPLC of fraction G19.1 (also representative for fraction G102.4); structures and descriptions of peaks 1–4 in Figure 76.4. Column: EC250/4 Nucleosil 100-5 C18, Macherey & Nagel, Germany. Solvent A: water + 0.1% trifluoroacetic acid, solvent B: acetonitrile + 0.1% trifluoroacetic acid, gradient 5–95% B in 45 min. (b) UV spectrum of peak 1 with maxima at 225.1 and 286.3 nm.

preparative HPLC: 1-[(3-methylbutyryl)phloroglucinyl]-β-D-glucopyranoside (**3**), named "*n-multifidol-glucoside*," and 5-[(2-methylbutyryl)phloroglucinyl]-β-D-glucopyranoside (**4**), named "*co-iso-multifidol-glucoside*." Whereas **1** and **3** are known compounds of hops, **2** was identified for the first time as a hops component and **4** is a new natural product.

To find structure activity relationships (SARs) we hydrolyzed compound (**1**) to yield the aglycon *co-multifidol* (**5**). Also, we included phloroglucinol (**6**) into our tests (Figure 76.4).

SAR Analyses

The isolated pure compounds as well as aglycon **5** and phloroglucinol (**6**) as a reference were tested for inhibition of Cox-1 activity. Dose–response curves for all compounds are given in Figure 76.5.

Aglycon **5** was equally effective as phloroglucinol (**6**) in inhibiting Cox-1 activity, with half-maximal inhibitory concentrations (IC_{50}s) of 4.0 ± 0.2 and $3.9 \pm 0.2\,\mu M$, respectively (summarized in Table 76.1). Addition of a glucose moiety at position C-1 or C-5 to yield the glucosides **1** and **4** significantly reduced the Cox-1 inhibitory potential, and we determined IC_{50} values of 23.7 ± 0.9 and $58.7 \pm 1.1\,\mu M$, respectively. Elongation of the acyl-side chain with a methyl group, as in compound **2** in comparison with compound **1**, further reduced the anti-inflammatory activity (IC_{50} $131.3 \pm 0.2\,\mu M$). Interestingly, with the second purification of compound **2**, the IC_{50} value was decreased to a value as low as $30.3 \pm 0.2\,\mu M$ (compound **2a** in Table 76.1). HPLC analyses of the two isolates revealed that compound **2** is not stable under extraction conditions and can lead to the formation of an additional peak, presumably the respective aglycon. Since aglycon **5** is about 6- and 15-fold more active than the glucosides **1** and **4**, we assume that impurities due to aglycon formation are responsible for the observed lower IC_{50} value. In contrast, derivative **3** was basically inactive with only 12% inhibition at a $100\,\mu M$ concentration ($IC_{50} > 100\,\mu M$).

From these data we concluded that:

(i) Phloroglucinol (**6**) is a good Cox-1 inhibitor.
(ii) Substitution with the short 2-methylpropanoyl moiety at position C-2 as in aglycon **5** does not reduce the inhibitory potential.
(iii) Addition of a sugar moiety in position C-1 reduces the IC_{50} value of **5** about 6-fold.
(iv) Glycosylation at position C-5 reduces the inhibitory potential more than addition of a sugar moiety at position C-1.
(v) Modifications of the acyl-side chain severely lower Cox-1 inhibitory potential.
(vi) For SAR analyses, stability and purity of the compounds have to be carefully monitored.

Outlook

The isolated phloroglucinol derivatives from hops showed a fairly good inhibition of Cox-1 activity. However, due to the relative high amount of nitrate, the native extract can not be used in significant amounts for the production of beer or other beverages. The nitrate content can be considerably reduced either by dialysis or by adsorption chromatography (Bohr and Becker, unpublished results). Such extracts with low nitrate content might contribute to taste and stability of beer as well as possess physiological effects if added in sufficient amounts. Until now it has not yet been tested if the above described phloroglucinol derivatives are present in beers that are either flavored with hop cones or with alcoholic extracts thereof.

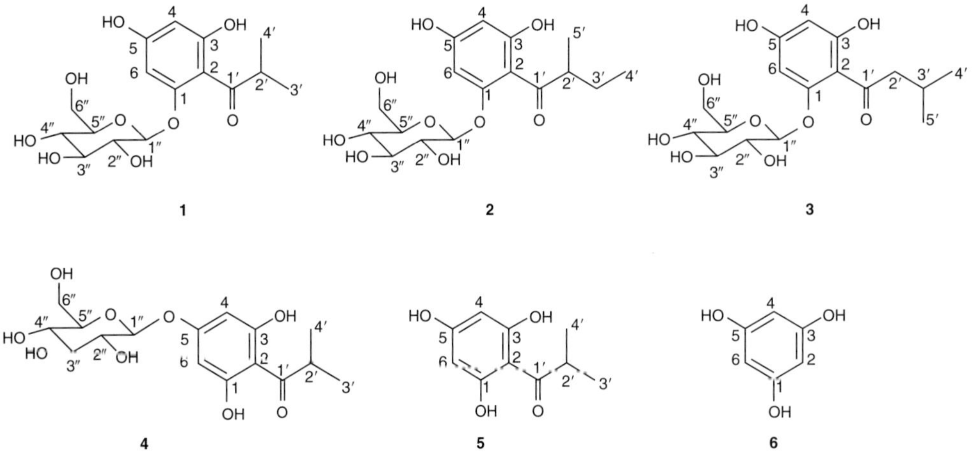

Figure 76.4 Chemical structures of compounds **1–6**. **1**: 1-[(2-methylpropanoyl)phloroglucinyl]-β-D-glucopyranoside = co-multifidol-glucoside; **2**: 1-[(2-methylbutyryl)phloroglucinyl]-β-D-glucopyranoside = ad-multifidol-glucoside; **3**: 1-[(3-methylbutyryl)phloroglucinyl]-β-D-glucopyranoside = *n*-multifidol-glucoside; **4**: 5-[(2-methylbutyryl)phloroglucinyl]-β-D-glucopyranoside = co-iso-multifidol-glucoside; **5**: (2-methylpropanoyl)phloroglucinol = co-multifidol; **6**: phloroglucinol.

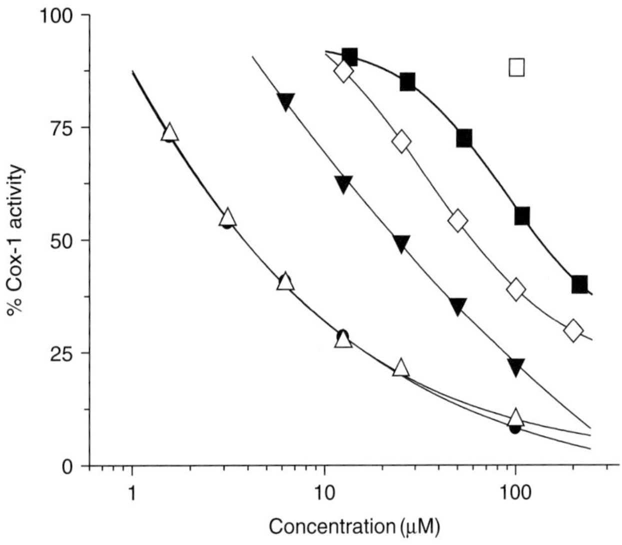

Figure 76.5 Dose-dependent inhibition of Cox-1 activity by acylphloroglucinol derivatives **1** (▼); **2** (■); **3** (□); **4** (◇); **5** (•) in comparison with phloroglucinol (**6**) (△); see Figure 76.4 for structures.

Summary Points

- Alcoholic hop extracts contain four multifidol-glucosides (acyl substituted phloroglucinol glucosides).
- The acyl-side chains are the same as found in hop bitter acids (humulones). Accordingly, the compounds were named with the prefix *n*-, co- and ad-.
- Phloroglucinol, the tested aglycon co-iso-multifidol (**5**) as well as one multifidol-glucoside (**1**) show fairly good anti-inflammatory (Cox-1 inhibitory) activity.
- A broader application of the alcoholic hops extract in brewery as well as in other areas of food industry may be obtained if the nitrate content of extract is reduced by adsorption chromatography or dialysis.

Table 76.1 Summary of Cox-1 inhibitory potential of isolated pure compounds in comparison with phloroglucinol

Compound	*% inhibition at 100 μM*	*IC_{50} (μM)**
(**1**) Co-multifidol-glucoside (G19.1.2. = G102.4.2)	78	23.7 ± 0.9
(**2**) Ad-multifidol-glucoside (G19.1.3)	46	131.3 ± 0.2
(**2a**) Ad-multifidol-glucoside (G102.4.3 with impurities of aglycon)	71	30.3 ± 0.2
(**3**) *n*-multifidol-glucoside (G102.4.4N)	12	>100
(**4**) Co-iso-multifidol-glucoside (G102.4.5)	61	58.8 ± 1.1
(**5**) Co-multifidol (G112.1.4)	92	4.0 ± 0.2
(**6**) Phloroglucinol	90	3.9 ± 0.2

*IC_{50}: concentration required to inhibit the activity of Cox-1 by 50%.

References

Albini, A., Dell'Eva, R., Vene, R., Ferrari, N., Buhler, D.R., Noonan, D.M. and Fascina, G. (2006). *FASEB J.* 20, 527–529.

Bertl, E., Klimo, K., Heiss, E., Klenke, F., Peschke, P., Becker, H., Eicher, T., Herhaus, C., Kapadia, G., Bartsch, H. and Gerhauser, C. (2004a). *Int. J. Cancer Prev.* 1, 47–61.

Bertl, E., Herhaus, C., Kapadia, G., Becker, H., Eicher, Th., Bartsch, H. and Gerhauser, C. (2004b). *Biochem. Biophys. Res. Commun.* 325, 287–295.

Bohr, G., Gerhauser, C., Knauft, J., Zapp, J. and Becker, H. (2005). *J. Nat. Prod.* 68, 1545–1548.

Furstenberger, G., Krieg, P., Muller-Decker, K. and Habenicht, A.J. (2006). *Int. J. Cancer* 119, 2247–2254.

Gerhauser, C., Alt, A., Heiss, E., Gamal-Eldeen, A., Klimo, K., Knauft, J., Neumann, I., Scherf, H.-R., Frank, N., Bartsch, H. and Becker, H. (2002a). *Mol. Cancer Ther.* 1, 959–969.

Gerhauser, C., Alt, A.P., Klimo, K., Knauft, J., Frank, N. and Becker, H. (2002b). *Phytochem. Rev.* 1, 369–377.

Jang, M., Cai, L., Udeani, G.O., Slowing, K.V., Thomas, C.F., Beecher, C.W., Fong, H.H., Farnsworth, N.R., Kinghorn, A.D., Mehta, R.G., Moon, R.C. and Pezzuto, J.M. (1997). *Science* 275, 218–220.

Ohshima, H., Tazawa, H., Sylla, B.S. and Sawa, T. (2005). *Mutat. Res.* 591, 110–122.

Pan, L., Becker, H. and Gerhauser, C. (2005). *Mol. Nutr. Food Res.* 49, 837–843.

77

Hops Derived Inhibitors of Nitric Oxide

Hajime Nozawa, Feng Zhao and Keiji Kondo Central Laboratories for Frontier Technology, Research Section for Applied Food Science, Kirin Holdings Co., Ltd., Takasaki, Gunma, Japan

Abstract

Nitric oxide (NO) plays an important role in many inflammatory responses and is also involved in carcinogenesis. In this chapter, the inhibitory effect of extracts from *Humulus lupulus* L. on both the production of NO and the expression of inducible NO synthase (iNOS) in mouse macrophage RAW 264.7 cells is discussed. The production of NO was induced by a combination of lipopolysaccharide (LPS) and IFN-γ, and determined by Griess assay. The expression of iNOS was detected by Western blotting. The LPS/IFN-γ-induced production of NO and expression of iNOS were significantly inhibited by the ethyl acetate soluble fraction of *Humulus lupulus* L. Through bioactivity-guided fractionation, humulene, five chalcones, 2,2-di-(3-methyl-2-butyleyl)-4,5-dihydroxy-cyclopent-4-en-1,3-dione, lupulone and three of its derivatives were isolated from the ethyl acetate soluble fraction. The chalcones, including xanthohumol, significantly inhibited the production of NO by suppressing the expression of iNOS and it is suggested that the double bond in α and β position of chalcones structure is important for the inhibitory activity of iNOS expression, by the comparison of the activities of these compounds and their chemical structures.

List of Abbreviations

Inos	Inducible nitric oxide synthase
NO	Nitric oxide
LPS	Lipopolysaccharide
DMSO	Dimethyl sulfoxide
NF-kB	Nuclear factor-kB

Introduction

Hops, the female inflorescences of the hop plant (*Humulus lupulus* L.), are widely used in the brewing industry to add bitterness and aroma to beer. Hop cones are also used in folk medicine as a tranquilizer or bitter stomachic. In the 1950s and 1960s, some papers reported the existence of substances with estrogen-like activity in hop cones (Chury, 1960; Bednar and Zenisek, 1961), and Kumai and his colleagues discovered that gonadotropin inhibitors were contained in hop cones (Kumai and Okamoto, 1984). Recently, some flavanones and chalcones with prenyl or geranyl groups have been identified in hops and beers, and their biological activities such as the inhibition of bone resorption (Tobe *et al.*, 1997), inhibition of diacylglycerol acyltransferase (Tabata *et al.*, 1997) and antimicrobial activities (Haas and Barsoumian, 1994) have been reported. Moreover, some constituents of hops have been reported to inhibit the growth of breast cancer cells in a dose-dependent manner (Miranda *et al.*, 1999). So, because of their potential anticancer properties, active agents from hops have received much recent attention. Xanthohumol, the principal flavonoid in hops, was reported to inhibit the proliferation of human breast cancer MCF-7 cells, colon cancer HT-29 cells and ovarian cancer A-2780 cells *in vitro* (Miranda *et al.*, 1999). Xanthohumol has also been shown to inhibit the ethoxyresorufin *O*-deethylase activity of recombinant human CYP1A1 and CYP1B1, and the acetanilide 4-hydroxylase activity of CYP1A2 (Miranda *et al.*, 2000). These findings suggest that further investigations on the biological activities of hops and on the active agents in this plant may be beneficial.

Nitric oxide (NO) is a gaseous free radical that is released by a family of enzymes, including a constitutive NO synthase and an inducible one (iNOS) (Vanvaskas and Schmidt, 1997). The excessive and prolonged NO generation mediated by iNOS has attracted attention because of its relevance to epithelial carcinogenesis (Tsuji *et al.*, 1996; Xie *et al.*, 1997). It has been reported that NO is also involved in the production of vascular epidermal growth factor (Xiong *et al.*, 1998), the overexpression of which induces angiogenesis and vascular hyperpermeability, and accelerates tumor development (Larcher *et al.*, 1998).

Beer in Health and Disease Prevention
ISBN: 978-0-12-373891-2

Nuclear factor-kB (NF-kB) and MAP kinase (including Erk1/2, SAPK/JNK, p. 38) are important regulators of iNOS expression in lipopolysaccharide (LPS)-induced macrophages (Bhat *et al.*, 1998; Pahl, 1999).

In this chapter, search for inhibitors of NO production in *Humulus lupulus* L. by activity-guiding fractionation and purification were performed, using an LPS/IFN-γ-induced NO production test in mouse macrophage RAW 264.7 cells. As a result, we have identified several compounds to be potent inhibitors of both the production of NO and the expression of iNOS.

Inhibitory Effects of the Ethyl Acetate Fraction, the *n*-Butanol Fraction and the Aqueous Fraction of Hops on NO Production Induced by LPS/IFN-γ in RAW 264.7 Cells

The hops CAS pellet (2.5 kg) was extracted with ethyl acetate to obtain a dark green extract (PEE, 329.17 g). The pellet was then extracted with 80% acetone (31 × three times), and the extract obtained was suspended in water and partitioned with *n*-butanol. Evaporation of the solvent yielded the *n*-butanol fraction (PEB, 84.19 g) and the aqueous fraction (PEW, 282.52 g).

RAW 264.7 cells were treated with LPS (100 ng/ml), IFN-γ (100 units/ml) and test samples dissolved in dimethyl sulfoxide (DMSO) (final DMSO concentration 0.2%, v/v). The levels of NO_2^- in the supernatant were measured by Griess assay after 16 h of incubation at 37°C. The inhibitory rate on NO production induced by LPS/IFN-γ was calculated by the NO_2^- levels as follows: Inhibitory rate (%) = 100 × (LPS/IFN−LPS/IFN/sample)/(LPS/IFN-untreated). Cytotoxicity was measured by the 3-(4,5-dimethylthiazol-2-yl)-2,5-diphenyltetrazolium bromide (MTT) assay. The percentage of suppression was calculated by comparing the absorbance of sample-treated cells with that of non-treated cells. The ethyl acetate soluble fraction, the *n*-butanol soluble fraction and the aqueous fraction of *Humuluslupulus* L. were tested for their inhibitory activities on the production of NO induced by LPS/IFN-γ. As shown in Figure 77.1, the ethyl acetate fraction exhibited the strongest inhibitory activity on NO production. The *n*-butanol fraction also inhibited NO production induced by LPS/IFN-γ; however, the aqueous fraction showed no inhibitory activity. These assay results suggested that the inhibitory agents in *Humuluslupulus* L. are low-polarity constituents.

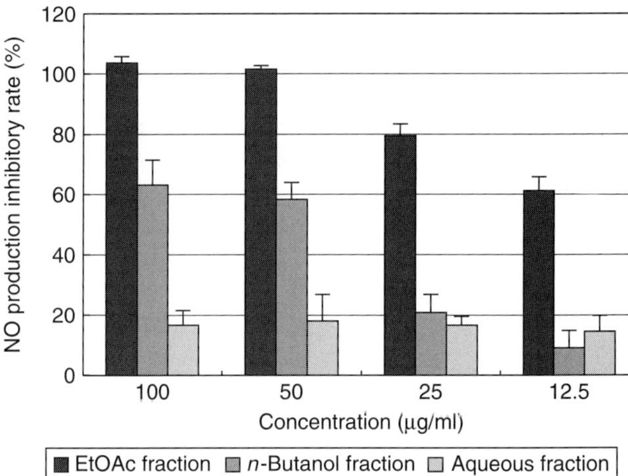

Figure 77.1 Inhibitory effects of the ethyl acetate fraction, the *n*-butanol fraction and the aqueous fraction of *Humulus lupulus* L. on NO production induced by LPS/IFN-γ. RAW 264.7 cells were treated with LPS/IFN-γ alone or together with the fractions at the concentrations indicated. After 16 h incubation, the supernatants were tested by Griess assay and the inhibitory rates were calculated. The experiment was performed independently twice and the data are expressed as mean ± SD values. An MTT assay was performed simultaneously, and the cell viabilities were more than 95%, except for 100 μg/ml PEE (6.4%) and for 50 μg/ml PEE (11.1%).

Mechanistic Examination for Inhibitory Effect of the Ethyl Acetate Fraction of Hops on NO Production

Inhibitors of NO production by macrophages act mainly through two mechanisms: the inhibition of iNOS expression and the inhibition of enzyme activity. Therefore, we examined the effect of the ethyl acetate fraction on iNOS protein expression by Western blotting. Cells were treated with LPS/IFN-γ alone or together with different doses of the ethyl acetate fraction. The treated and untreated cells were then collected and tested for their iNOS protein levels by Western blotting analysis. The results of Western blotting are shown in Figure 77.2. Although iNOS protein was undetectable in the untreated cells, it was significantly induced in cells stimulated with LPS/IFN-γ. Treatment with the ethyl acetate fraction inhibited the LPS/IFN-γ-induced iNOS protein expression in a dose-dependent manner. The results suggested that the ethyl acetate fraction of *Humulus lupulus* L. strongly inhibits the production of NO induced by LPS/IFN-γ by suppressing the expression of the iNOS protein.

Isolation and Characterization of Hops Derived Inhibitors for NO Production

Then the further bioassay-based fractionation has been performed: 262.7 g of the PEE fraction was separated by a silica gel column chromatography eluted with a hexane-ethyl acetate gradient (0→100%) of increasing polarity to give 15 fractions: PEE-1 (1.9 g), PEE-2 (5.1 g), PEE-3 (41.8 g), PEE-4 (19.1 g), PEE-5 (8.6 g), PEE-6 (39.1 g), PEE-7 (22.8 g), PEE-8 (13.6 g), PEE-9 (8.1 g), PEE-10 (33.1 g), PEE-11 (18.1 g), PEE-12 (21.6 g), PEE-13 (7.4 g), PEE-14 (5.2 g), PEE-15 (4.3 g). Fraction 1 inhibited NO production but concomitant cytotoxicity was observed.

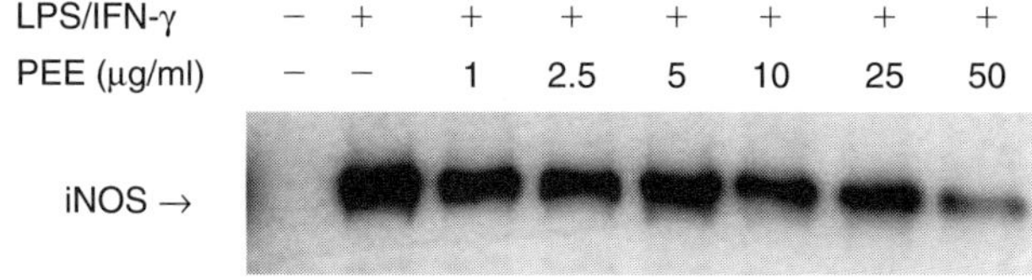

Figure 77.2 Inhibitory effects of the ethyl acetate fraction of *Humulus lupulus* L. on the iNOS expression induced by LPS/IFN-γ. Confluent RAW 264.7 cells were stimulated by the indicated conditions. The cells were collected and proteins were extracted, then, 10 μg of protein were separated on 7.5% SDS/PAGE and tested by Western blotting. The arrow signal indicates the 136 kDa iNOS-specific band.

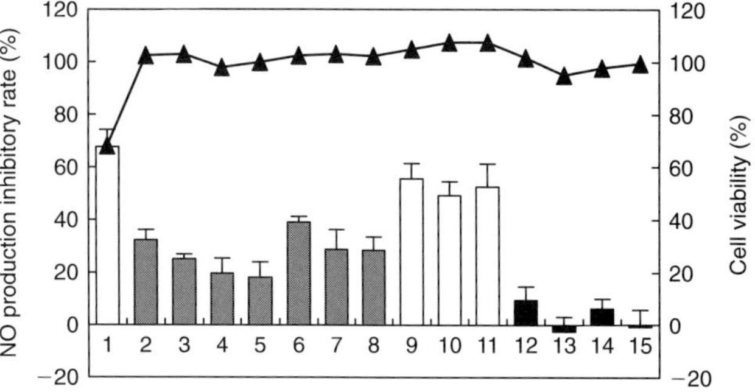

Figure 77.3 Inhibitory effects of the subfractions 1–15 of the ethyl acetate fraction of *Humulus lupulus* L. on the NO production induced by LPS/IFN-γ. RAW 264.7 cells were treated with LPS/IFN-γ alone or together with each fraction at a concentration of 10 μg/ml. After 16 h incubation, the supernatants were tested by Griess assay and the inhibitory rates were calculated. The experiment was performed independently in duplicate twice and the data are expressed as mean ± SD values. An MTT assay was performed simultaneously, and the solid line indicates the relative cell viability values.

Among the other fractions, fractions 9–11 also showed strong inhibitory activities with no cytotoxic effects. The inhibitory effects of other fractions were much weaker, especially the last four fractions (12–15), which contained the high-polarity constituents (Figure 77.3).

Fraction PEE-1 was separated by normal-phase silica gel column chromatography to obtain compound 1. Fraction PEE-9 was separated by a combination of normal-phase silica gel column chromatography, Sephadex LH-20 column chromatography and high-pressure liquid chromatography (HPLC) to obtain compound 2. Fraction PEE-10 was separated by a combination of normal-phase silica gel column chromatography, Sephadex LH-20 column chromatography and HPLC to obtain compounds 8–11. Fraction PEE-11 was separated by a combination of normal-phase silica gel column chromatography, Sephadex LH-20 column chromatography and HPLC to obtain compounds 3–7. Their chemical structures were determined by a combination of UV, IR, MS and NMR as shown in Figure 77.4. Chemical structures of known compounds 1 (humulene), 3 (xanthohumol), 4 (xanthohumol D), 5 (dihydroxanthohumol), 6 (xanthohumol B) and 8 (lupulone) were determined by comparison with the published data (Stevens *et al.*, 1997, 2000). Compound 2 was first isolated from a natural source, although its chemical synthesis has been reported. We consider it to be a type of biosynthesis product in *Humulus lupulus* L. Other structures were determined by a combination of UV, IR, MS and NMR spectral data (^{1}H-NMR, ^{13}C-NMR, HMBC, HMQC, ^{1}H-^{1}H COSY). Compound 7 is a new chalcone, an oxidation product of compound 3 (xanthohumol). So far, there has been no report of its isolation. Compounds 9–11 are derivatives of compound 8 (lupulone, a main β acid in hops), and are likely to be formed during the process of its oxidation.

Inhibitory Effects of Compounds 1–11 on the Production of NO Induced by LPS/INF-γ

The inhibitory activities of these isolated compounds were evaluated. Most of them exhibited significant inhibitory effects on the production of NO induced by LPS/IFN-γ. As shown in Table 77.1, the five chalcones (compounds 3–7) strongly inhibited NO production at low concentrations without showing cytotoxic effects. The inhibitory activities of chalcones (compounds 3–7) were much stronger than those of lupulone and its derivatives (compounds 8–11), suggesting that chalcones are the main inhibitors of NO production found in *Humulus lupulus* L. By comparing the inhibitory activities of these compounds and their chemical structures, we identified some interesting features that may affect the level of activity. Among the isolated chalcones, compound 5, which has no double bond between α and β position, inhibited NO production much more weakly than the other four compounds (3, 4, 6 and 7). This suggests that the double bond may be important for the inhibitory activity of chalcones. Compounds 4, 6 and 7 have the same backbone structure as xanthohumol (compound 3), but differ in the prenyl side chain. The inhibitory activities of these compounds are almost the same, which indicates that the prenyl chain is not necessary for inhibiting NO production. Compounds 9–11 are oxidative derivatives of lupulone (compound 8), with oxidation at different side-chain positions of lupulone. These compounds exhibited either much weaker inhibitory activities on NO production than lupulone (compound 9) or false inhibitions with strong cytotoxicity (compounds 10 and 11), meaning that oxidation may reduce the inhibitory activity of lupulone on NO production.

Inhibitory Effects of Compounds 1–8 on the Expression of iNOS Induced by LPS/IFN-γ

The effects of these isolated compounds on the expression of iNOS were also examined by Western blotting.

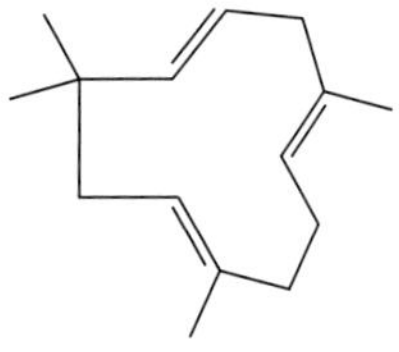

Figure 77.4 Chemical structures of compounds isolated from the ethyl acetate fraction of hops.

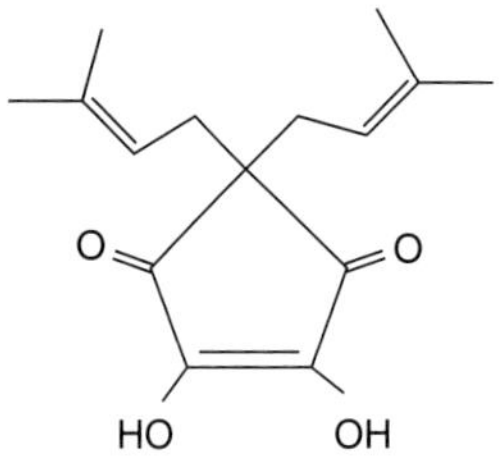

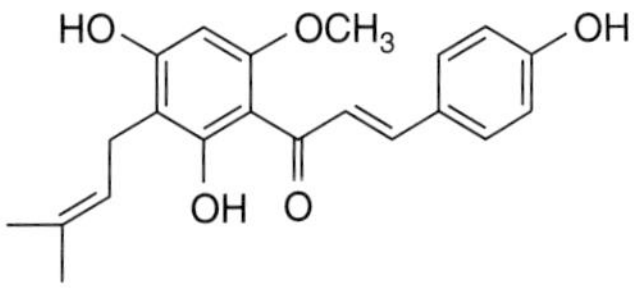

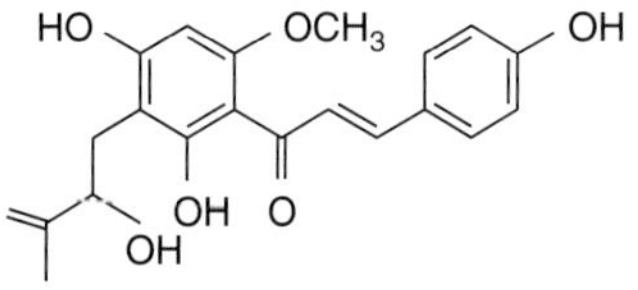

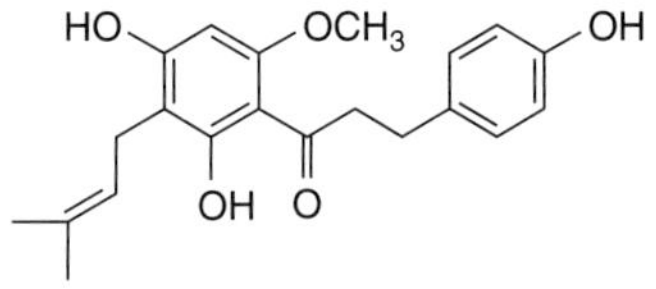

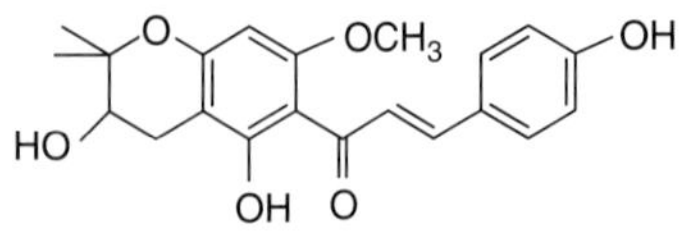

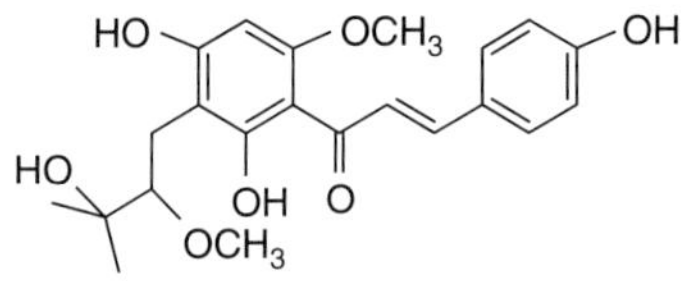

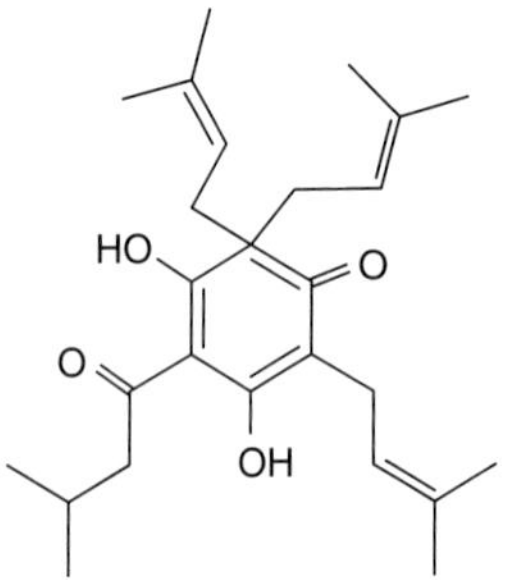

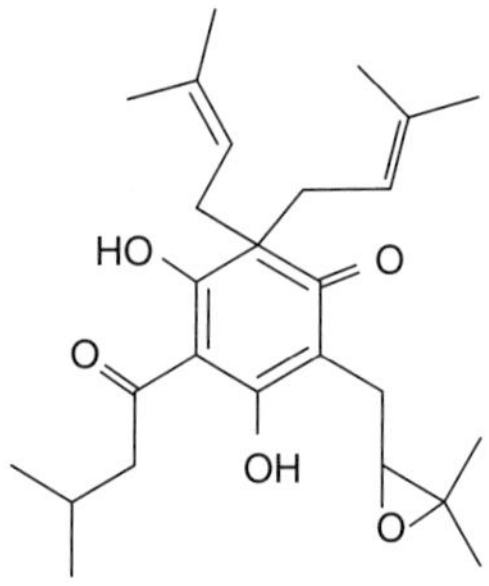

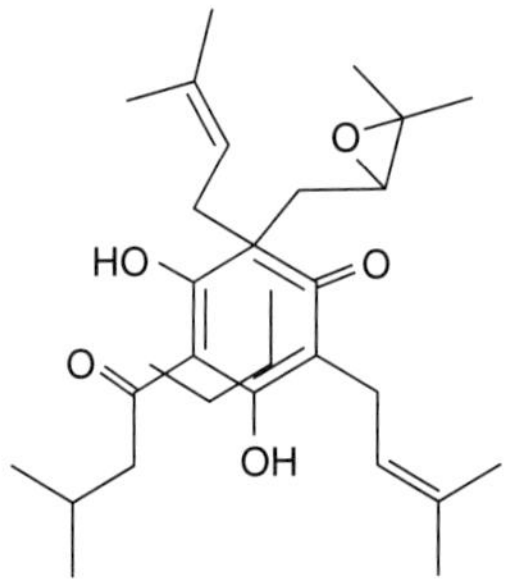

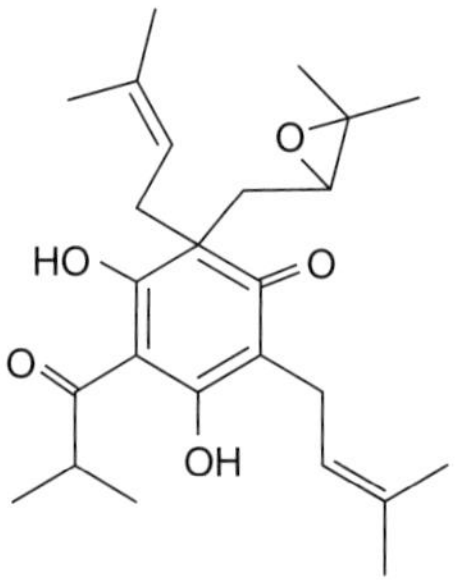

As shown in Figure 77.5, RAW 264.7 cells were treated with LPS/IFN-γ alone or together with isolated compounds 1–8 at 5 μg/ml, a concentration at which no cytotoxicity was observed. Compounds 3, 4, 6 and 7, which significantly inhibited NO production at 5 μg/ml, completely suppressed the expression of iNOS induced by LPS/IFN-γ. Other compounds (compounds 1, 2 and 8) did not inhibit iNOS expression at this concentration, whereas compound 5 slightly suppressed iNOS expression. Taken together, these results suggest that the chalcones, the main inhibitory agents of NO production in hops, inhibit NO production by suppressing the expression of iNOS protein induced by LPS/IFN-γ.

Macrophages play major roles in inflammation and host defense mechanisms against bacterial and viral infections (Adam and Hamilton, 1984). During acute and

Table 77.1 Inhibitory effects of compounds 1–11 on the production of NO induced by LPS/INF-γ

Compound	*Concentration (μg/ml)*	*NO P I R (%)*	*Cytotoxicity*
1	100	109.60 ± 3.0	+++
	50	106.91 ± 4.72	++
	10	34.98 ± 6.30	–
	5	15.70 ± 6.28	–
	1	2.69 ± 17.36	–
2	100	29.39 ± 8.95	–
	50	19.88 ± 3.92	–
	10	4.61 ± 5.73	–
	5	6.63 ± 3.31	–
	1	4.32 ± 5.01	–
3	100	94.83 ± 11.44	+++
	50	90.23 ± 15.38	+++
	10	91.67 ± 13.77	+++
	5	83.62 ± 10.08	–
	1	18.10 ± 13.55	–
4	100	104.90 ± 6.17	+++
	50	102.59 ± 6.72	+++
	10	103.75 ± 8.04	++
	5	76.37 ± 11.77	–
	1	8.07 ± 2.49	–
5	100	98.27 ± 1.45	+++
	50	98.56 ± 4.05	+++
	10	67.44 ± 11.62	+
	5	18.73 ± 3.92	–
	1	0.29 ± 12.25	–
6	100	101.21 ± 11.85	+++
	50	108.25 ± 4.75	+++
	10	103.18 ± 8.46	++
	5	91.97 ± 5.07	–
	1	34.98 ± 9.77	–
7	100	104.15 ± 9.56	+++
	50	103.63 ± 8.60	+++
	10	103.25 ± 8.09	–
	5	97.76 ± 8.60	–
	1	17.49 ± 6.45	–
8	100	101.72 ± 1.99	+++
	50	104.60 ± 3.25	+++
	10	74.14 ± 8.52	+
	5	35.34 ± 14.91	–
	1	22.41 ± 10.64	–
9	100	97.80 ± 1.69	+++
	50	88.99 ± 5.64	+++
	10	21.15 ± 11.72	–
	5	4.85 ± 11.95	–
	1	-21.15 ± 9.90	–
10	100	98.68 ± 3.01	+++
	50	101.32 ± 3.91	+++
	10	88.55 ± 14.71	+++
	5	55.90 ± 10.07	+++
	1	1.32 ± 2.50	+
11	100	102.46 ± 1.59	+++
	50	100.31 ± 2.54	+++
	10	98.00 ± 13.00	+
	5	35.38 ± 24.93	+
	1	2.15 ± 6.99	–

NO P I R (%): NO production inhibitory rate (%); +++, cell viability < 50%; ++, cell viability < 80%; +, cell viability < 95%; –, cell viability > 95%.

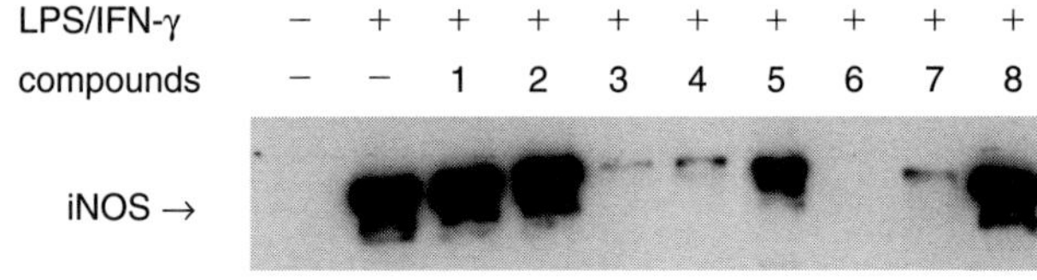

Figure 77.5 Inhibitory effects of compounds 1–8 on the expression of iNOS induced by LPS/IFN-γ. RAW 264.7 cells were stimulated with LPS/IFN-γ alone or together with a 5 μg/ml solution of each compound. The untreated and treated cells were collected and examined by Western blotting. The experiment was done independently twice and a representative result is shown. The arrow signal indicates the 136 kDa iNOS-specific band.

chronic inflammation, excessive production of NO may cause severe injury to host cells and tissues (Knowles and Moncada, 1994). iNOS, the enzyme responsible for the synthesis of NO in macrophages, is not expressed under normal conditions but is strongly induced upon exposure to LPS/IFN-γ. Through bioactivity-guided fractionation, we purified several NO production inhibitors from the ethyl acetate fraction of *Humulus lupulus* L. and compared their activities against their chemical structures. Xanthohumol (compound 3) and several other chalcones were found to be the major inhibitory constituents of hops. It has been recently reported that xanthohumol is the potent inducer of quinone reductase via activation of nrf2 by the reaction of its double bond between α and β position with Keap1 protein using matrix-assisted laser desorption time-of-flight mass spectrometry (Liu *et al.*, 2005). It is suggested from our results that xanthohumol and related chalcones might interact with the regulator for the iNOS expression.

Summary Points

- The ethyl acetate soluble fraction of hops (*Humulus lupulus* L.) inhibited LPS/IFN-γ-induced production of NO.
- The ethyl acetate soluble fraction of hops inhibited the expression of iNOS by Western blotting analysis.
- Eleven compounds (humulene, five chalcones, 2,2-di-(3-methyl-2-butyleyl)-4,5-dihydroxy-cyclopent-4-en-1,3-dione, lupulone and three of its derivatives) have been isolated from the ethyl acetate soluble fraction of hops.
- The chalcones, including xanthohumol, significantly inhibited the production of NO by suppressing the expression of iNOS and it is suggested that the double bond in α and β position of chalcones structure is important for the inhibitory activity of iNOS expression.

References

Adam, D.O. and Hamilton, T.A. (1984). *Annu. Rev. Immunol.* 2, 283–318.

Bednar, J. and Zenisek, A. (1961). *Brauwissenschaft* 14, 4–7.

Bhat, N.R., Zhang, P., Lee, J.C. and Hogan, E.L. (1998). *J. Neurosci.* 18, 1633–1641.

Chury, J. (1960). *Experientia* 16, 194–195.

Haas, G.J. and Barsoumian, R. (1994). *J. Food Protect.* 57, 59–61.

Henderson, M.C., Miranda, C.L., Stevens, J.F., Deinzer, M.L. and Buhler, D.R. (2000). *Xenobiotica* 30, 235–251.

Knowles, R.G. and Moncada, S. (1994). *Biochem. J.* 298, 249–258.

Kumai, A. and Okamoto, R. (1984). *Toxicol. Lett.* 21, 203–207.

Larcher, F., Murillas, R., Bolontrade, M., Conti, C.J. and Jorcano, J.L. (1998). *Oncogene* 17, 303–311.

Liu, G., Eggler, A.L., Dietz, B.M., Mesecar, A.D., Bolton, J.L., Pezzuto, J.M. and van Breemen, R.B. (2005). *Anal. Chem.* 77, 6407–6414.

Miranda, C.L., Stevens, J.F., Helmrich, A., Henderson, M.C., Rodriguez, R.J., Yang, Y.H., Deinzer, M.L., Barnes, D.W. and Buhler, D.R. (1999). *Food Chem. Toxicol.* 37, 271–285.

Miranda, C.L., Yang, Y.H., Henderson, M.C., Stevens, J.F., Santana-Rios, G., Deinzer, M.L. and Buhler, D.R. (2000). *Drug Metab. Dispos.* 28, 1297–1302.

Pahl, H.L. (1999). *Oncogene* 18, 6853–6866.

Stevens, J.F., Ivancic, M., Hsu, V.L. and Deinzer, M.L. (1997). *Phytochemistry* 44, 1575–1585.

Stevens, J.F., Taylor, A.W., Nickerson, G.B., Ivancic, M., Henning, J., Haunold, A. and Deinzer, M.L. (2000). *Phytochemistry* 53, 759–775.

Tabata, N., Ito, M., Tomoda, H. and Omura, S. (1997). *Phytochemistry* 46, 683–687.

Tobe, H., Muraki, Y., Kitamura, K., Komiyama, O., Sato, Y., Sugioka, T., Maruyama, H.B., Matsuda, E. and Nagai, M. (1997). *Biosci. Biotechnol. Biochem.* 61, 158–159.

Tsuji, S., Kawano, S., Tsujii, M., Takei, Y., Tanaka, M., Sawaoka, H., Nagano, K., Fusamoto, H. and Kamada, T. (1996). *Cancer Lett.* 108, 195–200.

Vanvaskas, S. and Schmidt, H.H.H.W. (1997). *J. Natl. Cancer Inst.* 89, 406–407.

Xie, K., Huang, S., Dong, Z., Juang, S.H., Wang, Y. and Fidler, I.J. (1997). *J. Natl. Cancer Inst.* 89, 421–427.

Xiong, M., Elson, G., Legarda, D. and Leibovich, S.J. (1998). *Am. J. Pathol.* 153, 587–598.

78

Non-specific Hydroxyl Radical Scavenging Properties of Melanoidins from Beer

Francisco J. Morales Instituto del Frío, Consejo Superior de Investigaciones Científicas, Madrid, Spain

Abstract

Melanoidins are widely distributed in western-countries diet, due to home or industrial processing of foods. In the past, melanoidins were considered as inert, brown-colored polymeric food constituents. However, recent research into their nutritional, physiological and functional properties has suggested that they have antioxidant properties. This chapter described the non-specific hydroxyl radical scavenging properties of melanoidins isolated from different styles of beer. During beer processing, melanoidins are formed mainly during kilning in a different yield according to the raw material and technological conditions applied. Melanoidins from pilsener beer, Belgium Abbeys style beer and dry-stout beer have shown hydroxyl radical scavenging properties in different extent. Beer melanoidins inhibit the 2-deoxy-D-ribose degradation competitively, showing that they are scavengers of hydroxyl radicals. Brewery companies should put more attention on those newly formed compounds since they may balance the overall antioxidant activity due to the loss of naturally occurring antioxidant substances.

List of Abbreviations

ESR	Electron spin resonance spectroscopy
LC	Liquid chromatography
TCA	Trichloroacetic acid
TBA	2-Thiobarbituric acid
DR	2-Deoxy-D-ribose
MR	Maillard reaction
MRP	Maillard reaction products
DPPH	2,2-Diphenyl-1-picrylhydrazyl
DMPD	*N,N*-Dimethyl-*p*-phenylenediamine
ABTS	2,2′-Azobis(3-ethylbenzothiazoline-6-sulfonic acid)
ROS	Reactive oxygen species
DTPA	Diethylenetriaminepentaacetic acid
Trolox	6-Hydroxy-2,5,7,8-tetramethylchroman-2-Carboxulic acid
CL	Chemiluminescence
DMPO	5,5-Dimethyl-1-pyrroline-*N*-oxide

Introduction

The beer production is an extremely complicated process since many variables are taking place and the chemistry and biochemistry involved in are highly complex. The compositions and concentrations of reducing substances are constantly changing throughout the process as well as raw material and treatment applied is a source of variation as well. Slight changes in structure, or even conformational changes, can alter the antioxidant activity of a compound. In this sense, the brewing industry is concerned with the stability of the beer under shelf-life. In recent years, there has been a general trend toward minimizing the use of added antioxidants in food in general and in beer production in particular (Pokorný, 1991). It is therefore desirable to prevent oxidation by maximizing the natural occurring reducing agent present in the raw materials and hence in the wort, as well as retaining newly formed heat-induced compounds which offer an overall reducing effect in the beer to increase its stability during storage (Galic *et al.*, 1994). This issue is greatly recognized by consumers and administrative bodies to keep the natural properties of this beverage.

But not only shelf-life is partly affected by the antioxidative status of the beer, it is known that antioxidants activity in beer plays a crucial role in providing flavor stability to beer (Bamforth *et al.*, 1993). Antioxidants formed during brewing are capable of delaying, retarding or preventing oxidation processes caused by activated or radical species and they are therefore thought to have a significant effect in malting and brewing as inhibitors of oxidative damage (Araki *et al.*, 1999). Furthermore, compounds with antioxidant activity play a crucial role maintaining the flavor stability of beer during storage by reducing the rate of lipid oxidation and thereby preventing the production of stale flavor compounds (Walters *et al.*, 1997; Goupy *et al.*, 1999). These components can inhibit lipoxygenase activity during malting and mashing and limit auto-oxidation during brewing and beer storage. Then protection of the natural polyphenols antioxidants of barley and the production of new antioxidants during malting are of great interest (Maillard and Berset, 1995).

Beer in Health and Disease Prevention
ISBN: 978-0-12-373891-2

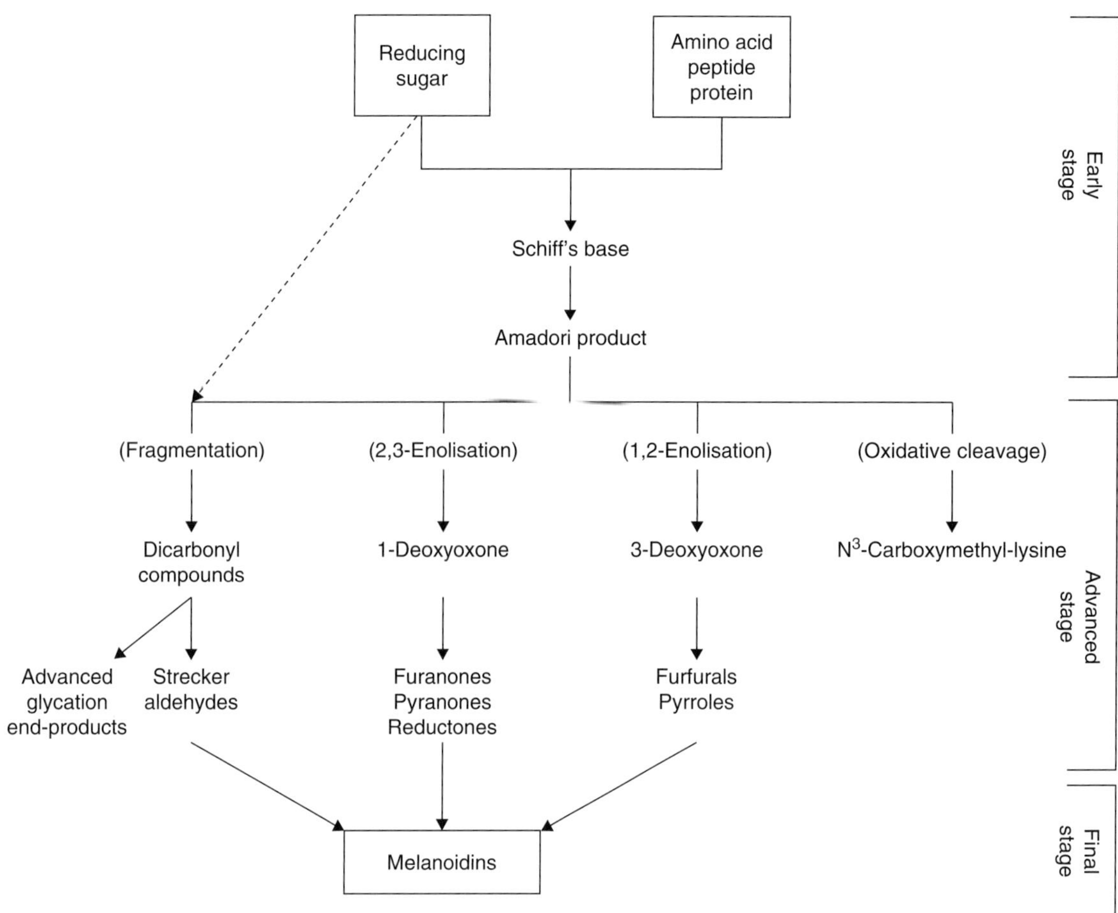

Figure 78.1 Schematic overview of the MR.

Formation of stable antioxidant compounds in beer is important from a technological point of view but from a health point of view as well. Beer is a low-alcohol beverage brewed from natural ingredients which may be involved in the prevention of cardiovascular and carcinogenesis diseases (Henderson *et al.*, 2000; Bamforth, 2002). One mechanism through which it may contribute to positive health effects is related to its antioxidant properties (Arimoto-Kobayashi *et al.*, 1999; Ghiselli *et al.*, 2000; Rivero *et al.*, 2005). An increase in plasma antioxidant capacity has been reported to occur following the consumption of certain types of beer and this increase can be associated with levels in plasma flavonoids in humans (Ghiselli *et al.*, 2000).

As reviewed by Chandra (2002), several reducing agents that are known to be important in malting and brewing include melanoidins and reductones, phenolics substances, thiols, non-fermentable reducing sugars and carotenoids and vitamins. Of these, melanoidins (formed during kilning throughout Maillard reaction (MR)) and polyphenols (natural from the barley, malt and hops) are the most significant sources of natural antioxidants in beer. On the other hand, a mixture of different types of antioxidants, which work via different mechanism, can often display a synergistic effect, for instance, a peroxide decomposer and a free radical inhibitor. The content of melanoidins and polyphenols in beer is largely influenced by the genetic factor of its raw materials and therefore by the environmental conditions in which they grow and it is also influenced by the technological brewing factors (Nicoli *et al.*, 1999; Lugasi, 2003).

Melanoidins are formed in the malt by both the thermal degradation of sugars and by the MR. MR occurs during heating of many foods of a typical Western diet which are heat processed and the resulting products have a direct impact on the organoleptic properties of the product (Ames, 2003). The MR is a complex network of reactions and is summarized in Figure 78.1. The initial stage involves the condensation of a carbonyl group, mostly form a reducing sugar, with a free amino group such as the epsilon amino group of lysine residue within peptides or proteins. This results in the formation of an unstable Schiff base, which spontaneously rearranges to form the more stable Amadori rearrangement product. Several Amadori products could be formed depending on the reactants taking place in the rearrangement, for instance, fructosyllysine is formed when initial sugar is glucose and amino group is lysine. Later, Amadori products can be degraded by several pathways, leading the formation of reductones and furfurals. These compounds can react further to give colored, low molecular mass products and melanoidins. On the other hand, Amadori products can also fragment to form various dicarbonyl compounds which are more reactive compounds and can lead to the formation of compounds that contribute to flavor such as Strecker aldehydes, pyrazines, thiophenes and furans. In the final stage of the MR, melanoidins are formed from reactive compounds formed in previous stages. Then melanoidins are formed by cyclizations, dehydrations, retroaldolizations, rearrangements, isomerizations and condensations of MR products, but none of them has been fully characterized. This final stage is not well characterized from a chemical and structural point of view yet.

During the brewing process, melanoidins are provided mainly from the malt, although they are also formed during mashing and wort boiling. It is known that MR products act as scavengers for reactive oxygen species (ROS) such as superoxide, peroxide and hydroxyl radicals. Melanoidins mainly consisted of compounds formed from carbohydrates and their degradation products. Besides proteins, other food constituents were incorporated in the melanoidin structure as well, such as lipid oxidation products and phenolics compounds in the case of beer and coffee as well. On the other hand, melanoidins comprise a substantial proportion of several food products apart from beer, such as coffee, roasted malt, breakfast cereals and bread, and are widely consumed with dietary components. In addition, melanoidins possess antioxidant activity (Manzocco *et al.*, 2001), are responsible for the development of color in heat-processed food products (Rizzi, 1997), may contribute to food texture and are likely to play a role in the binding of nutritionally important metals (O'Brien and Morrissey, 1997), potentially undesirable dietary compounds (Yen and Hsieh, 1994) and flavor compounds (Hofmann and Schieberle, 2002).

Concerning the natural phenolics substances present in the malt, they act as radical scavengers and are highly effective in inhibiting non-enzymatic lipid peroxidation as stated for a large number of studies. About 70–80% of the polyphenols in wort are malt-derived and 20–30% are from the hops (Chandra, 2002). Polyphenols are the most important antioxidant in pilsener malts; however, in dark malts MR products seem to be the major antioxidants. The most abundant polyphenols in malt are (+)-catechin, (−)-epicatechin, (+)-gallocatechin, ferrulic acid, *p*-coumaric acid and vanillic acid (McMurrough *et al.*, 1983). Traditionally, the use of colored malt is known to improve the stability of the finished beer, and it has also been shown that higher colored beers retain a greater reducing power during storage (Chapon *et al.*, 1971; Coghe and Delvaux, 2002). The final beer produced has a reducing power mainly dependent on melanoidin compounds and simple and polymerized polyphenols. It is likely that the polyphenols from these two sources are different, and the specific properties are highly dependent on the degree of polymerization. Furthermore, correlations between levels of (+)-catechin or ferrulic acid and antioxidant activity are poor, suggesting that other components, for example, polyphenols oligomers and MR products also contribute to the total antioxidant activity of beer (Woffenden *et al.*, 2002). An obvious effect will be a decrease in reducing power as oxidation gradually occurs over time. Oxygen in the head-space will therefore cause a problem during beer storage.

Kilning is the most important stage of malt production with regard to the formation of antioxidants since majority of reducing power come from the kilned malt. In fact, germination releases reducing sugars and amino acids. During the first step of kilning, the water at the surface layers of the grain is removed (the humidity falls from 0.45 to 0.12 g/g) and the MR is initiated. By altering the drying phase in a kiln or in a roasting cylinder, a wide assortment of dark specialty malts can be produced ranging in color from 5 to 1,600 European Brewery Convention (EBC) units. The final step of kilning (curing) involved temperatures up to 95°C causing the development of color, flavor and aroma (Woffenden *et al.*, 2002). Pale and larger malts are produced by kilning at 50–85°C over 28–32 h, but temperatures of 80–100°C are applied for up to 170 min for caramel malt production (Blenkinsop, 1991). Finally, classical colored malts are roasted at temperatures up to 240°C. Apart from the MR caramelization of sugars can also occur during the last stages of kilning, catalyzed by the low concentration of organic acids (Karakus, 1975). In general, pale malts contribute less reducing power to the wort and beer than higher color malts. Kilning involves drying of the malt for up to 30 h and results in a stable product that can be readily handled, stored and milled. The reducing power is associated with the higher temperatures involved in the production of color compounds, including both melanoidin and phenolics species (Woffenden *et al.*, 2002). As results of the higher temperatures applied for the production of dark specialty malts, higher levels of antioxidants (reductones and melanoidins) are formed during the MR. Consequently, beers with dark malts normally have a longer shelf-life than pale beers (Cantrell and Griggs, 1996).

Isolation of Water-Soluble Melanoidins from Commercial Beer Samples

There are several procedures to isolate the water-soluble high molecular weight (HMW) fraction from beer, named melanoidin. Dialysis has been widely used but some drawbacks concerning potential contamination and structural changes on the melanoidin have arisen since procedure usually takes 3 or 4 days. It is expected further that condensation of polymers structures during the dialysis and final structures could be different to the initial ones. High performance gel filtration chromatography is an efficient approach but the reduced amount of recovered melanoidin

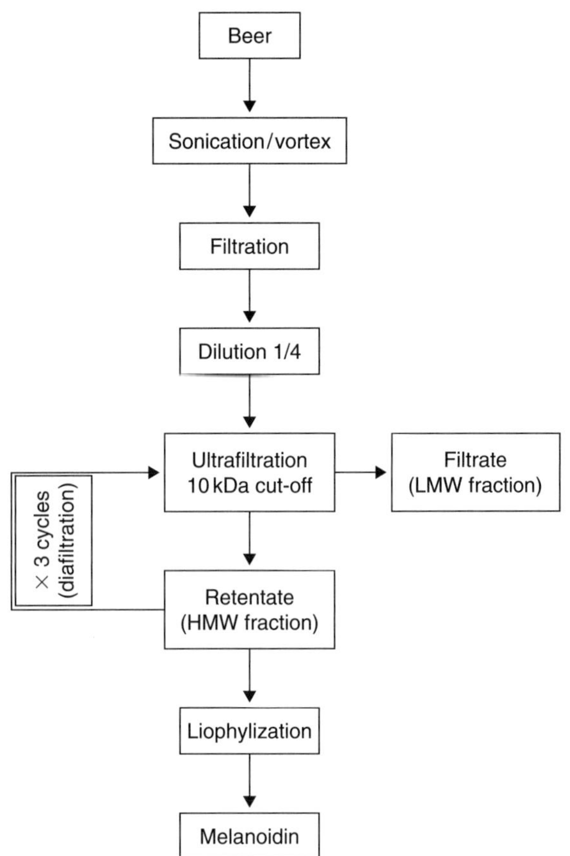

Figure 78.2 Flow diagram for isolation of soluble melanoidin fraction from beer.

is the limiting factor. Lately, ultrafiltration has been used by applying membranes with different cut-off, and provides a reliable and smart procedure for isolation in short time. A scheme of the procedure is depicted in Figure 78.2. Ultrafiltration combined a cost-effective, low time-consuming procedure with higher recoveries. Then, after sonication and appropriate dilution beer samples are subjected to ultrafiltration using an Amicon ultrafiltration cell model 8400 (Amicon, Beverly, MA, USA), equipped with a 10,000 Da nominal molecular mass cut-off membrane. The retentate was filled up to 200 ml with water and washed again. This washing procedure is repeated at least three times to ensure the absence of low molecular weight material (LMW). The HMW fraction corresponding to melanoidins can be freeze-dried and stored in a dessicator until analysis. Isolated beer melanoidins could be reanalyzed by gel filtration chromatography in absence of LMW compounds as described by Morales *et al.* (2005).

Antioxidant Activity of Maillard Reaction Products (MRP)

Most of the antioxidant properties of MR products have been evaluated on single model systems (sugar – amino acids) and latter on the different fractions according to their molecular weight. The main factors affecting the formation of antioxidant compounds are known to be pH (Lingnert and Eriksson, 1981), nature and molar ration of reactants (Kawashima *et al.*, 1977), water activity (Eichner, 1981) and temperature and heating time (Lingnert and Eriksson, 1980). But it is important to assess specific antioxidative activity of fractions of MRP for evaluating use in potential food processing strategies (Jing and Kitts, 2000). Several authors suggested that HMW fraction (⩾10 kDa, melanoidins) were responsible for the antioxidative efficiency of MR mixtures in water-soluble (Morales and Babbel, 2002) and water-insoluble matrices (Wagner *et al.*, 2002). Melanoidins, polymeric high molecular mass fraction of MRP, have traditionally been skipped from these studies since melanoidins have been considered as inert materials, associated to the concept of fiber.

Antioxidant activity of MRP from synthetic and food melanoidins, including beer, has been mainly related to determining peroxyl radical scavenging activity (Morales and Jiménez-Pérez, 2004) or quenching specific stable radicals, such as 2,2-diphenyl-1-picrylhydrazyl (DPPH) (Morales and Jiménez-Pérez, 2001) or *N,N*-dimethyl-*p*-phenylenediamine (DMPD) (Morales and Babbel, 2002). Few studies have reported the affinity of different model MRP to specifically scavenge hydroxyl radicals *in vitro* (Wijewickreme *et al.*, 1999). Since significant quantities of melanoidins enter in the human gut on daily basis (Ames *et al.*, 1999), it is important to assess the implication of these compounds on the overall antioxidant activity of foods. Studies focused on the antioxidant activity of melanoidins, and more specifically on the radical scavenging properties, are scarce in the literature. Furthermore, the effects of ROS and free radicals in producing tissue damage in human disorders are becoming increasingly well recognized. Active oxygen as superoxide ($O_2^{\bullet 2}$), hydrogen peroxide (H_2O_2) or hydroxyl radical ($^{\bullet}OH$) is a by-product of normal metabolism. It represents a potential toxic hazard to various biological molecules leading to tissue damage, cell injury or death (i.e. Yen and Chung, 1999). Hydroxyl radicals are short-lived, extremely reactive molecules that react by H-abstraction, electron addition or electron transfer with most organic compounds in a diffusion-limited reaction and thus cause the breakdown of essential cell constituents such as DNA, membrane lipids or cell wall polymers. Formation of $^{\bullet}OH$ or highly oxidizing species from H_2O_2 has been associated with transition metal ions such as iron and copper and reducing agents (at low concentrations) such as $O_2^{\bullet 2}$ and ascorbate. The damage induced by free radicals is often prevented by scavengers. The antioxidant activity of plasma has been shown to increase after consumption of foods high in antioxidants (Temple, 2000). Thus, phytochemicals may combat oxidative stress in the human body by maintaining a balance between oxidants and antioxidants (Temple, 2000). This is particularly important because under severe oxidative stress excessive formation of ROS and free radicals can damage biomolecules, such as DNA, proteins, lipids and carbohydrates, and lead to numerous disease conditions (Halliwell, 1996).

Methods for Assessing the Protective Effect of Molecules Toward Hydroxyl Radicals

In the past decades, scientific literature collected a huge number of procedures to assess the antioxidant activity of food constituents. Methods based on stable radicals have been criticized because these stable radicals are foreign to biological systems, in contrast to the short-lived radicals, like the hydroxyl and peroxyl radicals occurring as reaction intermediates in oxidative processes (Becker *et al.*, 2004). In general, •OH generation has three model systems, including ultraviolet photolysis of hydrogen peroxide, γ-irradiation of water (Tteiner and Babbs, 1990) and via chemical reactions. Fenton reaction is often used to generate •OH (Lloyd *et al.*, 1997). The hydroxyl radical is widely accepted to be generated when hydrogen peroxide reacts with Fe(II) (Fenton reaction).

$$Fe^{2+} + 2H_2O_2 \rightarrow Fe^{3+} + {}^{\bullet}OH + OH^-$$

There are several approaches for the detecting hydroxyl radicals or assessing the scavenging properties of substances toward hydroxyl radicals. One of these methods is the electron spin resonance spectroscopy (ESR), which measures the electron paramagnetic resonance spectrum of a spin adduct derivative after trapping (Geoffroy *et al.*, 2000; Domingues *et al.*, 2001; Mizuta *et al.*, 2002). But this method cannot be directly employed to acquire quantitative estimate of •OH production because the •OH adduct is a short-lived radical. Spin-traps are special designed molecules, which react readily with highly reactive radicals forming relatively stable spin-adducts. In the FRBR-assay (Fenton Reaction Based Radical assay), detection of hydroxyl radicals after reaction with the spin-trap 5,5-dimethyl-1-pyrroline-*N*-oxide (DMPO). But, the expensive instruments make it unsuitable for routine analysis.

Other approaches imply chemiluminescence (CL) (Parejo *et al.*, 2000; Tsai *et al.*, 2001), ultraviolet–visible and fluorescence spectrophotometry (Joseph *et al.*, 2001; Yang and Guo, 2001) or electrochemical detection (Zou *et al.*, 2002). Aromatic hydroxylation has also been applied, in which the hydroxylated products generated from the reaction of hydroxyl radicals with aromatic compounds, such as phenol, benzoic acid or salicylic acid (SA), are separated by gas chromatography or liquid chromatography (LC) by using different detectors (Coudara *et al.*, 1995; Vanhees *et al.*, 2001; Jurva *et al.*, 2002) but it presents some drawbacks (Li *et al.*, 1997). Methanesulfinic acid has also been adopted for determination of hydroxyl radicals by a spectrophotometric method (Babbs and Griffin, 1989) and LC (Fukui *et al.*, 1993). However, methanesulfinic acid is only an intermediate product, which also reacted rapidly with hydroxyl radicals leading to methanesulfonic acid and sulfate formation. Another highly sensitive method based on methyl radicals reacting with a fluorescamine-derivatized nitroxide forming a stable omethylhydroxylamine has been developed for the determination of hydroxyl radicals in biological systems (Li *et al.*, 1997). Another widely used approach in the reactions with SA to produce 2,3-dihydroxy benzoic acid (2,3-DHBA) and 2,5-dihydroxy-benzoic acid (2,5-DHBA). DHBA, as the probe of •OH, can be determined by LC.

Non-site-Specific Hydroxyl Radical (•OH) Scavenging Activity Assay

As described previously, hydroxyl radicals are easily generated by the Fenton reaction. However, the $Fe(II)/H_2O_2$ mixture has disadvantages in a scavenging assay because many antioxidants are also metal chelators. When the sample is mixed with Fe(II), it may alter the activity of Fe(II) by chelation. As a result, it is impossible to distinguish if the antioxidants are simply good metal chelators or •OH scavengers. The generation of radicals is not affected by iron chelators, such as diethylenetriaminepentaacetic acid (DTPA) or ethylenediaminetetraacetic acid (EDTA), bathophenanthroline disulfonic acid, phytic acid and bathocuprione disulfonic acid. EDTA prevent the uncontrolled generation of •OH and potential reducing effect of target substances is minimized.

Non-site-specific •OH radical scavenging activity of melanoidins can be measured according to the well-characterized method of Halliwell *et al.* (1987). Hydroxyl radical formation in a Fenton drive system in the absence or presence of melanoidins is evaluated by both time-course as to determine rate constants. Reaction mixture at a final volume of 1 ml contains 0.249 mM 2-deoxy-D-ribose (DR), 1 mM H_2O_2, 100 μM $FeCl_3$, 104 μM EDTA, 100 μM ascorbic acid, in 10 Mm NaH_2PO_4–$NaHPO_4$ buffer (pH 7.4). Solution containing EDTA and $FeCl_3$ is premixed the day before. All the solutions should be made up before use in de-aerated water. Several concentrations of melanoidins or reference antioxidant (trolox or chlorogenic acid) are tested in a final volume of 50 μl. Then reaction is initiated after the addition of hydrogen peroxide. Reaction media is incubated in a water bath at 37°C up to 120 min. The reaction is stopped by adding 100 μl of 28% (w/v) cold trichloroacetic acid (TCA) once incubation time is reached. The development of the chromogen is achieved by heating the reaction vessel in a boiling bath for 30 min before addition of 2-thiobarbituric acid (TBA) solution (1% w/v in 0.05 M NaOH). After cooling, the chromogen is determined spectrophotometrically at 532 nm against a blank containing phosphate buffer. The scavenger (melanoidin or reference antioxidant) rate constant (k_S) is determined from the plot $1/A$ vs. concentration of the scavenger (mg/ml), being A the absorbance at 532 nm of the experiment. Halliwell *et al.* (1987) proposed the reference value of 3.1×109/M/s

(0.0231 × 109 l/g/s) for the second rate constant of the reaction of DR with $^{\bullet}OH$ (k_{DR}), same value is applied for beer.

Hydroxyl Radical Scavenging Properties of Melanoidins from Beer

Hydroxyl radicals are formed in the mix by the Fenton reaction and are detected by their ability to degrade DR into fragments that on heating with TBA at low pH form a pink chromogen. TBA-adducts gave a maximum of absorbance at 532 nm which is named as positive control (Figure 78.3). The extent of the reaction can be determined by measuring the rate of inhibition of DR oxidation in the presence of the antioxidant molecule. Addition of hydroxyl radical scavengers competes with DR for hydroxyl radicals and diminishes chromogen formation at a defined time of reaction (Figure 78.3). Then, it is able to calculate a percentage of inhibition of the target molecule on the hydroxyl radicals. This approach cannot be directly applied when the aim is to evaluate the hydroxyl scavenging properties of different complex systems, where different molecules are expected. It is necessary to gain insight on the hydroxyl radical scavenging activity through a period of time.

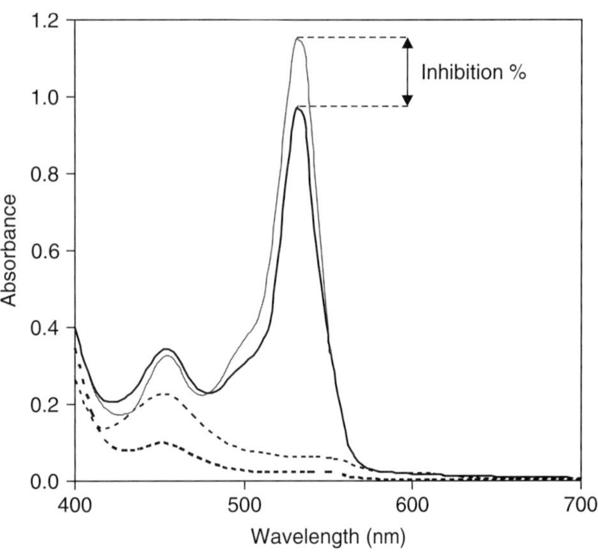

Figure 78.3 Classical spectrophotometric profile of a beer melanoidin sample after 30 min of reaction at 37°C with 0.337 mM deoxyribose. Deoxyribose positive control (absence of melanoidin, solid bold line), in the presence of beer melanoidin (solid line), blank assay (absence of deoxyribose, dotted line) and negative control (absence of both melanoidin and deoxyribose, bold dotted line).

Three widely distributed commercial brands of beer in Europe with different elaboration procedures were analyzed. A Pilsener style beer from a Spanish brewery, Abbeys style beer from a Belgian brewery, and a dry-stout beer from an Irish brewery were studied. Melanoidins isolated from these beers are used for assessing the antiradical activity. Table 78.1 shows the yield of melanoidin obtained from each sample.

Color is a classical attribute of melanoidins. Isolated melanoidins show an apparent absorbity (l/g/cm) of 0.014, 0.064 and 0.294 for pilsener, Abbey and dry-stout beers, respectively. The contribution of the color at the experimental conditions is always lower than 0.035 absorbance units at 532 nm. On the other hand, TBA reactive substances are not formed during the treatment of melanoidins in the absence of DR or are negligible to the contribution of the intrinsic color on the overall measurement at 532 nm at the range studied (Figure 78.3). The non-specific hydroxyl scavenging activities of melanoidins and reference material through a period of time are evaluated. The presence of EDTA–Fe(III) enhances the generation of hydroxyl radicals since keep it from attacking DR. Therefore, hydroxyl radicals generated attack DR in a non-site-specific manner (Halliwell *et al.*, 1987). Most of the melanoidins exerted inhibition effects on hydroxyl radical formation during the first part of the incubation period (up to 40 min) presumably due to the presence of residues acting as nucleophilic, and decreasing the activity after that. The hydroxyl radical scavenging activity is lost after 2 h of reaction for most of beer melanoidins. Trolox is able to keep the antiradical activity for at least 90 min. On the other hand, the efficiency to scavenge hydroxyl radical is significantly lower for melanoidins as compared with trolox (Table 78.2).

Table 78.1 Melanoidin content from three beer styles

Beer style	*Melanoidin content (g/l)*
Dry-stout beer	2.18
Abbeys style beer	2.36
Pilsener beer	1.63

Table 78.2 Rates of percentage of inhibition of the deoxyribose degradation by hydroxyl radicals in the presence of melanoidins (1 mg/ml) from three beer styles and coffee brew and trolox as reference material (0.05 mg/ml)

	Incubation time (min)						
Melanoidin	*10*	*20*	*30*	*40*	*60*	*90*	*120*
Pilsener beer	35.4	26.3	21.0	17.8	4.9	0.0	0.0
Abbey beer	33.2	29.4	24.6	23.1	10.6	2.1	0.0
Dry-stout beer	41.9	38.2	34.2	34.7	34.8	7.7	1.1
Coffee brew	24.2	29.0	28.4	26.8	23.5	8.7	0.4
Trolox	*81.9*	*81.4*	*81.8*	*83.1*	*79.6*	*84.8*	*71.9*

Since melanoidin structure is unknown, studies concerning the structure–activity relationships of melanoidins are limited (Jing and Kitts, 2000). Different hypotheses have been formulated on the structural backbone of these model melanoidins. A first hypothesis states that a melanoidin skeleton is constituted mainly from sugar degradation products, polymerized through aldol type condensations and probably branched via amino compounds (Yaylayan and Kaminsky, 1998; Cämmerer and Kroh, 1995). It was shown that, under water-free MR conditions, significant amounts of carbohydrates are incorporated as side chains, with an intact glycosidic bond, into the melanoidin skeleton (Cämmerer *et al.*, 2002). Tressl *et al.* (1998) proposed a complex macromolecular structure consisting of repeating units of furans and pyrroles, linked by polycondensation reactions. Hofmann (1998) identified low molecular weight chromophores and postulated the generation of melanoidin-type colorants by a crosslinking reaction between these LMW substances and non-colored HMW biopolymers, such as proteins.

It could be plausible that the antiradical effects of MRP could be correlated to their iron-chelating properties (Yoshimura *et al.*, 1997). Then it could be deactivated in iron Fenton-type reactions by chelating the iron and form an inactive complex with the melanoidin. It is known that melanoidins are able to quelate iron (Morales *et al.*, 2005), but this ability is drastically reduced in the presence of ascorbic acid. In the presence of ascorbic acid most of the iron was released from the melanoidin structure. Furthermore, EDTA eliminates the iron-chelating effects that may interfere with the accurate determination of hydroxyl radical scavenging activity in the system. On the other hand, ascorbic acid greatly increases the rate of $^{\bullet}OH$ generation by reducing iron and maintaining a supply of Fe^{2+}–EDTA quelate. Furthermore, the effect of melanoidins in the speciation of the iron during the time of incubation is not clear. Additional experiments are necessary to gain more insight on the iron-reducing ability of the beer melanoidins. The presence of the ascorbic acid ensures the rapid turn-over of Fe(II), if necessary. The ability of beer melanoidins to reduce Fe(III) at the reaction vessel concentrations is investigated by applying the ferrozine method. This effect imparts the pro-oxidant activity when catalytic transition metal ions are present. This fact is important to be evaluated when non-site-specific hydroxyl radicals scavenging ability assay is applied. Ferrozine was used to measure the levels of iron reduction in that it forms a stable complex with Fe(II) that can be measured by its absorbance at 562 nm. Beer melanoidins do not exert a change in the iron speciation for 2 h of incubation at 37°C in the reaction vessel (Morales, 2005).

A kinetic approach could be applied to assess the hydroxyl radical scavenging properties of beer melanoidins. The second order rate constants are obtained by competition kinetic method with DR whose product can be monitored (λ_{max} at 532 nm, ε of 153,000 l/mol/cm) (Gutteridge, 1981). Previously, it was confirmed that melanoidin did not scavenge hydrogen peroxide, and the intrinsic color did not show interferences with the DR assay at the concentration range tested (1.5–50 μg/ml in the reaction vessel). In agreement with Halliwell *et al.* (1987), the rate constant for the reaction of scavengers with hydroxyl radical can be determined based on the following equation:

$$1/A = 1/A_0(1 + k_M[M]/k_{DR}[DR])$$

where A is the absorbance in the presence of melanoidin (M) at concentration [M] and A_0 the absorbance in the absence of a scavenger; rate constants of reactions in the presence (k_M) or absence of melanoidin (k_{DR}), [DR] is the concentration of deoxyribose used in the experiment. A scheme of the competitive reactions involved is represented in Figure 78.3. It was represented by $1/A$ against melanoidin concentration to calculate the constant rates from the slope (Figure 78.4). The rate constant (k_M) was determined from the slope of the curve. Higher slope is related to a higher competition toward $^{\bullet}OH$ radicals, meaning a higher antihydroxyl radical activity (Figure 78.5).

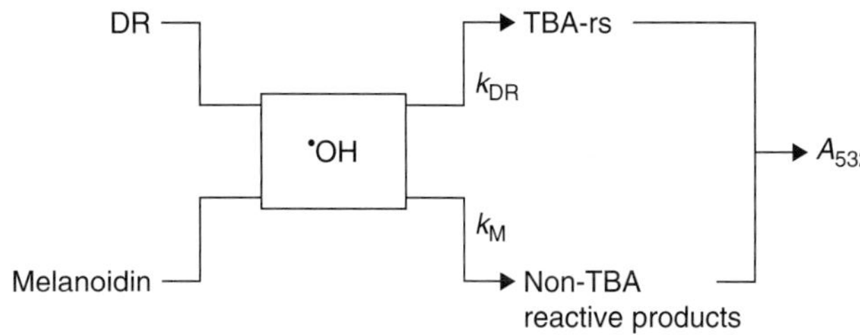

Figure 78.4 Scheme of the main chain reaction and rate constants involved in the competitive deoxyribose test for assessing hydroxyl radical scavenging properties of beer melanoidins.

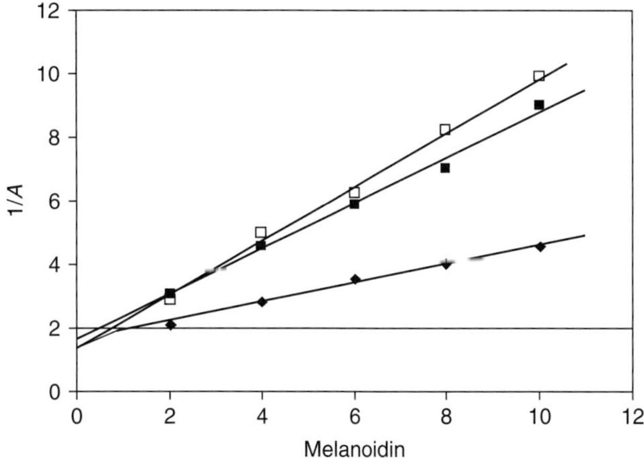

Figure 78.5 Competition curves of melanoidins (mg/ml) from Pilsener beer (◆), Abbey style beer (□) and dry-stout beer (■). Reaction was carried out in phosphate buffer (pH 7.4) at 37°C for 30 min. Data average of two independent assays.

Table 78.3 Second order rate constants (k_M) for trolox, melanoidins from beer and coffee brew determined by the competitive assay of the deoxyribose method

Melanoidin	*Range*	A_0	*r*	$k_M \times 10^6$	$SD \times 10^6$
Pilsener beer	2.0–10.0	0.627	0.997	3.02	0.33
Abbey beer	2.0–10.0	0.794	0.998	10.52	0.01
Dry-stout beer	2.0–10.0	0.635	0.996	7.22	0.35
Coffee brew	0.4–2.0	0.821	0.996	13.00	0.01
Trolox	*0.005–0.50*	*2,062*	*0.963*	*2,491.07*	*46.58*

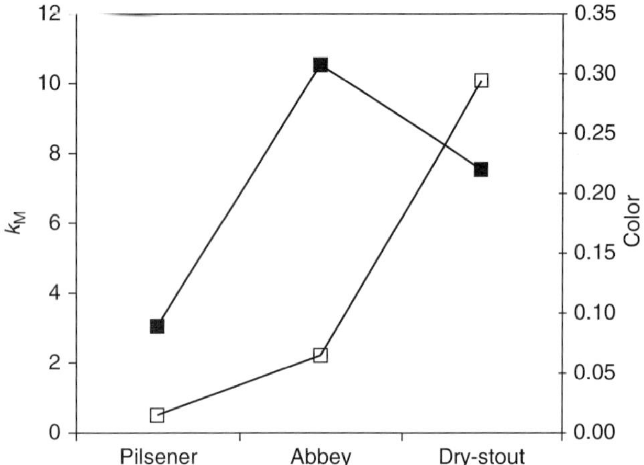

Figure 78.6 Relationship between color (apparent absorbity, l/g/cm, □) and hydroxyl radical scavenging properties (k_M, l/g/s, ■) for melanoidins isolated from Pilsener, Abbeys and dry-stout beer.

Based on the competition principle, the second order rate constants of OH radical of melanoidins are summarized in Table 78.3. Beer melanoidins are found to inhibit the DR degradation competitively, showing that they are scavengers of $^{\bullet}OH$ radicals. The efficiency to scavenge hydroxyl radicals could be applied for classification of the melanoidins reactivity. Traditional approaches did not give clear results where indirect methods are useful to get knowledge on the functional residues attached to the melanoidin skeleton. At present, the mechanism by which OH radicals react with melanoidins is not documented.

As previously mentioned, color is the most relevant external characteristic of the melanoidins. Many previous investigations tried to find a correlation between the browning and the antioxidant properties of several processed food (i.e. Anese *et al.*, 1999; Manzocco and Nicoli, 2003). It is noticed that a lack of correlation between beer melanoidins and color, meaning that chromophore residues linked to the melanoidin skeleton are not the main responsible for the hydroxyl scavenging properties of the melanoidins (Figure 78.6). These findings lead to the conclusion that both non-specific hydroxyl radical scavenging properties of beer melanoidins and the color increase with heating time to a maximum level, after which point antioxidant activity decreases while color levels off, in agreement as described by Samaras *et al.* (2005) for malt model systems. Thermally induced compounds produced at higher temperatures and/or long heating times may contribute to color development, but not to antioxidant activity. Also, some thermally induced compounds possessing antioxidant activity may degrade on prolonged heating. Manzocco and Nicoli (2003) stated that correlation of antioxidant activity and color is expected in food and model systems where MR is the sole or prevalent driving force, and content of thermolabile naturally occurring antioxidant is low. In a previous work, evaluating the antiperoxyl activity of melanoidins in watery fluids, a correlation with color melanoidins in watery fluids was found (Morales and Jiménez-Pérez, 2004). It could be plausible to state that residues involved in the scavenging of hydroxyl radicals by beer melanoidins are not necessarily colored.

Summarizing, many compounds are formed with antioxidant activity during the beer production process. Researchers and brewery companies should put much attention on the potential antioxidant activity of newly formed compounds since reduction of antioxidant activity due to loss of natural antioxidant compounds from malt at least could be balanced. Levels of phenolics compounds in malt do not explain the overall antioxidant activity in malts and beer. This effect is more pronounced in beer processed with severely roasted malts. Hence, it should be plausible that MRP and melanoidins should be taken into account to understand the overall antioxidant activity of beers. Future studies should be addressed to gain more insight on the structural characterization of melanoidins from beer as well as to clarify the main LMW substances involved in their formation during kilning. It has been reported that beer melanoidins protect against oxidation induced by hydroxyl radicals which is important for protecting beer against oxidation and therefore for beneficial health implications. In that sense, brewery companies could get more precise information to drive the process to obtain melanoidins with higher protective effect against different radical species.

Summary Points

- During brewery process a myriad of new compounds are formed and some of them exert a significant antiradical activity.

- Melanoidins are colored polymeric material newly formed at the final stage of the MR during kilning.
- Beer melanoidins exert hydroxyl radical scavenging properties *in vitro* as recorded by the DR test. Different brewing process may be classified according to their potential antiradical activity.
- Hydroxyl radical scavenging activity of beer melanoidins is not related to their color, meaning that colored structures are not involved in such antioxidant effect.

References

Ames, J.M. (2003). The Maillard reaction. In Hudson, B.J.F. (ed.), *Progress in Food Proteins – Biochemistry*, pp. 99–153. Elsevier Applied Science, London.

Ames, J.M., Wynne, A., Hofmann, A., Plos, S. and Gibson, G.R. (1999). *Br. J. Nutr.* 82, 489–495.

Anese, M., Manzocco, L., Nicoli, M.C. and Lerici, C.R. (1999). *J. Sci. Food Agric.* 79, 750–754.

Araki, S., Kimura, T., Shimizu, C., Furusho, S., Takashio, M. and Shinotsuka, K. (1999). *J. Am. Brew. Chem.* 57, 34–38.

Arimoto-Kobayashi, S., Sugiyama, C., Harada, N., Takeuchi, M., Takemura, M. and Hayatsu, H. (1999). *J. Agric. Food Chem.* 47, 221–230.

Babbs, C.F. and Griffin, D.W. (1989). *Free Radic. Biol. Med.* 6, 493–503.

Bamforth, C.W. (2002). *Nutr. Res.* 22, 227–237.

Bamforth, C.W., Muller, R.E. and Walker, M.D. (1993). *J. Am. Soc. Brew. Chem.* 51, 79–88.

Becker, E.M., Nissen, L.R. and Skibsted, L.H. (2004). *Eur. Food Res. Technol.* 219, 561–571.

Blenkinsop, P. (1991). *Tech. Q. Master Brew. Assoc. Am.* 28, 145–149.

Cämmerer, B. and Kroh, L. (1995). *Food Chem.* 53, 55–59.

Cämmerer, B., Jalyschko, W. and Kroh, L. (2002). *J. Agric. Food Chem.* 50, 2083–2087.

Cantrell, I.C. and Griggs, D.L. (1996). *Tech. Q. Master Brew. Assoc. Am.* 33, 82–86.

Chandra, S.G. (2002). *Melanoidins in Food and Health*, pp. 137–142. European Communities, Brussels.

Chapon, L., Louis, C. and Chapon, S. (1971). *Proc. Congr. Eur. Brew. Conv.* 13, 307–322.

Coghe, S. and Delvaux, F. (2002). *Cerevesia* 27, 20–26.

Coudara, C., Martin, M., Fatome, M. and Favier, A. (1995). *Anal. Biochem.* 227, 101–111.

Domingues, P., Domingues, M.R., Amado, F.M. and Ferrer-Correia, A.J. (2001). *J. Am. Soc. Mass Spectrom.* 12, 1214–1219.

Eichner, K. (1981). *Prog. Food Nutr. Sci.* 5, 441–451.

Fukui, S., Hanasaki, Y. and Ogawa, H. (1993). *J. Chromatogr. A* 630, 187–193.

Galic, K., Palic, A. and Cikovic, N. (1994). *Monastsschr Brauwiss* 47, 124–127.

Geoffroy, M., Lambelet, P. and Richert, P. (2000). *J. Agric. Food Chem.* 48, 974–978.

Ghiselli, A., Natella, F., Guidi, A., Montanari, L., Fantozzi, P. and Scaccini, C. (2000). *J. Nutr. Biochem.* 11, 76–80.

Goupy, P., Hughes, M., Boivin, P. and Amiot, M.J. (1999). *J. Sci. Food Agric.* 79, 1625–1634.

Gutteridge, J.M.C. (1981). *FEBS Lett.* 128, 343.

Halliwell, B. (1996). *Free Radic. Res.* 25, 57–74.

Halliwell, B., Gutteridge, J.M.C. and Aruoma, O. (1987). *Anal. Biochem.* 165, 215–219.

Henderson, M.D., Miranda, C.L., Stevens, J.F., Deinzer, M.L. and Buhler, D.R. (2000). *Xenobiotica* 30, 235–251.

Hofmann, T. (1998). *Z Lebensm Unters Forsch A* 206, 251–258.

Hofmann, T. and Schieberle, P. (2002). *J. Agric. Food Chem.* 50, 319–326.

Jing, H. and Kitts, D.D. (2000). *Food Res. Int.* 33, 509–516.

Joseph, J.M., Luke, T.L., Aravind, U.K. and Aravindakumar, C.T. (2001). *Water Environ. Res.* 73, 243–247.

Jurva, U., Wikstrom, H.V. and Bruins, A.P. (2002). *Rapid. Commun. Mass Spectrom.* 16, 1934–1940.

Karakus, M. (1975). Ph.D. Thesis, University of Nancy I, Nancy.

Kawashima, K., Itoh, H. and Chibata, I. (1977). *J. Agric. Food Chem.* 25, 202–204.

Li, B., Gutierrez, P.L. and Blough, N.V. (1997). *Anal. Chem.* 69, 4295–4302.

Lingnert, H. and Eriksson, C.E. (1980). *J. Food. Process. Preserv.* 4, 161–172.

Lingnert, H. and Eriksson, C.E. (1981). *Prog. Food Nutr. Sci.* 5, 453–466.

Lloyd, R.V., Hanna, P.M. and Mason, R.P. (1997). *Free Radic. Biol. Med.* 22, 885–888.

Lugasi, A. (2003). *Acta Alimen.* 32, 181–192.

Maillard, M.N. and Berset, C. (1995). *J. Agric. Food Chem.* 43, 1789–1793.

Manzocco, L. and Nicoli, M.C. (2003). In Vergarud, G. and Morales, F.J. (eds), *Melanoidins in Food and Health*, Vol. 4, pp. 114–119. Office for Official Publications of the European Communities, Luxemburg.

Manzocco, L., Calligaris, S., Mastrocola, D., Nicoli, M.C. and Lerici, C.R. (2001). *Trends Food Sci. Technol.* 11, 340–346.

McMurrough, I., Hennigan, G.P. and Loughrey, M.J. (1983). *J. Inst. Brew.* 89, 15–23.

Mizuta, Y., Masumizu, T., Kohno, M., Mori, A. and Packer, L. (2002). *J. Agric. Food Chem.* 50, 2772–2777.

Morales, F.J. (2005). *Anal. Chem. Acta* 534, 171–176.

Morales, F.J. and Jiménez-Pérez, S. (2001). *Food Chem.* 72, 119–125.

Morales, F.J. and Babbel, M.B. (2002). *J. Agric. Food Chem.* 50, 2788–2792.

Morales, F.J. and Jiménez-Pérez, S. (2004). *Eur. Food Res. Technol.* 218, 515–520.

Morales, F.J., Fernández-Fraguas, C. and Jiménez-Pérez, S. (2005). *Food Chem.* 90, 821–827.

Nicoli, M.C., Anese, M. and Manzocco, L. (1999). *Trends Food Sci. Technol.* 10, 94–100.

O'Brien, J. and Morrissey, P.A. (1997). *Food Chem.* 58, 17–27.

Parejo, I., Codina, C., Petrakis, C. and Kefalas, P. (2000). *J. Pharmacol. Toxicol. Meth.* 44, 507–512.

Pokorný, J. (1991). *Trends Food Sci. Technol.* 9, 223–227.

Rivero, D., Perez-Magariño, S., Gonzalez-Sanjose, M.L., Valls-Belles, V., Codoñer, P. and Muñiz, P. (2005). *J. Agric. Food Chem.* 53, 3637–3642.

Rizzi, G.P. (1997). *Food. Rev. Int.* 13, 1–28.

Samaras, T.S., Gordon, M.H. and Ames, J.M. (2005). *J. Agric. Food Chem.* 53, 4938–4945.

Temple, N.J. (2000). *Nutr. Res.* 20, 449–459.

Tressl, R., Wondrak, G.T., Garbe, L.-A., Krüger, R.-P. and Rewicki, D. (1998). *J. Agric. Food Chem.* 46, 1765–1776.

Tsai, C.H., Stern, A., Chiou, J.F., Chern, C.L. and Liu, T.Z. (2001). *J. Agric. Food Chem.* 49, 2137–2141.

Tteiner, M.G. and Babbs, C.F. (1990). *Arch. Biochem. Biophys.* 278, 478–481.

Vanhees, I., Van den Bergh, V., Schildermans, R., De Boer, R., Compernolle, F. and Vinckier, C. (2001). *J. Chromatogr. A* 915, 75–83.

Wagner, K.H., Derkits, S., Herr, M., Schuh, W. and Elmadfa, I. (2002). *Food Chem.* 78, 375–382.

Walters, M.T., Heasman, A.P. and Hughes, P.S. (1997). *J. Am. Soc. Brew. Chem.* 55, 91–98.

Wijewickreme, A.N., Krejpcio, Z. and Kitts, D.D. (1999). *J. Food Sci.* 64, 457–461.

Woffenden, H.M., Ames, J.A., Chandra, S., Anese, M. and Nicoli, M.C. (2002). *J. Agric. Food Chem.* 50, 4925–4933.

Yang, X.F. and Guo, X.Q. (2001). *Analyst* 126, 1800–1804.

Yaylayan, V.A. and Kaminsky, E. (1998). *Food Chem.* 63, 25–31.

Yen, G.C. and Hsieh, P.P. (1994). *J. Agric. Food Chem.* 42, 133–137.

Yen, G.C. and Chung, D.Y. (1999). *J. Agric. Food Chem.* 47, 1326–1332.

Yoshimura, Y., Iijima, T., Watanabe, T. and Nakazawa, H. (1997). *J. Agric. Food Chem.* 45, 4106–4109.

Zou, H., Tai, C., Gu, X.X., Zhu, R.H. and Guo, Q.H. (2002). *Anal. Bioanal. Chem.* 373, 111–115.

79

Anti-obesity Effects of a Dietary Isomerized Hop Extract Containing Isohumulones Generated via Peroxisome Proliferators-Activated Receptors

Hiroaki Yajima Central Laboratories for Frontier Technology, Kirin Holdings Co., Ltd., Yokohama, Japan

Abstract

Isomerized hop extract (IHE), which consists mainly of isohumulones and is required in the beer-brewing process, was investigated for its effects on diet-induced obesity. Supplementation of high fat-containing chow with IHE reduced body weight gain and improved glucose tolerance in C57BL/6N and KK-A^y mice. Reduced weight gain was also observed in C57BL/6N mice fed a standard diet containing IHE. IHE may induce its effects by inhibiting fat absorption through the intestines, and peroxisome proliferator-activated receptors (PPARs) may also be involved. Isohumulones activated PPARs α and γ. Diabetic KK-A^y mice treated with isohumulones showed reduced plasma glucose, triacylglycerol, and free fatty acid levels. Isohumulone treatment did not cause significant weight gain, though treatment with the PPARγ agonist pioglitazone did. C57BL/6N mice fed a high fat diet and treated with isohumulones showed improved glucose tolerance, reduced insulin resistance, increased liver fatty acid oxidation, and decreased hypertrophic adipocyte size. A study of diabetes patients suggested that IHE significantly decreased blood glucose and hemoglobin A1c levels. These results suggest that isohumulones can modulate insulin sensitivity in mice on a high fat diet that develop insulin resistance and in patients with type 2 diabetes.

Introduction

Obesity has been described as "a product of free society in which a multitude of food choices and job opportunities are available" (Grundy, 2004). It is also well recognized that obesity extracts social costs. Obesity, the abnormal excessive growth of adipose tissue and accumulation of abdominal fat, results from the combined effects of excess energy intake and reduced energy expenditure (Spiegelman and Flier, 2001). It is also known to be an underlying risk factor for cardiovascular disease (CVD). Obesity raises the risk for CVD because of its association with other risk factors such as hypertension, hyperglycemia, hypercholesterolemia (major risk factors) and atherogenic dyslipidemia, insulin resistance, proinflammatory state, and prothrombotic state (emerging risk factors). The majority of obese persons who develop CVD have a cluster of major and emerging risk factors known as "metabolic syndrome" (National Cholesterol Education Program (NCEP) Expert Panel on Detection, 2002; Grundy, 2004). It has been suggested that the increasing prevalence of obesity is mainly responsible for the rising prevalence of metabolic syndrome in the United States and worldwide (Ford *et al.*, 2002).

The Adult Treatment Panel III (ATP III) stated that the root causes of metabolic syndrome were overweight or obese status, physical inactivity, and genetic factors. The specific factors considered to be important included abdominal obesity, hypertension, glucose intolerance, and other conditions related to metabolic syndrome (Expert Panel on Detection, 2001; Reaven, 2006). In fact, it was reported that the components of metabolic syndrome occur more commonly in obese persons, but this relationship is not due to obesity itself. Rather, obesity increases the likelihood that a person will become insulin resistant (Abbasi *et al.*, 2002; McLaughlin *et al.*, 2003). Also, adiposity is only one of the variables determining whether a person is sufficiently insulin resistant to develop an adverse clinical outcome, and defects in insulin metabolism play a fundamental role in the development of CVD risk factors (metabolic syndrome) (Reaven, 2006). Therefore, we should pay attention to insulin resistance as an obesity-related CVD risk factor. Insulin resistance is defined as reduced insulin action in peripheral tissues such as skeletal muscle, adipose tissue, and liver. It is closely associated with type 2 diabetes (Pi-Sunyer, 2002).

While extensive research has gone into developing anti-obesity drugs (Schwartz *et al.*, 2000), the abilities of various factors present in foods derived from plant sources

Beer in Health and Disease Prevention
ISBN: 978-0-12-373891-2

to ameliorate obesity, such as caffeine in oolong tea and capsiate in sweet pepper, have also been investigated (Han *et al.*, 1999; Ohnuki *et al.*, 2001; Birketvedt *et al.*, 2002). Furthermore, attention has recently been focused on the potential use of constituents in plants and other foods for the treatment of diabetic symptoms (Fujita *et al.*, 2001). The treatment of type 2 diabetes with herbal plants, which was carried out generations ago in Europe, may have provided some benefit because they contained compounds that stimulated the activity of PPARs α and γ (Swanston-Flatt *et al.*, 1989; Takahashi *et al.*, 2002).

The transcriptional factor PPARγ is highly expressed in adipocytes, where it regulates genes responsible for growth and differentiation following its activation by both natural and synthetic ligands. Activation of PPARγ was shown not only to stimulate the differentiation of adipocytes but also to induce their apoptotic death, thereby preventing adipocyte hypertrophy (Yamauchi *et al.*, 2001). PPARα, another nuclear fatty acid receptor that is widely expressed in liver, muscle, kidney, and intestine, mediates the expression of genes involved in lipid metabolism. Activators of PPARα, such as fibrates, lower circulating lipid levels and are commonly used to treat hypertriglyceridemia and other dyslipidemic states. Abnormalities in fatty acid metabolism underlie the development of insulin resistance and alterations in glucose metabolism. Recent studies have suggested that the activation of PPARα helped to modulate insulin resistance that was triggered by the oversupply and accumulation of lipid (Guerre-Millo *et al.*, 2000; Ye *et al.*, 2001). It has also been reported that several novel compounds that act as co-ligands for PPARs α and γ can improve insulin sensitivity and correct diabetic dyslipidemia in obese diabetic animals (Ljung *et al.*, 2002; Ye *et al.*, 2003).

Hops, the female inflorescences of the hop plant (*Humulus lupulus* L.), are used as a preservative and flavoring agent in the beer-brewing process. Humulones, also called α acids, are the primary compounds responsible for imparting the bitter taste to hops. They have been shown to suppress the expression of cyclooxygenase-2 (COX-2), a key enzyme that is involved in inflammation and carcinogenesis, and that has been shown to inhibit angiogenesis (Shimamura *et al.*, 2001). During the beer-brewing process, humulones are converted to isohumulones, also called iso-α-acids, which are the actual compounds responsible for imparting the bitter taste to beer. The physiological effects of isohumulones, other than their anti-bacterial properties, have not been as fully investigated as those of humulones (Simpson and Smith, 1992). Isohumulones are composed primarily of isohumulone, isocohumulone, and isoadhumulone, and they exist in beer at concentrations of 20–40 ppm. Isomerized hop extract (IHE), which consists primarily of isohumulones, is made by extracting α acids from the other components in hops, and then heating them in an alkaline environment to induce isomerization.

Prevention of Diet-Induced Obesity by IHE

IHE (ISOHOPCO2N) was purchased from Botanix Limited. The purity of isohumulones in IHE is 79% and its isohumulone:isocohumulone:isoadhumulone ratio is 37:48:15. Male KK-A^y mice and female C57BL/6N mice were maintained on either a standard (AIN93G (Reeves *et al.*, 1993)) or high fat (60% of total calories (Ikemoto *et al.*, 1996)) diet, with or without added IHE.

Six C57BL/6N mice (three mice/cage) that were placed on the *ad libitum* diets described above had their average energy intake measured daily during the course of the study. Body weight gain in C57BL/6N mice fed a high fat diet containing 0.2% or 0.6% IHE was significantly reduced in a dose-dependent manner compared to mice fed a high fat diet without IHE (control group) (Figure 79.1a). Specifically, the body weights of mice fed a diet containing 0.2% or 0.6% IHE were reduced by 14.1% and 22.0%, respectively, compared to control animals after 6 weeks of feeding. No significant differences in energy intake were demonstrable between the groups (Table 79.1). Similarly, there were no significant differences in the weights of their heart, spleen, or liver. However, ingestion of IHE prevented the weight gain in subcutaneous, retroperitoneal, and parametrial adipose tissues and in the kidney in a dose-dependent manner (Table 79.1). Feeding C57BL/6N mice an AIN93G standard diet containing 0.2% or 0.6% IHE for 5 weeks resulted in body weights that were reduced by 9.9% and 13.1%, respectively, compared to the control group (Figure 79.1b). On the other hand, feeding these mice a high fat diet containing 0.2% or 0.6% IHE for 5 weeks resulted in body weights that were reduced by 14.0% and 21.3%, respectively, compared to the control group. Note that these reductions were greater than those seen in mice fed standard chow, and the differences measured for the animals fed 0.6% IHE-containing chow reached statistical significance.

Six KK-A^y mice (one mouse/cage) were fed restricted diets. Specifically, these mice received either 4.5 g of a high fat diet or 5.0 g of a normal (AIN) diet, with or without added IHE. These dietary amounts represent the maximum amount of chow that the animals were able to consume during a 24-h period. When 6-week-old KK-A^y mice were fed a high fat diet containing 0.2% and 1.2% IHE for 5 weeks, their body weights were reduced by 9.7% and 10.9% compared to controls, respectively (Figure 79.1c). Administration of IHE to their diet did not affect body weight gain in KK-A^y mice that were fed the normal AIN93G chow (Figure 79.1d).

These results showed that body weight gain in most of the groups fed a diet supplemented with IHE was reduced in a dose-dependent manner compared to control animals; this effect was more marked in animals fed a high

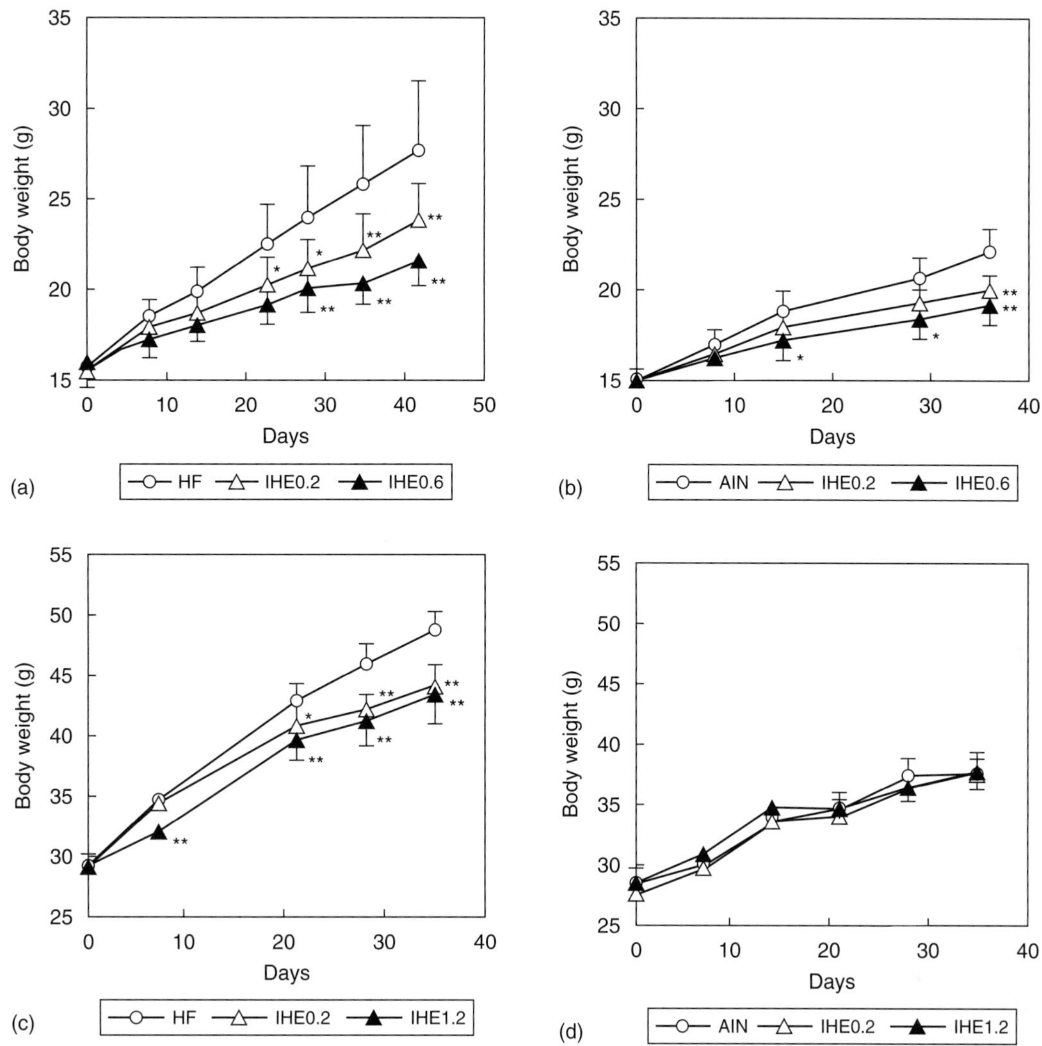

Figure 79.1 Effects of IHE on body weight in C57BL/6N and KK-A^y mice. Female C57BL/6N mice (n = 6, 3 mice/cage) were fed a high fat (a) or standard diet (b) that was supplemented with 0.2% or 0.6% (w/w) IHE. Male KK-A^y mice (n = 6, 1 mouse/cage) were fed a high fat (c) or standard diet (d) that was supplemented with either 0.2% or 1.2% IHE. The data represent the mean ± SD for 6–8 mice. *$p < 0.05$, **$p < 0.01$ for the high fat diet-fed group vs. the IHE-supplemented group on the same day.

Table 79.1 Tissue weights and energy intake of C57BL/6N mice fed a standard (AIN93G) diet or a high fat diet with or without IHE

	AIN control	*HF*	*IHE0.2*	*IHE0.6*
Heart (g)	0.13 ± 0.02	0.12 ± 0.02	0.12 ± 0.01	0.10 ± 0.01
Spleen (g)	0.076 ± 0.01	0.065 ± 0.01	0.071 ± 0.01	0.065 ± 0.008
Kidney (g)	0.24 ± 0.02	0.27 ± 0.01	0.25 ± 0.02*	0.24 ± 0.03**
Liver (g)	1.1 ± 0.08	1.0 ± 0.1	0.90 ± 0.4	0.95 ± 0.07
Adipose tissue (g)				
Subcutaneous	0.32 ± 0.1	1.9 ± 0.9	1.4 ± 0.4	0.87 ± 0.28**
Retroperitoneal	0.092 ± 0.03	0.44 ± 0.2	0.29 ± 0.1*	0.17 ± 0.06**
Parametrial	0.060 ± 0.03	0.37 ± 0.2	0.20 ± 0.07*	0.13 ± 0.04**
Energy intake (kJ/day)		38.8 ± 1.7	40.6 ± 1.3	38.1 ± 2.9

Notes: IHE was mixed with a high fat diet at 0.2 or 0.6 % (w/w). Tissue weights were measured after 6 weeks of feeding. Energy intake was measured daily during the course of the study. Results are represented as the means ± SD for six mice.

*$p < 0.05$ for the high fat diet-fed group vs. the IHE supplemented group.

**$p < 0.01$ for the high fat diet-fed group vs. the IHE supplemented group.

fat diet. The fact that there were no differences in food intake in C57BL/6N mice that were fed the various diets suggests that IHE had a direct effect in preventing body weight gain. The body weight-lowering effect of IHE was confirmed in genetically obese KK-A^y mice that were kept on a calorie-restricted diet. It is noteworthy that the body weight-lowering effect of IHE was not observed when KK-A^y mice were fed a regular diet. Although the results of studies involving female C57BL/6N and male KK-A^y mice are shown here, the weight-lowering effect of IHE was also observed in male C57BL/6N and female KK-A^y mice (data not shown), suggesting that the effects of IHE are sex-independent.

Adipose tissue mass in C57BL/6N and KK-A^y mice was significantly reduced by IHE supplementation in a dose-dependent manner. The reduction in kidney weight observed in IHE-supplemented C57BL/6N mice was likely due to the normalization of kidney hypertrophy that had been induced by the high fat diet, since the kidney weight in mice fed 0.6% IHE was almost the same as that found in mice fed the standard diet. A decrease in the weight of subcutaneous and epididymal adipose tissues, as well as the liver and kidney, was observed in the IHE diet-supplemented KK-A^y mice (Table 79.2). The mean weights of the liver and kidney in animals fed chow supplemented with 1.2% IHE were nearly identical to those of mice fed the AIN93G diet (liver; 2.5 ± 0.25 (g), and kidney; 0.52 ± 0.04 (g)), suggesting that the weights of the liver and kidney in animals fed IHE-containing high fat diet were normal. The concentration of triacylglycerols in the liver of IHE diet-supplemented animals was similarly reduced in a dose-dependent manner (Table 79.2).

Table 79.2 Tissue weights and liver triacylglycerol content of KK-A^y mice fed a high fat diet with or without IHE

	HF	*IHE0.2*	*IHE1.2*
Liver (g)	3.9 ± 0.3	3.3 ± 0.3**	2.6 ± 0.3**
Liver triacylglycerol (mmol/g liver)	0.21 ± 0.03	0.20 ± 0.05	0.10 ± 0.02**
Kidney (g)	0.72 ± 0.05	0.58 ± 0.06**	0.52 ± 0.06**
Adipose tissue (g)			
Subcutaneous	1.9 ± 0.2	1.4 ± 0.2**	1.4 ± 0.2**
Epididymal	2.0 ± 0.2	2.0 ± 0.2	0.9 ± 0.3

Notes: IHE was mixed with the diet at 0.2% and 1.2% (w/w). Tissue weight was determined after 5 weeks of feeding. Results are represented as the means ± SD for six mice.

**$p < 0.01$ for the high fat diet-fed group vs. the IHE supplemented group.

Inhibition of Intestinal Dietary Fat Absorption by IHE

Supplementation of the diet of Wistar rats with IHE significantly increased the lipid content of their feces compared to control rats fed the high fat diet alone. There was no significant difference in the total weight of feces produced by the two groups (Figure 79.2a).

The serial changes in plasma triacylglycerol levels of rats after oral administration of lipid emulsion are shown in Figure 79.2b. Plasma triacylglycerol levels in rats treated with IHE (100 and 150 mg/kg body weight) were significantly reduced compared to rats treated with vehicle at all time points up through 5 h after administration. At 2 h

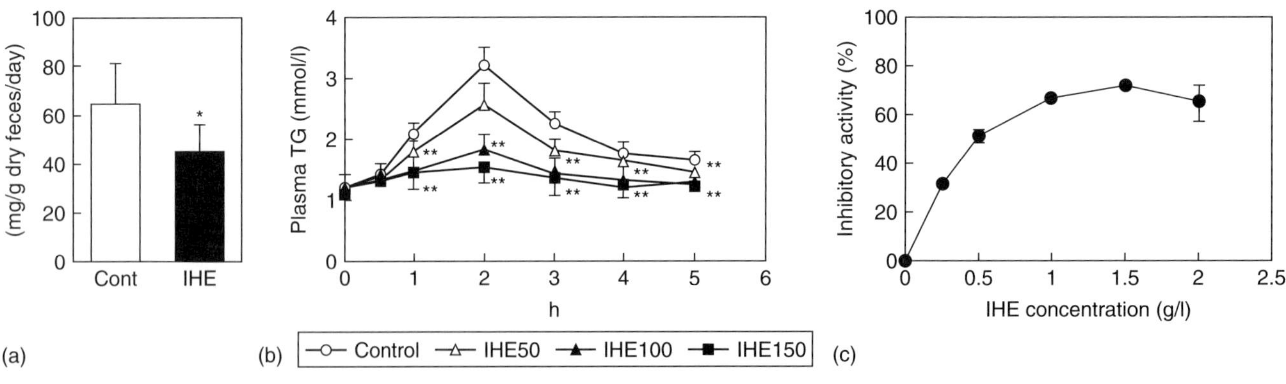

Figure 79.2 Effects of IHE on intestinal lipid absorption. (a) Fecal lipid content of Wistar rats. Feces of the rats fed a high fat diet with or without IHE were collected and weighed four times every 24 h from day 12 to day 15. They were then lyophilized and their lipids extracted and quantified gravimetrically. *$p < 0.05$ for the high fat diet-fed group vs. the IHE-supplemented group. (b) Wistar rats were orally administered lipid emulsion containing IHE at a concentration of 50, 100, or 150 mg/kg body weight. Plasma triacylglycerol (TG) levels were quantified at the indicated times after administration of lipid emulsion. The data represent the mean ± SD for six rats. **$p < 0.01$ for the high fat diet-fed group vs. the IHE-supplemented group at each indicated time. (c) Effect of IHE on pancreatic lipase activity. *In vitro* pancreatic triacylglycerol lipase activity was determined in the absence or presence of IHE. The inhibitory effect of IHE on pancreatic lipase was expressed as the relative percent suppression of enzymatic activity. The data represent the mean ± SD from three independent experiments.

after administration, the elevation in plasma triacylglycerol levels was suppressed by IHE in a dose-dependent manner; peak levels in rats treated with 50, 100, and 150 mg/kg IHE were reduced to 67.9%, 36.4%, and 20.1%, respectively, of the values seen in control animals. As shown in Figure 79.2c, IHE also inhibited pancreatic triacylglycerol lipase activity, which plays a crucial role in intestinal lipid absorption, in a dose-dependent manner; lipase activity was suppressed by about 50% in the presence of 0.5 g/l of IHE.

These results might suggest that inhibition of lipase activity by IHE contributed to the reduction in plasma triacylglycerols in these animals. The inhibitory effect of IHE on lipid absorption may have accounted for our data showing that the reduction in body weight gain induced by IHE in mice fed a high fat diet was greater than that seen in animals fed a standard diet. It has been reported that teasaponin, an inhibitor of pancreatic lipase activity that was isolated from oolong tea, suppressed the increase in body weight of mice fed a high fat diet (Han *et al.*, 2001). Accordingly, it is likely that the inhibition of intestinal lipid absorption by IHE was responsible to some extent for the effect of IHE in reducing body weight gain.

Modulation of Lipid Metabolism by IHE

Quantitative RT-PCR analysis of the mRNAs for the acyl-CoA oxidase (ACO), medium-chain acyl-CoA dehydrogenase (MCAD), and diacylglycerol *O*-acyltransferase 2 (DGAT2) genes in the liver of KK-A^y mice fed a standard diet with or without IHE was performed. Treatment of mice with IHE significantly increased the mRNA levels of the ACO and MCAD genes while significantly reducing the expression of the DGAT2 gene (Table 79.3).

Table 79.3 Effect of IHE on the expression of genes involved in fatty acid metabolism

	Control	*IHE*
Acyl-CoA oxidase	1.00 ± 0.11	1.55 ± 0.15*
Medium-chain acyl-CoA dehydrogenase	1.00 ± 0.21	1.31 ± 0.16**
Diacylglycerol acyltransferase	1.00 ± 0.16	0.720 ± 0.068*

Notes: Total RNA was isolated from KK-A^y mice fed a diet with or without 1.2% IHE. The RNA was subjected to quantitative RT-PCR to measure the mRNA levels of the indicated genes. Results are expressed as relative expression levels normalized to the expression of the control group (mean ± SD, $n = 6$).

*$p < 0.01$ for the standard diet-fed group (control) vs. the IHE supplemented group.

**$p < 0.05$ for the standard diet-fed group (control) vs. the IHE supplemented group.

ACO and MCAD are known to be regulated by PPARα and to be involved in β-oxidation in the liver (Schoonjans *et al.*, 1996). In contrast, the DGAT2 gene plays a vital role in the production of triacylglycerol (Meegalla *et al.*, 2002; Waterman and Zammit, 2002). These results suggest that IHE might accelerate lipid oxidation, while at the same time it suppresses triacylglycerol biosynthesis. This effect of IHE on lipid metabolism may be related to its effect on reducing body weight gain.

Activation of PPARs by IHE and the Active Ingredient Contained in IHE

The peroxisome proliferator-activated receptors (PPARs) are nuclear fatty acid receptors that have been implicated in obesity-related metabolic diseases such as insulin resistant-type 2 diabetes, hyperlipidemia, and coronary artery disease. To evaluate the ability of IHE to transactivate PPARs, reporter assays were performed.

An increase in luciferase activity was observed following the addition of IHE to HepG2 cells that were transfected with PPARα. The addition of 50 μg/ml of IHE significantly increased luciferase activity compared to the vehicle control, and this increase was smaller than that seen when 1 μM fenofibrate, a specific agonist for PPARα, was added to the cells. IHE also increased luciferase activity in CV-1 cells transfected with PPARγ. The effect of 50 μg/ml of IHE was almost the same as that of 1 μM pioglitazone, a specific agonist for PPARγ (Figure 79.3a).

Purification of the active component that induces PPAR-mediated transcription, resulted in the identification of isohumulones. Isohumulones, also called iso-α-acids, are the compounds that impart a bitter flavor to beer. Figure 79.4 shows the chemical structure of three major homologs of isohumulones, that is isohumulone, isocohumulone, and isoadhumulone. The effects of isohumulones and IHE on PPARs α and γ were evaluated in transient co-transfection assays.

A dose-dependent increase in luciferase activity was observed following the addition of isohumulones to cells transfected with PPARγ. The addition of either 10 μM isohumulone, isocohumulone, or isoadhumulone induced a 3.8-, 3.5-, and 2.8-fold increase in luciferase activity, respectively, compared to the vehicle control (Figure 79.3b). These activities were almost the same as those seen when 1 μM pioglitazone, a specific agonist of PPARγ, was added to the cells. Isohumulone and isocohumulone also activated the PPARα construct in a dose-dependent manner; 10 μM isohumulone and isocohumulone increased luciferase activity by about 3.2- and 1.9-fold, respectively, compared to the vehicle control (Figure 79.3c). Isoadhumulone had no effect on PPARα, suggesting that the side-chain of isohumulone may be involved in the activation of the PPARα receptor. The activity of isohumulone at 30 μM was almost the same as that of 3 μM fenofibrate, a PPARα-selective agonist.

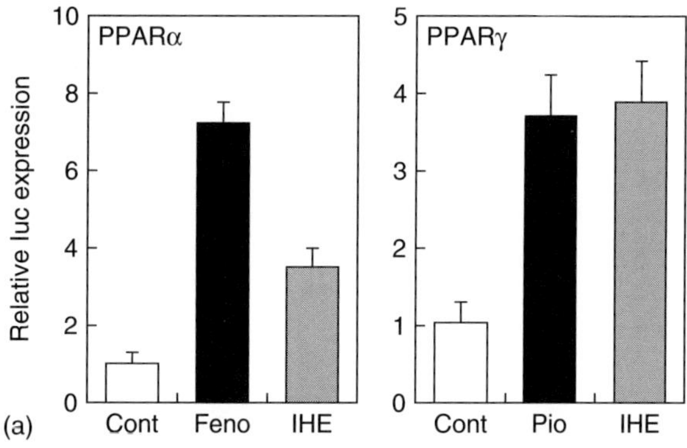

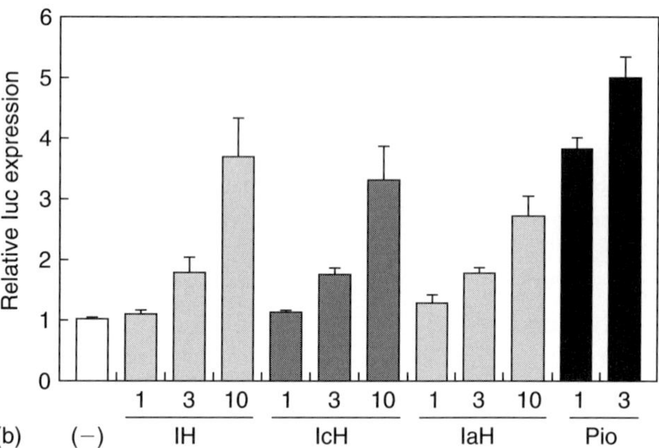

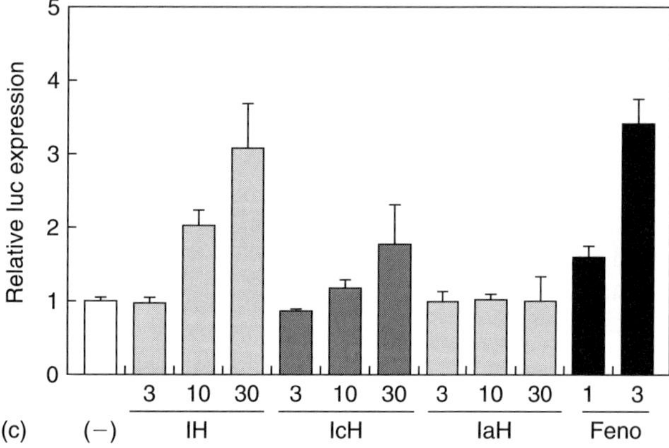

Figure 79.3 Transactivation of PPARs by IHE and isohumulones. (a) IHE activated transcription mediated by PPARs α and γ. Details of the assay are described below. (b) Activation of PPARγ by isohumulones. CV-1 cells were co-transfected with a luciferase reporter plasmid, pG5 luc (Promega), containing five copies of GAL4 UAS in the promoter region and an expression vector for the human PPARγ ligand-binding domain fused to the GAL4 DNA binding domain (DBD). Results show the relative luciferase expression levels normalized with the protein concentration of the cell lysates. (c) Activation of PPARα by isohumulones. HepG2 cells were co-transfected with pG5 luc and an expression vector for the human PPARα coding region fused to the GAL4 DBD. Isohumulone (IH), isocohumulone (IcH), and isoadhumulone (IaH) at the indicated concentrations were added to the transfected cells. Pioglitazone (Pio) and fenofibrate (Feno) were used as positive controls for PPARs γ and α transactivation, respectively.

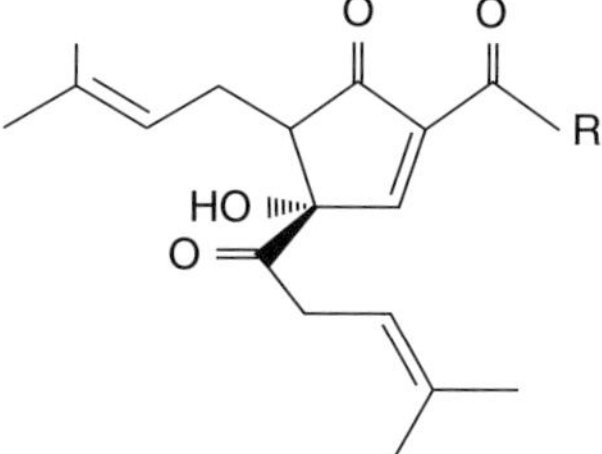

Figure 79.4 Structure of isohumulone. (R: $-CH_3CH(CH_3)_2$; 2-(3-methylbutanoyl)-5-(3-methyl-2-butenyl)-3,4-dihydroxy-4-(4-methyl-3-pentenoyl)-2-cyclopentenone), isocohumulone (R: $-CH(CH_3)_2$; 2-(2-methylpropanoyl)-5-(3-methyl-2-butenyl)-3,4-dihydroxy-4-(4-methyl-3-pentenoyl)-2-cyclopentenone), and isoadhumulone (R: $-CH(CH_3)C_2H_5$; 2-(2-methylbutanoyl)-5-(3-methyl-2-butenyl)-3,4-dihydroxy-4-(4-methyl-3-pentenoyl)-2-cyclopentenone).

These results indicate that isohumulones activated transcription that was mediated by PPARs α and γ, suggesting that isohumulones may modulate reactions that are regulated by these transcriptional activators. Metabolic syndrome, which is particularly relevant to insulin resistance, is characterized by glucose intolerance, hyperinsulinemia, dyslipidemia, and hypertension, and is frequently associated with visceral obesity. Pharmacological treatment of this syndrome aims to reduce insulin resistance and other risk factors by modulating PPARs. Fibrate drugs, which act as ligands for PPARα, and thiazolidinedione drugs, which are ligands for PPARγ, are often used to treat hyperlipidemia and hyperglycemia, respectively. Combination therapy using these medications is an attractive option for the treatment of obese, type 2 diabetics. Compounds that have dual agonistic activity on both of these receptors have been shown to reverse symptoms of insulin sensitivity and dyslipidemia in obese diabetic animals (Murakami *et al.*, 1998; Ljung *et al.*, 2002). Therefore, amelioration of hyperglycemia and hyperlipidemia by activating PPARs with isohumulones should be possible.

Isohumulones Reduce Insulin Resistance and Prevent the Development of Diabetes in Mice

Treatment of KK-A^y mice with isohumulones for 2 weeks significantly lowered their plasma triacylglycerol (62.6% for isohumulone, 76.4% for isocohumulone, respectively) and free fatty acid (FFA) (73.1% for isohumulone, 84.8% for isocohumulone, respectively) levels. These reductions were comparable to those seen in 0.05% pioglitazone-treated mice (60.5% and 69.9%, respectively) (Figure 79.5a and b). The non-fasting plasma glucose levels of isohumulones-treated mice were also reduced to 65.3% of controls for isohumulone and 87.1% of controls for isocohumulone, although these levels were higher than those seen in animals fed pioglitazone (35.1%) (Figure 79.5c). There was

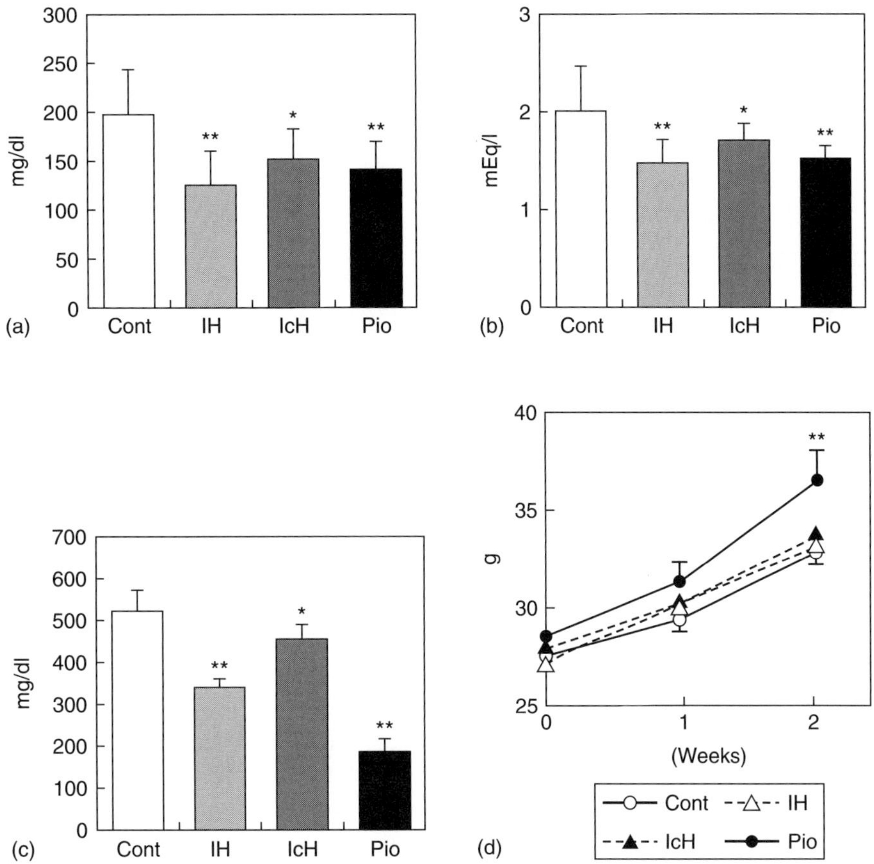

Figure 79.5 Isohumulone and isocohumulone prevented the development of diabetes in KK-A^y mice. Male KK-A^y mice were fed either a standard diet or a diet containing 0.18% isohumulone (IH), 0.18% isocohumulone (IcH), or 0.05% pioglitazone (Pio) for two weeks. Fasting blood samples were collected and plasma triacylglycerol and FFA levels were measured (a, b). Non-fasting plasma glucose levels were also determined (c), and body weights were measured weekly (d). Data are the means ± SD for six mice per group. $^*p < 0.05$, $^{**}p < 0.01$ vs. control.

a significant difference in body weight gain between these groups in spite of their equivalent caloric intake. Thus, pioglitazone induced a 10% increase in body weight, while isohumulones did not induce an increase in body weight compared to the control group (Figure 79.5d). As described above, IHE did not affect body weight gain in KK-A^y mice fed a normal diet. Therefore, the influence of isohumulones on body weight gain in mice seemed to be similar to that of IHE. These results suggest that isohumulones ameliorate the pathology of genetically diabetic KK-A^y mice without affecting body weight gain, whereas body weight increased after treatment with pioglitazone, an anti-diabetic PPARγ agonist.

Female C57BL/6N mice were fed a high fat diet for 12 weeks. During their last 14 days on the diet, they were orally administered isocohumulone. Oral glucose tolerance tests (OGTTs) and insulin tolerance tests (ITTs) were performed on their 10th and 14th day of isocohumulone treatment, respectively.

After glucose loading, plasma glucose levels in the mice treated with isocohumulone at 10 and 100 mg/kg/day were significantly reduced compared to mice treated with vehicle at all time points, except for the mouse treated with 100 mg/kg of isocohumulone at 120 min (Figure 79.6a). Fasting plasma insulin levels were significantly reduced in animals treated with 100 mg/kg isocohumulone (2,396 ± 520 and 1,605 ± 570 (pg/ml) for vehicle-treated and 100 mg isocohumulone-treated mice, respectively). Plasma insulin levels during the OGTT were also reduced in the isocohumulone-treated animals (Figure 79.6b). The insulin resistance indices (IR, (Mondon *et al.*, 1981)) of mice treated with isocohumulone (1,094.4 ± 259.2 and 1,034.0 ± 259.2 for 10 mg isocohumulone-treated and 100 mg isocohumulone-treated mice, respectively) were significantly ($p < 0.01$ using the Dunnett's test) lower than that of the control group (2,217.3 ± 792.9), indicating that isocohumulone improved insulin sensitivity in mice fed a high fat diet. Modulation of insulin sensitivity was also observed after treatment with isohumulone; a significant decrease in IR was observed in the group receiving 100 mg/kg of isohumulone (1,240.2 ± 259.5, $p < 0.01$ using the Dunnett's test, data not shown). Results of the ITT showed a greater

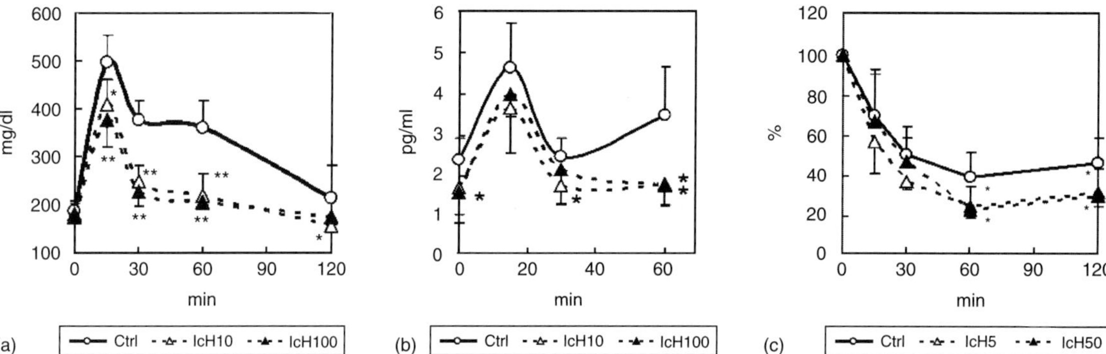

Figure 79.6 Isocohumulone ameliorated insulin resistance in high fat diet-fed C57BL/6N mice. Female C57BL/6N mice were fed a high fat diet for 10 weeks. For glucose tolerance testing, isocohumulone (IcH) was orally administered to mice at a dose of 10 or 100 mg/kg body weight for 14 days. Control mice received buffer alone. The mice were then subjected to an OGTT. For oral glucose testing, D-glucose (1 g/kg body weight) was administered by stomach tube after an overnight fast. Blood samples were collected from the orbital sinus before and 15, 30, 60, and 120 min after delivery of the glucose load, under light anesthesia. Control mice received buffer alone. (a) Plasma glucose and (b) insulin concentrations were plotted on the graph (mean ± SD, $n = 5$–6). For insulin tolerance testing, high fat diet-fed mice were administered IcH at a dose of 5 or 50 mg/kg body weight for 10 days. For insulin tolerance testing, human insulin was injected intraperitoneally (0.75 U/kg body weight) into non-fasted animals. Blood samples were collected from the tail vein before and 15, 30, and 60 min after insulin injection and blood glucose levels were determined. Blood glucose concentrations during the ITT were plotted on the graph (mean ± SD, $n = 6$) (c). $^{*}p < 0.05$ and $^{**}p < 0.01$ for vehicle vs. treatment with IcH at each indicated time.

glucose-lowering effect in mice treated with isocohumulone for 10 days than in vehicle-treated animals (Figure 79.6c). Plasma glucose levels in mice treated with 5 or 50 mg/kg of isocohumulone were significantly reduced to 76.8% and 69.3% of controls after 60 min and to 82.8% and 69.3% of controls after 120 min. These results indicated that insulin resistance and glucose intolerance in obese mice fed a high fat diet improved after short-term oral administration of isohumulones.

Effect of Isohumulones on Liver and White Adipose Tissue of Mice

Quantitative real time RT-PCR analysis of the mRNAs for ACO and fatty acid translocase/CD36 (FAT) genes in the liver of KK-A^y mice treated with isohumulone, isocohumulone, or pioglitazone was performed (Figure 79.7a). ACO and FAT, whose expression levels are regulated by PPARα, are involved in peroxisomal β-oxidation of fatty acids and in the uptake of long-chain fatty acids through the cell membrane, respectively (Motojima *et al.*, 1998; Memon *et al.*, 2000).

Treatment of mice with isohumulone, isocohumulone, or pioglitazone increased ACO and its mRNA levels by 1.6-, 1.7-, and 2.7-fold, and FAT mRNA levels by 2.9-, 3.3-, and 2.8-fold, compared to the control mice, respectively. The significant increase in ACO and FAT mRNA levels in the pioglitazone-treated mice was likely due to activation of PPARα by pioglitazone. An increase in the activity of ACO was observed in the liver of C57BL/6N mice treated with isohumulone or isocohumulone (Figure 79.7b). These results indicated that the effect of isohumulones on liver was similar to that of IHE.

Isohumulones treatment unexpectedly resulted in only a fairly small increase in the expression of PPARγ-regulated adipocyte differentiation related protein (adipocyte-ADRP/aP2) and lipoprotein lipase (LPL) genes. These proteins are involved in lipid uptake and storage in the white adipose tissue (WAT) (Tontonoz *et al.*, 1994) of KK-A^y mice; only the LPL mRNA level in the mice treated with isocohumulone increased significantly, by 1.2-fold, although treatment with pioglitazone did increase the aP2 and LPL mRNA levels by 2- and 1.7-fold, respectively (Figure 79.7c). Histological analysis of subcutaneous WAT of the high fat diet-fed C57BL/6N mice treated with isohumulone, isocohumulone, or pioglitazone for 10 days revealed an increase in the number of small adipocytes after treatment with all three of these compounds compared to vehicle-treated mice (Figure 79.7d). These results suggested that isohumulones affect WAT as well as liver.

The Effects of Oral Isohumulones in Type 2 Diabetics: A Placebo-Controlled Pilot Study

The ethics committee of KIRIN Brewery Co., Ltd. approved this study, and it complied with the principles outlined in the Declaration of Helsinki. Written informed consent was obtained from all subjects. Twenty volunteers with mild, type 2 diabetes (both males and females) were included in this study. Ten men and 10 women were randomized into one of two groups receiving either placebo or a capsule containing 100 mg of IHE.

Supplementation of 10 mild diabetic patients with IHE over 8 weeks resulted in a significant reduction in their

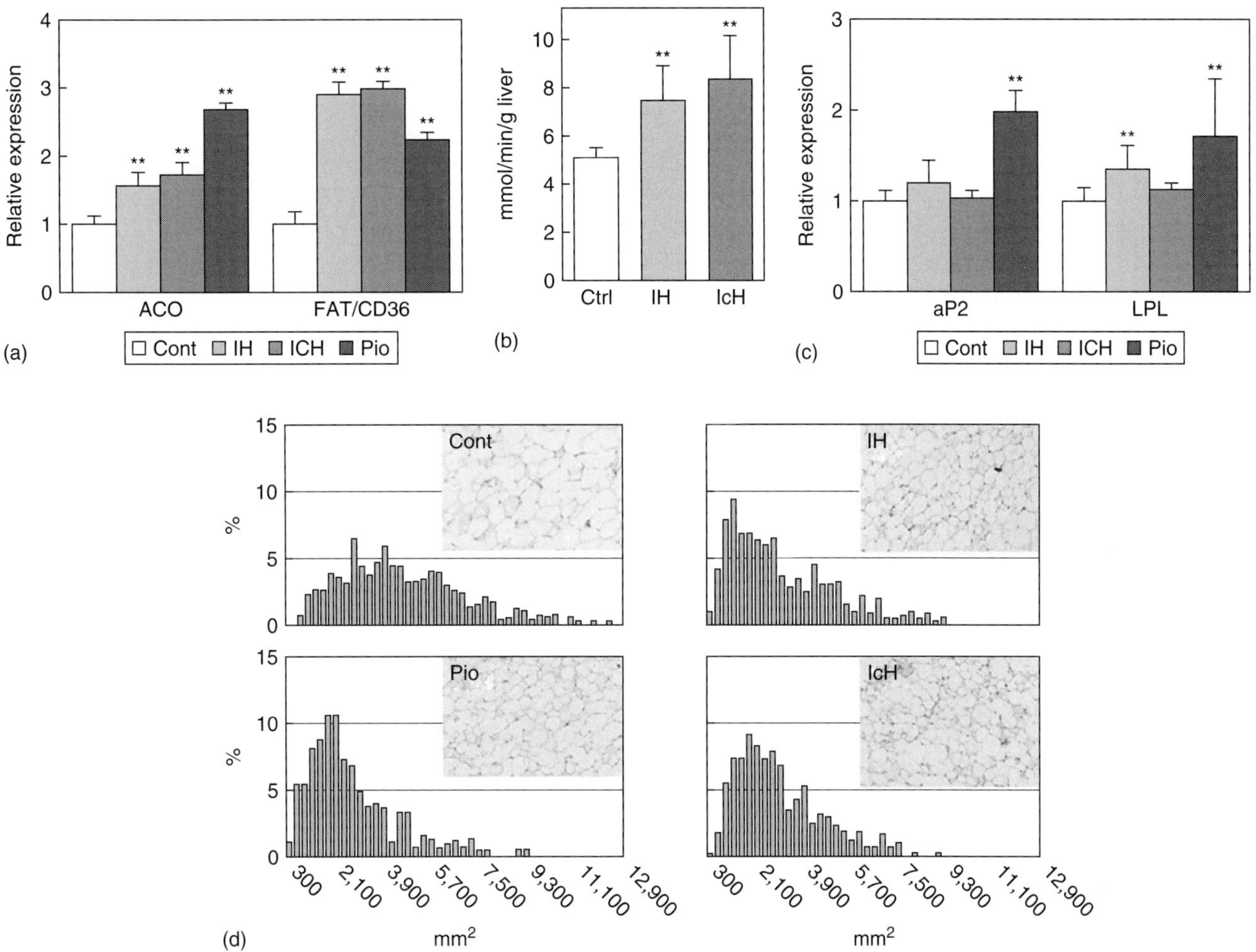

Figure 79.7 Effects of isohumulone and isocohumulone on liver and WAT. (a and c) Total RNA was isolated from liver and subcutaneous adipose tissue of KK-A^y mice fed diets containing 0.18% isohumulone (IH), 0.18% isocohumulone (IcH), or 0.05% pioglitazone (pio). Quantitative RT-PCR was performed to measure the mRNA levels of liver ACO and FAT (a), and aP2 and LPL in WAT (c). Results are presented as relative expression levels normalized to the expression level in the control group (mean ± SD, $n = 6$). (b) ACO activity in the liver of C57BL/6N mice treated with IH or IcH at 100 mg/kg weight for 6 days. Six-week-old female C57BL/6N mice fed a standard diet were orally administered isohumulone or isocohumulone for 6 days. Their livers were then isolated and homogenized. The homogenates were centrifuged and their supernatants were used as an enzyme source. Data are presented as the amount of hydrogen peroxide produced by oxidation of palmitoyl-CoA in the homogenates. **$p < 0.01$ vs. control. (d) Histological analysis and cell-size distribution of subcutaneous WAT in C57BL/6N mice. High fat diet-fed mice were orally administered vehicle (Cont), IH or IcH (100 mg/kg weight), or pioglitazone (Pio) (10 mg/kg weight) for 2 weeks. Their subcutaneous WAT was removed and fixed in 4% paraformaldehyde in phosphate-buffered saline (PBS). Fixed specimens were dehydrated, embedded in tissue-freezing medium, and frozen in liquid nitrogen. Sections (14 μm) were cut and stained with hematoxylin and eosin. More than 200 cells/mouse in each group were analyzed. Bar indicates 100 μm.

blood glucose and hemoglobin A1c levels by 10.1% and 6.4%, respectively; interestingly, a weak but significant reduction in blood glucose levels (7.3%) was also observed in the placebo control group. Furthermore, significant reductions in systolic blood pressure and blood levels of GPT, GOT, and γGPT were observed in the IHE-treated group (7.2%, 33.4%, 21.3%, and 25.6% reduction, respectively) (Table 79.4). These results indicated that isohumulones modulated insulin sensitivity in type 2 diabetic patients. Interestingly, in this latter study the patients also showed significant reductions in systolic blood pressure and in the levels of serum markers of liver disorder. The amount of daily isohumulone intake from IHE was about 80 mg, which is approximately the amount of IHE present in 20 l of beer. Since this study was preliminary and the minimum effective dose of isohumulones has not yet been determined, we do not recommend attempting to obtain therapeutic doses of isohumulones by drinking sufficient quantities of beer. However, these results indicate that isohumulones in beer are worth investigating further as therapeutic agents for the treatment of metabolic syndrome associated with insulin resistance.

Table 79.4 Results of the placebo-controlled pilot study of the effects of hop extract in type 2 diabetic patients

	IHE		*Placebo*	
	0 Week	*8 Weeks*	*0 Week*	*8 Weeks*
Blood glucose (mg/dl)	127.1 ± 10.9	114.3 ± 10.4*	130.5 ± 12.0	122.3 ± 8.37**
HbA1c (%)	7.14 ± 0.36	6.68 ± 0.68*	7.00 ± 0.38	6.76 ± 0.65
Systolic blood Pressure (mmHg)	137.1 ± 13.6	128.6 ± 15.5*	129.0 ± 16.4	127.5 ± 15.3
GPT (IU/l)	40.8 ± 26	27.2 ± 11.0*	25.4 ± 18.0	24.8 ± 23
GOT (IU/l)	28.6 ± 13	22.5 ± 6.30**	25.7 ± 10.0	27.0 ± 16
γGTP (IU/l)	48.1 ± 41	35.8 ± 26.0**	75.3 ± 91.0	78.3 ± 110

Notes: Twenty volunteers with mild, type 2 diabetes (both males and females) were included in this study. The subjects were between 45 and 65 years of age (mean=53 years) and had fasting blood glucose and hemoglobin A1c levels between 110 and 140 (mg/dl) and 6.4 and 8.0 (%), respectively. IHE containing isohumulones at a purity of 79% was used in this study. The subjects were randomized to one of two groups that received either a placebo or a capsule containing 100 mg of IHE (equivalent to about 80 mg of isohumulones) twice a day for 12 weeks. Laboratory tests were performed every 4 weeks for 12 weeks. Data are indicated as the means ± SD.

*$p < 0.01$ vs. 0 week of each group.
**$p < 0.05$ vs. 0 week of each group.

Summary Points

- IHE, which consists mainly of isohumulones and is a required component of the beer-brewing process, showed an inhibitory effect on diet-induced obesity in mice.
- Inhibition of intestinal lipid adsorption by IHE was responsible to some extent for the effect of IHE in reducing body weight gain.
- Isohumulones improve insulin sensitivity and prevent the development of diabetes in mice.
- IHE and isohumulones modulate lipid metabolism, accelerate lipid oxidation, and suppress triacylglycerol biosynthesis.
- The modulatory effect of IHE and isohumulones on lipid metabolism via nuclear receptor peroxisome PPARs may also, at least in part, be responsible for its beneficial effects on body weight gain.

Disclosure

The contents of this section were initially published in another journals (Yajima *et al.*, 2004; Yajima *et al.*, 2005).

References

Abbasi, F., Brown Jr., B.W., Lamendola, C., McLaughlin, T. and Reaven, G.M. (2002). *J. Am. Coll. Cardiol.* 40, 937–943.

Birketvedt, G.S., Travis, A., Langbakk, B. and Florholmen, J.R. (2002). *Nutrition* 18, 729–733.

Expert Panel on Detection, Evaluation, and Treatment of High Blood Cholesterol in Adults. (2001). *JAMA* 285, 2486–2497.

Ford, E.S., Giles, W.H. and Dietz, W.H. (2002). *JAMA* 287, 356–359.

Fujita, H., Yamagami, T. and Ohshima, K. (2001). *J. Nutr.* 131, 2105–2108.

Grundy, S.M. (2004). *J. Clin. Endocrinol. Metab.* 89, 2595–2600.

Guerre-Millo, M., Gervois, P., Raspe, E., Madsen, L., Poulain, P., Derudas, B., Herbert, J.M., Winegar, D.A., Willson, T.M., Fruchart, J.C., Berge, R.K. and Staels, B. (2000). *J. Biol. Chem.* 275, 16638–16642.

Han, L.K., Takaku, T., Li, J., Kimura, Y. and Okuda, H. (1999). *Int. J. Obes. Relat. Metab. Disord.* 23, 98–105.

Han, L.K., Kimura, Y., Kawashima, M., Takaku, T., Taniyama, T., Hayashi, T., Zheng, Y.N. and Okuda, H. (2001). *Int. J. Obes. Relat. Metab. Disord.* 25, 1459–1464.

Ikemoto, S., Takahashi, M., Tsunoda, N., Maruyama, K., Itakura, H. and Ezaki, O. (1996). *Metabolism* 45, 1539–1546.

Ljung, B., Bamberg, K., Dahllof, B., Kjellstedt, A., Oakes, N.D., Ostling, J., Svensson, L. and Camejo, G. (2002). *J. Lipid Res.* 43, 1855–1863.

McLaughlin, T., Abbasi, F., Cheal, K., Chu, J., Lamendola, C. and Reaven, G. (2003). *Ann. Intern. Med.* 139, 802–809.

Meegalla, R.L., Billheimer, J.T. and Cheng, D. (2002). *Biochem. Biophys. Res. Commun.* 298, 317–323.

Memon, R.A., Tecott, L.H., Nonogaki, K., Beigneux, A., Moser, A.H., Grunfeld, C. and Feingold, K.R. (2000). *Endocrinology* 141, 4021–4031.

Mondon, C.E., Dolkas, C.B. and Oyama, J. (1981). *Am. J. Physiol.* 240, E482–E488.

Motojima, K., Passilly, P., Peters, J.M., Gonzalez, F.J. and Latruffe, N. (1998). *J. Biol. Chem.* 273, 16710–16714.

Murakami, K., Tobe, K., Ide, T., Mochizuki, T., Ohashi, M., Akanuma, Y., Yazaki, Y. and Kadowaki, T. (1998). *Diabetes* 47, 1841–1847.

National Cholesterol Education Program (NCEP) Expert Panel on Detection, Evaluation, and Treatment of High Blood Cholesterol in Adults (Adult Treatment Panel III). (2002). *Circulation* 106, 3143–3421.

Ohnuki, K., Haramizu, S., Oki, K., Watanabe, T., Yazawa, S. and Fushiki, T. (2001). *Biosci. Biotechnol. Biochem.* 65, 2735–2740.

Pi-Sunyer, F.X. (2002). *Obes. Res.* 10, 97S–104S.

Reaven, G.M. (2006). *Am. J. Clin. Nutr.* 83, 1237–1247.

Reeves, P.G., Nielsen, F.H. and Fahey, Jr. G.C. (1993). *J. Nutr.* 123, 1939–1951.

Schoonjans, K., Staels, B. and Auwerx, J. (1996). *J. Lipid Res.* 37, 1939–1951.

Schwartz, M.W., Woods, S.C., Porte Jr., D., Seeley, R.J. and Baskin, D.G. (2000). *Nature* 404(6778), 661–671.

Shimamura, M., Hazato, T., Ashino, H., Yamamoto, Y., Iwasaki, E., Tobe, H., Yamamoto, K. and Yamamoto, S. (2001). *Biochem. Biophys. Res. Commun.* 289(1), 220–224.

Simpson, W.J. and Smith, A.R. (1992). *J. Appl. Bacteriol.* 72(4), 327–334.

Spiegelman, B.M. and Flier, J.S. (2001). *Cell* 104(4), 531–543.

Swanston-Flatt, S.K., Day, C., Flatt, P.R., Gould, B.J. and Bailey, C.J. (1989). *Diabetes Res.* 10(2), 69–73.

Takahashi, N., Kawada, T., Goto, T., Yamamoto, T., Taimatsu, A., Matsui, N., Kimura, K., Saito, M., Hosokawa, M., Miyashita, K. and Fushiki, T. (2002). *FEBS Lett.* 514(2-3), 315–322.

Tontonoz, P., Hu, E. and Spiegelman, B.M. (1994). *Cell* 79(7), 1147–1156.

Waterman, I.J. and Zammit, V.A. (2002). *Diabetes* 51(6), 1708–1713.

Yajima, H., Ikeshima, E., Shiraki, M., Kanaya, T., Fujiwara, D., Odai, H., Tsuboyama-Kasaoka, N., Ezaki, O., Oikawa, S. and Kondo, K. (2004). *J. Biol. Chem.* 279(32), 33456–33462.

Yajima, H., Noguchi, T., Ikeshima, E., Shiraki, M., Kanaya, T., Tsuboyama-Kasaoka, N., Ezaki, O., Oikawa, S. and Kondo, K. (2005). *Int. J. Obesity* 29(8), 991–997.

Yamauchi, T., Kamon, J., Waki, H., Murakami, K., Motojima, K., Komeda, K., Ide, T., Kubota, N., Terauchi, Y., Tobe, K., Miki, H., Tsuchida, A., Akanuma, Y., Nagai, R., Kimura, S. and Kadowaki, T. (2001). *J. Biol. Chem.* 276(44), 41245–41254.

Ye, J.M., Doyle, P.J., Iglesias, M.A., Watson, D.G., Cooney, G.J. and Kraegen, E.W. (2001). *Diabetes* 50(2), 411–417.

Ye, J.M., Iglesias, M.A., Watson, D.G., Ellis, B., Wood, L., Jensen, P.B., Sorensen, R.V., Larsen, P.J., Cooney, G.J., Wassermann, K. and Kraegen, E.W. (2003). *Am. J. Physiol. Endocrinol. Metab.* 284(3), E531–E540.

80

Moderate Beer Consumption: Effects on Silicon Intake and Bone Health

Ravin Jugdaohsingh & Jonathan J. Powell MRC Human Nutrition Research, Elsie Widdowson Laboratory, Fulbourn Road, Cambridge, UK

Abstract

Accumulated evidence suggests that dietary silicon (Si) is beneficial for bone and connective tissue health and that higher intakes of dietary Si are associated with higher bone mineral density (BMD) (a proxy for bone health). A major source of Si is whole grain cereals and their products, such as beer, which is brewed from macerated, malted whole grain barley. Beer is a top contributor to Si intake in men and is a source of highly bioavailable Si. Beer also has a modest alcohol content. It is well established that moderate ingestion of alcoholic beverages is associated with increased BMD but mechanisms are unknown. In a recent extensive review (Jugdaohsingh *et al.*, 2006) we have made a case for ethanol and Si as the two major constituents of alcoholic beverages that can positively influence BMD; the latter being nearly beer-specific. Indeed in a recent report, we showed that the association between moderate beer ingestion and BMD was significantly reduced when a correction was made for Si (Tucker *et al.*, 2004). This was not seen with the other types of alcoholic beverages (wine and liquor). In more recent detailed analyses (Tucker *et al.*, 2007 unpublished data) we confirmed these findings and showed that while the major positive effect of moderate beer ingestion on BMD is an ethanol effect, some could be attributed to Si. Thus *moderate* beer ingestion (1–4 UK units/day) could be advantageous to bone health by providing both an anti-resorptive and an anabolic component, namely ethanol and silicon, respectively.

List of Abbreviations

APOSS	Aberdeen Prospective Osteoporosis Screening Study
BMD	Bone mineral density
Si	Silicon
HRT	Hormone replacement therapy

Introduction

Silicon (Si) is a major, naturally occurring element in animal diets, including the human diet (Powell *et al.*, 2005). Accumulating evidence over the last 30 years strongly suggests that dietary Si is beneficial to bone and connective tissue health (Sripanyakorn *et al.*, 2005) and, with our collaborators, we recently reported strong positive associations between dietary Si intake and bone mineral density (BMD) in US and UK cohorts (Jugdaohsingh *et al.*, 2004; Macdonald *et al.*, 2005). BMD, at the population level, is a proxy for functional bone health. A major source of dietary Si is whole grain cereals and their products including beer which is a macerated product of malted whole grain barley (Sripanyakorn *et al.*, 2004; Powell *et al.*, 2005), and beer is a top contributor to dietary Si intake in men (Jugdaohsingh *et al.*, 2002, 2004). Women drink much less beer so it's not a major contributor to Si intake in this population. Beer is also a source of alcohol (ethanol), and alcohol consumption *per se* strongly influences BMD and bone health (Jugdaohsingh *et al.*, 2006). In a preliminary analysis (global linear regression) we recently reported that Si intake from beer ingestion may explain some of the positive association between moderate beer ingestion and BMD (Jugdaohsingh *et al.*, 2004). In a more recent detailed analysis (Tucker *et al.*, 2007 unpublished data) we dissected out and compared the individual effects of the alcoholic beverages (beer, wine and spirits) on BMD and determined the contribution of Si to these associations. These results support our previous published findings of a contributory effect of Si from beer ingestion on BMD although the effect (attributable benefit) is small compared to that derived from the moderate ethanol ingestion (Jugdaohsingh *et al.*, 2004). Nonetheless, this was not seen with the other types of alcoholic beverages (wine and liquor) that have lower levels of Si and this is the first time that the effect of a non-ethanol component has been shown to contribute to the health benefit of moderate ingestion

Beer in Health and Disease Prevention
ISBN: 978-0-12-373891-2

of alcoholic beverages. This chapter summaries these findings and, prior to this, gives a brief overview/description of what Si is and its effects on BMD and bone health.

What Is Si?

Silicon, a non-metallic element with an atomic weight of 28, is the second most abundant element of the Earth's crust after oxygen (Sjöberg, 1996). It is also one of the most abundant trace elements in the human body, found at similar levels to selenium and zinc (Dobbie and Smith, 1982; Geigy Scientific Tables, 1984). Although widely distributed in the environment, Si is rarely found in its free form as it readily reacts with oxygen and water to form insoluble oxides (e.g. quartz, cristobalite and tridymite) and silicates (e.g. Ca, Mg, Al silicates), respectively, which at 92%, are the most common minerals on Earth (Klein, 1993). Biological and chemical weathering of these minerals leaches/releases soluble silicates or "silicic acids" into soil solutions, and natural water bodies, where Si is present in the latter at concentrations between 1 and 15 mg/l in the form of orthosilicic acid [$Si(OH)_4$] (Farmer, 1986). Orthosilicic acid is a weak diprotic acid and the most stable Si species in aqueous solutions at low (≤2 mM) total Si concentrations (Iler, 1979; Glasser and Lachowski, 1980; Glasser, 1982). However, at concentrations above 2 mM and around neutral pH, orthosilicic acid polymerizes to form a range of silica species from soluble dimers through aquated oligomers, polymers and colloids to solid phase silica, reducing the solubility and hence bioavailability of Si (Iler, 1979; Glasser and Lachowski, 1980; Glasser, 1982; Sjöberg, 1996; Taylor *et al.*, 1997). Silicon is also present in silicones, which are synthetic (i.e. man-made) "organo-silicon" compounds, but these are rarely found in the diet or in nature in general.

Silicon, as orthosilicic acid, is neutrally charged at physiological pHs and is relatively chemically inert. Thus, until recently, it was suggested not to take part in any biochemical reactions/interactions in higher animals, even though it is known to be actively taken up and transported by some primitive organisms and plants to form elaborate silica exoskeletons and biogenic silica, respectively the formation of which is assisted and controlled by proteins and polysaccharides (Cha *et al.*, 1999; Kröger *et al.*, 1999; Perry and Keeling-Tucker, 2000). Recently, however, Kinrade *et al.* (1999, 2004) reported that $Si(OH)_4$ interacts readily with alkyl diols of sugars to form five- and six-coordinate Si complexes suggesting that interactions with organic bio-molecules is at least possible. Functional, biological binding sites for Si (orthosilicic acid) still remain elusive, however.

Where Is Si Found?

Humans are exposed to numerous sources of silica/Si including dust, pharmaceuticals, supplements, cosmetics and medical implants and devices. However, the major and most important source of exposure for the majority of the population is the diet, and typical Si intakes are 20–50 mg/day in Western countries (Pennington, 1991; National Academy of Science, 2001; Jugdaohsingh *et al.*, 2002; McNaughton *et al.*, 2005). Intakes in males (33.1 ± 19.4 mg/d) is higher than in females (25.0 ± 11.4 mg/d), which is mainly due to higher intake of beer in males (Pennington, 1991; Jugdaohsingh *et al.*, 2002, 2004; Sripanyakorn *et al.*, 2005); beer is a high natural source of Si (see below). Intake also decreases significantly with age in adults (0.1 mg for every additional year) (National Academy of Science, 2001; Jugdaohsingh *et al.*, 2002).

Food sources

Silicon is taken up and actively accumulated by some plants and deposited as solid amorphous silica (phytoliths) in the cell lumen and walls (Sangster and Hodson, 1986; Epstein, 1999). As such, plant-based foods tend to have higher levels of Si (1–23 mg/100 g) compared to foods of animal origin, which contain very little Si (<1 mg/100 g; Powell *et al.*, 2005; Table 80.1). Amongst plant-based foods, un-refined ("whole") cereal grains (oats, barley, wheat) and grasses (e.g. rice) have the highest Si levels (mean 8 ± 6 mg/100 g; Powell *et al.*, 2005). Up to 50% of the Si is present in the hulls and husks, which is lost in the refined/processed food. However, grain products such as breakfast cereals, flour and bread, biscuit, rice, pasta, cake and pastry, etc. are still high dietary sources of Si (Pennington, 1991; Jugdaohsingh *et al.*, 2002; Powell *et al.*, 2005). Naturally high levels of Si are also present in some vegetables, namely beans, spinach and root vegetables and some herbs (mean 1.79 ± 2.42 mg/100 g; Pennington, 1991; Powell *et al.*, 2005). Fruits generally contain low levels of Si except for bananas and dried fruits and nuts (mean 1.34 ± 1.30 mg/100 g; Powell *et al.*, 2005). However, very little Si is digested in the gut and made available from bananas (<2%; Jugdaohsingh *et al.*, 2002). As already stated earlier, animal and dairy products are low in Si (Powell *et al.*, 2005). Slightly higher levels of Si may be present in offals and the less popular eaten parts (Pennington, 1991) presumably due to the presence of large vessels, since Si is suggested to contribute to the integrity of blood vessels such as the aortic wall lining (the tunica intima) (Loeper *et al.*, 1979).

Silicon-containing additives, typically silicates, are added to manufactured and processed foods as anti-caking agents, hygroscopic agent, emulsifiers, thickeners, stabilizers, coating agent and anti-foaming agents; for example, in beverage mixes, salad dressings, snack foods and sugar substitutes (Anonymous, 1974; Villota and Hawkes, 1986; Hanssen and Marsden, 1987). As noted earlier, solid phase silicates are thought to be inert and generally not absorbed in the gastrointestinal tract (see below), and, under UK regulations, solid phase silicate additives are added at less than

Table 80.1 Silicon in the diet

	Si (mg/100g)			
Food Groups	*Range*	*Mean*	*N*	*Si (mg/portion)*
Cereal grains and products				
Breakfast cereals	1.34–23.36	7.79	16	2.92 (37.5g)
Breads/flour	0.34–6.17	2.87	15	1.45 (50.5g)
Biscuits	1.05–2.44	1.56	5	0.406 (26g)
Rice	0.88–3.76	1.54	8	1.85 (120g)
Pasta	0.62–1.84	1.11	7	2.55 (230g)
Fruits				
Raw and canned	0.1–4.77	1.34	33	1.35 (101g)
Dried	6.09–16.61	10.54	3	3.51 (33.3g)
Vegetables	0.1–8.73	1.79	49	1.25 (70g)
Legumes (lentils, pulses, etc.)	0.38–4.42	1.46	11	0.759 (52g)
Nuts and seeds	0.28–1.99	0.78	4	0.174 (22.3g)
Milk and milk products	0.07–0.47	0.31	3 + TDS	0.288 (93g)
Meat and meat products	0.1–1.89		TDS	0.125–2.36 (125g)
Beverages (non-alcoholic)				
Tap water	0.095–0.61	0.37	11	0.740 (200g)
Mineral and spring waters	0.24–1.46	0.55	14	1.82 (330g)
Tea and coffee	0.24–0.86	0.51	6	1.33 (260g)
Fruit juices	0.05–1.5	0.38	11	0.866 (228g)
Fizzy/carbonated	0.11–0.19	0.15	6	0.507 (338g)
Milk based	0.2–3.96	1.30	6	3.38 (260g)
Beverages (alcoholic)				
Beers	0.9–3.94	1.92	76	6.37 (can/bottle) 11.0 (1 pint)
Wines	0.68–2.31	1.35	3	1.69 (125g)
Port/sherries	1.24–1.26	0.13	2	0.62–0.63 (50g)
Liquor/spirits	0.06–0.20	0.13	1	0.052 (40g)

Note: Mean silicon (Si) levels (mg/100g and mg/portion) in the different food groups and in non-alcoholic and alcoholic beverages. Plant-based foods, in particular whole grain cereals and products (including beer), are high sources of dietary Si, while dairy and animal products contain negligible levels. For each food group the range, mean level and number of foods analyzed are given. Mean portion sizes are given in parentheses. Table is adapted from Powell *et al.* (2005). *N*: number of samples. TDS: sample from the Food Standard Agency Total Diet Study.

2% weight of the food (Anonymous, 1974; Dobbie and Smith, 1982).

Drinking water

Silicon in drinking water is derived from the weathering of rocks and soil minerals and since different types of minerals weather at different rates, the concentration of Si in drinking water is dependent on the surrounding geology (Farmer, 1986). Concentration ranges between 0.2 and 14 mg/l in tap water, although the majority tends to be at the lower/mid-end (2–6 mg/l) (Dobbie and Smith, 1982; Birchall and Chappell, 1989; Roberts and Williams, 1990; Parry *et al.*, 1998; Powell *et al.*, 2005). Concentrations in mineral waters are typically higher, especially those from volcanic sources, such as Volvic (16 mg/l), Spritzer (30 mg/l) and Fiji (40 mg/l) mineral waters, from France, Malaysia and Fiji, respectively (Jugdaohsingh *et al.*, 2006 unpublished data). Silicon levels in tea, coffee, squash, etc. are derived from the water used to prepare these beverages and potentially also from the silicate additives that are present in instant tea and coffee (Powell *et al.*, 2005).

Beer and other alcoholic beverages

Whole grain barley and hops are used in making beer and the maceration (mashing) process breaks down the phytolithic silica in the husks, etc. into soluble forms, so this beverage is high in Si (see Chapter 46; also: Pennington, 1991; Bellia *et al.*, 1994; Sripanyakorn *et al.*, 2004; Powell *et al.*, 2005; Table 80.1). We previously reported a mean (±SD) concentration of 19.2 ± 6.6 mg Si/l beer (Sripanyakorn *et al.*, 2004). Not surprisingly, therefore, beer can be a major contributor to Si intake in the Western diet, especially for men who consume considerably more beer than women (Pennington, 1991; Jugdaohsingh *et al.*, 2002; Sripanyakorn *et al.*, 2004; Powell *et al.*, 2005), contributing, on average, between 11% and 24% of total daily Si intake (Jugdaohsingh *et al.*, 2002, 2004). The consumption of beer in the United Kingdom was 173 pints per capita in 2004 (http://www.kirin.co.jp/english/ir/news_release051215_4.html), confirming beer as a significant dietary source of Si in the UK diet.

In contrast, levels of Si in wines are more varied and can be as high as some beers (see Chapter 46; Powell *et al.*, 2005; Table 80.1). Silicon levels in liquors/spirits is much lower being 1.3 ± 0.04 mg/l (Jugdaohsingh *et al.*, 2004).

Silicon Metabolism

Absorption

Recent studies have increased our understanding of the bioavailability of Si from food and other sources, but the mechanism(s) of absorption of Si from the gastrointestinal tract is/are yet to be established (Calomme *et al.*, 1998; Reffitt *et al.*, 1999; Van Dyck *et al.*, 1999; Jugdaohsingh *et al.*, 2002; Sripanyakorn *et al.*, 2004, 2005; Sripanyakorn *et al.*, 2005 unpublished data). Uptake from the gastrointestinal tract is primarily dependent on the speciation of Si, and soluble orthosilicic acid [$Si(OH)_4$] is the most bioavailable and readily absorbable species (Yokoi and Enomoto, 1979; Calomme *et al.*, 1998; Reffitt *et al.*, 1999; Van Dyck *et al.*, 1999; Jugdaohsingh *et al.*, 2002; Sripanyakorn *et al.*, 2004, 2005; Sripanyakorn *et al.*, 2005 unpublished data). Thus, drinking water, beer and other fluids/beverages can provide the most readily bioavailable source of Si in the diet, which, coupled with the fact that fluid ingestion can account for ≤20% of the total dietary intake of Si (Bellia *et al.*, 1994), makes these sources significant contributors to bio-active Si exposure (Reffitt *et al.*, 1999; Jugdaohsingh *et al.*, 2002). At least 55% of Si in beer is absorbed and much is then rapidly excreted in urine within 6–8 h of ingestion (Bellia *et al.*, 1994; Sripanyakorn *et al.*, 2004) (Figure 80.1). Absorption and excretion profiles were similar or slightly higher than for orthosilicic acid (Sripanyakorn *et al.*, 2004) (Figure 80.1a and b) suggesting that beer alcohol must only minimally affect the metabolism of Si and confirming that Si is present in beer as absorbable and bioactive orthosilicic acid (Sripanyakorn *et al.*, 2004).

Silicon is also readily absorbed from food sources (mean 41% of ingested dose) suggesting that much phytolithic silica is broken down to soluble species (e.g. orthosilicic acid) in the gastrointestinal tract, prior to absorption (Reffitt *et al.*, 1999; Jugdaohsingh *et al.*, 2002).

Excretion

The main route of elimination/excretion of absorbed Si is via the kidneys into urine (Berlyne *et al.*, 1986; Reffitt *et al.*, 1999). Indeed, renal function appears to be a good determinant of plasma Si concentration (Hosokawa and Yoshida, 1990; Roberts and Williams, 1990; D'Haese *et al.*, 1995; Sanz-Medel *et al.*, 1996; Parry *et al.*, 1998). Silicon is not associated with plasma proteins and thus it is readily filtered by the renal glomerulus (Adler and Berlyne, 1986; D'Haese *et al.*, 1995), and eliminated with little tubular reabsorption. Hence, urinary Si excretion is a good proxy for absorption, or of gastrointestinal uptake into serum (Reffitt *et al.*, 1999) and this is commonly used/exploited in Si absorption studies to study the bioavailability of Si from Si-containing foods and compounds.

Tissue Distribution, Function and Essentiality

Some absorbed Si is retained by the body and all tissues contain some Si, but highest levels are found in bone and

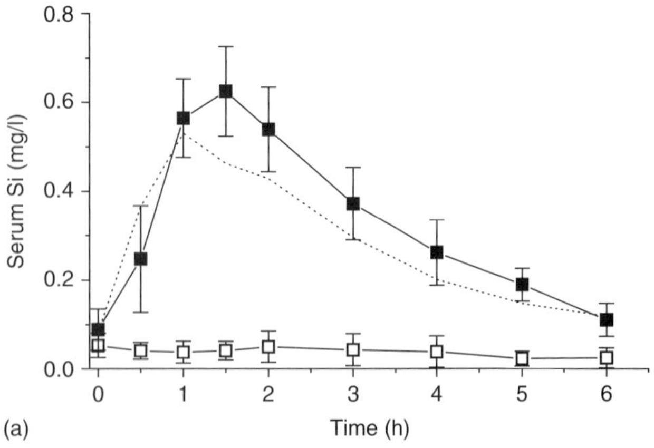

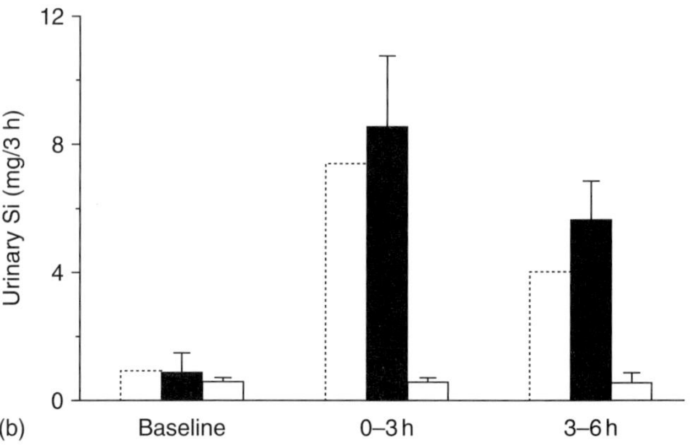

Figure 80.1 Bioavailability of silicon from beer. (a) Mean (± SD) serum silicon (Si) and (b) urinary Si excretion (mg/3 h), in eight subjects following the ingestion of 600 ml beer containing 22.5 mg Si and 4.6% alcohol (■–■, *black bars*), and 600 ml solution containing 4.6% ethanol and negligible amounts of Si <0.02 mg (□–□, *white bars*). For comparison, the absorption and urinary excretion profiles for orthosilicic acid are shown (*dotted line*). The results suggest that Si in beer is highly bioavailable. Further, speciation studies confirmed that Si is present as orthosilicic acid in beer (Sripanyakorn *et al.*, 2004).

other connective tissues, such as skin, nail, trachea, tendons and aorta and very much less (10- to 20-fold less) in soft tissues (Le Vier, 1975; Carlisle, 1986; Jugdaohsingh *et al.*, 2006 unpublished data). Silicon is suggested to be integrally bound to connective tissues and their components and to play an important structural role (Schwarz, 1973) as Si deprivation has detrimental effects on these tissues (Carlisle, 1972; Schwarz and Milne, 1972), as is also speculated to occur with normal aging with the decline in tissue Si levels (McCarty, 1997). *Vice versa*, increasing Si intake has been reported to have beneficial effects on these tissues, *especially* bone where much of current work has concentrated (Loeper *et al.*, 1979; Schiano *et al.*, 1979; Eisinger and Clairet, 1993; Hott *et al.*, 1993; Lassus, 1993, 1997; Rico *et al.*, 2000; Jugdaohsingh *et al.*, 2004; Barel *et al.*, 2005; Spector *et al.*, 2005; Calomme *et al.*, 2006). The potential importance of Si in bone health is thus discussed below.

Dietary Si and Bone

Mounting evidence over the last 30 years strongly supports a biological role for Si in bone and connective tissue health. This includes cellular, animal and human studies (see Sripanyakorn *et al.*, 2005 for a review of the evidence). Recent studies have shown that dietary Si, as soluble orthosilicic acid, has anabolic effects on human osteoblast-like cells and in animal models of post-menopausal osteoporosis (Hott *et al.*, 1993; Rico *et al.*, 2000; Calomme *et al.*, 2006). Increased type I collagen synthesis, osteocalcin secretion and alkaline phosphatase activity have been reported in human osteoblast-like cells (Reffitt *et al.*, 2003; Arumugam *et al.*, 2006). In animal studies, supplemental Si not only inhibits bone loss but also increases BMD above controls, suggesting Si may have both anti-resorptive and anabolic properties (Hott *et al.*, 1993; Rico *et al.*, 2000).

There are few studies of Si in humans, but these have also shown that supplemental Si has both anti-resorptive and anabolic properties (Schiano *et al.*, 1979; Eisinger and Clairet, 1993; Spector *et al.*, 2005). Additionally, in a recent cross-sectional study in the Framingham Offspring Cohort we reported that dietary Si intake was positively and significantly associated with BMD in pre-menopausal women, less so in men and not at all in post-menopausal women (Jugdaohsingh *et al.*, 2004). Large differences in BMD, up to 10%, were observed between the highest (>40 mg/d) and lowest (<14 mg/d) Si intake categories in men and pre-menopausal women with similar results obtained using a linear regression model. These results, in pre- and post-menopausal women, we recently confirmed in a cohort of the UK population (Macdonald *et al.*, 2005). Using the APOSS (Aberdeen Prospective Osteoporosis Screening Study) cohort we similarly showed that dietary Si intake was significantly positively associated with BMD at the hip and spine of pre-menopausal women. We also showed a similar correlation in post-menopausal women but only in those currently on hormone replacement therapy (HRT) (Macdonald *et al.*, 2005). A weaker (non-significant) correlation was found in past-HRT users and no correlation in those who had never taken HRT. These two studies strongly suggest that higher intake of dietary Si is associated with higher BMD, a marker of bone strength and bone quality, and also suggests a potential interaction between Si and hormonal status.

Altogether, the accumulated evidence suggests that Si plays an important role in bone health. However, although a number of possible mechanisms have been proposed the exact role/biochemical function of Si remains unknown.

Beer Ingestion and Bone Health

Moderate alcohol consumption (up to 14 g alcohol/d (1 serving/d) for women and up to 28 g/d (2 servings/d) men) seems to be beneficial to health *per se*, in contrast to excessive alcohol consumption/alcohol abuse that is associated with increased risk of morbidity and mortality (De Loromier, 2000). Thus moderate consumption of alcoholic beverages is associated with higher BMD, especially in post-menopausal and elderly women (Jugdaohsingh *et al.*, 2006); differences in BMD of 1–16% have been reported between drinkers and abstainers/minimal drinkers, with highest BMD in moderate drinkers (Feskanich *et al.*, 1999; Rapuri *et al.*, 2000; Tunner and Sibonga, 2001; Williams *et al.*, 2004; see also Jugdaohsingh *et al.*, 2006 for a review of current evidence). There are, however, few studies in men and pre-menopausal women and previous studies have used simple linear regression models to test for association when the relationship between alcohol consumption and health status is described as "J" or "U" shaped. In addition many have inconsistently adjusted for potential confounders of BMD. Hence there is still a need for well-controlled, robust studies, and the individual effects of the different classes of alcoholic beverages (beer, wine, liquor) on BMD has also not been studied or dissected out.

We have recently studied the effects of the different classes of alcoholic beverages (beer, wine and spirits) on BMD in men, pre- and post-menopausal women of the Framingham Osteoporosis cohort, using both continuous and categorical analyses with adjustment for all known potential confounding factors of BMD (Tucker *et al.*, 2004; Tucker *et al.*, 2006 unpublished data). From these analyses, linear regression analysis showed that alcohol intake was positively associated with adjusted BMD at the hip sites and lumbar spine in men and women. Categorical analysis by alcohol intake supported these findings, and showed differences in BMD of 4–6% at the trochanter between those ingesting moderate amounts of alcohol and abstainers/non-drinkers (Tucker *et al.*, 2007 unpublished data). Differences existed between men, pre- and post-menopausal women and between the different classes of alcoholic beverages. For men, associations (with BMD) for beer intake was > liquor > wine intake, while for post-menopausal women associations for wine intake ≥ beer = liquor. Our findings thus support current evidence that moderate consumption of alcohol may be beneficial to bone health, but also suggest that the different types of alcoholic beverages may have different effects on BMD and gender, that the other (non-alcoholic) components of the beverage may have additional/contributory effect on the association between alcohol intake and BMD. We have investigated one such component, namely Si, which is found almost exclusively in beer, compared to the other alcoholic beverages (see below).

Beer Silicon and Bone

The mechanism of action of moderate alcohol consumption on BMD is less clear. Although in our recent review (Jugdaohsingh *et al.*, 2006) a case was made for the acute suppression of bone resorption as the primary effect of moderate ethanol ingestion, the effect of minerals/nutrients obtained from moderate alcohol consumption has not been well studied. Indeed, as noted above these non-alcohol constituents may contribute to the effect/association between alcohol intake and BMD. Since beer is a major source of bioavailable Si, we have investigated whether the contribution of Si from beer ingestion could contribute to the positive effects of moderate alcohol consumption on bone. Firstly, one 300–574 ml size serving of beer would contribute between 3.8 and 16 mg Si/day (or 2–9 mg/d absorbed if bioavailability is taken into consideration), which could be enough to detect an association with BMD based on Si intake and BMD data (Jugdaohsingh *et al.*, 2004). Indeed, an increase in Si intake of 5–6 mg/d was associated with a 2–5% increase in BMD at the Trochanter in men and pre-menopausal women, respectively. Secondly, in previous work, we looked at the association between beer intake and BMD, with and without correcting for Si intake. Correcting for the Si contribution from beer attenuated the positive association and reduced or negated the significance between beer intake and BMD (Jugdaohsingh *et al.*, 2004). Similar investigations on the intake of non-beer alcohols showed no effect of Si correction on the alcohol-BMD association, due to the small contribution of Si intake from non-beer alcohols (Jugdaohsingh *et al.*, 2004). Thus these findings suggest that the Si component of beer may explain/contribute to some of the positive effects of moderate alcohol consumption on bone. However, as noted previously, these findings are based on basic regression models as an initial "global overview" and further, more detailed studies are required using categorical data to really dissect out the role of Si vs. that of ethanol and/or other components in the association of the intakes of different alcoholic beverages with bone health.

We recently completed these detailed analyses, that is, using both linear and categorical analysis of alcohol intake (Tucker *et al.*, 2006 unpublished data). We confirmed our previous findings, including that adjustment for Si intake reduces the magnitude and significance of the association between beer intake and BMD in men and pre-menopausal women but not post-menopausal women (Tucker *et al.*, 2006 unpublished data). Further, categorical analysis in men indicated that some of the effects for moderate beer consumption on BMD may be attributed to Si intake from beer ingestion. As previously reported, adjustment for Si intake had no effect on the associations between wine or liquor intake and BMD as expected since wine and liquor are lesser and negligible sources of dietary Si, respectively (Powell *et al.*, 2005). These results suggest that the main effect of moderate alcohol consumption on BMD is an ethanol effect, which is suggested to act on bone resorption (Rapuri *et al.*, 2000; Tunner and Sibonga, 2001; Jugdaohsingh *et al.*, 2006). However, these results also provide some evidence for a non-ethanol, bone active component in beer, namely Si. This is the first time a non-ethanol effect has been dissected out and reported. The Si effect is moderate and observed at the higher intake categories and in contrast to ethanol, Si is more likely to act on bone formation (Jugdaohsingh *et al.*, 2004; Sripanyakorn *et al.*, 2005). Thus moderate beer ingestion may not only inhibit bone resorption but also increase bone formation which could make beer unique amongst the other alcoholic beverages.

Summary Points

- Dietary Si is a major component of the daily diet; 20–50 mg/d in the Western diet.
- Higher intake of dietary Si is associated with higher BMD (a marker of bone strength and bone quality) in men, pre- and post-menopausal women on HRT.
- Major sources of dietary Si are whole grain cereals and their products including beer, a macerated product of whole grain barley.
- Beer is a top contributor to daily Si intake in men, who are typically beer drinkers and beer is one of the most highly bioavailable source of Si.
- *Moderate* ingestion of beer, up to 1 serving/d (or 14 g alcohol) for women and up to 2 servings/d (28 g alcohol) for men, is associated with increased BMD; an increase of 4–6% at the trochanter compared to abstainers (non-drinkers).
- This effect is mainly an alcohol (ethanol) effect, but at least a small proportion of the increased BMD in men, at the trochanter, could be attributed to Si intake from beer ingestion.
- Moderate ingestion of beer may provide both an anti-resorptive and an anabolic component, namely ethanol and Si, respectively.

Acknowledgments

We acknowledge The Frances and Augustus Newman Foundation, Food Standard Agency UK, US Department of

Agriculture (contract 53-3K06-5-10), National Institutes of Health (RO1 AR/AG 41398), the Framingham Heart Study (supported by NIH/NHLBI contract NO1-HC-38038), the Wellcome Trust, the Government of Thailand, Special Trustees of Guy's and St. Thomas' Hospitals, and the charitable foundation of the Institute of Brewing and Distilling for their support over the years with our research program.

References

Adler, A.J. and Berlyne, G.M. (1986). *Nephron* 44, 36–39.

Anonymous (1974). *Toxicological Evaluation of Some Food Additives Including Anticaking Agents, Antimicrobials, Antioxidants, Emulsifiers and Thickening Agents.* pp. 21–30. World Health Organization, Geneva.

Arumugam, M.Q., Ireland, D.C., Brooks, R.A., Rushton, N. and Bonfield, W. (2006). *Bioceramics* 18, 121–124. Pts 1 & 2 Key Engineering Materials 309–311.

Barel, A., Calomme, M., Timchenko, A., De Paepe, K., Demeester, N., Rogiers, V., Clarys, P. and Vanden Berghe, D. (2005). *Arch. Dermatol. Res.* 297, 147–153.

Bellia, J.P., Birchall, J.D. and Roberts, N.B. (1994). *Lancet* 343, 235.

Berlyne, G.M., Adler, A.J., Ferran, N., Bennett, S. and Holt, J. (1986). *Nephron* 43, 5–9.

Birchall, J.D. and Chappell, J.S. (1989). *The Lancet* p, 953.

Calomme, M., Geusens, P., Demeester, N., Behets, G.J., D'Haese, P., Sindambiwe, J.B., Van Hoof, V. and Vanden Berghe, D. (2006). *Calcif. Tissue Int.* 78, 227–232.

Calomme, M.R., Cos, P., D'Haese, P.C., Vingerhoets, R., Lamberts, L.V., De Broe, M.E., Van Hoorebeke, C. and Vanden Berghe, D.A. (1998). In Collery, P., Brätter, P., Negretti de Brätter, V., Khassanova, L. and Etienne, J.-C. (eds), *Metal Ions in Biology and Medicine, Volume 5*, pp. 228–232. John Libbey Eurotext, Paris.

Carlisle, E.M. (1972). *Science* 178, 619.

Carlisle, E.M. (1986). In Evered, D. and O'Connor, M. (eds), *Silicon Biochemistry, Ciba Foundation Symposium 121*, pp. 123–139. John Wiley and Sons Ltd, Chichester.

Cha, J.N., Shimizu, K., Zhou, Y., Christiansen, S.C., Chmelka, B.F., Stucky, G.D. and Morse, D.E. (1999). *Proc. Nat. Acad. Sci. USA* 96, 361–365.

D'Haese, P.C., Shaheen, F.A., Huraid, S.O., Djukanovic, L., Polenakovic, M.H., Spasovski, G., Shikole, A., Schurgers, M.L., Daneels, R.F., Lamberts, L.V., Van Landeghem, G.F. and De Broe, M.E. (1995). *Nephrol. Dial. Transpl.* 10, 1838–1844.

De Loromier, A.A. (2000). *Am. J. Surg.* 180, 357–361.

Dobbie, J.W. and Smith, M.J.B. (1982). *Scot. Med. J.* 27, 10–19.

Eisinger, J. and Clairet, D. (1993). *Magnesium Res.* 6, 247–249.

Epstein, E. (1999). *Ann. Rev. Plant Physiol. Plant Mol. Biol.* 50, 641–664.

Farmer, V.C. (1986). In Evered, D. and O'Connor, M. (eds), *Silicon Biochemistry, Ciba Foundation Symposium 121*, pp. 4–23. John Wiley and Sons Ltd, Chichester.

Feskanich, D., Korrick, S.A., Greenspan, S.L., Rosen, H.N. and Colditz, G.A. (1999). *J. Women Health* 8, 65–73.

Geigy Scientific Tables (1984). In Lentner, C. (ed.), *Physical Chemistry, Composition of Blood, Hematology, Somatometric Data Volume 1–3*, Ciba-Geigy Limited; International Medical and Pharmaceutical Information, Basle, Switzerland.

Glasser, L.S.D. (1982). *Chem. Bri.*, 36–40.

Glasser, L.S.D. and Lachowski, E.E. (1980). *J. Chem. Soc. Dalton Trans.*, 393–398.

Hanssen, M. and Marsden, J. (1987). *E for Additives.* HarperCollins Publishers, Glasgow.

Hosokawa, S. and Yoshida, O. (1990). *Int. Urol. Nephrol.* 22, 373–378.

Hott, M., de Pollak, C., Modrowski, D. and Marie, P.J. (1993). *Calcif. Tissue Int.* 53, 174–179.

Iler, R.K. (1979). *The Chemistry of Silica. Solubility, Polymerisation, Colloid and Surface Properties, and Biochemistry.* John Wiley & Sons, New York.

Jugdaohsingh, R., Anderson, S.H.C., Tucker, K.L., Elliott, H., Kiel, D.P., Thompson, R.P.H. and Powell, J.J. (2002). *Amer. J. Clin. Nutr.* 75, 887–893.

Jugdaohsingh, R., Tucker, K.L., Qiao, N., Cupples, L.A., Kiel, D.P. and Powell, J.J. (2004). *J. Bone Miner. Res.* 19, 297–307.

Jugdaohsingh, R., O'Connell, M.A., Sripanyakorn, S. and Powell, J.J. (2006). *Proc. Nutr. Soc.* 65, 291–310.

Kinrade, S.D., Balec, R.J., Schach, A.S., Wang, J. and Knight, C.T. (2004). *Dalton Trans.* 21, 3241–3243.

Kinrade, S.D., Del Nin, J.W. and Schach, A.S. (1999). *Science* 285, 1542–1545.

Klein, C. (1993). In Guthrie Jr., G.D. and Mossman, B.T. (eds), *Health Effects of Mineral Dust, Reviews in Mineralogy Vol. 28, Ineralogical Society of America*, p. 8. Bookcrafters Inc, Washington, DC.

Kröger, N., Deutzmann, R. and Sumper, M. (1999). *Science* 286, 1129–1132.

Lassus, A. (1993). *J. Inter. Med. Res.* 21, 209–215.

Lassus, A. (1997). *J. Inter. Med. Res.* 25, 206–209.

Le Vier, R.R. (1975). *Bioinorg. Chem.* 4, 109–115.

Loeper, J., Goy-Loeper, J., Rozensztajn, L. and Fragny, M. (1979). *Atherosclerosis* 33, 397–408.

Macdonald, H.M., Hardcastle, A.E., Jugdaohsingh, R., Reid, D.M. and Powell, J.J. (2005). *J. Bone Miner. Res.* 20, S393.

McCarty, M.F. (1997). *Med. Hypotheses* 49, 175–176.

McNaughton, S.A., Bolton-Smith, C., Mishra, G.D., Jugdaohsingh, R. and Powell, J.J. (2005). *Br. J. Nutr.* 94, 813–817.

National Academy of Sciences (2001). *Dietary Reference Intakes for Vitamin A, Vitamin K, Boron, Chromium, Copper, Iodine, Iron, Manganese, Nickel, Silicon, Vanadium and Zinc.* National Academy Press, Washington, DC.

Parry, R., Plowman, D., Delves, H.T., Roberts, N.B., Birchall, J.D., Bellia, J.P., Davenport, A., Ahmad, R., Fahal, I. and Altman, P. (1998). *Nephrol. Dial. Transpl.* 13, 1759–1762.

Pennington, J.A.T. (1991). *Food Addit. Contam.* 8, 97–118.

Perry, C.C. and Keeling-Tucker, T. (2000). *J. Biol. Inorg. Chem.* 5, 537–550.

Powell, J.J., McNaughton, S.A., Jugdaohsingh, R., Anderson, S., Dear, J., Khot, F., Mowatt, L., Gleason, K.L., Sykes, M., Thompson, R.P.H., Bolton-Smith, C. and Hodson, M.J. (2005). *Br. J. Nutr.* 94, 804–812.

Rapuri, P.B., Gallagher, J.C., Balhorn, K.E. and Ryschon, K.L. (2000). *Am. J. Clin. Nutr.* 72, 1206–1213.

Reffitt, D.M., Jugdoahsingh, R., Thompson, R.P.H. and Powell, J.J. (1999). *J. Inorg. Biochem.* 76, 141–147.

Reffitt, D.M., Ogston, N., Jugdaohsingh, R., Cheung, H.F., Evans, B.A., Thompson, R.P., Powell, J.J. and Hampson, G.N. (2003). *Bone* 32, 127–135.

Rico, H., Gallego-Largo, J.L., Hernández, E.R., Villa, L.F., Sanchez-Atrio, A., Seco, C. and Gérvas, J.J. (2000). *Calcif. Tissue Int.* 66, 53–55.

Roberts, N.B. and Williams, P. (1990). *Clin. Chem.* 36, 1460–1465.

Sangster, A.G. and Hodson, M.J. (1986). In Evered, D. and O'Connor, M. (eds), *Silicon Biochemistry, Ciba Foundation Symposium 121*, pp. 90–111. John Wiley and Sons Ltd, Chichester.

Sanz-Medel, A., Fairman, B. and Wróbel, K. (1996). In Caroli, S. (ed.), *Element Speciation in Bioinorganic Chemistry, Chemical Analysis Series, Vol. 135*, pp. 223–254. John Wiley and Sons Ltd, Chichester.

Schiano, A., Eisinger, F., Detolle, P., Laponche, A.M., Brisou, B. and Eisinger, J. (1979). *Rev. Rhum.* 46, 483–486.

Schwarz, K. (1973). *Proc. Nat. Acad. Sci. USA.* 70, 1608–1612.

Schwarz, K. and Milne, D.B. (1972). *Nature* 239, 333–334.

Sjöberg, S. (1996). *J. Non-crys. Sol.* 196, 51–57.

Spector, T.D., Calomme, M.R., Anderson, S., Swaminathan, R., Jugdaohsingh, R., Vanden-Berge, D.A. and Powell, J.J. (2005). *J. Bone Miner. Res.* 20, S172.

Sripanyakorn, S., Jugdaohsingh, R., Elliott, H., Walker, C., Mehta, P., Shouker, S., Thompson, R.P.H. and Powell, J.J. (2004). *Br. J. Nutr.* 91, 403–409.

Sripanyakorn, S., Jugdaohsingh, R., Thompson, R.P.H. and Powell, J.J. (2005). *Br. Nutr. Found. Nutr. Bull.* 30, 222–230.

Taylor, P.D., Jugdaohsingh, R. and Powell, J.J. (1997). Soluble silica with high affinity for aluminium under physiological and natural conditions. *J. Am. Chem. Soc.* 119, 8852–8856.

Tucker, K.L., Powell, J.J., Qiao, N., Cupples, L.A. and Kiel, D.P. (2004). *J. Bone Miner. Res.* 19, S85.

Tucker *et al.* (2007). (Unpublished data).

Tunner, R.T. and Sibonga, J.D. (2001). *Alcohol Res. Health* 25, 276–281.

Van Dyck, K., Van Cauwenbergh, R., Robberecht, H. and Deelstra, H. (1999). *Fresenius J. Anal. Chem.* 363, 541–544.

Villota, R. and Hawkes, J.G. (1986). *Crit. Rev. Food Sci. Nutr.* 23, 289–321.

Williams, F.M., Cherkas, L.F., Spector, T.D. and MacGregor, A.J. (2004). *BMC Cardiovas. Disord.* 4, 20.

Yokoi, H. and Enomoto, S. (1979). *Chem. Pharm. Bull. (Tokyo)* 27, 1733–1739.

81

Biolabeling of Xanthohumol in Hop Cones (*Humulus Lupulus* L., Cannabaceae) with Stable and Radioactive Precursors for Biosynthetic and Metabolic Studies

Hans Becker and Stefanie Berwanger Pharmakognosie und Analytische Phytochemie der Universität des Saarlandes, Saarbrücken, Germany
Norbert Frank German Cancer Research Center (DKFZ) Chemoprevention, Im Neuenheimer Feld, Heidelberg, Germany

Abstract

The biosynthesis of xanthohumol (Xn), a prenylated chalcone from hop cones has been studied by feeding ^{13}C labeled precursors to hop cuttings. Feeding of [ring-$^{13}C6$] phenylalanine resulted in incorporation of the B-ring of the chalcone. [1-^{13}C] acetate and [2-^{13}C] malonate were incorporated in the A-ring according to the established biosynthesis of chalcones. The biosynthetic pathway of the prenyl side chain was attributed to the deoxyxylulose or methylerythrothiol (MEP) pathway. Uniform labeled ^{13}C-glucose (2.5%) led to a 9-fold increase of ^{13}C abundance of every carbon atom of the molecule. These results prompted us to perform labeling studies with radioactive ^{14}C-glucose which resulted in Xn with a specific activity of up to 318 μCi/mmol. The radioactive Xn can be used for distribution and metabolic studies in experimental animals.

Introduction

According to the "German Reinheitsgebot," beer is exclusively made from water, malt and hops. Hops is used for more than 500 years in brewery due to its bitter acids which are located in specific glands of the female hops cones and which contribute to the bitter taste and to the stability of beer.

Besides these bitter acids, hops – and therefore even beer – contains other compounds, from which in recent years mainly the phenolic compounds have attracted attention because of their interesting physiological properties. Thus Gerhäuser *et al.* (2002a) isolated 51 compounds from unstabilized beer and tested them for potential cancer chemopreventive activities. Some of these compounds showed inhibitory effects on enzymes involved in carcinogen metabolism (inhibition of phase 1 cytochrome P450 1 A activity), induction of NAD(P)H:quinone oxidoreductase as well as anti-inflammatory properties (inhibition of lipopolysaccharide-mediated induction of inducible nitric oxide synthase, inhibition of cyclooxygenase 1). Among these phenolic compounds xanthohumol (Xn) has shown the most outstanding activities and was therefore chosen for further detailed tests on its chemopreventive potential (Gerhäuser *et al.*, 2002b).

Besides the above-mentioned activities Xn is able to scavange reactive oxygen species, including hydroxyl- and peroxyl radicals and to inhibit superoxide anion radical production. It demonstrates anti-inflammatory properties not only by inhibition of cyclooxygenase-1 but also by inhibition of cyclooxygenase-2 activity and it shows antiestrogenic potential. Antiproliferative mechanisms of Xn to prevent carcinogenesis in the progression phase include inhibition of DNA synthesis and induction of cell cycle arrest in S phase, apoptosis and cell differentiation. Xn at nanomolecular concentrations prevents carcinogen-induced preneoplastic lesions in mouse mammary gland organ culture. The anti-infective potential of Xn in comparison with other hop constituents and Xn-metabolites was summarized by Gerhäuser (2005).

Xn belongs to a group of prenylated chalcones and flavanones which are located in the glands of the female cones as well as the bitter acids (Stevens *et al.*, 1997). The amount of Xn in hop cones differs between the various varieties. It ranges from 0.23% (Hersbrucker Spalt) to 0.95% (Hallertauer Taurus) (Biendl, 2002/2003).

During the brewing process most of Xn is transformed into the flavanon iso-xanthohumol. Following only relative small amounts of Xn can be detected in beer. According to Stevens *et al.* (1999), American beers contain between 0.005 mg/l (wheaten beer) and 0.69 mg/l (porter). We analyzed

Beer in Health and Disease Prevention
ISBN: 978-0-12-373891-2

German beers with Xn ranging from 0.05 to 0.16 mg/l (Cernko and Becker, unpublished results).

Due to the promising results regarding the chemopreventive potential of Xn, new brewing techniques have been developed to increase the yield of Xn in beer recently (Wunderlich *et al.*, 2005). With these techniques and depending on the addition of roasted malt or special Xn-enriched roasted malt extracts, dark beers with more than 10 mg Xn/l were achieved.

Metabolites of Xn have been identified through transformation with rat liver microsomes (Yilmazer *et al.*, 2001) and in rat feces (Nookandeh *et al.*, 2004). *In vivo* tissue distribution and the bioavailability of Xn have still to be clarified for its future commercial or therapeutical use.

For bioavailability studies, radiolabeled compounds have been widely used (Vitrac *et al.*, 2003) because these compounds and their metabolites can be easily traced *in vivo*. Since no chemical synthesis of Xn has been published so far, biolabeling seemed to be an appropriate method for obtaining ^{13}C- and ^{14}C labeled Xn. The biolabeling method uses the plant metabolism for the incorporation of isotope into the respective natural compound by feeding labeled biosynthetic precursors of this compound to the plant. The choice of a suitable isotope depends on its stability in the molecule and on the commercial availability (and its price) of precursor compounds.

For tracing a radiolabeled compound and its metabolites *in vivo*, it is important to know the labeling position within the molecule as even fragments of the molecule could be included into radiodetection. It is not possible to precisely determine the incorporation pattern and ratio of ^{14}C into the molecules for each carbon. However by using the stable isotope ^{13}C, distinct labeling patterns can be obtained, as this isotope can easily be detected and quantified by using quantitative ^{13}C-NMR-technique. Therefore such experiments, using ^{13}C labeled precursors, are mainly carried out for biosynthesis studies, because the fate of a labeled precursor during plant metabolism can be easily traced.

To clarify the labeling positions and ratios in Xn for further ^{14}C experiments and to clarify the hitherto unknown biosynthesis of the prenyl side chain of Xn, we carried out experiments by feeding ^{13}C labeled potential known biosynthetic precursors (Berwanger *et al.*, 2005a) to hops. Studies on biosynthesis of bitter acids in hops were carried out by this method by Goese *et al.* (1999).

Biosynthesis of Xn

It is quite sure that the chalcone moiety is synthesized by a combination of the phenylpropane pathway (ring B) and the acetate/malonate pathway (ring A) (Heller and Forkmann, 1968). The prenyl side chain may be formed either by the classical acetate-mevalonate pathway or by the deoxyxylulose/methylerythrothiol (MEP) pathway (Eisenreich *et al.*, 1998; Rohmer, 1999). Direct labeled precursors to distinguish between the two pathways for the prenyl side chain were not available. Glucose is a universal nutrient for plants. For biosynthetic studies either uniform or 1-^{13}C labeled glucose was used in *in vitro* cultures (e.g. Adam *et al.*, 1998), *in vitro* crown plantlets (Umlauf *et al.*, 2004) or in cuttings from plants (e.g. Goese *et al.*, 1999). To distinguish between the two alternative pathways [1-^{13}C] glucose or uniform labeled [U-^{13}C] glucose has been successfully applied in various cases (Adam *et al.*, 1998; Eisenreich *et al.*, 1998). Whereas the classical mevalonate pathway leads to a symmetric labeling of the prenyl side chain (C-2″, C 4″, C-5″), the MEP-pathway will lead to the labeling of C-1″ and C-5″ (see Figure 81.1). With the latter precursor also a labeling of the two ring systems in specific positions and the connecting C-3 unit is expected.

Selection of potential precursors

To label specifically the B-ring ^{13}C labeled phenylalanine seemed to be a suitable precursor. It was expected that the amino acid is metabolized by phenylalanine-ammonium-lyase (Pal) to cinnamic acid, followed by hydroxylation in para position to *p*-coumaric acid. The activated form of this acid (*p*-coumaroyl-CoA) should then condensate successively with three molecules of acetate via malonate to yield the A-ring of Xn. 1-^{13}C-acetate or 2-^{13}C-malonate were the respective precursors which were commercially available.

Furthermore we fed glucose as general metabolite either as [U-^{13}C] glucose or as [1-^{13}C] glucose. The labeling pattern with [1-^{13}C] glucose should allow elucidation of the biosynthetic origin of the prenyl side chain. Incorporation was detected by means of quantitative ^{1}H and ^{13}C NMR spectrometry (Braun *et al.*, 1996).

Feeding conditions ^{13}C-experiments

For our feeding experiments a similar setup was used as described by Goese *et al.* (1999). Hop sprouts were obtained from a hop variety rich in Xn (Hallertauer Taurus). Fifteen short sprouts of approximately 2 cm containing 2–3 cones were cut from the plant using a razor blade. Their stems were immediately immersed into one of the following solutions in Gamborg B5 medium (Gamborg *et al.*, 1968):

0.5% [ring – $^{13}C6$] phenylalanine
0.5% [2-^{13}C] acetate
0.5% [2-^{13}C] malonate
1% [1-^{13}C] glucose
2.5% [U-13C] glucose

The stems were left for 6–11 days until wilting occurred. The cones were then cut, dried at 40°C and stored at −20°C until further use.

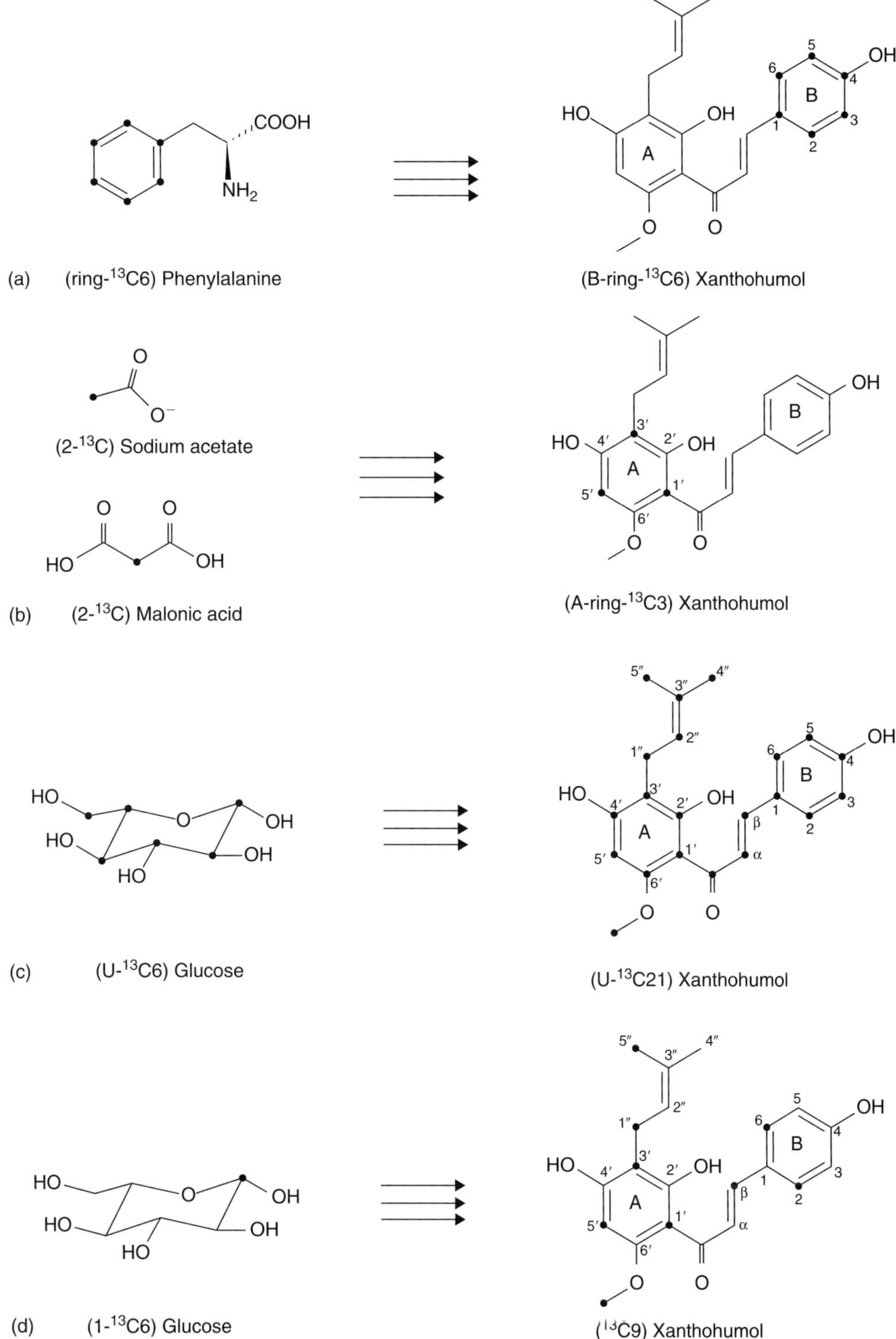

Figure 81.1 Labeling pattern of xanthohumol with ^{13}C precursors: (a) incorporation of [ring $^{13}C_6$]phenylalanine; (b) incorporation of [2-^{13}C] acetate or [2-^{13}malonate]; (c) incorporation of [U-$^{13}C_6$]glucose; (d) incorporation of [1-^{13}C]glucose. • = labeled carbon.

Isolation of Xn

The hop cones were minced and extracted with hot methanol under reflux for 1 h. After cooling, the extract was filtered and evaporated to dryness. Fractionation and isolation of Xn was achieved by column chromatography with a modified method according to Gardner (1972). About 1 g of the extract were applied to a small column (8 cm length,

Table 81.1 ^{13}C-NMR values and ^{13}C-abundance in % for the incorporation of ^{13}C-labeled precursors

C-atom	*δC (ppm)*	*Acetate (0.5%)*	*Malonate (0.5%)*	*Phenylalan (0.1%)*	*Phenylalan (0.1%)*	*Glucose (1%)*
1	127.3	1.13	1.19	**3.73**	**3.73**	1.30
2	130.0	0.95	0.98	**3.48**	**3.48**	**2.20**
3	115.7	0.99	1.07	**3.48**	**3.48**	1.15
4	158.9	1.11	1.16	**3.51**	**3.51**	1.28
5	115.7	0.99	1.07	**3.48**	**3.48**	1.15
6	130.0	0.95	0.98	**3.48**	**3.48**	**2.20**
1′	105.7	**1.84**	**1.77**	1.04	1.04	**2.67**
2′	164.6	0.98	1.06	0.86	0.86	0.97
3′	107.9	**1.81**	**1.77**	1.20	1.20	**2.56**
4′	161.7	1.08	1.08	1.02	1.02	1.28
5′	90.7	**1.81**	**1.70**	1.16	1.16	**2.59**
6′	160.8	1.01	1.10	0.92	0.92	1.28
1″	21.3	1.13	1.13	1.05	1.05	**2.42**
2″	122.5	1.01	1.19	1.12	1.12	1.04
3″	132.1	1.06	1.12	1.09	1.09	1.50
4″	25.5	1.12	1.13	1.02	1.02	1.23
5′	17.6	1.12	1.15	1.10	1.10	**2.66**
$-$O**C**H$_3$	55.4	1.07	1.09	1.04	1.04	1.81
C=O	192.8	0.99	1.19	1.11	1.11	1.43
α	124.8	0.96	1.03	1.12	1.12	1.12
β	132.1	1.12	1.08	1.07	1.07	**2.18**

Note: Bold values are labeled positions.

2 cm i.d.) filled with a mixture (1/1) of kieselgur and polyvinylpyrrolidone. Elution was by a gradient of 100% methanol to methanol/ethylacetate -0.1% formic acid (water saturated) 60:40. Fractions were monitored by thin layer- and high-performance-liquid-chromatography.

NMR-spectroscopy

NMR spectra were recorded in $CDCl_3/CD_3OD$ (92:8, v/v), [^{1}H-NMR (500 MHz), ^{13}C-NMR (125 MHz)] relative to $CDCl_3$ at $\delta_H = 7.24$, $\delta_C = 77.0$ using a Bruker DRX spectrometer. ^{13}C measurements were recorded with the inverse gated decoupling pulse sequence in the presence of 0.1 M Cr(acac)$_3$ (Braun *et al.*, 1996). For integration the signal-to-noise ratio was at least 40:1.

Incorporation of ^{13}C

The results of the experiments for the incorporation of ^{13}C labeled precursors for the chalcone core were in full agreement with the established data (Heller and Forkmann, 1968) (see Figure 81.1).

[2-^{13}C] acetate and [2-^{13}C] malonate led to a significant labeling of the expected positions C-1′, C-3′ and C-5′ in ring A. The presence of ^{13}C in these positions was at least 1.6-fold compared to the natural 1.11% of this isotope. [Ring-$^{13}C_6$] phenylalanine was nearly uniformly incorporated into ring B whereas the other carbon atoms seemed not to be affected.

The feeding of [1-^{13}C] glucose resulted in the enrichment of ^{13}C into the positions C-1″ and C-5″ thus proving that the MEP-pathway is active in the biosynthesis of the prenyl side chain. This is in agreement with hop bitter acids where the prenyl side chain is formed in the same way (Goese *et al.*, 1999).

In addition to the above-described experiments we carried out labeling with uniform labeled glucose ([U-$^{13}C_6$] glucose), which led to a 9-fold enrichment in nearly every carbon atom of the Xn-skeleton (Berwanger *et al.*, 2005a) (see Table 81.1).

Radioactive labeling of Xn

On the basis of these results it was possible to perform experiments (Berwanger *et al.*, 2005b) with uniform labeled radioactive glucose ([U-$^{14}C_6$]glucose) by feeding a solution containing 55 mCi [U-$^{14}C_6$]glucose to hop cones. This incorporation experiment resulted in radioactive Xanthohumol with a high specific activity of 318 μCi/mmol.

The experimental design was the same as for ^{13}C incubation. We conducted two different feeding experiments: (1) the total amount of radioactive glucose was fed on the first day of incubation and (2) the same amount was fed successively over 4 days. In both experiments 40 mg radiolabeled Xn of high chemical purity was isolated. The specific activity of Xn in the two experiments differed by a factor of 6. Whereas in experiment (1) the specific activity was 318 μCi/mmol, it was only 53.1 μCi/mmol in experiment (2). This big variation in ^{14}C incorporation may be explained by decreasing activity of the enzymes involved in the biosynthesis of secondary metabolites and/or by a reduction of the transport of the precursors.

Outlook

The resulting radioactive Xn can be used for bioavailability and distribution studies (Frank *et al.*, unpublished results) that are urgently needed to determine the target organs for its chemopreventive effects. Moreover future studies could be done *in vitro* and *in vivo* with specifically labeled B-ring Xn or A-ring Xn or even side chain labeled Xn by using the respective radiolabeled precursors.

The high efficacy of isotope incorporation and the easily feasibility of the incubation, is the main advantage of this biolabeling method. A further positive point of this method is the concurrently labeling of other pharmacologically interesting hop compounds, such as bitter acids and the phytoestrogen 8-prenlynaringenin, which could also be used for pharmacological *in vitro* tests or *in vivo* distribution studies.

Summary Points

- Xanthohumol shows various effects related to chemoprevention.
- Biosynthesis of xanthohumol was elucidated by feeding ^{13}C labeled precursors to hop cones, such as [ring-$^{13}C_6$] phenylalanine, [2-^{13}C] acetate, [2-^{13}C] malonate, [1-^{13}C] glucose, [U-^{13}C] glucose.
- The labeling pattern of the chalcone skeleton proved the well-established biosynthetic pathway. The biosynthesis of the prenyl side chain was attributed to the deoxyxylulose/methylerythrothiol pathway.
- Radioactive xanthohumol is obtained by feeding uniform labeled ^{14}C-glucose.
- Radioactive xanthohumol can be used for bioavailability and distribution studies.
- Feeding ^{14}C-glucose leads to other labeled hop compounds (e.g. 8-prenylnaringenin).

References

Adam, K.P., Thiel, R., Zapp, J. and Becker, H. (1998a). *Arch. Biochem. Biophys.* 354, 181–187.

Berwanger, S., Zapp, J. and Becker, H. (2005a). *Planta. Med.* 71, 530–534.

Berwanger, S., Frank, N., Knauft, J. and Becker, H. (2005b). *Mol. Nutr. Food Res.*, 821–823.

Biendl, M. (2002/2003). *Hopfenrundschau Int.*, 72–75.

Braun, S., Kalinowski, H.O. and Berger, S. (1996). *100 and More Basic NMR Experiments*, pp. 228–236. VHC-Wiley, Weinheim.

Eisenreich, W., Schwarz, M., Cartayrade, A., Arigoni, D., Zenk, M.H. and Bacher, A. (1998). *Chem. Biol.*, R221–R233.

Gamborg, O.L., Miller, R.A. and Ojima, K. (1968). *Exp. Cell Res.* 50, 151–158.

Gardner, D.J.S. (1972). *United States Patent* 3, 744–794.

Gerhäuser, C., Alt, A.P., Klimo, K., Knauft, J., Frank, N. and Becker, H. (2002a). *Phytochem. Rev.* 1, 369–377.

Gerhäuser, C., Alt, A.P., Heiss, E., Gamal-Eldee, A., Klimo, K., Knauft, J., Neumann, I., Scherf, H.J., Frank, N., Bartsch, H. and Becker, H. (2002b). *Mol. Cancer Ther.* 1, 959–969.

Gerhäuser, C. (2005). *Mol. Nutr. Food. Res.* 49, 827–831.

Goese, M., Kammhuber, K., Bacher, A., Zenk, M.H. and Eisenreich, W. (1999). *Eur. J. Biochem.* 263, 445–447.

Heller, W. and Forkmann, G. (1968). In Harborne, J.B. (ed.), *The Flavonoids. Advances in Research Since 1986*, pp. 499–508. Chapman & Hall, London.

Nookandeh, A., Frank, N., Steiner, F., Ellinger, R., Schneider, B., Gerhäuser, C. and Becker, H. (2004). *Phytochemistry* 65, 561–570.

Rohmer, M. (1999). *Nat. Prod. Rep.* 16, 565–574.

Stevens, J.F., Ivancic, M., Hsu, V.L. and Deinzer, M.L. (1997). *Phytochemistry* 44, 1575–1585.

Stevens, J.F., Taylor, A.W. and Deinzer, M.L. (1999). *J. Chromatogr.* A832, 97–107.

Umlauf, D., Zapp, J., Becker, H. and Adam, K.P. (2004). *Phytochemistry* 65, 2463–2470.

Vitrac, X., Desmouliere, A., Brouillard, B., Krisa, S., Deffieux, G., Barthe, N., Rosenbaum, J. and Merillon, J.M. (2003). *Life Sci.* 72, 2219–2233.

Wunderlich, S., Zürcher, A. and Back, W. (2005). *Mol. Nutr. Food Res.*, 874–881.

Yilmazer, M., Stevens, J.F., Deinzer, M.L. and Buhler, D.R. (2001). *Drug Metab. Dispos.* 29, 223–231.

(ii) Cardiovascular and Cancer

82

Epicatechin and Its Role in Protection of LDL and of Vascular Endothelium

Tankred Schewe Institute of Biochemistry and Molecular Biology I, Heinrich Heine University of Duesseldorf, Duesseldorf, Germany
Helmut Sies Institut fuer Biochemie und Molekularbiologie I, Duesseldorf, Germany

Abstract

(−)-Epicatechin is a dietary polyphenol exerting beneficial effects on the cardiovascular system as judged from epidemiological and clinical studies. Cocoa products, red wine as well as green and black tea are most prominent sources for (−)-epicatechin and related flavan-3-ols. The possible contribution of beer still remains to be substantiated. Comparison of the uptake and elimination kinetics as well as of plasma peak concentrations revealed that among dietary flavan-3-ols, (−)-epicatechin exhibits sufficient bioavailability. The catechol arrangement of the B ring in flavan-3-ols accounts for radical-scavenging, reducing and metal ion-chelating properties *in vitro*, which may play a protective role in the gastrointestinal tract, whereas for the metabolites in blood plasma these properties are largely lost if this grouping is blocked through glucuronidation and/or methylation. This fact may explain why flavan-3-ols and other flavonoids show strong antioxidant activities *in vitro* such as inhibition of low-density lipoprotein (LDL) oxidation, whereas the corresponding activities *in vivo* or *ex vivo* are only moderate. Flavan-3-ols serve antioxidant functions in a broader sense suppressing reactions of prooxidant enzymes such as myeloperoxidase, lipoxygenases and NADPH oxidases. High flavan-3-ol intake through a model meal or beverage gives rise to anti-atherosclerotic, anti-inflammatory and anti-platelet activities *in vivo* as well as improvement of endothelial function of arterial vessels, and lowering of blood pressure. Part of these actions is closely connected with modulation of nitric oxide metabolism of vascular endothelium. *In vitro*, (−)-epicatechin protects vascular endothelial cells against a number of cytotoxic and proapoptotic actions of oxLDL. Mechanistically, the protective actions involve prevention and scavenging of superoxide anion radical, peroxynitrite and nitrogen dioxide radical, collectively leading to elevation of bioavailability and bioactivity of nitric oxide and, in turn, to improvement of endothelial function.

List of Abbreviations

CVD	Cardiovascular diseases
FMD	Flow-mediated dilation
HPLC	High-performance liquid chromatography
HDL	High-density lipoprotein
LDL	Low-density lipoprotein
oxLDL	Oxidatively modified low-density lipoprotein
MPO	Myeloperoxidase
eNOS	Endothelial nitric oxide synthase
iNOS	Inducible nitric oxide synthase

Introduction

Epidemiological evidence accumulated showing that consumption of red wine, tea and cocoa products is inversely associated with the risk of cardiovascular diseases (CVD) and cardiac death, which is attributed to a high content of flavonoids and other dietary polyphenols (Maron, 2004; Buijsse *et al.*, 2006). Among flavonoids, (−)-epicatechin has found particular interest, because its bioavailability surpasses that of structurally related compounds such as (+)-catechin, (−)-catechin and other flavan-3-ols (Manach and Donovan, 2004; Donovan *et al.*, 2006, and references therein). Moreover, protective actions of (−)-epicatechin on the cardiovascular system are substantiated by a number of *in vivo* and *in vitro* studies. A recent study suggested that the *in vivo* effects are largely mediated by (−)-epicatechin (Schroeter *et al.*, 2006). (−)-Epicatechin also occurs in beer. Most knowledge on absorption, pharmacokinetics and biological activities of (−)-epicatechin and related polyphenols *in vivo* comes from studies with humans consuming red wine, tea or high-flavanol cocoa products.

Beer in Health and Disease Prevention
ISBN: 978-0-12-373891-2

Chemistry

(−)-Epicatechin is the prototype of flavan-3-ols (also termed catechins), a major subgroup of flavonoids of plant origin (besides flavonols, flavones, flavanones, isoflavones and anthocyanins). Further congeners are among others, the epimer (+)-catechin as well as (−)-epicatechin gallate, (−)-epigallocatechin and (−)-epigallocatechin gallate. Natural mixtures of flavan-3-ols contain not only monomeric compounds but also oligomers, the procyanidins, consisting of 2–10 monomer units linked through C—C bridges between the flavan ring systems. The catechol arrangement at the B ring is a crucial structural feature of flavan-3-ols, which determines several chemical properties such as reductant and free radical-scavenging activities and chelation of transition metal ions. (−)-Epicatechin monomer contains a total of five hydroxyl groups, which lend the lipophilic flavan system sufficient hydrophilicity as reflected by an octanol–water partition coefficient of 1.5 (Schroeder *et al.*, 2003), thus rendering the molecule soluble in both lipophilic and aqueous environment, and hence passively permeable through biomembranes. Unlike the flavonol quercetin, having the same number and positions of hydroxyl groups, in (−)-epicatechin the double bond systems of the three rings (A, B and C) are not conjugated with each other, which gives rise to distinct chemical and biological properties. Most importantly, (−)-epicatechin exhibits less prooxidant and cytotoxic properties at high concentrations than quercetin. The high degree of conjugation of the double bonds enables quercetin to be oxidized to an array of quinoid oxidation products, so-called quinone methides (Awad *et al.*, 2002), which cannot be expected to such an extent with (−)-epicatechin or related flavan-3-ols.

The chemical structures of some monomeric and oligomeric flavan-3-ols are shown in Figure 82.1. For details as to chemistry of flavonoids and related polyphenols the reader may refer to the respective monograph by Haslam (1998).

Absorption, Biotransformation and Biological Kinetics

Monomeric (−)-epicatechin is satisfactorily absorbed from the small intestine. Dependent on ingested dose and food source of flavan-3-ols (red wine, green or black tea or cocoa products in most studies) total plasma concentrations including conjugated metabolites between 0.2 and 6 μM have been reported (Manach and Donovan, 2004, and references therein). The peak level is usually reached 1–2 h after intake (Schroeter *et al.*, 2006). Its epimer (+)-catechin, although contained in most dietary sources in comparable amounts, gives rise to much lower plasma levels (∼0.1 μM) than (−)-epicatechin, possibly owing to faster metabolism, so that its bioavailability is considerably lower (Holt *et al.*, 2002). The same is true for galloylated flavan-3-ols, which exhibit faster renal elimination. In plasma, however, they are conjugated to a lesser extent than (−)-epicatechin. Procyanidins are not absorbed, except for possible trace amounts of the dimers procyanidin B_1 and B_2 (Holt *et al.*, 2002). The half-lives of monomeric flavan-3-ols range between 1.5–7 h and are shorter than that of the flavonol quercetin (for review, see Manach and Donovan, 2004).

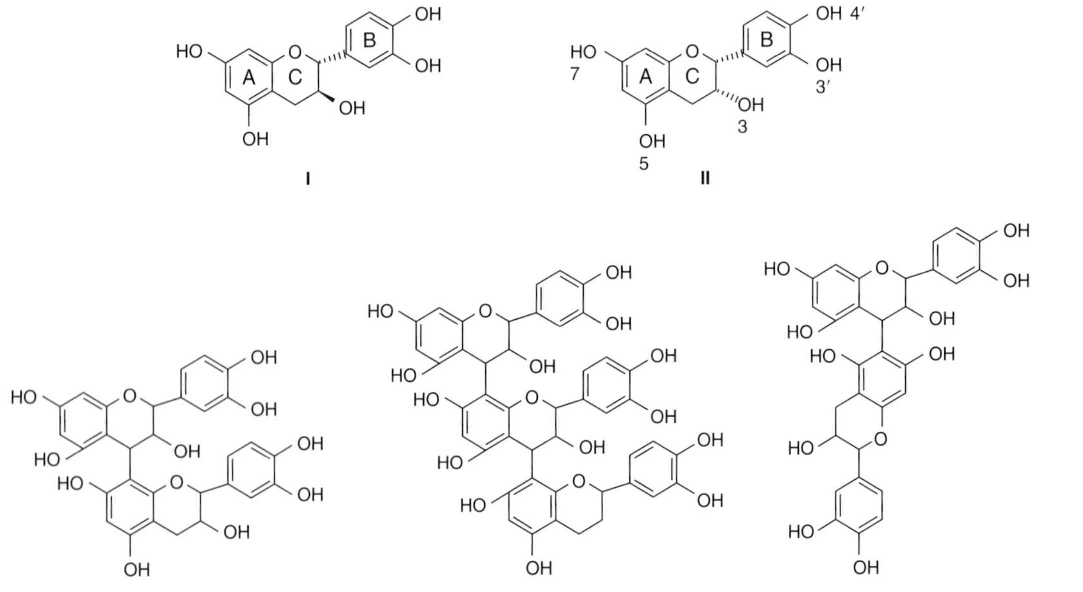

Figure 82.1 Major flavan-3-ols identified in beer (Weiß and Hofmann, 2006; modified). **I**, (+)-catechin; **II**, (−)-epicatechin; **III**, epicatechin(4β→8)-epicatechin (procyanidin B_2); **IV**, [epicatechin(4β→8)]$_2$-epicatechin (procyanidin C_1); **V**, epicatechin(4β→6)-epicatechin (procyanidin B_5). The stereochemistry in **III**, **IV** and **V** was not considered. The Arabic numerals in **I** designate the positions of OH groups.

While food rich in protein and lipid does not seemingly influence the absorption and elimination of flavan-3-ols, bread and sugar-containing test meals enhance the bioavailability of (−)-epicatechin and (+)-catechin to 140% of controls, which is thought to be due to decrease in elimination half-life (Schramm *et al.*, 2003). An opposite effect has been postulated for ethanol, which accelerates the urinary excretion of flavan-3-ols by virtue of its diuretic action (Donovan *et al.*, 2002). This effect of ethanol should be kept in mind in evaluating beer as source of flavan-3-ols. Thus, the (−)-epicatechin content of beer has been reported to be only about one-fourth of that of red wine (de Pascual-Teresa *et al.*, 2000), whereas the ethanol contents of the two beverages are comparable.

In human plasma the following (−)-epicatechin metabolites occurring 1 h after administration were identified in the order of decreasing average levels: epicatechin-3′-glucuronide > epicatechin > 4′-*O*-methyl-epicatechin-3′-glucuronide > 3′-*O*-methyl-epicatechin ≈ 4′-*O*-methyl-epicatechin-5-(or 7)-glucuronide, indicating that upon absorption a sizeable amount of (−)-epicatechin is conjugated involving both glucuronidation at B and A rings and selective methylation of 3′-OH or 4′-OH of the catechol arrangement of the B ring (Natsume *et al.*, 2003). Except for non-metabolized epicatechin and 3′-*O*-methyl-epicatechin, these compounds were also isolated from human urine (Natsume *et al.*, 2003), so that the metabolic fate of 3′-*O*-methyl-epicatechin remained unexplored. Sulfated metabolites were also reported.

The metabolic profile of (−)-epicatechin metabolites is possibly not limited to conjugative metabolism, but may also include oxidative conversions, which were not addressed so far. Oxidative conversions of flavonoids are known, however, for galangin, kaempferide and isoflavones via cytochrome P450 catalysis (Walle, 2004). Moreover, flavonoids are prone to non-enzymatic oxidations by reactive oxygen species, which are expected to be favored under pathophysiologic conditions.

A considerable part of dietary (−)-epicatechin is not absorbed as unchanged molecule, but is metabolized by the microflora of the large intestine yielding a number of absorbable phenolic acids such as 4-hydroxybenzoic, 3,4-dihydroxybenzoic, 3-methoxy-4-hydroxybenzoic and 3-methoxy-4-hydroxyhippuric acids as well as di-hydroxylated phenylvalerolactone, which were detected in human plasma in conjugated form (Rechner *et al.*, 2002; Rios *et al.*, 2003; Manach and Donovan, 2004). The total amount of these microbial metabolites in urine accounts for as much as 15% of the ingested dose. Procyanidins are also metabolized via this route yielding other phenolic acids. The efficiency of the intestinal microbial breakdown of procyanidins, however, decreases with increasing oligomer size, which may be due to some antibacterial activity of larger oligomers.

The fact that a number of dietary polyphenols, such as procyanidins and anthocyanins, among the compounds occurring in beer, are not or only poorly absorbed does not rule out beneficial biological actions for the human organism. In addition to serve as substrates for microbial conversions, they may also directly act in the gastrointestinal tract. Besides protection against development of gastrointestinal tumors such as colon cancer, they are capable of reducing and, thus, of detoxifying food-derived hydroperoxides, which are sometimes abundant in high-fat meals. By this mode, dietary polyphenols are expected to counteract postprandial oxidative stress (for review, see Sies *et al.*, 2005b).

An incomplete or retarded absorption of certain flavan-3-ols from the gastrointestinal tract may also be advantageous for their modulating effects on water and chloride secretion by the small intestine as suggested from mild inhibitory effects of cocoa flavan-3-ols on forskolin-stimulated cystic fibrosis transmembrane conductance regulator activity (Schuier *et al.*, 2005). This action may plausibly explain the known capability of cocoa products of alleviating diarrhea.

Flavan-3-ol content of beer

Data as for the content of (−)-epicatechin, (+)-catechin and total flavan-3-ols in beer (Table 82.1) vary by two orders of magnitude. Arts *et al.* (2000) detected sizeable amounts in various sorts of green tea, black tea and red wine as well as low amounts in white wine and chocolate milk, but failed to detect them in lager beer (Heineken), possibly owing to a too high detection limit of their analytical method. By contrast, de Pascual-Teresa *et al.* (2000) analyzed a broad array of Spanish foodstuffs and beverages and presented a complete pattern of flavan-3-ols of beer without specifying the sort of beer; the content of (−)-epicatechin was found to be 1.8 ± 0.6 mg/l and that of total flavan-3-ols 6.4 ± 1.9 mg/l, which is in fair agreement with recently reported data, where the high-performance liquid chromatography (HPLC) method was evaluated by recovery experiments, revealing recovery rate of >90% (Kusche, 2005).

De Pascual-Teresa *et al.* (2000) also reported that soluble cocoa, red wine and green tea have 3.3-, 4.2- and 69-fold, respectively, higher contents of (−)-epicatechin than beer.

Table 82.1 Content of flavan-3-ols in beer[1]

(−)-Epicatechin	*(+)-Catechin (mg/l)*	*Total flavan-3-ols*	*Reference*
<0.5	<1	<2	Arts *et al.* (2000)
1.8	7.3	6.4	de Pascual-Teresa *et al.* (2000)
132	–	–	Gorinstein *et al.* (1997a)
1.2	5.8	–	Kusche (2005)
11.1	60.5	–	Weiß and Hofmann (2006)

[1] Unpublished data for lager beer (mg/l): Epicatechin 0.6, catechin 1.8, dimer procyanidin B3 1.5, dimer gallocatechin–catechin 1.8, kindly provided by Dr. A. Scalbert, Unité de Nutrition Humaine, INRA, Centre de Recherche de Clermont-Ferrand/Theix, France (personal communication, with permission).

On the other hand, beer surpassed white wine and coffee 3-fold. Moreover, hardly any flavanols were found in vegetables, which usually contain, however, other polyphenols.

Gorinstein *et al.* reported an (−)-epicatechin content of 132 ± 2.5 mg/l in a special sort of beer and achieved in their clinical studies with this beer beneficial effects on some blood parameters (Gorinstein *et al.*, 1997a, b). In a variety of clinical studies using cocoa or chocolate, relevant beneficial effects were achieved with an intake of at least 40 mg (−)-epicatechin or 140 mg total flavan-3-ols, respectively (Ding *et al.*, 2006; Engler *et al.*, 2006, and references therein). Such an intake can be regarded as clue to evaluate whether a special sort or brand of beer may have a flavan-3-ol-related health benefit.

The phenolic constituents of beer including flavonoids originate from barley or wheat malt (70–80%) and hop (20–30%). The flavan-3-ol content of malts varies depending on barley cultivar and growing area. The flavan-3-ols of beer contribute to bitter-astringent taste of the beverage.

In general, the flavan-3-ol content of beverages and foodstuffs strongly depends on the source variety, stage of ripeness, post-harvesting conservation, and processing as well as on origin of the sample. The behavior of flavan-3-ols during beer processing has recently been studied in detail (Kusche, 2005). While the mashing program had no or only slight influence, the oxygen-sensitivity of beer polyphenols turned out to be strongly temperature-dependent. The sensitivity to heat increased in the order (+)-catechin < procyanidin B_3 < prodelphinidin B_3 (Kusche, 2005). Interestingly, (−)-epicatechin was not detected during the mashing process; it was formed, however, through depolymerization of procyanidins during wort boiling (Kusche, 2005).

Collectively, a conclusive appraisal of the (−)-epicatechin content of beer is not possible until a systematic study with a large variety of sorts and brands of beer using an evaluated analytical method will have been conducted.

Although in beer the content of (+)-catechin is at least four times higher than that of (−)-epicatechin, the following sections focus on (−)-epicatechin, since in human blood plasma (−)-epicatechin and its metabolites predominate due to a better bioavailability (Manach and Donovan, 2004, and references therein).

Flavan-3-ols and antioxidant capacity

Flavanols and other dietary polyphenols are capable of reducing oxidants and of scavenging injurious radicals *in vitro*. This capacity can be quantified in complex mixtures by various methodological approaches. The antioxidant capacity of a beverage is a useful parameter to evaluate both stability during storage and the protectant action against dietary oxidants during the gastrointestinal passage. For example, it has been estimated that 500 ml of beer has the same antioxidant capacity as 150 ml of red wine (Paganga *et al.*, 1999), which may roughly correlate with the (−)-epicatechin content of these beverages. The antioxidant capacity of red wine per serving is topped by cocoa drink (Lee *et al.*, 2003).

Estimation of the total antioxidant capacity of blood plasma upon intake of a polyphenol-rich diet, although assessed in numerous studies, does not provide useful information, since secondary metabolic effects by other plant constituents are mirrored rather than direct polyphenol effects (Lotito and Frei, 2006). The antioxidant capacity of plasma is mainly determined by endogenous antioxidants such as urate, which occurs in the millimolar range, whereas the plasma level of flavan-3-ols barely exceeds micromolar concentrations. By contrast, the plasma level of α-tocopherol (vitamin E) is a relevant parameter for the antioxidant function of plasma, because this natural antioxidant accumulates in plasma lipoproteins rendering them more resistant to oxidative modification (see below).

By virtue of their antioxidant capacity, flavan-3-ols are capable of counteracting oxidative stress. Oxidative stress has been defined as a shift in the balance between prooxidant and antioxidant processes of the organism toward prooxidants (Sies, 1985).

Flavan-3-ols and cardiovascular diseases (CVD)

CVD are prominent causes of death in industrial countries. The risk of CVD is strongly influenced by aspects of individual lifestyle, including nutrition. Epidemiological prospective cohort studies revealed that a general high intake of flavonoids from fruits, vegetables, tea, red wine and cocoa products is associated with a lowered risk of CVD mortality (Huxley and Neil, 2003, and references therein). The more specific contribution of flavan-3-ols, an important subgroup of flavonoids, to this health benefit is documented by respective studies on the intake of dark chocolate and other cocoa products, one of their most prominent dietary source. A recent meta-analysis of literature data revealed an inverse correlation between chocolate consumption and CVD mortality (Ding *et al.*, 2006). This conclusion is convincingly supported by a 15-year follow-up study on a cohort of 470 elderly men, in which high cocoa intake was significantly correlated with both lowered blood pressure and diminished CVD mortality (Buijsse *et al.*, 2006). It must be kept in mind, however, that this correlation is an association and does not prove cause–effect relationship, because it may also reflect a more general lifestyle favorable for cardiovascular health.

Although such extensive *in vivo* studies as with cocoa products were not conducted with beer, intake of beer may also be beneficial for cardiovascular health. Daily intake of 330 ml Israeli Maccabee beer by patients with coronary artery disease and atherosclerosis led to a significant increase in HDL cholesterol and plasma α-tocopherol as compared with a corresponding control group without intake of any alcoholic beverage (Gorinstein, 1997b). These changes are generally viewed as beneficial for cardiovascular health (see next sections), although in this study an improvement of other clinical parameters reflecting cardiovascular functions more directly was not observed.

Human studies on intake of high-flavanol cocoa products as well as respective *in vitro* investigations revealed antioxidant, anti-platelet and anti-inflammatory activities as well as improvement of endothelial function of blood vessels and lowering of blood pressure (Keen *et al.*, 2005; Engler *et al.*, 2006; Ding *et al.*, 2006, and references therein). Since (−)-epicatechin isolated from cocoa polyphenols produced similar biological responses (Schroeter *et al.*, 2006), this compound is concluded to play a key role. Its mode of action seems to involve more than one mechanism.

Epicatechin and plasma lipoproteins

Plasma lipoproteins play a pivotal role in atherosclerosis and, consequently, in CVD. While low-density lipoprotein (LDL) favors the development of atherosclerotic lesions, high-density lipoproteins (HDL) are protective against it, so that the LDL/HDL ratio of plasma is a determinant for the risk of CVD. This ratio appears to be favorably lowered by (−)-epicatechin and related flavan-3-ols by 2 ways: (i) elevation of HDL as measured as HDL cholesterol (Gorinstein, 1997b; Wan *et al.*, 2001; Mursu *et al.*, 2004), (ii) lowering of LDL through up-regulation of hepatic LDL receptor (Bursill *et al.*, 2007).

Recent atherosclerosis research revealed that biochemical modification of LDL, affecting its composition and, in turn, receptor affinities, greatly enhances the injurious potential of LDL in the pathogenesis of LDL in various disease states. Thus, the "oxidation hypothesis of atherosclerosis" predicts that the proatherogenic and proinflammatory role of LDL is mediated by oxidative modification of LDL. While cells take up native LDL via the well-regulated LDL receptor, thus preventing deleterious consequences, oxidized LDL (oxidatively modified low-density lipoprotein, oxLDL) is avidly taken up by vascular endothelial cells, macrophages and other cells via so-called scavenger receptors. In response to this oxLDL-mediated pathway, the cells are damaged by several ways. The impact of LDL oxidation implies the following sites of pharmacological or dietary intervention to counteract atherosclerosis and endothelial dysfunction: (i) generation of oxLDL, (ii) interaction of oxLDL with vascular endothelial cells. Recent research from this laboratory has provided ample evidence that (−)-epicatechin blocks both consecutive steps of this scenario (Steffen *et al.*, 2006a).

Impact of LDL Oxidation in Jeopardizing Cardiovascular Health: oxLDL The pathophysiologic role of oxidative modifications of LDL has been suggested from observations that oxLDL species are detectable in early and advanced atherogenic lesions in the arterial wall, whereas no such species occur in uninvolved areas of the same blood vessels. In these lesions, a cascade of events is initiated by oxLDL leading to vascular dysfunction and progression of the lesion and finally to plaque rupture and occlusion of the vessel, a key process responsible for myocardial infarction.

OxLDL is used in the literature as collective term for chemically modified species of LDL particles, which are heterogeneous in composition and biological activities. The modifications can include the lipid moiety and/or apoB-100, the protein component of LDL. Modification of the lipid moiety is brought about by lipid peroxidation and gives rise to a number of biologically active lipid oxidation products such as free and esterified polyunsaturated hydro(pero)xy fatty acids, oxygenated products of cholesterol and its esters (oxysterols), lysophospholipids, platelet-activating factor-like phospholipid cleavage products, F_2-isoprostanes and various aldehydes. Lipid-derived oxidation products are believed to contribute to proinflammatory events in the subendothelial space of arterial vessels such as activating expression of adhesion molecules, apoptosis of endothelial cells, recruitment and differentiation of monocytes and fibrous plaque formation. Modification of the protein moiety preferably includes oxidation-sensitive amino acid residues such as lysine, arginine, tyrosine, tryptophan, threonine and methionine. Oxidation of lysines or their masking by aldehydes (e.g. by malondialdehyde and 2-hydroxynonenal, which originate from lipid peroxidation) via Schiff base formation leads to loss of positive charges of the apoprotein, which renders the whole oxLDL particle more negative as detectable by electrophoresis.

A mildly oxidized form of oxLDL, "LDL-minus," becomes detectable in plasma about 2 h after intake of a fat and carbohydrate-rich, but polyphenol-poor meal (Ursini and Sevanian, 2002). This phenomenon, a consequence of postprandial oxidative stress (Sies *et al.*, 2005b), is due to a high oxidant load from the gastrointestinal tract to the blood plasma, which cannot be sufficiently compensated by the endogenous antioxidant systems of the organism.

Other pathways to generate oxLDL species *in vivo* are difficult to define, but may be a consequence of systemic or local oxidative stress. Local injury of the endothelium of the wall of arterial vessels facilitates LDL oxidation. Such loci enable both LDL and inflammatory cells such as monocytes to enter the subendothelial space of the vessel, where the monocytes differentiate to macrophages, and a cocktail of oxidants are released from activated inflammatory cells that promote LDL oxidation and other prooxidant and proinflammatory responses ("response-to-injury hypothesis of atherosclerosis").

Employing an enzyme-linked immunoassay on aldehyde-modified oxLDL, the plasma level of oxLDL was found to strongly correlate with coronary artery disease (Holvoet *et al.*, 1998). It turned out to be a prognostic biomarker of subclinical atherosclerosis development (Wallenfeldt *et al.*,

2004). Elevated plasma levels of oxLDL are predictive for a future coronary heart disease event such as myocardial infarction (Meisinger *et al.*, 2005; Johnston *et al.*, 2006). Similar conclusions have been drawn for the plasma level of myeloperoxidase (MPO) (Brennan *et al.*, 2003), a prooxidant enzyme that is recruited in atherosclerotic lesions and capable of modifying LDL (Schewe and Sies, 2005, and references therein). No studies were conducted until now to address the effect of dietary intake of flavan-3-ols on these parameters.

LDL oxidation *in vivo* can be mimicked in a number of *in vitro* models. A most common model is Cu^{2+}-catalyzed LDL oxidation owing to its methodological simplicity, although it does not reflect the *in vivo* situation, because plasma does not contain free Cu^{2+} ions. Modification of LDL by a reaction system MPO/H_2O_2/nitrite is preferable (Kostyuk *et al.*, 2003; Kraemer *et al.*, 2004, Schewe and Sies, 2005; Steffen *et al.*, 2006a), because it may mirror the *in vivo* process of LDL oxidation more closely. A number of other *in vitro* models can also be applied. They include spontaneous autoxidation (storage under air) as well as enzymatic (MPO, 15-lipoxygenase), non-enzymatic (transition metal ions, free radical-generating compounds, irradiation plus photosensitizers) and cellular reactions (vascular endothelial cells, macrophages). The oxLDL preparations thus obtained differ with respect to both chemical composition and biological activities, which needs to be considered when data are evaluated.

Epicatechin Protects Against LDL Oxidation Strongly *In Vitro*, but Only Marginally *Ex Vivo* While no data are available as to the effect of (−)-epicatechin on LDL oxidation *in vivo*, a universal protection against LDL oxidation *in vitro* is well documented (Table 82.2). Notably, all LDL oxidation systems, so far tested, proved to be inhibited by micromolar concentration of (−)-epicatechin or other flavonoids. As an example, the time-course of Cu^{2+}-elicited LDL oxidation is shown in Figure 82.2. (−)-Epicatechin increases dose-dependently the lag phase without affecting the propagation phase, thus shifting the time-curve to the right. In contrast, with lipid peroxidation of LDL catalyzed by the reaction system MPO/H_2O_2/nitrite, both lag phase and propagation phase are affected by (−)-epicatechin (Kraemer *et al.*, 2004). Interestingly, the MPO/nitrite system also evokes protein tyrosine nitration of LDL, forming 3-nitrotyrosine. This reaction may contribute to formation and progression of atherosclerotic lesions, since both MPO-derived products and 3-nitrotyrosine are accumulated in such lesions (Daugherty *et al.*, 1994; Leeuwenburgh *et al.*, 1997). An alternative route to protein-bound 3-nitrotyrosine is the reaction with peroxynitrite (Ischiropoulos, 2003). Peroxynitrite, formed in a diffusion-controlled reaction from nitric oxide ($^{\bullet}NO$) and superoxide anion radical ($O_2^{\bullet-}$), is both strong oxidant and nitrating agent. (−)-Epicatechin is known to protect against oxidant and nitrating reactions of peroxynitrite (Schroeder *et al.*, 2001; Wippel *et al.*, 2004). Since (−)-epicatechin in micromolar concentrations does not only abrogate MPO-catalyzed lipid peroxidation, but also tyrosine-protein nitration as well as chloride-dependent increase in relative electrophoretic mobility by MPO (Steffen *et al.*, 2006a), we conclude that this dietary polyphenol is a potent protectant against MPO-mediated proatherogenic modifications of both lipid and protein moieties of LDL *in vitro*. This quality may be one way by which (−)-epicatechin or its metabolites could limit oxidative modification of LDL *in vivo*.

A number of studies addressed the susceptibility of LDL to oxidation *ex vivo* (Table 82.3). The protective effects

Table 82.2 Effect of (−)-epicatechin on LDL modification *in vitro*

Oxidant system	*Parameter*	*Effect*	*Effective concentration (μM)*	*Reference*
MPO/nitrite	Conjugated dienes in lipids	Prolongation of lag phase	0.5–5	Kraemer *et al.* (2004)
MPO/nitrite	Conjugated dienes in lipids	Lowering of reaction rate	2–10	Kraemer *et al.* (2004)
MPO/tyrosine	Conjugated dienes in lipids	Lowering of reaction rate	2–10	Kraemer *et al.* (2004)
MPO/nitrite	Protein tyrosine nitration	Inhibition	0.1–1	Kraemer *et al.* (2004)
MPO/nitrite	Oxysterols	Inhibition	2–10	Steffen *et al.* (2006b)
MPO/chloride	Relative electrophoretic mobility	Shift to anode	1.5–6	Steffen *et al.* (2006a)
15-Lipoxygenase	Cholesteryl ester hydroperoxide	Inhibition	0.1	da Silva *et al.* (2000)
Human aortic endothelial cells	Conjugated dienes in lipids	Inhibition	0.08–5	Pearson *et al.* (1998)
Human aortic endothelial cells	Depletion of vitamin E	Protection	10	Zhu *et al.* (1999)
J774 murine macrophages	Conjugated dienes in lipids	Inhibition	0.5–1	Rifici *et al.* (2002)
Cu^{2+}	Conjugated dienes in lipids	Prolongation of lag phase	0.1–1	Kraemer *et al.* (2004)
Peroxynitrite	Protein tyrosine nitration	Inhibition	10	Pannala *et al.* (1997)
Peroxynitrite	Protein tyrosine nitration	Inhibition	0.1–3	Kraemer *et al.* (2004)

of flavan-3-ol intake, however, although being statistically significant in the majority of these studies, are rather marginal. Thus, extension of the length of the lag phase of LDL oxidation by as low as 8–15% cannot be regarded as relevant protection. It must be emphasized, however, that most previous studies employed Cu^{2+} oxidation, the biological relevance of which for the *in vivo* process is questionable. Further efforts are needed, therefore, to substantiate a role of LDL protection *in vivo*, including *ex vivo* susceptibility of LDL to MPO-elicited or cell-mediated modifications as well as measurement of oxLDL levels in plasma.

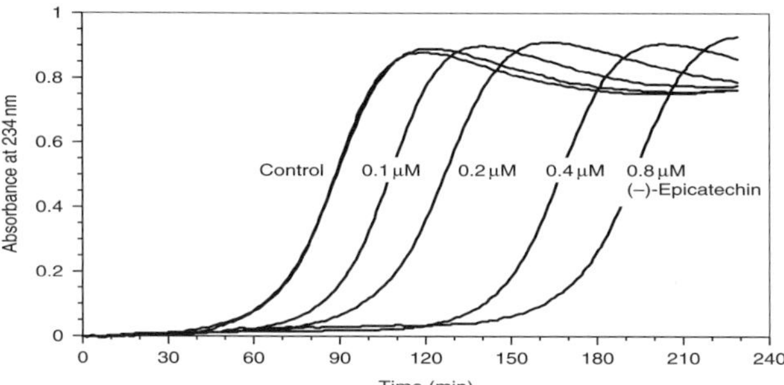

Figure 82.2 Dose-dependent effect of (−)-epicatechin on Cu^{2+}-catalyzed LDL oxidation. The time-course of conjugated dienes absorbing at 234 nm is shown in the absence (control) and presence of increasing concentrations of (−)-epicatechin. At reaction start the basal absorbance was adjusted to zero. The presence of conjugated dienes is a structural feature of peroxidized polyunsaturated fatty acids. Therefore, their concentration in LDL mirrors the degree of lipid peroxidation of LDL. As seen, the start of lipid peroxidation is strongly retarded (lag phase). During the lag phase LDL is protected by endogenous antioxidants such as vitamin E present in LDL. At the end of the lag phase vitamin E and other protectant compounds are destroyed by the Cu^{2+}-treatment, so that lipid peroxidation starts and continues with nearly linear rate (propagation phase). The reaction ceases, when all accessible polyenoic fatty acid residues of LDL lipids are peroxidized (termination phase). (−)-Epicatechin and related polyphenols selectively prolong the lag phase without affecting propagation and termination phases. This effect may be due to refilling of antioxidative capacity of LDL.

Epicatechin Protects Against oxLDL-Mediated Damage to Vascular Endothelial Cells As stated above, interaction of oxLDL with vascular endothelial cells is a key event leading to atherosclerotic lesions of arterial vessels, thus favoring CVD. Using cultured endothelial cells, this process can be studied *in vitro*. As numerous investigators have shown, oxLDL is highly toxic toward various endothelial cell lines. Notably, we have demonstrated that MPO/H_2O_2/nitrite-oxLDL is more cytotoxic than Cu^{2+}-oxLDL despite a lower extent of lipid peroxidation (Steffen *et al.*, 2005). Distinct patterns of oxysterols were recently identified as reason for this difference (Steffen *et al.*, 2006b). Since pure oxysterols or defined mixtures mimicked the behavior of oxLDL preparations, it may be concluded that oxysterols, in particular 7β-hydroxycholesterol, contribute to a sizeable part to the cytotoxicity of oxLDL. Another oxysterol, 7-ketocholesterol, attenuated the injurious effects of 7β-hydroxycholesterol (Steffen *et al.*, 2006b). As expected, formation of oxysterols during LDL oxidation was dose-dependently inhibited by (−)-epicatechin (Steffen *et al.*, 2006b).

The damage to vascular endothelial cells by oxLDL is complex and involves several targets, all of them being protected by (−)-epicatechin (Table 82.4). A key event of this multiple damage could be oxLDL-elicited activation of the endothelial nicotinamide adenine dinucleotide phosphate (NADPH) oxidase generating $O_2^{\bullet-}$, thus provoking

Table 82.3 Inhibition of LDL oxidation *ex vivo* upon intake of flavanol-rich food

Flavanol source	*LDL oxidation catalyst*	*Parameter*	*Effect*	*Reference*
Green and black tea extracts	Cu^{2+}	Conjugated dienes, lag phase	No effect	van het Hof *et al.* (1997)
Black tea	Cu^{2+}	Conjugated dienes, lag phase	No effect	O'Reilly *et al.* (2000)
Cocoa liquor	AMVN	Conjugated dienes, lag phase	Prolongation by 11%	Hirano *et al.* (2000)
Cocoa powder	AMVN[a]; Cu^{2+}	Conjugated dienes, lag phase	Significant prolongation	Osakabe *et al.* (2001)
Cocoa powder + chocolate	Cu^{2+}	Conjugated dienes, lag phase	Prolongation by 8% ($p = 0.01$)	Wan *et al.* (2001)
Dark chocolate	Cu^{2+}	Conjugated dienes, lag phase	Prolongation by 11% ($p < 0.05$)	Mathur *et al.* (2002)
Grape extract	Cu^{2+}	TBARS[b]	Inhibition by 15% ($p < 0.01$)	Vigna *et al.* (2003)
		Conjugated dienes, lag phase	Prolongation by 15% ($p < 0.05$)	

[a]AMVN, 2,2′-azobis(4-methoxy-2,4-dimethylvaleronitrile), an inducer of free radical-mediated oxidations.
[b]TBARS, thiobarbituric acid-reactive substances, an indirect measure for peroxidized polyenoic fatty acids.

oxidative stress. This assumption was corroborated through detection of oxLDL-induced, 2-deoxyglucose-sensitive $O_2^{\bullet -}$ generation in endothelial cells, which was inhibited by apocynin, a known NADPH oxidase inhibitor (Steffen *et al.*, 2007a). 2-Deoxyglucose blocks the oxidative pentose-phosphate pathway of glucose metabolism, a major source of NADPH generation. Notably, $O_2^{\bullet -}$ generation was also suppressed by (−)-epicatechin (Steffen *et al.*, 2007a), which may explain the universal protectant action of this polyphenol on endothelial cells. Some protectant actions required pretreatment of the cells with (−)-epicatechin. Therefore, it is conceivable that metabolites rather than the parent compound constitute the active agent(s). Murine aortic endothelial cells have been observed to accumulate (−)-epicatechin from the medium within 10 min followed by sizeable conversion of it after 1 h. The putative conversion products and their biological activities remain to be identified. (−)-Epicatechin (Cos *et al.*, 1998) as well as its plasma metabolites (Harada *et al.*, 1999) are known to scavenge $O_2^{\bullet -}$, which may additionally contribute to the counteraction of NADPH oxidase activation and to attenuate $O_2^{\bullet -}$ generation via pathways other than NADPH oxidase in endothelial cells. Taken together, these data argue in favor of NADPH oxidase as a prominent site of endothelium-protectant action of flavan-3-ols and/or their metabolites (see "Note" on page 812).

Epicatechin and bioavailability of nitric oxide

Structural and functional intactness of the endothelium of vascular walls is an important prerequisite for cardiovascular health. Thus, its ability to dilate enables an adequate transport of oxygen through blood stream via arterial conduit vessels and capillaries to organs and tissues, including heart and brain. An important mediator for endothelial dilation is $^{\bullet}$NO, which is formed in endothelial cells through an L-arginine pathway by endothelial NO synthase (eNOS). $^{\bullet}$NO is cofactor for soluble guanylate cyclase in smooth muscle cells forming cyclic guanosine monophosphate (cGMP) that in turn regulates smooth muscle tone by dilating the vessel. Besides this signal function, $^{\bullet}$NO at low concentration possesses antioxidant, anti-inflammatory and cytoprotective properties, making it a protectant for endothelial cells. Among others it inhibits LDL oxidation. This dual function requires the maintenance and functional adaptation of an adequate steady-state level of bioavailable $^{\bullet}$NO. Although being chemically relatively stable, $^{\bullet}$NO is short-lived in biological systems, mainly due to reactions with other molecules or oxidations. The steady-state level of $^{\bullet}$NO is lowered under conditions of oxidative stress, since more $^{\bullet}$NO is consumed due to a higher oxidant load. For review of the role of $^{\bullet}$NO for protection of the arterial wall against atherosclerosis the reader is referred to Napoli *et al.* (2006).

The crucial role of the bioavailability of $^{\bullet}$NO for vascular function has been demonstrated by measurement of flow-mediated dilation (FMD). With this method the dilation of the brachial conduit artery is measured *in vivo* after transient ischemia provoked by a cuff (Kelm, 2002). The FMD is mediated through the L-arginine/$^{\bullet}$NO pathway as evident from the effect of eNOS inhibitors. This response is markedly diminished with individuals at risk for CVD, a phenomenon known as endothelial dysfunction. Several studies demonstrated marked improvement of FMD 2 h after intake of a high-flavan-3-ol cocoa beverage or chocolate, but not of low-flavan-3-ol control diet (Heiss *et al.*, 2003; Schroeter *et al.*, 2006, and references therein). Elevation of FMD unequivocally coincided with an increase in plasma nitroso compounds and with the

Table 82.4 Adverse actions of MPO/H_2O_2/nitrite-oxLDL on endothelial cell lines

Target of damage	*Cell line*	*Assay*	*Protection by (−)-epicatechin*
Integrity of plasma membrane	HUVEC	LDH release	+
Mitochondrial energy conservation	BAEC, HUVEC, EA.hy926	MTT reduction	+
Cell proliferation	HUVEC	BrdU incorporation	+
Integrity of DNA	HUVEC	DNA fragmentation	+
Integrity of cellular proteins	BAEC, HUVEC	Protein carbonylation and nitration	+
Redox state	HUVEC	Glutathione level	+
Response to oxidant load	HUVEC	H_2DCF oxidation	+
Expression level of eNOS	BAEC, EA.hy926	Western blot, proteasomal degradation	+
Expression level of iNOS	BAEC, RAEC	Western blot; nitrite assay	(+)
Secondary $^{\bullet}$NO metabolism	RAEC	Nitrite/nitrate assay	+

Note: HUVEC, human umbilical vein endothelial cells; BAEC, bovine aortic endothelial cells; RAEC, rat aortic endothelial cells; EA.hy926, a human endothelial cell line originating from hydridization of HUVEC with a lung tumor cell line; LDH, lactate dehydrogenase; MTT, 3-[4,5-dimethylthiazol-2-yl]2,5-diphenyltetrazolium bromide; BrdU, 5-bromo-2′-deoxyuridine; H2DCF, 2′,7′-dichlorodihydrofluorescein.

Source: These data were compiled from Steffen *et al.* (2005, 2006a, b, 2007a).

maximum of plasma metabolites of (−)-epicatechin. These observations show that (−)-epicatechin ameliorates the bioavailability and bioactivity of •NO *in vivo*.

The effect of (−)-epicatechin on •NO metabolism was also studied with endothelial cells *in vitro* (see "Note" on page 812). Exposure of endothelial cells to MPO/H_2O_2/nitrite-oxLDL caused down-regulation of eNOS protein, which was prevented by pretreatment with (−)-epicatechin (Steffen *et al.*, 2005). This effect of (−)-epicatechin was brought about by suppression of the proteasomal degradation of eNOS protein, although proteasome activity of a cell-free system was not inhibited (Steffen *et al.*, 2007a). Notably, down-regulation by oxLDL of eNOS protein was accompanied by up-regulation of inducible •NO synthase (iNOS), an isoform of eNOS, the induction of which is paralleled, however, by proinflammatory events, so that through the iNOS pathway preferably peroxynitrite rather than bioavailable •NO is generated. (−)-Epicatechin partially suppressed both oxLDL-mediated up-regulation of iNOS protein and iNOS-dependent •NO formation and strongly abrogated the formation of nitrated and carbonylated proteins in endothelial cells, which were shown to be to a large part mediated by iNOS (Steffen *et al.*, 2007a). Notably, (−)-epicatechin significantly elevated the nitrite/nitrate ratio of the secondary oxidation products of •NO (Steffen *et al.*, 2007a), which may reflect a suppression of injurious peroxynitrite formation (see below). Since nitrate may be regarded as indicator of intermittent peroxynitrite formation (see next section), it appears that (−)-epicatechin "tames" the iNOS by converting it from deleterious to beneficial.

Molecular mechanisms of epicatechin

Previous investigators supposed that (−)-epicatechin and related dietary polyphenols would simply act as general antioxidant. If this assumption would be true, antioxidant vitamins such as vitamins C and E should exert similar effects. We have shown, however, that antioxidant vitamins do not share a number of protective actions of (−)-epicatechin (Steffen *et al.*, 2006a). Thus, MPO/H_2O_2/nitrite-elicited lipid peroxidation of LDL is strongly inhibited by (−)-epicatechin, but only weakly by vitamin E, another radical chain-breaking natural antioxidant. This type of lipid peroxidation involves the nitrogen dioxide radical (•NO_2) to start free radical chain reaction. Flavan-3-ols appear to possess high affinity to scavenge this short-lived radical, which is apparently not sufficiently accessible to vitamin E.

A general antioxidant activity would imply inhibition of lipid peroxidation *in vivo*. F_2-isoprostanes are a reliable parameter of *in vivo* lipid peroxidation, but upon intake of high-flavanol-cocoa products neither sizeable lowering of the plasma level (Wiswedel *et al.*, 2004) nor any effect on urinary excretion of F_2-isoprostanes (Mathur *et al.*, 2002) were observed. As already mentioned, lipid peroxidation of LDL *ex vivo* is only marginally affected under these conditions as well (Table 82.3). These observations are in sharp contrast to the potent inhibition of several types of LDL oxidation *in vitro* (Table 82.2). A plausible explanation for this discrepancy may be the chemical nature of the plasma metabolites of (−)-epicatechin, which are predominantly glucuronidated or methylated at the 3′ or 4′ hydroxyls of the catechol arrangement in the B ring (Natsume *et al.*, 2003), whereas the free radical-scavenging action requires a free catechol grouping. Indeed, flavonoid metabolites having a partially blocked catechol exhibit a strongly diminished antioxidant activity toward free radicals.

(−)-Epicatechin has antioxidant activity in a broader sense, which is reflected by the fact that reactions of prooxidant enzymes are also suppressed, even though they do not implicate free radicals. Thus, 5- and 15-lipoxygenase activities are inhibited by flavan-3-ols and other flavonoids directly at the enzyme level (Sies *et al.*, 2005a, and references therein). Since these lipoxygenases are involved in both inflammation and atherogenesis, a contribution of these enzyme inhibitions may be plausible. Here again, however, lipoxygenase inhibition requires a free catechol arrangement, and evidence for its occurrence *in vivo* is still lacking.

The flavonoid inhibition of NADPH oxidase, another prooxidant enzyme system important for oxidative stress, has already been reported for the leukocyte enzyme in older work (Tauber *et al.*, 1984) and was now demonstrated also for the endothelial enzyme (Steffen *et al.*, 2007a, b; 2008). Recent work on the mode of action of epicatechin and its methyl ethers on endothelial NADPH oxidase (see "Note" on page 812) make this target as prominent site of the action of epicatechin *in vivo* probable. It may afford a plausible explanation for the protection of the vascular endothelium by dietary flavan-3-ols, as substantiated by recent *in vivo* data. Through blockage of NADPH oxidase-mediated $O_2^{\bullet -}$ formation, generation of secondary reactive oxygen species such as H_2O_2 and •OH radical is prevented. Elimination of $O_2^{\bullet -}$ generation also preserves bioavailable •NO by shutting down the formation of peroxynitrite. By this mode, flavan-3-ols or their metabolites may sustain an adequate steady-state level of bioactive •NO necessary for both function as well as antioxidant and anti-inflammatory defense reactions of the vascular endothelium.

Summary Points

- Epicatechin belongs to the group of micronutrients thought to provide health benefit by preventing or alleviating CVD.
- Epicatechin is absorbed from the intestine as well as bioavailable and bioactive in humans.
- Cocoa, dark chocolate, red wine and tea are major known sources of epicatechin and related compounds, whereas beer as a source of flavonoids was studied less extensively.

- In addition to general antioxidant activities, recent studies reveal a modulation of the metabolism of nitric oxide and reactive nitrogen species, which results in preservation and improvement of endothelial function of arterial vessels.
- Metabolic conversion products of epicatechin such as methylated and glucuronidated species may contribute to the protectant action on the vascular endothelium.

Note

Recently, new aspects on the mode of action of (−)-epicatechin on endothelial NADPH oxidase were revealed (Steffen *et al.*, 2007b, 2008). Vascular endothelial cells convert (−)-epicatechin or the plasma metabolite (−)-epicatechin glucuronide to 3′- and 4′-*O*-methyl epicatechin via catechol-*O*-methyltransferase (COMT). These methyl ethers act as inhibitors of endothelial NADPH oxidase. This, in turn, spares $^{\bullet}$NO from its reaction with the superoxide anion radical, so that there is an elevation in the cellular level of $^{\bullet}$NO, as actually observed.

References

Arts, I.C.W., van de Putte, B. and Hollman, C.H. (2000). *J. Agric. Food Chem.* 48, 1752–1757.

Awad, H.M., Boersma, M.G., Boeren, S., van der Woude, H., van Zanden, J., van Bladeren, P.J., Vervoort, J. and Rietjens, I.M.C.M. (2002). *FEBS Lett.* 520, 30–34.

Brennan, M.L., Penn, M.S., van Lente, F., Nambi, V., Shishehbor, M.H., Aviles, R.J., Goormastic, M., Pepoy, M.L., McErlean, E.S., Topol, E.J., Nissen, S.E. and Hazen, S.L. (2003). *New Engl. J. Med.* 349, 1595–1604.

Buijsse, B., Feskens, E.J.M., Kok, F.J. and Kromhout, D. (2006). *Arch. Intern. Med.* 166, 411–417.

Bursill, C.A., Abbey, M. and Roach, P.D. (2007). *Atherosclerosis* 193, 86–93.

Cos, P., Ying, L., Calomme, M., Hu, J.P., Cimanga, K., van Poel, B., Pieters, L., Vlietinck, A.J. and van den Berghe, D. (1998). *J. Nat. Prod.* 61, 71–78.

da Silva, E.L., Abdallah, D.S.P. and Terao, J. (2000). *IUBMB Life* 49, 289–295.

Daugherty, A., Dunn, J.L., Rateri, D.L. and Heinecke, J.W. (1994). *J. Clin. Invest.* 94, 437–444.

de Pascual-Teresa, S., Santos-Buelga, C. and Rivas-Gonzalo, J.C. (2000). *J. Agric. Food Chem.* 48, 5331–5337.

Ding, E.L., Hutfless, S.M., Ding, X. and Girotra, S. (2006). *Nutr. Metab.* (London). 3:2, doi 10.1186/1743-7075-3-2.

Donovan, J.L., Kasim-Karakas, S., German, J.B. and Waterhouse, A.L. (2002). *Br. J. Nutr.* 87, 31–37.

Donovan, J.L., Crespy, V., Oliveira, M., Cooper, K.A., Gibson, B.B. and Williamson, G. (2006). *Free Radic. Res.* 40, 1029–1034.

Engler, M.B. and Engler, M.M. (2006). *Nutr. Rev.* 64, 109–118.

Gorinstein, S., Zemser, M., Lichman, I., Berebi, A., Kleipfish, A., Libman, I., Trakhtenberg, S. and Caspi, A. (1997a). *J. Intern. Med.* 241, 47–51.

Gorinstein, S., Zemser, M., Berliner, M., Goldstein, R., Libman, I., Trakhtenberg, S. and Caspi, A. (1997b). *J. Intern. Med.* 242, 219–224.

Harada, M., Kan, Y., Naoki, H., Fukui, Y., Kageyama, N., Nakai, M., Miki, W. and Kiso, Y. (1999). *Biosci. Biotechnol. Biochem.* 63, 973–977.

Haslam, E. (1998). *Practical Polyphenolics – From Structure to Molecular Recognition and Physiological Action.* Cambridge University Press, New York.

Heiss, C., Dejam, A., Kleinbongard, P., Schewe, T., Sies, H. and Kelm, M. (2003). *JAMA* 290, 1030–1031.

Hirano, R., Osakabe, N., Iwamoto, A., Matsumoto, A., Natsume, M., Takizawa, T., Igarashi, O., Itakura, H. and Kondo, K. (2000). *J. Nutr. Sci. Vitaminol. (Tokyo)* 46, 199–204.

Holt, R.R., Lazarus, S.A., Sullards, M.C., Zhu, Q.Y., Schramm, D.D., Hammerstone, J.F., Fraga, C.G., Schmitz, H.H. and Keen, C.L. (2002). *Am. J. Clin. Nutr.* 76, 798–804.

Holvoet, P., Vanhaecke, J., Janssens, S., van de Werf, F. and Collen, D. (1998). *Circulation* 98, 1487–1494.

Huxley, R.R. and Neil, H.A.W. (2003). *Eur. J. Clin. Nutr.* 57, 904–908.

Ischiropoulos, H. (2003). *Biochem. Biophys. Res. Commun.* 305, 776–783.

Johnston, N., Jernberg, T., Lagerqvist, B., Siegbahn, A. and Wallentin, L. (2006). *Int. J. Cardiol.* 113, 167–173.

Keen, C., Holt, R.R., Oteiza, P.I., Fraga, C.G. and Schmitz, H.H. (2005). *Am. J. Clin. Nutr.* 81, 298S–303S.

Kelm, M. (2002). *Am. J. Physiol. Heart Circ. Physiol.* 282, H1–H5.

Kostyuk, V.A., Kraemer, T., Sies, H. and Schewe, T. (2003). *FEBS Lett.* 537, 146–150.

Kraemer, T., Prakosay, I., Date, R.A., Sies, H. and Schewe, T. (2004). *Biol. Chem.* 385, 809–818.

Kusche, M. (2005). Kolloidale Trübungen in untergärigen Bieren – Entstehung, Vorhersage und Stabilisierungsmaßnahmen. Thesis, Technical University of Munich, Germany: Wissenschaftszentrum Weihenstephan.

Lee, K.W., Kim, Y.J., Lee, H.J. and Lee, C.Y. (2003). *J. Agric. Food Chem.* 51, 7292–7295.

Leeuwenburgh, C., Hardy, M.M., Hazen, S.L., Wagner, P., Oh-ishi, S., Steinbrecher, U.P. and Heinecke, J.W. (1997). *J. Biol. Chem.* 272, 1433–1436.

Lotito, S.B. and Frei, B. (2006). *Free Radic. Biol. Med.* 41, 1727–1746.

Manach, C. and Donovan, J. (2004). *Free Radic. Res.* 38, 771–785.

Maron, D.J. (2004). *Curr. Atheroscler. Rep.* 6, 73–78.

Mathur, S., Devaraj, S., Grundy, S.M. and Jialal, I. (2002). *J. Nutr.* 132, 3663–3667.

Meisinger, C., Baumert, J., Khuseyinova, N., Loewel, H. and Koenig, W. (2005). *Circulation* 112, 651–657.

Mursu, J., Voutilainen, S., Nurmi, T., Rissanen, T., Virtanen, J.K., Kaikkonen, J., Nyyssönen, K. and Salonen, J.T. (2004). *Free Radic. Biol. Med.* 37, 1351–1359.

Napoli, C., de Nigris, F., Williams-Ignarro, S., Pignalosa, O., Sica, V. and Ignarro, L.J. (2006). *Nitric Oxide* 15, 265–279.

Natsume, M., Osakabe, N., Oyama, M., Sasaki, M., Baba, S., Nakamura, Y., Osawa, T. and Terao, J. (2003). *Free Radic. Biol. Med.* 34, 840–849.

O'Reilly, J.D., Sanders, T.A. and Wiseman, H. (2000). *Free Radic. Res.* 33, 419–426.

Osakabe, N., Baba, S., Yasuda, A., Iwamoto, T., Kamiyama, M., Takizawa, T., Itakura, H. and Kondo, K. (2001). *Free Radic. Res.* 34, 93–99.

Paganga, G., Miller, N. and Rice-Evans, C.A. (1999). *Free Radic. Res.* 30, 153–162.

Pannala, A.S., Rice-Evans, C.A., Halliwell, B. and Singh, S. (1997). *Biochem. Biophys. Res. Commun.* 232, 164–168.

Pearson, D.A., Frankel, E.N., Aeschbach, R. and German, J.B. (1998). *J. Agric. Food Chem.* 46, 1445–1449.

Rechner, A.R., Kuhnle, G., Bremner, P., Hubbard, G.P., Moore, K.P. and Rice-Evans, C.A. (2002). *Free Radic. Biol. Med.* 33, 220–235.

Rifici, V.A., Schneider, S.H. and Khachadurian, A.K. (2002). *J. Nutr.* 132, 2532–2537.

Rios, L.Y., Gonthier, M.P., Remesy, C., Mila, I., Lapierre, C., Lazarus, S.A., Williamson, G. and Scalbert, A. (2003). *Am J. Clin. Nutr.* 77, 912–918.

Schewe, T. and Sies, H. (2005). *Biofactors* 24, 49–58.

Schramm, D.D., Karim, M., Schrader, H.R., Holt, R.R., Kirkpatrick, N.J., Polagruto, J.A., Ensunsa, J.L., Schmitz, H.H. and Keen, C.L. (2003). *Life Sci.* 73, 857–869.

Schroeder, P., Klotz, L.O., Buchczyk, D.P., Sadik, C.D., Schewe, T. and Sies, H. (2001). *Biochem. Biophys. Res. Commun.* 285, 782–787.

Schroeder, P., Klotz, L.O. and Sies, H. (2003). *Biochem. Biophys. Res. Commun.* 307, 69–73.

Schroeter, H., Heiss, C., Balzer, J., Kleinbongard, P., Keen, C.L., Hollenberg, N.K., Sies, H., Kwik-Uribe, C., Schmitz, H.H. and Kelm, M. (2006). *Proc. Natl. Acad. Sci. USA* 103, 1024–1029.

Schuier, M., Sies, H., Illek, B. and Fischer, H. (2005). *J. Nutr.* 135, 2320–2325.

Sies, H. (1985). In Sies, H. (ed.), *Oxidative Stress*, pp. 1–6. Academic Press, London, UK.

Sies, H., Schewe, T., Heiss, C. and Kelm, M. (2005a). *Am. J. Clin. Nutr.* 81, 304–312.

Sies, H., Stahl, W. and Sevanian, A. (2005b). *J. Nutr.* 135, 969–972.

Steffen, Y., Schewe, T. and Sies, H. (2005). *Biochem. Biophys. Res. Commun.* 331, 1277–1283.

Steffen, Y., Schewe, T. and Sies, H. (2006a). *Free Radic. Res.* 40, 1076–1085.

Steffen, Y., Wiswedel, I., Peter, D., Schewe, T. and Sies, H. (2006b). *Free Radic. Biol. Med.* 41, 1139–1150.

Steffen, Y., Jung, T., Klotz, L.O., Schewe, T., Grune, T. and Sies, H. (2007a). *Free Radic. Biol. Med.*, 42, 955–970.

Steffen, Y., Schewe, T. and Sies, H. (2007b). *Biochem. Biophys. Res. Commun.* 359, 828–833.

Steffen, Y., Gruber, C., Schewe, T. and Sies, H. (2008). *Arch. Biochem. Biophys.* 469, 209–219.

Tauber, A.I., Fay, J.R. and Marletta, M.A. (1984). *Biochem. Pharmacol.* 33, 1367–1369.

Ursini, F. and Sevanian, A. (2002). *Biol. Chem.* 383, 599–605.

van het Hof, K.H., de Boer, H.S., Wiseman, S.A., Lien, N., Westrate, J.A. and Tijburg, L.B. (1997). *Am. J. Clin. Nutr.* 66, 1125–1132.

Vigna, G.B., Costantini, F., Aldini, G., Carini, M., Catapano, A., Schena, F., Tangerini, A., Zanca, R., Bombardelli, E., Morazzoni, P., Mezzetti, A., Fellin, R. and Maffei Facino, R. (2003). *Metabolism* 52, 1250–1257.

Walle, T. (2004). *Free Radic. Biol. Med.* 36, 829–837.

Wallenfeldt, K., Fagerberg, B., Wikstrand, J. and Hulthe, J. (2004). *J. Intern. Med.* 256, 413–420.

Wan, Y., Vinson, A.A., Etherton, T.D., Proch, J., Lazarus, S. and Kris-Etherton, P.M. (2001). *Am. J. Clin. Nutr.* 74, 596–602.

Weiß, A. and Hofmann, T. (2006). http://www.wifoe.org/Berichte%20und%20Dokumente/B71-I.pdf.

Wippel, R., Rehn, M., Gorren, A.C., Schmidt, K. and Mayer, B. (2004). *Biochem. Pharmacol.* 67, 1285–1295.

Wiswedel, I., Hirsch, D., Kropf, S., Gruening, M., Pfister, E., Schewe, T. and Sies, H. (2004). *Free Radic. Biol. Med.* 37, 411–421.

Zhu, Q.Y., Huang, Y., Tsang, D. and Chen, Z.Y. (1999). *J. Agric. Food Chem.* 47, 2020–2025.

83

Isohumulones from Beer Modulate Blood Lipid Status

Aruto Yoshida Central Laboratories for Frontier Technology, Kirin Brewery Co., Ltd., Yokohama, Japan

Abstract

Isohumulones, which impart bitter flavor and an antibacterial property to beers, are generated from humulones (also known as alpha acids) in the hop plant (*Humulus lupulus* L.) during the brewing process. The three major types of isohumulones are isohumulone, isocohumulone, and isoadhumulone, all of which are structurally related. The presence of isohumulones has long been noted in beers, but their physiologic actions remained curiously obscure. However, their unexpected pleiotropic effects on glucose and lipid metabolism in the body have recently been uncovered due to the availability of isomerized hop extract (IHE) that primarily contains isohumulones. Oral administration of IHE or isohumulones to mice results in significantly decreased blood triglyceride and non-esterified free fatty acid (NEFA) levels, adipose tissue weight, and hepatic cholesterol content. Microarray analysis and quantitative real time PCR (QPCR) have indicated that IHE dose-dependently upregulated the expression of hepatic genes involved in microsomal co-oxidation and peroxisomal and mitochondrial β-oxidation. These effects are very similar to those that follow administration of hypolipidemic drugs with the potential of activating the peroxisome proliferator-activated receptor α (PPARα). Moreover, these effects are not seen in PPARα-deficient mice. An *in vitro* reporter assay also indicates the activation of PPARα by isohumulone and isocohumulone. These observations strongly suggest that isohumulones upregulate the expression of key genes in hepatic fatty acid oxidation, and that they ameliorate blood and hepatic lipid profiles through activation of PPARα. This review focuses primarily on the effects of isohumulones on lipid metabolism through PPARα activation. Several PPARα independent functions are also described. These physiologic actions of isohumulones may be potentially therapeutic for the prevention of dyslipidemia in metabolic syndrome and alcoholic fatty liver disease.

List of Abbreviations

3KT	3-Ketoacyl-CoA thiolase
ACO	Acyl-CoA oxidase
ACSL	Long-chain fatty acid CoA ligase
ApoCIII	Apolipoprotein CIII
CACT	Carnitine/acylcarnitine translocase
CAT	Carnitine acetyltransferase
Chol	Cholesterol
CPT2	Carnitine palmitoyltransferase 2
CTL	Control
Cyp	Cytochrome P450
DCI	Mitochondrial delta3-delta2-enoyl-CoA isomerase
DGAT2	Diacylglycerol acyltransferase 2
FABP	Fatty acid binding protein
FF	Fenofibrate
FLD	Fatty liver disease
HDL	High-density lipoprotein
IHE	Isomerized hop extracts
LCFA	Long-chain fatty acid
L-PBE	Peroxisomal enoyl-CoA hydratase/L-3-hydroxyacyl-CoA dehydrogenase bifunctional enzyme
LPL	Lipoprotein lipase
LDL	Low-density lipoprotein
MCFA	Medium-chain fatty acid
NAFLD	Non-alcoholic fatty liver disease
NEFA	Non-esterified free fatty acid
PECI	Delta3-delta2-enoyl-CoA isomerase
PPAR	Peroxisome proliferator-activated receptor
QPCR	Quantitative real time PCR
RXR	Retinoid X receptor
SCFA	Short-chain fatty acid
VLCFA	Very long-chain fatty acid
VLDL	Very-low density lipoprotein

Introduction

The recent increased consumption of foods containing high levels of sugar and saturated fats, in conjunction with reduced physical activity, have caused an explosive increase in the incidence of obesity worldwide. There has also been a

Beer in Health and Disease Prevention
ISBN: 978-0-12-373891-2

proportionate increase in obesity-associated metabolic disorders, including type 2 diabetes, dyslipidemia (high triglycerides and low high-density lipoprotein (HDL)-lipoproteins), hypertension, and non-alcoholic fatty liver disease (NAFLD) accompanied by insulin resistance. Thus, the prevention of this medical sequela is a very serious issue. Accordingly, improved food choices offer a promising approach to solve obesity-related health problems (Kopelman, 2000; Evans *et al.*, 2004). Accumulating evidence has demonstrated that peroxisome proliferator-activated receptors (PPARs) are potential molecular targets for drugs to treat metabolic syndrome. PPARs are members of the nuclear receptor superfamily of ligand-inducible transcription factors. They play a central role in carbohydrate and lipid metabolism and inflammation. PPARα is a target of hypolipidemic drugs, fibrates, and PPARγ is a target of insulin-sensitizing antidiabetic drugs, thiazolidinediones (Evans *et al.*, 2004). Recently, a report suggested that isohumulones, which are the bitter compounds in beer, activate both PPARα and PPARγ *in vitro* and that they also ameliorate insulin resistance, hyperglycemia, and dyslipidemia in diabetic mice (Yajima *et al.*, 2004). This is the first observation relating to the physiologic effect of isohumulones, which have long been known to be a component of beer. Several latest studies have also supported the possibility that isohumulones may be potentially therapeutic for the prevention of dyslipidemia in metabolic syndromes and fatty liver diseases (FLD) (Miura *et al.*, 2005; Shimura *et al.*, 2005; Yajima *et al.*, 2005). This review primarily discusses recent progress of the effects of isohumulones on lipid metabolism through PPARα activation.

Metabolic Syndrome and PPARα

Obesity and metabolic syndrome

Since the 1980s, increased consumption of more energy-dense, nutrient-poor foods with high levels of sugar and saturated fats, combined with reduced physical activity, have caused an explosive increase in the obese population. Nowadays, the obesity epidemic is not restricted to industrialized societies such as North America, Western Europe, and Japan. Obesity is growing at a much faster rate in developing countries than in the developed world. The World Health Organization recently announced that obesity has reached epidemic proportions globally. More than 1 billion adults are overweight, of which at least 300 million are clinically obese. Along with the increase in obesity and overweight status, there has been a proportionate increase in obesity-associated metabolic disorders, including type 2 diabetes, dyslipidemia (high triglycerides and low HDL-lipoproteins), and hypertension. This dangerous cluster of chronic diseases accompanied by insulin resistance is correctively referred to as metabolic syndrome, or syndrome X (Kopelman, 2000; Evans *et al.*, 2004). Recently, obesity and obesity-associated FLD have become global health problems, and NAFLD, defined as a significant accumulation of fat in the liver without alcohol consumption, is also considered one aspect of metabolic syndrome (Bugianesi *et al.*, 2005; Hamaguchi *et al.*, 2005). This medical sequela is currently one of the most serious global threats that reduces the overall quality of life. Effective weight management for people at risk of developing obesity involves a range of long-term strategies including prevention, weight maintenance, and management of co-morbidities. Several public health efforts to diminish food portion sizes, improve food choices, and increase physical activity represent promising approaches to solve this global problem.

Roles of PPARα in lipid metabolism

PPARs are members of the nuclear receptor superfamily of ligand-inducible transcription factors. They form a heterodimer complex with retinoid X receptors (RXRs). Since PPARs bind to a diverse set of saturated and unsaturated fatty acids, and their eicosanoid derivatives generated from dietary fat or cellular metabolism function as natural ligands, they seem to play a role as lipid sensors for modulating lipid metabolism, storage, and transport in the body (Kersten *et al.*, 2000; Kliewer *et al.*, 2001; Evans *et al.*, 2004). In contrast to other nuclear receptors, the ligand binding domain of PPARs accommodates a wide range of structurally diverse ligands. Ligand binding triggers a conformational change of the PPAR/RXR complex, recruits transcriptional regulators and basal transcriptional machinery, and results in activation of a series of target gene expressions (Xu *et al.*, 2001). So far, three PPAR isotypes, α, δ, and γ, have been found in mammals. Their possible roles in the regulation of glucose homeostasis and inflammation, as well as lipid and lipoprotein metabolism, have been indicated. Accumulating evidence has also intimated a possible link between these PPARs and metabolic syndrome (Evans *et al.*, 2004).

PPARα is highly expressed in liver and to a lesser extent in heart, skeletal muscles, and kidneys. This expression profile is considerably different from the patterns that PPARγ is primarily expressed in adipose tissue and PPARδ is present throughout the body. Consistent with their expression profiles, each PPAR plays a unique role in the regulation of energy metabolism. During prolonged fasting, the expression of hepatic PPARα is increased, and fatty acids released from adipose tissues are transported into the liver. As a result, the activation of PPARα by fatty acids promotes lipid utilization as an energy source instead of carbohydrate and protein (Kersten *et al.*, 2000; Duval *et al.*, 2002; Lefebvre *et al.*, 2006). This PPARα mediated regulation is a critical response during fasting, as indicated by the fact that PPARα-deficient mice display severe hypoglycemia, hypoketonemia, hyperlipemia, and fatty liver. These conditions are likely due to reduced capacity for hepatic fatty acid oxidation, which generates acetyl-CoA that is required for gluconeogenesis and ketogenesis on demand (Lee *et al.*, 1995; Kersten *et al.*, 1999; Leone *et al.*, 1999).

As well, PPARα is an important therapeutic target for hypolipidemic drugs, and a class of synthetic PPARα agonists such as fibrates (fenofibrate, benzafibrate, and ciprofibrate, gemfibrozil, among others) has been developed (Kersten *et al.*, 2000; Kliewer *et al.*, 2001). In a variety of mice models, these drugs commonly decrease triglyceride and increase HDL-cholesterol level in the blood, accompanying enhanced hepatic fatty acid oxidation systems including microsomal ω-oxidation and peroxisomal and mitochondrial β-oxidations (Schoonjans *et al.*, 1996; Kersten *et al.*, 2000; Reddy and Hashimoto, 2001; Ferre, 2004; Lefebvre *et al.*, 2006). In addition, fibrates may improve adiposity, hepatic and muscle steatosis, as well as insulin sensitivity (Guerre-Millo *et al.*, 2000; Chou *et al.*, 2002; Ip *et al.*, 2003; Kim *et al.*, 2003; Ide *et al.*, 2004; Tsuchida *et al.*, 2005; Haluzik *et al.*, 2006). Although PPARα activation leads to peroxisome proliferation, hepatomegaly, and hepatocarcinoma in rodents, these are not observed in humans. A recent study with PPARα-humanized mice demonstrated that species specific effects are due to structural differences between the receptors. Furthermore, the control of lipid metabolic pathways is separable from cell proliferation pathways (Lee *et al.*, 1995; Cheung *et al.*, 2004). Accordingly, several fibrate drugs have shown potent hypotriglycemic efficacy in hyperlipemic subjects without serious side effects, resulting in a subsequent reduction of cardiovascular morbidity (Staels *et al.*, 1998; Guay, 2002; Staels and Fruchart, 2005). Some clinical studies have suggested that fibrates may also improve insulin sensitivity in type 2 diabetic patients (Ferrari *et al.*, 1977; Murakami *et al.*, 1984; Kobayashi *et al.*, 1988; Haluzik and Haluzik, 2006).

Effects of Isohumulones Intake

Isohumulones

The hop plant (*Humulus lupulus* L.) has been used in brewing over the centuries to impart bitterness and aroma to beers. The bitter taste of beer is largely due to the presence of isohumulones (also known as iso-alpha acids), which are generated from humulones (also known as alpha acids) that exist within lupulin glands in hop cones. Although humulones in themselves are not particularly bitter and are poorly soluble, they are converted into the bitter-tasting and more soluble isohumulones by an isomerization reaction that occurs during the process of boiling wort in the brew (Malowicki and Shellhammer, 2005). Wort is an aqueous solution containing primarily hops and fermentable sugars (e.g. glucose, maltose, maltotriose) obtained by enzymatic hydrolysis of starch from malt, or from other sources such as wheat, corn, and rice. The three major compounds of isohumulones, isohumulone, isocohumulone, and isoadhumulone, are all structurally related. They are derived from humulone, cohumulone, and adhumulone, respectively (Figure 83.1a). The concentration of isohumulones in beers is generally up to 100 mg/l, and they are responsible for 70% of the observed sensory bitterness in beers (Techakriengkrai *et al.*, 2004). In traditional brewing, whole hops are added to wort; however, many brewers have taken to use hop pellets or hop extract to increase brewing efficiency. Also, isomerized hop extract (IHE), which primarily contains isohumulones, is sometimes used in the post-fermentation adjustment of beer bitterness.

The use of hops is also important for keeping beers in a bacteriostatic condition. While humulones show remarkable antibacterial properties against Gram-positive bacteria such as *Bacillus subtilis* and *Staphylococcus aureus*, isohumulones have

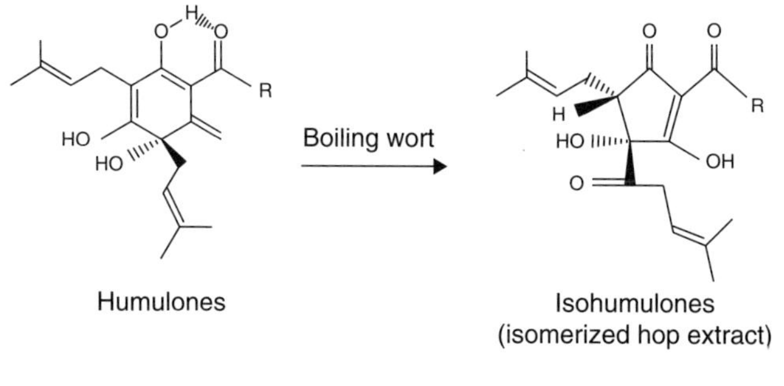

R	Humulones	Isohumulones
$-CH_2CH(CH_3)_2$	Humulone	Isohumulone
$-CH(CH_3)_2$	Cohumulone	Isocohumulone
$-CH(CH_3)CH_2CH_3$	Adhumulone	Isoadhumulone

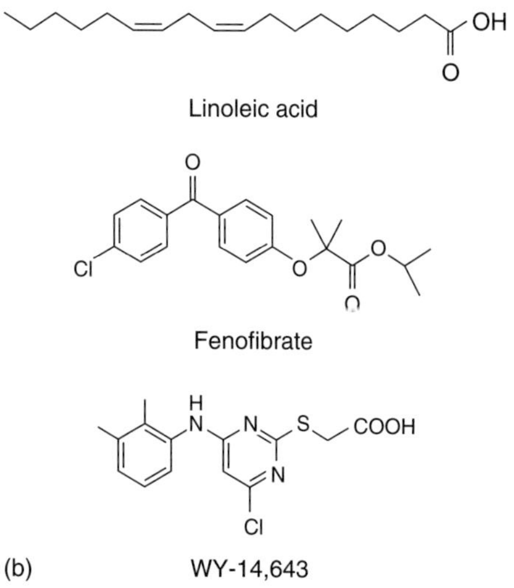

Figure 83.1 Structures of hop-derived compounds (a) and representative PPARα agonists (b). Humulones are converted into isohumulones during the process of boiling wort in the brewing.

much weaker effects under neutral pH condition (Teuber, 1970). Nevertheless, isohumulone seems to still be crucial for the prevention of the major beer spoiler lactic bacteria, since it exhibits 20 times greater antibacterial activity against *Lactobacillus brevis* than humulone under low pH condition, as is observed in beers (Simpson and Smith, 1992). However, neither isohumulones nor humulones substantially inhibit growth of Gram-negative bacteria. Although the presence of isohumulones in beer has long been noted, their physiologic actions have remained obscure. This might be due to the relatively low stability and limited commercial availability of purified isohumulone, isocohumulone, and isoadhumulone. However, their unexpected pleiotropic effects on the body have recently been uncovered due to the availability of IHE, which is used for beer manufacturing (Yajima *et al.*, 2004; Miura *et al.*, 2005; Shimura *et al.*, 2005; Yajima *et al.*, 2005). In particular, the aqueous type of IHE, such as ISOHOP CON2 (Botanix Ltd., UK), is superior in terms of purity, stability, and usability compared to the viscous kettle type. ISOHOP CON2 is a solution that is standardized to 30% w/w isohumulones. It is produced from a supercritical CO_2 hop extract and is isomerized under alkaline conditions in an all aqueous process. The purity of the isohumulones is approximately 80% and its isohumulone:isocohumulone: isoadhumulone ratio is 37:48:15. Several reports have shown good agreement regarding the physiologic effects of IHE and the purified isohumulones (Yajima *et al.*, 2004; Miura *et al.*, 2005).

Activation of PPARα *in vitro* reporter assay

An *in vitro* reporter assay is often used to evaluate the transient transcriptional activation of PPARs by ligands (Lehmann *et al.*, 1997). Interestingly, isohumulone dose-dependently activates PPARα in assays using a human hepatocellular carcinoma line, HepG2, and its specific activity is approximately one-tenth that of a PPARα agonist, fenofibrate (FF) (Yajima *et al.*, 2004). The crystal structure of the PPARα protein shows that it has a relatively large binding pocket that can accommodate diverse fatty acids and fibrates (Xu *et al.*, 2001). However, curiously, isohumulone has no marked similarity to these molecules (Figure 83.1a and b). This may suggest that isohumulone is a structurally unique PPARα agonist and that it may have potential as a candidate for a new lead compound for therapeutics. Also, isohumulones have drawn attention as food-derived PPARα activators, since few dietary factors having this activity other than lipids have been reported, to our knowledge (Rimando *et al.*, 2005). It is interesting that structural differences in the side chain of isohumulones affect the ligand binding and/or transactivation of PPARα. The activity of isocohumulone is approximately 10-fold lower than that of isohumulone, and isoadhumulone has no effect. This result is in stark contrast to the fact that all three isohumulones equivalently activate PPARγ, and that none of them activates PPARδ (Yajima *et al.*, 2004). However, this may not be so surprising, because the three PPAR subtypes show distinct selectivity against synthetic ligands, although there is a 60–70% sequence identity between their ligand binding domains. In particular, PPARδ has a narrower ligand binding domain that only accepts a limited set of ligands (Xu *et al.*, 2001). Further study will be necessary to elucidate why PPARα accepts the relatively long side chain of isohumulone but not the branching methyl group at the base of isocohumulone and isoadhumulone (Figure 83.1a).

Effects on body and tissue weights

Supplement of IHE in the diet dose-dependently suppresses body weight gain in the absence of a remarkable change of food intake in mice (Miura *et al.*, 2005; Shimura *et al.*, 2005; Yajima *et al.*, 2005). In male C57BL/6N mice, consumption of a basic diet containing 1% IHE suppresses body weight gain within 1 week, regardless of cholesterol content in the diet (Shimura *et al.*, 2005) (Figure 83.2a), whereas such an inhibition is only observed with a high-fat diet in male obese KK-A^y mice (Yajima *et al.*, 2005). In female C57BL/6N mice, 1% IHE significantly suppresses body weight gain within 2 weeks under cholesterol supplemented or atherogenic (high-fat and high-cholesterol) diet conditions (Figure 83.2b) while such an inhibition is not detected within 1 week when mice are placed on a chow diet (Miura *et al.*, 2005). Additionally, the preventive effect is observed even in 0.2% IHE within 3 weeks under high-fat diet conditions (Yajima *et al.*, 2005). Taken together, these data indicate that the inhibition of body weight gain by IHE is more distinct under high-fat diet and longer feeding conditions. It is noteworthy that the same repression is also observed in mice fed purified isohumulones (Figure 83.2b) (Miura *et al.*, 2005).

Although several reports have shown that a PPARα agonist, FF, inhibits body weight gain in male mice fed a high-fat diet (Guerre-Millo *et al.*, 2000; Yoon *et al.*, 2002; Jeong *et al.*, 2004), such an inhibition is not observed in female mice (Yoon *et al.*, 2002; Yoon *et al.*, 2003). Also, another PPARα agonist, WY-14,643, shows no obvious antiobesity effect even in male mice when they consume comparable amounts of diets (Ide *et al.*, 2004; Tsuchida *et al.*, 2005). Thus, it is likely that the effect of PPARα activation on body weight is not so significant, and it might require certain conditions such as a high-fat diet, long feeding periods, and/or genetically manipulated mice. In contrast, IHE shows a relatively clear suppression of body weight gain within a few weeks for both genders of mice. Since IHE induces less hepatic PPARα activation than FF *in vivo* (Shimura *et al.*, 2005) and represses the body weight gain even in PPARα-deficient mice (Figure 83.2c), the phenomenon is probably due to some other mechanisms.

Short-term supplementation of 1% IHE increases the relative liver weight in both male and female C57BL/6N mice (Figure 83.3a and b), which is reminiscent of the rodent specific hepatomegaly that has been reported as a result of PPARα activation (Akiyama *et al.*, 2001; Cheung *et al.*, 2004). The fact that the phenomenon disappears in PPARα-deficient mice suggests the involvement of PPARα (Figure 83.3c). However, it is curious that long-term feeding of 0.2% IHE in a high-fat diet rather decreases liver weight in obese mice (Yajima *et al.*, 2005). Since FF increases liver weight in mice fed a high-fat diet (Jeong *et al.*, 2004), the effect might be PPARα independent and related to hepatic lipid content, as described below. Interestingly, IHE significantly reduces the weights of subcutaneous, retroperitoneal, and parametrial adipose tissues in female C57BL/6N mice and the weights of subcutaneous and epididymal adipose tissues in male KK-A^y mice (Yajima *et al.*, 2005). These results are very similar to recent observations that FF (Guerre-Millo *et al.*, 2000; Haluzik *et al.*, 2006) and WY-14,643 (Tsuchida *et al.*, 2005) remarkably reduce the weights of various adipose tissues, suggesting the importance of PPARα activation. In addition, IHE tends to slightly decrease kidney weight in both male and female mice under high-fat diet conditions, although the basis for this effect is still unclear (Miura *et al.*, 2005; Yajima *et al.*, 2005). No significant change is detected in the weights of heart and spleen (Yajima *et al.*, 2005).

Effects on blood and hepatic lipids

Numerous studies have demonstrated that PPARα agonists decrease blood triglyceride and non-esterified free fatty

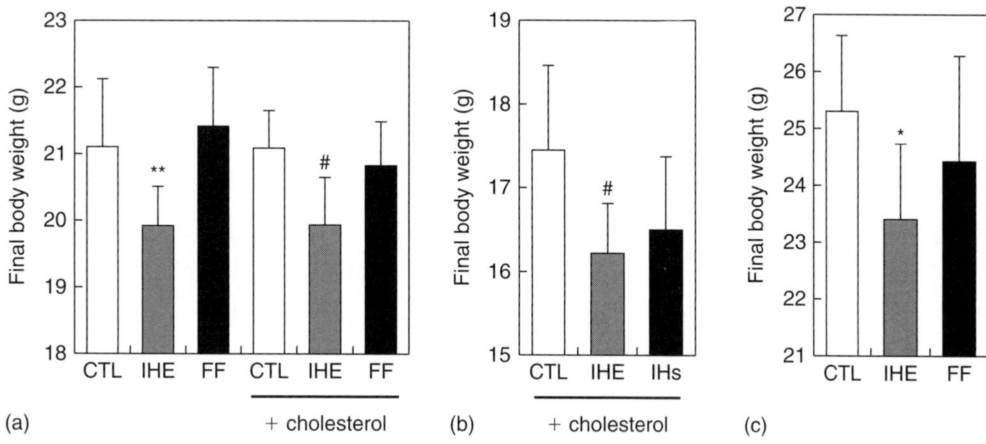

Figure 83.2 The effect of 1% isomerized hop extract (IHE), 0.05% fenofibrate (FF), or 0.3% isohumulones (IHs) intake for 1 week on final body weight in male C57BL/6N mice (a), in female C57BL/6N mice (b), and in male PPARα-deficient mice (c). Two types of basic diets (i.e. AIN-76A or AIN-76A + cholesterol (Chol)) were used. The results are expressed as the mean ± SD. $^{*}p < 0.05$ and $^{**}p < 0.01$ vs. AIN-76A diet; $^{\#}p < 0.05$ vs. AIN-76A + Chol diet. *Source*: Miura *et al.* (2005), Shimura *et al.* (2005).

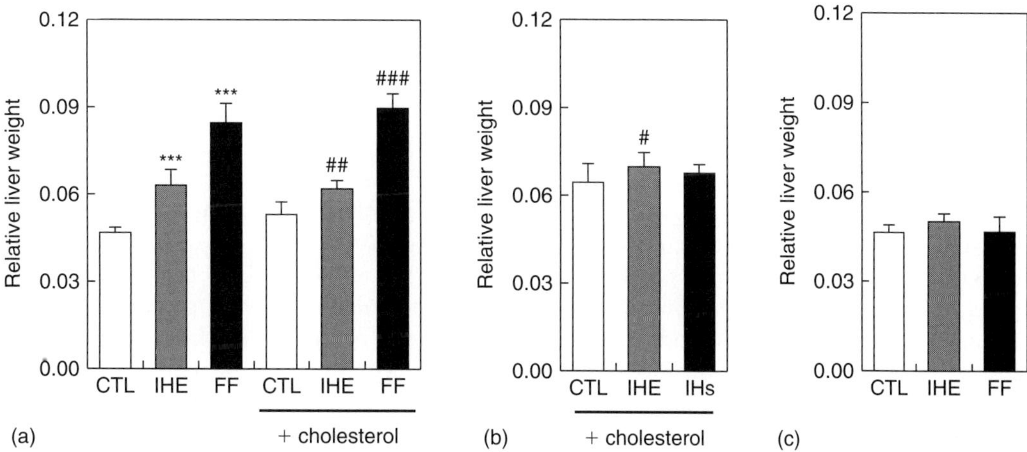

Figure 83.3 The effect of 1% isomerized hop extract (IHE), 0.05% fenofibrate (FF), or 0.3% isohumulones (IHs) intake for 1 week on relative liver weight in male C57BL/6N mice (a), in female C57BL/6N mice (b), and in male PPARα-deficient mice (c). Two types of basic diets (i.e. AIN-76A or AIN-76A + cholesterol (Chol)) were used. Relative tissue weight was calculated by dividing tissue weight (g) by body weight (g). The results are expressed as the mean ± SD. $^{***}p < 0.0001$ vs. AIN-76A diet; $^{\#}p < 0.05$, $^{\#\#}p < 0.001$, and $^{\#\#\#}p < 0.0001$ vs. AIN-76A + Chol diet. *Source*: Miura *et al.* (2005), Shimura *et al.* (2005) .

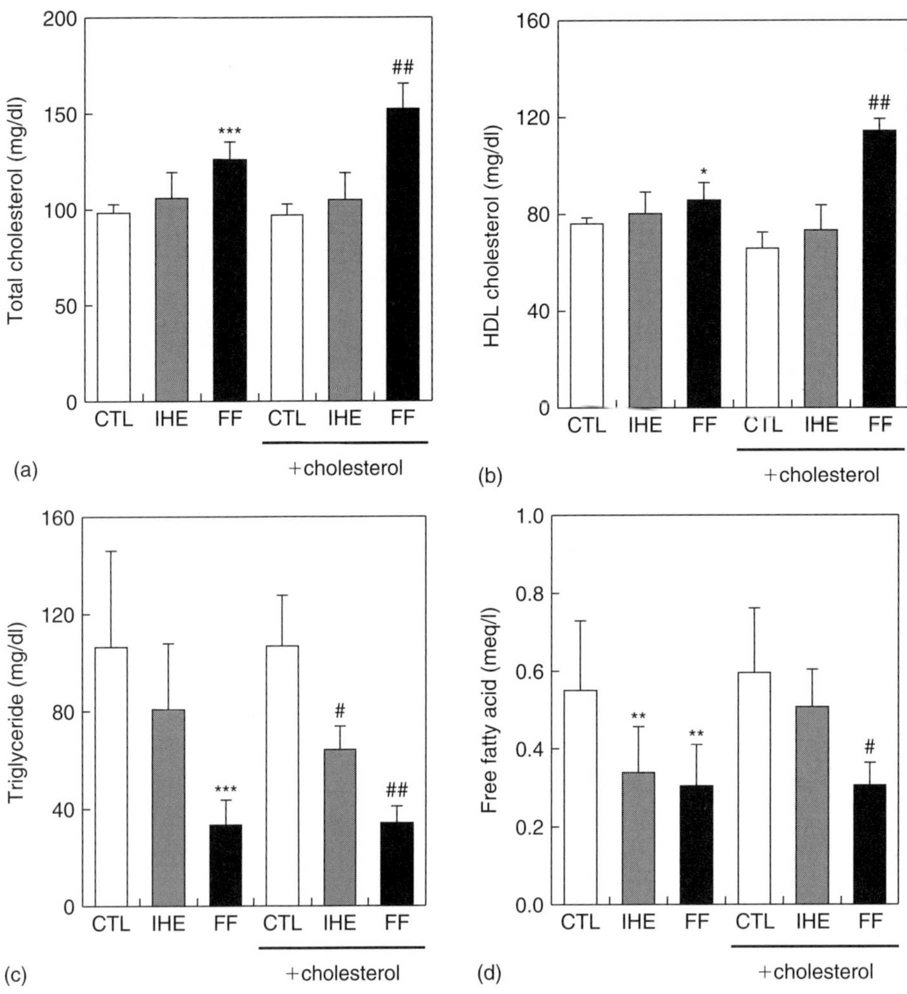

Figure 83.4 The effects of 1% isomerized hop extract (IHE) or 0.05% fenofibrate (FF) intake for 1 week on plasma total cholesterol (a), HDL-cholesterol (b), triglyceride (c), and NEFA (d) levels in male C57BL/6N mice. Two types of basic diets (i.e. AIN-76A and AIN-76A + cholesterol (Chol)) were used. The results are expressed as the mean ± SD. *$p < 0.05$, **$p < 0.01$, and ***$p < 0.0001$ vs. AIN-76A diet; $^{\#}p < 0.01$ and $^{\#\#}p < 0.0001$ vs. AIN-76A + Chol diet. *Source*: Shimura *et al.* (2005).

acid (NEFA) levels and increase HDL-cholesterol levels in rodents (Olivier *et al.*, 1988; Schoonjans *et al.*, 1996; Kersten *et al.*, 2000; Tsuchida *et al.*, 2005; Lefebvre *et al.*, 2006). Likewise, 1% IHE significantly decreases blood triglyceride level both in male (Figure 83.4c) and female mice (Miura *et al.*, 2005) within a few weeks, even when they are fed a standard diet. IHE also lowers NEFA in male mice (Figure 83.4d), regardless of whether or not the diet is supplemented with cholesterol. It is important to note that purified isohumulone and isocohumulone also reduce blood triglyceride and NEFA in male KK-A^y mice, and that the former shows a slightly stronger effect than the latter, consistent with their observed potency in PPARα activation in an *in vitro* reporter assay (Yajima *et al.*, 2005). While IHE slightly but insignificantly increases blood total and HDL-cholesterol levels in male mice fed a normal diet (Figure 83.4a and b), these parameters are more apparent when female mice are fed an atherogenic diet (Miura *et al.*, 2005). The plasma cholesterol profile analyzed by gel filtration chromatography has clearly indicated that the major contributor to increased total cholesterol is the rise in the number of HDL but not low-density lipoprotein (LDL) particles (Miura *et al.*, 2005). The fact that none of these alterations in blood lipid profile by IHE is observed in PPARα-deficient mice (Figure 83.5) indicates that they depend on PPARα activation.

The mice fed 1% IHE or a corresponding amount of isohumulones for 1 week show a significant decrease of cholesterol content in the liver. This is especially apparent in a cholesterol supplemented diet, and a similar effect is also observed for FF (Figure 83.6a) (Miura *et al.*, 2005). While there have been few reports on the action of PPARα agonists in hepatic cholesterol metabolism, a recent study has demonstrated that WY-14,643 lowers hepatic cholesterol levels, with a corresponding decrease in cholesterogenic carbon flux in mice; a similar reduction is not observed in PPARα-deficient mice (Knight *et al.*, 2005).

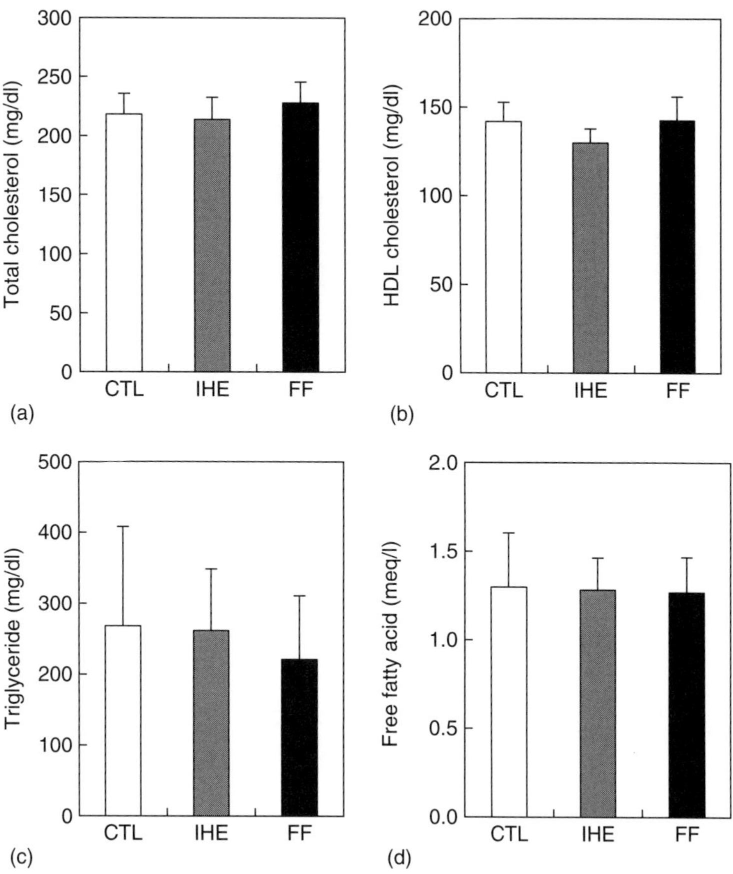

Figure 83.5 The effects of 1% isomerized hop extract (IHE) or 0.05% fenofibrate (FF) intake for 1 week on plasma total cholesterol (a), HDL-cholesterol (b), triglyceride (c), and NEFA (d) levels in male PPARα-deficient mice. AIN-76A was used as a basic diet. The results are expressed as the mean ± SD. *Source*: Shimura *et al*. (2005).

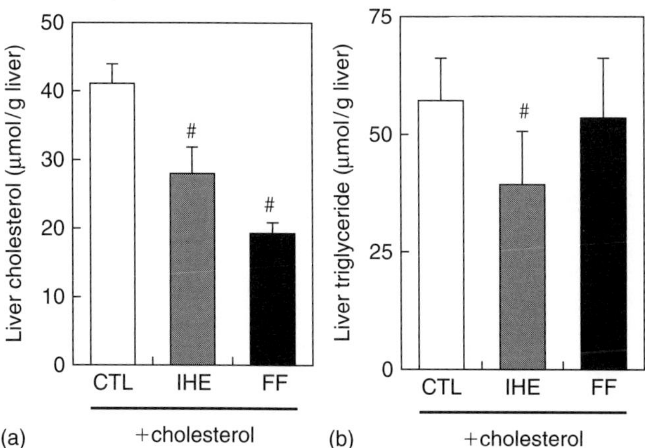

Figure 83.6 The effects of 1% isomerized hop extract (IHE) or 0.05% fenofibrate (FF) intake for 2 weeks on hepatic cholesterol (a) and triglyceride (b) contents in female C57BL/6N mice. AIN-76A + cholesterol (Chol) was used as a basic diet. The results are expressed as the mean ± SD. #p < 0.05 vs. AIN-76A + Chol diet. *Source*: Miura *et al*. (2005).

Thus, the decrease of hepatic cholesterol by isohumulones appears to be PPARα dependent. In contrast, IHE as well as isohumulones also reduces hepatic triglyceride, whereas such an effect is not observed for FF under the same conditions (Figure 83.6b). This suggests that isohumulones may have a unique and PPARα independent influence on triglyceride metabolism in the liver. The reason for this is currently unknown; however, it may be related to the significant decrease of diacylglycerol acyltransferase 2 (DGAT2) expression in the liver, which has been noted in male KK-A^y mice fed with IHE (Yajima *et al.*, 2005). Recent reports have demonstrated that the mice overexpressing hepatic DGAT2 exhibit a marked increase in hepatic triglyceride content (Yamazaki *et al.*, 2005) and that obese mice showing reduced hepatic DGAT2 expression following treatment with an antisense oligonucleotide show a significant reduction of triglyceride in the liver (Yu *et al.*, 2005).

Effects of hepatic gene expression and lipid metabolism

Alteration of hepatic gene expression in male C57BL/6N mice fed with diets containing either 1% IHE or 0.05% FF for 1 week has been analyzed by cDNA microarray and quantitative real time PCR (QPCR) (Shimura *et al.*, 2005). As shown in Table 83.1, IHE and FF specifically increase

Table 83.1 List of hepatic genes upregulated by IHE and FF in C57BL/6N male mice

Accession no.	Gene name	*Fold change*				
		IHE/CTL	*FF/CTL*	*Chol/CTL*	*IHE + Chol/CTL*	*FF + Chol/CTL*
AA106365	Cytochrome P450, 4a14 (Cyp4a14)	14.3	211.4	LI[a]	34.0	203.8
AA755385	Cytochrome P450, 4a10 (Cyp4a10)	12.7	78.3	0.7	11.2	59.3
AA718155	Peroxisomal bifunctional enzyme (L-PBE)	5.0	32.9	0.9	5.4	49.2
AI450521	Thioredoxin interacting factor (Vdup1)	LI	25.1	LI	LI	111.5
AA080270	Fatty acid binding protein 4, adipocyte (FABP4, aP2)	LI	20.6	LI	LI	13.5
AA739040	Lipoprotein lipase (LPL)	LI	16.9	LI	LI	19.4
AA656694	Cytochrome P450, 2b9	LI	14.4	LI	LI	14.7
AA755022	Mitochondrial uncoupling protein 2 (UCP2)	LI	8.2	LI	LI	7.3
AA260931	Peroxisomal biogenesis factor 11a	1.8	7.9	0.9	1.2	8.2
AA666595	Phospholipid transfer protein (PLTP)	LI	7.5	0.8	LI	2.7
AA511089	Glutathione *S*-transferase, theta 2	LI	7.0	LI	LI	6.0
AA473526	Carnitine acetyltransferase (CAT)	LI	6.9	LI	LI	7.4
AA726565	Cell division cycle 91-like 1	LI	6.9	LI	LI	13.1
AA606914	Mitochondrial delta3, delta2-enoyl-CoA isomerase (DCI)	2.4	6.1	0.9	1.9	4.8
AA067147	Malic enzyme, supernatant	4.2	5.8	0.8	2.4	8.0
AA066072	Phosphatidylcholine transfer protein	2.8	5.4	LI	2.1	4.6
AA624422	Adipose differentiation related protein	1.5	4.5	0.6	1.0	4.6
AI466451	Fatty acid binding protein 1, liver (FABP1)	1.0	4.4	0.8	1.0	3.0
AA612012	Acyl-coenzyme A oxidase (ACO)	1.2	4.3	0.7	1.1	4.0
AI789976	Acyl-CoA synthetase 1 (ACSL1)	2.0	3.8	1.1	1.7	4.4
AA619894	Diazepam binding inhibitor (acyl-CoA binding protein)	1.6	3.8	0.9	1.2	3.2
AI046529	Monocarboxylate transporter 1 (MCT1)	1.9	3.6	0.8	1.4	3.3
AA754922	Stearoyl-coenzyme A desaturase 1 (SCAD1)	1.3	3.2	1.8	1.8	3.8
AA738765	Malonyl-CoA decarboxylase	LI	3.2	0.9	LI	3.3
AA437485	Peroxisomal membrane protein 1 (PXMP1, Zwellweger syndrome 2)	1.9	3.1	0.7	1.1	3.1
AW210430	Peroxisomal delta3, delta2-enoyl-CoA isomerase (PECI)	1.2	3.1	0.9	1.3	2.5
AA638944	d-dopachrome tautomerase	1.6	3.1	1.1	1.5	2.5
AA529824	Fatty acid binding protein 2, intestinal (FABP2)	1.3	3.0	1.5	1.8	3.4
W82109	Kinesin light chain 1	1.5	3.0	0.8	1.3	2.5
AA217253	ATP binding cassette, sub-family G (WHITE), member 2	1.7	3.0	1.2	1.6	3.1
AA822067	Epoxide hydrolase 1, microsomal	4.8	2.9	1.2	4.7	3.5
AA212042	RAB9, member RAS oncogene family	LI	2.9	0.8	1.1	2.2
AW209706	Carnitine palmitoyltransferase 2 (CPT2)	LI	2.9	0.9	1.2	2.5
AA544212	Cellular repressor of E1A-stimulated genes	3.0	2.7	0.9	2.6	2.9

AA562563	Mitochondrial carnitine/acylcarnitine translocase (CACT)	1.5	2.7	0.8	1.3	3.0
AI892244	Cytochrome c, somatic	1.2	2.6	1.1	1.1	2.1
AA839264	2-Hydroxyphytanoyl-CoA lyase	1.6	2.5	0.8	1.3	2.2
W62765	Histone deacetylase 1	1.5	2.5	0.8	1.2	2.3
AA562548	Mitochondrial isocitrate dehydrogenase 2 (NADP+)	1.4	2.5	1.0	1.4	2.4
AA450526	Heat shock 10kDa protein 1 (chaperonin 10)	1.6	2.5	1.0	1.5	2.5
AA213107	Mitochondrial glycerol-3-phosphate acyltransferase	1.3	2.4	0.9	1.1	2.1
AA671231	Cystatin B	1.6	2.3	1.0	1.4	2.1
AA791665	Alcohol dehydrogenase family 1, subfamily A1 (ADH1)	2.5	2.2	1.0	2.4	2.3
AA106512	Monocarboxylate transporter 2 (MCT2)	2.0	2.2	LI	LI	2.5
AA049031	ATX1 (antioxidant protein 1) homolog 1 (yeast)	1.7	2.2	1.2	1.4	2.3
AA066694	Fatty acid transporter protein 2 (FATP2)	1.1	2.2	1.2	1.4	2.3
AI046504	Epoxide hydrolase 2, cytoplasmic	1.4	2.1	1.0	1.2	2.3
AI642230	Cyclic AMP phosphoprotein, 19kD	2.2	2.1	1.0	1.7	2.0
AI549621	Mitochondrial NADH dehydrogenase 4	1.5	2.1	1.6	1.5	2.1
AA607100	Keratin complex 2, basic, gene 8	1.8	2.1	1.3	1.7	2.3
AA683883	Mitochondrial dicarboxylate carrier	1.3	2.1	1.0	1.0	2.4
AA616998	Calcium binding protein A11	1.4	2.0	0.9	1.3	2.0
AI552897	Nicotinamide nucleotide transhydrogenase	1.6	2.0	1.2	1.6	2.1
AA008222	Smoothened homolog (drosophila)	1.6	2.0	1.5	1.5	2.1
	Number of genes upregulated more than 2-fold[b]	23	105	4	23	76

Notes: Male C57BL/6N mice at 6 weeks of age were fed basic diets containing either 1% IHE or 0.05% FF for 1 week. Two types of basic diets, AIN-76A and AIN-76 + 0.2% Cholesterol (Chol), were used. The pooled RNA from the liver of six mice was used for two-color cDNA microarray analysis.

[a] LI: Low intensity. The spot showed a low intensity signal (log 10(Cy3*Cy5) < 6).

[b] The number includes both annotated and functionally unknown genes.

Source: Shimura *et al*. (2005).

Table 83.2 QPCR analysis of the genes altered by IHE and FF in the liver of male C57BL/6N and PPARα-deficient mice

GeneBank Accession no.	KEGG Accession no.	Category / Gene name	Fold change[a] C57BL/6 IHE/CTL	FF/CTL	Chol/CTL	IHE + Chol/CTL	FF + Chol/CTL	PPARa (–/–) IHE/CTL	FF/CTL
		Microsomal v-oxidation							
AA755385	mmu13117	Cytochrome P450, 4a10 (Cyp4a10)	11.4	40.7	1	9.5	33.9	−1.4	−1.4
	mmu13118	Cytochrome P450, 4a12 (Cyp4a12)	4.1	19.8	1.1	4.0	14.5	1.0	1.0
AA106365	mmu13119	Cytochrome P450, 4a14 (Cyp4a14)	46.5	171.4	−2.5	28.1	131.7	−1.7	−1.8
		Peroxisomal β-oxidation							
AA066694	mmu26458	Fatty acid transporter protein 2 (FATP2)	1.0	1.8	1.2	1.2	1.4	1.0	1.0
AA612012	mmu11430	Acyl-CoA oxidase (ACO)	2.4	6.5	1.3	1.6	5.6	1.3	1.1
AA718155	mmu74147	Peroxisomal l-bifunctional enzyme (L-PBE)	6.0	46.5	1.4	6.6	39.3	1.1	1.0
	mmu113868	3-Ketoacyl-CoA thiolase (3KT)	2.9	7.5	1.6	2.8	7.1	1.1	1.1
AW210430	mmu23986	Peroxisomal delta3, delta2-enoyl-CoA isomerase (PECI)	1.3	2.6	1.0	1.3	2.2	1.0	1.0
		Mitochondrial β-oxidation							
AW209706	mmu12896	Carnitine palmitoyltransferase 2 (CPT2)	1.4	2.4	1.3	1.4	2.1	−1.1	−1.1
AA562563	mmu57279	Mitochondrial carnitine/acylcarnitine translocase (CACT)	1.5	3.4	1.2	1.4	3.1	−1.3	−1.2
AA473526	mmu12908	Carnitine acetyltransferase (CAT)	2.4	3.2	2.5	3.0	3.6	1.3	1.1
AA606914	mmu13177	Mitochondrial delta3, delta2-enoyl-CoA isomerase (DCI)	1.5	3.2	1.0	1.5	2.8	1.0	1.0
		Other enzymes and proteins							
AA739040	mmu16956	Lipoprotein lipase (LPL)	3.8	17.1	3.5	4.9	19.5	1.6	1.1
	mmu11814	Apolipoprotein CIII (ApoCIII)	−1.4	−2.0	1.1	−1.4	−2.5	−1.3	−1.1
AI789976	mmu14081	Acyl-CoA synthetase 1 (ACSL1)	1.7	3.3	1.2	1.3	2.6	−1.1	−1.1
	mmu50790	Acyl-CoA synthetase 4 (ACSL4)	1.5	2.6	1.7	1.0	2.6	−1.1	1.0
AK006541	mmu433256	Acyl-CoA synthetase 5 (ACSL5)	1.8	2.2	1.0	1.2	2.0	−1.2	1.0
AI466451	mmu14080	Fatty acid binding protein 1, liver (FABP1)	−1.1	2.1	−1.1	−1.4	1.6	−1.6	−1.4
AA529824	mmu14079	Fatty acid binding protein 2, intestinal (FABP2)	1.0	1.5	1.2	1.2	1.6	−1.8	−1.6
AA080270	mmu11770	Fatty acid binding protein 4, adipocyte (FABP4, aP2)	1.3	18.9	1.5	1.4	9.2	−1.4	1.0
AA755022	mmu22228	Mitochondrial uncoupling protein 2 (UCP2)	1.3	7.2	1.4	1.3	4.7	−1.2	1.0
AA666595	mmu18830	Phospholipid transfer protein (PLTP)	1.5	6.1	−1.1	−1.3	4.1	−1.1	1.2
AA067147	mmu17436	Malic enzyme, supernatant	3.7	4.7	1.1	2.3	4.4	−1.6	−1.2
AA754922	mmu20249	Stearoyl-coenzyme A desaturase 1 (SCAD1)	2.4	3.2	2.5	3.0	3.6	−1.7	1.2

Note: Male C57BL/6N mice at 6 weeks of age were fed basic diets containing either 1% IHE or 0.05% FF for 1 week. Two types of basic diets, AIN-76A and AIN-76A + 0.2% Cholesterol (Chol), were used. The pooled RNA from the liver of six mice was used to determine the expression of each gene by QPCR.

Source: Shimura *et al*. (2005).

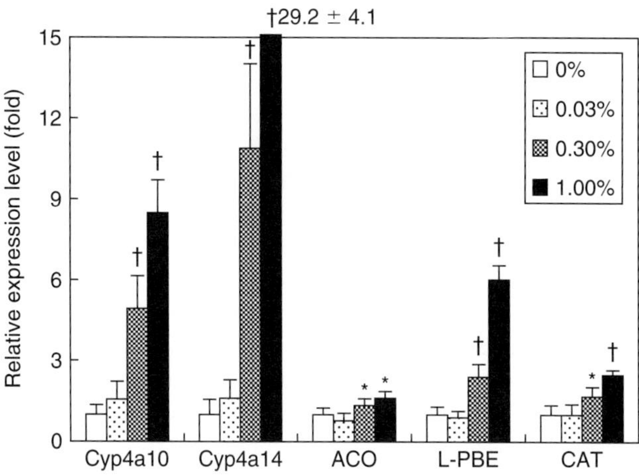

Figure 83.7 Dose-dependent induction of representative PPARα target genes in liver by isomerized hop extract (IHE). Male C57BL/6N mice were fed AIN-76A containing 0%, 0.03%, 0.3%, or 1% IHE for 1 week. The relative expression level of each gene was determined by QPCR. The results are expressed as the mean ± SD. *$p < 0.05$ and †$p < 0.0001$ vs. control diet (Shimura *et al.*, 2005). Cyp: cytochrome P450.

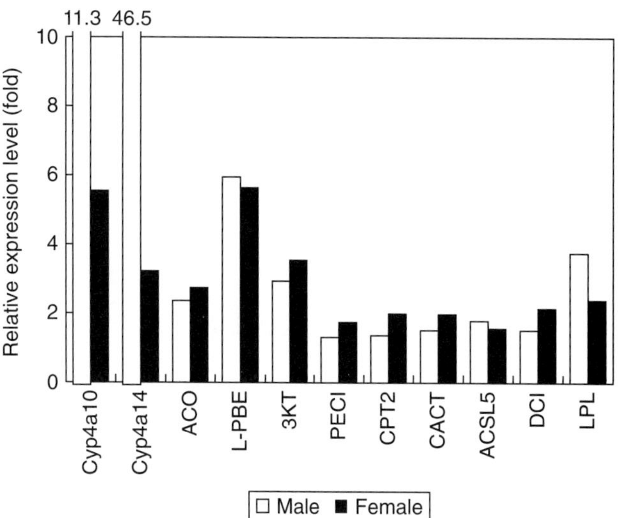

Figure 83.8 Gender differences in isomerized hop extract (IHE)-induced hepatic gene expression. Male and female C57BL/6N mice were fed AIN-76A containing 1% IHE for 1 week. The pooled RNA from six mice was used to determine the relative expression level of each gene by QPCR (Shimura *et al.*, 2005). Cyp: cytochrome P450.

the expression of approximately 20 and 100 genes among the 8,245 genes analyzed, respectively. These numbers are not significantly affected by supplementation of the diet with 0.2% cholesterol, as cholesterol alone does not significantly affect hepatic gene expression. The annotated genes upregulated more than 2-fold by FF are listed in Table 83.1, and the precise quantification of the selected genes by QPCR is shown in Table 83.2. The fold change values between the microarray analysis and QPCR correlate highly ($R^2 = 0.94$), indicating high reliability of the transcriptional profiles. FF greatly increases the expression of genes involved in microsomal ω-oxidation and peroxisomal and mitochondrial β-oxidation, which is a common feature induced by several different PPARα activators (Cherkaoui-Malki *et al.*, 2001; Yamazaki *et al.*, 2002; Frederiksen *et al.*, 2004). Likewise, but to a lesser extent, IHE upregulates most of these target genes of PPARα as follows (Tables 83.1 and 83.2). Both FF and IHE induce Cyp4a14 most strikingly (171.4- and 46.5-fold, respectively), and also significantly upregulate the other two members of the Cyp4a family (Cyp4a10 and Cyp4a12), suggesting an enhancement of microsomal ω-oxidation. In addition, they significantly increase a series of enzymes including peroxisomal enoyl-CoA hydratase/L-3 hydroxyacyl-CoA dehydrogenase bifunctional enzyme (L-PBE), acyl-CoA oxidase (ACO), 3-ketoacyl-CoA thiolase (3KT), and delta3-delta2-enoyl-CoA isomerase (PECI), which are involved in peroxisomal β-oxidation. It should be noted that increased enzymatic activity of ACO has also been reported in male C57BL/6N mice administered 100 mg/kg body weight of isohumulone or isocohumulone for 6 days (Yajima *et al.*, 2004). In contrast to these drastic changes in microsomal ω-oxidation and peroxisomal β-oxidation, elevations in the expression of genes involved in mitochondrial β-oxidation are small. Thus, FF clearly induces carnitine acetyltransferase (CAT), carnitine/acylcarnitine translocase (CACT), carnitine palmitoyltransferase 2 (CPT2), and mitochondrial delta3-delta2-enoyl-CoA isomerase (DCI) in the range from 2.4- to 3.4-fold, while the values for IHE range from 1.4- to 2.4-fold (Table 83.2). Additionally, IHE and FF weakly induce the expression of several long-chain fatty acid CoA ligases, ACSL1, 4, and 5, which are required for the activation of fatty acids to metabolize compounds in the two β-oxidation systems described above (Reddy and Hashimoto, 2001; Coleman *et al.*, 2002). It is noteworthy that FF and IHE significantly increase the expression of lipoprotein lipase (LPL) and reduce the expression of apolipoprotein CIII (ApoCIII), which is involved in triglyceride hydrolysis (Table 83.2).

The expression levels of representative hepatic genes (i.e. Cyp4a10, Cyp4a14, ACO, L-PBE, and CAT) increase in a dose-dependent fashion in response to IHE feeding (Figure 83.7). Statistically significant inductions for all of these genes are detected in male mice within 1 week at an IHE concentration of 0.3%. A comparable hepatic gene induction in fatty acid oxidation is also observed in female C57BL/6N mice (Figure 83.8). However, the induction of Cyp4a10 and Cyp4a14 genes in males is significantly higher than for female mice fed with IHE as well as FF. A similar gender specific high induction of the hepatic Cyp4 family by clofibrate has been also observed in rats (Sundseth and Waxman, 1992), but not all peroxisome proliferators induce increased gene expression of this gene family in males (Bell *et al.*, 1993). Additionally, the LPL

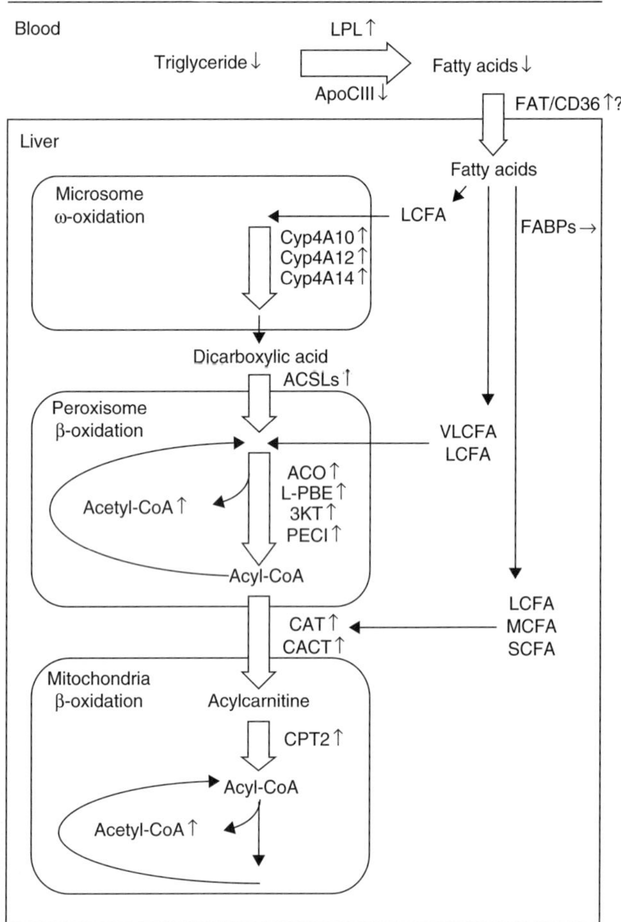

Figure 83.9 Schematic representation of hepatic lipid metabolism altered by isomerized hop extract (IHE) intake in C57BL/6 mice. Enhanced lipid hydrolysis and fatty acid oxidation pathways are indicated by thick arrows. The regulation of representative PPARα target genes is indicated with small arrows (Shimura *et al.*, 2005). Cyp: cytochrome P450; DGAT2: diacylglycerol acyltransferase 2; FABP: fatty acid binding protein; LCFA: long-chain fatty acid; MCFA: medium-chain fatty acid; SCFA: short-chain fatty acid; VLCFA: very long-chain fatty acid.

gene is induced to a greater extent in male than in female mice, which may be related to the greater reduction of blood triglyceride level in males (Figure 83.8).

Again, the genes significantly induced by IHE as well as by FF are mainly involved in microsomal ω-oxidation and peroxisomal and mitochondrial β-oxidation. These are typical hepatic PPARα target genes, and their induction for the most part is not seen in PPARα-deficient mice (Table 83.2). Thus, the results strongly indicate the alteration of gene expressions is mediated through PPARα activation (Lee *et al.*, 1995; Akiyama *et al.*, 2001; Reddy and Hashimoto, 2001).

Although IHE and FF induce most of the PPARα target genes in a similar manner, there are several exceptions. Distinct differences are found in the genes of the fatty acid binding protein (FABP) family, which is thought to bind to and transport fatty acids to various sites within the cell. FF increases the expression of FABP1, 2, and 4 (most notably FABP4), but IHE does not (Table 83.2). Since FABP1 is abundantly expressed in liver, it seems to be the most important member for hepatic lipid metabolism. However, FABP1-deficient mice show no significant change in serum and tissue lipid profiles and fatty acid distribution within hepatic complex lipid species. Rather, the increasing of hepatic triglyceride in respond to fasting is suppressed in the deficient mice (Newberry *et al.*, 2003). Therefore, a lack of induction of the FABP family by IHE might not have a significant impact on blood lipids. Instead, this phenomenon may be related to the lower hepatic triglyceride content in IHE fed mice, which is not observed for FF (Miura *et al.*, 2005). A recent report illustrates that the induction of FABP1 by PPARα agonists is markedly repressed by the expression of COUP-TFII through its binding to a complex of PPARα/RXRα (Spann *et al.*, 2006). Thus, isohumulones may specifically affect the recruitment of other transcriptional regulators. A similar different regulation mechanism for the human apolipoprotein A-I gene has been also observed when comparing effects of FF and gemfibrozil, which is due to a differential recruitment of coactivators to the promoters (Duez *et al.*, 2005).

In accordance with the changes in hepatic gene expression, the decreased blood triglyceride and NEFA and the increased blood HDL-cholesterol in response to IHE and FF are almost completely abolished in PPARα-deficient mice (Figure 83.5). Accordingly, these physiologic changes appear to be consequence of PPARα-dependent enhancement of lipolysis and fatty acids catabolism in liver (Figure 83.9). Since LPL hydrolyzes the triglyceride moiety of chylomicrons and very-low density lipoprotein (VLDL) particles, and ApoCIII effectively inhibits this hydrolysis, the upregulation of LPL and the downregulation of ApoCIII contribute to the reduction of blood triglyceride level cooperatively (Schoonjans *et al.*, 1996). The released fatty acids seem to be converted into acyl-CoA derivatives by the increased ACSLs, and they are further effectively degraded by coordination of three enhanced fatty acid oxidation systems as follows (Reddy and Hashimoto, 2001). The enzymes of the Cyp4a family are rate limiting in ω-oxidation, and they metabolize long-chain fatty acids to dicarboxylic acids. Although ω-oxidation is a minor pathway of fatty acid metabolism, significant amounts of dicarboxylic acids are generated under conditions of fatty acid overload in obesity and diabetes (Sanders *et al.*, 2005). In the peroxisomal β-oxidation pathway, ACO (Fan *et al.*, 1996), L-PBE (Qi *et al.*, 1999), 3KT (Chevillard *et al.*, 2004), and PECI (Geisbrecht *et al.*, 1999) preferentially degrade straight very long- and long-chain fatty acids in addition to dicarboxylic acids from the microsome. This reaction is likely to become more important during periods of increased influx of fatty acids into liver, since ACO-deficient mice exhibit severe microvesicular hepatic steatosis (Fan *et al.*, 1996). The acyl-CoAs with appropriately shortened chains in peroxisomes are then transported to mitochondria to complete their oxidation. Mitochondrial β-oxidation is the major process for degradation of short-, medium-, and long-chain fatty acids to generate energy. This results in shortening of fatty acids into acetyl-CoA subunits, which then either condense into ketone bodies or enter the tricarboxylic acid cycle for further oxidation to water and carbon dioxide. CAT, CACT, and CPT2 are involved in the rate-limiting carnitine shuttle system for the entry of fatty acids into mitochondria. CAT prefers short- and medium-chain acyl groups and catalyzes the reversible exchange of acyl groups between carnitine and coenzyme A. This enzyme may also be important for fatty acid transport processes from the peroxisome to mitochondria (Hsiao *et al.*, 2006). The resulting acylcarnitines are translocated into the mitochondrial matrix through CACT, and they are then converted back to the acyl-CoA by the action of CPT2 for the following β-oxidation (Longo *et al.*, 2006).

Prospective effects on health

Several recent reports have demonstrated that isohumulones upregulate the expression of key genes in hepatic fatty acid oxidation and ameliorate blood and hepatic lipid profiles through the activation of PPARα (Yajima *et al.*, 2004; Miura *et al.*, 2005; Shimura *et al.*, 2005). These results conjure up the image of their similar efficacy to the PPARα agonists, fibrates. Fibrates have been used as hypolipidemic drugs for several decades, and their safety and efficacy in patients have been extensively demonstrated (Staels *et al.*, 1998; Guay, 2002; Staels and Fruchart, 2005). Several clinical trials further indicate that fibrates reduce the progression of coronary atherosclerosis (Ericsson *et al.*, 1997; Frick *et al.*, 1997; Anonymous 2001) and the primary and secondary incidence of coronary heart disease (Frick *et al.*, 1987; Rubins *et al.*, 1997; Anonymous, 2000). Also, several lines of evidence suggest that fibrates reverse endothelial dysfunction, which is closely related to atherosclerosis and hypertension, in patients with type 2 diabetes (Evans *et al.*, 2000; Avogaro *et al.*, 2001; Playford *et al.*, 2002) and hypertriglyceridemia (Capell *et al.*, 2003). These results illustrate the fact that PPARα agonists are particularly useful to treat atherogenic dyslipidemia of prediabetic individuals and diabetic patients, who often also exhibit insulin resistance and obesity and are highly susceptible to cardiovascular morbidity. Accordingly, isohumulones may provide an alternative for the prevention and amelioration of dyslipidemia and endothelial dysfunction in metabolic syndrome. Indeed, a preliminary pilot study with mild type 2 diabetic subjects suggests a hypotensive effect of isohumulones (Yajima *et al.*, 2004)

The lipid-lowering action of isohumulones through activation of PPARα may also be good news for the prevention of FLD. In the past, excessive alcohol consumption accounted for the majority of FLD cases, but in recent years obesity-associated FLD has attracted considerable attention. Although FLD is now clinically categorized into two broad entities, alcoholic FLD and non-alcoholic FLD, both commonly encompass a morphological spectrum consisting of hepatic steatosis and steatohepatitis, which have an inherent propensity to progress toward the development of cirrhosis and hepatocellular carcinoma. In mice, chronic ethanol feeding deteriorates hepatic fatty acid degradation and promotes an accumulation of hepatic lipids with an accompanying increase of blood triglyceride and NEFA. This appears to include decreased DNA binding of PPARα in the liver, which is mainly caused by acetaldehyde generated during ethanol metabolism (Galli *et al.*, 2001; Fischer *et al.*, 2003). Treatment with a PPARα agonist, WY-14,643, significantly improves the DNA binding activity of PPARα and ethanol-induced steatosis, resulting in decreasing hepatic and blood triglyceride levels and blood NEFA levels in mice (Fischer *et al.*, 2003). Similarly, the PPARα agonists FF (Tsutsumi and Takase, 2001) and clofibrate (Nanji *et al.*, 2004) also ameliorate ethanol-induced steatosis in rats. In addition to these effects of fibrates on alcoholic FLD, several reports have shown that WY-14,643 reduces hepatic triglyceride accumulation, with a significant decrease of blood triglyceride levels, in different types of non-alcoholic FLD mouse models (Chou *et al.*, 2002; Ip *et al.*, 2003; Kim *et al.*, 2003; Ide *et al.*, 2004). Thus, isohumulones may play a role in protecting against the development of alcoholic and non-alcoholic FLD.

Isohumulones are only a few of the food-derived PPAR activators, and their presence has long been noted in beer. Our results suggest that they might be beneficial, not to mention cost effective, for the prevention and/or treatment of cardiovascular disease and FLD. However, further human study is necessary to confirm their potential benefits, since the effects shown so far are mostly based on animal studies. Simple arithmetic based on short-term animal studies indicates that we would need to drink more than 5 l/kg body weight of beer daily to obtain the optimal effects of these compounds (Miura *et al.*, 2005). However, a preliminary pilot study with mild type 2 diabetic subjects suggests that the daily intake of approximately 50 mg of isohumulones, which is generally contained in less than two litters of beer, may contribute to the prevention of hypertension. (Yajima *et al.*, 2004). Thus, it appears to be important to evaluate the possible utility of isohumulones from beer for prevention of metabolic syndrome by epidemiological studies. Further investigations will unravel whether the original idea of our mediaeval ancestors to use the hop plant in the production of beer actually has great medical merit.

Summary Points

- The major bitter compounds in beers are isohumulone, isocohumulone, and isoadhumulone, all of which are produced from the hop plant (*Humulus lupulus* L.) during the beer-making process.

- Isohumulone and isocohumulone activate PPARα in an *in vitro* reporter assay, while isoadhumulone does not.
- Supplementation with isohumulones suppresses body weight gain without an effect on food intake through a PPARα independent mechanism.
- Supplementation with isohumulones increases liver weight and decreases adipose tissue weight.
- Supplementation with isohumulones decreases triglyceride and NEFA and increases HDL-cholesterol in blood through the activation of PPARα.
- Supplementation with isohumulones decreases hepatic triglyceride and cholesterol contents.
- Supplementation with isohumulones dose-dependently induces hepatic gene expression mainly of proteins that are involved in fatty acid oxidation in a PPARα-dependent manner.
- Although the effects of isohumulones are generally observed both in male and female, subtle differences are detected in the biochemical parameters and gene expressions.
- Animal studies suggest a possibility that isohumulones provide an alternative for the prevention and amelioration of dyslipidemia in metabolic syndrome, whereas further human study is needed.

References

Akiyama, T.E., Nicol, C.J., Fievet, C., Staels, B., Ward, J.M., Auwerx, J., Lee, S.S., Gonzalez, F.J. and Peters, J.M. (2001). *J. Biol. Chem.* 276, 39088–39093.

Anonymous (2000). *Circulation* 102, 21–27.

Anonymous (2001). *Lancet* 357, 905–910.

Avogaro, A., Miola, M., Favaro, A., Gottardo, L., Pacini, G., Manzato, E., Zambon, S., Sacerdoti, D., de Kreutzenberg, S., Piliego, T., Tiengo, A. and Del Prato, S. (2001). *Eur. J. Clin. Invest.* 31, 603–609.

Bell, D.R., Plant, N.J., Rider, C.G., Na, L., Brown, S., Ateitalla, I., Acharya, S.K., Davies, M.H., Elias, E., Jenkins, N.A. *et al.* (1993). *Biochem. J.* 294, 173–180.

Bugianesi, E., McCullough, A.J. and Marchesini, G. (2005). *Hepatology* 42, 987–1000.

Capell, W.H., DeSouza, C.A., Poirier, P., Bell, M.L., Stauffer, B.L., Weil, K.M., Hernandez, T.L. and Eckel, R.H. (2003). *Arterioscler. Thromb. Vasc. Biol.* 23, 307–313.

Cherkaoui-Malki, M., Meyer, K., Cao, W.Q., Latruffe, N., Yeldandi, A.V., Rao, M.S., Bradfield, C.A. and Reddy, J.K. (2001). *Gene Expr.* 9, 291–304.

Cheung, C., Akiyama, T.E., Ward, J.M., Nicol, C.J., Feigenbaum, L., Vinson, C. and Gonzalez, F.J. (2004). *Cancer Res.* 64, 3849–3854.

Chevillard, G., Clemencet, M.C., Etienne, P., Martin, P., Pineau, T., Latruffe, N. and Nicolas-Frances, V. (2004). *BMC Biochem.* 5, 3.

Chou, C.J., Haluzik, M., Gregory, C., Dietz, K.R., Vinson, C., Gavrilova, O. and Reitman, M.L. (2002). *J. Biol. Chem.* 277, 24484–24489.

Coleman, R.A., Lewin, T.M., Van Horn, C.G. and Gonzalez-Baro, M.R. (2002). *J. Nutr.* 132, 2123–2126.

Duez, H., Lefebvre, B., Poulain, P., Pineda Torra, I., Percevault, F., Luc, G., Peters, J.M., Gonzalez, F.J., Gineste, R., Helleboid, S., Fruchart, J.C., Fievet, C., Lefebvre, P. and Staels, B. (2005). *Arterioscler. Thromb. Vasc. Biol.* 25, 585–591.

Duval, C., Chinetti, G., Trottein, F., Fruchart, J.C. and Staels, B. (2002). *Trends Mol. Med.* 8, 422–430.

Ericsson, C.G., Nilsson, J., Grip, L., Svane, B. and Hamsten, A. (1997). *Am. J. Cardiol.* 80, 1125–1129.

Evans, M., Anderson, R.A., Graham, J., Ellis, G.R., Morris, K., Davies, S., Jackson, S.K., Lewis, M.J., Frenneaux, M.P. and Rees, A. (2000). *Circulation* 101, 1773–1779.

Evans, R.M., Barish, G.D. and Wang, Y.X. (2004). *Nat. Med.* 10, 355–361.

Fan, C.Y., Pan, J., Chu, R., Lee, D., Kluckman, K.D., Usuda, N., Singh, I., Yeldandi, A.V., Rao, M.S., Maeda, N. and Reddy, J.K. (1996). *J. Biol. Chem.* 271, 24698–24710.

Ferrari, C., Frezzati, S., Romussi, M., Bertazzoni, A., Testori, G.P., Antonini, S. and Paracchi, A. (1977). *Metabolism* 26, 129–139.

Ferre, P. (2004). *Diabetes* 53, S43–S50.

Fischer, M., You, M., Matsumoto, M. and Crabb, D.W. (2003). *J. Biol. Chem.* 278, 27997–28004.

Frederiksen, K.S., Wulff, E.M., Sauerberg, P., Mogensen, J.P., Jeppesen, L. and Fleckner, J. (2004). *J. Lipid Res.* 45, 592–601.

Frick, M.H., Elo, O., Haapa, K., Heinonen, O.P., Heinsalmi, P., Helo, P., Huttunen, J.K., Kaitaniemi, P., Koskinen, P., Manninen, V. *et al.* (1987). *New Engl. J. Med.* 317, 1237–1245.

Frick, M.H., Syvanne, M., Nieminen, M.S., Kauma, H., Majahalme, S., Virtanen, V., Kesaniemi, Y.A., Pasternack, A. and Taskinen, M.R. (1997). *Circulation* 96, 2137–2143.

Galli, A., Pinaire, J., Fischer, M., Dorris, R. and Crabb, D.W. (2001). *J. Biol. Chem.* 276, 68–75.

Geisbrecht, B.V., Zhang, D., Schulz, H. and Gould, S.J. (1999). *J. Biol. Chem.* 274, 21797–21803.

Guay, D.R. (2002). *Cardiovasc. Drug Rev.* 20, 281–302.

Guerre-Millo, M., Gervois, P., Raspe, E., Madsen, L., Poulain, P., Derudas, B., Herbert, J.M., Winegar, D.A., Willson, T.M., Fruchart, J.C., Berge, R.K. and Staels, B. (2000). *J. Biol. Chem.* 275, 16638–16642.

Haluzik, M.M. and Haluzik, M. (2006). *Physiol. Res.* 55, 115–122.

Haluzik, M.M., Lacinova, Z., Dolinkova, M., Haluzikova, D., Housa, D., Horinek, A., Vernerova, Z., Kumstyrova, T. and Haluzik, M. (2006). *Endocrinology* 147, 4517–4524.

Hamaguchi, M., Kojima, T., Takeda, N., Nakagawa, T., Taniguchi, H., Fujii, K., Omatsu, T., Nakajima, T., Sarui, H., Shimazaki, M., Kato, T., Okuda, J. and Ida, K. (2005). *Ann. Intern. Med.* 143, 722–728.

Hsiao, Y.S., Jogl, G. and Tong, L. (2006). *J. Biol. Chem.* 281, 28480–28487.

Ide, T., Tsunoda, M., Mochizuki, T. and Murakami, K. (2004). *Med. Sci. Monit.* 10, BR388–BR395.

Ip, E., Farrell, G.C., Robertson, G., Hall, P., Kirsch, R. and Leclercq, I. (2003). *Hepatology* 38, 123–132.

Jeong, S., Kim, M., Han, M., Lee, H., Ahn, J., Song, Y.H., Shin, C., Nam, K.H., Kim, T.W., Oh, G.T. and Yoon, M. (2004). *Metabolism* 53, 607–613.

Kersten, S., Seydoux, J., Peters, J.M., Gonzalez, F.J., Desvergne, B. and Wahli, W. (1999). *J. Clin. Invest.* 103, 1489–1498.

Kersten, S., Desvergne, B. and Wahli, W. (2000). *Nature* 405, 421–424.

Kim, H., Haluzik, M., Asghar, Z., Yau, D., Joseph, J.W., Fernandez, A.M., Reitman, M.L., Yakar, S., Stannard, B., Heron-Milhavet, L., Wheeler, M.B. and LeRoith, D. (2003). *Diabetes* 52, 1770–1778.

Kliewer, S.A., Xu, H.E., Lambert, M.H. and Willson, T.M. (2001). *Recent Prog. Horm. Res.* 56, 239–263.

Knight, B.L., Hebbachi, A., Hauton, D., Brown, A.M., Wiggins, D., Patel, D.D. and Gibbons, G.F. (2005). *Biochem. J.* 389, 413–421.

Kobayashi, M., Shigeta, Y., Hirata, Y., Omori, Y., Sakamoto, N., Nambu, S. and Baba, S. (1988). *Diabetes Care* 11, 495–499.

Kopelman, P.G. (2000). *Nature* 404, 635–643.

Lee, S.S., Pineau, T., Drago, J., Lee, E.J., Owens, J.W., Kroetz, D.L., Fernandez-Salguero, P.M., Westphal, H. and Gonzalez, F.J. (1995). *Mol. Cell. Biol.* 15, 3012–3022.

Lefebvre, P., Chinetti, G., Fruchart, J.C. and Staels, B. (2006). *J. Clin. Invest.* 116, 571–580.

Lehmann, J.M., Lenhard, J.M., Oliver, B.B., Ringold, G.M. and Kliewer, S.A. (1997). *J. Biol. Chem.* 272, 3406–3410.

Leone, T.C., Weinheimer, C.J. and Kelly, D.P. (1999). *Proc. Natl. Acad. Sci. USA* 96, 7473–7478.

Longo, N., Amat di San Filippo, C. and Pasquali, M. (2006). *Am. J. Med. Genet. C Semin. Med. Genet.* 142, 77–85.

Malowicki, M.G. and Shellhammer, T.H. (2005). *J. Agric. Food Chem.* 53, 4434–4439.

Miura, Y., Hosono, M., Oyamada, C., Odai, H., Oikawa, S. and Kondo, K. (2005). *Br. J. Nutr.* 93, 559–567.

Murakami, K., Nambu, S., Koh, H., Kobayashi, M. and Shigeta, Y. (1984). *Br. J. Clin. Pharmacol.* 17, 89–91.

Nanji, A.A., Dannenberg, A.J., Jokelainen, K. and Bass, N.M. (2004). *J. Pharmacol. Exp. Ther.* 310, 417–424.

Newberry, E.P., Xie, Y., Kennedy, S., Han, X., Buhman, K.K., Luo, J., Gross, R.W. and Davidson, N.O. (2003). *J. Biol. Chem.* 278, 51664–51672.

Olivier, P., Plancke, M.O., Theret, N., Marzin, D., Clavey, V. and Fruchart, J.C. (1988). *Atherosclerosis* 74, 15–21.

Playford, D.A., Watts, G.F., Best, J.D. and Burke, V. (2002). *Am. J. Cardiol.* 90, 1254–1257.

Qi, C., Zhu, Y., Pan, J., Usuda, N., Maeda, N., Yeldandi, A.V., Rao, M.S., Hashimoto, T. and Reddy, J.K. (1999). *J. Biol. Chem.* 274, 15775–15780.

Reddy, J.K. and Hashimoto, T. (2001). *Annu. Rev. Nutr.* 21, 193–230.

Rimando, A.M., Nagmani, R., Feller, D.R. and Yokoyama, W. (2005). *J. Agric. Food Chem.* 53, 3403–3407.

Rubins, H.B., Robins, S.J., Collins, D., Fye, C.L., Anderson, J.W., Elam, M.B., Faas, F.H., Linares, E., Schaefer, E.J., Schectman, G., Wilt, T.J. and Wittes, J. (1999). *New Engl. J. Med.* 341, 410–418.

Sanders, R.J., Ofman, R., Valianpour, F., Kemp, S. and Wanders, R.J. (2005). *J. Lipid Res.* 46, 1001–1008.

Schoonjans, K., Staels, B. and Auwerx, J. (1996). *Biochem. Biophys. Acta* 1302, 93–109.

Shimura, M., Hasumi, A., Minato, T., Hosono, M., Miura, Y., Mizutani, S., Kondo, K., Oikawa, S. and Yoshida, A. (2005). *Biochem. Biophys. Acta* 1736, 51–60.

Simpson, W.J. and Smith, A.R. (1992). *J. Appl. Bacteriol.* 72, 327–334.

Spann, N.J., Kang, S., Li, A.C., Chen, A.Z., Newberry, E.P., Davidson, N.O., Hui, S.T. and Davis, R.A. (2006). *J. Biol. Chem.* 281, 33066–33077.

Staels, B. and Fruchart, J.C. (2005). *Diabetes* 54, 2460–2470.

Staels, B., Dallongeville, J., Auwerx, J., Schoonjans, K., Leitersdorf, E. and Fruchart, J.C. (1998). *Circulation* 98, 2088–2093.

Sundseth, S.S. and Waxman, D.J. (1992). *J. Biol. Chem.* 267, 3915–3921.

Techakriengkrai, I., Paterson, A., Taidi, B. and Piggott, J.R. (2004). *J. Inst. Brew.* 110, 51–56.

Teuber, M. (1970). *Appl. Microbiol.* 19, 871.

Tsuchida, A., Yamauchi, T., Takekawa, S., Hada, Y., Ito, Y., Maki, T. and Kadowaki, T. (2005). *Diabetes* 54, 3358–3370.

Tsutsumi, and Takase, S. (2001). *Alcohol. Clin. Exp. Res.* 25, 75S–79S.

Xu, H.E., Lambert, M.H., Montana, V.G., Plunket, K.D., Moore, L.B., Collins, J.L., Oplinger, J.A., Kliewer, S.A., Gampe Jr., R.T., McKee, D.D., Moore, J.T. and Willson, T.M. (2001). *Proc. Natl. Acad. Sci. USA* 98, 13919–13924.

Yajima, H., Ikeshima, E., Shiraki, M., Kanaya, T., Fujiwara, D., Odai, H., Tsuboyama-Kasaoka, N., Ezaki, O., Oikawa, S. and Kondo, K. (2004). *J. Biol. Chem.* 279, 33456–33462.

Yajima, H., Noguchi, T., Ikeshima, E., Shiraki, M., Kanaya, T., Tsuboyama-Kasaoka, N., Ezaki, O., Oikawa, S. and Kondo, K. (2005). *Int. J. Obesity (London)* 29, 991–997.

Yamazaki, K., Kuromitsu, J. and Tanaka, I. (2002). *Biochem. Biophys. Res. Commun.* 290, 1114–1122.

Yamazaki, T., Sasaki, E., Kakinuma, C., Yano, T., Miura, S. and Ezaki, O. (2005). *J. Biol. Chem.* 280, 21506–21514.

Yoon, M., Jeong, S., Nicol, C.J., Lee, H., Han, M., Kim, J.J., Seo, Y.J., Ryu, C. and Oh, G.T. (2002). *Exp. Mol. Med.* 34, 481–488.

Yoon, M., Jeong, S., Lee, H., Han, M., Kang, J.H., Kim, E.Y., Kim, M. and Oh, G.T. (2003). *Biochem. Biophys. Res. Commun.* 302, 29–34.

Yu, X.X., Murray, S.F., Pandey, S.K., Booten, S.L., Bao, D., Song, X.Z., Kelly, S., Chen, S., McKay, R., Monia, B.P. and Bhanot, S. (2005). *Hepatology* 42, 362–371.

84

Flavonoids in Beer and Their Potential Benefit on the Risk of Cardiovascular Disease

C-Y. Oliver Chen. and Jeffrey B. Blumberg Antioxidants Research Laboratory, Jean Mayer USDA Human Nutrition Research Center on Aging, Tufts University, Boston, MA, USA

Abstract

Beer is a popular alcoholic beverage and its consumption is characterized by a U- or J-shaped relation to the risk of cardiovascular disease (CVD). In addition to the ability of ethanol to elevate high-density lipoprotein–cholesterol, other constituents of beer, including flavonoids, may also contribute to its association with a reduced risk of CVD among moderate drinkers. Flavonoids are ubiquitous in plant-based foods and an integral part of any diet that includes fruits, vegetables, whole grains and/or beverages derived from them. Six classes of flavonoids, including 31 specific compounds, have been characterized in beer with a wide range of concentration, from 0.001 to 20 mg/l, likely due to variations in the barley and hops, brewing and stabilization processes, and duration of storage. The principal flavonoids in beer are isoxanthohumol, catechin, catechin gallate, epicatechin gallate, kaempferol, quercetin, procyanidin B3, and prodelphidins B3 and B9. Flavonoid intake has been demonstrated to impact an array of biochemical and functional actions in animal models and human studies that are associated with ameliorating CVD risk, such as reducing angiogenesis, cholesterol, inflammation, oxidative stress, and thrombogensis as well as promoting vascular reactivity. Nonetheless, definitive studies on the direct contribution of flavonoids to the benefit of moderate beer consumption on CVD remain to be undertaken.

Introduction

Alcoholic beverages, including beers, spirits, and wines, have been consumed for millennia and are an integral part of the daily diet among people in several societies. Average daily intake of beer in the USA is 227 ml per person (USDA, 2004), equivalent to 4% of energy intake (at 5% ethanol content) in a 2,000 kcal diet. While alcoholic beverages are consumed for pleasure and relaxation, observational studies reveal a U- or J-shaped relationship between their intake and overall morbidity and mortality (Camargo *et al.*, 1997; Keil *et al.*, 1997; Gaziano *et al.*, 2000; Gronbaek, 2006). These data suggest this potential health benefit is obtained at light to moderate consumption, that is, 10–19 and <10 g alcohol/day for men and women, respectively (Moore and Pearson, 1986; Fuchs *et al.*, 1995; Kannel and Ellison, 1996; Hendriks and van Tol, 2005; Mukamal *et al.*, 2006). While this health benefit appears independent of the type of alcoholic beverage, several reports have focused particularly on the value of red wine (Rimm *et al.*, 1996; Cleophas, 1999). In trying to elucidate the mechanism of action of alcoholic beverages on CVD risk, most attention has been directed to the ability of ethanol to elevate high-density lipoprotein (HDL)-cholesterol. However, other constituents may also contribute to reducing the incidence of CVD among drinkers either independently from or in a complementary manner to ethanol (Pace-Asciak *et al.*, 1995; Gasbarrini *et al.*, 1998; Serafini *et al.*, 1998). This chapter reviews the basis for a potential contribution of beer flavonoids to reduced CVD risk.

Beer Consumption and Risk of CVD

CVD, including coronary heart disease, cerebrovascular disease, and peripheral artery disease, is the leading cause of morbidity and mortality in the industrialized world (World Health Organization, 2006). The pathogenesis of CVD involves injury to vascular endothelial cells, stimulation of inflammatory responses, adhesion of lymphocytes to vessel walls and migration into the intima, oxidation of LDL, formation of lipid-laden foam cells, development of plaque, and thrombosis (De Caterina *et al.*, 2006). Numerous risk factors of CVD have been identified (Table 84.1). Most of these factors are modifiable through lifestyle changes and pharmacotherapy, except age, male sex, and ethnicity/genetics (Scott, 2004).

Importantly, the impact of drinking alcoholic beverages on CVD risk can be positive or negative depending on amount and pattern of consumption (Hendriks and

Beer in Health and Disease Prevention
ISBN: 978-0-12-373891-2

Table 84.1 Risk factors of CVD[a]

Modifiable risk factors	*Impact of moderate consumption of alcoholic beverages*
Clinical and lifestyle risk factors	
Visceral obesity	?[b]
Hypertension	↑
Smoking	–[d]
Excessive alcohol intake	–[d]
Physical inactivity	–[d]
Dietary patterns high in saturated fats and cholesterol; low in fruits, vegetables, soluble fiber, and whole grains	–[d]
Psychosocial stress	?[c]
Biochemical risk factors	
Dyslipidemia (high triglycerides and LDL-cholesterol; low HDL cholesterol)	↓
Lipoprotein(a)	–[d]
Hyperglycemia	–[d]
Platelet aggregation	↓
Oxidative stress	↓
Chronic inflammation	↓
Hyperhomocysteinemia	↓
Endothelial dysfunction	↓

[a] Funatsu *et al.* (2005); Hawkins (2004); Hendriks and van Tol (2005); Homma (2004); Scott (2004); Zilkens *et al.* (2005).
[b] Heavy drinking can substantially increase caloric intake but the impact of moderate intakes is not clear.
[c] Heavy drinking is associated with mood and anxiety disorders but the impact of moderate consumption is less well characterized but often considered a relaxant.
[d] No association.

van Tol, 2005). Regular and moderate consumption of alcoholic beverages can ameliorate some CVD risk factors such as elevating HDL-C via reducing hepatic lipase and increasing lipoprotein lipase and lecithin:cholesterol acyltransferase activity (Gaziano *et al.*, 1993; Hendriks and van Tol, 2005). In addition, ethanol can improve antioxidant capacity by raising HDL paraoxonase 1 activity (Van der Gaag *et al.*, 1999; Sierksma *et al.*, 2002a); promote vascular reactivity via increasing nitric oxide availability (Puddey *et al.*, 2001); decrease platelet aggregation by lowering the concentration of fibrinogen (Dimmitt *et al.*, 1998; Sierksma *et al.*, 2002b; De Lange *et al.*, 2003); and blunt inflammation (Sierksma *et al.*, 2002b). In contrast, heavy drinking can elevate blood pressure and psychosocial stresses as well as promote visceral obesity, thereby contributing to the development of metabolic syndrome, diabetes, and CVD.

While ethanol is the principal ingredient shared among beer, wine, and spirits, their impact on CVD risk may vary substantially due to quantity and quality of phytochemicals. Some observational studies indicate a significant inverse relationship between CVD and red wine consumption but weak or null associations with beer and spirits (Truelsen *et al.*, 1998; Gronbaek, 1999; Di Castelnuovo *et al.*, 2002; Ruf, 2003). However, other larger cohort studies demonstrate comparable protection from beer, wine, and spirits (Rimm *et al.*, 1991; Keil *et al.*, 1997). The conflicts between these reports can be attributed to unknown confounding factors as well as to established factors such as socioeconomic status (Nielsen *et al.*, 2004). When examining only beer consumption among Czech men, Bobak *et al.* (2000) found that 4–9 l/week was associated with the lowest risk of CVD. In a study of 312 patients with clinically stable, angiographically confirmed coronary heart disease and 479 healthy controls, Brenner *et al.* (2001) found an odds ratio (OR) of 0.55 (95% confidence interval (CI) = 0.37–0.83) for coronary heart disease in drinkers compared with non-drinkers, with particularly strong reduction among participants drinking predominantly beer. In a prospective study of 24,523 Danish participants, Gronbaek *et al.* (2000) found that for coronary heart disease OR were 0.78 (95% CI = 0.67–0.91), 0.74 (0.63–0.86), and 0.97 (0.83–1.12) for beer, wine, and spirits drinkers with alcohol intake at 1–7 drinks/week compared with non-drinkers. A health benefit from moderate consumption of beer has also been suggested by a clinical trial in which 330 ml/day for 30 days was found to lower thrombogenic activity in 28 coronary heart disease patients (Gorinstein *et al.*, 1997). In addition to its alcohol content, beer may possess other bioactive constituents, particularly flavonoids, derived from its two principal plant ingredients, barely and hops (Gronbaek, 2006).

Nomenclature and Chemistry of Flavonoids

Flavonoids, a subfamily of polyphenols, are secondary metabolites involved in plant growth, reproduction, protection against pathogens and predators, and seed germination (Treutter, 2005). They are products of the shikimate pathway from phenylalanine and the acetate pathway (Aherne and O'Brien, 2002). The shared structure defining flavonoids is a diphenylpropane (C6-C3-C6) consisting of three phenolic rings (Figure 84.1). The A ring is usually derived from resorcinol or phloroglucinol synthesized via the acetate pathway and the B ring is derived from the shikimate pathway. Flavonoids are typically divided into eight subclasses: anthocyanin, chalcone, dihydroflavonol, flavan-3-ol (or catechin), flavanone, flavone, flavonol, and isoflavone based on the connection position of the B and C rings as well as the degree of oxidation and hydroxylation of the C ring. The majority of plant flavonoids have a conjugated moiety linked to the hydroxyl group via glycosylation, malonylation, methylation, and/or sulfation, with glucoside as the most frequently occurring form (Bravo, 1998).

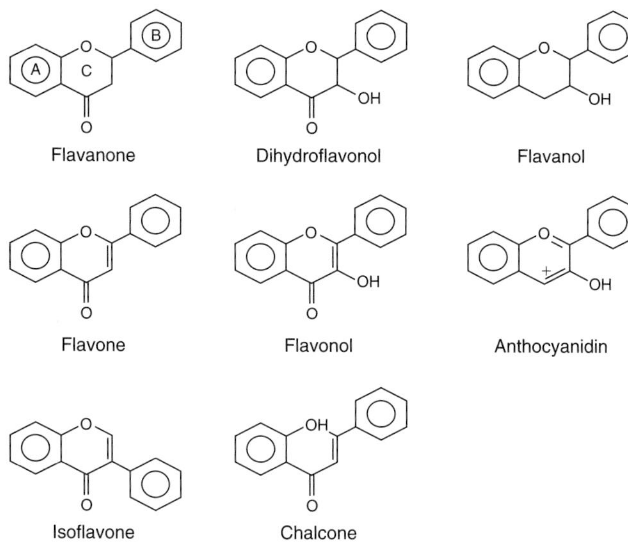

Figure 84.1 Molecular structures of typical flavonoids.

Dietary Sources of Flavonoids

Flavonoids are ubiquitous in common plant foods, for example, with the flavonols quercetin, kaempferol, and myricetin found in onions, curly kale, leeks, broccoli, blueberries, red wine, and tea; the flavones, apigenin and luteolin, found in parsley, celery, and cereals; the flavanones naringenin, hesperetin, and eriodictyol found in tomatoes, mint, grapefruit, oranges, and lemons; the isoflavones genistein, daidzein, and glycetin found in soy foods; the flavan-3-ols catechin and epicatechin found in green tea, red wine, and cocoa; the anthocyanins cyanidin and malvidin found in red wine, grapes, beans, onions, and berries (Manach *et al.*, 2004). Their distribution in plants is dependent in part on the degree of accessibility of the plant's parts to light and other environmental stresses (Aherne and O'Brien, 2002); thus, most flavonoids tend to be prevalent and most concentrated in the outer parts of plants, for example, leaves, flowers, and the skin or peel of fruit (Aherne and O'Brien, 2002). Although flavonoids are an integral part of our daily diet, intakes have not been accurately or fully determined for nutrient databases because of the several thousand individual flavonoids present and their marked variation due to the impact of environmental, seasonal, agricultural production, and other factors, including differences between varietals of the same species. Nevertheless, daily average intakes have been estimated to range between 14 and 72 mg/day, though individual differences may be substantially less or greater (Graf *et al.*, 2005; USDA, 2006).

Flavonoids in Beer

Beer is produced in a simple fermentation process using barley (*Hordeum vulgare* L.), dried flowers of hops (*Humulus lupulus* L.), water, and yeast. In addition to being rich in amino acids, peptides, and B vitamins, beer contains phenolic acids and flavonoids derived principally from barley and hops, with most of these compounds from barley (Boivin *et al.*, 1993). Barley contains flavanols, flavonols, and proanthocyanidins with total polyphenols at 1.2–1.5 g/kg (Madigan *et al.*, 1994) (Table 84.2). Hops, added to

Table 84.2 Maximum possible concentrations of flavonoids in beers, determined by HPLC[a]

Flavonoid	*Beer (mg/l)*	*Hop (mg/kg)*	*Barley (mg/kg)*
Chalcone			
Xanthohumol	≤1.2	4,800	
Flavanone			
Isoxanthohumol	≤3.44	80	
Naringenin	≤0.007		
6-Prenylnaringenin	≤0.056		
6-Granylnaringenin	≤0.074		
8-Prenylnaringenin	≤0.240	20	
Flavan-3-ol			
Catechin	≤7.3	260	30–95
Catechin gallate	≤20.0		
Catechin-7-*O*-glucoside	≤0.195		
Epicatechin	≤1.8	194	
Epicatechin gallate	≤ 20.0		
Gallocatechin	≤1.0		
3′-O-methylcatechin	≤0.053		
Flavone			
Apigenin	≤0.012		
Apigenin-6-*C*-glucoside	≤0.032		
Apigenin-6-*C*-glucoside-7-*O*-glucoside	≤0.038		
Flavonol			
Kaempferol	≤16.4		109
Kaempferol-3-glucoside		310–620	
Kaempferol-3-rhamnosid	≤1.0		231
Kaempferol-3-rutinoside		600–1,160	
Myricetin	≤0.5		
Quercetin	≤10.0		
Quercetin-glucoside		80–1,040	
Quercitrin	≤2.3		
Isoquercitrin	≤1.0		
Rutin	≤1.8	130–910	
Isoflavone			
Biochanin A	≤0.001		
Daidzein	≤0.001		
Formononetin	≤0.004		
Genistein	≤0.002		
Proanthocyanidin			
Procyanidin B3	≤3.6		63–350
Prodelphidin B3	≤4.5		48–450
Prodelphidin B9	≤3.9		
Prodelphidin C	≤0.076		
Prodelphidin C2			40–105

[a] Achilli *et al.* (1993); Andersen *et al.* (2000); Arts *et al.* (2000); Clarke *et al.* (2004); Cortacero-Ramírez *et al.* (2004); de Pascual-Teresa *et al.* (2000); Garciía *et al.* (2004); Gerhauser (2005); Goupy *et al.* (1999); Hertog *et al.* (1993b); Jandera *et al.* (2005); Lapcik *et al.* (1998); Li and Deinzer (2006); Madigan *et al.* (1994); McMurrough (1981); McMurrough and Baertt (1994); Milligan *et al.* (1999); Stevens *et al.* (1999); Tekel' *et al.* (1999); USDA (2006).

enhance bitterness and flavor to beer, contain polyphenols at 3–6% dry weight comprised largely of proanthocyanidins, flavanols, and flavonols (De Keukeleire *et al.*, 1999). Large variations in the flavonoid composition and content of both barley and hops are due to plant varieties, methods of cultivation and harvesting, and degree of aging. Tedesco *et al.* (2005) and Vinson *et al.* (2003) determined the range of total phenolics in commercially available beers from 187 to 2,504 μmol/l (32–426 mg/l) using the Folin–Ciocalteu assay. The rank of total phenolic content among different types of beers was ales > lagers > low calorie > non-alcoholic (Vinson *et al.*, 2003).

Using a more specific HPLC determination of phenolic compounds, individual flavonoids in beer have been identified and quantitated, including those from the anthocyanin, chalcone, flavonol, flavan-3-ol, procyanidin, and isoflavone classes (Table 84.2). The concentration of individual flavonoids is expressed according to their possible maximum value because of relatively large variations in reported concentrations of individual flavonoid among beers analyzed by laboratories in different countries. The major reported flavonoids are catechin, catechin gallate, epicatechin gallate, isoxanthohumol, kaempferol, quercetin, procyanidin B3, and prodelphidin B3 and B9 (see structures in Figure 84.2). Interestingly, flavones, isoflavones, and catechin gallate have not been identified in barely or hops. These flavonoids may be created during brewing process from related compounds, for example, xanthohumol, a prenylflavonoid chalcone found in hops. Xanthohumol may be converted into isoxanthohumol via thermal isomerization (Stevens and Page, 2004). There are not only four prenylflavonoids in beer, principally isoxanthohumol, but also 6-prenylnaringenin, 6-granylnaringenin, and 8-prenylnaringenin (8-PN) (Stevens and Page, 2004). Although 8-PN is a negligible component of beer at 0.24 mg/l, it appears beer is a unique dietary source of this flavonoid. While isoflavones are found principally in soy foods, genistein, biochanin A, daidzein, and formononetin are found as well in beer (Lapcik *et al.*, 1998). The natural concentration of flavonoids in freshly brewed beer is reduced through the use of polyvinylpolypyrrolidone (a stabilizer) which adsorbs flavanols and tannins as well as through subsequent filtration steps employed to prevent haze formation (McMurrough *et al.*, 1995). Further, flavonoid content declines during the storage of beer through conversion to tannoids (flavonoid polymers) (McMurrough and O'Rourke, 1997).

Although their calculations must be considered as a rough estimate, Vinson *et al.* (2003) have estimated total phenol intake from beer at 42 mg catechin equivalents/day/person, based on the average consumption of beer at 225 ml/day and 64 mg catechin from a serving (341 ml or 12 oz.). Flavonoid intake from consumption of red wine has been

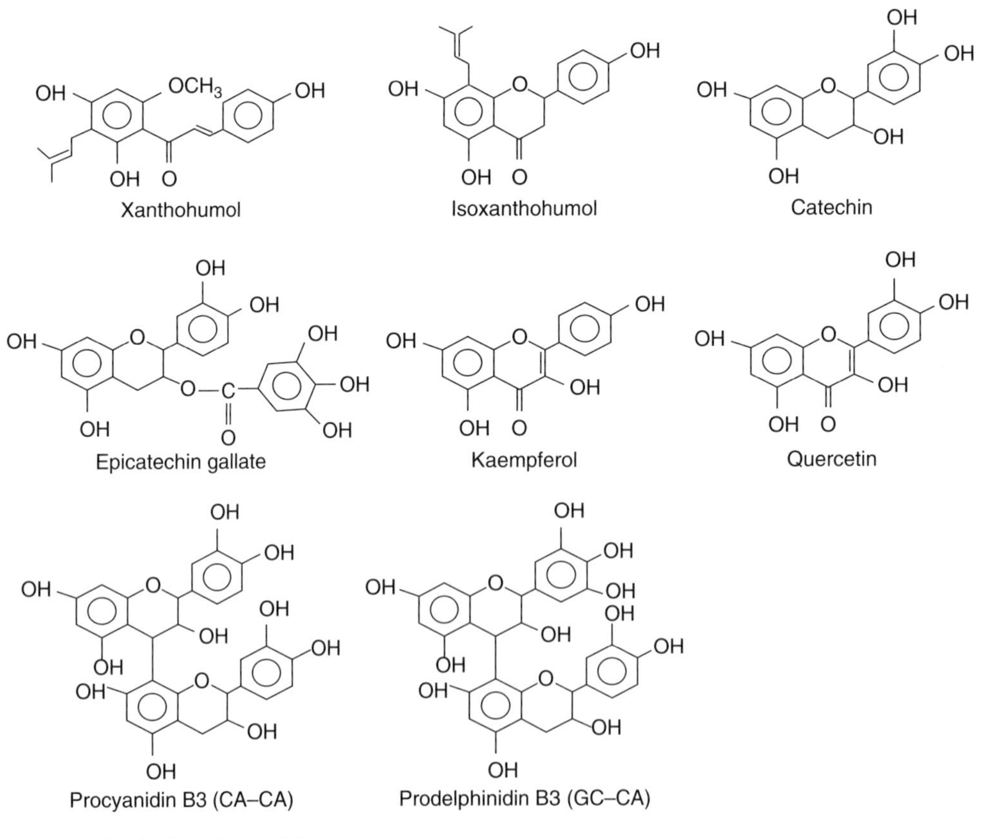

Xanthohumol

Isoxanthohumol

Catechin

Epicatechin gallate

Kaempferol

Quercetin

Procyanidin B3 (CA–CA)

Prodelphinidin B3 (GC–CA)

Figure 84.2 Structures of major beer flavonoids.

estimated at 21 mg/day (Vinson and Hontz, 1995; Vinson, 1998). Thus, depending on one's dietary pattern, consumption of beer or wine can contribute significantly to flavonoid intake.

Absorption and Metabolism of Flavonoids

Flavonoids are absorbed throughout the gastrointestinal tract and excreted in the feces or urine (Figure 84.3). The site and rate of absorption depend in part on the specific flavonoid and its conjugation with sugar, degree of polymerization, and solubility (Bravo, 1998; Scalbert and Williamson, 2002). Sugar moieties are generally cleaved by lactase phlorizin hydrolase or β-glucosidase prior to absorption. In the colon, flavonoids can be degraded into phenolic acids by gut microflora (Bravo, 1998). Flavonoids can enter enterocytes via active transportation (Walle, 2004). Once absorbed, glucuronide, sulfate, and/or methyl groups are added to hydroxyl moieties via phase II pathways in enterocytes, liver, and kidney (Manach *et al.*, 2004). Subsequently, flavonoid metabolites are transported to extrahepatic tissues and eventually to the kidneys where they are excreted in the urine or incorporated into bile and recycled to the gut and eventually excreted in the feces (Bravo, 1998). The maximum concentration of most flavonoids in human plasma is reached 1–6 h after ingestion. The elimination half-life of most flavonoids ranges from 1 to 18 h depending on the flavonoid class and specific compound (Manach *et al.*, 2005b). The acute bioavailability and kinetics of flavan-3-ols, flavones, flavonols, and isoflavones have been partly characterized though little information is available regarding these parameters during chronic consumption or their interactions with other food components (Manach *et al.*, 2005b). Much less is known about the bioavailability of proanthocyanidins though it has been suggested little can be absorbed as the intact parent form and, thus, their bioactivity may be a result of the phenolic acids absorbed after their breakdown by gut microflora (Gonthier *et al.*, 2003). Xanthohumol, a prenylchalcone present in hops, has been detected in rat plasma in the form of two monoglucuronides with a maximum concentration reached 4 h after ingestion (Yilmazer *et al.*, 2001). The bioavailability of isoxanthohumol and 8-prenylnaringenin has not been characterized.

Mechanisms of Beer Flavonoids in CVD Reduction

As noted, ethanol is generally considered the most significant contributor in alcoholic beverages to the reduction in CVD risk via increasing HDL-C and fibrinolysis and decreasing platelet aggregation. Nonetheless, due to a relevant array of bioactivities, flavonoids have also been suggested to contribute to this benefit of moderate drinking (Langer *et al.*, 1992; Renaud and Ruf, 1996; Dimmitt *et al.*, 1998; Mann and Folts, 2004). Observational data from the Zutphen Elderly Study (Hertog *et al.*, 1993a; Keli

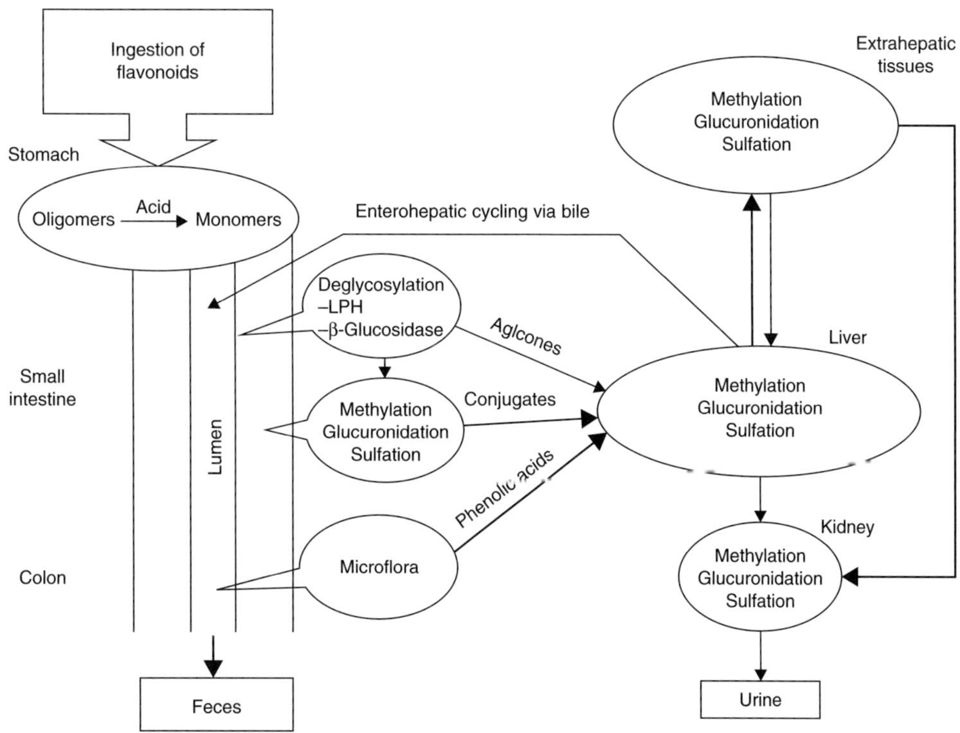

Figure 84.3 Absorption, metabolism, and excretion of flavonoids. LPH, lactase phlorizin hydrolase.

et al., 1996), Rotterdam Study (Geleijnse *et al.*, 1999), and Iowa Study (Yochum *et al.*, 1999) suggest flavonoid intake reduces CVD risk. While direct evidence regarding the impact of beer flavonoids on health remains to be determined, flavonoids present in beer have been shown to have anti-inflammatory, antioxidant, and hypocholesterolemic actions as well as work to maintain homeostasis and endothelial function via several different pathways important to the pathogenesis of chronic disease (Figure 84.4).

Anti-inflammatory activity

Atherosclerosis is substantially a chronic inflammatory response to injured endothelium (Ross, 1999; Libby, 2002). C-reactive protein (CRP), an acute-phase protein and useful biomarker of inflammation, has been established as a significant predictive factor of CVD (Ridker *et al.*, 2001; Albert *et al.*, 2003). Indeed, the relationship between CRP and consumption of alcohol is consistent with the U-shaped relation between CVD risk and drinking (Imhof *et al.*, 2001; Stewart *et al.*, 2002; Albert *et al.*, 2003; Volpato *et al.*, 2004). Sierksma *et al.* (2002b) conducted a cross-over trial in 10 men and 9 women providing 4 and 3 glasses of beer with dinner daily (providing 40 and 30 g ethanol/day, respectively) for 3 weeks and found a 35% reduction in plasma CRP compared to a similar intervention with non-alcohol beer. While this study did not evaluate flavonoid intake or status, flavonoids have been shown to reduce biomarkers of inflammation, including CRP, tumor necrosis factor-α, monocyte chemoattractant protein, and nuclear factor-κB. For example, Estruch *et al.* (2004) found that 30 g ethanol from flavonoid-rich red wine daily for 28 days decreased CRP by 21% as compared to an equivalent amount of ethanol from gin in 40 healthy men (mean age = 37.6 years). However, results from other human studies with flavonoid-rich foods indicate equivocal or null outcomes regarding CRP (de Maat *et al.*, 2000; Mathur *et al.*, 2002; Fukino *et al.*, 2005). Thus, additional studies are warranted with particular attention provided to the flavonoid composition and content of both the beer and other foods in the diet.

Antioxidant activity

Reactive oxygen species generated during normal aerobic metabolism can damage DNA, lipids, and proteins if not adequately protected by the antioxidant defense network. Low-density lipoproteins (LDL) are particularly susceptible to free radical attack. Oxidized LDL contributes to atherogenesis by promoting inflammation, stimulating

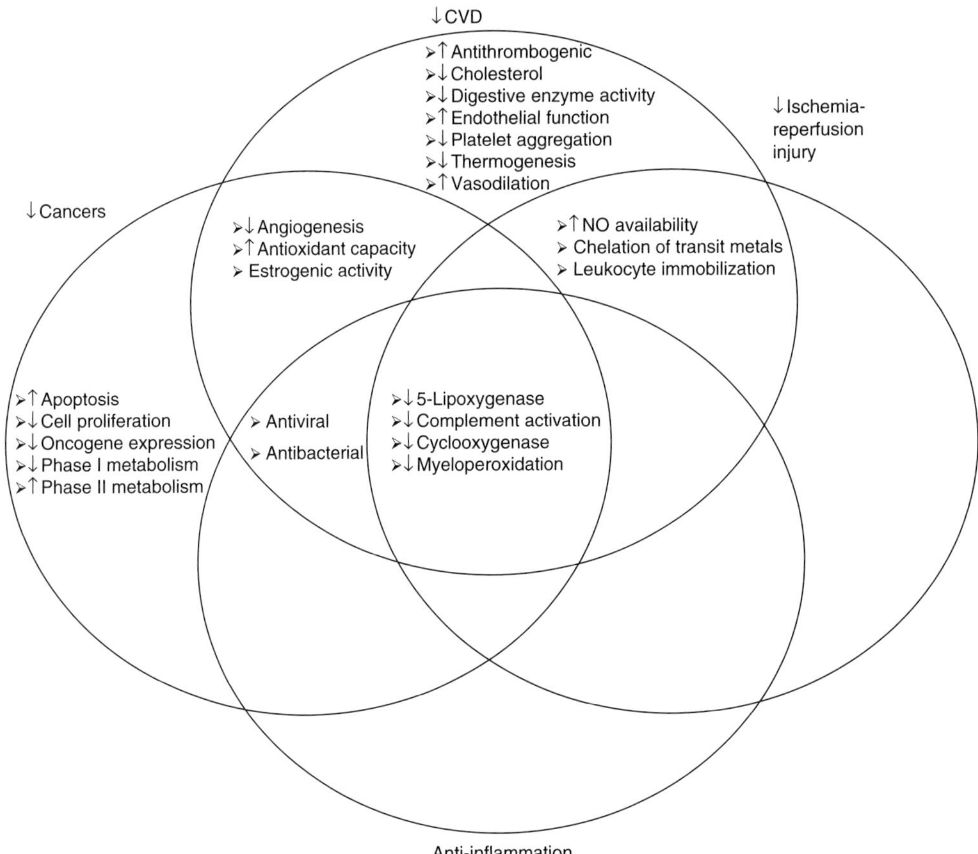

Figure 84.4 Putative preventive mechanisms of flavonoids against chronic disease.

smooth muscle cell proliferation, impairing endothelial function, and provoking platelet aggregation (Esper *et al.*, 2006). Flavonoids, including those from beer, may act to increase the resistance of LDL to oxidation by scavenging both reactive oxygen and nitrogen species, chelating transition minerals like copper and iron, and up-regulating endogenous antioxidant defenses (Torel and Cillard, 1986; Robak and Gryglewski, 1988; Hu *et al.*, 1995; Nijveldt *et al.*, 2001). While there are no reports examining the effect of beer flavonoids on biomarkers of oxidative stress *in vivo*, Vinson *et al.* (2003) and Miranda *et al.* (2000) found LDL resistance against oxidation was enhanced *in vitro* by beer with its potency greater than α-tocopherol but less than quercetin.

The antioxidant capacity of beer against lipoprotein oxidation has been examined in animal models. Even though ethanol can act as a pro-oxidant via action on hepatic cytochrome P450-2E1 (Nagy, 2004), Gasbarrini *et al.* (1998) reported that chronic beer consumption increased lipoprotein resistance against oxidation *ex vivo* in rats. In another rat study, Gasowski *et al.* (2004) found an inverse association between the antioxidant capacity of beer and the reduction of plasma malondialdehyde, a biomarker of lipid peroxidation. Using hamsters, Vinson *et al.* (2003) found that lager or dark beer containing 2% ethanol enhanced lipoprotein resistance against *ex vivo* oxidation by ≥1-fold as compared to ethanol only. This experimental evidence implicates flavonoids and/or other phenolic compounds as contributors to the antioxidant actions of beer.

Several assays have been employed to evaluate the "total antioxidant capacity" of foods and beverages, including the oxygen radical absorbance capacity (ORAC), total reactive antioxidant potential (TRAP), trolox equivalent antioxidant capacity (TEAC), and ferric reducing antioxidant power (FRAP) assays. Using the TEAC assay assays, Gasowski *et al.* (2004) reported the antioxidant capacity of four beers (from Bulgaria, Czech Republic, Israel, and the Netherlands) ranged from 1.65 to 2.07 mmol Trolox equivalents/l. Using the FRAP assay, Tedesco *et al.* (2005) determined the antioxidant capacity of 48 commercial beers without ethanol ranged from 112.2 to 637.5 μmol quercetin equivalents/l. The antioxidant capacity of beer is attributed to its polyphenol content due to its strong correlation with H-donating capacity (Lugasi, 2003). In addition to acting as an antioxidant in simple chemical reactions *in vitro*, constituents in beer have been shown to increase total antioxidant capacity in plasma. Using the TRAP assay, Ghiselli *et al.* (2000) found a bolus of 500 ml beer (4.5% ethanol) elevated total plasma antioxidant capacity by 17% in healthy adults but the same volume of dealcoholized beer or 4.5% ethanol were without an effect on this parameter. In contrast, Van der Gaag *et al.* (2000) found no effect of beer (40 g alcohol/day) consumed for 3 weeks on total antioxidant capacity in 11 healthy, non-smoking middle-aged men with the TEAC assay; however, this outcome may have been confounded by a 15% reduction in plasma concentrations of vitamin C and β-carotene (but not other carotenoids, vitamin E, or glutathione). Further study of the kinetics of beer flavonoids under acute and chronic conditions of intake would help resolve the discrepancy among these studies.

Red wine appears to have the highest polyphenol content of alcoholic beverages, about 8-fold greater than that of beer (Gorinstein *et al.*, 1998a; Lugasi, 2003). However, lyophilized dry substances from 6 ml beer and 2 ml red wine had comparable efficacy inhibiting lipid peroxide formation by 50% in rats, suggesting the bioavailability and/or bioactivity of antioxidants from beer might be more potent than those from red wine (Gorinstein *et al.*, 1998b). Again, more studies directly examining beer flavonoids *in vivo* are necessary to clarify their actions and putative health benefits.

Cholesterol lowering activity

Dyslipidemia, that is, elevated total cholesterol (TC), triglyceride (TG), and LDL-C and/or low HDL-C, is a significant CVD risk factor. Evidence from animal models, observational studies, and clinical trials indicate that flavonoids derived from tea, virgin olive oil, cocoa, soybean, and red clover possess hypocholesterolemic activity due to their inhibition of cholesterol and fatty acid absorption, apoB-100 production, and very low-density lipoprotein (VLDL) secretion (Zern and Fernandez, 2005). Thus, the flavan-3-ols, flavanones, and isoflavones in beer share the capacity for this action, though consideration must be given to their content per serving with regard to achieving a similar magnitude of effect (Zern and Fernandez, 2005; Manach *et al.*, 2005a). Nonetheless, beer flavonoids may act in an additive or synergistic manner with ethanol to improve lipid profiles. While there is no direct evidence demonstrating a hypocholesterolemic action of beer *in vivo*, dried beer substances (6 ml beer equivalent/day), including flavonoids, phenolic acids, minerals, vitamins, and amino acids, fed to rats fed a diet containing 5% sunflower oil and 1% cod liver oil decreased TC, TG, and LDL-C (Gorinstein *et al.*, 1998a). The magnitude of improvement in lipid profiles was comparable to rats fed 2 ml red wine dried substances. A beneficial effect of ethanol-free beer constituents on cholesterol metabolism and accumulation in aorta was observed in a study using LDLr−/− apoB100/100 mice (Degrace *et al.*, 2006). Using hamsters, an animal model in which cholesterol metabolism is similar to that of humans, Vinson *et al.* (2003) also found that constituents other than ethanol in lager and dark beer decreased TC by 57% and 70% and TG by 76% and 51%, respectively, as well as inhibited atherosclerotic foam cell formation by 62% and 71%. However, null results were observed in apoE−/− mice fed ethanol, mild beer, dark beer, or ethanol-free beer (Escola-Gil *et al.*, 2004). The influence of genomics on flavonoid action remains to be determined.

Hemostasis and endothelial function

Vascular hemostasis involves a delicate balance between the formation and degradation of blood clots within an interacting network of coagulation factors and vessel walls (Lefevre *et al.*, 2004). Impaired hemostasis is associated with increased risk of CVD (Willoughby *et al.*, 2002). The effect of alcoholic beverages on hemostasis may partially explain the U- or J-shaped relation between moderate drinking and CVD. Hendricks *et al.* (1994) found that moderate consumption of beer, wine, or spirits (40 g alcohol/day) with dinner for 4 days temporarily increased plasminogen activator inhibitor activity, in a manner sufficient to increase fibrinolysis. Similarly, Gorinstein *et al.* (1997) provided 22 patients with coronary artery disease with 330 ml beer (20 g alcohol) daily for 30 days and found a decrease in thrombogenic activity. As noted above, these studies do not demonstrate a specific effect of beer flavonoids but such results are consistent with reports of other interventions with flavonoids showing improved hemostasis, including increased bleeding time and reduced platelet aggregation (Freedman *et al.*, 2001; Murphy *et al.*, 2003; Hubbard *et al.*, 2004).

Endothelial cells serve not only as a physical barrier between blood and smooth muscles in the vessel wall but participate dynamically in both anti- and pro-atherogenic actions, including the regulation of vasomotor tone, adhesion and aggregation of platelets, adhesion and migration of monocytes, and proliferation of smooth muscle cells (Esper *et al.*, 2006). Endothelial dysfunction predisposed by smoking, hypercholesterolemia, hypertension, diabetes, and/or hyperhomocystinemia plays a critical role in the development of atherosclerosis (Ross, 1999; Kinlay and Ganz, 2000). Endothelial function can be assessed using a non-invasive measure of flow-mediated dilation (FMD) in the brachial artery. FMD is regulated substantially by nitric oxide (NO) release following the endothelial response to sheer stress and consequent relaxation of the underlying smooth muscle (Kinlay and Ganz, 2000). Moderate intake of alcoholic beverages may enhance this vascular reactivity due to the effect of ethanol to increase NO production as well as HDL-C (Puddey *et al.*, 2001). The increase of FMD induced by both red wine and alcohol-free red wine suggests that flavonoids can directly improve endothelial function (Karatzi *et al.*, 2004, 2005). Other flavonoid-rich foods, including grape juice, black tea, soy, and cocoa, have also shown a beneficial effect on endothelial function in healthy adults and/or patients with coronary heart disease (Manach *et al.*, 2005a). While beer flavonoids may also act in a similar manner, studies have yet to test this hypothesis.

Summary Points

- Flavonoids possess a variety of biological actions, particularly as demonstrated *in vitro* and in short-term studies *in vivo*. However, their bioactivity in humans remains to be fully examined, particularly in "real-life" conditions with a mixed diet of foods and beverages consumed in usual amounts.
- Consumption of beer and other alcoholic beverages in excess is associated with increases in blood pressure and psychosocial stress which are risk factors for CVD.
- Beer consumption in moderation appears to reduce CVD risk via the beneficial action of ethanol and perhaps other constituents, particularly flavonoids, on hemostasis, inflammation, oxidative stress, and/or vascular reactivity.
- Beer has been characterized as containing 31 flavonoids derived principally from barley and hops. Major beer flavonoids are isoxanthohumol, catechin, catechin gallate, epicatechin gallate, kaempferol, quercetin, procyanidin B3, and prodelphidins B3 and B9.
- The concentrations of flavonoids in beer vary widely from 0.001 to 20 mg/l depending on the plant ingredients, brewing techniques, stabilization process, and duration of storage.
- Beer consumption has been associated with an increase in HDL-C. In addition to this action of ethanol, beer flavonoids may contribute independently or in conjunction with ethanol to an improved lipid profile and an associated reduction in atherogenesis.
- Acute, moderate beer consumption can increase total antioxidant capacity in plasma, an effect attributed to its polyphenol content. Dry matter from red wine and beer has a comparative ratio of antioxidant potency *in vitro* of 1:3.

Acknowledgments

Support was provided by the US Department of Agriculture (USDA) Agricultural Research Service under Cooperative Agreement No. 58-1950-4-401. The contents of this publication do not necessarily reflect the views or policies of the USDA nor does mention of trade names, commercial products, or organizations imply endorsement by the US government.

References

Achilli, G., Cellerino, G.P., Gamache, P.H. and Melzi D'Eril, G.V. (1993). *J. Chromatogr.* 632, 111–117.

Andersen, M.L., Outtrup, H. and Skibsted, L.H. (2000). *J. Agric. Food Chem.* 48, 3106–3111.

Aherne, S.A. and O'Brien, N.M. (2002). *Nutrition* 18, 75–81.

Albert, M.A., Glynn, R.J. and Ridker, P.M. (2003). *Circulation* 107, 443–447.

Arts, I.C., van De Putte, B. and Hollman, P.C. (2000). *J. Agric. Food Chem.* 48, 1752–1757.

Bobak, M., Skodova, Z. and Marmot, M. (2000). *BMJ* 320, 1378–1379.

Boivin, P., Malanda, M., Maillard, M.N., Berset, C., Richard, H., Hugues, M., Richard-Forget, F. and Nicolas, J. (1993). *Proc. Congr. Eur. Brew. Conv.* 24, 397–404.

Bravo, L. (1998). *Nutr. Rev.* 56, 317–333.

Brenner, H., Rothenbacher, D., Bode, G., Marz, W., Hoffmeister, A. and Koenig, W. (2001). *Epidemiology* 12, 390–395.

Camargo Jr., C.A., Hennekens, C.H., Gaziano, J.M., Glynn, R.J., Manson, J.E. and Stampfer, M.J. (1997). *Arch. Int. Med.* 157, 79–85.

Clarke, D.B., Barnes, K.A. and Lloyd, A.S. (2004). *Food Addit. Contam.* 21, 949–962.

Cleophas, T.J. (1999). *Biomed. Pharm.* 53, 417–423.

Cortacero-Ramírez, S., Segura-Carretero, A., Cruces-Blanco, C., Romero-Romero, M.L. and Fernández-Gutiérrez, A. (2004). *Anal. Bioanal. Chem.* 380, 831–837.

De Caterina, R., Zampolli, A., Del Turco, S., Madonna, R. and Massaro, M. (2006). *Am. J. Clin. Nutr.* 83, 421S–426S.

De Keukeleire, D., De Cooman, L., Rong, H., Heyerick, A., Kalita, J. and Milligan, S.R. (1999). *Basic Life. Sci.* 66, 739–760.

De Lange, D.W., Van Golden, P.H., Scholman, W.L., Kraaijenhagen, R.J., Akkerman, J.W. and Van De Wiel, A. (2003). *Eur. J. Int. Med.* 14, 361–366.

de Maat, M.P., Pijl, H., Kluft, C. and Princen, H.M. (2000). *Eur. J. Clin. Nutr.* 54, 757–763.

de Pascual-Teresa, S., Santos-Buelga, C. and Rivas-Gonzalo, J.C. (2000). *J. Agric. Food Chem.* 48, 5331–5337.

Degrace, P., Moindrot, B., Mohamed, I., Gresti, J. and Clouet, P. (2006). *Atherosclerosis.* [Epub ahead of print] doi:10.1016/j.atherosclerosis.2006.01.012.

Di Castelnuovo, A., Rotondo, S., Iacoviello, L., Donati, M.B. and De Gaetano, G. (2002). *Circulation* 105, 2836–2844.

Dimmitt, S.B., Rakic, V., Puddey, I.B., Baker, R., Oostryck, R., Adams, M.J., Chesterman, C.N., Burke, V. and Beilin, L.J. (1998). *Blood Coagul. Fibrin.* 9, 39–45.

Escola-Gil, J.C., Calpe-Berdiel, L., Ribas, V. and Blanco-Vaca, F. (2004). *Nutr. J.* 3, 1.

Esper, R.J., Nordaby, R.A., Vilarino, J.O., Paragano, A., Cacharron, J.L. and Machado, R.A. (2006). *Cardiovasc. Diabetol.* 5, 4.

Estruch, R., Sacanella, E., Badia, E., Antúnez, E., Nicolás, J.M., Fernández-Solá, J., Rotilio, D. and Urbano-Márquez, A. (2004). *Atherosclerosis* 175, 117–123.

Freedman, J.E., Parker III, C., Li, L., Perlman, J.A., Frei, B., Ivanov, V., Deak, L.R., Iafrati, M.D. and Folts, J.D. (2001). *Circulation* 103, 2792–2798.

Fuchs, C.S., Stampfer, M.J., Colditz, G.A., Giovannucci, E.L., Manson, J.E., Kawachi, I., Hunter, D.J., Hankinson, S.E., Hennekens, C.H. and Rosner, B. (1995). *New Engl. J. Med.* 332, 1245–1250.

Fukino, Y., Shimbo, M., Aoki, N., Okubo, T. and Iso, H. (2005). *J. Nutr. Sci. Vitaminol. (Tokyo)* 51, 335–342.

Funatsu, K., Yamashita, T. and Nakamura, H. (2005). *Hypertens. Res.* 28, 521–527.

García, A.A., Grande, B.C. and Gándara, J.S. (2004). *J. Chromatogr. A.* 1054, 175–180.

Gasowski, B., Leontowicz, M., Leontowicz, H., Katrich, E., Lojek, A., Ciz, M., Trakhtenberg, S. and Gorinstein, S.T. (2004). *J. Nutr. Biochem.* 15, 527–533.

Gasbarrini, A., Addolorato, G., Simoncini, M., Gasbarrini, G., Fantozzi, P., Mancini, F., Montanari, L., Nardini, M., Ghiselli, A. and Scaccini, C. (1998). *Dig. Dis. Sci.* 43, 1332–1338.

Gaziano, J.M., Buring, J.E., Breslow, J.L., Goldhaber, S.Z., Rosner, B., VanDenburgh, M., Willett, W. and Hennekens, C.H. (1993). *New Engl. J. Med.* 329, 1829–1834.

Gaziano, J.M., Gaziano, T.A., Glynn, R.J., Sesso, H.D., Ajani, U.A., Stampfer, M.J., Manson, J.E., Hennekens, C.H. and Buring, J.E. (2000). *J. Am. Coll. Cardiol.* 35, 96–105.

Geleijnse, J.M., Launer, L.J., Hofman, A., Pols, H.A. and Witteman, J.C. (1999). *Arch. Int. Med.* 159, 2170–2174.

Gerhauser, C. (2005). *Eur. J. Cancer* 41, 1941–1954.

Ghiselli, A., Natella, F., Guidi, A., Montanari, L., Fantozzi, P. and Scaccini, C. (2000). *J. Nutr. Biochem.* 11, 76–80.

Gonthier, M.P., Donovan, J.L., Texier, O., Felgines, C., Remesy, C. and Scalbert, A. (2003). *Free Radical Biol. Med.* 35, 837–844.

Gorinstein, S., Zemser, M., Lichman, I., Berebi, A., Kleipfish, A., Libman, I., Trakhtenberg, S. and Caspi, A. (1997). *J. Int. Med.* 241, 47–51.

Gorinstein, S., Zemser, M., Weisz, M., Haruenki, R. and Trakhtenberg, S. (1998a). *J. Nutr. Biochem.* 9, 131–135.

Gorinstein, S., Zemser, M., Weisz, M., Halevy, S., Martin-Belloso, O. and Trakhtenberg, S. (1998b). *J. Nutr. Biochem.* 9, 682–686.

Gronbaek, M. (1999). *Food Chem. Toxicol.* 37, 921–924.

Gronbaek, M., Becker, U., Johansen, D., Gottschau, A., Schnohr, P., Hein, H.O., Jensen, G. and Sorensen, T.I.A. (2000). *Ann. Int. Med.* 133, 411–419.

Gronbaek, M. (2006). *Curr. Opin. Lipidol.* 17, 17–21.

Goupy, P., Hugues, M., Boivin, P. and Amiot, M.J. (1999). *J. Sci. Food Agric.* 79, 1625–1634.

Graf, B.A., Milbury, P.E. and Blumberg, J.B. (2005). *J. Med. Food* 8, 281–290.

Hawkins, M.A. (2004). *Obes. Res.* 12, 107S–114S.

Hendriks, H.F. and van Tol, A. (2005). *Alcohol Handbook Exp. Pharmacol.* 170, 339–361.

Hendriks, H.F., Veenstra, J., Velthuis-te, Wierik, E.J., Schaafsma, G. and Kluft, C. (1994). *BMJ* 308, 1003–1006.

Hertog, M.G., Feskens, E.J., Hollman, P.C., Katan, M.B. and Kromhout, D. (1993a). *Lancet* 342, 1007–1011.

Hertog, M.G., Hollman, P.C.H. and van de Putte, B. (1993b). *J. Agric. Food Chem.* 41, 1242–1246.

Homma, Y. (2004). *J. Atheroscler. Thromb.* 11, 265–270.

Hu, F.B. and Willett, W.C. (2002). *JAMA* 288, 2569–2578.

Hu, J.P., Calomme, M., Lasure, A., DeBruyne, T., Pieters, L., Vlietinck, A. and Vanden Berghe, D.A. (2002). *Biol. Trace Elem. Res.* 47, 327–331.

Hubbard, G.P., Wolffram, S., Lovegrove, J.A. and Gibbins, J.M. (2004). *J. Thromb. Haemost.* 2, 2138–2145.

Imhof, A., Froehlich, M., Brenner, H., Boeing, H., Pepys, M.B. and Koenig, W. (2001). *Lancet* 357, 763–767.

Jandera, P., Skeifikova, V., Rehova, L., Hajek, T., Baldrianova, L., Skopova, G., Kellner, V. and Horna, A. (2005). *J. Sep. Sci.* 28, 1005–1022.

Kannel, W.B. and Ellison, R.C. (1996). *Clin. Chim. Acta.* 246, 59–76.

Karatzi, K., Papamichael, C., Aznaouridis, K., Karatzis, E., Lekakis, J., Matsouka, C., Boskou, G., Chiou, A., Sitara, M., Feliou, G., Kontoyiannis, D., Zampelas, A. and Mavrikakis, M. (2004). *Coron. Artery Dis.* 15, 485–490.

Karatzi, K.N., Papamichael, C.M., Karatzis, E.N., Papaioannou, T.G., Aznaouridis, K.A., Katsichti, P.P., Stamatelopoulos, K.S., Zampelas, A., Lekakis, J.P. and Mavrikakis, M.E. (2005). *Am. J. Hypertens.* 18, 1161–1167.

Keil, U., Chambless, L.E., Doring, A., Filipiak, B. and Stieber J. (1997). *Epidemiology* 8, 150–156.

Keli, S.O., Hertog, M.G., Feskens, E.J. and Kromhout, D. (1996). *Arch. Int. Med.* 156, 637–642.

Kinlay, S. and Ganz, P. (2000). *Am. J. Cardiol.* 86, 10J–14J.

Langer, R.D., Criqui, M.H. and Reed, D.M. (1992). *Circulation* 85, 910–915.

Lapcik, O., Hill, M., Hampl, R., Wahala, K. and Adlercreutz, H. (1998). *Steroids* 63, 14–20.

Lefevre, M., Kris-Etherton, P.M., Zhao, G. and Tracy, R.P. (2004). *J. Am. Diet. Assoc.* 104, 410–419.

Li, H.J. and Deinzer, M.L. (2006). *J. Agric. Food Chem.* 54, 4048–4056.

Libby, P. (2002). *Nature* 420, 868–874.

Lugasi, A. (2003). *Acta. Alim.* 32, 181–192.

Madigan, D., McMurrough, I. and Smyth, M.R. (1994). *Analyst* 119, 863–868.

Manach, C., Scalbert, A., Morand, C., Remesy, C. and Jimenez, L. (2004). *Am. J. Clin. Nutr.* 79, 727–747.

Manach, C., Mazur, A. and Scalbert, A. (2005a). *Curr. Opin. Lipidol.* 16, 77–84.

Manach, C., Williamson, G., Morand, C., Scalbert, A. and Remesy, C. (2005b). *Am. J. Clin. Nutr.* 81, 230S–242S.

Mann, L.B. and Folts, J.D. (2004). *Pathophysiology* 10, 105–112.

Mathur, S., Devaraj, S., Grundy, S.M. and Jialal, I. (2002). *J. Nutr.* 132, 3663–3667.

McMurrough, I. (1981). *J. Chromatogr.* 218, 683–693.

McMurrough, I. and Baertt, T. (1994). *J. Inst. Brew.* 100, 409–416.

McMurrough, I., Madigan, D. and Smyth, M.R. (1995). *J. Agric. Food Chem.* 43, 2687–2691.

McMurrough, I. and O'Rourke, T. (1997). *Tech. Q. Master Brew. Assoc. Am.* 34, 271–277.

Milligan, S.R., Kalita, J.C., Heyerick, A., Rong, H., De Cooman, L. and De Keukeleire, D. (1999). *J. Clin. Endocrinol. Metab.* 84, 2249–2252.

Miranda, C.L., Stevens, J.F., Ivanov, V., McCall, M., Frei, B., Deinzer, M.L. and Buhler, D.R. (2000). *J. Agric. Food. Chem.* 48, 3876–3884.

Moore, R.D. and Pearson, T.A. (1986). *Medicine* 65, 242–267.

Mukamal, K.J., Chung, H., Jenny, N.S., Kuller, L.H., Longstreth Jr., W.T., Mittleman, M.A., Burke, G.L., Cushman, M., Psaty, B.M. and Siscovick, D.S. (2006). *J. Am. Geriatr. Soc.* 54, 30–37.

Murphy, K.J., Chronopoulos, A.K., Singh, I., Francis, M.A., Moriarty, H., Pike, M.J., Turner, A.H., Mann, N.J. and Sinclair, A.J. (2003). *Am. J. Clin. Nutr.* 77, 1466–1473.

Nagy, L.E. (2004). *Annu. Rev. Nutr.* 24, 55–78.

Nielsen, N.R., Schnohr, P., Jensen, G. and Grønbæk, M. (2004). *J. Int. Med.* 255, 280–288.

Nijveldt, R.J., van Nood, E., van Hoorn, D.E., Boelens, P.G., van Norren, K. and van Leeuwen, P.A. (2001). *Am. J. Clin. Nutr.* 74, 418–425.

Pace-Asciak, C.R., Hahn, S., Diamandis, E.P., Soleas, G. and Goldberg, D.M. (1995). *Clin. Chim. Acta.* 235, 207–219.

Puddey, I.B., Zilkens, R.R., Croft, K.D. and Beilin, L.J. (2001). *Clin. Exp. Pharmacol. Physiol.* 28, 1020–1024.

Renaud, S.C. and Ruf, J.C. (1996). *Clin. Chim. Acta.* 246, 77–89.

Ridker, P.M., Stampfer, M.J. and Rifai, N. (2001). *JAMA* 285, 2481–2485.

Rimm, E.B., Giovannucci, E.L., Willett, W.C., Colditz, G.A., Ascherio, A., Rosner, B. and Stampfer, M.J. (1991). *Lancet* 338, 464–468.

Rimm, E.B., Klatsky, A., Grobbee, D. and Stampfer, M.J. (1996). *Br. Med. J.* 312, 731–736.

Robak, J. and Gryglewski, R.J. (1988). *Biochem. Pharmacol.* 37, 837–841.

Ross, R. (1999). *New Engl. J. Med.* 340, 115–149.

Ruf, J.C. (2003). *Drugs Exp. Clin Res.* 29, 173–179.

Scalbert, A. and Williamson, G. (2002). *J. Nutr.* 130, 2073S–2078S.

Scott, J. (2004). *Curr. Opin. Genet. Dev.* 14, 271–279.

Sareen, J., McWilliams, L., Cox, B. and Stein, M.B. (2004). *J. Affect. Disord.* 82, 113–118.

Serafini, M., Maiani, G. and Ferro-Luzzi, A. (1998). *J. Nutr.* 128, 1003–1007.

Sierksma, A., van der Gaag, M.S., van Tol, A., James, R.W. and Hendriks, H.F. (2002a). *Alcohol Clin. Exp. Res.* 26, 1430–1435.

Sierksma, A., van der Gaag, M.S., Kluft, C. and Hendriks, H.F. (2002b). *Eur. J. Clin. Nutr.* 56, 1130–1136.

Stevens, J.F. and Page, J.E. (2004). *Phytochemistry* 65, 1317–1330.

Stevens, J.F., Taylor, A.W. and Deinzer, M.L. (1999). *J. Chrom. A.* 832, 97–107.

Stewart, S.H., Mainous III, A.G. and Gilbert, G. (2002). *J. Am. Board Fam. Pract.* 15, 437–442.

Tedesco, I., Nappo, A., Petitto, F., Iacomino, G., Nazzaro, F., Palumbo, R. and Russo, G.L. (2005). *Nutr. Cancer* 52, 74–83.

Tekel', J., De Keukeleire, D., Rong, H., Daeseleire, E. and Van Peteghem, C. (1999). *J. Agric. Food Chem.* 47, 5059–5063.

Torel, J. and Cillard, P. (1986). *Phytochemistry* 25, 383–387.

Truelsen, T., Gronbaek, M., Schnohr, P. and Boysen, G. (1998). *Stroke* 29, 2467–2472.

Treutter, D. (2005). *Plant Biol.* 7, 581–591.

US Department of Agriculture, Economic Research Service. Washington, DC, 2004; US per capita food consumption Beverages (individual). http://www.ers.usda.gov/Data/Food-Consumption (accessed March 10, 2006).

US Department of Agriculture, Agricultural Research Service. USDA Database for the Flavonoid Content of Selected Foods, Release 2 (2006). http://www.ars.usda.gov/Services/docs.htm?docid=6231 (accessed June 10, 2006).

Vinson, J.A. and Hontz, B.A. (1995). *J. Agric. Food Chem.* 43, 401–403.

Vinson, J.A. (1998). *Adv. Exp. Med. Biol.* 439, 151–164.

Vinson, J.A., Mandarano, M., Hirst, M., Trevithick, J.R. and Bose, P. (2003). *J. Agric. Food Chem.* 51, 5528–5533.

van der Gaag, M.S., van Tol, A., Scheek, L.M., James, R.W., Urgert, R., Schaafsma, G. and Hendriks, H.F. (1999). *Atherosclerosis* 147, 405–410.

van der Gaag, M.S., Ubbink, J.B., Sillanaukee, P., Nikkari, S. and Hendriks, H.F. (2000). *Lancet* 355, 1522.

Volpato, S., Pahor, M., Ferrucci, L., Simonsick, E.M., Guralnik, J.M., Kritchevsky, S.B., Fellin, R. and Harris, T.B. (2004). *Circulation* 109, 607–612.

Walle, T. (2004). *Free Radical. Biol. Med.* 36, 829–837.

Willoughby, S., Holmes, A. and Loscalzo, J. (2002). *Eur. J. Cardiovasc. Nurs.* 1, 273–288.

World Health Organization. The Atlas of Heart Disease and Stroke. Internet: http://www.who.int/cardiovascular_diseases/resources/atlas/en/ (accessed March 10, 2006).

Yilmazer, M., Stevens, J.F. and Buhler, D.R. (2001). *FEBS Lett.* 491, 252–256.

Yochum, L., Kushi, L.H., Meyer, K. and Folsom, A.R. (1999). *Am. J. Epidemiol.* 149, 943–949.

Zern, T.L. and Fernandez, M.L. (2005). *J. Nutr.* 135, 2291–2294.

Zilkens, R.R., Burke, V., Hodgson, J.M., Barden, A., Beilin, L.J. and Puddey, I.B. (2005). *Hypertension* 45, 874–879.

85
Vasoactivity of Flavonols, Flavones and Catechins

Owen L. Woodman School of Medical Sciences, RMIT University, Victoria, Australia

Abstract

Flavonols, flavones and catechins are three families amongst the very large group of biologically active plant-derived compounds known as flavonoids. These compounds have in common that they are all vasoactive and antioxidant, and through these actions it has been proposed that they may offer protection against cardiovascular disease. Each of these compounds is found in significant levels in barley and hops, the two important plant ingredients in beer, and therefore beer is one of the dietary sources of these flavonoids. The flavonols and flavones cause purely vasorelaxation *in vitro*, whereas catechins can cause contraction or relaxation depending on the individual compound and the concentration. By contrast, all of these compounds are reported to improve endothelium-dependent dilation in humans that may result from their common ability to preserve nitric oxide (NO) activity. This arises from the antioxidant actions of these flavonoids resulting in reduced inactivation of NO by the superoxide anion. Oxidant stress is an important contributor to the pathogenesis of cardiovascular disease and this chapter will review the growing evidence that flavonols, flavones and catechins through their direct and indirect actions on the vasculature are able to prevent the development of hypertension and ischemia/reperfusion injury.

List of Abbreviations

ACE	Angiotensin converting enzyme
DNA	Deoxyribonucleic acid
ECg	Epicatechin gallate
eNOS	Endothelial nitric oxide synthase
HUVEC	Human umbilical vein endothelial cell
LDL	Low-density lipoprotein
NO	Nitric oxide
SOD	Superoxide dismutase
TUNEL	Terminal deoxynucleotidyl transferase mediated dUTP nick end labeling
ACh	Acetylcholine
DiOHF	3′,4′-dihydroxy flavonol
EC	Epicatechin
EGC	Epigallocatechin
EGCg	Epigallocatechin gallate
MDA	Malondialdehyde
SHR	Spontaneously hypertensive rat
TBARS	Thiobarbituric acid-reactive substances

Introduction

The flavonoids are a large group of plant-derived compounds that are known to exhibit biological effects, including lowering plasma levels of low-density lipoproteins (LDLs), inhibiting platelet aggregation and reducing cell proliferation. In addition, many flavonoids have been reported to modulate vascular tone and to exert antioxidant activity. Flavonoids are based on the structure of 2-phenylbenzopyrone, differing from one another in the orientation of hydroxylation or methylation, the position of the benzenoid substituent, the degree of unsaturation and the types of sugar attached. Of the many classes of flavonoids of particular interest to this review are the flavonols, flavones and catechins (which are also referred to as flavanols or flavan-3-ols). Flavones and flavonols are structurally very similar with a 2,3-double bond conjugated with the 4-oxo group in ring C, with flavonols having an extra hydroxyl substitution at the carbon 3 position (Figure 85.1). By contrast, the catechins lack the double bond in the middle ring (Figure 85.2). Flavonoids are ubiquitous to green plant cells, including in barley and hops, leading to their ingestion through the consumption of beer in addition to many other foodstuffs. The phenolic content of beer depends on both the raw materials and the brewing process (Vinson *et al.*, 2003).

Fitzpatrick *et al.* (1993) demonstrated that wine and grape products such as quercetin and tannic acid cause endothelium-dependent relaxation in rat thoracic aorta and there have been several subsequent reports of the pharmacological actions of flavonoids on vascular smooth muscle tone. Duarte *et al.* (1993b) compared the relaxant effects of examples of compounds from the different structural subgroups of flavonoids. They reported that the order of potency for relaxation was flavonols > flavones > catechins. In addition these three groups of compounds exert significant antioxidant activity through a variety of mechanisms. This review

Beer in Health and Disease Prevention
ISBN: 978-0-12-373891-2

will focus on the direct vascular actions of these three groups of flavonoids including the ability of these polyphenols to preserve endothelial function as a result of their antioxidant effects, potentially offering protection against cardiovascular disease. In particular the evidence that flavonols, flavones and catechins may offer protection against hypertension and ischemia/reperfusion injury is explored.

	R_1	R_2	R_3	R_4	R_5
Flavones					
Apigenin	–	OH	–	OH	OH
Chrysin	–	–	–	OH	OH
Luteolin	OH	OH	–	OH	OH
Flavonols					
Fisetin	OH	OH	OH	–	OH
Quercetin	OH	OH	OH	OH	OH
Kaempferol	–	OH	OH	OH	OH
3′,4′-dihydroxyflavonol	OH	OH	OH	–	–

Figure 85.1 Flavonols and flavones. The general chemical structures of flavonols and flavones. Flavonols differ from flavones by the extra hydroxyl substitution at the C_3 position on the C ring.

Quantity of Flavones, Flavonols and Catechins in Beer

The two important plant ingredients in beer, barley and hops, both act as sources of the flavonoids and other polyphenolic compounds found in beer. Barley is a particularly good source of the catechins, epicatechin and epigallocatechin (EGC) but flavonols have also been identified (Goupy *et al.*, 1999), as have flavones (Markham and Mitchell, 2003). Hops also provides a source of both flavonols and flavones that are then found in beer (Stevens *et al.*, 2002). Vinson (1998) suggested that the most common phenols found in beer are "flavonols, phenolic acids, catechins, procyanidins and tannins" but there are only a few reports of quantitative analysis of distinct phenols found in beer. McMurrough *et al.* (1996) reported that a lager beer contained 56 mg/l of total polyphenols with flavonols contributing 19.5 mg/l. After examination of nine non-alcoholic beers from Spain, Alonso Garcia *et al.* (2004) reported that the total polyphenol content ranged from 0.8 to 8.6 mg/l with catechin contributing 0–4.5 mg/l and EC 0–0.22 mg/l. There was no detectable level of the flavonol quercetin. In an analysis of the catechin content of a variety of Spanish foodstuffs, De Pascual-Teresa *et al.* (2000) reported that a beer had a total flavonol content of 6.4 mg/l including catechin (7.3 mg/l), EC (1.8 mg/l) and gallocatechin (3.1 mg/l).

Vinson *et al.* (2003) have made an estimate of the average phenol intake from beer compared to wine in the United States based on consumption statistics for the year 2000 provided by the US Department of Agriculture. They

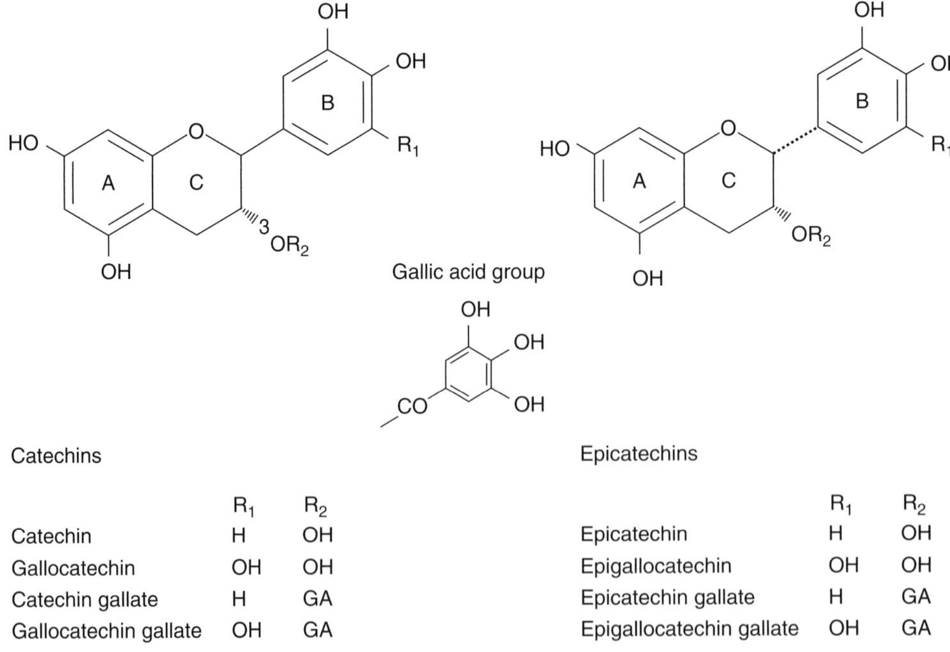

	R_1	R_2
Catechin	H	OH
Gallocatechin	OH	OH
Catechin gallate	H	GA
Gallocatechin gallate	OH	GA

	R_1	R_2
Epicatechin	H	OH
Epigallocatechin	OH	OH
Epicatechin gallate	H	GA
Epigallocatechin gallate	OH	GA

Figure 85.2 Catechins. The general chemical structures of the most common catechins. The third hydroxyl substitution on the B ring forms a gallate group and a gallic acid group may be attached to the oxygen at the C_3 position on the C ring.

concluded that if lager beer were consumed, containing 677 μM phenols, at the average volume of 225 ml/day the phenol intake, expressed as catechin equivalents, would be 42 mg/day. This is twice the amount of phenol obtained from the average of 20.7 ml of red and white wine per day based on a phenol concentration of 3,397 μM (Vinson, 1998). Thus, whilst wine is often referred to as an important source of cardioprotective flavonols, in societies where beer is more widely consumed than wine, it too should be recognized as an important source of flavonoids together with other beverages such as tea, in addition to foodstuffs, particularly fruits and vegetables.

Vascular Activity of Flavonols and Flavones

The observations of the vascular effects of extracts of wine, fruit and vegetables have provoked considerable interest in the potential activity of flavones and flavonols. Particular attention has been paid to quercetin, the most abundant of the naturally occurring flavonols. Several studies have demonstrated relaxant effects of quercetin, predominantly in rat isolated aorta (Duarte *et al.*, 1993a, b; Fitzpatrick *et al.*, 1993; Chen and Pace-Asciak, 1996; Flesch *et al.*, 1998; Chan *et al.*, 2000; Perez-Vizcaino *et al.*, 2002) also in coronary arteries from rabbits (Rendig *et al.*, 2001) and pigs (Taubert *et al.*, 2002). Although one of the initial studies indicated that the mechanism of quercetin-induced relaxation involved the release of a dilator from the endothelium, the same study also reported the contrary finding that the responses were unaffected by inhibition of nitric oxide synthase (NOS) (Fitzpatrick *et al.*, 1993). A number of subsequent studies reported that quercetin acted in an endothelium-dependent manner (Duarte *et al.*, 1993a, b; Flesch *et al.*, 1998; Perez-Vizcaino *et al.*, 2002), whereas in our laboratory removal of the endothelium decreased the sensitivity to quercetin without altering the maximum relaxation (Chan *et al.*, 2000). Chen and Pace-Asciak (1996) also noted that whilst low concentrations of quercetin acted in an endothelium-dependent manner, higher concentrations caused relaxation in the absence of the endothelium. Furthermore inhibition of NOS reversed relaxation in response to low but not high concentrations of quercetin. Taking into account all of these observations it appears that quercetin predominantly acts by direct relaxation of vascular smooth muscle and in addition it stimulates the release of endothelium-derived NO. Similar observations have been made with other flavonols such as leukocyanidol, fisetin, galangin and 3′,4′-dihydroxy flavonol (DiOHF) (Andriambeloson *et al.*, 1997; Chan *et al.*, 2000; Morello *et al.*, 2006).

Flavonols differ from flavones by the presence of a hydroxyl group at the 3 position of the C ring (Figure 85.1). It appears that it is this structural feature that leads to the endothelium-dependent component of flavonol-induced relaxation. The ability of flavonols to acutely stimulate the release of endothelium-derived NO is supported by the studies of Taubert *et al.* (2002) who measured NO release from porcine coronary arteries in response to 28 phenols commonly occurring in plant foods. The flavonols quercetin, myricetin and fisetin were very effective stimulants of NO release, whereas the flavones apigenin, luteolin and naringenin caused much less effect (Taubert *et al.*, 2002). Flavones, without the hydroxyl substitution at the 3 position, are most commonly reported to act in an entirely endothelium-independent manner (Duarte *et al.*, 1993b; Herrera *et al.*, 1996; Chan *et al.*, 2000; Ajay *et al.*, 2003) although apigenin has been reported to show some sensitivity to NOS inhibition (Zhang *et al.*, 2002).

Of the flavonoids studied, flavonols and flavones appear to demonstrate the greatest level of vasorelaxant (Duarte *et al.*, 1993a) and antioxidant activity (Rice-Evans *et al.*, 1996; Pietta, 2000). The extra hydroxyl group present in the flavonols at the C_3 position (Figure 85.1) is important for vascular activity as they are more potent vasodilators than flavones (Duarte *et al.*, 1993a). The pattern of substitution of hydroxyl groups on the A and B rings of these compounds also influences activity, particularly substitution on the B ring, as flavonols with a $C_{2',4'}$ diOH or $C_{3',4',5'}$ triOH orientation are weak vasodilators (Herrera *et al.*, 1996), while a catechol group, comprising OH groups at $C_{3'}$ and $C_{4'}$, is associated with strong vasorelaxant activity (Herrera *et al.*, 1996). In contrast, OH substitution on the A ring reduces the relaxant actions of flavonols (Chan *et al.*, 2000). Similar to vascular activity, the antioxidant activity of flavones is enhanced by the C_3 OH group, indicating that flavonols are better antioxidants than the flavones (Figure 85.1) (Cao and Li, 2004; Kim and Lee, 2004). On ring B, the presence of a catechol group is reported to be a major determinant for high radical scavenging activity (Burda and Oleszek, 2001; Kim and Lee, 2004), and an additional OH at $C_{5'}$ results in even higher activity (Cos *et al.*, 1998).

In studies from our laboratory the flavonols 3′-hydroxyflavonol, DiOHF and 7,4′-dihydroxy flavonol tended to be more potent at causing vasodilation than DiOHF, consistent with the observations of Duarte *et al.* (1993b) who reported that flavonols, with the additional OH substitution at the C_3 position of the C ring, are the more potent vasodilators of the two groups. Although the B ring catechol group has been proposed as an important determinant for vasodilator activity (Herrera *et al.*, 1996), we found that, DiOHF was equally potent at impairing Ca^{2+}-contraction and less potent at impairing PE-contraction than 3′-hydroxyflavonol. This suggests that the C_3' OH group on the B ring could be the main determinant for maximal vascular activity, while the presence of an additional OH group at C_4 results in unchanged or even lessened activity. The higher potencies observed in flavonols and flavones with the C_3' OH group (Duarte *et al.*, 1993a) further support this proposition. The C_4' OH group may be less important than the C_3' OH as 7,4′-dihydroxy flavonol tended to be less active than 3′-hydroxyflavonol at reducing vascular tone, although the reduced activity may also be due to the C_7 OH, which has been previously proposed to be associated with lessened activity (Chan *et al.*, 2000). Duarte *et al.* (1993b) demonstrated that flavonols were more active vasodilators than flavones; however, this may only be true for flavonols with other substitutions on the A or B ring, as flavonol with only the C_3 OH group and unsubstituted flavone were equally weak at reducing vascular tone (Woodman *et al.*, 2005). Moreover results of this study indicate that although substituted flavonols are more potent than flavones, it appears that the C_3 OH alone contributes little to activity. However the C_3 OH group may aid in the ability of OH substitutions on the A and B rings to increase vascular activity of the flavonol. The substitution of methoxy groups at positions C_3' and C_4' on the B ring abolished the high vascular activity of the catechol group, as 3′,4′-dimethoxyflavonol was observed to exhibit very weak vascular activity (Woodman *et al.*, 2005). A limitation to our understanding of structure–activity relationships is that there are relatively few flavonols and flavones available with three or less hydroxyl substitutions or substitutions other than hydroxy or methoxy. Synthesis of flavonols and flavones with a wider variety of substitutions would facilitate the further investigation of the vascular structure–activity relationships of these compounds.

The mechanism of the endothelium-independent component of flavone- and flavonol-induced relaxation remains uncertain. Mechanisms that have been proposed include an inhibitory effect on protein kinase C, which is involved in contraction (Duarte *et al.*, 1993a), or in the activity of phosphodiesterases, which inactivate cyclic nucleotides that are involved in relaxation (Herrera *et al.*, 1996). Alternatively, flavonols and flavones may interfere with the utilization of calcium in the contractile process in vascular smooth muscle cells that may involve a reduced influx of extracellular calcium (Duarte *et al.*, 1994) and impairment of release of intracellular calcium stores (Chan *et al.*, 2000). There is also some evidence of the involvement of calcium-activated and ATP-sensitive potassium channels in flavone and flavonol-induced relaxation (Calderone *et al.*, 2004).

Vascular Activity of Catechins

There have been several reports of the vasoactivity of the catechins, predominantly in rat isolated aorta, but the mechanism of their vascular effects remains uncertain. The most common catechins are shown in Figure 85.2. Of the eight most common catechins, EC, epicatechin gallate (ECg), EGC and epigallocatechin gallate (EGCg) are the compounds most frequently investigated in regard to their vascular activity. In contrast to the flavones and flavonols, which universally cause vascular relaxation, those catechins that possess vascular activity have been observed to induce both contraction and relaxation which is related to both structure and concentration.

The earliest reports of the vascular activity of catechins were that they were relaxants (Andriambeloson *et al.*, 1997; Huang *et al.*, 1998, 1999; Chen *et al.*, 2000, 2001) which generally acted in an endothelium-independent manner (Andriambeloson *et al.*, 1997, 1998; Chen *et al.*, 2002) although it was also reported that the relaxation could be partially inhibited by endothelium removal, inhibition of endothelial NOS (eNOS) with L-NAME and by iberiotoxin, an inhibitor of large conductance, calcium-activated potassium channels. In all of these studies, rat aorta was employed for the assays.

Subsequently Sanae *et al.* (2002) in a more thorough investigation of the structure–activity relationships of all of the eight common catechins shown in Figure 85.2 reported that, in rat aortae precontracted with phenylephrine, EGC and EGCg enhanced phenylephrine-induced contraction at low concentrations that did not on their own cause any effect. Relaxation was only observed at the high concentrations of 100 μM. The contraction appeared to arise due to the impairment of the activity of endothelium-derived NO as contraction was abolished by endothelium removal and EGC and EGCg both inhibited relaxant responses to acetylcholine (ACh). Removing the endothelium did not affect the EGCg-induced relaxation and enhanced the relaxation to EGC (Sanae *et al.*, 2002).

Later studies confirmed the biphasic responses to EGCg (Shen *et al.*, 2003; Lorenz *et al.*, 2004; Alvarez *et al.*, 2006). In our laboratory we compared the responses to catechin, EC, ECg, EGC and EGCg in rat isolated carotid artery rings (Figure 85.3). Catechin and EC had no effect in the

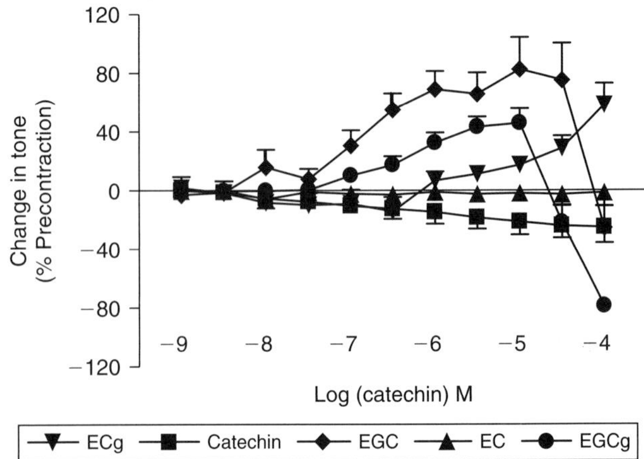

Figure 85.3 Vascular actions of catechins. Cumulative concentration–response curves to catechin, EC, EGC, ECg and EGCg in rat carotid artery rings. The artery rings were contracted with phenylephrine to produce approximately 50% of their maximal tone before addition of the catechins. Only EGCg showed significant relaxation at the highest concentration although EGC also showed reversal of previous contraction at that concentration. Data is shown as mean ± SEM, n = 6–9. *Source*: Lee and Woodman (unpublished observations).

submaximally constricted rat aorta, whereas ECg and EGC caused only contraction. EGCg caused concentration-dependent contraction at concentrations up to 10 μM but this was reversed at higher concentrations with a marked relaxation at the highest concentration tested (100 μM). The mechanism of contraction remains uncertain with a variety of mechanisms proposed such as release of H_2O_2 (Shen *et al.*, 2003) and promotion of calcium entry (Alvarez-Castro *et al.*, 2004). The role of the endothelium in the relaxant responses is not clear as there are reports supporting (Chen *et al.*, 2002; Lorenz *et al.*, 2004) and opposing (Alvarez-Castro *et al.*, 2004) a role of the endothelium. Lorenz *et al.* (2004) provided evidence that EGCg was able to increase eNOS activity when bovine aortic endothelial cells were exposed to the catechin for 15 min, but the level of eNOS protein expression was not affected by catechin treatment for 72 h. Anter *et al.* (2004, 2005) also reported that polyphenols derived from black tea acutely enhanced eNOS activity. Unfortunately the contents of the black tea polyphenols were not identified but it is likely that catechins were the major components of the extract.

Preservation of Endothelial Function by Flavones, Flavonols and Catechins

In addition to direct relaxation of vascular smooth muscle, an important action of the flavonols and flavones may be their ability to enhance responses to other vasodilator stimuli. There is epidemiological evidence that the consumption of polyphenols, in particular flavonols, flavones and catechins, in foods and beverages offers protection against cardiovascular disease (Arts and Hollman, 2005; Stangl *et al.*, 2006). The mechanisms of any beneficial effects of dietary polyphenols on the cardiovascular system are uncertain but are the focus of considerable interest. In particular, a number of studies have investigated the possibility that flavones, flavonols and catechins may increase the bioactivity of endothelium-derived NO.

Maintenance of release of endothelium-derived NO is critical for normal cardiovascular function. Endothelium-derived NO, in addition to acting as a vasodilator contributing to the local regulation of blood flow, is a potent inhibitor of platelet aggregation and platelet adhesion to endothelial cells (Tziros and Freedman, 2006). In addition, NO inhibits the expression of surface adhesion molecules that promote leukocyte adhesion to endothelial cells and migration into the vascular wall (Kubes *et al.*, 1991).

There is a range of mechanisms by which the bioactivity of endothelium-derived NO might be increased (Figure 85.4), for example, an increase in synthesis resulting from an increase in expression of eNOS. Alternatively interventions that attenuate the rate of inactivation of NO, for example by reducing the interaction with superoxide anions, would also increase NO activity. Considerable attention has been paid to the possible antioxidant activity of flavones and flavonols (Cos *et al.*, 1998; De Groot and Rauen, 1998; Vinson, 1998). Several mechanisms of flavonoid antioxidant activity have been reported including suppression of synthesis of reactive oxygen species

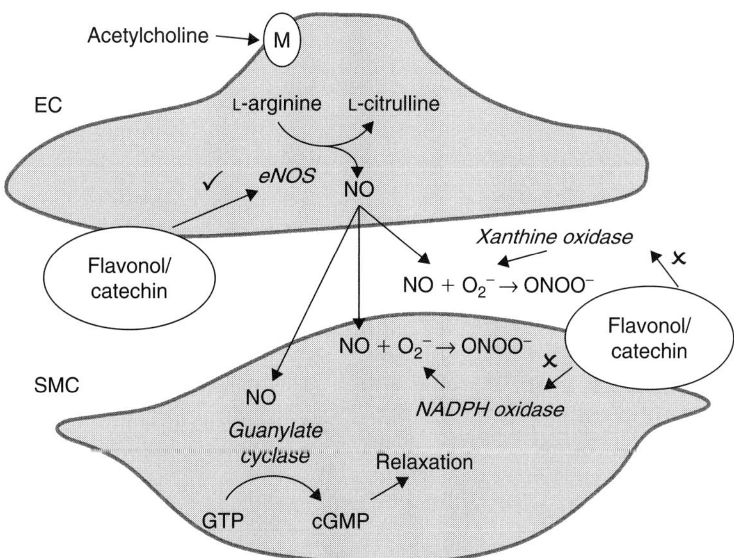

Figure 85.4 Sites of action of flavonols and catechins. Diagram illustrating possible sites at which flavonols and catechins may act to enhance the release or activity of endothelium-derived NO. The release of NO can be increased by increasing the expression or activity of eNOS. Alternatively the bioactivity of NO once released may be increased by reducing the interaction with superoxide anions (O_2^-). There is evidence that flavonols and catechins may inhibit the activity of two important enzymatic sources of superoxide, that is xanthine oxidase and NADPH oxidase. In addition they may act as radical scavengers directly inactivating superoxide.

(ROS) by inhibiting enzymes such as xanthine oxidase and NADPH oxidase or by chelating trace metals that play an important role in oxygen metabolism (Pietta, 2000). Structure–activity studies of flavones and flavonols indicate that the presence of a 3-hydroxyl group in the heterocyclic ring and a catechol group in ring B favors antioxidant activity (Pietta, 2000). Furthermore the structural features of the flavonols that result in their effective scavenging of superoxide also favor their ability to attenuate the toxic effects of peroxynitrite (Santos and Mira, 2004). Endothelium-derived NO rapidly reacts with superoxide anions (rate constant $2 \times 10^{10} M^{-1} s^{-1}$) to form peroxynitrite (Kissner *et al.*, 1997), which then reduces the relaxant activity of NO. Superoxide dismutase (SOD) also reacts rapidly with superoxide (rate constant $1\text{–}2 \times 10^{10} M^{-1} s^{-1}$) and in so doing enhances NO bioavailability (Ferrer-Sueta *et al.*, 2002) and may enhance endothelium-dependent relaxation (Jackson *et al.*, 1998). We have demonstrated that flavonols with demonstrated antioxidant activity, such as DiOHF, are able to mimic the actions of SOD and significantly improve endothelium-dependent dilation in the presence of oxidant stress (Figure 85.5) (Chan *et al.*, 2003; Woodman *et al.*, 2005). Similarly,

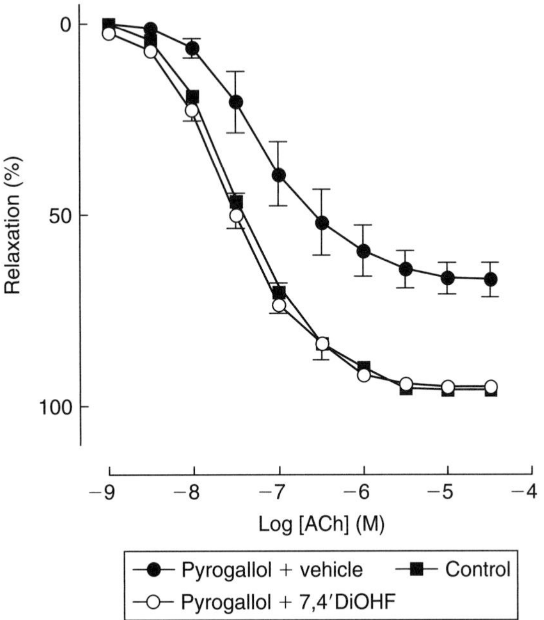

Figure 85.5 Flavonol protection against oxidant stress. Concentration–response curves to ACh in the absence or presence of pyrogallol (2×10^{-5}M) in endothelium-intact rat aortic rings. Pyrogallol auto-oxidizes to generate superoxide resulting in impaired endothelium-dependent relaxation. 7,4′-dihydroxy flavonol (7,4′DiOHF) was able to acutely enhance endothelium-dependent relaxation in the presence of the oxidant stress indicating an ability to rapidly scavenge superoxide anions. Data is shown as mean ± SEM, $n = 6$. *Source*: Modified from Woodman *et al.* (2005).

Girard *et al.* (1995) demonstrated the ability of a synthetic flavone to preserve endothelium-dependent relaxation in the presence of oxidant stress caused by pyrogallol. However antioxidant capacity alone does not guarantee the ability to enhance endothelium-dependent relaxation. For example, the well-known antioxidant ascorbic acid does not enhance endothelium-dependent relaxation in arteries when endogenous superoxide levels are elevated by inhibiting the activity of endogenous SOD (Jackson *et al.*, 1998). This is probably due to the relatively slow rate of reaction between ascorbic acid and superoxide anions (rate constant $2 \times 10^{5} M^{-1} s^{-1}$) (Gotoh and Niki, 1992). Butkovic *et al.* (2004) also investigated the effect of flavonoid structure on the reaction rate with superoxide and concluded that flavonols such as kaempferol and quercetin reacted very rapidly with free radicals. Thus it is likely that flavones and flavonols have the potential to promote vascular NO activity by attenuating the interaction with superoxide.

The antioxidant activity of flavonols and flavones may also be important in contributing to an anti-apoptotic action (Pryor *et al.*, 2006). Apoptosis was induced in human umbilical vein endothelial cells (HUVECs) by incubation with oxidized LDL. The flavonols quercetin and myricetin effectively attenuated lipid peroxidation and decreased deoxyribonucleic acid fragmentation measured by terminal deoxynucleotidyl transferase mediated dUTP nick end labeling staining. Apoptosis in HUVECs exposed to oxidized LDL was confirmed by increased expression of Bax and activated caspase-3 and decreased levels of Bcl-2, whereas the flavonols attenuated the changes in these markers of apoptosis. The flavones luteolin and apigenin, which demonstrated less antioxidant activity than the flavonols, were also less effective in preserving cell viability in the presence of oxidant stress (Jeong *et al.*, 2005).

There is also some limited direct evidence that flavonols can increase NO synthesis. Benito *et al.* (2002) supplemented the diet of rats with quercetin for 10 days and then demonstrated an increase in eNOS activity in the aorta together with elevated levels of cGMP. This elevation of NO synthesis was not accompanied by any change in eNOS protein expression. Wallerath *et al.* (2005) also reported that several flavonols did not affect the expression of eNOS protein or mRNA in human endothelial cells and that quercetin decreased the level of eNOS protein. Taken together with the functional data, indicating the involvement of endothelium-derived NO in flavonol-induced relaxation, it appears that a non-genomic activation of eNOS is most likely to contribute to the vascular actions of flavonols.

Catechins also efficiently scavenge a variety of ROS and nitrogen species such as superoxide, NO and peroxynitrite (Jovanovic and Simic, 2000; Paquay *et al.*, 2000; Boveris *et al.*, 2002; Stangl *et al.*, 2006). Of the catechins the ability to scavenge superoxide is favored by the presence of a gallate group, that is, EGCg, gallocatechin gallate and ECg

(Nakagawa and Yokozawa, 2002) and by the catechol group on the B ring (Figure 85.2). In addition to radical scavenging, catechins can chelate metal ions thereby reducing the generation of oxygen radicals (Guo *et al.*, 1996; Seeram *et al.*, 2002). There do not appear to be any reports that the ability to scavenge superoxide is able to preserve endothelium-dependent relaxation in the presence of oxidant stress. Catechins have, however, been reported to exert a number of effects linked to their antioxidant activity that are likely to result in preservation or improvement of endothelial function. EC, EGCg and catechin have all been reported to protect endothelial cells from injury caused by exposure to oxidized LDL (Jeong *et al.*, 2005; Steffen *et al.*, 2006) and EC was demonstrated to inhibit the oxidation of LDL (Kostyuk *et al.*, 2003).

Flavonols and Flavones in Hypertension

An increase in total peripheral resistance resulting from both structural and functional changes in the arterioles is a characteristic of hypertension, and endothelial dysfunction is an important contributor to the increase in arteriolar tone. This may involve impaired release of NO (Yang and Kaye, 2006) and/or a decrease in NO bioavailability due to increased inactivation by superoxide anions (Paravicini and Touyz, 2006). As flavones and flavonols both enhance NO activity and exert antioxidant effects, they are logical candidates for investigation for the treatment or prevention of hypertension. The efficacy of the flavonol quercetin has been investigated in a variety of models of hypertension in rats (Table 85.1). Duarte and colleagues reported that quercetin reduces systolic blood pressure in spontaneously hypertensive rats (Duarte *et al.*, 2001; Sanchez *et al.*, 2006) as well as in rats where hypertension is induced by NOS inhibition (Duarte *et al.*, 2002), DOCA salt (Galisteo *et al.*, 2004) or impaired renal perfusion (Garcia-Saura *et al.*, 2005). In each of these studies, together with that by another research group (Jalili *et al.*, 2006), quercetin failed to alter arterial pressure in normotensive control animals. There is clear evidence that the antihypertensive actions of quercetin are associated with an improvement in endothelial function together with a reduction in oxidant stress. Quercetin treatment improves endothelium-dependent relaxation in aortae from hypertensive rats without affecting endothelium-independent relaxation (Duarte *et al.*, 2001, 2002; Ajay *et al.*, 2003, 2006; Galisteo *et al.*, 2004; Garcia-Saura *et al.*, 2005; Sanchez *et al.*, 2006). In addition quercetin exerts a number of actions suggesting that antioxidant activity may contribute to the antihypertensive outcomes. Several studies report that quercetin lowers biomarkers of oxidant stress such as urinary isoprostane, plasma malondialdehyde, and plasma and liver thiobarbituric acid-reactive substances (Duarte *et al.*, 2001; Galisteo *et al.*, 2004; Garcia-Saura *et al.*, 2005; Jalili *et al.*, 2006). Sanchez *et al.* (2006) also demonstrated that the significantly greater superoxide generation by aortae from spontaneously hypertensive rats, in comparison to normotensive Wistar–Kyoto controls, was lowered by quercetin treatment, an effect that was accompanied by a decreased expression of the NADPH oxidase subunit $p47^{phox}$. There is considerable evidence supporting a critical role for NADPH oxidase-derived ROS in hypertension (Paravicini and Touyz, 2006). This is the first evidence that quercetin might target an important mechanism in the pathogenesis of hypertension.

Despite these positive findings with quercetin, there is an absence of human intervention studies using flavonols to test their potential antihypertensive activity. Whilst two studies report that quercetin did not alter arterial pressure, in both cases the subjects had normal blood pressure and, given the observation that quercetin does not affect arterial pressure in normotensive rats, the outcome of those studies is predictable. The efficacy of quercetin as an antihypertensive in humans awaits an intervention trial using a suitable group of hypertensive subjects.

Catechins as Antihypertensives

Although the antihypertensive actions of flavonols are well established in animal models there has been very little investigation of catechins. Negishi *et al.* (2004) examined the effects of mixed polyphenols derived from green or black tea in spontaneously hypertensive stroke prone rats. The treatments were provided in the rats drinking water and the green tea polyphenols were predominantly catechins (3.5 g/l) but there were also flavonols (0.5 g/l) and polymetric flavonoids (1 g/l). The rats consuming the green tea polyphenols for 3 weeks achieved a plasma total catechin concentration of 200 nM and had significantly lower systolic and diastolic blood pressures compared to controls. A possible mechanism for this antihypertensive action includes inhibition of angiotensin converting enzyme (ACE). Actis-Goretta *et al.* (2003) demonstrated that EC caused concentration-dependent inhibition of rabbit lung ACE. Further investigation indicated that EGC was the most active ACE inhibitor of the catechins tested and that the flavonols quercetin and kaempferol did not share the ability to inhibit the enzyme activity (Actis-Goretta *et al.*, 2006). Further investigation of the mechanism of the antihypertensive actions of the catechins is clearly warranted.

In clinical studies the potential antihypertensive actions of catechins have been investigated by the inclusion of catechin-rich dark chocolate or cocoa in the diet. There have been mixed outcomes in healthy, normotensive subjects where decreases in arterial pressure were reported in two studies from the same group of researchers (Grassi *et al.*, 2005a, b), whereas others reported no change in arterial pressure (Fisher *et al.*, 2003; Engler *et al.*, 2004; Fisher and Hollenberg, 2006). It should be noted that, even in the

Table 85.1 Studies that have investigated the antihypertensive actions of quercetin and flavone

Treatment	*Model of hypertension*	*Biomarkers significantly affected*	*Biomarkers not significantly affected*	*Reference*
Quercetin (10 mg/kg/day, oral, 5 weeks)	Spontaneously hypertensive rat	SBP, DBP, HR[a] LV weight index[b] Kidney weight index[c] Endothelium-dependent relaxation (ACh) of aorta Urinary isoprostane Plasma MDA[d]	Endothelium-independent relaxation (SNP) Aortic constriction to noradrenaline or KCl	Duarte *et al*. (2001)
Quercetin (5 or 10 mg/kg/day, oral, 6 weeks)	NOS inhibition (l-NAME 75 mg/100 ml drinking water)	SBP LV weight index Kidney weight index Proteinuria	Endothelium-dependent relaxation (ACh) of aorta Endothelium-independent relaxation (SNP) Aortic constriction to noradrenaline or KCl	Duarte *et al*. (2002)
Quercetin (10 mg/kg/day, oral, 5 weeks)	Uninephrectomy and DOCA salt (12.5 mg/week sc, 5 weeks)	SBP Endothelium-dependent relaxation (ACh) of aorta Heart and plasma TBARS		Galisteo *et al*. (2004)
Quercetin (10 mg/kg/day, oral, 4 weeks)	Spontaneously hypertensive rat	SBP Endothelium-dependent relaxation (ACh) of aorta	Endothelium-independent relaxation (SNP)	Ajay and Mustafa (2005)
Flavone (10 mg/kg/day, oral, 4 weeks)	Spontaneously hypertensive rat	SBP Endothelium-dependent relaxation (ACh) of aorta Endothelium-independent relaxation (SNP)		Ajay and Mustafa (2005)
Quercetin (10 mg/kg/day, oral, 5 weeks)	Two-kidney, one clip Goldblatt rats	SBP Proteinuria Endothelium-dependent relaxation (ACh) of aorta Plasma TBARS Liver glutathione peroxidase	Endothelium-independent relaxation (SNP) Aortic constriction to noradrenaline or KCl	Garcia-Saura *et al*. (2005)
Quercetin (10 mg/kg/day, oral, 13 weeks)	Spontaneously hypertensive rat	SBP, mean AP, HR LV weight index Endothelium-dependent relaxation (ACh) of aorta eNOS activity, protein expression of eNOS and caveolin-1 aortic superoxide $p47^{phox}$ expression	Kidney weight index Endothelium-independent relaxation (SNP) TXB_2 synthesized by aorta	Sanchez *et al*. (2006)
Quercetin (1.5 g/kg chow)	Abdominal aortic constriction in rats	SBP, DBP Heart weight index Aortic hypertrophy Endothelium-dependent relaxation (ACh) of aorta Liver TBARS	Endothelium-dependent relaxation (ACh) of mesenteric and coronary arteries Endothelium-independent relaxation (SNP) Aortic constriction to noradrenaline or potassium chloride	Jalili *et al*. (2006)

Notes: The flavonol quercetin has been demonstrated to reduce arterial pressure, and to exert a number of other beneficial cardiovascular outcomes, in a variety of rat models of hypertension. Flavone has also shown a similar decrease in SBP in spontaneously hypertensive rats.

[a] SBP, systolic blood pressure; DBP, diastolic blood pressure; HR, heart rate.
[b] Left ventricle to body weight ratio.
[c] Kidney to body weight ratio.
[d] Malondialdehyde.

latter studies where there was no significant change in arterial pressure, there was an improvement in endothelium-dependent dilation. In another study, a range of doses (90–400 mg) of EGCg were administered to normotensive men and it was found that there was a significant elevation of diastolic pressure in the following 24 h (Berube-Parent *et al.*, 2005). However the catechin was given in combination with caffeine that may have caused the pressor effect. Grassi *et al.* (2005b) also reported that the intake of 88 mg catechins per day for 15 days decreased systolic and diastolic pressure in patients with essential hypertension, once again accompanied by an improvement in endothelial function. The results of these clinical studies using mixed catechins contained in foodstuffs suggest that the further investigation of individual catechins is warranted in animal studies to investigate mechanism of action and structure–activity relationships.

Prevention of Injury Due to Ischemia and Reperfusion

As described earlier there is considerable epidemiological evidence that dietary intake of flavonols, flavones and catechins may reduce the incidence of cardiovascular disease. The dilator actions of these compounds may contribute to their protective effects as well as their antioxidant activity (Vinson, 1998). ROS such as the free radicals superoxide anion (O_2^-) and hydroxyl radical (OH^-) and non-radicals hydrogen peroxide (H_2O_2), peroxynitrite ($ONOO^-$) and hypochlorous acid (HOCl) all contribute to oxidant stress. NO reacts very rapidly with superoxide anion to produce peroxynitrite anion. Thus ROS can disturb endothelial function by enhancing degradation of NO and in addition by oxidizing lipids, in particular LDL, resulting in impaired endothelium-dependent relaxation (Cominacini *et al.*, 2000). In a number of disease states, such as atherosclerosis, hypertension and diabetes, the impairment of endothelium-dependent relaxation has been associated with enhanced degradation of NO by ROS (Cai and Harrison, 2000).

In addition to the contribution of long-term oxidant stress to chronic disease such as hypertension and atherosclerosis, an acute exacerbation in the generation of ROS is important in reperfusion injury of organs after a period of ischemia. There is a well-established link between reperfusion injury and the generation of oxygen radicals (Becker, 2004), and there are many studies demonstrating that oxygen radical scavengers reduce cardiac injury (Sobey and Woodman, 1993). In experimental animals inhibition of the effects of ROS has also proved to be an effective means of preserving coronary vasodilator capacity after ischemia and reperfusion. For example, treatment with the xanthine oxidase inhibitor, allopurinol preserves endothelium-dependent vasodilation *in vivo* and *in vitro* (Sobey and Woodman, 1993). There is also clinical evidence that antioxidants improve outcomes after ischemia and reperfusion. Antioxidants administered in the period immediately after myocardial infarction reduce infarct size and cardiac events (Tribble, 1999; Becker, 2004). In addition ascorbate, α-tocopherol and other antioxidants given before and continued after coronary angioplasty reduce the incidence of restenosis (Tribble, 1999).

Although there has been only limited investigation of the anti-ischemic actions of flavonols the observations have been consistently positive. There are several reports that flavonols and flavones are able to improve cardiac function after ischemia and reperfusion of rabbit and rat isolated hearts (Rump *et al.*, 1994; Schussler *et al.*, 1995; Lebeau *et al.*, 2001; Brookes *et al.*, 2002) as well as reducing ischemia–reperfusion injury to other organs such as kidney (Inal *et al.*, 2002; Singh *et al.*, 2004) and stomach (Mojzis *et al.*, 2001). In addition daflon a purified micronized flavonoid fraction containing 90% diosmin (flavone) and 10% hesperidin (flavanone) improved microvascular function after ischemia and reperfusion in the hamster cheek pouch (Bouskela *et al.*, 1997). The protective actions of daflon may be due to inhibition of expression of leukocyte adhesion molecules (Korthuis and Gute, 1999) and subsequently reduced adhesion of leukocytes to endothelial cells (Bouskela *et al.*, 1999).

We have investigated the protective action of DiOHF on vascular dysfunction caused by ischemia and reperfusion (Chan *et al.*, 2003). DiOHF was administered at one of two times, either prior to ischemia or during ischemia but before reperfusion. ACh- and sodium nitroprusside (SNP)-induced vasodilation was then assessed in the previously ischemic and reperfused rat hindquarters. Similar to SOD, DiOHF administered before ischemia or before reperfusion significantly enhanced vasodilation to both ACh and SNP in rats subjected to ischemia–reperfusion. Thus, we demonstrated that the synthetic flavonol DiOHF preserves vasodilator reactivity normally impaired by ischemia and reperfusion of the hindquarters vasculature. This indicates that DiOHF, like SOD, reduces vascular plugging caused by ischemia and reperfusion and, thus, preserves vasodilator reserve. We have also demonstrated that DiOHF is able to reduce infarct size after myocardial ischemia and reperfusion in anesthetized sheep (Wang *et al.*, 2004). DiOHF also reduced superoxide generation by myocardium in the ischemic zone, increased levels of NO metabolites in the venous outflow and improved coronary blood flow on reperfusion. Thus it appears that the antioxidant activity of this synthetic flavonol does result in improved endothelial function after ischemia and reperfusion in addition to the reduction in infarct size suggesting that it has clinical potential for improving recovery from myocardial infarction and other ischemic syndromes.

Recently considerable attention has been paid to the potential for flavones and flavonols to protect neurones against injury resulting from ischemia of the brain. There is now an established association between brain injury caused by ischemic or hemorrhagic stroke and the presence of oxidant stress. Acute brain injury increases the levels of excitotoxic amino acid neurotransmitters, such as glutamate, which in turn stimulate the generation of ROS. This suggests that antioxidants should prevent propagation of tissue injury, improve survival and reduce morbidity after stroke. Unfortunately, whilst a few antioxidants have shown efficacy in animal models of cerebral ischemia, none are yet to demonstrate a positive outcome in large scale clinical trials (Gilgun-Sherki *et al.*, 2002). Thus a number of groups have targeted flavonoids toward this elusive goal. Both flavones and flavonols have demonstrated neuroprotection in a variety of models of ischemic brain injury. When injury was induced by permanent occlusion of the middle cerebral artery in rats, infarct size was reduced by nictoflorin, a rutinoside of the flavonol kaempferol (Li *et al.*, 2006), or the flavone wogonin (Cho and Lee, 2004). Infarct size after transient ischemia–reperfusion is also reduced by quercetin (Cho *et al.*, 2006), morin (Gottlieb *et al.*, 2006) or wogonin (Lee *et al.*, 2003). In addition amentoflavone reduces infarct size in a rat model of hypoxic-ischemic brain injury where rat pups at post-natal day 7 had one common carotid artery ligated and were then exposed to 8% oxygen for 2.5 h (Shin *et al.*, 2006). In addition to their antioxidant activity there is evidence that the flavones and flavonols exert other protective actions such as preventing the activation of the apoptotic protein caspase-3 (Kang *et al.*, 2004; Shin *et al.*, 2006) or inhibiting matrix metalloproteinases (Cho *et al.*, 2006).

There has been even less investigation of the ability of catechins to prevent ischemic injury despite some promising observations. Chan *et al.* (1996) reported that catechin possesses significant antioxidant activity, an effect that was confirmed to occur *in vivo* with a mixture of catechins (Maffei Facino *et al.*, 1999). The antioxidant action of this catechin preparation was suggested to explain its ability to reduce ischemia-induced damage of rat isolated hearts (Maffei Facino *et al.*, 1999). Similarly catechin treatment was found to reduce injury to subsequent renal ischemia and reperfusion. The protective actions of catechin were associated with reduced oxidant injury and maintenance of the activity of renal antioxidant enzymes (Singh *et al.*, 2005). EGCg (Fiorini *et al.*, 2005) and mixed catechins extracted from green tea (Muia *et al.*, 2005) have also been reported to attenuate ischemia–reperfusion injury of the liver and gastrointestinal tract, respectively.

Sutherland *et al.* (2006) have recently reviewed the evidence that catechins may also prevent ischemic damage to the brain. EGCg is reported to be protective against injury caused by transient or permanent cerebral ischemia (Lee *et al.*, 2000, 2003; Nagai *et al.*, 2002; Choi *et al.*, 2004; Rahman *et al.*, 2005; Sutherland *et al.*, 2005). There have been both positive (Matsuoka *et al.*, 1995; Inanami *et al.*, 1998) and negative (Dajas *et al.*, 2003; Rivera *et al.*, 2004) outcomes with catechin. Protection has been associated with antioxidant activity in some studies (Inanami *et al.*, 1998; Choi *et al.*, 2004) but other actions of catechins such as an inhibition of calcium entry to nerve cells (Sutherland *et al.*, 2006) and inhibition of the expression of pro-apoptotic genes (Mandel and Youdim, 2004) have also been implicated.

Thus flavonols, flavones and catechins have all demonstrated some capacity to attenuate ischemia/reperfusion injury. Although it is often suggested that it is their antioxidant activity that leads to the beneficial effects, the precise mechanism of action is yet to be determined. In particular, it is not known whether their vascular actions might also contribute to their efficacy. A possible argument against that hypothesis is the similar protective capacities of the flavonols and catechins despite the limited vasodilator actions of the catechins. The earlier failure to demonstrate efficacy of antioxidants in clinical trials, after positive outcomes from animal experiments, means that any interpretation of the possible benefits of these agents needs to be cautious.

Summary Points

- Flavonols, flavones and catechins are found in significant levels in beer as well as other beverages, fruits and vegetables.
- Flavonols and flavones are able to exert direct relaxant effects that are predominantly endothelium-independent. By contrast, catechins show quite variable vascular effects ranging from no effect to pure constriction to constriction at low doses and vasodilation at high doses.
- Through their antioxidant activity flavonols, flavones and catechins are all able to improve endothelial function by protecting endothelium-derived NO from inactivation by ROS.
- Animal studies suggest that these compounds can protect against hypertension and ischemia/reperfusion injury. While the antioxidant activity of these flavonoids contributes to those benefits, the mechanism of action remains to be fully elucidated.
- Animal studies support the epidemiological evidence that flavonols, flavones and catechins may be useful in the prevention or treatment of cardiovascular disease but this needs to be supported by further clinical trials.

References

Actis-Goretta, L., Ottaviani, J.I., Keen, C.L. and Fraga, C.G. (2003). *FEBS Lett.* 555, 597.

Actis-Goretta, L., Ottaviani, J.I. and Fraga, C.G. (2006). *J. Agric. Food Chem.* 54, 229–234.

Ajay, M. and Mustafa, M.R. (2005). *J. Cardiovasc. Pharmacol.* 46, 36–40.

Ajay, M., Gilani, A.U. and Mustafa, M.R. (2003). *Life Sci.* 74, 603–612.

Ajay, M., Achike, F.I., Mustafa, A.M. and Mustafa, M.R. (2006). *Diabetes Res. Clin. Prac.* 73, 1–7.

Alonso Garcia, A., Cancho Grande, B. and Simal Gandara, J. (2004). *J. Chromatogr. A Food Sci.* 1054, 175–180.

Alvarez, E., Campos-Toimil, M., Justiniano-Basaran, H., Lugnier, C. and Orallo, F. (2006). *Br. J. Pharmacol.* 147, 269–280.

Alvarez-Castro, E., Campos-Toimil, M. and Orallo, F. (2004). *Naunyn Schmiedebergs Arch. Pharmacol.* 369, 496–506.

Andriambeloson, E., Magnier, C., Haan-Archipoff, G., Lobstein, A., Anton, R., Beretz, A., Stoclet, J.C. and Andriantsitohaina, R. (1998). *J. Nutr.* 128, 2324–2333.

Andriambeloson, E., Kleschyov, A.L., Muller, B., Beretz, A., Stoclet, J.C. and Andriantsitohaina, R. (1997). *Br. J. Pharmacol.* 120, 1053–1058.

Anter, E., Thomas, S.R., Schulz, E., Shapira, O.M., Vita, J.A. and Keaney Jr., J.F. (2004). *J. Biol. Chem.* 279, 46637–46643.

Anter, E., Chen, K., Shapira, O.M., Karas, R.H. and Keaney Jr., J.F. (2005). *Circ. Res.* 96, 1072–1078.

Arts, I.C.W. and Hollman, P.C.H. (2005). *Am. J. Clin. Nutr.* 81, 317S–325S.

Becker, L.B. (2004). *Cardiovasc. Res.* 61, 461–470.

Benito, S., Lopez, D., Saiz, M.P., Buxaderas, S., Sanchez, J., Puig-Parellada, P. and Mitjavila, M.T. (2002). *Br. J. Pharmacol.* 135, 910–916.

Berube-Parent, S., Pelletier, C., Dore, J. and Tremblay, A. (2005). *Br. J. Nutr.* 94, 432–436.

Bouskela, E., Cyrino, F.Z.G.A. and Lerond, L. (1997). *Br. J. Pharmacol.* 122, 1611–1616.

Bouskela, E., Cyrino, F.Z.G.A. and Lerond, L. (1999). *J. Vasc. Res.* 36, 11–14.

Boveris, A., Valdez, L. and Alvarez, S. (2002). *Ann. NY Acad. Sci.* 957, 90–102.

Brookes, P.S., Digerness, S.B., Parks, D.A. and Darley-Usmar, V. (2002). *Free Radic. Biol. Med.* 32, 1220–1228.

Burda, S. and Oleszek, W. (2001). *J. Agric. Food Chem.* 49, 2774–2779.

Butkovic, V., Klasinc, L. and Bors, W. (2004). *J. Agric. Food Chem.* 52, 2816–2820.

Cai, H. and Harrison, D.G. (2000). *Circ. Res.* 87, 840–844.

Calderone, V., Chericoni, S., Martinelli, C., Testai, L., Nardi, A., Morelli, I., Breschi, M.C. and Martinotti, E. (2004). *Naunyn Schmiedebergs Arch. Pharmacol.* 370, 290–298.

Cao, Z. and Li, Y. (2004). *Eur. J. Pharmacol.* 489, 39–48.

Chan, E.C.H., Pannangpetch, P. and Woodman, O.L. (2000). *J. Cardiovasc. Pharmacol.* 35, 326–333.

Chan, E.C.H., Drummond, G.R. and Woodman, O.L. (2003). *J. Cardiovasc. Pharmacol.* 42, 727–735.

Chan, P., Juei-Tang, C., Chiung-Wen, T., Chiang-Shan, N. and Chuang-Ye, H. (1996). *Life Sci.* 59, 2067–2073.

Chen, C.K. and Pace-Asciak, C.R. (1996). *Gen. Pharmacol.* 27, 363–366.

Chen, J.W., Zhu, Z.Q., Hu, T.X. and Zhu, D.Y. (2002). *Acta Pharmacol. Sin.* 23, 667–672.

Chen, Z.Y., Law, W.I., Yao, X.Q., Lau, C.W., Ho, W.K. and Huang, Y. (2000). *Acta Pharmacol. Sin.* 21, 835–840.

Cho, J. and Lee, H.K. (2004). *Biol. Pharm. Bull.* 27, 1561–1564.

Cho, J.Y., Kim, I.S., Jang, Y.H., Kim, A.R. and Lee, S.R. (2006). *Neurosci. Lett.* 404, 330–335.

Choi, Y.B., Kim, Y.I., Lee, K.S., Kim, B.S. and Kim, D.J. (2004). *Brain Res.* 1019, 47–54.

Cominacini, L., Pasini, A.F., Garbin, U., Davoli, A., Tosetti, M.L., Campagnola, M., Rigoni, A., Pastorino, A.M., Lo Cascio, V. and Sawamura, T. (2000). *J. Biol. Chem.* 275, 12633–12638.

Cos, P., Ying, L., Calomme, M., Hu, J.P., Cimanga, K., Van Poel, B., Pieters, L., Vlietinck, A.J. and Vanden Berghe, D. (1998). *J. Nat. Prod.* 61, 71–76.

Dajas, F., Rivera-Megret, F., Blasina, F., Arredondo, F., Abin-Carriquiry, J.A., Costa, G., Echeverry, C., Lafon, L., Heizen, H., Ferreira, M. and Morquio, A. (2003). *Braz. J. Med. Biol. Res.* 36, 1613–1620.

De Groot, H. and Rauen, U. (1998). *Fundam. Clin. Pharmacol.* 12, 249–255.

De Pascual-Teresa, S., Santos-Buelga, C. and Rivas-Gonzalo, J.C. (2000). *J. Agric. Food Chem.* 48, 5331–5337.

Duarte, J., Perez-Vizcaino, F., Zarzuelo, A., Jimenez, J. and Tamargo, J. (1993a). *Eur. J. Pharmacol.* 239, 1–7.

Duarte, J., Vizcaino, F.P., Utrilla, P., Jimenez, J., Tamargo, J. and Zarzuelo, A. (1993b). *Gen. Pharmacol.* 24, 857–862.

Duarte, J., Perez-Vizcaino, F., Zarzuelo, A., Jiminez, J. and Tamargo, J. (1994). *Eur. J. Pharmacol.* 262, 149–156.

Duarte, J., Perez-Palencia, R., Vargas, F., Ocete, M.A., Perez-Vizcaino, F., Zarzuelo, A. and Tamargo, J. (2001). *Br. J. Pharmacol.* 133, 117–124.

Duarte, J., Jimenez, R., O'valle, F., Galisteo, M., Perez-Palencia, R., Vargas, F., Perez-Vizcaino, F., Zarzuelo, A. and Tamargo, J. (2002). *J. Hypertens.* 20, 1843–1854.

Engler, M.B., Engler, M.M., Chen, C.Y., Malloy, M.J., Browne, A., Chiu, E.Y., Kwak, H.-K., Milbury, P., Paul, S.M., Blumberg, J. and Mietus-Snyder, M.L. (2004). *J. Am. Coll. Nutr.* 23, 197–204.

Ferrer-Sueta, G., Quijano, C., Alvarez, B. and Radi, R. (2002). *Method. Enzymol.* 349, 23–37.

Fiorini, R.N., Donovan, J.L., Rodwell, D., Evans, Z., Cheng, G., May, H.D., Milliken, C.E., Markowitz, J.S., Campbell, C., Haines, J.K., Schmidt, M.G. and Chavin, K.D. (2005). *Liver Transpl.* 11, 298–308.

Fisher, N.D. and Hollenberg, N.K. (2006). *J. Hypertens.* 24, 1575–1580.

Fisher, N.D., Hughes, M., Gerhard-Herman, M. and Hollenberg, N.K. (2003). *J. Hypertens.* 21, 2281–2286.

Fitzpatrick, D.F., Hirschfield, S.L. and Coffey, R.G. (1993). *Am. J. Physiol.* 265, H774–H778.

Flesch, M., Schwarz, A. and Bohm, M. (1998). *Am. J. Physiol.* 275, H1183–H1190.

Galisteo, M., Garcia-Saura, M.F., Jimenez, R., Villar, I.C., Zarzuelo, A., Vargas, F. and Duarte, J. (2004). *Mol. Cell Biochem.* 259, 91–99.

Garcia-Saura, M.F., Galisteo, M., Villar, I.C., Bermejo, A., Zarzuelo, A., Vargas, F. and Duarte, J. (2005). *Mol. Cell Biochem.* 270, 147–155.

Gilgun-Sherki, Y., Rosenbaum, Z., Melamed, E. and Offen, D. (2002). *Pharmacol. Rev.* 54, 271–284.

Girard, P., Sercombe, R., Sercombe, C., Le Lem, G., Seylaz, J. and Potier, P. (1995). *Biochem. Pharmacol.* 49, 1533–1539.

Gotoh, N. and Niki, E. (1992). *Biochim. Biophys. Acta* 1115, 201–207.

Gottlieb, M., Leal-Campanario, R., Campos-Esparza, M.R., Sanchez-Gomez, M.V., Alberdi, E., Arranz, A., Delgado-Garcia, J.M., Gruart, A. and Matute, C. (2006). *Neurobiol. Dis.* 23, 374–386.

Goupy, P., Hugues, M., Boivin, P. and Amiot, M. (1999). *J. Sci. Food Agric.* 79, 1625–1634.

Grassi, D., Lippi, C., Necozione, S., Desideri, G. and Ferri, C. (2005a). *Am. J. Clin. Nutr.* 81, 611–614.

Grassi, D., Necozione, S., Lippi, C., Croce, G., Valeri, L., Pasqualetti, P., Desideri, G., Blumberg, J.B. and Ferri, C. (2005b). *Hypertension* 46, 398–405.

Guo, Q., Zhao, B., Li, M., Shen, S. and Xin, W. (1996). *Biochim. Biophys. Acta* 1304, 210–222.

Herrera, M.D., Zarzuelo, A., Jiminez, J., Marhuenda, E. and Duarte, J. (1996). *Gen. Pharmacol.* 27, 273–277.

Huang, Y., Zhang, A., Lau, C.W. and Chen, Z.Y. (1998). *Life Sci.* 63, 275–283.

Huang, Y., Chan, N.W., Lau, C.W., Yao, X.Q., Chan, F.L. and Chen, Z.Y. (1999). *Biochim. Biophys. Acta* 1427, 322–328.

Inal, M., Altinisik, M. and Bilgin, M.D. (2002). *Cell Biochem. Funct.* 20, 291–296.

Inanami, O., Watanabe, Y., Syuto, B., Nakano, M., Tsuji, M. and Kuwabara, M. (1998). *Free Radic. Res.* 29, 359–365.

Jackson, T.S., Xu, A., Vita, J.A. and Keaney Jr., J.F. (1998). *Circ. Res.* 83, 916–922.

Jalili, T., Carlstrom, J., Kim, S., Freeman, D., Jin, H., Wu, T.C., Litwin, S.E. and David Symons, J. (2006). *J. Cardiovasc. Pharmacol.* 47, 531–541.

Jeong, Y.J., Choi, Y.J., Kwon, H.M., Kang, S.W., Park, H.S., Lee, M. and Kang, Y.H. (2005). *Br. J. Nutr.* 93, 581–591.

Jovanovic, S.V. and Simic, M.G. (2000). *Ann. NY Acad. Sci.* 899, 326–334.

Kang, S.S., Lee, J.Y., Choi, Y.K., Kim, G.S. and Han, B.H. (2004). *Bioorg. Med. Chem. Lett.* 14, 2261–2264.

Kim, D.O. and Lee, C.Y. (2004). *Crit. Rev. Food Sci. Nutr.* 44, 253–273.

Kissner, R., Nauser, T., Bugnon, P., Lye, P.G. and Koppenol, W.H. (1997). *Chem. Res. Toxicol.* 10, 1285–1292.

Korthuis, R. and Gute, D.C. (1999). *J. Vasc. Res.* 36, 15–23.

Kostyuk, V.A., Kraemer, T., Sies, H. and Schewe, T. (2003). *FEBS Lett.* 537, 146–150.

Kubes, P., Suzuki, M. and Granger, D.N. (1991). *PNAS* 88, 4651–4655.

Lebeau, J., Neviere, R. and Cotelle, N. (2001). *Bioorg. Med. Chem. Lett.* 11, 23–27.

Lee, H., Kim, Y.O., Kim, H., Kim, S.Y., Noh, H.S., Kang, S.S., Cho, G.J., Choi, W.S. and Suk, K. (2003a). *FASEB J.* 17, 1943–1944.

Lee, S.-R., Suh, S.-I. and Kim, S.-P. (2000). *Neurosci. Lett.* 287, 191–194.

Lee, S.Y., Kim, C.Y., Lee, J.J., Jung, J.G. and Lee, S.R. (2003b). *Brain Res. Bull.* 61, 399–406.

Li, R., Guo, M., Zhang, G., Xu, X. and Li, Q. (2006). *Biol. Pharm. Bull.* 29, 1868–1872.

Lorenz, M., Wessler, S., Follmann, E., Michaelis, W., Dusterhoft, T., Baumann, G., Stangl, K. and Stangl, V. (2004). *J. Biol. Chem.* 279, 6190–6195.

Maffei Facino, R., Carini, M., Aldini, G., Berti, F., Rossoni, G., Bombardelli, E. and Morazzoni, P. (1999). *Life Sci.* 64, 627–642.

Mandel, S. and Youdim, M.B.H. (2004). *Free Radic. Biol. Med.* 37, 304.

Markham, K.R. and Mitchell, K.A. (2003). *Z Naturforsch [C]* 58, 53–56.

Matsuoka, Y., Hasegawa, H., Okuda, S., Muraki, T., Uruno, T. and Kubota, K. (1995). *J. Pharmacol. Exp. Ther.* 274, 602–608.

McMurrough, I., Madigan, D. and Kelly, R.J. (1996). *J. Am. Soc. Brew. Chem.* 54, 141–148.

Mojzis, J., Hviscova, K., Germanova, D., Bukovicova, D. and Mirossay, L. (2001). *Physiol. Res.* 50, 501–506.

Morello, S., Vellecco, V., Alfieri, A., Mascolo, N. and Cicala, C. (2006). *Life Sci.* 78, 825–830.

Muia, C., Mazzon, E., Di Paola, R., Genovese, T., Menegazzi, M., Caputi, A.P., Suzuki, H. and Cuzzocrea, S. (2005). *Naunyn Schmiedebergs Arch. Pharmacol.* 371, 364–374.

Nagai, K., Jiang, M.H., Hada, J., Nagata, T., Yajima, Y., Yamamoto, S. and Nishizaki, T. (2002). *Brain Res.* 956, 319–322.

Nakagawa, T. and Yokozawa, T. (2002). *Food Chem. Toxicol.* 40, 1745–1750.

Negishi, H., Xu, J.W., Ikeda, K., Njelekela, M., Nara, Y. and Yamori, Y. (2004). *J. Nutr.* 134, 38–42.

Paquay, J.B., Haenen, G.R., Stender, G., Wiseman, S.A., Tijburg, L.B. and Bast, A. (2000). *J. Agric. Food Chem.* 48, 5768–5772.

Paravicini, T.M. and Touyz, R.M. (2006). *Cardiovasc. Res.* 71, 247.

Perez-Vizcaino, F., Ibarra, M., Cogolludo, A.L., Duarte, J., Zaragoza-Arnaez, F., Moreno, L., Lopez-Lopez, G. and Tamargo, J. (2002). *J. Pharmacol. Exp. Ther.* 302, 66–72.

Pietta, P.G. (2000). *J. Nat. Prod.* 63, 1035–1042.

Pryor, W.A., Houk, K.N., Foote, C.S., Fukuto, J.M., Ignarro, L.J., Squadrito, G.L. and Davies, K.J.A. (2006). *Am. J. Physiol.* 291, R491–R511.

Rahman, R.M.A., Nair, S.M., Helps, S.C., Shaw, O.M., Sims, N.R., Rosengren, R.J. and Appleton, I. (2005). *Neurosci. Lett.* 382, 227–230.

Rendig, S.V., Symons, J.D., Longhurst, J.C. and Amsterdam, E.A. (2001). *J. Cardiovasc. Pharmacol.* 38, 219–227.

Rice-Evans, C.A., Miller, N.J. and Paganga, G. (1996). *Free Radic. Biol. Med.* 20, 933–956.

Rivera, F., Urbanavicius, J., Gervaz, E., Morquio, A. and Dajas, F. (2004). *Neurotox. Res.* 6, 543–553.

Rump, A.F.E., Schussler, M., Acar, D., Cordes, A., Theisohn, M., Rosen, R., Klaus, W. and Fricke, U. (1994). *Gen. Pharmacol.* 25, 1137–1142.

Sanae, F., Miyaichi, Y., Kizu, H. and Hayashi, H. (2002). *Life Sci.* 71, 2553–2562.

Sanchez, M., Galisteo, M., Vera, R., Villar, I.C., Zarzuelo, A., Tamargo, J., Perez-Vizcaino, F. and Duarte, J. (2006). *J. Hypertens.* 24, 75–84.

Santos, M.R. and Mira, L. (2004). *Free Radic. Res.* 38, 1011.

Schussler, M., Holzl, J., Rump, A.F.E. and Fricke, U. (1995). *Gen. Pharmacol.* 26, 1565–1570.

Seeram, N.P., Schutzki, R., Chandra, A. and Nair, M.G. (2002). *J. Agric. Food Chem.* 50, 2519–2523.

Shen, J.Z., Zheng, X.F., Wei, E.Q. and Kwan, C.Y. (2003). *Clin. Exp. Pharmacol. Physiol.* 30, 88–95.

Shin, D.H., Bae, Y.C., Kim-Han, J.S., Lee, J.H., Choi, I.Y., Son, K.H., Kang, S.S., Kim, W.K. and Han, B.H. (2006). *J. Neurochem.* 96, 561–572.

Shutenko, Z., Henry, Y., Pinard, E., Seylaz, J., Potier, P., Berthet, F., Girard, P. and Sercombe, R. (1999). *Biochem. Pharmacol.* 57, 199–208.

Singh, D., Chander, V. and Chopra, K. (2005). *Pharmacol. Rep.* 57, 70–76.

Sobey, C.G. and Woodman, O.L. (1993). *Trend. Pharmacol. Sci.* 14, 448–453.

Stangl, V., Lorenz, M. and Stangl, K. (2006). *Mol. Nutr. Food Res.* 50, 218–228.

Steffen, Y., Schewe, T. and Sies, H. (2006). *Free Radic. Res.* 40, 1076.

Stevens, J.F., Miranda, C.L., Wolthers, K.R., Schimerlik, M., Deinzer, M.L. and Buhler, D.R. (2002). *J. Agric. Food Chem.* 50, 3435–3443.

Sutherland, B.A., Shaw, O.M., Clarkson, A.N., Jackson, D.N., Sammut, I.A. and Appleton, I. (2005). *FASEB J.* 19, 258–260.

Sutherland, B.A., Rahman, R.M. and Appleton, I. (2006). *J. Nutr. Biochem.* 17, 291–306.

Taubert, D., Berkels, R., Klaus, W. and Roesen, R. (2002). *J. Cardiovasc. Pharmacol.* 40, 701–713.

Tribble, D.L. (1999). *Circulation* 99, 591–595.

Tziros, C. and Freedman, J.E. (2006). *Curr. Drug Targ.* 7, 1243–1251.

Vinson, J.A. (1998). In Manthey, J.A. and Buslig, B.S. (eds), *Flavonoids in the Living System*. Plenum Press, New York.

Vinson, J.A., Mandarano, M., Hirst, M., Trevithick, J.R. and Bose, P. (2003). *J. Agric. Food Chem.* 51, 5528–5533.

Wallerath, T., Li, H., Godtel-Ambrust, U., Schwarz, P.M. and Forstermann, U. (2005). *Nitric Oxide* 12, 97.

Wang, S., Dusting, G.J., May, C.N. and Woodman, O.L. (2004). *Br. J. Pharmacol.* 142, 443–452.

Woodman, O.L., Meeker, W.F. and Boujaoude, M. (2005). *J. Cardiovasc. Pharmacol.* 46, 302–309.

Yang, Z. and Kaye, D.M. (2006). *Trend. Cardiovasc. Med.* 16, 118.

Zhang, Y.H., Park, Y.S., Kim, T.J., Fang, L.H., Ahn, H.Y., Hong, J.T., Kim, Y., Lee, C.K. and Yun, Y.P. (2002). *Gen. Pharmacol.* 35, 341–347.

86

The Anti-invasive and Proapoptotic Effect of Xanthohumol: Potential Use in Cancer

Barbara Vanhoecke and Marc Bracke Laboratory of Experimental Cancer Research, Department of Radiotherapy and Nuclear Medicine, Ghent University Hospital, Ghent, Belgium
Jerina Boelens, Sofie Lust and Fritz Offner Department of Hematology, Ghent University Hospital, Ghent, Belgium

Abstract

In recent years, a lot of attention has been paid to phytochemicals such as flavonoids with anticancer effects since they may interact with cellular signaling pathways controlling proliferation, differentiation, apoptosis and invasion. Invasion is the hallmark of malignancy, and the search for anti-invasive agents remains a challenge. A number of studies reported a promising role for xanthohumol (X) as a chemopreventive agent, since it can modulate the carcinogen metabolism and act by cytotoxic/-static mechanisms. Recently, X was investigated for its anti-invasive activity on human breast cancer cell lines and shown to inhibit the invasion of breast cancer cells in different invasion assays. One of the possible mechanisms of the anti-invasive effect of X includes the involvement of the E-cadherin/catenin invasion-suppressor complex. Another mechanism by which X influences the invasive behavior is by reducing the number of invasive cells (i.e. by promoting cell death). Recent data demonstrate that X induces a specific stress reaction (i.e. endoplasmic reticulum stress) followed by the unfolded protein response and programmed cell death (apoptosis). In this overview, we highlight the effect of X on invasion and survival of breast cancer cells and the mechanisms associated with these effects.

List of Abbreviations

8PN	8-Prenylnaringenin
APAF-1	Apoptotic protease activating factor 1
ATF6	Activating transcription factor 6
BiP	B-cell immunoglobulin heavy-chain binding protein
bZIP	Basic leucine zipper
CHI	Chick heart invasion assay
CHOP	C/EBP homologous protein-10, also known as GADD153
CI	Collagen invasion assay
CNX	Calnexin
COX	Cyclooxygenase
CRT	Calreticulin
cyt c	Cytochrome c
ECM	Extracellular matrix
eIF2α	α Subunit of eukaryotic translation initiation factor 2
ER	Endoplasmic reticulum
ERAD	Endoplasmic reticulum-associated degradation
ERSE	Endoplasmic reticulum-stress-responsive element
FAA	Fast aggregation assay
GRP	Glucose-regulated protein
IRE1	Inositol-requiring enzyme 1
NO	Nitrogen oxide
PCD	Programmed cell death
PDI	Protein-disulphide isomerase
PERK	Doublestranded RNA-activated protein kinase-like ER kinase
PG	Prostaglandin
PHF	Precultured heart fragment
PPI	Peptidyl–prolyl isomerases
QR	Quinone reductase
ROS	Reactive oxygen species
S1P	Site-1 protease
S2P	Site-2 protease
TF	Transcription factor
UPR	Unfolded protein response
UPRE	Unfolded protein response-responsive element
X	Xanthohumol
XBP1	X-box-binding protein 1

Introduction

A typical Asian diet contains approximately 150–200 mg flavonoids per day. These compounds are of particular interest, since they may interact with cellular signaling

Beer in Health and Disease Prevention
ISBN: 978-0-12-373891-2

pathways controlling proliferation, differentiation, apoptosis and invasion of cancer cells. Moreover, flavonoids have different targets in the cancer cell, in the normal host cell or in the extracellular matrix (ECM). This review focuses on the anticancer effect of the prenylated chalcone, xanthohumol (X). From a medical point of view, the prenylated flavonoids are most notable since they add unique health-beneficial properties to beer (Gerhaüser *et al.*, 2002). Prenylated flavonoids can be divided into two major groups: prenylated chalcones and prenylated flavanones. The most abundant prenylated flavonoid in the hop cones is X, which generally accounts for *ca.* 90% of the prenylated flavonoids in the hop plant (Stevens *et al.*, 1997). The structure of X was already described in 1957 as 6′-*O*-methyl-3′-prenylchalconaringenin (Verzele *et al.*, 1957). However, only during the last decade, X has gained attention as a promising cancer chemopreventive agent.

Recent studies reported that X can inhibit carcinogenesis at the initiation, promotion and progression stages of cancer. Consistent with its anti-initiating potential, X efficiently modulates the carcinogen metabolism at the level of carcinogen activation by CYP450 enzymes and at the level of detoxification by Phase II detoxifying enzymes like quinone reductase (QR) (Miranda *et al.*, 2000; Gerhaüser *et al.*, 2002). In addition, it contributes to the prevention of oxidative damage by scavenging reactive oxygen species (ROS) and nitrogen oxide (NO) production (Miranda *et al.*, 2000; Gerhaüser *et al.*, 2002; Zhao *et al.*, 2003). In the present review, we will note that X can also induce ROS formation (oxidative stress) which is associated with endoplasmic reticulum (ER) stress that ultimately results in selective cancer cell death.

Potential anticancer-promoting mechanisms include anti-inflammatory properties by inhibition of cyclooxygenase (COX) activity and anti-estrogenic activities. Excessive production of prostaglandins (PGs), endogenous mediators of inflammation, is associated with carcinogenesis. PGs are thought to stimulate proliferation and promote angiogenesis, essential for tumor growth (Subbaramaiah *et al.*, 1997). X was characterized as an effective anti-inflammatory agent by inhibiting the activity of COX-1 and COX-2 (Chi *et al.*, 2001; Gerhaüser *et al.*, 2002). Similar to PGs, hormones like estradiol are regarded as endogenous tumor promotors, stimulate tumor growth via interaction with estrogen receptors, and increase the risk for breast and uterine cancer (Reid *et al.*, 1996). X was identified as an anti-estrogen without intrinsic estrogenic potential, as demonstrated by the dose-dependent inhibition of estrogen-mediated induction of alkaline phosphatase activity and by a weak inhibition of cell growth in a human endometrial cell bio-assay for estrogenic activity (Gerhaüser *et al.*, 2002).

The progression phase of cancer cells is characterized by an uncontrolled cell proliferation independent of hormonal or growth factor stimulation. During this phase, important mechanisms regulating tissue homeostasis, such as apoptosis and terminal cell differentiation, are impaired (King and Cidlowski, 1995; Compagni and Christofori, 2000). X appeared to be the most effective anti-proliferative agent of six prenylated hop flavonoids in human breast cancer (MCF-7), colon cancer (HT-29) and ovarian cancer (A-2780) cells *in vitro* (Miranda *et al.*, 1999). Furthermore, X was found to inhibit DNA polymerase that can initiate *de novo* DNA synthesis (Gerhaüser *et al.*, 2002). Inhibition of DNA synthesis may be one of the mechanisms by which X exerts its anti-proliferative effect in cancer cells. However, additional mechanisms have been proposed. For example, X may cause growth arrest at more than one stage of the cell cycle (Miranda *et al.*, 1999). Gerhaüser *et al.* (2002) found that X causes a significant dose-dependent accumulation of breast cancer cells in the S-phase of the cell cycle and induces apoptosis of cancer cells after 48 h. In addition, X has been demonstrated to induce terminal differentiation in human promyelocytic leukemia cells (Gerhaüser *et al.*, 2002). In this review, the mechanisms associated with the proapoptotic effect of X will be described in detail.

Invasion and Progression

During the progression phase of cancer, new clones of cancer cells with increased proliferative capacity, invasiveness and metastatic potential arise and increase the malignancy of the disease. Invasion and metastasis are multistep processes (Figure 86.1) and result from the cross-talk between cancer cells and the microenvironmental elements of the host, that is, the ECM, fibroblastic cells (myofibroblasts), lymphocytes, macrophages, dentritic cells and endothelial cells. Paget's "seed and soil hypothesis" according to which the microenvironment of each organ (the soil) influences the survival and growth of the cancer cells (the seed) is still valid today (Paget, 1889). It implicates the destructive entry of the cancer cells into normal tissue by attachment to the ECM, proteolysis of these components, loss of cell–cell contacts, and subsequent migration through the ECM (Liotta and Kohn, 2001; Friedl, 2004). After survival in the circulation and arrest of metastatic cells in the vasculature, degradation of the basement membrane surrounding the blood vessels and extravasation occur. Survival and growth of the cancer cells at the site of extravasation results from interactions with the host cells and the ECM including activities like cell–cell adhesion, cell–matrix adhesion, proteolysis and motility. Like growth, survival and angiogenesis, invasion is the result of a balance between stimulatory and inhibitory factors.

Cellular activities associated with the invasive phenotype comprise cell–cell adhesion, cell–matrix adhesion, ectopic survival, migration and proteolysis. Based on previous reports that flavonoids possess potential anti-invasive properties *in vitro* (Bracke *et al.*, 1994, 1996; Rong *et al.*, 2001), the effect of X on cancer cell invasion has recently been

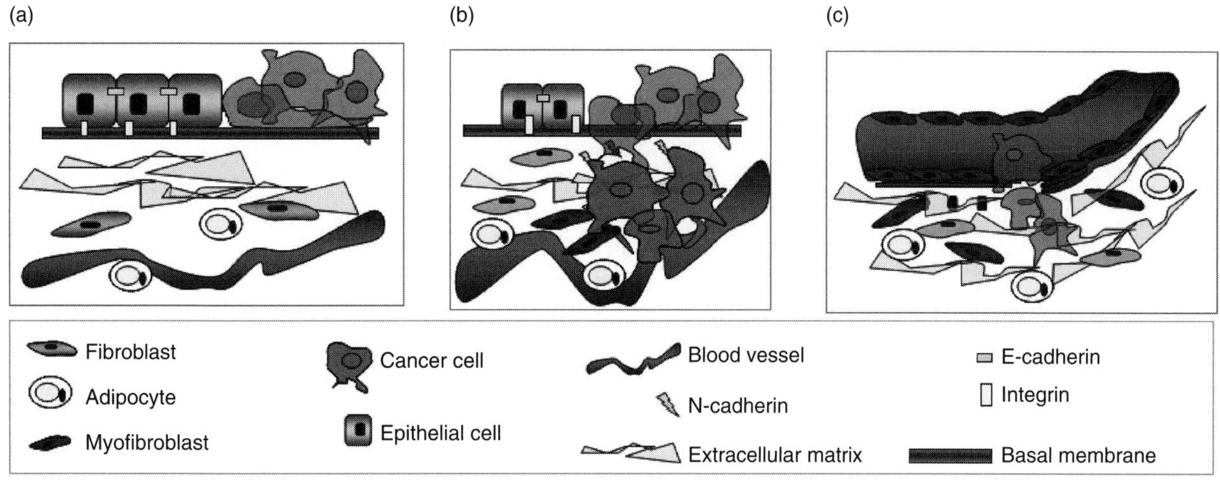

Figure 86.1 The multistep process of cancer: (a) During tumor progression, a series of cumulative genomic alterations modulate the transition from a normal to a malignant state. (b) During the multistep invasion process of metastasis, cancer cells invade from the primary tumor tissue through the basement membrane into the surrounding tissue. (c) They can enter the blood circulation (intravasation) (b) so that they can reach distant organs where they can form secondary tumors (metastasis) after extravasation, survival and growth. A continuous molecular cross-talk between tumor cells, host and environmental factors has an impact on a series of cellular activities such as growth, differentiation, ECM production and degradation, invasion, ectopic survival and metastasis. The success of the invasive process depends how cells interact with one another and with the other elements of the ecosystem.

investigated. By using the chick heart invasion assay (CHI) (Figure 86.2a), proven to be a valuable tool for evaluation of invasion (Bracke *et al.*, 2001), evidence was provided that X inhibits invasion of breast cancer cells into normal chick heart tissue (Vanhoecke *et al.*, 2005). This anti-invasive effect was confirmed in another invasion assay (i.e. the collagen invasion assay, CI) (Bracke *et al.*, 2001) (Figure 86.2b). Collagen type I is the most abundant protein in humans and the fibers are extremely stable structures. During cancer invasion, the rates of collagen type I and of other ECM elements degradation are accelerated. Native collagen type I is degraded by matrix-metalloproteinases which are zinc-dependent endopeptidases expressed at low levels in normal adult tissues and upregulated during normal and pathological remodeling processes, embryonic development, inflammation, tumor invasion and metastasis (Birkedal-Hansen, 1995; Egeblad and Werb, 2002). Pericellular breakdown of ECM components generates localized matrix defects and remodeling along migration tracks. However, cancer cells do not always rely on proteolytic matrix remodeling for migration, but rather acquire a shape change to allow gliding and squeezing through gaps and trails present in connective tissues (Friedl and Wolf, 2003). To invade the surrounding tissue and to metastasize at the secondary site, cancer cells must cross the ECM barrier which comprises the basement membrane and the interstitial stroma. Collagen type IV, laminin, entactin and heparan sulfate proteoglycans are the major constituents of the basement membrane while collagen type I and III, elastin, vitronectin, proteoglycans and glycoproteins are the major constituents of the interstitial stroma.

Effect of X on Invasion of Breast Cancer Cells

To screen a potential anti-invasive effect of X, three cell lines derived from human mammary carcinomas (MCF-7/6, MCF-7/AZ and T47-D) were used. These cell lines were selected because they have retained many morphological and biochemical characteristics of their mammary origin, such as the expression of the estrogen receptor α (Bracke *et al.*, 1991) and their striking differences in invasive properties in the CHI model (Vanhoecke *et al.*, 2005). MCF-7/6 cells spontaneously invade into the chick heart tissue, whereas MCF-7/AZ and T47-D formed a non-invasive multilayered epithelium covering the heart fragments. Earlier studies also demonstrated the existence of invasive and non-invasive variants of the MCF-7 cell population (Rong *et al.*, 2001).

The effect of X on invasion of MCF-7/6 cells into chick heart fragments was examined during 8 days of treatment using varying concentrations (0.1, 1, 5, 10, 20, 50 and 100 μM); 5 μM X inhibited invasion of MCF-7/6 cells completely, and the effect could be described as Grade I. Immunohistochemical staining with 5D10, a specific anti body against the MCF-7 cells, confirmed that no cancer cells had invaded the chick heart (Figure 86.2c right panel), in contrast to the untreated cells (Figure 86.2c left panel). Lower concentrations (<1 μM) only partially inhibited invasion whereas higher concentrations (10, 20, 50 and 100 μM) were toxic both for MCF-7/6 cells and the chick heart tissue. The anti-invasive effect was not due to irreversible cytotoxicity or increased resistance of the chick

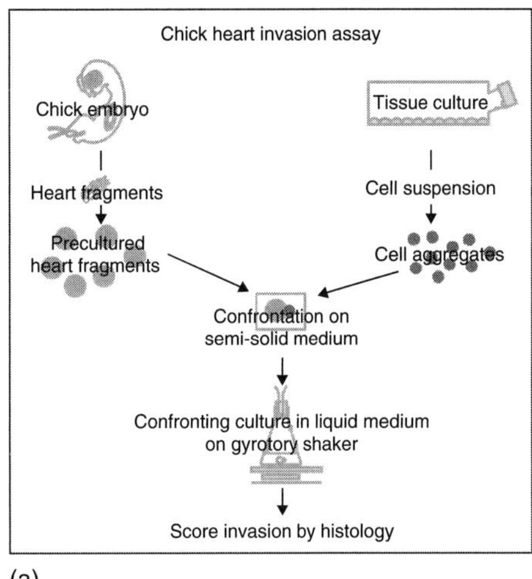

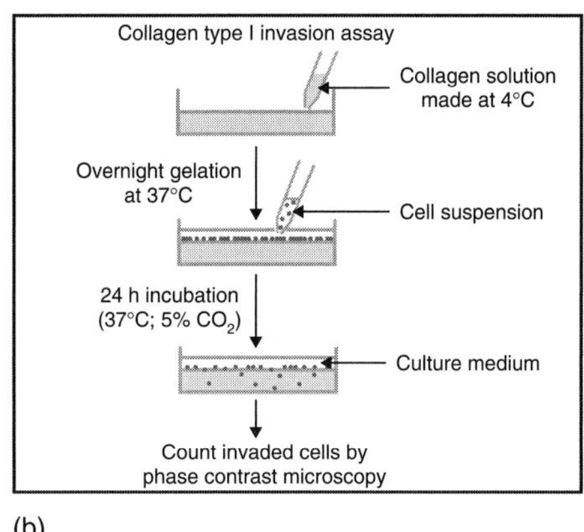

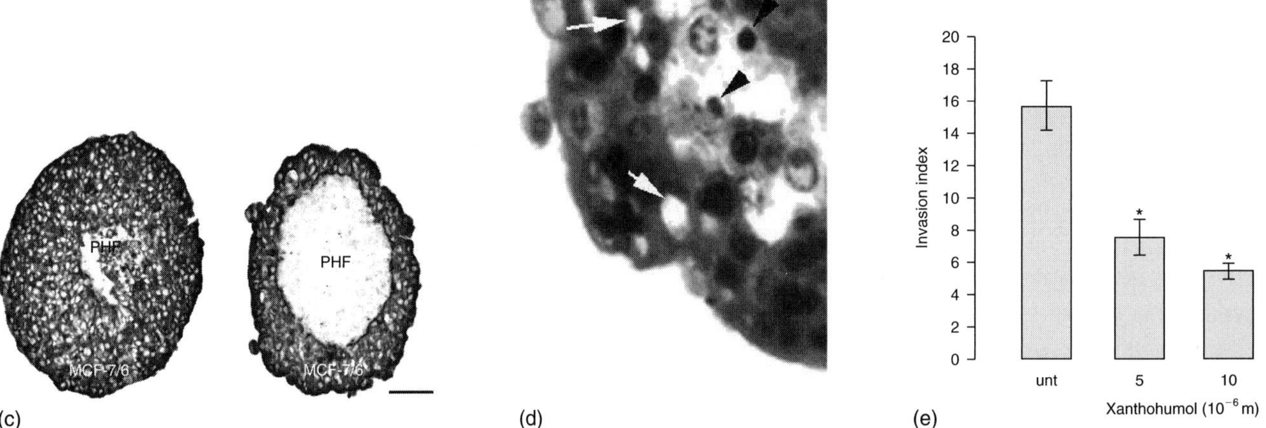

Figure 86.2 The effect of X on invasion: (a) Chick heart invasion assay. In CHI, heart tissue fragments are dissected from 9-day-old chicken embryos and precultured to obtain living spheroids with a standard diameter of 0.4 mm. These precultured heart fragments (PHFs) are mainly composed by cardiomyocytes, but fibroblasts and endothelial cells are present as well. The ECM contains laminin, fibronectin, collagen type IV and collagen type I. These PHFs are confronted with standard volume aggregates (diameter 0.2 mm) of invasive test cells, such as human MCF-7/6 breast cancer cells (Soule *et al.*, 1973). The aggregates become attached to PHFs by incubation on a semi-solid agar bed overnight and are then transferred as individual pairs into mini-Erlenmeyer flasks for suspension culture in liquid medium. After 8 days of incubation on a gyratory shaker, the cultures are fixed and imbedded for histology. After serial sectioning and staining of the sections with hematoxylin–eosin, the interaction of the cancer cells with the PHF can be reconstructed tri-dimensionally from microscopic analysis of all sections. Although automated image analysis systems are available, the results can be classified along a 5-grades objective scale: Grade 0: Only PHF is found. No confronting cells can be observed. Grade I: The confronting test cells are attached to the PHF and do not occupy the heart tissue. Grade II: Occupation of the PHF is limited to the outer fibroblast-like and myoblast cell layers. Grade III: The confronting cells have occupied the PHF, but have left more than half of the original amount of heart tissue intact. Grade IV: The confronting cells have occupied more than half of the original volume of the PHF. The assay has proven to be relevant to cancer invasion in cancer patients for multiple reasons: Invasion is progressive in time and space as it is in natural tumors, the histological pattern of invasion resembles the one observed in the tumor of origin, and the assay discriminates between benign (non-invasive) and malignant (invasive) tumors. However, the assay does not cover all aspects of invasion, as it does not take into account the contribution of immune cells. (b) Collagen invasion assay. Collagen gels, with a minimum thickness of 250 μm, are prepared in a 6-well plate (Nunc, Roskilde, Denmark), from a collagen type I solution (Upstate Biotechnology, Lake Pacid, NY), and polymerized overnight at 37°C. Cancer cells are incubated on top of these collagen gels for 24 h at 37°C in presence or absence of a test compound. The number of cells penetrating into the gel or remaining at the surface can be counted using an inverted-microscope controlled by a computer program. Invasion indices (%) are ratios between the number of invaded cells inside the collagen gel and the total number of cells, counted in at least 12 microscopic fields and determined with a computer-assisted-inverted-microscope (Bracke *et al.*, 2001; Vakaet *et al.*, 1991). (c) Light micrographs of sections from 8-days-old confronting cultures of PHFs and MCF-7/6 cells. Untreated confrontations (left panel) are compared with confrontations treated with 5 μM X (right panel). MCF-7/6 cells were stained immunohistochemically with the monoclonal antibody 5D10 and appear dark. Scale bar = 50 μm. (d) Detailed morphological analysis of the confronting cultures revealed a selective effect of X on the MCF-7/6 cells. Nuclear pyknosis (arrowheads, black) and vacuolization (arrows, white) could be observed in the MCF-7/6 cells but not in the heart cells. Scale bar = 50 μm. (e) Effect of X on invasion of T47-D cells into collagen type I gel. Cells were treated with varying concentrations for 24 h. Results are presented as percentage (%) of invasion (percentage of penetrating cells divided by the total number of cells; mean ± standard deviation). The % of invasion of X-treated T47-D cells is compared with the % of invasion of solvent-treated cells (unt). Asterisks: ρ value ≤ 0.001.

heart tissue against the invasive behavior of the MCF-7/6. Moreover, the effect of X appeared to be selective for the cancer cells as signs of nuclear pyknosis and vacuolization were present in the MCF-7/6 cells but not in the chick heart cells (Figure 86.2d).

Furthermore, the CI assay was performed to evaluate if the anti-invasive effect of X was restricted to MCF-7/6 cells. Invasiveness of MCF-7/6, MCF-7/AZ and T47-D cells was assessed and MCF-7/6 and MCF-7/AZ cells were considered non-invasive (1–2%) whereas T47-D strongly invaded the collagen gel (10–15%). Consequently, T47-D cells were chosen to test varying X concentrations (5, 10 and 30 μM) and a significant concentration-dependent anti-invasive effect could be observed after 24 h (Figure 86.2e).

An anti-invasive effect can be based either on a reduction of the number of invasive cancer cells, on a decreased invasiveness per cell or on an increased resistance toward invasion (Parmar *et al.*, 1997). However, a number of data suggested that the target of X resides in the cancer cells. Morphological analysis of the confronting cultures and growth assays with aggregates and cell cultures, clearly depicted a cytotoxic effect of X on the cancer cells while normal cells remained unaffected. Therefore, X could target specific activities implicated in breast cancer progression, like cell–cell adhesion *via* the E-cadherin/catenin complex, as reported for other flavonoids like 8-prenylnaringenin (8PN) (Rong *et al.*, 2001), genistein and daidzein (Maubach *et al.*, 2003). Cell–cell adhesion has a critical role in morphogenesis, establishment of tissue architecture, cell–cell communication and normal cell growth and ensures tissue integrity. During malignant transformation and invasion of epithelial tumors, cell–cell adhesion is often disrupted. The prototype of homotypic cell–cell adhesion (this is between cells of the same type) is the invasion-suppressor molecule E-cadherin, the major cadherin present in polarized epithelial cells (Bracke *et al.*, 1996; Mareel *et al.*, 1997). Cadherins form a family of cell-surface glycoproteins that function in promoting calcium-dependent cell–cell adhesion and serve as the transmembrane components of adherens junctions. Cell–cell adhesions are formed through the stable calcium-dependent binding of a dimer of another cell. Intracellularly, the E-cadherin molecule is attached to the actin cytoskeleton via the catenins that interact with transmembrane or cytoplasmic proteins (Figure 86.3). Disruption of the E-cadherin/catenin complex or one of its components may therefore promote invasion and is a common feature of carcinoma cells. Yet, mutations of the genes of these molecules are rare in human cancer. Therefore, agents that influence positively or negatively E-cadherin-mediated cellular responses, may stimulate or inhibit invasion. As the complex appears to be amenable to hormonal modulation by (anti-)estrogens, resulting in the upregulation of E-cadherin expression (Blaschuk and Farookhi, 1989) or function in mammary cancer cells (Bracke *et al.*, 1994),

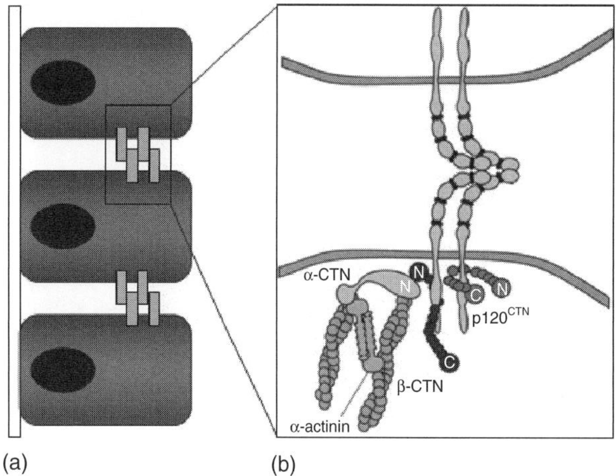

Figure 86.3 The E-cadherin/catenin complex (simplified scheme): E-cadherin is a calcium-dependent transmembrane protein involved in adhesion junctions of epithelial cells. It typically connects epithelial cells, reducing their invasion potential. (a) Its extracellular domain mediates homophilic interaction with E-cadherin expressed by adjacent cells. The association of E-cadherin cytoplasmic domain to cytoplasmic proteins called catenins is necessary for strong cell adhesion. E-cadherin C-terminus interacts directly with β-catenin (β-CTN/PLAKO), which in turn binds α-catenin (α-CTN) and α-actinin to provide a link between E-cadherin and the actin cytoskeleton. p120ctn is a catenin which binds directly to the juxtamembrane region of E-cadherin (B). *Abbreviation list*: CTN, catenin.

Rong *et al.* (2001) evaluated if the hop phytoestrogen 8PN was able to influence the cell–cell aggregation of MCF-7/6 cells, which have a defective E-cadherin/catenin complex. Indeed, they found that aggregates treated with 8PN were larger than their untreated counterparts and that increased cell–cell adhesion and cell number contributed to this phenomenon. In parallel, our group showed that X stimulates cell–cell adhesion in an E-cadherin-mediated manner in an aggregation assay (Figure 86.4a). The assay is based on the preparation of a single-cell suspension in E-cadherin-saving conditions followed by quantification of cell aggregation in a calcium-containing medium (Boterberg *et al.*, 2001). Subsequently, the suspension was treated with varying X concentrations for 30 min at 4°C and incubated at 37°C for 30 min under continuous shaking, while untreated cells were incubated with 0.1% EtOH. Cells were fixed in 2.5% paraformaldehyde at the start of the incubation and after 30 min and the particle size distribution was measured with a Coulter Particle Size Counter LS 200 (Coulter Company, Miami, FL, USA). Thus, using human MCF-7/6 breast cancer cells with a functionally defective E-cadherin/catenin complex, we demonstrated that X was able to stimulate aggregation of MCF-7/6 cells in suspension thereby restoring the function of the complex (Figure 86.4b) (Vanhoecke *et al.*, 2005). The implication of E-cadherin was indicated by a neutralizing monoclonal antibody, MB2, which functionally blocks the molecule. Co-treatment with X and MB2 during

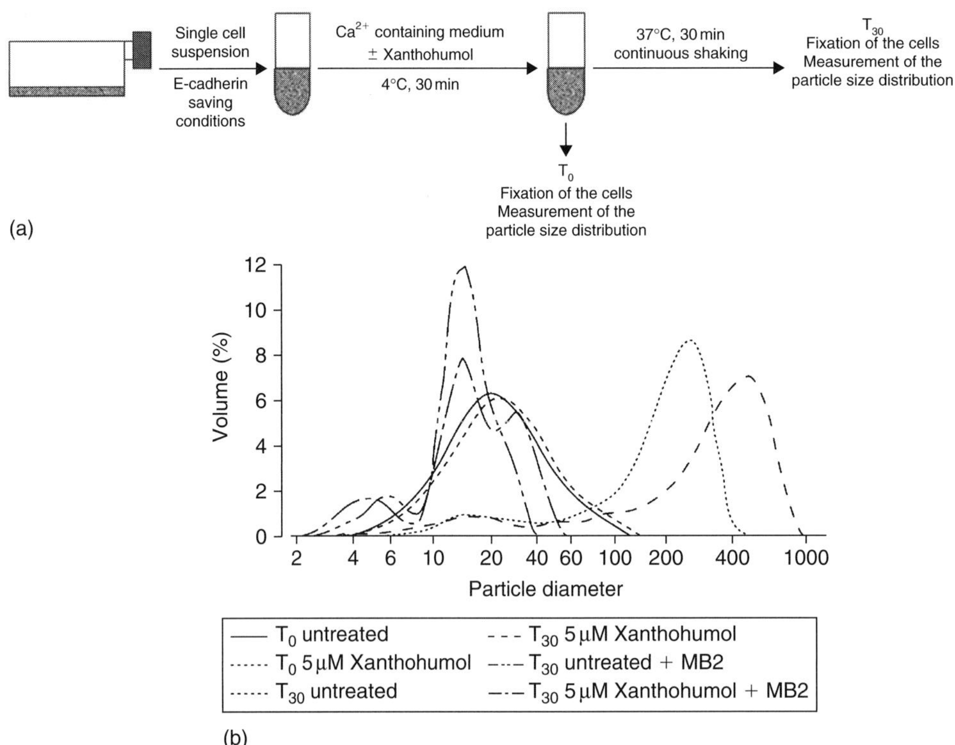

Figure 86.4 The effect of X on cell–cell adhesion: (a) The aggregation assay is based on the preparation of a single-cell suspension in E-cadherin-saving conditions followed by quantification of cell aggregation in a calcium-containing medium. The suspension is treated with the test compound for 30 min at 4°C and incubated at 37°C for 30 min under continuous shaking. Cells are fixed in 2.5% paraformaldehyde at the start of the incubation (N_0) and after 30 min (N_{30}) and the particle size distribution is measured with a Coulter Particle Size Counter LS 200 (Coulter Company, Miami, FL, USA). (b) Breast cancer cells (MCF-7/6) were pretreated for 24 h with varying X concentrations followed by trypsinization in E-cadherin-saving conditions to preserve E-cadherin-mediated cell–cell adhesion during the assay. In the presence of a calcium-containing aggregation buffer, cells were allowed to aggregate for 30 min in the presence or the absence of varying X concentrations. The initial mean particle diameter of the MCF-7/6 cells at time zero was 27.65 μm for solvent-treated cells (T_0 untreated) and 30.27 μm for the 5 μM X-treated cells (T_0 5 μM X), indicating suspensions of single cells or cell doublets in both conditions. After 30 min, the mean particle diameter shifted toward 177.4 μm for solvent-treated cells indicating aggregates of around 6 cells (T_{30} untreated). However, for X-treated cells aggregates of around 11 cells were formed and the mean particle diameter shifted toward 328.2 μm (T_{30} 5 μM X). The implication of E-cadherin was indicated by a neutralizing monoclonal antibody, MB2, which functionally blocks the molecule. Co-treatment with X and MB2 (T_{30} 5 μM X + MB2) during aggregation completely abrogated the effect of 5 μM X (T_{30} 5 μM X). *Abbreviation list*: MB2, monoclonal antibody 2.

aggregation completely abrogated the effect of X. However, the molecular mechanisms underlying this stimulated E-cadherin-mediated cell–cell adhesion have not yet been unraveled.

Recently, Albini *et al.* (2006) showed that X inhibited proliferation of both endothelial and KS-IMM tumor cells and strongly reduced their invasion in different *in vitro* invasion models. Moreover, they demonstrated that X was able to reduce solid tumor growth and angiogenesis *in vivo*. These observations suggest that X interferes with the molecular mechanisms of migration and survival as was evidenced by the inhibitory effects of X on NF-κB and Akt pathways both involved in the regulation of invasion, migratory and prosurvival signaling pathways.

Apart from its effect on cell–cell adhesion, X might also influence factors like cytokines and growth factors present in the microenvironment of the confronting cultures that are associated with cancer cell invasion (Rolland *et al.*, 1980; Rozic *et al.*, 2001; Wülfing *et al.*, 2003). Indeed, X has been reported to reduce inflammation by inhibiting the activity of COXs and the production of PGs via this route (Gerhaüser *et al.*, 2002), and may, directly or indirectly, affect the invasive potential of the cancer cells.

ER Stress, Survival and Apoptosis

In eukaryotic cells, the ER is the principal site for folding and maturation of transmembrane, secretory and ER-resident proteins. Functions of the ER are affected by various intracellular and extracellular stimuli, which include inhibition of glycosylation, reduction of disulfide bonds, calcium depletion from the ER lumen, impairment of protein transport to the Golgi and expression of mutated proteins in the ER.

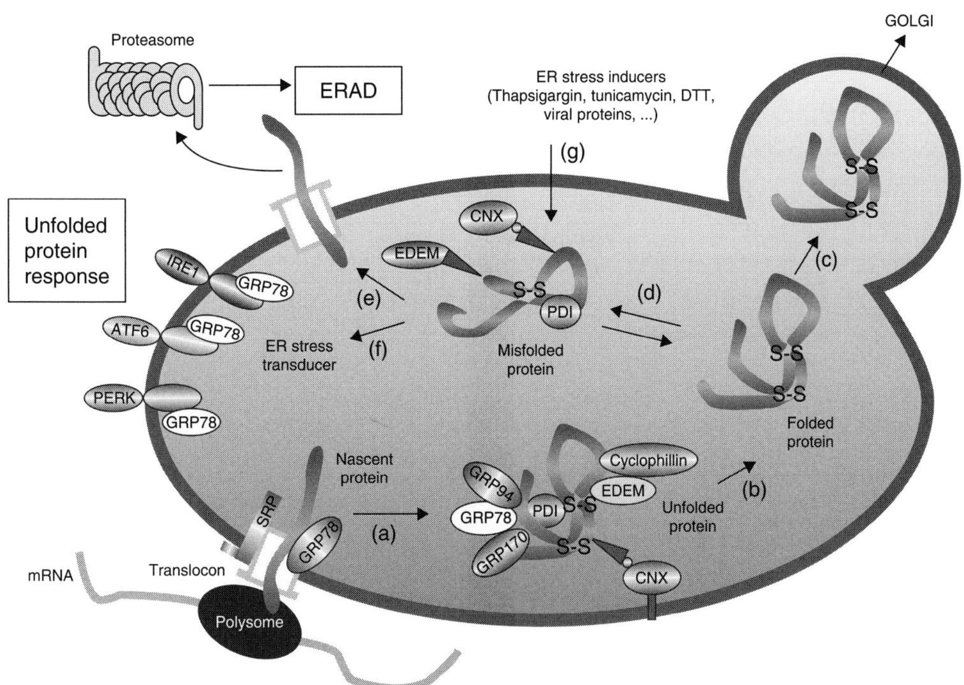

Figure 86.5 ER functions under non-stress conditions. (a) Proteins that are destined for synthesis in the ER are recognized, through signal peptides, by the signal recognition particle (SRP), which associates with the ribosome. The complex diffuses to the translocon, where the SRP docks with the SRP receptor (SR). GRP78 is the chaperone responsible for maintaining the permeability barrier of the ER translocon, the proteinaceous channel in the ER-membrane to which a nascent peptide is transferred for folding and assembly in the ER, during the early stages of protein translocation. Once the nascent peptide chains reache a length of 70 amino acids, GRP78 is released from the translocon, opening the channel to allow translocation of the protein into the luminal space. (b) As the nascent peptide is entering the ER, it is often modified by addition of *N*-linked glycans before folding. In the extremely crowded, calcium-rich, oxidizing environment of the ER lumen, resident chaperones like GRP78, GRP94, GRP170, CNX, CRT, PDI and ER-degradation-enhancing α-mannosidase-like protein (EDEM) serve to facilitate proper folding of the nascent protein by preventing its aggregation, monitoring the processing of the highly branched glycans, and forming disulfide bonds to stabilize the folded protein. (c) Once correctly folded and modified, the protein will exit the ER through coat protein (COP) II-coated vesicles and move to the Golgi apparatus through the secretory pathway. (d) Misfolded proteins can associate with CNX, PDI and EDEM (e) for retrotranslocation to the cytosol, ubiquitination and digestion by the proteasome via a process called the ERAD. (f) Perturbations that alter the ER homeostasis disrupt folding, and lead to the accumulation of unfolded proteins and protein aggregates, which are detrimental to cell survival. As a consequence, the cell has evolved an adaptive coordinated response to limit further accumulation of unfolded proteins in the ER. This signaling pathway is termed as the UPR and is associated with the activation of three ER-stress transducers, namely the PERK, the IRE1 and ATF6. GRP78 is the master regulator of the activation of the ER-stress transducers. In non-stress conditions, the ER-stress sensors are associated with GRP78, which keeps them in their inactive state. (g) The functions of the ER can be affected by various extracellular stimuli, so called ER stress. ER stress can be induced by agents that interfere with protein glycosylation (i.e. glucose starvation, tunicamycin, calcium balance (i.e. thapsigargin), disulfide bond formation (i.e. dithiotreitol (DTT)), and/or by a general protein overload of the ER (i.e. viral and non-viral oncogenesis). *Abbreviation list*: pATF6, cleaved ATF6.

Under ER stress, unfolded/misfolded proteins accumulate in the ER lumen, which induces conflicting cellular activities: survival and apoptosis. To cope with this stress, cells activate intracellular signaling pathways such as the unfolded protein response (UPR) and the ER-associated degradation (ERAD). However, under conditions of severe ER stress or when the UPR has been compromised, the cell may be incapable of maintaining ER homeostasis, which may eventually activate programmed cell death (PCD) pathways.

To assist in the folding of nascent polypeptides and to prevent aggregation of folding intermediates, the ER contains a high concentration of chaperones including the glucose-regulated proteins (GRPs), calnexin (CNX), calreticulin (CRT), peptidyl–prolyl isomerases (PPI), and protein-disulphide isomerase (PDI) (Gething and Sambrook, 1992). In addition to their role in folding, some of these chaperones act as a quality control system to ensure that only correctly folded proteins proceed to the Golgi apparatus for further processing and secretion (Kuznetsov *et al.*, 1997; Ellgaard *et al.*, 1999) (Figure 86.5). Of particular interest is the chaperone GRP78, which has been characterized in B-cells as part of the immunoglobulin secretory machinery and is also known as B-cell immunoglobulin heavy-chain binding protein (BiP), due to its association with incompletely assembled subunits of antibody

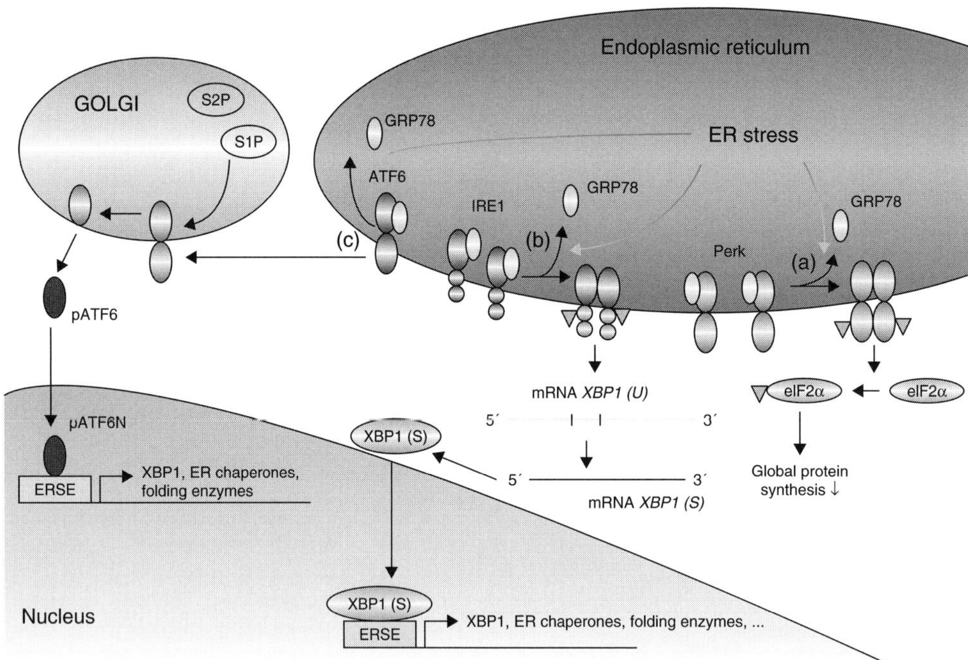

Figure 86.6 ER functions under stress conditions. (a) On accumulation of unfolded proteins in the ER lumen, GRP78 releases from PERK is activated to phosphorylate eIF2 on the α-subunit at Ser51. As phosphorylation of eIF2α reduces the functional level of eIF2α, the general rate of translation initiation is reduced. (b) In parallel, IRE1 dimerizes and activates its endoribonuclease activity after its release from GRP78. It splices its substrate XBP1 mRNA to remove a small intron, which changes the translational reading frame of XBP1 to yield a potent transcriptional activator that activates the transcription of responsive genes, including XBP1, ER chaperones and folding enzymes. (c) At the same time, ATF6 moves to the Golgi compartment, where it is cleaved by the S1P and S2P to yield a cytosolic fragment. This p50ATF6 fragment (pATF6) migrates to the nucleus to activate the transcription of responsive genes, including XBP1, ER chaperones and folding enzymes. *Abbreviation list*: XBP1(u), X-box-binding protein 1 (unspliced); XBP1(s), X-box-binding protein 1 (spliced).

molecules (Haas and Wabl, 1983; Bole *et al.*, 1986). GRP78 resides primarily within the ER (Munro and Pelham, 1986; Haas, 1994; Little *et al.*, 1994) and although it is constitutively expressed, its expression is enhanced up to 20-fold in cells under a variety of stressful conditions or agents that interfere with protein glycosylation, folding, transport, and disrupt calcium homeostasis (Lee, 1992; Li *et al.*, 1993).

The functions of the ER can be affected by various intra- or extracellular stimuli. Agents that interfere with protein glycosylation, calcium balance, disulfide bond formation and/or by a general protein overload of the ER are well-known inducers of ER stress (Kaufman, 1999; Pahl, 1999; Lee, 2001), therefore disrupt folding and lead to the accumulation of unfolded proteins and protein aggregates. As a consequence, the cell has evolved an adaptive coordinated response to limit further accumulation of unfolded proteins in the ER which are detrimental for cell survival. This signaling pathway is termed as the UPR and consists of three different mechanisms: (1) translational attenuation to further limit the synthesis of misfolded proteins (Harding *et al.*, 1999); (2) transcriptional activation of genes encoding ER-resident chaperones (Gething and Sambrook, 1992) and (3) ERAD, which serves to reduce the stress and thereby restores the folding capacity by directing misfolded proteins in the ER back into the cytosol for degradation by the 26S proteasome (reviewed by Meusser *et al.*, 2005). This integrated intracellular signaling pathway transmits information about the protein folding status in the ER lumen to the cytoplasm and the nucleus via the activation of three ER-stress sensor molecules namely the doublestranded RNA-activated protein kinase-like ER kinase (PERK), the inositol-requiring enzyme 1 (IRE1) and activating transcription factor 6 (ATF6) (Figure 86.6).

PERK is an ER-resident transmembrane serine/threonine protein kinase, which consists of an ER luminal stress-sensing domain, a transmembrane domain, and a cytosolic domain with kinase activity that phosphorylates the α subunit of eukaryotic translation initiation factor 2 (eIF2α) in response to ER stress (Shi *et al.*, 1998; Harding *et al.*, 1999; Liu *et al.*, 2000). Phosphorylation of eIF2α reduces formation of translation initiation complexes and thus translation.

IRE1 is an ER-transmembrane glycoprotein consisting of a *N*-terminal ER luminal stress-sensing domain, a transmembrane domain, and a cytosolic domain with both serine/threonine kinase and *C*-terminal endoribonuclease activities (Tirasophon *et al.*, 1998; Wang *et al.*, 1998). ER stress initiates its dimerization and autophosphorylation

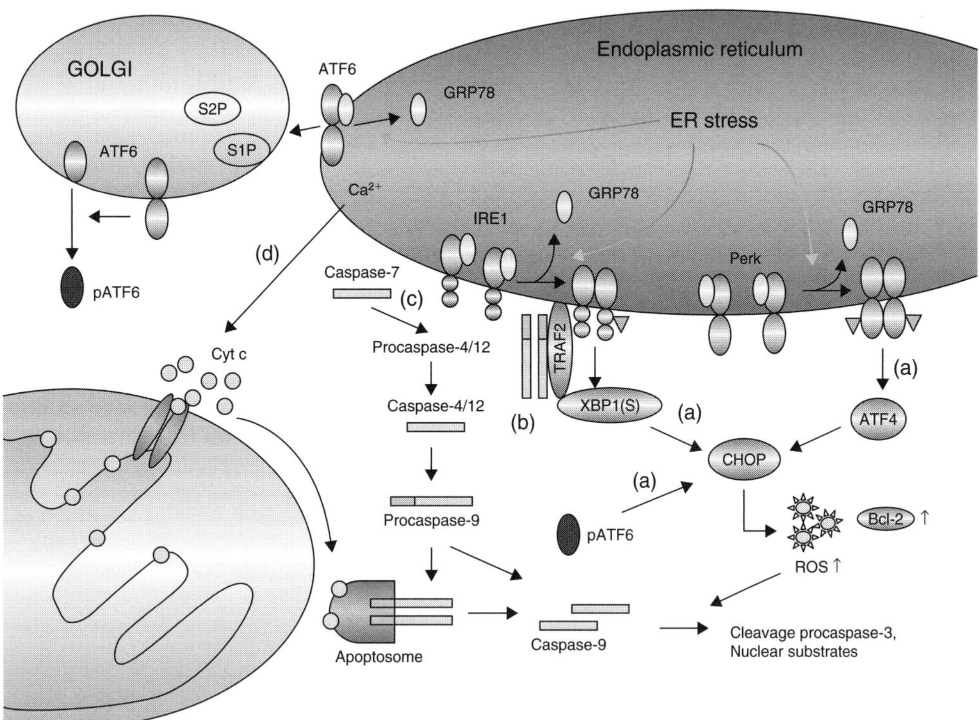

Figure 86.7 ER stress and apoptosis (simplified scheme): (a) Activation of PERK can result in the preferential translation of selective mRNAs under ER stress. Translational upregulation of ATF4 yields a potent transcriptional activator that activates the transcription of responsive genes, including CHOP. CHOP can also be induced by activation of ATF6 and IRE1. Upregulation of CHOP results in the downregulation of the anti-apoptotic proteins bcl-2 and bcl-xL and in ROS accumulation. The disturbed balance between proapoptotic proteins, for example, bad, bak and bax, and the anti-apoptotic bcl-2 proteins and the increase in oxidative stress activate the intrinsic apoptotic pathway. (b) By sequestering IRE1, TNF-receptor-activating factor 2 (TRAF2) promotes clustering of and release from ER-localized procaspase-12/-4 upon ER stress. Procaspase-12/-4 is then converted to caspase-12/-4 which initiates a caspase cascade through cleavage of procaspase-9 and -3. This pathway is independent of APAF-1 and mitochondrial cyt c release. (c) Furthermore, procaspase-12 can be activated by caspase-7 after its relocation from the cytosol to the ER. (d) Calcium released from the ER is rapidly taken up by the mitochondria, where it may lead to collapse of the inner membrane potential, cytochrome (cyt c) release and subsequent initiation of the caspase cascade.

to activate its kinase and RNase activities. The splicing of its substrate, the mRNA of X-box-binding protein 1 (XBP1), a basic leucine zipper (bZIP)-containing transcription factor (TF), removes a 26-nucleotide intron leading to a potent TF that binds to the unfolded protein response-responsive element (UPRE) and ER-stress-responsive element (ERSE) sequence of many ER stress and UPR-target genes (Yoshida *et al.*, 2001; Lee *et al.*, 2002).

p90/p110ATF6 is an ER-resident ATF consisting of a cytosolic *N*-terminal (bZIP) domain, a transmembrane domain and a *C*-terminal ER luminal stress-sensing domain (Haze *et al.*, 1999). Upon ER stress, ATF6 transits to the Golgi compartment where it is cleaved by Golgi site 1 and site-2 proteases (S1P and S2P) to generate a fragment, namely p50ATF6 (Brown and Goldstein, 1997; Yoshida *et al.*, 1998; Haze *et al.*, 1999; Kaufman, 1999; Li *et al.*, 2000; Wang, 2000; Ye *et al.*, 2000; Sakai and Rawson, 2001). p50ATF6 then translocates to the nucleus where it binds to the ERSE of target genes.

GRP78 is the master regulator of the activation of the ER-stress sensors. Under normal conditions, GRP78 serves as a negative regulator of IRE1, PERK and ATF6. However, upon ER stress, GRP78 releases from the transducers and binds to unfolded proteins. GRP78 release from IRE1 and PERK permits their homodimerization and activation (Bertolotti *et al.*, 2000; Liu *et al.*, 2000). GRP78 release from ATF6 permits its transport to the Golgi compartment (Ye *et al.*, 2000; Shen *et al.*, 2005).

For many years, two major pathways of PCD were believed to induce apoptosis namely the intrinsic pathway, which is mainly controlled at the level of the mitochondria, and the extrinsic pathway, which is regulated by binding of specific death ligands to their receptors on the cell surface. However, a number of recent studies have now provided convincing evidence that PCD cascades can be initiated also at other sites within the cell, in particular, organelles such as the ER and the Golgi apparatus. Indeed, although the UPR is a cytoprotective response, prolonged ER stress can activate PCD through mitochondria-dependent or mitochondria-independent pathways (Rao *et al.*, 2002; Breckenridge *et al.*, 2003) (Figure 86.7). While attenuating global protein synthesis, phosphorylation of eIF2α by PERK promotes preferential translation of ATF4 mRNA, which results in transcriptional induction of a proapoptotic protein, namely CHOP (C/EBP homologous protein-10, also known as GADD153) (Wang *et al.*, 1998; Harding *et al.*, 2000). CHOP is able to transcriptionally downregulate the levels of the anti-apoptotic bcl-2 and upregulate DR5, a ember of the death receptor protein family (Yamaguchi and Wang, 2004). In addition, CHOP leads to a depletion of the cellular glutathione levels (Marciniak *et al.*, 2004) and it increases the levels of ROS in the cell (McCullough *et al.*, 2001). This results in leakage of mitochondrial cytochrome c (cyt c), activation of cytosolic apoptotic protease activating factor 1 (APAF-1), and stimulation of caspase-9 and -3.

ER stress can also activate general regulators of apoptosis, including the bcl-2 and caspase families of proteins. Several BH3-only proapoptotic members of the bcl-2 family, including bim (Morishima *et al.*, 2004), bik (Germain *et al.*, 2002, 2005; Mathai *et al.*, 2002, 2005), PUMA (Reimertz *et al.*, 2003; Li *et al.*, 2006), bax and bak (Nutt *et al.*, 2002a, b; Scorrano *et al.*, 2003; Zong *et al.*, 2003; Oakes *et al.*, 2005) can be involved. Accumulation of these proapoptotic members may antagonize ER-membrane-resident anti-apoptotic members such as bcl-xL and bcl-2, resulting in structural changes of the ER, ER calcium release and/or caspase-12 activation (Breckenridge *et al.*, 2003; Zong *et al.*, 2003). Caspases are required for apoptosis, and certain members of this family of cysteine proteinases associate with the ER-like caspase-12/-4. Although caspase-12 may play an important role during ER stress-induced apoptosis, it has recently been shown that its expression is not required for apoptosis, as cells lacking caspase-12 were not protected from apoptosis after treatment with ER-stress agents (Obeng and Boise, 2005). Procaspase-12 can also be cleaved by caspase-7. Rao *et al.* (2002) demonstrated that ER stress induces translocation of cytosolic caspase-7 to the ER surface followed by cleavage of procaspase-12.

Also stress-activated protein kinases such as JNK and p38MAPK can be activated during ER stress through signaling from the ER-stress transducers to the cell nucleus (Urano *et al.*, 2000) and are involved during apoptosis.

The ability of the cell to detoxify ROS and thus oxidative stress is crucial for homeostasis and survival. Indeed, free radical production has been implied in development of cancer, progression of neurodegenerative diseases and in ageing processes (Hayes and Pulford, 1995; Richter *et al.*, 1995; Hayes *et al.*, 1999). Intracellular glutathione levels serve as buffer of oxidative stress and reduced glutathione plays an active role in removal of toxic compounds via binding and promoting ROS export (Richter *et al.*, 1995). ER stress can induce oxidative stress due to the formation of ROS (Rushmore *et al.*, 1991). The cellular response to ROS is the induction of genes that encode proteins that function as antioxidants and enzymes involved in glutathione biosynthesis (Rushmore *et al.*, 1991; Hayes and Pulford, 1995; Hayes *et al.*, 1999).

Effect of X on Survival of Breast Cancer Cells

Chemical ER-stress inducers like tunicamycin, thapsigargin and brefeldin A are well reported to induce cell death via a disturbance of the ER homeostasis. Recently, our laboratory discovered that X induces ER stress and apoptosis in various human breast cancer cell lines but not in human primary normal breast epithelial cells (unpublished data). In T47-D breast cancer cells, X stimulates the transcription (evidenced by quantitative RT-PCR) and translation (evidenced by Western blotting) of the ER chaperone GRP78, the marker for ER stress. During the X-induced ER stress, the ER-stress transducers PERK, IRE1 and ATF6 are activated. X stimulated the phosphorylation of eIF2α, the splicing of XBP1 and the cleavage of ATF6. Furthermore, sustained ER stress eventually resulted in apoptotic events like activation of caspase-9 and -3, downregulation of expression of anti-apoptotic proteins bcl-xL and mcl-1, upregulation of the proapoptotic CHOP and ATF4, accumulation of ROS and stimulated poly(ADP)ribose-polymerase (PARP) cleavage, a marker of late apoptosis (Figure 86.8). Interestingly, susceptibility to the X-induced apoptosis appeared to correlate with the GRP78 expression levels as MCF-7/6 cells in which GRP78 expression levels were unaltered after treatment with X, were shown to be most sensitive to apoptosis.

Thus – and in contrast to what is published about the molecular mechanisms of flavonoid-induced apoptosis – the proapoptotic effect of X appeared to be associated with a chronic stress condition in the cancer cells. In that respect, we note that flavonoids can initiate, apart from an oxidative stress response, an ER-stress response, that ultimately results in apoptosis and cell death. As the ER-stress response is characterized by an upregulation of the ER-stress chaperone, GRP78 and based on the observations that X induced in some, but not all, breast cancer cell lines GRP78 upregulation, it is interesting to unravel the role of this chaperone in the resistance of breast cancer cells to X.

In conclusion, X has multiple effects on human breast cancer cells *in vitro*. It elicits both a direct and an indirect effect on invasion through a stimulation of the E-cadherin-mediated cell–cell adhesion and a decrease in the number of invasive cells by promoting a chronic stress condition and PCD (Scheme 86.1). Agents that inhibit cancer cell invasion by selective killing of cancer cells, inhibiting their growth or stimulating cell–cell adhesion between cancer

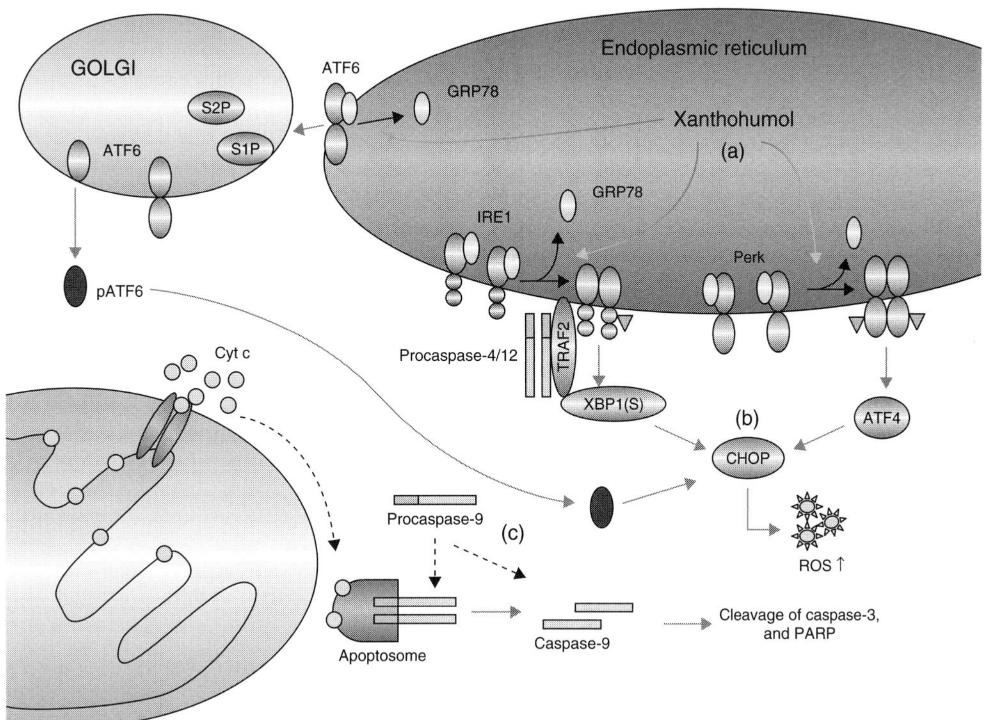

Figure 86.8 Signaling pathways involved during X-induced ER stress and apoptosis (a) X induces ER stress which triggers the UPR. All three ER-stress sensor molecules IRE1, PERK and ATF6 are involved. Activation of PERK results in the phosphorylation of eIF2α (not shown), the activation of IRE1 in the spicing of XBP1 (XBP1(S)), and the activation of ATF6 in a 50kD cleavage fragment, pATF6. (b) Activation of the UPR results in the translational upregulation of ATF4 which yields the potent proapoptotic protein CHOP, and in oxidative stress through the accumulation of ROS. (c). The X-induced sustained ER-stress is followed by the activation of the intrinsic apoptotic pathway, accompanied by the activation of caspase-9, caspase-3 and the cleavage of the nuclear protein PARP. ER-associated caspases (caspase-4/-12 and -7) are not involved. (d).

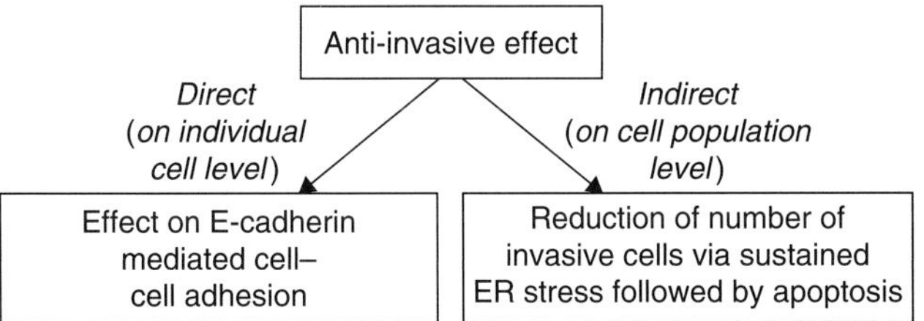

Scheme 86.1

cells should be considered as potential therapeutic drugs in cancer.

Summary Points

- X inhibits invasion of human breast cancer cells.
- X stimulates E cadherin mediated cell cell adhesion.
- X induces a chronic stress response in the cell, namely ER-stress.
- ER-stress induces a specific response, namely the UPR.
- Sustained ER-stress results in the activation of the intrinsic apoptotic pathway and cell death.
- Therefore, X induces ER-stress and cell death by activation of the UPR and apoptosis of human breast cancer cells.

References

Albini, A., Dell'Eva, R., Vené, R., Ferrari, N., Buhler, D.R., Noonan, D.M., and Fassina, G. (2006). *FASEB J.*, 20, 527–529.

Bertolotti, A., Zhang, Y., Hendershot, L.M., Harding, H.P. and Ron, D. (2000). *Nat. Cell Biol.* 2, 326–332.

Birkedal-Hansen, H. (1995). *Curr. Opin. Cell Biol.* 7, 728–735.

Blaschuk, O.W. and Farookhi, R. (1989). *Dev. Biol.* 136, 564–567.

Bole, D.G., Hendershot, L.M. and Kearney, J.F. (1986). *J. Cell Biol.* 102, 1558–1566.

Boterberg, T., Bracke, M.E., Bruyneel, E.A. and Mareel, M.M. (2001). In Brooks, S.A. and Schumacher, U. (eds.), *Methods in Molecular Medicine, Vol. 58: Metastasis Research Protocols, Vol. 2: Cell Behavior In Vitro and In Vivo*, pp. 33–45. Humana Press, Totowa NJ.

Bracke, M.E., Van Larebeke, N.A., Vyncke, B.M. and Mareel, M.M. (1991). *Br. J. Cancer* 63, 867–872.

Bracke, M.E., Charlier, C., Bruyneel, E.A., Labit, C., Mareel, M.M. and Castronovo, V. (1994). *Cancer Res.* 54, 4607–4609.

Bracke, M.E., Van Roy, F.M. and Mareel, M.M. (1996). In *Attempts to Understand Metastasis Formation I* (eds.) Günthert, U. and Birchmeier, W. , Springer-Verlag, Berlin pp. 123–161.

Bracke, M.E., Boterberg, T., Bruyneel, E.A. and Mareel, M.M. (2001). In Brooks, S.A. and Schumacher, U. (eds), *Methods in Molecular Medicine: Metastasis Research Protocols Col 58*, Humana Press, NJ, pp. 81–89.

Breckenridge, D.G., Germain, M., Mathai, J.P., Nguyen, M., and Shore, G.C. (2003). *Oncogene* 22, 8608–8618.

Brown, M.S., and Goldstein, J.L. (1997). *Cell* 2, 331–340.

Chi, Y.S., Jong, H.G., Son, K.H., Chang, H.W., Kang, S.S. and Kim, H.P. (2001). *Biochem. Pharmacol.* 62, 1185–1191.

Compagni, A. and Christofori, G. (2000). *Br. J. Cancer* 83, 1–5.

Egeblad, M. and Werb, Z. (2002). *Nat. Rev. Cancer* 2, 161–174.

Ellgaard, L., Molinari, M. and Helenius, A. (1999). *Science* 286, 1882–1888.

Friedl, P. (2004). *Curr. Opin. Cell Biol.* 16, 14–23.

Friedl, P. and Wolf, K. (2003). *Biochem. Soc. Symp.* 70, 277–285.

Gerhaüser, C., Alt, A., Heiss, E., Gamal-Eldeen, A., Klimo, K., Knauft, J., Neumann, I., Scherf, H.-R., Frank, N., Bartsch, H. and Becker, H. (2002). *Mol. Cancer Ther.* 1, 959–969.

Germain, M., Mathai, J.P. and Shore, G.C. (2002). *J. Biol. Chem.* 277, 18053–18060.

Germain, M., Mathai, J.P., McBride, H.M. and Shore, G.C. (2005). *EMBO J.* 24, 1546–1556.

Gething, M.J. and Sambrook, J. (1992). *Nature* 355, 33–45.

Haas, I.G. (1994). *Experientia* 50, 1012–1020.

Haas, I.G. and Wabl, M. (1983). *Nature* 306, 387–389.

Harding, H.P., Zhang, Y. and Ron, D. (1999). *Nature* 397, 271–274.

Hayes, J.D. and Pulford, D.J. (1995). *Crit. Rev. Biochem. Mol. Biol.* 30, 445–600.

Hayes, J.D., Ellis, E.M., Neal, G.E., Harrison, D.J. and Manson, M.M. (1999). *Biochem. Soc. Symp.* 64, 141–168.

Haze, K., Yoshida, H., Yanagi, T., Yura, K. and Mori, K. (1999). *Mol. Biol. Cell* 10, 3787–3799.

Kaufman, R.J. (1999). *Genes Dev.* 13, 1211–1233.

King, K.L. and Cidlowski, J.A. (1995). *J. Cell Biochem.* 158, 175–180.

Kuznetsov, G., Chen, L.B. and Nigam, S.K. (1997). *J. Biol. Chem.* 272, 3057–3063.

Lee, A.S. (1992). *Curr. Opin. Cell Biol.* 4, 267–273.

Lee, A.S. (2001). *Trends Biochem. Sci.* 26, 504–510.

Lee, K., Tirasophon, W., Shen, X., Michalak, M., Prywes, R., Okada, T., Yoshida, H., Mori, K. and Kaufman, R.J. (2002). *Genes Dev.* 16, 452–466.

Li, J., Lee, B., Lee, A.S. (2006). *J. Biol. Chem.* 281, 7760–7270.

Li, M., Baumeister, P., Roy, B., Phan, T., Foti, D., Luo, S. and Lee, A.S. (2000). *Mol. Cell Biol.* 20, 5096–5106.

Li, W.W., Alexandre, S., Cao, X. and Lee, A.S. (1993). *J. Biol. Chem.* 268, 12003–12009.

Liotta, L.A. and Kohn, E.C. (2001). *Nature* 411, 375–379.

Little, E., Ramakrishnan, M., Roy, B., Gazit, G. and Lee, A.S. (1994). *Crit. Rev. Eukaryot. Gene Expr.* 4, 1–18.

Liu, C.Y., Schroder, M. and Kaufman, R.J. (2000). *J. Biol. Chem.* 275, 24881–24885.

Marciniak, S.J., Yun, C.Y., Oyadomari, S., Novoa, I., Zhang, Y., Jungreis, R., Nagata, K., Harding, H.P., and Ron, D. (2004). *Genes Dev.* 18, 3066–3077.

Mareel, M.M., Bracke, M.E., Van Roy, F.M. and De Baetselier, P. (1997). In Bertino, J.R. (ed.), *Encyclopedia of Cancer, Vol. II*, pp. 1072–1083. Academic Press, San Diego.

Mathai, J.P., Germain, M., Marcellus, R.C. and Shore, G.C. (2002). *Oncogene* 21, 2534–2544.

Mathai, J.P., Germain, M. and Shore, G.C. (2005). *J. Cell Biol.* 162, 587–597.

Maubach, J. (2003). A study of *in vitro* and *in vivo* biological effects of soy- and hop-derived phyto-oestrogens. Ph.D. Thesis, Faculty of Pharmaceutical Sciences, Ghent University.

McCullough, K.D., Martindale, J.L., Klotz, L.O., AW, T.Y. and Holbrook, N.J. (2001). *Mol. Cell Biol.* 21, 1249–1259.

Meusser, B., Hirsch, C., Jarosch, E. and Sommer, T. (2005). *Nat. Cell Biol.* 7, 766–772.

Miranda, C.L., Stevens, J.F., Helmrich, A., Henderson, M.C., Rodriguez, R.J., Deinzer, M.L., Barnes, D.W. and Bühler, D.R. (1999). *Food Chem. Toxicol.* 37, 271–285.

Miranda, C.L., Aponso, G.L.M., Stevens, J.F., Deinzer, M.L. and Bühler, D.R. (2000). *Cancer Lett.* 149, 21–29.

Morishima, N., Nakanishi, K., Tsuchiya, K., Shibata, T. and Seiwa, E. (2004). *J. Biol. Chem.* 279, 50375–50381.

Munro, S. and Pelham, H.R. (1986). *Cell* 46, 291–300.

Nutt, L.K., Chandra, J., Pataer, A., Fang, B., Roth, J.A., Swisher, S.G., O'Neil, R.G. and McConkey, D.J. (2002a). *J. Biol. Chem.* 277, 20301–20308.

Nutt, L.K., Pataer, A., Pahler, J., Fang, B., Roth, J., McConkey, D.J. and Swisher, S.G. (2002b). *J. Biol. Chem.* 277, 9219–9225.

Oakes, S.A., Scorrano, L., Opferman, J.T., Bassik, M.C., Nishino, M., Pozzan, T. *et al.* (2005). *Proc. Natl. Acad. Sci. USA* 102, 105–110.

Obeng, E.A. and Boise, L.H. (2005). *J. Biol. Chem.* 280, 29578–29587.

Paget, S. (1889). *Lancet* 1, 571–573.

Pahl, H.L. (1999). *Physiol. Rev.* 79, 683–701.

Parmar, V.S., Bracke, M.E., Philippé, J., Wengel, J., Jain, S.C., Olsen, C.E., Bisht, K.S., Sharma, N.K., Courtens, A., Sharma, S.K., Vennekens, K., Van Marck, V. *et al.* (1997). *Bioorg. Med. Chem.* 5, 1609–1619.

Rao, R.V., Castro-Obregon, S., Frankowski, H., Schuler, M., Stoka, V., del Rio, G., Bredesen, D.E., and Ellerby, H.M. (2002). *J. Biol. Chem.* 277, 21836–21842.

Reid, S.E., Murthy, M.S., Kaufman, M. and Scanlon, E.F. (1996). *Br. J. Surg.* 83, 1037–1046.

Reimertz, C., Kogel, D., Rami, A., Chittenden, T. and Prehn, J.H. (2003). *J. Cell Biol.* 162, 587–597.

Richter, C., Gogvadze, V., Laffranchi, R., Schlapbach, R., Schweizer, M., Suter, M., Walter, P. and Yaffee, M. (1995). *Biochim. Biophys. Acta* 1271, 67–74.

Rolland, P.H., Martin, P.M., Jacquemier, J., Rolland, A.M. and Toga, M. (1980). *J. Natl. Cancer Inst.* 64, 1061–1070.

Rong, H., Boterberg, T., Maubach, J., Stove, C., Depypere, H., Van Slambrouck, S., Serreyn, R., De Keukeleire, D., Mareel, M. and Bracke, M. (2001). *Eur. J. Cell Biol.* 80, 580–585.

Rozic, J.G., Chakraborty, C. and Lala, P.K. (2001). *Int. J. Cancer* 93, 497–506.

Rushmore, T.H., Morton, M.R. and Pickett, C.B. (1991). *J. Biol. Chem.* 266, 11632–11639.

Sakai, J. and Rawson, R.B. (2001). *Curr. Opin. Lipidol.* 12, 261–266.

Scorrano, L., Oakes, S.A., Opfermann, J.T., Cheng, E.H., Sorcinelli, M.D. and Pozzan, T. (2003). *Science* 300, 135–139.

Shen, J., Snapp, E.L., Lippincott-Schwartz, J. and Prywes, R. (2005). *Mol. Cell Biol.* 25, 921–932.

Shi, Y., Vattem, K.M., Sood, R., An, J., Liang, J., Stramm, L. and Wek, R.C. (1998). *Mol. Cell. Biol.* 18, 7499–7509.

Soule, H.D., Vazquez, J., Long, A., Albert, S. and Brennan, M. (1973). *J. Natl. Cancer Inst.* 51, 1409–1416.

Stevens, J.F., Ivanicic, M., Hsu, V.L. and Deinzer, M.L. (1997). *Phytochemistry* 44, 1575–1585.

Subbaramaiah, K., Zakim, D., Weksler, B.B. and Dannenberg, A.J. (1997). *Proc. Soc. Exp. Biol. Med.* 216, 201–210.

Tirasophon, W., Welihinda, A.A. and Kaufman, R.J. (1998). *Genes Dev.* 12, 1812–1824.

Urano, F., Wang, X., Bertolotti, A., Zhang, Y., Chung, P., Harding, H.P. and Ron, D. (2000). *Science* 287, 664–666.

Vakaet, L. Jr., Vleminckx, K., Van Roy, F. and Mareel, M. (1991). *Invasion Metastasis* 11, 249–260.

Vanhoecke, B., Derycke, L., Van Marck, V., Depypere, H., De Keukeleire, D. and Bracke, M. (2005). *Int. J. Cancer* 117, 889–895.

Verzele, M., Stockx, J., Fontijn, F. and Anteunis, M. (1957). *Soc. Chim. Belges* 66, 452–475.

Wang, X.Z., Harding, H.P., Zhang, Y., Jolicoeur, E.M., Kuroda, M. and Ron, D. (1998). *EMBO J.* 17, 5708–5717.

Wang, Y., Shen, J., Arenzana, N., Tirasophon, W., Kaufman, R.J. and Prywes, R. (2000). *J. Biol. Chem.* 275, 27013–27020.

Wülfing, P., Diallo, R., Müller, C., Wülfing, C., Poremba, C., Heinecke, A., Rody, A., Greb, R.R., Böcker, W. and Kiesel, L. (2003). *J. Cancer Res. Clin. Oncol.* 129, 375–382.

Yamaguchi, H., and Wang, H.G. (2004). *J. Biol. Chem.* 279, 45495–45502.

Ye, J., Rawson, R.B., Komuro, R., Chen, X., Dave, U.P., Prywes, R., Brown, M.S. and Goldstein, J.L. (2000). *Mol. Cell* 6, 1355–1364.

Yoshida, H., Haze, K., Yanagi, H., Yura, T. and Mori, K. (1998). *J. Biol. Chem.* 273, 33741–33749.

Yoshida, H., Matsui, T., Yamamoto, A., Okada, T. and Mori, K. (2001). *Cell* 107, 881–891.

Zhao, F., Nozawa, H., Daikonnya, A., Kondo, K. and Kitanaka, S. (2003). *Biol. Pharmaceut. Bull.* 26, 61–65.

Zong, W.X., Li, C., Hatzivassiliou, G., Lindsten, T., Yu, Q.C., Yuan, J. and Thompson, C.B. (2003). *J. Cell Biol.* 162, 59–69.

87

Anti-cancer Property of Epicatechin Gallate in Colon Cancer Cells

Seung Joon Baek and Seong-Ho Lee Laboratory of Environmental Carcinogenesis, Department of Pathobiology, College of Veterinary Medicine, University of Tennessee, Knoxville, TN, USA

Abstract

There is persuasive epidemiological and experimental evidence that dietary polyphenolic plant-derived compounds have anti-cancer activity. Many laboratories, including ours, have reported such an effect in cancers of the gastrointestinal tract, lung, skin, prostate, and breast. The catechins are a group of polyphenols found in many beverages, including beer. While the preponderance of the data strongly indicates significant anti-tumorigenic benefits from catechins, the potential molecular mechanisms involved remain obscure. Although most studies are from epigallocatechin gallate (EGCG), much effort has recently been paid to epicatechin gallate (ECG) regarding the identification of its biological properties, including anti-cancer activity. ECG has been shown to alter the expression of several genes that are involved in apoptosis, cell cycle arrest, and angiogenesis. For examples, non-steroidal anti-inflammatory drug-activated gene and activating transcription factor 3 are induced, whereas basic fibroblast growth factor is down-regulated in the presence of ECG. Thrombospondin, an anti-angiogenic factor, is also increased by ECG treatment in human colorectal cancer. Several biological activities of ECG have been described and discussed. Therefore, this chapter attempts to highlight the biological activities of ECG in human colorectal cancer, and emphasize the pro-apoptosis and anti-angiogenesis that may play a role in chemopreventive activity of ECG.

Introduction

During the last half century, extensive research has identified various dietary compounds found in vegetables, fruits, and beverages, compounds that can potentially be used not only for the prevention of cancer but also for other diseases. Beer, a low-alcohol beverage, is one of the most commonly consumed alcoholic beverages in the world. It has not only plenty of nutrients, but also beneficial non-nutrient compounds such as phenolic acids, flavonoids, chalcones, proanthocyanidins, and catechins (Gerhauser, 2005). Although heavy alcohol consumption is one of the leading causes of preventable death related to coronary heart and liver disease, low or moderate alcohol consumption was associated with a beneficial effect on cancer-related mortality in middle age (35–69), compared with non-drinking and heavy drinking groups (Thun *et al.*, 1997). Epidemiological studies also suggested that moderate consumption of alcoholic beverages including beer is significantly associated with a reduction in coronary heart disease mortality (Rimm *et al.*, 1991; Gronbaek *et al.*, 1995). It has also been known that drinking beer can significantly decrease cholesterol and triglyceride level, and inhibit atherosclerosis compared to a control group that drinks 2% alcohol only (Vinson *et al.*, 2003). The protective effects of beer may be the result of non-alcoholic phenolic compounds abundantly present in beer. Furthermore, several animal studies examined beer's antioxidative and anti-tumorigenic properties in liver and colorectal carcinogenesis. Intake of beer significantly increased antioxidant capacity of plasma, for example, as a protective agent against the oxidation of ascorbic acid and unsaturated fatty acids (Pulido *et al.*, 2003; Gasowski *et al.*, 2004). Beer consumption decreased liver DNA adducts, induced by several heterocyclic amines (Arimoto-Kobayashi *et al.*, 1999) and reduced the incidence of dimethylhydrazine- or azoxymethane-induced colonic carcinogenesis (Nelson and Samelson, 1985; Nozawa *et al.*, 2004). Moderate beer intake was also associated with higher bone mineral density in postmenopausal elderly women (Rapuri *et al.*, 2000) and lowered the risk of type-2 diabetes (Conigrave *et al.*, 2001) as well as dementia (Ruitenberg *et al.*, 2002). Thus, non-nutrient components found specifically in beer, rather than the alcohol, may play an important role in beer's beneficial effects on several diseases.

Beer has a complex mixture of polyphenols ranging from 150 to 300 mg/l in concentration (Bendelow, 1977). Since the average per capita consumption of beer in the United States in 2004 was 224 ml/day (USDA, 2005), we can assume a consumption of 34–67 mg/day of polyphenolic compounds. Polyphenols in beers are present in the malt (70–80%) and hops (20–30%) used to make beer, and have an impact on the quality of flavor, colloidal

Beer in Health and Disease Prevention
ISBN: 978-0-12-373891-2

stability, and haze formation by oxidative polymerization (Gerhauser, 2005; Lopez and Edens, 2005). Because phenolic compounds can act as antioxidants in the human body, polyphenols in beer appear to be responsible for the benefits of beer. Among the numerous polyphenols isolated from unstabilized beer, total catechins, which have been detected in concentrations of <15 mg/l, account for approximately 70% of the polyphenolic compounds of beer (Gerhauser *et al.*, 2002). The major catechin substances are epicatechin (EC), epicatechin gallate (ECG), epigallocatechin (EGC), and epigallocatechin gallate (EGCG). Catechin gallates such as ECG and EGCG are esters of a catechin and gallic acid (GA). Although ECG is not the major catechin in beer, it shows a strong biological activity in several aspects, including apoptosis, transport, and growth inhibition in colorectal cancer cells (Okabe *et al.*, 1997; Vaidyanathan and Walle, 2003; Baek *et al.*, 2004a). However, ECG has not been studied in detail regarding how this compound affects several disease statuses. Several studies have shown that EGCG induces apoptosis in cancer cells, but little effort has been directed at evaluating the induction of apoptosis by ECG. Thus, the precise molecular mechanisms by which the other ester forms of ECG-induced anti-cancer activity remain to be elucidated. This chapter will provide the value of ECG present in beer as an antioxidant and potential cancer chemopreventive agent and its application in cancer prevention.

Biological Activities of ECG in General

ECG [(−)-epicatechin-3-gallate] is a 3-gallate ester form of (−)-epicatechin, as shown in Figure 87.1. The health benefits of ECG are mainly attributable to its antioxidant properties and contribution to the reduced risk of cancer, obesity, and cardiovascular disease as well as to its anti-hypertensive effect, antibacterial and antiviral activity, ultraviolet protection to skin, and neuroprotective power (Zaveri, 2006).

Kinetic analysis of the antioxidation process demonstrates that ECG is a strong antioxidant for microsomal peroxidation and synergizes the effect of endogenous alpha-tocopherol (Cai *et al.*, 2002). As an alpha-tocopheroxyl radical scavenger, ECG was the most effective catechin among the catechins tested, including EGCG, EC, EGC, and GA (Liu *et al.*, 2000). In addition to its antioxidant effects, ECG is studied for its effect on cellular and molecular targets in signal transduction pathways associated with cell death and survival in cancer chemoprevention. Studies in animal models of carcinogenesis clearly demonstrate anti-cancer activities against various tumor models. As summarized in Table 87.1, ECG inhibits the growth of tumors in the colon (Hong *et al.*, 2001; Weyant *et al.*, 2001; Baek *et al.*, 2004a), breast (Liao *et al.*, 1995; Bigelow and Cardelli, 2006), prostate (Ahmad *et al.*, 1997; Chung *et al.*, 2001), head and neck (Lim *et al.*, 2006), lung (Yang *et al.*, 1998), and skin (Ahmad *et al.*, 1997; Huang *et al.*, 2005). Intake of catechin-rich green tea prevented an increase in body weight in an obese animal model (Kao *et al.*, 2000) and inhibited adipocyte proliferation (Hung *et al.*, 2005; Wu *et al.*, 2005). ECG also inhibited development of insulin resistance and hyperglycemia (Wu *et al.*, 2004), as well as coronary artery disease and atherogenesis (Miura *et al.*, 2000). ECG inhibited fatty acid synthase, which is a potential therapeutic target of obesity (Tian, 2006; Zhang

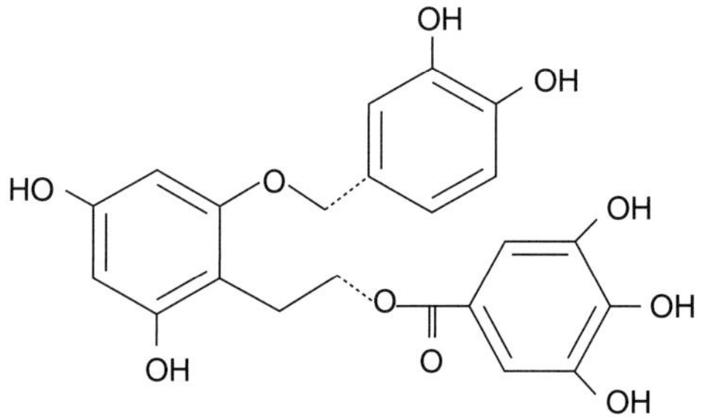

Figure 87.1 Chemical structure of ECG.

Table 87.1 The beneficial effects of ECG on human disease

Beneficial effects	*Possible mechanism(s)*	*References*
Oxidation	?	Cai *et al.* (2002); Liu *et al.* (2000)
Colon cancer	NAG-1↑, COX-2↓, ATF3↑ FAK↓	Baek *et al.* (2004a); Hong *et al.* (2001); Weyant *et al.* (2001)
Breast cancer	AKT, ERK↑	Bigelow and Cardelli (2006); Liao *et al.* (1995)
Prostate cancer	?	Ahmad *et al.* (1997); Chung *et al.* (2001)
Head and neck cancer	Cyclin D1↓	Lim *et al.* (2006)
Lung cancer	?	Yang *et al.* (1998)
Skin cancer	UV-induced ERK↓	Ahmad *et al.* (1997); Huang *et al.* (2005)
Lymphoma	?	Ahmad *et al.* (1997)
Angiogenesis	PDGFβ-indcued PI3K↓ TSP↑	Sachinidis *et al.* (2002); Baek *et al.* (2004a)
Obesity, diabetes	FAS↓	Kao *et al.* (2000); Tian (2006); Zhang *et al.* (2006)
	ERK↓, Cdk2↓ cyclin D1↓	Hung *et al.* (2005); Wu *et al.* (2005)
	t-BHP-induced oxidative stress	Rizvi *et al.* (2005)
Cardiovascular diseases	MMP-2↓	El Bedoui *et al.* (2005)
	VCAM-1↓	Ludwig *et al.* (2004)
Microbial infection	?	Yanagawa *et al.* (2003)
Neurodegeneration	6-OHDA-induced apoptosis↓	Nie *et al.* (2002)

et al., 2006). In addition, ECG protected the development of diabetes by suppression of oxidative stress (Rizvi *et al.*, 2005), and directly inhibited synthesis of new blood vessels by inhibition of matrix metalloproteinases and vascular cell adhesion molecules, the physiological activators of angiogenesis (Ludwig *et al.*, 2004; El Bedoui *et al.*, 2005), and inhibited the growth of vascular smooth muscle cells, which play an important role in the development of proliferative cardiovascular diseases (Sachinidis *et al.*, 2002). ECG showed anti-helicobacter pylori activity as effective as the EGCG effect (Yanagawa *et al.*, 2003). In addition, age-associated diseases such as Parkinson's disease (Nie *et al.*, 2002; Mandel *et al.*, 2004) were inhibited by ECG intake. Therefore, the multiple biological pathways involved in human diseases could be modulated by ECG and further represent an important target of chemoprevention research.

ECG-Induced Apoptosis in Colorectal Cancer

Cancer is second only to heart disease as the leading cause of death in the United States, and colorectal cancer is one of the most prevalent causes of cancer-related mortality in the Western world. Further development of therapeutic and preventative means of controlling this disease are clearly needed, particularly as they pertain to gastrointestinal cancer (Lamprecht and Lipkin, 2003). Since colorectal cancer progresses for 10–40 years, several approaches could attack this heterogeneous disease (Figure 87.2). Among these, prevention studies are the most promising from the public health point of view. Chemoprevention is one of the most rapidly growing fields, and apoptosis induction is a target of this chemoprevention research.

Apoptosis can be induced by a wide variety of physical, chemical, and biological stimuli, and two very distinct apoptotic pathways have been identified: the death receptor pathway involving activation of caspase-8, and the mitochondrial pathway involving caspase-9. These two independent apoptotic pathways converge on the activation of downstream caspase-7, -6, and -3, key proteins that mediate apoptosis. Cellular stress, including that generated by many chemotherapeutic agents, stimulates the p53/p73/p14^{ARF} pathway, which is thought to act by increasing expression of pro-apoptotic proteins such as Bcl-2 family members Bax, Bak, and Bcl-XS. These in turn, stimulate mitochondrial release of cytochrome c, which causes Apafl to bind to procaspase-9 and activate this apoptotic pathway. To date, there have been few reports on whether ECG affects apoptosis in colon cancer cells by modifying expression of key regulatory proteins, or whether apoptosis occurs through caspase-8 and/or mitochondria (caspase-9)-dependent mechanisms in colorectal cancer cells.

The similarity of the biochemical events during apoptosis is reflected by a high uniformity of morphological

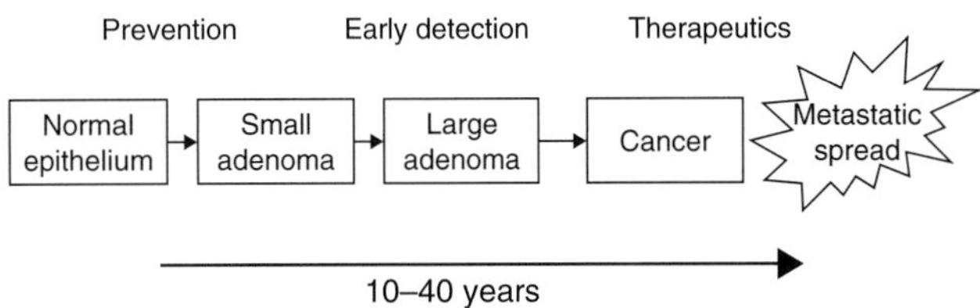

Figure 87.2 Schematic diagram of colorectal tumorigenesis.

changes in many situations of naturally occurring or experimentally induced cell death. As shown in Figure 87.3, ECG obviously increases apoptosis in human colorectal cancer cells as assessed by cell morphology. ECG-treated HCT-116 cell culture contained many cells with condensed DNA and fragmented apoptotic bodies, whereas treatment with vehicle or 50 μM EGCG did not produce the same observations. In addition to changing morphology and biochemical pathways, there have also been reports that several apoptotic-related genes at the molecular levels are affected by ECG. In this section, we focus on two apoptosis-related genes, NAG-1 and ATF3, which are induced by ECG.

NAG-1

NAG-1 (non-steroidal anti-inflammatory drug-activated gene-1) was identified by PCR-based subtractive hybridization from an NSAID-induced library in cyclooxygenase (COX)-negative cells as a divergent member of the TGF-β superfamily (Baek *et al.*, 2001). The induction of NAG-1 by NSAIDs is an important COX-independent mechanism by which some of these proven anti-inflammatory compounds mediate their effects (Baek *et al.*, 2002b). NAG-1 protein has broad activity in inflammation, cancer, and differentiation. Although the molecular mechanisms responsible for these functions have yet to be determined in detail, experimental evidence suggests that NAG-1 may share at least some of the common functions of TGF-β superfamily cytokines (Baek and Eling, 2006). It is highly expressed in mature intestinal epithelial cells, but is significantly reduced in human colorectal carcinoma samples and neoplastic intestinal polyps of *Min* mice (Kim *et al.*, 2002). In addition, it has been reported that NAG-1 overexpression from a recombinant adenoviral vector results in up to an 80% reduction of MDA-MB-468 and MCF-7 breast cancer cell viability (Li *et al.*, 2000), and treatment of prostate cancer cells with purified NAG 1 induces apoptosis (Liu *et al.*, 2003).

To obtain further support for *in vitro* results, we have made a transgenic mouse (NAG-Tg) that expressed the human form of NAG-1 in all tissues, including the intestinal tract, and then investigated intestinal tumor development. The transgenic mice appeared to be normal but were smaller in weight (Baek *et al.*, 2006). The mice were either treated with a carcinogen that induces intestinal tumors or a genetic mutation that results in intestinal tumors was

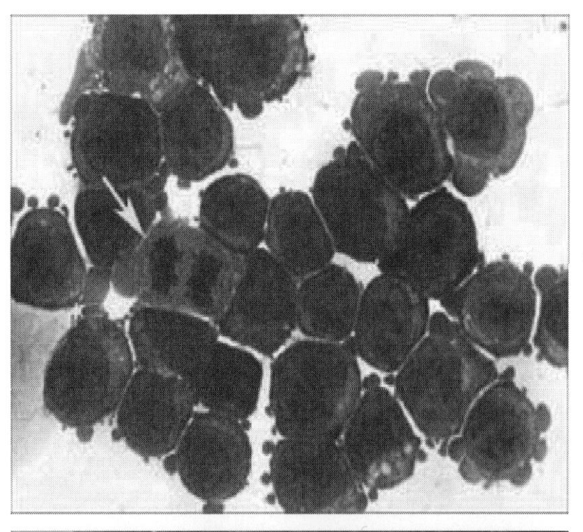

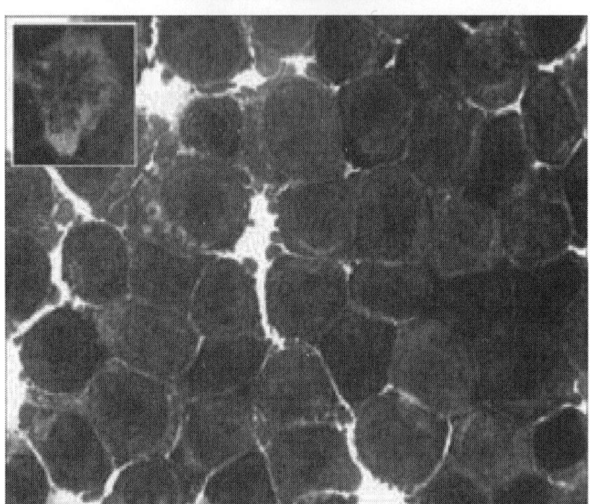

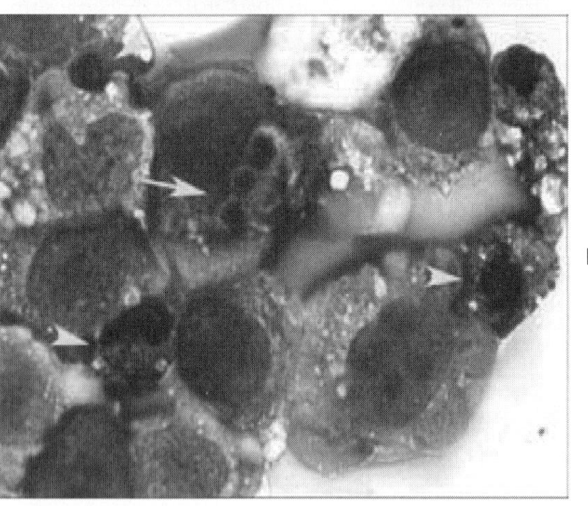

Figure 87.3 ECG induces apoptosis in HCT-116 cells. Representative photomicrographs of cytospin preparations from HCT-116 cell cultures treated with vehicle (0.2% DMSO), EGCG (50 μM), or ECG (50 μM) for 48 h. Mitotic figures were obvious in vehicle (arrow) and EGCG-treated cells (inserted), but not apparent in ECG-treated cells. In contrast, ECG-treated cells (arrow) more often had morphologic features of apoptosis, with condensation of nuclear chromatin and cytoplasmic structure, and fragmentation into smaller, discrete bodies. Wright-Giemsa stain, 600×.

introduced into the NAG-Tg mice. Compared to control mice, the NAG-Tg mice had a greater than 50% reduction in intestinal cancer, confirming the tumor suppression activity of NAG-1. These data support the evidence that NAG-1 is linked to apoptosis and that its reduced expression may enhance tumorigenesis.

NAG-1 expression is up-regulated in a prostaglandin-independent manner in human colorectal cancer cells by several NSAIDs (Baek *et al.*, 2002b), as well as by anti-tumorigenic compounds such as resveratrol (Baek *et al.*, 2002a), genistein (Wilson *et al.*, 2003), ECG (Baek *et al.*, 2004a), indole-3-carbinol (Lee *et al.*, 2005), PPARγ ligands (Baek *et al.*, 2004b; Yamaguchi *et al.*, 2006a), horehound extracts (Yamaguchi *et al.*, 2006b), 5F-203 (Monks *et al.*, 2003), and retinoid 6-[3-(1-adamantyl)-4-hydroxyphenyl]-2-naphthalene carboxylic acid (AHPN) (Newman *et al.*, 2003). While some dietary compounds, including resveratrol and genistein, induce NAG-1 expression through the p53 tumor suppressor protein, NSAIDs, ECG, and indole-3-carbinol induce NAG-1 in a p53-independent manner. Thus, several pathways are involved in NAG-1 expression. ECG seems to be one of the strongest NAG-1 inducers among the other catechins. Unlike EGCG, ECG induces NAG-1 expression in a p53-independent manner. Therefore, ECG induces NAG-1 expression in cells lacking p53, and a NAG-1 promoter that lacks the p53 binding site is activated in the presence of ECG (Baek *et al.*, 2004a). Furthermore, p53 protein expression is not induced by ECG. Since most of colorectal cancer cells were mutated in a p53 locus, any compound like ECG that does not mediate p53 expression will be beneficial.

ATF3

ATF3 (activating transcription factor) is designated as a stress-inducible gene and several genes have been implicated as the targets of ATF3. The ATF3 homodimer functions as a repressor for most of the target genes such as gadd153/Chop10, E-selectin, and phosphoenolpyruvate carboxylase (Chen *et al.*, 1996; Hai and Hartman, 2001). However, the heterodimeric complex of ATF3 with c-Jun, for instance, has been demonstrated to function as a transcriptional activator (Hai and Hartman, 2001). ATF3 binds to the AP-1 family, and its transcriptional activity differs according to its counterpart. ATF3, in combination with c-Jun, activates specific promoters containing AP-1 and CRE sites, but in contrast, ATF3 in combination with JunB potently represses activation of these promoters (Hsu *et al.*, 1992). In addition, Hai and colleagues proposed mechanisms by which ATF3 can perform the opposite functions of gene repression or activation (Chen *et al.*, 1994). The functional consequence of ATF3 thus varies in stress signals and cell types. ATF3 is induced by camptothecin and etoposide, agents known to induce apoptosis (Hai *et al.*, 1999; Hai and Hartman, 2001). Furthermore, ATF3 is highly expressed after sulindac sulfide treatment and may also play an important role in sulindac sulfide-induced apoptosis and anti-tumorigenic activity (Iizaka *et al.*, 2002). Tetracycline-inducible overexpression of ATF3 suppresses cell growth and slows cell cycle progression from the G_1 to the S phase (Fan *et al.*, 2002).

ATF3 has been postulated to be a tumor suppressor gene because it coordinates the expression of genes that may be linked to cancer (Fawcett *et al.*, 1999). Moreover, the expression of ATF3 was repressed in human colorectal tumors compared to normal adjacent tissue (Bottone *et al.*, 2003). Interestingly, it has been reported that both ATF3 and NAG-1 were co-induced by treatment with the 5F-203 anti-tumorigenic compound (Monks *et al.*, 2003) and sulindac (Iizaka *et al.*, 2002). We also found that ATF3 expression is induced by ECG or indole-3-carbinol treatment, supporting the concept that ATF3 expression has a role in compound-induced apoptosis (Baek *et al.*, 2004a; Lee *et al.*, 2005). However, the exact molecular mechanisms of ATF3 action and gene regulation in carcinogenesis need to be elucidated further.

Down-regulation of β-catenin signaling

Many signaling pathways play a pivotal role in colorectal tumorigenesis. Specifically, the Wnt/β-catenin signaling pathway is important in development and tumorigenesis (Polakis, 2000; Widelitz *et al.*, 2000). In an unstimulated cell, most of the endogenous β-catenin interacts with adenomatous polyposis coli (APC), glycogen synthase kinase (GSK)-3β, casein kinase 1α, axin, or the closely related factor conductin/Axil, and is found at epithelial cell adherens junctions, where it interacts with E-cadherin and α-catenin to help mediate cell adhesion. However, binding of the Wnt ligand to its receptor complex triggers a series of events that ultimately disrupt the β-catenin/APC/Axin/GSK3β complex. This, in turn, results in the nuclear accumulation of β-catenin and to the increased transcription of Wnt-β-catenin target genes. In the nucleus, β-catenin acts as a transcriptional activator in conjunction with the LEF/TCF DNA binding proteins. The transcription of Wnt-β-catenin target genes is further modulated by a variety of different co-activators and co-repressors that have been identified in the past decade. Among the target genes of the β-catenin/TCF complex, several cell growth related genes have been identified, including cyclin D1 (Shtutman *et al.*, 1999; Tetsu and McCormick, 1999), c-myc (He *et al.*, 1998), and PPAR-δ (He *et al.*, 1999). Indeed, ECG down-regulates cyclin D1 expression by the suppression of β-catenin signaling (Lim *et al.*, 2006). Like other polyphenols that suppress the β-catenin signaling pathway, the inhibition of β-catenin signaling by ECG should be considered as a molecular target in colorectal cancer. Although the exact mechanisms have not been elucidated, down-regulation of β-catenin signaling plays an important role in chemopreventive compound-induced anti-cancer activity.

ECG-Induced Anti-angiogenesis

Angiogenesis, the generation of new capillaries by sprouting of pre-existing microvessels, is a tightly regulated process that is restricted to a few conditions, including normal reproductive function and wound healing (Whisenant and Bergsland, 2005). However, aberrant angiogenesis is a crucial factor in the pathogenesis of numerous diseases, including cancer. In this section, we will focus on the alteration of pro-angiogenesis factor bFGF and anti-angiogenesis factor TSP-1, mediated by ECG treatment.

TSP-1

Thrombospondin-1 (TSP-1) is an extracellular glycoprotein first recognized as an inhibitor of angiogenesis more than a decade ago. Since then, much has been learned about its ability to regulate vascular growth in several angiogenesis models, functional domains have been identified, and mechanisms of action determined. TSP-1 is a potent inhibitor of angiogenesis and effectively inhibits a wide variety of angiogenic stimuli, including VEGF, proteins that act via tyrosine kinase receptors, G proteins, serine/threonine kinase receptors and lipids. To examine other potential pathways by which ECG induces anti-tumorigenic activity, we performed superarray analysis to characterize the mRNA expression profile of cancer-related genes in HCT-116 cells. After incubation with or without 50 μM ECG, cellular RNA was extracted, and cancer-related gene expression was analyzed using Superarray™ membranes. TSP-1 is a gene that was up-regulated >3.0-fold by ECG (Table 87.2). Oligonucleotide primers were designed for TSP1, and RT-PCR was performed. TSP1 transcription was markedly up-regulated with ECG treatment, whereas the levels of transcription of GAPDH were not affected. We then performed Western analysis to confirm that ECG induces TSP1 protein expression. TSP-1 is induced by ECG treatment as early as 1 h after treatment, with increased expression following 24–48 h of treatment. Taken together, these results showed that ECG may alter several genes in HCT-116 cells, including TSP1, which probably account for apoptotic and/or anti-tumorigenic activities.

TSP-1 is an inhibitor of invasion but also an inhibitor of angiogenesis and its suppression is crucial for the angiogenic switch in many tumor models. The cellular mechanism is not well known, but TSP-1 can inhibit endothelial cell growth via the apoptotic pathway (Hamano *et al.*, 2004). TSP 1 inhibits the activity of matrix metalloproteinase 9, which causes a release of vascular endothelial growth factor (VEGF) sequestered in the extracellular matrix, thereby increasing invasion potential (Rodriguez-Manzaneque *et al.*, 2001). Moreover, TSP-1 can promote secretion of PAI-1, which was shown to inhibit the invasiveness of human lung carcinoma cells (Albo *et al.*, 1999). Thus, ECG induces TSP-1, followed by the induction of anti-tumorigenic activity mediated by anti-angiogenesis.

Table 87.2 ECG altered gene expression in human colorectal cancer cells

Gene name	*Description*	*GeneBank*	*Up/down*
Bcl-x	Bcl2-like 1	NM_138578	Up
CDC25A	Cell division cycle 25A	NM_001789	Up
E-Cadherin	E-Cadherin	NM_004360	Up
IFNA1	Interferon α 1	NM_024013	Up
IL-8	Interleukin 8	NM_000584	Up
IKBA/MAD-3	NF-κB inhibitor, α	NM_020529	Up
uPA	Plasminogen activator, urokinase	NM_002658	Up
uPAR	Plasminogen activator, urokinase receptor	NM_002659	Up
DNA-PK	Protein kinase	NM_006904	Up
PAI-1	Plasminogen activator inhibitor type 1	NM_000602	Up
TSP1	Thrombospondin 1	NM_003246	Up
TIMP1	Tissue inhibitor of metalloproteinase 1	NM_003254	Up
TNFA	Tumor necrosis factor	NM_000594	Up
Apaf-1	Apoptotic protease activating factor	NM_001160	Down
RB1	Retinoblastoma 1	NM_000321	Down

Note: HCT-116 cells were seeded into plates 100mm in diameter. Once they reached 60–80% confluency, vehicle or 50μM ECG was added and treated for 24h. Total RNA was extracted and cDNA was labeled from 5μg of total RNA in a reverse-transcription (RT) reaction with biotin-16-dUTP (Roche Diagnostics GmbH). RT reaction was performed using MMLV reverse transcriptase (Promega, WI). The labeled cDNA was hybridized to GEArray Q Series Human Cancer PathwayFinder Gene Array (HS-006, SuperArray Bioscience) overnight at 60°C. The membrane used in the present study contained 96 genes that were closely related to cancer, in addition to four positive control genes (glyceraldehyde-3-phosphate dehydrogenase, cyclophillin A, ribosomal protein L13A, and β-actin) and one negative control (pUC18). The list of genes identified by up- and down-regulation by ECG, compared to the vehicle treated samples, is shown.

bFGF

Basic fibroblast growth factor (bFGF, also known as FGF-2) is a well-documented angiogenic growth factor that induces endothelial cell replication, migration, and extracellular proteolysis (Chen *et al.*, 2004). The bFGF protein is produced by several normal, tumor, and endothelial cells, and has autocrine activities in angiogenesis and may promote angiogenesis both by a direct effect on endothelial cells and indirectly by the up-regulation of VEGF in endothelial cells. Thus, bFGF and VEGF have a synergistic effect in the induction of angiogenesis both *in vitro* and *in vivo*. Basic FGF belongs to the FGF superfamily, which contains at least 20 distinct FGFs (Dow and deVere White, 2000). Four different bFGF polypeptides of 18–24.2kDa can be formed from one *fgf-2* gene. The bFGF peptide does not code for a signal sequence required for vectorial translocation into endoplasmic reticulum and can be released through a yet unknown mechanism of exocytosis independent of the ER-Golgi pathway. Mechanical damage such as wounding has also been proposed as one mechanism for release of biologically active bFGF from endothelial cells. In the extracellular matrix and on the cell surface, bFGF is bound to heparan-like glycosaminoglycans (HLGAGs). The association to HLGAGs may afford bFGF protection from proteolysis, besides creating a localized and persistent reservoir of the growth factor. Like VEGF, bFGF also inhibits apoptosis of endothelial cells, and it is a well-characterized fibroblast growth factor that induces mitogenic and chemotactic activity and differentiation of some other cell types of mesodermal and neuroectodermal origin.

Our recent results with human colorectal cancer cells indicated that either ECG or EGCG treatment suppressed bFGF expression at both transcriptional and translational levels (unpublished results). While transcriptional regulation by ECG is not clear, ECG clearly suppressed bFGF protein expression via degradation. ECG activates ubiquitinase-dependent protein degradation in human colorectal cancer cells, followed by the selective degradation of bFGF. It has been demonstrated that ester bond-containing polyphenols such as EGCG and ECG potently and specifically inhibit the chemotrypsin-like activity of the proteasome *in vitro* (Wan *et al.*, 2005). However, our data suggest that ECG promotes proteasome machinery and facilitates protein degradation. Therefore, the precise mechanisms by which catechins affect protein degradation need to be elucidated.

Concluding Remarks

The appropriate use of a chemopreventive agent that includes catechins ultimately depends on the understanding of catechin's mechanism of action at all levels. Based on such knowledge, the trend in the field of chemoprevention has been to develop new agents based on their mechanism of action. With the rapid progress in molecular medicine and development of the state-of-the-art technologies applied to biomedical research in general, we are now better aware of the intracellular events associated with chemopreventive compounds. Despite this progress, the identification of molecular and cellular targets of chemopreventive phytochemicals remains still incomplete. In this regard, catechins, especially EGCG and ECG, have received much attention by the pharmacological and nutritional scientists, who demonstrated that cancer chemoprevention by catechins, can be achieved by signaling transduction blockade.

Most results regarding catechin effects on chemopreventive activity are from EGCG. Few studies were performed using ECG, although ECG has been shown to be more potent in some aspects. ECG is a strong apoptosis inducer, and NAG-1/ATF3 expressor in HCT-116 cells, compared to other catechins. ECG also suppresses bFGF as illustrated in Figure 87.4. In this chapter, we have further shown that EGCG and ECG may affect different mechanisms regarding

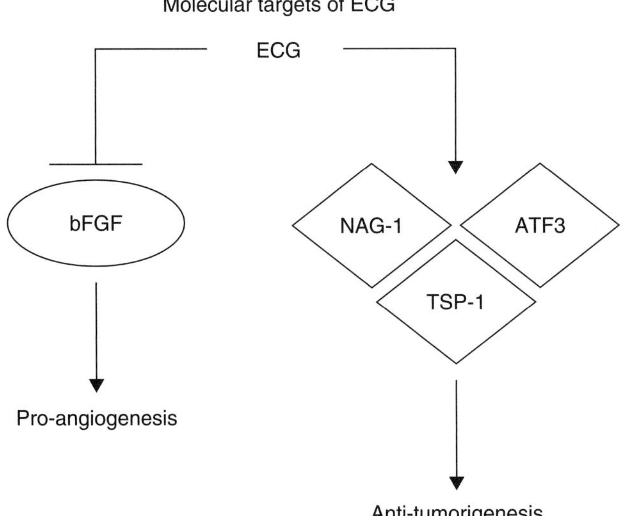

Figure 87.4 Schematic diagram of molecular targets of ECG. ECG enhances pro-apoptotic protein and anti-angiogenic protein, but suppresses angiogenic protein.

chemopreventive activity. Although ECG differs from EGCG only by the lack of one hydroxyl group on the B-ring, ECG is more biologically active than EGCG in some aspects. Although further studies are required to recommend using ECG as a supplementary compound, ECG could be a potential agent for the chemoprevention of colorectal cancer.

Acknowledgment

Research described in this chapter was supported by the grant R21CA109423 from NCI/NIH, and the authors thank Ms. Misty R. Bailey for her editorial assistance.

References

Ahmad, N., Feyes, D.K., Nieminen, A.L., Agarwal, R. and Mukhtar, H. (1997). *J. Natl. Cancer Inst.* 89, 1881–1886.

Albo, D., Berger, D.H., Vogel, J. and Tuszynski, G.P. (1999). *J. Gastrointest. Surg.* 3, 411–417.

Arimoto-Kobayashi, S., Sugiyama, C., Harada, N., Takeuchi, M., Takemura, M. and Hayatsu, H. (1999). *J. Agric. Food Chem.* 47, 221–230.

Baek, S.J. and Eling, T.E. (2006). *Prog. Lipid Res.* 45, 1–16.

Baek, S.J., Kim, J.S., Jackson, F.R., Eling, T.E., McEntee, M.F. and Lee, S.H. (2004a). *Carcinogenesis* 25, 2425–2432.

Baek, S.J., Kim, J.S., Nixon, J.B., DiAugustine, R.P. and Eling, T.E. (2004b). *J. Biol. Chem.* 279, 6883–6892.

Baek, S.J., Kim, K.S., Nixon, J.B., Wilson, L.C. and Eling, T.E. (2001). *Mol. Pharmacol.* 59, 901–908.

Baek, S.J., Okazaki, R., Lee, S.-H., Martinez, J.M., Kim, J.S., Yamaguchi, K., Mishina, Y., Martin, W.D., Shoieb, A., McEntee, J.F. and Eling, T.E. (2006). *Gastroenterology* 131, 1553–1560.

Baek, S.J., Wilson, L.C. and Eling, T.E. (2002a). *Carcinogenesis* 23, 425–432.

Baek, S.J., Wilson, L.C., Lee, C.H. and Eling, T.E. (2002b). *J. Pharmacol. Exp. Ther.* 301, 1126–1131.

Bendelow, V. (1977). *ASBC J.* 35, 150–152.

Bigelow, R.L. and Cardelli, J.A. (2006). *Oncogene* 25, 1922–1930.

Bottone Jr., F.G., Martinez, J.M., Collins, J.B., Afshari, C.A. and Eling, T.E. (2003). *J. Biol. Chem.* 278, 25790–25801.

Cai, Y.J., Ma, L.P., Hou, L.F., Zhou, B., Yang, L. and Liu, Z.L. (2002). *Chem. Phys. Lipid* 120, 109–117.

Chen, B.P., Liang, G., Whelan, J. and Hai, T. (1994). *J. Biol. Chem.* 269, 15819–15826.

Chen, B.P., Wolfgang, C.D. and Hai, T. (1996). *Mol. Cell Biol.* 16, 1157–1168.

Chen, C.H., Poucher, S.M., Lu, J. and Henry, P.D. (2004). *Curr. Vasc. Pharmacol.* 2, 33–43.

Chung, L.Y., Cheung, T.C., Kong, S.K., Fung, K.P., Choy, Y.M., Chan, Z.Y. and Kwok, T.T. (2001). *Life Sci.* 68, 1207–1214.

Conigrave, K.M., Hu, B.F., Camargo Jr., C.A., Stampfer, M.J., Willett, W.C. and Rimm, E.B. (2001). *Diabetes* 50, 2390–2395.

Dow, J.K. and deVere White, R.W. (2000). *Urology* 55, 800–806.

El Bedoui, J., Oak, M.H., Anglard, P. and Schini-Kerth, V.B. (2005). *Cardiovasc. Res.* 67, 317–325.

Fan, F., Jin, S., Amundson, S.A., Tong, T., Fan, W., Zhao, H., Zhu, X., Mazzacurati, L., Li, X., Petrik, K.L. *et al.* (2002). *Oncogene* 21, 7488–7496.

Fawcett, T.W., Martindale, J.L., Guyton, K.Z., Hai, T. and Holbrook, N.J. (1999). *Biochem. J.* 339, 135–141.

Gasowski, B., Leontowicz, M., Leontowicz, H., Katrich, E., Lojek, A., Ciz, M., Trakhtenberg, S. and Gorinstein, S. (2004). *J. Nutr. Biochem.* 15, 527–533.

Gerhauser, C. (2005). *Eur. J. Cancer.* 41, 1941–1954.

Gerhauser, C.A.A., Klimo, K., Knauft, J., Frank, N. and Becker, H. (2002). *Phytochem. Rev.* 1, 369–377.

Gronbaek, M., Deis, A., Sorensen, T.I., Becker, U., Schnohr, P. and Jensen, G. (1995). *BMJ* 310, 1165–1169.

Hai, T. and Hartman, M.G. (2001). *Gene* 273, 1–11.

Hai, T., Wolfgang, C.D., Marsee, D.K., Allen, A.E. and Sivaprasad, U. (1999). *Gene Expr.* 7, 321–335.

Hamano, Y., Sugimoto, H., Soubasakos, M.A., Kieran, M., Olsen, B.R., Lawler, J., Sudhakar, A. and Kalluri, R. (2004). *Cancer Res.* 64, 1570–1574.

He, T.C., Chan, T.A., Vogelstein, B. and Kinzler, K.W. (1999). *Cell* 99, 335–345.

He, T.C., Sparks, A.B., Rago, C., Hermeking, H., Zawel, L., da Costa, L.T., Morin, P.J., Vogelstein, B. and Kinzler, K.W. (1998). *Science* 281, 1509–1512.

Hong, J., Smith, T.J., Ho, C.T., August, D.A. and Yang, C.S. (2001). *Biochem. Pharmacol.* 62, 1175–1183.

Hsu, J.C., Bravo, R. and Taub, R. (1992). *Mol. Cell Biol.* 12, 4654–4665.

Huang, C.C., Fang, J.Y., Wu, W.B., Chiang, H.S., Wei, Y.J. and Hung, C.F. (2005). *Arch. Dermatol. Res.* 296, 473–481.

Hung, P.F., Wu, B.T., Chen, H.C., Chen, Y.H., Chen, C.L., Wu, M.H., Liu, H.C., Lee, M.J. and Kao, Y.H. (2005). *Am. J. Physiol. Cell Physiol.* 288, C1094–C1108.

Iizaka, M., Furukawa, Y., Tsunoda, T., Akashi, H., Ogawa, M. and Nakamura, Y. (2002). *Biochem. Biophys. Res. Commun.* 292, 498–512.

Kao, Y.H., Hiipakka, R.A. and Liao, S. (2000). *Am. J. Clin. Nutr.* 72, 1232–1234.

Kim, K.S., Baek, S.J., Flake, G.P., Loftin, C.D., Calvo, B.F. and Eling, T.E. (2002). *Gastroenterology* 122, 1388–1398.

Lamprecht, S.A. and Lipkin, M. (2003). *Nat. Rev. Cancer* 3, 601–614.

Lee, S.H., Kim, J.S., Yamaguchi, K., Eling, T.E. and Baek, S.J. (2005). *Biochem. Biophys. Res. Commun.* 328, 63–69.

Li, P.X., Wong, J., Ayed, A., Ngo, D., Brade, A.M., Arrowsmith, C., Austin, R.C. and Klamut, H.J. (2000). *J. Biol. Chem.* 275, 20127–20135.

Liao, S., Umekita, Y., Guo, J., Kokontis, J.M. and Hiipakka, R.A. (1995). *Cancer Lett.* 96, 239–243.

Lim, Y., Lee, S.-H., Song, M.-H., Yamaguchi, K., Yoon, J.-H., Choi, E.C. and Baek, S.J. (2006). *Eur. J. Cancer.* 42, 3260–3266.

Liu, T., Bauskin, A.R., Zaunders, J., Brown, D.A., Pankhurst, S., Russell, P.J. and Breit, S.N. (2003). *Cancer Res.* 63, 5034–5040.

Liu, Z., Ma, L.P., Zhou, B., Yang, L. and Liu, Z.L. (2000). *Chem. Phys. Lipid* 106, 53–63.

Lopez, M. and Edens, L. (2005). *J. Agric. Food Chem.* 53, 7944–7949.

Ludwig, A., Lorenz, M., Grimbo, N., Steinle, F., Meiners, S., Bartsch, C., Stangl, K., Baumann, G. and Stangl, V. (2004). *Biochem. Biophys. Res. Commun.* 316, 659–665.

Mandel, S., Maor, G. and Youdim, M.B. (2004). *J. Mol. Neurosci.* 24, 401–416.

Miura, Y., Chiba, T., Miura, S., Tomita, I., Umegaki, K., Ikeda, M. and Tomita, T. (2000). *J. Nutr. Biochem.* 11, 216–222.

Monks, A., Harris, E., Hose, C., Connelly, J. and Sausville, E.A. (2003). *Mol. Pharmacol.* 63, 766–772.

Nelson, R.L. and Samelson, S.L. (1985). *Dis. Colon Rectum* 28, 460–462.

Newman, D., Sakaue, M., Koo, J.S., Kim, K.S., Baek, S.J., Eling, T. and Jetten, A.M. (2003). *Mol. Pharmacol.* 63, 557–564.

Nie, G., Jin, C., Cao, Y., Shen, S. and Zhao, B. (2002). *Arch. Biochem. Biophys.* 397, 84–90.

Nozawa, H., Yoshida, A., Tajima, O., Katayama, M., Sonobe, H., Wakabayashi, K. and Kondo, K. (2004). *Int. J. Cancer* 108, 404–411.

Okabe, S., Suganuma, M., Hayashi, M., Sueoka, E., Komori, A. and Fujiki, H. (1997). *Jpn. J. Cancer Res.* 88, 639–643.

Polakis, P. (2000). *Gene. Dev.* 14, 1837–1851.

Pulido, R., Hernandez-Garcia, M. and Saura-Calixto, F. (2003). *Eur. J. Clin. Nutr.* 57, 1275–1282.

Rapuri, P.B., Gallagher, J.C., Balhorn, K.E. and Ryschon, K.L. (2000). *Am. J. Clin. Nutr.* 72, 1206–1213.

Rimm, E.B., Giovannucci, E.L., Willett, W.C., Colditz, G.A., Ascherio, A., Rosner, B. and Stampfer, M.J. (1991). *Lancet* 338, 464–468.

Rizvi, S.I., Zaid, M.A., Anis, R. and Mishra, N. (2005). *Clin. Exp. Pharmacol. Physiol.* 32, 70–75.

Rodriguez-Manzaneque, J.C., Lane, T.F., Ortega, M.A., Hynes, R.O., Lawler, J. and Iruela-Arispe, M.L. (2001). *Proc. Natl. Acad. Sci. USA* 98, 12485–12490.

Ruitenberg, A., van Swieten, J.C., Witteman, J.C., Mehta, K.M., van Duijn, C.M., Hofman, A. and Breteler, M.M. (2002). *Lancet* 359, 281–286.

Sachinidis, A., Skach, R.A., Seul, C., Ko, Y., Hescheler, J., Ahn, H.Y. and Fingerle, J. (2002). *Faseb J.* 16, 893–895.

Shtutman, M., Zhurinsky, J., Simcha, I., Albanese, C., D'Amico, M., Pestell, R. and Ben-Ze'ev, A. (1999). *Proc. Natl. Acad. Sci. USA* 96, 5522–5527.

Tetsu, O. and McCormick, F. (1999). *Nature* 398, 422–426.

Thun, M.J., Peto, R., Lopez, A.D., Monaco, J.H., Henley, S.J., Heath Jr., C.W. and Doll, R. (1997). *New Engl. J. Med.* 337, 1705–1714.

Tian, W.X. (2006). *Curr. Med. Chem.* 13, 967–977.

USDA (2005). www.ers.usda.gov/data/foodconsumption/.

Vaidyanathan, J.B. and Walle, T. (2003). *J. Pharmacol. Exp. Ther.* 307, 745–752.

Vinson, J.A., Mandarano, M., Hirst, M., Trevithick, J.R. and Bose, P. (2003). *J. Agric. Food Chem.* 51, 5528–5533.

Wan, S.B., Landis-Piwowar, K.R., Kuhn, D.J., Chen, D., Dou, Q.P. and Chan, T.H. (2005). *Bioorg. Med. Chem.* 13, 2177–2185.

Weyant, M.J., Carothers, A.M., Dannenberg, A.J. and Bertagnolli, M.M. (2001). *Cancer Res.* 61, 118–125.

Whisenant, J. and Bergsland, E. (2005). *Curr. Treat. Option Oncol.* 6, 411–421.

Widelitz, R.B., Jiang, T.X., Lu, J. and Chuong, C.M. (2000). *Dev. Biol.* 219, 98–114.

Wilson, L.C., Baek, S.J., Call, A. and Eling, T.E. (2003). *Int. J. Cancer* 105, 747–753.

Wu, B.T., Hung, P.F., Chen, H.C., Huang, R.N., Chang, H.H. and Kao, Y.H. (2005). *J. Agric. Food Chem.* 53, 5695–5701.

Wu, L.Y., Juan, C.C., Ho, L.T., Hsu, Y.P. and Hwang, L.S. (2004). *J. Agric. Food Chem.* 52, 643–648.

Yamaguchi, K., Lee, S.H., Eling, T.E. and Baek, S.J. (2006a). *Mol. Cancer Ther.* 5, 1352–1361.

Yamaguchi, K., Liggett, J.L., Kim, N.C. and Baek, S.J. (2006b). *Oncol. Rep.* 15, 275–281.

Yanagawa, Y., Yamamoto, Y., Hara, Y. and Shimamura, T. (2003). *Curr. Microbiol.* 47, 244–249.

Yang, G.Y., Liao, J., Kim, K., Yurkow, E.J. and Yang, C.S. (1998). *Carcinogenesis* 19, 611–616.

Zaveri, N.T. (2006). *Life Sci.* 78, 2073–2080.

Zhang, R., Xiao, W., Wang, X., Wu, X. and Tian, W. (2006). *Biotechnol. Appl. Biochem.* 43, 1–7.

88

Use of Quercetin in Prostate Cancer Cell

Charles Y. F. Young Department of Urology, Mayo Clinic/Foundation, Rochester, MN, USA

Abstract

The anti-cancer activity of beers is believed residing in its non-alcoholic portion containing phyto-polyphenols that comes from the raw materials including hops and malt, used for making beers. Although a recent study indicated that beers and red wines may have a trend of reduction of prostate cancer risk, more studies with a large population are required to demonstrate its potency. Quercetin, a major polyphenol existing in many fruits and vegetables, is one of the polyphenols found in beers that shows anti-prostate cancer activities in cell culture and animal models. In addition to its strong antioxidant/detoxification activities, quercetin can derail cell cycle progression by causing various cell phase arrests, therefore exhibiting anti-proliferative activities and inducing apoptosis. Alterations in expression levels or activities of a number of cell cycle regulatory related genes including Cdc2/Cdk-1, cyclin B1, phosphorylated pRb and p21 were observed by quercetin treatment. Similarly, the expression or activities of apoptotic-related proteins like anti-apoptotic proteins Bcl-2 and Bcl-X-L and pro-apoptotic proteins Bax and caspase-3 are also found to be changed by quercetin. Quercetin may also affect a number of signaling molecules or transcription factors including the androgen receptor, the signal transducer and activator of transcription 3 (STAT3), c-Jun, Sp1, etc. in prostate cancer cells in response to stimulation by hormones or growth factors/cytokines. Finally, it has been shown in several studies that a combining use of quercetin with other agents (e.g. ellagic acid, tamoxifen, etc.) may enhance the anti-prostate cancer effects of quercetin.

List of Abbreviations

ACF	Aberrant crypt foci
AR	Androgen receptor
ARE	Androgen responsive element
CYP	Cytochrome P450 enzyme
FAS	Fatty acid synthase
GSP	Glutathione *S*-transferase
HSP70	Heat shock protein 70
IGFs	Insulin-like growth factors
IGFBP-3	IGF binding protein-3
IL-6	Interleukin 6
IP3	Inositol 1, 4, 5-triphosphate
QR	Quinone reductase
STAT3	The signal transducer and activator of transcription 3
SULT	Sulfotransferase
UGT	Uridine diphosphate-glucuronyltransferase
VEGF	Vascular endothelial growth factor

Introduction

It is well established the seriousness of alcohol abuse to the health of individuals (Fothergill and Ensminger, 2006). It has been a long time that there was a suspicion that use of alcoholic beverages may have a positive impact on prostate cancer risk. However, many recent studies (Jain *et al.*, 1998; Sesso *et al.*, 2001; Albertsen and Gronbaek, 2002; Platz *et al.*, 2004; Chang *et al.*, 2005; Schoonen *et al.*, 2005) seem to indicate that alcohol intake from beer, wine or liquor may not be a strong contributor to prostate cancer risk, except possibly in men who drink large quantities. For example, a large prospective cohort study of 47,843 US men with 2,497 men developing prostate cancer revealed no positive association between alcohol consumption and cancer risk (Platz *et al.*, 2004). Another relative large cohort study also showed no association of neither amount nor type of alcohol consumed with the risk of prostate cancer (Albertsen and Gronbaek, 2002). A Harvard Alumni Health study showed only liquor, but not wine or beer, consumption was positively associated with prostate cancer (Sesso *et al.*, 2001). On the other hand, it was suggested that drinking red wine may relatively reduce prostate cancer risk (Schoonen *et al.*, 2005). Interestingly, another study showed that beer may have trends to decrease risk of prostate cancer (Jain *et al.*, 1998). Clearly more in-depth studies will be required to clarify the issue. Regardless, excessive alcohol consumption can seriously damage general health of individuals and should be avoided.

Recently, an animal study (Nozawa *et al.*, 2004) demonstrated that azoxymethane (AOM)-induced colonic

Beer in Health and Disease Prevention
ISBN: 978-0-12-373891-2

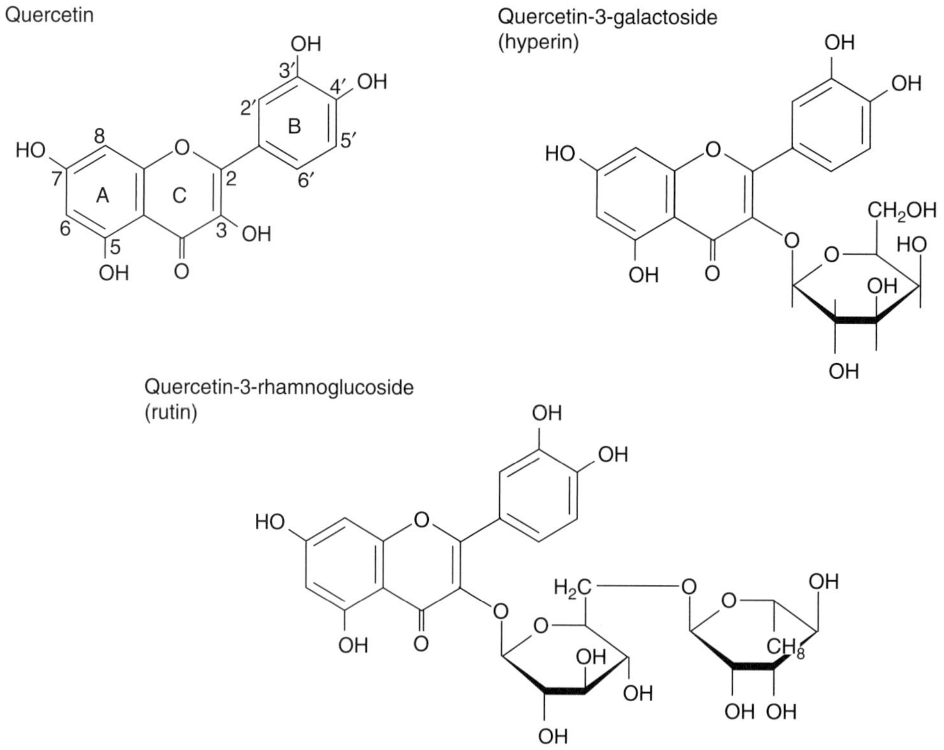

Figure 88.1 Chemical structures of quercetin and some derivatives.

carcinogenesis in male Fischer 344 rats can be repressed by intake of beer. This investigation showed that freeze-dried beer, but not alcohol can significantly inhibit the formation of aberrant crypt foci (ACF), suggesting that non-alcohol components of beer could be responsible for the inhibition. A long-term (42 weeks) of beer intake decreased tumor incidence by 22% and decreased the number of neoplastic lesions by 44%. In an *in vitro* study (Tedesco *et al.*, 2005), the authors selected a particular brand of beer containing high antioxidant polyphenols for investigating cell proliferation effects of lyophilized beer materials in comparison with that from another brand of beer with low polyphenol contents on a leukemia cell line, HL-60. The lyophilized beer material containing high polyphenol content showed much higher anti-proliferation effect than that from low polyphenol containing beer. The important point is that these studies seem to suggest that certain non-alcoholic components, perhaps particularly polyphenols, in beer may have chemopreventive effects and that intake of beer might contribute to a reduction in the risk of cancer development. Again, more *in vitro* and human clinical studies may be required to further investigate any chemopreventive effects of beer on cancers.

It has been shown that a main type of substances in beer presenting potential anti-cancer activities is plant phenolics (Gorinstein *et al.*, 2000; Gerhauser, 2005; Nardini *et al.*, 2006). These plant phenolics or polyphenols possess antioxidant properties which are thought to have anti-cancer activity. Paganga *et al.* (1999) estimated that the antioxidant activities of plant polyphenols in 500 ml beer are equivalent to 4 apples, 2 cups of tea or 500 g of fresh onion. The beer phenolics are mainly from hop (20–30%) and malt (70–80%), the two major raw materials for making beer. One of the major forms of poly-phenols in beer is quercetin and its glycosyl-derivatives (Figure 88.1 and Table 88.1).

Quercetin Actions in Prostate Cancer Cells

Prostate cancer is among the top cancer killers for men in several western or highly industrialized countries, such as United States, United Kingdom, etc. It has been suggested that the much higher rates of prostate cancer incidents in these countries than that in those less-developed countries may be largely attributable to life styles, especially diets (Kamangar *et al.*, 2006; Klein, 2006). In general agreement, prostate cancer is one of cancer types most suitable for chemoprevention modalities, in part, because it requires decades to develop or progress (Kamangar *et al.*, 2006; Klein, 2006).

Structure of quercetin

Quercetin is one of the most abundant flavonoids present in various fruits, vegetables and beverages (Aherne and

Table 88.1 Glycosyl derivatives of quercetin

	Source (example)
Quercetin-3-arabinoside (avicularin)	Apple, onion
Quercetin-3-galactoside (hyperin)	Apple
Quercetin-3-glucoside (isoquercitrin)	Apple, onion
Quercetin-3, 4′-glucoside	Onion
Quercetin-3-rhamnoglucoside (rutin)	Onion, apple, black tea
Quercetin-3-rhamnoside (quercitrin)	Cherry
Quercetin-3-xyloside (reynoutrin)	Apple, berries
Quercetin-3-pentoside	Berries

Source: Amaral *et al.* (2004); Erlund (2004); Häkkinen *et al.* (1999); Hertog *et al.* (1992); Hertog *et al.* (1993); Lu and Foo (1997); Vvedenskaya *et al.* (2004).

Table 88.2 Quercetin content in fruits and vegetables

	mg/100g
Apple	2–26
Apricot	2.5–5.3
Bilberry	10.5–16
Black currant	3.7–6.8
Broad bean	2–134
Broccoli	0.6–3.7
Cabbage, red	0.19–0.62
Cauliflower	0–3.1
Chives	10.4–30
Cranberry	149
Elderberry	10.5–24
Endive	0.1–2.6
Onion, white	18–63
Fresh bean	3.2–4.5
Grape, red	1.5–37
Grape, white	0.2–1.2
Kale	1.2–11
Leak	1.0–2.5
Lettuce	0.2–47
Pear	0.3–4.5
Plum	0–1.5
Raspberry	0.5–2.9
Red currant	0.2–2.7
Sour cherry	2.3–8
Sweet cherry	0.6–2.4
Tomato, cherry	0.4–7.4
Tomato, red	0.16–43
White currant	0.3–2.8

Source: This table is reproduced with some modifications from Aheme and O'Brien (2002), Elsevier Science Inc.

Table 88.3 Quercetin content in beverages

Beverage	*mg/100 ml*
Apple juice	0.25
Grape juice	0.44
Grapefruit juice	0.49
Lemon juice	0.74
Orange juice	0.34–0.57
Tomato juice	1.1–1.3
Tea, black bags	1.7–2.5
Tea, black loose	1.0–1.6
Tea, green	0.11–2.3
Tea, oolong	1.3
Wine, red	0–1.6
Beer	0.095

Source: This table is reproduced with some modifications from Aheme and O'Brien (2002), Elsevier Science Inc.

O'Brien, 2002, Mertens-Talcott *et al.*, 2003; Erlund, 2004; Manach *et al.*, 2004) (Tables 88.2 and 88.3). The basic nucleus structure of flavonoids consists of two benzene rings (A and B) connected by an oxygen containing pyrene ring (C). With a various substitution pattern in these three rings it forms a large numbers of subgroups. Basically, flavonoids can be divided into several classes (e.g. anthocyanidins, flavanols/catechins, flavones, flavonols, flavanones and isoflavones, etc.) depending on oxidation levels on the C-ring. Quercetin belongs to a class of flavonoids, called flavonols, which carry a carbonyl group on C-4 (4-oxo) of the C-ring. So far quercetin is one of the most commonly investigated plant phenolics for its biological functions, maybe because it possesses much higher anti-radical activities toward hydroxyl radical, peroxyl and superoxide anion than many other flavonoids (Morel *et al.*, 1993; Skibola and Smith, 2000). Interestingly, quercetin also exists in many different glycosidic forms in their natural sources. The glycoside moiety is linked through hydroxyl group at C3 position of the C-ring as seen in the examples of Figure 88.1. Some examples (Sagesser and Deinzer, 1996; Aherne and O'Brien, 2002; Mertens-Talcott *et al.*, 2003; Manach *et al.*, 2004; Chen *et al.*, 2005; Lee *et al.*, 2005) (Table 88.1) of quercetin glycosides are quercetin-3-rhamnoglucoside (or rutin) in black tea, guercetin-4′-glucoside and guercetin-3, 4′-glucoside in onion, quercetin galactoside in apples, and quercetin arabinosides in berries. The glycoside moieties may facilitate absorption in human intestine.

Anti-carcinogenesis of quercetin by antioxidative/detoxification effects

Oxidative stress can cause cellular damage at protein, lipid and DNA levels. Accumulative damages of those cellular components may be linked to cancer development. It has been proposed that certain reactive oxygen species may be related to prostate cancer development in that male hormones/androgens are shown to be an important agent to produce such oxygen species in the prostate (Ripple *et al.*, 1997, 1999). Note, androgens via the nuclear androgen receptor (AR) are absolutely required for development and maintenance of normal human and rodent prostates. In addition, oxidative species such as reactive oxygen, nitrogen and lipid species as well as other environmental reactive agents derived from consumption of red meat, fats/oils and exposures to pollutants may be more or less contributed to prostate cancer development (Hsieh and Albertsen, 2003; Kamangar *et al.*, 2006; Colli and Colli, 2006; Klein, 2006; Moon *et al.*, 2006; Rodriguez *et al.*, 2006). Quercetin has been shown as one of the strong antioxidants *in vitro* (Morel *et al.*, 1993; Skibola and Smith, 2000). Potentially it might act as a scavenger to remove some reactive oxygen species generated by androgens or other sources. However, whether quercetin could actually exert its antioxidative activities effectively in the body remains elusive.

Quercetin could act at least two ways to ward off reactive oxidants (Nagata *et al.*, 1999; Aherne and O'Brien, 2002; Mertens-Talcott *et al.*, 2003; Erlund, 2004; Manach *et al.*, 2004; Moon *et al.*, 2006). In principle, the phenolic group of polyphenols including quercetin can accept an electron from or be oxidized by radicals to form a more stable, less reactive phenoxyl radical, and thus disrupting further chain oxidative reactions. Secondly quercetin can be an effective phase II detoxifying enzyme inducer or a direct phase I enzyme inhibitor to indirectly reduce formation of carcinogens activated by endogenous metabolism pathways (Nagata *et al.*, 1999; Aherne and O'Brien, 2002; Mertens-Talcott *et al.*, 2003; Erlund, 2004; Manach *et al.*, 2004; Moon *et al.*, 2006). For example, it was reported that quercetin can inhibit human cytochrome CYP1 enzymes (a phase I enzyme) at 50% inhibition concentration of 4.1 uM in a prostate cancer cell (Chaudhary and Willett, 2006). The CYP1B1 enzyme can metabolize polycyclic aromatic hydrocarbons to active carcinogenic metabolites (Chaudhary and Willett, 2006). Sun *et al.* (1998) found that several flavonoids including quercetin can induce activity of a phase II enzyme, UDP-glucuronyltransferase (UGT), in a human prostate cancer cell line, whose enzyme activity can enhance the removal of androgens like testosterone from body, implying that the flavonoids tested may be used to modulate hormone metabolism and therefore for prevention or treatment of prostate cancer. Table 88.4 lists some examples of phase I and II enzymes that can be affected by quercetin in both non-prostate and prostate tissues or *in vitro* cell culture conditions. It is assumed that the detoxifying effects of those phase I and II enzymes outside of the prostate (e.g. liver) may benefit in protecting from prostate cancer formation. However, whether all of these enzymes are expressed and can be affected by quercetin in the prostate remains to be further studied.

Table 88.4 Known effects of quercetin on expression or activities of phase I and II enzymes

Enzyme	*effect*	*References*
Phase I		
CYP1A1	Increases mRNA expression	Ciolino *et al.* (1999)
CYP1A2	Inhibitor	Tsyrlov *et al.* (1994)
CYP3A4	Inhibitor	Obach (2000)
Phase II		
UGT	Increases enzyme activity	van der Logt *et al.* (2003)
UGT1A1	Increases enzyme activity	Williams *et al.* (2002)
GSTP1-1	Inhibitor	van Zanden *et al.* (2003)
QR	Increases enzyme activity	Uda *et al.* (1997); Valerio *et al.* (2001)
SULT1A1	Inhibitor	Mesia-Vela and Kauffman (2003)
SULT1E1	Inhibitor	Schrag *et al.* (2004)

Notes: Related to carcinogenesis, although phase I enzymes can activate procarcionogens and phase II enzymes are used to detoxify potential carcinogens, either one can sometimes also do opposite actions, depending on substrates and varying conditions.

CYP, cytochrome P450 enzymes; UGT, uridine diphosphate-glucuronyltransferase; GSP, glutathione *S*-transferase; QR, quinone reductase; SULT, sulfotransferase.

Anti-androgen receptor effects

As mentioned above, androgens are not only important to the normal prostate but also implicated in the development and progression of prostate cancer (Scher *et al.*, 2004; Dehm and Tindall, 2005). The androgen action is mediated by a specific nuclear receptor protein or AR. In fact, the AR is a member of nuclear receptor superfamily of transcription factors (Scher *et al.*, 2004; Dehm and Tindall, 2005), and is activated by androgens to regulate gene expression and proliferation of prostatic cells. Upon androgen binding, the AR will be translocated from cytoplasm to nucleus and then binds a specific DNA sequence, termed androgen responsive element or ARE, in the promoter area of androgen target/regulated genes. Activated AR may undergo some chemical modification such as phosphorylation and acetylation and recruit other non-DNA-binding proteins named co-activators to enhance gene transcription. Androgen deprivation or ablation can cause prostate epithelial apoptosis, therefore prostate regression, and is the basis for androgen or hormonal therapy of prostate cancer (Scher *et al.*, 2004; Dehm and Tindall, 2005). As aforementioned, androgens via the receptor may enhance oxidation stress which would increase genomic mutation rates. Properly modulating androgen actions in the prostate might be an effective means to prevent prostate cancer development and progression.

Like several other dietary factors (Ren *et al.*, 2000; Bektic *et al.*, 2004; Cho *et al.*, 2004; Dong *et al.*, 2004; Gao *et al.*, 2004; Lee *et al.*, 2004; Jiang *et al.*, 2006; Morris *et al.*, 2006), quercetin has been shown to exhibit activity of inhibiting the expression and function of the AR in prostate cancer cells (Xing *et al.*, 2001; Morris *et al.*, 2006). Further, the functional repression of the AR by quercetin is due to prolonged overexpression of c-Jun which has been shown to be able to physically interact with the AR (Yuan *et al.*, 2004, 2005). c-Jun is a transcription factor but acts as a co-repressor of the AR in quercetin-treated prostate cancer cells. Further studies (Palapattu *et al.*, 2005) showed that quercetin can reduce phosphorylation of the AR and increase interaction of AR with Sp1, the latter is another transcription factor, but in this case acting as a co-activator to enhance AR's function. The repression effect of quercetin could be due to the combination of hypophosphorylation and increased interactions of AR with c-Jun and Sp1 (published data). More in-depth studies will be needed to understand how quercetin could facilitate the formation of the above protein complex to inhibit AR action in prostate cancer cells.

Anti-inflammatory effects

This section will only focus on the relevance in prostate cancer. The recent realization of association of inflammatory lesions with prostatic cancerous tissues suggests the potential involvement of local inflammation in prostate carcinogenesis (Ho *et al.*, 2004; Hodge *et al.*, 2005; Mauri *et al.*, 2005; Palapattu *et al.*, 2005). It has been shown that quercetin has anti-inflammation effects (Di Carlo *et al.*, 1999). Whether this effect has any influence on repressing prostate carcinogenesis is not clear at present time. Preliminary studies seemed to indicate the possibility, because inflammation-related factors can be produced in infiltrated immune cells as well as prostate cells (Shariat *et al.*, 2001; Lee *et al.*, 2003; Sivashanmugam *et al.*, 2004; Hodge *et al.*, 2005; Mauri *et al.*, 2005; Zhu *et al.*, 2006). These factors may modify endocrine response and enhance prostate cell proliferation. For instance, pro-inflammatory cytokine factors including interleukin 6 (IL-6) may be overexpressed in pre-cancerous and cancerous areas of the prostate and stimulate prostate cell proliferation and increase immune cell filtration. Interestingly, IL-6 and other cytokines may activate AR without the presence of or at very low concentrations of androgens. This could provide an additional way to enhance AR functions (e.g. cell proliferation and oxidative stress). Preliminary data shown in Figures 88.2 and 88.3 indicate that quercetin may be able to inhibit IL-6 mediated activities (e.g. AR activation without androgens) in prostate cancer cells. Moreover, it has been shown that quercetin can inhibit NO production in prostate cancer cells. NO may be related to induction of inflammation (Kampa *et al.*, 2000). Interestingly, quercetin has been suggested to treat prostatitis, an inflammatory form of the prostate (Shoskes and Manickam, 2003).

Effects on cell proliferation, cell cycle and apoptosis

A major hallmark of cancer cells is their deregulated cell cycle compared to a stringent cell cycle control of their normal counterparts (Hermeking and Benzinger, 2006). Basically, cancer cells will allow themselves to proliferate continuously if nutrients and space are not restricted, which is mainly because of aberrant expression of extracellular factors

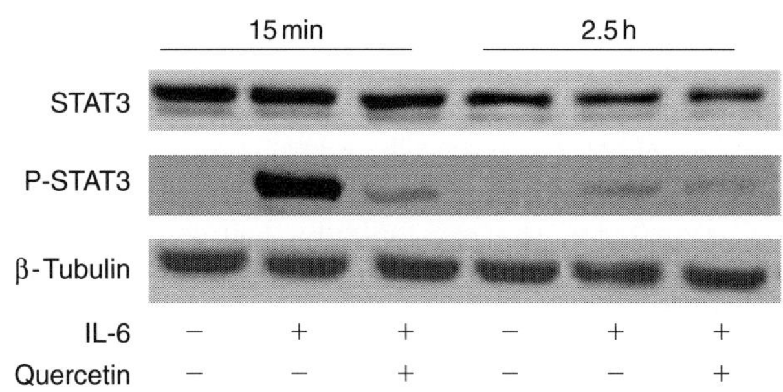

Figure 88.2 Quercetin inhibits activation of STAT3 stimulated by interleukin 6 (IL-6) in human prostate cancer cell line, LNCaP. LNCaP cells were treated with or without IL-6 (50 ng/ml) ± quercetin (50 uM) for 15 min or 2.5 h. Thirty microgram proteins from cell extracts prepared from the above cells were used for immunoblotting analysis for phosphorylated STAT3 and total STAT3 with specific antibodies. Phosphorylated STAT3 represents the activation of STAT3 by IL-6. This study shows that IL6 activates STAT3 by inducing phosphorylation of STAT3 but not changing the levels of STAT3 after short incubation of cells with IL-6. Quercetin can inhibit phosphorylation of STAT3. Tubulin was used as internal controls for equal loading.

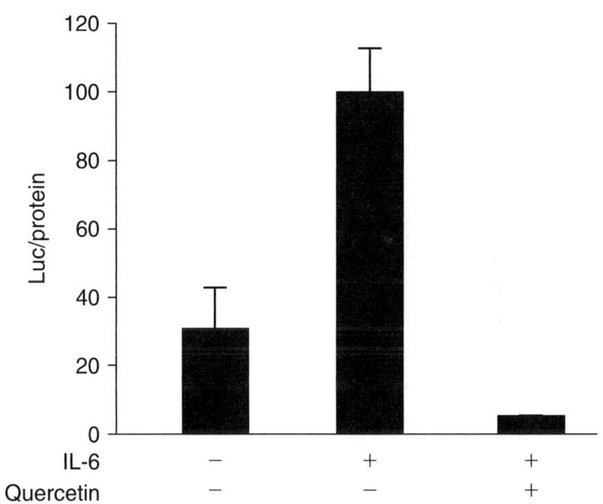

Figure 88.3 Quercetin inhibits IL-6 induced AR activation of luciferase reporter expression via the prostate-specific antigen (PSA) promoter in a transfection assay. IL-6 activates STAT3 which in turn interacts and activates the AR. The expression of PSA is mediated via AR activated by androgens or IL6. In this figure, LNCaP cells that express AR were used for transfection with a PSA promoter-luciferase plasmid construct (1 μg) and then treated with (+) or without (−) IL6 (50 ng/ml)) ± quercetin (50 uM) overnight. Cell extracts were prepared for luciferase and protein assays. Luciferase activities were normalized with protein contents and used to present AR function activated by IL-6 which can be inhibited by quercetin.

(e.g. growth factors) and/or intracellular factors (e.g. cyclins, cyclin-dependent kinases and kinase inhibitors, etc.) related to regulation of the cell cycle in cancer cells or tissues.

Quercetin may inhibit cancer cell proliferation by stalling cell cycle progression at particular stages of the cell cycle, which may result in cell death or apoptosis, depending on cell types or concentrations of quercetin used. For instance, quercetin at 100 uM can induce G0/G1 phase arrest of bladder cancer cell and subsequently apoptosis (Ma *et al.*, 2006). Interestingly, this study showed that quercetin may possess anti-DNA methyltransferase activity, and, therefore, re-activate the expression of tumor suppressors. However, quercetin can cause G2/M phase arrest in human PC-3 prostate cancer cells followed by apoptosis (Vijayababu *et al.*, 2005). The induced apoptosis could be related to inhibition of multiple intracellular signaling pathways involving tyrosine kinase activity (Wang *et al.*, 2003). Also, substantial decrease in the expression of cell cycle related proteins such as Cdc2/Cdk-1, cyclin B1 and phosphorylated pRb and increase in p21 were observed (Vijayababu *et al.*, 2005). Quercetin may inhibit PC-3 cell proliferation by reducing insulin-like growth factors (IGFs) and IGF binding protein-3 (IGFBP-3) secretion (Vijayababu *et al.*, 2006a) or reducing the expression of ErbB-2 and ErbB-3 to prevent proliferative stimulation by transforming growth factor alpha and epidermal growth factor (Huynh *et al.*, 2003). It was reported (Vijayababu *et al.*, 2006b) that quercetin can downregulate matrix metalloproteinases 2 and 9 proteins expression in PC-3 cells, which may reduce cell migration and metastasis ability. In addition, anti-apoptotic proteins like Bcl-2 and Bcl-X-L were significantly decreased and pro-apoptotic proteins Bax and caspase-3 were increased. Quercetin induced G2/M phase arrest can be seen in another prostate cancer cell line, LNCaP (Shenouda *et al.*, 2004). Another study (Knowles *et al.*, 2000) reported that quercetin at 25 uM blocks PC-3 cells at G2/M transition, but at 100 uM it causes an increase in S-phase, whereas neither concentration induces apoptosis. The discrepancy between this latter study and the above study regarding the detection of apoptosis in the same cell line is not clear.

Furthermore, it was suggested (Brusselmans *et al.*, 2005) that in both prostate and breast cancer cells, fatty acid synthesis by fatty acid synthase (FAS) inhibited by flavonoids including quercetin may play a critical role of inducing apoptosis. This notion seems to be supported by reversal of apoptosis by addition of palmitate, the end product of FAS.

Synergistic effects with other chemical or physical factors

Obviously when consuming quercetin-containing foods and/or beverages, inevitably many phytochemicals possessing anti-cancer activities would be partaken with quercetin. However, there are only few studies showing some phytochemicals can synergistically enhance anti-carcinogenesis activities of quercetin. For example, ellagic acid, a type of flavonoids, can synergistically increase anti-proliferation ability of quercetin at low concentrations in human leukemia cells (Mertens-Talcott *et al.*, 2005). This study indicated that ellagic acid can enhance expression of tumor suppressors like p21waf1/cip1 and p53 as well as signaling molecules, MAP kinases induced by quercetin. The same group of the authors (Mertens-Talcott and Percival, 2005) demonstrated that when quercetin and another flavonoid, resveratrol, work together, they can induce transient cell cycle arrest and largely increase apoptosis of human leukemia cells. Other study (Chen *et al.*, 2005) showed that quercetin can act synergistically with vitamins C and E to block oxidation of low-density lipoprotein.

It has been realized that combination chemotherapy is increasingly practiced for more effective treatment of advanced prostate cancers. Synergistic effects of a combining use of quercetin and other agents have been studied to explore therapeutic potentials in treating prostate cancer. An early study (Li *et al.*, 1999) showed that quercetin and a synthetic drug called ribavirin in combination can produce a synergistic anti-proliferative action against myeloma 8,226 cell line and ovarian carcinoma OVCAR-5 cell line due to the synergistic reduction of an oncogenic signal transduction (i.e. IP3 concentration). Another intriguing observation is that Fujita *et al.* (2004) reported that a combination of quercetin and heat treatment can increase cytotoxic effect in a lymphoid cell line. In xenograft mouse model, Asea *et al.* (2001) demonstrated that quercetin can dramatically enhance the effects of hyperthermia on inhibiting tumor growth of two human prostate cancer cell lines, PC-3 and DU145. Another *in vitro* study (Nakanoma *et al.*, 2001) using human prostate cancer lines JCA-1 and LNCaP showed that quercetin can reduce heat shock protein 70 (HSP70) induced by heat shock treatment and increase cell number in G1 phase. The authors concluded that quercetin can enhance heat shock-induced apoptosis in both JCA-I and LNcap cells. Further study (Jones *et al.*, 2004) concluded that indeed HSP70 plays a role in protection of prostate tumor cells from apoptosis because depletion of HSP70 by using anti-sense oligonucleotide approach can induce cell apoptosis without any additional treatments. This probably explains why quercetin treatment can synergistically enhance apoptosis of human prostate cancer cells treating with heat shock *in vitro* or a hyperthermia procedure to xenograft models.

Furthermore, a human prostate cancer CWR22-xenograft model was used to determine therapeutic efficacy of tamoxifen (a synthetic non-steroidal antiestrogen), quercetin or a combined tamoxifen and quercetin for 28 days (Ma *et al.*, 2004a). The results showed either tamoxifen or quercetin alone only exhibited a moderate anti-tumor growth effect, whereas the combined tamoxifen and quercetin showed synergistic reduction of tumor weight and volume. The authors showed that angiogenesis-related molecular events including the vascular endothelial growth factor (VEGF) and microvessel density in tumor areas are largely reduced, suggesting quercetin may potentiate the tamoxifen effects on repressing tumor angiogenesis. Owing to low potency of quercetin for treating prostate cancer, Paliwal *et al.* (2005) showed if prostate and skin cancer cells pre-treated with low-frequency ultrasound (20 kHz, $2\,W\,cm^{-2}$, 60 s) can exhibit strong cytotoxicity in the presence of quercetin. Interestingly the combined effects only affect cancer cells but not their normal counterparts. However, at present time, there is no clear explanation of how ultrasound selectively sensitizes cancer cells to amplify cytotoxic effects of quercetin.

Recently a 5 reductase inhibitor finastride, which can reduce androgen concentrations in the prostate, has been shown to be possibly used in humans for preventing prostate cancer (Zeliadt *et al.*, 2005). In animal model, male rats received finasteride showed lower serum androgen and prostate weight, whereas in quercetin treated male rats, serum androgen levels were increased and prostate weight was also slightly increased (Ma *et al.*, 2004b). However, co-administration of quercetin and finasteride reduced prostate weight much higher than finasteride alone. It was shown that quercetin enhances finasteride to cause a wide range of changes in cell cycle regulatory proteins including lower levels of cyclin D1, CDK-4, cdc-2, and phospho-cdc-2 at tyrosine 15, phospho-MEK1/2, phospho-MAP kinase, phospho-pRb and higher levels of tumor suppressors p53, and p15, p21 and p27 when compared to non-treated prostate. The authors concluded that quercetin synergizes with finasteride to reduce the wet prostate weight through a cell cycle-related pathway. This study seems to warrant future investigations to test if quercetin may be used in combination with finasteride for effective prevention or even treatment of prostate cancer.

Quercetin in human or animal studies

Results from numerous *in vitro* studies strongly suggest quercetin exerts anti-cancer activities. Animal model data seem to support the notion that quercetin possesses anti-carcinogenesis activities in some studies but are not confirmed by others. A recent study (Volate *et al.*, 2005) showed that quercetin (being the most potent one among the tested) and other flavonoids can reduce formation of ACF in an AOM-induced rat colon cancer model. However, an earlier study (Femia *et al.*, 2003) using onion or tomatoes fortified with quercetin glycosides did not show any obvious anti-carcinogenesis effects. Another earlier study (Mahmoud *et al.*, 2000) used C57BL/6J-Min/+(Min/+) mice bearing a germline mutation in the Apc gene and capable of spontaneously developing numerous intestinal adenomas by 15 weeks of age to investigate anti-tumor efficacy of quercetin. This study also failed to show anti-cancer effect of quercetin. On the other hand, Verma *et al.* (1988) were able to demonstrate that quercetin can inhibit both the incidence and the number of palpable rat mammary tumors in both 7,12-dimethylbenz(a)anthracene (DMBA)- and *N*-nitrosomethylurea-induced mammary cancer in female Sprague-Dawley rats. Moreover, Jin *et al.* (2006) in a very recent report showed that quercetin can effectively repress formation of lung cancer induced by benzo[a]pyrene in mice. Yuan *et al.* (2006) reported that liposomal quercetin can effectively inhibit growth of several types of tumor in mouse models. Asea *et al.* (2001) showed that quercetin can significantly inhibit the growth of human prostate cancer cells in athymic mice.

Similar to animal models, human studies of quercetin effects on cancer development are also relatively scarce and results are not necessarily consistent. Recently Neuhouser (2004) comprehensively reviewed data from 4 cohort studies and 6 case-control studies focusing on dietary flavonoids and cancer risk. The author concluded that the most consistent results from those studies was that high intake of dietary flavonoids especially quercetin may reduce lung cancer risk. Some of the studies described in this report also found no association of quercetin and the risk of prostate cancer. In an average of 6.1 year follow-up of the alpha-tocopherol, beta-carotene cancer prevention (ATBC) cohort study of 27,100 Finnish male smokers, intake of flavonols and flavones was reported (Hirvonen *et al.*, 2001) to be inversely associated with the risk of lung cancer but not with other cancers including prostate cancer. Another Finnish study (Knekt *et al.*, 2002) investigating flavonoid intake and the risk of chronic diseases of 10,054 men and women showed that men with higher quercetin intakes has a lower lung cancer risk. These above studies seem to confirm the earlier study that high intakes of quercetin-containing foods might lower the risk of lung cancer. However, Spanish studies (Garcia-Closas *et al.*, 1998; Garcia-Closas *et al.*, 1999) showed that quercetin does not reduce lung cancer risk in women but does have a trend to reduce gastric cancer risk. A recent study (Adebamowo *et al.*, 2005) reported that no overall association between intake of flavonols including quercetin and risk of breast cancer is found. Interestingly, a case-control study (McCann *et al.*, 2005) of diet and prostate cancer in Western New York involving 433 men with primary, histologically confirmed prostate cancer and 538 population-based controls, frequency matched to cases on age and county of residence was conducted. When compared with men in the lowest quartile of intake, reduced risks were observed for men in the highest quartile of intake of quercetin as well as several other phytochemicals studied.

Clearly the above studies are not sufficient to conclude whether quercetin can effectively reduce prostate cancer risk. Incorporating the measurements of bioavailable quercetin in the study subjects into designs of the future epidemiologic studies may be helpful in the evaluation (Lambert *et al.*, 2005). Intervention study could also be useful to determine the efficacy of quercetin in prostate cancer prevention.

Concluding Remarks

Non-alcoholic portion of beers has been shown to have anti-cancer activities on human cancer cells in culture vessels and chemical-induced tumor in laboratory animal models. A human survey study seemed to suggest that drinking beer and some wines may have trends to reduce prostate cancer risk; of course, more studies will be required to verify that in the near future. Quercetin is a major antioxidant polyphenolic molecule found in many vegetables and fruits as well as in beers and red wines. It has been shown that quercetin possesses anti-prostate cancer cells activities for example, proliferation inhibition, apoptosis, anti-androgen receptor and inhibiting other growth regulatory related cellular factors in prostate cancer cell culture and/or animal systems. However, whether quercetin can really reduce human prostate cancer risk remains to be rigorously studied.

References

Adebamowo, C.A., Cho, E., Sampson, L., Katan, M.B., Spiegelman, D., Willett, W.C. and Holmes, M.D. (2005). *Int. J. Cancer* 114, 628–633.

Aherne, S.A. and O'Brien, N.M. (2002). *Nutrition* 18, 75–81.

Albertsen, K. and Gronbaek, M. (2002). *Prostate* 52, 297–304.

Amaral, J.S., Seabra, R.M., Andrade, P.B., Valentao, P., Pereira, J.A. and Ferreres, F. (2004). *Food Chem.* 88, 373–379.

Asea, A., Ara, G., Teicher, B.A., Stevenson, M.A. and Calderwood, S.K. (2001). *Int. J. Hyperther.* 17, 347–356.

Bektic, J., Berger, A.P., Pfeil, K., Dobler, G., Bartsch, G. and Klocker, H. (2004). *Eur. Urol.* 45, 245–251.

Brusselmans, K., Vrolix, R., Verhoeven, G. and Swinnen, J.V. (2005). *J. Biol. Chem.* 280, 5636–5645.

Chang, E.T., Hedelin, M., Adami, H.O., Gronberg, H. and Balter, K.A. (2005). *Cancer Cause Control* 16, 275–284.

Chaudhary, A. and Willett, K.L. (2006). *Toxicology* 217, 194–205.

Chen, C.Y., Milbury, P.E., Lapsley, K. and Blumberg, J.B. (2005). *J. Nutr.* 135, 1366–1373.

Cho, S.D., Jiang, C., Malewicz, B., Dong, Y., Young, C.Y.F., Kang, K.S., Lee, Y.S., Ip, C. and Lu, J.X. (2004). *Mol. Cancer Ther.* 3, 605–611.

Ciolino, H.P., Daschner, P.J. and Yeh, G.C. (1999). *Biochem. J.* 340, 715–722.

Colli, J.L. and Colli, A. (2006). *Urol. Oncol.* 24, 184–194.

Dehm, S.M. and Tindall, D.J. (2005). *Expert Rev. Anticancer Ther.* 5, 163–174.

Di Carlo, G., Mascolo, N., Izzo, A.A. and Capasso, F. (1999). *Life Sci.* 65, 337–353.

Dong, Y., Lee, S.O., Zhang, H.T., Marshall, J., Gao, A.C. and Ip, C. (2004). *Cancer Res.* 64, 19–22.

Erlund, I. (2004). *Nutr. Res.* 24, 851–874.

Femia, A.P., Caderni, G., Ianni, M., Salvadori, M., Schijlen, E., Collins, G., Bovy, A. and Dolara, P. (2003). *Eur. J. Nutr.* 42, 346–352.

Fothergill, K.E. and Ensminger, M.E. (2006). *Drug Alcohol Depend.* 82, 61–76.

Fujita, M., Nagai, M., Murata, M., Kawakami, K., Irino, S. and Takahara, J. (2004). *Leuk. Res.* 21, 139–145.

Gao, S., Liu, G.Z. and Wang, Z.X. (2004). *Prostate* 59, 214–225.

Garcia-Closas, R., Agudo, A., Gonzalez, C.A. and Riboli, E. (1998). *Nutr. Cancer* 32, 154–158.

Garcia-Closas, R., Gonzalez, C.A., Agudo, A. and Riboli, E. (1999). *Cancer Cause Control* 10, 71–75.

Gerhauser, C. (2005). *Eur. J. Cancer* 41, 1941–1954.

Gorinstein, S., Caspi, A., Zemser, M. and Trakhtenberg, S. (2000). *Nutr. Res.* 20, 131–139.

Häkkinen, S.H., Kärenlampi, S.O., Heinonen, I.M., Mykkänen, H.M. and Törrönen, A.R. (1999). *J. Agric. Food Chem.* 47, 2274–2279.

Hermeking, H. and Benzinger, A. (2006). *Semin. Cancer Biol.* 16, 183–192.

Hertog, M.G.L., Hollman, P.C.H. and Katan, M.B. (1992). *J. Agric. Food Chem.* 40, 2379–2383.

Hertog, M.G.L., Hollman, P.C.H. and van de Putte, B. (1993). *J. Agric. Food Chem.* 41, 1242–1246.

Hirvonen, T., Virtamo, J., Korhonen, P., Albanes, D. and Pietinen, P. (2001). *Cancer Cause Control* 12, 789–796.

Ho, E., Boileau, T.W.M. and Bray, T.M. (2004). *Arc. Biochem. Biophys.* 428, 109–117.

Hodge, D.R., Hurt, E.M. and Farrar, W.L. (2005). *Eur. J. Cancer* 41, 2502–2512.

Hsieh, K. and Albertsen, P.C. (2003). *Urol. Clin. N. Am.* 30, 669.

Huynh, H., Nguyen, T.T.T., Chan, E. and Tran, E. (2003). *Int. J. Oncol.* 23, 821–829.

Jain, M.G., Hislop, G.T., Howe, G.R., Burch, J.D. and Ghadirian, P. (1998). *Int. J. Cancer* 78, 707–711.

Jiang, C., Lee, H.J., Li, G.X., Guo, J.M., Malewicz, B., Zhao, Y., Lee, E.O., Lee, J.H., Kim, M.S., Kim, S.H. and Lu, J.X. (2006). *Cancer Res.* 66, 453–463.

Jin, N.Z., Zhu, Y.P., Zhou, J.W., Mao, L., Zhao, R.C., Fang, T.H. and Ng, X.R. (2006). *Basic Clin. Pharmacol. Toxicol.* 98, 593–598.

Jones, E.L., Zhao, M.J., Stevenson, M.A. and Calderwood, S.K. (2004). *Int. J. Hyperther.* 20, 835–849.

Kamangar, F., Dores, G.M. and Anderson, W.F. (2006). *J. Clin. Oncol.* 24, 2137–2150.

Kampa, M., Hatzoglou, A., Notas, G., Damianaki, A., Bakogeorgou, E., Gemetzi, C., Kouroumalis, E., Martin, P.M. and Castanas, E. (2000). *Nutr. Cancer* 37, 223–233.

Klein, E.A. (2006). *Ann. Rev. Med.* 57, 49–63.

Knekt, P., Kumpulainen, J., Jarvinen, R., Rissanen, H., Heliovaara, M., Reunanen, A., Hakulinen, T. and Aromaa, A. (2002). *Am. J. Clin. Nutr.* 76, 560–568.

Knowles, L.M., Zigrossi, D.A., Tauber, R.A., Hightower, C. and Milner, J.A. (2000). *Nutr. Cancer* 38, 116–122.

Lambert, J.D., Hong, J., Yang, G.Y., Liao, J. and Yang, C.S. (2005). *Am. J. Clin. Nutr.* 81, 284S–291S. bioavailable.

Lee, H.H., Ho, C.T. and Lin, J.K. (2004). *Carcinogenesis* 25, 1109–1118.

Lee, J.H., Kim, S.D., Lee, J.Y., Kim, K.N. and Kim, H.S. (2005). *Food Sci. Biotech.* 14, 171–174.

Lee, S.O., Lou, W., Hou, M., de Miguel, F., Gerber, L. and Gao, A.C. (2003). *Clin. Cancer Res.* 9, 370–376.

Li, W., Shen, F. and Weber, G. (1999). *Oncol. Res.* 11, 243–247.

Lu, Y.R. and Foo, L.Y. (1997). *Food Chem.* 59, 187–194.

Ma, L., Feugang, J.M., Konarski, P., Wang, J., Lu, J.Z., Fu, S.J., Ma, B.L., Tian, B.Q., Zou, C.P. and Wang, Z.P. (2006). *Front. Biosci.* 11, 2275–2285.

Ma, Z.S., Huynh, T.H., Ng, C.P., Do, P.T., Nguyen, T.H. and Huynh, H. (2004a). *Int. J. Oncol.* 24, 1297–1304.

Ma, Z.S., Nguyen, T.H., Huynh, T.H., Do, P.T. and Huynh, H. (2004b). *J. Endocri.* 181, 493–507.

Mahmoud, N.N., Carothers, A.M., Grunberger, D., Bilinski, R.T., Churchill, M.R., Martucci, C., Newmark, H.L. and Bertagnolli, M.M. (2000). *Carcinogenesis* 21, 921–927.

Manach, C., Scalbert, A., Morand, C., Rémésy, C. and Jimenez, L. (2004). *Am. J. Clin. Nutr.* 79, 727–747.

Mauri, D., Pentheroudakis, G., Tolis, C., Chojnacka, M. and Pavlidis, N. (2005). *Urol. Oncol.* 23, 318–322.

McCann, S.E., Ambrosone, C.B., Moysich, K.B., Brasure, J., Marshall, J.R., Freudenheim, J.L., Wilkinson, G.S. and Graham, S. (2005). *Nutr. Cancer* 53, 33–41.

Mertens-Talcott, S.U. and Percival, S.S. (2005a). *Cancer Lett.* 218, 141–151.

Mertens-Talcott, S.U., Talcott, S.T. and Percival, S.S. (2003). *J. Nutr.* 133, 2669–2674.

Mertens-Talcott, S.U., Bomser, J.A., Romero, C., Talcott, S.T. and Percival, S.S. (2005b). *J. Nutr.* 135, 609–614.

Mesia-Vela, S. and Kauffman, F.C. (2003). *Xenobiotica* 33, 1211–1220.

Morris, J.D.H., Pramanik, R., Zhang, X., Carey, A.M., Ragavan, N., Martin, F.L. and Muir, G.H. (2006). *Cancer Lett.* 239, 111–122.

Moon, Y.J., Wang, X.D. and Morris, M.E. (2006). *Toxicol. Vitro* 20, 187–210.

Morel, I., Lescoat, G., Cogrel, P. *et al.* (1993). *Biochem. Pharmacol.* 45, 13–19.

Nakanoma, T., Ueno, M., Iida, M., Hirata, R. and Deguchi, N. (2001). *Int. J. Urol.* 8, 623–630.

Nardini, M., Natella, F., Scaccini, C. and Ghiselli, A. (2006). *J. Nutr. Biochem.* 17, 14–22.

Nagata, H., Takekoshi, S., Takagi, T., Honma, T. and Watanabe, K. (1999). Tokai. *J. Exp. Clin. Med.* 24, 1–11.

Neuhouser, M.L. (2004). *Nutr. Cancer* 50, 1–7.

Nozawa, H., Yoshida, A., Tajima, O., Katayama, M., Sonobe, H., Wakabayashi, K. and Kondo, K. (2004). *Int. J. Cancer* 108, 404–411.

Obach, R.S.J. (2000). *Pharmacol. Exp. Therap.* 294, 88–95.

Paganga, G., Miller, N. and Rice-Evans, C.A. (1999). *Free Radical Res.* 30, 153–162.

Palapattu, G.S., Sutcliffe, S., Bastian, P.J., Platz, E.A., De Marzo, A.M., Isaacs, W.B. and Nelson, W.G. (2005). *Carcinogenesis* 26, 1170–1181.

Paliwal, S., Sundaram, J. and Mitragotri, S. (2005). *Br. J. Cancer* 92, 499–502.

Platz, E.A., Leitzmann, M.F., Rimm, E.B., Willett, W.C. and Giovannucci, E. (2004). *Am. J. Epidemiol.* 159, 444–453.

Ren, F.G., Zhang, S.B., Mitchell, S.H., Butler, R. and Young, C.Y.F. (2000). *Oncogene* 19, 1924–1932.

Ripple, M.O., Henry, W.F., Rago, R.P. and Wilding, G. (1997). *J. Natl. Cancer Inst.* 89, 40–48.

Ripple, M.O., Henry, W.F., Schwarze, S.R., Wilding, G. and Weindruch, R. (1999). *J. Natl. Cancer Inst.* 91, 1227–1232.

Rodriguez, C., McCullough, M.L., Mondul, A.M., Jacobs, E.J., Chao, A., Patel, A.V., Thun, M.J. and Calle, E.E. (2006). *Cancer Epidemiol. Biomarkes Prev.* 15, 211–216.

Sagesser, M. and Deinzer, M. (1996). *J. Am. Soc. Brew. Chem.* 54, 129–134.

Scher, H.I., Buchanan, G., Gerald, W., Butler, L.M. and Tilley, W.D. (2004). *Endocr.-Relat. Cancer* 11, 459–476.

Schoonen, W.M., Salinas, C.A., Kiemeney, L.A.L.M. and Stanford, J.L. (2005). *Int. J. Cancer* 113, 133–140.

Schrag, M.L., Cui, D.H., Rushmore, T.H., Shou, M.G., Ma, B. and Rodrigues, A.D. (2004). *Drug Metab. Dispos.* 32, 1299–1303.

Sesso, H.D., Paffenbarger, R.S. and Lee, I.M. (2001). *Int. J. Epidemiol.* 30, 749–755.

Shariat, S.F., Andrews, B., Kattan, M.W., Kim, J., Wheeler, T.M. and Slawin, K.M. (2001). *Urology* 58, 1008–1015.

Shenouda, N.S., Zhou, C., Browning, J.D., Ansell, P.J., Sakla, M.S., Lubahn, D.B. and MacDonald, R.S. (2004). *Nutr. Cancer* 49, 200–208.

Shoskes, D.A. and Manickam, K. (2003). *World J. Urol.* 21, 109–113.

Sivashanmugam, P., Tang, L. and Daaka, Y. (2004). *J Biol. Chem.* 279, 21154–21159.

Skibola, C.F. and Smith, M.T. (2000). *Free Radical Biol. Med.* 29, 375–383.

Sun, X.Y., Plouzek, C.A., Henry, J.P., Wang, T.T.Y. and Phang, J.M. (1998). *Cancer Res.* 58, 2379–2384.

Tedesco, I., Nappo, A., Petitto, F., Iacomino, G., Nazzaro, F., Palumbo, R. and Russo, G.L. (2005). *Nutr. Cancer* 52, 74–83.

Tsyrlov, I.B., Mikhailenko, V.M. and Gelboin, H.V. (1994). *Biochim. Biophys. Acta.* 1205, 325–335.

Uda, Y., Price, K.R., Williamson, G. and Rhodes, M.J. (1997). *Cancer Lett.* 120, 213–216.

Valerio, L.G., Kepa, J.K., Pickwell, G.V. and Quattrochi, L.C. (2001). *Toxicol. Lett.* 119, 49–57.

van der Logt, E.M.J., Roelofs, H.M.J., Nagengast, F.M. and Peters, W.H.M. (2003). *Carcinogenesis* 24, 1651–1656.

van Zanden, J.J., Ben Hamman, O., van Lersel, M.L., Boeren, S., Cnubben, N.H., Lo Bello, M., Vervoort, J., van Bladeren, P.J. and Rietjens, I.M. (2003). *Chemico-Biological Interactions* 145, 139–148.

Verma, A.K., Johnson, J.A., Gould, M.N. and Tanner, M.A. (1988). *Cancer Res.* 15, 5754–5758.

Vijayababu, M.R., Kanagaraj, P., Arunkumar, A., Ilangovan, R., Aruldhas, M.M. and Arunakaran, J. (2005). *Cancer Res. Clin. Oncol.* 131, 765–771.

Vijayababu, M.R., Arunkumar, A., Kanagaraj, P. and Arunakaran, J. (2006a). *J. Carcinog.* 5(10).

Vijayababu, M.R., Arunkumar, A., Kanagaraj, P., Venkataraman, P., Krishnamoorthy, G. and Arunakaran, J. (2006b). *Mol. Cell Biochem.* 287, 109–116.

Volate, S.R., Davenport, D.M., Muga, S.J. and Wargovich, M.J. (2005). *Carcinogenesis* 26, 1450–1456.

Vvedenskaya, I.O., Rosen, R.T., Guido, J.E., Russell, D.J., Mills, K.A. and Vorsa, N. (2004). *J. Agric. Food Chem.* 52, 188–195.

Wang, S.H., DeGroff, V.L. and Clinton, S.K. (2003). *J. Nutr.* 133, 2367–2376.

Williams, J.A., Ring, B.J., Cantrell, V.E., Campanale, K., Jones, D.R., Hall, S.D. and Wrighton, S.A. (2002). *Drug Metab. Dispos.* 30, 1266–1273.

Xing, N., Chen, Y., Mitchell, S.H. and Young, C.Y. (2001). *Carcinogenesis* 22, 409–414.

Yuan, H., Pan, Y. and Young, C.Y. (2004). *Cancer Lett.* 213, 155–163.

Yuan, H.Q., Gong, A.Y. and Young, C.Y.F. (2005). *Carcinogenesis* 26, 793–801.

Yuan, Z.P., Chen, L.J., Fan, L.Y., Tang, M.H., Yang, G.L., Yang, H.S., Du, X.B., Wang, G.Q., Yao, W.X., Zhao, Q.M., Ye, B., Wang, R., Diao, P., Zhang, W., Wu, H.B., Zhao, X. and Wei, Y.Q. (2006). *Clin. Cancer Res.* 12, 3193–3199.

Zhu, P., Baek, S.H., Bourk, E.M., Ohgi, K.A., Garcia-Bassets, I., Sanjo, H., Akira, S., Kotol, P.F., Glass, C.K., Rosenfeld, M.G. and Rose, D.W. (2006). *Cell* 124, 615–629.

Zeliadt, S.B., Etzioni, R.D., Penson, D.F., Thompson, I.M. and Ramsey, S.D. (2005). *Am. J. Med.* 118, 850–857.

89

Beer and Prevention of Heterocyclic Amine-Induced DNA Adducts and O^6-methylguanine

Sakae Arimoto-Kobayashi Graduate School of Medicine, Dentistry and Pharmaceutical Sciences, Okayama University, Okayama, Japan

Abstract

Non-volatile dissolved materials in beer amount to as much as about 5% (w/w) on freeze-drying of beer samples. These dissolved components should be taken into account for any study of the biological effects of beer. We have described here inhibitory effects of beer on the formation of O^6-methylguanine (O^6-meG) by *N*-methyl-*N'*-nitro-*N*-nitrosoguanidine (MNNG) in the DNA of Salmonella YG7108 when beer was added to bacteria in the presence of MNNG. We have also evaluated the *in vivo* effects of beer components on the formation of DNA adducts by Trp-P-2, MeIQx and PhIP under conditions reflecting human dietary habits. The protective effects were found in liver and lung, the target organ for MeIQx tumorigenesis in mice, with a drinking solution containing beer components and also by adding beer components to the diet to simulate intake of food additives. We also investigated the inhibitory effects of a solution of beer components on DNA damage in mice liver with single and continuous administration of Trp-P-2. Furthermore, we evaluated the *in vivo* protective effect of beer samples in relation to PhIP-induced DNA adduct formation in the colon (the target organ associated with PhIP tumorigenesis) and other important organs (liver, lung and kidney) of mice fed with a beer solution or by the addition of beer components to the diet.

List of Abbreviations

CMBA	2-Chloro-4-methylthiobutanoic acid
EROD	7-Ethylresorufin *O*-deethylase
MeIQx	2-Amino-3,8-dimethylimidazo[4,5-*f*]quinoxaline
MROD	7-Methoxyresorufin *O*-demethylase
MNNG	*N*-methyl-*N'*-nitro-*N*-nitrosoguanidine
O^6-meG	O^6-methylguanine
PhIP	2-Amino-1-methyl-6-phenylimidazo[4,5-*b*]pyridine
RAL	relative adduct labeling
Trp-P-2	3-Amino-1-methyl-5*H*-pyrido[4,3-*b*]indole
Trp-P-2(NHOH)	3-Hydroxyamino-1-methyl-5*H*-pyrido[4,3-*b*]indole

Introduction

Antimutagenic and anticarcinogenic effects of dietary components are being studied extensively (IARC, 1996; Ohigashi *et al.*, 1997; World Cancer Research Fund, 1997). Many epidemiological studies have demonstrated reduced mortality from coronary heart diseases among moderate alcohol consumers in comparison to abstainers (Rimm *et al.*, 1991). On the other hand, there is evidence that alcohol itself increases the risk of mouth, esophageal and primary liver cancers (World Cancer Research Fund, 1997). There are conflicting reports concerning the relationship between beer consumption and the risk of cancer. For example, Riboli *et al.* (1991) did not find an association between beer consumption and colon cancer, whereas Kato *et al.* (1990) have shown that beer drinkers have an increased risk to colorectal cancer. Swanson *et al.* (1993) suggested an inverse association between moderate beer consumption and endometrial cancer. However, Potter *et al.* (1992) suggested a relationship between beer consumption and lung cancer. Non-volatile dissolved materials in beer amount to as much as about 5% (w/w) on freeze-drying of beer samples, as shown in our previous report (Arimoto-Kobayashi *et al.*, 1999). Therefore, these dissolved components should be taken into account for any study of the biological effects of beer.

The carcinogenicity and anticarcinogenicity of dietary components is currently receiving a great deal of attention (Dashwood, 2002; Knasmuller, 2002). Heterocyclic amines, including 2-amino-3,8-dimethylimidazo[4,5-*f*]quinoxaline (MeIQx), 2-amino-1-methyl-6-phenylimidazo[4,5-*b*]pyridine (PhIP) and 3-amino-1-methyl-5*H*-pyrido[4,3-*b*]indole (Trp-P-2), which have been identified as potent mutagens and carcinogens in rodents, are produced in foods during the

Beer in Health and Disease Prevention
ISBN: 978-0-12-373891-2

process of cooking (Felton *et al.*, 2000; Sugimura, 2000). Since humans are frequently exposed to cooked-food carcinogens such as heterocyclic amines, these compounds are suspected of being human carcinogens (Sugimura, 2000). Epidemiological studies have established an apparent association between the consumption of well-cooked red meat and certain types of cancer. Ohgaki *et al.* (2000) showed that Trp-P-2 at 0.02% in the diet induced a high incidence of hepatocellular tumors in female CDF1 mice, and that mice fed MeIQx at 0.06% in the diet developed liver tumor, lymphoma and leukemia in males and liver and lung tumors in females. Mice fed with PhIP at 0.04% in the diet had a higher incidence of lymphoma and leukemia than control mice, and rats fed with PhIP at 0.00125–0.01% in the diet developed colon and prostate carcinomas in males, while mammary gland carcinomas appeared in females.

We have previously investigated the inhibitory effects of beer on bacterial mutagenicity of preactivated heterocyclic amines (3-hydroxyamino-1-methyl-5*H*-pyrido[4,3-*b*]indole (Trp-P-2(NHOH)) and 2-hydroxyamino-6-methyldipyrido [1,2-*a*:3′,2′-*d*]imidazole (Glu-P-1(NHOH)) (Arimoto-Kobayashi *et al.*, 1999)), 2-chloro-4-methylthiobutanoic acid (CMBA) (Kimura *et al.*, 1999) and *N*-methyl-*N*′-nitro-*N*-nitrosoguanidine (MNNG) (Yoshikawa *et al.*, 2002). Beer also inhibited the mutagenicity of Trp-P-2, IQ, MeIQx and PhIP in the presence of metabolic activation (Arimoto-Kobayashi *et al.*, 2006). Beer prevented radiation-induced chromosome aberrations in human lymphocytes (Monobe *et al.*, 2003), and genotoxicity of PhIP in V79 cells measured by the comet assay (Edenharder *et al.*, 2002).

We have also isolated and identified pseudouridine from beer as an antimutagenic substance against MNNG (Yoshikawa *et al.*, 2002), and glycine betaine, a compound present in beer and known to be distributed widely in plants and animals, which inhibits CMBA, the sanma-fish mutagen (Kimura *et al.*, 1999) (Figure 89.1). Pseudouridine and glycine betaine did not inhibit the mutagenicity of heterocyclic amines. There must therefore be another component(s) in beer that is responsible for the antimutagenicity toward heterocyclic amines.

We have described here an investigation of the effects of beer on the formation of O^6-methylguanine (O^6-meG) by MNNG in the DNA of Salmonella YG7108 when beer was added to bacteria in the presence of MNNG. We have also evaluated the *in vivo* effects of beer components on the formation of DNA adducts by Trp-P-2, MeIQx and PhIP under conditions reflecting human dietary habits. The protective effects were studied in liver and lung, the target organ for MeIQx tumorigenesis in mice, with a drinking solution containing beer components and also by adding beer components to the diet to simulate intake of food additives. We also investigated the effects of a solution of beer components on DNA damage in mice liver with single and continuous administration of Trp-P-2. Furthermore,

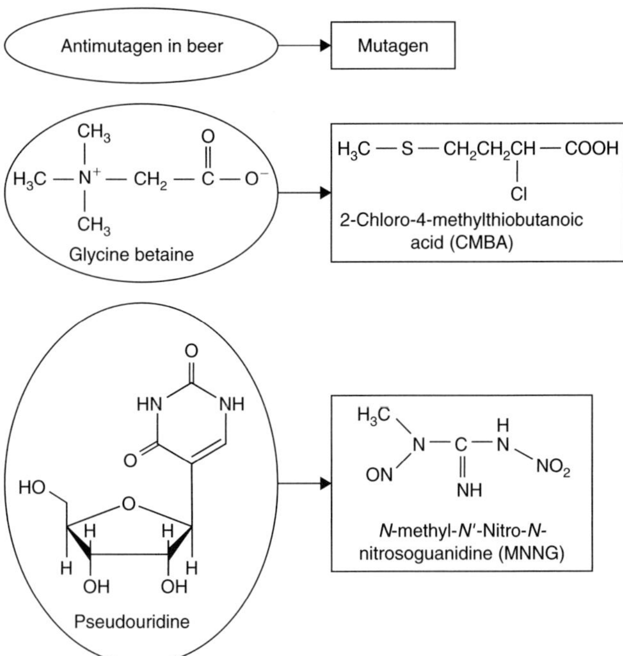

Figure 89.1 Structures of mutagen and corresponding antimutagenic compounds in beer.

we evaluated the *in vivo* protective effect of beer samples in relation to PhIP-induced DNA adduct formation in the colon (the target organ associated with PhIP tumorigenesis) and other important organs (liver, lung and kidney) of mice fed with a beer solution or by the addition of beer components to the diet.

Abstracted with permission from *J. Agric. Food Chem.*, 47, 221–230, 1999 and *J. Agric. Food Chem.*, 53, 812–815, 2005. Copyright 2006 American Chemical Society. Abstracted with permission from *Biol. Pharm. Bull.*, 29, 67–70, 2006. Copyright 2006 the Pharmaceutical Society of Japan.

Materials and Animals

MNNG (CAS 70-25-7), Trp-P-2 (CAS 62450-07-1), MeIQx (77500-04-0) and PhIP (CAS 105650-23-5) were obtained from Wako Chemicals (Osaka, Japan). O^6-meG was obtained from Sigma (St. Louis, MO). The diet for mice (MF powder) was purchased from Oriental Yeast (Tokyo, Japan). *Salmonella typhimurium* TA100 was a gift from Dr. B.N. Ames of the University of California, Berkeley, and strain YG7108 was provided by Dr. Yamada of the National Institute of Public Health, Tokyo (Yamada *et al.*, 1995). CDF1 mice (male, 6-weeks old) and C57BL/6N mice (male, 6-weeks old) were obtained from Charles River Japan (Atsugi, Japan) and housed one or two mice per cage with access to food and water *ad libitum*, unless indicated otherwise.

All experiments were carried out in accordance with the Safety Guidelines of Okayama University and the Japanese

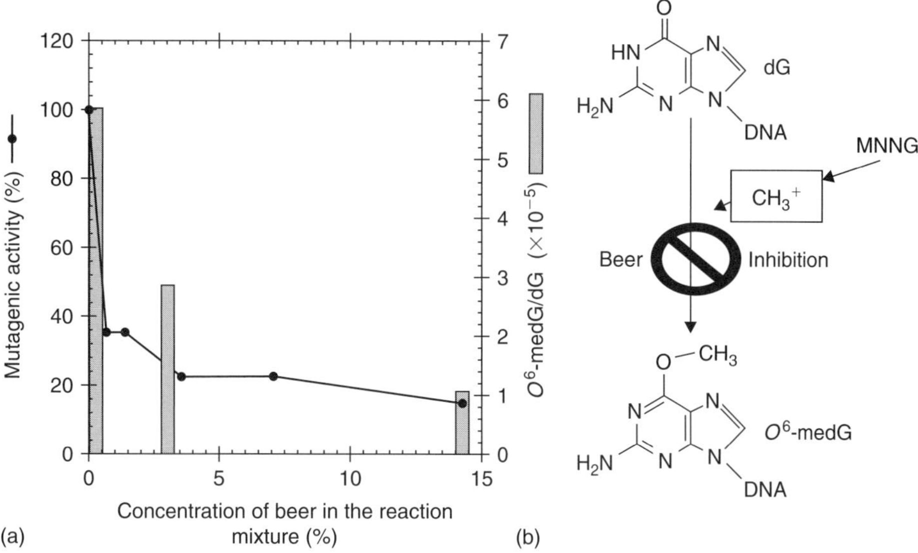

Figure 89.2 Inhibitory effects of beer on the formation of O^6-meG in DNA of *S. typhimurium* YG7108 treated with MNNG. (a) Inhibitory effects of beer in the Ames test (circle) and the formation of O^6-medG in Salmonella treated with MNNG (square) (Arimoto-Kobayashi *et al.*, 1999). (b) Scheme of inhibitory mechanisms of beer components on genotoxicity of MNNG. Abstracted with permission from Arimoto-Kobayashi *et al.* (1999). Copyright 2006 American Chemical Society.

Government Management Law for toxic chemicals (No. 303). Animal experiments were carried out in accordance with the Guidelines for Animal Experiments at Okayama University Advanced Science Research Center, Japanese Government Animal Protection and Management Law (No. 105), and Japanese Government Notification on Feeding and Safekeeping of Animals (No. 6). Statistical analyses were performed using ANOVA analysis and the unpaired Student's t-test with KaleidaGraph (Sydney Software, Reading, PA, USA). Results were considered significant at $p < 0.05$.

Preparation of Beer Samples

Two different samples of beer (beer-A and beer-B) produced in Japan were examined. Beer-A was a stout beer and beer-B was a lager beer, both of which were purchased in local stores in Okayama. Beer samples were freeze-dried to remove ethanol, unless indicated otherwise. The solid obtained was dissolved in a volume of water representing a fifth, a half or an equal volume of the original sample, designated as "beer solution (×5)," "beer solution (×2)" and "beer solution (×1)," respectively. "μL eq." represents the amount of beer equivalent to a corresponding volume of beer.

Effects of Beer on the Formation of O^6-meG in DNA from *S. typhimurium* YG7108 Treated with MNNG

An overnight culture of *S. typhimurium* YG7108 (50 ml) was mixed with MNNG (final concentration, 0.014 mM) and beer (beer-A, 0–50 ml) in 0.07 M Na-phosphate (pH 7). The beer used was not freeze-dried, but an original sample. Total volume was 350 ml. The concentration of beer in the reaction mixture was 0%, 2.85% (10 ml of beer in 350 ml of mixture) and 14.3% (50 ml of beer in 350 ml of mixture). The possibility of any effects due to ethanol was eliminated by inclusion of ethanol to a fixed concentration (1.1%) in these treatments. The mixture was incubated for 30 min at 37°C with continuous mechanical shaking. The treated bacteria were then collected by centrifugation at 500 rpm for 10 min at 4°C. The genomic DNA of Salmonella was prepared using a previously described method (Wilson, 1997). The DNA obtained was dissolved in 0.1 ml of 0.1 N HCl and heated at 70°C for 30 min. The mixture was then cooled in ice before the addition of ethanol (2 volume). Precipitates were removed from the mixture by centrifugation and the supernatant obtained was concentrated under a reduced pressure. The residue was dissolved in 0.05 ml water and analyzed using high performance liquid chromatography (HPLC) on a Waters system (USA) coupled to a fluorescence detector (Arimoto-Kobayashi *et al.*, 1997). HPLC was performed with an ODS-80Ts column (4.6 × 250 mm; Tosoh, Japan): column temperature 40°C; eluent 0.1 M NH_4OAc (pH 5.0)–methanol (95:5); flow rate 0.8 ml/min; fluorescence (287 nm excitation and 362 nm emission) of O^6-meG and 247 nm absorbance of dG were detected.

As shown in Figure 89.2, the beer sample (beer-A) inhibited O^6-meG formation by MNNG in the DNA of *S. typhimurium* YG7108. The decrease in O^6-meG was dependent on the dose of beer. Beer-A (original, not freeze-dried) showed inhibition of MNNG mutagenicity in the Ames test using *S. typhimurium* TA100 (Figure 89.2). The concentration of beer in this experiment, 50 ml of beer in 350 ml of the reaction mixture (i.e. 14.3%), corresponds to 0.1 ml of beer in 0.7 ml of the preincubation mixture of the Ames assay described in Figure 89.3, in which the mutagenicity of MNNG was decreased to 16.4%. The decrease in the formation of O^6-meG to 16% by this beer concentration was consistent with the decreased level of mutagenicity.

Beer-A inhibited the MNNG-mediated methylation of guanine residues in the DNA of *S. typhimurium* (Figure 89.2). It is likely that the inhibitory effect of beer upon the mutagenicity of MNNG is a result of this suppression of alkylation of DNA.

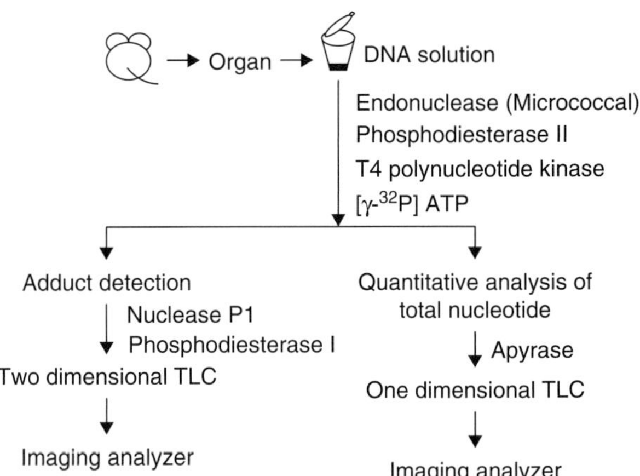

Figure 89.3 Brief scheme of the ^{32}P-postlabeling methods.

Effects of a Beer Solution on Formation of Trp-P-2-DNA Adducts in Mice

Experiment 1 (single administration of Trp-P-2 with gavage, and beer-A components in drink for 4 days)

The effects of a beer solution (beer-A) on Trp-P-2-DNA adducts were investigated with CDF_1 mice. Mice were divided into five groups, each composed of three mice kept in a cage. Treatments were started from 3 p.m. of day 1. They were given normal food and a drinking solution consisting of either plain water (group 1), the "beer solution (×2)" (group 2), the "beer solution (×1)" (group 3), or the "beer solution (×2)" (group 4), all of which were provided *ad libitum*. After 72 h, an aqueous solution of Trp-P-2 (30 mg/kg b.w.) was administered orally to each animal of groups 1–3. The volume of the Trp-P-2 solution was about 0.2 ml. One mouse was used as a no-treatment control, fed only a normal diet with plain water, and was given no Trp-P-2. After an additional 24 h of feeding with the beer solutions, the animals were sacrificed and their livers were removed for analysis. DNA was isolated from the liver by phenol extraction and analyzed by the ^{32}P-postlabeling method using the intensification protocol described previously (Sugiyama *et al.*, 1996). Briefly, as detailed in Figure 89.3, the DNA was digested with micrococcal nuclease and spleen phosphodiesterase, and the digest was then labeled with ^{32}P under adduct-intensification conditions (Ochiai *et al.*, 1993) using T4 polynucleotide kinase and [γ-^{32}P]ATP. The labeled mixture was further digested with nuclease P1 and phosphodiesterase I. The digest was subjected to ODS-TLC (thin-layer chromatography), contact-transferred to polyethyleneimine cellulose TLC (Randerath *et al.*, 1984) and the plate was developed four times, as described elsewhere (Sugiyama *et al.*, 1996). The radio activities of adduct spots were analyzed using a Bio-Imaging Analyzer (BAS 2000, Fuji Photo Film, Tokyo) with an exposure time of 2 h. The adduct level was determined with relative adduct labeling (RAL) (Randerath *et al.*, 1985), namely, "RAL in the modified adduct-intensification method" = [(count rate in adduct nucleotides)/(count rate in total nucleotides)] × (IF)−1, where IF (intensification factor) is the value obtained in a Trp-P-2-only experiment, such that IF = [RAL in the modified adduct-intensification method]/[RAL in the modified standard method]. The detection limit was 1.0 adduct/10^7 nucleotides.

Experiment 2 (single administration of Trp-P-2, and beer-A components in the diet for 4 days)

The effects of beer-A (original, not freeze-dried) and beer-A solution (×5) on Trp-P-2-DNA adducts were also investigated with C57BL/6N mice. Trp-P-2 (30 mg/kg) was given to mice by gastric intubation in a single dose dissolved in sterile water on day 3. For controls, solvent (water) was given to mice not receiving Trp-P-2 by intubation (group 4). A diet mixed with water or a beer sample was given to mice for 3 days. A diet mixed with water and Trp-P-2 was given to mice in group 1, while a diet mixed with beer-A (original, not freeze-dried) and Trp-P-2 was given to mice in group 2. Group-3 mice received a diet mixed with beer-A solution (×5) and Trp-P-2, and mice in group 4 were given a diet mixed with water alone. Mice were sacrificed on day 4.

Experiment 3 (continuous feeding with Trp-P-2 in the diet for 3 days, and beer-A components in a diet paste for 5 days)

Trp-P-2 and beer solution-A were mixed with an equal weight of the control diet (MF powder, Oriental Yeast, Tokyo, Japan) to form a paste, which was given to C57BL/6N mice for 5 days. The total amount of Trp-P-2 given was 30 mg/kg. Diets mixed with either water (groups 1 and 4), beer-A solution (×1) (group 2) or beer-A solution (×5) (group 3) were given to mice for 2 days. Diets mixed with Trp-P-2 (group 1), Trp-P-2 and beer-A solution

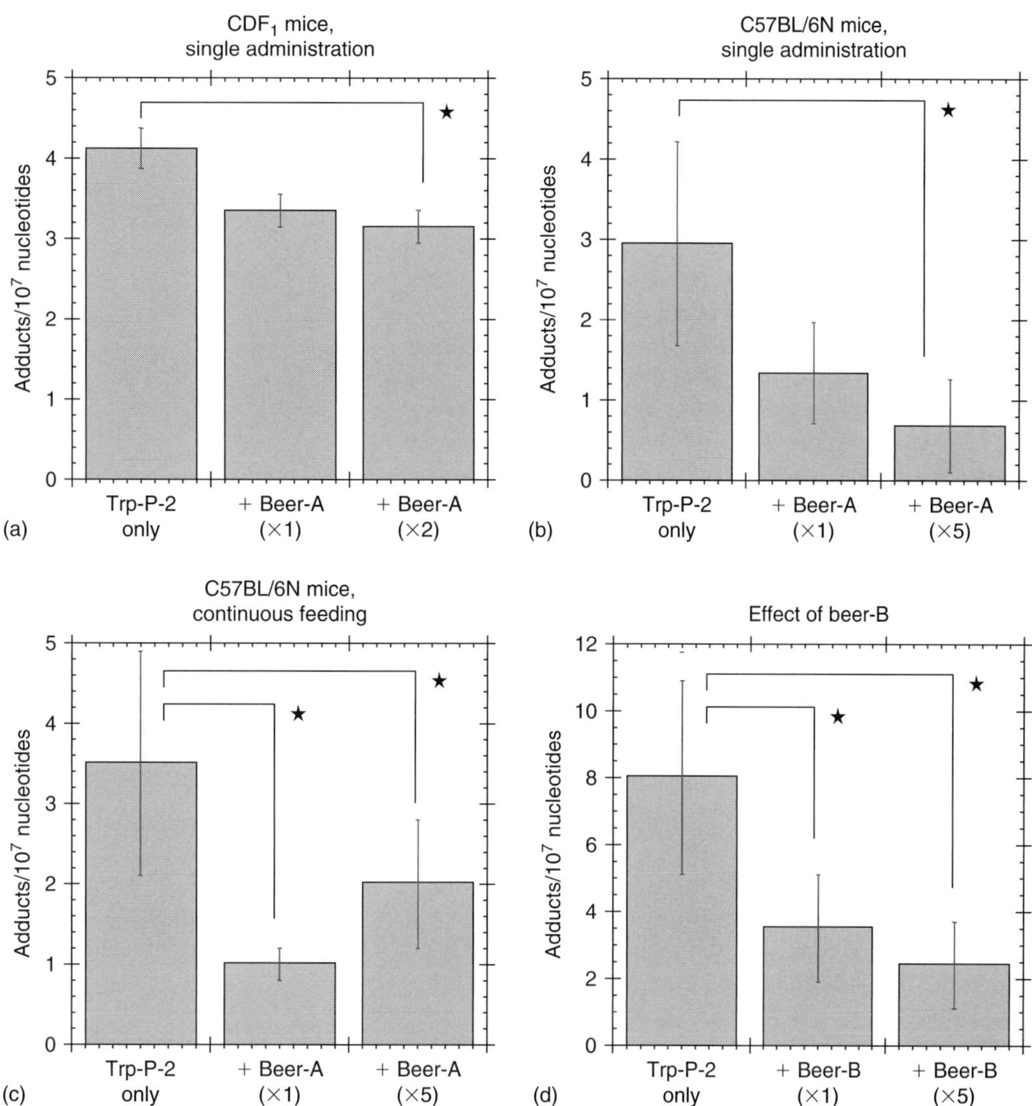

Figure 89.4 Inhibitory effects of a beer solution on DNA adduct formation in mice fed Trp-P-2. Formation of Trp-P-2-DNA adduct in the liver in mice treated with (a) single administration of Trp-P-2 with gavage, and beer-A components in drink for 4 days, (b) single administration of Trp-P-2, and beer-A components in the diet for 4 days, (c) continuous feeding with Trp-P-2 in the diet for 3 days, and beer-A components in a diet paste for 5 days, (d) continuous feeding with Trp-P-2 in the diet for 3 days, and beer-B components in a diet paste for 5 days (Arimoto-Kobayashi *et al.*, 1999, 2005). *Significantly different at $p < 0.05$.

(×1) (group 2), Trp-p-2 and beer-A solution (×5) (group 3) or water only (group 4) were given for 5 days. Mice were sacrificed on day 8.

Experiment 4 (continuous feeding with Trp-P-2 in the diet for 3 days, and beer-B components in a diet paste for 5 days)

Beer-B solution was given to C57BL/6N mice. The concentration of Trp-P-2 in the diet was 0.005%. A diet mixed with beer-B solution was given for 2 days, and then a diet containing Trp-P-2 with beer solution was given for 3 days. Mice were sacrificed on day 5. Other procedures were similar to those of Experiment 3. Providing 0.005% of Trp-P-2 in the diet for 3 days was equivalent to the administration of a total of 25 mg/kg body weight.

As shown in Figure 89.4a, adduct formation in the liver DNA of CDF1 mice given Trp-P-2 on day 3 decreased significantly by the continuous administration of twice the concentrated beer (freeze-dried beer-A) constituents for 4 days, compared with that of mice given Trp-P-2 without beer (Experiment 1, Figure 89.4a). No adducts were observed in the tested organs of mice fed on a control diet (group 4; data not shown).

Reproducibility of the protective effect with another mouse strain (C57BL/6N) was investigated, and results revealed that adduct formation in the liver DNA of mice given Trp-P-2 with a single administration on day 3 also decreased significantly by the continuous administration of beer-A solution (×5) in the diet for 4 days, compared with that of mice given Trp-P-2 without a beer solution (Experiment 2, Figure 89.4b). Formation of DNA adducts in liver DNA in C57BL mice receiving administration of Trp-P-2 at 0.005% in the diet was observed with an amount of Trp-P-2 that was lower than that recorded for carcinogenicity in CDF_1 mice. Adducts of Trp-P-2 produced in the liver DNA of mice that were continuously given Trp-P-2 in the diet for 5 days decreased following the addition of beer-A solution (×1) and beer-A solution (×5) in the form of a diet paste (Experiment 3, Figure 89.4c). Reproducibility of the protective effect of beer constituents in another kind of beer sample, the lager type, was investigated with beer-B solution (Experiments 4, Figure 89.4d). Adduct formation in liver DNA of mice fed Trp-P-2 for 5 days decreased significantly with addition of beer-B solution (×1) and beer-B solution (×5) in the diet, compared to that of mice fed with Trp-P-2-only.

Trp-P-2 in the diet induced a high incidence of hepatocellular tumors in female CDF_1 mice. Previously, we reported that beer samples inhibited the mutagenicity of both Trp-P-2 and Trp-P-2(NHOH) in the Ames test. We also observed in an earlier study that a direct-acting mutagenicity emerges in the serum of mice that have been administered Trp-P-2 intravenously, and that this direct-acting mutagenicity persists for a period of 0.5–6 h after the administration (Aji *et al.*, 1994). Trp-P-2(NHOH) is known to be a primary metabolite of Trp-P-2 (Ishii *et al.*, 1980). Since Trp-P-2 itself is an indirect mutagen, the direct activity detected in the serum has been ascribed to the presence of Trp-P-2(NHOH), the metabolically activated form of Trp-P-2. The present study demonstrated that the administration of freeze-dried beer in drinking water and in the diet inhibited Trp-P-2-DNA adduct formation in the liver. The antimutagenic and Trp-P-2(NHOH)-degrading component(s) of beer may work after being absorbed through the digestive tract.

The genotoxicity of Trp-P-2 in mice also depends on the induction of phase I cytochrome P450 (CYP) enzymes and phase II enzymes. We have already demonstrated that Trp-P-2(NHOH) production from Trp-P-2 through *in vitro* metabolic activation was inhibited by the presence of beer components (Arimoto-Kobayashi *et al.*, 2005). The suppression of the metabolic conversion from Trp-P-2 to Trp-P-2(NHOH) indicated that the antimutagenic effects of beer components on Trp-P-2 were linked with the inhibition of metabolic activation. Therefore, the results suggest that steps involved in the activation of Trp-P-2 and binding of Trp-P-2(NHOH) to DNA are the targets of the antimutagenicity of beer (Figure 89.5).

DNA adduct formation in the livers of mice receiving a single administration (*p.o.*) or continuous supply of Trp-P-2 was significantly inhibited by the addition of beer-A solution to the diet (Experiments 2 and 3, Figure 89.4b and c).

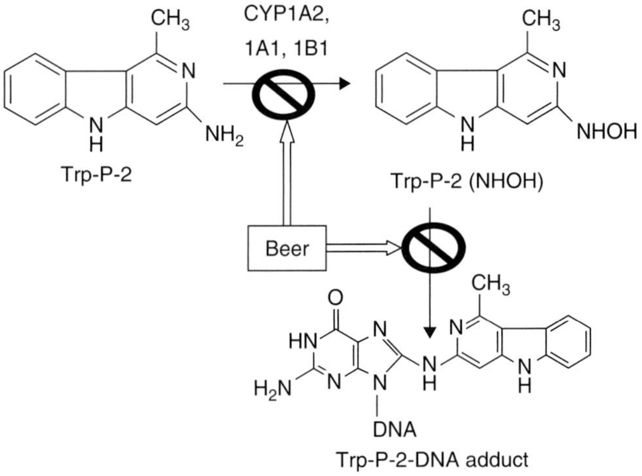

Figure 89.5 Scheme of the antigenotoxic mechanisms of beer components on Trp-P-2-DNA adduct formation.

It is interesting that beer inhibited DNA adduct formation in the target organ of Trp-P-2 tumorigenesis, the liver. This observation suggests that protective effects can also be anticipated in humans when beer components are consumed on a daily basis with occasional or periodic intake of fried fish and meats. Both stout-type beer (beer-A) and lager-type beer (beer-B) solutions inhibited DNA adduct formation by Trp-P-2 *in vivo* (Experiment 4, Figure 89.4d). The effects of both types of beer components (beer-A and beer-B solutions) were similar in relation to the preventive effects on DNA adduct formation by Trp-P-2. The results suggest that antigenotoxic components might be present in beer.

Effects of a Beer Solution on Formation of MeIQx-DNA Adducts in Mice

Experiment 5 (beer-A components in drink for 5 days, and MeIQx in a diet paste for 3 days)

For an investigation of the influence of beer on MeIQx-DNA adducts, beer-A solution was given to C57BL/6N mice as a replacement for drinking water for 5 days, and a diet containing MeIQx (0.005%) was given for the subsequent 3 days. MeIQx was dissolved and mixed with diet powder to form a diet paste. Four groups of mice received the diet paste mixture with either MeIQx (group 1), MeIQx and beer-A solution (×1) in water (group 2), MeIQx and beer-A solution (×2) in water (group 3) or the paste alone as a control (group 4). The calorie content of the diet was adjusted with maltose. Mice were sacrificed on day 6 by cervical dislocation. Tissues were collected, washed with ice-cold KCl (0.15 M), and frozen in liquid nitrogen. Samples were stored at −80°C until use. The amount of heterocyclic amine-DNA adduct in the DNA of treated mouse tissue was determined using the modified adduct-intensification analysis in the ^{32}P-postlabeling method, as described above.

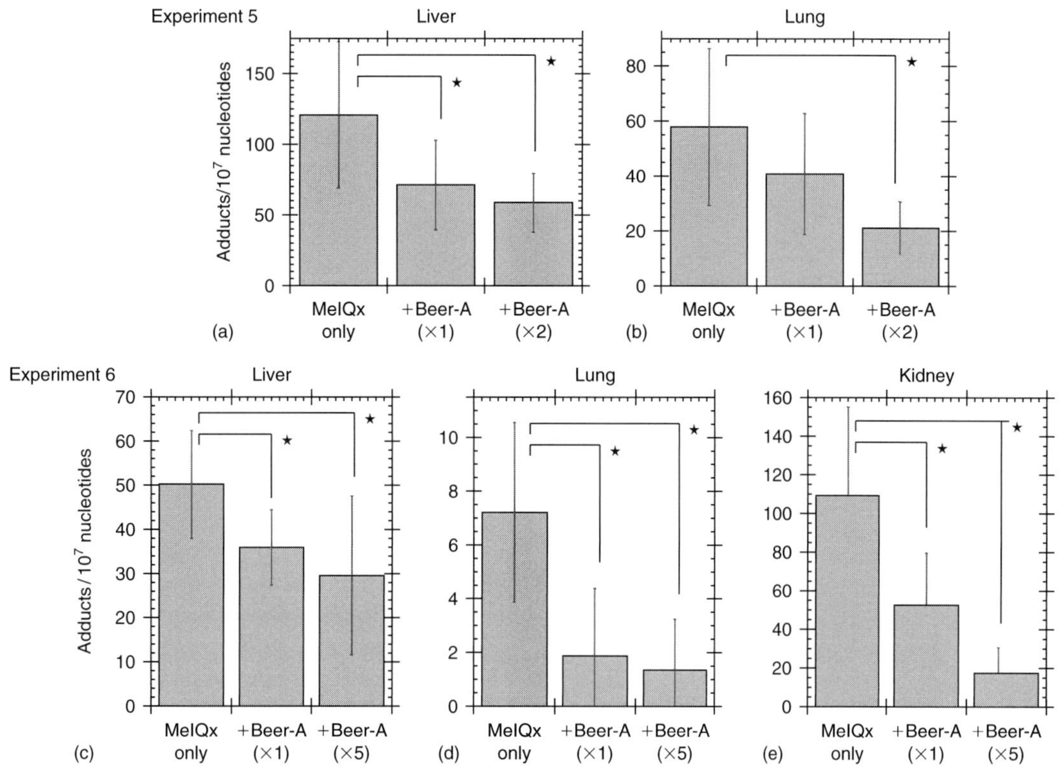

Figure 89.6 Inhibitory effects of a beer solution on DNA adduct formation in mice fed MeIQx. Formation of MeIQx-DNA adduct in (a, c) liver, (b, d) lungs and (e) kidney in mice treated with (a, b) beer-A components in drink for 5 days, and MeIQx in a diet paste for 3 days or (c–e) beer-A components in the diet for 5 days and MeIQx in the diet for 3 days (Arimoto-Kobayashi *et al.*, 2005). *Significantly different at $p < 0.05$.

Experiment 6 (beer-A components in the diet for 5 days and MeIQx in the diet for 3 days)

Beer solution-A and a MeIQx solution (final level of 0.005%) were mixed with an equal weight of powdered diet to form a paste, which was given to C57BL/6N mice. Mice received a control diet mixed with water for 2 days (groups 1 and 4), a diet mixed with beer-A solution (×1) (group 2), or a diet mixed with beer-A solution (×2) (group 3). Then, the mice were given a diet mixed with MeIQx (group 1), beer-A solution (×1) and MeIQx (group 2), beer-A solution (×2) and MeIQx (group 3) or a control diet (group 4), for 3 days. Mice were sacrificed on day 6. Other procedures were similar to those used for Experiment 5.

As shown in Figure 89.6, DNA adducts of MeIQx were formed in the liver, lung and kidney of mice given MeIQx at 0.005% in the diet (Experiments 5 and 6). No adducts were observed in the tested organs of mice fed a control diet (group 4) (Figure 89.7). The addition of beer-A solution to the drinking water significantly decreased the formation of DNA adducts in the liver and lung of mice given MeIQx in the diet, compared with that of mice given MeIQx without a beer solution (Experiment 5). The amounts of DNA adducts in the liver, lung and kidney of mice given MeIQx in the diet also decreased significantly when beer-A solution (×1) and (×5) were added to the diet (Experiment 6). Typical examples of MeIQx adduct spots on a PEI sheet are shown in Figure 89.7. The intensity of MeIQx adduct spots obtained from the liver of a mouse given MeIQx and beer in the diet was lower than that obtained for a mouse given MeIQx alone (Experiment 6).

The effects of a beer solution in the form of a drinking beverage were investigated because of its relevance to the human situation. The presence of beer-A solution in drinking water decreased the level of DNA adduct formation in the liver and lung of mice fed with MeIQx (0.005%) in the diet (Figure 89.6a and b). The addition of beer-A solution in the diet to mimic intake of food additives also decreased DNA adduct formation in the liver, lung and kidney of mice given MeIQx in the diet (Figure 89.6c–e). Ohgaki *et al.* (2000) showed that mice fed MeIQx at 0.06% in the diet developed liver tumors, lymphomas and leukemia in males, and liver and lung tumors in females. The results of our investigation suggest that beer components both in drinking water and in the diet could suppress DNA adducts of MeIQx in target organs of tumorigenesis (liver and lung) and in a non-target organ (kidney).

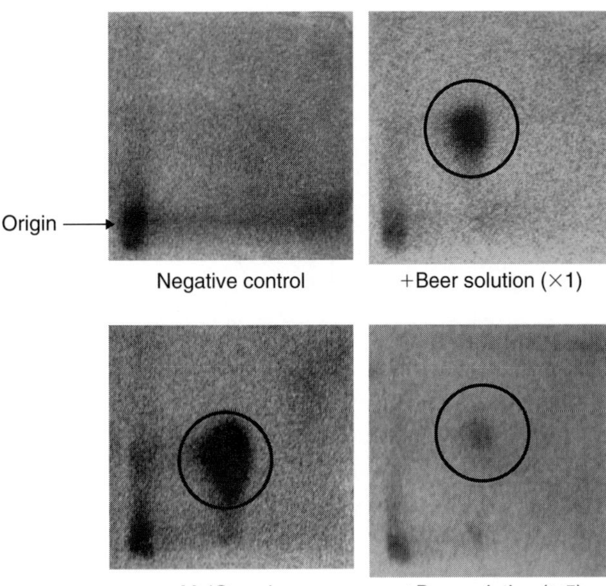

Figure 89.7 Inhibitory effects of a beer solution on DNA adduct formation in the liver in mice fed MeIQx detected by ^{32}P-postlabeling. Examples of MeIQx adduct spots on a PEI sheet. A spot of MeIQx-DNA adduct is marked by a circle.

Effects of a Beer Solution on Formation of PhIP-DNA Adducts in Mice

Experiment 7 (beer-A components in drink for 5 days and PhIP in the diet for 3 days)

C57BL/6N mice were housed singly or in pairs in a cage with access to food and water *ad libitum*. The diet was prepared by mixing 3 g of feed with 3 ml of 0.005% PhIP solution or 3 ml of water (for the control diet) to form a diet paste (final weight, 6 g). The calorie content of the diet was adjusted using maltose. Investigations concerning the influence of beer on PhIP-induced DNA adduct formation involved continuously providing beer-A components (beer-A solution) to mice instead of drinking water for 5 days. Diet paste (6 g) carrying 0.005% PhIP was given for three subsequent days at 3 p.m. Four groups of mice received a diet mixed with either PhIP (group 1), PhIP in the diet and a beer-A solution (×1) in water (group 2), PhIP in the diet and a beer-A solution (×2) in water (group 3) or a control diet (group 4). Mice were sacrificed on day 6 by cervical dislocation. Tissues were excised, washed with ice-cold 0.15 M KCl, frozen in liquid nitrogen, and then stored at −80°C until use. The amount of PhIP-DNA adducts in treated mouse tissue was determined using a modified adduct-intensification analysis of the ^{32}P-postlabeling method (Fukutome *et al.*, 1994). Each detection and quantitative analysis of PhIP-DNA adducts was carried out in triplicate and the reproducibility was confirmed.

Experiment 8 (beer-A components in diet for 5 days and PhIP in diet for 3 days)

C57BL/6N mice were fed with a paste formed by mixing beer-A components (beer-A solution) and 0.005% PhIP with an equal weight of the control diet (powder). For 2 days, mice received a control diet mixed with either water (groups 1 and 4), the beer-A solution (×1) (group 2) or the beer-A solution (×5) (group 3). For the subsequent 3 days, mice were given a diet mixed with PhIP (group 1), the beer-A solution (×1) and PhIP (group 1), the beer-A solution (×5) and PhIP (group 3) or a control diet (group 4). Mice were sacrificed on day 6. Subsequent procedures were similar to those outlined for Experiment 7.

As shown in Figures 89.8 and 9, PhIP-induced DNA adducts were formed in the colon, liver, lung and kidney of mice given 0.005% PhIP in the diet. No adducts were observed in the tested organs of mice fed a control diet (group 4; data not shown). The formation of DNA adducts in the colon and lungs of mice given PhIP in the diet decreased significantly with administration of drinking beer-A solution (×2) *ad libitum*, compared with mice given PhIP without beer-A solution (Figure 89.8). Beer-A solution (×1) and (×5) administered in the diet also significantly decreased the amount of DNA adducts in the liver and lung of mice given PhIP in the diet (Figure 89.9).

Beer-A solution in drinking water decreased the amount of DNA adducts formed in the colon and lung of mice fed with PhIP (Figure 89.8). This result suggested that beer components in drinking water could suppress the formation of PhIP-DNA adducts in target organs (colon) associated with carcinogenesis in male rats. The addition of beer-A solution in the diet also decreased the amount of DNA adducts formed in the liver and lung of mice given PhIP; however, this effect was not observed for the colon (Figure 89.9). The observed differences in the suppression of DNA adduct formation in the liver and colon between Experiments 7 and 8 could be explained by the differences in feeding method employed in each experiment. It is known that enterohepatic circulation is important for PhIP metabolism. Watkins *et al.* (1991) reported that fecal excretion was the major route of elimination of PhIP, and suggested biliary excretion of PhIP. Buonarati *et al.* (1992) reported that urinary and fecal excretion over 24 h accounted for 16% and 42–56% of the dose, respectively, in mice administered [^{14}C]PhIP (i.p.). This suggested that colon cells had been exposed to PhIP for over 24 h following administration. The diet paste given to mice in Experiment 8 was completely eaten by 9 a.m. the following day. Mice in Experiment 7 were given beer-A solution throughout the experimental period as drinking water, while mice in Experiment 8 received a diet mixed with beer-A solution between 3 p.m. and 9 a.m. the following day, but then received a diet mixture without beer-A solution from 9 a.m. to 3 p.m. The continuous presence of beer components

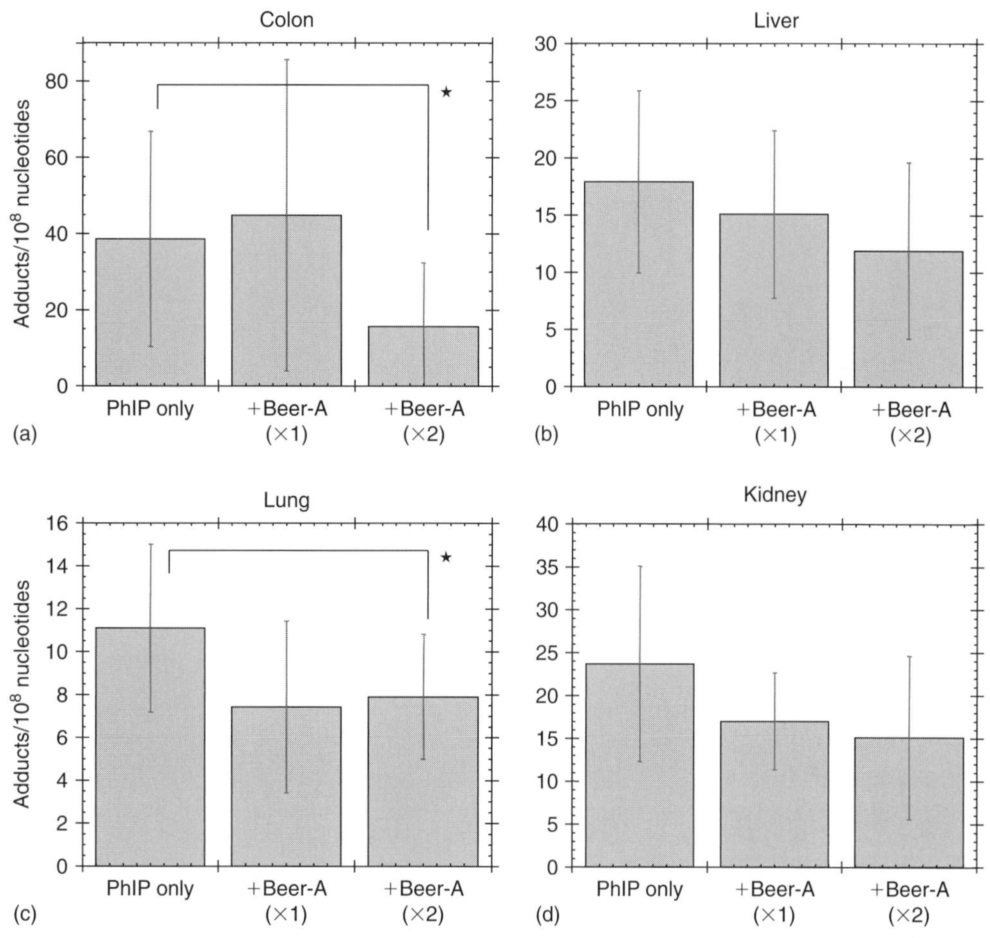

Figure 89.8 Effects of a beer solution in the drinking water on DNA adduct formation in mice fed PhIP. Formation of PhIP-DNA adduct in (a) colon, (b) liver, (c) lungs and (d) kidney in mice treated with beer-A components in drink for 5 days and PhIP in the diet for 3 days (Arimoto-Kobayashi *et al.*, 2006). *Significantly different at $p < 0.05$.

throughout an experimental period might be more effective in providing protection against PhIP-induced DNA damage in the colon. In contrast, administration of beer with PhIP in the diet might be more effective in suppressing the activation of PhIP by CYP enzymes during the first pass through the liver of mice.

Results obtained from the Ames test showed that certain beer samples could inhibit the mutagenicity of heterocyclic amines (PhIP, MeIQx, IQ and Trp-P-2) that were present in cooked food (Arimoto-Kobayashi *et al.*, 2006). The present study revealed that the amount of DNA adducts in mice fed with MeIQx and PhIP decreased significantly with administration of beer-A solution mixed in drinking water, as well as in the diet (Figures 89.6–9). A common mechanism concerning the inhibitory effect of components in beer-A toward mutagenicity in the Ames test and DNA adduct formation induced by PhIP and MeIQx might be involved. The metabolism of mutagens represents one protection mechanism associated with the use of certain chemopreventive agents (Nelson *et al.*, 2001; Walters *et al.*, 2004). PhIP was metabolically activated by CYP1A1, CYP1A2 and CYP1B1 through a process involving *N*-hydroxylation (Boobis *et al.*, 1994; Hammons *et al.*, 1997). The CYP1A2-catalyzed *N*-hydroxylation pathway was shown to account for 70% of the overall elimination of a PhIP dose ingested by human volunteers, and 91% of ingested MeIQx (Boobis *et al.*, 1994). Relative enzyme activity in the presence of beer has been demonstrated (Arimoto-Kobayashi *et al.*, 2006). 7-Methoxyresorufin *O*-demethylase (MROD) activity was significantly inhibited by the presence of beer solutions (beer-A and -B). The amount of beer sample needed for a 50% inhibition (IC_{50}) of demethylase activity was approximately 60 and 200 μl eq./ml for beer-A and -B, respectively. 7-Ethylresorufin *O*-deethylase (EROD) activity was slightly enhanced by the presence of a small amount of beer solution, and was then inhibited. The differences were significant at $p < 0.05$. The amount of beer solution needed for 50% inhibition (IC_{50}) values of deethylase activity were 80 and 200 μl eq./ml for beer-A and beer-B, respectively. Suppression of CYP1A2 and CYP1A1 activities suggested that the antimutagenicity observed with the Ames test was related to the inhibition of metabolic activation. The inhibition of DNA adduct formation might also be linked with the inhibition of metabolic activation.

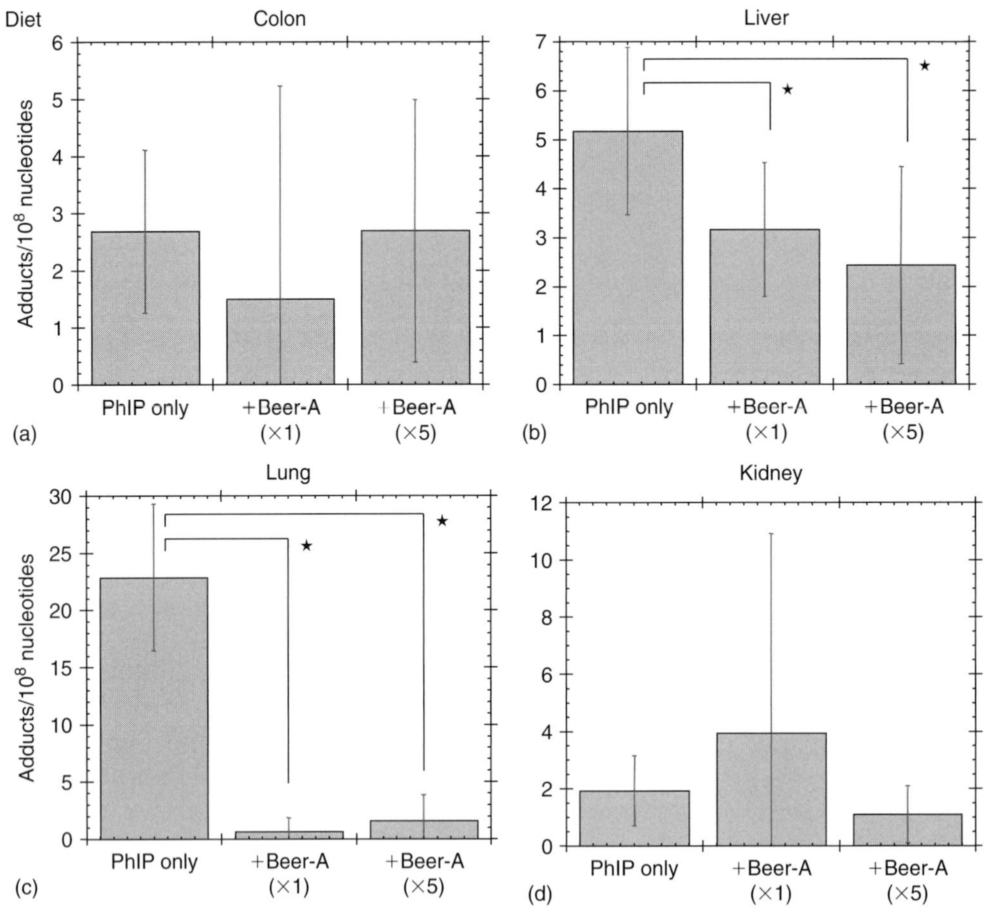

Figure 89.9 Effects of a beer solution mixed in the diet on DNA adduct formation in mice fed with PhIP. Formation of PhIP-DNA adduct in (a) colon, (b) liver, (c) lungs and (d) kidney in mice treated with beer-A components in diet for 5 days and PhIP in diet for 3 days (Arimoto-Kobayashi *et al.*, 2006). *Significantly different at $p < 0.05$.

Components from hops could be responsible for the inhibition of CYP enzymes by beer. For example, 8-prenylnaringenin and xanthohumol from hops inhibited the mutagenic activation of CYP1A2-mediated IQ (Miranda *et al.*, 2000). Although an antimutagenic effect against heterocyclic amines remains to be determined, it is assumed that beer components have at least one target associated with the observed antimutagenicity, namely, the inhibition of the activity of CYP enzyme activities for PhIP. The formation of DNA adducts and associated genetic changes play critical roles in processes involved in carcinogenesis (Nagao *et al.*, 2001). The results of the present study have provided candidates that might act as potential modulators of heterocyclic amine-induced carcinogenesis. Due to the wide-spread consumption of beer in human populations, its potential protective effects against mutagens are worthy of further investigation.

Summary Points

- Beer inhibits the formation of O^6-meG by MNNG in the DNA of Salmonella YG7108 when beer was added to bacteria in the presence of MNNG.
- Beer components inhibit the formation of DNA adducts in mice fed with Trp-P-2, MeIQx and PhIP under conditions reflecting human dietary habits, that is, with a drinking solution containing beer components and also by adding beer components to the diet to simulate intake of food additives.
- Inhibitory effects of a solution of beer components were found on DNA damage in mice liver with single and continuous administration of Trp-P-2.
- The *in vivo* protective effect of beer samples were found in relation to PhIP-induced DNA adduct formation in the colon (the target organ associated with PhIP tumorigenesis) and other important organs (liver, lung and kidney) of mice fed with a beer solution or by the addition of beer components to the diet.

References

Aji, T., Matsuoka, H., Ishii, A., Arimoto, S. and Hayatsu, H. (1994). *Mutat. Res.* 305, 265–272.

Arimoto-Kobayashi, S., Kaji, K., Sweetman, G.M.A. and Hayatsu, H. (1997). *Carcinogenesis* 18, 2429–2433.

Arimoto-Kobayashi, S., Sugiyama, C., Harada, N., Takeuchi, M., Takemura, M. and Hayatsu, H. (1999). *J. Agric. Food Chem.* 47, 221–230.

Arimoto-Kobayashi, S., Takata, J., Nakandakari, N., Fujioka, R., Okamoto, K. and Konuma, T. (2005). *J. Agric. Food Chem.* 53, 812–815.

Arimoto-Kobayashi, S., Ishida, R., Nakai, Y., Idei, C., Takata, J., Takahashi, E., Okamoto, K., Negishi, T. and Konuma, T. (2006). *Biol. Pharm. Bull.* 29, 67–70.

Boobis, A.R., Lynch, A.M., Murray, S., de la Torre, R., Solans, A., Farre, M., Segura, J., Gooderham, N.J. and Davis, D.S. (1994). *Cancer Res.* 54, 89–94.

Buonarati, M.H., Roper, M., Morris, C.J., Happe, J.A., Knize, M.G. and Felton, J.S. (1992). *Carcinogenesis* 13, 621–627.

Dashwood, R.H. (2002). *Mutat. Res.* 511, 89–112.

Edenharder, R., Sager, J.W., Glatt, H., Muckel, E. and Platt, K.L. (2002). *Mutat. Res.* 521, 57–72.

Felton, J.S., Jagerstad, M., Knize, M.G., Skog, K. and Wakabayashi, K. (2000). In Nagao, M. and Sugimura, T. (eds), *Food Borne Carcinogens Heterocyclic Amines*, pp. 198–228. Chichester, Wiley.

Fukutome, K., Ochiai, M., Wakabayashi, K., Watanabe, S., Sugimura, T. and Nagao, M. (1994). *Jpn. J. Cancer Res.* 85, 113–117.

Hammons, G.J., Milton, D., Stepps, K., Guengerich, F.P., Tukey, R.H. and Cadlubar, F.F. (1997). *Carcinogenesis* 18, 851–854.

IARC (1996). In Stewart, B.W., McGregor, D. and Kleihues, P. (eds), *Principles of Chemoprevention*, pp. 1–332. Lyon, IARC Scientific Publications.

Ishii, K., Yamazoe, Y., Kamataki, T. and Kato, R. (1980). *Cancer Res.* 40, 2596–2600.

Kato, I., Tominaga, S. and Ikari, A. (1990). *Jpn. J. Cancer Res.* 81, 115–121.

Kimura, S., Hayatsu, H. and Arimoto-Kobayashi, S. (1999). *Mutat. Res.* 439, 267–276.

Knasmuller, S., Steinkellner, H., Majer, B.J., Nobis, E.C., Scharf, G. and Kassie, F. (2002). *Food Chem. Toxicol.* 40, 1051–1062.

Miranda, C.L., Yang, Y.-H., Henderson, M.C., Stevens, J.F., Santana-Rios, G., Deinzer, M.L. and Buhler, D.R. (2000). *Drug Metabol. Dispos.* 28, 1297–1302.

Monobe, M., Arimoto-Kobayashi, S. and Ando, K. (2003). *Mutat. Res.* 538, 93–99.

Nagao, M., Ochiai, M., Okochi, E., Ushijima, T. and Sugimura, T. (2001). *Mutat. Res.* 477, 119–124.

Nelson, C.P., Kidd, L.C.R., Sauvageot, J., Isaacs, W.B., De Marzo, A.M., Groopman, J.D., Nelson, W.G. and Kensler, T.W. (2001). *Cancer Res.* 61, 103–109.

Ochiai, M., Nagaoka, H., Wakabayashi, K., Tanaka, Y., Kim, S.-B., Tada, A., Nukaya, H., Sugimura, T. and Nagao, M. (1993). *Carcinogenesis* 14, 2165–2170.

Ohgaki, H. (2000). In Nagao, M. and Sugimura, T. (eds), *Food Borne Carcinogens Heterocyclic Amines*, pp. 198–228. Chichester, Wiley.

Ohigashi, H., Osawa, T., Terao, J., Watanabe, S. and Yoshikawa, T. (1997). *Food Factors for Cancer Prevention.* Springer, Tokyo. pp. 1–677.

Potter, J.D., Sellers, T.A., Folsom, A.R. and McGovern, P.G. (1992). *Ann. Epidemiol.* 2, 587–595.

Randerath, E., Agrawal, H.P., Weaver, J.A., Bordelon, C.B. and Randerath, K. (1985). *Carcinogenesis* 6, 1117–1126.

Randerath, K., Haglund, R.E., Phillips, D.H. and Reddy, M.V. (1984). *Carcinogenesis* 5, 1613–1622.

Riboli, E., Cornee, J., Macquart-Moulin, G., Kaaks, R., Casagrande, C. and Guyader, M. (1991). *Am. J. Epidemiol.* 134, 157–166.

Rimm, E.D., Giovannucci, E.L., Willett, W.C., Colditz, G.A., Ascherio, A., Rosner, B. and Stampfer, M.J. (1991). *Lancet* 338, 464–468.

Sugimura, T. (2000). *Carcinogenesis* 21, 387–395.

Sugiyama, C., Shinoda, A., Hayatsu, H. and Negishi, T. (1996). *Jpn. J. Cancer Res.* 87, 325–328.

Swanson, C.A., Wilbanks, G.D., Twiggs, L.B., Mortel, R., Berman, M.L., Barrett, R.J. and Brinton, L.A. (1993). *Epidemiology* 4, 530–536.

Walters, D.G., Young, P.J., Agus, C., Knize, M.G., Boobis, A.R., Gooderham, N.J. and Lake, B.G. (2004). *Carcinogenesis* 25, 1659–1669.

Watkins, B.E., Esuni, H., Wakabayashi, K., Nagao, M. and Sugimura, T. (1991). *Carcinogenesis* 12, 1073–1078.

Wilson, K. (1997). In Ausubel, F.M., Brent, R., Kingston, R.E., Moore, D.D., Seidman, J.G., Smith, J.A. and Struhl, K. (eds), *Current Protocols in Molecular Biology*, Vol. I, pp. 241–245. New York, John Wiley & Sons, Inc.

World Cancer Research Fund (1997). *Food, Nutrition and the Prevention of Cancer: A Global Perspective.* American Institute of Cancer Research, Washington, D.C. pp. 1–670

Yamada, M., Sedwick, B., Sofuni, T. and Nohmi, T. (1995). *J. Bacteriol.* 177, 1511–1519.

Yoshikawa, T., Kimura, S., Hatano, T., Okamoto, K., Hayatsu, H. and Arimoto-Kobayashi, S. (2002). *Food Chem. Toxicol.* 40, 1165–1170.

90

Techniques for Assessing Anti-cancer Effects of Beer

Clarissa Gerhäuser German Cancer Research Center, Division Toxicology and Cancer Risk Factors, Workgroup Chemoprevention, Heidelberg, Germany

Abstract

The development of cancer (carcinogenesis) is a multi-stage process which is generally divided into initiation, promotion and progression phases. Carcinogenesis offers a variety of targets for intervention at every stage. These include modulation of xenobiotics metabolism, antioxidant and radical-scavenging activity, anti-mutagenic, anti-inflammatory and anti-hormonal mechanisms, anti-proliferative activities, induction of terminal cell differentiation and apoptosis (programmed cell death) as well as inhibition of angiogenesis. For each of these mechanisms, *in vitro* test systems have been described that allow the identification of potential anti-cancer activity. This chapter will give a brief overview of the mechanisms and describe the basic principle of the test systems, as well as instrumental requirements.

Introduction: Carcinogenesis and Targets for Anti-cancer Activity

The development of cancer is a multi-stage process which is generally divided into initiation, promotion and progression phases, as depicted in Scheme 90.1. Carcinogenesis can be regarded as an accumulation of genetic or biochemical cell damage which offers a variety of targets for chemopreventive agents to prevent or inhibit the slow progression from early genetic lesions to tumor development (Hanahan and Weinberg, 2000). During the initiation phase, a carcinogen, either directly or after metabolic activation to a reactive molecule, interacts with intracellular macromolecules (DNA, proteins). This may cause DNA damage, which, if not repaired, can result in mutations and genetic damage. These mutations eventually lead to an altered expression of oncogenes and tumor suppressor genes or, for example continuous activation of protein kinases during the promotion phase, and finally result in modified cell structure, uncontrolled cell proliferation, tumor growth and metastases (De Flora and Ferguson, 2005). This cascade of events offers a variety of targets for chemopreventive intervention at every stage.

As indicated in Scheme 90.1, well-established molecular mechanisms of chemoprevention include modulation of xenobiotics metabolism, antioxidant and radical-scavenging activity, anti-mutagenic, anti-inflammatory and anti-hormonal mechanisms, anti-proliferative activities, induction of terminal cell differentiation and apoptosis (programmed cell death) as well as inhibition of angiogenesis, the tumor-induced formation of new blood vessels (De Flora and Ferguson, 2005; Aggarwal and Shishodia, 2006).

Techniques

For the mechanisms and targets described above, various *in vitro* methods have been described which are suitable to assess anti-cancer effects of beer and beer-derived constituents.

Modulation of xenobiotics metabolism

Compounds effective at the initiation stage of carcinogenesis are described as blocking agents; that is, they block carcinogen interaction with DNA. An important mechanism of blocking agents is the modulation of xenobiotics metabolism, that is inhibition of metabolic activation of carcinogens by phase 1 cytochrome P450 (CYP) enzymes, and induction of phase 2 drug-detoxification enzymes to enhance excretion of reactive metabolites (Kohle and Bock, 2006). Phase 1 enzymes such as Cyp1A1, CYP1A2, CYP1B1, CYP2E1 and CYP3A4 activate xenobiotics by addition of functional groups which render these compounds more water-soluble (Nebert and Dalton, 2006). Then, phase 2 enzymes like glutathione *S*-transferase, *N*-acetyl transferase, sulfotransferases or UDP-glucuronosyl transferase conjugate the activated compounds to endogenous ligands, thus facilitating their excretion in the form of these conjugates. Although phase 1 enzymatic activity may be required for complete detoxification, it frequently contributes to the activation of carcinogens (Table 90.1). Moreover, the activity of phase 1 enzymes is often induced by carcinogens and xenobiotics *via* the action of the so-called aryl hydrocarbon (A*h*) receptor, which binds these compounds and stimulates the expression of several phase 1 and phase 2 enzymes (Bock and Kohle, 2006; Brauze *et al.*, 2006). Consequently, inhibition of the

Beer in Health and Disease Prevention
ISBN: 978-0-12-373891-2

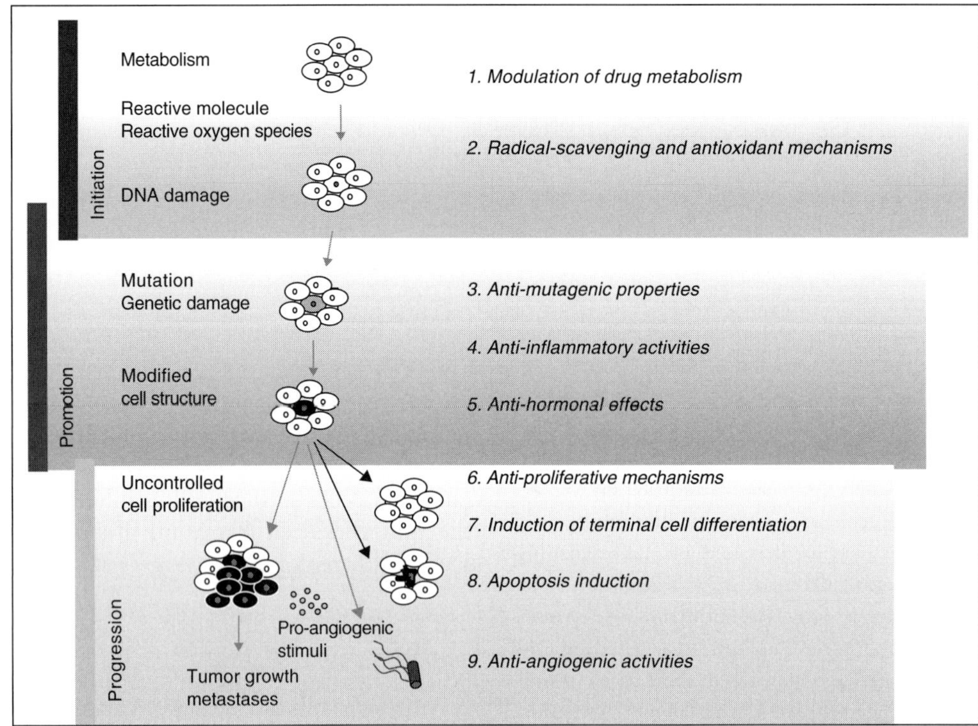

Scheme 90.1 Carcinogenesis (left) and mechanisms of anti-cancer activity (right).

Table 90.1 Methods to determine inhibition of cytochrome P450 (CYP) activities

Enzyme	*Responsible for the activation of*	*Enzyme source*	*Activity*	*Substrate*	*Determination*
CYP1A1	Polycyclic aromatic hydrocarbons	Human recombinant CYP1A1[a]	EROD[a]	7-Ethoxyresorufin	Fluorimetric[b] Ex. 530 nm, Em. 585 nm
Cyp1A	Polycyclic aromatic hydrocarbons	β-NF-induced rat H4IIE cell homogenates	Dealkylase	7-Cyano-ethoxycoumarin	Fluorimetric[c] Ex. 408 nm, Em. 460 nm
CYP1A2	Heterocyclic aromatic amines	hrCYP1A2	AC-4-OH	Acetanilide	HPLC[b]
CYP1A2	Aflatoxin B1 (AFB1)	hrCYP1A2	AFB1 metabolism	AFB1	HPLC[b]
CYP1B1	Polycyclic aromatic hydrocarbons, hormones (estradiol)	hrCYP1B1	EROD	7-Ethoxyresorufin	Fluorimetric[b] Ex. 530 nm, Em. 585 nm
CYP2E1	Alcohol, nitrosamines, chlorinated hydrocarbons	hrCYP2E1	Chloroxazone 6-hydroxylase	Chloroxazone	HPLC[b]
CYP3A4	Aflatoxin B1	hrCYP3A4	Nifedipine oxidase	Nifedipine	HPLC[b]

[a]AC-4-OH, acetanilide-4-hydroxylase; AFB1, aflatoxin B1; β-NF, β-naphthoflavone; CYP, cytochrome P450; Em, emission; EROD, ethoxyresorufin *O*-deethylase; Ex., excitation; hr, human recombinant.
[b]Henderson *et al.* (2000).
[c]Gerhauser *et al.* (2003).

enhanced activity of phase 1 enzymes concomitantly with induction of detoxifying phase 2 enzymes is considered a logical strategy in chemoprevention (Moon *et al.*, 2006). Agents that selectively induce phase 2 enzymes are so-called monofunctional inducers, whereas less desirable bifunctional inducers lead to simultaneous induction of phase 1 and phase 2 enzyme activities (Kohle and Bock, 2006).

Methods for the Determination of Phase 1 Enzyme Activities Phase 1 enzymes are often monooxygenases and dealkylate or hydroxylate their substrates to render them more hydrophilic.

A standard substrate for various phase 1 enzymes is 7-ethoxyresorufin, which is de-ethylated by 7-ethoxyresorufin *O*-deethylase (EROD) activity to form 7-hydroxyresorufin. To determine inhibition of the activity of phase 1 enzymes, substrate conversion is monitored fluorimetrically or by high-performance liquid chromatography (HPLC). Suitable enzyme sources are liver microsomes or S9 supernatants of liver homogenates prepared from rodents pretreated with an enzyme inducer such as Aroclor 1254, homogenates from cultured H4IIE rat hepatoma cells induced with 10 μM β-naphthoflavone for 38 h (for Cyp1A activity), or microsomes of insect cells expressing human recombinant enzymes (supersomes), respectively. Enzymes are incubated with suitable substrates and the rate of product formation is monitored over a period of time with linear enzyme kinetics, as summarized in Table 90.1 (Henderson *et al.*, 2000; Gerhauser *et al.*, 2003). Beer constituents have been shown to inhibit the activities of CYP1A1, CYP1A2 and CYP1B1, whereas potential to inhibit CYP2E1 and CYP3A4 was negligible (Henderson *et al.*, 2000; Gerhauser *et al.*, 2003).

Methods to Measure Phase 2 Enzyme Induction For the identification of inducers of phase 2 enzymes, Prochaska and Santamaria, (1988) have developed a rapid and direct assay of NAD(P)H:(quinone-acceptor) oxidoreductase (QR; EC 1.6.99.2) activity in cultured Hepa1c1c7 murine hepatoma cells. QR catalyzes the two-electron reduction of menadione (2-methyl-1,4-naphthoquinone) to menadiol by NADPH. In parallel, MTT [3-(4,-5-dimethylthiazo-2-yl)-2,5-diphenyltetrazolium bromide] is reduced non-enzymatically by menadiol, resulting in the formation of a blue formazan which can be quantitated on a microtiter plate absorbance reader (Scheme 90.2).

Although QR does not catalyze a conjugation reaction, it is induced coordinately with other phase 2 enzymes and therefore used as a marker enzyme (Kohle and Bock, 2006). Use of the BP^{r}c1 cell line, a mutant of Hepa1c1c7 cells defective in A*h* receptor-mediated induction, allows the distinction of mono- and bifunctional enzyme inducers (Seidel and Denison, 1999). Prenylated chalcones and flavanones from hop and beer have been shown to induce QR activity in Hepa1c1c7 cells (Miranda *et al.*, 2000a; Gerhauser *et al.*, 2002a).

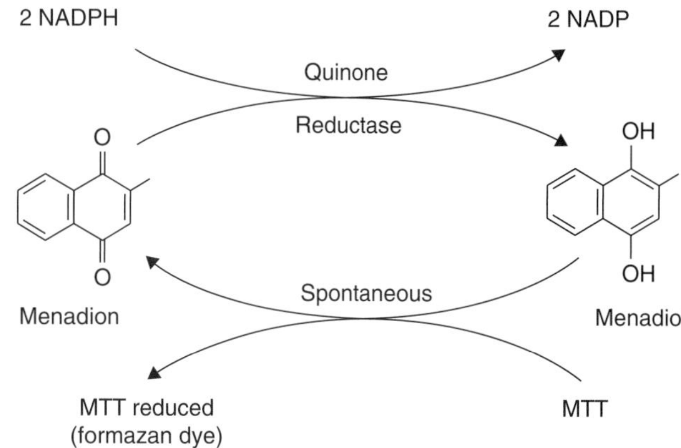

Scheme 90.2 Determination of NAD(P)H:quinone reductase activity according to Prochaska and Santamaria (1988).

Antioxidant activity

Generally, in a healthy organism several physiological processes lead to the formation of reactive oxygen species (ROS) (Valko *et al.*, 2007). Insufficient oxygen consumption in mitochondria during fat metabolism (lipid peroxidation) might result in the production of ROS. Also, manifestation of oxidative stress (e.g. by immune diseases, chronic inflammation and infection) disturbs the intracellular homeostasis of pro- and antioxidants. Overproduction of ROS leads to the formation of highly reactive oxidation products, activation of carcinogens, formation of oxidized DNA bases and DNA strand breaks. These then cause mistakes during DNA replication and genetic alterations, increased transformation frequencies, induced transcription of redox-regulated proteins and ultimately result in enhanced cell proliferation and tumor promotion/progression (Valko *et al.*, 2007).

In a biological system there are multiple free radical and oxidant sources (e.g. $O_2^{\bullet -}$, $^1O_2$, $HO^\bullet$, $NO^\bullet$, $ONOO^-$, HOCl, $RO(O)^\bullet$, $LO(O)^\bullet$) which are controlled by at least four general sources of antioxidants: (i) enzymes, such as superoxide dismutase, glutathione peroxidase and catalase; (ii) large proteins including albumin and ferritin; (iii) small molecules (glutathione, ascorbic acid, tocopherol, carotenoids, (poly)phenols) and (iv) some hormones (estrogen, angiotensin, melatonin, etc.) (Prior *et al.*, 2005). Assays to determine antioxidant capacity (AOC) are manifold. Since both oxidants and antioxidants have different chemical and physical characteristics, no single assay will accurately reflect all antioxidants and all radical sources in a complex biological system.

Techniques to Assess AOC Prior *et al.* (2005) and Huang *et al.* (2005) have recently reviewed and evaluated the most common techniques to assess antioxidant activities and have described the chemistry behind these assays. Methods distinguish between hydrogen atom transfer (HAT) and single electron transfer (SET) reactions. HAT-based methods measure the classical ability of an antioxidant to quench free radicals by hydrogen donation, whereas SET-based methods detect the ability of a potential antioxidant to transfer one electron to reduce another compound.

- HAT-based reactions:

$X^{\bullet} + AH \rightarrow XH + A^{\bullet}$
with $X^{\bullet}$ (free radical) and AH (any H donor)

HAT reactions are solvent- and pH-independent and rapid. However, the presence of reducing agents such as metals can disturb the reaction.

- SET-based reactions:

$X^{\bullet} + AH \rightarrow X^{-} + AH^{\bullet +}$
$AH^{\bullet +} + H_2O \rightarrow A + H_3O^{+}$
$X^{-} + H_3O^{+} \rightarrow XH + H_2O$
$M(III) + AH \rightarrow AH^{+} + M(II)$ with M (metal)

Reactivity in SET methods is based on deprotonation and ionization potential of the reactive functional group; therefore, SET methods are pH-dependent. Notably, SET-methods are very sensitive to ascorbic acid and uric acid, which maintain the plasma redox potential (Prior *et al.*, 2005).

The most common methods for the assessment of AOC, including a categorization of the simplicity of the assay, instrumentation required, biological relevance, mechanisms, endpoints, quantitation method as well as whether the assay is suitable to measure lipophilic and hydrophilic antioxidants are summarized in Table 90.2 (adapted from Prior *et al.*, 2005).

AOC methods using HAT reaction mechanisms include the oxygen radical absorbance capacity (ORAC) assay, the total radical-trapping antioxidant parameter (TRAP) assay, the total oxygen scavenging capacity (TOSC) assay, and low-density lipoprotein (LDL) oxidation. The ferric reducing antioxidant power (FRAP) assay and copper reduction assay (CUPRAC) belong to the SET-based methods, whereas the trolox equivalent antioxidant capacity (TEAC) and the 2,2-diphenyl-1-picrylhydrazyl (DPPH) assay utilize both HAT- and SET mechanisms.

For a description of the test systems as well as advantages/disadvantages of each system refer to Prior *et al.* (2005). The authors recommend to use a combination of the ORAC assay (modified with fluorescein instead of the originally descried β-phycoerythrin) based on a HAT-mechanism and the TEAC assay as a SET-based method together with the Folin–Ciocalteu (FC) assay, which is commonly used as a measure of total phenolics in natural products. The FC assay may be regarded as an oxidation/reduction reaction and thus represents another simple, sensitive and precise method to determine AOC (improved modification of Singelton and Rossi (1965) with gallic acid as a reference standard).

Numerous studies have investigated the AOC of beer and beer constituents using the test systems described above or modification thereof. It is generally accepted that the AOC of beer correlates with its polyphenol content (Lugasi and Hovari, 2003).

Anti-mutagenic potential

Several activated carcinogens and ROS lead to DNA damage, which will result in mutations if not repaired. A well-established test system to detect mutagens is the Ames

Table 90.2 Comparison of techniques for assessing antioxidant capacity (based on Prior *et al.*, 2005)

Assay	*Simplicity*	*Instrumentation required*	*Biological relevance*	*Endpoint*	*Quantitation*	*Lipophilic and hydrophilic AOC*
HAT-based methods						
ORAC	+++[a]	+	+++	Fixed time	AUC[b]	+++
TRAP	−−−	−− (specialized)	+++	Lag phase	IC_{50} lag time	−−
TOSC	−	−	++	IC_{50}[c]	AUC	−−−
LDL Oxidation	−	+++	+++	Lag phase	Lag time	−−−
SET-based methods						
FRAP	+++	+++	−−	Time	ΔOD[d] fixed time	−−−
CUPRAC	+++	+++		Time	ΔOD fixed time	−−−
Methods utilizing both HAT- and SET-based mechanisms						
TEAC	+	+	−	Time	ΔOD fixed time	+++
DPPH	+	+	−	IC_{50}	ΔOD fixed time	−

[a]From highly undesirable (−−−) to highly desirable (+++).
[b]AUC: area under curve.
[c]IC50: half-maximal inhibitory concentration.
[d]OD: optical density.

assay, initially described by Ames *et al.* (1973a, b). The test uses various *Salmonella typhimurium* strains as sensitive indicators for DNA damage caused by structurally diverse mutagens, and mammalian liver extracts for metabolic conversion of carcinogens to their active mutagenic forms. The Ames assay has been utilized to demonstrate anti-mutagenic activity of beer and prenylflavonoids from hops against the food-derived mutagenic heterocyclic amine 2-amino-1-methyl-6-phenlyimidazole[4,5-*b*]pyridine (PhIP) (Miranda *et al.*, 2000b; Arimoto-Kobayashi *et al.*, 2006) and other heterocyclic amines (Arimoto-Kobayashi *et al.*, 1999). Anti-mutagenic potential was partly attributed to the inhibition of metabolic activation of these mutagens.

To counteract mutagenic and lethal effects of DNA damage, healthy organisms have developed DNA repair pathways (Salles *et al.*, 1999). The two most important processes are the nucleotide excision repair (NER) and the base excision repair (BER) pathway. *In vitro* eukaryotic DNA excision repair assays have been described (Salles *et al.*, 1995), but so far, not effects of beer on DNA repair have been reported.

Anti-inflammatory mechanisms

It is assumed that up to 18% of all cancer cases are related to chronic inflammatory processes as for example chronic gastritis, esophagitis, pancreatitis, ulcerative colitis and Crohn's disease (Ohshima *et al.*, 2005).

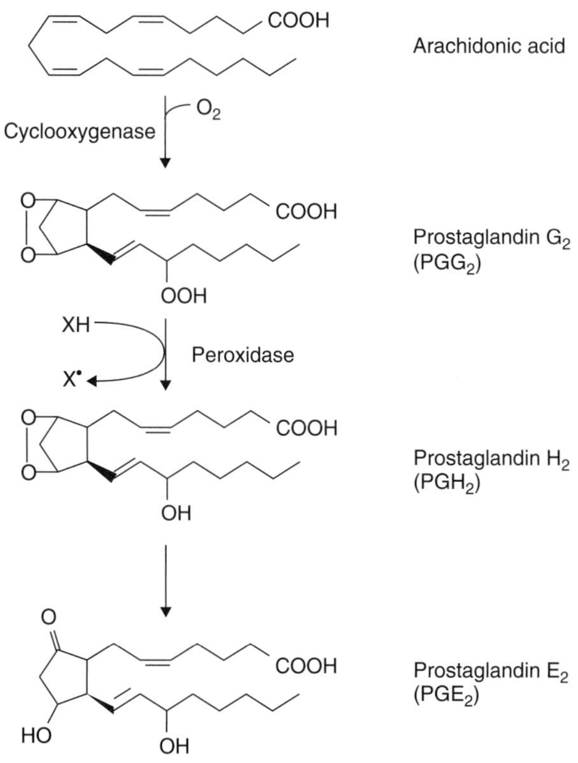

Scheme 90.3 Formation of prostaglandin PGE_2 from arachidonic acid by cyclooxygenases.

Inhibition of Cyclooxygenases Excessive production of prostaglandins, that is hormone-like endogenous mediators of inflammation, is thought to be a causative factor of cellular injury and may ultimately lead to carcinogenesis. Cyclooxygenase (Cox) 1 and 2 enzymes play a substantial role in the biosynthesis of prostaglandins from arachidonic acid as depicted in Scheme 90.3. Cox enzymes contain two catalytic sites, the Cox site, which exists as a long hydrophobic channel within the core of the protein, and a peroxidase site containing a heme moiety.

Since prostaglandin levels are often elevated in tumor tissue in comparison to normal tissue, and Cox-2 activity is inducible during the development of tumor cells, inhibitors of the arachidonic acid cascade are regarded as promising chemopreventive agents.

Methods to Detect Anti-inflammatory Activity Various test systems have been developed to identify anti-inflammatory agents. These systems are based on (i) the measurement of oxygen consumption, which occurs during the first step of Cox activity, (ii) monitoring direct binding of the inhibitor to the enzyme, or (iii) the quantification of arachidonic acid and the resulting prostaglandin metabolites (summarized in Table 90.3).

Enzyme sources for Cox-1 are sheep seminal vesicles or bovine aortic endothelial cells (BAECs), whereas Cox-2 can be enriched from sheep placental cotyledons or phorbol myristate acetate (PMA) treated BAECs. Alternatively, both human enzymes are commercially available as recombinant proteins expressed and purified from insect cells or *E. coli.*

Inhibition of Inducible Nitric Oxide Synthase Nitric oxide (NO) is an important signaling molecule and is involved in the immune defense against pathogens and certain tumor cells. Chronic inflammation and infection, however, result in the induction of the inducible form of NO synthase (iNOS) and consequently, in an overproduction of NO. Long-term elevated levels of NO have been linked to early steps in carcinogenesis *via* nitrosative desamination of DNA bases, accumulation of reactive nitrogen oxide species, DNA adduct formation and consequent DNA damage (Ohshima *et al.*, 2005; Lechner *et al.*, 2005).

Assay to Determine iNOS Acitivity To identify inhibitors of iNOS induction, the murine macrophage cell line Raw 264.7 can be utilized and stimulated with bacterial lipopolysaccharides (LPS) to mimic a state of infection and inflammation. Raw cells are plated in 96 well plates and incubated overnight. Cells are then treated with test compounds and stimulated with LPS for 24 h to induce iNOS. NO production is determined via quantification of nitrite levels in cell culture supernatants according to the Griess reaction. Briefly, 100-μl aliquots of cell culture supernatants are incubated with an equal volume of Griess reagent (1% sulfanilamide/ 0.1% naphthylethylene diamine dihydrochloride/2.5%

Table 90.3 Summary of test systems for the detection of cyclooxygenase inhibitors

Assay	*Cox-1/Cox-2*	*Simplicity*	*Throughput*	*Instrumentation required*	*Endpoint*	*Reference*
Cyclooxygenase reaction						
Oxygen consumption	Cox-1/Cox-2	+++	–	Clark-type electrode	Slope of O_2 consumption	Jang and Pezzuto (1997)
Ultrafiltration LC-MS	Cox-2	–	– –	HPLC-MS	Ligand binding[a]	Nikolic *et al.* (2000)
Metabolite production						
Radiodetection	Cox-1/Cox-2	++	+	HPLC with radiodetector	Detection of radiolabeled PGE_2	Redl *et al.* (1994)
Bovine aortic coronary endothelial cell assay	Cox-1/Cox-2[b]	–	+	Cell culture HPLC-DAD	UV-detection of 6-keto $PGF_{1}\alpha$ and 12-HHT[c]	Dannhardt and Ulbrich (2001)
ELISA[d]	Cox-1/Cox-2	+++	+++	Microplate reader	PGE_2 quantification	Cuendet *et al.* (2006)

[a]Allows immediate identification of known enzyme ligands.
[b]Cox-2 after stimulation.
[c]12-HHT: 12-L-hydroxy-5,8,10-heptadecatrienoic acid, derived non-enzymatically/enzymatically from PGH_2.
[d]Kits and enzyme sources commercially available (compare Reininger and Bauer, 2006).

H_3PO_4) at room temperature for 10 min. The absorbance at 550 nm is determined in a microplate reader, and nitrite levels are quantified in comparison with a nitrite standard curve (Heiss *et al.*, 2001). Using this model, inhibitors of NO production have been identified in hops (Zhao *et al.*, 2003, 2005) and beer (Gerhauser *et al.*, 2002b).

Anti-hormonal effects

Similar to prostaglandins, hormones like estradiol are regarded as endogenous tumor promoters, stimulate cell growth via interaction with estrogen receptors, and increase the risk for breast and uterine cancer (Yager and Davidson, 2006). In addition, estrogen metabolites may directly react with DNA to form adducts. Release of these adducts from DNA and repair of the resulting damage may lead to DNA mutations that can initiate various types of hormone-related cancers. Hops has repeatedly been reported to possess estrogenic properties. Therefore, evaluation of estrogenic and potential anti-estrogenic properties of hops and beer is important.

Measurement of Estrogenic and Anti-estrogenic Properties Estrogenic and anti-estrogenic effects can be determined at several levels: (i) interaction with the estrogen receptors α and β; (ii) estrogen-induced gene transcription; (iii) estrogen-induced enzyme activity and (iv) estrogen-induced cell proliferation in estrogen-responsive mammary cancer cell lines (overview of test systems in Table 90.4). All systems can be used to detect estrogenic effects, but also to measure anti-estrogenic properties, when test compounds are applied simultaneously with estrogens. Indirectly, anti-estrogenic effects can be achieved by inhibition of aromatase (CYP 19), which converts male testosterone into female estrogen.

To monitor the relevance of *in vitro* findings, the uterotrophic assay is a generally accepted short-term *in vivo* screening assay for estrogenicity or anti-estrogenicity. Immature prepubertal or adult ovariectomized female rats or mice are used. Administration of an estrogenic compound will lead primarily to an increase in the uterine weight besides effects on other estrogen-dependent parameters. Anti-estrogenic compounds diminish this estrogen-dependent weight increase (Kanno *et al.*, 2001).

Anti-proliferative activity

The survival of multicellular organisms involves a balance between cell proliferation and cell death. Overexpression of hormone/growth factors and their receptors might present a growth advantage to pre-neoplastic cells. Also, continuous accumulation of genetic damage and mutations during carcinogenesis can result in uncontrolled cell proliferation and cell growth.

Test to Determine Anti-proliferative Activity A simple test system to monitor the effects of test compounds on proliferation of cultured cancer cells is the sulforhodamine B (SRB) assay, developed by Skehan *et al.* (1990). The SRB assay is based on the ability of the protein dye SRB to bind

Table 90.4 Summary of *in vitro* test systems to determine estrogenic and anti-estrogenic activity

Assay	*Material*	*Instrumentation required*	*Reference*
Direct estrogenic and anti-estrogenic activity			
Estrogen receptor (ER) binding assay	Human recombinant ER-α/-β combined with use of fluorescent non-steroidal estrogen	Fluorescence polarization instrument	Bolger *et al.* (1998)
Yeast ER cytosensor assay	Yeast strains expressing human ER-α, -β or both, and ER-controlled yeast enhanced green fluorescence protein	Microplate fluorescence reader	Bovee *et al.* (2004a, b)
MVLN assay	Bioluminescent MCF-7-derived cell line, expressing ER-controlled firefly luciferase	Luminescence reader or photon-counting camera	Pons *et al.* (1990); Demirpence *et al.* (1993)
Ishikawa Var-1 bioassay	Human endometrial cell line with estrogen-dependent alkaline phosphatase activity	Microplate photometer	Littlefield *et al.* (1990); Markiewicz *et al.* (1992)
Proliferation of MCF-7 cells	Human hormone-dependent breast cancer cell line expressing functional ER	Microplate photometer	Katzenellenbogen *et al.* (1987); Skehan *et al.* (1990)
Indirect anti-estrogenic activity			
Aromatase inhibition	Human recombinant CYP19 (aromatase) and *O*-benzylfluorescein benzyl ester as a substrate	Microplate fluorescence reader	Stresser *et al.* (2000)

electrostatically and pH-dependent to protein basic amino acid residues of trichloroacetic acid-fixed cells. Under mild basic conditions the dye can be extracted from cells and quantified by photometric or fluorescent determination. The assay is non-destructive and fixed/stained cells are indefinitely stable. These practical advances make the SRB assay an appropriate and sensitive tool to measure drug-induced inhibition of cell proliferation even at large-scale application. Miranda *et al.* (1999) have used this model to detect anti-proliferative and cytotoxic activity of several hop flavonoids.

Induction of cell differentiation

Differentiation refers to the ability of cancer cells to escape from uncontrolled cell proliferation and to revert to their normal counterparts. Its induction represents an important non-cytotoxic therapy for leukemia, and also breast, prostate and other solid malignancies.

Cell System to Monitor Differentiation-Inducing Capacity Terminal differentiation of human promyelocytic leukemia (HL-60) cells can be induced by a variety of chemical agents (Suh *et al.*, 1995). This process can be monitored by the generation of functionally mature granulocytes and monocytes/macrophages. HL-60 cells undergo growth arrest while they terminally differentiate. Consequently, cell proliferation and an arrest of cell growth are determined by cell counting. Differentiation along the granulocytic lineage is based on the ability of phagocytic cells to generate superoxide upon stimulation with PMA, which is detectable by reduction of nitroblue tetrazolium (NBT). NBT-positive cells are counted as a marker for differentiation.

Induction of differentiation to monocytes/macrophages is determined by evaluation of the expression of non-specific/specific acid esterase by cell staining (Suh *et al.*, 1995).

Induction of apoptosis

Apoptosis (programmed cell death) is a genetically controlled response for cells to commit suicide. Apoptosis represents an innate cellular defense mechanism against carcinogen-induced cellular damage by inhibiting survival and growth of altered cells and removing them at different stages of carcinogenesis. Accordingly, deregulation of apoptosis has been implicated in the onset and progression of cancer. Apoptotic cells are characterized by specific morphological and biochemical changes. The morphological features of apoptosis consist of chromatin condensation, cell shrinkage and membrane blebbing, which can be clearly observed by light microscopy. The biochemical changes during apoptosis induction include (i) the appearance of phosphatidylserine on the cell membrane surface, (ii) increased mitochondrial membrane permeability, (iii) activation of caspases, (iv) DNA fragmentation and (v) protein cleavage at specific locations.

Methods to Detect Induction of Apoptosis Based on these characteristics of apoptotic cells, multiple methods have been described to detect the induction of apoptosis.

Basically all methods have some limitations and are not completely specific and quantitative (Sgonc and Gruber, 1998; Hall, 1999).

(i) Phosphatidylserine is normally situated on the inner surface of the cytoplasmic membrane. During apoptosis, phosphatidylserine is translocated to the outer surface. Annexin V, a highly conserved 35 kDa protein, has a high affinity to phosphatidylserine and can be used, as a fluorescent conjugate, to detect phosphatidylserine externalization by flow cytometry or fluorescent microscopy.

(ii) Breakdown of the mitochondrial transmembrane potential can be measured by fluorochromes that are sensitive to the electrochemical potential within the mitochondria, such as JC-1. These changes can be detected by flow cytometry or fluorescent microscopy.

(iii) The caspases are a group of aspartic acid-specific cysteine proteases which are activated during apoptosis. These unique proteases, which are synthesized as inactive pro-forms, are involved in the initiation and execution of apoptosis once activated by proteolytic cleavage. Caspase assays are based on the measurement of caspase processing to an active enzyme (detected by Western blotting) and of their proteolytic activity using suitable peptide substrates which yield fluorescent or colored products after cleavage. A number of commercial kits and reagents are available to assess apoptosis based on caspase function.

(iv) During the execution phase of apoptosis, nucleases are activated which cleave DNA into 180–200 bp increments. This DNA fragmentation (DNA laddering) can be detected by gel electrophoresis. At the single cell level, the TUNEL (TdT-mediated dUTP nick-end labeling) assay measures the fragmented DNA of apoptotic cells by catalytically incorporating fluorescein-12-dUTP(a) at 3′-OH DNA ends using the enzyme "terminal deoxynucleotidyl transferase." The fluorescein-12-dUTP-labeled DNA can then be visualized directly by fluorescence microscopy or quantified by flow cytometry. Alternatively, biotinylated nucleotides can be incorporated and detected via streptavidin-coupled horseradish peroxidase with suitable colorimetric substrates. DNA fragmentation is also detectable by flow cytometry after propidium iodine staining of fixed cells via the occurrence of a subG1 peak in cell cycle analyses.

(v) Poly(ADP-ribose)polymerase (PARP) is a zinc-dependent eukaryotic DNA-binding protein that specifically recognizes DNA-strand breaks produced during apoptosis induction. The 113 kD protein serves as a substrate for effector caspases and is cleaved during apoptosis into 89-kD and 24-kD fragments, which can be detected by Western blotting as specific markers of apoptosis.

For more in-depth mechanistic evaluation of apoptosis induction, changes in the expression and phosphorylation of pro- and anti-apoptotic proteins can be detected by Western blotting. Some relevant mechanisms observed during the induction of apoptosis by dietary factors have been summarized by Khan *et al.* (2007).

Inhibition of angiogenesis

Angiogenesis – the formation of new blood vessels from already established vessels – plays an essential role in tumor survival and growth. Without adequate blood supply, a tumor cannot grow beyond a critical size of 1–2 mm^2 due to lack of oxygen and nutrients (Carmeliet, 2000). The process of angiogenesis is regulated by various factors and includes multiple steps, which may be targets for anti-angiogenic agents, such as (i) production of growth factors, (ii) activation of endothelial cells, (iii) production of lytic enzymes to digest the basement membrane and extracellular matrix, (iv) endothelial cell migration, proliferation and tube formation.

Test Systems for Anti-angiogenic Activity Current test systems for anti-angiogenic research have been summarized by Auerbach *et al.* (2003). Cell-based systems using endothelial cells only investigate single steps of angiogenesis, for example proliferation, migration or differentiation to microtubules.

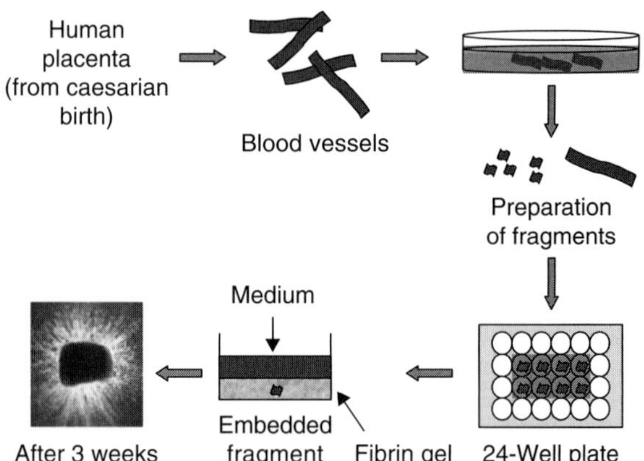

Scheme 90.4 Scheme of the human *in vitro* anti-angiogenesis assay. Superficial arterial or venular vessels are pulled from human placentas and immersed immediately in tissue culture medium. Fragments of 1–2 mm^2 are prepared by cutting, placed in the eight center wells of a 24-well plate and embedded in 1-ml fibrin gel. The gel is overlaid with 1 ml medium containing the test compound at one test concentration (three wells), a solvent control (three wells) and a positive control inhibitor at a concentration giving 40–60% inhibition of vessel growth (two wells). Medium is changed twice weekly. Experiments are terminated after 21 days, when microvessel density reaches a plateau phase. Microvessel density is quantified by acquisition of standardized digital images and densitometric evaluation. Details are described in Bertl *et al.* (2004, 2006).

Therefore, these assays are useful only for mechanistic elucidation. The chorio-allantoic membrane (CAM) assay is an *in vivo* assay using fertilized chicken eggs. Test compounds are placed on carriers, and inhibitory potential can be assessed either on normal CAM vasculature or on growth factor-induced angiogenesis. The rabbit cornea assay is an animal model for angiogenesis. Since all these assays have some limitations for screening, we have developed a human *in vitro* anti-angiogenic model, which covers a broad range of angiogenic key steps, starting from the production of growth factors up to endothelial cell proliferation, migration and tube formation (Bertl *et al.*, 2004, 2006). The main principle of the test is described in Scheme 90.4.

The model has been used to investigate anti-angiogenic activity of several potential cancer chemopreventive agents, including isoxanthohumol (Bertl *et al.*, 2004). Recently, humulone as well as xanthohumol have been described as anti-angiogenic agents (Shimamura *et al.*, 2001; Gerhauser, 2005; Albini *et al.*, 2006).

Summary Points

- Cancer is a complex process that offers various targets for inhibition.
- Multiple test systems have been developed that are suitable to detect anti-cancer agents. These are either simple chemical or biochemical (enzyme) models or involve the *in vitro* culture of primary cells, cancer cell lines, or tissues. Short-term *in vivo* models allow, for example the detection of anti-estrogenic agents.
- Mechanisms of anti-cancer agents include modulation of xenobiotics metabolism, anti-oxidant and radical-scavenging activity, anti-mutagenic, anti-inflammatory and anti-hormonal mechanisms, anti-proliferative activities, induction of terminal cell differentiation and apoptosis (programmed cell death) as well as inhibition of angiogenesis.
- Care should be taken when selecting a test system for a certain mechanism, for example antioxidant activity, since these models are often not equally relevant for the human situation.
- When a potential anti-cancer agent has been identified, proof of anti-cancer efficacy (either preventive or therapeutic) can only be obtained in suitable animal models, which reflect parameters such as absorption, bioavailability, tissue distribution, metabolism and excretion and monitor whether a compound or extract is truly capable to reduce cancer burden *in vivo*. These models are however not included in this chapter.

References

Aggarwal, B.B. and Shishodia, S. (2006). *Biochem. Pharmacol.* 71, 1397–1421.

Albini, A., Dell'Eva, R., Vene, R., Ferrari, N., Buhler, D.R., Noonan, D.M. and Fassina, G. (2006). *FASEB J.* 20, 527–529.

Ames, B.N., Durston, W.E., Yamasaki, E. and Lee, F.D. (1973a). *Proc. Natl. Acad. Sci. USA* 70, 2281–2285.

Ames, B.N., Lee, F.D. and Durston, W.E. (1973b). *Proc. Natl. Acad. Sci. USA* 70, 782–786.

Arimoto-Kobayashi, S., Sugiyama, C., Harada, N., Takeuchi, M., Takemura, M. and Hayatsu, H. (1999). *J. Agric. Food. Chem.* 47, 221–230.

Arimoto-Kobayashi, S., Ishida, R., Nakai, Y., Idei, C., Takata, J., Takahashi, E., Okamoto, K., Negishi, T. and Konuma, T. (2006). *Biol. Pharm. Bull.* 29, 67–70.

Auerbach, R., Lewis, R., Shinners, B., Kubai, L. and Akhtar, N. (2003). *Clin. Chem.* 49, 32–40.

Bertl, E., Klimo, K., Heiss, E., Klenke, F., Peschke, P., Becker, H., Eicher, T., Herhaus, C., Kapadia, G., Bartsch, H. and Gerhauser, C. (2004). *Int. J. Cancer Prev.* 1, 47–61.

Bertl, E., Bartsch, H. and Gerhauser, C. (2006). *Mol. Cancer Ther.* 5, 575–585.

Bock, K.W. and Kohle, C. (2006). *Biochem. Pharmacol.* 72, 393–404.

Bolger, R., Wiese, T.E., Ervin, K., Nestich, S. and Checovich, W. (1998). *Environ. Health Perspect.* 106, 551–557.

Bovee, T.F., Helsdingen, R.J., Koks, P.D., Kuiper, H.A., Hoogenboom, R.L. and Keijer, J. (2004a). *Gene* 325, 187–200.

Bovee, T.F., Helsdingen, R.J., Rietjens, I.M., Keijer, J. and Hoogenboom, R.L. (2004b). *J. Steroid. Biochem. Mol. Biol.* 91, 99–109.

Brauze, D., Widerak, M., Cwykiel, J., Szyfter, K. and Baer-Dubowska, W. (2006). *Toxicol. Lett.* 167, 212–220.

Carmeliet, P. (2000). *Nat. Med.* 6, 389–395.

Cuendet, M., Mesecar, A.D., DeWitt, D.L. and Pezzuto, J.M. (2006). *Nat. Protocol* 1, 1915–1921.

Dannhardt, G. and Ulbrich, H. (2001). *Inflamm. Res.* 50, 262–269.

De Flora, S. and Ferguson, L.R. (2005). *Mutat. Res.* 591, 8–15.

Demirpence, E., Duchesne, M.J., Badia, E., Gagne, D. and Pons, M. (1993). *J. Steroid. Biochem. Mol. Biol.* 46, 355–364.

Gerhauser, C. (2005). *Eur. J. Cancer* 41, 1941–1954.

Gerhauser, C., Alt, A.P., Klimo, K., Knauft, J., Frank, N. and Becker, H. (2002a). *Phytochem. Rev.* 1, 369–377.

Gerhauser, C., Alt, A., Heiss, E., Gamal-Eldeen, A., Klimo, K., Knauft, J., Neumann, I., Scherf, H.R., Frank, N., Bartsch, H. and Becker, H. (2002b). *Mol. Cancer Ther.* 1, 959–969.

Gerhauser, C., Klimo, K., Heiss, E., Neumann, I., Gamal Eldeen, A., Knauft, J., Liu, G., Sitthimonchai, S. and Frank, N. (2003). *Mutat. Res.* 523, 163–172.

Hall, P.A. (1999). *Endocr. Relat. Cancer* 6, 3–8.

Hanahan, D. and Weinberg, R.A. (2000). *Cell* 100, 57–70.

Heiss, E., Herhaus, C., Klimo, K., Bartsch, H. and Gerhauser, C. (2001). *J. Biol. Chem.* 276, 32008–320015.

Henderson, M.C., Miranda, C.L., Stevens, J.F., Deinzer, M.L. and Buhler, D.R. (2000). *Xenobiotica* 30, 235–251.

Huang, D., Ou, B. and Prior, R.L. (2005). *J. Agric. Food Chem.* 53, 1841–1856.

Jang, M.S. and Pezzuto, J.M. (1997). *Method Cell Sci.* 19, 25–31.

Kanno, J., Onyon, L., Haseman, J., Fenner-Crisp, P., Ashby, J. and Owens, W. (2001). *Environ. Health Perspect.* 109, 785–794.

Katzenellenbogen, B.S., Kendra, K.L., Norman, M.J. and Berthois, Y. (1987). *Cancer Res.* 47, 4355–4360.

Khan, N., Afaq, F. and Mukhtar, H. (2007). *Carcinogenesis* 28, 233–239.

Kohle, C. and Bock, K.W. (2006). *Biochem. Pharmacol.* 72, 795–805.

Lechner, M., Lirk, P. and Rieder, J. (2005). *Semin. Cancer Biol.* 15, 277–289.

Littlefield, B.A., Gurpide, E., Markiewicz, L., McKinley, B. and Hochberg, R.B. (1990). *Endocrinology* 127, 2757–2762.

Lugasi, A. and Hovari, J. (2003). *Nahrung* 47, 79–86.

Markiewicz, L., Hochberg, R.B. and Gurpide, E. (1992). *J. Steroid. Biochem. Mol. Biol.* 41, 53–58.

Miranda, C.L., Stevens, J.F., Helmrich, A., Henderson, M.C., Rodriguez, R.J., Yang, Y.H., Deinzer, M.L., Barnes, D.W. and Buhler, D.R. (1999). *Food Chem. Toxicol.* 37, 271–285.

Miranda, C.L., Aponso, G.L., Stevens, J.F., Deinzer, M.L. and Buhler, D.R. (2000a). *Cancer Lett.* 149, 21–29.

Miranda, C.L., Yang, Y.H., Henderson, M.C., Stevens, J.F., Santana-Rios, G., Deinzer, M.L. and Buhler, D.R. (2000b). *Drug Metabol. Dispos.* 28, 1297–1302.

Moon, Y.J., Wang, X. and Morris, M.E. (2006). *Toxicol. In Vitro* 20, 187–210.

Nebert, D.W. and Dalton, T.P. (2006). *Nat. Rev. Cancer* 6, 947–960.

Nikolic, D., Habibi-Goudarzi, S., Corley, D.G., Gafner, S., Pezzuto, J.M. and van Breemen, R.B. (2000). *Anal. Chem.* 72, 3853–3859.

Ohshima, H., Tazawa, H., Sylla, B.S. and Sawa, T. (2005). *Mutat. Res.* 591, 110–122.

Pons, M., Gagne, D., Nicolas, J.C. and Mehtali, M. (1990). *Biotechniques* 9, 450–459.

Prior, R.L., Wu, X. and Schaich, K. (2005). *J. Agric. Food Chem.* 53, 4290–4302.

Prochaska, H.J. and Santamaria, A.B. (1988). *Anal. Biochem.* 169, 328–336.

Redl, K., Breu, W., Davis, B. and Bauer, R. (1994). *Planta Med.* 60, 58–62.

Reininger, E.A. and Bauer, R. (2006). *Phytomedicine* 13, 164–169.

Salles, B., Frit, P., Provot, C., Jaeg, J.P. and Calsou, P. (1995). *Biochimie* 77, 796–802.

Salles, B., Rodrigo, G., Li, R.Y. and Calsou, P. (1999). *Biochimie* 81, 53–58.

Seidel, S.D. and Denison, M.S. (1999). *Toxicol. Sci.* 52, 217–225.

Sgonc, R. and Gruber, J. (1998). *Exp. Gerontol.* 33, 525–533.

Shimamura, M., Hazato, T., Ashino, H., Yamamoto, Y., Iwasaki, E., Tobe, H., Yamamoto, K. and Yamamoto, S. (2001). *Biochem. Biophys. Res. Commun.* 289, 220–224.

Singelton, V.L. and Rossi, J.A. (1965). *Am. J. Enol. Vitic.* 16, 144–158.

Skehan, P., Storeng, R., Scudiero, D., Monks, A., McMahon, J., Vistica, D., Warren, J.T., Bokesch, H., Kenney, S. and Boyd, M.R. (1990). *J. Natl. Cancer Inst.* 82, 1107–1112.

Stresser, D.M., Turner, S.D., McNamara, J., Stocker, P., Miller, V.P., Crespi, C.L. and Patten, C.J. (2000). *Anal. Biochem.* 284, 427–430.

Suh, N., Luyengi, L., Fong, H.H., Kinghorn, A.D. and Pezzuto, J.M. (1995). *Anticancer Res.* 15, 233–239.

Valko, M., Leibfritz, D., Moncol, J., Cronin, M.T., Mazur, M. and Telser, J. (2007). *Int. J. Biochem. Cell. Biol.* 39, 44–84.

Yager, J.D. and Davidson, N.E. (2006). *New Engl. J. Med.* 354, 270–282.

Zhao, F., Nozawa, H., Daikonnya, A., Kondo, K. and Kitanaka, S. (2003). *Biol. Pharm. Bull.* 26, 61–65.

Zhao, F., Watanabe, Y., Nozawa, H., Daikonnya, A., Kondo, K. and Kitanaka, S. (2005). *J. Nat. Prod.* 68, 43–49.

Part IV

Assay Methods and Techniques Used for Investigating Beer and Related Compounds

91

The Evaluation of Beer Aging

María Purificación Hernández-Artiga and Dolores Bellido-Milla Department of Analytical Chemistry, Faculty of Sciences, University of Cádiz, Cádiz, Spain

Abstract

Beer contains certain components, which act as protective agents in relation to consumers' health, such as antioxidants, which decrease over time. The shelf life of package beer is determined to a large extent by the appearance of haze or deterioration of the flavor. A comprehensive understanding of the mechanisms involved in beer instability has yet to be achieved. The raw materials are considered the main source of haze precursors, although the brewing process also has effects. Flavor stability depends on the oxygen content of the packaged beer, which gives rise to active oxygen species. The process of beer aging in the package is discussed with the aim of evaluating the various methods found in the literature for the detection of beer aging. These methods have been classified according to the methodology used, as follows: methodologies to measure one compound or groups of similar compounds, methodologies to detect the time elapsed for appearance of $OH^{\bullet}$ radicals, simulations adding exogenous free radicals to beer, and other methods related to the general properties of sensory analysis and sensors. Correlations between sensory analysis and chemical analysis are emphasized. Attention is given to controversial opinions of authors in relation to compounds with antioxidant properties which retard beer aging. The complexity of the mechanisms and the amount of compounds involved in beer aging is pointed out. The methods that follow the evolution of general properties are considered more closely related to beer aging than those following a single compound. A secondary aim is to shed light on a more holistic understanding of beer aging, the mechanisms of which are at present only poorly understood.

List of Abbreviations

ABTS	2,2′-Azino-bis(3-ethylbenzothiazoline-6-sulfonic acid)
CEAC	Vitamin C equivalent antioxidant capacity
EN	Electronic nose
ESR	Electron spin resonance
FID	Flame ionization detector
GC	Gas chromatography
HPLC	High performance liquid chromatography
MEK	Methyl ethyl ketone
MRP	Maillard reaction product
MS	Mass spectrometry
SPE	Solid phase extraction
TAA	Total antioxidant activity
TEAC	Trolox equivalent antioxidant capacity
UV–Vis	Ultraviolet–visible

Introduction

Besides their gustatory and nutritional properties, beers contain some components that have been recognized in epidemiological studies as acting as protective agents. This is the case of natural antioxidants (Nicoli *et al.*, 1997). It has been reported that the intake of beer significantly increases plasma antioxidant capacity, since beer is able to transfer its phenolic compounds to body fluids (Montanari *et al.*, 1999). It is well known that many antioxidants are lost during storage, producing beer aging. These compounds can also react with other beer components, which make beer aging a complicated process involving many components and mechanisms, which at present are not very well understood.

It is not clear whether Maillard reaction products (MRPs) exhibit predominantly mutagenic or antimutagenic activity. The antimutagenic activity has been attributed to the fact that certain MRPs can act as antioxidants (i.e., chain breakers) oxygen scavengers and metal chelating agents (Nicoli *et al.*, 1997).

In epidemiological studies with Spanish people groups, it has been found an inadequate intake of riboflavin and niacin (B vitamins) that can be normalized along with minerals and proteins by moderate beer consumption (Serra-Majen and Aranceta, 2003; Bamforth, 2004).

Chemical methods to evaluate antioxidant capacity provide information on beer stability, but they may not

Beer in Health and Disease Prevention
ISBN: 978-0-12-373891-2

be correlated with the health effects, which are evaluated by biological methods. The information obtained by both methods is required (Gonzalez-San José *et al.*, 2001).

Maturation (commercial aging) at the final stage in the brewery followed by filtration is carried out to develop desirable flavors and aromas and to diminish off-flavors. It also allows time for proteins and polyphenols to precipitate, which contribute to a haze in the final beer if not removed. In spite of this, the finished beer continues changing and a new period of aging starts. Compared to most other alcoholic beverages, beer is unique because it is unstable when in the final package (Stewart, 2004). The shelf life of packaged beer is essentially determined by either the appearance of haze (colloidal instability) or deterioration of the flavor. Both of these phenomena are the result of non-biological oxidation processes that involve active oxygen species (Andersen *et al.*, 2000). This implies a wide range of complex chemical processes, including proteins, carbohydrates, polyphenols, metal ions, thiols, sulfur dioxide and carbonyl compounds. However, in spite of the scientific progress in this field during the last decades, a complete understanding of the mechanisms involved in beer instability is still lacking.

When beer is stored for an extended time period, permanent haze is formed. Although the brewing process does affect colloidal stability, raw materials are considered the source of haze precursors. The colloidal instability of beer is mainly caused by the formation of insoluble complexes between proteins and oxidized polyphenols (Andersen *et al.*, 2000). Therefore, the balance between these two groups of compounds largely dictates colloidal stability (Andersen *et al.*, 2000). Haze formation is increased mainly by storage temperature and the presence of oxygen (closely related to flavor instability). Iron at trace levels indirectly promotes the haze formation due to its catalytic role in oxidation reactions. The movement of beer accelerates haze formation (due to the rapid interaction of colloids) and light encourages oxidation and haze formation (Stewart, 2004).

The flavor stability depends on the oxygen content of the packaged beer. It is critical that the oxygen level in beer be as low as possible immediately prior to packaging (less than 100 mg/l) and that oxygen accumulation during filling is minimized. The oxidative reaction of beer has been recognized as the most important cause of the staling of flavor development. Molecular oxygen, O_2, is itself relatively unreactive (Bamforth and Parsons, 1985), but the activated forms of oxygen (O_2^-, O_2^{2-}, H_2O_2, $OH^\bullet$), which are called "active oxygen" species in beer oxidation, have been indicated to participate in the aging process (Uchida and Ono, 1996) (Figure 91.1).

The oxidation reactions involve Fenton reactions, which are dependent on oxygen and iron or copper ions, and minimizing these contents in the packaged beer has a positive effect on flavor stability (Andersen *et al.*, 2000). However, it is now clear that flavor stability is in fact influenced by all stages of the brewing process. In many foods, staling is

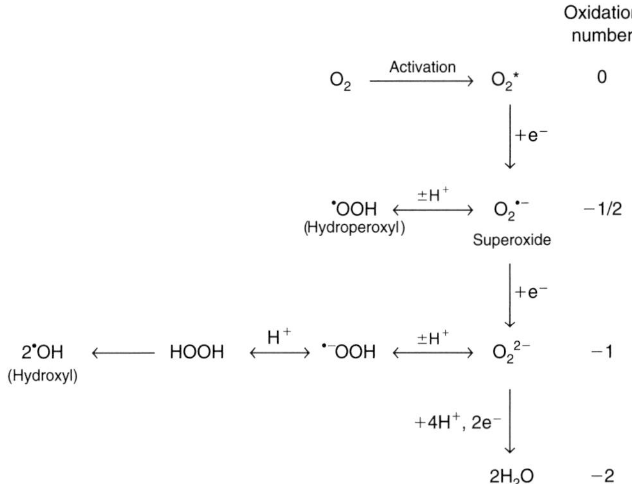

Figure 91.1 Reactive oxygen species. Schematic showing generation from molecular oxygen. The hydroxyl radical ($OH^\bullet$) and hydroperoxyl (OOH) are considered to be the most reactive.

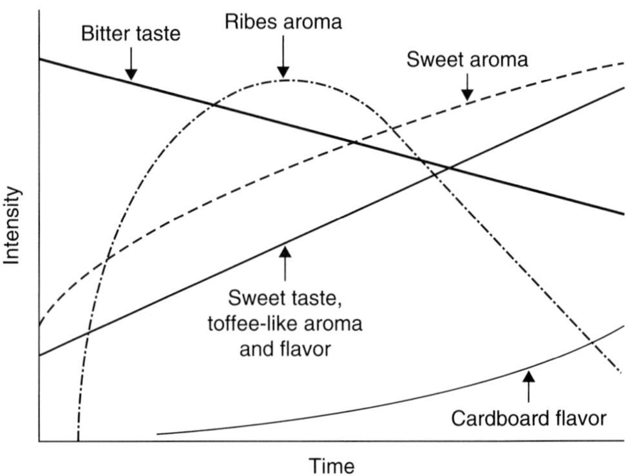

Figure 91.2 The Dalgliesh plot. Changes in various flavors in beer as the beer is stored over time.

caused by the appearance of various unwanted unsaturated carbonyl compounds. The same is true in beer staling (Bamforth, 2000). The actual compounds responsible for stale flavor vary during prolonged storage, as evidenced by the changes in the flavor profile of beers (Figure 91.2).

It is known that the development of certain carbonyl compounds (oxidation products) plays an essential role in the loss of taste stability (Varmuza *et al.*, 2002). The compounds causing the "sweetish, leathery character" of very old beers have not been identified. However, there is evidence that the "papery cardboard character" of 2–4-month-old beer is due to unsaturated aldehydes. The most flavor-active is *trans*-2-nonenal, with a very low stale flavor threshold. Other aldehydes such as nonadienal, decadienal and undecadienal, may also exceed threshold levels (Stewart, 2004). Other compounds have been found to increase in concentration during beer aging and include: β-damascenona, methional dimetyltrisulfide (Chevance *et al.*, 2002; Guido *et al.*, 2004) and furfuryl ethyl ether (Vanderhaegen, 2004). It is known that beer flavor stability is determined by the endogenous antioxidant activity of beer itself, which is affected by each step in the brewing process (Uchida and Ono, 1996). Beers contain compounds with antioxidant properties such as reducing sugars, sulfur dioxide, phenolic compounds, vitamins and MRPs. A considerable number of phenolic compounds may act as antioxidants, with mechanisms involving both free radical scavenging and metal chelation (Fantozzi *et al.*, 1998). The beer phenolic compound content described in the bibliography oscillates between 50 and 350 mg/l. On the other hand, the role of phenols as antioxidants is controversial. In fact, contradictory results have been reported on the effectiveness of some phenolic compounds as potential antioxidants, pointed out the sulfite as relevant antioxidant in beer (Kaneda and Takashio, 1996; Uchida and Ono, 1996; Foster *et al.*, 1999).

Methods to Evaluate Beer Aging

Although off-flavors are easily identifiable by sensory analysts trained in the assessment of beer flavor, there is a definite requirement for analytical methods that may detect the specific compounds responsible for these flavors and thereby enable quantitative determination of beer staling. It is possible to find in the literature numerous methodologies to evaluate beer aging; they refer mainly to flavor instability, which has become the most important factor in determining the shelf life of packaged beer (Uchida and Ono, 1996). We can classify them as follows:

(a) Methodologies to measure one compound or groups of similar compounds.
(b) Methodologies to detect the time elapsed for the appearance of OH radicals.
(c) Simulations adding an exogenous free radical to beer.
(d) Other methods related to a variety of general properties.
(e) Sensory analysis and sensors (electronic nose (EN) and electronic tongue).

Methodologies to measure one compound or groups of similar compounds

There are numerous studies indicating that volatile long-chain unsaturated aldehydes are the main compounds responsible of the initial stale flavor of beer.

E-2-nonenal is believed to be the major source of the "cardboard" character of (appearing in) stale beer. Simultaneous determination of *E*-2-nonenal and β-damascenone by reverse phase liquid chromatography with UV detection is reported (Guido *et al.*, 2004). This entails steam distillation, passage of the distillate through a C_{18} solid phase extraction (SPE) column, and analysis by high performance liquid chromatography (HPLC) with UV detection. The results were confirmed by gas chromatography with a mass spectrometry detector (GC–MS). *E*-2-nonenal at 0.06–0.07 μg/l in fresh beer and 0.16–0.20 μg/l in aged beer. β-damascenone was found at 1.8 μg/l in fresh beer and at 2.8–2.9 μg/l in aged beers. Both compounds are proposed as markers of beer aging.

The increase of β-damascenone content during aging has been reported in commercial Belgian beers (Chevance *et al.*, 2002). The methodology used consists of an extraction; passage through a resin and injection in a gas chromatographer with a flame ionization detector (FID) and olfactometry detector. In fresh commercial beers, β-damascenone was detected below 25 ng/g and in aged beers up to 210 ng/g.

Furfuryl ethyl ether, detected by gas chromatography, has also been proposed as a marker of aging (Vanderhaegen, 2003, 2004). Concentrations between 76 and 216.7 μg/l were found in 4-year-old aged beers. It is concluded that the aging of ale beers differs significantly from that of lager beers.

Dimetyltrisulfide is a key flavor in beers; the detection of precursors of this compound has also been investigated (Gijs *et al.*, 2000) by means of extractions followed by gas chromatography.

Chromatographic techniques (GC–MS after steam distillation and HPLC) have been used to determine aldehydes, ketones and esters relevant in beer aging, both in fresh beers and in artificially aged samples (Varmuza *et al.*, 2002). A chemometric evaluation shows that the concentration profiles in artificially aged beer samples are clearly distinguishable from those of fresh samples.

The behavior of sulfites in beers during fermentation and storage after packaging was studied using HPLC with a fluorescence detector to determine aldehyde–bisulfite adducts. Acetaldehyde–bisulfite and free sulfite decreased during beer storage, indicating that they are oxidized by free radical reactions during beer storage and inhibit the oxidation of the other beer components. They proposed that the contribution of sulfite to beer flavor stability is not based on a masking effect on stale flavor through adduct formation, but rather on an antioxidative action, a radical scavenging action (Kaneda and Takashio, 1996).

A method for the evaluation of beer aging measuring acetaldehyde and sulfite voltammetric peaks is reported. The ratio of acetaldehyde and SO_2 currents correlates well with those given by an expert sensory panel (Guido *et al.*, 2003). These results are supported by the theory of an adduct acetaldehyde – SO_2 formation with a high constant (compared with other carbonyl compounds – SO_2), and furthermore, acetaldehyde is the main component of the carbonyl compounds in beers. These adducts are not flavor actives. Other authors had previously accepted the mechanism of the adduct formation (Illet *et al.*, 1996) as responsible for the SO_2 contribution to beer stability.

In a review (Illet, 1995) of sulfur dioxide in beers the methods to determine SO_2 have been presented based on a variety of methodologies. They are classified as follows: distillation followed by titration, iodometric titration with visual or electronic end point determination, ultraviolet–visible (UV–Vis) spectrophotometry (based on the reaction between SO_2, *p*-rosaniline and formaldehyde or on the reaction with the tetradichloromercurate (II) ion or on the use of dithiobis(2-nitrobenzoic acid) after distillation), selective electrodes, enzymic determination, chromatographic methods (gas chromatography, ion chromatography, ion exclusion and high performance liquid chromatography). The total concentration of SO_2 typically ranges from 1 to 30 mg/l.

Methodologies to detect the time elapsed for the appearance of OH$^{\bullet}$ radicals

Partially reduced forms of oxygen (notably superoxide and hydroxyl radicals) are the responsible species that cause flavor instability due to oxidation. Free radicals were observed after a definite period during an oxidative forcing test. The detected free radicals were identified as hydroxyl radicals (OH$^{\bullet}$) using a spin trapping method with electron spin resonance (ESR) spectroscopy (Uchida and Ono, 1996). It was found that the OH$^{\bullet}$ was not always generated just after starting the forcing test, but was generated after a definite time period the authors called the "lag time" of OH$^{\bullet}$-radical generation. The lag time was considered to be related to the endogenous antioxidant activity of beer. Beer itself has endogenous antioxidant activity to prevent free radical generation and free radicals are generated only after the antioxidants in beer are deactivated. The effect of the catalytic role of the ferrous ion was investigated and it was concluded that it contributes to the generation of free radicals. The same authors demonstrated that the method to detect the endogenous antioxidant activity by ESR exhibited a good correlation with sensory analysis by experimental panelists (Uchida *et al.*, 1996).

A number of potential antioxidants have been evaluated for their effect on the formation of radicals in beer using the ESR lag phase method (Andersen *et al.*, 2000). Sulfite was found to be the only one able to delay radical formation, whereas phenolic compounds had no effect. Ascorbate, cystein and cysteamin were, on the other hand, found to be prooxidants which reduce iron and copper ions to Fe(II) and Cu(I) that catalyze free radical formation. Other authors (Foster *et al.*, 1999) obtained similar results studying flavor stability using ESR to detect free radicals, which support the theory that phenolic compounds do not contribute to the antioxidant capacity but SO_2 does increase the lag time.

In terms of the sulfite contribution to beer stabilization, two mechanisms have been proposed (Kamiura and Kaneda, 1993). First, sulfite inhibits beer oxidation during storage by acting as an antioxidant. Second, sulfite masks staling flavors via adduct formation between aldehydes and bisulfite.

The results obtained using ESR support the first mechanism (Uchida and Ono, 1996; Foster *et al.*, 1999; Andersen *et al.*, 2000), since the sulfite inhibits the generation of radicals, it extends the lag time and retards beer flavor staling. These results are supported by the ones obtained by HPLC with fluorescence detection (Kaneda and Takashio, 1996), which indicated sulfite has an extremely poor reactivity with *trans*-2-nonenal (responsible for the cardboard flavor with a very low threshold). Furthermore, in the same article it is reported that acetaldehyde bisulfite and free sulfite decrease during beer storage, indicating they are oxidized by free radical reactions during beer storage and inhibit the oxidation of other components.

Simulations adding an exogenous free radical to beer

These simulations are based on the determination of the total antioxidant activity (TAA) by measuring the capacity of beer to capture free radicals. It is possible to measure all of the antioxidant components known in a sample individually, but this is time-consuming and expensive. In addition, since there seems to be cooperation between antioxidants during oxidative stress, examining one in isolation may not accurately reflect their combined activity (Cano *et al.*, 1998). Interest has, therefore, been focused by many researchers on the measurement of TAA. Beer generally contains a range of antioxidants, the most important of which are the polyphenols, phenolic acids, sulfur dioxide, reducing sugars, vitamins and products of the Maillard reaction.

The methods used to determine the total antioxidant capacity are based on the addition of an exogenous free radical and measurement of the decrease in absorbance (by UV–Vis spectrophotometry) produced by the addition of beer.

Method of the 2,2-Diphenyl-1-picryl Hydrazyl Radical (Kaneda *et al.*, 1995) This method is limited by low reproducibility when it is applied to beers.

Method of the *N,N*-dimethyl-*p*-phenylenediamine (Gonzalez-San José *et al.*, 2001) This method has previously been applied to wine. The corresponding cation radical is obtained by oxidation with Fe(III) chloride at pH 5.25. The absorbance is measured by UV–Vis spectrophotometry at 505 nm. A small volume of beer is added and the absorbance decreases due to free radical scavenging capacity of the sample is measured. The absorbance difference is related to the antioxidant capacity. It is expressed as TEAC (trolox equivalent antioxidant capacity) using a calibration curve plotted with different amounts of trolox or as CEAC (vitamin C equivalent antioxidant capacity). It is a rapid, reproducible and inexpensive method. It was applied to 80 commercial beers grouped in four types: lager, stout, alcohol-free and special (fruit, wheat and ecological). Beers containing red fruits exhibited the maximum activity. The values obtained were between 2–56 mg CEAC and 20–190 mg TEAC (in a package of 333 ml). These ranges were similar in the four types.

Method of the 2,2′-Azino-bis(3-ethylbenzothiazoline-6-sulfonic acid) Recently, the 2,2′-Azino-bis(3-ethylbenzothiazoline-6-sulfonic acid) ABTS method (Millar *et al.*, 1993) was presented as an excellent tool for determining the antioxidant activity of plant materials and beverages (Arnao *et al.*, 1996; Cano *et al.*, 1998; Cano-Lario *et al.*, 1998). The procedure to determine the antioxidant capacity is as follows: The $ABTS^{\bullet+}$ is prepared by enzymatic oxidation of ABTS with H_2O_2 and peroxidase. It (shows) displays the spectrum that can be observed in Figure 91.3.

One hundred microliters of distilled water are added to 2.5 ml of $ABTS^{\bullet+}$ and the absorbance is measured by UV–Vis spectrophotometry at 414 nm. Subsequently, 100 μl of beer is added into the spectrophotometer cuvette that contains 2.5 ml of $ABTS^{\bullet+}$ and the new absorbance is measured. The absorbance difference is recorded. This is called the "end point" method (Cano *et al.*, 1998). Another strategy with ABTS has been described for citric fruit juices and is known as "lag time." This is based on the addition of the antioxidant to the ABTS peroxidase/H_2O_2 system to retard the formation of the $ABTS^{\bullet+}$ (Arnao *et al.*, 1996). This method is longer and prone to interference, which affects radical formation compared to the end point method.

The authors applied to beers the described "end point method" (Oñate-Jaén *et al.*, 2006) and found that the absorbance difference was not stable and the absorbance value for $ABTS^{\bullet+}$ plus beer continues slowly decreasing for approximately 30 min, after which a tendency to stabilize was observed. The correlation coefficient between the absorbance decrease at $t = 0$ (measured immediately after mixing) and the absorbance decrease at $t = 90$ min was $r = 0.938$, therefore, the absorbance decrease at $t = 0$ was proposed as a measure of the antioxidant capacity of beer. Furthermore, this measurement of the immediate absorbance decrease represents the group of beer antioxidants acting with a rapid mechanism when free radicals are formed naturally in this beverage. The slow antioxidants are of less interest since a slow radical scavenger reaction allows the oxidation of the beer compounds. This method provides a rank order of antioxidant capacity.

The quantitative evaluation using ascorbic acid or trolox proposed by some authors was considered troublesome and unnecessary. Therefore, the authors propose this precise methodology as an index to compare the antioxidant capacity of beers that really is related to the taste and stability of this beverage, since it represents antioxidants with rapid kinetics.

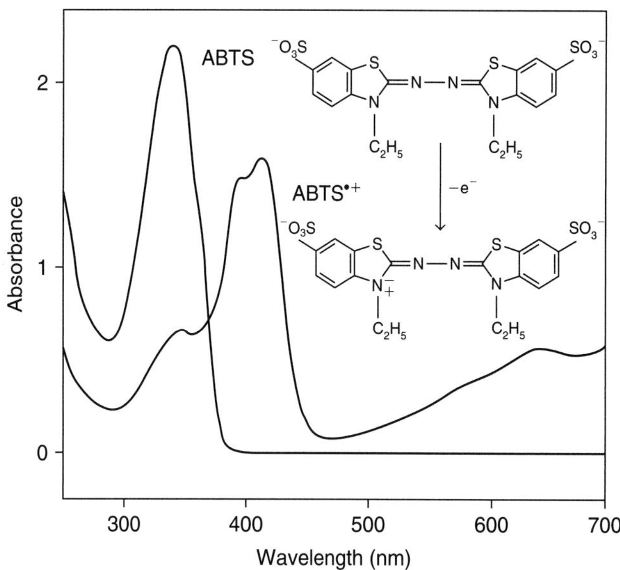

Figure 91.3 UV–Vis spectrum of the ABTS and $ABTS^{\bullet+}$. The $ABTS^{\bullet+}$ absorbance measured at $\lambda_{max} = 414$ nm.

Other methods related to general properties

Many of the carbonyl compounds that play an essential role in the loss of taste stability exhibit a characteristic absorption in the UV region 240–310 nm. The absorption integral for this region has been successfully used as an easy parameter for characterizing the quality and aging status of beer (Klein *et al.*, 2000). The same authors had found that this values correlates well with furanic aldehydes.

A simple and direct method to evaluate beer aging based on liquid–liquid extraction and UV–Vis spectrophotometric measurement has been developed (Oñate-Jaén *et al.*, 2006). The procedure is as follows: 20 ml of fresh beer after being degasified was extracted with methyl ethyl ketone (MEK) after 5 min shaking. The organic phase spectrum was registered and it showed a broad band with a maximum at $\lambda = 333$ nm. It is shown in Figure 91.4.

As is well known, beers develop compounds that end up producing haze since the colloidal stability is broken down; therefore, the extraction with a solvent of low polarity can isolate the compounds with low solubility in the aqueous medium of beer. A search of the literature was used to identify the groups of compounds extracted with MEK. Hydroxycinnamic derivatives (phenolic compounds) were found to exhibit a very similar band with a maximum around 330 nm (Maillard *et al.*, 1996). In a previous work (Bellido-Milla *et al.*, 2004), the authors identified phenolic acid in beers by UV–Vis spectrophotometry at 333 nm with a previous extraction or separation by high pressure liquid chromatography. Reports were also found on methods able to identify MRPs in the extract, since soluble premelanoidins absorb between 320 and 350 nm (Morales and Jimenez-Pérez, 2001), MRPs of low polarity are also found at 334.4 nm (Billaud *et al.*, 2004) by HPLC with UV–Vis spectrophotometry detector.

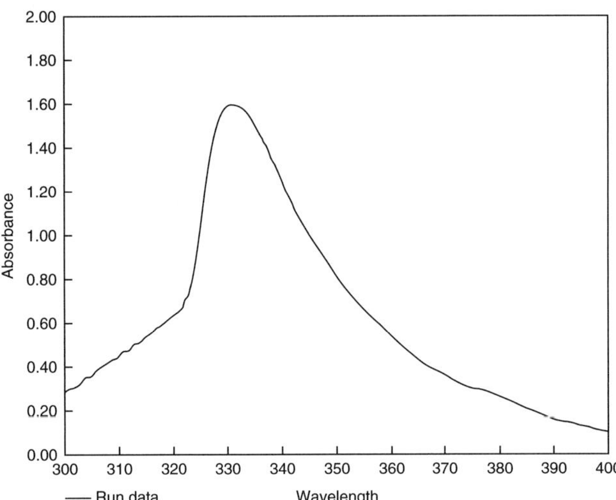

Figure 91.4 UV–Vis spectrum of the MEK extract for pilsner beer.

Certain experiments, heating and measuring the antioxidant capacity of beers before and after extraction with EMK have confirmed the presence of both groups of compounds in the extract. The ABTS method and the extraction method were checked for a group of beers (control) and for the same beers after natural and forced aging. The forced aging test at 60°C is carried out to save analytical time, since qualitatively similar results have been found compared to natural aging (Uchida and Ono, 1996) (when higher temperatures are used the changes undergone are not comparable to a natural aging). The results are shown in Table 91.1.

In all cases, the values were observed to diminish with aging. Pilsner beer in both aging methods exhibits a higher decrease, probably due to the traditional brewing process without additives by which it is obtained. A similar behavior for natural and forced aging (60°C) has been observed by other authors when ESR is used (Uchida *et al.*, 1996). The decrease of absorbance for EMK extract might be due to the transformation of the extracted compounds (mainly polyphenols) by aging.

In order to study the utility of the two methods mentioned above, 34 beers were analyzed. They were obtained from local stores and represent the types of beers readily available to consumers. The antioxidant capacity and the absorbance of the EMK extract were obtained in fresh and aged beers (60°C) during a week. The correlation coefficient (r) between both groups of data for the 34 fresh beers is 0.896. This allows predicting the antioxidant capacity by means of the mathematical model $A = 0.234 + 0.424\ E$. Therefore, with a simple extraction and a measurement by UV–Vis spectrophotometry the antioxidant capacity can be predicted avoiding the use of an organic reagent and the development of the corresponding free radical. The correlation coefficients between fresh and aged beers for the antioxidant capacity and the EMK extract are 0.939 and 0.995, respectively. It means that it is possible to predict the antioxidant capacity for aged beers from fresh beers.

With the aim of differentiating groups of beers the analysis of variance was applied to the results obtained from the 34 beer samples analyzed. Statistically significant differences were found between ecological and non-ecological beers. Lager and weizen were also differentiated from stout beers.

Reductones are a type of antioxidants which can bind oxygen or be oxidized in the presence of oxygen and transition metals acting as prooxidants. They are powerful reducing agents. Different types of reductones have a considerable influence on the stability of beers. An automated voltammetric method for the determination of the reducing power of beer has been reported (Sobiech *et al.*, 1998). The reductones are determined indirectly using the redox dyestuff 2,6-dichlorophenol-indophenol. Its reduced form is electrochemically reoxidized. The highest reductone contents were observed with dark beers. This is due to a higher melanoidin content (MRP) resulting from the higher kilning temperature. This is the reason for the persistent flavor stability of dark beer. The values of strongly hopped pilsner beers were considerably higher than those of conventional pale lager beers, as hop bitter acids and hop polyphenols can also react as reductones. The lowest values were obtained for alcohol-free beers. It is possible to take the different reactivity of reductones into consideration. A "reductone distribution" with repeated measurement at several reaction times could be achieved. This would extend the

Table 91.1 Results of natural and forced aging

	EMK extract absorbance			*Absorbance decrease of ABTS$^{\bullet+}$*		
Beers	Control beer	Natural aging	Forced aging	Control beer	Natural aging	Forced aging
Carlsberg	0.840	0.766	0.783	0.580	0.493	0.346
Pilsner	1.666	1.328	1.273	0.719	0.600	0.303
Leffe	1.707	1.526	1.673	0.814	0.517	0.623
Negra modelo	0.963	1.025	0.938	0.552	0.394	0.293

Note: Comparison of EMK extract absorbance and absorbance decrease of ABTS$^{\bullet+}$ for natural and forced aging in different types of beers.

range of possible applications of the method, as reductones of different reactivity can have a different influence on the stability of beer. The authors propose future investigations about the correlation of reductone content and composition with colloidal and flavor stability.

Chemiluminiscence has been reported to be observed during beer storage, probably due to MRPs (Morales and Jimenez-Pérez, 2001). The changes produced patterns during beer storage that show a good correlation with the degree of stale flavor in panel scores. The deterioration rates of beers might be assessable by measuring the chemiluminiscence. However, the precision needed for the accurate prediction of beer flavor stability is as yet a subject of research (Kaneda *et al.*, 1990, 1991, 1994).

Sensory analysis and sensors

It is quite possible for a beer to have physical and chemical properties well within generally accepted levels and yet be completely unacceptable in taste. Sensory data are therefore also necessary to complement the chemical analysis. In order to obtain this data, the use of a highly trained sensory panel is necessary. The members of this panel are trained in identifying the various characteristics associated with the aroma, taste, mouth feel and aftertaste of the product (McKellar *et al.*, 2002). The major problems with flavor components typically found in beer arise primarily as a result of flavor instability during storage. Perhaps, the best known tool for sensory beer flavor detection is the construction of the beer flavor wheel (Hughes and Baxter, 2001), which brings together the main descriptors associated with taste and odors for many beers produced commercially. It can be seen in Figure 91.5.

A modification has been suggested to incorporate aspects of texture and mouth feel (Hughes and Baxter, 2001). Reliable and statistically well-founded tests are available which can provide authoritative and semiquantitative information that can be applied to make decisions about beer quality (Bamforth, 1998). These methods can be divided into difference tests and descriptive tests. For the descriptive tests a wide terminology is used. The individual attributes are scored by the tasters (usually from 0 to 10). It takes real ability to be able to separate out the various terms and recognize them individually. Once the scoring is completed, the findings may be reported in the form of a spider diagram (Figure 91.6).

A spindle represents each flavor. The shape is characteristic of a product. This test is usually applied to fresh beers but they could be used also to detect beer aging due to sensory changes in beer flavor during the aging process.

The determination of foodstuff quality is usually carried out with the help of sample preparation and rather complex and expensive instrumentation. These types of analysis may ultimately be profound and reliable but the procedures can hardly be done rapidly and, moreover, on-site

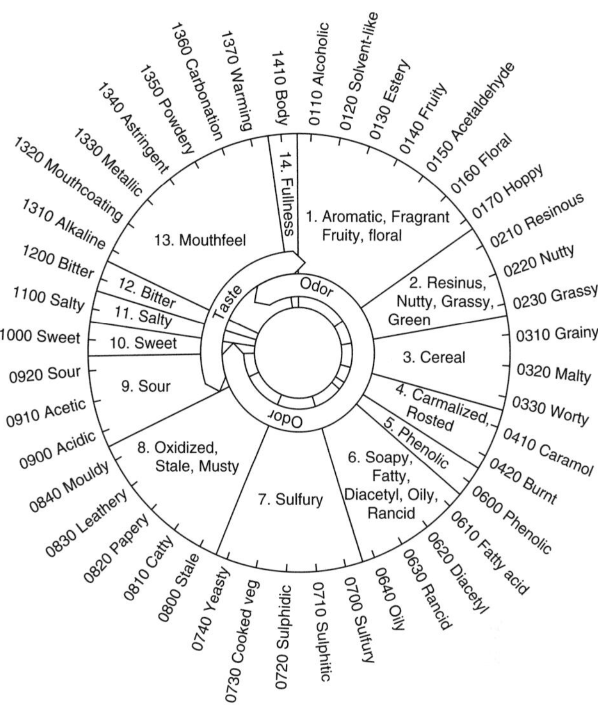

Figure 91.5 The meilgaard beer flavor wheel. Sensory assessment of beer.

or on-line. For quality control it is necessary to monitor the evolution of a group of certain components that accurately reflect the process of aging and spoilage. These components can be numerous or unknown and the problem appear to be quite difficult. Besides, it is very complex at present to compare the results of instrumental analysis to biological sensing. One of the promising directions of development of different analytical methods implies the use of artificial sensors combined with advanced statistical methods. Electronic nose, devices constructed according to the principles of the human olfactory system, based on sensor arrays and application of pattern recognition tools are at present capable of distinguishing between very complex and rather similar gas mixtures, such as the odors of certain beverages, sometimes even odors containing up to several hundreds of components (Legin *et al.*, 1997). The EN is one of the most promising techniques for rapid analysis of volatiles. Generally, it consists of a semiselective metal oxide sensor array that reacts with volatile chemicals in the sample headspace. Data are analyzed using computer based pattern recognition algorithms. The result is a "fingerprint" characteristic of the headspace volatiles, which allows qualitative comparisons. EN systems have recently been applied to the analysis of beer. Instruments based on ion-conducting polymer sensors have been applied to the differentiation of beers brands, identification of hops and monitoring of fermentation. Recently, a sensor was used to establish the influence of aging time in the brewery (maturation) and on the development of the aroma characteristics of beer (McKellar *et al.*, 2002). The results were

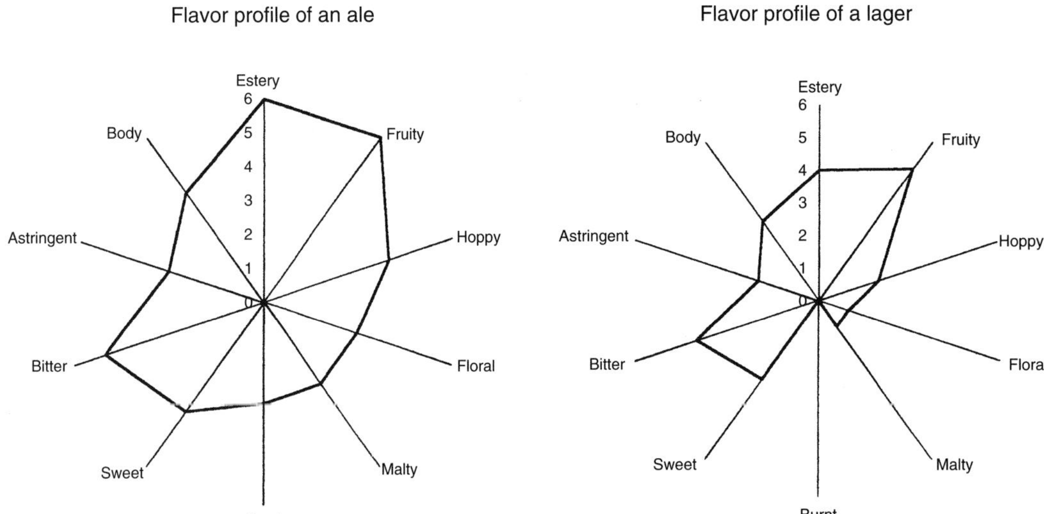

Figure 91.6 The spider diagram. The flavor of beer represented by spider diagram. Each flavor term is represented by a spindle.

compared to data obtained from a trained sensory panel and by headspace analysis with GC–MS. The EN was able to distinguish finished beer made after different periods of maturation, while the sensory panel was not. The results suggest that the EN can complement traditional chemical and sensory approaches to the optimization of beer maturation (McKellar *et al.*, 2002).

However, there is too little evidence that gas phase composition is always perceptibly dependent on the evolution of the liquid phase composition. There is not sufficiently clear reasons to assume that all changes taking place in liquid are reflected adequately by the detectable changes in the gas phase and hence by EN output. The development and evolution of a set of devices for liquids has been reported (Legin *et al.*, 1997). It is based on a wide range of potentiometric chemical sensors and methods of complex signal processing. Such a system mimics significantly the organization (but not the actual appearance) of human sense and, also using the analogy with the EN can be called a prototype of electronic tongue. It has been used to distinguish between different sorts of the same type of beverages (tea, coffee, juice, soft drinks and beers) and to monitor the aging process of juice.

The application of an EN or electronic tongue to follow beer aging in the package was not found upon literature search, but it could be an appropriate tool to study beer staling.

Conclusions

There are a great number of published methods for evaluating the process of beer aging based on different instrumental techniques. The aging process is closely related to the antioxidant capacity. The retarding role of sulfite in the beer aging process is more relevant than the role of polyphenols. The sulfite acts as an antioxidant by radical scavenging rather than adduct formation, which mask flavor staling. The amount of O_2 present when beer is in its final package is an important factor in that an increase in O_2 gives rise to a more rapid aging through the formation of active oxygen species. Since sensory analysis obviously has the final word, more research needs to be conducted on the development and application of sensors (EN and electronic tongue) to beer aging, since such technologies appear to hold the greatest promise to imitate the detection of flavors by the actual consumers.

Summary Points

- The beer aging mainly depends on the raw materials, the oxygen present and the brewing process. So, polyphenols and proteins form insoluble complexes that provoke colloidal instability in the final beer. Also, the active oxygen species act in non-biological oxidation process, they increase the haze formation (colloidal instability) and they are the most important cause of the staling of flavor development (flavor instability). On the other hand, the flavor instability is determined by endogenous antioxidant activity of beer itself, which is affected by each step in the brewing process.
- Two different methodologies are available for evaluating beer aging. The first requires analytical methods to detect the compounds responsible for these flavors and enable quantitative determination. The second implies trained sensory panel to assess the beer flavor.
- Chromatographic techniques have been used to determine aldehydes, ketones and esters relevant in beer aging. Some of these compounds are responsible for the initial

stale flavor of beer ("sweetish leathery character" and "papery cardboard character").

- ESR spectroscopy technique have been utilized to detect and to identify the free radicals coming from active oxygen species. These free radicals are responsible for flavor instability due to oxidation of beer. The results obtained with ESR have proved that the SO_2 is the only one able to delay the radical formation.
- The measurement of the capacity of beer constituents to capture free radicals is recognized as TAA. The UV–Vis spectrophotometry is the technique more widely applied to determine the TAA through the addition of an exogenous free radical and measurement of the decrease in absorbance. This methodology evaluates the cooperation among endogenous antioxidants of beer during oxidative stress.
- The reductones (a type of antioxidants) have been determined indirectly by voltammetric methods. With this methodology it is possible to evaluate the reducing power of different type of beers. The changes observed during beer storage have been assessable by chemiluminiscence. These changes produced patterns that show a good correlation with the degree of stale flavor in panel scores.
- Sensory analysis performed by trained sensory panel, is necessary to complete the data obtained by analytical methods. The results of sensory analysis provide semi-quantitative information about beer quality. The methodology is based on difference and descriptive tests and the testers score the individual attributes of beers.
- The development of artificial sensors, such as EN and electronic tongue, is a promising direction to evaluate the process of aging and spoilage of beers. The advantages of this methodology are the rapidity (analysis on-site or on-line), the accurate analysis for quality control, and the inexpensive and simple instrumentation and in the present, these sensors are the complement to the traditional chemical and sensory analysis.

References

Andersen, M.L., Outtrup, H. and Skibsted, L.H. (2000). *J. Agric. Food Chem.* 48, 3106–3111.

Arnao, M.B., Cano, A., Hernández-Ruiz, J., García-Cánovas, F. and Acosta, M. (1996). *Anal. Biochem.* 236, 255–261.

Bamforth, C.W. (1998). *Beer Tap into the Art and Science of Brewing*. pp.171–186. Plenum Press, New York.

Bamforth, C.W. (2000). *MBAA TQ* 37, 165 171.

Bamforth, C.W. (2004). Beer Health and Nutrition, In Blackwell Publishing (ed.), pp. 71–90. Blackwell Publishing, Oxford.

Bamforth, C.W. and Parsons, R. (1985). *J. Am. Soc. Brew. Chem.* 43, 197–202.

Bellido-Milla, D., Oñate-Jaén, A., Palacios-Santander, J.M., Palacios-Tejero, D. and Hernández-Artiga, M.P. (2004). *Microchim. Acta* 144, 183–190.

Billaud, C., Brun-Mèrimee, S., Louarme, L. and Nicolas, J. (2004). *Food Chem.* 84, 223–233.

Cano, A., Hernández-Ruiz, J., García-Cánovas, F., Acosta, M. and Arnao, M.B. (1998). *Phytochem. Anal.* 9, 196–202.

Cano-Lario, A., Acosta-Echevarria, M. and Bañon-Arnao, M. (1998). *Alimentaria. Septiembre*, 73–76.

Chevance, F., Guyot-Declerck, C., Dupont, J. and Collin, S. (2002). *J. Agric. Food Chem.* 50, 3818–3821.

Fantozzi, P., Montanari, L., Manzini, F., Gasbarrini, A., Addolorato, G. and Simmoncini, M. (1998). *Lebensm. Wiss. Technol. – Food Sci. Technol.* 31, 221–227.

Foster, C., Schwieger, J., Narzib, L., Back, W., Uchida, M., Ono, M. and Yanagi, K. (1999). *Monatsschrift für Brauwissenschaft* 5/6, 86–93.

Gijs, L., Perpète, Ph., Timmermans, A. and Collin, S. (2000). *J. Agric. Food Chem.* 48, 6196–6199.

Gonzalez-San José, M.L., Muñiz-Rodriguez, P. and Valls-Belles, V. (2001). Actividad Antioxidante de la Cerveza: Estudios in Vitro e in Vivo. In Centro de Información Cerveza y salud (ed.), pp. 1–57. Centro de Información Cerveza y salud, Madrid.

Guido, L.F., Fortunato, N.A., Rodrigues, J.A. and Barros, A.A. (2003). *J. Agric. Food Chem.* 51, 3911–3915.

Guido, L.F., Carneiro, J.R., Santos, J.R., Almeida, P.J., Rodrigues, J.A. and Barros, A.A. (2004). *J. Chromagr.* 1032, 17–22.

Hughes, P.S., Baxter, E.D. (2001). Beer Quality, Safety and Nutritional Aspects, The Royal Society of Chemistry (ed.), p. 68. The Royal Society of Chemistry, Cambridge.

Illet, D.R. (1995). *MBAA TQ* 32, 213–221.

Illet, D.R., Burke, S. and Simpson, W.J. (1996). *J. Sci. Food Agric.* 70, 337–340.

Kamiura, M. and Kaneda, H. (1993). *Shelf – life Studies of Foods and Beverages*, Elsevier (ed.), pp. 821–889. Elsevier, New York.

Kaneda, H. and Takashio, M. (1996). *J. Am. Soc. Brew. Chem.* 54, 115–120.

Kaneda, H., Kano, Y., Kamimura, M., Kawasaki, S., Osawa, T. and Koshino, S. (1990). *J. Food Sci.* 55, 1361–1364.

Kaneda, H., Kano, Y., Kamimura, M., Kawasaki, S. and Osawa, T. (1991). *J. Inst. Brew.* 97, 105–109.

Kaneda, H., Kano, Y., Osawa, T. and Kawasaki, S. (1994). *J. Am. Soc. Brew. Chem.* 52, 70–75.

Kaneda, H., Kobayashi, N., Furusho, S., Sahara, H. and Koshino, S. (1995). *Master Brew. Assoc. Am. Tech. Q* 32, 90–94.

Klein, H., Glinsner, T., Natter, M. and Steiner, I. (2000). *Monatsschrift für Brauwissen schaft* 53, 217.

Legin, A., Rudnitskaya, A., Vlasov, Y., Di Natale, C., Davide, F. and Dámico, A. (1997). *Sensor and Actuators* 44, 291–296.

Maillard, M.N., Soum, M.H., Boivin, P. and Berset, C. (1996). *Lebensm-Wiss. Technol – Food Sci. Tecnol.* 29, 238–244.

McKellar, R.C., Young, J.C., Johnston, A., Knight, K.P., Lu, X. and Buttenham, S. (2002). *MBBAA TQ.* 39, 99–105.

Millar, N.J., Rice-Evans, C., Davies, M.J., Gopinathan, V. and Milner, A. (1993). *Clin. Sci.* 84, 407–412.

Montanari, L., Perretti, G., Natella, F., Guidi, A. and Fantozzi, P. (1999). *Lebensm-Wiss. u-Technol.* 32, 535–539.

Morales, F.J. and Jimenez-Pérez, S. (2001). *Food Chem.* 72, 119–125.

Nicoli, M.C., Anese, M., Parpinel, M.T., Franceschi, S. and Lerici, C.R. (1997). *Cancer Lett.* 114, 71–74.

Oñate-Jaén, A., Bellido-Milla, D. and Hernández-Artiga, M.P. (2006). *Food Chem.* 97, 361–369.

Serra-Majen, L. and Aranceta, J. (2003). La cerveza en la alimentación de los españoles: Relación entre el consumo de cerveza y el consumo de energía y nutrientes, el índice de masa corporal y la actividad física en la población adulta española. In Centro de Información Cerveza y salud (ed.), pp. 1–89. Centro de Información Cerveza y salud, Madrid

Sobiech, R.M., Neumann, R. and Wabner, D. (1998). *Electroanalysis* 10, 969–975.

Stewart, G.G. (2004). *J. Chem. Educ.* 81, 963–968.

Uchida, M. and Ono, M. (1996). *J. Am. Soc. Brew. Chem.* 54, 198–204.

Uchida, M., Suga, S. and Ono, M. (1996). *J. Am. Soc. Brew. Chem.* 54, 205–211.

Vanderhaegen, B., Neven, H., Coghe, S., Verstrepen, K.J., Verachtert, H. and Derdelinckx, G. (2003). *J. Agric. Food Chem.* 51, 6782–6790.

Vanderhaegen, B., Neven, H., Daenen, L., Verstrepen, K.J., Verachtert, H. and Derdelinckx, G. (2004). *J. Agric. Food Chem.* 52, 1661–1668.

Varmuza, K., Steiner, I., Glinsner, T. and Klein, H. (2002). *Eur. Food Res. Technol.* 215, 235–239.

92

Use of Electrospray Ionization Mass Spectrometry to Fingerprint Beer

Rodrigo R. Catharino Thomson Mass Spectrometry Laboratory, Institute of Chemistry, State University of Campinas, UNICAMP, Campinas, SP, Brazil
Alexandra C.H.F. Sawaya Program for Post-graduate Studies in Pharmacy, Bandeirante University of São Paulo, UNIBAN, São Paulo, SP, Brazil
Marcos N. Eberlin Thomson Mass Spectrometry Laboratory, Institute of Chemistry, State University of Campinas, UNICAMP, Campinas, SP, Brazil

Abstract

Mass spectrometry constitutes one of the most encompassing instrumental techniques in science, widely applied in the fields of chemistry, biology, medical science and technology. Direct insertion electrospray ionization mass spectrometry (ESI-MS) is a fast and sensitive method which differentiates diverse types of beer, in both positive and negative ion modes, characterizing their main constituents. Although the basic ingredients of beer (water, malt, hops and yeast) have not changed much since the dark ages, variations in these ingredients and in the manufacturing process result in diverse types of beer. The spectra or fingerprints of each type of beer permit not only the separation of samples according to their main characteristics, but also further information through the ESI-MS/MS fragmentation of the diagnostic ions of each type, adding another dimension to the analytical results. Fast and characteristic beer fingerprint mass spectra were obtained by ESI-MS in both the negative and positive modes. A total of 29 samples of ale produced in Brazil and other countries were divided into three groups by visual analysis of the positive [ESI(+)-MS] and negative [ESI(−)-MS] mode fingerprints as well as by chemometric analysis of the data. Many of the marker ions in both modes were found to be simple sugars and oligosaccharides, although their intensities varied depending on the type of ale (pale colored, dark colored and sweetened). This shows that direct infusion ESI-MS could distinguish between samples of ale with different compositions and is promising as a fast and efficient method of beer characterization.

List of Abbreviations

APCI	Atmospheric pressure chemical ionization
CO	Carbon monoxide
CO_2	Carbon dioxide
CI	Chemical ionization
CID	Collision-induced dissociation
D	Dark beer
DIOS	Desorption ionization on silicon
EI	Electron ionization
ESI	Electrospray ionization
ESI-MS	Electrospray ionization mass spectrometry
ESI-MS/MS	Electrospray ionization with sequential (tandem) mass spectrometry
ESI(+)-MS	Positive ion mode electrospray ionization mass spectrometry
ESI(−)-MS	Negative ion mode electrospray ionization mass spectrometry
FAB	Fast atom bombardment
GABA	δ-Aminobutyric acid
H_2O	Water
ICP–AES	Inductively coupled plasma atomic emission spectrometry
IEM	Ion evaporation model
M	Malt beer
MALDI	Matrix assisted laser desorption ionization
MS	Mass spectrometry
$[M + H]^+$	Protonated molecule
$[M - H]^-$	Deprotonated molecule
$[M + K]^+$	Potassium adduct of a molecule
$[M + Na]^+$	Sodium adduct of molecule
m/z	Mass to charge ratio
NH_3	Ammonia
P	Pale beer
PCA	Principal component analysis
RCM	Residual charge model
TOF	Time of flight

Introduction

Recent advances in instrumentation and development of new and revolutionary techniques have revitalized mass spectrometry (MS) which constitutes one of the most

Beer in Health and Disease Prevention
ISBN: 978-0-12-373891-2

encompassing instrumental techniques in science, widely applied in the fields of chemistry, biology, medical science and technology. Opening new horizons and ample perspectives for future development, MS has consolidated its position as an extremely versatile and essential scientific tool for both fundamental and applied research. In the field of beverages, MS has been increasingly applied with excellent results for complex compositions such as beer.

Direct insertion electrospray ionization mass spectrometry (ESI-MS) is a fast and sensitive method which differentiates diverse types of beer, characterizing their main constituents. The spectra or fingerprints of each type of beer permit not only the separation of samples according to their main characteristics, but also further information through the ESI-MS/MS fragmentation of the diagnostic ions of each type, adding another dimension to the analytical results. As ESI-MS shows such great potential for the analysis of different types of beer, it can be applied to both research and development as well as quality control during the manufacturing procedure and in the final product.

Manufacturing and Composition of Beer

Beer is an aqueous solution of complex composition containing CO_2, ethyl alcohol, several inorganic salts and multiple organic compounds. Inorganic salts come primarily from the brewing grains (such as barley and other cereals) and water. The mineral composition of water in natural reservoirs depends on the minerals found in the region. In areas where rocks are harder, water will not penetrate through them into the soil, therefore will be "softer" with a lower concentration of dissolved salts. Many of the organic compounds come from the brewing materials but others are by-products of yeast metabolism and are responsible for most of the flavor characteristics that are so unique to beer.

The most important stages of beer processing are malting, brewing and fermentation, followed by maturation, filtering and bottling (Hardwick, 1995). During the malting and mashing procedures that produce the wort, polysaccharides and starches from the cereals are hydrolyzed to low molecular weight sugars (such as glucose, sucrose and maltose) as well as malt oligosaccharides (consisting of 3–10 glucose units). Most of the low molecular weight sugars are converted into alcohol during the fermentation process, whereas maltotetraose and higher oligosaccharides are not fermented by most yeast strains (Berlitz *et al.*, 2004; Mauri *et al.*, 2004).

Beers throughout the world have distinctive tastes, although brewed from similar materials, their uniqueness comes from the mineral content of the water used, small variations in the ingredients employed and differences in the brewing methods. In a strict sense, there are two classical beer styles, ales and lagers. Ales are fermented using *Saccharomyces cerevisiae* in a process frequently denominated "high fermentation" at temperatures normally between 16°C and 24°C. Lagers are fermented using a different species of yeast and at lower temperatures (Berlitz *et al.*, 2004). Commercially available brands of beer in Brazil are produced exclusively by the high fermentation process, therefore are all ales. Three different types can be found: pale colored ales, dark colored ales and sweetened dark-colored ales known as malt beer.

At the present time, beer is produced in modern high technology equipment, although many traditional artisan concepts are taught in renowned beer master courses. The use of modern analytical techniques, which are fast and efficient, will permit the optimization of the manufacturing process, resulting in a higher quality product.

Chemical Characterization of Beer

The characterization of beer samples according to their mineral content has been carried out using inductively coupled plasma atomic emission spectrometry (ICP–AES) in 32 samples of lager, dark and low alcoholic content beers (Alcázar *et al.*, 2002). Several papers relate the identification of classes of compounds in beer by ESI-MS associated with liquid chromatography (Hofte *et al.*, 1998; Degelmann *et al.*, 1999; Whittle *et al.*, 1999) and capillary electrophoresis (Klampfl *et al.*, 2002). Recently, the sugars in beer were analyzed directly by ESI-MS, without previous chromatographic separation (Mauri *et al.*, 2004).

ESI is a soft and wide-ranging ionization technique that has revolutionized the way the molecules are ionized and transferred to mass spectrometers for mass and property measurements as well as structural characterization. ESI has therefore greatly expanded the applicability of MS to a variety of new classes of molecules with thermal instability, high polarity and mass (Cole, 1997). Although ESI mass (and tandem or sequential mass) spectrometry has been most successfully applied to the analysis of biomolecules (Kotiaho *et al.*, 2000; Cooks *et al.*, 2001; Rioli *et al.*, 2003), ESI-MS has also been proven to be a powerful technique for the structural characterization of organic, inorganic and organometallic compounds. Direct infusion ESI-MS has also been applied as a fast fingerprint method for complex mixtures such as plant extracts, propolis and wine (Catharino *et al.*, 2006). ESI, with direct sample introduction, is also a convenient technique for the direct introduction of beer into a mass spectrometer, as most molecules bearing acidic or basic sites will be detected and MS/MS with collision-induced dissociation (CID) of ionized molecules can be used for structural elucidation studies.

Mass Spectrometry

According to John B. Fenn, Nobel prize winner in 2002 and pioneer in the use of ESI-MS for biological molecules, MS is "The art of measuring atoms and molecules to

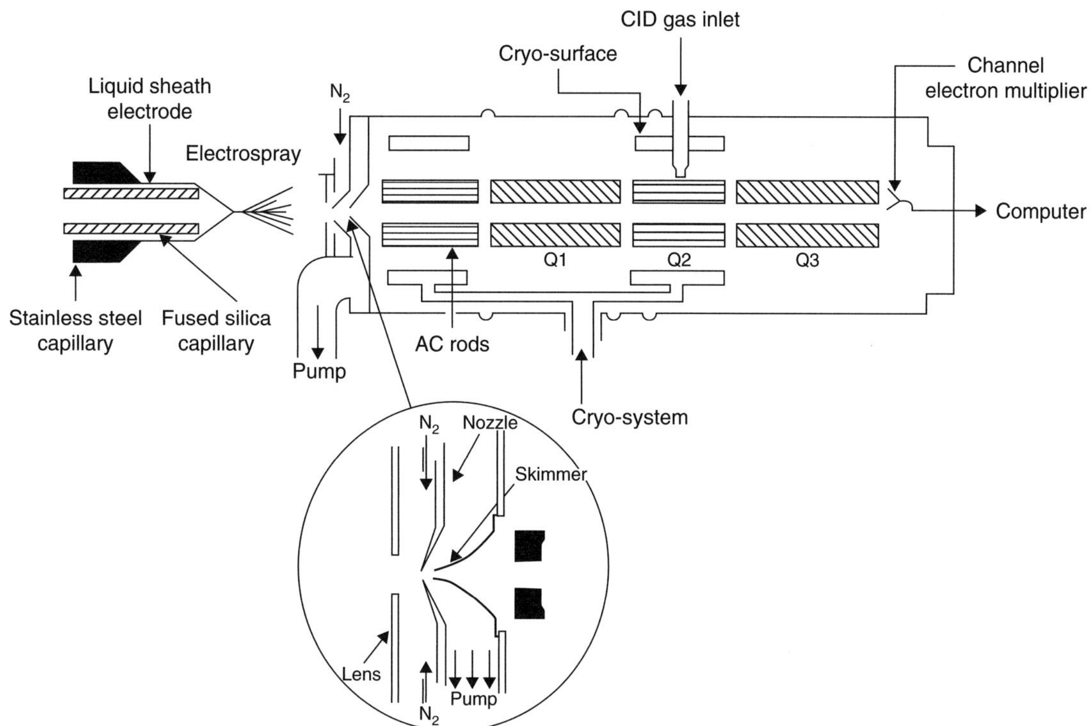

Figure 92.1 Schematic drawing of an electrospray ionization, triple quadrupole, mass spectrometer. Samples are introduced via the capillary, where molecules are ionized and transferred to the gas state through the electrospray process, which are attracted into the mass spectrometer through a difference in potential. The nitrogen gas between the orifice and nozzle prevents the entrance of neutral molecules into the mass analyzer (Q1). To obtain the dissociation patterns of marker compounds, these are mass selected in Q1, dissociated by collision against a gas in Q2 and the fragments analyzed in a second mass analyzer (Q3).

determine their molecular mass. This mass information is often sufficient, frequently necessary and always useful for determining the identity and structure of a compound. To carry out this art, a charge is added to sample of interest (analyte). The trajectory of the resultant ion is then measured under vacuum, under diverse electronic and magnetic fields. In this way, the basic condition for this method is the transformation of molecules into ions. The ionization of low molecular weight compounds is rapidly carried out in the gas phase by the collision of the neutral molecules with electrons, photons or other ions. In the last years, various researchers have made efforts toward producing ions from high molecular weight compounds (>1000 Da) which are too complex to be vaporized without decomposing."

Mass spectrometers have been described as the smallest scales in the world, not due to the size of the equipment, but due to the fact that it "weighs" molecules. For the last decade, mass spectrometry has gone through great technological advances, permitting its application to the analysis of proteins, peptides, carbohydrates, DNA, drugs and several other relevant biological molecules. Using ionization sources such as electrospray ionization (ESI) and matrix assisted laser desorption ionization (MALDI), mass spectrometry has become an irreplaceable tool in biological science, for example. Mass spectrometers determine molecular weight of ions by measuring their mass to charge ratio (*m/z*). The same basic components are found in practically all mass spectrometers (Figure 92.1). After introducing the sample, ions are formed by the loss or gain of an electric charge, when parting from a neutral molecule. Once the ions are formed, they are directed toward a mass analyzer (molecular scale), by a difference in potential, where they are separated according to their *m/z* relation and finally detected (Siuzdak, 2005).

There are different kinds of ionization sources, such as electron ionization (EI), chemical ionization (CI), fast atom bombardment (FAB), matrix assisted laser desorption ionization (MALDI), desorption ionization on silicon (DIOS), atmospheric pressure chemical ionization (APCI) and electrospray ionization (ESI), used in the following study.

Electrospray ionization mass spectrometry

The principle of ESI-MS is the transference of ions existing in solution directly to the gas phase, in a mild manner. This versatility has significantly increased the number of substances that can be analyzed by mass spectrometry, permitting polypeptides, which would be instable in the analytic conditions necessary for EI or CI, to be analyzed without decomposing. ESI involves forming an electrolytic spray of a solution, which produces electrically charged droplets, from which the ions are then liberated. The structure of an ESI source is quite simple, compared to other sources for mass spectrometry. A source of high voltage (1.0–7.0 kV) in contact with a solution containing polar substances is necessary. This solution is pumped through a micro-capillary (i.e. 50 to 100 μm) at a flow rate of 1–20 μl/min, or less (at flow rates of less than 1 μl/min, it is usually called nanoelectrospray). When a positive potential is applied to the solution, the positively charged ions tend to move away, toward a less positively charged region, that is, toward the counter electrode. Therefore, the droplet formed at the tip of the capillary is enriched with cations. As the charge density increases in the droplet, the electric field formed between the capillary and the counter electrode causes a deformation of the droplet in contact with the capillary tip. The droplet becomes cone shaped and called a Taylor cone. This cone-shaped droplet remains "stuck" to the tip of the capillary until the charge density and the repulsion between the ions present in the droplet overcome the surface tension, resulting in small, highly charged droplets breaking away from the tip of the capillary. The frequency of this process depends on the magnitude of the electric field, the surface tension of the liquid and the conductivity of the solution (Cole, 1997).

As reported above, electrospray can generate ionic species through an electrolytic process, similar to an electrolytic cell with two electrodes. The metal capillary, or a metallic wire in contact with the solution, is one of the electrodes of the cell, which can be considered the work electrode, because the main reactions which alter the initial chemical system occur on its surface. The second electrode is the counter electrode, which is usually earthed. Due to the difference of potential applied and the closeness of these two electrodes, there is a high electric field in this region, resulting in the Taylor cone. The electrospray system functions as a special type of electrolytic cell, because movement of ions between electrodes does not happen without interruption in the solution, as in conventional cells, but part of it happens in the gas phase (Cole, 1997).

After the highly charged droplets are liberated from the Taylor cone and pass through the region between the tip of the capillary and the counter electrode, they go through dessolvation. The mass of solvent in the droplets is reduced by evaporation, aided by a flow of inert dessolvation gas, normally nitrogen, at a temperature between 30°C and 100°C. As the amount of solvent in the droplet decreases, the charge density increases to the point where the repulsion between ions overcomes the surface tension and smaller droplets are formed. This process is known as Columbic explosions and is illustrated in Figure 92.2. The maximum charge, *Q*, which a drop with a ray of *R* can maintain before fragmenting into smaller droplets is given by equation 92.1:

$$Q = 8\pi(\varepsilon_0 \gamma R^3)^{1/2} \qquad (92.1)$$

where ε_0 is the permissiveness in space and γ is the surface tension of the drop. This deduction was proposed by Lord Rayleigh and is known as the Rayleigh limit. The dessolvation process has been studied by various groups, for example, Tang and co-workers observed that the droplets do not necessarily have to reach the Rayleigh limit to break up (Russel, 1994). Rupture actually occurs at around 80% of the limit, resulting in droplets with 2–3% of the mass of

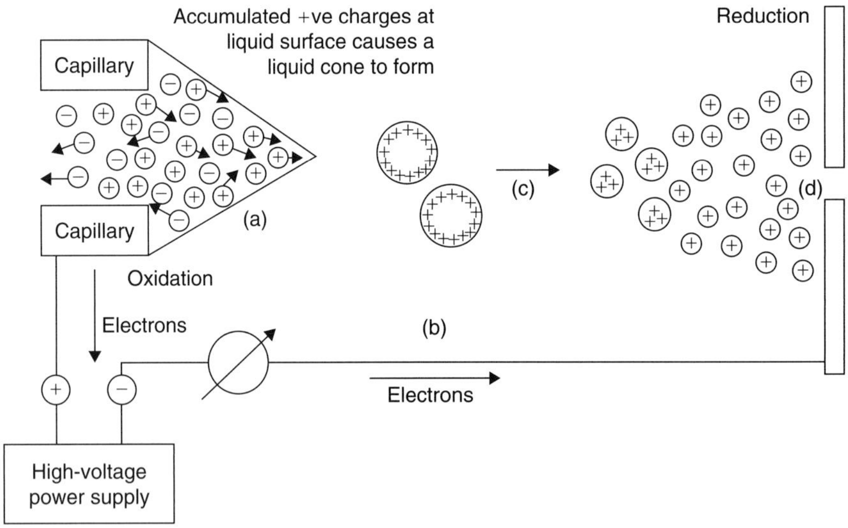

Figure 92.2 Schematic drawing of the Taylor cone on the tip of the capillary (ESI source) and the Columbic explosions forming smaller droplets. The accumulated charges on the tip of the capillary result in the Taylor cone, and the expulsion of small, highly charged droplets, which through Columbic explosions form even smaller droplets.

the original drop, but containing 10–18% of the original charge. In this way, the droplets formed are much smaller but have a much higher *m/z*.

Two models of mechanisms for the final transfer of the ions to the gas phase have been proposed. One was proposed by Dole in 1968 and named the residual charge model (RCM), and depends on the formation of extremely small charged droplets, generated by successive Columbic explosions, containing only one ion. When the solvent evaporates, the ion will be left alone in the gas phase. The other mechanism, proposed by Thomson and Iribarne, named the ion evaporation model (IEM), suggests that the emission of ions occurs directly from these small, highly charged droplets, from which the ions are ejected due to the electrostatic repulsion between ions of the same charge.

After they are formed, the ions reach the sampling cone, which has a very small orifice with a diameter of 1 μm, and then pass into a low pressure area. At the atmospheric pressure/vacuum interface, a series of pumps and optical lenses lead the ions to the mass analyzer. The region between the sampling cone, the skimmer and the lenses or hexapoles is very important for, in this area, CID can occur. The ions formed by electrospray are present, along with the drying gas (nitrogen). There is a difference of potential which accelerates these ions, leading to a physical collision with the drying gas. Therefore, if a solvated ion enters this area, it can collide and fragment. The CID process is interesting in fragmentation studies, but it can make visualization of the species that were in the original solution difficult. To minimize the CID effect, the difference in potential between sampling cone and the skimmer must be reduced.

The CID process used in tandem or sequential mass spectrometry (MS/MS) has an important role in the structural determination of ions and the analysis of complex mixtures. Used together with ionization such as FAB, MALDI and ESI, which generate ions with high molecular mass but with little or no fragmentation, the activation and dissociation of the molecules by CID furnish fragmentation patterns that give important structural information about the ions, frequently necessary for their identification and characterization. The CID process can be considered as a two-step process: activation through collision, where a fraction of the kinetic energy of the ion (M_1) is transferred to its internal energy, followed by the uni-molecular dissociation of the internally excited ion. This process is illustrated in equations 92.2 and 92.3.

$$M_1^+ + M_2 \rightarrow M_1^{+*} + M_2 \tag{92.2}$$

$$M_1^{+*} \rightarrow M_3^+ + M_4 \tag{92.3}$$

Raftery and Geczy (2002) used the technique of low energy CID together with ESI and MALDI for the study of polypeptides with cross-linking bonds with protonated sulfonamides, proving, through the observed dissociations, the formation of sulfonamide links through the oxidative processes which resulted between thiols and amines, which can both stabilize or modify the function of the protein. Williams *et al.* (2003) used CID in a high precision ESI–TOF system for the sequencing of a mixture of peptides. Biological molecules have been successfully analyzed through electrospray systems and (MS/MS) (Cooks *et al.*, 2001; Koch *et al.*, 2002; Rioli *et al.*, 2003). This system permits molecules, such as peptides for example, which would not be stable in EI or CI conditions, to be analyzed without decomposing. ESI-MS has also been applied to the identification and structural characterization of organic (Eberlin *et al.*, 2003), inorganic and organometallic compounds, precursors of nanomaterials and identification of nanoclusters (Gaumet and Strouse, 2000).

A series of electrochemical processes occur during ESI, the importance of these processes in relation to this ionization source and the advances toward a better understanding of the process were the subjects of discussions between researchers such as la Mora, Fenn, Cole, Enke, Berkel and Martinez-Sanchez (Cole, 2000; de la Mora *et al.*, 2000). For an ion accelerated by a voltage *V*, the resulting speed of *v* relates to its mass/charge (*m/z*) ratio. In time of flight (TOF) mass analyzers, ions are separated according to their TOF and the mass/charge ratio is determined by measuring the time taken to complete a given distance (*L*) to the detector. These variables are correlated in equation 92.4:

$$m/z = 2eEs(t/L)^2 \tag{92.4}$$

where *E* is the extraction pulse, *s* is the length of the tube on which *E* is applied, *t* is the TOF measured for the ion. In this way, all the ions receive the same initial kinetic energy through the extraction pulse (*E*) and then fly along the tube with length (*L*) where they are separated according to their *m/z*, as the lighter ions take less time to reach the end. One advantage of TOF mass analyzers is their sensitivity, resulting from two instrumental characteristics: high transmission rates – due to the lack of ray defining fends and separation of ions by TOF – which, differently form spatial separation, does not direct some of the ions away from the detector. In view of the advances in the data acquisition instruments, it is possible to acquire spectra referring to the total mass range analyzed. The resolution of the TOF mass analyzers can be increased by the use of reflectrons or ion mirrors, with the function of compensating for differences in the initial kinetic energy of identical ions. After passing through the tube, the ions go into a retardation field, defined by a series of grids and they are turned back into the tube. The principle behind the reflectron is that the ions with the greatest kinetic energy will penetrate more deeply in this retardment field, taking more time to return to the tube, whereas those with less energy (but the same mass) will penetrate less, and finally both will reach the detector simultaneously. The reflectron results in a loss of signal due to the grid, therefore gridless reflectrons are being developed.

Fingerprinting samples with a complex composition

The ease with which ESI-MS provides spectra of samples with a complex composition in a short time (few minutes) in an ample *m/z* range, where each spectrum has unique characteristics, permits the use of ESI-MS as a fingerprinting technique. ESI-MS has been used as fingerprinting system for: the analysis of molecular species of triacylglycerols extracted from lipids (Hans and Gross, 2001), the analysis and characterization of 52 synthetic substances with the application of principal component analysis (PCA) to determine the differences and similarities within the compounds used in the pharmaceutical industry (Schoonjans *et al.*, 2002), the analysis of ethanolic extracts of different types of propolis from different geographic regions, providing spectra containing diagnostic ions for each type (Sawaya *et al.*, 2004), the analysis of subproducts resulting from the chlorine added to potable water (Zhang *et al.*, 2004), proof of authenticity and origin of whisky samples, being able to prove if a sample is false or authentic in a matter of minutes (Möller *et al.*, 2005) and in the analysis of different samples of beer, separating them into classes, identifying the diagnostic ions for each type, with MS/MS analysis of the characteristic ions adding a further dimension to the fingerprints obtained (Araújo *et al.*, 2005).

Mass Spectrometry Fingerprinting of Beer

The advantages offered by ESI-MS permit this technique to be used in different areas, including analysis of beer, as reported above. This was the first study where the ESI-MS fingerprints of different types of beer, the classification of the samples according to their main diagnostic ions and the study of these diagnostic ions were carried out. The following procedure was standardized: 10 ml of the beer sample was placed in a 100 ml beaker and placed in an ultrasonic bath, to de-gas the sample, with minimum loss of volatile substances. The choice of this procedure was based on the reproducibility of the ESI-MS fingerprints obtained, considering the quantity and the intensity of the ions. A solution can contain ions resulting from dissolution (of salts, for example), by adding a proton ($[M + H]^+$) or subtracting a proton ($[M - H]^-$) from a neural molecule, or by forming complexes with cations, anions, acidic or basic compounds of a wide variety of molecular masses. A Q-TOF mass spectrometer (Micromass, Manchester, UK) was used for fingerprint ESI-MS analysis. The conditions used were: source temperature 100°C, capillary voltage 3.0 kV and cone voltage used 40 V. An aliquot of 250 μl of each de-gassed beer sample was diluted in a flask with a 1:1 solution of water:methanol to a final volume of 1.0 ml. In positive mode analysis [ESI(+)-MS] 2 μl of formic acid was added to each sample and in negative mode analysis [ESI(−)-MS] 2 μl of ammonium hydroxide solution were added. The samples were infused at a flow rate of 15 μl/min using a syringe pump (Harvard Apparatus). Mass spectra were acquired over a *m/z* range of 50–1000.

Although beer has a complex composition, direct insertion ESI-MS, without previous chromatographic separation, proved to be a convenient technique for the analysis of beer. In beer, many molecules possess acidic or basic sites, can be observed in the fingerprint as a singly charged ion of the monoprotonated $[M + H]^+$ or deprotonated $[M - H]^-$ form. Several different makes and varieties of beer were selected and analyzed, to obtain fingerprints in both the positive and negative ion modes, containing a set of diagnostic ions which are characteristic for each type of beer. The variability observed in the diagnostic ions results from variations in the raw materials used as well as the fabrication process. The storage conditions and the age of the beverage can also influence the composition of the samples, that is, the presence absence of determined substances; therefore, the Brazilian samples of beer were analyzed within 1 or 2 months of fabrication, which is the normal shelf life of beer in supermarkets. The samples of beer from other countries were between 4 and 6 months old (Araújo *et al.*, 2005). The type of beer, brand name and place of origin of the beer samples can be seen in Table 92.1.

The visual analysis of the fingerprints obtained by ESI-MS in both the positive [ESI(+)-MS] and negative ion [ESI(−)-MS] modes, and the observation of the most intense ions, permits the division of these beer samples into three distinct groups, corresponding to three well-defined beer types, being: P = pale (lager, pilsner, draft); D = dark (bock, stout, dunkel) and M = malt (malt beer).

Positive ion mode fingerprints

In the positive ion mode fingerprints, substances can be observed as protonated neutral molecules, or adducts of cations found in the solution. Figure 92.3a shows a typical ESI(+)-MS fingerprint for a pale (P) beer with intense ions observed in the *m/z* range from 70 to 705. Several similarities can be observed with Figure 92.3c, presenting a typical fingerprint for dark (D) beer; however, some ions are absent or present with different intensities. As to Figure 92.3b, presenting a typical fingerprint of malt beer, no ions can be observed in the region above *m/z* 400. This type of beer is known for its sweet taste, resulting from the addition of sugar and caramel, which give the beer its dark color and reduce the bitter taste of hops.

Table 92.1 Origin, brand name and abbreviation used for the samples of beer analyzed

Origin	*Brand name*	*Abbreviation*
Brazil	Schincariol	P1
Brazil	Primus	P2
Brazil	Dado	P3
Brazil	Antarctica	P4
Brazil	Brahma	P5
Brazil	Skol	P6
Brazil	Heineken	P7
Brazil	Budweiser	P8
Europe	Warsteiner	P9
Europe	Sapporo Draft	P10
Brazil	Miller	P11
Brazil	Summer Draft	P12
Brazil	Antarctica Malzbeer	M1
Brazil	Schincariol Malzbeer	M2
Brazil	Brahma Malzbeer	M3
Brazil	Xingu	M4
Europe	Sweetheart	D1
Europe	Warsteiner Premium Dunkel	D2
Brazil	Schincariol Munich	D3
Europe	Ruddles County	D4
Europe	Murphy's	D5
Europe	Abbot Ale	D6
Brazil	Baden Baden Bock	D7
Brazil	Baden Baden Stout	D8
Brazil	Bohemia Escura	D9
Brazil	Caracu	D10
Europe	Guiness	D11
Brazil	Kaiser Bock	D12

Notes: Samples of ale analyzed by ESI-MS in both negative and positivesion modes.

P = pale; D = dark; M = malt beer.

Source: Adapted from Araújo *et al.* (2005).

To derive more information from the fingerprints, the most intense ions were fragmented by CID. The resulting MS/MS fragmentation patterns were analyzed and compared with standards and data in literature, resulting in the identification of diagnostic ions such as sugars and maltose oligomers, among others. Therefore, in Figure 92.3a, the fingerprint of pale beer, the ions of *m/z* 365, 527 and 689 are the sodium adducts $[M + Na]^+$ of maltose, maltotriose and maltotetraose, respectively, whereas *m/z* 381, 543 and 705 are the potassium adducts $[M + K]^+$ of the same carbohydrates. Similar to the pale (P) beers, the dark (D) beers also present the potassium adducts of these carbohydrates. It is interesting to note that in the dark beers, only the potassium adducts (*m/z* 381, 543 and 705) are clearly visible in the fingerprint, and the sodium adducts are practically imperceptible. This demonstrates the capacity of ESI-MS fingerprinting to show the concentration ratio of $[K^+]/[Na^+]$ in D and P type beers. Dark beers have a more intense ion of *m/z* 219 (which is the potassium adduct of glucose) in their fingerprints than in pale beer. For malt (M) beer fingerprints the most intense ions are *m/z* 203, 219, which the MS/MS fragmentation patterns show to be the sodium and potassium adducts of glucose, respectively, and a potassium adduct of a dimer of glucose at *m/z* 399. The potassium and sodium adducts of the other malt oligosaccharides are not observed in the fingerprint of malt beer. Considering that malt beer differs from pale beer mainly in respect to the addition of sugar and caramel at the end of the manufacturing process, clearly the presence of large amounts of glucose inhibits the detection of the other malt oligosaccharides due to matrix suppression. In ESI-MS, matrix suppression results from the presence of more and less polar substances in the same droplet. This suppression can occur as the result of competition between different components to become ionized, competition to reach the surface of the droplet, differences in the polarity of the compounds resulting in different solvation effects, among others (Annesley, 2003).

Other ions present in the fingerprints are *m/z* 163 and 325, referent to anhydrohexose and a potassium adduct of a dimer of anhydrohexose, respectively. Ions of *m/z* 116 and 118 are present in all spectra, and for the dark beers *m/z* 116 is the base peak (the most intense ion present). According to their MS/MS and searches in the NIST database, compared to substances known to be present in beer, *m/z* 116 is probably the protonated amino acid, proline, and *m/z* 118 a protonated amino acid with the formula $C_5H_{11}NO_2$ (2-amino-3-methylbutanoic acid). The MS/MS of the intense ion of *m/z* 104 shows neutral losses that may correspond to NH_3, H_2O, CO and CO_2, and typical fragmentation may be attributed to GABA, δ-aminobutyric acid.

Negative ion mode fingerprints

The presence of ions in the negative mode fingerprints is due to the abstraction of protons from neutral molecules with the aid of ammonium hydroxide, as well as adducts of the neutral molecules with anions present in solution. The negative ion mode [ESI(−)-MS] fingerprints show a large variety of ions, which was to be expected, given the low pH value of this beverage. Acid compounds ionize preferably in the negative ion mode. As observed previously in relation to the positive ion mode fingerprints, the ESI(−)-MS fingerprints separate the samples into three groups, which correspond to the main types of beer. Figure 92.4a shows a fingerprint of a typical pale (P) beer sample. The most intense ions appear in the *m/z* range between 75 and 925. The most intense ions of *m/z* 161, 179, 341, 503, 665 and 827 correspond to the deprotonated forms of anhydrohexose, glucose, maltose, maltotriose, maltotetraose and maltopentaose (respectively) as determined by their MS/MS. Pairs of anions of *m/z* 377 and 379, 539 and 541, 701 and 703 are the chloride adducts of maltose, maltotriose, and maltotetraose (typical isotopic pattern of 3:1 between $_{35}Cl$ and $_{37}Cl$). Other intense ions present in the fingerprint that are characteristic of pale beer are *m/z* 439 (adduct of *m/z*

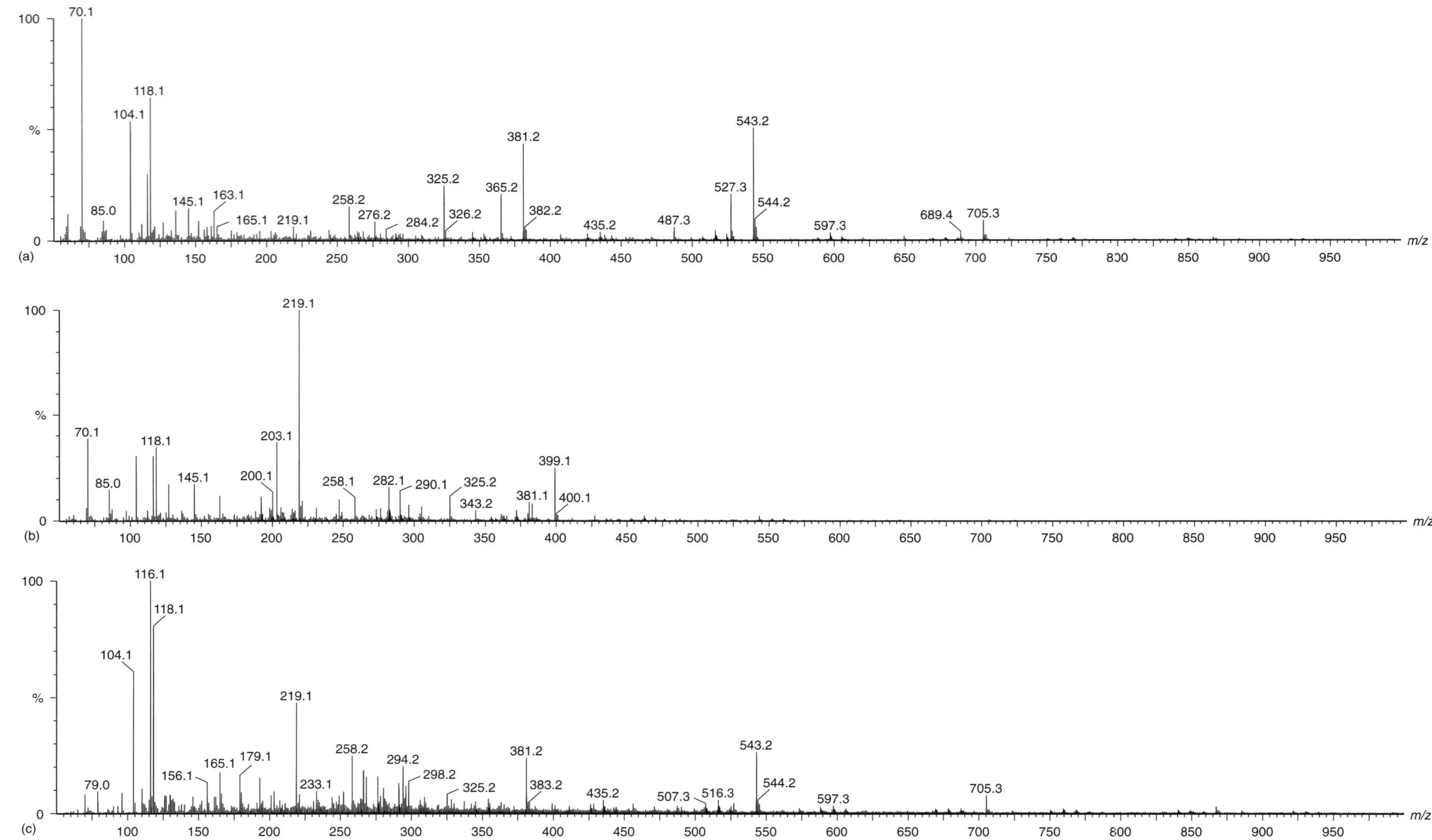

Figure 92.3 Positive ion mode electrospray mass spectrometry fingerprints of beer. *Source*: Adapted from Araújo *et al.* (2005). ESI(+)-MS mass spectra characteristic of (a) pale colored ale, (b) malt beer and (c) dark colored ale. Differences in the presence and intensity of the positively charged ions observed in the fingerprints are the result of differences in composition between these types of beer.

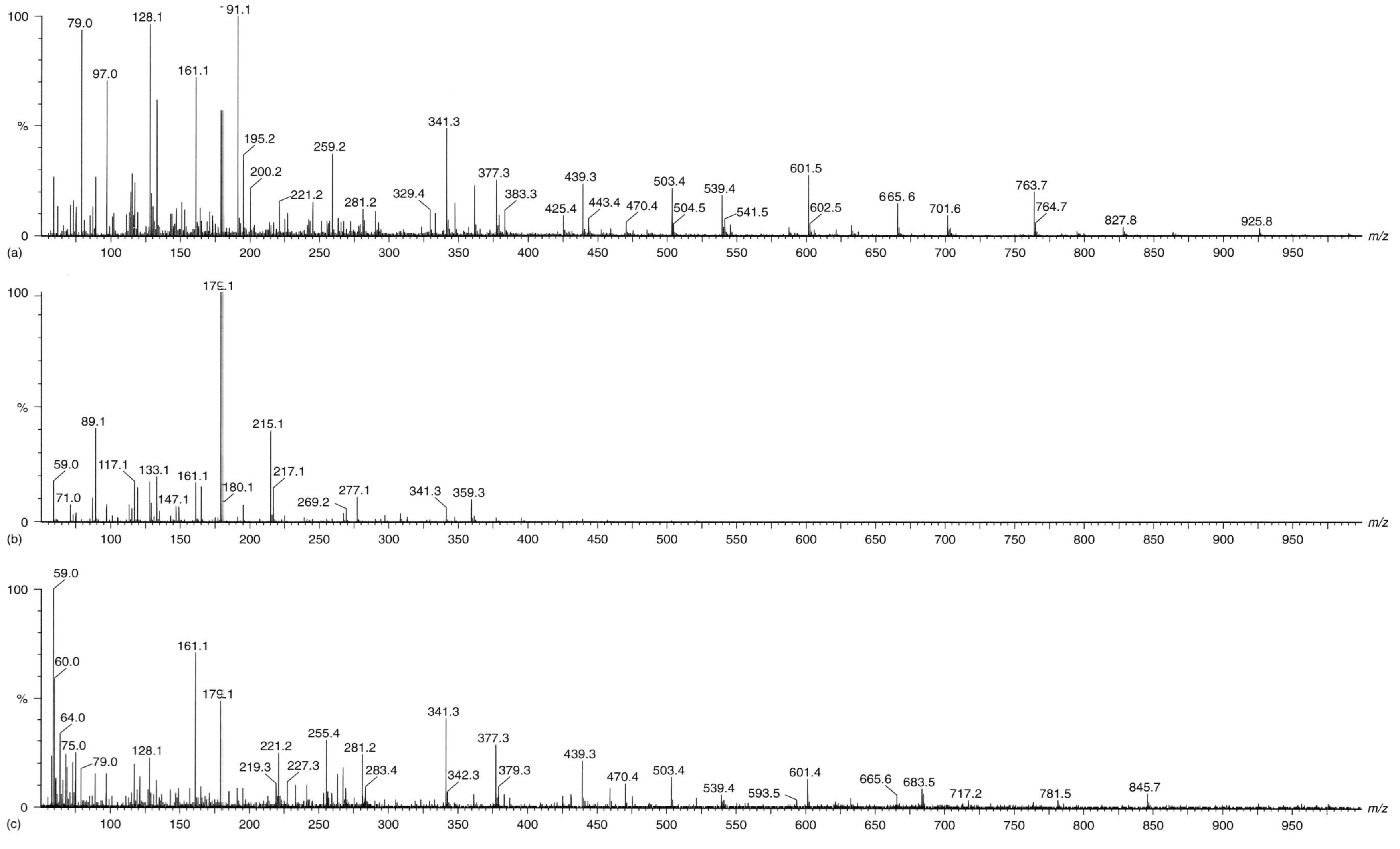

Figure 92.4 Negative ion mode electrospray mass spectrometry fingerprints of beer. *Source*: Adapted from Araújo *et al.* (2005). ESI(−)-MS mass spectra characteristic of (a) pale colored ale, (b) malt beer and (c) dark colored ale. Differences in the presence and intensity of the negatively charged ions observed in the fingerprints are the result of differences in composition between these types of beer.

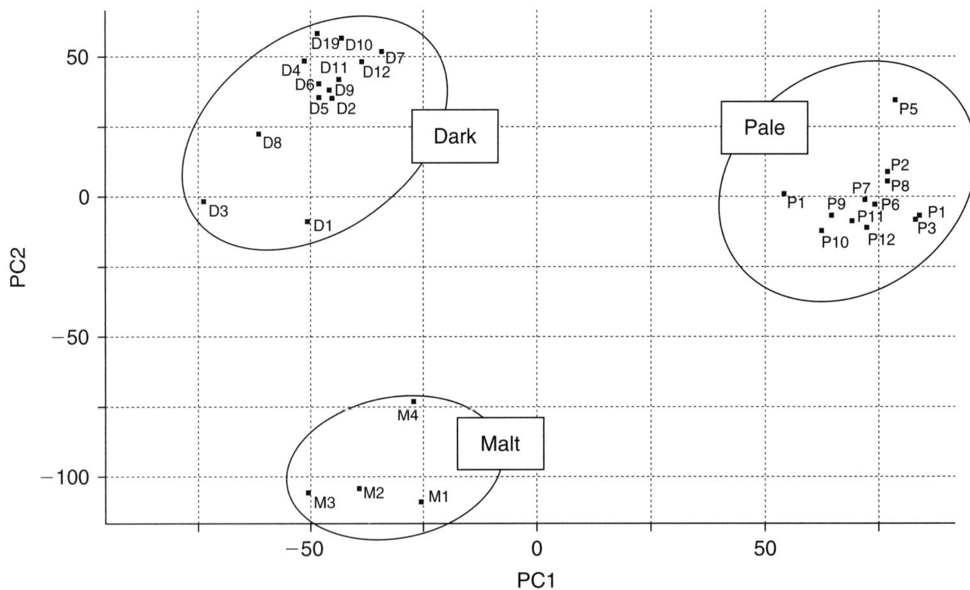

Figure 92.5 Statistical grouping of beer samples according to their positive ion mode fingerprints. *Source*: Adapted from Araújo *et al.* (2005). Scores of principal component analysis of the positive ion mode fingerprints ions of the 29 samples of beer (for abbreviations see Table 92.1). Samples were clearly grouped according to their type (P = pale, M = malt beer, D = dark).

259 with glucose), *m/z* 601 (adduct of *m/z* 259 with maltose) and *m/z* 763 (adduct of *m/z* 259 with maltotriose). *m/z* 259 itself is an adduct of *m/z* 79 with maltose.

Figure 92.4b shows the typical ESI(−)-MS fingerprint of malt beer (M). As noted before, the addition of caramel during the manufacturing process of this type of beer makes the ion of *m/z* 179 (deprotonated glucose) the base peak of the fingerprint, followed by the chloride adducts of glucose at *m/z* 215 and 217. The ion of *m/z* 359 appears only in fingerprints of malt beer and is the dimer of deprotonated glucose. Once again, the effect of matrix suppression in relation to the ions corresponding to the other oligosaccharides can be observed.

The fingerprint of a typical sample of dark (D) beer can be observed in Figure 92.4c, which is quite similar to that of pale beer (Figure 92.4a), with the high mass ions in lesser intensity and the pair of ions of *m/z* 161 and 179, standing out. As with pale beer, *m/z* 161 corresponds to deprotonated anhydrohexose and *m/z* 179 to deprotonated glucose. Other characteristic ions for this dark beer are *m/z* 255 and 683, the latter is the dimer of deprotonated maltose (Araújo *et al.*, 2005).

Statistical Analysis of Results

Simple sugars and oligosaccharides stand out in the positive and negative fingerprints of beer, while the relative intensity of marker ions varies according to the type of ale analyzed. This variability made the grouping of samples according to their composition possible in both ion modes, as well as other characteristic ions, mainly in the lower mass range of 50–200. Statistical analysis of results by PCA permitted the clear grouping of samples according to the results in both the negative and positive ion modes. Data matrixes were constructed using the information of the mass spectra obtained in both ESI(+)-MS and ESI(−)-MS modes. The groups formed by the 20 major peaks of each of the 29 samples analyzed were the variables. The exploratory data analysis was applied to the data matrix constituted by the 29 samples (as the rows) and this group of variables (as the columns). Einsight and Pirouette, both from Infometrix (Seattle, WA), were used to perform the PCA using Mean Center as data pre-treatment.

Figure 92.5 shows a scatter plot of PC1 and PC2 from the data matrix obtained from positive mode fingerprints. In this case, PC1 has 42% and PC2 has 27% of the variance. The pale colored ales are placed on the right side of the figure while the dark colored ales and Malzbier are divided in two groups on the left side. For the pale ales the variables that characterize them are the ions of *m/z* 70, 118, 206, 258 and 325. For malt beer the most influent variables are the ions of *m/z* 70, 203 and 219. For dark colored ales the most important ions are *m/z* 116, 381 and 399. Most of these ions stand out in the positive mode fingerprints and have already been discussed.

In the negative mode, chemometric analysis also divides the samples in three groups (Figure 92.6); PC1 has 57% and PC2 has 17% of the variance in the original data matrix. The pale colored ales are on the right side of the figure but divided into two subgroups. Most Brazilian samples (P1, P2, P3, P4, P5, P11, P12) are in one while the foreign samples and one Brazilian sample (P6) are in another. The

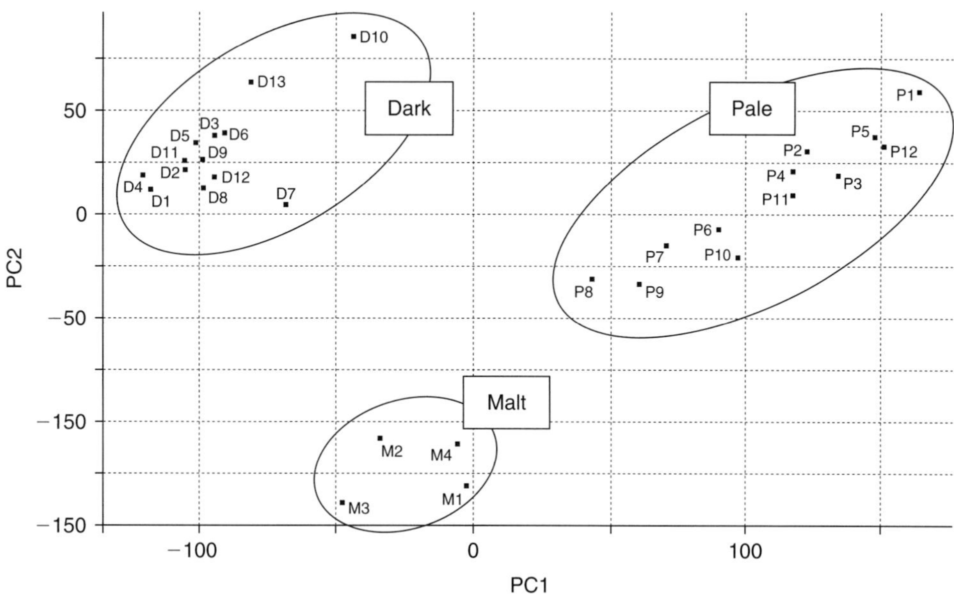

Figure 92.6 Statistical grouping of beer samples according to their negative ion mode fingerprints. *Source*: Adapted from Araújo *et al.* (2005). Scores of principal component analysis of the negative ion mode fingerprints ions of the 29 samples of beer (for abbreviations see Table 92.1). Samples were clearly grouped according to their type (P = pale, M = malt beer, D = dark).

ions that have the most influence on the grouping of these samples are the ions of *m/z* 79, 97, 101, 128, 133, 161, 191, 259, 341 and 363. The samples of dark ales and malt beer are found on the left side of the figure and the most influent ions for dark ales are *m/z* 59, 161, 221, 341 and 377. For malt beer, the most important ions are *m/z* 89, 179, 215, 217 and 277.

Simple sugars and oligosaccharides stand out in the positive and negative fingerprints of beer, while the relative intensity of marker ions varies according to the type of ale analyzed. This variability made the grouping of samples according to their composition possible in both positive and negative ion modes.

The results obtained showed that ESI-MS fingerprinting, both in the negative and positive ion modes, is a fast, robust and selective method for high throughput screening of beer samples. PCA was a useful tool for the grouping of samples and the identification of marker ions for each type of sample. Further studies are being undertaken to identify other beer components that influence the taste and odor of this beverage.

Acknowledgment

This work has been partially supported by the São Paulo State Research Foundation (FAPESP) and the National Research Council (CNPq).

Summary Points

- Mass spectrometry constitutes one of the most encompassing instrumental techniques in science, widely applied in the fields of chemistry, biology, medical science and technology.
- A brief review of the theoretical basis of mass spectrometry and ESI is presented.
- Direct insertion ESI-MS is a fast and sensitive method which differentiates diverse types of beer, characterizing their main constituents.
- Further information about the composition and type of beer can be obtained through the ESI-MS/MS fragmentation of the diagnostic ions of each sample.
- A total of 29 samples of ale produced in Brazil and other countries were divided into three groups by visual analysis of the positive [ESI(+)-MS] and negative [ESI(−)-MS] mode fingerprints as well as by chemometric analysis of the data.
- Many of the marker ions in both modes were found to be simple sugars and oligosaccharides, although their intensities varied depending on the type of ale (pale colored, dark colored and sweetened).
- A statistical analysis of results, PCA, confirmed the visual evaluation of the MS beer fingerprints obtained.

References

Alcázar, A., Pablos, F., Martín, M.J. and González, A.G. (2002). *Talanta* 57, 45–52.

Annesley, T.M. (2003). *Clin. Chem.* 49, 1041–1044.

Araújo, A.S., Rocha, L.L.R., Tomazela, D.M., Sawaya, A.C.H.F., Almeida, R.R., Catharino, R.R. and Eberlin, M.N. (2005). *Analyst* 130, 884–889.

Berlitz, H.D., Grosch, W. and Schieberle, P. (2004). *Food Chemistry* (3rd edn). Springer-Verlag, Germany.

Catharino, R.R., Sawaya, A.C.H.F., Cunha, I.B.S., Fogaça, A.O., Facco, E.M.P., Godoy, H.T., Daudt, C.E. and Eberlin, M.N. (2006). *J. Mass Spectrom.* 41, 185–190.

Cole, R.B. (1997). *Electrospray Ionization Mass Spectrometry*. John Wiley & Sons Inc., New York.

Cole, R.B. (2000). *J. Mass Spectrom.* 35, 763–772.

Cooks, R.G., Zhang, D.X., Koch, K.J., Gozzo, F.C. and Eberlin, M.N. (2001). *Anal. Chem.* 73, 3646–3655.

Degelmann, P., Becker, M., Herderich, M. and Humpf, H.U. (1999). *Chromatographia* 49, 543–546.

Eberlin, M.N., Meurer, E., Santos, L.S. and Pilli, R.A. (2003). *Org. Lett.* 5, 1391–1394.

Gaumet, J.J. and Strouse, G. (2000). *J. Am. Soc. Mass Spectrom.* 11, 338–344.

Hans, X.L. and Gross, R.W. (2001). *Analytic. Biochem.* 265, 88–100.

Hardwick, W.A. (1995). *Handbook of Brewing*. Marcel Dekker, New York.

Hofte, A.J.P., Van der Hoeven, R.A.M., Fung, S.Y., Verpoorte, R., Tjaden, U.R. and Van der Greef, J. (1998). *J. Am. Soc. Brew. Chem.* 56, 118–122.

Klampfl, C.W., Himmelsbach, M., Buchberger, W. and Klein, H. (2002). *Anal. Chim. Acta* 454, 185–191.

Koch, K.J., Gozzo, F.C., Nanita, S.C., Takats, Z., Eberlin, M. N. and Cooks, R.G. (2002). *Angew. Chem. Int. Ed. Engl.* 41, 1721.

Kotiaho, T., Eberlin, M.N., Vainiotalo, P. and Kostiainen, R. (2000). *J. Am. Soc. Mass Spectrom.* 11, 526–535.

Mauri, P., Minoggio, M., Simonetti, P., Gardana, C. and Pietta, P. (2002). *Rapid Commun. Mass Spectrom.* 16, 743–748.

Möller, J.K., Catharino, R.R. and Eberlin, M.N. (2005). *Analyst* 130, 890–897.

de la Mora, J.F., Berkel, G.J.V., Enke, C.G., Cole, R.B., Sanchez, M.M. and Fenn, J.B. (2000). *J. Mass Spectrom.* 35, 939–952.

Raftery, M.J. and Geczy, C.L.J. (2002). *J. Am. Soc Mass Spectrom.* 13, 709–718.

Rioli, V., Gozzo, F.C., Shida, C.S., Krieger, J.E., Heimann, A.S., Linardi, A., Almeida, P.C., Hyslop, S., Eberlin, M.N. and Ferro, E.S. (2003). *J. Biol. Chem.* 278, 8547–8555.

Russel, D.H. (1994). *Experimental Mass Spectrometry*. Plenum Press, New York.

Sawaya, A.C.H.F., Tomazela, D.M., Cunha, I.B.S., Bankova, V.S., Marcucci, M.C., Custódio, A.R. and Eberlin, M.N. (2004). *Analyst* 129, 739–744.

Schoonjans, V., Taylor, N., Hudson, B.D. and Massart, D.L. (2002). *J. Pharm. Biomed. Anal.* 28, 537–548.

Siuzdak, G. (2005). *An Introduction to Mass Spectrometry Ionization: An Excerpt from the Expanding Role of Mass Spectrometry in Biotechnology*, 2nd edn. MCC Press, San Diego, CA.

Whittle, N., Eldridge, H., Bartley, J. and Organ, G. (1999). *J. Inst. Brew.* 105, 89–99.

Williams, J.D., Flanagan, M., Lopez, L., Fischer, S. and Miller, L.A.D. (2003). *J. Chromatogr. A.* 1020, 11–26.

Zhang, X.R., Minear, R.A., Guo, Y.B., Hwang, C.J., Barret, S.E., Ikeda, K., Shimizu, Y. and Matsui, S. (2004). *Water Res.* 38, 3920–3930.

93

Methods for the Characterization of Beer by Nuclear Magnetic Resonance Spectroscopy

A.M. Gil Department of Chemistry-CICECO, University of Aveiro, Campus de Santiago, 3810-193 Aveiro, Portugal
J. Rodrigues Department of Chemistry-CICECO, University of Aveiro, Campus de Santiago, 3810-193 Aveiro, Portugal

Abstract

The use of high-resolution nuclear magnetic resonance (NMR) spectroscopy in the characterization of beer is described, making reference to site-specific natural fractionation (SNIF) NMR methods, NMR characterization of beer extracts and, finally, of whole beer. Qualitative analysis of specific components in beer usually requires the tandem use of NMR and other analytical techniques for sample extraction/concentration and complementary characterization. For whole beer, a range of newly developed NMR-based methods have been applied, showing promise in widening the range of detectable compounds and lowering detection limits. NMR quantitative analysis has also been applied successfully for specific compound families in beer extracts and in whole beer. Practical applications accommodating large sample numbers require the use of multivariate analysis and the existing applications of this strategy are reviewed.

List of Abbreviations

Ala	Alanine
DOSY	Diffusion ordered spectroscopy
GABA	γ-Aminobutyric acid
His	Histidine
HPAEC-PAD	High-performance anion-exchange chromatography with pulsed amperometric detection
Ile	Isoleucine
IRMS	Isotopic ratio mass spectrometry
LC	Liquid chromatography
Leu	Leucine
MALDI-TOF MS	Matrix-assisted laser desorption/ ionization-time of flight mass spectrometry
M_r	Molecular mass
MS	Mass spectrometry
NMR	Nuclear magnetic resonance
PCA	Principal component analysis
Phe	Phenylalanine
PLS	Partial least squares
Pro	Proline
RT	Retention time
SNIF	Site-specific natural fractionation
TOCSY	Total correlation spectroscopy
Tyr	Tyrosine
Un.	Unassigned
Val	Valine

Introduction

The characterization of the chemical composition of beer and its relation to quality is of great importance for efficient quality control and to improve the properties of the final product. The complex chemical composition of beer depends on many factors including water quality, malt, hop, yeasts and the precise recipe and timing of the brewing process. An adequate characterization of chemical composition might, thus, give important indications about the nature and history of the beer sample and have significant implications for the quality control of the product.

Nuclear magnetic resonance (NMR) spectroscopy is a technique of increasing promise in the chemical characterization of complex mixtures such as beer, wine, fruit juices and many other foodstuffs. NMR is based on the magnetic moments of some atomic nuclei (e.g. the nuclei of ^{1}H, ^{13}C, ^{15}N) which enable them to reorient when exposed to a fixed external magnetic field and absorb radiofrequency energy (Table 93.1). The exact value of the radiofrequency absorbed is exquisitely dependent on the chemical environment of the nucleus in a molecule, so that each compound gives, in the case of proton (^{1}H) NMR, a well-defined set of ^{1}H absorption peaks. In addition, the intensity of each absorption peak reflects the number of nuclei therefore

Beer in Health and Disease Prevention
ISBN: 978-0-12-373891-2

Table 93.1 Summary of principles and some applications of NMR spectroscopy

Principle	NMR is based on the magnetic moments (μ) of some atomic nuclei (e.g. the nuclei of ^{1}H, ^{13}C, ^{15}N) which enable them to reorient when exposed to a fixed external magnetic field (B_0) and absorb radiofrequency energy. The exact value of energy absorbed depends on the chemical environment of the nucleus in a molecule, hence, each compound gives, in the case of proton (^{1}H) NMR, a well-defined set of ^{1}H absorption peaks.
Some applications	• Determination of chemical structure and quantitation of compounds in solution. • Determination of secondary and tertiary structures of proteins in solution. • Determination of chemical structure and molecular interactions in the solid state. • Determination of overall compositional profile in complex mixtures. • Determination of product origin for quality control.

enabling quantitative as well as qualitative studies. The principles and methods of NMR spectroscopy are described in detail in several publications (Harris, 1983; Derome, 1987).

NMR-based methods have long been recognized as valuable in the monitoring of quality of many alcoholic drinks and beverages. The first applications involved the use of site-specific natural isotope fractionation (SNIF) NMR. This technique measures the isotopic ratios, for example D/H or $^{12}C/^{13}C$ of ethanol by NMR (Cordella *et al.*, 2002). These ratios are very sensitive to many aspects of the history of the drink: geographical origin, specific materials and methods employed. An alternative approach is the recording of high-resolution NMR spectra of abundant nuclei such as ^{1}H, a method which has the ability of simultaneously detecting several families of compounds over a wide range of concentrations ($>$ μmolar). This has, traditionally, been applied to the detection of particular compounds or families of compounds in concentrated food extracts, however, an increasing number of applications for the direct analysis of foods has been noted in the last few years. Requiring minimal or no sample preparation, a direct high-resolution NMR spectrum of a complex mixture such as beer or wine presents the challenge of interpretation of multiple compound profiles in one spectrum. Spectral assignment normally relies on the so-called bidimensional (or 2D) NMR methods to disentangle spectral information to some extent but, when the analysis of large sample numbers is considered, the use of multivariate analysis methods is required. Indeed, the richness of information made available in direct 1D and 2D NMR spectra of a mixture poses the problem of extensive signal overlap and, hence, great difficulty in extracting fully detailed compositional information, particularly for a large number of samples. The tandem use of NMR and multivariate analysis methods such as principal component analysis (PCA) or partial least squares (PLS) regression enables large sample groups to be tackled and meaningful compositional variations to be detected. This approach has been the basis of numerous NMR-based methods for classification and origin determination of foods (Belton *et al.*, 1998; Sacchi *et al.*, 1998; Le Gall *et al.*, 2001; Brescia *et al.*, 2002; Charlton *et al.*, 2002; Košir and Kidrič, 2002; Brescia *et al.*, 2003; Duarte *et al.*, 2004), providing the possibility of pinpointing specific compounds responsible for the occurrence and/or intensity of a particular property of the final product.

NMR Applications to the Study of Beer

SNIF NMR of beer

Isotopic ratios such as D/H, $^{12}C/^{13}C$, $^{16}O/^{18}O$ found in naturally occurring molecules are not constant and depend on biochemical pathways and reaction mechanisms. In food science, this has been exploited to assign the origin of food components and, hence, detect food adulteration (Rossmann, 2001). This strategy is now routinely applied in the wine industry, mainly with basis on D/H measurements by ^{2}H NMR and often used in tandem with other methods (e.g. isotopic ratio mass spectrometry (IRMS)). In the case of beer, a limited number of applications have been carried out, to our knowledge. ^{2}H NMR has been applied to beer to determine the origin of malt from several grain species (Martin *et al.*, 1985). Also, the D/H ratio of the methylene group in beer ethanol and the $^{16}O/^{18}O$ ratio of beer water have been suggested to correlate to regional origin. The D/H and ^{13}C abundance values have been measured by NMR and MS, respectively, for the ethanol from a set of commercial beers, as well as ethanol from grain spirit, beet sugar and wheat malt (Rossmann, 2001). The authors of this work noted the narrow range of D/H values and ^{13}C abundance observed for beers from different regions within the same country (Germany).

High-resolution NMR of beer extracts

This section summarizes the work carried out so far on the analysis of beer extracts by NMR, often in tandem with other analytical techniques. Many of these studies have addressed the characterization of the carbohydrate constituents of beer. The most abundant carbohydrates in beer are those derived from starch during the mashing step (Baxter and Hughes, 2001) with the resulting wort containing glucose, maltose, some branched non-fermentable dextrins and some residual straight-chain dextrins. Beer also contains non-starch polysaccharides such as arabinoxylans and β-glucan which, although depolymerized to some extent, remain present in beer and may be the cause of undesirable precipitation and filtration problems. An early study of barley β-D-glucan has been carried out by ^{1}H and ^{13}C NMR and resulted in the assignment of several oligosaccharides produced by the treatment of barley flour with a fungal β-D-glucanase (Bock *et al.*, 1991).

A 1D and 2D NMR study, in tandem with matrix-assisted laser desorption/ionization-time of flight mass spectrometry (MALDI-TOF MS), on chromatographically separated carbohydrate fractions of beer has resulted in the identification of several new derivatives of trehalose, sucrose, maltooligosaccharides and linear glucose oligomers with α(1→3) and α(1→4) linkages (Vinogradov and Bock, 1998). The same work comprised a study of the branching pattern of beer dextrins by enzymatic degradation and subsequent NMR analysis. Beer arabinoxylans have also been investigated using NMR methods (Bock *et al.*, 1991; Broberg *et al.*, 2000; Ferré *et al.*, 2000). One of these studies describes the characterization of nanomole amounts of arabinoxylan oligosaccharides, fractionated by high-performance anion-exchange chromatography with pulsed amperometric detection (HPAEC-PAD) (Broberg *et al.*, 2000). This was achieved by a specific NMR probe adapted for measurement of low sample amounts by the use of a smaller diameter NMR tube and magic angle spinning technology. The authors employed a range of 2D NMR experiments for the detailed assignment of oligosaccharides in the samples. Figure 93.1 shows the anomeric regions of the ^{1}H NMR spectra of arabinoxylan subfractions obtained firstly by size-exclusion chromatography (UF4, UF5 and UF6) and further fractionated by HPAEC-PAD (fractions a to e). Some NMR assignments are shown for fractions UF5, demonstrating the specificity of the method. The same NMR tools were used for the characterization of the substrate preference and specificity of an arabinoxylan arabinofuranohydrolase newly isolated from germinated barley (Ferré *et al.*, 2000). More recently, water-soluble high molar mass arabinoxylans from barley have been obtained by size-exclusion fractionation and characterized by ^{1}H NMR, amongst other techniques (Dervilly *et al.*, 2002).

Since hops determine the taste and flavor of beer, the analysis of hop components and their derivatives is of great importance in the brewing industry. The major components responsible for bitterness are the hop bitter acids: the α- and the β-acids. During brewing, the former give rise to iso-α-acids and these and their derivatives are known to impart the typical bitter taste of beer. NMR characterization of α-acids, iso-α-acids and their reduced products (isohumulones) has been achieved by several ^{1}H and ^{13}C NMR studies of hop extracts as well as of standard compounds (Pusecker *et al.*, 1997; Pusecker *et al.*, 1999,

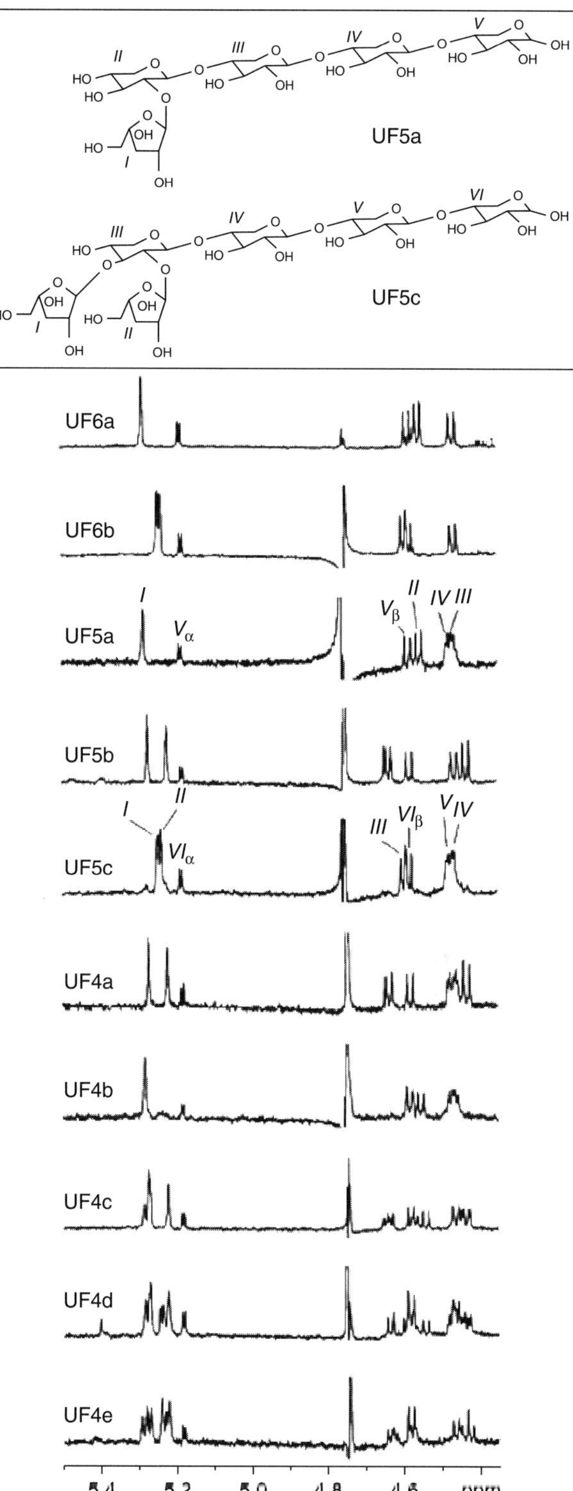

Figure 93.1 Anomeric regions of 1D ^{1}H NMR spectra of arabinoxylan subfractions. The anomeric regions of 1D ^{1}H NMR spectra of subfractions UF6a–b, UF5a–c and UF4a–e (arabinoxylan fractions) recorded with 256 scans at 500 MHz with a 4-mm ^{1}H-observe nano NMR probe on approximate sample amounts between 3 and 26 nmol (3 and 18 μg, respectively). The assignments of some characteristic signals of the novel oligosaccharides in subfractions UF5a and UF5c are indicated in the figure (reprinted from Broberg *et al.* (2000); Copyright 2000, with permission from Elsevier).

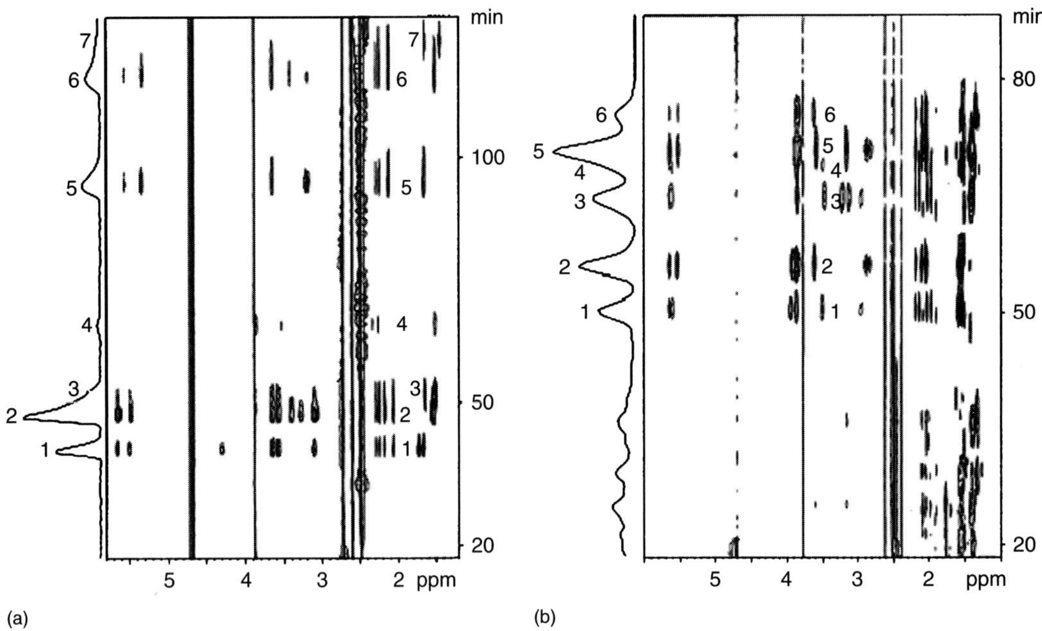

Figure 93.2 LC-NMR contour plots for a CO_2 hop extract and for isohumulones. LC-NMR contour plots with NMR projection (left side) of (a) CO_2 hop extract: 1 = co-humulone, 2 = humulone, 3 = ad-humulone, 4 = unknown, 5 = colupulone, 6 = lupulone, 7 = adlupulone; (b) isohumulones: 1 = *trans*-iso-co-humulone, 2 = *cis*-iso-co-humulone, 3 = *trans*-isohumulone, 4 = *trans*-iso-ad-humulone, 5 = *cis*-iso-humulone, 6 = *cis*-iso-ad-humulone (reprinted from Pusecker *et al.* (1999); Copyright 1999, with permission from Elsevier).

Hoek *et al.*, 2001; Nord *et al.*, 2003). The qualitative analysis of these compounds was shown to benefit greatly from the on-line coupling of LC with NMR (LC-NMR), as shown by a study of hop extracts and isohumulones in which unambiguous identification of many components was achieved (Pusecker *et al.*, 1999). Figure 93.2 shows the LC-NMR plots obtained for a CO_2 hop extract and for isohumulones. In another study, the components of isohumulone mixtures have been fully characterized by ^{1}H and ^{13}C NMR (Nord *et al.*, 2003). Following initial quantitative NMR studies for these compounds, to aid in hop extract analysis and standardization (Pusecker *et al.*, 1997), an improved quantitative NMR method has been proposed based on the integration of selected signals in the NMR spectrum (Hoek *et al.*, 2001). In an attempt to better control beer properties related to hops, a method for predicting the acidity of iso-α-acids in beer based on ^{13}C NMR was proposed (Friedrich and Galensa, 2002). Indeed, a relationship between ^{13}C chemical shift and iso-α-acids acidity was found, enabling the estimation of the solubility and stability properties of these compounds.

Many compounds other than carbohydrates and hop acids play extremely important roles in beer quality, and the value of NMR spectroscopy to detect many different compound types simultaneously has been recognized as useful for rapid beer evaluation. This approach has been applied to 2-butanol beer extracts (Khatib *et al.*, 2006), making use of multivariate analysis, namely PCA, to detect differences in the aromatic compounds present. It was shown that PCA applied to 2D *J*-resolved NMR spectra gave good separation between the extracts of different beers. Such separation was interpreted in terms of the contents of nucleic acid derivatives, amino acids, organic acids, alcohols, cholines and carbohydrates.

Other works on beer extracts have used a different perspective, exploiting hops as potential source of new bioactive compounds and using NMR for structural determination (Chadwick *et al.*, 2004; Stavri *et al.*, 2004). For instance, a bioassay-guided fractionation of a hexane hop extract was carried out in order to identify antimycobacterial constituents, using the mycobacterial species *Mycobacterium fortutium* (Stavri *et al.*, 2004). Another example is the full NMR characterization of the constituents of a hop extract obtained by supercritical CO_2 separation, aiming at identifying compounds with estrogenic activity (Chadwick *et al.*, 2004).

Attempting to investigate the role of specific components on the brewing process, an NMR study has enabled the identification of a new flavanol glucoside from barley and malt (Friedrich and Galensa, 2002) and the evaluation of its quantitative change during malting. This type of compound is believed to be involved in the formation of beer haze and, possibly, also in beer flavor stability. A different and more practical approach was taken to measure NMR T_2 relaxation times, which reflect molecular mobility, for mash, spent grain suspensions, worts and carbohydrate solutions, to investigate a possible correlation with the rheological properties of such systems (Gotz *et al.*, 2003).

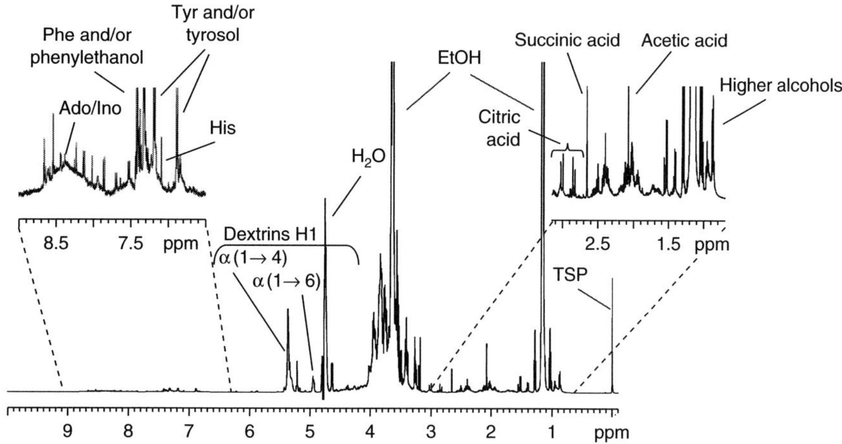

Figure 93.3 Typical 1D ^{1}H NMR spectrum of whole beer. Typical 1D ^{1}H NMR spectrum of a whole beer sample after degassing in an ultrasound bath for 10 min. The sample was inserted into an NMR tube with 10% D_2O and 0.02% TSP-d_4 (sodium 3-(trimethylsilyl)propionate-d_4), as a reference for ^{1}H chemical shift (δ). The inserts show vertical expansions of the high field (right) and low field (left) regions of the spectrum and some assignments are shown (Phe, Tyr, His correspond to the 3-letter codes of phenylalanine, tyrosine and histidine).

The authors concluded that the characteristic viscosities of those materials may be measured through NMR T_2, in relatively short times and avoiding, in some cases, the errors of conventional rheometric methods.

High-resolution NMR of whole beer

The direct characterization of beer by NMR presents the attractive feature of being simple, rapid and non-invasive since the only sample preparation required is degassing for a few minutes. Figure 93.3 shows a typical ^{1}H NMR spectrum of intact beer, where the high number of peaks is clear, as is the problem of signal overlap in all regions of the spectrum. Overlap with broad components is evident in all regions reflecting the presence of large M_r compounds, as well as the expected mixture of low M_r compounds. Over the past few years, a number of strategies have been applied to attempt (1) the continuously increasing assignment of new compounds in intact beer and (2) to find a user-friendly method for spectral interpretation and analysis of large numbers of samples, for practical use to be made of the methods. The first approach for disentangling 1D ^{1}H NMR information is to carry out 2D NMR experiments. These experiments spread the 1D information in 2D and, the use of a range of different experiments based on homonuclear (^{1}H/^{1}H) (Figure 93.4) and heteronuclear (usually, ^{1}H/^{13}C) correlation, have enabled the assignment of about 30 compounds in intact beer (Duarte *et al.*, 2003a). However, when sample complexity is high, such as in beer, this does not suffice and complementary methods are required. Hyphenated methods such as LC-NMR have proven useful, not only for the analysis of beer extracts but also for intact beer (Duarte *et al.*, 2003a; Duarte *et al.*, 2003b; Gil *et al.*, 2003). Making use of the addition of an MS dimension, in the form of LC-NMR/MS, has enabled the identification of many

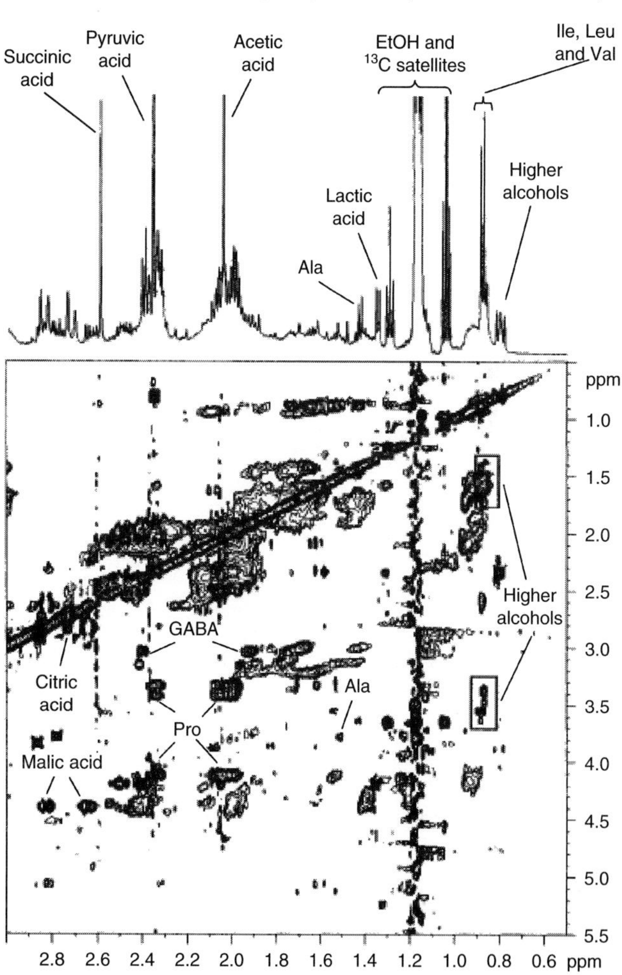

Figure 93.4 Expansion of a 2D homonuclear (^{1}H/^{1}H) correlation NMR spectrum recorded for whole beer. Expansion of a 2D total correlation spectroscopy (TOCSY) spectrum recorded for whole beer. The 1D NMR projection is shown at the top and some assignments are shown at the bottom. Ala, Ile, Leu, Pro and Val correspond to the 3-letter codes of alanine, isoleucine, leucine, proline and valine; GABA correspond to γ-aminobutyric acid.

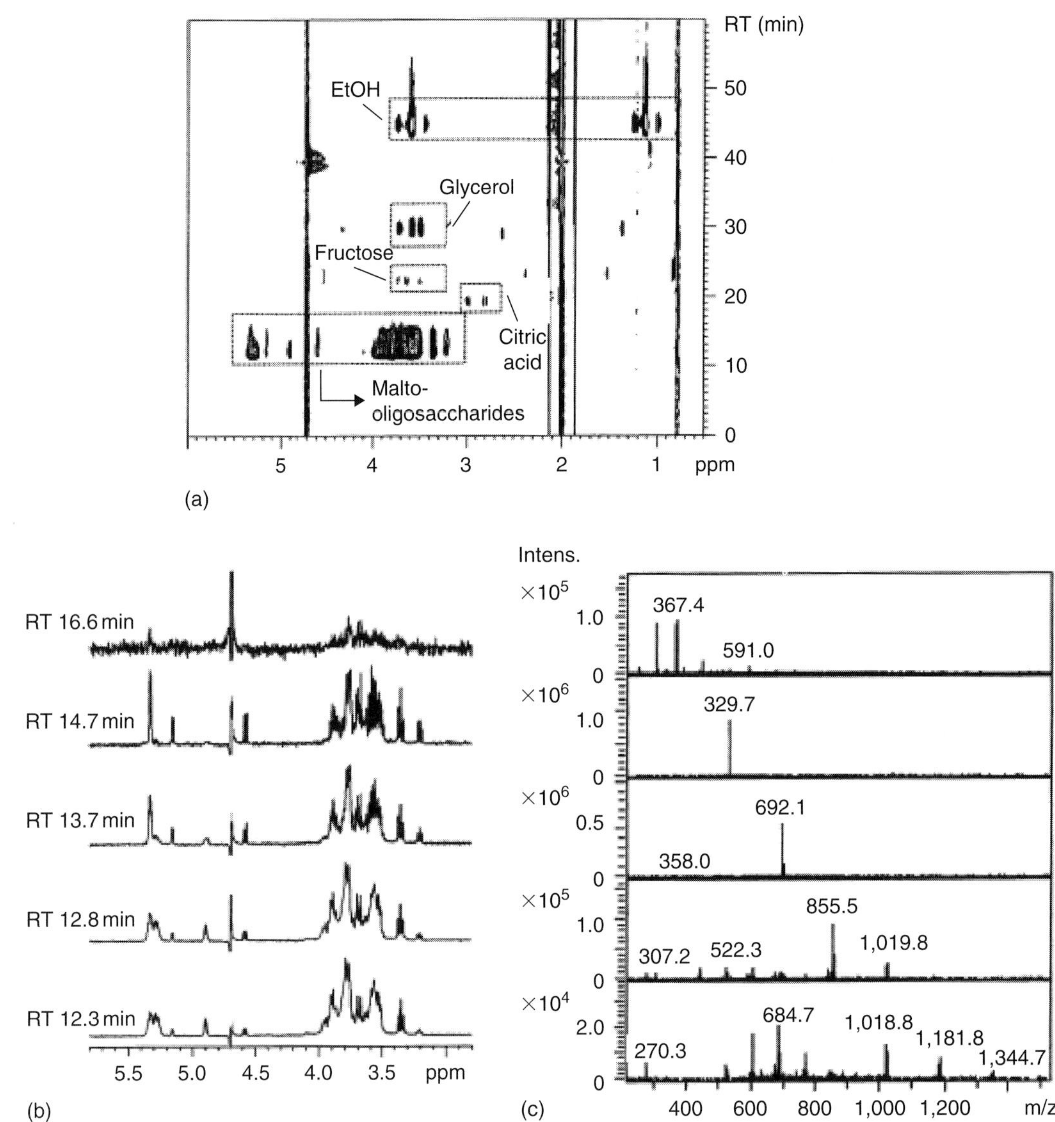

Figure 93.5 LC-NMR plot, selected NMR spectra and corresponding MS spectra obtained for an ale beer. (a) LC-NMR on-flow record obtained for an ale beer (whole sample). The labels identify the main fractions separated; (b) rows extracted from the on-flow record shown in (a); (c) MS spectra acquired concurrently with the NMR data, using positive-ionization. RT indicate LC retention time (reprinted with permission from *Journal of Agriculture and Food Chemistry*, 51, Duarte et al. (2003b); Copyright 2003 American Chemical Society).

aromatic compounds and of oligosaccharides differing in size and branching degree. Figure 93.5 shows the LC-NMR plot obtained for a beer, using an ion-exchange resin. Examples of the ^{1}H NMR spectra taken across the LC-NMR plot are shown, together with the corresponding MS spectra. Their analysis enabled several oligosaccharide fractions to be characterized in terms of average size and degree of branching. Another NMR-based tool of great value for the qualitative analysis of beer is diffusion ordered spectroscopy or DOSY, a technique which results in a representation of 1D NMR spectra as a function of compound diffusivity. This leads to a 2D plot such as that shown in Figure 93.6. In spite of signal overlap not allowing accurate diffusivity information to be obtained, the DOSY method presents considerable promise for (1) identification of both low and high M_r compounds through the knowledge of their diffusivity properties and (2) detection of unexpected interactions or bonding between different moieties, detected through their common diffusivity. Comparison of the DOSY spectra of different beers has enabled a clearer picture of the aromatic composition to be obtained, unveiling new compounds for which molecular size could be estimated and some evidence of slow-diffusing polyaromatic species (Gil *et al.*, 2004).

The aid offered by multivariate analysis for NMR interpretation and tackling large sample groups has become increasingly clear over the last few years. The work carried out has mainly employed PCA and some applications have comprised

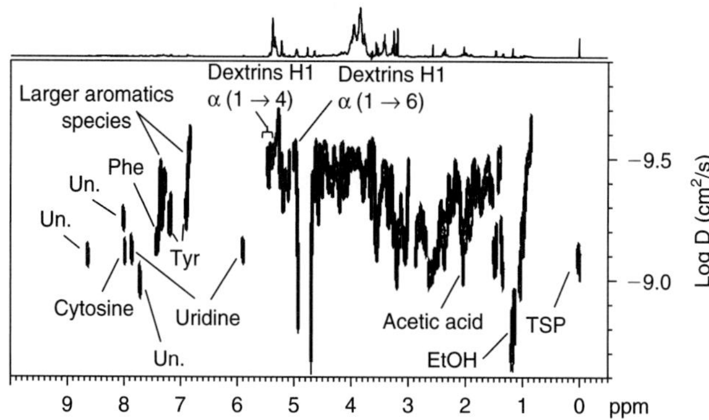

Figure 93.6 Typical 2D DOSY plot obtained for a whole beer sample. Some assignments are shown for lower and higher M_r compounds. Amino acids are identified by their 3-letter codes; Un: unassigned compound.

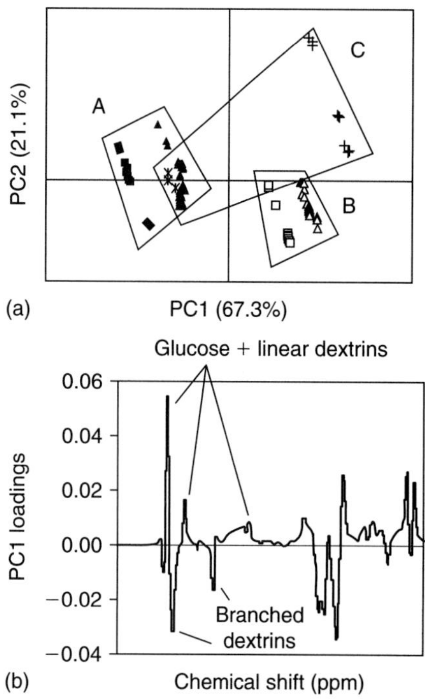

Figure 93.7 PCA of the sugar regions (3.1–5.8 ppm) of the ^{1}H NMR spectra of a set of beers. Results of PCA of the sugar regions (3.1–5.8 ppm) of the ^{1}H NMR spectra of a set of beers: (a) scores scatter plot of PC1 vs. PC2 for spectra processed with line broadening 10 Hz and (b) corresponding PC1 loadings profile. Labels A, B and C indicate different brewing sites situated in different countries; for each site, beers produced in different dates are shown as: (◆) A1, (■) A2, (▲) A3; (◇) B1, (□) B2, (△) B3 and (*) C1, (−) C2, (+) C3. Grouping shapes were drawn manually in the scores scatter plots to aid the eye. Negative and positive PC1 values correspond, respectively, to signals from branched dextrins and from glucose and linear dextrins.

the separation of beer samples in terms of type: ales, lagers and alcohol free (Duarte *et al.*, 2002; Duarte *et al.*, 2004). Beer types were found to differ particularly in terms of their aromatic composition, as a reflection of the different types of fermentation procedures employed. In addition, the NMR/PCA method enabled sample groups differing in carbohydrate composition to be identified. In a subsequent work, the high throughput of a flow injection NMR system has been used and PCA of the NMR spectra of a large set of beers showed that (1) beers from barley malt may be distinguished from those from wheat malt, (2) beers from the same brewing sites tend to cluster together and (3) beers with some degree of deterioration may be identified (Lachenmeier *et al.*, 2005). The effect of different brewing sites on the composition of beer has been further investigated through the NMR/PCA strategy (Almeida *et al.*, 2006), indicating that considerable compositional changes affect some organic acids, dextrins and aromatic compounds, even when beer type and recipe are, in principle, kept unchanged. This should reflect fine differences in hardware setup, materials and even local uses and culture. Figure 93.7 shows an example of the separation of lager beers produced in different countries (sites A, B and C), in terms of their dextrin characteristics. This opens the possibility of using NMR and multivariate analysis for the rapid monitoring of the brewing process.

Besides PCA, PLS also has found useful applications in the analysis of beer (Nord *et al.*, 2004; Lachenmeier *et al.*, 2005). This method has been used to calibrate the NMR method against specific reference methods and this has been applied to the quantitation of organic and amino acids in intact beer (Nord *et al.*, 2004) and to the determination of reference parameters such as original gravity or ethanol and lactic acid contents (Lachenmeier *et al.*, 2005). A short review has recently summarized the use of state of the art NMR in several issues of beer production and characterization (Duus, 2005).

Summary Points

- NMR spectroscopy is perhaps the most powerful method for the full structural analysis of compounds in concentrated extracts; in this respect, applications to beer comprise mainly the study of hop components and of carbohydrates.
- New NMR technology like nano-probes or hyphenated techniques have promising potential for extract analysis at low nanomolar concentrations and for unveiling structurally similar compounds.
- Direct NMR analysis of intact beer has added attractiveness for simple and rapid applications at the industrial level.
- Direct qualitative analysis is made possible by exploiting state of the art methods like hyphenated NMR and DOSY.
- Handling of large-sample groups with a view to routine practical applications requires the use of multivariate analysis for NMR interpretation and validation of results; PCA and PLS regression are powerful tools applied until now for the discrimination of beers according to several different parameters.

References

Almeida, C., Duarte, I.F., Barros, A., Rodrigues, J., Spraul, M. and Gil, A.M. (2006). *J. Agric. Food Chem.* 54, 700–706.

Baxter, E.D. and Hughes, P.S. (2001). *Beer Quality Safety and Nutritional Aspects.* Royal Society of Chemistry, Cambridge.

Belton, P.S., Colquhoun, I.J., Kemsley, E.K., Delgadillo, I., Roma, P., Dennis, M.J., Sharman, M., Holmes, E., Nicholson, J.K. and Spraul, M. (1998). *Food Chem.* 61, 207–213.

Bock, K., Duus, J.Ø., Norman, B. and Pedersen, S. (1991). *Carbohydr. Res.* 211, 219–233.

Brescia, M.A., Caldarola, V., De Giglio, A., Benedetti, D., Fanizzi, F.P. and Sacco, A. (2002). *Anal. Chim. Acta* 458, 177–186.

Brescia, M.A., Košir, I.J., Caldarola, V., Kidrič, J. and Sacco, A. (2003). *J. Agric. Food Chem.* 51, 21–26.

Broberg, A., Thomsen, K.K. and Duus, J.Ø. (2000). *Carbohydr. Res.* 328, 375–382.

Chadwick, L.R., Nikolic, D., Burdette, J.E., Overk, C.R., Bolton, J.L., van Breemen, R.B., Fröhlich, R., Fong, H.H.S., Farnsworth, N.R. and Pauli, G.F. (2004). *J. Nat. Prod.* 67, 2024–2032.

Charlton, A.J., Farrington, W.H.H. and Brereton, P. (2002). *J. Agric. Food Chem.* 50, 3098–3103.

Cordella, C., Moussa, I., Martel, A.C., Sbirrazzuoli, N. and Lizzani-Cuvelier, L. (2002). *J. Agric. Food Chem.* 50, 1751–1764.

Derome, A.E. (1987). In *Modern NMR Techniques for Chemistry Research: Organic Chemistry Series*, Vol. 6 (ed. J.E. Baldwin), Pergamon Press, Oxford.

Dervilly, G., Leclercq, C., Zimmermann, D., Roue, C., Thibault, J.F. and Saulnier, L. (2002). *Carbohydr. Polym.* 47, 143–149.

Duarte, I.F., Barros, A., Belton, P.S., Righelato, R., Spraul, M., Humpfer, E. and Gil, A.M. (2002). *J. Agric. Food Chem.* 50, 2475–2481.

Duarte, I.F., Spraul, M., Godejohann, M., Braumann, U. and Gil, A.M. (2003a). In Belton, P.S., Gil, A.M., Webb, G.A. and Rutledge, D. (eds), *Magnetic Resonance in Food Science: Latest Developments*, pp. 151–157. Royal Society of Chemistry, Cambridge.

Duarte, I.F., Godejohann, M., Braumann, U., Spraul, M. and Gil, A.M. (2003b). *J. Agric. Food Chem.* 51, 4847–4852.

Duarte, I.F., Barros, A., Almeida, C., Spraul, M. and Gil, A.M. (2004). *J. Agric. Food Chem.* 52, 1031–1038.

Duus, J.Ø. (2005). In Engelson, S., Belton, P.S. and Jakobsen, H.J. (eds), *Magnetic Resonance in Food Science: the Multivariate Challenge*, pp. 91–95. Royal Society of Chemistry, Cambridge.

Ferré, H., Broberg, A., Duus, J.Ø. and Thomsen, K.K. (2000). *Eur. J. Biochem.* 267, 6633–6641.

Friedrich, W. and Galensa, R. (2002). *Eur. Food Res. Technol.* 214, 388–393.

Gil, A.M., Duarte, I.F., Godejohann, M., Braumann, U. and Spraul, M. (2003). *Anal. Chim. Acta* 488, 35–51.

Gil, A.M., Duarte, I., Cabrita, E., Goodfellow, B., Spraul, M. and Kerssebaum, R. (2004). *Anal. Chim. Acta* 506, 215–223.

Gotz, J., Schneider, J., Forst, P. and Weisser, H. (2003). *J. Am. Soc. Brew. Chem.* 61, 37–47.

Harris, R.K. (1983). *Nuclear Magnetic Resonance Spectroscopy: A Physicochemical View.* Longman Scientific & Technical, Essex.

Hoek, A., Hermans-Lokkerbol, A.C.J. and Verpoorte, R. (2001). *Phytochem. Anal.* 12, 53–57.

Khatib, A., Wilson, E.G., Kim, H.K., Lefeber, A.W.M., Erkelens, C., Choi, Y.H. and Verpoorte, R. (2006). *Anal. Chim. Acta* 559, 264–270.

Košir, I.J. and Kidrič, J. (2002). *Anal. Chim. Acta* 458, 77–84.

Lachenmeier, D.W., Franck, W., Humpfer, E., Schäfer, H., Keller, S., Mörtter, M. and Spraul, M. (2005). *Eur. Food Res. Technol.* 220, 215–221.

Le Gall, G., Puaud, M. and Colquhoun, I.J. (2001). *J. Agric. Food Chem.* 49, 580–588.

Martin, G.J., Benbernou, M. and Lantier, F. (1985). *J. Inst. Brew.* 91, 242–249.

Nord, L.I., Sorensen, S.B. and Duus, J.Ø. (2003). *Magn, Reson. Chem.* 41, 660–670.

Nord, L.I., Vaag, P. and Duus, J.Ø. (2004). *Anal. Chem.* 76, 4790–4798.

Pusecker, K., Holtzel, A., Albert, K., Bayer, E., Wildenauer, M. and Rust, U. (1997). *Monatsschr. Brauwiss.* 50, 70–74.

Pusecker, K., Albert, K. and Bayer, E. (1999). *J. Chromatogr.* A836, 245–252.

Rossmann, A. (2001). *Food Rev. Int.* 17, 347–381.

Sacchi, R., Mannina, L., Fiordiponti, P., Barone, P., Paolillo, L., Patumi, M. and Segre, A. (1998). *J. Agric. Food Chem.* 46, 3947–3951.

Stavri, M., Schneider, R., O'Donnell, G., Lechner, D., Bucar, F. and Gibbons, S. (2004). *Phytother. Res.* 18, 774–776.

Vinogradov, E. and Bock, K. (1998). *Carbohydr. Res.* 309, 57–64.

94

Methods for the Vibrational Spectroscopy Analysis of Beers

Salvador Garrigues and Miguel de la Guardia Department of Analytical Chemistry, University of Valencia, Valencia, Spain

Abstract

The main possibilities and drawbacks of vibrational spectroscopy techniques, infrared (both in the middle and near infrared ranges) and Raman, for the analysis of beers have been reviewed taking into consideration methods proposed in the scientific literature for the determination of as many as possible compounds and parameters of beers. Details about the procedures available and comments on the future developments in this field have been based on the experience of authors and extended checking of the characteristics of the procedures published till now.

List of Abbreviations

ANN	Artificial neuronal networks
ASBC	American Society of Brewing Chemistry
ATR	Attenuated total reflectance
DR	Dynamic range
EBC	European Brewery Convention
FA	Flow analysis
FTIR	Fourier transform infrared
GC	Gas chromatography
ICP-MS	Inductively coupled plasma-mass spectrometry
IR	Infrared
LD	Limit of detection
LED	Light emitting diode
MIR	Middle infrared
MLR	Multiple linear regression
MS	Mass spectrometry
NIR	Near infrared
NMR	Nuclear magnetic resonance
PARAFAC	Parallel factor analysis
PCA	Principal component analysis
PLS	Partial least squares
SEC	Standard error of calibration
SEP	Standard error of prediction
SIA	Sequential injection analysis

Introduction

Vibrational spectroscopy covers a vast wavenumber range, from 12,500 to 10 cm^{-1}, between the visible and the microwave frequencies and offers interesting information about the transitions between the fundamental and excited vibrational stages of molecules.

Infrared (IR) and Raman spectroscopy are the main vibrational techniques and, on considering IR, middle infrared (MIR) and near infrared (NIR) must be evaluated separately with regard to functional differences in instrumentation and nature of the bands obtained from the interactions between IR radiation and molecules.

Nowadays, based on the developments in instrumentation and software for data treatment, vibrational spectroscopy has become an important tool for quantitative analysis in addition to its traditional applications in qualitative analysis.

Taking into consideration the aqueous nature of beer samples and the tremendous absorption of water in the MIR and NIR ranges, it is clear that old filter-based and dispersive instruments and classical materials used to build cells were scarcely suitable to obtain data about these samples. However, the new developments in fast techniques based on diode array detectors and Fourier transform-based instruments offer exciting possibilities to cumulate hundreds of scans per spectrum in a short time and thus provide an excellent signal-to-noise ratio, absolutely necessary to obtain spectra in the presence of water as a solvent and/or matrix.

The possibilities offered by vibrational spectrometry to measure transmission and reflectance modes together with its flexibility to obtain spectra from solid, liquid, and gas samples, can be considered as their major advantage for applied analysis (Cadet and de la Guardia, 2000).

However incorporation of flow analysis (FA) strategies to the measurements in both, IR and Raman, increases clearly the features of the procedures based on vibrational spectrometry, increasing the speed and precision of

Beer in Health and Disease Prevention
ISBN: 978-0-12-373891-2

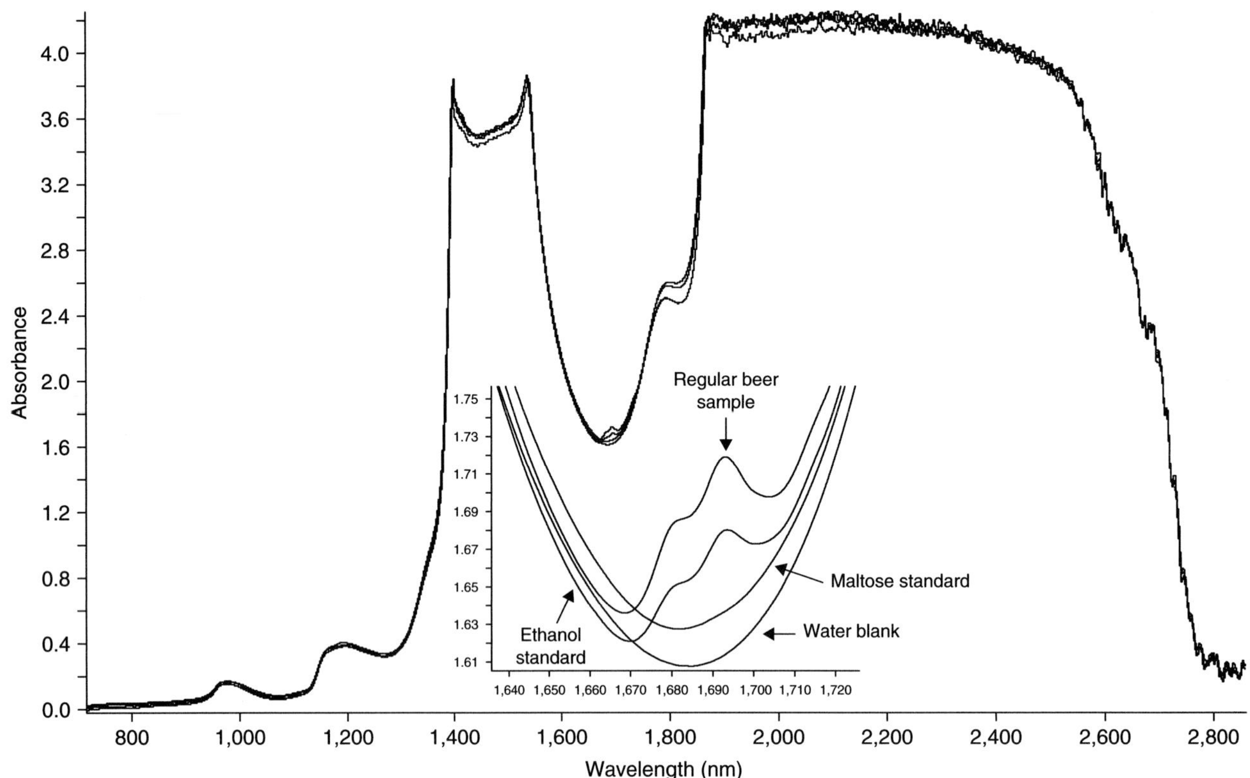

Figure 94.1 Transmittance NIR spectra of water, an ethanol standard, a maltose standard and regular beer using air as a reference.

determinations and reducing drastically the reagent's consumption and waste generation, thus, contributing to the development of environment friendly methodologies (Garrigues and de la Guardia, 2002).

In this chapter, we will consider the main applications that can be found in the literature for the analysis of beers by IR and Raman spectroscopy, and we will look to the future developments in this field.

Vibrational Spectra of Beers

The water content of beers is approximately 90–92% m/m, so the characteristic vibrational spectra of beers are strongly dominated by water and affected by the contribution of two other main constituents: ethanol and carbohydrates.

We can consider maltose as the representative carbohydrate in beers because it is the major sugar in malt and cereals used in the brewing process and the main building block for dextrins.

Briefly, to interpret vibrational spectra of beers it is necessary to consider the spectra of water, ethanol, and maltose.

In the NIR interval between 700 and 2,500 nm (approximately 18,285–4,000 cm^{-1}), water presents four intense absorption bands which increasing order of intensity correspond to 970 nm a combination band ($2\nu_1 + \nu_3$), 1,200 nm combination band ($\nu_1 + \nu_2 + \nu_3$), 1,450 nm corresponding to ($\nu_1 + \nu_3$), and 1,930 nm due to the combination ($\nu_1 + \nu_2$), where ν_1 is the vibration corresponding to symmetric stretching mode, ν_2 the bending mode, and ν_3 an asymmetric stretching one (Maeda *et al.*, 1995). For a pathlength of 0.2 mm, the band at 1,930 nm presents an absorbance intensity of approximately 1.1 absorbance units, whereas the absorbance at 1,450 nm is around 0.25 units. Pathlengths higher than 3 mm provide a saturation of the aforementioned two bands as can be seen in Figure 94.1, which corresponds to NIR spectra obtained by transmittance measurements in a glass vial with an optical pathlength of 6.5 mm. Under these conditions, water bands at 1,200 and 970 nm can be clearly seen.

Figure 94.1 also shows the NIR spectrum of ethanol and maltose standards and the signal corresponding to a regular beer. It can be appreciated that in the region between 1,550 and 1,800 nm water absorbs less than ethanol, maltose, and beer. For a pathlength equal or lower than 1 mm, this behavior can also be observed in the region between 2,000 and 2,400 nm. Then, if we use water as a reference apart from a complete transparency below 1,350 nm, the aforementioned two spectral windows can be used for determination of ethanol and maltose.

The spectral range between 1,550 and 1,820 nm is shown in Figure 94.2a, in which the characteristic spectra of ethanol, maltose and those of three different types of beer can be observed: regular, low-alcohol content (below 1% v/v) and alcohol-free beer. As it can be seen, ethanol presents

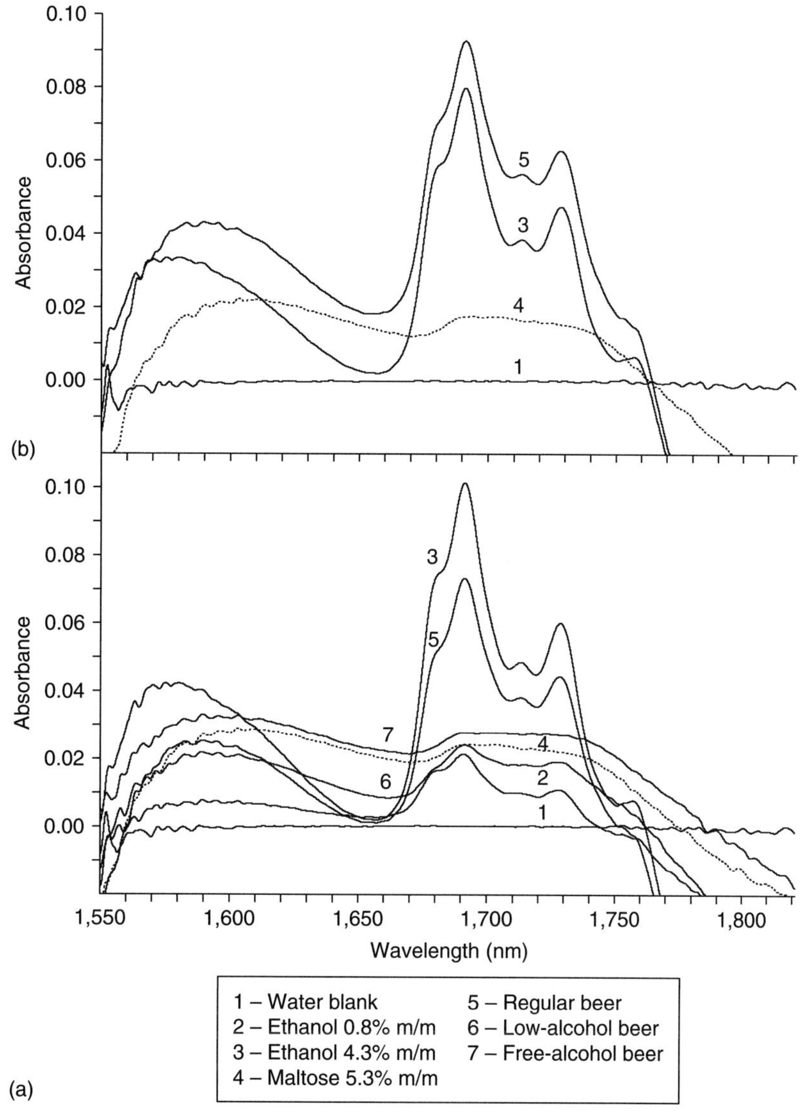

Figure 94.2 Transmittance NIR spectra using water as a reference.

a band at 1,570 nm whereas maltose occurs at 1,590 nm. Both bands correspond to the first overtones of the OH vibration of alcohols. Approximately 1,700 nm bands corresponding to first overtones of CH stretch-vibration can be seen. For ethanol, bands at 1,684 and 1,692 nm are due to the first overtone of the two —CH_3 asymmetric stretching modes and bands at 1,714 and 1,729 nm to the —CH_2— and —CH_3 asymmetric stretching, respectively, whereas maltose exhibits a wide band probably due to the highly varying environment of the different CH bands within the carbohydrate molecule (Adachi *et al.*, 2002).

In the region between 2,200 and 2,400 nm, three peaks for ethanol – 2,260, 2,300 and 2,350 nm – can be observed. Maltose exhibits a broad band between 2,050 and 2,200 nm that can be assigned to combination bands of the OH vibrations of alcohols. Two less intense peaks are present around 2,280 and 2,320 nm.

Water presents a high absorption in the middle range (4,000–300 cm^{-1}), and because of that the pathlength value used for transmission measurements markedly affects terribly the spectra obtained.

Water has two intense bands around 3,400 and 1,600 cm^{-1}, which correspond to fundamental vibrations of —OH groups. Owing to the high absorbance of water in the MIR, attenuated total reflectance (ATR) technique or transmittance with a pathlength of the order of 0.01–0.05 mm are required to obtain an adequate transparent region using water as a reference. Figure 94.3 shows ATR spectra of water, also for ethanol, maltose standards and a regular beer.

Spectra shown in Figure 94.3 is evidence of the differences between ethanol, beer and maltose as compared with water in the regions around 3,000 and 1,000 cm^{-1}. Inset figures correspond to MIR spectra obtained using a blank

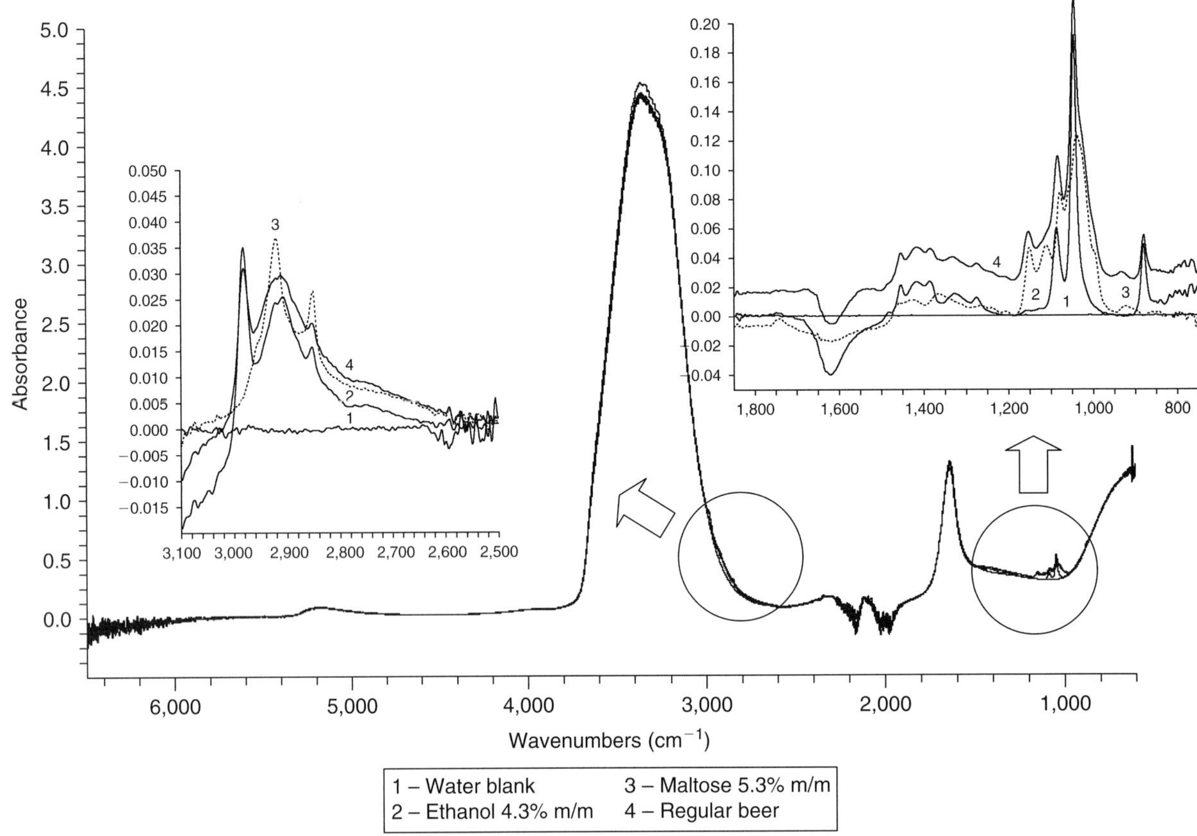

Figure 94.3 ATR-MIR spectra of water, an ethanol standard, a maltose standard and regular beer using air as a reference. Inset figures: detailed selected regions of the spectra using water as a reference.

of water. As it has been indicated in the Introduction section of this chapter, Fourier transform-based spectrometers enable a fast recording of the whole spectrum and final spectra is obtained by accumulating a significant number of scans to increase the signal-to-noise ratio.

It can be appreciated that both, ethanol and maltose, present absorption bands in the selected regions: ethanol strongly absorbs at 877, 1,052 (phase C—C—O stretch), 1,086, 2,850, 2,900 and 2,970 cm^{-1}, whereas maltose shows several overlapping bands ranging from 998 to 1,155 cm^{-1}, also the bands at 2,850 and 2,900 cm^{-1}.

As compared with the NIR region, the MIR ethanol and maltose spectra present an important degree of overlap and thus, for direct analysis of beer, the use of derivative spectra and/or chemometric data treatment is necessary.

Figure 94.4 shows typical ATR–FTIR (Fourier transform infrared) spectra of ethanol and maltose standards, and those of three different beer samples (alcohol-free, low content and regular), all of them in absorbance mode together with the first- and second-order derivative signals. It is noticeable how ethanol can be then clearly distinguished from the maltose contribution.

Raman spectroscopy has been proposed for the analysis of ethanol in beverages (Galloway, 1992; Mendes *et al.*, 2003; Nordon *et al.*, 2005) and also in ethanol-fuel (Mendes *et al.*, 2003), because Raman spectrum of ethanol presents well-defined emission bands.

The most important Raman band of ethanol is presented at 883 cm^{-1} shift and corresponds to the symmetric C—C—O stretching. Other typical bands are located at 1,097 cm^{-1} (CH_3 bending), 1,053 cm^{-1} (asymmetric C—C—O stretching), 1,276 cm^{-1} (CH_2 wagging) and 1,455 cm^{-1} (C—OH bending). Additionally, three bands are present between 3,000 and 2,800 cm^{-1} corresponding to CH stretching modes. As compared with Raman spectra of beers, the main signal differences are due to the contribution of maltose, also providing in some cases a shift of the spectral baseline due to the sample fluorescence.

Vibrational Analysis of Beers

Traditional techniques such as NIR, MIR or Raman spectroscopy could be applied to the determination of the main analytes present in beers.

It is clear that, based on the characteristic bands present in untreated samples reported in the previous section, analytes such as ethanol or maltose could be determined directly in previously degassed samples by transmittance or reflectance measurements.

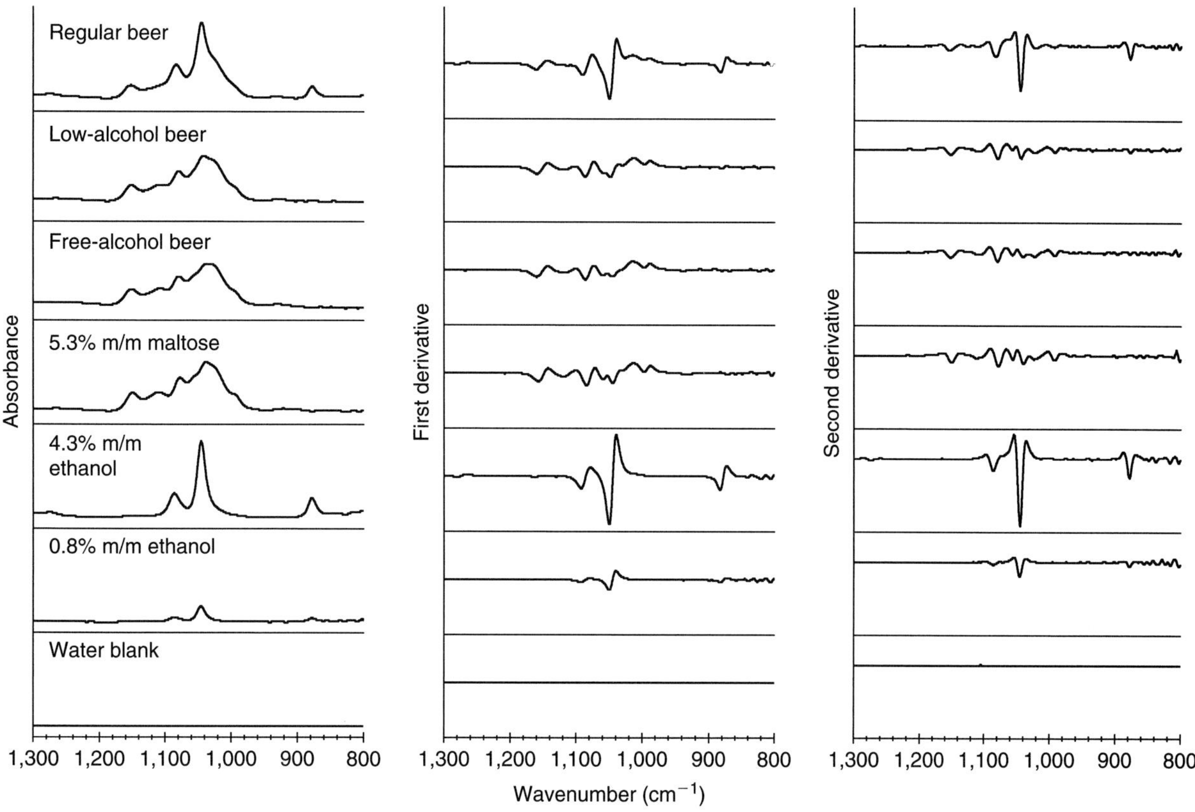

Figure 94.4 Selected regions in the ATR spectra: zero order, first derivative and second derivative.

In this section, we will detail the methodology found in the literature for beer analysis based on the selection of the most appropriate bands in zero-order or first-order spectra and the use of external calibrations built from pure standard solutions or previously analyzed samples.

We have not considered the multivariate-based calibration techniques, which will be commented in the next section devoted to chemometric methods.

NIR spectroscopy

Table 94.1 summarizes papers found in the literature concerning transmission, reflectance, or transflectance measurements in the NIR range.

The main part of studies concern the determination of ethanol (Coventry and Hunston, 1984; Halsey, 1985; Gallignani *et al.,* 1993; Luo and Liu, 1998; Schropp *et al.*, 2002; Engelhard *et al.*, 2004) or ethanol and maltose (Gallignani *et al.,* 1994a), ethanol and extract (Schropp *et al.,* 2002) or ethanol and original gravity (Halsey and Buckee, 1985).

Beer samples, previously analyzed, are used to look for specific bands in the NIR, suitable for ethanol determination; and Coventry and Hunston (1984), established that absorbance measurements at 1,386 nm in the zero-order spectra and measurements at 1,672 nm in the first-order derivative were the most adequate for direct determination of ethanol; it was confirmed that first derivative data provided the best regression coefficient and the lowest standard error for analysis of samples not used to build the calibration.

However, Halsey (1985) confirmed that transmittance measurements provide more accurate results for ethanol determination than transflectance ones.

We confirmed that using peak-to-valley measurements between 1,680 and 1,703 nm in the first derivative spectra of degassed beers, an accurate determination of ethanol in the range 0.3–25% v/v, with a limit of detection of 0.1% v/v and using aqueous standards of ethanol for calibration (Gallignani *et al.*, 1993) can be done.

The aforementioned results were extended to the determination of both maltose and ethanol, using zero-order measurements at 1,414 nm and 1,693 nm (with a baseline established between 1,657 and 1,720 nm), respectively, a limit of detection of 0.07% v/v ethanol using water as a reference being obtained. However, the use of a 4.5% m/v maltose solution as a reference offers a simplified procedure for ethanol determination with a sampling frequency of 120 h^{-1} (Gallignani *et al.*, 1994a).

Luo and Liu (1998) also proposed external calibration with pure ethanol standards in water and the use of water as a blank for determination of ethanol up to 24% v/v

Table 94.1 NIR methods employed for beer analysis

Measurement mode instrument	*Data treatment calibration*	*Analyte*	*Band/spectral range considered*	*Figures of merit*	*Comments*	*Reference*
Dispersive (transmission) Varian Cary 500	Linear regression 5 ethanol/water standards (water as a reference)	Ethanol	1,692 nm (ethanol) and 1,719 nm (maltose presents the same absorption than 1,692 nm)	DR = 0–8% v/v LD = 0.07% v/v Correlation coefficient = 0.9995 (34 samples)	• Pathlength = 10 mm, resolution = 1 nm • Interpretative difference spectroscopy: measurement of the difference at two wavelengths • Valid for normal and low-alcohol content beers	Engelhard *et al.* (2004)
Dispersive (transmission) Anton Para Analyzer	Instrument calibration with water and a 10% v/v ethanol solution	Alcohol Real extract Original extract	1,150–1,200 nm	DR = 0.01–14.40% v/v, *P* = 0.02% v/v, R^2 = 0.9997 DR = 2.03–11.35% m/m, *P* = 0.01% m/m, R^2 = 0.9999 DR = 4.78–28.30% m/m, *P* = 0.02% v/v, R^2 = 0.9997	• Samples degassing by shaking and filtration • Analysis of 119 samples and comparing results obtained with those obtained by a distillation reference method • Original and real extract calculations require the determination of density using the DMA 4500 (Anton Paar)	Schropp *et al.* (2002)
Dispersive transmittance	External calibration Water as a blank	Ethanol	Absorbance at 1,382 + 1,691 + 1,730 nm	DR = up to 24% v/v *P* (*n* = 6) = 2.5–4%	• Sample diluted to 25 ml • Multiwavelength overlapping spectrometry	Luo and Liu (1998)
Dispersive transmittance (*b* = 10 mm) Perkin Elmer Lambda 9	External calibration using water as a reference	Ethanol Maltose	1,693 nm (baseline 1,657–1,720 nm) for ethanol 1,414 nm for maltose	For ethanol LD = 0.07% v/v *P* = 0.2% (regular beers) and 2.0% (low-alcohol beers)	• Degassing by filtration • Stopped flow strategy for a fast filling and cleaning of measurement cell • Comparison of different baseline corrections	Gallignani *et al.* (1994a)
	Simplified stopped flow method using 4.5% m/m maltose as reference	Ethanol		*P* = 0.5% (regular beers) and 1.1% (low-alcohol beers) Sampling frequency: 120 h^{-1}		
Dispersive transmittance Perkin Elmer Lambda 9	Simple regression External calibration: ethanol/water standards	Ethanol	First derivative Peak to valley lecture between 1,680 and 1,703 nm	DR = 0.3 – 25% v/v LD = 0.1% v/v *P* = 0.3%	• Sample degassing by filtration	Gallignani *et al.* (1993)
Transmittance Transflectance		Ethanol Original gravity			• Direct analysis of beers by NIR • Transmittance measurements more accurate than transflectance ones • Presented at the European Brewing Committee 20th Congress, Helsinki	Halsey and Buckee (1985)
Transmittance Neotec 6350 MKII (Pacific Scientific Gardner)	Absorbance and first derivative Beer samples: 30 for calibration and 114 for prediction	Ethanol	1,100–2,500 nm (30 scans per sample) Absorbance: 1,386 nm 1st derivative: 1,672 nm	Absorbance: SEC = 0.86, SEP = 1.08, *R* = 0.82 First derivative: SEC = 0.29, SEP = 0.54, *R* = 0.99	• Degassing by filtration	Coventry and Hunston (1984)

b, pathlength; DR, dynamic range; LD, limit of detection; *P*, precision; *R*, coefficient of regression; SEC, standard error of calibration; SEP, standard error of prediction.

using the sum of the absorbance data obtained at 1,302 + 1,691 + 1,730 nm in zero-order spectra.

Engelhard *et al.* (2004) have proposed the use of the technique called interpretative difference spectroscopy to compare the absorbance of ethanol and maltose at 1,692 nm with that of maltose at 1,719 nm. A limit of detection of 0.07% v/v is obtained using a pathlength of 10 mm with a series of five external standards of ethanol in water.

It can be concluded that NIR permits the direct measurement of ethanol in all types of beers without the need of a previous distillation or the use of multivariate calibrations.

MIR spectroscopy

Simple regression and external calibration from MIR spectra have been proposed for the determination of ethanol (Gallignani *et al.*, 1994b, c; Maudoux *et al.*, 1998; Gallignani *et al.*, 2005; Armenta *et al.*, 2006), maltose (Gallignani *et al.*, 1994c), dissolved CO_2 (Wilks, 1988) and oils (Skinner, 1996); the possibilities to determine carbohydrates (Haberkorn *et al.*, 2002) by using the standard addition approach is also evident.

For details about methods employed for MIR analysis of beers see Table 94.2. In the case of CO_2 determination, in-line measurements can be made by ATR measurements obtained at 4.26 μm (Wilks, 1988).

The method proposed for oils in beers is based on data at 2,930 cm^{-1} after beer filtration through polytetrafluoroehylene (PTFE) membranes or stirring with diatomeus earth followed by extraction with freon (Skinner, 1996), thus providing a methodology comparable to that employed for oil and grease determination in waters. It is interesting to note that contents up to 0.2 mg/l oil were found in beers, probably due to contamination from engines used in the brewing process.

Preliminary studies about ethanol determination were based on transmission measurements using 0.029 mm pathlength cells and first-order derivative measurements between 1,052 and 1,040 cm^{-1} after smoothing of the signals; a limit of detection of 0.025% v/v is reported (Gallignani *et al.*, 1994b). The aforementioned limit of detection provides a good tool for the analysis of low-alcohol content beers for which a maltose correction by measurements between 1,160 and 1,144 cm^{-1} in the first-order derivative spectra must be done (Gallignani *et al.*, 1994c). However, for beer samples with alcohol content equal or higher than 1% v/v, second order derivative measurements at 1,046 cm^{-1} corrected with a baseline established between 1,055 and 1,037 cm^{-1} does not require a maltose correction and provides a limit of detection of 0.035% v/v.

In recent years it has been proposed that ethanol can be determined by absorbance measurements at 871 cm^{-1}, corrected with a baseline established between 844 and 929 cm^{-1}, after online liquid–liquid extraction with chloroform (Gallignani *et al.*, 2005).

The use of vapor phase-FTIR, based on the direct injection of 1 μl degassed sample in a carrier stream of nitrogen gas at 90°C, provided a limit of detection of 0.07% (v/v) from measurements of the peak area between 1,150 and 950 cm^{-1} for a gas cell with a pathlength of 3.2 m and a volume of 110 ml (Perez-Ponce *et al.*, 1996). Recently, it has been evidenced that a low-cost device of 38 mm pathlength and 470 μl internal volume, which provides a limit of detection of 0.15% v/v (Armenta *et al.*, 2006) can be used.

Haberkorn *et al.* (2002) have developed a mid-IR flow through sensor for carbohydrate determination by sequential injection analysis (SIA) using 4% agarose polymer beads (Gelatin Sheparose 4B) with immobilized amyloglucosidase and based on differences between absorbance measurements at 1,049 cm^{-1} and the maximum absorbance in the range 1,090–1,070 cm^{-1} in the spectra obtained before and after enzymatic reaction. Beer samples were analyzed by standard addition approach.

On comparing methods proposed for beer analysis in the NIR and MIR range, it can be concluded that MIR provides a sensitive and versatile tool for direct measurements and to use simple external calibration lines in most of the proposed applications.

Chemometric Methods in Beer Analysis

Complex data treatment of spectra offers unique tools for multiparametric determination, and taking into account the great number of data provided by vibrational spectra is not at all surprising, MIR and NIR spectra have been used to obtain as much as possible information from untreated samples.

In the case of beer analysis, transmission and ATR data in the MIR and transmission and transflectance data in NIR, in addition to Raman spectra, have been employed to determine ethanol (Maudoux *et al.*, 1998; Norgaard *et al.*, 2000; Mendes *et al.*, 2003; Iñón *et al.*, 2005, 2006; Llario *et al.*, 2006; Lachenmeier, 2007); original extract (Norgaard *et al.*, 2000; Westad and Martens, 2000; Iñón *et al.*, 2005, 2006; Llario *et al.*, 2006); original gravity (Maudoux *et al.*, 1998; Lachenmeier, 2007), and, in some cases, other parameters like relative density, pH, lactic acid, bitterness and color (Lachenmeier, 2007), or nitrogen and polyphenols (Maudoux *et al.*, 1998).

Multivariate calibration strategies, from principal component analysis (PCA) to artificial neuronal networks (ANN) and, specially, partial least squares (PLS) have been employed for vibrational data treatment of beers.

PCA was used to classify beers based on their ethanol content; MIR data obtained in ATR mode together with nuclear magnetic resonance (NMR) data (Duarte *et al.*, 2004) were employed.

Table 94.3 shows a brief summary of applications found in the literature for multivariate analysis of beers based on

Table 94.2 MIR methods employed for beer analysis

Measurement mode instrument	*Data treatment calibration*	*Analyte*	*Band/spectral range considered*	*Figures of merit*	*Comments*	*Reference*
FTIR transmission (b = 38 mm) Bruker Tensor 27	Simple regression External calibration: ethanol/water mixtures	Alcohol	Peak area between 1,130 and 992 cm^{-1} (baseline: 1,158–957 cm^{-1})	LD = 0.15% v/v P = 0.2% Volume sample = 1 µl Sample frequency = 30 h^{-1}	• Ultrasonic sample degassing • Simple and low cost device for FTIR-vapor phase • Comparison with head space-GC	Armenta *et al.* (2006)
FTIR transmission (b = 0.5 mm) Perkin Elmer Spectrum 2000	Simple regression External calibration: 0.05–15% v/v ethanol/water	Ethanol	Absorbance at 877 cm^{-1} (baseline: 844–929 cm^{-1})	LD = 0.03% v/v P = 1.3% Volume sample = 1 ml Sample frequency = 25 h^{-1}	• Ultrasonic sample degassing • On-line liquid–liquid extraction with chloroform • Flow analysis	Gallignani *et al.* (2005)
FTIR transmission (b = 50 µm) Bruker IFS 88	Standard addition	Carbohydrate (expressed as maltose)	Difference between the absorbance at 1,049 cm^{-1} and the maximum absorbance value in the range from 1,090 to 1,070 cm^{-1} in the difference spectra before and after enzymatic reaction		• Ultrasonic degassing beers and diluted 1:10 with water • Mid-IR flow-through sensor for carbohydrate measurement in beers • Sequential injection analysis (SIA) • 4% agarose polymer beads with immobilized amyloglucosidase	Haberkorn *et al.* (2002)
FTIR transmission	Simple regression External calibration	Oils in beers	2,930 cm^{-1}	Contents found up to 0.2 mg/l	• Beer filtration through PTFE (pclytetrafluoroethylene) membranes or stirring with diatomeus earth and extraction with 1,1,2 trichlorotrifluoroethane (Freon 113)	Skinner (1996)

FTIR transmission (b = 3.2 m) Nicolet Magna 550	Simple regression External calibration: ethanol/water mixtures	Ethanol	1,150–950 cm^{-1} peak area	LD = 0.07% v/v P = 2.05% Sample volume = 1 μl Sampling frequency = 51 h^{-1}	• Vapor phase with a 3.2 m pathlength cell • Beer degassing by filtration and ultrasonic.	Perez-Ponce *et al.* (1996)
FTIR transmission (b = 0.029 mm) Perkin Elmer 1750	Simple regression External calibration: ethanol/water and maltose/water mixtures	Ethanol Maltose	Beers with ethanol > 1%: Second derivative at 1,046 cm^{-1} (baseline: 1,055–1,037 cm^{-1}) Low-alcohol beers < 1% First derivative + 13 points smoothing: 1,052–1,040 cm^{-1} (maltose correction: 1,160–1,144 cm^{-1})	LD = 0.035% v/v (second derivative) LD = 0.025% v/v (first derivative) Coefficient of regression = 0.991 Dynamic range: 0.5–12% v/v P: 0.7%	• Beer degassing by filtration • Micro-flow cell for measurements	Gallignani *et al.* (1994c)
FTIR transmission (b = 0.029 mm) Perkin Elmer 1750	Linear regression External calibration: ethanol/water mixtures	Ethanol	First derivative + 13 points smoothing: 1,052–1,040 cm^{-1}	LD = 0.025% v/v Dynamic range: 0.2–15% v/v Precision (n = 5): 0.5%	• Sample degassing by filtration and ultrasonic • The method can be applied to all types of alcoholic beverages • High sugar content beverages require a correction between 1,052 and 140 cm^{-1}.	Gallignani *et al.* (1994b)
Reflectance (ATR) LAN-1	In-line measurements	Dissolved CO_2	4.26 m		• MIR-ATR sensor for monitoring dissolved CO_2	Wilks (1988)

b, pathlength; GC, gas chromatography; LD: limit of detection; P, precision.

Table 94.3 Chemometrics methods applied to vibrational spectrometry analysis of beers

Technique measurement mode	*Data treatment standards number*	*Analyte*	*Factors or PC*	*RMSEC*	*RMSEP*	*Comments*	*Reference*
FTIR transmittance	PLS	Ethanol Original gravity Relative density pH Lactic acid Bitterness unit EBC color	3 2 4 5 6 6 7		0.21% v/v 0.44 m/m 0.0006 g/ml 0.11 78.52 mg/l 5.18 19.10	• 461 samples • No details about calibration and/or validation set	Lachenmeier (2007)
FT-NIR (transmission) combined with FTIR (ATR)	PLS C = 15, V = 28	Ethanol Original extract Real extract	4 3 4	0.103% v/v 0.211% m/m 0.208% m/m	0.121% v/v 0.192% m/m 0.095% m/m	• Cluster analysis for sample classification and selection of the calibration set • Combination of MIR and NIR spectra	Iñón *et al.* (2006)
	PCA–ANN	Ethanol Original extract Real extract	3 (N = 2) 9 (N = 4) 2 (N = 2)	0.092% v/v 0.059% m/m 0.141% m/m	0.091% v/v 0.145% m/m 0.046% m/m		
FTIR (ATR)	PLS C = 12, V = 11	Ethanol Original extract Real extract	2 3 3	0.12% v/v 0.17% m/m 0.069% m/m	0.14% v/v 0.20% m/m 0.075% m/m	• Cluster analysis for sample classification and selection of the calibration set • Combination of MIR and NIR spectra	Llario *et al.* (2006)
	PLS C = 12, V = 21	Ethanol Original extract Real extract	2 3 3	0.12% v/v 0.17% m/m 0.069% m/m	0.12% v/v 0.17% m/m 0.069% m/m		
	PLS C = 23, V = 21	Ethanol Original extract Real extract	2 3 3	0.32% v/v 0.19% m/m 0.077% m/m	0.12% v/v 0.20% m/m 0.103% m/m		
FT-NIR (transmission)	PLS C = 15, V = 28	Ethanol Original extract Real extract	3 4 4	0.10% v/v 0.18% m/m 0.13% m/m	0.08% v/v 0.14% m/m 0.12% m/m	• Cluster analysis for sample classification and selection of the calibration set • Sample introduction comparison: glass vials 6.5 mm and • Flow cell 1 mm	Iñón *et al.* (2005)
	PLS C = 30, V = 13	Ethanol Original extract Real extract	3 4 4	0.08% v/v 0.16% m/m 0.13% m/m	0.10% v/v 0.14% m/m 0.09% m/m		

FTIR (ATR) and NMR	PCA classification (also with NMR analysis)	Classification based in ethanol content: ale, large and alcohol-free				• Golden gate accessory (1 reflection) • 49 samples	Duarte *et al.* (2004)
FT-NIR (transflectance)	PLS External calibration $C = 12$, $V = 12$	Ethanol	4	0.425% v/v	0.324% v/v	• Band assignation for Raman spectra • Second derivative for Raman	Mendes *et al.* (2003)
FT-Raman	PLS 2nd derivative External calibration $C = 12$, $V = 12$	Ethanol	4	1.9% v/v	0.548% v/v		
Dispersive NIR (transmission)	Interval-PLS $C = 40$, $V = 20$	Original extract	2	0.15% Plato	0.17% Plato	• Pathlength = 10 mm • Range: 400–2,500 nm	Norgaard *et al.* (2000)
Dispersive NIR (transmission)	Jackknife PLS $C = 40$, $V = 20$	Original extract	4	0.14% Plato	0.17% Plato	• Quartz cell: 10 mm • Range: 400–2,500 nm	Westad and Martens (2000)
NIR (transmission) NIR (reflection, dried extract technique)	PLS $C = 70$, $V = 40$ Dispersive MLR – second derivative PLS	Alcohol Real extract original gravity nitrogen (ppm) Polyphenols	6 7 5	R: CV = 5.12% R: CV = 3.67% R: CV = 6.00% T: CV = 3.66% R: CV = 5.13% T: CV = 3.72% R: CV = 5.39%	CV = 5.94% CV = 6.19% CV = 6.07% T: CV = 6.06% R: CV = 9.03% T: CV = 4.74% R: CV = 8.04%	• Transmission (pathlength = 1 mm) • Reflection (dried extract technique)	Maudoux *et al.* (1998)

C, calibration; CV, coefficient of variation; PC: principal component; R, reflectance; RMSEC, root mean standard error of calibration; RMSEP, root mean standard error of prediction; T, transmittance; V, validation.

vibrational spectra and, as it can be seen, there are many alternatives based on the use of different data sets and software programs.

However, for a critical evaluation of the different strategies proposed, the size and selection criteria must be considered to establish the calibration set and the use or not of a validation sample set.

Pioneering studies of Maudoux *et al.* (1998) were based on NIR spectra obtained by transmission or reflectance after drying 800 μl of beer at 50°C in a glass filter. On using the spectral information in the range 1,100–2,500 nm, it was confirmed that reflectance mode was better than transmittance in all cases. Multiple linear regression (MLR) data treatment on second derivative spectra provided the best results for ethanol and original gravity prediction, PLS being the best treatment to obtain accurate data on real extract, total nitrogen, and total polyphenols.

Studies made by Martens *et al.* for PLS–NIR determination of original extract on transmission data obtained using a dispersive instrument and a pathlength of 10 mm evidenced that interval-PLS provided better results than the use of full spectra. Jackknife (Westad and Martens, 2000) and PC forwarded stepwise selection and recursively weighted regression (Norgaard *et al.*, 2000) were used for variable selection, being the best procedure, for a working range between 1,202 and 1,298 nm (49 variables). They provided the same predictive features for just 2 factors as compared with the jackknife, which requires 4 factors working in the wavelength range 1,152–1,330 nm (9 selected variables).

Mendes *et al.* (2003) selected the wavelength ranges 7,824–9,113 cm^{-1} and 5,529–6,025 cm^{-1} to determine ethanol by PLS–NIR using transflectance measurements and 12 pure standards as a calibration set. The method provided better features than the use of second derivative Raman spectra.

On considering our contribution in the field of beer analysis using chemometrics (Iñón *et al.*, 2005, 2006; Llario *et al.*, 2006), we can conclude that both NIR and MIR offer excellent tools for ethanol, original, and real extract determination in beers. For each measurement technique and measurement mode, specific wavenumber ranges must be selected to enhance the analytical results. It is also necessary to move from a spectral range to another on modifying the bandpass and, thus, for NIR transmission measurements the use of flow cells of 1 mm involves the selection of spectral windows between 2,298–2,337 nm, 2,259–2,348 nm and 2,249–2,303 nm for ethanol, original extract, and real extract, respectively, being selected for a 6.5 mm bandpass at 1,667–1,742 nm, 1,667–1,686 nm and 1,162–1,684 nm (Iñón *et al.*, 2005). The simultaneous treatment of MIR and NIR data involves the need to consider nonlinear relationships and thus ANN offers the best performance (Iñón *et al.*, 2006).

Lachenmeier (2007) used a Wine Scan instrument to obtain FTIR transmittance data, which, treated off-line by PLS considering full spectral range, provided good prediction features for ethanol and original gravity, and relatively good results for lactic acid and relative density. The instrument does not seem adequate for pH, bitterness, and color determination.

From published studies it is clear that chemometric and vibrational spectroscopy offers a great combination to evaluate major components in beer samples. However, in our opinion additional studies are required to extract as much possible information from vibrational spectra of beers and it could be also convenient to combine IR data with those obtained by other methodologies such as inductively coupled plasma-mass spectrometry (ICP-MS) and mass spectrometry (MS), which could incorporate information concerning elemental composition and trace organic compounds to create chemometric tools suitable to control all the parameters involved in both the origin of raw materials and the brewing process.

Beer Analyzers Based on Vibrational Spectroscopy

Ales and lager are two major categories of beers. Yeasts used in fermentation determine the differences between these types. Color, bitterness, and gravity are additional variables that further describe all beers. Color is determined by the type and amount of malt; bitterness depends on the type and amount of grain and hops used in the beer's production; and gravity refers to the beer density, related to dissolved sugars and alcohol content.

Local and global beer producers need to produce vast quantities of highly reproducible and comparable beer at many different sites and, because of this and legal requirements related with alcohol taxes, it is absolutely necessary to ensure the quality of the final product.

Beer analysis traditionally involves methods such as catalytic oxidation, fractional distillation, and gas chromatography. The high number of analysis to ensure the quality of the final product and the need for a fast response to detect changes in the production process have encouraged the commercialization of specific instruments for beer analysis.

One of the more popular and accurate beer analyzers has been the SCABA by Foss. From a degassed beer or wort sample this instrument determines, by U-shaped oscillator measures, the specific gravity and, using a catalytic sensor, the alcohol vapor in equilibrium with sample. pH and color of all beer types can also be measured. This analyzer requires only 50 ml of sample and has a capacity to do 20 determinations per hour. However, in the year 2000 the production of this instrument was stopped and 2007 was the last date for parts availability of the SCABA model 5610.

As it has been described in previous sections of this chapter, vibrational techniques, especially NIR-based ones, offer tremendous possibilities for direct alcohol measurement in liquid samples and because of this, in the past years, many of the commercialized beer analyzers incorporated NIR units for an accurate and fast determination of ethanol and other parameters such as original gravity and extract content.

Some examples of beer analyzers based on vibrational procedures are shown in Table 94.4. As it can be seen, most of them use transmittance measurements. Old fiber-based systems have been replaced by scanning monochromators, solid-state diode array detectors, or interferometer systems based on Fourier transform. A spectral range between 850 and 1,050 nm is commonly used but an extended range to 570 nm is required when these instruments incorporate color measurement modules.

In some cases, NIR spectrometers have been adapted for beer analysis, such as the Perkin Elmer Brewer's assistant, by incorporating a flow cell with an autosampler unit. Also specific software permits the determination of parameters such as alcohol content, original and present gravity from FT-NIR spectra and to estimate other properties as real or apparent extract, degree of fermentation, and energy value. This instrument requires only 5 ml of sample volume and can process 50 beers per hour.

Beer analyzer calibration is made, usually, by means of beer samples previously characterized by reference methods; complex mathematical routines based on the use of chemometrics for calculations are required.

In the past years, Anton Paar has commercialized a beer analyzer that combines a NIR alcoholyzer with an oscillating U-tube density meter. Using a high-resolution spectrometer and a patented selective alcohol measurement approach based on a narrow highly alcohol-specific range of the NIR spectrum, the alcohol contents is precisely determined. From density measurement the extract density is calculated. Original extract, degree of fermentation, and calories are also determined. One of the main advantages of this instrument is that it does not require chemometric calibration procedures needed by traditional NIR-based instruments: the system is simply adjusted with air and water and, occasionally, with an ethanol/water solution. Some details of this instrument, about the measuring range for the different parameters controlled and repeatability characteristics can be seen in Table 94.4. Only 30 ml degassed beer is required per measurement and studies comparing this instrument with the distillation method have shown no significant deviation of the mean values, the reproducibility being 0.025% v/v for alcohol determination.

In a collaborative study for ethanol determination in low alcohol and nonalcohol beers, 10 beer samples covering 5 ethanol levels were analyzed by 17 participant laboratories. Fourteen of these participants used the Anton Paar NIR analyzer and the results reported a repeatability of 0.022% and a reproducibility of 0.103% that was achieved for this instrument (Toivola *et al.*, 2005). For accurate determination of alcohol in low-alcohol content beer samples (>0.37% v/v) the NIR method was recommended.

NIR analyzers designed for reflectance measurement of solids and used for quality control of malt and other grains, incorporate in some cases a liquid module that permits the routine analysis of beer.

Among the different beer analyzers shown in Table 94.4, it is important to comment on the Infratec^{TM} 1256 beverage Analyzer (Foss). This system, suitable for analysis of different types of alcoholic beverages, permits a direct measurement of the samples into their bottles without sample preparation in less than 45 s. This high throughput analysis makes the use of this instrument to control the production at-line possible. The analyzer incorporates a selection of ready-to-use calibrations (regression programs) for different types of beverages, based on PLS and artificial neural network. Alcohol content, original extract, and color can be directly predicted and other calculated parameters are real extract, apparent extract, degree of fermentation, energy, specific gravity, original gravity, present gravity, extract gravity, spirit indication, and refractive index.

All beer analyzers performed accurately when samples were analyzed under controlled conditions, and any of them is adequate for online measurements.

Infrared Engineering (Essex, UK) developed an industrial beer analyzer, namely Liquidata, based on transmittance measurements using a 1 mm path length sensor probe that is inserted into the beer stream. This system works in the 750–3,000 nm range, among which five key wavelengths were identified for water in beer, eight are significant to ethanol, and five relevant to sugars. Eleven beers, covering alcohol content from 0% to 12% v/v and original gravity between 20° and 90°, were used for instrument calibration. The differences between the Liquidata results and those obtained by reference methods are adequate with the tolerance levels specified by brewers and a standard error of prediction lower than 0.04% ethanol was achieved for any beer analyzed with this system (Benson, 1996).

McNab Inc. also presented at the 107th Master Brewers Association of the Americas (Anniversary Convention, Cincinnati, Ohio, USA) a NIR probe (KSA monitor) for online alcohol determination in beer production by transmission measurements. This instrument is appropriate for brewing plants that produce multiple brands and identifies in-line brand changes.

VitalSensors Technologies developed a sensor for online determination of CO_2 in beer streams, based on ATR MIR measurements. This sensor is a solid-state device and operates at a wavelength of 4.27 µm. Errors due to density are eliminated and the sensor requires no maintenance. Other potential applications for using MIR-based sensors are the determination of ethanol, carbohydrates, and dissolved sugars.

However, in spite of the high number of specific instruments available for beer analysis and their applicability to solve real problems of production and control, there is a lack of information regarding the fundamentals and validation of results reported and, because of this, additional

Table 94.4 Examples of commercial beer analyzers based on the use of vibrational spectroscopy

Instrument	*Technique*	*Parameter: range (precision/accuracy)* *Calculated parameters*	*Details/remarks*
Quik-Check 10L (Leco Corporation)	NIR-transmission	Alcohol: 3–6% (*A* = ±0.035%) Original gravity: 30–60°S (*A* = ±0.2%)	• Requires calibration against known standards (well-characterized samples) • Electronic temperature controlled cell • Sample aspirated with an internal pump
Rapitec 5665 Beer Analyzer (Foss)	NIR dispersive: fast scanning monochromator (1,100–2,500 nm)	AlcoholExtract	• Source: tungsten lamp • Detector: lead sulphide • Analysis time: 60 samples/h • Sample size: 50 ml/min • Supplied with a selection of a beer calibrations • Last year of production: 2001 (parts availability until 2008)
Infratec™ 1256 Beverage Analyzer (Foss)	NIR dispersive: scanning (850–1,050 nm/ 570–1,100 nm with color module)	Alcohol Original extract Color *Real extract, apparent extract, degree of fermentation, energy, specific gravity, present gravity, extract gravity, refractive index*	• At-line operating • Without sample preparation: beer inside bottle • Regression programs: PLS and ANN • Analysis time: <45 s • Sample volume: min 215 ml
Infratec™ 1241 Grain Analyzer with Sample Transport/Beer Module (Foss)	NIR (transmission) dispersive: scanning (850–1,050 nm/ 570–1,100 nm with color module)	Barley malt: protein, moisture, extract and soluble protein Green malt: moisture contentBeer: alcohol and real extract *Original extract, real degree of fermentation, calories*	• Source: Tungsten halogen lamp • Detector: silicon • Resolution: 2 nm • Regression programs: PLS and ANN • Sample preparation: degassing
Brewer's Assistant (Perkin Elmer)	FT-NIR with autosampler	Alcohol content: 0–12% v/v Original gravity: 1,019–1,095 Kg/l (19–95°S) Present gravity: 0,998–1,030 Kg/l (−1.8 to 26°S) Other properties: real extract, apparent extract, degree of fermentation, energy value	• Quartz NIR cell with auto sampler • Pathlength: 0.5 mm • Sample volume: 5 ml • Analysis time: approximately 50 samples/h • Regression program: PLS
Alcolyzer Plus Beer Analyzing System (Anton Paar)	NIR dispersive: high resolution scanning	Alcohol content: 0–12% v/v (*P* = 0.01% v/v) Density (with an oscillating U-tube density meter): 0–3 g/ml *Real extract: 0–20% m/m (P = 0.01% m/m)* *Original extract: 0–30% Plato (P = 0.03% Plato)* *Degree of fermentation (%)* *Calories (Kcal/Kg)*	• Does not require chemometric calibration • Sample volume: 30 ml • Analysis time: 15 samples/h
Series 1000 Alcohol Analyzer (NIR Technology Systems)	NIR transmission: solid-state diode array (860–1,020 nm)	Alcohol content	• Pathlength: 30 mm • Calibration using standard samples
LIQUIDATA Infrared Engineering	NIR (transmission) dispersive: 750–3,000 nm	Alcohol (SEP <0.04% v/v)	• On-line measurements • 1 mm pathlength probe
VS-1000C (VitalSensors Technologies)	NIR (attenuated total reflectance)	CO_2 dissolved	• Wavelength: 4.27 μm • Measurement directly in the product stream
KSA monitor (McNab, Inc.)	NIR-absorbance	Alcohol	• On-line measurements • Does not require recalibration per beer brand • Alcohol reading not affected by changes in color, turbidity or presence of sugars

A: accuracy; FT: Fourier transform; *P*: precision.

research must take place to clearly show the users the ways to improve their analysis based on vibrational spectroscopy and this is the reason for the continuous publication of methodologies that involve adaptation of MIR, NIR, or Raman general instruments to the determination of, as much as possible, beer parameters based on the use of different measurement modes and chemometric approaches (see section "Chemometric Methods in Beer Analysis").

Vibrational Spectroscopy for Control of Brewing Process

In addition to final beer analysis, vibrational spectroscopy has been applied to the different stages of the brewing process and, as for example, Meurens and Yan (2002) in the *Handbook of Vibrational Spectroscopy* include a specific chapter devoted to the applications of vibrational spectroscopy in brewing.

Figure 94.5 shows the main phases of brewing process from malting to milling, mashing, brewing, fermentation, maturation, and packaging; and it is clear that many of the main beer parameters need to be controlled in several of these steps.

Table 94.5 shows some of the contributions that can be found in the literature devoted to the use of vibrational spectroscopy for analytical purposes during the brewing process. NIR spectroscopy, in the reflectance mode, seems to be a common technique used for the quality control of dry raw materials for brewing.

Control of the barley malting process is not only important for the final quality of beer, but it is also necessary to ensure the characteristics of other raw materials such as hop, yeast, and obviously, water.

Barley is a major component of the brewing process, and parameters such as moisture, protein, β-glucan, and malt extract require a rigorous control that can be made by NIR spectroscopy as it can be seen in Table 94.5.

The Analysis Committee of the European Brewery Convention (EBC) proposed a comparative study between laboratories for determination of moisture and nitrogen content of barley and malt by NIR spectroscopy. Laboratory participants in this trial used their own calibrations and the measurements were carried out in either transmission and/or reflectance mode using whole kernels or ground samples. In this study, relative standard deviation values of NIR data were much higher than those found for the reference methods, probably due to the different calibration procedures and methodologies used by participants (Angelino, 1996). The American Society of Brewing Chemistry (ASBC) in a posterior collaborative trial (Munar *et al.*, 1998) concluded that values of moisture and protein in whole grain barley obtained by NIR did not differ significantly from those obtained with conventional techniques, and recommended the inclusion of NIR spectroscopy as analytical methods for the control of the aforementioned parameters.

In a collaborative study using the InfraAlyzer 400, Carnielo *et al.* (1985) concluded that transfer of centrally prepared calibrations to other reflectance instruments was

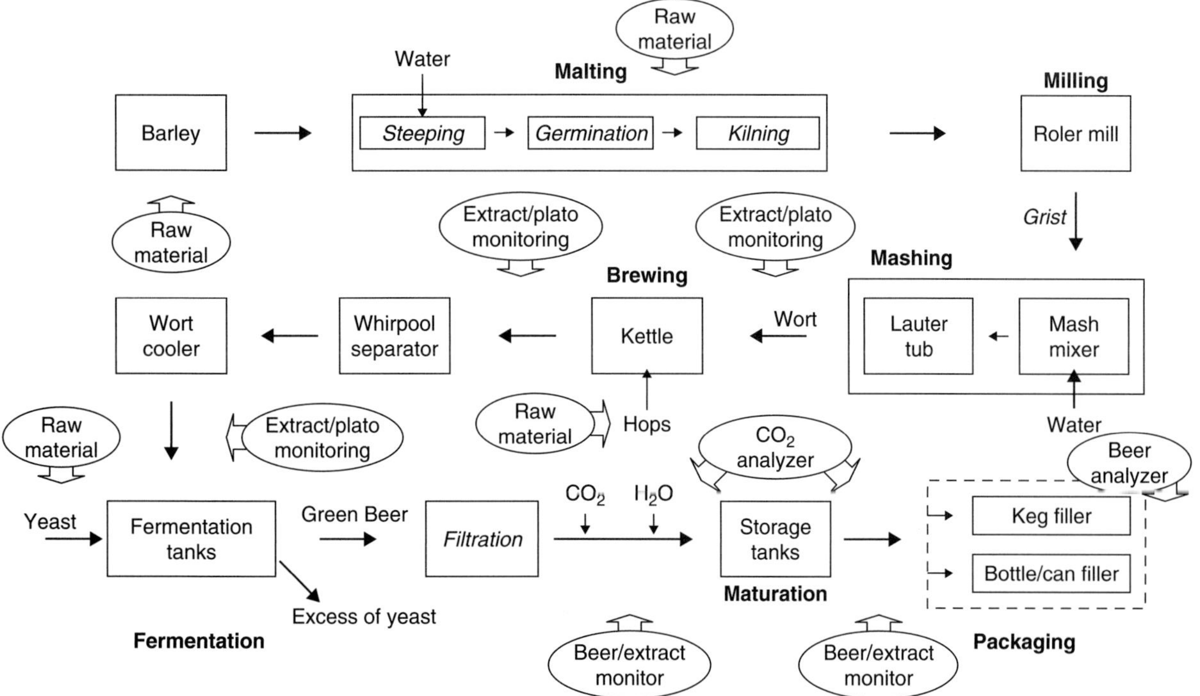

Figure 94.5 Possibilities of the use of vibrational techniques during the brewing process.

Table 94.5 The use of vibrational spectroscopy in the brewing process

Technique	*Analyte/parameter*	*Brewing process step*	*Reference*
NIR reflectance	Malt extract	Malting (barley)	McGuire (1982)
NIR reflectance	Malting potential of barley: moisture, malt extract, protein and β-glucan	Malting (barley)	Henry (1985a)
NIR reflectance	Barley and malt quality	Malting	Carnielo *et al.* (1985)
NIR reflectance	α- and β-glucans	Malting (barley)	Henry (1985b)
NIR transmittance	Maltose, glucose, maltotriose, total carbohydrates, fermentable sugars, total soluble nitrogen, free α-amino nitrogen and β-glucan	Mashing (wort)	Halsey (1986)
NIR reflectance	Moisture, nitrogen, hot water extract, total carbohydrates, fermentable sugars, total soluble nitrogen and fermentability	Malting (malt)	Halsey (1987)
NIR reflectance	Moisture, protein	Malting (barley)	Yan *et al.* (1991)
NIR transmission MIR transmission	Maltose, glucose, total fermentable sugars, maltotriose, nitrogen and free α-amino nitrogen	Mashing (wort)	Tenhunen *et al.* (1994)
NIR reflectance	Glycogen in yeast	Fermentation (yeast)	Mochaba *et al.* (1994)
NIR reflectance MIR transmittance	Trehalose in yeast	Fermentation (yeast)	Moonsamy *et al.* (1995)
NIR transmission MIR reflectance	Moisture and N content in barely and malt	Malting (barley and malt)	Angelino (1996)
Transmission NIR	Wort fermentability	Mashing (wort)	Sjoholm *et al.* (1996)
NIR transmission	Fermentable sugar	Mashing (wort)	Wilke and Parthey (1996)
NIR reflectance	Total protein in yeast	Fermentation (yeast)	Majara *et al.* (1998)
NIR reflectance	Soluble substances, β-glucan and moisture	Malting (barley)	Allosio *et al.* (1997)
NIR reflectance (ATR)	Maltose, glucose and fermentable sugars	Mashing (wort)	Eberl *et al.* (1998)
MIR reflectance diffuse	Yeast strains	Fermentation (yeast)	Timmins *et al.* (1998)
NIR transflectance	Wort parameters	Mashing (wort)	Ratcliffe and Panozzo (1999)
NIR reflectance	α-Acid content, β-acid content and hop storage index	Brewing (hop)	Garden *et al.* (2000)
NIR reflectance	Protein content in barley and malt	Malting (barley and malt)	Fox *et al.* (2002)
NIR reflectance	Fermentability wort Apparent degree of fermentability. Final attenuation apparent extract	Mashing (wort)	Samp *et al.* (2003)
NIR transmission	Barley quality: germination vigour	Malting (barley)	Moller (2004)

found to be possible for the determination of moisture and protein content in barley and malt, but not in malt extract or modified malt.

Malting quality of barley is related to the amount of β-glucan dissolved at low pH under defined conditions. Malt hot water extract is another parameter used in assessment of malting quality of barley and it is a function of the amount of sugar and low-molecular-weight dextrans produced during mashing by action of α-amylase on the barley starch. Conventional methods to control the aforementioned parameters are tedious and poorly adapted to rapid screening of early generation breeding lines. Thus, NIR reflectance could be an alternative for rapid control of barley and to predict the quality of malt obtained; it was most successful when the malt was produced without additives or addition of water during the germination process (Henry, 1985a).

The study of Moller (2004) using NIR transmittance measurements has evidenced the capability of this technique for the prediction and viability of barley. To do this, PCA and PLS regression must be combined, using the jack-knife validation to calculate the important variables to be considered and measured.

Parallel factor analysis (PARAFAC), a three-way factor analysis technique, has also been applied to the barley transformation in malt (monitoring the malting process). Appearance of soluble substances, β-glucan degradation, and moisture modification are parameters that can be controlled by PARAFAC–NIR to differentiate batches of barley during the malting process (Allosio *et al.*, 1997).

The possibilities of NIR spectroscopy to control the evolution of the content of *S*-methylmethionine during the killing process have been studied by Yan *et al.* (1991), having obtained standard errors of prediction of 3.5 ppm for the validation set of samples.

Garden *et al.* (2000) studied the application of NIR spectroscopy for the determination of α-acid content, β-acid content, and hop storage index in baled hop samples.

During the mashing process, the extraction of maltose and other fermentable sugar from solubilized starch occurs, and then the wort is obtained. This extract can be measured by transmittance or reflectance measurement.

Halsey (1986) studied the analysis of extracted wort by transmittance measurements, using a pathlength of 3 mm, after sampling, filtering, and thermostating of this extract. In a posterior study, Halsey (1987) evaluated the possibility of direct reflectance measurement of whole malt to predict wort composition (hot water extract, total carbohydrates, fermentable sugars, total soluble nitrogen, free amino nitrogen, and fermentability) from spectra on whole malt, without the need for mashing, and in less than 2 min.

Tenhunen *et al.* (1994) compared the use of transmission measurements in the NIR and MIR ranges and used Fourier transform instruments for the determination of maltose, glucose, total fermentable sugars, maltotriose, nitrogen, and free α-amino nitrogen in worts, requiring only the sample filtration. A CaF_2 transmission cell with a 0.5 mm pathlength was used for NIR in the range 2,000–2,440 nm, whereas a 0.025 mm pathlength and a spectral range 900–1,600 cm^{-1} was employed for MIR. The use of a transmission cell in MIR provided better results than a ZnSe ATR cell due to the possible deposition of some wort compounds on the ATR crystal. MIR spectroscopy provides slightly better results than NIR but sample handling by the first technique was more difficult. This negative aspect can be overcome by using FA technique (Garrigues and de la Guardia, 2002).

Eberl *et al.* (1998) proposed the use of ATR measurements for in-line NIR determination of maltose, glucose, and fermentable sugars during the mashing process; the method requiring only a few seconds to obtain the results.

Wilke and Parthey (1996) proposed the use of a NIR-based sensor for in-line measurements of fermentable sugars during the mashing process.

An enhanced method for calibration of NIR reflectance determination of fermentability wort, based on the application of an orthogonal signal correction algorithm before the use of PLS calibration was developed by Samp *et al.* (2003). This algorithm removed almost 60% of the variance in the NIR spectra, which was independent or orthogonal to the fermentability measures and the standard error of prediction; apparent degree of fermentability and final attenuation of the apparent extract were improved by 50% and 90%, respectively.

Garden *et al.* (2000) studied the application of NIR spectroscopy for the determination of α- and β-acid content, also hop storage index, in baled hop samples.

Active yeast is important for brewing high-quality beer, and traditional methods are based on fermentation performance. Content of protein, trehalose, and glycogen are parameters also used to asses the viability of yeast employed in brewing. Majara *et al.* (1998) have proposed a NIR method for the determination of protein in brewers' yeast that requires only 30 min per sample (25 min correspond to sample preparation). Moonsamy *et al.* (1995) have obtained acceptable results, as compared with enzymatic methods or by the cell dry weigh method, for a rapid NIR measurement of yeast trehalose for both dried yeast and slurry samples containing 30% m/m. Direct slurry measurements by transmittance NIR provide more accurate results than reflectance NIR on dried yeast, probably due to the absence of the drying stage. Mochaba *et al.* (1994) propose the use of NIR spectroscopy for measurement of yeast glycogen.

It can be seen that vibrational spectroscopy is highly valuable to study solid or suspended materials in addition to control wort and beer, and thus efforts must be made to not only improve the capabilities of MIR and NIR, but also to incorporate Raman measurements to evaluate the steps of the brewing process.

Concluding Remarks and Future Developments

The details of the methods available in the literature for beer analysis through IR and Raman spectroscopy are evidence of the validity of these techniques for the fast and accurate determination of major and minor components of beer together with their capability to extract information about the main characteristics of these samples.

However, additional efforts must be made to extend the applicability of vibrational spectroscopy-based techniques to obtain data about trace compounds of beer.

However, the new technology of light emitting diodes (LEDs) can offer possibilities for the development of low cost, compact, and portable devices suitable for use in the brewing process for sensoring the fermentation of malt extracts and alcohol formation.

Advances in automation, especially those based on modern flow methodologies, such as SIA (Haberkorn *et al.*, 2002) and multicommutation (Ródenas-Torralba *et al.*, 2004), could also increase the practical features of vibrational spectroscopy-based methods by increasing the sampling throughput and reducing the consumption of samples and reagents, also by minimizing the waste generation. In this sense, advances could be expected in the coming years in the automation of vapor-phase IR spectroscopy by the incorporation of minipumps and pinch valves, which could provide continuous sensitive measurements of volatile beer components without any previous sample preparation.

Finally, the tremendous growth of chemometrics and the availability of software packages for PLS and ANN will encourage the people working in this field to model vibrational data, individually or together, with other techniques to obtain a complete picture of processes and samples. In this sense, the classical approach based on the addition of sample information and matrix treatment will also be improved by the use of second- or third-order methodologies involving the hypermatrix data treatment of spectra coming from different techniques or from a single technique but incorporating the evolution of samples with time.

Thus, we can conclude that we are at the beginning of a long trip in which the molecular information of beers obtained by IR and Raman will be of a great value for beer analysis.

Summary Points

- Infrared spectra of beers reflect the characteristics bands of their main constituents: water, ethanol, and carbohydrates (maltose).
- Ethanol presents characteristic bands in the NIR region at 1,570, 1,684, 1,692, 1,714, 1,729, 2,260, 2,300, and 2,350 nm.
- Maltose, the main carbohydrate in beers, presents broad bands at 1,590 nm, also between 2,050 and 2,200 nm, and two less intense peaks around 2,280 and 2,320 nm.
- In the MIR range, ethanol presents characteristic bands at 877, 1,052, 1,086, 2,850, and 2,970 cm^{-1}, whereas maltose has several overlapped peaks between 998 and 1,155 cm^{-1} and characteristic bands at 2,850 and 2,900 cm^{-1}.
- Ethanol and/or maltose can be determined directly in beer samples by infrared transmittance or reflectance measurements using univariate external calibrations.
- Modern beer analyzers are based on infrared (NIR) and density measurements and permit to determine several parameters in each sample in less than 1 min.
- Combined use of infrared measurements and chemometrics offers a powerful tool for beer control analysis.
- Vibrational spectroscopy can be used at-line and/or in-line for quality control of the different stages of brewing process.

References

Adachi, D., Katsumoto, Y., Sato, H. and Ozaki, Y. (2002). *Appl. Spectros.* 56, 357–361.

Allosio, N., Boivin, P., Bertrand, D. and Courcoux, P. (1997). *J. Near Infrared Spectros.* 5, 157–166.

Angelino, S.A.G.F. (1996). *J. Inst. Brew.* 102, 73–74.

Armenta, S., Esteve-Turrillas, F.A., Quintas, G., Garrigues, S., Pastor, A. and de la Guardia, M. (2006). *Anal. Chim. Acta* 569, 238–243.

Benson, I.B. (1996). In Davies, A.M.C. and Williams, P. (eds), *NIRS: The Future Waves*, pp. 239–248. NIR publications, Chichester.

Cadet, F. and de la Guardia, M. (2000). Infrared quantitative analysis. In Meyers, R.A. (ed.), *Encyclopedia of Analytical Chemistry*, pp. 10879–10909. John Wiley & Sons, Chichester.

Carnielo, M., Grandclerc, J., Muller, P., Moll, M., Grandvoinet, P., Berger, M., Simiand, J.P., Lemaitre, M., Mari, D., Lhommel, F., Leboeuf, J.P., Rouiller, M. and Mabille, M. (1985). *J. Inst. Brew.* 91, 174–179.

Coventry, A.G. and Hunston, M.J. (1984). *Cereal Foods World* 29, 715–718.

Duarte, I.F., Barros, A., Almeida, C., Spraul, M. and Gil, A.M. (2004). *J. Agric. Food Chem.* 52, 1031–1038.

Eberl, R., Parthey, B. and Wilke, J. (1998). *J. Near Infrared Spectros.* 6, A133–aA140.

Engelhard, S., Lohmannsroben, H.G. and Schael, F. (2004). *Appl. Spectros.* 58, 1205–1209.

Fox, G.P., Onley-Watson, K. and Osman, A. (2002). *J. Inst. Brew.* 108, 155–159.

Gallignani, M., Garrigues, S. and de la Guardia, M. (1993). *Analyst* 118, 1167–1173.

Gallignani, M., Garrigues, S. and de la Guardia, M. (1994a). *Anal. Chim. Acta* 296, 155–161.

Gallignani, M., Garrigues, S. and de la Guardia, M. (1994b). *Anal. Chim. Acta* 287, 275–283.

Gallignani, M., Garrigues, S. and de la Guardia, M. (1994c). *Analyst* 119, 1773–1778.

Gallignani, M., Ayala, C., Brunetto, M.D., Burguera, J.L. and Burguera, M. (2005). *Talanta* 68, 470–479.

Galloway, D.B. (1992). *J. Chem. Educ.* 69, 79–83.

Garden, S.W., Pruneda, T., Irby, S. and Hysert, D.W. (2000). *J. Am. Soc. Brew. Chem.* 58, 73–82.

Garrigues, S. and de la Guardia, M. (2002). Flow-injection analysis-Fourier transform infrared spectrometry (FIA/FT-IR). In Chalmers, J.M. and Griffiths, P.R. (eds), *Handbook of Vibrational Spectroscopy*, pp. 1661–1675. John Wiley & Sons, Chichester.

Halsey, S.A. (1985). *J. Inst. Brew.* 91, 306–312.

Halsey, S.A. (1986). *J. Inst. Brew.* 92, 387–393.

Halsey, S.A. (1987). *J. Inst. Brew.* 93, 407–412.

Halsey, S.A. and Buckee, G.K. (1985). *J. Inst. Brew.* 91, 126.

Haberkorn, M., Hinsmann, P. and Lendl, B. (2002). *Analyst* 127, 109–113.

Henry, R.J. (1985a). *Carbohydr. Res.* 14, 13–19.

Henry, R.J. (1985b). *J. Sci. Food Agric.* 36, 249–254.

Iñón, F.A., Llario, R., Garrigues, S. and de la Guardia, M. (2005). *Anal. Bioanal. Chem.* 382, 1549–1561.

Iñón, F.A., Garrigues, S. and de la Guardia, M. (2006). *Anal. Chim. Acta* 571, 167–174.

Lachenmeier, D.W. (2007). *Food Chem.* 101, 825–832.

Llario, R., Iñón, F.A., Garrigues, S. and de la Guardia, M. (2006). *Talanta* 69, 469–480.

Luo, H.Q. and Liu, S.P. (1998). *Fenxi Huaxue* 26, 97–99.

Maeda, H., Ozaki, Y., Tamaka, M., Hayashi, N. and Kajima, T. (1995). *J. Near Infrared Spectros.* 3, 191–201.

Majara, M., Mochaba, F.M., O'Connor-Cox, E.S.C., Axcell, B.C. and Alexander, A. (1998). *J. Inst. Brew.* 104, 143–146.

Maudoux, M., Yan, S.H. and Collin, S. (1998). *J. Near Infrared Spectros.* 6, A363–A366.

McGuire, C.F. (1982). *Cereal Chem.* 59, 510–511.

Mendes, L.S., Oliveira, F.C.C., Suarez, P.A.Z. and Rubim, J.C. (2003). *Anal. Chim. Acta* 493, 219–231.

Meurens, M. and Yan, S.H. (2002). Applications of vibrational spectroscopy in brewing. In Chalmers, J.M. and Griffiths, P.R. (eds), *Handbook of Vibrational Spectroscopy*, pp. 3363–3671. John Wiley & Sons, Chichester.

Mochaba, F., Tortline, P. and Axcell, B. (1994). *J. Am. Soc. Brew. Chem.* 52, 145–147.

Moller, B. (2004). *J. Inst. Brew.* 110, 18–33.

Moonsamy, N., Mochaba, F., Majara, M., O'Connor-Cox, E.S.C. and Axcell, B.C. (1995). *J. Inst. Brew.* 101, 203–2006.

Munar, M., Christopher, D., Edney, M., Habernicht, D., Joy, R., Laycock, G., Sieben, R., Swenson, W. and Casey, G. (1998). *J. Am. Soc. Brew. Chem.* 56, 189–194.

Nordon, A., Mills, A., Burn, R.T., Cusick, F.M. and Littlejohn, D. (2005). *Anal. Chim. Acta* 548, 148–158.

Norgaard, L., Saudland, A., Wagner, J., Nielsen, J.P., Munck, L. and Engelsen, S.B. (2000). *Appl. Spectrosc.* 54, 413–419.

Perez-Ponce, A., Garrigues, S. and de la Guardia, M. (1996). *Analyst* 121, 923–928.

Ratcliffe, M. and Panozzo, J.F. (1999). *J. Inst. Brew.* 105, 85–88.

Ródenas-Torralba, E., Ventura-Gayete, J., Morales-Rubio, A., Garrigues, S. and de la Guardia, M. (2004). *Anal. Chim. Acta* 512, 215–221.

Samp, E.J., Sedin, D. and Foster, A. (2003). *J. Inst. Brew.* 109, 16–26.

Schropp, P., Bruder, T. and Forstner, A. (2002). *Monatsschr. Brauwissen.* 55, 212–216.

Sjoholm, K., Tenhunen, J., Tammisola, J., Pietila, K. and Home, S. (1996). *J. Am. Soc. Brew. Chem.* 54, 135–140.

Skinner, K.E. (1996). *J. Am. Soc. Brew. Chem.* 54, 191–197.

Tenhunen, J., Sjoholm, K., Pietila, K. and Home, S. (1994). *J. Inst. Brew.* 100, 11–15.

Timmins, E.M., Quain, D.E. and Goodacre, R. (1998). *Yeast* 14, 885–893.

Toivola, A., Varju, P. and Torrent, J. (2005). *J. Inst. Brew.* 111, 241–244.

Westad, F. and Martens, H. (2000). *J. Near Infrared Spectros.* 8, 117–124.

Wilke, J. and Parthey, B. (1996). *Monatsschr. Brauwissen.* 49, 115–118.

Wilks, P.A. (1988). *Tech. Q. Master Brew. Assoc. Am.* 25, 113–116.

Yan, S.H., Meurens, M., Maudoux, M., Derdelinckx, G. and Dufour, J.P. (1991). *Proceedings of the 23rd European Brewery Convention*, pp. 489–499. Lisbon.

95

Fluorescence Methods for Analysis of Beer

Ewa Sikorska Faculty of Commodity Science, Poznań University of Economics, Poznań, Poland
Igor Khmelinskii Universidade do Algarve, FCT, DQBF, Campus de Gambelas, Faro, Portugal
Marek Sikorski Faculty of Chemistry, A. Mickiewicz University, Poznań, Poland

Abstract

Autofluorescence of beer probed by conventional and multidimensional fluorescence techniques – total luminescence and synchronous scanning fluorescence spectroscopy – is discussed. The spectra of beers reveal the presence of similar fluorescent components in beers of various brands, exhibiting a relatively intense short-wavelength emission ascribed to aromatic amino acids, and a less intense emission in the long-wavelength region, which may originate from the group B vitamins and polyphenolics. Application of multivariate methods to emission data treatment enables quantitative and qualitative analysis of beers based on fluorescence measurements. Examples are provided for application of the techniques to classification of beers, controlling changes during storage, and determination of bitterness of beers and their vitamin B_2 contents. The performance of fluorescence in beer analysis is compared with that of other spectroscopic methods. The potential of these methods in food analysis, screening, and quality control is discussed.

List of Abbreviations

ANN	Artificial neural network
CCD	Charge coupled device
EBC	European Brewery Convention
EEM	Excitation–emission matrix
FAD	Flavin adenine dinucleotide
FTIR	Fourier transform–infrared
ATR-FTIR	Attenuated total reflectance Fourier transform–infrared
HPLC	High performance liquid chromatography
IBU	International bitter units
IR	Infrared
kNN	k-nearest neighbors
LDA	Linear discriminant analysis
MBT	3-Methyl-2-butene-1-thiol
NAD	Nicotinamide adenine dinucleotide
NADH	Reduced form of nicotinamide adenine dinucleotide
NADP	Nicotinamide adenine dinucleotide phosphate
NADPH	Reduced form of nicotinamide adenine dinucleotide phosphate
NIR	Near-infrared
FMN	Flavin mononucleotide
NMR	Nuclear magnetic resonance
PC	Principal component
PCA	Principal component analysis
PLS	Partial least squares
RMSECV	Root mean square error of cross-validation
Rf	Riboflavin
TLS	Total luminescence spectroscopy
UV	Ultraviolet
VIS	Visible

Introduction

Beer analysis is important for evaluation of its organoleptic characteristics, quality, nutritional aspects, and safety. A wide variety of analytical methods and chemical measurements are usually implemented to characterize and quantify various beer properties and constituents. For example, bitterness units and European Brewery Convention color are assessed by photometry, organic acids are analyzed using liquid chromatography or enzymatic methods, higher alcohols and other volatile compounds are determined using gas chromatography. In most cases, analytic methods require pre-treatment of samples to separate and concentrate the target compounds. Such techniques are expensive, time-consuming, involve the use of undesirable organic solvents, and require highly trained laboratory personnel. Moreover, fractionation and separation procedures may alter the nature of the sample, and cause loss or dilution of certain compounds.

Beer in Health and Disease Prevention
ISBN: 978-0-12-373891-2

The development of fast analytical methods, which may be applied directly to the analyzed material and thus make extensive sample pre-treatment unnecessary, is of great interest in food and beverage analysis. Spectroscopic techniques are particularly useful in such applications (Oldham *et al.*, 2000), as they enable rapid and non-invasive characterization of the samples. In contrast to conventional methods, which usually focus on the analysis of a single, or of a selected few compounds or properties, spectroscopy may provide information about a very wide range of different compounds in a single measurement. This feature is especially important in food analysis because sensory properties of products and their quality are usually determined by a variety of components and their interactions. The potential of spectroscopic methods is expanded by application of multivariate methods for data analysis.

Nuclear magnetic resonance (NMR) (Duarte *et al.*, 2002; Duarte *et al.*, 2004; Nord *et al.*, 2004; Lachenmeier *et al.*, 2005; Almeida *et al.*, 2006; Khatib *et al.*, 2006), near-infrared (NIR) (Engelhard *et al.*, 2006; Inon *et al.*, 2006), and infrared (IR) (Duarte *et al.*, 2004; Llario *et al.*, 2006; Lachenmeier, 2007) spectroscopy have been proved useful for direct beer analysis. Recently, fluorescence spectroscopy has been receiving an increasing attention in food analysis (Christensen *et al.*, 2006). Fluorescence is a type of photoluminescence, a process in which a molecule, promoted to an electronically excited singlet state by absorption of UV (ultraviolet), VIS (visible), or NIR radiation, decays back to its ground state by emission of a photon. Among the benefits of fluorescence spectroscopy are its enhanced selectivity as compared to other spectroscopic methods, its high sensitivity to a wide array of potential analytes, and in general, the avoidance of consumable reagents and of extensive sample pre-treatment (Oldham *et al.*, 2000). The fluorescent analysis may take advantage of the presence of natural fluorescent food components or contaminants. On the other hand, fluorescence can be induced in food by adding fluorophores or by producing specific fluorescent derivatives of the analytes.

Conventional fluorescence techniques, relying on measurements of single emission or excitation spectra, are often insufficient in the direct analysis of complex systems. In such cases, total luminescence or synchronous scanning fluorescence techniques may improve the analytic potential of the fluorescence measurements (Ndou and Warner, 1991). Total luminescence spectroscopy (TLS) involves simultaneous acquisition of multiple excitation and emission wavelengths to increase the method selectivity. The resulting emission–excitation data matrix (EEM) provides a total intensity profile of the sample over the range of excitation and emission wavelengths scanned (Ndou and Warner, 1991; Christensen *et al.*, 2006). Synchronous fluorescence spectrometry takes advantage of the ability to vary both the excitation and emission wavelengths during the analysis: in this method excitation and emission monochromators are scanned simultaneously, synchronized so that a constant wavelength difference is maintained between the two (Ndou and Warner, 1991).

Several papers reported investigations and applications of intrinsic beer fluorescence. Fluorescence lifetimes and spectral data have been explored in diluted beers (Apperson *et al.*, 2002). Beer autofluorescence and europium-induced delayed fluorescence with multivariate data evaluation were used for determination of bitterness in beer (Christensen *et al.*, 2005); other authors developed a simple, sensitive fluorometric method for precise quantification of riboflavin in beer (Duyvis *et al.*, 2002). Total fluorescence spectroscopy and synchronous fluorescence spectroscopy were applied for characterization and differentiation of various brands of beers, for monitoring changes occurring in beer during storage under different conditions, and for quantification of vitamin B_2 (Sikorska *et al.*, 2003, 2004a, b, 2006).

In this chapter we characterize the autofluorescence of beers and present an analytical application of the fluorescence measurements.

Fluorescence Characteristics of Beer

The characteristics of beer autofluorescence are expected to be quite complex due to overlapping emissions from numerous species. Therefore, it is necessary to apply multidimensional fluorescence techniques to obtain a comprehensive description of the fluorescent components. Three-dimensional spectra are known as excitation–emission matrices or total luminescence spectra, in which one axis represents the excitation wavelength, another – the emission wavelength, and the third – the intensity (Ndou and Warner, 1991; Guilbault, 1999). Alternatively, three-dimensional spectra may be transformed into two-dimensional contour maps, in which one axis represents the emission and another – the excitation wavelength. The contours are plotted by linking points of equal fluorescence intensity. Such a presentation is more practical for visual analysis of the fluorescence patterns.

A total luminescence spectrum gives a comprehensive description of the fluorescent components of the mixture, incorporating all the information present in the absorption and fluorescence spectra of fluorescent constituents. Due to these features, the total luminescence contour map may serve as a unique fingerprint for identification and characterization of the sample studied. The spectral resolution of an excitation–emission matrix depends on the number of conventional emission scans at different excitation wavelengths, used to construct the contour plot. Acquisition of contour maps of sufficient resolution on conventional spectrofluorometers requires a large number of emission scans for each sample. The analysis may be speeded up with charge coupled device or video-spectrofluorometers; however, such instruments are not widely accessible in laboratories (Guilbault, 1999).

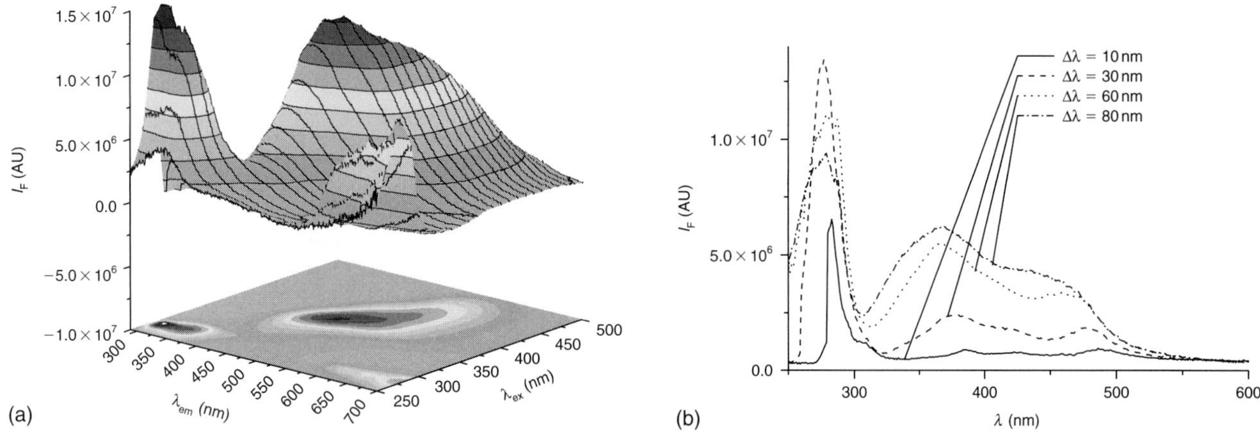

Figure 95.1 (a) Three-dimensional plot and contour map of total luminescence spectra of a lager beer measured for undiluted sample using front-face geometry. (b) Synchronous-scan fluorescence spectra of a lager beer measured for undiluted sample using front-face geometry, Δλ (10, 30, 60, 80 nm).

For analytical purposes, the synchronous fluorescence techniques may be used instead of the TLS (Ndou and Warner, 1991). Synchronous scanning fluorescence spectroscopy is a very useful technique for the analysis of mixtures of fluorescent compounds. Both excitation and emission characteristics are included in the spectrum by simultaneously scanning both excitation and emission wavelengths, keeping a constant difference between them. As a result, the selectivity for individual components is considerably improved and much additional information on mixtures of fluorescent compounds is gained. The synchronous scanning fluorescence method is a very simple and effective means of simultaneously obtaining data for several compounds present in a mixture. Although it provides less information than the TLS, it may present a viable alternative in many cases due to its inherent simplicity and rapidity.

Undiluted beers exhibit high UV–VIS absorption, thus fluorescence measured using the conventional arrangement, the right-angle geometry, is severely distorted due to primary and secondary inner-filter effects, which may be eliminated by diluting the samples. On the other hand, dilution reduces fluorescence intensities arising from such components that are either present in low concentrations or have low fluorescence quantum yields. Measurements for undiluted samples may be performed using front- or back-face geometry (Sikorska *et al.*, 2003, 2004b, 2006). Front-face geometry avoids filter effects, although other phenomena including energy transfer and collisional quenching remain active. In the back-face geometry, due to using a triangular cell the optical path length of the exciting radiation is considerably reduced, resulting in a reduction of the primary inner-filter effect. The emitted light is still absorbed, as the optical path length for the emission is ca. 0.5 cm in a typical cell; however, the absorption at longer emission wavelengths is considerably lower than that at shorter excitation wavelengths. All of these three geometries were used in beer fluorescence measurements: front face and back face for bulk samples and right angle for diluted samples.

The most complete fluorescent characteristics of beers were obtained in the front-face geometry (Sikorska *et al.*, 2004b). The spectra of undiluted beer (Figure 95.1a), measured using the front-face geometry, exhibit a relatively intense band with excitation at about 250 nm and emission at 350 nm. Additionally, a distinct emission band with excitation at 350 nm and emission at 420 nm, and a less intense emission band with excitation at 450 nm and emission at 520 nm are observed. In the spectra of diluted beer samples (3.2% v/v in water) the short-wavelength fluorescence with excitation at 250 nm and emission at 350 nm is present, while only a very weak emission band exists with excitation at 350 nm and emission at 420 nm, and almost no fluorescence above 400 nm in excitation and 500 nm in emission is observed. The short-wavelength emission is completely removed in spectra of undiluted beer measured using back-face geometry, while the longer-wavelength emission retains a reasonable intensity.

The emission characteristics for several lager beers studied are quite similar, indicating the presence of similar fluorescent components (Sikorska *et al.*, 2004b). On the other hand, differences in band positions, shapes, and relative intensities for various beers are easily noticeable. TLS can be used for fingerprinting of the respective beers, and may, for example, allow beer identification and quality monitoring.

The shape and intensity of synchronous spectra depend on the offset between the excitation and emission wavelengths, $\Delta\lambda$, which defines the preferred wavelength interval between the absorption and emission bands (Figure 95.1b). Generally an effective bandwidth reduction is observed at small $\Delta\lambda$ when compared to a conventionally recorded emission band, at a cost of some sensitivity reduction.

Table 95.1 Fluorescent properties of selected beer components and their concentration in beer

	Fluorescence properties			
Fluorophore	*Solvent*	λ_{ex} *(nm)*	λ_{em} *(nm)*	*Concentration in beer*
Amino acids				
Phenylalanine	Water	258	284 (Christensen *et al.*, 2006)	5.9 mg/100 g (Moller *et al.*, 2002), 20–105.3 mg/dm^3 (Erbe and Bruckner, 2000)
Tyrosine	Water	276	302 (Christensen *et al.*, 2006)	14.9 mg/100 g (Moller *et al.*, 2002), 5.7–71.3 mg/dm^3 (Erbe and Bruckner, 2000)
Tryptophan	Water	280	357 (Christensen *et al.*, 2006)	3.1 mg/100 g (Moller *et al.*, 2002)
Vitamins				
Vitamin B_2 Riboflavin	Water	270, 382, 448	518 (Christensen *et al.*, 2006)	0.020–0.040 mg/100 g (Moller *et al.*, 2002), 0.0156–0.0278 mg/100 g (Vinas *et al.*, 2004), 0.169–0.508 mg/dm^3 (Andres-Lacueva *et al.*, 1998), 0.210–0.312 mg/dm^3 (Duyvis *et al.*, 2002), 0.130–0.280 mg/dm^3 (Su *et al.*, 2004)
FAD	Water	262, 370, 450	540 (Islam *et al.*, 2003)	0.019–0.065 mg/dm^3 (Andres-Lacueva *et al.*, 1998), 0.0014–0.0053 mg/100 g (Vinas *et al.*, 2004)
FMN	Water	265, 370, 450	540 (Islam *et al.*, 2003)	0.081 mg/dm^3 (Andres-Lacueva *et al.*, 1998), nd (Vinas *et al.*, 2004)
Vitamin B_3 NAD(P)H	Water	340	470 (Friedrich, 1988)	0.65–1.1 mg/100 g (Moller *et al.*, 2002)
Vitamin B_6 Pyridoxine	Water	328	393 (Christensen *et al.*, 2006)	0.03–0.08 mg/100 g (Moller *et al.*, 2002)
Phenolics				
Epicatechin	Water	280	320–324 (Cho and Mattice, 1990)	65.5 mg/dm^3 (Gorinstein *et al.*, 2000), 0.9–1.9 mg/dm^3 (Shahidi and Naczk, 2003)
Catechin	Water	280	320–324 (Cho and Mattice, 1990)	3.4–6.3 mg/dm^3 (Shahidi and Naczk, 2003)
p-Coumaric acid	Water pH = 10.7	330	435 (Sanchez *et al.*, 1988)	2.1 mg/dm^3 (Gorinstein *et al.*, 2000), 0.6–1.1 mg/dm^3 (Sanchez *et al.*, 1995), 1.06 mg/dm^3 (Nardini *et al.*, 2006), 0.026–0.129 mg/dm^3 (Montanari *et al.*, 1999), 6.01–6.97 mg/dm^3 (Sanchez *et al.*, 1988)
		330	443 (Gorinstein *et al.*, 2000)	
Ferulic acid	Water pH = 11.2	340	460 (Gorinstein *et al.*, 2000)	6.8 mg/dm^3 (Gorinstein *et al.*, 2000), 0.131 ng/ml (Sanchez *et al.*, 1996), 13.50 mg/dm^3 (Nardini *et al.*, 2006), 0.116–0.274 mg/dm^3 (Montanari *et al.*, 1999)
Gallic acid	Water	260	339 (Polewski *et al.*, 2002)	2.9 mg/dm^3 (Gorinstein *et al.*, 2000), 0.008–0.034 mg/dm^3 (Montanari *et al.*, 1999)
	Water pH = 4.63	260	357 (Gorinstein *et al.*, 2000)	

λ_{ex}, λ_{em}: wavelength of fluorescence excitation and emission maxima; NAD(P)H: reduced forms of dinucleotide (NAD) and nicotinamide adenine dinucleotide phosphate (NADP); FAD: flavin adenine dinucleotide; FMN: flavin mononucleotide.

Synchronous fluorescence spectra of an undiluted beer in the front-face geometry obtained at $\Delta\lambda = 10$ nm show a sharp, intense band with a maximum at 283 nm and a weak broad emission with maxima at 385, 426, and 488 nm (Sikorska *et al.*, 2004b). The short-wavelength emission band is broadened in spectra measured at $\Delta\lambda = 30$ nm and its maximum is shifted to 275 nm, accompanied by an increased intensity of both this band and of the broad emission between 300 and 500 nm. Further increasing the $\Delta\lambda$ values to 60 and 80 nm led to a decrease of the fluorescence intensity in the short-wavelength region; simultaneously, the long-wavelength broad bands grew in intensity and their maxima were shifted to the blue.

In analogy to total luminescence spectra, the synchronous fluorescence spectra of a lager beer diluted in water (3.2% v/v) exhibit mainly the short-wavelength fluorescence. No short-wavelength emission is observable in the synchronous spectra of undiluted beer samples recorded using the back-face geometry.

Fluorescent Beer Components

The major beer components, water, ethanol, and carbohydrates, are non-fluorescent; however, beers contain a very wide range of minor components, including proteins, amino acids, vitamins, and phenolic compounds, some of which exhibit fluorescence. Thus, the intrinsic emission of beers originates from numerous fluorescent species. Consequently, a complete assignment of the spectral features is problematical. Some tentative qualitative assignments could be made, based on comparison of the observed characteristic features with the well-known fluorescent properties of the particular beer constituents.

Fluorescence properties of selected beer components are summarized in Table 95.1, along with some examples of their measured concentrations. Note that the concentrations may vary widely, depending on the beer type, reproducing diversity of the raw materials and brewing conditions.

As evident from Table 95.1, compounds exhibiting natural fluorescence belong to at least three distinct groups of beer constituents: amino acids, vitamins, and distinct phenolic compounds. The relatively intense band, observed in each beer, with the excitation at ca. 250–300 nm and the emission at ca. 300–400 nm, has been ascribed to amino acids (Apperson *et al.*, 2002; Sikorska *et al.*, 2004b; Christensen *et al.*, 2005). Beer contains a variety of amino acids, however, only three of them are fluorescent, tryptophan, tyrosine, and phenylalanine, all having aromatic character. The emission in the short-wavelength region may also originate from catechin or epicatechin – the proanthocyanidin monomers. However, it was shown that contribution of polyphenols at this spectral zone is minimal since their removal by polyvinylpolypyrrolidone had not affected the observed fluorescence significantly (Apperson *et al.*, 2002).

The broad emission at longer wavelengths originates presumably from several fluorescent components, including compounds of the vitamin B group and phenolic compounds (Sikorska *et al.*, 2004b; Christensen *et al.*, 2005). Indeed, beer contains many phenolic compounds, which include a wide range of structures from simple monophenols to polymeric polyphenols of varying complexity. Beer is also a rich source of water-soluble B vitamins. The emission band at ca. 450/500–600 nm could be ascribed to vitamin B_2 emission (Friedrich, 1988). The principal forms of vitamin B_2 found in nature are riboflavin, flavin mononucleotide (FMN), and flavin adenine dinucleotide (FAD), although beer contains mainly riboflavin. Vitamin B_3 (niacin) includes nicotinic acid, nicotinamide, and their coenzyme forms: nicotinamide adenine dinucleotide (NAD) and nicotinamide adenine dinucleotide phosphate (NADP). Reduced forms NAD(P)H are fluorescent (Friedrich, 1988). Vitamin B_6 group includes pyridoxine, pyridoxal, pyridoxamine, pyridoxic acid, and pyridoxal 5′-phospate, all of these compounds emit in the 385–400 nm range (Friedrich, 1988; Ramanujam, 2000). According to some authors (Apperson *et al.*, 2002), iso-α-acids may also contribute to beer autofluorescence.

The intense short-wavelength emission band observed in the synchronous fluorescence spectra of diluted beer samples was attributed to amino acid fluorescence, mainly that of tyrosine, in analogy to the total luminescence spectra (Sikorska *et al.*, 2004b). The long-wavelength emission in the synchronous spectra of bulk beers should originate from the vitamin B group of compounds. The existence of more than one band suggests that several substances emit in this region, possibly including phenolic compounds.

Figure 95.2 shows spectra of aromatic amino acids and vitamin B_2 recorded at $\Delta\lambda = 10$ nm. Phenylalanine, tyrosine, and tryptophan exhibit single narrow bands in the short-wavelength region with the respective maxima at 263, 283, and 296 nm. Riboflavin emission occurs in the long-wavelength region with a maximum at 489 nm. The very good match between fluorescence of tyrosine and riboflavin and the respective emission bands of beers supports the identification of these two fluorophores (Sikorska *et al.*, 2004b). Further studies are needed to confirm assignments of the other fluorescent bands and to establish a quantitative relationship between the chemical composition of a beer and its fluorescence characteristics. Such study could be of great interest because fluorescent compounds present in beer have a strong impact on both the beer properties and its nutritional value and stability. For example, the concentration of amino acids in beer may serve as an indicator for the fermentation performance. Free amino acids present in wort are metabolized by yeast during fermentation, therefore content of amino acids in beer is determined by wort and yeast metabolism (Nord *et al.*, 2004).

Phenolic compounds may contribute either beneficially or harmfully to several of the beer properties (Shahidi and Naczk, 2003). They are involved in physical and chemical stability, shelf life, and foam maintenance. They contribute to flavor because they cause both bitterness and astringency. Polyphenols are well known for their participation in protein–polyphenol haze development. Some beer phenolics may also act as antioxidants in the human body, contributing beneficially to the health of the consumer.

The vitamins present in beer contribute to its nutritional value. The active form of vitamin B_2, FMN, and FAD serve as prosthetic groups of oxidoreductase enzymes, which catalyze essential oxidation/reduction steps in almost every metabolic pathway (Nollet, 2004). It was shown that riboflavin possesses some disease prevention and health promotion functions, including protection against malaria, vascular disease, and certain cancers. Recently riboflavin has gained a renewed interest after it was shown to protect

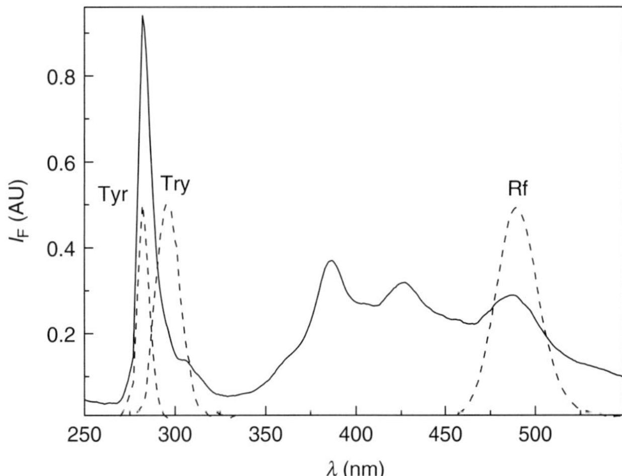

Figure 95.2 Synchronous fluorescence spectra, recorded at $\Delta\lambda = 10$ nm, of beer, tyrosine (Tyr), tryptophan (Try), and riboflavin (Rf) in water, at pH = 4; fluorescence intensity of standard compounds was normalized.

vital tissues from ischemia-induced oxidative injury resulting from heart attack or stroke (Foraker *et al.*, 2003).

Apart from its nutritional value, riboflavin have been postulated to contribute to the development of flavor changes: the sunstruck and stale flavor (Sakuma *et al.*, 1991; Burns *et al.*, 2001; Goldsmith *et al.*, 2005; Huvaere *et al.*, 2005; Huvaere *et al.*, 2006).

Niacin participates in oxidation–reduction systems and plays an essential role in the enzyme systems responsible for the metabolism of carbohydrates, fatty acids, and amino acids. Nicotinic acid and nicotinamide are used for treating cardiovascular disease, insulin-dependent mellitus, and certain cancers (Nollet, 2004).

Vitamin B_6 acts as an essential coenzyme involved in amino acid, carbohydrate, and fat metabolism. Among other roles, it is required for the formation of hemoglobin (Nollet, 2004).

Classification of Beers Using Synchronous Fluorescence Spectra

Despite their general similarity, the profiles of synchronous fluorescence spectra of individual beers vary significantly, producing unique spectral patterns (Sikorska *et al.*, 2004b). The synchronous fluorescence spectrum can serve as a spectral signature of the particular sample and may be used, for example, in qualitative analysis, quality monitoring, for beer identification, or for authentication purposes. For such applications multivariate statistical methods should be applied. Exploratory analysis of synchronous fluorescence spectra of different beers was performed using principal component analysis (PCA) (Wold *et al.*, 1987). PCA is an unsupervised multivariate method, used to analyze the inherent structure of the data. PCA reduces dimensionality of the dataset by finding principal components (PCs) which are linear combinations of the original variables. PCs are orthogonal to each other and designed in such a way that each one successively accounts for the maximum variability of the dataset. A plot of the PC scores reveals relations existing between the samples, such as natural clustering in the data or outlier samples.

PCA modeling for undiluted and water-diluted beer samples was performed for synchronous fluorescence spectra measured at $\Delta\lambda = 10$ and 60 nm, respectively, with back-face and right-angle geometry. The resulting scores are shown in Figure 95.3. The PCA analysis reveals sample clustering reflecting the beer brands. Larger dispersion seen for diluted samples results from errors introduced by the dilution procedure, and additional noise appearing in measurements of week signals from the diluted samples.

The possibility of discriminating different beers on the basis of their synchronous fluorescence spectra was investigated by using two statistical methods: the *k*-nearest neighbors (*k*NN) method and the linear discriminant analysis (LDA) (Sikorska *et al.*, 2004b). The *k*NN method is a non-parametric classification method, which allows to analyze entire spectra, without any reduction of the datasets (Wu and Massart, 1997). In principle, the test object is assigned to a cluster, which is most represented in the set of *k*-nearest training objects. For each data point, the closest data points, called "nearest neighbors" are searched for, and then decision is made according to the values of these neighbors. *k*NN is one of the simplest learning techniques – the learner only needs to store the examples, while the classifier does its work by observing the examples most similar to the one to be classified. The *k*-values were chosen in the range of $k = 1, \ldots, 10$.

Additionally, LDA was performed on simplified datasets. For this purpose, six wavelengths were extracted from each synchronous spectrum measured at a particular $\Delta\lambda$ and analyzed.

Classification of various beer samples using *k*NN method was very good, with zero or very low classification error and low standard deviation values (Sikorska *et al.*, 2004b). The best discrimination was achieved for bulk beers using synchronous fluorescence spectra measured at $\Delta\lambda = 10$ and 60 nm and for diluted beers using spectra measured at $\Delta\lambda = 10$ nm. LDA also produced a satisfactory discrimination between different beers. The results show that to discriminate between beers, instead of recording entire spectra, the fluorescence intensity could be measured at selected excitation–emission wavelength pairs and then subjected to LDA.

The results confirmed that both the short-wavelength UV-emission and the long-wavelength visible emission can be applied to discriminate various beers. Although both techniques could be applied for beer discrimination, the spectra of bulk samples appear to be more reliable than

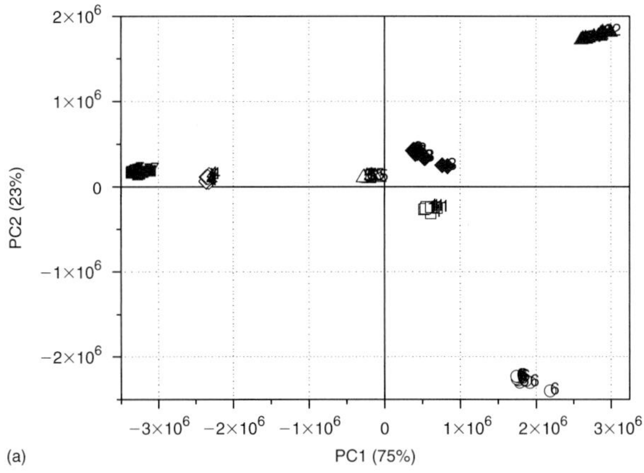

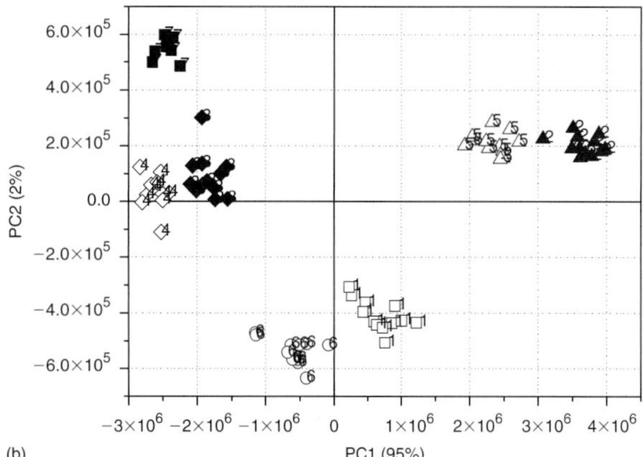

Figure 95.3 Score plots for PCA model of synchronous-scan fluorescence spectra measured at $\Delta\lambda$ = 10 nm, of bulk (a) and diluted (b) lager beers of seven different brands.

those of diluted beers. Apart from qualitative distinctions, the samples also differ in fluorescence intensities of particular components. These differences should reflect variation in the contents of fluorescent compounds and might be used for quantitative evaluation of beer components.

Monitoring Beer During Storage by Fluorescence Spectroscopy

Fluorescence spectroscopy allows monitoring changes in the chemical composition of beers during storage. Recently fluorescence spectroscopy has been applied to the samples of two lager beers of various brands stored in clear glass bottles in different conditions: in darkness at 4°C, and at 22°C, one in darkness and the other one under diffuse light, for 21 days (Sikorska *et al.*, 2006). The samples were analyzed by means of various fluorescence techniques for both diluted and bulk samples.

The total luminescence spectra of fresh beer and beer stored in light differ mainly in the band occurring at 450 nm in excitation and between 500 and 600 nm in emission, in the zone characteristic for vitamin B_2 (riboflavin) and, in general, attributed to flavins present in beer. This emission disappears in beer exposed to light, result of flavin photodegradation (Heelis, 1982). The total luminescence characteristics of beers stored in the dark at 4°C and 22°C (not shown) were almost identical to those of fresh beers. Generally the changes occurring during storage are more pronounced in bulk rather than in diluted samples.

It has been shown that synchronous spectra allow discrimination between differently stored beer samples. Two lager beers A and B of different brands were used for the study. Because significant changes in fluorescence characteristics of beer during storage occurred mainly in the long-wavelength emission region, synchronous spectra of bulk beers were chosen for the multivariate analysis, with the exploratory data analysis performed using PCA (Wold *et al.*, 1987).

Two PCA models were analyzed for synchronous fluorescence spectra of beers that were either fresh or stored in different conditions (Figure 95.4) (Sikorska *et al.*, 2006). The first model includes all the storage conditions, while the second model excludes the samples exposed to light. The distribution of samples in the score plots for both models clearly displays clustering of beer samples according to freshness and storage conditions. The samples exposed to light are clearly distinct from both fresh beer and samples stored in the dark by the negative values of the first principal component PC1, which explains 83% of the total variance. The loading for this component shows the importance of the bands attributed to flavins, with a maximum at 489 nm, and also of the short-wavelength bands at 375–450 nm. PC2 explains 15% of the total variance and is related to the changes in the 350–440 nm bands. This component differentiates the samples stored in the dark at 22°C from all other samples.

In the second PCA model the samples exposed to light were excluded. In this model, PC1 and PC2 describe 90% and 7% of the total variance, respectively. PC1 corresponds to variations in the bands with maxima at 428, 400, and 380 nm, while PC2 describes changes in the bands with maxima at 367 and 380 nm. It is important to note that convincing discrimination between samples stored in darkness at different temperatures was achieved by the PCA analysis, which we found impossible to achieve by visual inspection of the same spectra.

Comparison of the two PCA models shows that the main difference between beers stored in darkness and under light corresponds to changes in the spectral zone around 490 nm, which is characteristic to the riboflavin emission. These observations confirm riboflavin photodecomposition and its stability in the absence of light (Heelis, 1982; Andres-Lacueva *et al.*, 1998; Duyvis *et al.*, 2002). The differences

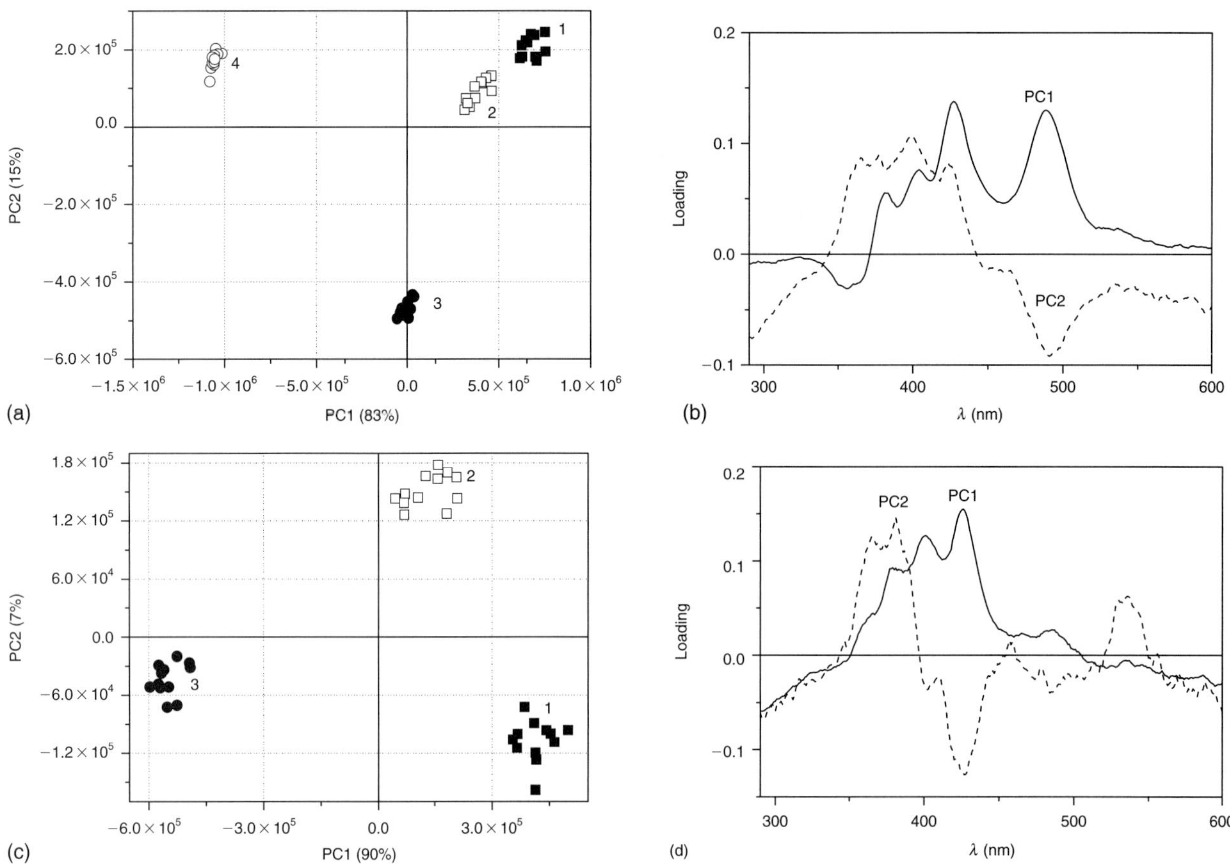

Figure 95.4 Score (a, c) and loading (b, d) plots for two PCA models of synchronous-scan fluorescence spectra of bulk beer A stored in different conditions, recorded for $\Delta\lambda$ = 10 nm; 1 – fresh beer and samples stored for 21 days; 2 – darkness, 4°C; 3 – darkness, 22°C; 4 – exposed to diffuse light, 22°C. Series 4 was only included in the model represented in (a, b). *Source*: Reprinted from Sikorska *et al.* (2006), with permission from Elsevier.

in riboflavin emission are insignificant in samples protected from light.

Similar clustering of samples according to storage conditions was observed for synchronous fluorescence spectra recorded for $\Delta\lambda = 60$ nm with all four series of samples, and the importance of the emission originating from flavins in differentiating samples exposed to light from those stored in darkness was confirmed.

With respect to quality monitoring, it is desirable to separate products into classes, such as fresh and aged samples. To test the feasibility of such classification based on the fluorescence spectra, the *k*NN and LDA methods were employed. All differently stored samples of beer A could be correctly classified by *k*NN using synchronous fluorescence spectra recorded both for $\Delta\lambda = 10$ and 60 nm, and appropriate *k*-values. The classification errors increased at higher *k*-values and the misclassification rates were generally higher for the spectra measured for $\Delta\lambda = 60$ nm. LDA provided 100% classification for both sets of synchronous spectra. The *k*NN analysis of synchronous spectra of beer B for $\Delta\lambda = 10$ nm led to 3.4–5.2% classification error depending on the *k*-value, as a consequence of poor separation between fresh beers and beers stored in darkness at 4°C. Much better classification was achieved in the analysis of $\Delta\lambda = 60$ nm spectra. With LDA, the fraction of correct classification was about 88% for $\Delta\lambda = 10$ nm spectra and 100% for $\Delta\lambda = 60$ nm spectra.

Alterations of intrinsic beer fluorescence occurring during aging refer directly to subtle and minor chemical changes of beer components. A comprehensive picture of mixtures of fluorescent compounds is obtained, although further studies are needed to identify specific molecules. It is feasible that stored and validated fluorescence spectra can serve as references for beer quality control purposes. Fluorescence may also be used as a tool for investigating the processes occurring in beer upon light exposure.

It is well known that beers exposed to visible light may develop a flavor known as "lightstruck," due mainly to formation of 3-methyl-2-butene-1-thiol (MBT) (Sakuma *et al.*, 1991; Burns *et al.*, 2001; Huvaere *et al.*, 2006). The mechanism of this process has been intensively studied. It is believed that the primary photophysical event that leads to the formation of the lightstruck flavor is the excitation of riboflavin to its triplet state followed by electron transfer from iso-α-acids (Huvaere *et al.*, 2004).

Evaluation of light-induced degradation of beers focused mainly on formation of sulfur-containing degradation products, in particular MBT. However, quantitative analysis of MBT in beer represents a significant challenge because of its low flavor threshold, chemical reactivity, relatively high boiling point (126°C), and propensity to adsorb onto surfaces. The methods for analysis of MBT include headspace gas chromatography (Gunst and Verzele, 1978; Peppard, 1985), gas chromatography and mass spectrometric detection (Goldstein *et al.*, 1993), solid-phase microextraction and gas chromatography with pulsed flame photometric detection (Hill and Smith, 2000), gas chromatography–mass spectrometry (Masuda *et al.*, 2000), and a purge-and-trap method with gas chromatography–mass spectrometric detector (Sakuma *et al.*, 1991). Recently Pozdrik *et al.* (2006) have shown that disappearance of riboflavin absorbance at 445 nm from beers exposed to light is directly linked to formation of the lightstruck flavor. The authors proposed simple spectrophotometric methods for determining lightstruck susceptibility based on measurement of riboflavin concentration in beer. The measurements of riboflavin fluorescence may offer an alternative to this method, providing higher sensitivity and selectivity as compared to absorption. Moreover, fluorescence may enable a simultaneous analysis of catechin and tryptophan, proven riboflavin triplet state quenchers, which provide some protection against lightstruck flavor formation (Goldsmith *et al.*, 2005).

Analysis of Vitamin B_2 Using Intrinsic Beer Fluorescence

The concentration of vitamin B_2 in beer is an important factor in assessing its nutritional value and flavor stability. The methods used for flavin quantification include high performance liquid chromatography (HPLC), enzymatic, microbiological, and fluorometric techniques. In most cases, these methods require pre-treatment of samples to separate and concentrate the target compounds.

Recently a method has been proposed for determination of vitamin B_2 in beer using its native fluorescence (Duyvis *et al.*, 2002). Briefly, the method is based on the riboflavin standard addition directly to the diluted beer. Subsequent titration with the apo-form of riboflavin-binding protein, which is efficiently and specifically quenching the riboflavin fluorescence, allows subtracting of the background fluorescence of beers, due to fluorescent species other than riboflavin. It has been proved that the fluorescence observed enables to determine riboflavin quantitatively, as other flavins only occur in beers in negligible amounts. Duyvis *et al.* (2002), using this same method, have obtained riboflavin content for lager beers in the range of 0.56–0.83 μmol/dm^3, comparable to riboflavin content in beer in the range of 0.45–1.35 μmol/dm^3 determined by Andres-Lacueva *et al.* (1998) using the HPLC method.

Alternatively, the concentration of riboflavin in beer may be determined by direct measurements of fluorescence spectra combined with multivariate regression method (Sikorska, 2006).

The front-face emission spectrum of beer measured at $\lambda_{exc} = 450\,\text{nm}$ exhibits a single band with its maximum at 550 nm ascribed to the riboflavin fluorescence (Duyvis *et al.*, 2002; Sikorska *et al.*, 2004b, 2006). In the synchronous fluorescence spectra taken at $\Delta\lambda = 30$ and 60 nm, the longest-wavelength emission band belongs to riboflavin (Sikorska *et al.*, 2004b, 2006). The linear regression analysis between fluorescence intensity at the peak of riboflavin emission and real vitamin B_2 content in beers provides fairly good results. The correlation coefficients of 0.839, 0.860, and 0.858, respectively, for the readings extracted from the emission spectra ($\lambda_{max} = 550\,\text{nm}$), and from the synchronous fluorescence spectra recorded at $\Delta\lambda = 30\,\text{nm}$ ($\lambda_{max} = 478\,\text{nm}$) and $\Delta\lambda = 60\,\text{nm}$ ($\lambda_{max} = 464\,\text{nm}$), respectively. However, the analysis of entire spectra instead of intensity at one wavelength should improve the results, as the model based on multivariate input data should be more robust against possible matrix interferences and differences in background fluorescence.

Partial least squares (PLS) regression was used for testing correlation between the emission and synchronous fluorescence spectra (X) and the real riboflavin concentration (Y) in beers. PLS is a method used for relating the variations in one or several response variables (Y-variables) to the variations of several predictors (X-variables), with explanatory or predictive purposes (Brereton, 2000). PLS models both the X- and Y-matrices simultaneously to find such latent variables in X that will best predict the latent variables in Y.

Emission spectra ($\lambda_{ex} = 450\,\text{nm}$), and the synchronous fluorescence spectra recorded at $\Delta\lambda = 30$ and 60 nm were used for the analysis (Sikorska, 2006). Riboflavin concentration was determined by fluorometric titration in beer samples, including untreated and irradiated beers and beers with addition of riboflavin. The riboflavin concentrations were in the range of 0.22–3.03 μmol/dm^3, the global mean riboflavin concentration was 0.84 ± 0.71 μmol/dm^3.

All regression models were validated using full cross-validation. Cross-validation is a strategy for validating calibration models based on systematically leaving out groups of samples in the modelling, and testing the left-out samples in the model based on the remaining samples. The regression models were evaluated using the correlation coefficient (r), and the root mean square error of cross-validation (RMSECV) parameter, as a term indicating the prediction error of the model. The RMSECV is defined by:

$$\text{RMSECV} = \sqrt{\frac{\sum_{i=1}^{N}\left(y_i^{\text{pred}} - y_i^{\text{ref}}\right)^2}{N}}$$

Table 95.2 Results of the PLS regression of riboflavin, Rf, content and the fluorescence spectra

PLS model	*Spectra range and transformation*	*Number of samples*	*Number of latent variables*	*r*	*RMSECV (μmol/dm³)*
Emission spectra	465–700 nm full range	34	5	0.971	0.15
Synchronous fluorescence spectra. $\Delta\lambda = 30\,nm$	250–600 nm full range	36	4	0.974	0.15
	440–520 nm Rf band	36	2	0.967	0.17
Synchronous fluorescence spectra. $\Delta\lambda = 60\,nm$	250–600 nm full range	35	3	0.959	0.20
	440–520 nm Rf band	35	2	0.960	0.19

r: correlation coefficient; RMSECV: root mean square error of cross-validation.

Source: Reprinted from Sikorska (2006), with permission from Springer Science and Business Media.

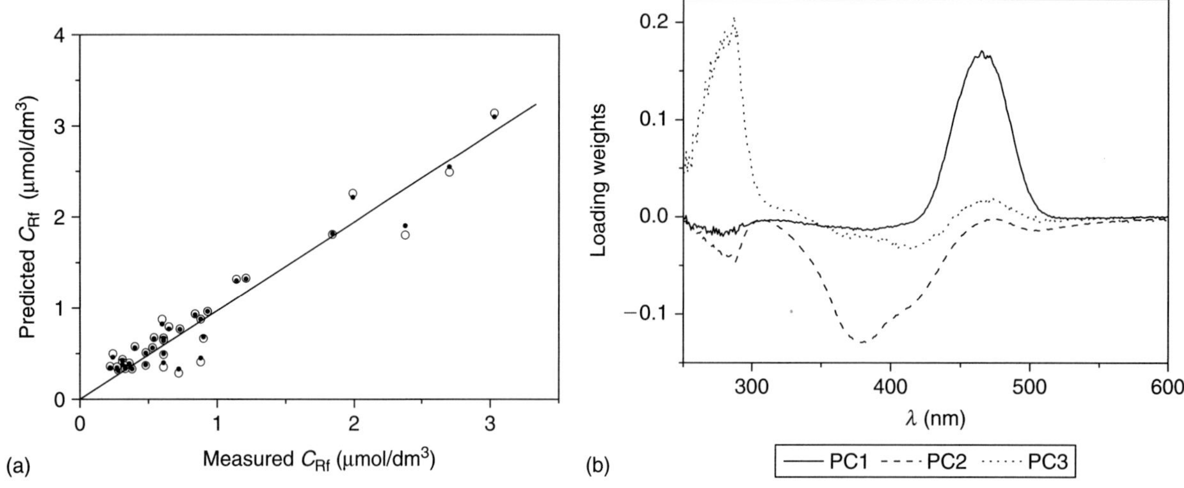

Figure 95.5 Results of the PLS regression based on the entire front-face synchronous fluorescence spectra of beers measured at $\Delta\lambda = 60\,nm$ and the riboflavin concentration obtained by fluorometric titration. (a) Plot of the riboflavin concentration predicted by the PLS model vs. the concentration measured by reference analysis. (b) Loading weights for the first three PCs of the PLS analysis.

where y_i^{pred} is the predicted concentration value for a sample in the cross-validation procedure, y_i^{ref} is the reference value, and N is the number of samples.

The calibration results are summarized in Table 95.2 and Figure 95.5. Figure 95.5a shows a typical plot of the riboflavin content predicted by the PLS model based on the synchronous fluorescence spectra taken at $\Delta\lambda = 60\,nm$ vs. the concentration obtained using the reference analysis. The linearity of the plot indicates good performance of the model in predicting the concentration of riboflavin (Sikorska, 2006).

All of the obtained PLS models underline a strong correlation between the fluorescence spectra and the riboflavin concentration. The best fitting parameters were obtained using the emission spectra and the synchronous fluorescence spectra measured at $\Delta\lambda = 30\,nm$.

The changes in the spectral range analyzed did not affect significantly the PLS results. The models analyzing full spectra performed very similarly to those restricted to the spectral zone corresponding to the riboflavin band. However, the number of latent variables was lower for the restricted model. Analysis of the loading weights for PLS regression analysis performed on synchronous fluorescence spectra recorded at $\Delta\lambda = 60\,nm$ (Figure 95.5b) shows that the PC1, which explains the majority of the Y variance (78%), corresponds to the long-wavelength band with the maximum at 464 nm, with only minor contributions of other spectral ranges, with PC2 and PC3, respectively, explaining 15% and 1% of the total Y variance. Similar results were obtained for PLS regression using synchronous fluorescence spectra recorded at $\Delta\lambda = 30\,nm$.

These results and the rather good correlation between the riboflavin concentration and the single-wavelength fluorescence intensity obtained in univariate regression indicate that the interferences affecting riboflavin quantification are rather insignificant even in undiluted beer samples. The values of RMSECV error for the obtained models corresponded to about 20% of the average riboflavin content over the entire set of beers studied. The relatively high error values may result from analyzing a diversity of beers, 10 different brands, including both untreated and irradiated beers with a wide range of the riboflavin content and diverse matrix constituents. We believe these error values will be significantly reduced in brand-specific models.

Method for Determination of Bitterness in Beer

Bitterness in beer is dependent primarily on the amount of iso-α-acids, which originate from the hop. Determination of these properties in beer and wort is a routine analysis in the brewing industry because bitterness is an essential quality parameter. Christensen *et al.* (2005) proposed two fluorescence methods for quantitative determination of bitterness in beer. One method was based on excitation–emission matrices of beer autofluorescence. The method requires only dilution and degassing of beer prior to measurements. Multivariate PLS regression models to bitterness expressed in international bitter units (IBU) using six PLS components for 21 beer samples, including light and dark beers. The prediction error (RMSECV) of 2.77 IBU was obtained. The RMSECV was reduced to 1.81 IBU when analysis was performed only on the light beer samples.

An alternative method used the analysis of delayed fluorescence induced by adding lanthanide ions to the beer sample (Christensen *et al.*, 2005). The delayed fluorescence results from the selective chelation of the lanthanide, europium, by the carbonyl structure in the iso-α-acids and the unique fluorescent properties of the resultant europium complex. PLS models yielded an RMSECV error of 2.65 IBU for all beers, while a model for the light beer samples gave an RMSECV of 1.75 IBU.

Comparison Between Fluorescence and Other Spectroscopic Methods in Beer Analysis

Spectroscopic methods applied for direct beer analysis include NMR (Duarte *et al.*, 2002, 2004; Nord *et al.*, 2004; Lachenmeier *et al.*, 2005; Almeida *et al.*, 2006; Khatib *et al.*, 2006), mid-IR (Fourier transform–infrared, FTIR) (Duarte *et al.*, 2004; Llario *et al.*, 2006; Lachenmeier, 2007), and NIR (Engelhard *et al.*, 2006; Inon *et al.*, 2006) spectroscopy. Table 95.3 provides some examples of direct beer analysis using spectroscopic methods.

All discussed techniques require little or no sample preparation. The IR, NIR, and fluorescence methods mostly use relatively inexpensive and simple instrumentation and enable faster spectral measurements, as compared to NMR. Therefore, they are attractive methods for routine measurements and can be used to screen samples and generate preliminary data that allow the analyst to decide whether a sample requires detailed characterization, perhaps by a more expensive and complex technique. FTIR, NIR, and fluorescence spectroscopy are cheaper, simpler, and faster methods of obtaining compositional information on foodstuffs, compared to NMR.

Much richer information concerning chemical components is provided using ^{1}H NMR as compared to other spectroscopic techniques. Analysis of ^{1}H NMR spectra of beers enables the identification of a wide variety of compounds ranging from organic acids, amino acids, and alcohols to higher molecular weight compounds such as lipids and large aromatic compounds like polyphenolics. NIR spectroscopy due to its low sensitivity is limited to the major beer constituents (e.g. alcoholic strength, original gravity). The spectra are more specific in the mid-IR range as compared to NIR, and clear response bands can be observed. The analysis of minor components is possible using FTIR spectroscopy, as for example required in bitterness evaluation and lactic acid quantification in beers. Fluorescence is restricted by its nature to emitting compounds only. This represents both a limitation and a possibility, whereas the multidimensional character enhances the selectivity of fluorescence in comparison to other methods. Moreover, its superior advantage is the highest sensitivity among the spectroscopic methods, which enables analysis of beer components inaccessible by other techniques.

Conclusions

Summarizing, the autofluorescence of beer was characterized, and the potential of fluorescence spectroscopy for qualitative and quantitative analysis of beers was demonstrated. It was shown that several classes of compounds may contribute to beer fluorescence, including vitamins, amino acids, and phenolics. The presented results demonstrated that rapid fluorescence measurements conducted directly on the beer samples and combined with multivariate data analysis can be used for qualitative and quantitative analysis. This method can be applied for beer discrimination according to the brand and freshness. It seems that fluorescence could be used as a simple and sensitive tool for monitoring changes in beer related to the sunstruck flavor formation. Quantitative determination of vitamin B_2 and bitterness is also possible after an appropriate calibration. Further studies are needed to resolve various issues that are important for practical application of the fluorescence techniques, among which are the method verification for specific kinds of beer, and its applicability for quantification of other fluorescent constituents, such as phenolic compounds and amino acids. Such studies will contribute to creation of convenient and widely applicable fluorescence-based methods for beer quality assurance.

Table 95.3 Examples of application of spectroscopic methods for direct analysis of beer

Spectroscopic methods	*Technique*	*Method of data analysis*	*Application*
NMR			
	^{1}H NMR	PCA	Discrimination between ale and lager beers (Duarte *et al.*, 2002) and according to content of dextrins, maltose, and glucose (Duarte *et al.*, 2004)
	^{1}H NMR	PLS	The quantification of organic acids and amino acids (Nord *et al.*, 2004)
	Flow-Injection ^{1}H NMR	PCA, PLS	Discrimination of beers made with barley malt and wheat malt, clustering of beers from the same brewing sites, discrimination of beers with deteriorated quality Quantitative determination of original gravity, ethanol, and lactic acid (Lachenmeier *et al.*, 2005)
	^{1}H NMR	PCA	Discrimination of beers differing in production site and date. Identification of lactic and pyruvic acid, linear dextrins, adenosine/inosine, uridine, tyrosine/tyrosol, and 2-phenylethanol (Almeida *et al.*, 2006)
	2D *J*-resolved NMR	PCA	Differentiation of beer. Identification of adenine, uridine, xanthine, tyrosine, proline, succinic acid, lactic acid, tyrosol, isopropanol, cholines, carbohydrates (Khatib *et al.*, 2006)
IR			
	FTIR-ATR	PCA	Discrimination of beers according to alcohol contents (Duarte *et al.*, 2004)
	FTIR-ATR	PLS	Determination of original and real extracts and alcohol content (Llario *et al.*, 2006)
	FTIR	PLS	Quantitative determination of ethanol, density, original gravity, and lactic acid. Semi-quantitative determination of pH, bitterness, and EBC color – screening analysis (Lachenmeier, 2007)
NIR			
	NIR	Difference absorption	Determination of ethanol (Engelhard *et al.*, 2006)
Combined FTIR–NIR			
	ATR-FTIR and NIR	PLS, ANN	Determination of real extract, original extract, and ethanol (Inon *et al.*, 2006)
Fluorescence spectroscopy			
	Synchronous fluorescence spectra	PCA	Discrimination of beers of different brands and stored under different conditions (Sikorska *et al.*, 2004b, 2006)
	Synchronous fluorescence spectra, emission spectra	PLS	Determination of vitamin B_2 (Sikorska, 2006)
	Excitation–emission matrix	PLS	Determination of bitterness (Christensen *et al.*, 2005)

EBC: European Brewery Convention; FTIR: Fourier transform–infrared; FTIR-ATR: attenuated total reflectance Fourier transform–infrared; ANN: artificial neural network.

Summary points

- Autofluorescence of beer was characterized, and the potential of fluorescence spectroscopy for qualitative and quantitative analysis of beers demonstrated.
- Several classes of compounds may contribute to beer fluorescence, including vitamins, amino acids, and phenolics.
- Rapid fluorescence measurements conducted directly on the beer samples and combined with multivariate data analysis can be used for:
  - qualitative and quantitative analysis;
  - beer discrimination according to the brand and freshness.

- Fluorescence may be used as a simple and sensitive tool for monitoring changes in beer related to the sunstruck flavor formation.
- Quantitative determination of vitamin B_2 and bitterness is possible after an appropriate calibration.
- Further studies are needed to resolve important practical issues, including:
  - method verification for specific kinds of beer,
  - its applicability for quantification of other fluorescent constituents, including:
    - phenolic compounds, and
    - amino acids.
  - this will allow to create convenient and widely applicable fluorescence-based methods for beer quality assurance.

References

Almeida, C., Duarte, I.F., Barros, A., Rodrigues, J., Spraul, M. and Gil, A.M. (2006). *J. Agric. Food Chem.* 54, 700–706.

Andres-Lacueva, C., Mattivi, F. and Tonon, D. (1998). *J. Chromatogr. A* 823, 355–363.

Apperson, K., Leiper, K.A., McKeown, I.P. and Birch, D.J.S. (2002). *J. Inst. Brew.* 108, 193–199.

Brereton, R.G. (2000). *Analyst* 125, 2125–2154.

Burns, C.S., Heyerick, A., De Keukeleire, D. and Forbes, M.D.E. (2001). *Chem. Eur. J.* 7, 4553–4561.

Cho, D. and Mattice, W.L. (1990). *J. Phys. Chem.* 94, 3847–3851.

Christensen, J., Ladefoged, A.M. and Norgaard, L. (2005). *J. Inst. Brew.* 111, 3–10.

Christensen, J., Norgaard, L., Bro, R. and Engelsen, S.B. (2006). *Chem. Rev.* 106, 1979–1994.

Duarte, I.F., Barros, A., Belton, P.S., Righelato, R., Spraul, M., Humpfer, E. and Gil, A.M. (2002). *J. Agric. Food Chem.* 50, 2475–2481.

Duarte, I.F., Barros, A., Almeida, C., Spraul, M. and Gil, A.M. (2004). *J. Agric. Food Chem.* 52, 1031–1038.

Duyvis, M.G., Hilhorst, R., Laane, C., Evans, D.J. and Schmedding, D.J.M. (2002). *J. Agric. Food Chem.* 50, 1548–1552.

Engelhard, S., Kumke, M.U. and Lohmannsroben, H.G. (2006). *Anal. Bioanal. Chem.* 384, 1107–1112.

Erbe, T. and Bruckner, H. (2000). *J. Chromatogr. A* 881, 81–91.

Foraker, A.B., Khantwal, C.M. and Swaan, P.W. (2003). *Adv. Drug Deliver. Rev.* 55, 1467–1483.

Friedrich, W. (ed.) (1988). *Vitamins.* Walter de Gruyter, Berlin, New York.

Goldsmith, M.R., Rogers, P.J., Cabral, N.M., Chiggino, K.P. and Roddick, F.A. (2005). *J. Am. Soc. Brew. Chem.* 63, 177–184.

Goldstein, H., Rader, S. and Murakami, A.A. (1993). *J. Am. Soc. Brew. Chem.* 51, 70–74

Gorinstein, S., Caspi, A., Zemser, M. and Trakhtenberg, S. (2000). *Nutr. Res.* 20, 131–139.

Guilbault, G.G. (1999). *Practical fluorescence.* Marcel Dekker, New York.

Gunst, F. and Verzele, M. (1978). *J. Inst. Brew.* 84, 291–292.

Heelis, P.F. (1982). *Chem. Soc. Rev.* 11, 15–39.

Hill, P.G. and Smith, R.M. (2000). *J. Chromatogr. A* 872, 203–213.

Huvaere, K., Olsen, K., Andersen, M.L., Skibsted, L.H., Heyerick, A. and De Keukeleire, D. (2004). *Photochem. Photobiol. Sci.* 3, 337–340.

Huvaere, K., Andersen, M.L., Skibsted, L.H., Heyerick, A. and De Keukeleire, D. (2005). *J. Agric. Food Chem.* 53, 1489–1494.

Huvaere, K., Andersen, M.L., Storme, M., Van Bocxlaer, J., Skibsted, L.H. and De Keukeleire, D. (2006). *Photochem. Photobiol. Sci.* 5, 961–969.

Inon, F.A., Garrigues, S. and de la Guardia, M. (2006). *Anal. Chim. Acta* 571, 167–174.

Islam, S.D.M., Susdorf, T., Penzkofer, A. and Hegemann, P. (2003). *Chem. Phys.* 295, 137–149.

Khatib, A., Wilson, E.G., Kim, H.K., Lefeber, A.W.M., Erkelens, C., Choi, Y.H. and Verpoorte, R. (2006). *Anal. Chim. Acta* 559, 264–270.

Lachenmeier, D.W. (2007). *Food Chem.* 101, 825–832.

Lachenmeier, D.W., Frank, W., Humpfer, E., Schafer, H., Keller, S., Mortter, M. and Spraul, M. (2005). *Eur. Food Res. Technol.* 220, 215–221.

Llario, R., Inon, F.A., Garrigues, S. and de la Guardia, M. (2006). *Talanta* 69, 469–480.

Masuda, S., Kikuchi, K. and Harayama, K. (2000). *J. Am. Soc. Brew. Chem.* 58, 152–154.

Moller, A., Saxholt, E., Christensen, A.T., and Hartkopp, H.B. (2002). Danish Food Composition Databank, version 5.0. Food Informatics, Institute of Food Safety and Nutrition, Danish Veterinary and Food Administration.

Montanari, L., Perretti, G., Natella, F., Guidi, A. and Fantozzi, P. (1999). *Food Sci. Technol.-Leb.* 32, 535–539.

Nardini, M., Natella, F., Scaccini, C. and Ghiselli, A. (2006). *J. Nutr. Biochem.* 17, 14–22.

Ndou, T. and Warner, I.M. (1991). *Chem. Rev.* 91, 493–507.

Nollet, L.M.L. (ed.) (2004). In *Handbook of Food Analysis.* Marcel Dekker, Inc., New York.

Nord, L.I., Vaag, P. and Duus, J.O. (2004). *Anal. Chem.* 76, 4790–4798.

Oldham, P.B., McCarroll, M.E., McGown, L.B. and Warner, I.M. (2000). *Anal. Chem.* 72, 197R–209R.

Polewski, K., Kniat, S. and Slawinska, D. (2002). *Curr. Top. Biophys.* 26, 217–227.

Pozdrik, R., Roddick, F.A., Rogers, P.J. and Nguyen, T. (2006). *J. Agric. Food Chem.* 54, 6123–6129.

Peppard, T.L. (1985). *J. Inst. Brew.* 91, 364–369.

Ramanujam, N. (2000). Fluorescence spectroscopy in vivo. In Meyers, R.A. (ed.), *Encyclopedia of Analytical Chemistry*, pp. 20–56. John Wiley, Chichester, UK.

Sakuma, S., Rikimaru, Y., Kobayashi, K. and Kowaka, M. (1991). *J. Am. Soc. Brew. Chem.* 49, 162–165.

Sanchez, F.G., Carnero, C. and Heredia, A. (1988). *J. Agric. Food Chem.* 36, 80–82.

Sanchez, F.G., Diaz, A.N. and Garcia, J.A.G. (1995). *Anal. Chim. Acta* 310, 399–406.

Sanchez, F., Navas, D. Lovillo, I. Feria, L.S. (1996). *Anal. Chim. Acta.* 328, 73–79.

Shahidi, F. and Naczk, M. (2003). In *Phenolics in Food and Nutraceuticals.* CRC Press, Boca Raton, FL.

Sikorska, E. (2006). *Eur. Food Res. Technol.* 225, 43–48.

Sikorska, E., Chmielewski, J., Koziol, J., Khmelinskii, I.V., Herance, R., Bourdelande, J.L. and Sikorski, M. (2003). *Polish J. Food Nutr. Sci.* 53, 113–118.

Sikorska, E., Gorecki, T., Khmelinskii, I.V. and Sikorski, M. *et al.* (2004a). In Rong, W. (ed.), *Focusing New Century – Commodity Trade Environment*, Vol. 1, pp. 167–171. China Agriculture Press, Beijing.

Sikorska, E., Gorecki, T., Khmelinskii, I.V., Sikorski, M. and De Keukeleire, D. (2004b). *J. Inst. Brew.* 110, 267–275.

Sikorska, E., Gorecki, T., Khmelinskii, I.V., Sikorski, M. and De Keukeleire, D. (2006). *Food Chem.* 96, 632–639.

Su, A.K., Chang, Y.S. and Lin, C.H. (2004). *Talanta* 64, 970–974.

Vinas, P., Balsalobre, N., Lopez-Erroz, C. and Hernandez-Cordoba, M. (2004). *J. Agric. Food Chem.* 52, 1789–1794.

Wold, S., Esbensen, K. and Geladi, P. (1987). *Chemometr. Intell. Lab.* 2, 37–52.

Wu, W. and Massart, D.L. (1997). *Anal. Chim. Acta* 349, 253–261.

96

Capillary Electrophoresis Methods Used for Beer Analysis

Antonio Segura-Carretero, Sonia Cortacero-Ramírez and Alberto Fernández-Gutiérrez Department of Analytical Chemistry, Faculty of Sciences, University of Granada, Granada, Spain

Abstract

In this chapter, an overview of capillary electrophoretic methods developed for determining different components of beer samples is presented. The different electrophoretic methods for the analysis of carbohydrates, alcohols, amino acids, amines, nucleic derivatives, inorganic and organic anions, vitamins, phenolic acids, bitter acids, aldehydes and sulfur compounds have been chronologically classified and the experimental and instrumental conditions of the electrophoretic method proposed are described in detail. The last section is dedicated to multicomponent analysis by capillary electrophoresis.

Introduction

Beer is a beverage which contains a great number of components, and their determination requires a potent analytical technique such as capillary electrophoresis (CE). CE is a versatile analytical tool that has emerged as a highly promising technique which needs an extremely small amount of sample and reagents and is capable of rapid and high-resolution separations and, what is more, the use of different detectors give an important potential for the analysis of beer components.

This technique permits the direct injection of samples almost without pre-treatment using pressure, vacuum or electrokinetics. Once injected, the sample components move differentially through the capillary under the influence of a high voltage, resulting in a rapid separation. CE is a very versatile technique, mainly because different methods are available such as capillary zone electrophoresis (CZE), micellar electrokinetic chromatography (MEKC), isotacophoresis (ITP), capillary electrochromatography (CEC), capillary gel electrophoresis (CGE) and capillary isoelectric focusing (CIEF) (Marina *et al.*, 2005) allowing the analysis of charged and uncharged compounds, almost all molecules and even whole organisms.

The physical and chemical properties of beer components also influence the different detectors selected. Nowadays, many detection systems can be used, such as ultraviolet (UV)–vis absorption, fluorimetry, phosphorimetry, mass spectrometry (MS), electrochemistry, conductivity and nuclear magnetic resonance, among others. The different detection systems described for CE, and the analytes in beer which can be analyzed are summarized in Table 96.1 (Khun and Hoffstetter-Kuhn, 1993; Fernández-Gutiérrez *et al.*, 2005).

Therefore, the development of CE methods for beer analysis has greatly increased which is reflected in the number of published reports, (Lindeberg, 1996; Sadecka and Polonsky, 2000; Cortacero-Ramírez *et al.*, 2003a). Figure 96.1 shows the number of publications about CE methods for beer analysis.

Analysis of Beer Components by CE

Beer, which is composed of around 8,000 compounds, is a complex sample. In this section, we describe the analysis of the different types of compounds and the possibility of multicomponent analysis using CE.

Analysis of carbohydrates

Carbohydrates are the main non-volatile components of beer (3.3–4.4%) and therefore monitoring the carbohydrates in wort and bottled beers is very important to modern brewing technology, particularly in the development of new kinds of beer and in the selection of raw materials and yeast strains. Three polysaccharides, starch, pentosan (arabinoxilan) and β-glucan together with sucrose are the primary sources of carbohydrates in beer (Vinogradov and Bock, 1998). The main monosaccharides are glucose and fructose, the disaccharides are maltose (14% of total wort carbohydrate) and sucrose (5% total wort carbohydrate)

Beer in Health and Disease Prevention
ISBN: 978-0-12-373891-2

Table 96.1 Different detection systems for capillary electrophoresis used in the analysis of beer components

Detection mode	*Approximately LOD (mol)*	*Advantages*	*Disadvantages*	*Analytes*
Optic techniques				
Spectrophotometry				
Direct	10^{-13}–10^{-15}	Easy to use and relatively universal	Relatively low sensitivity	Hop acids, phenolic acid, purines and pyrimidines
Indirect	10^{-12}–10^{-15}			Carbohydrates, inorganic and organic anions
Spectrofluorimetry				
Direct	10^{-15}–10^{-17}	Higher sensitivity than UV detection, high selectivity	Not universally usable	Vitamins
Indirect	10^{-14}–10^{-16}	Universal and rather high sensitivity	Restrictions in the choice of buffers	Amines, amino acids
Pre-column derivatization	10^{-18}–10^{-21}			Amines, amino acids
Post-column derivatization	10^{-17}			
Laser-induced fluorescence	10^{-18}–10^{-20}	The highest sensitivity	Types of analytes restricted	Amines, amino acids
Raman Spectroscopy	10^{-15}	High specificity	Types of analytes restricted	
Refraction index	10^{-14}–10^{-16}	High specificity		Carbohydrates
Electrochemistry techniques				
Conductometry	10^{-15}–10^{-16}	Peak area correlates linearly with migration time	Relatively low sensitivity not universally usable	Alditols, alcohols, amino acids
Amperometry	10^{-18}–10^{-19}	Very high sensitivity and selectivity	Limited to electroactive compounds, difficult to establish	Alditols, alcohols
Other techniques				
Mass spectrometry	10^{-16}–10^{-17}	Universal	Cost of equipment	Hop acids, iso-α-acids
Radiochemistry method	10^{-17}–10^{-19}	Specificity	Highly restricted	

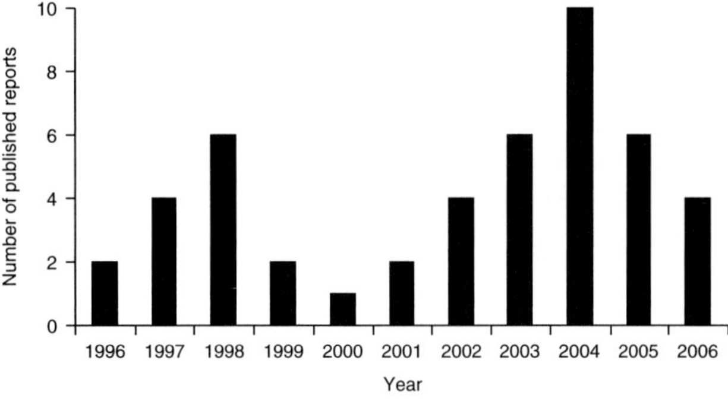

Figure 96.1 Evolution of use of the capillary electrophoretic method in beer analysis.

and the principal trisaccharide is maltotriose. Many of the carbohydrates emanate from the malt itself and others are produced during mashing (Hornsey, 1999).

CE has great potential for the separation of complex carbohydrate samples, but two major difficulties have to be overcome. Firstly, with the exception of a few naturally charged mono- and oligosaccharides, most carbohydrates molecules lack readily ionizable charged functions, a condition which excludes their direct differential migration and, in turn, separation with CE. Secondly, most carbohydrates neither absorb nor fluoresce, hindering their sensitive detection. These difficulties have lead to the use of the inherent properties of carbohydrates including: (i) the ease with which these molecules can be readily converted *in situ* to charged species by complex formation with other ions, such as borate and metal cations, which then ensure their differential electromigration and, in turn, separation in an electric field and (ii) the reactivity of the reducing end and other functional groups of sugar molecules (i.e. carboxylic acid groups and amino groups) which can be readily labeled with UV-absorbing or fluorescent tags, thus providing the centers for sensitive detection. In addition, the electrochemical oxidation of carbohydrates at the surface of metallic electrodes provides another means by which underivatized carbohydrates can be sensitively detected (Rassi El, 1996).

Among the methods published for the analysis of carbohydrates, we can find the research of Guttman *et al.* (1996) who proposed a method for determining carbohydrates in the biopharmaceutical and food and beverage industries (brewing) by CE fingerprinting.

Another method is the pre-column derivatization of carbohydrates with *p*-aminobenzoic acid and their separation as borate complexes by means of CZE, using a capillary tube of fused silica containing 20 mM borate buffer, pH

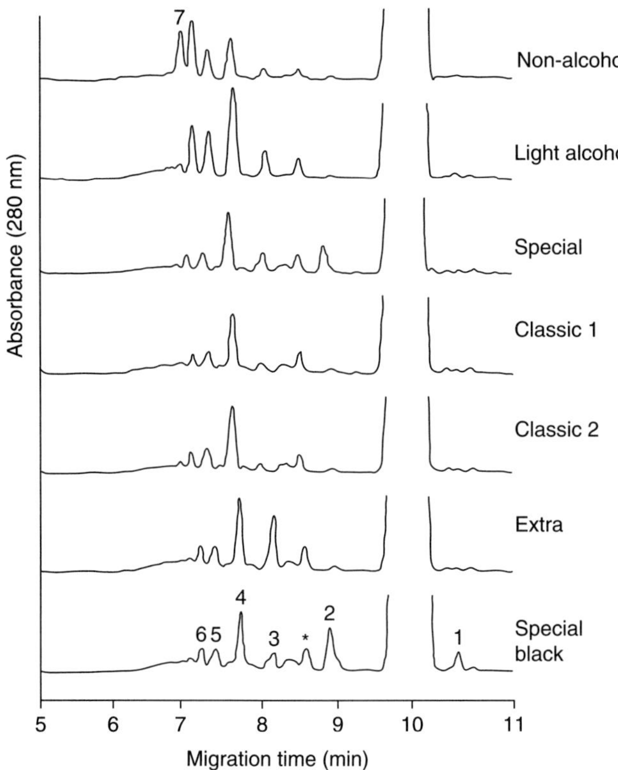

Figure 96.2 Electropherograms of PABA-carbohydrate from different beer samples. Peak assignment: (1) glucose, (2) maltose, (3) maltotriose, (4) maltotetraose, (5) maltopentaose, (6) maltohexaose, (7) maltoheptaose and R, derivatization reagent (*p*-aminobenzoic acid). Operation conditions: 20 mM sodium tetraborate, pH 10.2, capillary LT 57 cm, LD 50 cm, ID 75 μm; 20 kV, 8 s hydrodynamic injection. *Source*: Reproduced from Elsevier, Cortacero-Ramírez *et al*. (2004a).

10.2, as carrier. In this method, on-column UV-monitoring at 280 nm allows the detection of carbohydrates with a reducing end. This has been successfully applied to different types of beer (see Figure 96.2) (Cortacero-Ramírez *et al.*, 2004a).

Sucrose, galactose, fructose, glucose and maltose have also been analyzed in beer using microchip CE and a nickel amperometric detector. For this separation 35 mM NaOH in deionized water is used; the injections are carried out by applying the desired potential for 3 s and the voltage applied is 1,000 V (Wang *et al.*, 2004).

Cortacero-Ramírez *et al.* (2005a) use CE with indirect detection for the separation of five carbohydrates: sucrose, maltotriose, maltose, glucose and fructose. Indirect detection is an easy procedure that avoids the need for pre- or post-column labeling. This procedure can be used universally, and it is particularly useful for compounds that do not possess the necessary physical properties to allow direct detection. It is based on the displacement of a running electrolyte (chromophore or fluorophore) usually containing a co-ion with functions that can be detected through a decrease in the measurement signal. The method has been used to determine carbohydrates during the brewing process of a non-alcoholic beer.

Alditols and alcohols

In beers the most important alcohol is ethanol, which is present in most beers at levels in at least twice as high as other alcohols. This important fraction is formed during beer fermentation. Its formation is linked to yeast protein synthesis and is formed from keto-acids, which in turn may be formed by transamination or deamination of the amino acids in the wort, or synthesized from wort carbohydrates.

For the analysis of these compounds, Chen and Huang (1995, 1997) have developed an end-column amperometric detector for CE based on an incorporated Ni-microelectrode used for the determination of 10 alditols and alcohols, obtaining satisfactory performance with respect to the stability of the background current, lowering of detection limit (down to the sub-fmole level) and reproducibility. Its application demonstrates the presence of ethanol, glycerol, myo-inositol, erythritol, xylitol, arabitol and mannitol in two Taiwan beers.

Wang *et al.* (2004) have used a nickel electrode to detect alcohols in beer. Nickel is deposited directly at the end of an electrophoretic glass microchip using an electroless deposition procedure leading to a sensitive amperometric detector for alcohols. They have evaluated the integrated CE–electrochemical detection microsystem for the separation of ethanol and methanol in different beer samples.

Simonet *et al.* (2004) propose a method using CZE and a capillary containing the immobilized enzymes (alcohol dehydrogenase and lactate dehydrogenase) to enhance the sensitivity for the determination of ethanol. The running buffer used is a mixture of 15 mM β-NAD$^+$ in 50 mM phosphate buffer at pH 7.0. Separation is accomplished by using an applied voltage of 10 kV and a capillary temperature of 20°C, and the sample is injected under high pressure (20 psi) for 10 s with detection performed at 340 nm.

Amino acids

Beer contains an average of between 0.2 and 0.6 g/100 ml of protein-derived material. The amino acids are modulators of the flavor of beer and are responsible for the organoleptic quality. The lack of a strong chromophore for aliphatic amino acids has certainly been one of the limitations in the analysis of most natural amino acids by CE, but a common option is determination by direct UV detection at 185 nm or indirect UV detection using background electrolytes (BGEs).

Underivatized amino acids (lysine, histidine, arginine, glycine, alanine, serine, tryptophane, phenylalanine, tyrosine and proline) are determined in beer samples by CE with direct UV detection at 185 nm using a 10 mM phosfate buffer containing 30 mM octanesulfonic acid (pH

2.36) (Klampfl *et al.*, 1998; Klampfl, 1999). The main advantages are the simplicity and the speed of the method, allowing a fast screening of the amino acid patterns. No pre-treatment or derivatization steps are necessary, but the limits of detection (LODs) are relatively high for the aliphatic amino acids (10–50 mg/l). Bednar *et al.* (2001) proposed a method to determine aspartic and glutamic acids enantiomers in beer by CE with indirect detection using 10 mM sorbic acid/histidine, pH 5 and 10 mM of vancomycin.

High-voltage contactless conductivity detection (CCD) of underivatized amino acids in both acidic and basic media has been demonstrated (Tanyanyiwa *et al.*, 2003). The method determines 12 amino acids using buffer solutions at pH values of about 2.5. Lactic acid as BGE gives the best results in terms of LODs for arginine, lysine and histidine, which are approximately 2×10^{-7}, 3×10^{-7} and 4×10^{-7} M, respectively. The use of basic conditions at pH 10–11 generally produces more stable baselines and more consistent sensitivities allowing the determination of a range of 20 amino acids. In beer samples 11 amino acids are identified by this method. Coufal *et al.* (2003) also analyzed 20 underivatized essential amino acids using CZE with CCD. A simple acidic BGE containing 2.3 M acetic acid and 0.1% w/w hydroxyethylcellulose (HEC) allows the electrophoretic separation and sensitive detection of all 20 essential amino acids in their underivatized cationic form. The addition of HEC to the BGE suppressed both the electroosmotic flow and the analyte adsorption on the capillary surface, resulting in an excellent migration time reproducibility and a very good analyte peak symmetry.

To achieve better sensitivities, two alternative detection strategies are frequently used: derivatization of amino acids with a strong chromophore or suitable fluorophore labeling.

Tivesten *et al.* (1997) have developed a method for chiral determination of aspartic and glutamic acid. These compounds are derivatized using a fluorogenic reagent, *o*-phthaldialdehyde-2,3,4,6-tetra-*O*-acetyl-1-thiol-β-D-glucopyranose. With a neutral surfactant, octylglucoside, the D- and L-aspartic and glutamic acid derivatives are resolved outside the micellar retention window creating a high selectivity toward other amino acids. The method is applied for both aspartic and glutamic acid in their D- and L-forms in beer samples. The precapillary derivatization of 20 amino acids with naphthalene-2,3-dicarboxaldehyde (NDA) has been investigated by Dong *et al.* (2002). CZE with electrochemical detection is used for the analysis of these amino acids. The optimum conditions of separation and detection are borate, pH 9.48, for the electrolyte, 18 kV for the separation voltage and 1.15 V vs. a saturated calomel electrode for the detection potential. LODs of concentration for individual amino acids are between 1.7×10^{-7} and 1.8×10^{-6} M for injection voltage of 6 kV and injection time of 10 s. The relative standard deviation (RSD) is between 0.80% and 2.3% for the migration times and 1.4% and 6.4% for the electrophoretic peak currents. Only 10 amino acids can be well separated. This method is applied to the determination of amino acids in beer by the standard addition method. The recovery for the amino acids in beer is 91–109%.

Table 96.2 shows the experimental and instrumental conditions for analyzing amino acids in beer samples by CE.

Amines

Beer has been commonly reported to be a health risk for some consumers due to the biogenic amines it contains. Volatile amines originate from the malt and the hops used, and the conditions during mashing and boiling influence their concentration in beer.

Preston *et al.* (1997) introduced a method using CE with simultaneous UV–vis, and LIF detection was applied to identify and quantify selected amines (ammonia, ethylamine, isoamylamine and dibutylamine) in beer following derivatization with 7-chloro-4-nitrobenzo-2-oxa-1,3-diazole. The fluorescence detection method is more selective and sensitive for the determination of aliphatic amines in beer than UV–vis absorbance detection.

Sodium citrate buffer at pH 2.5 and sodium phosphate buffer at a concentration of 25 mM (pH 6.5) is used for determination of histamine in non-alcoholic malt beer and beer samples (Mahendradatta and Schwedt, 1998). Two types of extractions, solid-phase extraction (SPE) and liquid–liquid extraction (LLE) are carried out, best results being obtained with SPE.

Zhang *et al.* (2002) used CZE for the determination of histamine using end-column amperometric detection with a carbon fiber microelectrode, at a constant potential. The optimum conditions of separation and detection are 10 mM phosphate buffer, pH 5.6 for the buffer solution, 15 kV for the separation voltage and 1.35 V for the detection potential. The linear range is from 6.3×10^{-7} to 1.5×10^{-5} M with the regression coefficient of 0.9997, and the detection limit is 4.0×10^{-7} M (signal to noise ratio (S/N) = 3). The proposed method has been successfully applied to the direct determination of histamine in beer samples without any sample clean-up procedures.

To increase sensitivity and selectivity other authors use CE with LIF for the analysis of amines. Zhang and Sun (2004) developed a rapid and sensitive method for the simultaneous determination of histamine and histidine by CZE with LIF detection. A fluorogenic derivatization reagent, NDA is successfully applied to label the histamine and histidine, respectively. The optimal derivatization reaction is performed with 1.0 mM NDA, 20 mM NaCN and 20 mM borate buffer, pH 9.1 for 15 min. The separation of NDA-tagged histamine and histidine can be achieved in less than 4 min with 40 mM phosphate buffer (pH 5.8) as the running buffer. The detection limits for histamine and

Table 96.2 Method for determining amino acids in beer samples by CE

Detection	*Mode and detection system*	*Experimental conditions*	*Sample preparation*	*Reference*
Direct	MECK-UV	10 mM phosphate, 30 mM octanesulfonic, 5% AcN, pH 2.36 Voltage 30 kV Capillary, 92 cm × 50 μm Hydrostatic injection 10 cm for 15 s UV 185 nm	Degassed and diluted	Klampfl *et al.* (1998)
Indirect	CZE-UV	10 mM sorbic acid/histidine, 10 mM vancomycin, pH 5 Voltage, –10 kV Polyacrylamide-coated capillary, 35 (30.5) cm × 50 μm Hydrodinamic injection 10 psi.s UV 254 nm	Centrifuged, diluted with HCl (1:1), passed through the SPE column. Washing the column with 6 ml of water and 6 ml of 8 M ammonia solution were used to elute the amino acids. The elute was evaporated and the solution reconstituted by adding 1 ml of water	Bednar *et al.* (2001)
	ECZ-CCD	6 mM lactic acid, pH 2.4 Voltage, –25 kV Capillary, 60 cm × 25 μm Injection, electrokinetic: 7 s at 5 kV Detection, 450 Vp-p, 100 kHz	Degassed and diluted	Tanyanyiwa *et al.* (2003)
	CZE-CCD	2.3 M acetic acid, pH 2.1 and 0.1% w/w HEC Voltage, 30 kV Capillary, 66.5 cm × 50 μm Injection, 300 mbar.s, Temperature, 25°C	Sonicated for 10 min	Coufal *et al.* (2003)
Derivatization	MECK-UV or fluorescence	40 mM phosphate, 100 mM octylglucoside, 5% AcN, pH 6.5 Voltage 15 kV Capillary 40 cm × 50 μm Hydrodinamic injection 20 mbar for 8 s UV230 nm or fluorescence (He–Cd 325 nm)	Centrifuged, diluted and derivatized	Tivesten *et al.* (1997)
	ECZ-electrochemical detection	Borate, pH 9.48 Voltage 18 kV	Derivatized	Dong *et al.* (2002)

histidine are 5.5×10^{-9} and 3.8×10^{-9} M, respectively ($S/N = 3$). The RSD for migration time and peak height of derivatives are less than 1.5% and 5.0%, respectively. The method has been successfully applied to the analysis of histamine and histidine in beer samples.

Cao *et al.* (2005) have studied the analytical potential of a fluorescein analog, 6-oxy-(*N*-succinimidyl acetate)-9-(2′-methoxycarbonyl) fluorescein (SAMF), as a new labeling reagent for the determination of amino compounds by CE with LIF detection. The derivatization is performed at 30°C for 6 min in boric acid buffer at pH 8.0. The derivatives are baseline-separated in 15 min with 25 mM boric acid running buffer (pH 9.0), containing 24 mM sodium dodecyl sulphate (SDS) and 12.5% v/v acetonitrile. LOD for biogenic amines reaches 8×10^{-11} M ($S/N = 3$). The method has been applied to the determination of biogenic amines in three different beer samples with satisfactory recoveries varying from 92.8% to 104.8%.

Casado-Terrones *et al.* (2006), have compared the performance of two CE instruments, one commercial and one homemade device, for the determination of derivatized aminated compounds with fluorescein isothiocyanate (FITC). The commercial CE system first uses an argon ion laser as excitation source; the homemade CE device uses an inexpensive blue light-emitting diode (LED) as the light source and a charge-coupled device (CCD) as the detection system. After fine optimization of several separation parameters in both devices, a co-electroosmotic flow CE methodology is achieved in coated capillary tubing with 0.001% hexadimetrine bromide (HDB), and 50 mM sodium borate at pH 9.3 with 20% 2-propanol for the determination of several amines and aminoacids. Both systems have been applied to beer samples.

A sensitive CE method has been developed by Cortacero-Ramírez *et al.* (2007) for the simultaneous determination of 10 biogenic amine using LIF. Sample amines are first derivatized with FITC and filtered, and then separated with an uncoated capillary tubing in the presence of 50 mM sodium borate and 20% acetone at pH 9.3 at 30 kV. It is possible to analyze biogenic amines in brewing-process samples and in beer samples in less than 30 min, obtaining detection limits between 0.3 μg/l for ethylamine and 11.9 μg/l for 1,6-hexanodiamine.

Nucleic acid derivatives

Few methods exist for the determination of nucleic acid derivatives in beer by CE. Klampfl *et al.* (2002) have presented a quick and simple method for the determination of five purine bases (adenosine, guanosine, adenine, hypoxanthine and xanthine) and five pyrimidine bases (cytosine, cytidine, uridine, thymine and uracil) in beer samples using CZE with direct UV detection at 254 nm as well as MS detection using an electrospray ionization (ESI) interface. For this purpose, a carrier electrolyte and composition compatible with both methods of detection containing 300 mM diethylamine (DEA) is selected. LOD are in the range between 0.1 and 0.3 mg/l and calibration plots are found to be linear over at least two orders of magnitude.

Cortacero-Ramírez *et al.* (2003b, c, 2004b, c, d), have also determined purine and pyrimidine bases among other components by CZE-DAD and MEKC-DAD (for more detail see section "Multicomponent analysis").

Inorganic and organic anions

The measurement of the concentrations of inorganic and organic anions, in all phases of beer production, can be used to help track metabolic products of fermentation and correlate beer flavor trends. For the determination of these types of components CZE is normally used with indirect detection.

DeVries (1993) has determined organic acids (malate, citrate, succinate, pyruvate, acetate and lactate) by CE with indirect UV detection at pH 5.5 and the levels of organic acids in beer are tracked from cold wort to packaged beer.

Soga and Ross (1997) and Soga and Wakaura (1997) have determined three inorganic anions (chloride, sulfate and phosphate) and nine organic anions (oxalate, formate, malate, citrate, succinate, pyruvate, acetate, lactate and pyroglutamate) in beer using 2,6-pyridinedicarboxylic acid (pH 5.6) containing 0.5 mM cetyltrimethylammonium bromide, as BGE and indirect UV detection at 350 nm in less than 7 min. The LODs for all analytes are in the range of 0.9–2.5 mg/l. The method described allows the quantitative analysis of low-molecular-mass ionic components in beer using indirect UV detection as well as conductivity detection, providing RSD between 0.5% and 6.6% for the peak areas and excellent LODs ranging from 0.02 mg/l for chloride to 0.41 mg/l for phosphate.

For the determination of inorganic and organic anions in different types of beer, Klampfl and Katzmayr (1998) and Klampfl (1999), found it to be advantageous to use CZE with conductivity detection in series with UV detection at 254 nm. With a running buffer composed of 7.5 mM 4-aminobenzoic acid and 0.12 mM tetradecyltrimethylammonium bromide (pH 5.75 adjusted by the addition of histamine), conductivity detection proved to be more sensitive for the faster migrating anions, whereas UV detection was found to be superior for analytes with mobilities similar to that of 4-aminobenzoic acid. The combination of direct conductivity detection and indirect UV detection is useful for CZE analysis of samples such as beer containing both inorganic anions and organic low-molecular-mass anionic solutes, such as carboxylic acids. Using this technique, low LODs and LOQs can be obtained over a wide range of analyte mobilities. Conductivity detection is more suitable for ions with mobilities that are highly different from those of the carrier electrolyte co-ion, whereas indirect UV detection is superior for analytes showing the same or only small differences in mobility. This has been demonstrated for different varieties of beer samples, including fast migrating solutes, that is, chloride, sulfate and oxalate, as well as slowly migrating ingredients such as lactate, phosphate and pyroglutamate. Carbonate is determined in beer samples using on-line gas diffusion coupled to CE in a flow arrangement (Kuban and Karlberg, 1998).

The use of highly absorbing anionic dyes as probes and isoelectric ampholytes as buffers in BGEs combined with the use of an LED as a light source has been studied for ultrasensitive indirect photometric detection in CE (Johns *et al.*, 2000). Two dyes, tartrazine and naphthol yellow S, with histidine as the ampholytic buffer, were selected for detailed investigation. For the naphthol yellow *S*-histidine BGE, linearity and reproducibility were also evaluated, with excellent linearity being observed over a range of 5–500 mM, and reproducibility less than 1% for migration times and 2–8% for normalized peak areas. The approach has been successfully applied to several real samples including tap water, mineral waters and beer.

Masar *et al.* (2003), have used a poly(methylmethacrylate) CE chip, provided with a high sample load capacity separation system (a 8,500 nl separation channel combined with a 500 nl sample injection channel) and a pair of on-chip conductivity detectors, for CZE determination of oxalate in beer. Hydrodynamic and EOFs of the solution in the separation compartment of the chip are suppressed and electrophoresis is a dominant transport process in the separations performed on the chip. A low pH of the carrier electrolyte (3.8), implemented by aspartic acid and bis-tris propane, provides an adequate selectivity in the separation of oxalate from anionic beer constituents and, at the same time, a sufficient sensitivity in its conductivity detection. Under these working conditions, this anion can be detected at a 0.5 μM concentration in samples containing chloride (a major anionic constituent of beer) at a 1,800 higher concentration. Such a favorable analyte/matrix concentration ratio allows accurate and reproducible (typically, 2–5% RSD values of the peak areas of the analyte depending on its concentration in the sample) determination of oxalate in 500 nl volumes of 20–50 fold diluted beer samples. Short analysis times (about 4 min), minimum sample preparation and reproducible migration times of this analyte (0.5–1.0% RSD values) are characteristic for the CZE chip.

CZE with direct detection have been used when the components absorb. Therefore, a separation and determination of a mixture of 19 low-molecular-mass organic acids usually present in beer samples (oxalic acid, fumaric acid, ketoglutaric acid, mesaconic acid, malic acid, pyruvic acid, phthalic acid, benzoic acid, pyroglutamic acid, sorbic acid, 4-aminobenzoic acid, 4-hydroxybenzoic acid, protocatechuic acid, gallic acid, *p*-coumaric acid, homovanillic acid, syringic acid, ferulic acid and sinapinic acid) has been carried out by Cortacero-Ramírez *et al.* (2005b) using CZE electrophoresis. A polycation (HDB) is added to the electrolyte, which dynamically coats the inner surface of the capillary and causes a fast EOF. The main factors affecting reversal of the EOF such as the type of modifier and concentration and influence of organic solvents have been studied. Other modifiers, such as cetyltrimethylammonium bromide and tetradecyltrimethylammonium bromide have also been investigated. The composition of the running buffer is 25% 2-propanol, 0.001% HDB and 50 mM sodium phosphate (pH 8). The different instrumental parameters affecting the capillary electrophoretic separation used as optimum are a −15 kV voltage with a hydrodynamic injection for 7 s with UV detection at 210 nm. Figure 96.3 shows an electropherogram in the condition previously described.

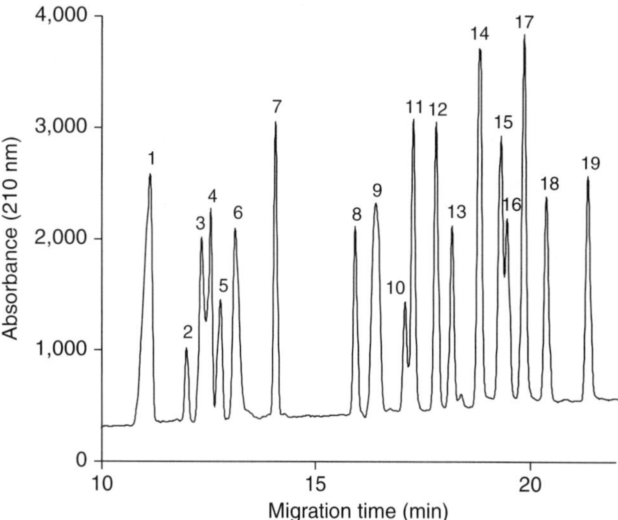

Figure 96.3 Separation of aliphatic and aromatic acids by co-electroosmotic CZE. Peaks: (1) oxalic acid (300 mg/l), (2) fumaric acid (10 mg/l), (3) ketoglutaric acid (100 mg/l), (4) mesaconic acid (10 mg/l), (5) malic acid (300 mg/l), (6) pyruvic acid (100 mg/l), (7) phthalic acid (10 mg/l), (8) benzoic acid (10 mg/l), (9) pyroglutamic acid (50 mg/l), (10) sorbic acid (10 mg/l), (11) 4-aminobenzoic acid (10 mg/l), (12) 4-hydroxybenzoic acid (10 mg/l), (13) protocatechuic acid (10 mg/l), (14) gallic acid (10 mg/l), (15) *p*-coumaric acid (10 mg/l), (16) homovanillic acid (10 mg/l), (17) syringic acid (10 mg/l), (18) ferulic acid (10 mg/l), (19) sinapinic acid (10 mg/l). Electrophoretic conditions: 50 mM sodium phosphate (pH 8), 0.001% HDB and 25% 2-propanol, hydrodynamically injection for 7 s, voltage −15 kV. *Source*: Reproduced from Elsevier, Cortacero-Ramírez *et al.* (2005b).

Vitamins

Beer contains small amounts of vitamins and a moderate intake can make a contribution to the daily vitamin requirements for health (http://www.beerandhealth.com).

L-Ascorbic acids are often added to beer as antioxidants, D-erythorbic acids have the same antioxidative properties as L-ascorbic acid and are sometimes substituted for L-ascorbic acid because they are cheaper. Marshall *et al.* (1995) have achieved baseline separation of L-ascorbic acid and D-erythorbic acid using a buffer consisting of 50 mM SDS and 5 mM dipotassium hydrogenorthophosphate (pH 9.2). Ten beers were analyzed for total L-ascorbic acids using this buffer. Baseline separation of L-ascorbic and D-erythorbic acids are also maintained when SDS is used for the separation. Replacing the 5 mM phosphate buffer (pH 9.2) with a 1:1 mixture of 20 mM tetraborate and 20 mM phosphate buffer (pH 8.6) results in enhanced separation of the two isomeric acids and a much shorter run time (6 min).

Klampfl *et al.* (2002) and Cortacero-Ramírez *et al.* (2003b, c, 2004b, c, d) determined adenine (vitamin B4) together with other analytes by CE with direct UV detection in different beer samples, finding that their content in beers with a reduced alcohol content, such as non-alcoholic beers and the light beers is higher than in other beers.

Su *et al.* (2004) described a simple, inexpensive and reliable method for the routine analysis of riboflavin in beer by CE–LED detection. A simple and straightforward sample preparation is involved and the method is based on an inexpensive blue LED as the light source combined with an on-line sample concentration technique. For this detection system, using a normal MEKC, stacking-MEKC and dynamic pH junction techniques, the LOD are found to be 480, 20 and 1 mg/l, respectively. In addition, the number of theoretical plates for riboflavin is determined to be 3.8×10^4 by means of a dynamic pH junction and this is improved to 3.2×10^6 when the dynamic pH junction-sweeping mode is applied. The concentrations of riboflavin in 12 samples of different types of commercial beer were found to be in the range of 130–280 mg/l.

The application of a UV-LED to on-line sample concentration/fluorescence detection in CE is described by Chang *et al.* (2006). The utility of a UV-LED (peak emission wavelength at 380 nm) is demonstrated by examining riboflavin. LOD for riboflavin is determined to be 0.2 mg/l by the normal MEKC mode, which improves to 3–7 μg/l when the dynamic pH-junction technique is applied. With this system, the concentration of riboflavin in beer can be determined.

Phenolic acids

Beverages of plant origin contain significant amounts of phenolic acids, these compounds have been well-described during recent years for their properties as antioxidants and scavengers of reactive oxygen and nitrogen species (Bourne *et al.*, 2000). In beer, phenolic acids are extracted into boiling wort; these compounds emanate from both malt and hops.

CE using amperometric detection has been used to detect phenolic acids in beer samples (Moane *et al.*, 1998). The electrophoretic separation requires the phenolic acids to be charged and therefore the pH is above their pK_as. However, electrochemical detection is optimum when the pH is 7.2. Cationic and neutral compounds in the beer samples interfere with electrochemical detection by passivating the electrode surface. These compounds are removed using a reversed-polarity injection technique to elute them from the separation capillary into the sample reservoir prior to electrophoretic separation. Electrophoretic peaks in the samples are identified by both matching their migration time and electrochemical properties with standards. The use of voltametric characterization provides improved peak identification for complex samples. Holland *et al.* (1999) have determined ferulic acid in beer by CE using an integrated on-capillary dual electrode electrochemical detector.

Rapid separation of a group of eight antioxidants by co-electroosmotic CE and their preliminary determination in foods (cereal, wine and beer) is described by Hernández-Borges *et al.* (2005). The compounds studied were protocatechuic acid, salicylic acid, *p*-hydroxybenzoic acid, vanillic acid, syringic acid, *p*-coumaric acid, ferulic acid and sinapinic acid. The best separation is achieved by the use of a running buffer consisting of 125 mM boric acid, 49 mM disodium hydrogen phosphate, 0.002% (w/v) HDB and 2.5 mM α-cyclodextrin, at pH 7.5; the analysis time is less than 3.5 min. Migration time and peak area reproducibility, studied on the same day ($n = 4$) and on three different days ($n = 12$), shows the method is reproducible. Antioxidants are extracted from beer samples by SPE with C-18 cartridges. This study shows that five of the eight compounds can be detected in beer samples.

Cortacero-Ramírez *et al.* (2005b) have also determinated 12 phenolic acids together with 7 organic acids using CE electrophoresis (see details in section "Inorganic and organic anions").

Beer bitter acids

The organoleptic characteristics of beer are mainly determined by the bitter-tasting iso-α-acids, which, in the brewing process, are formed from the α-acids occurring in hops. Quantification of the individual iso-α-acids is not straightforward, but recent results obtained by MEKC are promising. This capillary separation technique combines electrophoretic propulsion with chromatographic partitioning. The separation medium is a fused silica capillary, typically 50–75 μm ID filled with a buffer containing a surfactant that forms a micellar microphase (Van Ginkel *et al.*, 1992).

Vindevogel *et al.* (1991) have used MEKC-UV for the separation of six iso-α-acids using 30 mM phosphate buffer (pH 7.6) containing 40 mM SDS at 254 nm. Similar electrophoretic conditions are used to determine the total iso-α-acids previously preconcentrated by SPE (Szücs *et al.*, 1993). However, this method is labor intensive and difficult to automate. Therefore, a second approach, involving direct injection of beer with on-column focusing, has been investigated. Finally, 40 mM SDS, 65 mM phosphate and a 25 s injection time were selected for quantitative analysis. McLaughlin *et al.*, (1996) have also optimized a separation of iso-α-acids and β-acids from hop extracts by MEKC-UV at 214 nm, using a buffer 25 mM sodium tetraborate adjusted to pH 8.55 with 100 mM boric acid with 100 mM SDS.

MEKC has been used by Royle *et al.* (2001) for the separation of a sample of iso-α-acids and samples of reduced iso-α-acids (rho-, tetrahydro- and hexahydro-derivatives). Separation is performed in a fused silica capillary (64.5 cm total length and 56 cm to the detector, 50 μm ID) using 50 mM borate buffer containing 40 mM SDS at pH 9.3. Separations are monitored at 200 nm, with full spectral collection from 190–600 nm. Cortacero-Ramírez *et al.* (2004c) have also used MEKC-UV, to determine iso-α-acids among other components of beer. A buffer of 25 mM sodium borate and 110 mM SDS at pH 10.5 is selected as optimum.

Recently, CE has been coupled to MS. In general, if a separation technique is coupled with MS, the detection limits are better than those using UV detection, and the interpretation of the analytical results is more straightforward and more information is obtained because MS detection provides molecular weight and structural information. On-line coupling of CZE-ESI-MS for the separation and characterization of iso-α-acids in beer was investigated for the first time by García-Villalba *et al.* (2006). The CE-ESI-MS separation method consists of a running buffer 160 mM ammonium carbonate/ammonium hydroxide, pH 9, voltage 20 kV, 7 s injection time, sheath liquid 2-propanol/water 50:50 (v/v) with 0.1% TEA delivered at a flow ratio of 3 μl/min, a drying gas flow ratio at 4 l/min and at 150°C, nebulizing gas pressure 6 psi and MS analyses carried out using a compound stability of 25%. Figure 96.4 shows an electropherogram and mass spectra of an extra beer.

Aldehyde and ketone compounds

Acetaldehyde is determined in beer samples using capillary pieces containing immobilized enzymes (alcohol

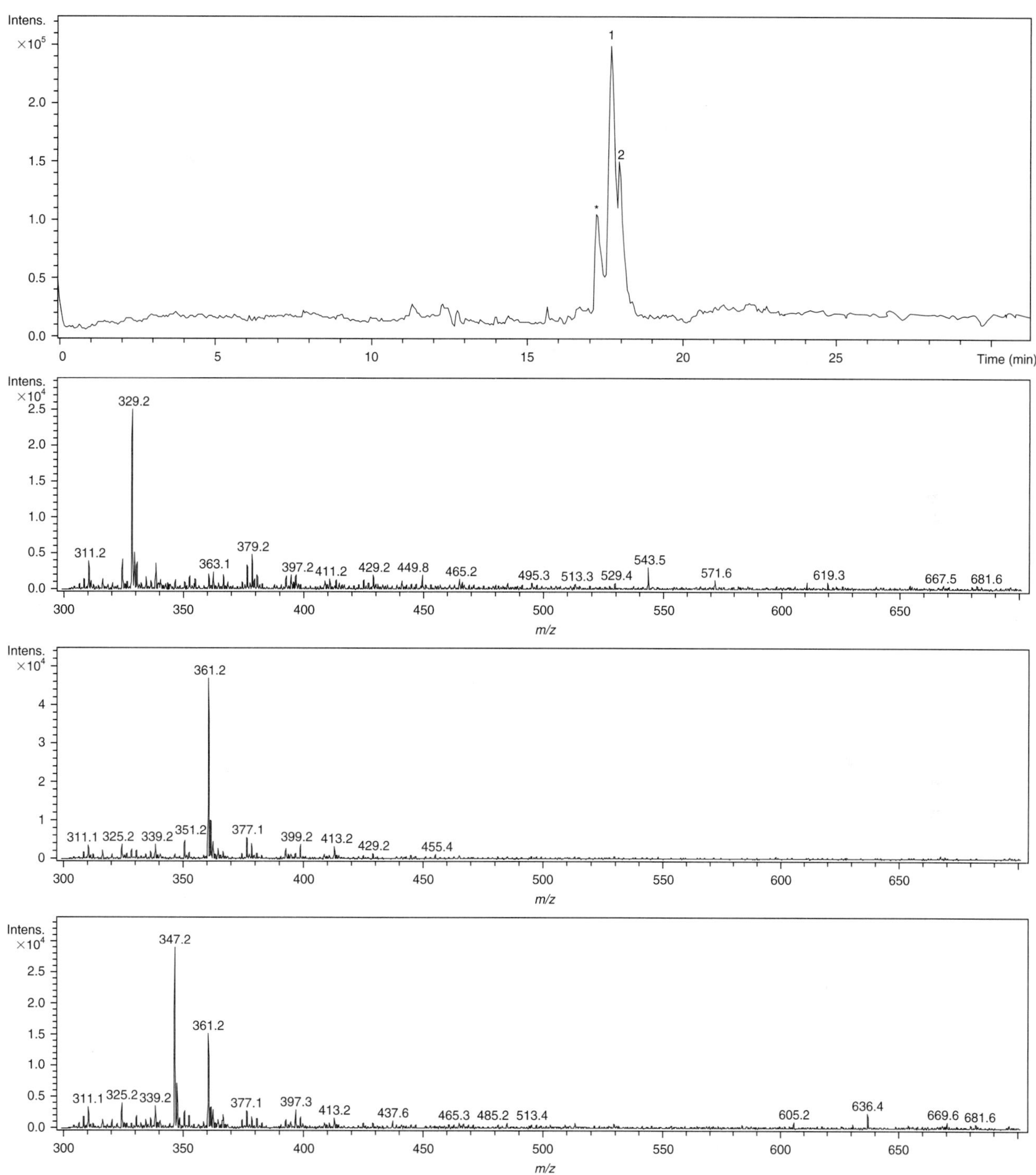

Figure 96.4 Electropherogram and mass spectra of an extra beer. Separation conditions were buffer ammonium carbonate/ammonium hydroxide 160 mM at pH 9; 50 μm ID fused silica capillary, 100 cm detector and total length, 20 kV, 7 s of hydrodynamic injection at 0.5 psi. Sheath liquid: 2-propanol/water 50:50 (v/v) containing 0.1% TEA, flow rate of 3 μl/min. Dry gas: 4 l/min, 150°C. Nebulizing gas pressure 6 psi. MS analysis was carried out using negative polarity. Compound stability: 25%. Peak numbers: *Unknown peak; 1, *trans* iso-humulone and *trans* iso-adhumulone (*m/z* 361.2); 2, iso-cohumulone (*m/z* 347.2). *Source*: Reproduced from American Chemical Society, García-Villalba *et al*. (2006).

Table 96.3 Analysis of beer samples

		Concentration (mg/l)						
Peak Number	*Analytes*	*Belgian origin*	*Abbey beer*	*Red malt beer*	*Trapense beer*	*Double malt beer*	*Extra lager beer*	*Wheat beer*
1	Tryptamine	12.8 ± 3.2	24.6 ± 2.5	14.0 ± 1.6	12.8 ± 3.2	15.1 ± 0.9	3.2 ± 0.3	11.5 ± 1.5
2	Tyramine	n.d.	n.d.	n.d.	n.d.	n.d.	n.d.	n.d.
3	Tyrosol	14.0 ± 2.4	14.9 ± 1.1	21.6 ± 2.9	10.9 ± 3.2	14.7 ± 0.3	31.6 ± 1.1	12.1 ± 1.8
4	Cytidine	28.7 ± 1.6	34.0 ± 4.4	48.3 ± 1.0	27.2 ± 3.5	39.8 ± 7.1	30.6 ± 0.6	23.2 ± 1.4
5	Adenosine	11.8 ± 2.0	7.3 ± 1.6	8.7 ± 1.5	14.0 ± 3.8	15.3 ± 2.2	4.8 ± 0.2	9.6 ± 1.9
6	Tryptophan	n.d.	n.d.	31.9 ± 1.4	n.d.	n.d.	5.3 ± 0.7	n.d.
7	Thymine	n.d.	n.q.	37.9 ± 0.7	n.d.	n.d.	n.d.	n.q.
8	Adenine	n.d.	n.q.	n.d.	n.d.	n.d.	n.d.	n.q.
9	Phenylalanine	35.5 ± 2.1	35.2 ± 2.8	17.9 ± 2.2	n.d.	n.d.	n.d.	30.9 ± 4.8
10	Rutin	n.d.	n.d.	n.d.	n.d.	n.d.	n.d.	n.d.
11	Maltol	n.d.	n.d.	n.d.	n.d.	n.d.	n.d.	n.d.
12	Tyrosine	n.d.	28.4 ± 5.3	28.6 ± 0.6	26.1 ± 2.4	41.2 ± 7.6	23.3 ± 1.5	50.1 ± 7.1
13	Uracil	24.8 ± 1.3	13.1 ± 2.4	14.0 ± 0.8	8.4 ± 3.2	n.d.	n.d.	n.d.
14	Epicatechin	n.d.	n.d.	n.d.	3.8 ± 0.5	n.d.	n.d.	n.d.
15	Catechin	6.8 ± 0.9	n.d.	n.d.	5.9 ± 0.9	10.1 ± 0.6	5.5 ± 0.2	n.d.
16	Guanosine	78.2 ± 1.2	87.4 ± 7.7	97.5 ± 3.9	71.3 ± 4.3	96.8 ± 4.9	38.1 ± 1.0	51.2 ± 7.5
17	Uridine	48.8 ± 5.3	52.3 ± 8.0	60.0 ± 3.4	31.9 ± 1.7	62.8 ± 8.5	40.2 ± 1.4	41.8 ± 6.9
18	Xanthine	94.0 ± 5.1	95.9 ± 3.6	116.6 ± 5.5	77.6 ± 6.0	99.0 ± 6.7	34.7 ± 1.1	35.3 ± 5.9

n.d., non-detected; n.q., non-quantified.

Source: Reproduced from Springer-Verlag, Cortacero-Ramírez *et al.* (2004b).

dehydrogenase and lactate dehydrogenase). On reaching the enzyme, the analyte is converted into a product with a high electrophoretic mobility, the migration time for which is a function of the position of the enzyme reactor. The running buffer is 12.5 mM β-NADH in 50 mM phosphate buffer at pH 7.0, voltage of 10 kV, capillary temperature of 20°C, hydrodynamic injection at 20 psi for 10 s and detection at 340 nm (Simonet *et al.*, 2004).

Do Rosario *et al.* (2005) have described a method for the determination of methylglyoxal (aldehyde form of pyruvic acid) in beer and yeast cells suspension matrices using *o*-phenylenediamine as derivatizing agent and SPE followed by CZE-DAD. 25 mM sodium phosphate running buffer at pH 2.2, 30 kV and 25°C gives the best instrumental conditions for the optimum separation of methylglyoxal in a suitable analytical time (<0 min), using an uncoated fused silica capillary of 75 μm inner diameter and an effective length of 45.1 cm with an extended light path and the wavelength set to 200 nm. Under optimized instrumental conditions, good reproducibility of the migration time (<1.1%), precision (<5%), an excellent linear dynamic range from 0.1 to 3.6 mg/l ($r^2 = 0.9997$), and low LODs (7.2 μg/l) are obtained for methylglyoxal measurements, using the internal standard system. This system could be used for routine quality control analysis as it is very cost-effective.

Sulfur compounds

The importance of numerous volatile sulfur compounds in the overall flavor of beer and in control of processing operations has long been recognized. The occurrence of hydrogen sulfide in fermentation gas has led to many surveys on the mechanisms of the formation of this compound and of mercaptans.

On-line gas diffusion coupled to CE system in a flow arrangement is a suitable technique for automated pre-treatment of samples with a complicated matrix composition (Kuban and Karlberg, 1998). The sample is merged with a modifying solution, that is a strong acid, in a flow system to transform the analytes of interest into their respective gaseous forms. With this method sulfite is not found in beer samples.

Multicomponent analysis

Breweries are an important branch of the food and beverage industries, and a large number of analytical determinations for processing as well as quality control are carried out in breweries every year. CE is a versatile technique and permits the analysis of a great number of components. Simultaneous determination of alcohols, amines, amino acids, flavonoids, and purine and pyrimidine bases in bottled beer samples directly without any pre-treatment has been carried out by CZE-DAD (Cortacero-Ramírez *et al.*, 2003a, b, c, 2004b). The best separation of the cited analytes is achieved in 70 mM sodium tetraborate solution and pH 10.25. LODs are from 2.1 to 5.6 mg/l for the 18 compounds studied. The developed method is rapid, sensitive and quantitative and has been applied to seven types of international bottled beers of different origins bought locally (see Table 96.3 and Figure 96.5).

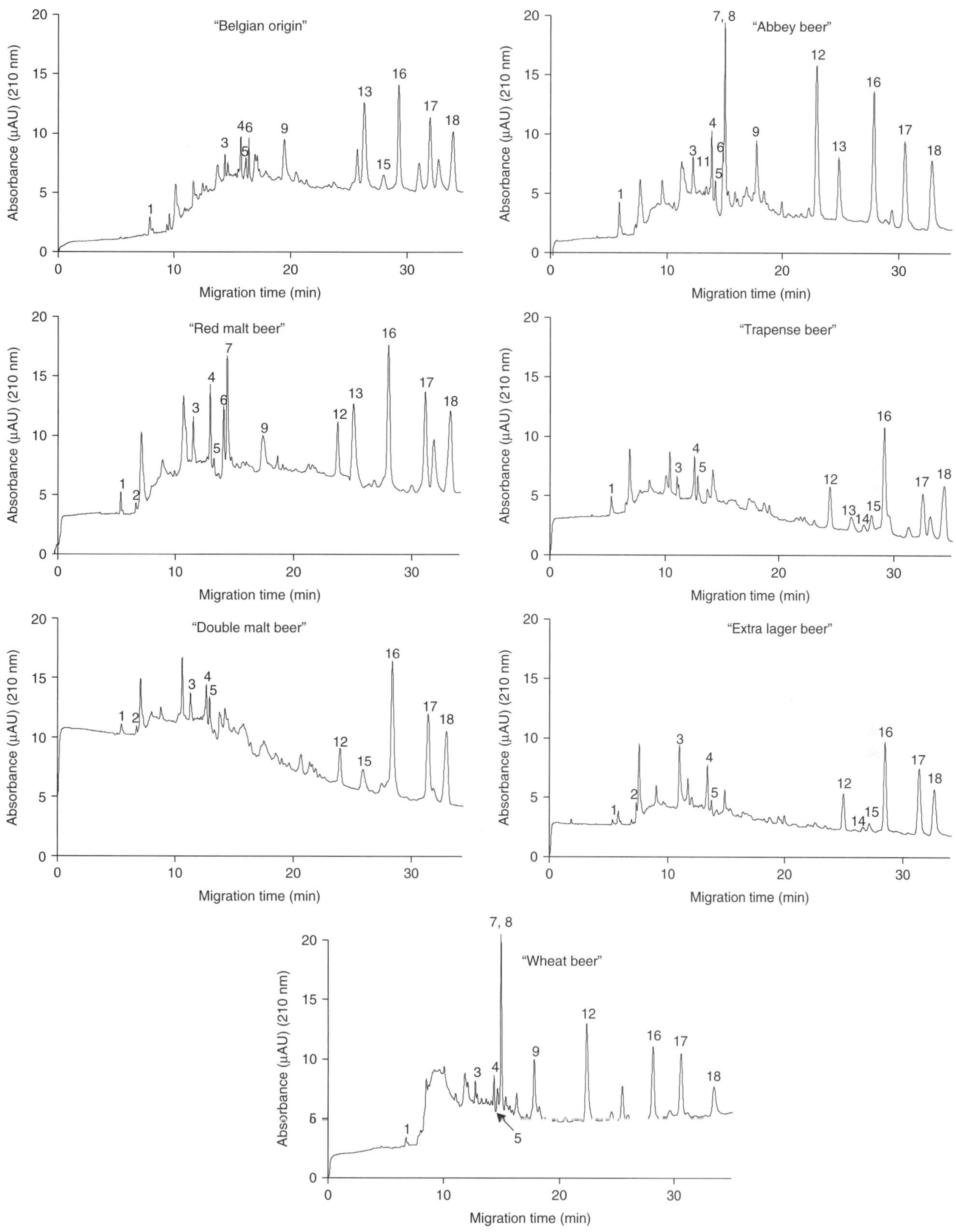

Figure 96.5 Electropherogram of beer samples of different origins. Conditions: 70 mM sodium borate buffer; pH 10.5; separation voltage, 20 kV; detection at 210; capillary, 50 cm × 75 μm ID (separation length, 50 cm); hydrodynamic injection, 5 s. Peak identification: 1 = tryptamine, 2 = tyramine, 3 = tyroso,; 4 = cytidine, 5 = adenosine, 6 = tryptophan, 7 = thymine, 8 = adenine, 9 = phenylalanine, 10 = rutin, 11 = maltol, 12 = tyrosine, 13 = uracil, 14 = epicatechin, 15 = catechin, 16 = guanosine, 17 = uridine, 18 = xanthine. *Source*: Reproduced from Springer-Verlag, Cortacero-Ramírez *et al.* (2004b).

Cortacero-Ramírez *et al.* (2004c, d) have developed a capillary electrophoretic method using MEKC-DAD to simultaneously analyze 26 beer constituents in a single procedure, including alcohols (furfuryl alcohol, maltol, tyrosol and 2-phenylethanol), iso-α-acids (iso-humulone, iso-cohumulone and iso-adhumulone), amino acids (phenylalanine, tryptophan and tyrosine), flavonoids (rutin, epicatechin and catechin) isoflavonoids (daidzein and genistein), vitamins (thymine and nicotinic acid), purine and pyrimidine bases (cytidine, adenosine, adenine, uracil, guanosine, hypoxanthine, uridine, adenosine-3′-monofosfate and xanthine).

After filtration, sample components are separated with uncoated capillary tubing and a 25 mM sodium borate and 110 mM SDS buffer at pH 10.5. Analyses are run at 14 kV and 8 s of hydrodynamic injection with UV detection at 210 and 270 nm that permits the resolution and determination of these compounds in beer samples. The method has been successfully applied to the direct determination of beer constituents without any sample clean-up procedures.

Summary Points

- This chapter has been written with the aim of summarizing all the publications on the use of CE in beer, and to investigate increasing the use of this technique in breweries routine analysis.
- Beer analysis is very important for quality control. In CE beer samples can often be directly injected into the separation capillary or require only minimal pre-treatment, such as dilution, derivatization or filtration.
- Solutes, which cannot be determined by direct sample injection have to be extracted and often concentrated. For extraction, the SPE procedures are typically used which have advantages of simplicity, rapidity, solvent elimination, high sensitivity, small sample volume, lower cost and simple automatization.
- Beer also contains many important components beneficial for health and the prevention of diseases, which can be analyzed by CE.
- Quantitative analysis is possible and the performance is comparable to that achieved with chromatographic techniques.

References

Bednar, P., Aturki, Z., Stransky, Z. and Fanali, S. (2001). *Electrophoresis* 22, 2129–2135.

Bourne, L., Paganga, G., Baxter, D., Hughes, P. and Rice-Evans, C. (2000). *Free Radic. Res.* 32, 273–280.

Cao, L.W., Wang, H. and Zhang, H.S. (2005). *Electrophoresis* 26, 1954–1962.

Casado-Terrones, S., Cortacero-Ramírez, S., Carrasco-Pancorbo, A., Segura-Carretero, A. and Fernández-Gutiérrez, A. (2006). *Anal. Bioanal. Chem.* 63, 2–3. (DOI 10.1007/s00216-006-0731-8)

Chang, Y.S., Shih, C.M. and Lin, C.H. (2006). *Anal. Sci.* 22, 235–240.

Chen, M.Ch. and Huang, H.J. (1995). *Anal. Chem.* 67, 4010–4014.

Chen, M.Ch. and Huang, H.J. (1997). *Anal. Chim. Acta* 341, 83–90.

Cortacero-Ramírez, S., Segura-Carretero, A., Cruces-Blanco, C., Hernáinz-Bermúdez de Castro, M. and Fernández-Gutiérrez, A. (2003a). *Trends Anal. Chem.* 22, 440–455.

Cortacero-Ramírez, S., Segura-Carretero, A., Cruces Blanco, C., Hernáinz Bermúdez, M. and Fernández-Gutiérrez, A. (2003b). *Proceedings of the 29th EBC Congress, 97*, ISBN 90-70143-22-4, pp. 993–1001.

Cortacero-Ramírez, S., Segura-Carretero, A., Cruces Blanco, C., Hernáinz-Bermúdezde Castro, M. and Fernández-Gutiérrez, A. (2003c). *Cerveza y Malta*, Dublin, 160, 41–44.

Cortacero-Ramírez, S., Segura-Carretero, A., Cruces-Blanco, C., Hernáinz-Bermúdez, M. and Fernández-Gutiérrez, A. (2004a). *Food Chem.* 87, 471–476.

Cortacero-Ramirez, S., Segura-Carretero, A., Cruces-Blanco, C., Romero-Romero, M. and Fernandez-Gutierrez, (2004b). *Anal. Bioanal. Chem.* 380, 831–837.

Cortacero-Ramírez, S., Segura-Carretero, A., Cruces-Blanco, C., Hernáinz Bermúdez, M. and Fernández-Gutiérrez, A. (2004c). *Cerveza y Malta* 163, 31–34.

Cortacero-Ramírez, S., Segura-Carretero, A., Cruces-Blanco, C., Hernáinz-Bermúdez, M. and Fernández-Gutiérrez, A. (2004d). *Electrophoresis* 25, 1867–1871.

Cortacero-Ramírez, S., Segura-Carretero, A., Cruces-Blanco, C., Hernáinz-Bermúdez, M. and Fernández-Gutiérrez, A. (2005a). *J. Sci. Food Agric.* 85, 517–521.

Cortacero-Ramirez, S., Segura-Carretero, A., Hernáinz-Bermúdez, M. and Fernandez-Gutierrez, A. (2005b). *J. Chromatogr. A* 1064, 115–119.

Cortacero-Ramírez, S., Arráez-Román, D., Segura-Carretero, A. and Fernández-Gutiérrez, A. (2007). *Food Chem.* 100, 383–389.

Coufal, P., Zuska, J., Van de Goor, T., Smith, V. and Gas, B. (2003). *Electrophoresis* 24, 671–677.

DeVries, K.J. (1993). *J. Am. Soc. Brew. Chem.* 51, 155–159.

Do Rosario, P.M.A., Cordeiro, C.A.A., Freire, A.P. and Nogueira, J.M.F. (2005). *Electrophoresis* 26, 1760–1767.

Dong, Q., Jin, W.R. and Shan, J.H. (2002). *Electrophoresis* 23, 559–564.

Fernández-Gutiérrez, A., Segura-Carretero, A. and Carrasco-Pancorbo, A. (2005). Fundamentos teóricos y modos de separation. In Fernández-Gutiérrez, S. and Segura-Carretero, S. (eds), *Electroforesis capilar: aproximación según la técnica de detección*, pp. 11–54. Universidad de Granada, Granada, España.

García-Villalba, R., Cortacero-Ramírez, S., Segura-Carretero, A. and Fernández-Gutiérrez, A. (2006). *J. Agric. Food Chem.* 54, 5400–5409.

Guttman, A., Brunet, S. and Cooke, N. (1996). *LC GC North American* 14, 788–791.

Hernández-Borges, J., Borges-Miquel, T., González-Hernández, G. and Rodríguez-Delgado, M.A. (2005). *Chromatographia* 62, 271–276.

Holland, L.A., Harmony, N.M. and Lunte, S.M. (1999). *Electroanalysis* 11, 327–330.

Hornsey, I.S. (1999). In Hornsey, I.S. (ed.), *Brewing*, pp. 45–46. The Royal Society of Chemistry, Cambridge, UK.

http://www.beerandhealth.com.

Johns, C., Macka, M. and Haddad, P.R. (2000). *Electrophoresis* 21, 1312–1319.

Khun, R. and Hoffstetter-Kuhn, S. (1993). Detection for capillary electrophoresis. In Springer-Verlag, (ed.), *Principles and Practice*, p. 151. Springer-Verlag, Berlin, Heidelberg, Germany.

Klampfl, C.W. (1999). *J. Agric. Food Chem.* 47, 987–990.

Klampfl, C.W. and Katzmayr, M.U. (1998). *J. Chromatogr. A* 822, 117–123.

Klampfl, W., Buchberger, W., Turner, M. and Fritz, J.S. (1998). *J. Chromatogr. A* 804, 349–355.

Klampfl, C.W., Himmelsbach, M., Buchberger, W. and Klein, H. (2002). *Anal. Chim. Acta* 454, 185–191.

Kuban, P. and Karlberg, B. (1998). *Talanta* 45, 477–484.

Lindeberg, J. (1996). *Food Chem.* 55, 73–94.

Mahendradatta, M. and Schwedt, G. (1998). *Z. Lebensm. Unters. Forsch. A* 206, 246–251.

Marina, M.A., Ríos, A. and Valcárcel, M. (2005). Fundamentals of capillary electrophoresis. In Barceló, D. (ed.), *Analysis and Detection by Fundamentals of capillary Electrophoresis*, pp. 19–21. Wilson & Wilson's, Elsevier, Amsterdam.

Marshall, P.A., Trenerry, V.C. and Thompson, C.A. (1995). *J. Chromatogr. Sci.* 33, 426–430.

Masar, M., Zuborova, M., Kaniansky, D. and Stanislawski, B. (2003). *J. Sep. Sci.* 26, 647–652.

McLaughlin, G.M., Weston, A. and Hauffe, K.D. (1996). *J. Chromatogr. A* 744, 123–134.

Moane, S., Park, S., Lunte, C.E. and Smyth, M.R. (1998). *Analyst* 123, 1931–1936.

Preston, L.M., Weber, M.L. and Murray, G.M. (1997). *J. Chromatogr. B* 695, 175–180.

Rassi El, Z. (1996). *High Performance Capillary Electrophoresis of Carbohydrates.* Beckman Instrument, p. 2. Fullerton, CA.

Royle, L., Ames, J.M., Hill, C.A. and Gardner, D.S.J. (2001). *Food Chem.* 74, 225–231.

Sadecka, J. and Polonsky, J. (2000). *J. Chromatogr. A* 880, 243–279.

Simonet, B.M., Rios, A. and Valcárcel, M. (2004). *Electrophoresis* 25, 50–56.

Soga, T. and Ross, G.A. (1997). *J. Chromatogr. A* 767, 223–230.

Soga, T. and Wakaura, M. (1997). *J. Am. Soc. Brew. Chem.* 55, 44–46.

Su, A.K., Chang, Y.S. and Lin, C.H. (2004). *Talanta* 64, 970–974.

Szücs, R., Vindevogel, J., Sandra, P. and Verhagen, L.C. (1993). *Chromatographia* 36, 323–329.

Tanyanyiwa, J., Schweizer, K. and Hauser, P.C. (2003). *Electrophoresis* 24, 2119–2124.

Tivesten, A., Lundqvist, A. and Folestad, S. (1997). *Chromatographia* 44, 623–630.

Van Ginkel, L.A., Stephany, R.W., Van Rossum, H.J. and Zoontjes, P.W. (1992). *Trends Anal. Chem.* 11, 275–280.

Vindevogel, J., Szücs, R., Sandra, P. and Verhagen, L.C. (1991). *J. High. Resolut. Chromatogr.* 14, 584–586.

Vinogradov, E. and Bock, K. (1998). *Carbohydr. Res.* 309, 57–64.

Wang, J., Chen, G. and Chatrathi, M.P. (2004). *Electroanalysis* 16, 1603–1608.

Zhang, L.Y. and Sun, M.X. (2004). *J. Chromatogr. A* 1040, 133–140.

Zhang, L.Y., Huang, W.H., Wang, Z.L. and Cheng, J. (2002). *Anal. Sci.* 18, 1117–1120.

97

Manual and Robotic Methods for Measuring the Total Antioxidant Capacity of Beers

Justin A. Fegredo, Max C.Y. Wong, Helen Wiseman and Victor R. Preedy Department of Nutrition and Dietetics, King's College London, London, UK

Abstract

It is well known that antioxidants are able to confer some protective effect against numerous pathologies such as cardiovascular disease. Alcoholic beverages such as red wine have thus attracted particular attention in recent years due to their high concentration of antioxidants such as phenolic compounds. However, research and information on the *in vitro* total antioxidant capacity (TAC) of beer has been limited, despite human studies suggesting that antioxidants in such beverages are bioavailable.

In this chapter, we provide comprehensive protocols for four commonly used assays for TAC: the oxygen radical absorbance capacity (ORAC), ferric reducing ability of plasma (FRAP), Trolox® equivalent antioxidant capacity (TEAC) and total phenols by Folin–Ciocalteu reagent (TP-FCR) assays. We have tested these assays for linearity and precision, finding excellent correlations and coefficients of variation, and furthermore applied these assays to measure the TAC of beers, red wines and orange juices. We found that the mean TAC of a number of ales (mean TEAC, 7.02 ± 0.08 mM Trolox® equivalents (TE); FRAP, 2.71 ± 0.18 mM; ORAC, 7,516 ± 404 μM TE; TP-FCR, 398 ± 30 mg/l) was several-fold lower than that of red wines (mean TEAC, 36.87 ± 1.04 mM TE; FRAP, 19.77 ± 1.25 mM; ORAC, 27,963 ± 908 μM TE; TP-FCR, 1,807 ± 94 mg/l) but comparable to that of commercially available orange juices (mean TEAC, 6.86 ± 0.28 mM TE; FRAP, 2.88 ± 0.94 mM; ORAC, 5,662 ± 630 μM TE; TP-FCR, 648 ± 45 mg/l). In addition, all of the assays showed strong linear correlations with one another (mean r^2 = 0.96, range 0.91–0.99).

The availability of comprehensive protocols for these assays will enhance research into TAC of beers and augment the evidence base for their benefit in health and wellbeing.

List of Abbreviations

6-FAM	6-Carboxyfluorescein
AAPH	2,2′-Azobis(2-amidinopropane)
ABTS	2,2′-Azino-bis(3-ethylbenzthiazoline-6-sulfonic acid)
AUC	Area under curve
FRAP	Ferric reducing ability of plasma
ORAC	Oxygen radical absorbance capacity
QC	Quality control
TAC	Total antioxidant capacity
TEAC	Trolox® equivalent antioxidant capacity
TP-FCR	Total phenols by Folin–Ciocalteu reagent
TPTZ	2,4,6-Tripyridyl-*s*-triazine
Trolox®	6-Hydroxy-2,5,7,8-tetramethylchroman-2-carboxylic acid
β-PE	β-Phycoerythrin

Introduction

The physiological activity of antioxidants has long been recognized as conferring some protective effect against numerous pathologies (Halliwell and Gutteridge, 1999). Although there are several endogenous antioxidant defense mechanisms, low-molecular-mass radical scavenging agents available as dietary antioxidants have received particular attention (Halliwell and Gutteridge, 1999). Beverages with a high antioxidant capacity, such as red wine and beer (Frankel *et al.*, 1995; Montanari *et al.*, 1999; Pellegrini *et al.*, 2000), have thus received special interest, and indeed it is their antioxidant component which is thought to account for some of their protective properties (Frankel *et al.*, 1993). *In vivo* studies in human volunteers have furthermore demonstrated that these antioxidants are bioavailable, and a significant increase in total antioxidant capacity (TAC) of plasma has been observed following ingestion of both red wine (Fernandez-Pachon *et al.*, 2005) and beer (Ghiselli *et al.*, 2000). It can therefore be concluded that the *in vitro* measurement of TAC of such beverages is of direct biological relevance.

Total Antioxidant Capacity As a Tool for Measuring Antioxidant Protection

Measurement of TAC (i.e. the total antioxidant protection provided by a sample) is both less costly and arguably of

Beer in Health and Disease Prevention
ISBN: 978-0-12-373891-2

greater biological relevance than measurement of individual antioxidants (e.g. individual polyphenols) since it takes into account both synergistic interactions (Huang *et al.*, 2005) and the contribution of presently unidentified antioxidant components (Rice-Evans *et al.*, 1996). Historically, assays for TAC have been classified according to their mathematical foundation (as either endpoint or area-under-curve (AUC) methods), although recently a newer classification has evolved according to whether the assays involve hydrogen atom transfer or electron transfer (Huang *et al.*, 2005). Hydrogen atom transfer-based assays, such as the oxygen radical absorbance capacity (ORAC) assay, typically involve monitoring competitive reaction kinetics – antioxidants compete with an oxidizable molecular probe to reduce free radicals; by monitoring oxidation of the probe, the degree of antioxidant protection for the probe (and hence TAC) can be derived (Huang *et al.*, 2005). Electron transfer-based assays, such as the ferric reducing ability of plasma (FRAP), Trolox® equivalent antioxidant capacity (TEAC) and total phenols by Folin–Ciocalteu reagent (TP-FCR) assay, involve one redox reaction (i.e. the transfer of an electron between two chemical species); TAC is then quantified by using the oxidant (i.e. the electron acceptor) as an indicator of reaction endpoint (Huang *et al.*, 2005). The mechanism behind these four assays is summarized in Table 97.1. Nevertheless, regardless of the assay employed, due consideration needs to be given to accuracy, precision (repeatability and reproducibility), linearity and limits of detection and quantification (see Table 97.2 for definitions).

Table 97.1 Commonly used assays for TAC

Assay	*Mechanism*
TEAC	Antioxidants present in the substrate promote reduction of an $ABTS^{\bullet +}$ radical cation which absorbs light at wavelength 734 nm. As in the ORAC assay, Trolox® is commonly used as an antioxidant standard (Re *et al.*, 1999).
FRAP	Antioxidants present in the substrate promote reduction of a ferric-2,4,6-tripyridyl-*s*-triazine (TPTZ) complex to its ferrous counterpart. Absorbance of the Fe^{2+}–TPTZ complex at 593 nm is monitored and correlated with TAC. Ascorbic acid is commonly used as an antioxidant standard (Benzie and Strain, 1996).
ORAC	Antioxidants present in the substrate compete with a 6-carboxyfluorescein (6-FAM) probe for reduction of thermally generated free radicals derived from 2,2′-azobis(2-amidinopropane) (AAPH). TAC is assessed by monitoring fluorescence of the 6-FAM probe. 6-Hydroxy-2,5,7,8-tetramethylchroman-2-carboxylic acid (Trolox®) is commonly used as an antioxidant standard (Naguib, 2000).
TP-FCR	The mechanism behind this assay is unclear. However, the presence of antioxidants results in a blue species (possibly $(PMoW_{11}O_{40})^{4-}$ which absorbs light at 760 nm and can be used to quantify TAC (Huang *et al.*, 2005). Gallic acid is commonly used as an antioxidant standard (Singleton *et al.*, 1999).

Table 97.2 Definition of assay parameters

Assay parameter	*Definition*
Accuracy	Accuracy refers to the closeness of agreement between actual test results and those expected according to true, accepted or reference values.
Coefficient of variation (CV)	CV quantifies the variability of a set of measurements around their arithmetic mean. It is calculated as (standard deviation/mean) and often multiplied by 100 to be expressed as a percentage. CV below 10–15% is generally regarded as acceptable.
Limit of detection and quantification	Limit of detection (blank plus three standard deviations of the blank) is defined as the minimum assay signal that can be *qualitatively* distinguished from noise. Limit of quantification is more stringent (blank plus nine standard deviations of the blank) and is the level above which a *quantitative* determination can be reliably made.
Linearity	An assay is said to be linear if the output is proportional to the input (e.g. in the FRAP assay, absorbance at 593 nm is proportional to concentration of ascorbic acid).
Repeatability	Repeatability refers to the precision (variation in repeated measurements taken from a single system) under consistent conditions (i.e. using the same instrumentation, the same operator and measuring repeats over short time periods). Often expressed as CV (see above) between measurements.
Reproducibility	Reproducibility refers to the precision (variation in repeated measurements) when using the same measurement procedure under inconsistent conditions (i.e. different instrumentation, operators or measuring repeats over longer time periods). Often expressed as CV (see above) between measurements.

Note: Assay parameters such as accuracy, linearity, limit of detection and quantification, and precision (repeatability and reproducibility) are important indicators of method reliability and due consideration should be given to such measures before the assays are employed.

Feasibility of the Assays in Determining Total Antioxidant Capacity

The assays outlined in Table 97.1 are commonly used both *in vitro*, that is, with beers (Montanari *et al.*, 1999) and *in vivo*, that is, with plasma after consumption of beer (Ghiselli *et al.*, 2000) for the assessment of TAC. They are easy to perform manually (using cuvettes and a spectrophotometer or fluorimeter) and furthermore are all amenable to high-throughput analysis; we have adapted these methods for use with the Biomek® FX Laboratory Automation Workstation (a liquid handling robot) and the BioTek® Synergy™ HT Multi-Detection Microplate Reader. Moreover, we have tested both manual and automated moieties of these assays for linearity (Figure 97.1) and repeatability (Table 97.3), with good results. In all four assays (both

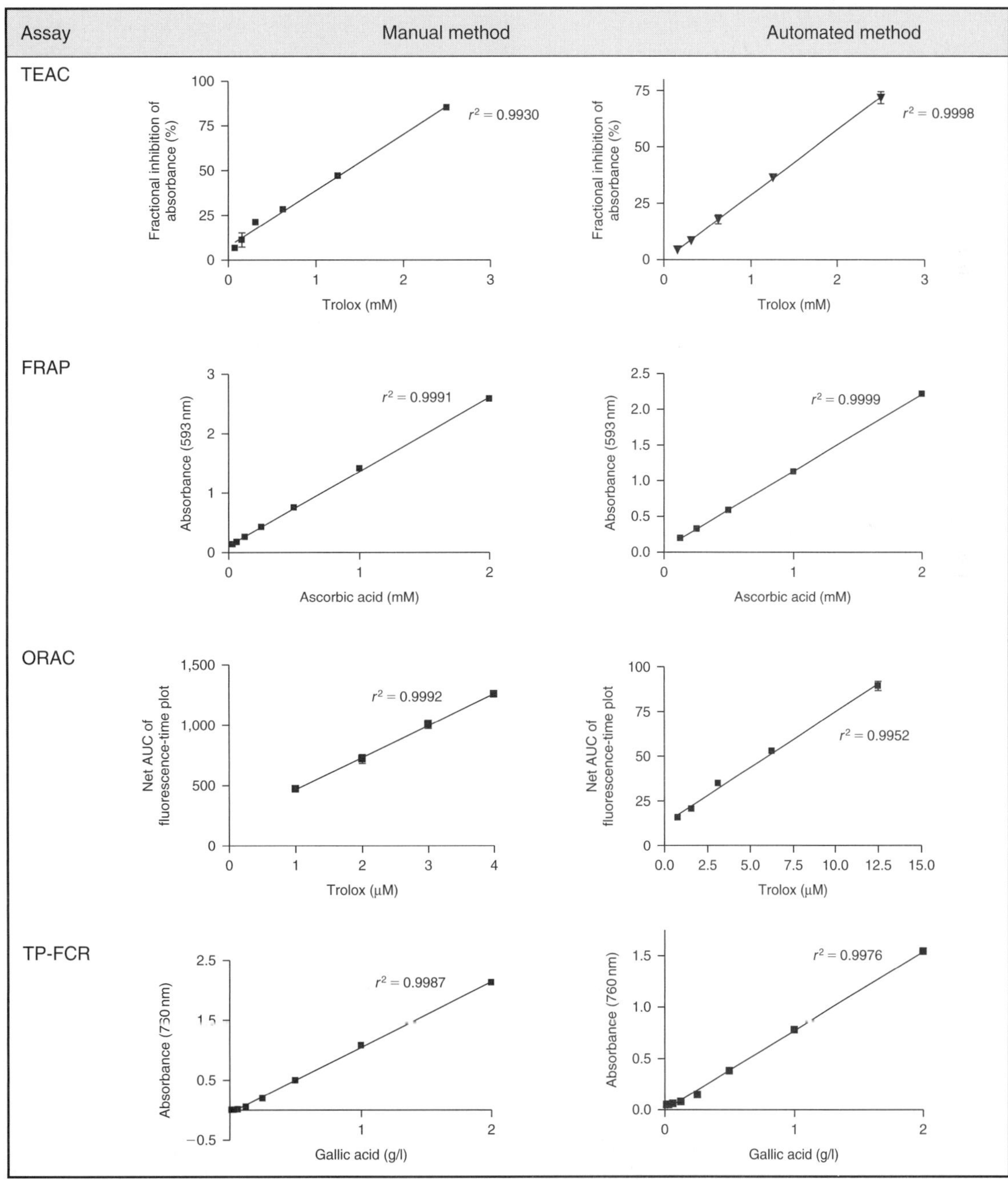

Figure 97.1 Linearity of some commonly used assays. Data are expressed as mean ± SEM (n = 3, error bars are too small to see). Both manual and automated methods of performing four common assays for TAC demonstrate good linearity when assessed using antioxidant standard solutions.

Table 97.3 Inter- and intra-assay precision of some commonly used assays

Assay	*Inter-assay variation Manual (%)*	*Automated (%)*	*Intra-assay variation Manual (%)*	*Automated (%)*
TEAC	11	10	6	5
FRAP	6	9	1	5
ORAC	4	8	2	1
TP-FCR	1	<1	<1	1

Note: Data are expressed as coefficients of variation (%) for the inter- and intra-assay variation of four assays for total antioxidant capacity, performed by either manual or automated techniques. Inter-assay variation refers to disparity in the value of an unchanged sample tested in different runs of an assay; intra-assay variation refers to disparity in the value of an unchanged sample tested in the same run of an assay.

Table 97.4 Preparation of beer samples

Assay	*Diluent*	*Dilution strength*[a]
TEAC[b]	5 mM phosphate buffered saline (0.9% w/v), pH 7.0	12.5%, 25%, 50%
FRAP	None necessary	None
ORAC	75 mM phosphate buffer, pH 7.0	5%
TP-FCR	None necessary	None

Notes: Each of the assays for total antioxidant capacity requires dilution with a different diluent and dilution factor.

[a] These dilution strengths are variable depending on the antioxidant capacity of beer samples tested; pilot assays may be necessary. In the case of the TEAC assay, concentrations of sample should be such that they produce between an inhibition of absorbance which is 20–80% that of the blank.

[b] For the TEAC assay, at least three dilutions of sample should be prepared for a dose–response curve to be constructed.

manual and automated), the measured TAC of beers is well above their limits of quantification and these tests can therefore be seen as accurate and reliable. In the next section, we present detailed laboratory protocols for performing these assays using both manual and automated techniques. Universal laboratory health and safety precautions must be adopted when following any of the procedures outlined in these protocols.

Laboratory Protocols

The samples for each assay should be prepared as shown in Table 97.4.

Blank measures are necessary to control for the effect of assay reagents in the absence of sample (reagent blanks), or sample in the absence of assay reagents (sample blanks). For reagent blanks, the sample will be replaced by an equivalent volume of diluent which is specific to each assay, for example, distilled water is used as a blank in the FRAP assay; 75 mM phosphate buffer (pH 7.0) in the ORAC assay, etc. For sample blanks, the reagents rather than samples are replaced with the appropriate diluent.

In addition to blank measures, a suitable sample must be chosen for use as an assay quality control (QC); this is necessary to ensure homogeneity between different batches of results. The QC used should not be changed between assays but should be demonstrated to return consistent results over time. For uniformity, the QC chosen should be prepared and assayed in the same way as the samples (see Table 97.4). In addition, employing the QC at several concentrations will contribute to providing a robust data set, as this will serve to confirm assay linearity.

Laboratory Protocol for the TEAC Assay

This is adapted from previous publications (Miller *et al.*, 1993; Re *et al.*, 1999).

Antioxidant standard preparation

- Prepare 25 ml of 2.5 mM 6-hydroxy-2,5,7,8-tetramethylchroman-2-carboxylic acid, or Trolox® (0.6257 g/l), in 5 mM phosphate buffered saline (pH 7.4) as a stock solution of antioxidant standard by which to calibrate the data. Dissolution may be facilitated by gentle sonication. This stock solution is stable for 4 weeks when stored at 4°C or 6 months at −20°C in the dark.
- Prepare fresh working standard solutions of concentration 2.5, 1.25, 0.625, 0.3125 and 0.15625 mM by serially diluting the stock Trolox® solution with 5 mM phosphate buffered saline (pH 7.4). Of each concentration, one run requires 3 × 10 μl (manual) or 3 × 70 μl (automated).

Reagent preparation

- Prepare 1 l of 5 mM phosphate buffered saline (0.9% w/v, pH 7.4) by mixing equal volumes of 1.12 mM NaH_2PO_4 (0.1343 g/l) and 3.88 mM Na_2HPO_4 (0.5509 g/l) and adding 9 g/l of NaCl. Use a magnetic stirrer to ensure proper mixing, and verify pH with a pH meter. Adjust as

Table 97.5 Measures required for each run in the TEAC assay

Measure	*Repeat*	*Volume[a] of test reagent*	*Volume[a] of working ABTS$^{\bullet+}$*
Reference	Single	1,010 μL DW[b]	None
Sample blank	Triplicate	10 μl sample	None (replaced with 1.0 ml DW[b])
Reagent blank	Triplicate	10 μl 5 mM PBS[b], pH 7.4	1.0 ml
Standard[c]	Triplicate	10 μl Trolox®	1.0 ml
Sample[c]	Triplicate	10 μl sample	1.0 ml
QC	Triplicate	10 μl QC	1.0 ml

Notes: For the TEAC assay, each run involves comparing absorbance at 734 nm at 6 min of a blank, several concentrations of standard, several concentrations of sample and a QC.

[a] Refers to volume required for the manual assay. In the automated assay the total volume will be scaled down from 1,010 μl to the size of the microplate well volume (i.e. 3 μl of test reagent plus 300 μl of working ABTS$^{\bullet+}$).

[b] DW, distilled water; PBS, phosphate buffered saline.

[c] This should be performed in triplicate at *all* working concentrations. That is, standard, three repeats at 2.5 mM plus three at 1.25 mM, etc.; sample, three repeats at 25%, three at 12.5%, etc.

necessary by adding solid NaH_2PO_4 or Na_2HPO_4 powder directly to buffer solution.

- Prepare 25 ml 14 mM 2,2′-azino-bis(3-ethylbenzthiazoline-6-sulfonic acid) diammonium salt solution, or ABTS (7.6816 g/l), in 5 mM phosphate buffered saline (pH 7.4).
- Prepare 25 ml 4.9 mM $K_2S_2O_8$ (1.3246 g/l) in 5 mM phosphate buffered saline (pH 7.4).
- Mix equal volumes of 14 mM ABTS and 4.9 mM $K_2S_2O_8$ to produce a stable ABTS$^{\bullet+}$ stock solution. A dark blue-green solution should be formed immediately; allow this to stand in the dark at room temperature for 12–16 h before use. The stock solution is stable for 2 days when stored in the dark at room temperature.
- Prepare a working ABTS$^{\bullet+}$ solution by diluting ABTS$^{\bullet+}$ (approximately 1/40 dilution) stock solution to an absorbance of 0.70 ± 0.02 AU at 734 nm and 30°C using 5 mM phosphate buffered saline (pH 7.4). One run requires 12 × 1.0 ml (manual) or 96 × 300 μl (automated for 96-well microplate). Verify absorbance using an absorbance spectrophotometer and store in the dark.

Performing the TEAC assay

Table 97.5 shows the measures required for each run in the TEAC assay.

The manual TEAC assay

1. Pre-incubate *all* reagents (including samples, standards, etc.) at 30°C.
2. Prepare 2 ml, 1 cm light path visible range cuvettes for each measure by adding 10 μl test reagent (as shown in Table 97.5). Note the purpose of the reference cuvette is simply to zero the absorbance of the spectrophotometer; it contains only distilled water.
3. Start the reaction by adding 1.0 ml ABTS$^{\bullet+}$ to each cuvette and mix well, according to Table 97.5.
4. Incubate the cuvettes at 30°C and record absorbance at 734 nm at 6 min (or other chosen endpoint).

The automated TEAC assay

1. Pre-incubate *all* reagents (including samples, standards, etc.) at 30°C.
2. Prepare a stock plate containing each test reagent (Table 97.5) at a minimum well volume of 70 μl (e.g. 3 wells with 70 μl of QC). The robot will later transfer 3 μl to a separate test plate in which the absorbance is to be measured.
3. Prepare the test plate by adding 300 μl of distilled water to all wells which will contain a *sample blank*. The distilled water is added to make up the volume which would otherwise be occupied by ABTS$^{\bullet+}$ radical solution.
4. Set the robot to pipette 300 μl of ABTS$^{\bullet+}$ radical solution into each well of the test plate (except those containing sample blanks).
5. Set the robot to then transfer 3 μl of test reagent (e.g. phosphate buffered saline, Trolox® standard, sample or QC) from the stock plate to test plate, and to mix the well contents by aspirating fluid from the bottom of the well and dispensing it at the surface.
6. Transfer the test plate to the microplate reader and incubate at 30°C; absorbance at 734 nm is read at 6 min (other endpoints can be chosen).
7. The absorbance data can be imported into Microsoft Excel for analysis.

Calculation of TEAC

- Preliminary data handling: check coefficients of variation (CV) for sample/standard repeats within assays and QC between assays. Exclude CV > 10–15%.

- Calculate fractional inhibition (FI) of $ABTS^{\bullet+}$ radicals using mean raw absorbance (A) data at 6 min (or chosen endpoint):

$$FI = \frac{\left[\begin{array}{l}A_{734} \text{ of reagent blank } - A_{734} \text{ of test solution} \\ - A_{734} \text{ of sample blank}\end{array}\right]}{A_{734} \text{ of reagent blank at 6 min}}$$

- Plot dose–response (DR) curves (i.e. concentration vs. fractional inhibition) for (1) Trolox® and (2) each sample.

$$\text{TEAC (mM)} = \frac{\text{Gradient of sample DR curve}}{\text{Gradient of Trolox DR curve}}$$

Laboratory Protocol for the FRAP Assay

This is adapted from a previous publication (Benzie and Strain, 1996).

Antioxidant standard preparation

- Prepare (fresh) 100 ml of 2 mM ascorbic acid (0.3522 g/l) in distilled water as a stock solution of antioxidant standard by which to calibrate the data. An ascorbic acid standard curve can be prepared by serial dilution down to 1.00, 0.50 and 0.25 mM. Of each concentration, one run requires $3 \times 100\,\mu l = 300\,\mu l$ (manual) or $3 \times 70\,\mu l = 210\,\mu l$ (automated). Ascorbic acid solution is both light and air sensitive, and should be stored in a sealed brown bottle and covered with foil (at room temperature).

Reagent preparation

- Prepare 20 ml of 40 mM HCl solution.
- Prepare 20 ml of 10 mM 2,4,6-tripyridyl-*s*-triazine, or TPTZ (3.1230 g/l), in 40 mM HCl.
- Prepare 20 ml of 20 mM $FeCl_3 \cdot 6H_2O$ (5.4060 g/l) in distilled water.
- Prepare 1 l of 300 mM sodium acetate buffer, pH 3.6 as follows: add 3.1 g sodium acetate trihydrate ($C_2H_3NaO_2 \cdot 3H_2O$) to 16 ml glacial acetic acid ($C_2H_4O_2$) and make up to 1,000 ml with distilled water.
- Prepare FRAP reagent ($12 \times 3.0 = 36$ ml for one manual run; $96 \times 300\,\mu l = 28.8$ ml for one automated run) by mixing together the sodium acetate buffer, TPTZ and $FeCl_3 \cdot 6H_2O$ solutions in a volumetric ratio of 10:1:1, respectively. FRAP reagent is light sensitive; cover with foil.

Performing the FRAP assay

Table 97.6 shows the measures required for each run in the FRAP assay.

The manual FRAP assay

1. Pre-incubate *all* reagents (including samples, standards, etc.) at 37°C.
2. Prepare 4 ml, 1 cm light path visible range cuvettes for each measure by adding the test reagent to distilled water (as shown in Table 97.6). Note the purpose of the reference cuvette is simply to zero the absorbance of the spectrophotometer; it contains distilled water.
3. Start the reaction by adding FRAP reagent to each cuvette and mix well, according to Table 97.6.
4. Incubate the cuvettes at 37°C and record absorbance at 593 nm at 6 min (or other chosen endpoint; we have found greater stability of absorbance after 30 min).

The automated FRAP assay

1. Pre-incubate *all* reagents (including samples, standards, etc.) at 37°C.
2. Prepare a stock plate containing each test reagent (Table 97.6) at a minimum well volume of 70 μl (e.g. 3 wells

Table 97.6 Measures required for each run in the FRAP assay

Measure	*Repeat*	*Volume[a] of reagents* *Test reagent*	*Distilled water*	*FRAP reagent*
Reference	Single	None	3.4 ml	None
Sample blank	Triplicate	100 μl sample	3.3 ml	None
Reagent blank	Triplicate	100 μl distilled water	300 μl	3.0 ml
Standard curve[b]	Triplicate	100 μl ascorbic acid	300 μl	3.0 ml
Sample	Triplicate	100 μl sample	300 μl	3.0 ml
QC	Triplicate	100 μl QC	300 μl	3.0 ml

Notes: For the FRAP assay, each run involves comparing absorbance at 593 nm at 6 min of a blank, standard, sample and a QC.

[a] Refers to volume required for the manual assay. In the automated assay the total volume will be scaled down from 3.4 ml to the size of the microplate well volume (e.g. 10 μl of sample plus 30 μl of distilled water plus 300 μl of FRAP reagent).

[b] This should be performed in triplicate at *all* working concentrations. That is, three repeats at 2 mM, three at 1 mM, etc.

with 70 μl of QC). The robot will later transfer 10 μl to a separate test plate in which the absorbance is to be measured.
3. Prepare the test plate by adding 330 μl distilled water to all wells which will contain a *sample blank*. The distilled water is added to make up the volume which would otherwise be occupied by the 30 μl of distilled water and 300 μl of FRAP reagent.
4. Set the robot to pipette 30 μl of distilled water and 300 μl of FRAP reagent into all wells of the test plate (except those containing *sample blanks*).
5. Set the robot to then transfer 10 μl of distilled water (reagent blank), ascorbic acid standard, sample and QC from the stock plate to test plate, and to mix the well contents by aspirating fluid from the bottom of the well and dispensing it at the surface.
6. Transfer the test plate to the microplate reader and incubate at 37°C; absorbance at 593 nm is read at 6 min (other endpoints can be chosen; we have found greater stability of absorbance after 30 min).
7. The absorbance data can be imported into Microsoft Excel for analysis.

Calculation of FRAP

- Preliminary data handling: check coefficients of variation (CV) for sample/standard repeats within assays and QC between assays. Exclude CV > 10–15%.
- Calculate net absorbance (A) of each sample and each standard, using mean raw absorbance (A) data at 6 min (or chosen endpoint):

$$\text{Net } A_{593} \text{ of sample} = A_{593} \text{ of sample} - A_{593} \text{ of sample blank} - A_{593} \text{ reagent blank}$$

$$\text{Net } A_{593} \text{ of standard} = A_{593} \text{ of standard} - A_{593} \text{ of reagent blank}$$

- Produce a standard dose–response curve (i.e. concentration of ascorbic acid vs. net absorbance). Interpolation of net absorbance of an unknown sample will thus give TAC in *ascorbic acid equivalents*.
- Since ascorbic acid can accept two electrons while the reduction from Fe^{3+} to Fe^{2+} ions requires one, the *ferric* reducing antioxidant power is obtained by:

$$\text{FRAP} = \text{Ascorbic acid equivalents} \times 2$$

Laboratory Protocol for the ORAC Assay

This is adapted from previous publications (Cao *et al.*, 1993; Naguib, 2000; Huang *et al.*, 2002).

Antioxidant standard preparation

- Prepare 25 ml 2.5 mM Trolox® (0.6257 g/l) in 75 mM sodium phosphate buffer (pH 7.0) as a stock solution of antioxidant standard by which to calibrate the data. Dissolution may be facilitated by gentle sonication. This stock solution is stable for 4 weeks when stored at 4°C or 6 months at −20°C in the dark.
- Prepare fresh working standard solutions of concentration 100, 200, 300 and 400 μM by diluting the stock Trolox® solution with 75 mM sodium phosphate buffer (pH 7.0) at dilution factors of 1:25, 2:25, 3:25 and 4:25, respectively. These will form 1, 2, 3 and 4 μM Trolox® solutions in final concentration; one ORAC unit is defined as the net protection provided by 1 μM Trolox® in final concentration. Of each concentration, one run requires 3 × 30 = 90 μl (manual) or 3 × 70 = 210 μl (automated).

Reagent preparation

- Prepare 1 l of 75 mM sodium phosphate buffer (pH 7.0) by mixing equal volumes of 31.5 mM NaH_2PO_4 (3.7803 g/l) and 43.5 mM Na_2HPO_4 (6.1742 g/l). Use a magnetic stirrer to ensure proper mixing, and verify pH with a pH meter. Adjust as necessary by adding solid NaH_2PO_4 or Na_2HPO_4 powder directly to buffer solution.
- Prepare fresh 12 mM 2,2′-azobis(2-amidinopropane), or AAPH (3.2542 g/l), in 75 mM phosphate buffer (pH 7.0); this is a free radical generating solution. One run requires 12 × 1.5 = 18 ml (manual) or 96 × 150 μl = 14.4 ml (automated). The radicals are thermally generated, thus AAPH solution should be stored in an ice bath and discarded within 8 h.
- Prepare 25 ml of 6.0×10^{-4} M 6-carboxyfluorescein, or 6-FAM (0.2258 g/l), in 75 mM phosphate buffer (pH 7.0) for use as a fluorescent probe stock solution. This can last several months at 4°C in the dark.
- Prepare a fresh working 6-FAM solution of concentration 6.0×10^{-8} M by diluting the stock solution with 75 mM sodium phosphate buffer (pH 7.0) at a dilution factor of 1:10,000. One run requires 12 × 750μl = 9 ml (manual) or 96 × 75 μl = 7.2 ml (automated). This should be prepared daily and stored in the dark.

Performing the ORAC assay

Table 97.7 shows the measures required for each run in the ORAC assay.

The manual ORAC assay

1. Pre-incubate all reagents (including samples, standards, etc.) at 37°C, *except for* the 12 mM AAPH; this must remain in the ice bath.
2. Prepare 4 ml, 1 cm light path fluorescence cuvettes for each measure by adding 30 μl test reagent (as shown

Table 97.7 Measures required for each run in the ORAC assay

Measure	*Repeat*	*Volume[a] of reagents* *Test reagent*	*6-FAM (μl)*	*75 mM PB[b], pH 7.0 (μl)*	*AAPH (ml)*
Sample blank	Triplicate	30 μl sample	None	2,970	None
Reagent blank	Triplicate	30 μl 75 mM PB[b], pH 7.0	750	720	1.5
Standard curve[c]	Triplicate	30 μl Trolox®	750	720	1.5
Sample	Triplicate	30 μl sample	750	720	1.5
QC	Triplicate	30 μl QC	750	720	1.5

Notes: For the ORAC assay, each run involves comparing fluorescent emission of a blank, standard, sample and a QC.

[a] Refers to volume required for the manual assay. In the automated assay the total volume will be scaled down from 3.0 ml to the size of the microplate well volume (e.g. 3 μl of sample, 75 μl of 6-FAM, 72 μl of 75 mM PB (pH 7.0) and 150 μl of AAPH; total volume 300 μl).

[b] PB, phosphate buffer.

[c] This should be performed in triplicate at *all* working concentrations. That is, three repeats at 100 μM, three at 200 μM, etc.

in Table 97.7) to 750 μl working 6-FAM solution and 720 μl 75 mM phosphate buffer (pH 7.0). Mix well by inversion.

3. Initiate the reaction by adding 1.5 ml AAPH solution and continue to incubate the reaction mixture at 37°C.
4. Measure initial fluorescence (emission wavelength 520 nm, bandpass 20 nm; excitation wavelength 495 nm, bandpass 15 nm) at the start of the reaction, and subsequently every 60 s, until a plateau is reached in fluorescent emission; at this point the reaction is complete.

The automated ORAC assay

1. Pre-incubate all reagents (including samples, standards, etc.) at 37°C, *except for* the 12 mM AAPH; this must remain in the ice bath.
2. Prepare a stock plate containing each test reagent (Table 97.7) at a minimum well volume of 70 μl (e.g. 3 wells with 70 μl of QC). The robot will later transfer 3 μl to a separate test plate in which the absorbance is to be measured.
3. Prepare the test plate by adding 297 μl of 75 mM phosphate buffer (pH 7.0) to all wells which will contain a *sample blank*. The phosphate buffer is added to make up the volume which would otherwise be occupied by 6-FAM and AAPH.
4. Set the robot to pipette 75 μl of 6-FAM, 72 μl of 75 mM phosphate buffer (pH 7.0) and 3 μl of test reagent into all wells of the test plate (note *sample blank* wells will only receive the test reagent).
5. Remove AAPH solution from the ice bath and set the robot to pipette 150 μl into all wells (except for *sample blank* wells) of the test plate and mix by aspiration and dispensing.
6. Transfer the test plate to the microplate reader and incubate at 37°C. Measure initial fluorescence (emission wavelength 520 nm, bandpass 20 nm; excitation wavelength 495 nm, bandpass 15 nm) at the start of the reaction and subsequently every 2 min for approximately 3 h (or until each well has reached a plateau in fluorescent emission). At this point the reaction is said to be complete.
7. The kinetic curve for fluorescent emission can be imported into Microsoft Excel for analysis.

Calculation of ORAC

- For each measure (please refer to Table 97.7), a kinetic curve for time vs. raw fluorescent emission can be plotted to completion – this should be converted to relative fluorescent emission (where maximum and minimum intensities are given nominal values of 1 and 0, respectively).
- Calculate AUC of the time vs. relative fluorescence plots, for each cuvette/well.
- Data should be screened at this point: check coefficients of variation (CV) for sample/standard repeats within assays and QC between assays. Exclude CV $>$ 10–15%.
- Calculate the net AUC of standards, samples and QC as follows:

$$\text{Net AUC} = \text{mean AUC}_{\text{standard/sample/QC}} - \text{mean AUC}_{\text{reagent blank}} - \text{mean AUC}_{\text{sample blank}}$$

- Produce a standard dose–response curve (i.e. final concentration of Trolox® vs. net AUC). Note that a working 100 μM Trolox® standard is actually 1 μM in final concentration; this is important because one ORAC unit is defined as the net protection area provided by 1 μM Trolox® in *final concentration*. Interpolation of net AUC of an unknown sample on this standard curve will thus give TAC in Trolox® equivalents (TE).

Laboratory Protocol for the TP-FCR Assay

This is adapted from a previous publication (Singleton *et al.*, 1999).

Table 97.8 Measures required for each run in the TP-FCR assay

Measure	*Repeat*	*Volume[a] of reagents* *Test reagent*	*DW[b] (ml)*	*2N FCR (μl)*	*20% Na_2CO_3 (μl)*	*DW[b] (μl)*
Reference	Single	None	3.0	None	None	None
Sample blank	Triplicate	30 μl sample	1.8	None	None	1,170
Reagent blank	Triplicate	30 μl DW[b]	1.8	150	450	570
Standard curve[c]	Triplicate	30 μl gallic acid monohydrate	1.8	150	450	570
Sample	Triplicate	30 μl sample	1.8	150	450	570
QC	Triplicate	30 μl QC	1.8	150	450	570

Notes: For the TP-FCR assay, each run involves comparing absorbance at 760 nm at 2 h of a blank, standard, sample and a QC.

[a] Refers to volume required for the manual assay. In the automated assay the total volume will be scaled down from 3.0 ml to the size of the microplate well volume (e.g. 3 μl of sample, 180 μl of distilled water, 15 μl of 2N FCR, 45 μl of 20% Na_2CO_3 and finally 57 μl of distilled water to make up volume to 300 μl).

[b] DW, distilled water.

[c] This should be performed in triplicate at *all* working concentrations. That is, three repeats at 2 g/l, three at 1 g/l, etc.

Antioxidant standard preparation

- Prepare 50 ml 2 g/l gallic acid (or 2.2117 g/l gallic acid monohydrate – more water soluble) in distilled water as a stock solution of antioxidant standard by which to calibrate the data. This stock solution is stable for 1–2 days at 4°C, or can be frozen for several months in aliquots of usable size.
- Prepare fresh working standard solutions of concentration 2, 1, 0.5, 0.25, 0.125 and 0.0625 g/l by serial dilution of the stock gallic acid solution with water. Of each concentration, one run requires 3 × 30 = 90 μl (manual) or 3 × 70 = 210 μl (automated).

Reagent preparation

- Prepare 100 ml 20% Na_2CO_3 (200 g/l) in distilled water using a magnetic stirrer to ensure proper mixing (one run requires 12 × 450 μl = 5.4 ml (manual) or 96 × 45 μl = 4.32 ml (automated)). *TAKE CARE: dissolution of Na_2CO_3 in water is exothermic; the solution will become hot.*
- Prepare 50 ml 2N Folin–Ciocalteu's phenol reagent according to Singleton *et al.* (1999) – we used a commercially available version. One run requires 12 × 150 μ = 1.8 ml (manual) or 96 × 45 μl = 1.44 ml (automated). This working reagent is light sensitive.

Performing the TP-FCR assay

Table 97.8 shows the measures required for each run in the TP-FCR assay.

The manual TP-FCR assay

1. Prepare 4 ml, 1 cm light path visible range cuvettes for each measure by adding 30 μl test reagent (as shown in Table 97.8). Note the purpose of the reference cuvette is simply to zero the absorbance of the spectrophotometer; it contains distilled water.
2. To each cuvette, add 1.8 ml of distilled water and 150 μl of 2N Folin–Ciocalteu's reagent (Table 97.8); mix well. After 1 min and before 8 min, add 450 μl of 20% Na_2CO_3 and 570 μl of distilled water (Table 97.8); this will produce a final volume of 3.0 ml.
3. Allow these cuvettes to stand in the dark at room temperature, and record absorbance at 760 nm at 2 h (or other chosen endpoint).

The automated TP-FCR assay

1. Prepare a stock plate containing each test reagent (Table 97.8) at a minimum well volume of 70 μl (e.g. 3 wells with 70 μl of QC). The robot will later transfer 3 μl to a separate test plate in which the absorbance is to be measured.
2. Prepare the test plate by adding distilled water to all wells which will contain a *sample blank*. The distilled water is added to make up the volume which would otherwise be occupied by Folin and Ciocalteu's reagent and Na_2CO_3 solution.
3. Set the robot to pipette 180 μl of distilled water, 3 μl of test reagent and 15 μl of Folin–Ciocalteu's phenol reagent into each well, and to mix the well contents by aspirating fluid from the bottom of the well and dispensing it at the surface. Remember that distilled water and Folin–Ciocalteu's reagent are not added to *sample blank* wells. Program the robot to then pause for 180 s, and then to subsequently add 45 μl of 20% Na_2CO_3 followed by 57 μl of distilled water to each well (except for *sample blank* wells). This will produce a total volume of 300 μl per well, which should again be mixed by aspiration and dispensing.

4. Allow the test plate to stand in the dark at room temperature for 2 h (or chosen endpoint), then transfer to the microplate reader and read absorbance of each well at 760 nm.
5. The absorbance data can be imported into Microsoft Excel for analysis.

Calculation of TP-FCR

- Preliminary data handling: check coefficients of variation (CV) for sample/standard repeats within assays and QC between assays. Exclude CV > 10–15%.
- Calculate net absorbance (A) of each sample and each standard, using mean raw absorbance (A) data at 2 h (or chosen endpoint):

$$\text{Net } A_{760} \text{ of sample} = A_{760} \text{ of sample} - A_{760} \text{ reagent blank} - A_{760} \text{ sample blank}$$

$$\text{Net } A_{760} \text{ of standard} = A_{760} \text{ of standard} - A_{760} \text{ of reagent blank}$$

- Produce a standard dose–response curve (i.e. concentration of gallic acid vs. net absorbance). Interpolation of net absorbance of an unknown sample will thus give TAC in *gallic acid equivalents*.

Use of the Assays in Assessing the Total Antioxidant Capacity of Beers

We have tested several beverages, including draft and bottled ales, red wines and orange juices for TEAC, FRAP, ORAC and TP-FCR (Table 97.9). Draft ales appeared to have a marginally higher TAC than bottled ales in all four assays, although this was not significant. However, ales in general appear to have higher radical quenching ability than orange juices (ORAC assay: ales, 7,515 ± 404 μM TE; orange juices, 5,662 ± 630 μM TE; $p < 0.05$) but lower reducing capacity (TP-FCR assay: ales, 398 ± 30 mg/l; orange juices, 648 ± 45 mg/l; $p < 0.01$). As expected from previous studies (Pellegrini *et al.*, 2000) red wines demonstrate the highest TAC in all four assays.

Practical Aspects in the Determination of Total Antioxidant Capacity

The experimental protocols that we have included in this chapter are comprehensive and have been used in our laboratory with great success. Whilst we have found these assays

Table 97.9 Total antioxidant capacity of various beverages

	Assay			
Beverage	*TEAC (mM TE)*	*FRAP (mM)*	*ORAC (μM TE)*	*TP-FCR (mg/l)*
Draft ales				
Fuller's London Pride	7.11	2.86	7,580	418
Timothy Taylor's Landlord	7.05	2.73	8,369	400
Old Speckled Hen	7.68	3.05	8,857	461
Premium Spitfire	7.10	2.87	7,529	398
Guinness	6.82	2.86	6,459	407
Bottled ales				
Whitechapel Porter	7.09	3.76	9,119	576
Bishops Finger	7.19	3.49	9,554	517
Master Brew	6.94	2.02	6,853	306
Whitstable Bay	6.70	1.92	6,722	257
Spitfire	6.75	2.15	6,415	266
1698	6.84	2.11	5,216	375
Red wines				
Los Torunos Merlot, Chile (2004)	38.82	21.51	28,239	1,891
Cabernet Sauvignon, Prahora Valley (2002)	35.28	17.34	26,271	1,620
Cono Sur Pinot Noir, Chile (2004)	36.51	20.45	29,380	1,911
Orange juices				
Waitrose Freshly Squeezed	7.23	3.92	5,253	674
Sainsburys Pure	7.04	3.71	4,834	709
Costcutter	6.31	1.00	6,899	560

Note: Data are values for the TAC of several beverages as assessed by the TEAC, FRAP, ORAC and TP-FCR assays. Red wines have the greatest TAC, several-fold higher than ales and orange juices, which are comparable.

to be effective, many of the practical aspects will depend on the instrumentation and other resources available. For example, microplates are available in several configurations, with variable material, color and pre-treatment. In our assays we have chosen to use clear, untreated, polystyrene flat-bottomed 96-well microplates (Corning catalog *#9017*). However, solid black plates are available; these serve to minimize well-to-well crosstalk and are particularly useful in fluorescence-based assays such as the ORAC assay. Careful consideration should be given to choice of assay reagents, especially those used during sample preparation. For example, use of a phosphate buffer as a diluent is entirely acceptable in the TEAC and ORAC assays; however, samples to be assessed by FRAP should be diluted using water, since phosphate buffer forms a precipitate with FRAP reagent. Aside from the diluents, the active reagents in each assay can be modified; indeed newer generations have subtly different requirements. For example, the original TEAC assay employed metmyoglobin which in the presence of hydrogen peroxide catalyzed oxidation of ABTS to form the $ABTS^{\bullet+}$ radical cation (Miller *et al.*, 1993). The improved TEAC assay combines ABTS with potassium persulfate, producing a stock $ABTS^{\bullet+}$ radical solution which is thought to possess greater stability (Re *et al.*, 1999). In the ORAC assay, the choice of fluorescent probe is flexible: several probes have been employed including β-phycoerythrin (β-PE) (Cao *et al.*, 1993) and 6-carboxyfluorescein (Naguib, 2000). Of these the latter appears to be of greater use due to both stability and absence of interaction with polyphenols in the test substrate (Ou *et al.*, 2001). Choice of antioxidant standards by which to calibrate the data is also variable, although the standards of choice appear to be Trolox® (TEAC and ORAC), gallic acid (TP-FCR) and ascorbic acid (FRAP).

We reiterate that experimental procedure should be adapted with respect to the equipment available. For example, our liquid handling robot allows different handling protocols for liquids of different viscosity, thus plasma (used for *in vivo* TAC assays) will be pipetted differently to less viscous fluids (such as beer). In addition, although most absorbance-based assays use standard maximal wavelengths to monitor reaction kinetics, fluorescence-based assays such as the ORAC assay have employed variable emission and excitation wavelengths and bandpass sizes.

Inherent Limitations in Assays for Total Antioxidant Capacity

It is well known that the various assays for TAC are not directly comparable and may demonstrate only weak correlations with one another (Cao and Prior, 1998). One reason for this is the differential sensitivity of each assay toward specific antioxidants in the test substrate. For example, proteinaceous substances have a relatively low contribution to TAC when assessed by FRAP, compared to other assays (Cao *et al.*, 1998). Another important explanation is that assays such as FRAP and TP-FCR measure only the reducing capacity of a sample *without exposing it to radical species* (cf. TEAC in which samples are exposed to $ABTS^{\bullet+}$ and ORAC in which samples are exposed to peroxyl radicals), thus no indication is given of radical scavenging ability. We reiterate that the conditions under which these assays are performed are non-physiological, for example, temperature (TEAC, 30°C; TP-FCR, room temperature) and pH (FRAP, pH = 3.6; TP-FCR, pH ≈ 10). Handling of antioxidants and free radicals under physiological conditions is likely to differ somewhat and consequently when performed *in vitro* these assays have only limited biological relevance.

One final but fundamental methodological consideration in the TEAC, FRAP and TP-FCR assays is the use of an arbitrary "endpoint" or definitive moment at which the reaction is said to be complete. This underestimates TAC because it does not allow the reaction to reach full completion and in addition does not allow for antioxidants which exhibit a lag phase (Huang *et al.*, 2005). In contrast, assays such as ORAC employ an AUC technique to reaction completion, allowing both degree and length of inhibition to be combined into a single quantity (Cao and Prior, 1998). It has been proposed that TP-FCR be used as the definitive test for reducing ability, whilst ORAC be used as an indicator of radical scavenging ability (Huang *et al.*, 2005).

Conclusion and Future Directions

This chapter presents comprehensive protocols for the *in vitro* measurement of TAC. Given that the antioxidant component of such beverages is bioavailable and would thus help to reduce oxidative stress, we anticipate that the application of these assays to beers will serve to provide a stronger basis for the function of beer in health and wellbeing.

Summary Points

- Antioxidants are protective against numerous pathologies, such as cardiovascular disease.
- Assessing the TAC of a sample is more useful than assaying individual antioxidants as it can be seen as a "holistic" measure of antioxidant protection.
- Assays for TAC demonstrate good linearity and repeatability, and can be automated for high-throughput analysis of samples.
- *In vitro* antioxidant capacity has some biological relevance as the antioxidants in beer have been shown to be bioavailable.
- TAC of ales is comparable to that of orange juices but several-fold lower than that of red wines. TAC of draft ales is marginally but non-significantly higher than that of bottled ales.
- Wider application of these assays will undoubtedly have an important function in the fields of nutrition and

pathology, and provide further evidence for the use of beer in maintenance of health and wellbeing.

Acknowledgments

The authors would also like to thank the staff of the Department of Nutrition and Dietetics, and Dr. Matt Arno of the Genomics Centre, King's College London. We also extend our gratitude to The Wellington (351 The Strand, London, WC2R 0HS, UK) for providing the draft beers, and Ian Dixon of Shepherd Neame Limited (17 Court Street, Faversham, Kent, ME13 7AX, UK) for supplying many of the bottled beers free of charge.

References

Benzie, I.F. and Strain, J.J. (1996). *Anal. Biochem.* 239, 70–76.

Cao, G. and Prior, R.L. (1998). *Clin. Chem.* 44, 1309–1315.

Cao, G., Alessio, H.M. and Cutler, R.G. (1993). *Free Radic. Biol. Med.* 14, 303–311.

Cao, G., Russell, R.M., Lischner, N. and Prior, R.L. (1998). *J. Nutr.* 128, 2383–2390.

Fernandez-Pachon, M.S., Villano, D., Troncoso, A.M. and Garcia-Parrilla, M.C. (2005). *J. Agric. Food Chem.* 53, 5024–5029.

Frankel, E.N., Kanner, J., German, J.B., Parks, E. and Kinsella, J.E. (1993). *Lancet* 341, 454–457.

Frankel, E.N., Waterhouse, A.L. and Teissedre, P.L. (1995). *J. Agric. Food Chem.* 43, 890–894.

Ghiselli, A., Natella, F., Guidi, A., Montanari, L., Fantozzi, P. and Scaccini, C. (2000). *J. Nutr. Biochem.* 11, 76–80.

Halliwell, B. and Gutteridge, J.M.C. (1999). *Free Radicals in Biology and Medicine*. Clarendon Press, Oxford, UK.

Huang, D., Ou, B., Hampsch-Woodill, M., Flanagan, J.A. and Prior, R.L. (2002). *J. Agric. Food Chem.* 50, 4437–4444.

Huang, D., Ou, B. and Prior, R.L. (2005). *J. Agric. Food Chem.* 53, 1841–1856.

Miller, N.J., Rice-Evans, C., Davies, M.J., Gopinathan, V. and Milner, A. (1993). *Clin. Sci. (London)* 84, 407–412.

Montanari, L., Perretti, G., Natella, F., Guidi, A. and Fantozzi, P. (1999). *Lebensmittel-Wissenschaft und-Technologie* 32, 535–539.

Naguib, Y.M. (2000). *Anal. Biochem.* 284, 93–98.

Ou, B., Hampsch-Woodill, M. and Prior, R.L. (2001). *J. Agric. Food Chem.* 49, 4619–4626.

Pellegrini, N., Simonetti, P., Gardana, C., Brenna, O., Brighenti, F. and Pietta, P. (2000). *J. Agric. Food Chem.* 48, 732–735.

Re, R., Pellegrini, N., Proteggente, A., Pannala, A., Yang, M. and Rice-Evans, C. (1999). *Free Radic. Biol. Med.* 26, 1231–1237.

Rice-Evans, C.A., Miller, N.J. and Paganga, G. (1996). *Free Radic. Biol. Med.* 20, 933–956.

Singleton, V.L., Orthofer, R. and Lamuela-Raventós, R.M. (1999). *Meth. Enzymol.* 299, 152–178.

98

Methods for the HPLC Analysis of Phenolic Compounds and Flavonoids in Beer

Pavel Jandera Department of Analytical Chemistry, Faculty of Chemical Technology, University of Pardubice, Pardubice, Czech Republic

Abstract

A variety of high-performance liquid chromatography (HPLC) methods are available for the determination of the individual phenolic acids, polyphenols, flavonoids and related compounds contributing to the antioxidant activity of beer. Successful separation of the individual compounds requires appropriate selection of columns, mobile phases and optimization of the operation conditions. Ultraviolet/visible, fluorimetric and electrochemical detection techniques for HPLC determination of phenolic compounds are compared with special attention to the highly sensitive and selective coulometric array detectors. Hyphenated techniques employing coupling of HPLC with mass spectrometry or with nuclear magnetic resonance are valuable tools for identification and structure elucidation of phenolic and related compounds in beer, hops and malt extracts. Finally, sample pre-treatment for HPLC of natural antioxidants is addressed.

List of Abbreviations

APCI	Atmospheric pressure chemical ionization
CE	Capillary electrophoresis
CoulArray	Coulometric electrode array detector
ESI	Electrospray ionization
F_m	Flow-rate of the mobile phase, in ml/min
GC	Gas chromatography
H	Normalized peak height
HPLC	High-performance liquid chromatography
LC	Liquid chromatography
MEKC	Micellar electrokinetic chromatography
MIP	Molecularly imprinted polymer
NMR	Nuclear magnetic resonance
PB	Particle beam
PDA	Photodiode array
R_s	Resolution of the pairs of compounds with adjacent peaks
SIM	Selected-ion monitoring
SPE	Solid-phase extraction
UV	Ultraviolet
VIS	Visible
cav	Caffeic acid
cat	Catechin
chlor	Chlorogenic acid
fer	Ferulic acid
gal	Gallic acid
4hpac	4-Hydroxyphenylacetic acid
phba	4-Hydroxybenzoic acid
pro	Protocatechuic acid
van	Vanillin

Introduction

Beer contains many phenols, the greater part of which comes from the malt, the remaining from the hop. Natural compounds present in beer include great variety of monomeric phenolic compounds and polyphenols, including phenolic acids (hydroxybenzoic acid derivatives, hydroxycinnamic acid derivatives), quercetin, campherol and other flavonoid types, flavanones, flavonol aglycones, flavonol glycosides, prenylated and non-prenylated chalcones, proanthocyanidins, catechins, coumarins, etc. Phenolic acids occur in germinated barley either in the free form or bound to the cell wall. Phenolic compounds have an important effect on the oxidative stability and microbial safety of beer and not only influence the stability of beer taste, smell and color, but also exhibit important biological activity and may act as antioxidants in human body, for example reducing the concentration of free radicals and acting as protective agents against oxidation of unsaturated fatty acids. Their potential preventive protection against cardiovascular diseases and cancer is attributed mainly to increasing the antioxidant capacity of plasma. Radical-scavenging and antioxidant mechanisms inhibit DNA damage and lead to anti-microbial,

Beer in Health and Disease Prevention
ISBN: 978-0-12-373891-2

anti-inflammatory and anti-tumor effects (Holasová *et al.*, 2002; Saija *et al.*, 1995; Choi *et al.*, 2002; Erlund, 2004; Gerhauser, 2005).

Generally, similar analytical methods can be used for the analysis of antioxidants in beer, wine, fruit juices or plant extracts, the main difference being in sample preparation and treatment prior to analysis, which depends on the matrix. The traditional methods of determination of the antioxidant activity of a sample such as beer rely on the determination of the induction period before the start of auto-oxidation reaction in presence of oxygen, such as NTZ/hypoxanthine superoxide assay or ferric thiocyanate method (Antolovich *et al.*, 2002).

However, such tests do not provide information on the contributions of the individual natural antioxidants to the antioxidant activity of beer. The need for profiling and identifying individual phenolic compounds triggered replacement of traditional methods by analytical separation techniques. The limited volatility and thermal instability of many phenolic compounds have restricted the application of gas chromatography (GC) and GC/MS to their analysis, unless suitable derivatization such as trimethylsilylation is used prior to the analysis. High-performance liquid chromatography (HPLC) currently is the most popular and reliable technique for analysis of phenolic acids, polyphenols and flavonoid natural antioxidants, even though capillary zone electrophoresis (CE) (Sádecká and Polonský, 2000; Minussi *et al.*, 2003), micellar electrokinetic chromatography (Cortacero-Ramirez *et al.*, 2004) or thin-layer chromatography (Simonovska *et al.*, 2003) are also occasionally used.

HPLC has been applied for relatively long time for the analysis of isohumulones (bitter-tasting iso-α-acids) in beer and hops. Applications of HPLC to the profiling or determination of the individual antioxidants in fruit, vegetables, plant extracts, tea, wine, beer and hop extracts has attracted continuously increasing attention since the early 1990s (Hertog *et al.*, 1992, 1993; Tsuchiya *et al.*, 1997; Dalluge *et al.*, 1998). Especial attention was focused on the target analysis of specific compounds, which are believed to have especial chemo-preventive activities, namely xanthohumol (a prenylated chalcone from hop) (Miranda *et al.*, 2000), quercetin and rutin (Careri *et al.*, 2000) or *trans*-resveratrol, occurring not only in wine, but also in hop and beer (Callemien *et al.*, 2005). On the other hand, new methods are being continuously developed for simultaneous analysis of various polyphenols and related antioxidants. For example, biologically active isoflavonoids genistein, biochanin A, daidzein and formononetin in various samples of bottled beer were determined using the combination of reversed-phase HPLC and radioimmunoassay in concentrations ranging from 0.1 to 10 nmol/l (Lapčík *et al.*, 1998). The advances in the development of new methods for the determination of bioactive phenols were recently reviewed (Robards, 2003).

HPLC of Antioxidants with Spectrophotometric and Fluorimetric Detection

Routine detection in HPLC based on the monitoring of the absorption of radiation in the near ultraviolet (UV) or visible (VIS) region was almost exclusively used in the early applications of HPLC for the analysis of natural antioxidants. All phenolic compounds possess a strong chromophore system, therefore UV–VIS detection often provides good results with the detection limits in the low ppm level for real samples, especially in routine HPLC analyses aimed at the determination of target compounds (McMurrough, 1980, 1981). However, no single wavelength is ideal for all classes of phenolic and flavonoid antioxidants, as various classes display absorbance at distinctly different wavelengths. Single-wavelength UV absorption detection is usually performed at the wavelengths providing maximum detection sensitivity (Careri *et al.*, 2000): 280 nm is used most frequently for phenolic acids and flavanones, whereas better sensitivity was found at 265 nm for flavones and flavonols, or at higher wavelengths in the VIS region for anthocyanidins (360 nm). Even though the detection at a low wavelength (e.g. 225 nm) is more general, it often has problems with high background absorption and the detection at higher wavelengths often enables to overcome interferences caused by impurities absorbing at lower wavelengths (Amakura *et al.*, 2000; Revilla and Ryan, 2000). Detection limits in 1–50 ng ranges were reported for HPLC with single-wavelength detection (Bocchi *et al.*, 1996), but they vary for the individual compounds, which differ significantly in molar absorptivities. To overcome the problems in quantitation due to these differences, Tsimidou *et al.* (1992) suggested classifying various phenols into four groups and using a single calibration standard for the members of each group.

Photodiode array (PDA) spectrophotometric detection has become very popular in HPLC of natural antioxidants, as it not only allows easy selection of suitable detection wavelength providing best sensitivity of determination, but also UV spectra can be obtained on-line. This is a very useful feature of the PDA detection, as the UV spectra of the individual phenolic and flavonoid antioxidants provide considerable structural information that can distinguish the type of compounds such as simple phenol, flavone, xanthone, etc. and provides valuable clues for the identification of the individual compounds (Escarpa *et al.*, 2002). The spectra of eluting peaks at the apex and both inflexion points can be compared and used as the indicator of peak purity (possible coelution). HPLC with UV detection was used for monitoring the profile of caffeic, sinapic, syringic and vanillic acids as antioxidants in human plasma after intake of beer. This method is used to identify the impact of brewing technology on minor components with antioxidant activity present in beer (Ghiselli *et al.*, 2000).

Concentrations of (+)-catechin and ferulic acid as the markers for flavor stability of beer were measured using an HPLC/UV method (Walters *et al.*, 1997). HPLC with UV detection served as the basis of an automatic analyzer for the determination of the total polyphenols contents in beer and wort (Sakuma *et al.*, 1995).

Rapid HPLC methods with UV/VIS detection are available for screening and determination of natural antioxidants in beer after pre-column or post-column derivatization of target classes of compounds. Derivatization not only increases the sensitivity and the selectivity of determination, but also may improve the possibilities for identification of separated compounds. Post-column chemical reaction with *p*-dimethylaminocinnamaldehyde after HPLC separation was applied for the determination of phenolic compounds and flavanols, including catechin, epicatechin, gallocatechins, procyanidin B-2 and other procyanidins and prodelphinidins (de Pascual-Teresa *et al.*, 2000). The absorbance ratio at 640 and 280 nm combined with the retention time and the whole UV/VIS spectrum were used for characterization of the separated compounds (de Pascual-Teresa *et al.*, 1998).

Fluorescence detection in HPLC is more selective and sensitive than UV-absorbance detection and may be used for sensitive determination of some antioxidants shoving natural fluorescence, such as *trans*-resveratrol (Rodriguez-Delgado *et al.*, 2001, 2002). The intensity of fluorescence of some phenolic acids (*p*-hydroxybenzoic, ferulic, vanillic, etc.) is enhanced by formation of inclusion complexes with cyclodextrins. This phenomenon was utilized for the determination of the phenolic compounds in beer at ng/ml level using reversed-phase HPLC with fluorimetric detection and the buffered mobile phase containing 0.01 mol/l α-cyclodextrin (García Sánchez *et al.*, 1996).

Electrochemical Detection in HPLC of Phenolic and Flavonoid Compounds

Significantly improved detection sensitivity and selectivity for natural antioxidants taking the advantage of their reducing properties was achieved using HPLC with electrochemical detection, either amperometric or coulometric, usually with an octadecyl silica column and aqueous–organic mobile phases containing acidic buffers to suppress the dissociation of weakly acidic phenolic compounds. HPLC with electrochemical detection allows achieving detection limits in low pg levels (Bocchi *et al.*, 1996). In an early application, Roston and Kissinger (1981) determined six phenolic acids in ethyl acetate beer extracts using a dual-electrode amperometric detector with glassy carbon electrode. Lunte (1987) analyzed nine flavonoids in beverages and Hayes *et al.* (1987a, b) identified and determined 11 phenolic compounds and flavonoids in beer using reversed-phase HPLC with amperometric detection.

Coulometric detection with a porous graphite electrode through which the effluent from the chromatographic column passes (Figure 98.1) increases considerably the contact area of the electrode with sample compounds, so that nearly 100% of the analyte is subject to electrochemical reaction, in comparison with less than 10% typical with amperometric detection. The porous electrode design also increases significantly the signal stability with respect to the amperometric detection. Furthermore, coulometric detection in HPLC also greatly simplifies sample preparation as the phenolic compounds are the only electroactive substances in beer oxidizable at a low potential. Hence other compounds in beer do not interfere and the extraction of phenolic compounds from beer and wort matrices is not needed. Because of high selectivity, sensitivity and signal stability, HPLC with coulometric detection is ideally suited for the analysis of phenolic compounds and has become increasingly popular for the analysis of natural antioxidants in food, beer and other beverages.

The Coulochem II electrochemical detector with two coulometric detection cells in series, each containing a porous graphite measuring and a hydrogen–palladium reference electrode, was used for HPLC analysis of phenolic compounds and flavonoids in beer (Hayes *et al.*, 1987a, b; Nardini and Ghiselli, 2004). Dual-channel coulometric detection improves significantly stability, accuracy and reliability in comparison with single-channel detection, as the signal of the compounds of interest can be enhanced and the signal of interfering compounds can be eliminated by appropriate setting of the operating electrode potentials in the two channels (McMurrough and Baert, 1994). Nardini and Ghiselli (2004) used this method for comparison of the contents of 13 free phenolic acids and phenolic acids bound in glycosides and complexes after alkaline hydrolysis and found that 3–10 times more acids are present in the bound than in the free form in beer. Two dimeric and three trimeric proanthocyanidins (McMurrough and Baert, 1994) and flavanols prodelphinidin B3, procyanidin B3, (+)-catechin and (−)-epicatechin (Madigan *et al.*, 1994) were identified and determined in beer using a dual-electrode coulometric detector.

Unfortunately, neither amperometric nor coulometric electrochemical detection is generally compatible with the gradient elution mode, which is necessary for separation of complex mixtures of phenolic compounds. This problem has been solved by the development of a multi-channel detector with the arrays of 4, 8, 12 or 16 three-electrode electrochemical cells connected in series. The electrochemical detection with an electrode array (CoulArray) is not only very sensitive and highly selective, but also provides different and reproducible signal responses to the sample compounds at the reduction or oxidation potentials applied across the individual flow-through cells connected in series (in 4, 8, 12 or 16 channel arrays). Hence, the ratios of the areas of the dominant peak (recorded in the channel providing the

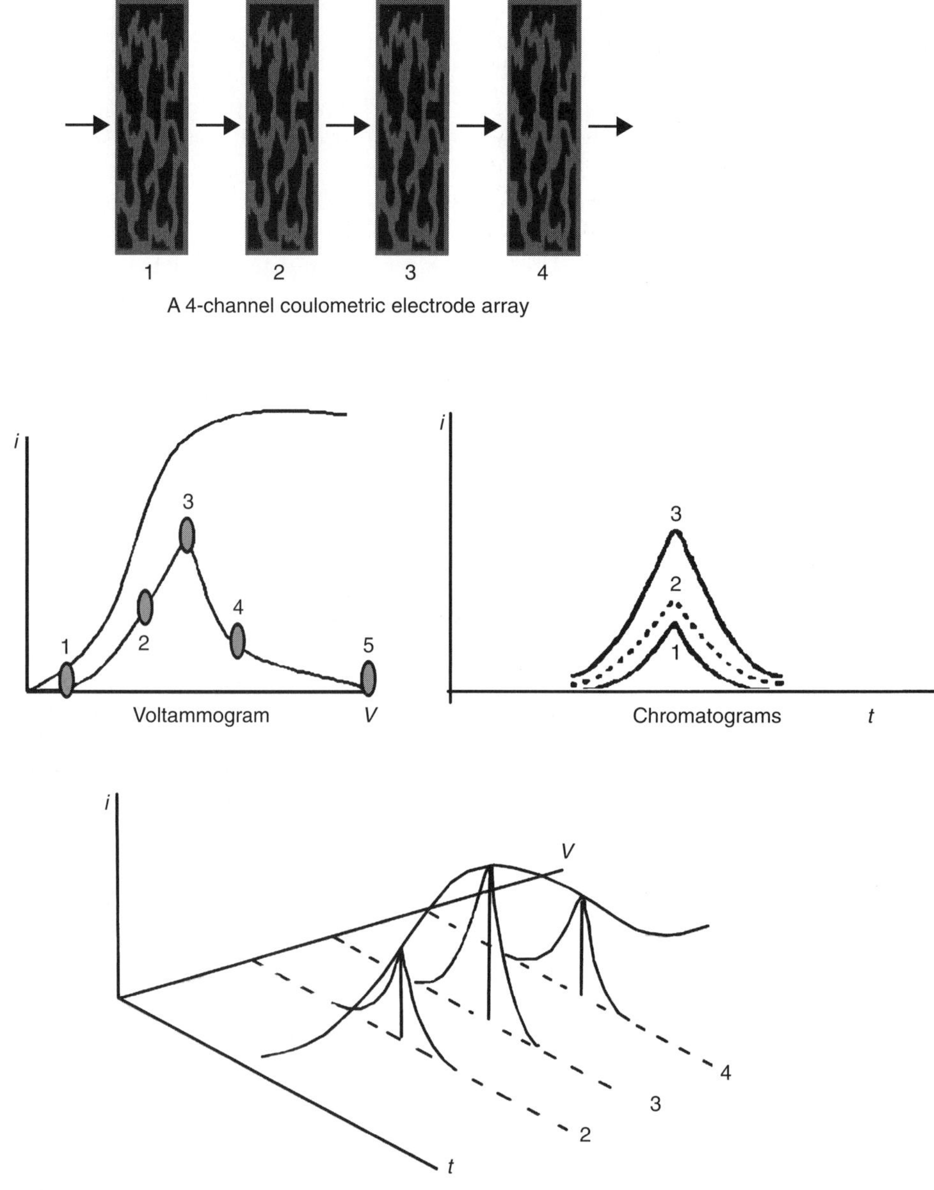

Figure 98.1 Schematics of a 4-channel coulometric electrode array detector. The numbers at the signals in voltammograms and chromatograms correspond to the order of the electrodes arranged in series.

highest response) to the areas of the so-called pre-dominant and the post-dominant peaks (in the channels just before and after the dominant peak channel, respectively) can be used to confirm the identification of sample compounds (Figure 98.1). Further, inverse proportionality was found between the dominant peak potential corresponding to the maximum detector response and the antioxidant activity of phenolic acids (Peyrat-Maillard *et al.*, 2000). Phenolic acids show maximum detector response at low oxidation potentials (100–450 mV), whereas flavonoids have two maxima, at 0–300 mV and at 600–900 mV. Further, the CoulArray detector is controlled by the software compensating for the baseline drift during a gradient run, which may cause serious problems when gradient HPLC is attempted with other electrochemical detection systems. Finally, hydrodynamic voltammograms can be recorded as the plots of the response (peak areas) vs. several potentials applied on the measuring electrode and used as an aid in assignment of peaks to the individual phenolic compounds, in analogy to the UV spectra recorded by PDA detectors (Careri *et al.*, 2000; Rodtjer *et al.*, 2006). Signals recorded in the individual channels with different applied potentials can also be used to resolve

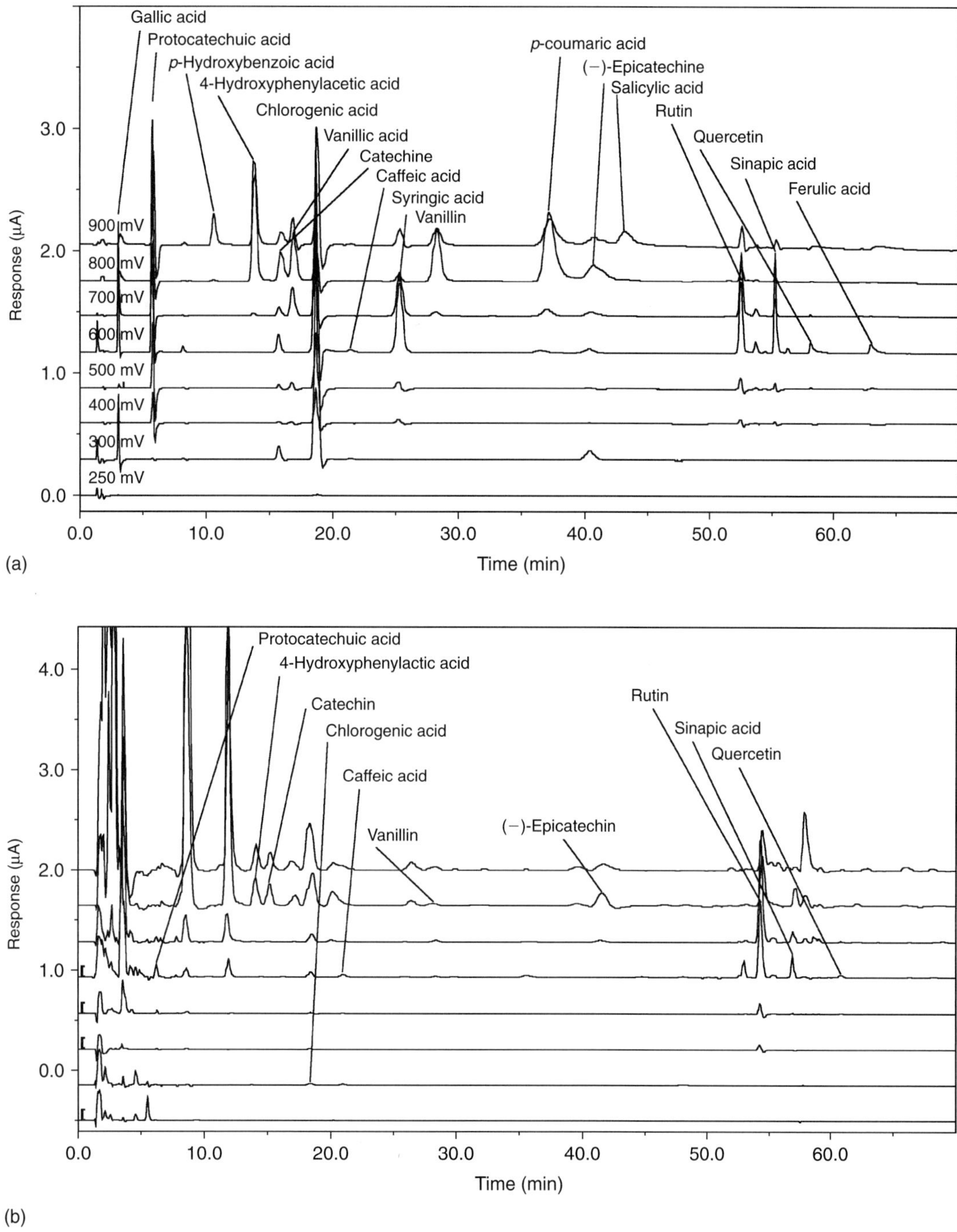

Figure 98.2 Chromatograms of phenolic compounds (0.001 mg/l each). (a) Standards and (b) a beer sample (diluted 1:4). Gradient elution on a C18 column with CoulArray detection.

coeluting peaks (Floridi *et al.*, 2003). Hence, electrochemical coulometric array detection is a powerful tool for the selective and sensitive detection of natural antioxidants.

Achilli *et al.* (1993) and Gamache *et al.* (1993) reported applications of a 16-channel CoulArray detector for the analysis of more than 30 phenolic compounds and flavonoids in fruit juice, wine, beer and other beverages. Guo *et al.* (1997) used similar conditions and a 12-channel detector for the analysis of 31 phenolic compounds and flavonoids in fruit and vegetables. An 8-channel CoulArray detector was used for the analysis of phenolic compounds and flavonoids in wort and beer using gradient (Floridi *et al.*, 2003; Škeříková *et al.*, 2004). Figure 98.2 shows chromatograms illustrating the separation of standard compounds and of the phenolic antioxidants in beer. Montanari *et al.* (1999) found some differences in the concentrations of free phenolic acids in beer samples determined by direct sample injection in HPLC with an 8-channel CoulArray detector and the results of HPLC with PDA spectrophotometric detection at the concentration levels 0.01–0.2 mg/l.

HPLC/MS and HPLC/NMR of Phenolic and Related Compounds

On-line coupling of liquid chromatography with mass spectrometry (LC/MS) has revolutionized the analysis of non-volatile compounds in food products, which usually are complex mixtures containing miscellaneous naturally occurring compounds. In this connection, the mass spectrometer may be used as a highly selective and sensitive detector, but, above all, it provides valuable information to confirm positively the identity of separated phenolic and related natural antioxidants. Further, HPLC/MS offers bi-dimensional resolution of complex samples, allowing compounds with overlapping chromatographic peaks to be distinguished. Tandem MS/MS techniques are useful for structural elucidation. Careri *et al.* (1998) presented an overview of the early applications of LC/MS methods in food analysis, including flavonoids, phenolic and related compounds.

LC/MS interfacing is less straightforward than coupling of gas chromatography with mass spectrometry (GC/MS) and various technical solutions to this problem have been suggested. Using particle-beam electron-impact interface (PB-EI-MS) in combination with HPLC, library-searchable EI mass spectra can be obtained. Using a bonded nitrile column in the normal-phase mode and gradient hexane–diethyl ether–propan-2-ol–formic acid, detection limits comparable with UV detection (2–50 ng) were achieved for phenolic acids in the selected ion monitoring (SIM) mode (Bocchi *et al.*, 1996). With a narrow-bore reversed-phase packed capillary column connected to a capillary-scale PB interface, the detection limits were reduced to the low pg range (Cappiello *et al.*, 1999).

The real success in LC/MS interfacing was achieved after the introduction of atmospheric pressure "soft" ionization techniques necessary to analyze thermally labile and highly polar natural compounds in MS. Electrospray/ionspray–mass spectrometric interface for LC rapidly supplanted thermospray ionization used in the 1980s, brought breakthrough advantages in terms of sensitivity and has been widely applied in LC/MS of phenolic compounds and flavonoids (Careri *et al.*, 1998). The electrospray ionization (ESI) technique in the negative-ion mode provides mass spectra of phenolic acids containing mainly the ions of deprotonated molecules and the ions corresponding to the losses of CO_2. Flavonol and flavone glycosides provide both the deprotonated molecules of the glycosides and the ions corresponding to the deprotonated aglycones, which are due to the loss of the sugar part of the molecule (Sanchez-Rabaneda *et al.*, 2003a). In the SIM mode, detection limits in the sub-nanogram range were found (Careri *et al.*, 1999). HPLC with another soft ionization interface, atmospheric pressure chemical ionization (APCI), is useful for identification of flavones, flavonols and flavanones, which provide characteristic pseudomolecular anions in the negative-ion mode (Justesen *et al.*, 1998).

The APCI LC/MS technique has been applied to the analysis of iso-α-acids (bitter acids) in hop extracts and beer (Vanhoenacker *et al.*, 2004) and for the determination of *trans*-resveratrol in beer and hop extracts after preliminary removal of hydrophobic bitter compounds; 0.5 ppm *trans*-resveratrol was found in hop pellets, from which it is transferred to beer in the brewing process (Callemien *et al.*, 2005). HPLC in combination with ESI–MS detection in the negative-ion mode has been used to identify proanthocyanidins extracted from malt (Friedrich *et al.*, 2000) and from beer (Whittle *et al.*, 1999). Catechin, epicatechin, gallocatechin, epigallocatechin and several phenolic acids and proanthocyanidin dimers and trimers were identified in beer and their contents were used to distinguish various beer types.

LC coupled with tandem MS (LC/MS/MS) in the negative-ion mode is very useful for structure elucidation (Sanchez-Rabaneda *et al.*, 2003b). The collisional activation energy can be adjusted to provide different fragmentation patterns in both the sugar and aglycone parts of the molecules of phenolic and flavonoid compounds in the MS/MS product ion scans, with fragment ions characteristic for each family of natural antioxidants (Poon, 1998). Reversed-phase HPLC–MS/MS using a triple-quadrupole mass spectrometer equipped with a heated nebulizer–APCI interface was used for identification and determination of xanthohumol and six other prenylflavonoids in methanolic hop extracts and commercial beer samples by positive-ion multiple-reaction monitoring (Stevens *et al.*, 1999). LC/MS/MS was used for stable isotope dilution analysis of polyphenols (pyrogallol, catechin, epicatechin, various phenolic acids, etc.) in various matrices, including beer samples, with quantification limits 10–30 nmol/l (Lang *et al.*, 2006).

Nuclear magnetic resonance (NMR) spectrometry is a powerful complementary technique if the mass spectral data are insufficient for structural assignment. However, the disadvantage of NMR is its limited sensitivity and need for isolation of relatively large quantities of pure substances, so that on-line coupling of HPLC with NMR is only at the early stage development. The NMR spectra of phenols are often complex and do not allow unambiguous identification of the isolated compounds, therefore HPLC is usually simultaneously coupled to both NMR and MS. Large sample quantities are injected (often using a semi-preparative column) and ^{1}H NMR spectra are acquired more frequently in the stop-flow mode than under the real-time separation conditions. Further, the selection of mobile phase is limited and deuterated solvents should be used where possible to avoid signal interferences, for example, mixtures of acetonitrile and D_2O with small amount of formic acid. HPLC/NMR coupling was employed for the analysis of hop bitter acids (Pusecker *et al.*, 1999) and of phenolic acids and related compounds in beer (Gil *et al.*, 2003).

Selectivity and Optimization of HPLC Separation of Phenolic and Flavonoid Compounds in Beer

Phenolic acids, polyphenols and both glycoside and aglycone flavonoids are almost exclusively separated in reversed-phase HPLC mode. Many natural antioxidants are strongly polar compounds, requiring highly aqueous mobile phases for successful separation. On the other hand, some flavonoids are rather non-polar and mobile phases with a higher concentration of organic modifier are necessary to accomplish their elution. Most phenolic compounds are weak acids, which are more or less dissociated in the mobile phases depending on their structure and – to a lesser extent – on the concentration of the organic solvent(s) in the mobile phase. The retention in reversed-phase HPLC generally decreases with increasing concentration and decreasing polarity of the organic modifier in the aqueous–organic mobile phase and with increasing polarity and degree of dissociation of the analytes. Gallic acid with three phenolic –OH groups elutes first, followed by dihydroxy- and monohydroxybenzoic acids. Flavonoid compounds generally elute later than simple phenolic compounds; as a rule, aglycones are retained more strongly than the corresponding glycosides. To improve the separation of compounds strongly differing in polarities in a single run, gradient elution with increasing concentration of the organic modifier (usually acetonitrile or methanol) is often used.

The non-dissociated form of a phenolic acid is more or less retained on an alkyl silica gel column, depending on the number of hydroxyl groups and other polar substituents and on the hydrocarbon matrix, whereas the ionic form is usually very little retained, if at all. Moreover, the peaks of the acid anions are often asymmetrical, may show strong tailing and sometimes even splitting. Hence, aqueous–organic mobile phases containing acidic buffers are typically used to suppress the dissociation, to increase the retention and to improve the peak symmetry of phenolic compounds in reversed-phase HPLC. Alternatively, ion-pairing reagents can be added to the mobile phases, such as tetraalkylammonium salts, which form more strongly retained neutral ion associates with the anions of phenolic acids.

Not only the retention, but also the separation selectivity, resolution and sensitivity strongly depend on the pH of the mobile phase, which should be optimized to obtain best separation of polar phenolic compounds. Figure 98.3 shows the dependence of the resolution and of the signal response of phenolic acids occurring in beer on the pH of the mobile phase. Another important point in the selection of the mobile phase for HPLC is the compatibility with the detection technique used: non-volatile buffers and salts should be avoided in HPLC/MS of phenolic compounds (ammonium acetate with acetic or formic acid in aqueous acetonitrile is usually suitable mobile phase). Sensitive electrochemical detection requires mobile phases composed of high-purity components, which should not contain

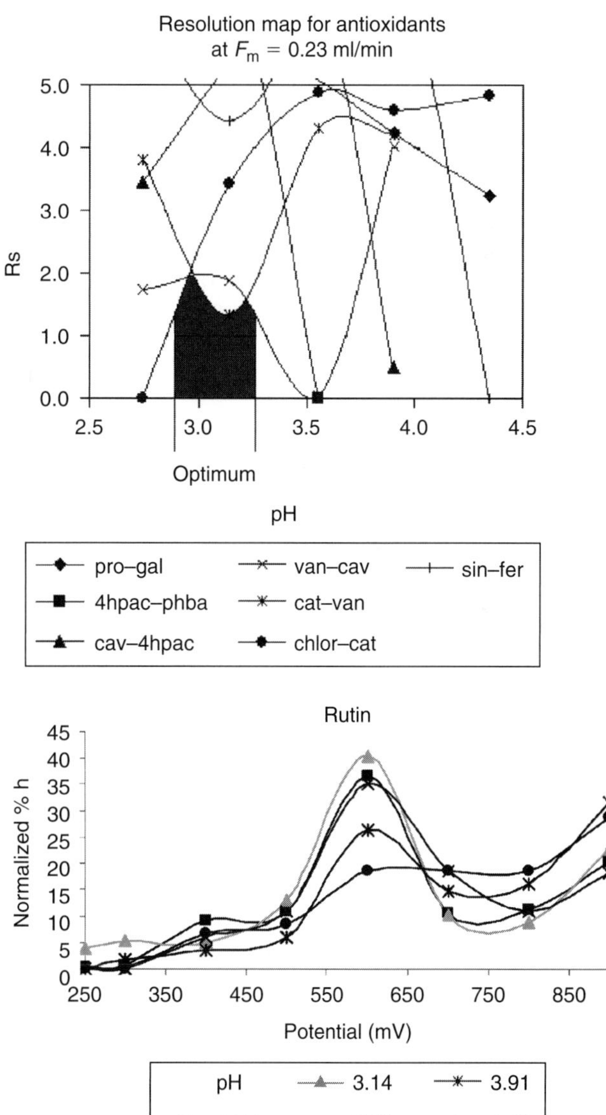

Figure 98.3 pH effect on the chromatographic resolution and sensitivity. R_s – resolution of the pairs of compounds with adjacent peaks. pro – protocatechuic acid, gal – gallic acid, 4hpac – 4-hydroxyphenylacetic acid, phba – 4-hydroxybenzoic acid, cav – caffeic acid, van – vanillin, cat – catechin, chlor – chlorogenic acid, sin – sinapic acid, fer – ferulic acid. F_m – flow-rate of the mobile phase, in ml/min, h – normalized peak height of rutin. Multichannel coulometric detection.

even traces of electrochemically active impurities and acetonitrile is preferred to methanol as the organic modifier. To decrease the baseline noise using coulometric detection, the whole LC system should be passivated by flushing with diluted nitric acid for a short time before the first analysis.

Generally, an alkyl silica column, such as C18, is used most frequently for HPLC of phenolic compounds in beer. In the earlier isocratic applications, mobile phases contained ammonium phosphate (Lunte, 1987), or acetate buffer and citric acid (Kenyherz and Kissinger, 1977). The use of mixed ternary mobile phases containing methanol, 1-propanol and water was also reported (Roston and Kissinger, 1981). For simultaneous analysis of a larger number (more than 30) phenolic compounds in beer in a single run, linear or segmented gradients were applied with increasing concentration of methanol or acetonitrile in aqueous mobile phases containing various ionic additives, such as sodium dihydrogenphosphate and phosphoric acid (Floridi *et al.*, 2003), ammonium acetate and formic acid (Řehová *et al.*, 2004), sodium dodecylsulfate, sodium phosphate and phosphoric acid (Achilli *et al.*, 1993) or nitriloacetic acid (Gamache *et al.*, 1993). The method was used for comparison of the concentrations of the individual antioxidants in various types of beer (Škeříková *et al.*, 2004). Figure 98.4 compares the average probability of occurrence and concentrations of some phenolic and flavonoid natural antioxidants found in Czech lager (pivo L) and draft (pivo T) beers.

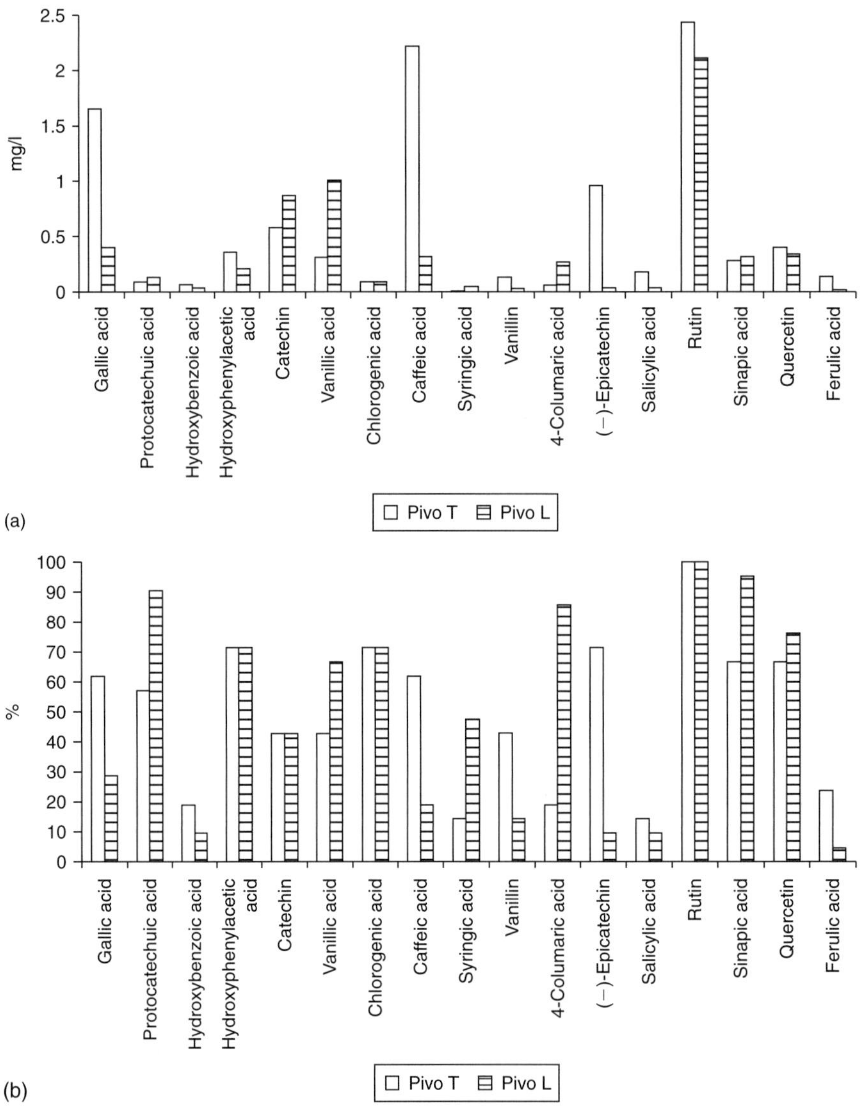

Figure 98.4 Mean concentrations and probability of occurrence of phenolic antioxidants in Czech beer. (a) Mean concentrations of antioxidants as the average for all beer types; pivo T – draft beer, 14 different types; pivo L – lager beer, 14 different types. Three repeated analyses for each type of beer. (b) Average probability of occurrence in % of beer samples where the compound was found above the limits of determination.

Recently, five different C18 columns were compared and for each column optimum gradients were designed for the analysis of natural phenolic and flavonoid antioxidants in various samples, including beer, wort, hop extracts, wine, tea and yacon extracts (Jandera *et al.*, 2005) in connection with the electrode-array coulometric detection. Some non-alkyl chemically bonded stationary phases provide different selectivity for phenolic compounds in comparison with C18 columns, such as polyethyleneglycol silica (Blahová *et al.*, 2006) or phenyl silica (Cacciola *et al.*, 2006) bonded stationary phases, which were applied for two-dimensional serial or parallel separations of phenolic compounds in beer, wine and other samples. ZR-carbon stationary phase with a carbon layer deposited on zirconia dioxide support also provides the selectivity for phenolic acids widely differing from C18 columns. This stationary phase has outstanding temperature stability and can be used for high-temperature separations, unlike most alkyl silica columns; unfortunately this column retains too strongly flavones (Cacciola *et al.*, 2006).

Using a combination of stationary phases with different selectivities in two-dimensional HPLC is potentially promising method for increasing the peak capacity in the analysis of phenolic compounds in beer and other samples. In the so-called "comprehensive" LC × LC setup (Figure 98.5), the whole sample is analyzed on-line on each of the two columns connected via a 10-port switching valve. Figure 98.6 shows an example of contour-plot presentation of a two-dimensional LC × LC chromatogram of phenolic compounds in beer with a bonded phenyl stationary phase in the first dimension and a short chromolith monolithic C18 column in the second dimension.

Sample Treatment and Enrichment in HPLC of Natural Antioxidants

HPLC with coulometric detection is sensitive and selective enough for the detection and quantitation of phenolic compounds in beer without special sample pre-treatment. However, some flavonoids are present in low concentrations in beer and other natural samples and because of the complexity of the sample matrices, selective sample preparation

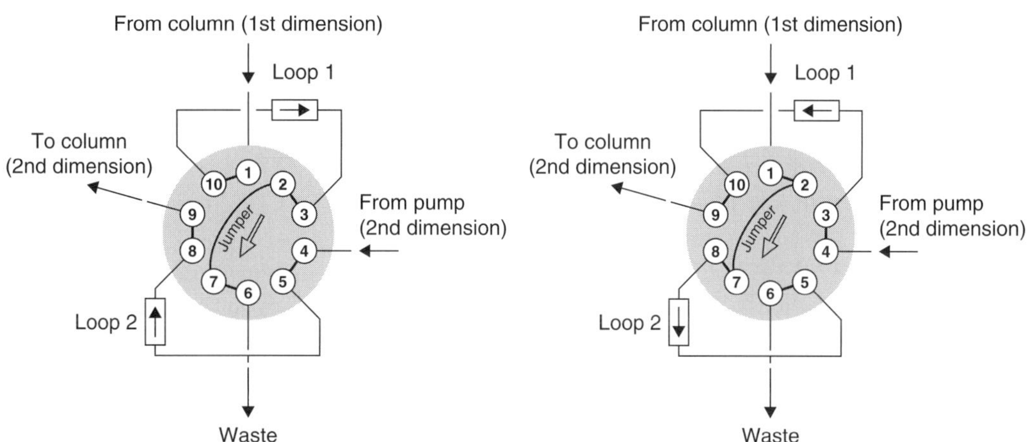

Figure 98.5 LC × LC setup with a 10-port switching valve interface and two sampling loops. Separation of a fraction trapped in one sampling loop in the second LC dimension while the next fraction from the first LC dimension fills the other loop.

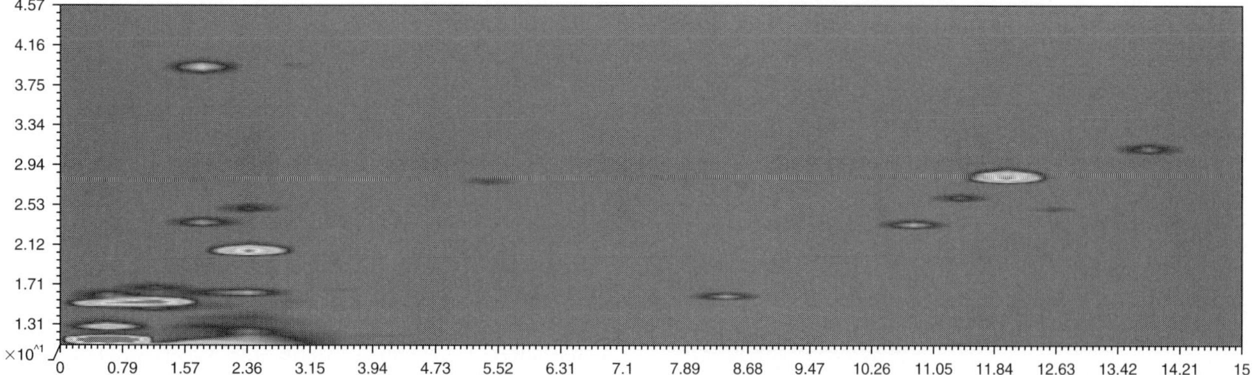

Figure 98.6 Two-dimensional LC × LC separation of antioxidants in a beer sample. Contour-plot presentation of a two-dimensional chromatogram. First dimension: a phenyl silica column (*x*-axis); second dimension: a monolithic C18 silica column (*y*-axis).

methods are sometimes applied to increase the selectivity and sensitivity of prior to chromatographic analysis using other detection techniques. Pre-concentration and/or isolation of compounds are frequently performed using solid-phase extraction (SPE) (Sakkiadi *et al.*, 2001; Alonso-Salces *et al.*, 2005). Montanari *et al.* (1999) used SPE and re-extraction with ethyl acetate/methanol prior to the HPLC analysis of phenolic acids in beer samples with PDA spectrophotometric detection at the concentration levels 0.01–0.2 mg/l.

Among various flavonoids, quercetin and rutin are becoming now the topic of increasing interest due to their natural antioxidant activity. The determination of quercetin and its glycosylated analog, rutin, is typically performed with HPLC using diode array or MS detectors, with sample pre-concentration using SPE (Sakkiadi *et al.*, 2001; Ishii *et al.*, 2003; Dubber *et al.*, 2005; Molnar-Perl and Fuzfai, 2005). Polymeric sorbents with molecularly imprinted target compound templates (MIPs) were applied as materials for the selective SPE and pre-concentration of rutin and quercetin from beer and other beverages before the analysis by high-pressure LC (Theodoridis *et al.*, 2006).

Summary Points

- Phenolic compounds and flavonoids are important sources of antioxidant activity of beer.
- HPLC methods with various detection techniques are well suited for the determination of the individual compounds contributing to the antioxidant activity of beer.
- Spectrophotometric detection methods are not very sensitive, but the diode array detector allows measuring UV spectra, which are unique characteristics of phenolic and flavonoid compounds.
- Fluorescence and electrochemical detection techniques provide improved sensitivity for the determination of phenolic compounds with fluorophore groups or electrochemical activity.
- Coulometric detection, especially with a multi-channel electrode array, is ideally suited for HPLC of phenolic compounds in beer: It is highly sensitive, provides selective response for natural antioxidants, which are all electrochemically active compounds, and offers possibilities for their identification on the basis of the hydrodynamic voltammograms and on the ratios of the peak areas of the dominant, pre-dominant and post-dominant peaks recorded at various potentials applied to the individual electrochemical cells.
- HPLC/MS with ESI and APCI techniques provides valuable information on the molar mass of phenolic compounds for their identification.
- For more detailed structural information, collisionally induced LC/MS/MS spectra can be measured.
- Most frequently, HPLC in reversed-phase mode is used for the separation of phenolic compounds.
- The separation of more complex mixtures of phenolic and flavonoid compounds in beer, wine or plant extracts usually requires gradient elution with increasing concentration of methanol or acetonitrile to be used.
- For best separation selectivity and resolution, pH of the mobile phase should be optimized, usually in weakly acidic range to suppress the dissociation of weak phenolic acids.
- Limitations concerning the purity or volatility of components imposed by the electrochemical or MS detection should be considered when selecting the optimum mobile phase of phenolic compounds.
- In addition to most frequently used C18 columns, other silica gel-based chemically bonded phases such as polyethylene glycol, phenyl or carbon deposited on zirconia dioxide provide useful complementary selectivity, which can be used in two-dimensional separations to increase the number of compounds separated in a single run.
- Coulometric detection is selective enough so that other compounds present in beer do not interfere in the determination of phenolic compounds and beer samples can be analyzed directly without special requirements on sample pre-treatment.
- With other less selective or less sensitive detection methods, SPE is the technique of choice for beer sample pre-separation and enhancement.

Acknowledgment

A part of the material presented in this review is based on the research supported by the Ministry of Education of the Czech Republic under the project number MSM0021627502.

References

Achilli, G., Cellerino, G.P., Gamache, P.H. and Melzi d'Eril, G.V. (1993). *J. Chromatogr.* 632, 111–117.

Alonso-Salces, R.M., Barranco, A., Corta, E., Berrueta, L.A., Gallo, B. and Vicente, F. (2005). *Talanta* 65, 654–662.

Amakura, Y., Okada, M., Tsuji, S. and Tonogai, Y. (2000). *J. Chromatogr. A* 891, 183–188.

Antolovich, M., Prenzler, P.D., Patsalides, E., McDonald, S. and Robards, K. (2002). *Analyst* 127, 183–198.

Bocchi, C., Careri, M., Groppi, F., Mangia, A., Manini, P. and Mori, G. (1996). *J. Chromatogr. A* 753, 157–170.

Blahová, E., Jandera, P., Cacciola, F. and Mondello, L. (2006). *J. Sep. Sci.* 29, 555–566.

Cacciola, F., Jandera, P., Blahová, E. and Mondello, L. (2006). *J. Sep. Sci.* 29, 2500–2513.

Callemien, D., Jerkovic, V., Rozenberg, R. and Collin, S. (2005). *J. Agric. Food Chem.* 53, 424–429.

Cappiello, A., Famiglini, G., Mangani, F., Careri, M., Lombardi, P. and Mucchino, C. (1999). *J. Chromatogr. A* 855, 515–527.

Careri, M., Mangia, A. and Musci, M. (1998). *J. Chromatogr. A* 794, 263–297.

Careri, M., Elviri, L. and Mangia, A. (1999). *Rapid Com. Mass Spect.* 13, 2399–2405.

Careri, M., Elviri, L., Mangia, A. and Musci, M. (2000). *J. Chromatogr. A* 881, 449–460.

Choi, C.V.W., Kim, S.C., Hwang, S.S., Choi, B.K., Ahn, H.J., Lee, M.Y., Park, S.H. and Kim, S.K. (2002). *Plant Sci.* 163, 1161–1168.

Cortacero-Ramirez, S., Segura-Carretero, A., Cruces-Blanco, C., de Castro, M.H.B. and Fernandez-Gutierez, A. (2004). *Electrophoresis* 25, 1867–1871.

Dalluge, J.J., Nelson, B.C., Thomas, J.B. and Sander, L.C. (1998). *J. Chromatogr. A* 793, 265–274.

Dubber, M.J., Sewram, V., Mshicileli, N., Shephard, G.S. and Kanfer, I. (2005). *J. Pharm. Biomed. Anal.* 37, 723–731.

Erlund, I. (2004). *Nutr. Res.* 24, 851–874.

Escarpa, A., Morales, M.D. and Gonzáles, M.C. (2002). *Anal. Chim. Acta* 460, 61–72.

Floridi, S., Marconi, O., Montanari, L. and Fantozzi, P. (2003). *J. Agric. Food Chem.* 51, 1548–1554.

Friedrich, W., Eberhardt, A. and Galensa, R. (2000). *Eur. Food Res. Technol.* 211, 56–64.

Gamache, P., Ryan, E. and Acworth, I.N. (1993). *J. Chromatogr.* 635, 143–150.

García Sánchez, F., Díaz, A.N., Lovillo, J. and Feria, L.S. (1996). *Anal. Chim. Acta* 328, 73–79.

Gerhauser, C. (2005). *Eur. J. Cancer* 41, 1941–1954.

Ghiselli, A., Natella, F., Guidi, A., Montanari, L., Fantozzi, P. and Scaccini, C. (2000). *J. Nutr. Biochem.* 11, 76–80.

Gil, A.M., Duarte, I.F., Godejohann, M., Braumann, U., Maraschin, M. and Spraul, M. (2003). *Anal. Chim. Acta* 488, 35–51.

Guo, C., Cao, G., Sofic, E. and Prior, R.L. (1997). *J. Agric. Food Chem.* 45, 1787–1796.

Hayes, P.J., Smyth, M.R. and McMurrough, I. (1987a). *Analyst* 112, 1197–1204.

Hayes, P.J., Smyth, M.R. and McMurrough, I. (1987b). *Analyst* 112, 1205–1207.

Hertog, M.G.L., Hollman, P.C.H. and Katan, M.B. (1992). *J. Agric. Food Chem.* 40, 2379–2386.

Hertog, M.G.L., Hollman, P.C.H. and Van de Putte, J. (1993). *J. Agric. Food Chem.* 41, 1242–1250.

Holasová, M., Fiedlerová, V., Smrčinová, H., Orsak, M., Lachman, J. and Vavreinová, S. (2002). *Food Res. Int.* 35, 207–211.

Ishii, K., Furuta, T. and Kasuya, Y. (2003). *J. Chromatogr. B* 794, 49–56.

Jandera, P., Škeříková, V., Řehová, L., Hájek, T., Baldriánová, L., Škopová, G., Kellner, V. and Horna, A. (2005). *J. Sep. Sci.* 28, 1005–1022.

Justesen, U., Knuthsen, P. and Leth, T. (1998). *J. Chromatogr. A* 799, 101–110.

Kenyhercz, T.M. and Kissinger, P.T. (1977). *J. Agric. Food Chem.* 25, 959–961.

Lang, R., Mueller, C. and Hofmann, T. (2006). *J. Agric. Food Chem.* 54, 5755–5762.

Lapčík, O., Hill, M., Hampl, R., Wahala, K. and Adlecreutz, H. (1998). *Steroids* 63, 14–20.

Lunte, S.M. (1987). *J. Chromatogr.* 384, 371–382.

Madigan, D., McMurrough, I. and Smyth, M.R. (1994). *J. Am. Soc. Brew. Chem.* 52, 152–155.

McMurrough, I. (1980). *Brauwissenschaft* 33, 328.

McMurrough, I. (1981). *J. Chromatogr.* 218, 683–693.

McMurrough, I. and Baert, T. (1994). *J. Inst. Brew.* 100, 409–416.

Minussi, R.C., Rossi, M., Bologna, L., Cordi, L., Rotilio, D., Pastore, G.M. and Durán, N. (2003). *Food Chem.* 82, 409–416.

Miranda, C.L., Stevens, J.F., Ivanov, V., McCall, M., Frei, B., Deinzer, M.L. and Buhler, D.R. (2000). *J. Agric. Food Chem.* 48, 3876–3884.

Molnar-Perl, I. and Fuzfai, Z. (2005). *J. Chromatogr. A* 1073, 201–227.

Montanari, L., Perretti, G., Natella, F., Guidi, A. and Fantozzi, P. (1999). *Food Sci. Technol. (Lebensm-Wiss. U. Technol.)* 32, 535–539.

Nardini, M. and Ghiselli, A. (2004). *Food Chem.* 84, 137–143.

de Pascual-Teresa, S., Treutter, D., Rivas-Gonzalo, J.C. and Santos-Buelga, C. (1998). *J. Agric. Food Chem.* 46, 4209–4213.

de Pascual-Teresa, S., Santos-Buelga, C. and Rivas-Gonzalo, J.C. (2000). *J. Agric. Food Chem.* 48, 5331–5337.

Peyrat-Maillard, N., Bonnely, S. and Berset, C. (2000). *Talanta* 51, 709–716.

Poon, G.K. (1998). *J. Chromatogr. A* 794, 63–74.

Pusecker, K., Albert, K. and Bayer, E. (1999). *J. Chromatogr. A* 836, 245–252.

Řehová, L., Škeříková, V. and Jandera, P. (2004). *J. Sep. Sci.* 27, 1345–1359.

Revilla, E. and Ryan, J.-M. (2000). *J. Chromatogr. A* 881, 461–469.

Robards, K. (2003). *J. Chromatogr. A*, 657–691.

Rodriguez-Delgado, M.A., Malovaná, S., Pérez, J.P., Borges, T. and Montelongo, F.J.G. (2001). *J. Chromatogr. A* 912, 249–253.

Rodriguez-Delgado, M.A., González-Hernández, G., Conde-González, J.E. and Pérez-Trujillo, J.P. (2002). *Food Chem.* 78, 523–532.

Rodtjer, A., Skibsted, L.H. and Andersen, M.L. (2006). *Eur. Food Res. Technol.* 223, 663–668.

Roston, D.A. and Kissinger, P.T. (1981). *Anal. Chem.* 53, 1695–1699.

Sádecká, J. and Polonský, J. (2000). *J. Chromatogr. A* 880, 243–279.

Saija, A., Scalese, M., Lanza, M., Marzullo, D., Bonina, F. and Castelli, F. (1995). *Free Radic. Biol. Med.* 19, 481–486.

Sakkiadi, A.-V., Stavrakakis, M.N. and Haroutounian, S.A. (2001). *Lebens.-Wissen. Technol.* 34, 410–413.

Sakuma, S., Kikuchi, C. and Kowaka, M. (1995). *J. Am. Soc. Brew. Chem.* 53, 29–32.

Sanchez-Rabaneda, F., Jauregui, O., Casals, I., Andres-Lacueva, C., Izquierdo-Pulido, M. and Lamuela-Raventos, R.M. (2003a). *J. Mass Spect.* 38, 35–42.

Sanchez-Rabaneda, F., Jauregui, O., Lamuela-Raventos, R.M., Bastida, J., Viladomat, F. and Codina, C. (2003b). *J. Chromatogr. A* 1008, 57–72.

Simonovska, B., Vovk, I., Andrenšek, S., Valentová, K. and Ulrichová, J. (2003). *J. Chromatogr. A* 1016, 89–98.

Škeříková, V., Grynová, L. and Jandera, P. (2004). *Chem. Listy* 98, 343–348.

Stevens, J.F., Taylor, A.W. and Deinzer, M.L. (1999). *J. Chromatogr. A* 832, 97–107.

Theodoridis, G., Lasáková, M., Škeříková, V., Tegou, A., Giantsiou, N. and Jandera, P. (2006). *J. Sep. Sci.* 29, 2310–2321.

Tsimidou, M., Papadopoulos, G. and Boskou, D. (1992). *Food Chem.*, 44, 53–60.

Tsuchiya, H., Sato, M., Hirotsugu, K., Okubo, T., Juneja, L.R. and Kim, M. (1997). *J. Chromatogr. B* 703, 253–258.

Vanhoenacker, G., De Keukeleire, D. and Sandra, P. (2004). *J. Chromatogr. A* 1035, 53–61.

Walters, M.T., Heasman, A.P. and Hughes, P.S. (1997). *J. Am. Soc. Brew. Chem.* 55, 83–89.

Whittle, N., Eldridge, H., Bartley, J. and Organ, G. (1999). *J. Inst. Brew.* 105, 89–99.

99

Methods for the Assay of Iso-α-acids and Reduced Iso-α-acids in Beer

Gerd Vanhoenacker and Pat Sandra Research Institute for Chromatography, Kennedypark, Kortrijk, Belgium

Abstract

Iso-α-acids or isohumulones are hop-derived beer constituents which are formed in the brewing process. The qualitative and quantitative analysis of iso-α-acids and reduced iso-α-acids is an important element in the quality control of beers because of the distinctive influence these compounds have on beer bitterness and foam stability. Iso-α-acids are light sensitive and play a key role in the origin of the well-known lightstruck "skunky" flavor of beer. Therefore, beers are generally stored in lightproof cans or dark bottles and reduced iso-α-acids are often added to the beer to stabilize taste and foam.

An overview is presented on the current state-of-the-art in the analysis of iso-α-acids and reduced iso-α-acids in beer using analytical separation methods. The various sample preparation techniques are summarized and the application of stir bar sorptive extraction (SBSE) is highlighted. This extraction/clean-up was successfully applied for the quantitative analysis of iso-α-acids and the qualitative analysis of reduced iso-α-acids in beer. Liquid chromatography (LC) is by far the most popular analytical separation method for the assay of these compounds. In addition to the widespread liquid chromatography–ultraviolet detection (LC–UV) methods, the application of liquid chromatography–mass spectroscopy (LC–MS) and capillary electrophoresis (CE) for the analysis of bitter acids in beer is demonstrated.

List of Abbreviations

APCI	Atmospheric pressure chemical ionization
CE	Capillary electrophoresis
CEC	Capillary electrochromatography
EIC	Extracted ion chromatogram
ESI	Electrospray ionization
IBUs	International Bittering Units
LC	Liquid chromatography
LC–UV	Liquid chromatography–ultraviolet detection
LC–MS	Liquid chromatography–mass spectroscopy
MEEKC	Microemulsion electrokinetic chromatography
MEKC	Micellar electrokinetic chromatography
MM	Molecular mass
PDMS	Polydimethylsiloxane
RSD	Relative standard deviation
SBSE–LD	Stir bar sorptive extraction–liquid desorption

Introduction

The main ingredients in the brewing process are water, malted barley, yeast, and hops or hop extracts. The result is a complex collection of compounds in a water–ethanol mixture that we call beer. A schematic representation of the brewing process is depicted in Figure 99.1. The characteristic bitter taste of beer is due to the presence of hop-derived substances, the so-called iso-α-acids or isohumulones, which are formed from the almost tasteless hop α-acids during the boiling of sweet wort with hops (*Humulus lupulus* L.) in the brewery (Verzele, 1986). The analysis of hop acids, which include, in addition to α-acids, also β-acids is an important criterion to assess the quality of hops and hop extracts. During brewing, the relatively insoluble hop β-acids (lupulones) are removed or oxidized, while each hop α-acid (humulone) is transformed into its corresponding mixture of epimeric bitter-tasting iso-α-acids (*cis* and *trans* isomers) (Verzele, 1986). As a result, six iso-α-acids (isohumulones) originate from the three main hop α-acids. These compounds are not only responsible for the bitter taste of beer, but they also exhibit bacteriostatic properties and, furthermore, play an essential role in enhancing the foam stability of beer as well as in the formation of off-flavors like the lightstruck flavor (Kuroiwa *et al.*, 1963; De Keukeleire *et al.*, 1992; Smith *et al.*, 1998).

Reduced iso-α-acids such as dihydroiso-α-acids (dihydroisohumulones, also known as rho-isohumulones), tetrahydroiso-α-acids (tetrahydroisohumulones) are often used in the brewing process to enhance both the light and

Beer in Health and Disease Prevention
ISBN: 978-0-12-373891-2

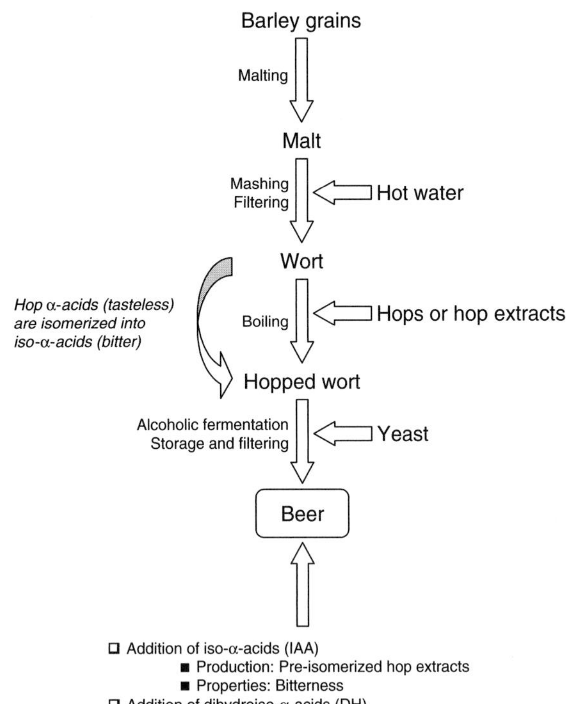

Figure 99.1 The brewing process. Schematic presentation of the various steps in the brewing process. Hops are added during the boiling of the wort. During this step, the tasteless hop α-acids are transformed into bitter-tasting iso-α-acids. At the end of the brewing process, a known amount of iso-α-acids and/or reduced iso-α-acids (dihydro- and tetrahydroiso-α-acids) can be added to control bitterness, taste, and foam and light stability.

the foam stability of beer. The structures of the main hop acids, the beer iso-α-acids, and the reduced iso-α-acids (tetrahydro- and dihydroiso-α-acids) are shown in Figure 99.2. Tetrahydroiso-α-acids also exist as *cis* and *trans* isomeric pairs resulting in six stereomers. Reduction of iso-α-acids to dihydroiso-α-acids introduces an additional chiral center, leading to two epimeric reaction products for each iso-α-acid. The group of dihydroiso-α-acids, thus, consists of 12 stereomeric members. A combination of both reduction processes leads to the formation of 12 additional hexahydroiso-α-acids (hexahydroisohumulones), which are not discussed here because of their limited use.

Quantitation of isohumulones and reduced isohumulones in beer is an important parameter in the quality control of beers because of their key role in the flavor characteristics of beer. Moreover, specific conventions regarding their use in some parts of the world stress accurate qualitative and quantitative determination. Addition of, for example, non-natural reduced forms of iso-α-acids is not allowed in German beers due to the "Reinheitsgebot" stating that only natural hop compounds may be used in the brewing process. Analytical methods for detection and quantitation of both iso-α-acids and reduced iso-α-acids are, therefore, of utmost importance.

Chromatographic separation of all 24 structurally similar compounds (isohumulones and reduced isohumulones) in a single analysis represents a daunting task. However, for quality control purposes only part of these compounds usually need to be analyzed (e.g. isohumulones and tetrahydroisohumulones) and often complete separation/quantitation of all individual bitter acids is not required. In general, the quantitation is performed of a group (e.g. quantity of isohumulones) but superior individual separation will enhance the characterization of the typical bitter taste.

LC and LC–MS Analysis

(Partially reprinted from Vanhoenacker et al. (2004), Copyright 2004, with permission from Elsevier B.V.)

The quantitation of the bitter acids during the brewing process or in the final product can be performed mainly by two procedures. The result can then be expressed as IBUs (International Bittering Units), a value for the beer bitterness. One IBU corresponds with 1 mg/l (ppm) of isohumulone. Lager beers, for example, will have values ranging from 15 to 25 IBUs.

The first possibility is to extract the bitter acids by liquid–liquid extraction using a solvent (e.g. isooctane) and analyzing the extract with UV–Vis spectrophotometry. The obvious disadvantage of this technique is the errors generated by UV-absorbing contaminants in the extract since this technique lacks selectivity. The method also does not provide any information regarding the relative amounts of the individual bitter acids and the quantity of reduced isohumulones added during the brewing process.

To have a more detailed analysis on the relative and absolute quantities of individual bittering compounds in beer, the solutes need to be separated from each other. Liquid chromatography (LC) is intensively used for the analysis of α- and β-acids in hops (Verzele and van de Velde, 1987; Hermans-Lokkerbol and Verpoorte, 1994; Harms *et al.*, 2001) and iso-α-acids in beer (Verzele *et al.*, 1990; De Keukeleire *et al.*, 1992; Harms *et al.*, 2001). The LC analysis of iso-α-acids and reduced iso-α-acids in beer is generally preceded by a pre-concentration/clean-up step, either by liquid–liquid extraction or by solid-phase extraction on reversed-phase material (Vindevogel *et al.*, 1991; Szücs *et al.*, 1993; Clark *et al.*, 1998). Recently, a new solventless extraction method named stir bar sorptive extraction (SBSE) has been described (Baltussen *et al.*, 1999). SBSE is normally combined with thermal desorption–capillary gas chromatography analysis and the sensitivity and simplicity of SBSE have been demonstrated for the analysis of volatiles and semi-volatiles in a variety of sample matrices like water (Peñalver *et al.*, 2003), beverages (Tredoux *et al.*,

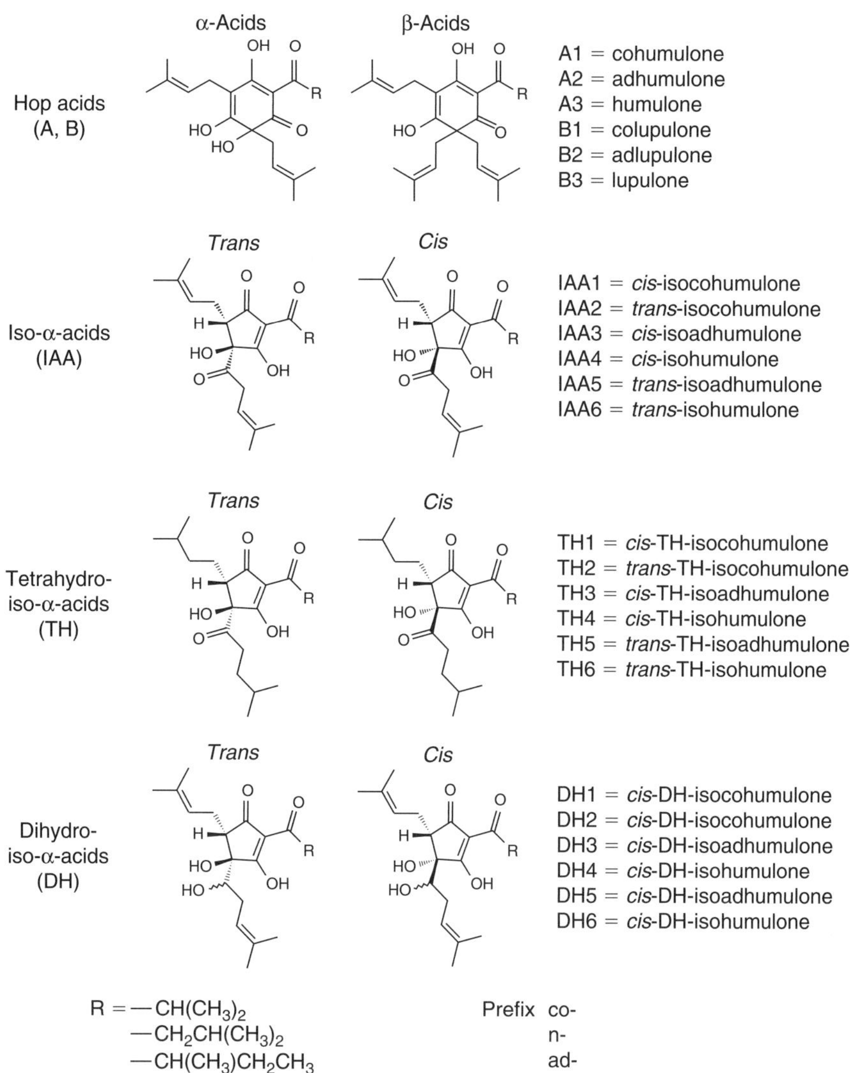

Figure 99.2 Structures and peak codes of the compounds of interest. Overview of the various hop acids (A, B), iso-α-acids (IAA), tetrahydroiso-α-acids (TH), and the *cis*-dihydroiso-α-acids (DH). Each type of acid exists as a co-, n-, and ad-homolog.

2000), biological fluids (Tienpont *et al.*, 2003), fruits, and vegetables (Sandra *et al.*, 2003). SBSE, however, can also be combined with liquid desorption (LD), which opens perspectives for the analysis of thermally labile compounds. Harms *et al.* presented the first application of SBSE–LD for the profiling of iso-α-acids in beer by LC (Harms *et al.*, 2001). However, state-of-the-art instrumentation also allows the direct analysis of the bitter compounds in beer, that is direct injection without enrichment/clean-up.

All routine LC methods use involatile buffer additives such as phosphate and citrate for the separation of iso-α-acids and reduced iso-α-acids (Burroughs and Williams, 1999; Harms and Nitzsche, 2001). These mobile phases are not compatible with mass spectroscopic (MS) detection. Only few reports have been published on LC–MS analysis of hop acids and no literature is available on the analysis of iso-α-acids and reduced iso-α-acids by LC–MS. Using ammonium acetate or acetic acid as mobile-phase additives and electrospray ionization (ESI) in the negative mode, hop acids were analyzed in beer after direct injection (Hofte *et al.*, 1998). Humulones (α-acids) were found to be present in beer at concentration levels of 150–200 μg/l (ppb), while lupulones (β-acids) were absent. Isohumulones and reduced isohumulones were not analyzed. Another report focused on the quantitation of 8-prenylnaringenin, a potent phytoestrogen, in hops, hop products, and beers. Reversed-phase LC was carried out on a C18 column using formic acid as a buffer additive and ESI MS in the positive mode for detection (Rong *et al.*, 2000). No quantitation was performed for the hop and beer bitter acids.

The following LC method enables simultaneous analysis of iso-α-acids and reduced iso-α-acids in beer without sample pre-concentration using an alkaline, MS compatible mobile phase (Vanhoenacker *et al.*, 2004). The method can be fine-tuned for fast separation of iso-α-acids and tetrahydroiso-α-acids in typical European beers.

Experimental

The calibration extract containing hop α- and β-acids (ICE 1) was from "Versuchsstation Schweizerischer Brauereien" (Zürich, Switzerland). Pre-isomerized hop extract containing iso-α-acids was obtained from Hopstabil GmbH (Wolnzach, Germany). The dihydroiso-α-acids standard (all-*cis*, DCHA-Rho, ICS-R1) was from Labor Veritas (Zürich, Switzerland) and the standard for tetrahydroiso-α-acids from Kalsec (Kalamazoo, MI, USA). The standards were dissolved separately in methanol to a concentration of 1 mg/ml. These stock solutions were stored at –20°C and used to prepare standard solutions.

Beers were bought at local stores, kept at room temperature, and freshly opened prior to analysis. They were degassed by ultrasonication and a portion was filtered through a syringe filter (0.2 μm, PTFE) prior to injection.

Analyses were performed on an Agilent 1100 LC equipped with a binary pump, vacuum degasser, autosampler, column thermostat, and a diode array detector (DAD) (Agilent Technologies, Waldbronn, Germany). For complete separation two Zorbax Extend C18 columns, 150 mml × 4.6 mm ID, packed with 5 μm particles were coupled in series (Agilent Technologies, Waldbronn, Germany). The mobile phase consisted of 5 mM ammonium acetate in 20% (v/v) ethanol adjusted to an apparent pH of 9.95 with ammonia (solvent A) and acetonitrile/ethanol 60/40 (v/v) (solvent B). The flow rate was set at 1 ml/min and gradient elution was performed. The gradient was the following: 0–3 min, 0% B isocratic; 3–4 min, 0–16% B; 4–54 min, 16–40% B; 54–57 min, 40–95% B; 57–65 min, 95% B isocratic. The column temperature was maintained at 35°C; 100 μl of a degassed and filtered beer sample was injected. Detection was performed with a DAD set at 256 nm (iso-α-acids and reduced iso-α-acids) and at 330 nm (α- and β-acids). The mass spectrometer was an Agilent 1100 Series Trap version SL with an atmospheric pressure chemical ionization (APCI) source (Agilent Technologies, Waldbronn, Germany). Negative ionization was performed in the scan mode (*m/z* 150–600). The target mass was set at *m/z* 350 and maximum accumulation time at 300 ms. Interface settings were: N_2 drying gas temperature 330°C, N_2 drying gas flow 5 l/min, APCI vaporizer temperature 450°C, nebulizer 60 psi, capillary voltage 4,000 V.

The fast separation was carried out on one Zorbax Extend C18 column, 150 mmL × 3 mm ID, packed with 3.5 μm particles (Agilent Technologies, Waldbronn, Germany). The mobile phase consisted of 10 mM ammonium acetate in water adjusted to pH 8 with ammonia (solvent A) and acetonitrile (solvent B). The flow rate was set at 0.6 ml/min and gradient elution was performed. The gradient was the following: 0–5 min, 28% B isocratic; 5–11 min, 28–40% B; 11–12 min, 40–95% B; 12–15 min, 95% B isocratic. The column temperature was maintained at 30°C; 20 μl of a degassed and filtered beer sample was injected. UV detection was performed at 256 nm.

Results and discussion

LC of iso-α-acids and reduced iso-α-acids is commonly carried out in the reversed-phase mode with a C18 or a C8 stationary phase. Problems related with interaction of solutes with trace metals present in the reversed-phase material have been reported (Verzele *et al.*, 1990; De Keukeleire *et al.*, 1992). Buffers are added to the mobile phase to improve separation and reproducibility. The buffer is usually acidic (phosphate) or neutral (citrate). Here, a high-pH mobile phase was opted for, because this enhanced peak shape and efficiency. As an example, the resolution for the iso-α-acids IAA3, IAA4, IAA5, and IAA6, the most critical part of the separation, improves significantly when the pH of the mobile phase is raised from neutral to alkaline. This is caused by the increased efficiency and the enhanced selectivity for these acidic solutes at elevated pH. It was the aim to develop a method compatible with MS detection and a volatile mobile-phase additive was therefore chosen. Ammonium acetate was selected and the appropriate pH was attained using ammonia. The optimum apparent pH (in 20% v/v ethanol) was found to be 9.95. Care should be taken to accurately control the pH, since small variations cause significant changes in chromatographic selectivity. The high pH mandates selection of a stationary phase that is stable in basic media. The columns used (Zorbax Extend) are stable up to pH 11.5. Ethanol was preferred over methanol, because it consistently provided a better separation.

The mass spectra of the co-homologs, obtained by LC–MS in the negative APCI ionization mode, are shown in Figure 99.3. A distinctive fragmentation pattern is observed for each group of hop-derived acids. Iso-α-acids and reduced iso-α-acids fragment similarly via dehydration and loss of a side chain. For iso-α-acids and tetrahydroiso-α-acids, dehydration is followed by loss of a 4-methyl-3-pentenoyl or a 4-methylpentanoyl side chain, respectively. Dihydroiso-α-acids are characterized by cleavage of the 1-hydroxy-4-methyl-2-pentenyl side chain followed by dehydration. Splitting off water from α-acids sets the stage for ring opening and loss of a ring carbon together with a hydroxyl group and a 3-methyl-2-butenyl side chain. Reclosure furnishes a five-membered ring. β-Acids are marked by loss of a 3-methyl-2-butenyl side chain only.

Figure 99.4 shows an LC–DAD–MS analysis of a standard solution containing ca. 10 mg/l (ppm) of each group of hop-derived acids. For UV detection, iso-α-acids and reduced iso-α-acids are monitored at 256 nm and α- and β-acids at 330 nm. In UV detection, co-elution occurs between a

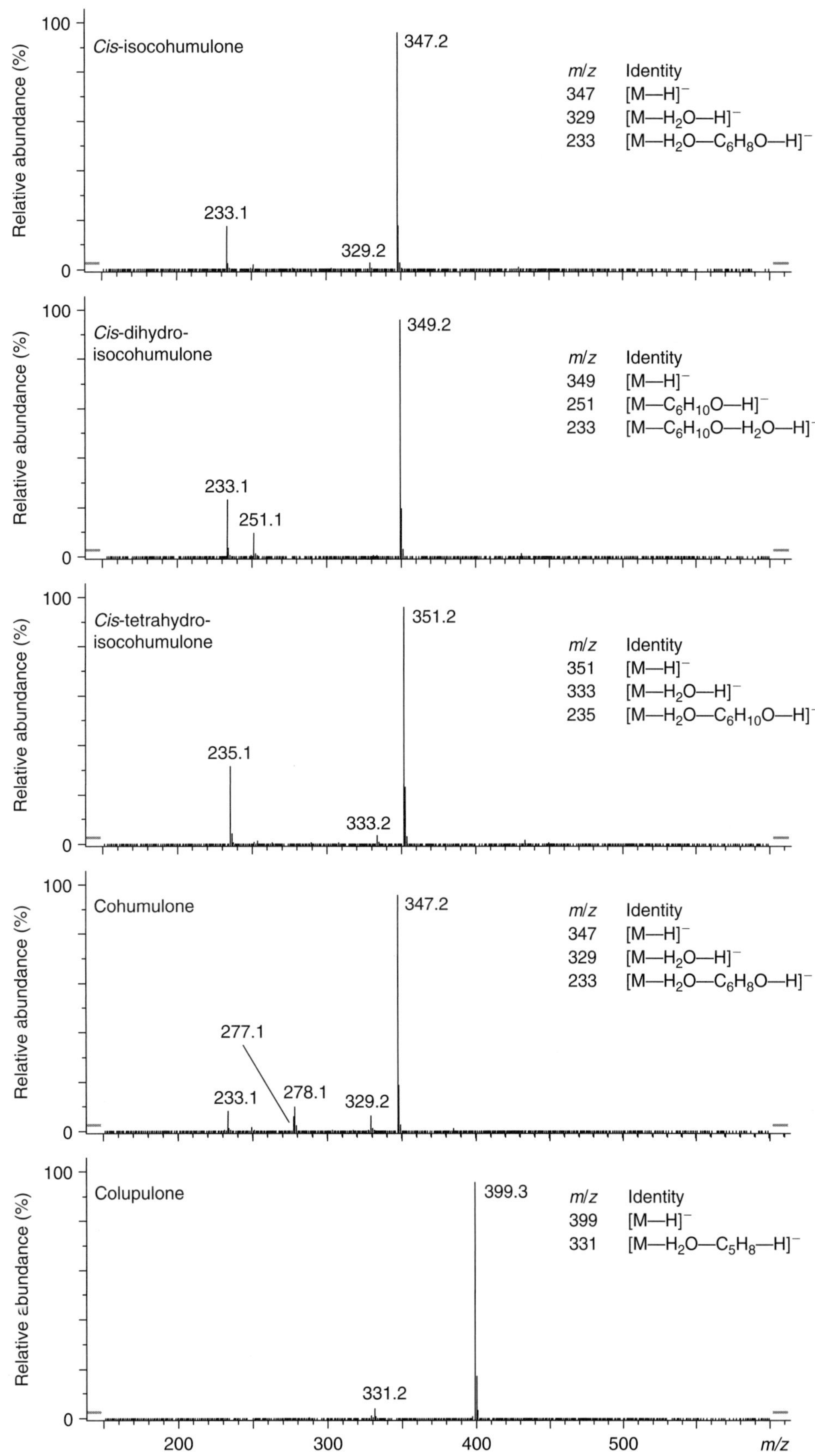

Figure 99.3 Mass spectra of the co-homologs of iso-α-acids, reduced iso-α-acids, and hop α- and β-acids. MS was performed using APCI in the negative mode. Distinctive fragmentation patterns are observed for each group of hop-derived acids. Molecular and fragment ions were selected for each compound to construct the chromatograms in reversed-phase LC–MS.

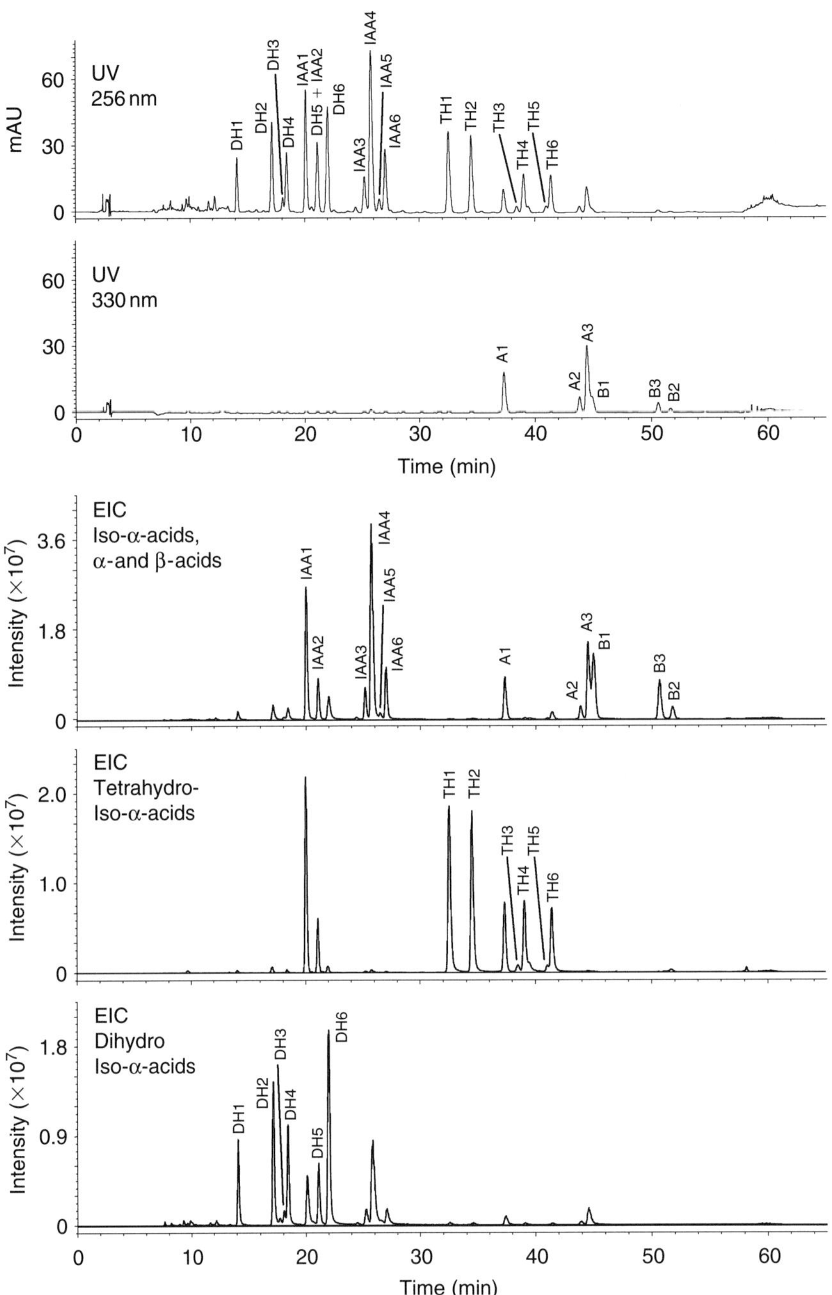

Figure 99.4 LC–UV and LC–MS chromatograms of a standard mixture of hop-derived acids. Chromatograms for the analysis of a standard mixture of hop-derived acids (10 mg/l of each group). EIC (selected ions: see Table 99.1). MS was performed using APCI in the negative mode. IAA, iso-α-acids; TH, tetrahydroiso-α-acids; DH, dihydroiso-α-acids; A, α-acids; B, β-acids. Peak numbers: see Figure 99.2.

cis-dihydroisoadhumulone epimer (DH5) and *trans*-isocohumulone (IAA2). The MS traces are extracted ion chromatograms (EIC) composed of the molecular ions and the most important fragments. The selected ions were also used for quantitative analyses (Table 99.1). Iso-α-acids and dihydroiso-α-acids share an identical fragment ion (*m/z* 233 for co-forms and *m/z* 247 for n- and ad-forms). Also, isocohumulone, tetrahydroisohumulone, and tetrahydroisoadhumulone have a common ion (*m/z* 347). However, these compounds are chromatographically sufficiently separated to avoid interference. Co-elution of DH5 and IAA2 is not problematic for MS detection, as the *m/z* values differ. MS selectivity, thus, enables to resolve both compounds and to quantify them correctly.

Four point calibration graphs in the range of 5–50 mg/l (ppm) were constructed by analyses of standard solutions. Because of co-elution of DH5 and IAA2 in UV detection, two separate calibration series were made, the first

Table 99.1 Molecular ions and fragment ions used for constructing LC–MS EIC for the various groups of compounds

Compound		*MM*	*Selected ions*
IAA	co	348	233, 329, 347
	n/ad	362	247, 343, 361
DH	co	350	233, 251, 349
	n/ad	364	247, 265, 363
TH	co	352	235, 333, 351
	n/ad	366	249, 347, 365
A	co	348	233, 277, 278, 329, 347
	n/ad	362	247, 291, 292, 343, 361
B	co	400	331, 399
	n/ad	414	345, 413

Note: A number of ions were selected for each compound to construct the chromatograms in reversed-phase LC–MS. MS was performed using APCI in the negative mode. IAA, iso-α-acids; TH, tetrahydroiso-α-acids; DH, dihydroiso-α-acids; A, α-acids; B, β-acids; MM, molecular mass.

series containing the reduced iso-α-acids and the second series the iso-α-acids and α- and β-acids. Repeatability of injection was performed by six consecutive injections of the calibration solution of both series at a concentration of ca. 10 mg/l (ppm) for each group of acids. The obtained relative standard deviations (RSDs) for the iso-α-acids and reduced iso-α-acids were all below 0.3% for UV detection, while these values varied between 5% and 9% for MS detection. Since UV and MS are performed on-line, the difference in repeatability is only caused by the detection. It is known that MS performs inferior in this respect compared to UV or DAD (Lazou *et al.*, 2000) and the rather high RSDs for MS detection are not unusual for ion trap MS. Poor results for the α- and β-acids are due to instability of those sensitive solutes in the injection vial. Their impact on the bitterness of beer, however, is not important; hence, they were not determined. Results for calibration and repeatability are summarized in Table 99.2.

A selection of 14 beers was analyzed by LC–UV–MS and the iso-α-acids and reduced iso-α-acids contents were quantified (Table 99.3). For iso-α-acids, the ratio of n-, co-, and ad-isohumulones and the *cis*/*trans* ratios were calculated for each beer. Beers that contain larger amounts of n- and ad-isohumulones are characterized by a more subtle bitterness, while the *cis*/*trans* ratio is relevant with respect to the flavor stability. Representative chromatograms of LC–UV analyses at 256 nm are shown in Figure 99.5.

Lager 1 is a German beer that is devoid of reduced iso-α-acids. The very high *cis*/*trans* ratio (>10) can be attributed to the use of advanced pre-isomerized hop products. In the other beers, this ratio varies between 2 and 5. The profile of Lager 5 is typical for a Western-European pilsner-type beer. In current brewing practice, beers (Lagers 3–6) contain a small portion of tetrahydroiso-α-acids, mainly to improve foam stability. Smaller breweries often still use natural hop cones (Lager 2, non-alcoholic lager, Belgian Trappist). The difference between the two beers contained in clear bottles is striking. Because they are not protected from light, it could be expected that measures were taken to stabilize their flavor and bitterness. In Lager clear bottle 2, dihydro- and tetrahydroiso-α-acids have been applied, resulting in a much lower concentration of iso-α-acids. Conversely, in Lager clear bottle 1, only iso-α-acids are detected, while a high content of isocohumulone is found compared to isoadhumulone and isohumulone. Light stable beers 1 and 2 do not contain iso-α-acids, the bitterness being delivered by dihydro- and tetrahydroiso-α-acids. Wheat beers are much less bitter than lager beers, which are reflected by their low iso-α-acid contents.

The quantitative values obtained with LC–MS are close to those found with LC–UV. The only clear trend in the results is that the recovered amount of dihydroiso-α-acids is consistently higher in LC–MS compared to LC–UV. Other discrepancies in recovered amounts and calculated ratios between LC–MS and LC–UV appear at random. The significant difference between the ratios of co-, n-, and ad-isohumulones in the second lager in a clear bottle is due to co-elution of a *cis*-dihydroisoadhumulone epimer and *trans*-isocohumulone. The LC–MS chromatogram of this beer is shown in Figure 99.6. The peak area for *trans*-isocohumulone was not included in the calculations by LC–UV analysis. The peak was regarded as *cis*-dihydroisoadhumulone leading to inaccurate quantitation. The iso-α-acid content is underestimated and the dihydroiso-α-acids are overestimated. This also explains, for this particular beer, why the isocohumulone content in LC–UV is significantly lower compared to LC–MS and why the difference between the recovered amounts of dihydroiso-α-acids is small. Thus, for this particular case, results for the co-, n-, and ad-isohumulones ratios obtained with LC–MS are more reliable than those obtained with LC–UV.

A similar method can be used for fast LC–UV analysis of isohumulones and tetrahydroisohumulones in beers. Main goals in this analysis are speed and accuracy. A complete separation of all individual acids is no longer essential. Therefore, the pH can be lowered and the mobile-phase composition and gradient can be adapted to meet the specific needs of the brewer. An example of such an analysis is shown in Figure 99.7. Using these conditions, the iso-α-acids are separated from the tetrahydroiso-α-acids and can be quantified separately in ca. 12 min.

CE Analysis

(Partially reprinted from De Villiers et al. (2004), Copyright 2004, with permission from Wiley-VCH Verlag GmbH & Co. KgaA.)

An alternative to the LC separation of the bitter acids is capillary electrophoresis (CE). Electrodriven separation techniques such as micellar electrokinetic chromatography

Table 99.2 Comparison of the calibration data and repeatability of injection for LC–UV and LC–MS

	IAA (5.85, 11.70, 23.40, 58.50 ppm)		*TH (5.28, 10.55, 21.11, 52.76 ppm)*		*DH (5.18, 10.35, 20.70, 51.75 ppm)*		*A/B (4.33, 8.67, 17.34, 43.34 ppm)*	
	UV	*MS*	*UV*	*MS*	*UV*	*MS*	*UV*	*MS*
Calibration (R^2)	1.0000	0.9994	1.0000	0.9987	1.0000	0.9992	0.9994	0.9946
Repeatability (RSD, %)	0.26	8.94	0.19	6.44	0.18	7.08	4.76	22.70

Note: The linearity of the method was evaluated by four consecutive injections of standard mixtures at different concentration levels (ca. 5, 10, 20, and 50 mg/l of each group). Repeatability of injection was performed by six consecutive injections of a standard mixture (10 mg/l of each group). IAA, iso-α-acids; TH, tetrahydroiso-α-acids; DH, dihydroiso-α-acids; A, α-acids; B, β-acids; R^2, correlation coefficient; RSD, relative standard deviation.

Table 99.3 LC–UV and LC–MS quantitative results for various beers

	IAA concentration (ppm)		*IAA % co/ad/n*		*IAA ratio cis/trans*		*TH concentration (ppm)*		*DH concentration (ppm)*	
Beer	*UV*	*MS*	*UV*	*MS*	*UV*	*MS*	*UV*	*MS*	*UV*	*MS*
Lager 1	23.23	22.48	33.3/13.5/53.2	31.8/15.4/52.8	10.2	12.4	–	–	–	–
Lager 2	29.81	27.70	33.3/12.9/53.8	33.4/14.2/52.4	2.9	2.9	–	–	–	–
Lager 3	18.04	19.81	30.9/13.6/55.5	32.2/15.0/52.8	2.3	2.4	4.79	5.31	–	–
Lager 4	20.98	22.18	37.4/11.7/50.9	36.4/14.0/49.5	3.1	3.0	3.71	3.91	–	–
Lager 5	24.57	23.56	32.1/12.2/55.7	32.1/12.9/55.0	3.1	3.2	4.98	4.98	–	–
Lager 6	23.91	21.60	40.1/10.8/49.1	39.4/12.3/48.3	2.9	2.8	3.16	3.06	–	–
Non-alcoholic lager	33.65	27.14	30.6/12.5/56.9	31.0/13.6/55.4	3.4	3.2	–	–	–	–
Lager clear bottle 1	20.47	20.96	45.3/10.5/44.2	43.2/10.7/46.1	3.7	4.4	–	–	–	–
Lager clear bottle 2	6.25	6.25	21.7/15.0/63.3	38.3/12.5/49.2	2.2	1.5	5.42	4.83	5.42	5.47
Light stable beer 1	–	–	–	–	–	–	4.29	4.47	11.68	14.30
Light stable beer 2	–	–	–	–	–	–	0.81	0.70	23.43	27.94
Belgian Trappist	24.10	23.30	40.9/12.5/46.6	39.6/14.6/45.8	5.0	5.0	–	–	–	–
Wheat beer 1	8.55	8.76	43.5/15.9/40.6	42.8/13.2/44.0	3.9	4.8	–	–	–	–
Wheat beer 2	11.89	12.34	37.7/12.5/49.8	35.3/14.2/50.5	3.1	3.1	–	–	–	–

Note: LC–UV and LC–MS data for the analysis of iso-α-acids and reduced iso-α-acids in beers after direct injection. The concentration of each group of compounds is measured. For the iso-α-acids the *cis/trans* ratio and the ratio of co-, ad-, and n-iso-α-acids are also calculated. IAA, iso-α-acids; TH, tetrahydroiso-α-acids; DH, dihydroiso-α-acids.

(MEKC) (Vindevogel *et al.*, 1990; Vindevogel and Sandra, 1991), microemulsion electrokinetic chromatography (MEEKC) (Szücs *et al.*, 1996), and capillary electrochromatography (CEC) (Vanhoenacker *et al.*, 2001) have been evaluated for the analysis of hop acids while iso-α-acids were successfully separated by MEKC (Vindevogel *et al.*, 1991; Royle *et al.*, 2001). Contrary to LC, a pre-concentration step (solid-phase extraction, liquid–liquid extraction) prior to the CE analysis of iso-α-acids and reduced iso-α-acids in beer is favorable, although direct injection of beers with stacking has been described (Szücs *et al.*, 1993).

SBSE–LD is applied here for quantitative analysis of iso-α-acids and for detection of reduced iso-α-acids in various beers by MEKC (De Villiers *et al.*, 2004). The iso-α-acid content of several beers was determined and compared with results obtained with the LC method using direct beer injection.

Experimental

The buffer for MEKC analyses was filtered through a disposable syringe filter (0.45 μm, Nylon). Polydimethylsiloxane(PDMS)-coated stir bars (Twister™) were supplied by Gerstel (Mülheim a/d Ruhr, Germany). Beers were bought at local stores, kept at room temperature, and freshly opened prior to analysis. Pre-isomerized hop extract containing iso-α-acids was obtained from Hopstabil GmbH (Wolnzach, Germany). Dihydroiso-α-acids (DCHA-Rho, ICS-R1) were from Labor Veritas (Zürich, Switzerland) and tetrahydroiso-α-acids from Kalsec (Kalamazoo, MI, USA).

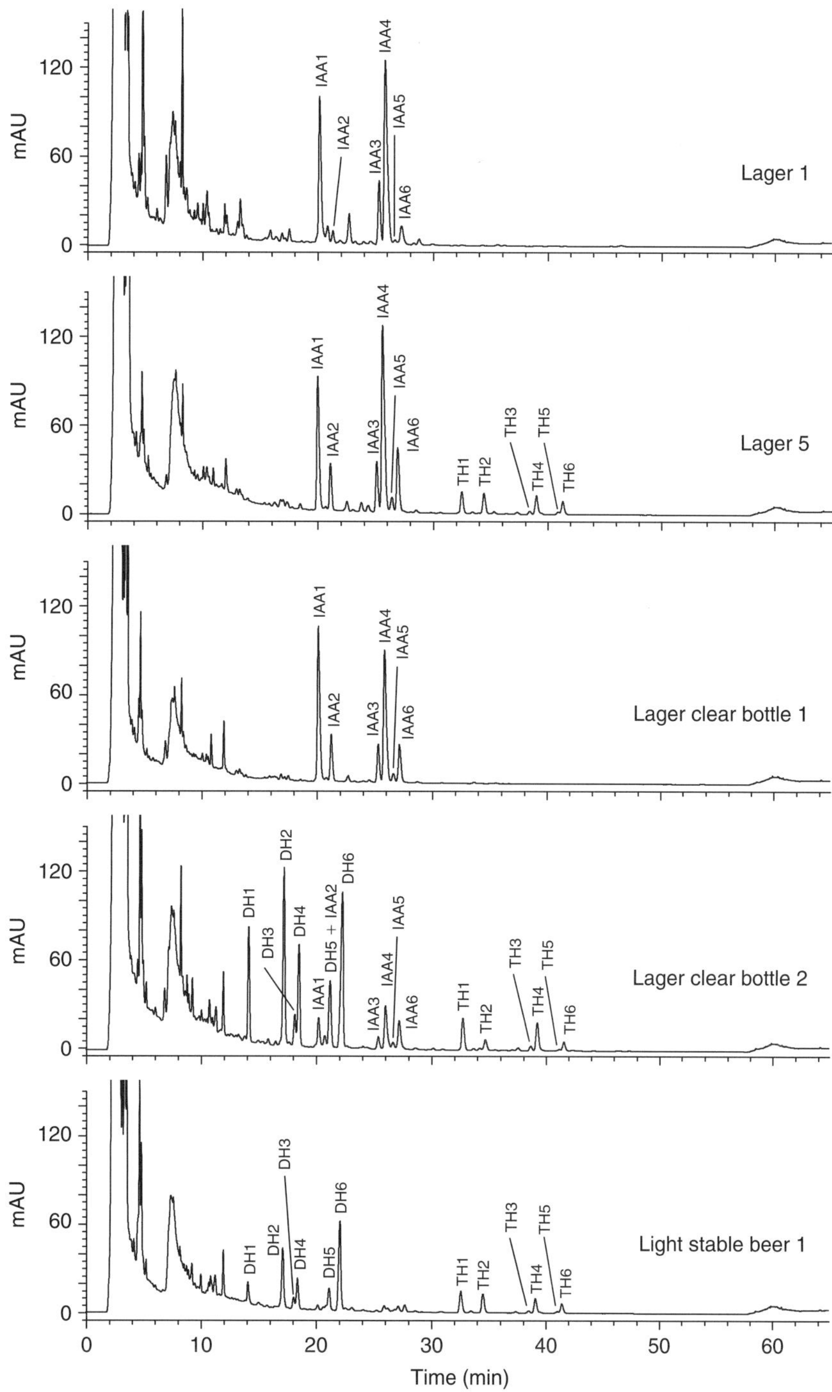

Figure 99.5 LC–UV analyses of various beers. Chromatograms for the analysis of a selection of beers after direct injection with detection at 256 nm. Significant differences can be observed between the various beers. IAA, iso-α-acids; TH, tetrahydroiso-α-acids; DH, dihydroiso-α-acids. Peak numbers: see Figure 99.2.

LC analyses for the investigation of the sorption and desorption process were performed in collaboration with A. De Villiers at the University of Stellenbosch (South Africa). For analytical conditions we refer to De Villiers *et al.* (2004). The beer samples were also analyzed by LC after direct injection. Full details of the method are described above.

MEKC analyses were performed on an HP^{3D}CE Capillary Electrophoresis System equipped with a DAD (Agilent Technologies, Waldbronn, Germany). An extended lightpath bare fused-silica capillary (Agilent Technologies, Waldbronn, Germany) with an ID of 50 μm and a total length of 64.5 cm (effective length is 56 cm) was used.

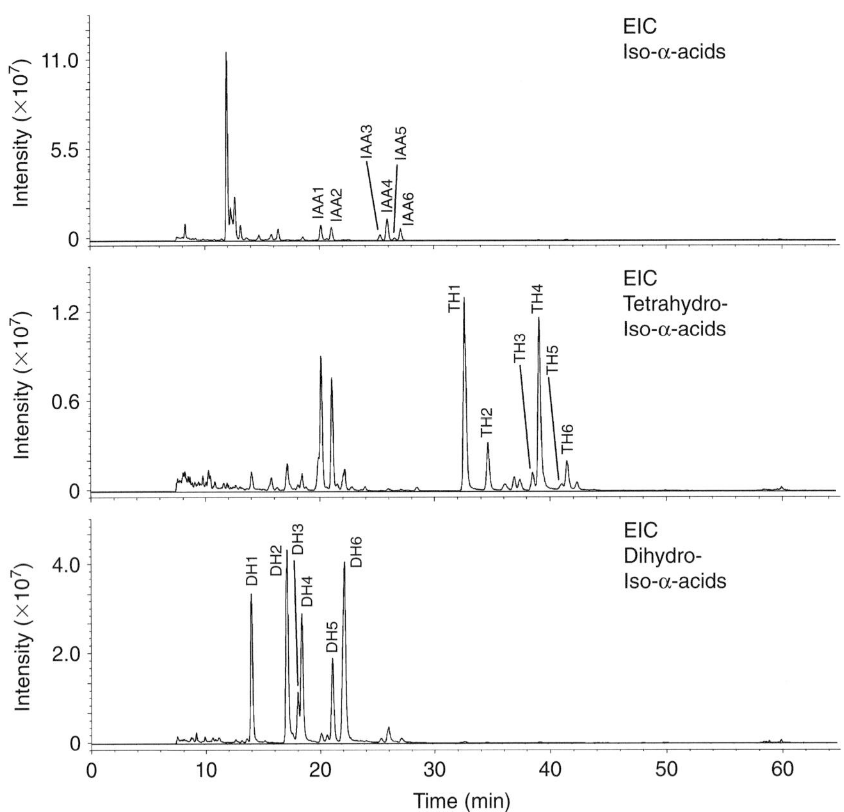

Figure 99.6 LC–MS analysis of "Lager clear bottle 2." Chromatograms for the LC–MS analysis after direct injection of "Lager clear bottle 2." The beer flavor and bitterness are stabilized with dihydro- and tetrahydroiso-α-acids. EIC (selected ions: see Table 99.1). MS was performed using APCI in the negative mode. IAA, iso-α-acids; TH, tetrahydroiso-α-acids; DH, dihydroiso-α-acids. Peak numbers: see Figure 99.2.

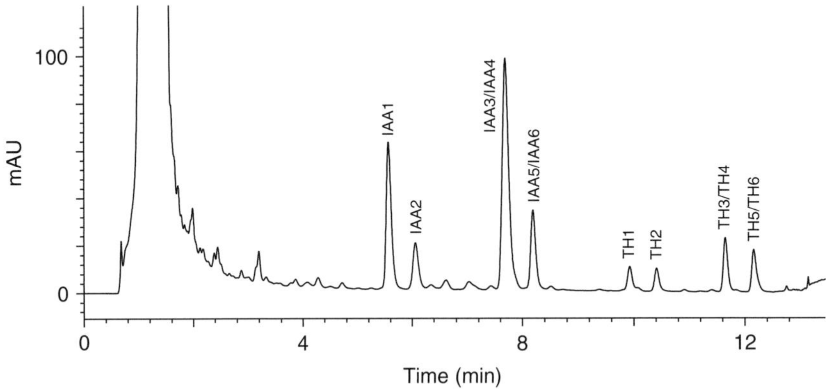

Figure 99.7 Fast LC–UV analysis of a typical Western-European pilsner-type beer. Chromatogram for the fast LC–UV analysis of a typical Western-European pilsner-type beer after direct injection with detection at 256 nm. IAA, iso-α-acids; TH, tetrahydroiso-α-acids. Peak numbers: see Figure 99.2.

The buffer consisted of 40 mM phosphate (pH 10.2 with NaOH) containing 80 mM sodium dodecyl sulfate. Injection was performed hydrodynamically at 50 mbar for 10 s for the SBSE-enriched samples and for 15 s for direct injection of beer. The separation voltage was 25 kV and detection was performed at 255 nm. The capillary temperature was set at 25°C. Between runs, the capillaries were conditioned by flushing with NaOH (0.1 M) for 2 min, water for 1 min, and buffer for 3 min, consecutively.

Different sample preparation parameters, that is for sorption and desorption, were studied. The final SBSE–LD–MEKC procedure is as follows; 20 ml beer is poured in a headspace vial of 40 and 1 ml HCl (1 M) is added. A stir bar containing 24 μl PDMS is introduced and the sample is stirred at 1,500 rpm and 25°C for 60 min. The stir bar is dipped in bidistilled water and dried on a tissue paper. The stir bar is then placed in 2 ml acetonitrile and stirred at 1,500 rpm and 25°C for 60 min. A 1 ml portion is withdrawn and evaporated to dryness under a nitrogen stream. The residue is dissolved in 0.5 ml bidistilled water and the sample is injected.

Results and discussion

Sorption and desorption kinetics were studied using LC because of its greater sensitivity compared to MEKC. The sorption step was investigated using only one stir bar. The stir bar was added to 20 ml beer acidified with 1 ml HCl (1 M). Magnetic stirring at different time intervals took place in a closed vial covered with aluminum foil. After each sorption step, the stir bar was removed and rinsed with water before being placed in 2 ml acetonitrile for 60 min (stirred as for sorption); 30 μl of the desorption liquid was then directly analyzed by LC. The stir bar was cleaned between samplings by thermal desorption for 60 min at 300°C. The results are summarized in Figure 99.8. Equilibrium between the PDMS coating and the aqueous phase was not reached after 120 min. The long equilibration time can be accounted for by slow diffusion rates of the molecules into PDMS. Since the diffusion time is proportional to the square of the film thickness of the coating, the equilibration time can be greatly reduced by decreasing the thickness of the coating. The short equilibration times found when using solid-phase microextraction demonstrates this statement (Pawliszyn, 1997). However, loss of sensitivity resulting from a thinner coating would make the analysis of the iso-α-acids impossible. For reasons of convenience, 60 min was chosen as the practical sorption time.

To study desorption, the sorption time was kept constant at 60 min. Acetonitrile was chosen as desorption solvent, because of its efficiency in desorbing relatively polar compounds from the stir bar without causing excessive swelling of the PDMS coating. Sorption took place in acidified beer. After removal and rinsing, the stir bar was placed in 2 ml acetonitrile; 10 μl of the desorption liquid was analyzed directly by LC in function of time. From the desorption graph in Figure 99.8, it can be observed that equilibrium between the two phases was reached after 60 min, and this time frame was chosen as optimum desorption time in subsequent analyses.

Next, a comparison was made between a "dry" stir bar and a stir bar saturated with a specific solvent. One stir bar was used and it was regenerated between experiments by thermal desorption (60 min at 300°C). The same beer was analyzed consecutively with a dry (thermally desorbed), acetonitrile-, and isooctane-saturated stir bar. Stirring in solvent for 20 min was applied to saturate the stir bar. Using sorption and desorption times of 60 min, the same beer was extracted as above and analyzed using MEKC. It

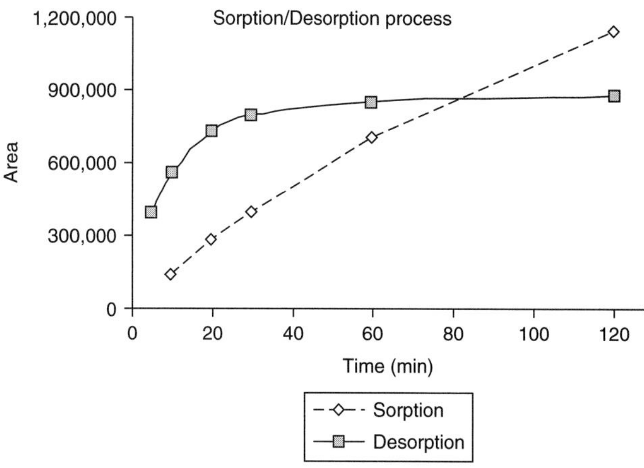

Figure 99.8 SBSE–LD sorption and desorption graphs for iso-α-acids. Investigation of sorption and desorption step for the iso-α-acids in the SBSE–LD sample preparation. For desorption, the equilibrium between the beer and the stir bar is reached at ca. 60 min. The equilibrium of the sorption process has not been reached after 120 min. A 60 min sorption time was chosen as a compromise.

was found that the amount of iso-α-acids absorbed into the stir bar increased in the order: dry stir bar < acetonitrile-saturated stir bar < isooctane-saturated stir bar. The effect of isooctane saturation can be explained by a swelling effect of the solvent on PDMS, which should facilitate diffusion into the phase. Further, the desorption equilibrium conditions also differ significantly, as the PDMS phase should be more hydrophobic, hence the equilibrium concentration of the acids in the desorbing acetonitrile is expected to increase. For an acetonitrile-saturated stir bar (almost no swelling), an increase in polarity of the coating caused by saturation with acetonitrile translates into improved sorption efficiency. The desorption efficiency might decrease in this case. The net effect is, however, an increase in overall extraction efficiency. Although higher recoveries were obtained compared to dry sampling for the same period of time (ca. 1.1 for acetonitrile and 1.8 for isooctane), the reproducibility was lower.

In further experiments, it was demonstrated that the desorption equilibration process could be accelerated, by either heating or sonication of the desorption liquid. This results from increased diffusion rates at elevated temperatures, as well as from possible temperature dependence of the relevant distribution coefficients. For the SBSE–LD–MEKC analysis of beer, sensitivity and reproducibility were found to be adequate and sorption and desorption were subsequently performed at 25°C without sonication.

Although iso-α-acids are generally present in sufficiently large concentrations (typically 20–50 mg/l) in beers, direct injections of beer followed by MEKC analysis is not feasible for the analysis of these compounds due to interference of matrix components. Application of SBSE–LD prior to

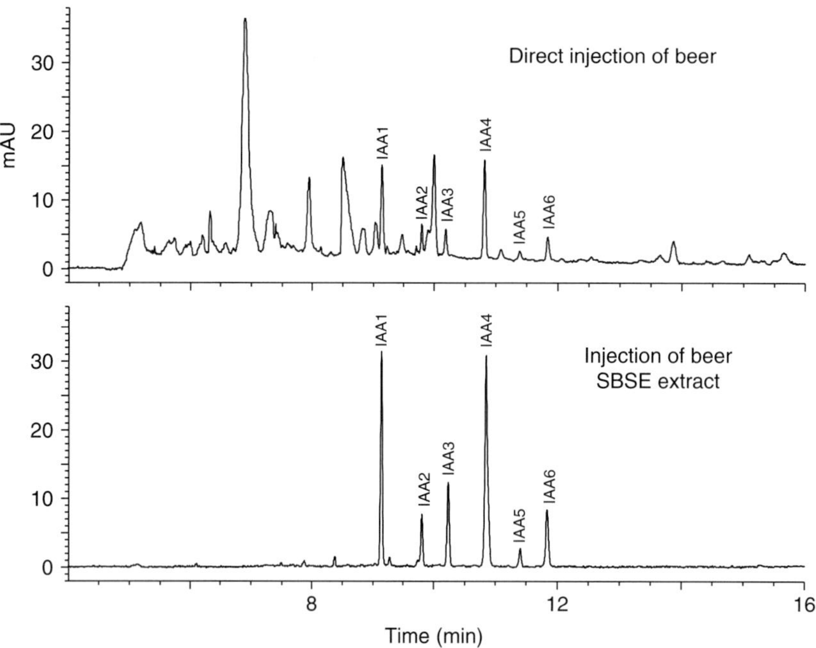

Figure 99.9 Comparison of MEKC analysis of direct injection of beer and injection after SBSE–LD. Result of MEKC analysis of direct injection of beer and injection after SBSE–LD. The sample preparation yields clean extracts free of most interfering compounds. IAA, iso-α-acids. Peak numbers: see Figure 99.2.

injection leads to isolation of iso-α-acids and reduced iso-α-acids from the matrix, hence, clean extracts are obtained. The comparison between direct injection and injection after SBSE–LD is shown in Figure 99.9. The more polar beer constituents (eluting before the iso-α-acids in the electropherogram) are not extracted by SBSE.

The MEKC method allows simultaneous determination of iso-α-acids and reduced iso-α-acids. A calibration graph was constructed by SBSE analysis of four simulated beer samples (5% ethanol) containing a standard solution of iso-α-acids (5.85, 14.62, 29.25, and 58.50 mg/l, respectively). Each level was analyzed in triplicate. Good linearity (correlation coefficient of 0.9985) was obtained in this concentration range. The reproducibility of the method was evaluated by six analyses of the same beer using six fresh stir bars. Each sample was injected in duplicate. RSDs on migration time and time-corrected area (area/migration time) ranged from 0.14% to 0.26% and from 2.33% to 5.76%, respectively.

A selection of local and foreign beers was analyzed using the methodology described above. Results were compared for the total iso-α-acid content and for the presence or absence of reduced iso-α-acids. Some representative electropherograms of extracts of beers are shown in Figure 99.10. As expected the German beer (Lager 1 in Figure 99.10) does not contain reduced isohumulones. The profile of the non-German lager (Lager 6 in Figure 99.10) is typical for a Western-European lager beer that usually contains iso-α-acids to which a portion of tetrahydroiso-α-acids is added to improve foam stability. The procedure is more common in large breweries when compared to smaller ones. As already seen in the LC analyses, the difference between the two beers that are contained in clear bottles is striking. Because they are not protected from light, the taste-active compounds should be stabilized in some way. One beer is composed mainly of dihydro- and tetrahydroiso-α-acids (Lager clear bottle 2 in Figure 99.10). The concentration of iso-α-acids is significantly lower in comparison to the other beers. In the second beer presented in a clear bottle, only iso-α-acids are detected (Lager clear bottle 1 in Figure 99.10). This beer is also characterized by a relatively high content of isocohumulone.

Whereas reduced iso-α-acids were only qualitatively investigated, iso-α-acids were quantified in various beers using the constructed calibration graph. Results were compared with the results obtained by the described LC method after direct injection of the beers. The recovered amounts in MEKC are in good agreement with the amounts found by direct injection of beers by LC (Table 99.4).

SBSE–LD LC Analysis

The SBSE–LD extracts analyzed by MEKC were also applied to the LC–UV method. For this comparison, the desorption liquid (acetonitrile) was diluted 10-fold with water prior to injection to reconstitute the sample to its original concentration (for a recovery of 100%). A comparison of LC–UV analyses by direct injection and by injection

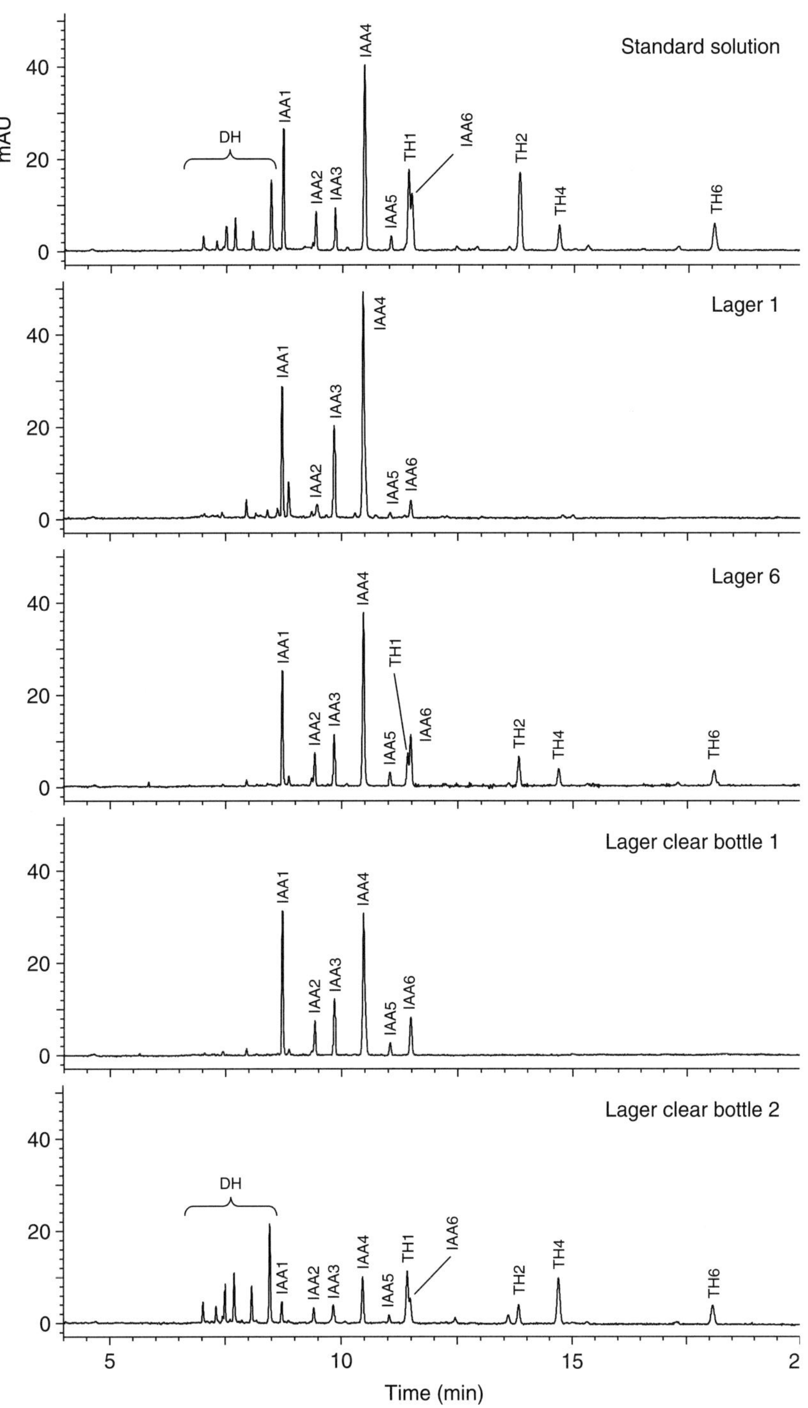

Figure 99.10 MEKC analyses of a standard solution and various beers. Results for MEKC analyses of a standard mixture of hop-derived acids (20 mg/l of each group) and various beers after SBSE–LD. Significant differences can be observed between the various beers. IAA, iso-α-acids; TH, tetrahydroiso-α-acids; DH, dihydroiso-α-acids. Peak numbers: see Figure 99.2.

after SBSE–LD is shown in Figure 99.11. The peak areas obtained for the injections of the diluted extracts were compared with the peak areas obtained after direct injection of the same beer. The averaged recoveries were ca. 19.4% for iso-α-acids, ca. 43.1% for tetrahydroiso-α-acids, and ca. 8.5% for dihydro-α-acids. Using log p values calculated with the software program KowWIN (Meylan, 2000) and the known phase ratio β, the theoretical recovery of iso-α-acids from beer (with the assumption that $K_{PDMS/beer} >> K_{o/w}$) was determined to be 45% (for log p = 2.9). It should be noted that these recoveries are not obtained under the conditions employed in this study for the beer analyses

Table 99.4 MEKC results for various beers

	IAA concentration (ppm)			
Beer	*MEKC* (after SBSE–LD)	*LC–UV* (direct injection)	*TH*	*DH*
Lager 1	25.50	23.23	–	–
Lager 3	19.98	18.04	+	–
Lager 4	17.52	20.98	+	–
Lager 6	23.74	23.91	+	–
Lager clear bottle 1	22.63	20.47	–	–
Lager clear bottle 2	6.39	6.25	+	+
Light stable beer 1	0.00	0.00	+	+
Belgian Trappist	25.61	24.10	–	–

Note: MEKC data for analysis of iso-α-acids (quantitative) and reduced iso-α-acids (qualitative) in various beers after SBSE–LD sample preparation. For the iso-α-acids, the concentration is compared with the result obtained with LC–UV after direct injection of the beers. IAA, iso-α-acids; TH, tetrahydroiso-α-acids; DH, dihydroiso-α-acids; +/−, detected/not detected.

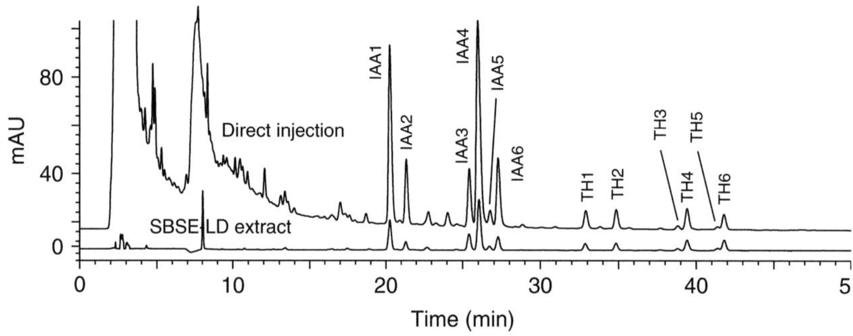

Figure 99.11 Comparison of LC–UV analysis of direct injection of beer and injection after SBSE–LD. Overlay of chromatograms for LC–UV of beer after direct injection and injection after SBSE–LD sample preparation. The SBSE–LD extract was diluted 10 times prior to analysis. The sample preparation yields clean extracts free of most interfering compounds. IAA, iso-α-acids; TH, tetrahydroiso-α-acids. Peak numbers: see Figure 99.2.

(i.e. 60 min sorption time), since equilibrium was not established. The significant difference in recovery between the different groups of hop-derived acids can be explained by the considerable variations in polarity of these compounds, as can be deduced from the chromatograms.

Summary Points

LC–UV and LC–MS were successfully applied for the simultaneous analysis of iso-α-acids and reduced iso-α-acids in beers by direct injection. Volatile mobile-phase additives enable hyphenation to MS operated in the APCI mode.

- An alkaline mobile-phase pH improves peak shape and selectivity.
- All major bitter acids are separated within 65 min, with the exception of the pair *cis*-dihydroisoadhumulone/*trans*-isocohumulone. Thus, quantitation of iso-α-acids in the presence of dihydroiso-α-acids using UV detection is questionable. With MS detection these compounds could be differentiated according to their *m*/*z* value.

Both UV and MS detection are sufficiently sensitive to analyze beers without sample pre-concentration. The performance in terms of quantification of bitter acids by LC–UV and LC–MS is compared for standard solutions and a selection of 14 beers.

- The values obtained with LC–MS are similar to those obtained with LC–UV, except for the dihydroiso-α-acids. The recovered amounts of dihydroiso-α-acids were consistently higher in LC–MS compared to LC–UV.
- MS detection proved superior to UV detection in view of enhanced sensitivity and selectivity, notwithstanding higher RSDs.
- The method can easily be adapted for fast routine LC–UV analysis of iso-α-acids and tetrahydroiso-α-acids in beer without sample pre-concentration.

SBSE–LD followed by MEKC separation represents a simple, efficient, and reproducible new method for the analysis of beer iso-α-acids. Parameters affecting both sorption and desorption were studied.

- Very clean extracts free of most interfering compounds were obtained.
- The developed MEKC method is fast and enables analysis of both iso-α-acids and reduced iso-α-acids.
- Quantitative results are in good agreement with results obtained by LC using direct beer injection.

References

Baltussen, E., Sandra, P., David, F. and Cramers, C. (1999). *J. Microcol. Sep.* 11, 737–747.

Burroughs, L.J. and Williams, P.D. (1999). *Proceedings of the 27th European Brewery Convention*, Cannes, May 25–28, pp. 283–290.

Clark, J., Burroughs, L. and Guzinski, J. (1998). *J. Am. Soc. Brew. Chem.* 56, 76–79.

De Keukeleire, D., Vindevogel, J., Szücs, R. and Sandra, P. (1992). *Trends Anal. Chem.* 11, 275–280.

De Villiers, A., Vanhoenacker, G., Lynen, F. and Sandra, P. (2004). *Electrophoresis* 25, 664–669.

Harms, D. and Nitzsche, F. (2001). *J. Am. Soc. Brew. Chem.* 59, 28–31.

Harms, D., Nietzsche, F., Hoffmann, A., David, F. and Sandra, P. (2001). http://www.gerstel.comwww.gerstel.com, Gerstel Application Note 5.

Hermans-Lokkerbol, A.C.J. and Verpoorte, R. (1994). *J. Chromatogr. A* 669, 65–73.

Hofte, A.J.P., van der Hoeven, R.A.M., Fung, S.Y., Verpoorte, R., Tjaden, U.R. and van der Greef, J. (1998). *J. Am. Soc. Brew. Chem.* 56, 118–122.

Kuroiwa, Y., Hashimoto, N., Hashimoto, H., Kokubo, E. and Nakgawa, K. (1963). *Proc. Am. Soc. Brew. Chem.* 28, 181–193.

Lazou, K., De Geyter, T., De Reu, L., Zhao, Y. and Sandra, P. (2000). *LC-GC Europe* 13, 340–356.

Meylan, W. (2000). Software KowWIN Version 1.66, SRC-LOGKOW, SRC-ESC, Syracuse, USA.

Pawliszyn, J. (1997). *Solid Phase Microextraction: Theory and Practice*. Wiley-VCH, Weinheim, Germany.

Peñalver, A., García, V., Pocurull, E., Borrull, F. and Marcé, R. (2003). *J. Chromatogr. A* 1007, 1–9.

Rong, H., Zhao, Y., Lazou, K., De Keukeleire, D., Milligan, S.R. and Sandra, P. (2000). *Chromatographia* 51, 545–552.

Royle, L., Ames, J., Hill, C. and Gardner, D. (2001). *Food Chem.* 74, 225–231.

Sandra, P., Tienpont, B. and David, F. (2003). *J. Chromatogr. A* 1000, 299–310.

Smith, R., Davidson, D. and Wilson, R. (1998). *J. Am. Soc. Brew. Chem.* 56, 52–57.

Szücs, R., Vindevogel, J., Sandra, P. and Verhagen, L. (1993). *Chromatographia* 36, 323–329.

Szücs, R., Van Hove, E. and Sandra, P. (1996). *J. High Resolut. Chromatogr.* 19, 189–192.

Tienpont, B., David, F., Benijts, T. and Sandra, P. (2003). *J. Pharm. Biomed. Anal.* 32, 569–579.

Tredoux, A., Lauer, H., Heideman, T. and Sandra, P. (2000). *J. High Resolut. Chromatogr.* 23, 644–646.

Vanhoenacker, G., Dermaux, A., De Keukeleire, D. and Sandra, P. (2001). *J. Sep. Sci.* 24, 55–58.

Vanhoenacker, G., De Keukeleire, D. and Sandra, P. (2004). *J. Chromatogr. A* 1035, 53–61.

Verzele, M. (1986). *J. Inst. Brew.* 92, 32–48.

Verzele, M. and van de Velde, N. (1987). *J. Chromatogr. A* 387, 473–480.

Verzele, M., Steenbeke, G., Verhagen, L.C. and Strating, J. (1990). *J. High Resolut. Chromatogr.* 13, 826–831.

Vindevogel, J. and Sandra, P. (1991). *J. High Resolut. Chromatogr.* 14, 795–801.

Vindevogel, J., Sandra, P. and Verhagen, L. (1990). *J. High Resolut. Chromatogr.* 13, 295–298.

Vindevogel, J., Szücs, R., Sandra, P. and Verhagen, L. (1991). *J. High Resolut. Chromatogr.* 14, 584–586.

100

Methods for Determining Biogenic Amines in Beer

Anastasia Zotou Department of Chemistry, Laboratory of Analytical Chemistry, Aristotle University of Thessaloniki, Thessaloniki, Greece
Zacharenia Loukou General Chemical States Laboratory, Kavala Division, Karaoli Square, Kavala, Greece

Abstract

The objective of this chapter is to provide information about the analytical methods used so far for the determination of biogenic amines in beer. Only a limited number of publications describing such methods appear in the literature and most of them include the use of high-performance liquid chromatography, with either pre- or post-column derivatization, or recently the use of capillary electrophoresis. Depending on the applied method, sample pretreatment ranges from simple degassing and dilution of the samples to tedious extraction procedures. The biogenic amines commonly found in beers are: histamine, tyramine, tryptamine, 2-phenylethylamine, putrescine, cadaverine, spermine, spermidine and agmatine at varying levels, which are affected mainly by raw materials, brewing techniques and hygiene conditions during brewing and storage.

List of Abbreviations

BNZ-Cl	Benzoyl chloride
CE	Capillary electrophoresis
DBS-Cl	Dabsyl chloride
DNS-Cl	Dansyl chloride
FITC	Fluorescein isothiocyanate
GC	Gas chromatography
GC–MS	Gas chromatography–mass spectrometry
HPLC	High-performance liquid chromatography
HPTLC	High-performance thin-layer chromatography
IEC	Ion-exchange chromatography
LLE	Liquid–liquid extraction
NBD-Cl	7-Chloro-4-nitro-benzo-2-oxa-1,3-diazole
NDA	Naphthalene-2,3-dicarboxaldehyde
ODS	Octadecyl silica
OPA	*o*-Phthalaldehyde
PNZ-Cl	*p*-Nitrobenzyloxycarbonyl-chloride
POLE	Polyoxyethylene-10-lauryl ether
RSD	Relative standard deviation
SAMF	6-Oxy-(*N*-succinimidyl acetate)-9-(2′-Methoxycarbonyl) fluorescein
SIM	Single-ion monitoring
SPE	Solid-phase extraction
TLC	Thin-layer chromatography
UV	Ultraviolet
UV–VIS	Ultraviolet–visible

Introduction

Biogenic amines are low relative molecular mass organic bases that possess biological activity and can occur in animals, plants and fermented or non-fermented food as a result of normal metabolic activity. They are usually derived from microbial decarboxylation of the corresponding amino acids or by transamination of aldehydes by amino acid transaminases (Kalač *et al.*, 1997).

Taking into account their structure and possible consequences to the human physiology, biogenic amines, mostly abundant in beers, can be divided into three groups (see also Table 100.1):

1. Aromatic, heterocyclic amines – such as histamine, tyramine, 2-phenylethylamine and tryptamine – to which some toxicity is attributed, with symptoms such as nausea, headaches, etc.
2. Aliphatic, di-, tri- and polyamines – such as putrescine, cadaverine, spermine, spermidine and agmatine – which belong to the same metabolic cycle and they increase the toxicity of the aromatic and heterocyclic amines.
3. Aliphatic volatile amines – such as methylamine, ethylamine and isoamylamine – for which no toxic effects have been reported, but whose determination is important because they can alter the organoleptic characteristics of food (Moret and Conte, 1996).

The metabolic routes of biogenic amines and ingested alcohol proceed by the same enzyme system, so it is necessary

Beer in Health and Disease Prevention
ISBN: 978-0-12-373891-2

Table 100.1 Classification of biogenic amines found in beer

Classes of biogenic amines	*Biogenic amines found in beer*	
	Trivial name	*Systematic name*
Aromatic heterocyclic amines	Histamine	4-(2-Aminoethyl)-1,3-diazole
	Tyramine	4-Hydroxy-phenethylamine
	Tryptamine	3-(2-Aminoethyl)indole
	2-Phenylethylamine	–
Aliphatic polyamines*	Putrescine	Butane-1,4-diamine
	Cadaverine	Pentane-1,5-diamine
	Spermine	*N,N′*-bis (3-aminopropyl)butane-1,4-diamine
	Spermidine	*N*-(3-aminopropyl)butane-1,4-diamine
	Agmatine	(4-Aminobutyl) guanidine
Aliphatic volatile amines	Methylamine	–
	Dimethylamine	–
	Ethylamine	–
	Butylamine	–
	Dibutylamine	–

*Polyamine = any of a group of organic compounds, composed of only carbon, nitrogen and hydrogen and containing two or more amino groups.

to pay special attention to fermented alcoholic beverages such as beer, where the presence of ethanol has a synergistic interaction that can increase the toxic effect of some biogenic amines (Peatfield, 1995).

The types and levels of biogenic amines in beers are affected mainly by raw materials, brewing techniques and hygiene conditions during brewing and storage (Halász *et al.*, 1994). Biogenic amines present in beers can be divided into three groups according to their source of origin. High levels of putrescine, agmatine, spermine and spermidine are usually found in malt. Tyramine, 2-phenylethylamine and other polyamines have been determined in hop, but it has little influence on the total content of biogenic amines in beer, since the amount used in brewing is small. The second group is related to amines that are generated during mashing and wort boiling, for example tyramine, agmatine and cadaverine. The last group consists of tyramine and tryptamine that can be synthesized during mashing and fermentation (Izquierdo-Pulido *et al.*, 1994; Hannah *et al.*, 1988; Beatriz *et al.*, 1999). The entire amount and the spectrum of biogenic amines arising in beers could be associated mainly with the hygiene conditions during brewing and to a lesser extent during further processing and storage. Wort contamination by microorganisms possessing specific amino acid decarboxylases, such as lactic acid bacteria or wild yeast, lead to the formation of characteristic amines like tyramine and histamine (Izquierdo-Pulido *et al.*, 1995). Due to high consumption of beer and the possible harmful effects of biogenic amines, it is important to determine their levels. Moreover, biogenic amine levels could be used as an indicator of raw material quality, correct conditions of brewing and final product freshness. The levels of amines in North and South American, and European beers have been investigated. The various structures of amines commonly found in beers of different type and origin are given in Figure 100.1. Data on the levels of the commonly found biogenic amines in beers, analyzed over the past few years, are presented in Tables 100.2 and 100.3.

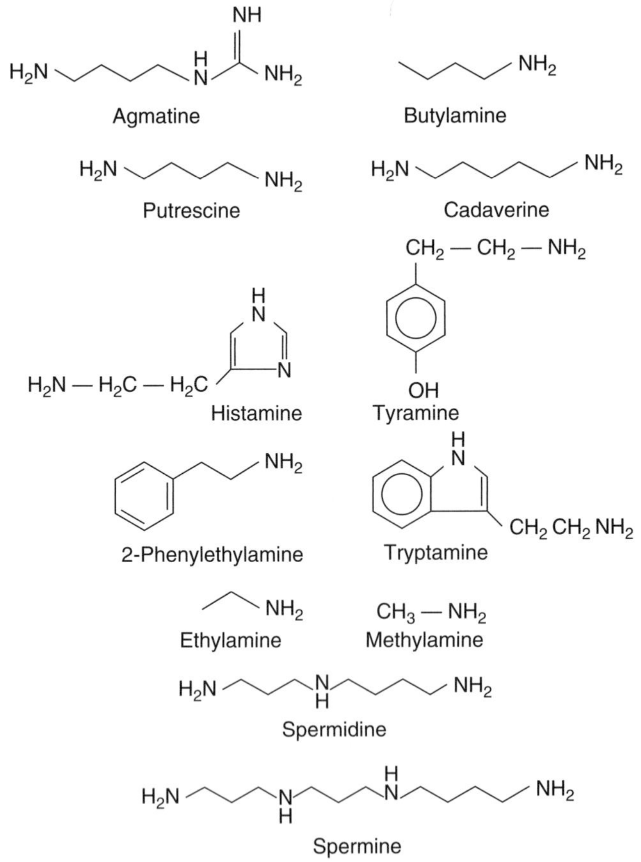

Figure 100.1 Structure of biogenic amines commonly found in beer.

Table 100.2 Aromatic biogenic amines commonly found in beer

Country/continent of beer origin	Concentration range* (mg/l)				Reference
	Histamine	Tyramine	Tryptamine	2-Phenylethylamine	
Brazil	<0.2–1.5	0.3–36.8	<0.4–10.1	< 0.2–1.7	Beatriz *et al.* (1999)
Czech Republic	0.30–1.19	4.68–12.70	–	–	Kalač*et al.* (1997)
Europe	<0.3–21.6	0.5–67.5	< 0.3–5.4	< 0.3–8.3	Izquierdo-Pulido *et al.* (1996a)
Greece	0.47–2.14	1.41–7.09	–	ND	Zotou *et al.* (2003)
	0.57–2.30	1.51–6.06	–	–	Loukou and Zotou (2003)
Italy	ND	0.6–17.2	ND–2.6	ND–1.6	Buiatti *et al.* (1995)
Spain	0.38–1.49	3.48–7.68	–	–	Izquierdo-Pulido *et al.* (1991)
	0.4–0.9	3.2–8.6	0.1–2.7	0.3–0.4	Izquierdo-Pulido *et al.* (1996b)
	ND–4.82	0.26–20.47	ND–5.03	–	Romero *et al.* (2003)
	<0.2–0.6	<0.2–0.6	–	–	Cortacero-Ramirez *et al.* (2005)
Poland	0.44–0.72	0.86–1.19	0.93–2.09	ND–0.67	Slomkowska and Ambroziak (2002)
Portugal	0.03–0.14	0.47–1.65	–	0.01–0.06	Fernandes *et al.* (2001)

*Ranges of mean values of biogenic amine concentrations (in mg/l) found in beers of different types and origin, based on varying numbers of observations; ND, not detected.

Table 100.3 Polyamines commonly found in beer

Country/continent of beer origin	Concentration range* (mg/l)					Reference
	Putrescine	Cadaverine	Spermine	Spermidine	Agmatine	
Brazil	0.9–9.8	<0.2–2.6	<0.2–2.1	<0.2–6.0	2.1–46.8	Beatriz *et al.* (1999)
Bulgaria	1.01–3.02	0.19–6.23	0.02–0.08	0.02–0.35	–	Lozanov *et al.* (2004)
Czech Republic	6.67–11.50	12.1–14.7	–	–	–	Kalač*et al.* (1997)
Europe	1.5–15.2	<0.3–39.9	<0.3–3.9	<0.3–6.8	0.5–40.9	Izquierdo-Pulido *et al.* (1996a)
Greece	3.11–4.78	0.26–2.10	0.20–1.44	1.13–4.54	–	Zotou *et al.* (2003)
	3.21–5.23	–	0.20–1.41	1.20–4.45	–	Loukou and Zotou (2003)
Italy	1.4–4.2	ND–0.8	ND	0.3–1.4	–	Buiatti *et al.* (1995)
Spain	3.2–6.4	0.3–1.4	ND–0.4	0.6–1.7	4.7–13.0	Izquierdo-Pulido *et al.* (1996b)
	3.46–7.15	0.35–1.07	0.49–1.19	0.26–2.62	–	Linares *et al.* (2001)
	1.44–8.41	0.17–8.41	ND–0.33	ND–0.63	–	Romero *et al.* (2003)
	8.3–22.4	<0.2–13.6	–	–	0.2–5.7	Cortacero-Ramirez *et al.* (2005)
Poland	1.25–2.09	0.62–0.83	5.21–11.58	1.20–4.00	–	Slomkowska and Ambroziak (2002)
Portugal	1.35–6.85	0.19–0.81	–	–	–	Fernandes *et al.* (2001)

*Ranges of mean values of biogenic amine concentrations (in mg/l) found in beers of different types and origin, based on varying numbers of observations; ND, not detected.

Methods for the determination of biogenic amines in foods are not numerous and only a few of these have been applied to beer. Methods that have been used throughout the years include spectrofluorometric and enzymatic techniques, the use of amino acid analyzer, thin-layer chromatography (TLC), gas chromatography (GC), ion exchange chromatography (IEC), high-performance liquid chromatography (HPLC), being the preferred technique, and in recent years capillary electrophoresis (CE).

Due to the lack of an easily detectable common chromophore group in amines, it is necessary to increase the sensitivity of the method by pre- or post-column derivatization. Some of the reagents used are *o*-phthalaldehyde (OPA), dansyl-chloride (DNS-Cl), dabsyl-chloride (DBS-Cl), benzoyl-chloride (BNZ-Cl), *p*-nitrobenzyloxycarbonyl-chloride (PNZ-Cl), 7-chloro-4-nitro-benzo-2-oxa-1,3 diazole (NBD-Cl), fluorescein isothiocyanate (FITC), 6-oxy-(-*N*-succinimidyl acetate)-9-(2′-methoxycarbonyl) fluorescein (SAMF) and naphthalene-2,3-dicarboxaldehyde (NDA). Information about the employed techniques, the derivatization reagents and the detection systems is included in Table 100.4.

Regardless of the analytical method and the derivatizing agent used, clean-up and preconcentration steps (e.g. liquid–liquid extraction (LLE), solid-phase extraction (SPE)) before and/or after the derivatization are often required, to determine the biogenic amines at the low levels, that they are present in beers, with no interferences from other compounds (e.g. amino acids, phenolic compounds). These steps are summarized in Table 100.5.

Table 100.4 Analytical techniques, derivatization reagents and detection systems used for the determination of biogenic amines in beer

Amine	*Analytical technique*	*Derivatization reagent*	*Detection system*	*Reference*
Histamine	Spectrofluorimetry	OPA	λ_{ex} = 350 nm, λ_{em} = 430 nm	Izquierdo-Pulido *et al.* (1991, 1995)
Tyramine	Spectrofluorimetry	α-Nitroso-β-napthol	λ_{ex} = 450 nm, λ_{em} = 540 nm	
Ten amines	Ion-pair HPLC	Post-column with OPA	λ_{ex} = 340 nm, λ_{em} = 445 nm	Beatriz *et al.* (1999), Izquierdo-Pulido *et al.* (1993, 1996a, b, 2000)
Six amines	RP-HPLC	Pre-column with OPA	λ_{ex} = 345 nm, λ_{em} = 440 nm	Petridis and Steinhart (1995)
Eight amines	RP-HPLC	Pre-column DNS-Cl	UV = 254 nm	Buiatti *et al.* (1995)
Eight amines	RP-HPLC	Pre-column DNS-Cl	UV = 340 nm	Slomkowska and Ambroziak (2002)
Eleven amines	RP-HPLC	Pre-column DNS-Cl	UV = 254 nm	Zotou *et al.* (2003)
Eleven amines	RP-HPLC	Pre-column DNS-Cl	λ_{ex} = 320 nm, λ_{em} = 523 nm	Loukou and Zotou (2003)
Eight amines	RP-HPLC	Pre-column DBS-Cl	UV = 445 nm	Romero *et al.* (2003)
Five amines	RP-HPLC	Pre-column benzoyl-Cl	UV = 254 nm	Kalač *et al.* (1997)
Four amines	MECC	Pre-column 7-chloro-4-nitrobenzo-2-oxa-1,3-diazole	λ_{ex} = 488 nm, λ_{em} = 540 nm	Preston *et al.* (1997)
Six amines	MECC	Pre-column benzoyl-Cl	UV = 200 nm	Kalač *et al.* (2002)
Histamine	CZE	–	Amperometric 1.35 V vs. SCE	Zhang *et al.* (2002)
Seven amines	CZE	Pre-column SAMF	LIF ($\lambda_{ex}/\lambda_{em}$ = 488/520 nm)	Cao *et al.* (2005)
Ten amines	CE	Pre-column FITC	LIF ($\lambda_{ex}/\lambda_{em}$ = 488/520 nm)	Cortacero-Ramirez *et al.* (2005)
Four amines	HP-TLC	DNS-Cl	FL ($\lambda_{ex}/\lambda_{em}$ = 338/505 nm)	Linares *et al.* (2001)
Twenty-two amines	GC	Pre-column isobutyl chloroformate	MS at SIM	Fernandes *et al.* (2001)

CE, capillary electrophoresis; CZE, capillary zone electrophoresis; DBS-Cl, dabsyl chloride; DNS-Cl, dansyl chloride; FITC, fluorescein isothiocyanate; FL, fluorescence; GC, gas chromatography; HP-TLC, high-performance thin-layer chromatography; LIF, laser induced fluorescence; MECC, micellar electrokinetic chromatography; MS, mass spectrometry; OPA, *o*-Phthalaldehyde; RP-HPLC, reversed-phase high-performance liquid chromatography; SAMF, 6-oxy-(*N*-succinimidyl acetate)-9-(2′-methoxycarbonyl) fluorescein; SIM, single ion monitoring; UV, ultraviolet.

Table 100.5 Procedures described in the literature for the analysis of biogenic amines in beer

Amines	*Sample preparation*	*Liquid–liquid extraction*	*Solid-phase extraction*			*Reference*
			Conditioning	*Washing*	*Elution*	
Histamine	Alkalization	For histamine: *n*-butanol, re-extracted with HCl (0.1 M)	–	–	–	Izquierdo-Pulido *et al.* (1991, 1995)
Tyramine		For tyramine: ethyl acetate, re-extracted with HCl (0.1 M)				
Ten amines	Homogenization, decarbonation and filtration	–	–	–	–	Beatriz *et al.* (1999), Izquierdo-Pulido *et al.* (1993, 1996a, b, 2000)
Eight amines	Saturation, degassing	With 10 ml of *n*-butanol – chloroform 1:1 (v/v). Mixture blending for 30 min. 1 ml of the organic phase + 2 drops of HCl, taken to dryness at room temperature. Dissolved with 1 ml of saturated sodium dicarbonate.	–	–	–	Buiatti *et al.* (1995)
Eight amines	Degassing	–	ODS cartridges MeOH/H_2O	20 ml 40% MeOH + 6 ml 40% MeOH	10 ml 100% MeOH	Slomkowska and Ambroziak (2002)
Eleven amines	Degassing and PVP treatment	–	DSC-18 cartridges MeOH/H_2O	Two volumes water/acetone (80:20 v/v)	3 ml ACN	Loukou and Zotou (2003a, b) Zotou *et al.* (2003)
Five amines	Degassing	With 10 ml of diethyl ether; 5 ml of the extract evaporated with a warm air stream and the residue dissolved in 0.4 ml of 71% (v/v) MeOH.	–	–	–	Kalač *et al.* (1997)
Six amines	–	With diethylether after evaporation of the solvent and dissolved in methanol.	–	–	–	Kalač *et al.* (2002)

ACN, acetonitrile; MeOH, methanol; ODS, octadecyl; PVP, polyvinylpyrrolidone.

Methods of Analysis

One of the first procedures developed focused on the most toxicologically important amines namely histamine and tyramine. Izquierdo-Pulido *et al.* (1991, 1995) used a different extraction method for each amine. Histamine was extracted with *n*-butanol after sample alkalization, re-extracted with hydrochloric acid (0.1 M) and determined as a fluorescent complex with OPA. The emission and excitation wavelengths were 350 and 430 nm, respectively. Tyramine extraction similarly occurred in an alkaline sample and was carried out with ethyl acetate. After re-extraction with hydrochloric acid, the tyramine complex with α-nitroso-β-napthol was measured again by spectrofluorimetry ($\lambda_{ex} = 450$ nm and $\lambda_{em} = 540$ nm). As other biogenic amines are also of interest, comprehensive and more selective methods were developed.

Liquid chromatographic methods

Ten amines – histamine, tyramine, serotonin, phenylethylamine, tryptamine, cadaverine, putrescine, agmatine, spermidine and spermine – were separated in one run using ion-pair partition chromatography on a reversed-phase column by Izquierdo-Pulido *et al.* (1993). After separation, the amines were detected as fluorescent OPA derivatives. Determination limits of the method ranged from 0.3 to 0.4 mg/l, except for serotonin and spermine, which were slightly higher. Based on this work, Beatriz *et al.* (1999) determined the levels of biogenic amines in Brazilian beers. This method was also used to provide data on the contents of biogenic amines in different types of European beers (Izquierdo-Pulido *et al.*, 1996a). Since biogenic amine levels could be used as an indicator of raw material quality, correct conditions of brewing and final product freshness, Izquierdo-Pulido *et al.* (1996b) used their previous work (Izquierdo-Pulido *et al.*, 1993) to locate differences among breweries. In recent years, Izquierdo-Pulido *et al.* (2000) tried to determine the effect of tyrosine on tyramine formation during beer fermentation. Loret *et al.* (2005) also used ion-pair chromatography with OPA post-column derivatization to measure the quality of the beer fermentation process in Belgian samples.

Though post-column derivatization is more common when OPA is used, Petridis and Steinhart (1995) described a simple and selective HPLC method for determining biogenic amines in beers and other beverages with pre-column OPA derivatization. Sample preparation was based on a rapid amine extraction using 10% trichloroacetic acid and a cation exchange column for extract purification. For the RP-HPLC analysis, OPA/2-mercaptoethanol was used for the pre-column derivatization, followed by fluorescence detection ($\lambda_{ex} = 345$ nm, $\lambda_{em} = 440$ nm). A separation of 15 biogenic amines was achieved within 70 min. The recoveries for histamine, tyramine, putrescine, cadaverine, tryptamine and 2-phenylethylamine were higher than 95%. The detection limits lied between 0.1 and 0.5 pmol/injection (20 μl), depending on the amine and a good linearity was achieved in the range 0.5–500 pmol ($r > 0.99$).

Arlorio *et al.* (1999) combined an extraction pre-separation step with ion-pair chromatography. The extraction steps were carried out with either butanol or an ionic exchanger. The authors concluded that many interfering compounds were eliminated by the pre-separation step. However, this procedure appeared to be laborious and detection limits were not given.

Buiatti *et al.* (1995) separated eight amines (histamine, tyramine, 2-phenylethylamine, tryptamine, cadaverine, putrescine, spermidine and spermine) using 1,7-diaminoheptane as internal standard. Amine derivatives, prepared prior to HPLC analysis with dansyl chloride, were eluted from a reversed-phase column by an acetonitrile/dipotassium hydrogen-phosphate system, adjusted to pH 7 with orthophosphate/water. The acetonitrile concentration increased linearly from 65% to 90% during 0–6 min. UV detection was carried out at 254 nm. The amines were extracted from beers using liquid–liquid extraction (LLE). When saturated with anhydrous sodium carbonate, degassed beer samples were submitted to extraction using 10 ml of *n*-butanol–chloroform 1:1 (v/v) . The mixture was blended for 30 min. An aliquot of 1 ml of the organic phase was introduced into a screw-capped tube and two drops of hydrochloric acid were added. After the sample was taken to dryness at room temperature, it was dissolved with 1 ml of saturated sodium dicarbonate. Dansylation was performed by adding 1 ml of DNS-Cl reagent (5 mg/ml in acetone). The reaction mixture was left for 1 h at 40°C. A different approach was proposed by Slomkowska and Ambroziak (2002) who also used pre-column dansylation to determine the content of eight biogenic amines in Polish beers. Degassing of the beer samples was the only step prior to dansylation procedure. The preparation of dansyl derivatives was as follows: A 1-ml volume of the working standard solution or the degassed beer sample was pipetted into a screw-capped vial. Subsequently, the following reagents were added to the tube: 1 ml of 5% trichloroacetic acid, 250 μl internal standard, 1 ml of 5% Na_2CO_3 and finally 1 ml DNS-Cl in acetone. The mixture was left in the dark for 90 min at 50°C. SPE was used as a clean-up step prior to chromatographic separation, using C18 cartridges. Washing was carried out with 20 ml of 40% methanol and then with an additional volume of 6 ml. The elution of dansyl derivatives was performed with 10 ml of 100% methanol. UV detection at 340 nm was used. The method showed satisfying recoveries while the detection limits ranged from 0.19 mg/l for spermidine to 0.49 mg/l for 2-phenylethylamine.

Dansylation with UV detection after separation on an octadecyl silica (ODS) column was used to determine the levels of 11 amines (histamine, tyramine, methylamine, ethylamine, 2-phenylethylamine, isoamylamine, tryptamine, cadaverine, putrescine, spermidine and spermine) in Greek beers by Zotou *et al.* (2003). The method involved pre-column derivatization of the amines with dansyl chloride and subsequent SPE of the derivatives through C18 cartridges. The pH of 5-ml beer aliquots was adjusted to 9.5 with borate buffer. A 2-ml volume of the resulting solutions was transferred to reaction vials and 400 μl of the 1,7-diaminoheptane internal standard solution and 800 μl of a 1% w/v DNS-Cl solution were then added and the mixtures were brought to a total volume of 4 ml with acetone–water (3:1). Vigorous agitation followed and the reaction mixtures were left in darkness for 30 min at 65°C. After derivatization, the reaction vials were left to cool at room temperature and acetone was removed under a stream of nitrogen. The remaining aqueous phase of the derivatized sample was then applied to an SPE clean-up procedure, using Supelco DSC-18 cartridges (500 mg/3 ml). The cartridges were activated with two volumes of methanol followed by two volumes of water. After the samples had passed through, the cartridges were washed with two volumes of water–acetone (80:20 v/v) and dried under vacuum. The samples were finally eluted with 3 ml of acetonitrile and the eluates were evaporated to dryness under nitrogen. The residues were reconstituted with acetonitrile and the resulting solutions were injected to the chromatograph. The separation was achieved on an Inertsil ODS-3 column (250 × 4 mm ID, 5 μm) using a 35-min gradient elution method with a binary system of acetonitrile–water, a flow rate of 1 ml/min with UV detection at 254 nm. Before analysis samples were degassed by ultrasonication for 15 min followed by the removal of polyphenols with polyvinylpyrrolidone (PVP). Limits of detection ranged from 0.1 ng for methylamine and ethylamine to 1.5 ng for tryptamine injected on-column. The method showed good linearity, satisfactory recovery results and high levels of sensitivity and precision.

Dansyl derivatives combine the unique feature of being both fluorescent and detectable in the UV region. Taking advantage of this feature and also of the fact that DNS-Cl reacts with both primary and secondary amino groups providing very stable derivatives, in contrast to OPA, which reacts only with primary amines yielding unstable derivatives, Loukou and Zotou (2003a) proposed quantification of the dansylamides of 11 biogenic amines in beer by fluorescence detection, at $\lambda_{ex} = 320$ nm and $\lambda_{em} = 523$ nm. Sample pretreatment, derivatization process, SPE clean-up and chromatographic conditions were identical to those reported previously by Zotou *et al.* (2003). Linearity was obtained for concentrations ranging from 0.008 to 40.0 mg/l. The limits of detection were found to be 0.08 ng for methylamine and ethylamine to 2.0 ng for histamine injected on-column. A comparison between UV and fluorescence detection of the dansyl derivatives was performed by means of significance *t*-tests, at the 5% level, using the results obtained from the analysis of beer samples (Loukou and Zotou, 2003b). Statistically significant differences were found only for ethylamine and spermine.

Eight biogenic amines, as dabsyl derivatives, were determined in beer samples, intermediate products and raw materials (malt and maize) by Romero *et al.* (2003). Beers and worts were filtered through a 0.20-μm millipore membrane filter, prior to the derivatization process. If necessary, worts were centrifuged before filtration to eliminate yeast remains and solid materials. An aliquot of 1.5 ml of diluted beer or hydrochloric extract was transferred to a vial, adjusted to pH 8.2 with reaction buffer and water was added to 3.8 ml. After thorough mixing on a vortex-mixer, 1.6 ml of dabsyl chloride solution was added and it was mixed again. The mixture was heated in a water bath for 21 min at 70°C, shaking at 1 and 15 min. Then, a 4.6-ml volume of the dilution solution was added and allowed to stand for approximately 20 min in the water bath, shaking from time to time. The C18 column was equilibrated at 40°C and the dabsyl derivatives were separated at a flow rate of 1 ml/min, using gradient elution, with a binary system of eluent A (sodium acetate + 10% v/v dimethylformamide + 0.23% v/v triethylamine, at pH 5.0 with dilute acetic acid) and eluent B (87.5% v/v acetonitrile + 10% v/v *tert*-butylmethylether + 2.5% v/v water). The detection wavelength was 446 nm. Bottled and canned beers representing different types of Spanish-produced beers (non-alcoholic, low alcohol, lager, special and extra) were studied. To study the amine contents throughout the brewing process, the same batch from two breweries of the same trademark, which use traditional (Brewery A) and modern (Brewery B) technologies, respectively, was monitored. Samples of raw materials and semi-products were collected at the different stages: maceration, fermentation, maturation and bottling. The results of the analysis indicate that in brewing, technology and hygiene are the decisive factors that determine the amine concentrations in the final product and not their levels in the raw materials.

Pre-column derivatization of five beer amines in Czech beers was reported by Kalač *et al.* (1997) based on the work of Křížek and Hlavatá (1995). Biogenic amines in beer and in solid raw materials were determined after their derivatization with benzoyl-chloride as *N*-benzamides by an HPLC method with isocratic elution. The *N*-benzamides were monitored at 254 nm. Two parallel analyses were necessary. Histamine and tyramine were determined by the first and the other three amines by the second. Histamine and tyramine were determined in 35-ml aliquots of beer, degassed under vacuum, to which 1,7-diaminoheptane was added as an internal standard. The mixture was alkalized with sodium hydroxide solution; benzoylchloride was added followed by sonication. The procedure continued with acidification to pH 6.0 with perchloric acid, addition of a phosphate buffer and sodium chloride and mixing. The *N*-benzamides formed were extracted into 10 ml of diethyl ether. A 5-ml aliquot of the extract was evaporated with a warm air stream and the residue was dissolved in 0.4 ml of mobile phase (71% v/v methanol in water).

A 10-μl aliquot of the extract was then injected for HPLC analysis. Cadaverine, putrescine and tryptamine were determined in 40-ml aliquots of degassed beer. A solution of 1,6-diaminohexane was used as an internal standard. The sample pretreatment was the same as that described above, but only a 1-ml aliquot of diethyl ether extract was evaporated and dissolved in 0.3 ml of 63.5% (v/v) methanol in water. The injected volume was again 10 μl. The detection limits (approximately 0.3 mg/l) were similar for all amines. No significant differences were observed between beer types (pale/dark, original extract of wort 10%/12%) and amine concentrations. Testing three batches for changes in the amine concentration during the brewing process showed that the formation of amines occurred principally during the main fermentation.

The reagent *p*-nitrobenzyloxycarbonyl chloride (PNZ-Cl) has also been used for pre-column derivatization of biogenic amines in fermented beverages and vinegars (Kirschbaum *et al.*, 1999). This method was applied to the determination of histamine, tyramine, 2-phenylethylamine, tryptamine, cadaverine, putrescine, spermidine, spermine and serotonin in beer with UV detection at 265 nm. More recently, an HPLC method for the simultaneous analysis of amino acids and biogenic polyamines, using a new procedure for pre-column derivatization of amino groups with *N*-(9-fluorenylmethoxycarbonyloxy) succinimide and fluorometric detection at $\lambda_{ex} = 262$ nm and $\lambda_{em} = 630$ nm was described (Lozanov *et al.*, 2004). The separation of 20 amino acids and 4 biogenic polyamines (putrescine, cadaverine, spermine and spermidine) was achieved within 32 min on a sequence of three short (50 mm) reversed-phase C18, 5-μm columns with elution buffers based on dibutylamine phosphate. The method linearity, calculated for each amino acid and polyamine, had a correlation coefficient higher than 0.991, in concentrations ranging from 0.2 to 50 μM, except for spermine and methionine, where the correlation coefficients were $r = 0.984$ and $r = 0.979$, respectively. The stability of derivatives in acidified samples at 4°C and room temperature was demonstrated. The limit of quantification was estimated to be around 50 pM in 50-μl sample injection. The repeatability of the method, expressed as relative standard derivation (RSD), ranged from 1.1% to 6.7%

CE methods

In recent years, CE has evolved into an interesting alternative to HPLC, because of the higher efficiencies, faster separation times, ease of operation and the low sample volumes required. The attractive features of CE include also the almost zero solvent consumption, the high speed and the high-throughput chemical analysis of a wide variety of substances.

CE with simultaneous ultraviolet absorbance and laser-induced fluorescence (LIF) detection was applied to identify and quantify selected amines in beer, following derivatization with 7-chloro-4-nitrobenzo-2-oxa-1,3-diazole (NBD-Cl). Quantification was performed using the method of standard addition to avoid pH-dependent variations in the reactivity of the derivatizing agent with the added benefit of verifying peak identity. An inexpensive and "easy-to-use" on-column fiber optic fluorescence detection cell was built using two optical fibers, a 125-μm excitation and a 400-μm collector fiber, positioned against the bare capillary wall using commercial HPLC fittings. The alignment and positioning provided a detection limit of 1 pmol for dibutylamine using a modest laser power of 5 mW (Preston *et al.*, 1997). The pH of the beer was adjusted to 9.0 with 0.1 M NaOH prior to derivatization. For standard addition and peak identification, beer samples were spiked using concentrated amine solutions. Samples were derivatized by adding equal volumes of the beer sample, methanol saturated with sodium acetate and a solution of 10 mg/ml NBD-Cl in methanol. The mixture was then heated at 60°C for 2 h in a sealed container. The derivatized material was diluted 1:4 prior to injection.

Formation of six biogenic amines in bottled beers was investigated in seven laboratory experiments (Kalač *et al.*, 2002). Amines were determined as *N*-benzamides by micellar electrokinetic capillary chromatography. Biogenic amines were derivatized by benzoylchloride in 40-ml aliquots of beer sample. The amines were thus converted to *N*-substituted benzamides, which were extracted in a further step by diethylether; after evaporation of the solvent they were dissolved in methanol. Analyses were carried out on a fully automated system for capillary zone electrophoresis, equipped with a multi-wavelength UV–VIS scanning detector. Separations were achieved using a plain fused silica capillary column, 43 cm total length (36 cm effective length to the detector) and 75 mm inner diameter. The procedure was described in detail by Křížek and Pelikanova (1998). Detection limits were 0.6, 0.8, 0.8, 0.8, 1.0 and 4.1 mg/l for cadaverine, putrescine, tyramine, tryptamine, histamine and spermidine, respectively. Reproducibility of the analytical procedure was tested by parallel analyses of seven beer samples from one bottle.

Histamine in beers has also been determined by capillary zone electrophoresis with an end-column amperometric detection using a carbon fiber microelectrode, at a constant potential (Zhang *et al.*, 2002). The optimum conditions of separation and detection were 10 mmol/l phosphate buffer, pH 5.6 for the buffer solution, 15 kV for the separation voltage and 1.35 V (vs. an SCE reference electrode) for the detection potential. The linear range was between 6.3×10^{-7} and 1.5×10^{-5} mol/l with a regression coefficient of 0.9997, and a detection limit of 4.0×10^{-7} mol/l. This method did not require any sample clean-up procedures or derivatization for the determination of histamine to beer samples.

Zhang and Sun (2004) introduced a rapid and sensitive method for the simultaneous determination of histamine and histidine by capillary zone electrophoresis with lamp-induced fluorescence detection. A fluoregenic derivatization reagent,

NDA was successfully applied to label the histamine and histidine, respectively. The optimal derivatization reaction was performed with 1.0 mM NDA, 20 mM NaCN and 20 mM borate buffer, pH 9.1 for 15 min at room temperature. The separation of NDA-tagged histamine and histidine could be achieved in less than 200 s with 40 mM sodium dihydrogen phosphate adjusted to pH 5.8 with H_3PO_4 as the running buffer. Sample injection was performed in the hydrodynamic mode with sampling height at 9 cm for 30 s. Separations were carried out at a constant voltage of 18 kV. Beer samples were diluted with water before derivatization. The detection limits for histamine and histidine were 5.5×10^{-9} and 3.8×10^{-9} M, respectively. The RSDs for migration time and peak height of derivatives were less than 1.5% and 5.0%, respectively.

The analytical potential of a fluorescein analog, SAMF as a labeling reagent for the labeling and determination of amino compounds by CE with LIF detection ($\lambda_{ex}/\lambda_{em}$ = 488/520 nm) was investigated (Cao *et al.*, 2005). Biogenic monoamines and amino acids were chosen as model analytes to evaluate the analytical possibilities of this approach. The derivatization conditions and separation parameters for the biogenic amines were optimized in detail. The derivatization was performed at 30°C for 6 min in boric acid buffer (pH 8.0). The derivatives were baseline-separated in 15 min with 25 mM boric acid running buffer (pH 9.0), containing 24 mM SDS and 12.5% v/v acetonitrile. The concentration detection limit for biogenic amines reaches 8×10^{-11} mol/l. The proposed method was applied to the determination of biogenic amines in three different beer samples with satisfying recoveries varying from 92.8% to 104.8% and RSDs from 0.2% to 4.9%. The samples were diluted with water prior to derivatization. Under these conditions no interference from amino acids was observed. Finally, comparison of several fluorescein-based probes for amino compounds was discussed. With good labeling reaction, excellent photo-stability, pH-independent fluorescence (pH 4–9) and the resultant widely suited running buffer pH, SAMF has a great prospect in the determination of amino compounds in CE.

Cortacero-Ramirez *et al.* (2005) developed a sensitive capillary electrophoretic method for the simultaneous determination of 10 biogenic amines (agmatine, 1,6-hexanodiamine, cadaverine, putrescine, dibutylamine, histamine, tyramine, butylamine, dimethylamine and ethylamine), which usually appear in beer samples (special and non-alcoholic), using LIF. Sample amines were first derivatized and filtered and then separated with an uncoated capillary tubing in the presence of 50-mM sodium borate and 20% acetone at pH 9.3, at 30 kV. An 800-μl aliquot of each sample, previously degassed by ultrasonication, was derivatized using 495 μl of 0.2 M carbonate buffer at pH 9, 1,000 μl of FITC solution (10 mM), 1,000 μl of acetone and doubly deionized water to a final volume of 5 ml in a test tube. This solution was put into a thermostated bath for 2 h at 50°C and 2 ml of the resulting solution was diluted to a final volume of 10 ml with doubly deionized water before the analysis by CE. In the case of extra, special and non-alcoholic beer, a 1,500-μl aliquot was taken for the derivatization. After the derivatization procedure, the sample was passed through a 0.45 μm membrane filter prior to injection. It was possible to analyze biogenic amines in brewing-process samples and in beer samples in less than 30 min, obtaining detection limits between 0.3 μg/l for ethylamine and 11.9 μg/l for 1,6-hexanodiamine.

Other methods of analysis

Another technique for beer amine determination is the amino acid analyzer. This procedure employs a potassium citrate buffer system and a post-column ninhydrin reaction (Halász *et al.*, 1999). Samples (0.6 M perchloric acid extract of malt and previously decarbonated beer) were pre-separated on a column-packed Dowex 50WX8 cation-exchange resin (4×1 cm ID) to eliminate free amino acids and to concentrate amines. The eluate was evaporated to dryness on a water bath and the dry residue was redissolved in 0.01 M HCl and filtered through a 0.45-mm membrane filter. Analysis of amines (putrescine, histamine, cadaverine, agmatine, spermidine and spermine) was carried out by an amino acid analyzer. A potassium citrate buffer system was required to eluate the amines at a flow rate of 40 ml/h. The column temperature was maintained at 67°C. Colorimetric detection was accomplished at 570 nm after ninhydrin reaction.

Derivatives with DNS-Cl have also been separated by a high-performance thin-layer chromatographic method (HPTLC). The effects of non-ionic surfactants as mobile phase additives on the fluorescence intensity of dansyl derivatives of biogenic amines in HPTLC were investigated. Beer samples were degassed prior to dansylation. To a 2-ml aliquot of amine-solution (1 mg/ml) or beer, a 2-ml volume of saturated sodium hydrogen carbonate solution and 3 ml of DNS-Cl reagent (5 mg/ml) were added. The solution was mixed for 1 min and transferred quantitatively into microwave dansylation vessels. The vessels were closed and introduced into the microwave cavity. The reaction was carried out at 40% power (252 W) for 5 min, maintaining a maximum pressure of 3.4 bar inside the reactor. When the vessel was cold, the mixture was extracted with two portions of 2 ml of toluene and diluted to 10 ml with this solvent. This microwave assisted dansylation reduced analysis time. The dansyl derivatives of putrescine, cadaverine, spermidine and spermine were separated by HPTLC, with silica gel as stationary phase and an eluent consisting of chloroform–triethylamine (2 + 1 v/v) containing 5% m/v of polyoxyethylene-10-lauryl ether (POLE). A fiber-optic-based fluorescence instrument for *in situ* scanning was used for quantitative measurements ($\lambda_{ex}/\lambda_{em}$ = 338/505 nm). The compounds were determined over the range 0.5–85 ng, with RSDs between 0.44% and 1.16%. The detection limits of the amines ranged between

0.28 and 0.39 ng. It is shown that the presence of POLE in the mobile phase enhances both the fluorescence intensity and the signal-to-noise ratio of the chromatographed dansyl derivatives (Linares *et al.*, 2001).

A gas chromatography–mass spectrometry (GC–MS) method was developed by Fernandes *et al.* (2001) for simultaneous measurement of the concentrations of 22 volatile and non-volatile biogenic amines (methylamine, dimethylamine, ethylamine, diethylamine, propylamine, isopropylamine, butylamine, isobutylamine, amylamine, isoamylamine, 2-methylbutylamine, hexylamine, pyrrolidine, piperidine, morpholine, 1,3-diaminopropane, putrescine, cadaverine, 1,6-diaminohexane, 2-phenylethylamine, tyramine and histamine) in alcoholic beverages. The method was based on a previously reported two-phase derivatization procedure with isobutyl chloroformate, which reacted quantitatively with all the amines in 10 min. After eliminating excess reagent, by treatment with alkaline methanol or by evaporation (tyramine and histamine determination), the derivatized extracts were analyzed by GC–MS with single-ion monitoring (SIM). Quantification of amines was achieved by the use of a set of eight different internal standards, including five deuterated isotopic analogs. The method has excellent analytical characteristics. It has been used to assay the concentrations of these biogenic amines in 13 samples of commercially available beers. Eleven biogenic amines were found in all the samples; putrescine (maximum 6.9 mg/l) and tyramine (maximum 1.7 mg/l) were the most abundant. Histamine was found in all samples at very low levels (maximum 147 mg/l).

An enzyme sensor array for the simultaneous determination of the three biogenic amines (histamine, tyramine and putrescine) by pattern recognition using an artificial neural network and its application to different food samples, among them beer, was described by Lange and Wittmann (2002). A combination of a monoamine oxidase, a tyramine oxidase and a diamine oxidase (with specific activities sufficient for rapid detection) are immobilized each on a separate screen-printed thick-film electrode via *trans*-glutaminase and glutaraldehyde to compare these cross-linking reagents with regard to their suitability. To calculate the amount of a specific biogenic amine, the raw data from multichannel software were transferred to a neural network. The sensor array takes 20 min to complete (excluding statistical data analysis) with only one extraction and subsequent neutralization step required prior to sensor measurement. However, the lower detection limits with this sensor (range between 5 and 10 mg/kg) compared to chromatographic methods appeared to lack sensitivity.

Summary Points

- There is currently much work ongoing globally, as researchers try to better understand the impact of biogenic amines and polyamines in our foods.
- In beer, bacterial contamination is a key source of biogenic amines and this is a source that can be controlled to ensure that the beer meets all quality and safety standards.
- Better methods of analysis for biogenic amines are being developed which allows for better monitoring.
- Liquid chromatographic methods with pre- or post-column derivatization followed by UV or fluorescence detection are the preferred methods of analysis, while in recent years CE methods are gaining ground.
- Sample pretreatment is usually simple, consisting only of degassing, though post-derivatization clean-up steps using SPE are usually needed.

References

Arlorio, M., Coisson, J.D. and Martelli, A. (1999). *Ital. J. Food Sci.* 11, 355–360.

Beatriz, M., Gloria, A. and Izquierdo-Pulido, M. (1999). *J. Food Comp. Anal.* 12, 129–136.

Buiatti, S., Boschelle, O., Mozzon, M. and Battistutta, F. (1995). *Food Chem.* 52, 199–202.

Cao, L., Wang, H. and Zhang, H. (2005). *Electrophoresis* 26, 1954–1962.

Cortacero-Ramirez, S., Arraez-Roman, D., Segura-Carretero, A. and Fernandez-Gutierrez, A. (2005). *Food Chem.* 100, 383–389.

Fernandes, J.O., Judas, I.C., Oliveira, M.B., Iferreira, I.M.P.L. and Ferreira, M.A. (2001). *Chromatogr. Suppl.* 53, S327–S331.

Halász, A., Baráth, A., Simon-Sarkadi, L. and Holzapfel, W. (1994). *Trend Food Sci. Technol.* 5, 42–49.

Halász, A., Baráth, Á. and Holzapfel, W.H. (1999). *Z. Lebensm. Unters. Forsch.* 201, 418–423.

Hannah, P., Glover, V. and Sandler, M. (1988). *Lancet* 1, 879.

Izquierdo-Pulido, M., Vidal-Carou, M.C. and Marine-Font, A. (1991). *Food Chem.* 42, 231–237.

Izquierdo-Pulido, M., Vidal-Carou, M.C. and Marine-Font, A. (1993). *J. AOAC Int.* 76, 1027–1032.

Izquierdo-Pulido, M., Marine-Font, A. and Vidal-Carou, M.C. (1994). *J. Food Sci.* 44, 1104–1107.

Izquierdo-Pulido, M., Font-Fabregas, J. and Vidal-Carou, M.C. (1995). *Food Chem.* 54, 51–54.

Izquierdo-Pulido, M., Hernandez-Jover, T., Marine-Font, A. and Vidal-Carou, M.C. (1996a). *J. Agric. Food Chem.* 44, 3159–3163.

Izquierdo-Pulido, M., Albala-Hurtado, S., Marine-Font, A. and Vidal-Carou, M.C. (1996b). *Z. Lebensm. Unters. Forsch.* 203, 507–511.

Izquierdo-Pulido, M., Marine-Font, A. and Vidal-Carou, M.C. (2000). *Food Chem.* 70, 329–332.

Kalač, P., Hlavatá, V. and Křížek, M. (1997). *Food Chem.* 58, 209–214.

Kalač, P., Savel, J., Křížek, M., Pelikova, T. and Prokopova, M. (2002). *Food Chem.* 79, 431–434.

Křížek, M. and Hlavatá, V. (1995). *Kvasny Prulm.* 41, 265–269 (in Czech).

Křížek, P. and Pelikanova, T. (1998). *J. Chromatography* A815, 243–250.

Kirschbaum, J., Meier, A. and Bruckner, H. (1999). *Chromatographia* 49, 117–124.

Lange, J. and Wittmann, C. (2002). *Anal. Bioanal. Chem.* 372, 276–283.

Linares, R.M., Ayala, J.H., Afonso, A.M. and Gonzales, V. (2001). *JPC – J. Planar. Chromatogr.* 14, 4–7.

Loret, S., Deloyer, P. and Dandrifosse, G. (2005). *Food Chem.* 89, 519–525.

Loukou, Z. and Zotou, A. (2003a). *J. Chromatogr. A* 996, 103–113.

Loukou, Z. and Zotou, A. (2003b). *Chromatographia* 58, 579–585.

Lozanov, V., Petrov, S. and Mitev, V. (2004). *J. Chromatogr. A* 1025, 201–208.

Moret, S. and Conte, L.S. (1996). *J. Chromatogr. A* 729, 363–369.

Peatfield, R.C. (1995). *Headache* 35, 355–357.

Petridis, K.D. and Steinhart, H. (1995). *Z. Lebensm. Unters. Forsch.* 201, 256–260. (in German).

Preston, L.M., Weber, M.L. and Murray, G.M. (1997). *J. Chromatogr. B* 695, 175–180.

Romero, R., Bagur, M.G., Sanchez-Vinas, M. and Gazquez, D. (2003). *Anal. Bioanal. Chem.* 376, 162–167.

Slomkowska, A. and Ambroziak, W. (2002). *Eur. Food Res. Technol.* 215, 380–383.

Zhang, L., Huang, W., Wang, Z. and Cheng, J. (2002). *Anal. Sci.* 18, 1117–1120.

Zhang, L.Y. and Sun, M.X. (2004). *J. Chromatogr. A* 1040, 133–140.

Zotou, A., Loukou, Z., Soufleros, E. and Stratis, I. (2003). *Chromatographia* 57, 429–438.

101

Beer and ESR Spin Trapping

Kevin Huvaere and Mogens L. Andersen Food Chemistry, Department of Food Science, University of Copenhagen, Frederiksberg C, Denmark

Abstract

The exposure of beer to light, heat, and oxygen negatively affects flavor properties and causes a reduced storage stability of bottled beer. As the deteriorating processes involve short-lived highly reactive radicals, methods to detect the presence of these intermediates have gained significant attention. In particular, detection of radicals in beer and beer-related model systems by the technique of spin trapping followed by electron spin resonance (ESR) spectroscopy has become an important tool for unraveling the mechanisms of degradation reactions in beer, for evaluating the flavor stability, and for predicting shelf life of beer.

List of Abbreviations

CIDEP	Chemically induced electron spin polarization
DMPO	5,5-Dimethyl-1-pyrroline *N*-oxide
EPR	Electron paramagnetic resonance
ESR	Electron spin resonance
MBT	3-Methylbut-2-ene-1-thiol
MNP	2-Methyl-2-nitrosopropane
PBN	*N-tert*-butyl-α-phenylnitrone
POBN	α-(4-Pyridyl 1-oxide)-*N-tert*-butylnitrone
RF	Riboflavin
TEMPO	2,2,6,6-Tetramethylpiperidine 1-oxyl
TR-ESR	Time-resolved electron spin resonance

Introduction

Lager beer is a product with a delicate aroma that can be altered by exposure to light, oxygen, and heat (Vanderhaegen *et al.*, 2006). These external factors are capable of initiating redox reactions in beer, which eventually are perceived by the consumer as changes in taste and flavor, and, in more severe cases, as the presence of turbidity due to haze formation. In recent years, it has become clear that the main intermediates in these reactions are radicals, that is, molecules that bear unpaired electrons and that are very reactive toward most types of organic molecules. The knowledge of the mechanisms how radicals destroy beer components is essential for optimizing production steps in view of improved beer quality, but also for predicting beer stability in relation to its shelf life.

Radical Detection

ESR spectroscopy

Electron spin resonance (ESR) spectroscopy detects radicals and, as these compounds show paramagnetic behavior, the technique is also referred to as electron paramagnetic resonance (EPR) spectroscopy. Since an electron is a charged particle spinning around its axis (next to orbiting around the nucleus), it generates a magnetic dipole. When placed in an external magnetic field two energetically different spin states (α and β) result, a phenomenon known as the Zeeman effect. The corresponding energy separation, E, is proportional to the strength of the magnetic field, H, as expressed by the fundamental equation $E = g\beta H$ (where β is the Bohr magneton and g is the Landé factor, which depends on the structure of the radical) (Figure 101.1).

Furthermore, from $E = h\nu$ (where h is Planck's constant and ν is the frequency of the electromagnetic radiation), it follows that $h\nu = g\beta H$ and transitions between the two states, if present in a magnetic field of constant strength, are induced by interaction of the electron with electromagnetic radiation of a discrete frequency. This is, in fact, the basic principle for ESR spectroscopy. However, most commercial ESR spectrometers are equipped with a fixed-frequency microwave source (between 9 and 10 GHz, X-band) and, consequently, samples are placed in a magnetic field with varying strength. Continuous wave ESR instruments, which are the most common type, record the signal, which originates from microwave absorption, as its first derivative and display it as a function of the strength of the applied magnetic field (Figure 101.1). Most organic radicals (including spin adducts) have g factors around 2, and their X-band ESR spectra are, therefore, observed at $H \sim 3{,}300$ G.

Beer in Health and Disease Prevention
ISBN: 978-0-12-373891-2

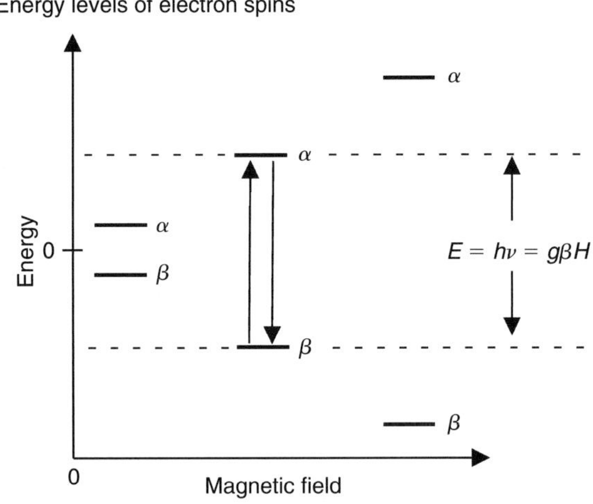

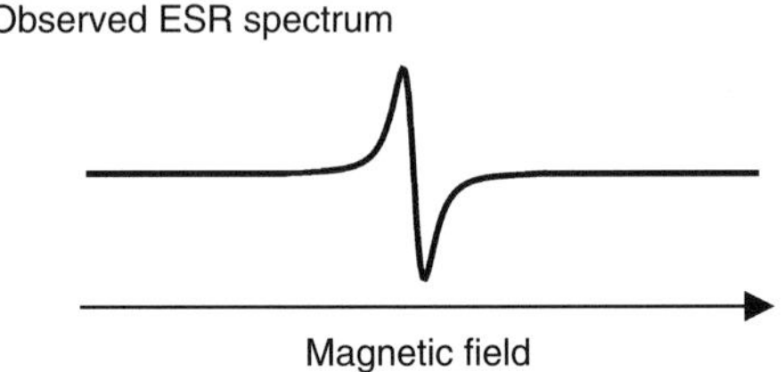

Figure 101.1 Energy separation between the two spin states of an electron (α and β) induced by applying an external magnetic field (the Zeeman effect). When resonance occurs, the corresponding signal is detected by continuous wave ESR and recorded as a first-derivative spectrum.

Spin trap
Spin adduct
Nitroso moiety
Nitroxyl radical
MNP
Nitrone moiety
β-hydrogen
DMPO
PBN
POBN

Figure 101.2 Overview of important spin traps and their resulting spin adducts after radical (R•) addition.

As the resonance of an unpaired spin is limited to the transitions between the β- and the α-state of the electron, only one line will appear in the resulting ESR spectrum (Figure 101.1). However, in view of deciphering radical structures, it is important to note that electron delocalization leads to interaction of the unpaired spin with other paramagnetic nuclei, such as ^{1}H and ^{14}N. Thus, hyperfine couplings arise and the ESR signal is split into additional lines. Both the number of lines and the magnitude of the couplings are essential for obtaining valuable information about the radical structure, as will be seen in following paragraphs.

Detection of radicals in beer

Although ESR spectroscopy allows radical detection in concentrations down to 1 μM under normal conditions, steady-state concentrations of radicals in beer, as a result of oxidation reactions, remain too low for direct detection. However, indirect detection can be aimed at by the technique of spin trapping, whereby highly reactive radicals are converted into stable radicals that accumulate to concentrations detectable by ESR (Rosen *et al.*, 1999). Such reaction is carried out by adding a so-called spin trap, a diamagnetic molecule that captures reactive radicals to form a stable spin adduct (Figure 101.2). Most spin traps contain either a nitrone or a nitroso moiety, structural features which, after radical addition, result in a nitroxyl radical with unique stability. Practically every ESR study of beer, wort or related model systems has applied spin trapping for detection of radicals (Kaneda *et al.*, 1988; Uchida and Ono, 1996; Andersen and Skibsted, 1998).

Oxidation in Beer

Shelf life prediction

Uchida *et al.* demonstrated that the spin trapping technique could be used to predict the stability of lager beer (Uchida *et al.*, 1996). In an oxygen-rich atmosphere, spin adduct formation after heating of beer in the presence of a spin trap was observed to follow a two-phase course (Figure 101.3). Initially, during the so-called lag phase or lag time, the formation of radicals was slow and, as a consequence, the level of generated spin adducts was very low. After the lag phase, the rate of radical formation increased and signals of spin adducts intensified linearly with time. It was proposed that the low rate of radical formation during the lag phase is caused by the presence of antioxidants, which quench radicals prior to initiating autooxidation cycles or, in the experimental setup, prior to adding to a spin trap. Thus, the length of the lag phase is the result of the competition

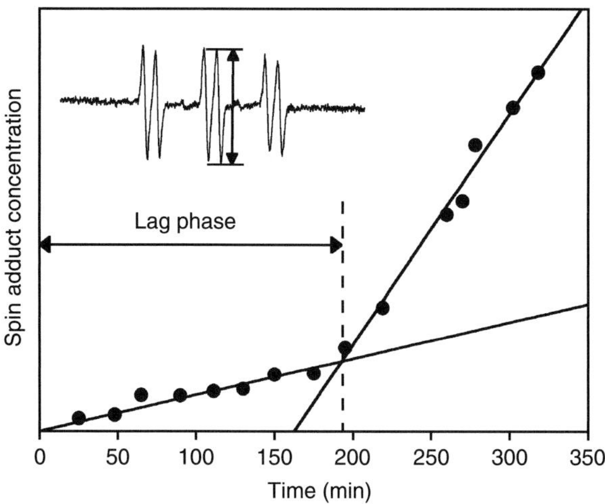

Figure 101.3 The determination of a lag time or lag phase during oxidation of beer is based on the intensity of ESR signals of the observed spin adducts.

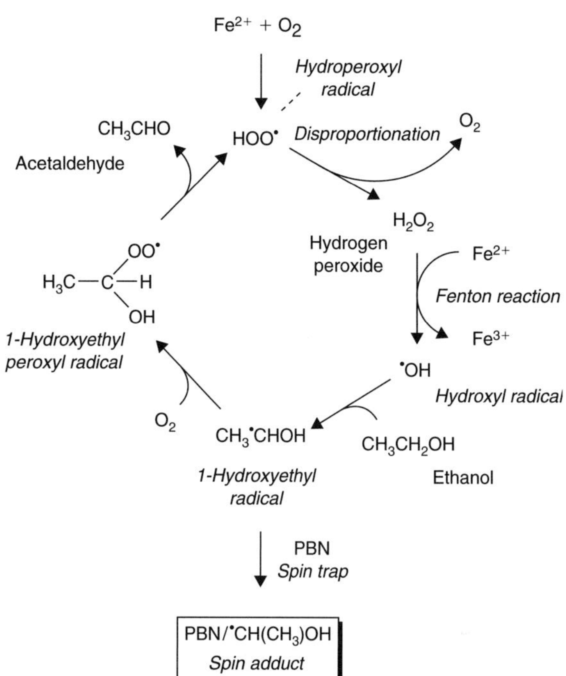

Figure 101.4 The mechanism of ethanol oxidation in an aerated beer matrix involves a 1-hydroxyethyl radical, resulting from hydrogen abstraction by a hydroxyl radical ($^\bullet OH$). This reactive intermediate originates from a Fenton-type reaction involving hydrogen peroxide and iron or copper ions.

between formation of radicals caused by the action of prooxidants and the quenching of radicals by antioxidants. A long lag phase indicates a high antioxidants-to-prooxidants ratio, while a short or absent lag phase suggests a small or negligible level of antioxidants compared to that of the prooxidants. Consequently, the lag time has been used as a criterion for endogenous antioxidant activity in beer, also referred to as EA value (Uchida *et al.*, 1996). In this respect, sulfite is suggested as one of the most important antioxidants in beer (Kaneda *et al.*, 1996; Uchida and Ono, 1999; Andersen *et al.*, 2000) and correlations between sulfite concentrations and lag times for radical formation in beer, as determined by ESR spin trapping, have been reported in several cases (Uchida *et al.*, 1996; Forster *et al.*, 1999; Nøddekær and Andersen, 2007). Obviously, different types of beer are expected to give different correlations, as levels of prooxidants and antioxidants may vary significantly.

As the length of the lag phase measured for fresh beer was found to correlate with the shelf life of beer during storage under normal conditions, spin trapping followed by ESR detection has become a fast and powerful tool for evaluating the flavor stability and for controlling quality during the production of beer (Uchida *et al.*, 1996; Forster *et al.*, 1999; Uchida and Ono, 2000).

Radicals observed during aerobic oxidative processes in beer

Spin trapping has become an important tool for studying the course of aerobic oxidative processes in beer, as such mechanisms involve several radicals and reactive oxygen species. The suggested intermediates are highly reactive and they participate in numerous reactions with various beer constituents. Eventually, the resulting reaction products are responsible for the changes in taste and aroma that are observed by the beer consumer.

One of the major oxidative reactions in beer includes the conversion of ethanol into acetaldehyde and, according to spin trapping experiments, a mechanism as depicted in Figure 101.4 was proposed. A 1-hydroxyethyl radical, $^\bullet CH(CH_3)OH$, has been identified (by using different spin traps; PBN: $a_N \sim 16.0\,G$; $a_H \sim 3.3\,G$, DMPO: $a_N \sim 15.9\,G$; $a_H \sim 22.9\,G$) as the radical that is predominantly leading to formation of ESR-detectable spin adducts (Andersen and Skibsted, 1998). This species is produced when a hydroxyl radical abstracts a hydrogen atom from ethanol, which is the most prevalent organic compound in beer. Indeed, the reactive hydroxyl radical shows little selectivity and, in this particular matrix, reacts preferentially with the relatively high-concentrated ethanol. Spin adducts of hydroxyl radicals are, therefore, only observed at high concentrations of spin trap molecules, which then efficiently compete with ethanol as a reaction partner (Andersen and Skibsted, 1998).

Hydroxyl radicals in beer are, most likely, generated by a Fenton-type reaction, in which hydrogen peroxide is reduced by iron(II) or copper(I):

$$H_2O_2 + Fe^{2+} + H^+ \rightarrow {}^\bullet OH + Fe^{3+} + H_2O$$

$$H_2O_2 + Cu^+ + H^+ \rightarrow {}^{\bullet}OH + Cu^{2+} + H_2O$$

Evidence for the pivotal role of iron and copper in radical formation followed from the observation of increased levels of spin adducts after addition of metal ions to beer (Uchida and Ono, 1996; Andersen and Skibsted, 1998; Uchida and Ono, 1999), whereas a reduced formation of spin adducts resulted from the presence of metal chelating agents (Uchida and Ono, 1996).

The substrate for Fenton reactions, hydrogen peroxide, originates from the disproportionation of superoxide, $O_2^{\bullet-}$, or its corresponding acidic form, the hydroperoxyl radical, $HOO^{\bullet}$. The formation and accumulation of hydrogen peroxide during aerobic oxidation of beer have been demonstrated by direct chemiluminescence spectroscopy (Uchida and Ono, 1999). Furthermore, it was shown by spin trapping experiments that the addition of hydrogen peroxide to beer led to an increased formation of radicals, whereas the presence of catalase, a peroxide-consuming enzyme, hampered radical formation (Uchida and Ono, 1996). Moreover, hydrogen peroxide levels in beer decreased after addition of sulfite (Uchida and Ono, 1999) and, referring to its role of main antioxidant in beer, it was suggested to be the result of a two-electron non-radical process with hydrogen peroxide (Andersen *et al.*, 2000).

Unlike for beer, the use of the spin trapping technique for detecting radicals in different types of wort has been less successful. Oxidation reactions are, most likely, also occurring in wort, but, apparently, the resulting radicals give rise to unstable spin adducts that do not accumulate into detectable amounts (Andersen and Skibsted, 2001).

Light-induced Oxidation of Beer

Lightstruck flavor

It is commonly known among brewers and beer lovers that exposure of beer to light results in significant quality loss, characterized by the development of an offensive taste and obnoxious odor. The phenomenon was first reported by Lintner back in 1875 and was referred to as lightstruck flavor (Lintner, 1875). The resulting off-flavor was principally attributed to the formation of 3-methylbut-2-ene-1-thiol (MBT) (Gunst and Verzele, 1978), also called *skunky thiol* due to its resemblance to compounds that prevail in the anal gland secretions of a skunk. Human scent is particularly sensitive to MBT and few nanograms per liter are sufficient to make lager beers unpalatable (Irwin *et al.*, 1993).

Increasing quality demands forced breweries to tackle the problem and scientists were involved to investigate the harmful effect of light on beer. As such, in 1963, research conducted under the supervision of Kuroiwa at the Kirin Brewery in Japan led to a breakthrough in the elucidation of the mechanism for lightstruck flavor formation in beer (Kuroiwa *et al.*, 1963). Remarkably, MBT was not observed on irradiation of unhopped beers, imputing hop-derived compounds a pivotal role in its formation mechanism (Kuroiwa and Hashimoto, 1961). In particular, isohumulones (Figure 101.5) were under suspicion, as their structural features allowed formation of a 3-methylbut-2-enyl

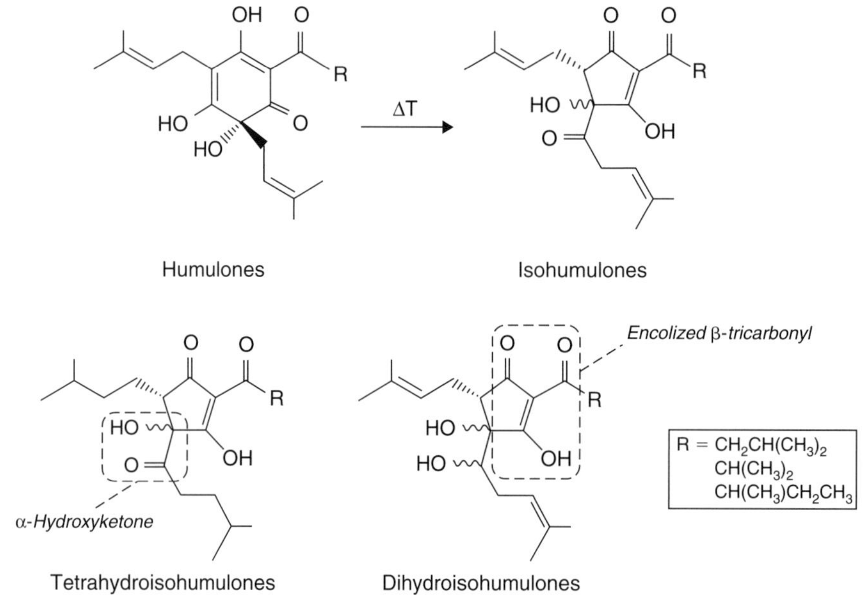

Figure 101.5 Isohumulones result from thermal isomerization of humulones. Reduced derivatives of isohumulones include tetrahydroisohumulones (side-chain double bonds reduced) and dihydroisohumulones (α-hydroxyketone moiety reduced to a vicinal diol).

radical, which, on interaction with a suitable sulfur source, would eventually lead to the formation of MBT. Resulting from thermal isomerization of hop-derived humulones during wort boiling, isohumulones occur in concentrations varying from 10 to 100 mg/l beer and are largely responsible for the typical bitter taste. Although the intervention of isohumulones seemed straightforward, degradation appeared to occur by an intricate mechanism. Indeed, the blue part of the visible spectrum (350–500 nm) was found most active in developing lightstruck flavor, but isohumulones are transparent in this wavelength region. Therefore, riboflavin (RF, vitamin B_2), which is naturally present in beer (few hundreds of micrograms per liter) (Andrés-Lacueva *et al.*, 1998; Duyvis *et al.*, 2002) and shows a strong absorption around 375 nm and around 445 nm, was put forward to act as a sensitizer. Upon irradiation, energy harvested by RF was suggested to be transferred to isohumulones, provoking disintegration of the α-hydroxyketone moiety with formation of a 4-methylpent-3-enoyl radical (Figure 101.6). Subsequent decarbonylation produces a 3-methylbut-2-enyl radical, which, after capture by a suitable sulfur source, would finally produce MBT, the compound characterizing lightstruck flavor. Although interpretation of the reaction mechanism was largely based on hypotheses, supported by minor experimental evidence, the formalism soon became established in the brewing community. As a consequence, further research stagnated and details about the consecutive reaction steps, essential for verifying the validity of the proposed mechanism, remained elusive. Moreover, the premature insights served as a basis for the development of the so-called light-stable derivatives of isohumulones. As the α-hydroxyketone moiety in isohumulones was suspected to be particularly vulnerable, reducing this moiety to a vicinal diol, as in dihydroisohumulones (Figure 101.5), was thought to inhibit photochemical degradation. On the other hand, reduction of the side-chain double bonds, as in tetrahydroisohumulones, would eventually prevent formation of a 3-methylbut-2-enyl radical, the main precursor of MBT.

To finally establish the underlying chemistry of lightstruck flavor formation and to evaluate the claimed stability of the reduced isohumulones, the photodegradation process was reinvestigated using modern spectroscopic techniques, including EPR spectroscopy that served as a powerful tool in unraveling the details of the mechanism.

Photochemistry of isohumulones

In view of photochemical reactivity, isohumulones consist of an enolized β-tricarbonyl chromophore, which shows a maximum absorbance around 255 nm with a shoulder around 270–280 nm (Maye *et al.*, 1999). The high molar extinction coefficient ($\varepsilon > 10^4 M^{-1} cm^{-1}$ at 275 nm) indicates a π–π^* transition, which leaves the n–π^* absorption of the isolated carbonyl in the 4-methylpent-3-enoyl side chain negligible (for structural features, see Figures 101.5 and 101.6). Consequently, isohumulones were found prone to photochemical breakdown on exposure to UV-B light (280–320 nm), but not to visible light (Blondeel *et al.*, 1987; Heyerick *et al.*, 2003). A detailed mechanistic study, involving excitation by a 308-nm laser pulse followed by time-resolved ESR (TR-ESR) spectroscopy, allowed direct detection of short-lived radicals with high spectral resolution (Burns *et al.*, 2001). The presence of

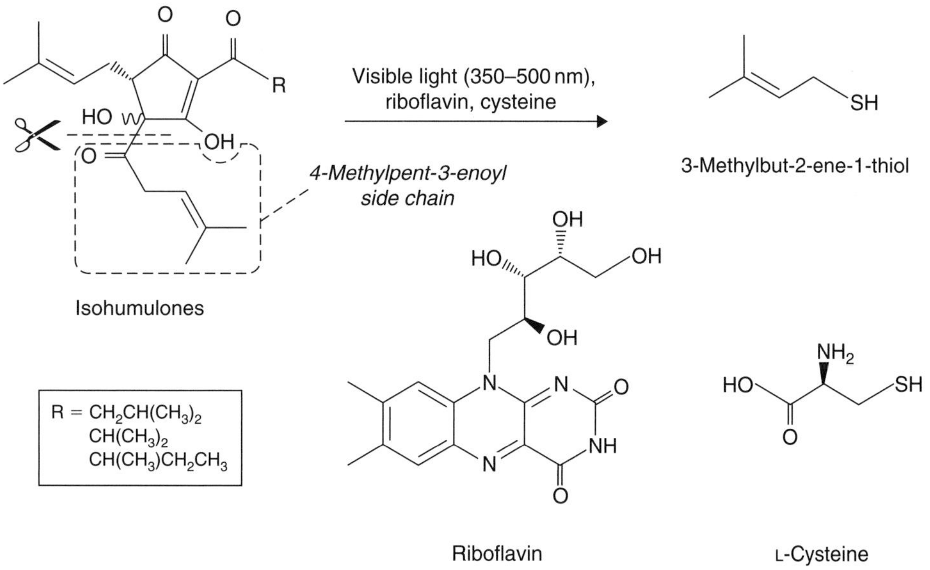

Visible light (350–500 nm), riboflavin, cysteine

4-Methylpent-3-enoyl side chain

Isohumulones

3-Methylbut-2-ene-1-thiol

R = $CH_2CH(CH_3)_2$, $CH(CH_3)_2$, $CH(CH_3)CH_2CH_3$

Riboflavin

L-Cysteine

Figure 101.6 The essential elements that are involved in the development of lightstruck flavor, as proposed by Kuroiwa (the Kuroiwa premise). Cleavage of the α-hydroxyketone moiety is pivotal in the formation of radical intermediates that eventually produce MBT.

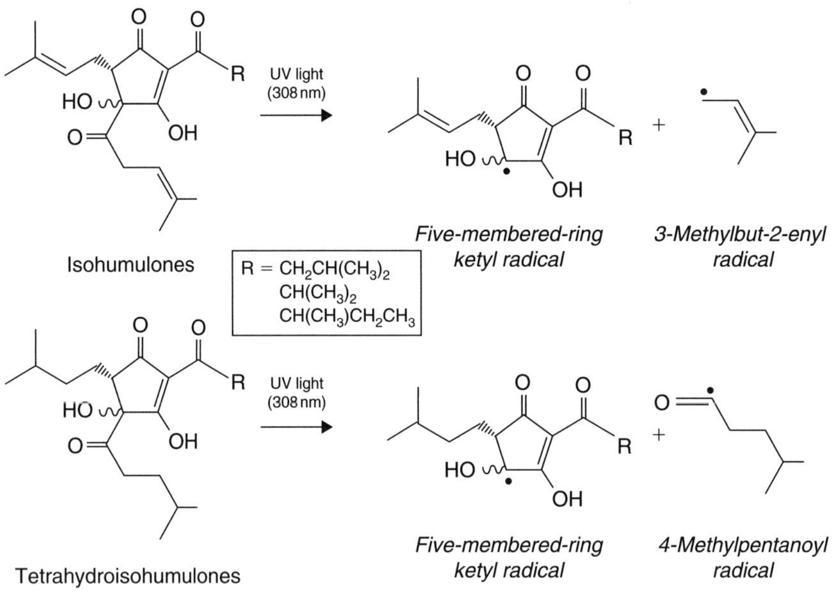

UV light (308 nm)

Isohumulones

R = $CH_2CH(CH_3)_2$
$CH(CH_3)_2$
$CH(CH_3)CH_2CH_3$

Five-membered-ring ketyl radical

3-Methylbut-2-enyl radical

UV light (308 nm)

Tetrahydroisohumulones

Five-membered-ring ketyl radical

4-Methylpentanoyl radical

Figure 101.7 Radicals derived from isohumulones and tetrahydroisohumulones, respectively, as observed after a 308-nm laser flash and subsequent detection by time-resolved ESR spectroscopy.

hyperfine couplings furnished essential structural information for characterizing reactive intermediates, hence it was found that direct photodegradation of isohumulones produced a strong emissive signal that was ascribed to the presence a five-membered-ring ketyl radical and a 3-methylbut-2-enyl radical (Figure 101.7). Indeed, the incipient 4-methylpent-3-enoyl radical, resulting from homolytic cleavage of the α-hydroxyketone moiety (Norrish Type I cleavage), should be rapidly decarbonylated. As spin density in the 3-methylbut-2-enyl radical is spread by extensive delocalization, the large number of hyperfine interactions (originating from coupling to multiple hydrogen atoms) decreased the intensity of the observed signal. On the other hand, tetrahydroisohumulones, which have both side-chain double bonds reduced with respect to isohumulones (Figure 101.7), showed a significantly different TR-ESR spectrum. Although radicals were still produced on cleavage of the unaltered α-hydroxyketone moiety, the resulting 4-methylpentanoyl failed to decarbonylate on a μs-timescale (Vollenweider and Paul, 1986). Thus, an acyl radical was observed and the lack of hyperfine couplings resulted in a more intense ESR signal. Reducing the side-chain carbonyl group, as in dihydroisohumulones, inhibited radical formation after a 308-nm laser flash and corroborated the mechanism of cleavage of the α-hydroxyketone moiety (as was observed for isohumulones and tetrahydroisohumulones). Although dihydroisohumulones did not directly lead to fragmentation, TR-ESR investigations still provided valuable mechanistic information. Indeed, on irradiation of these reduced derivatives in a frozen matrix, a net emissive signal arising from the triplet mechanism of chemically induced electron spin polarization (CIDEP) could be observed. This β-tricarbonyl triplet was not observed with isohumulones or tetrahydroisohumulones, probably due to instantaneous cleavage reactions, but its interference was indirectly deduced from the net emissive polarization of the observed spectra. Further evidence for formation of the triplet state of the β-tricarbonyl moiety followed from addition of the spin probe 2,2,6,6-tetramethylpiperidine 1-oxyl (TEMPO) to a solution of dihydroisohumulones. Although TEMPO does not exhibit any polarization on its own, the resulting spectrum showed an emissive signal. This particular polarization was ascribed to the magnetic interaction between the excited β-tricarbonyl triplet and the unpaired spin on the TEMPO molecule. From these observations, it was concluded that formation of the triplet-excited state of the β-tricarbonyl chromophore is the early photochemical event on absorption of UV-B light. Ensuing energy transfer to the isolated side-chain carbonyl moiety eventually induces a Norrish Type I cleavage, producing a ketyl radical and an acyl radical which, in the case of isohumulones, is readily decarbonylated to form a 3-methylbut-2-enyl radical. As dihydroisohumulones have the α-hydroxyketone moiety reduced to a vicinal diol, energy transfer fails and radicaloid decomposition is averted. In accordance with the findings from irradiation with UV light, these compounds are marketed and sold as a fully light-stable alternative for natural isohumulones.

The Kuroiwa model revisited

Although exposure of isohumulones to UV-B light produced a 3-methylbut-2-enyl radical, according to the Kuroiwa formalism (visible) blue light accounts for the formation of lightstruck flavor. Furthermore, beers packed in green bottles are particularly prone to photodegradation, yet colored glass is impenetrable for UV light (Sakuma *et al.*, 1991). Therefore, the intervention of RF in the photoreaction was thought to induce degradation by energy transfer, but this mechanism was later refuted due to unfavorable thermodynamics (Hastings *et al.*, 1992). As the interaction between RF and isohumulones remained an apparent discrepancy, a comprehensive insight of the underlying chemistry was aimed at. Therefore, model systems were investigated using a combination of TR-ESR and spin trapping followed by continuous wave ESR spectroscopy. After excitation of a solution containing isohumulones and flavin mononucleotide (an RF derivative used in model systems due to its enhanced water solubility) with a 355-nm laser pulse, the TR-ESR spectrum resulted in broad signal with a prominent emissive component (Heyerick *et al.*, 2005). The line width of ~19.0 G suggested a significant delocalization of the unpaired spin and was indicative of a reduced flavin semiquinone radical (Kay *et al.*, 1999). Detection of such species referred to an electron or hydrogen transfer mechanism which, obviously, would imply the occurrence of radicals derived from isohumulones (or derivatives). Indeed, superimposed signals were detected in the spectra produced by irradiation of isohumulones and tetrahydroisohumulones in the presence of flavin mononucleotide, but unambiguous identification was hampered by overlap with the intense flavin radical signal. Still, valuable mechanistic information was retrieved when the spin probe TEMPO was added to solutions containing isohumulones and flavin mononucleotide. Excitation by a 355-nm laser pulse, followed by TR-ESR analysis, resulted in a strongly emissive three-line spectrum which was ascribed to transfer of spin polarization when a triplet-excited state encounters an unpaired electron. This observation suggested the interference of triplet-excited flavin mononucleotide in the reaction mechanism, a finding which was in agreement with results that were obtained from laser flash photolysis coupled to transient absorption spectroscopy (Huvaere *et al.*, 2004a; Goldsmith *et al.*, 2005).

But, to claim deeper insight in the mechanism of lightstruck flavor formation, characteristic information about the radicals derived from isohumulones and reduced analogs was essential. Therefore, model solutions containing isohumulones (or derivatives) and a flavin compound were irradiated in the presence of spin traps, such as 5,5-dimethyl-1-pyrroline *N*-oxide (DMPO) and 2-methyl-2-nitrosopropane (MNP) (Huvaere *et al.*, 2005). Under these conditions, radicals arising from photooxidation of isohumulones add to the spin trap, giving rise to a relatively stable radical (Figure 101.2). Although only indirect information can be deduced from simulating the signals corresponding to these spin adducts, the coupling constants of the unpaired spin to nitrogen (a_N) and (if present) to hydrogen (a_H) have characteristic values and allow identification of the incipient radical. In this respect, the use of MNP provides direct structural information as the multiplicity of the splitting pattern is directly related to the number of hydrogens prevailing on the radical center to be trapped. However, MNP fails to trap oxygen-centered radicals, as the resulting spin adducts are highly unstable and readily decompose. Therefore, radical trapping experiments were also carried out using DMPO as spin trap, as it produces detectable spin adducts with various types of radicals (carbon-, oxygen-, and sulfur-centered). Still, collecting information on the nature of the trapped radical is complicated, as the triplet arising from the nitroxyl radical is doubled by the presence of the DMPO β-hydrogen (Figure 101.2).

Preliminary experiments including photooxidation of isohumulones by triplet-excited flavins in the presence of DMPO furnished readily detectable spin adducts, but elucidation of the structural features of the trapped radical(s) announced as an intricate exercise. However, as oxidation of isohumulones was presumed, their behavior under oxidizing conditions was first examined by electrolysis in an electrochemical cell (Huvaere *et al.*, 2003). As no flavins were involved, the simplified model system allowed various functionalities in the isohumulones (and also in its derivatives) to be fully explored. Remarkably, it was found from applying cyclic voltammetry that these compounds could only be oxidized when present in their salt (anionic) form, whereas the corresponding undissociated (acidic) form remained electrochemically inactive. Since the salt form, which prevails in the beer matrix, is characterized by ionization of the enolized β-tricarbonyl chromophore (which, as seen in Figure 101.5, is present in isohumulones as well as in its derivatives and consists of a delocalized π-system spread over four carbon and three oxygen atoms), electron release and concurrent formation of radicals, obviously either carbon- or oxygen-centered, was suggested to arise from this moiety. Addition of DMPO to a solution of salts of isohumulones in acetonitrile, followed by electrolysis, produced a single spin adduct with $a_N \sim 13.2$ G and $a_H \sim 8.9$ G that was assigned to trapping of an oxygen-centered radical (Figure 101.8). Addition of MNP showed a distinctly different picture, as adducts with two radicals ($a_N \sim 13.6$ G and $a_N \sim 7.9$ G, respectively) were observed. Both MNP adducts should originate from carbon-centered radicals and, as they only show coupling to nitrogen, no hydrogens are bond to the radical center. Indeed, the value of $a_N \sim 7.9$ G is characteristic for trapping of an acyl radical that possibly results from secondary stabilization pathways. On the other hand, the value of $a_N \sim 13.6$ G suggests trapping of a tertiary carbon with low-electron density, as a similar value has been reported for trapping of a trichloromethyl radical by MNP (Buettner, 1987). Consequently, the incipient radical was identified as a carbon-centered triacylmethyl radical (for structure, see Figure 101.9). Substituting dihydroisohumulones for isohumulones resulted in a similar adduct with MNP ($a_N \sim 15.3$ G),

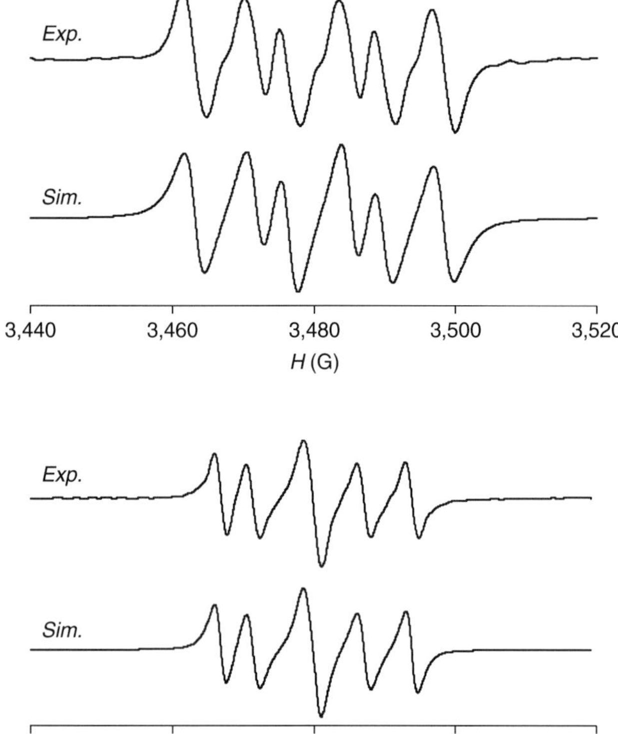

Figure 101.8 Experimental (*Exp.*) and simulated (*Sim.*) spin patterns of radicals derived from isohumulones after electrolysis (under a nitrogen atmosphere) and trapping by DMPO (*upper panel*) and MNP (*lower panel*), respectively.

as could be expected from oxidation of the ionized β-tricarbonyl moiety. Failure to observe a spin adduct with an acyl radical (as in the case of isohumulones) should be attributed to the presence of the diol moiety instead of an α-hydroxyketone. Spin trapping with DMPO gave rise to a spin adduct with $a_N \sim 13.1$ G and $a_H \sim 9.5$ G, which was very similar to the observations made for the electrolysis of isohumulones. However, two extra spin adducts were formed ($a_N \sim 14.5$ G; $a_H \sim 20.2$ G and $a_N \sim 14.7$ G; $a_H \sim 25.7$ G, respectively) that were ascribed to the trapping of carbon-centered radicals, most likely resulting from secondary reactions of the incipient oxygen-centered radical.

Thus, experiments involving electrolysis and subsequent spin trapping coupled to ESR analysis have demonstrated that the ionized β-tricarbonyl chromophore in isohumulones and its derivatives is a suitable target for oxidation. In this respect, it was investigated whether this moiety showed a similar reactivity in the presence of oxidizing species such as triplet-excited flavins (Huvaere *et al.*, 2005). In the case of tetrahydroisohumulones, radical addition to DMPO produced a characteristic spin adduct ($a_N \sim 14.8$ G; $a_H \sim 18.1$ G) that was ascribed to the trapping of an acyl radical. Furthermore, an extra species with $a_N \sim 15.4$ G; $a_H \sim 22.7$ G appeared in the ESR spectrum and a similar adduct resulted after photooxidation of isohumulones or dihydroisohumulones. Such spin adduct was previously observed in an analogous model system, but was, in that particular case, ascribed to the trapping of a 1-hydroxyethyl radical (Laane *et al.*, 1999).

Since DMPO generally furnishes poor structural information when investigating carbon-centered radicals, experiments were repeated with MNP as a spin trap. Thus, the spectrum observed after irradiation of a solution containing isohumulones (or derivatives) and RF showed a signal ($a_N \sim 16.5$ G) that was attributed to a spin adduct resulting from photochemical interaction between RF and MNP. Unless this extensive background signal, characterization of radicals derived from photooxidation of hop-derived compounds was not compromised. Indeed, irradiation in the presence of isohumulones resulted in an MNP adduct with a value of $a_N \sim 14.1$ G, while photooxidation of dihydroisohumulones resulted in an adduct with $a_N \sim 15.2$ G. As the values of the respective coupling constants were in good agreement with the values observed on electrochemical oxidation, these spin adducts were, likewise, ascribed to the trapping of low-electron density triacylmethyl radicals (Figure 101.9). A similar adduct ($a_N \sim 14.2$ G) resulted from irradiation of tetrahydroisohumulones, while an additional species with $a_N \sim 8.1$ G, corresponding to the trapping of an acyl radical, was ascribed to the trapping of a 4-methylpentanoyl radical (for structure, see Figure 101.7). This finding was in agreement with spin trapping experiments with DMPO, as well as with detailed product analyses identifying 4-methylpentanal as a major degradation product (Huvaere *et al.*, 2004b). Since a 4-methylpentanoyl radical results from cleavage of the α-hydroxyketone moiety, its unsaturated counterpart, a 4-methylpent-3-enoyl radical, would be expected to arise from photooxidation of isohumulones. However, no such radical was added to MNP, as decarbonylation to a stabilized 3-methylbut-2-enyl radical readily occurred (Figure 101.9) and eventually led to the formation of 2-methylbut-2-ene as major reaction product (Huvaere *et al.*, 2004b). Still, traces of an adduct with a 4-methylpent-3-enoyl radical could be observed when DMPO was used as spin trap.

From these spin trapping experiments, followed by ESR spectroscopy, it was clearly demonstrated that isohumulones release an electron in the presence of oxidizing species such as triplet-excited flavins. The resulting radicals are highly reactive and stabilization pathways induce fragmentation that eventually furnishes a 3-methylbut-2-enyl radical, the main precursor of MBT. This radical cannot be formed from reduced derivatives of isohumulones and, according to the definition, these compounds do not lead to light-struck flavor formation. However, the observation of spin adducts after (photo)oxidation of tetrahydroisohumulones and dihydroisohumulones, respectively, indicates that these compounds produce reactive radicals as well, which possibly

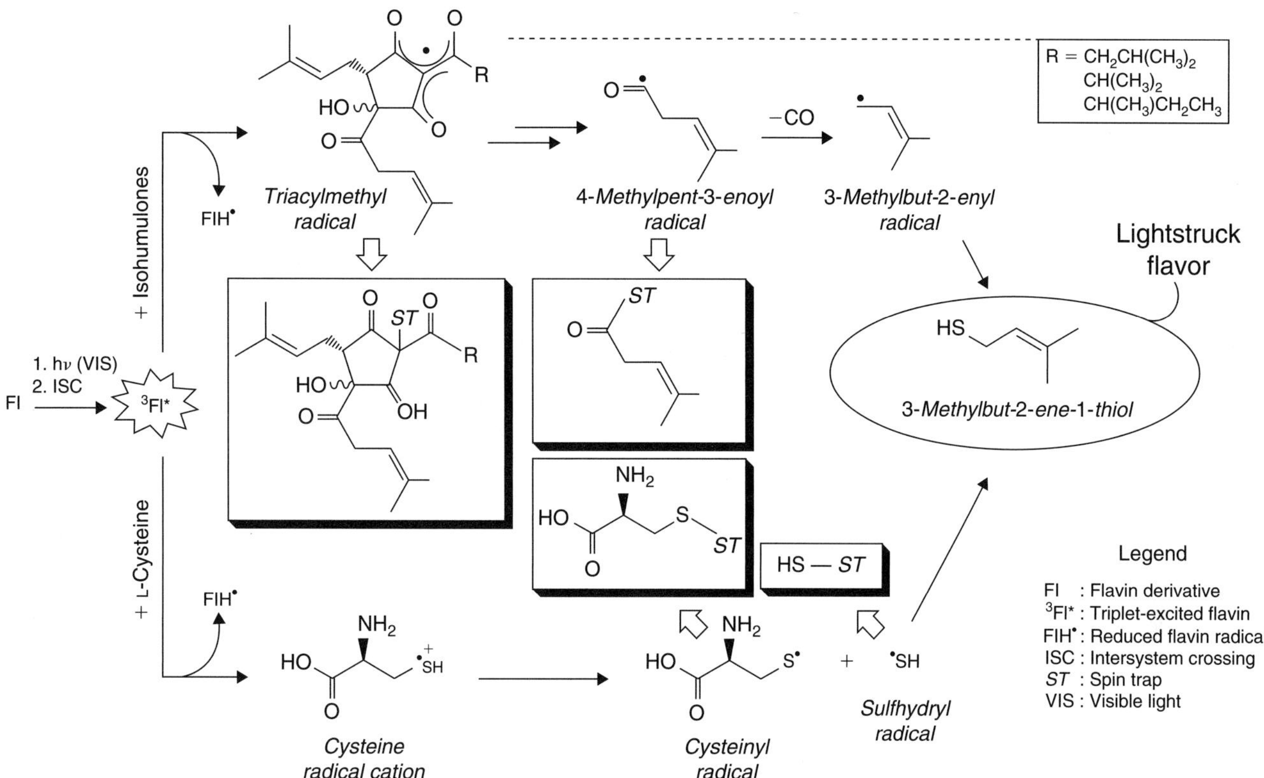

Figure 101.9 The mechanism of lightstruck flavor formation as a result of visible-light irradiation. Radicals that are identified by spin trapping followed by ESR spectroscopy are depicted in a box as their respective spin adducts.

lead to formation of flavor-active volatile compounds (Huvaere *et al.*, 2004b). Thus, it was concluded that, despite the structural modifications, reduced isohumulones are not resistant toward flavin-mediated photodecomposition.

The role of sulfur radicals

Although research into the photochemical degradation of isohumulones produced evidence for the formation of a 3-methylbut-2-enyl radical as a precursor of MBT, still the origin of the thiol group (—SH) remained obscure. However, the presence of this particular sulfur moiety is pivotal, as it is largely responsible for the repulsive odor that MBT produces. In this respect, cysteine, as well as sulfur-containing peptides and proteins occurring in the beer matrix, has been suggested to act as sulfur donor (Sakuma *et al.*, 1991). Details about a possible reaction mechanism remained forthcoming, until it was found from experiments with laser flash photolysis that these sulfur-containing compounds strongly affected the triplet lifetime of the excited flavin (Cardoso *et al.*, 2004). This effect could not be observed for compounds such as alanine, hence, it was concluded that the presence of the sulfur atom was pivotal for interaction. Moreover, detailed fundamental insights in the reaction mechanism were obtained from combining ESR spectroscopy with comprehensive product analyses by mass spectrometry (Huvaere *et al.*, 2006). Indeed, during irradiation of cysteine (and derivatives thereof) in the presence of flavin mononucleotide, a broad ESR signal (line width ~18.5 G) corresponding to the reduced flavin radical could be observed, indicating that an electron transfer (coupled to instant proton migration) mechanism was operative. Structural information about cysteine-derived intermediates only followed from addition of spin traps to the reaction mixture. Remarkably, MNP failed to produce detectable adducts after photooxidation of cysteine, but DMPO resulted in the formation of two adducts with $a_N \sim 15.2$ G; $a_H \sim 17.2$ G and $a_N \sim 15.0$ G; $a_H \sim 15.7$ G, respectively. The coupling constants of the former adduct were characteristic of a trapped cysteinyl radical (Davies *et al.*, 1987; Mottley *et al.*, 1987), which was formed by photooxidation and subsequent deprotonation of the resulting cysteine radical cation (Figure 101.9). The second adduct was not identified before but it was suggested to arise from addition of a sulfur-centered radical to DMPO, as coupling constants were very similar to those reported for a sulfenyl radical (RS•). Moreover, since a comprehensive study by mass spectrometry revealed hydrogen sulfide (H_2S) as the major reaction product derived from photooxidation of cysteine, the intervention of a sulfhydryl radical (•SH) was suggested and, consequently, the second DMPO adduct was ascribed to the trapping of •SH (Huvaere *et al.*, 2006). The feasibility of a C—S bond cleavage was confirmed when *S*-methylcysteine was substituted for cysteine, as photooxidation resulted in trapping of a thiomethyl radical ($a_N \sim 15.3$ G; $a_H \sim 18.0$ G observed for the DMPO adduct). This finding was in agreement with the detection of methanethiol and dimethyl disulfide as major reaction products.

The mechanism of lightstruck flavor formation unraveled

The observation of a sulfhydryl radical (•SH) after photooxidation of cysteine, in combination with the knowledge that, under similar conditions, isohumulones decompose to produce a 3-methylbut-2-enyl radical, strongly supported the premise that radical recombination leads to lightstruck flavor formation. The mechanism was corroborated by the detection of MBT after visible-light irradiation of model systems containing isohumulones, cysteine, and a flavin derivative (Huvaere *et al.*, 2006). As a result of these findings, details about the reactions leading to lightstruck flavor formation may now be considered as fully unraveled.

Summary Points

- Spin trapping and ESR spectroscopy is a powerful tool for studying oxidation reactions that occur in the beer matrix.
- Spin trapping and ESR spectroscopy can be used for predicting the flavor stability of beer and for quality control during the production of beer.
- Fenton reactions most likely initiate radical formation in beer and give rise to the reactive (but unselective) hydroxyl radical, •OH, that attacks beer constituents with formation of (flavor-active) degradation products.
- The most important radical adducts observed in an aerated beer matrix result from trapping of a 1-hydroxyethyl radical, •CH(CH_3)OH.
- Light-induced reactions in beer, leading to the formation of MBT as the principal contributor to lightstruck flavor, are the result of radicaloid breakdown of hop-derived compounds.
- Irradiation with UV light causes direct decomposition of isohumulones, eventually furnishing a 3-methylbut-2-enyl radical (the main precursor of MBT).
- Visible-light irradiation of isohumulones in the presence of a flavin derivative produces a 3-methylbut-2-enyl radical, as a result of electron abstraction (by triplet-excited flavins) and subsequent radical stabilization pathways.
- Triplet-excited flavins oxidize cysteine (and derivatives), generating a sulfhydryl radical (•SH) as an important intermediate in the formation of lightstruck flavor in beer.
- From spin trapping experiments followed by ESR spectroscopy, it was demonstrated that dihydroisohumulones, which are claimed to be light-stable, do not resist photooxidation by triplet-excited flavins and disintegrate upon interaction.

References

Andersen, M.L. and Skibsted, L.H. (1998). *J. Agric. Food Chem.* 46, 1272–1275.

Andersen, M.L. and Skibsted, L.H. (2001). *J. Agric. Food Chem.* 49, 5232–5237.

Andersen, M.L., Outtrup, H. and Skibsted, L.H. (2000). *J. Agric. Food Chem.* 48, 3106–3111.

Andrés-Lacueva, C., Mattivi, F. and Tonon, D. (1998). *J. Chromatogr. A* 823, 355–363.

Blondeel, G.M.A., De Keukeleire, D. and Verzele, M. (1987). *J. Chem. Soc. Perkin Trans. I* 1, 2715–2717.

Buettner, G.R. (1987). *Free Radic. Biol. Med.* 3, 259–303.

Burns, C.S., Heyerick, A., De Keukeleire, D. and Forbes, M.D.E. (2001). *Chem. Eur. J.* 7, 4553–4561.

Cardoso, D.R., Franco, D.W., Olsen, K., Andersen, M.L. and Skibsted, L.H. (2004). *J. Agric. Food. Chem.* 52, 6602–6606.

Davies, M.J., Forni, L.G. and Shuter, S.L. (1987). *Chem. Biol. Interact.* 61, 177–188.

Duyvis, M.G., Hilhorst, R., Laane, C., Evans, D.J. and Schmedding, D.J.M. (2002). *J. Agric. Food. Chem.* 50, 1548–1552.

Forster, C., Schwieger, J., Narziss, L., Back, M., Uchida, M., Ono, M. and Yanagi, K. (1999). *Monatsschrift für Brauwissenschaft* 52, 86–93.

Goldsmith, M.R., Rogers, P.J., Cabral, N.M., Ghiggino, K.P. and Roddick, F.A. (2005). *J. Am. Soc. Brew. Chem.* 63, 177–184.

Gunst, F. and Verzele, M. (1978). *J. Inst. Brew.* 84, 291–292.

Hastings, J.D., McGarrity, M.J., Bordeleau, L. and Thompson, J.D. (1992). *Abstracts of the Brewing Congress of the Americas*, September 1992, St. Louis, MO, USA, p. 97.

Heyerick, A., Zhao, Y., Sandra, P., Huvaere, K., Roelens, F. and De Keukeleire, D. (2003). *Photochem. Photobiol. Sci.* 2, 306–314.

Heyerick, A., Huvaere, K., Forbes, M.D.E. and De Keukeleire, D. (2005). *Photochem. Photobiol. Sci.* 4, 412–419.

Huvaere, K., Andersen, M.L., Skibsted, L.H., Heyerick, A. and De Keukeleire, D. (2003). *Chem. Eur. J.* 9, 4693–4699.

Huvaere, K., Olsen, K., Andersen, M.L., Skibsted, L.H., Heyerick, A. and De Keukeleire, D. (2004a). *Photochem. Photobiol. Sci.* 3, 337–340.

Huvaere, K., Sinnaeve, B., Van Bocxlaer, J. and De Keukeleire, D. (2004b). *Photochem. Photobiol. Sci.* 3, 854–858.

Huvaere, K., Andersen, M.L., Skibsted, L.H., Heyerick, A. and De Keukeleire, D. (2005). *J. Agric. Food Chem.* 53, 1489–1494.

Huvaere, K., Andersen, M.L., Storme, M., Van Bocxlaer, J., Skibsted, L.H. and De Keukeleire, D. (2006). *Photochem. Photobiol. Sci.* 5, 961–969.

Irwin, A.J., Bordeleau, L. and Barker, R.L. (1993). *J. Am. Soc. Brew. Chem.* 51, 1–3.

Kaneda, H., Kano, Y., Osawa, T., Ramarathnam, N., Kawakishi, S. and Kamada, K. (1988). *J. Food Sci.* 53, 885–888.

Kaneda, H., Takashio, M., Osawa, T., Kawakishi, S. and Tamaki, T. (1996). *J. Am. Soc. Brew. Chem.* 54, 115–120.

Kay, C.W.M., Feicht, R., Schulz, K., Sadewater, P., Sancar, A., Bacher, A., Möbius, K., Richter, G. and Weber, S. (1999). *Biochemistry* 51, 16740–16748.

Kuroiwa, Y. and Hashimoto, H. (1961). *Rep. Res. Lab Kirin Brew. Co. Ltd.* 4, 35–40.

Kuroiwa, Y., Hashimoto, N., Hashimoto, H., Kobuko, E. and Nakagawa, K. (1963). *Proc. Am. Soc. Brew. Chem.*, 181–193.

Laane, C., de Roo, G., van den Ban, E., Sjauw-En-Wa, M.-W., Duyvis, M.G., Hagen, W.A., van Berkel, W.J.H., Hilhorst, R., Schmedding, D.J.M. and Evans, D.J. (1999). *J. Inst. Brew.* 105, 392–397.

Lintner, C. (1875). *Lehrbuch der Bierbrauerei.* Verlag Vieweg und Sohn, Braunschweig, Germany. p. 343.

Maye, J.P., Mulqueen, S., Weiss, S., Xu, J. and Priest, M. (1999). *J. Am. Soc. Brew. Chem.* 57, 55–59.

Mottley, C., Toy, K. and Mason, R.P. (1987). *Mol. Pharmacol.* 31, 417–421.

Nøddekær, T. and Andersen, M.L. (2007). *J. Am. Soc. Brew. Chem.* 65, 15–20.

Rosen, G.M., Britigan, B.E., Halpern, H.J. and Pou, S. (1999). *Free Radicals. Biology and Detection by Spin Trapping.* Oxford University Press, New York.

Sakuma, S., Rikimaru, Y., Kobayashi, K. and Kowaka, M. (1991). *J. Am. Soc. Brew. Chem.* 49, 162–165.

Uchida, M. and Ono, M. (1996). *J. Am. Soc. Brew. Chem.* 54, 198–204.

Uchida, M. and Ono, M. (1999). *J. Am. Soc. Brew. Chem.* 57, 145–150.

Uchida, M. and Ono, M. (2000). *J. Am. Soc. Brew. Chem.* 58, 8–13.

Uchida, M., Suga, S. and Ono, M. (1996). *J. Am. Soc. Brew. Chem.* 54, 205–211.

Vanderhaegen, B., Neven, H., Verachtert, H. and Derdelinckx, G. (2006). *Food Chem.* 95, 357–381.

Vollenweider, J.K. and Paul, H. (1986). *Int. J. Chem. Kinet.* 18, 791–800.

102

Methods for Determining Ethanol in Beer

Domenica Tonelli Department of Physical and Inorganic Chemistry, University of Bologna, Viale Risorgimento, Bologna, Italy

Abstract

Ethanol, together with water and carbohydrates, is one of the main components of beer. Its concentration ranges from 0.05% (v/v) in alcohol free beers to about 12.5% in the strongest ones. An accurate and rapid determination of ethanol in beer is important for regulatory applications and process control in brewing industries, and on-line continuous monitoring is often desired. Classical methods such as refractometry, densitometry, or redox titration of the distilled sample, as well as gas chromatography, are routinely used in industry and in government control laboratories, but they are time- and labor-consuming procedures. To replace these techniques efforts have been made to develop methods with low-cost instrumentation and/or without complex sample pre-treatment. Biosensors based on alcohol oxidase and alcohol dehydrogenase enzymes have been fabricated and successfully applied to ethanol determination in alcoholic beverages. Furthermore, infrared spectroscopy in the mid- and near-infrared region as well as techniques such as flow injection have provided interesting possibilities to also automate ethanol determination.

List of Abbreviations

ADH	Alcohol dehydrogenase
AOX	Alcohol oxidase
ATR–FTIR	Attenuated total reflectance–Fourier transform infrared
CoPC	Cobalt phthalocyanine
CPE	Carbon paste electrodes
FIA	Flow injection analysis
GC	Gas chromatography
FID	Flame ionization detector
GD	Gas diffusion
GLC	Gas–liquid chromatography
HPLC	High performance liquid chromatography
HRP	Horseradish peroxidase
IR	Infrared
MB	Meldola's Blue
MGD	Membraneless gas diffusion
MIR	Mid-infrared
NAD	Nicotinamide adenine dinucleotide
NIR	Near-infrared
PAD	Pulsed amperometric detection
PV	Analytical pervaporation
SPE	Screen printed electrodes

Introduction

Beer is one of the oldest known alcoholic beverages, and is obtained by fermentation of cereals germinated in water in the presence of yeast. Fruits, herbs, and spices may also be used to give beer a particular character (Varnam and Sutherland, 1996). By 6000 BC, when the ancient cities of Mesopotamia were built, the brewing of beer was established. These beers would probably have been quite thick, higher in protein, lower in alcohol, and sweeter than those we are accustomed to today (Hughes and Baxter, 2001). The different combinations of ingredients, production processes, and storage conditions give rise to an enormous variety of beers – ales and lagers being defined as the two main types according to the conditions of their fermentation processes (Hughes and Baxter, 2001). There has been great interest in studying the chemical composition of beer, as this information is valuable for the assessment of beer quality and the development of new products. The main components of beers are water, carbohydrates, and ethanol. Ethanol content is an organoleptic parameter affecting both the beer classification (in term of taxes) and its taste (Varnam and Sutherland, 1996; Council Directive 92/84/EEC: OJ L 316, 1992, 31.10.1992 Bulletin, 10-1992). It is usually expressed in % (v/v). A range of other alcohols affect the flavor of beer, but they are present at levels at least two orders of magnitude lower than that of ethanol. Across the world, the alcohol content in beers ranges from less than 0.05% in alcohol free beers to a maximum of about 12.5% in the strongest beers. It has been recognized for a very long time that beer can make an important contribution to the diet. Beer contains an average of 0.2–0.6 g/100 ml of

Beer in Health and Disease Prevention
ISBN: 978-0-12-373891-2

protein-derived material, which is substantially more than other alcoholic beverages, such as wine (Pueyo *et al.*, 1993). Proteins and some amino acids are partially responsible for the nutritional value and stability of beer. In fact, they influence beer foam and haze stability. In addition, there are carbohydrates (3.3–4.4%) (Gallignani *et al.*, 1994), which have a marked influence on sweetness and can influence mouthfeel and sour and bitter perceptions, phenolic compounds such as cinnamic acids, benzoic acids, catechins, and flavonols which are responsible for beer flavor, physical stability, and antioxidant activity, organic acids (e.g. acetic, formic acids), bitter acids (isohumulones), and inorganic ions (Engelhard *et al.*, 2004). The range of inorganic compounds in beer is 0.5–2 g/l. It has been established that these minerals, which include major cations, trace metals and anions, influence both the taste and the clarity of the finished beer. The salt taste of beer is a direct consequence of the presence of inorganic anions and cations. Beer contains small amounts of vitamins of the B-group together with vitamins A, C, D, E, and K. Beer analysis is important for the evaluation of (i) organoleptic characteristics, (ii) quality, (iii) nutritional aspects, and (iv) safety, since beer is a biotechnological product having extraordinary economic implications. To optimize the brewing process, breweries have a strong interest in fast and easy quantification methods for the most important process and product parameters. Ethanol content is the single most important parameter for beer characterization. Nowadays, rapid and reliable determination of ethanol in a variety of samples has received much attention, since this compound plays an important role in clinical, food, and industrial analysis. Ethanol is the most common toxic substance involved in medical-legal cases, and is frequently a contributory factor in a variety of accidents. Usually, the pharmacological effects are observed at blood ethanol concentrations of about 10 mmol/l whereas lethal levels are 10 times this concentration (Liden *et al.*, 1998). The determination of ethanol in alcoholic beverages is a very important task due to its social and economical implications, particularly in relation to the taxes imposed in different countries on its use. This analysis is carried out in many laboratories, not only by producers, but also in government and customs laboratories.

Properties

The properties of ethanol are well known. It is a flammable liquid, its vapor concentrations being explosive in the range 3.3–19% (v/v) in air. Ethanol is clear and colorless with an odor and taste which are generally considered pleasant. It is reported to be detectable by nose at 350 ppm, while higher levels of about 5,000–10,000 ppm can cause irritation to the eyes and mucous membranes of the upper respiratory tract. Poisoning from ethanol normally comes from the consumption of alcoholic beverages, rather than from inhalation. Ethanol has marked hypnotic properties and depressive activity in the upper brain, which leads to changes in behavior including motor coordination, tolerance, dependence, and aggression even though it gives the initial impression of being a stimulant (Hunt, 1996). It can be toxic if consumed in excess (the lethal dose in rats is 13.7 g/kg) even if its toxicity is much lower than the superior homologs (Criddle, 1995). Its physical properties are reported in Table 102.1 and derive mainly from the presence of the hydroxyl group, which also determines the chemical properties of the compound.

Table 102.1 Physical and chemical properties of ethanol

Property	*Data*
Boiling point (1 atm)	78.5°C
Freezing point	−114.1°C
Flash point	9–11°C
Density (d_4^{20})	0.789 g/ml
Viscosity (20°C)	1.17 cP
Refractive index (n_D^{20})	1.361
Molecular weight	46.07
Solubility (water)	∞
pK_a	16

From the analytical point of view, the most important property is the ease by which the molecule can be oxidized to give acetaldehyde and, in some cases, acetic acid according to the pathway: $CH_3CH_2OH \rightarrow CH_3CHO \rightarrow CH_3COOH$.

Analysis of Ethanol

Many methods have been reported for ethanol determination. Traditionally, government legal requirements, taken together or separately, usually determine the choice of the method. These methods are essentially based on the following techniques: (i) distillation followed by physical or chemical measurements, (ii) chromatography, (iii) infrared spectrometry, (iv) enzyme methods, and (v) flow injection. Some of them are relatively expensive, time consuming, complex to perform and require laborious sample pre-treatment. Thus, there is an increasing demand for inexpensive, rapid, and reliable methods for ethanol determination. Electrochemical techniques, especially those employing sensitive amperometric biosensors, are particularly suited to this kind of analysis.

Distillation

The current official methods approved by the Excise authorities in most countries for determining alcohol content are based on physical measurements (usually, density or refractive index) carried out after a previous distillation of the sample, to separate the alcohol. As an example, the procedure adopted by the Analytical Division of the European

Brewery Convention for the determination of ethanol is based on the distillation of the beer, which has been first shaken and then filtered to remove dissolved CO_2, and the measurement of the density (D), after making up to a standardized final volume, of the distillate (European Brewery Convention, 1987). The density of the distillate is usually measured by traditional methods, such as the density bottle, pycnometer or hydrometer, or more frequently using electromagnetically induced oscillation techniques. These techniques are based on the principle that when a column of a liquid, at constant temperature, is electromagnetically excited, its period of oscillation (T), determined by comparison with a reference frequency produced by a crystal oscillator, is related to its density by the relationship: $D = A(T^2 - B)$, where A and B are calibration constants. The results of this method are unaffected by viscosity, volatility, or turbidity of the sample (Criddle, 1995). In case refractometry is used to quantitate ethanol, calibration curves are obtained from readings carried out on solutions with different alcohol percentages, against doubly distilled water (Gales, 1990). These methods are usually time consuming, require some kind of sample preparation and often well-trained laboratory staff, and are slow and difficult to automate. Moreover, they are macro-major methods and require a large sample and a quite high alcoholic degree. Alternatively, ethanol content can be estimated by chemical methods, such as simple volumetric redox titrations based on oxidation with chromium(VI) (Pilone, 1985) or xenon trioxide (Jaselskis and Warriner, 1966) or spectrophotometric assays (Caputi Jr. *et al.*, 1968; Hart and Fisher, 1971; Lau and Luk, 1994). It is common knowledge that potassium dichromate oxidizes ethanol to acetic acid. This reaction is used in the analysis of wines and beverages followed by the titrimetric dosage of the acetic acid formed (or of the excess of added dichromate with ferrous ammonium sulfate), but the above-mentioned problems of rapidity, specificity, and sensitivity are not resolved. Spectrophotometric methods for the determination of ethanol, being more sensitive, require a smaller quantity of sample (e.g. 1 ml) and allow to quantitate a lower alcohol content in beverages (e.g. less than 1%). However, these methods are also not selective and, requiring the distillation of the sample, are subject to the quantitative recovery of distillate. Magrì *et al.* (1997) described a spectrophotometric method based on the measure of chromium(VI) consumed by the reaction with ethanol, estimated by the decrease of the absorbance at 267 nm. The reaction is complete in about 15 min at room temperature and the method was successfully applied to the analysis of micro-samples of commercial beverages (beers, wines, and spirits) without the previous distillation of ethanol.

Chromatography

Various instrumental methods have been proposed to provide a direct determination of ethanol, based on gas chromatography (GC) (Caputi Jr. and Mooney, 1983; Cutaia, 1984) and liquid chromatography (Morawski *et al.*, 1983; Iwachido, 1986; Calull *et al.*, 1992). The use of gas–liquid chromatography (GLC) as a general analytical technique is now well established and it is rare to find a modern analytical laboratory without such equipment. Due to its volatility, ethanol lends itself to analysis by GLC with flame ionization detector (FID) since this detection is insensible to water. Polar columns of poly(ethyleneglycol) are generally used, and quantitation is performed by the internal standard technique using one of the propanols as standard (Gales, AOAC, 1990). Advantages of GLC are selectivity and high speed of analysis, compared with distillation. Furthermore, accuracy and precision are the same or even better than distillation. GLC is now accepted as a standard procedure for beer analysis in the United States and is the most common preferred method used for ethanol determination (Ough and Amerine, 1988). However, GLC equipment is still relatively expensive, requires skilled operators and often laboratory sample pre-treatment. Since a rapid method with a high degree of automation and cost-effectiveness is of considerable importance in the beverage mass-production industry, several techniques, aimed to simplify the complex and time-consuming classical procedures for analysis of alcoholic content, have been elaborated in the last few years.

Infrared spectroscopy

Quantitative analysis using optical spectroscopy is based on the Beer-Lambert Law, which states that there is a linear relationship between how much light is absorbed by a sample and the product of the concentration of the absorbing species and its pathlength. Infrared (IR) spectrometry in the mid-infrared (MIR) and the near-infrared (NIR) provides interesting possibilities for the direct determination of ethanol in beverages. By using the transmission mode, NIR spectroscopy offers the possibility of carrying out the determination employing ordinary glass or quartz cells. On the other hand, in the mid-range, it is necessary to use cells equipped with water-resistant windows and very small pathlengths ($b \leq 50\,\mu m$), to reduce the high absorption of infrared radiation by water (Gallignani *et al.*, 2005). Beers are aqueous solutions: as a consequence, only the spectral region in which water does not present significant absorption can be used for analytical purposes. In the mid-range, this region ranges between 3,050 and 800 cm^{-1}, except the CO_2 region comprised between 2,382 and 2,314 cm^{-1} (Llario *et al.*, 2006).

Figure 102.1 shows the spectrum obtained by attenuated total reflectance Fourier transform infrared spectroscopy (ATR–FTIR) of four different types of beers. They were recorded with samples of beer degassed for 5 min and filtered before filling the ATR cell.

In the spectrum of the beer without alcohol a series of bands between 1,200 and 950 cm^{-1} can be observed,

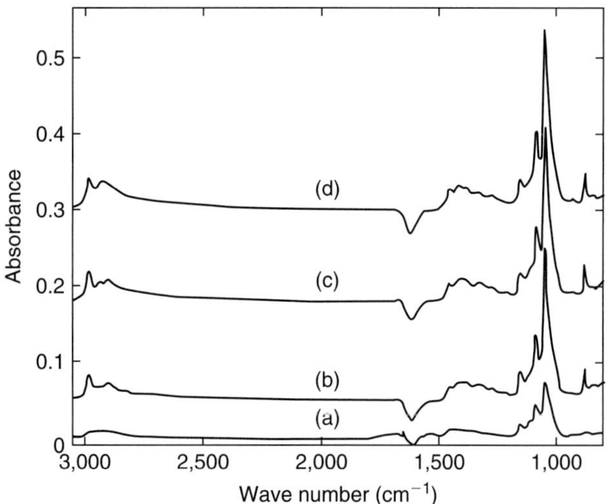

Figure 102.1 ATR–FTIR spectra of main types of beer samples: (a) beer without alcohol; (b) normal beer; (c) 100% malt beer; and (d) German beer. Spectra were shifted in the absorbance axis for clarity purposes. Reprinted with permission from Llario *et al.* (2006). Copyright: Elsevier.

corresponding to C—C and C—O vibration in carbohydrates, which may be correlated to the real and original extracts. The German beer is the sample with the highest extract value, and it can be seen that the band in the sugar region is the highest one. On the other hand, the sample without alcohol has the lowest extract value, and accordingly it has the lowest absorption in the aforementioned spectral region. In the region above 2,600 cm^{-1} the bands observed correspond to aliphatic vibrations, which are ascribed to stretching fundamental and deformation combination bands of methylene groups. When comparing the spectrum of the beer without alcohol to that of a normal beer, it can be observed that the main differences correspond to the bands located at 875 cm^{-1} (in-phase C—C—O stretching), 1,052 cm^{-1} (out-of-phase C—C—O stretching), 1,800 cm^{-1} (C—C skeletal stretching), and 2,970 cm^{-1} (asymmetric stretching band of methyl group), due to the absorbance of ethanol. Therefore, in all instances, special attention has to be paid to the presence of sugars in the sample, which leads to an important interfering effect on the analytical bands of ethanol. To solve this analytical problem, different strategies have been proposed, for example, based on the use of derivative FTIR. The method is based on first-order derivative FTIR measurements between the peak at 1,052 cm^{-1} and the valley at 1,040 cm^{-1} (see Figure 102.1) by using a micro-flow transmittance cell with ZnSe windows. It provides accurate results in the determination of ethanol in beer without requiring any previous chemical treatment of the sample or previous separation or extraction step. The limit of detection corresponds to 0.025% (v/v) and results obtained in the analysis of real samples of beer agree with those found by different reference procedures. For the determination of ethanol in beverages containing high concentrations of sugars, it is necessary, previously, to determine the sugar content by measuring the derivative value between 1,164 and 1,147 cm^{-1} and, subsequently, to correct the negative interference of sugars on the determination of ethanol between 1,052 and 1,040 cm^{-1} (Gallignani *et al.*, 1994).

With the purpose to definitively avoid the interfering effect of sugars, a new approach has been proposed by Gallignani *et al.* (2005), which involves the separation of the analyte from the matrix by means of a liquid–liquid extraction. The methodological proposal for the determination of ethanol in all types of alcoholic beverages includes the quantitative on-line liquid–liquid extraction of ethanol with chloroform, through a sandwich type cell equipped with a poly(tetraflu oroethylene) membrane, using a two-channel manifold and direct measurement of the analyte in the organic phase, by means of FTIR. The quantification is carried out by measuring the ethanol absorbance at 877 cm^{-1}, corrected by means of a baseline established between 844 and 929 cm^{-1}. The procedure, which does not require any sample pre-treatment, except for the simple degassing of beer, has been applied to determine ethanol in different alcoholic beverages such as beers, wines, and spirits. The results obtained highly agree with those obtained by a derivative FTIR spectrometric procedure and by headspace-GC with FID detection. Moreover, the consumption of chloroform is very low (about 20 ml/h) and the solvent could be easily recycled through its distillation. This method is simple, fast, precise, and accurate, and it can be easily adapted to any infrared spectrometer equipped with a standard transmission infrared cell. As a consequence, it represents a valid alternative for the determination of ethanol in alcoholic beverages, and could be suitable for routine control analysis.

In the last decade, NIR spectroscopy has become an important analytical tool as it normally requires little sample preparation, is inexpensive, and can be performed quickly. Infrared quantitative analyses typically involve the measurement of many samples with varying concentrations, known as the training set. A calibration is calculated from these spectra. This may be a simple curve, or may involve chemometric procedures like partial least square regression or multilinear regression to build up the calibration models. The calibration is normally based on the correlation between the absorbances of the samples at certain wavelengths and the target molecule concentrations in the calibration set, usually obtained by reference analysis.

From this calibration, the concentration of the substance in an unknown sample may be predicted. A calibration set is needed because the presence of another component can affect the spectrum of the compound of interest, and these procedures account for the resulting non-linearity in spectral response. A chemical case where this non-linearity is most pronounced, and therefore whose analysis needs special care, is in hydrogen-bonded systems, for instance, alcohols and water, as it occurs in beer. The absorption properties

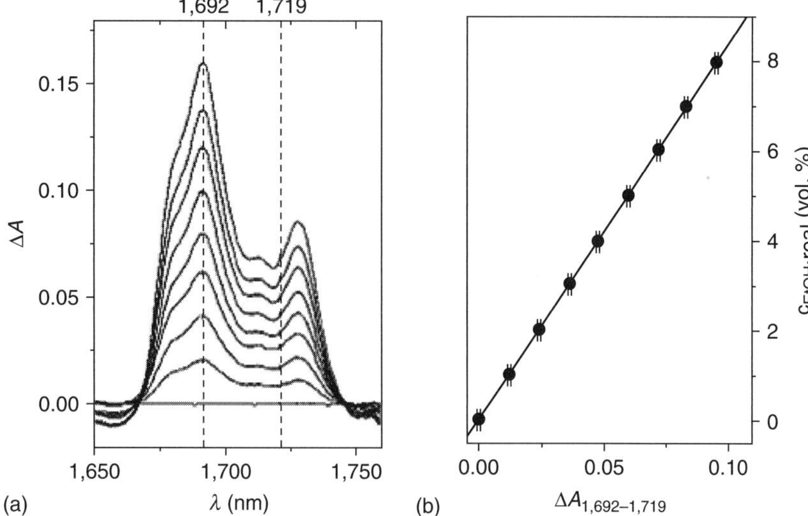

Figure 102.2 (a) NIR absorption difference spectra of ethanol/water mixtures with ethanol concentration of 0–8% (reference: water, d = 1 cm). (b) Correlation of the difference of absorbances at 1692 and 1719 nm, $\Delta A_{1,692-1,719}$, with $c_{EtOH,real}$. Reprinted with permission from Engelhard *et al.* (2004). Copyright: Society for Applied Spectroscopy.

of beer in the NIR spectral range are strongly dominated by the absorption of water and the other two main constituents, namely ethanol and carbohydrates. Maltose is considered as the representative carbohydrate because it is the major sugar in beer and the main building block for dextrins, which are the most important class of carbohydrates. Thus, for the interpretation of the NIR absorption spectra of beer, the knowledge of the NIR spectra of water, ethanol, and maltose is essential. The work of Engelhard *et al.* (2004) provides an interesting review on the assays used for alcohol determination and proposes a quantification method based on the interpretative difference of the absorption of radiation in the NIR spectral region using univariate statistics. The so-called "interpretative spectroscopy" has gained interest in recent years. Workman Jr. (1996) described several conditions to be fulfilled by an analytical method based on interpretative spectroscopy.

The bands used for the quantification of the analyte should have a known molecular assignment and the measured signal must be highly correlated with the analyte without interference. Furthermore, independence from other sample properties is essential.

Engelhard *et al.* (2004) validated their method by analyzing various beer samples with an ethanol concentration range between 0.5% and 8%. The method requires less expense in calibration and spectrometric equipment. The absorption was evaluated in the region of the first overtone of CH vibrations. For ethanol the two peaks at 1,684 and 1,692 nm are caused by the first overtone of the two CH_3 asymmetric stretching modes, whereas the features at 1,714 and 1,719 nm are assigned to CH_2 asymmetric stretching and CH_3 symmetric stretching vibrations, respectively. It is of particular advantage that the overall absorbance here is low enough (typically 2.5 with an optical pathlength of 1 cm) that samples of beer as such can be investigated in standard 1 cm cuvettes, which facilitates sample handling in routine analysis. To distinguish ethanol absorption from the carbohydrate background, measurements at a minimum of two wavelengths are necessary.

The two wavelengths were selected according to the assignment of the absorption bands of the main substances contained in beer in the NIR region, that is water, ethanol, and maltose, and the difference between the absorbances at these wavelengths was used for ethanol quantification. The wavelength pair at 1,692 and 1,719 nm was chosen: at 1,692 nm ethanol displays an absorbance maximum significantly over the 1,719 nm level, whereas the maltose absorption is equal at both wavelengths. The difference of absorbances between these wavelengths is proportional to the ethanol content of beer, but independent of its carbohydrate content.

As an example, Figure 102.2 shows the NIR absorption difference spectra of ethanol/water mixtures with ethanol concentration ranging from 0% to 8% used by Engelhard *et al.* (2004) to perform calibration. The limit of detection was 0.07 vol. %.

As the calibration is independent of the individual properties of the respective kinds of beer, this NIR spectroscopic method is very well suited to supplement fast process control in breweries.

Enzyme methods

For the analysis of ethanol in alcohol free and low alcohol beers, enzymatic procedures using different detection techniques such as fluorimetry, spectrophotometry or electrochemistry provide very sensitive and accurate methods. Enzymes, being essential components of living systems, catalyze almost all chemical reactions that take place in biological processes: they are flexible protein biocatalysts with very well-defined binding sites for the substrate. Many enzymes require the presence of a cofactor that may be firmly attached to the protein or may be added, in which case it is termed coenzyme. In food analysis, enzymatic assays are often carried out because of their high specificity. Furthermore, the ability of a single enzyme molecule to catalyze the conversion of a lot of substrate molecules provides an amplification effect, which enhances the sensitivity of the analysis. Enzymes are the most commonly employed catalytic reagents in analytical chemistry. They are usually used in an immobilized form so that they can be repeatedly used, with a consequent decrease in the cost of the analysis. When an enzyme or a biologically derived sensing element is either integrated or in intimate contact with a physicochemical transducer, the device is named a biosensor. The biochemical transducer converts the analyte into a chemical and/or physical property which is sensed and converted into a proper signal by the physical transducer. Enzymatic redox reactions are particularly related to electrochemical transducers, since an electron transfer is involved in the reaction mechanism of the enzyme. The physical combination of immobilized enzymes and electrodes can be accomplished in several ways: the enzyme is (i) immobilized in a membrane which is held in close proximity to the electrode surface, (ii) immobilized directly on the electrode surface, (iii) immobilized in an electrically conducting matrix, such as carbon–oil mixture, known as the carbon paste electrode (CPE). The enzyme substrate diffuses from the solution to the electrode surface, reaching the enzyme active site where it undergoes the enzymatic reaction. The product of the reaction will in turn diffuse to the electrode surface where the analytical reaction will take place. The determination of ethanol in beverages is carried out both by addition of the enzyme to the sample solution (commercial kits) and, more frequently, by means of a biosensor. Biosensors can be considered a big group of devices used to simplify methods of alcohol determination in beverages. Besides sensitivity and selectivity, biosensors have some advantages such as a simple measurement procedure and a short response time, which allow measurements both in batch and in flow conditions. Many reports on immobilized enzyme alcohol biosensors have appeared after Nanjo and Guilbault (1975) developed the first amperometric alcohol biosensor. In addition to the above-mentioned features, electrochemical amperometric biosensors have low cost and potential for miniaturization (Santos *et al.*, 2003). The great number of commercially available enzymes together with many kinds of immobilization techniques of several reagents and biological catalysts over different supports have contributed to the development of enzymatic electrodes (Gorton, 1995). Two enzymes are extensively used in the determination of ethanol, namely alcohol oxidase (AOX) and alcohol dehydrogenase (ADH), and alcohol oxidase–peroxidase coupled enzyme systems and biosensors based on microbial or plant tissue materials have also been developed, as reported in the literature (Akyilmaz and Dinckaya, 2003).

ADH Biosensors Ethanol is oxidized to acetaldehyde using nicotinamide adenine dinucleotide (NAD^+) and ADH, according to the reaction:

$$CH_3CH_2OH + NAD^+ \rightleftarrows CH_3CHO + NADH + H^+$$

The equilibrium lies toward ethanol but it is easily displaced to acetaldehyde formation by increasing the pH or removing acetaldehyde. The produced NADH is generally determined by measuring its absorbance at 334, 340, or 365 nm, or amperometrically. Alcohol biosensors based on ADH usually exhibit high selectivity and are oxygen independent; however, due to the need to add the coenzyme NAD^+ to the sample, ethanol determination is quite expensive with such biosensors. Moreover, NAD^+ needs to be close to the enzyme, without becoming irreversibly entrapped or linked (Azevedo *et al.*, 2005). Even more important, ADH-based sensors show limited operational stability and require high overpotential for the electrochemical oxidation of NADH to occur, as reported by Rebelo *et al.* (1994). These high potentials can cause interference from other electroactive substances present in beer samples. Furthermore, the intermediates produced during the oxidation can lead to electrode fouling. For this reason, various inorganic and organic mediators have been proposed for the electrochemical oxidation of NADH (Santos *et al.*, 2002). The above-mentioned problems can lead to a decrease in sensitivity, although it has been demonstrated that incorporation of NAD^+ into the conductive matrix of carbon paste overcomes the problems for some biosensors based on ADH. Santos *et al.* (2003) have described a reagentless amperometric biosensor for direct measurement of ethanol in a great variety of alcoholic beverages, including beer. The sensor was based on a CPE modified with ADH, NAD^+ cofactor, and Meldola's Blue (MB) adsorbed on silica gel coated with niobium oxide. The MB mediator showed excellent stability, improvement in the electrochemical activity, allowing the electro-oxidation of NADH at an applied potential of 0.0 V vs. saturated calomel electrode. Furthermore, the biosensor showed a wide linear response range (from 0.1 to 10 mM), an excellent operational stability (95% of the activity was maintained after 300 determinations) and storage stability (more than 3 months, when stored in a refrigerator).

AOX Biosensors In case of AOX, a flavoprotein, ethanol is oxidized in the presence of oxygen to give hydrogen peroxide according to the reaction:

$$CH_3CH_2OH + O_2 \rightarrow CH_3CHO + H_2O_2$$

AOX is an oligomeric enzyme consisting of eight identical sub-units arranged in a quasi-cubic geometry, each containing a strongly bound cofactor, flavin adenine dinucleotide molecule. AOX exhibits an inherent non-selectivity since other primary alcohols are enzymatically converted. For the analysis of beer, this property is not limitative because of the high concentration ratio of ethanol in respect to other alcohols. Due to the strong oxidizing character of oxygen, the oxidation of alcohols by AOX is irreversible. The classical way to follow a reaction catalyzed by AOX is to monitor the production of hydrogen peroxide or the consumption of O_2 (Azevedo *et al.*, 2005). The consumption of oxygen can be measured by optical detection but, more commonly, it is estimated amperometrically with a Clark-type O_2 electrode (Clark Jr. and Lyons, 1962). The cell consists of a platinum disk cathodic electrode inserted in a centrally located cylindrical insulator, which is surrounded by a ring-shaped Ag anode, at its bottom. The insulator and the electrodes are mounted inside a second cylinder which contains a buffered solution of potassium chloride. A thin gas permeable membrane, through which O_2 diffuses, is held at the bottom end of the tube by an *O*-ring. When the platinum electrode is poised at −600 mV (vs. Ag/AgCl), the reduction of oxygen occurs and a current proportional to its concentration is recorded. The first AOX-based biosensor for measuring ethanol concentration consisted in a Clark-type electrode covered by a membrane onto which AOX was immobilized by cross-linking with glutaraldehyde (Nanjo and Guilbault, 1975). The signal output of the electrode is the difference between the value recorded for base O_2 level and the decreased value, obtained after the enzymatic reaction has occurred. The amperometric biosensors which are based on the measurement of the depletion of oxygen do not suffer from the interference of other sample constituents. The major drawback is related to the dependence on oxygen which reduces the accuracy and reproducibility of the measurement, and to the fact that the minimum detectable concentration is not very low since the background signal of the device is high. The Clark-type electrode can be used also to monitor the production of H_2O_2. In such a case, the Pt working electrode is poised at a positive potential (+600 mV vs. Ag/AgCl) to oxidize hydrogen peroxide (see Figure 102.3).

Enzyme electrodes based on the direct detection of H_2O_2 constitute the so-called first generation of biosensors (see Figure 102.4a). After the pioneering work by Guilbault and Lubrano (1974) many other sensors were developed based on the direct detection of H_2O_2 using enzyme-membrane electrodes. More recently, carbon paste electrodes and screen printed electrodes have been developed using different immobilization procedures. These kinds of biosensors have many advantages such as the relative ease of manufacturing, wide linear range of response, but suffer from the interference of other reducing compounds present in the samples to be analyzed, due to the rather high working potential

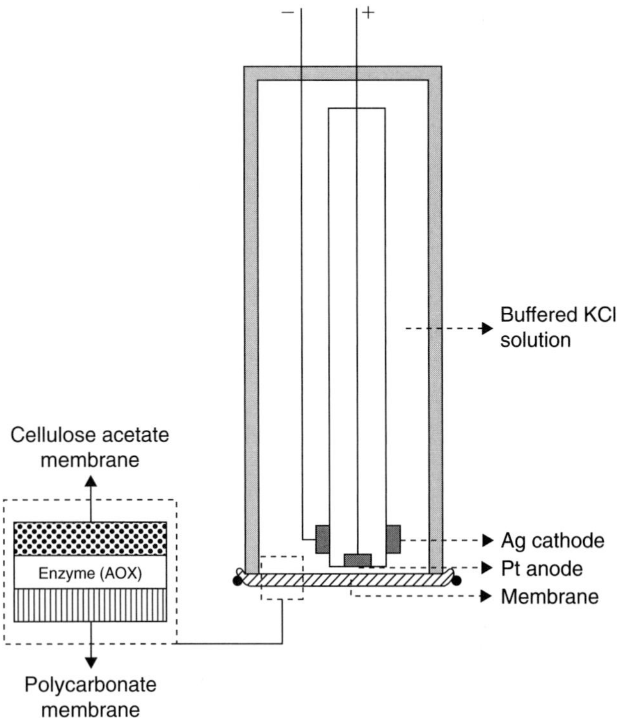

Figure 102.3 Schematic representation of an AOX-based biosensor of the first generation which exploits the production of H_2O_2 detected by a Clark-type electrode, modified with a membrane containing the enzyme, used to monitor the production of H_2O_2.The Pt working electrode is poised at a positive potential (+600 mV vs. Ag/AgCl) to oxidize hydrogen peroxide according to: $H_2O_2 \rightarrow O_2 + 2H^+ + 2e^-$.

that has to be applied for the oxidation of the enzymatically generated H_2O_2. A way to overcome the problem related to the direct detection of H_2O_2 is to decrease the applied potential by modifying the electrode with an electrocatalyst for the oxidation of H_2O_2 (see Figure 102.4b) or to use a bienzymatic electrode construction. In the latter approach AOX is used in combination with horseradish peroxidase (HRP), an enzyme capable of catalyzing the electroreduction of H_2O_2 to H_2O at low applied potentials (0 to +200 mV), even in the presence of soluble oxygen, as demonstrated by Kulis *et al.* (1981). Since then many other bienzyme electrodes with oxidases and peroxidases have been proposed using either direct or mediated electron transfer. Boujtita *et al.* (2000) have fabricated a disposable amperometric biosensor for the measurement of ethanol in beer based on a cobalt phthalocyanine (CoPC) modified screen printed carbon electrode coated with AOX and a permselective membrane (polycarbonate or nitrocellulose acetate). CoPC acts as electrocatalyst for the oxidation of H_2O_2 produced by the enzymatic reaction, and the reduced form of Co is oxidized at +400 mV vs. Ag/AgCl. The electrochemical regeneration of Co^{2+} provides the analytical signal, the magnitude of which is directly related to the amount of ethanol in the beer sample. The permselective

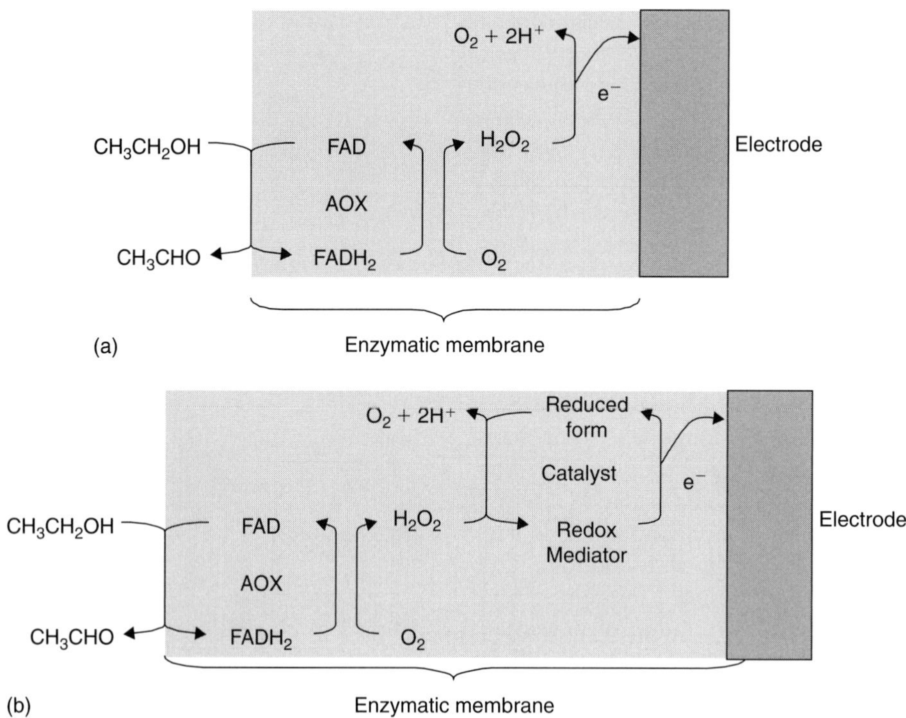

Figure 102.4 Reaction scheme for the catalytic oxidation of ethanol by AOX with (a) direct and (b) mediated hydrogen peroxide detection.

membrane on the surface of the biosensor acts as a barrier to interferents present in solution. The measurement procedure consist of a simple dilution of the sample in phosphate buffer and the determination of ethanol was carried out from a pre-constructed calibration graph, by recording the steady-state current. To test the possibility of using the device in the field, that is outside of the laboratory, the authors also tested chronoamperometry to determine ethanol in the same samples of beer, obtaining good results. In such a case, small volumes of beer samples were deposited on the printed strip to cover both the working and the reference electrode, and the response was recorded, applying the same potential of +400 mV vs. Ag/AgCl. It is worth mentioning that screen printed technology is gaining popularity in biosensors construction since it offers the possibility of mass-producing biosensors at low cost. Taking into account that robust, durable, and reusable biosensors are highly desired for the determination of alcohols in food and beverages, Guzmán-Vázques de Prada *et al.* (2003) have proposed composite graphite–Teflon electrodes incorporating the AOX enzyme coupled with HRP as well as the redox mediator ferrocene. These were constructed by simple and rapid physical inclusion of the enzymes and ferrocene in the bulk of rigid cylindrical pellets of the mixture graphite–70% Teflon, which are easily renewable by polishing with SiC paper. Furthermore, the absence of membranes on the electrode surface and the closeness of the enzymes and redox mediator to the electrode material allow fast responses both in batch and in flow-through conditions. The bienzymatic electrode operates by applying to the working electrode a potential of 0.00 V vs. Ag/AgCl/KCl (3 M) and recording the steady-state current in stirred solutions of diluted samples of beer. The time needed for the analysis of each sample is about 5 min. An interference study was carried out taking into account the substances that may be present, such as lactic and ascorbic acid (added as antioxidant), and citric, malic, and acetic acids which are used in some beers as flavoring agents. Neither malic acid nor citric acid affected the ethanol amperometric response of the bienzyme sensor, while a negative error was found for lactic and acetic acids, due to the fact that AOX catalyzes their oxidation also. Ascorbic acid also affects the ethanol response, but in this case the interference arises from its electrochemical oxidation at the applied potential. Nevertheless, the usual concentrations of these substances in beer are much lower than those necessary to produce a significant error in ethanol determination. The composite electrode was used for the analysis of different kinds of beer at low, medium, and high ethanol concentration, working both in batch and in flow modes, and the results were in agreement with those obtained with a commercial enzymatic kit using a colorimetric detection. The same bienzymatic system has been used in the development of commercial colorimetric alcohol sensors to estimate blood ethanol by detection of alcohol in breath or saliva (Adams, 1988). Other cases that require fast and reliable methods for ethanol determination will surely

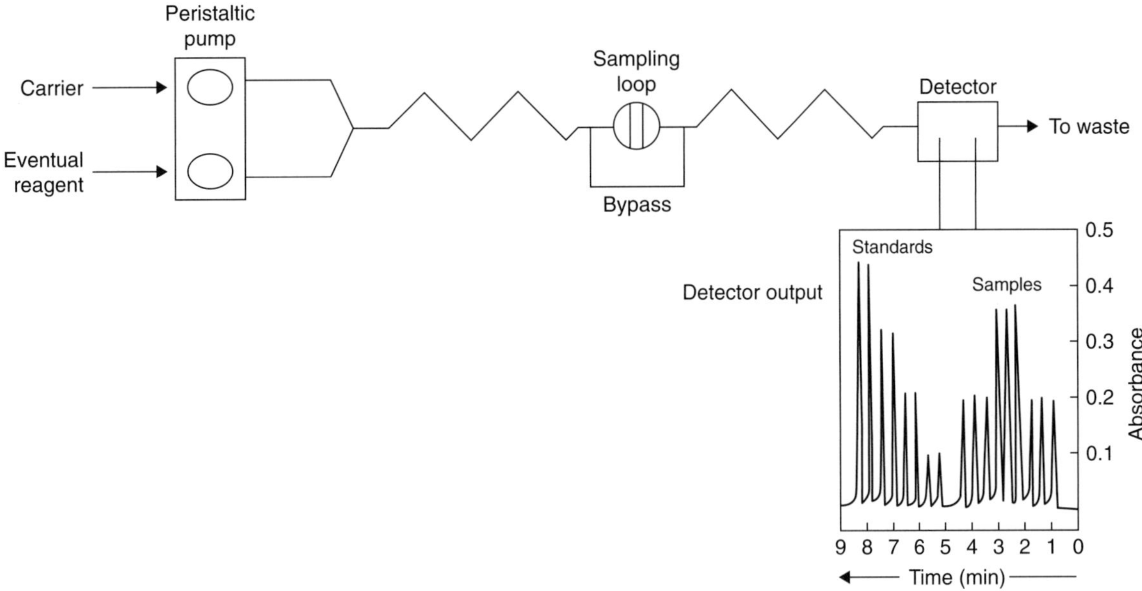

Figure 102.5 Schematic diagram of a flow injection apparatus. Samples and eventual reagents are transported through flexible plastic tubing by the action of a peristaltic pump. The most satisfactory injection systems are based on sampling loops similar to those used in liquid chromatography. The quantitative determination of the analyte is performed by injecting fixed volumes of standards and samples.

benefit from the commercial development of more AOX-based sensors.

Flow injection

A great deal of effort has been devoted to the automation of ethanol determination by flow analysis techniques. A simple scheme of a flow injection apparatus with the recorder output is reported in Figure 102.5.

Amperometric detection in flow systems is an appealing approach due to its high sensitivity, low cost, and high speed of analysis. During the last two decades of the previous century, much work has been carried out to develop electrochemical detectors for liquid chromatography with high sensitivity and low detection limits. Various metal electrodes can be used for the oxidation of ethanol, but they suffer from a rapid loss of activity due to a fouling of the surface by accumulation of reaction products. Pulsed amperometric detection (PAD) after dual-pulse clean-up of the electrode has been widely used for detection of alcohols in high performance liquid chromatography (HPLC). The PAD technique applies brief oxidative and reductive potential pulses to the working electrode to clean and activate the surface between steps to an intermediate potential for detection. Fung and Mo (1996) described a procedure for ethanol determination in beer based on flow injection dual-pulse staircase voltammetry with a Pt electrode in 0.1 M sodium hydroxide. Amperometric detection of ethanol in several alcoholic beverages by anodic oxidation in alkaline media on a copper/copper oxide electrode in flow injection systems has been reported by Paixão *et al.* (2002). It was verified to be in a good agreement with the results obtained by an alternative GC technique and labeled data, and the method has been found suitable for industrial applications. Recently, many reports on the application of chemically modified electrodes as amperometric detectors in flow systems have been published. As an example, Warriner *et al.* (2002) have proposed a Pt reagentless electrochemical sensor with a poly-L-lysine and PVC overlaying membrane, based on PAD, for monitoring ethanol formation during fermentation process. By using this configuration, problems associated with pH dependency of ethanol oxidation and interference from electroactive sugars were addressed. Biological recognition has been also successfully utilized in analytical flow techniques to increase selectivity. The enzymes have been commonly immobilized on a solid support contained in a small column or bound onto an electrode to be used as biosensors with electrochemical transduction. The linear range of enzymatic measurements is limited by the saturation kinetics of the respective enzyme. For this reason, most of the samples have to be diluted prior to analysis: this is an additional source of error, especially for gas-containing beverages such as beer. A further source of error is the interference caused by other chemical compounds within the sample. This drawback can be overcome by a separation technique. For volatile or semi-volatile compounds, separation of these species from the matrix is conveniently performed in flow injection using two types of membrane-based apparatus: gas diffusion (GD) or analytical pervaporation (PV) unit. Inside the GD unit, a hydrophobic membrane is normally fitted to allow passive transfer of gaseous compound from one side (donor stream) to the other side of the membrane (acceptor stream). In this way, selective detection of partially diffusible volatiles is accomplished (Pacey and Karlberg, 1989). Baadenhuisen and Seuren Jacobs (1979) introduced GD via hydrophobic membranes to flow injection analysis (FIA) and thus minimized interferences. Kindervater *et al.* (1990) optimized an amperometric FIA system and modified GD membranes to determine ethanol in beverages, without prior dilution. In all cases, the specificity of the detection system used was significantly increased by the use of a GD unit. PV is also a membrane-based kit for on-line separation of volatile compounds from donor to acceptor stream and is perfectly compatible with flow-based measurements. Pervaporation is a non-chromatographic membrane-based separation technique which has been employed for a long time in the industrial field: it selectively separates a liquid mixture by partial vaporization through a nonporous polymeric membrane. The separation is not based on relative volatilities, as in the case of distillation, but rather on the relative rates of permeation through the membrane. PV can be defined as the combination of evaporation and GD in a single module. Although the principle of PV is similar to GD, a constant volume of air gap is usually maintained between the level of donor solution and the membrane (Luque De Castro and Papaefstathiou, 1988). PV offers some advantages over GD, when applied to liquid suspension samples, because the membrane does not come into direct contact with samples. This prolongs the lifetime of the membrane. Recently, a flow analysis-pervaporation method for the determination of ethanol in beverages using vibrating tube density detector has been described, reporting a sample throughput of 15 samples/h (Gonzales *et al.*, 2003). In the case of the vibrating tube density detector either a straight or more usually a U-shaped tube causes mechanical resonant vibrations. The square of the resonance frequency is inversely proportional to the sum of the mass of tube and tube content. As both the tube mass and the tube inner volume are known values, the vibrating tube method allows the density of unknown fluids to be determined in a single measurement, after the instrument has been calibrated with two fluids, usually water and air, which give low and high tones for high and low density, respectively. The U-tube is kept oscillating continuously at the characteristic frequency, which depends on the density of the filled-in sample. The oscillation period is measured and converted into density by the equation of the mass-spring model: $f = 1/2\pi\sqrt{[c/(M + \rho V)]}$, where f, frequency; c, spring constant; M, mass; ρ, density; and V, volume. Although GD and PV units are very useful for selective analysis of volatile species, they are rather expensive, especially when membranes have to often be changed. In a very recent paper, Choengchan *et al.* (2006) have presented a new diffusion unit, named membraneless gas diffusion (MGD), since it does not employ a hydrophobic membrane, for the separation and collection of ethanol. In the MGD method the reaction between ethanol vapor and dichromate in acidic solution leads to the production of chromium (III), which is monitored spectrophotometrically at 590 nm. The MGD unit provides a greater mass transfer than GD unit and, having no membrane, it does not suffer from membrane malfunction caused by exposure to reagents, and its cost is lower. The authors have demonstrated the validity of the MGD unit for quantitative analysis of ethanol in alcoholic beverages.

Summary Points

- It is well known that beer can make an important contribution to the diet.
- Ethanol has marked hypnotic properties and depressive activity in the upper brain, even though it gives the initial impression of being a stimulant.
- The determination of ethanol in alcoholic beverages is a very important task, due to its social and economical implications.
- Classical methods of analysis are based on distillation followed by chemical titrations, or by measurements of density or refractive index.
- Nowadays, an instrumental technique, GC, is generally preferred for direct determination of ethanol, since classical methods are more time consuming.
- Rapid and cheap methods with a high degree of automation are especially desired by the brewery industry and by government and customs laboratories.
- Infrared spectrometry, especially in NIR and MIR regions, is a more recent technique which provides interesting possibilities for the direct determination of ethanol.
- Methods based on enzymatic reactions in solution are rapid and selective, but expensive.
- Biosensors based on different detection techniques, such as fluorimetry, spectrophotometry or electrochemistry, are tools which allow sensitive, accurate, and cheaper determinations.
- Flow analysis technique with amperometric or spectrophotometric detection is an appealing approach for the automation of ethanol analysis in beer.

References

Adams, E.C. (1988). Methods of preparing a test strip for alcohol testing. Patent No. 4 786 569, USA.

Akyilmaz, E. and Dinckaya, E. (2003). *Talanta* 61, 113–118.

Azevedo, A.M., Prazeres, D.M.F., Cabral, J.M.S. and Fonseca, L.P. (2005). *Biosens. Bioelectron.* 21, 235–247.

Baadenhuisen, H. and Seuren Jacobs, H.E. (1979). *Clin. Chem.* 25, 443–445.

Boujtita, M., Hart, J.P. and Pittson, R. (2000). *Biosens. Bioelectron.* 15, 257–263.

Calull, M., Lopez, E., Marce, R.M., Olucha, J.C. and Borrull, F. (1992). *J. Chromatogr.* 589, 151–158.

Caputi Jr., A. and Mooney, D.P. (1983). *J. Assoc. Off. Anal. Chem.* 66, 1152–1157.

Caputi Jr., A., Veda, M. and Brown, T. (1968). *Am. J. Enol. Vitic.* 19, 160–165.

Choengchan, N., Mantim, T., Wilairat, P., Dasgupta, P.K., Motomizu, S. and Nacapricha, D. (2006). *Anal. Chim. Acta* 579, 33–37.

Clark Jr., L.C. and Lyons, C. (1962). *Ann. NY Acad. Sci.* 102, 29–45.

Criddle, W.J. (1995). In Townshend, A. (ed.), *"Ethanol". Encyclopedia of Analytical Science*, Vol. 2. Academic Press, London.

Cutaia, A.J. (1984). *J. Assoc. Off. Anal. Chem.* 67, 192–193.

Engelhard, S., Löhmannsröben, H.G. and Schael, F. (2004). *Appl. Spectros.* 58, 1205–1209.

European Brewery Convention (1987). *Analytica EBC*, 4th edn. Brauerei und Getränke Rundschau, Zurich.

Fung, Y.S. and Mo, S.Y. (1996). *Analyst* 121, 369–372.

Gales, P.W. (1990). Malt beverages and brewing materials. In Helrich K. (ed.), *Official Methods of Analysis of the Association of Analytical Chemists*, Associate Chapter, p. 711, Chapter 27, Washington, DC; Vol. 2, 15th edn, p. 710, Arlington, VA

Gallignani, M., Garrigues, S. and de la Guardia, M. (1994). *Anal. Chim. Acta* 287, 275–283.

Gallignani, M., Ayala, C., del Rosario Brunetto, M., Burguera, J.L. and Burguera, M. (2005). *Talanta* 68, 470–479.

Gonzales-Rodriguez, J., Prez-Juan, P. and Luque de Castro, M.D. (2003). *Talanta* 59, 691–696.

Gorton, L. (1995). *Electroanalysis* 7, 23–45.

Guilbault, G.G. and Lubrano, G.J. (1974). *Anal. Chim. Acta* 69, 189–194.

Guzmán-Vázques de Prada, A., Peña, N., Mena, M.L., Reviejp, A.J. and Pingarrón, J.M. (2003). *Biosens. Bioelectron.* 18, 1279–1288.

Hart, F.L. and Fisher, M.J. (1971). *Modern Food Analysis*, Springer, New York.

Hughes, P.S. and Baxter, E.D. (2001). An overview of the Malting and Brewing Processes. *Beer: Quality, Safety and Nutritional Aspects*. The Royal Society of Chemistry, pp. 1–13, Cambrigde, UK.

Hunt, W.A. (1996). *Alcohol* 13, 147–151.

Iwachido, T., Ishimaruk, K. and Toei, K. (1986). *Anal. Sci.* 2, 495–496.

Jaselskis, B. and Warriner, J.P. (1966). *Anal. Chem.* 38, 563–564.

Kindervater, R., Künnecke, W. and Schmid, R.D. (1990). *Anal. Chim. Acta* 234, 113–117.

Kulis, J.J., Pesliakiene, M.V. and Samalius, A.S. (1981). *Bioelectrochem. Bioenerg.* 8, 81–88.

Lau, O.W. and Luk, S.F. (1994). *Int. Food Sci. Technol.* 29, 469–472.

Liden, H., Vijayakumar, A.R., Gorton, L. and Marko-Varga, G. (1998). *J. Pharm. Biomed. Anal.* 17, 1111–1128.

Llario, R., Inón, F.A., Garrigues, S. and de la Guardia, M. (2006). *Talanta* 69, 469–480.

Luque De Castro, M.D. and Papaefstathiou, I. (1998). *Trends Anal. Chem.* 17, 41–49.

Magrì, A.D., Magrì, A.L., Balestrieri, F., Sacchini, A. and Marini, D. (1997). *Fresenius J. Anal. Chem.* 357, 985–988.

Morawski, J., Dincer, A.K. and Ivie, K. (1983). *Food Technol.* 37, 57–60.

Nanjo, M. and Guilbault, G.G. (1975). *Anal. Chim. Acta* 75, 169–180.

Ough, C.S. and Amerine, M.A. (1988). *Methods for Analysis of Musts and Wines*, 2nd edn. Wiley-Interscience, New York.

Pacey, G.E. and Karlberg, B. (1989). *Flow Injection Analysis: A Practical Guide*. Elsevier Science Publisher, New York.

Paixão, T.R.L.C., Corbo, D. and Bertotti, M. (2002). *Anal. Chim. Acta* 472, 123–131.

Pilone, G.J. (1985). *J. Assoc. Off. Anal. Chem.* 68, 188–190.

Pueyo, E., Dizy, M. and Carmen-Polo, M. (1993). *Am. J. Enol. Vitic.* 44, 255–260.

Rebelo, M.J.F., Compagnone, D., Guilbault, G.G. and Lubrano, G.J. (1994). *Anal. Lett.* 27, 3027–3037.

Santos, A.A., Gorton, L. and Kubota, L.T. (2002). *Electroanalysis* 14, 805–812.

Santos, A.S., Freire, R.S. and Kubota, L.T. (2003). *J. Electroanal. Chem.* 547, 135–142.

Varnam, A.H. and Sutherland, J.P. (1996). *Bebidas: Tecnología, Química y Microbiología*, Acribia, S.A., Zaragoza.

Warriner, K., Morrissey, A., Alderman, J., King, G., Treloar, P. and Vadgama, P.M. (2002). *Sens. Actuators B* 84, 200–207.

Workman Jr., J.J. (1996). *Appl. Spectrosc. Rev.* 31, 251–320.

103

Quantification of Beer Carbohydrates by HPLC

Isabel M.P.L.V.O. Ferreira REQUIMTE, Serviço de Bromatologia, Faculdade de Farmácia, Universidade do Porto, R. Aníbal Cunha, Porto, Portugal

Abstract

Methods for quantification of carbohydrates in beer are summarized. Quantification of total sugars in beer is usually performed by spectrophotometric methods that give an approximate value of sugar content. Enzymatic methods are generally specific for only one or more sugars in a sample. Gas chromatographic methods are sensitive but require derivatization and are laborious when compared to liquid chromatographic techniques.

High performance liquid chromatography (HPLC) methods can provide qualitative and quantitative analysis of beer carbohydrates. The main chromatographic systems used are anion-exchange column with water containing bases or salts as the eluent; cation-exchange column with water as the eluent; alkyl-bonded silica gel column with water as the eluent and amine-bonded silica gel column with water–acetonitrile as the eluent. High performance anion-exchange chromatography is widely used; it is based on the fact that carbohydrates in a strongly alkaline environment will ionize, thereby rendering them amenable to separation on an ion-exchange column. However, of these systems, HPLC using an amine-bonded silica gel column coupled with evaporative light scattering detection is the one mostly used, it requires no derivatization, is sensitive and works well with gradients. Other detectors can be used, such as, refractive index, pulsed amperometric detection, mass spectrometry and nuclear magnetic resonance spectroscopy/mass spectrometry. Fluorescence-assisted carbohydrate electrophoresis of glucose, fructose, saccharose, maltose, and maltotriose in beer is also described.

HPLC/ELS methods were validated for quantification of glucose, fructose, maltose, maltotriose and maltotetraose in beer. The chromatographic analyses were carried out using an amino-bonded silica column. Identification of the carbohydrates in beers was performed by comparison with the retention times of the standards. The reliability of the methods in terms of precision, accuracy and detection limit values was verified. The methods were used to study the effect of mashing methods on carbohydrate content and to compare the carbohydrate patterns of beers produced in 10 different countries.

List of Abbreviations

HPLC	High performance liquid chromatography
LC	Liquid chromatographic
HPAEC	High performance anion-exchange chromatography
RI	Refractive index
ELS	Evaporative light scattering
PA	Pulsed amperometric
NMR/MS	Nuclear magnetic resonance spectroscopy/ mass spectrometry
FACE	Fluorescence-assisted carbohydrate electrophoresis

Introduction

Beer is a very complex mixture, major beer components are water, ethanol and carbohydrates comprising fermentable sugars (i.e. fructose, glucose, maltose and maltotriose) as well as glucose oligosaccharides and arabinoxylans (Brandolini *et al.*, 1995; De Keukeleire, 2000; Hughes and Baxter, 2001; Caballero *et al.*, 2003; Duarte *et al.*, 2003; Briggs *et al.*, 2004).

Monitoring of beer carbohydrate composition may therefore be an important tool for modern brewing technology, particularly in the selection of raw materials and yeast strains, product development and quality control. Quantitative evaluation of malto-oligosaccharides provides a useful control of the complex enzymatic system in beer brewing, particularly when changes in procedure are contemplated (Plaga *et al.*, 1989; Duarte *et al.*, 2003; Montanari *et al.*, 2005). In this respect it is important to control not only the total amount of fermentable carbohydrates formed but also the relative amounts of the different sugars.

Beer in Health and Disease Prevention
ISBN: 978-0-12-373891-2

Table 103.1 Summary of methodologies applied to analysis of beer carbohydrates

Method	*Type of carbohydrates assayed*	*Advantages/disadvantages*
Spectrophotometric	Total sugars	Classic method with long history of use/provide an approximate value
Enzymatic	Glucose, fructose, saccharose, galactose and polysaccharides	Specific/expensive
Gas chromatography	Monosaccharides	Very sensitive/laborious, requires derivatization
Liquid chromatography	Mono, di, oligo and low molecular weight polysaccharides	Does not require derivatization, different detectors can be used/some detectors lack sensitivity
Electrophoresis	Glucose, fructose, saccharose, maltose, maltotriose and low molecular weight polysaccharides	Requires derivatization to be used with fluorescence detector

Source: Adapted from *Analytica-EBC* (1998), Ramirez *et al*. (2005), Eliasson (2006).

Analyses of beer carbohydrates can be performed by different methodologies, including spectrophotometric, enzymatic, chromatographic and electrophoretic methods (Table 103.1).

Methods for Analysis of Beer Carbohydrates

Carbohydrates have been determined in some beers by chemical and enzymatic analysis. Spectrophotometric are classic methods with a long history, used for quantification of total sugars in beer; however, they provide only an approximate value of sugar content, because different sugars in solution react differently with the colorimetric reagent anthrone in 85% sulfuric acid (*Analytica-EBC*, 1998). On the other hand enzymatic methods are generally specific for only one or more sugars in a sample (Shanta-Kumara *et al.*, 1995). There are available enzymatic methods for quantification of glucose, fructose, saccharose, lactose, galactose and polysaccharides.

Gas chromatographic methods can also be used; however, since carbohydrates are not volatile, they must be derivatized, for example, into alditol acetates, prior to analysis. It is very sensitive, however it is laborious when compared to high performance liquid chromatography (HPLC) techniques.

Liquid chromatographic (LC) methods play an important role in determining carbohydrates, especially fermentable carbohydrates (Eliasson, 2006). HPLC methods can provide not only the qualitative analysis but also the quantitative determination (Honda, 1984; Anumula, 2000; Wei and Ding, 2000). The main chromatographic systems used for the separation of underivatized carbohydrates can be generalized as anion-exchange column with water containing bases or salts as the eluent (Torto *et al.*, 1995; Cataldi *et al.*, 2000); cation-exchange column with water as the eluent (Clement *et al.*, 1992); alkyl-bonded silica gel column with water as the eluent (Rajakyla, 1986) and amine-bonded silica gel column with water–acetonitrile as the eluent (Macrae and Dick, 1981; Macrae *et al.*, 1982; Nikolov *et al.*, 1985; Clement *et al.*, 1992; Ferreira and Ferreira, 1997; Ferreira *et al.*, 1998, 2005; Nogueira *et al.*, 2005). Column choice is based on the specific samples and the type of eluents to be used. High performance anion-exchange chromatography (HPAEC) is widely used, it is based on the fact that carbohydrates in a strongly alkaline environment will ionize, thereby rendering them amenable to separation on an ion-exchange column. However, of these systems, HPLC using an amine-bonded silica gel column is the one mostly used.

Carbohydrates analysis historically has used refractive index (RI) detection because of the lack of chromophores in the analytes, which are required for ultraviolet detection. RI (Boumahraz *et al.*, 1982; Nikolov *et al.*, 1985; Rajakyla, 1986; Gotsick and Benson, 1991; Clement *et al.*, 1992; Ferreira and Ferreira, 1997; Ferreira *et al.*, 1998; Castellari *et al.*, 2001) measurement is the most popular detection method for carbohydrates. However, it has many disadvantages, such as lacking sensitivity, baseline instability, temperature and flow-rate dependent, and incompatibility with gradient elution. Evaporative light scattering (ELS) detection requires no chromophores and works well with gradients. HPLC analysis of carbohydrates using gradient elution is desirable due to its decrease in analysis times. This detector is widely used as a semi-universal mass detector for HPLC (Mengerink *et al.*, 1991; Ferreira *et al.*, 2005; Nogueira *et al.*, 2005). It is based on the detection of solute molecules by light scattering after nebulization and evaporation of the mobile phase, so it is suitable to detect the nonvolatile compounds such as lipids (Marcato and Cecchin, 1996; Chang and Harris, 1998) and carbohydrates (Macrae and Dick, 1981; Macrae *et al.*, 1982; Clement *et al.*, 1992; Floridi *et al.*, 2001, 2005; Nogueira *et al.*, 2005).

Other detectors can be used such as pulsed amperometric (PA) detection which is directly compatible with the high ionic strength of alkali eluents (Klein and Leubolt, 1993; Gey *et al.*, 1996; Yan *et al.*, 1997) and MS detection for peak identification according to their mass to charge ratio. These two detectors can be installed in series or in parallel depending on the type of column (Bruggink *et al.*, 2005).

Direct analysis of beer by LC–NMR/MS (nuclear magnetic resonance spectroscopy/mass spectrometry) enables

Table 103.2 Summary of liquid chromatography methods applied to separation of beer carbohydrates

Chromatographic system	*Type of sugar*	*Eluent*	*Detector*	*References*
Anion-exchange column	Fermentable sugars	Sodium hydroxide	PA	Klein *et al.* (1993) Yan *et al.* (1997) Gey *et al.* (1996)
Anion-exchange column	Fermentable sugars and dextrins	Sodium hydroxide Sodium acetate	PA MS	Bruggink *et al.* (2005)
Amine-bonded silica	Fermentable sugars	Water–acetonitrile	RI	Gotsick and Benson (1991)
Amine-bonded silica	Fermentable sugars	Water–acetonitrile	Light scattering	Floridi *et al.* (2001) Ferreira *et al.* (2005) Nogueira *et al.* (2005) Montanari *et al.* (2005)
Sulfonated divinyl benzene–styrene copolymer	Fermentable sugars	0.0045N Sulfuric acid and acetonitrile	Refractive index	Castellari *et al.* (2001)
Cation-exchange column	Dextrins with degree of polymerization	0.0085 sulfuric acid in D_2O	Diode array	Duarte *et al.* (2003)
		Sodium acetate	NMR/MS	Vinogradov and Bock (1998)

Source: Adapted from cited literature.

the identification of dextrins with degree of polymerization of up to nine monomers. The use of hyphenated NMR spectroscopy for the rapid characterization of the carbohydrate composition of beers may be the basis of a useful tool for the quality control of beer (Vinogradov and Bock, 1998; Duarte *et al.*, 2003).

Electrophoretic separation of carbohydrates, glucose, fructose, saccharose, maltose and maltotriose in beer is also described (Thomas *et al.*, 2000). Saccharides labeled with the dye 8-amino-1,3,6-naphthalene trisulfonic acid can be separated by electrophoresis and detected with fluorescence-assisted carbohydrate electrophoresis (FACE). Oligosaccharides in beer can be identified in FACE assays based on comigration with standards (e.g. oligosaccharides derived from purified starch, β-glucan and pentosan). A variety of beers, including lager, light, ale, porter and stout, demonstrated distinct saccharide patterns in FACE analysis (Ramirez *et al.*, 2005).

Some of the LC methods mentioned above were applied to separation, identification and quantification of beer carbohydrates as summarized in Table 103.2.

HPLC/ELS for Quantification of Beer Carbohydrates

As mentioned above ELS is widely used for HPLC to obtain efficient and reproducible performance of carbohydrate analysis. This detector performs excellently with gradients. HPLC analysis of carbohydrates using gradient elution is desirable due to its decrease in analysis times. Column choice also plays a large role in carbohydrate analyses. The speed of analysis as well as the overall separation is based on column factors such as length, phase type and loading. A comparison of six different types of HPLC columns, namely, a silica based amino, a polymer based amino, two ion-exchange columns, a polyamine and a zirconia based column was performed for the separation of monosaccharides and oligosaccharides in beer and other drinks (Wilcox *et al.*, 2001). Columns were obtained from several manufacturers. Samples were simply filtered prior to analysis. The system included isocratic and binary LC pumps, an autosampler, mobile phase degasser and an ELS detector. Column choice should be based on the specific samples and the type of eluents to be used. Amino-bonded silica columns should be used with low water concentration mobile phases due to their inherent hydrolytic instability.

Floridi *et al.* (2001) described separation of fermentable and non-fermentable carbohydrates of up to 15 glucose units in wort, mashed malt and beer was obtained in 40 min by direct injection on an amino-bonded silica column, aqueous/acetonitrile gradient elution profile at room temperature and an HPLC–ELS apparatus. No chemical manipulation was involved and no derivatization was needed. The external standard method was used to calibrate the chromatographic system for carbohydrates quantification. According to authors the results were comparable with those found with the official HPLC–RI procedure and with chemical determination with Fehlung's reagent. This method was used to study the effect of mashing methods, namely, the effect of double decoction mashing method and the single decoction plus infusion mashing method on beer carbohydrates was compared (Montanari *et al.*, 2005).

An HPLC method with an ELS detector was validated for quantification of glucose, fructose, maltose, maltotriose and maltotetraose in beer (Nogueira *et al.*, 2005). The chromatographic analysis was carried out using an amino-bonded silica column. Gradient elution was carried out with a mixture of two solvents. Solvent A consisted of acetonitrile and solvent B consisted of water. Carbohydrates were eluted increasing the proportion of solvent B from 19% to 25% over 40 min: 0–19 min, 19% B; 20–40 min, 25% B. The flow rate was 1 ml/min. The temperature of the heated drift tube was 45°C, the gas pressure was 3.0 bar and gain 5. The beer samples were degassed for 15 min in an ultrasonic bath, diluted (1:2) in acetonitrile and filtered. Identification of the carbohydrates in beers was performed by comparison with the retention times of the standards (Figures 103.1 and 103.2). Sugar standard solutions with different concentrations were used, according to the quantity of these compounds in the beer matrix (0.05–5.0 g/l for fructose; 0.05–5.0 g/l for glucose; 0.05–15.0 g/l for maltose; 0.05–10.0 g/l for maltotriose and 0.05–5.0 g/l for maltotetraose). The detection limit values were estimated as the concentration providing a signal three times higher than the standard deviation of the background noise and were 0.005 g/l for fructose, 0.008 g/l for glucose and 0.01 g/l for maltose, maltotriose and maltotetraose. The reliability of the method in terms of precision and accuracy was verified in three different beer matrices, including free alcohol beer, beer with 100% malt and beer with adjuncts (Nogueira *et al.*, 2005).

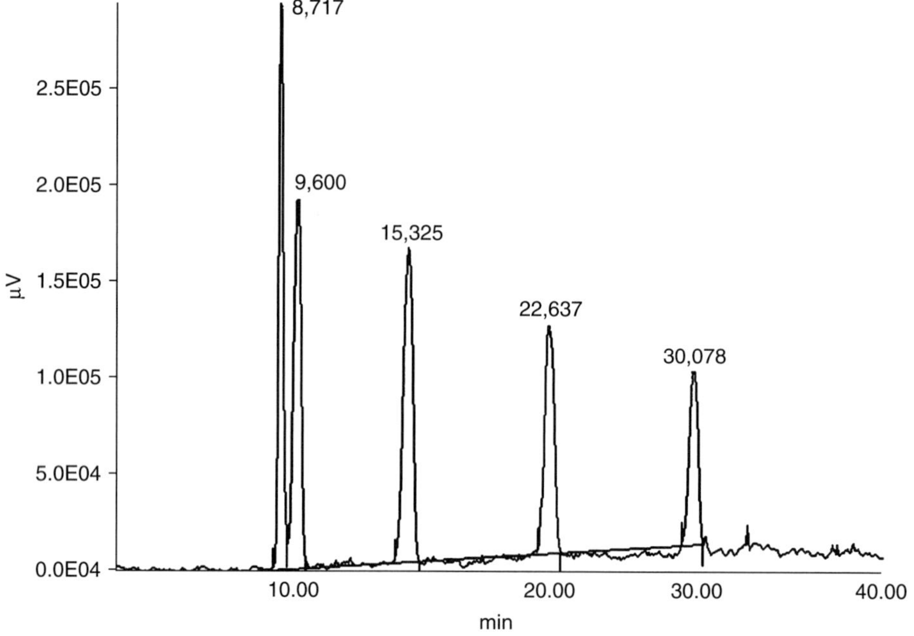

Figure 103.1 Typical chromatogram for separation of five carbohydrates in a standard solution. Fructose (t_R 8.717 min), glucose (t_R 9.600 min), maltose (t_R 15.325 min), maltotriose (t_R 22.637 min), maltotetraose (t_R 30.078 min) 2 g/l each. Chromatographic conditions: Spherisorb NH_2 column, 5 μm, 250 × 4.6 mm ID.

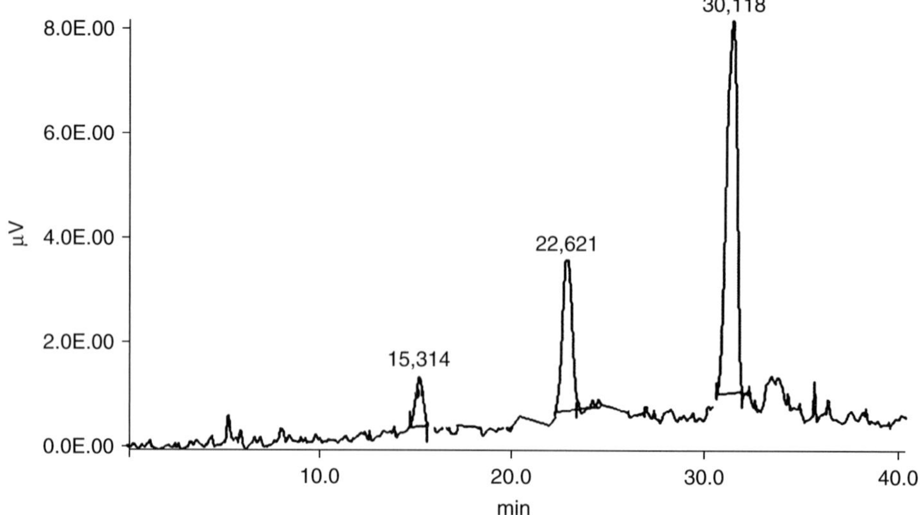

Figure 103.2 Typical chromatogram for separation of five carbohydrates in a lager beer sample. Maltose (t_R 15.314 min), maltotriose (t_R 22.621 min), maltotetraose (t_R 30.118 min). The beer samples were degassed for 15 min in an ultrasonic bath, diluted (1:2) in acetonitrile and filtered. Chromatographic conditions: Spherisorb NH_2 column, 5 μm, 250 × 4.6 mm ID.

The HPLC/ELS method validated for quantification of glucose, fructose, maltose, maltotriose and maltotetraose in beer (Nogueira *et al.*, 2005) was used to analyze beers produced in 10 different countries (Ferreira and Martins, 2007) (see Table 103.3). General inspection of the data was carried out for each type of beer (alcohol free, lager and ale) and each carbohydrate individually, using box-and-whisker plot. Box-and-whisker plots are helpful in interpreting the distribution of data. The median (or second quartile) of a set of data separates the data into two equal parts. Data can be further separated into quartiles. Quartiles separate the original set of data into four equal parts. Each of these parts contains one-fourth of the data. The first quartile is the median of the lower part of the data. The third quartile is the median of the upper part of the data. This procedure, which is suitable for skewed data, enabled the construction of Figures 103.3, 103.4 and 103.5, where results are displayed to favor mutual comparisons, the minimum and maximum

Table 103.3 Summary of beer samples analyzed by Ferreira and Martins (2007) and grouped according to beer type and ingredients mentioned in labels

Beer type	*Number of samples*	*Ingredients mentioned on the labels*	*Countries of origin*
Alcohol free	4	Water, malt, hop, unmalted cereals	Portugal Spain
	3	Water, malt, unmalted cereals, sugars, hop, antioxidant (E224)	Portugal Brazil
Lager	6	Water, malt, hop	Portugal Denmark Germany Holland Czech Republic Brazil
	12	Water, malt, unmalted cereals or glucose syrup, hop, antioxidant (E224)	Portugal Denmark Holland Belgium Spain Brazil
Ale	4	Water, malt, hop	UK Germany Belgium Irland

Source: Ferreira and Martins (2007).

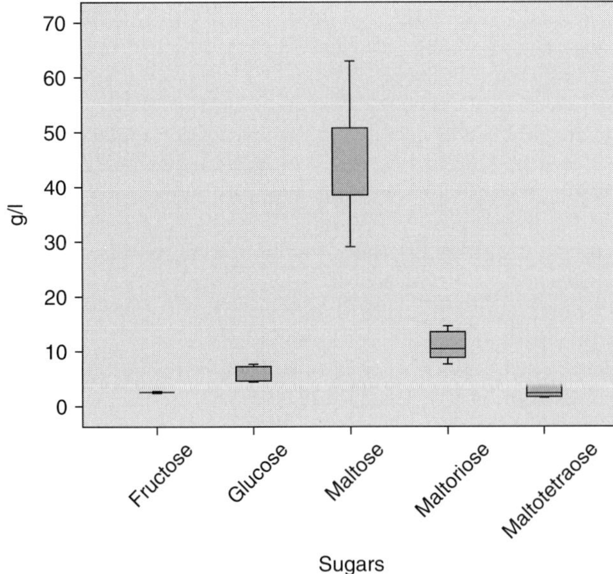

Figure 103.3 Box-and-whisker plots, obtained via non-metric univariate statistics, for monosaccharides and malto-oligosaccharides contents expressed in g/l for free alcohol beers.

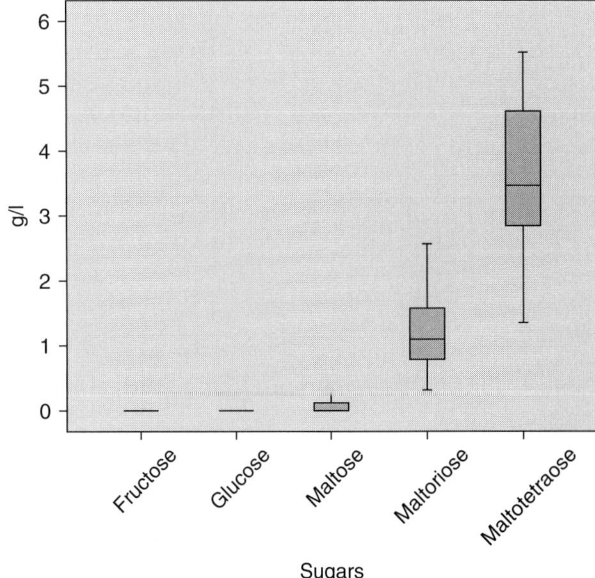

Figure 103.4 Box-and-whisker plots, obtained via non-metric univariate statistics, for monosaccharides and malto-oligosaccharides contents expressed in g/l for lager beers.

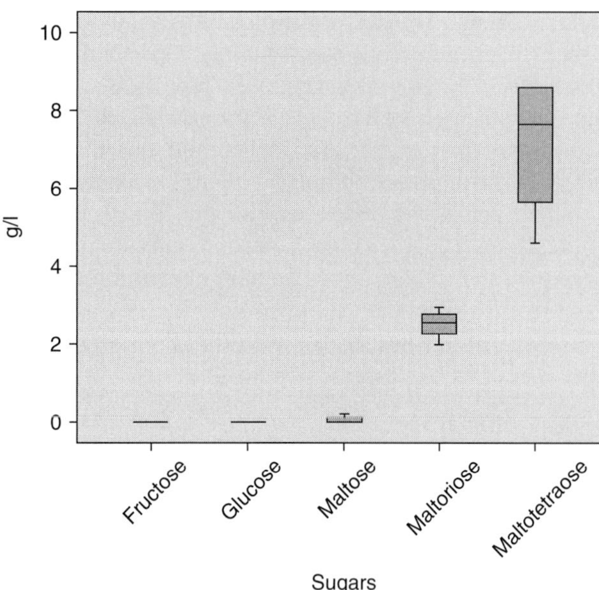

Figure 103.5 Box-and-whisker plots, obtained via non-metric univariate statistics, for monosaccharides and malto-oligosaccharides contents expressed in g/l for ale beers.

values observed, as well as the first quartile, the median and the third quartile are presented.

Figure 103.3 presents the concentration of fructose, glucose, maltose, maltotriose and maltotetraose in alcohol free beer samples. Similar qualitative profile was obtained for the six beer samples. However, within brands quantitative differences were observed for glucose, maltose and maltotriose contents. These samples suffered short fermentation; thus, great part of fructose, maltose, maltotriose and maltotetraose remained in beer.

As expected lager and ale beers presented significantly lower sugar content owing to an extended fermentation process (Figures 103.4 and 103.5). During fermentation the yeast absorbs and ferments first all the glucose and then maltose. Some yeasts, can also utilize maltotriose. Lagers were in general more fully fermented than ales and contained less residual carbohydrates. In conclusion, strong differences between the compositions in terms of carbohydrates were observed when analyzed by HPLC/ELS.

Summary Points

- Methods for quantification of carbohydrates in beer are summarized.
- HPLC methods for qualitative and quantitative analysis of beer carbohydrates, including anion-exchange column with water containing bases or salts as the eluent; cation-exchange column with water as the eluent; alkyl-bonded silica gel column with water as the eluent and amine-bonded silica gel column with water–acetonitrile as the eluent.
- HPLC detectors for carbohydrate analyses include ELS detection, the one mostly used, RI, PA detection, MS and NMR/MS.
- HPLC/ELS methods were validated for quantification of glucose, fructose, maltose, maltotriose and maltotetraose in beer. The chromatographic analyses were carried out using an amino-bonded silica column. The methods were used to study the effect of mashing methods on carbohydrate content and to compare the carbohydrate patterns of beers produced in 10 different countries
- Sugar composition of lager, ale and free alcohol beers was evaluated by HPLC/ELS.

References

Analytica-EBC (1998). *European Brewery Convention*, 5th edn. Verlag Hans Carl Getränke – Fachverlag, Nürnberg, Germany.

Anumula, K.R. (2000). *Anal. Biochem.* 283, 17–26.

Boumahraz, M., Davydov, V.Y. and Kiselev, A.V. (1982). *Chromatographia* 15, 751–756.

Brandolini, V., Menziani, E., Mazzotta, D., Cabras, P., Tosi, B. and Lodi, G. (1995). *J. Food Compos. Anal.* 8, 336–343.

Briggs, D.E., Boulton, C.A., Brookes, P.A. and Roger, S. (2004). *Brewing: Science and Practice.* pp. 1–290. Woodhead Publishing Limited and CRC Press, Boca Raton, USA.

Bruggink, C., Maurer, R., Herrmann, H., Cavalli, S. and Hoefler, F. (2005). *J. Chromatogr. A* 1085, 104–109.

Caballero, B., Trugo, L.C. and Finglas, P.M. (2003). *Encyclopedia of Food Sciences and Nutrition.* pp. 418–451. Academic Press Inc, USA.

Castellari, M., Sartini, E., Spinabelli, U., Riponi, C. and Galassi, S. (2001). *J. Chromatogr. Sci.* 39, 235–238.

Cataldi, T.R.I., Campa, C. and de Benedetto, G.E. (2000). *Fresenius J. Anal. Chem.* 368, 739–758.

Chang, C.D. and Harris, D.J. (1998). *J. Liq. Chromatogr. Rel. Technol.* 21, 1119–1134.

Clement, A., Young, D. and Brechet, C. (1992). *J. Liq. Chromatogr.* 15, 805–817.

De Keukeleire, D. (2000). *Quim. Nova* 23, 108–112.

Duarte, I.F., Godejohann, M., Braumann, U., Spraul, M. and Gil, A.M. (2003). *J. Agric. Food Chem.* 51, 4847–4853.

Eliasson, A.C. (2006). *Carbohydrates in Food*, 2nd edn. pp. 68–104. CRC Press, London, New York.

Ferreira, I.M.P.L.V.O and Ferreira, M.A. (1997). *J. Liq. Chromatogr. Rel. Technol.* 20, 3419–3429.

Ferreira, I.M.P.L.V.O. and Martins, F. (2007). *Alim. Hum.* 13, 26–31.

Ferreira, I.M.P.L.V.O., Gomes, A.M.P. and Ferreira, M.A. (1998). *Carbohydr. Polym.* 37, 225–229.

Ferreira, I.M.P.L.V.O., Jorge, K., Nogueira, L.C., Silva, F. and Trugo, L.C. (2005). *J. Agric. Food Chem.* 53, 4976–4981.

Floridi, S., Miniati, E., Montanari, L. and Fantozzi, P. (2001). *Monatsschrift fur Brauwissenschaft* 54, 209–215.

Gey, M.H., Unger, K.K. and Battermann, G. (1996). *Fresenius J. Anal. Chem.* 356, 339–343.

Gotsick, J.T. and Benson, R.F. (1991). *J. Liq. Chromatogr.* 14, 1887–1901.

Honda, S. (1984). *Anal. Biochem.* 140, 1–47.

Hughes, P.S. and Baxter, E.D. (2001). *Beer: Quality, Safety and Nutritional Aspects*. pp. 41–44. Royal Society of Chemistry, Cambridge, UK.

Klein, H. and Leubolt, R. (1993). *J. Chromatogr.* 640, 259–270.

Macrae, R. and Dick, J. (1981). *J. Chromatogr.* 210, 138–145.

Macrae, R., Trugo, L.C. and Dick, J. (1982). *Chromatographia* 15, 476–478.

Marcato, B. and Cecchin, G. (1996). *J. Chromatogr. A* 730, 83–90.

Mengerink, Y., Man, H.C.J.D. and Wal, S.V.D. (1991). *J. Chromatogr. A* 552, 593–604.

Montanari, L., Floridi, S., Marconi, O., Tironzelli, M. and Fantozzi, P. (2005). *Eur. Food Res. Technol.* 221, 175–179.

Nikolov, Z.L., Meagher, M.M. and Reilly, P.J. (1985). *J. Chromatogr.* 319, 51–54.

Nogueira, L.C., Silva, F., Ferreira, I.M.P.L.V.O. and Trugo, L.C. (2005). *J. Chromatogr. A* 1065, 207–210.

Plaga, A., Stumpfel, J. and Fiedler, H. (1989). *Appl. Microbiol. Biotechnol.* 32, 45–49.

Rajakyla, E. (1986). *J. Chromatogr.* 353, 1–12.

Ramirez, S.C., Carretero, A.S., Blanco, C.C., Castro, M.F.B. and Gutierrez, A.F. (2005). *J. Sci. Food Agric.* 85, 517–521.

Shanta-Kumara, H.M.C., Iserentant, D. and Verachtert, H. (1995). *Cerevisia Belgian J. Brew. Biotechnol.* 20, 47–53.

Thomas, B.R., Brandley, B.K. and Rodriguez, R.L. (2000). *J. Am. Soc. Brew. Chem.* 58, 124–127.

Torto, N., Buttler, T., Gorton, L., Marko-Varga, G., Stalbrand, H. and Tjerneld, F. (1995). *Anal. Chim. Acta* 313, 15–24.

Vinogradov, E. and Bock, K. (1998). *Carbohydr. Res.* 309, 57–64.

Wei, Y. and Ding, M. (2000). *J. Chromatogr. A* 904, 113–117.

Wilcox, M., Hefley, J.R. and Walsh, J.W. (2001). *IFT Annual Meeting*, 59A-25, New Orleans, Louisiana.

Yan, Z., Zhang, X.D. and Niu, W.J. (1997). *Mikrochim. Acta* 127, 189–194.

INDEX

B

C

D

F

N

O

Q

R

T